Discover electronic resources for the home and for the classroom

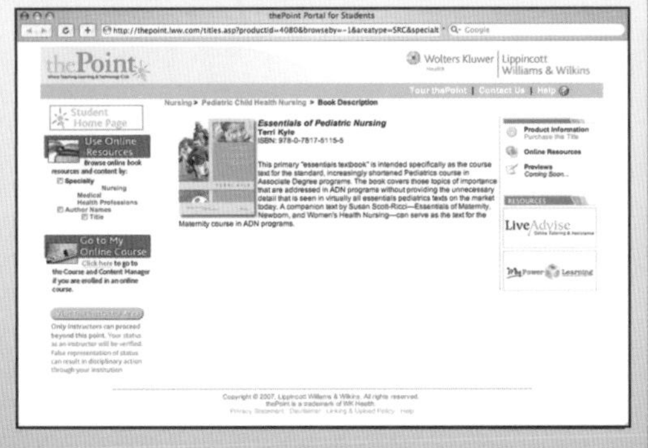

Online Study Guide for Essentials of Pediatric Nursing

By **Terri Kyle**

This exciting new resource, built for use on thePoint Course and Content Manager, or in WebCT or Blackboard Learning Management Systems, combines all the helpful activities found in print study guides with additional interactive resources only an online guide can provide. Packed with knowledge-based, application-level, and NCLEX-style review questions, as well as video vignette-based case studies, it's a great new way to help assess mastery of information and proficiency.

ISBN: 978-0-7817-6108-6
Visit http://thepoint.lww.com/kyle to learn more!

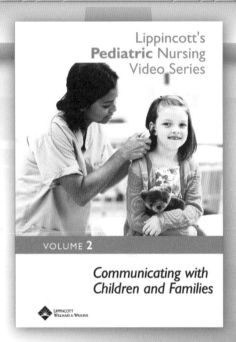

Lippincott's Pediatric Nursing Video Series

Each 45-minute documentary style video focuses on nursing care of children and families. Each video addresses a critical element of pediatric nursing care, and focuses on issues specific to five age groups—Infant (28 days to 1 year); Toddler (1-3 years); Pre-School (3-6 years); School Age (6-12 years); and Adolescent (12-18 years)—highlighted by nurse, patient, and family interviews.

- Module 1: Growth and Development
- Module 2: Communicating with Children and Families
- Module 3: Care of the Hospitalized Child

VHS, DVD and Streaming Video formats available
VHS Complete Set of 3 (Programs 1-3), 0-7817-6110-7
DVD Complete Set of 3 (Programs 1-3), 0-7817-9172-3
For Institutional Purchase only.
Call 1-800-399-3110 to speak to an Electronic Media Specialist.

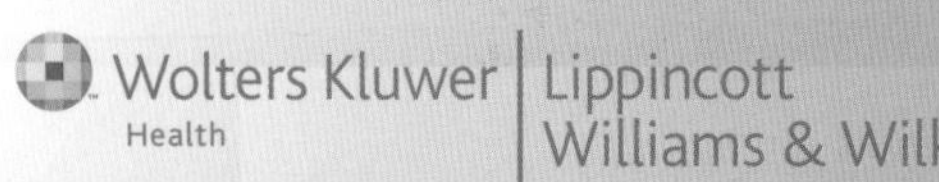

Put these skill-builders to work for you...

ORDER YOURS TODAY!

Essentials *of* Pediatric Nursing

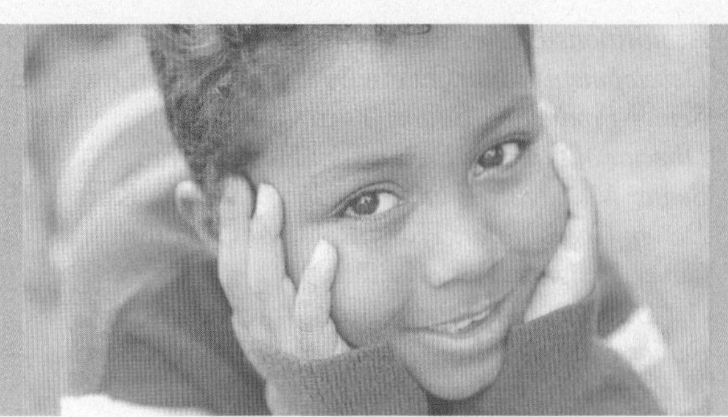

Essentials *of* Pediatric Nursing

Terri Kyle, MSN, CPNP

Associate Professor
Florida Hospital College of Health Sciences
Orlando, Florida

Wolters Kluwer Health | Lippincott Williams & Wilkins

Philadelphia • Baltimore • New York • London
Buenos Aires • Hong Kong • Sydney • Tokyo

Acquisitions Editor: Elizabeth Nieginski/Jean Rodenberger
Development Editor: Danielle DiPalma/Erin Sweeney
Senior Production Editor: Tom Gibbons
Director of Nursing Production: Helen Ewan
Senior Managing Editor / Production: Erika Kors
Design Coordinator: Holly Reid McLaughlin
Cover Designer: Bess Kiethas
Art Director, Illustration: Brett MacNaughton
Senior Manufacturing Manager: William Alberti
Indexer: Kathy Pitcoff
Compositor: Circle Graphics

ISBN-13: 978-0-7817-5115-5
ISBN-10: 0-7817-5115-2

10 9 8 7 6 5 4 3

Printed in China
Library of Congress Cataloging-in-Publication Data

Kyle, Terri.
Essentials of pediatric nursing / Terri Kyle.
p. ; cm.
Includes bibliographical references and index.
ISBN-13: 978-0-7817-5115-5 (hardcover : alk. paper)
ISBN-10: 0-7817-5115-2 (hardcover : alk. paper) 1. Pediatric nursing. I. Title.
[DNLM: 1. Nursing Care—methods. 2. Child. 3. Infant. 4. Nursing Assessment—methods. 5. Pediatric Nursing. WY 159 K99e 2008]
RJ245.K95 2008
618.92'00231—dc22

2007025968

Care has been taken to confirm the accuracy of the information presented and to describe generally accepted practices. However, the authors, editors, and publisher are not responsible for errors or omissions or for any consequences from application of the information in this book and make no warranty, expressed or implied, with respect to the currency, completeness, or accuracy of the contents of the publication. Application of this information in a particular situation remains the professional responsibility of the practitioner; the clinical treatments described and recommended may not be considered absolute and universal recommendations.

The authors, editors, and publisher have exerted every effort to ensure that drug selection and dosage set forth in this text are in accordance with the current recommendations and practice at the time of publication. However, in view of ongoing research, changes in government regulations, and the constant flow of information relating to drug therapy and drug reactions, the reader is urged to check the package insert for each drug for any change in indications and dosage and for added warnings and precautions. This is particularly important when the recommended agent is a new or infrequently employed drug.

Some drugs and medical devices presented in this publication have Food and Drug Administration (FDA) clearance for limited use in restricted research settings. It is the responsibility of the health care provider to ascertain the FDA status of each drug or device planned for use in his or her clinical practice.

LWW.COM

RRS0809

This book is dedicated to my incredible family, without whom I could never have accomplished this monumental task. My husband John has unfailingly stood by my side, providing continuous positive affirmation and infinite support for this project. My son Christian and my daughter Caitlin have blessed me with their patience and faith in me, as well as the opportunity for me to experience all the stages of growth and development first-hand. The book is also dedicated to the wonderful babies born during this project: Natalie, Ben, Grace, and Ella.

ACKNOWLEDGMENTS

The thrilling and challenging experience of authoring this textbook would not have been possible without the tremendous support of the Lippincott Williams & Wilkins family. In particular I want to thank Michelle McIlvain (Regional Sales Manager) for initially querying me about this idea that had long been a secret goal of mine; Elizabeth Nieginski (Senior Acquisitions Editor) for believing so strongly in my ideas and never letting me give up; and Danielle DiPalma (Senior Development Editor) for her vision and organization, but especially for her patience with me. I would like to express immense gratitude to Sarah Kyle (Development Editor) for so clearly being able to see what I wanted and her tireless attention to detail even up through the ninth month of pregnancy and while moving her family across continents. Thank you to Maryann Foley (Development Editor) for stepping in and filling the gaps, Erin Sweeney for assisting with transmission of the manuscript, Brett MacNaughton (Art Director) and the entire art team for the beautiful illustrations, as well as Tom Gibbons (Senior Production Editor) and the production team for their diligent efforts. My good friend and colleague, Susan Carman, deserves special thanks for her significant contribution not only to writing chapters and case studies as well as being involved in the development of the online study guide, but also for always listening to, supporting, and encouraging me. Special thanks to Amy Gellerman (Producer), Gus Freedman (Photographer), Newton-Wellesley Hospital pediatric department, and Boston Shriner's Hospital for the beautiful photography they contributed. I would also like to thank all of the pediatric nurses who contributed their wealth of knowledge and expertise to developing chapters for this book. This would not have been possible without all of you.

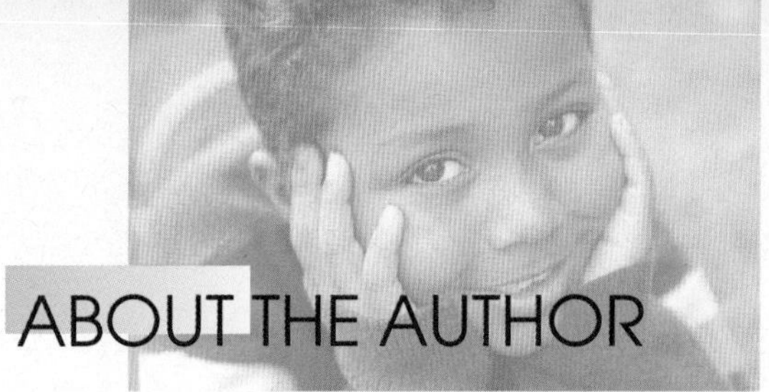

ABOUT THE AUTHOR

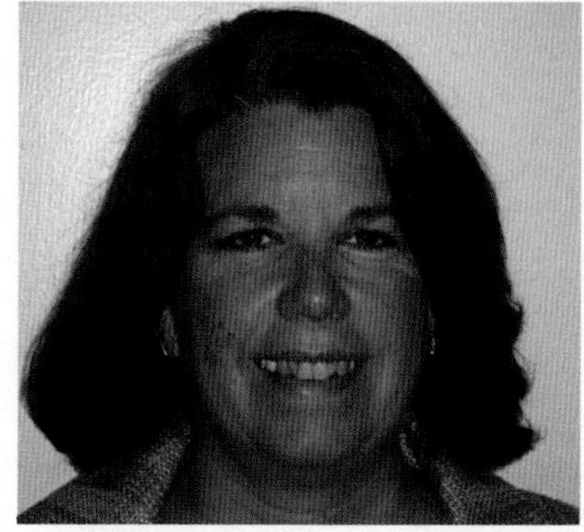

Terri Kyle earned a Bachelor of Science in Nursing from the University of North Carolina at Chapel Hill and a Master of Science in Nursing from Emory University in Atlanta, Georgia. She is a certified pediatric nurse practitioner and is currently enrolled in the Doctor of Nursing Practice program at the University of Florida. Practicing pediatric nursing for over 20 years, Terri has had the opportunity to serve children and their families in a variety of diverse settings.

She has experience in inpatient pediatrics in pediatric and neonatal intensive care units, newborn nursery, specialized pediatric units, and community hospitals. She has worked as a pediatric nurse practitioner in pediatric specialty clinics and primary care. She has been involved in teaching nursing for over 15 years with experience in both undergraduate and graduate nursing education. Terri is a fellow in the National Association of Pediatric Nurse Practitioners and a member of Sigma Theta Tau International Honor Society of Nursing, the National League for Nursing, the Society of Pediatric Nurses, and the Association of Camp Nurses.

With the limited time allotted in schools to the topic of pediatric nursing, Terri recognized the need for a textbook that "got to the point." She strongly believes in a concepts-based approach for learning nursing—that is, to teach the basics to students in a broad contextual format so that they can apply that knowledge in a variety of situations. The concepts-based approach to nursing education is time-efficient for nursing educators and fosters the development of critical thinking skills in student nurses.

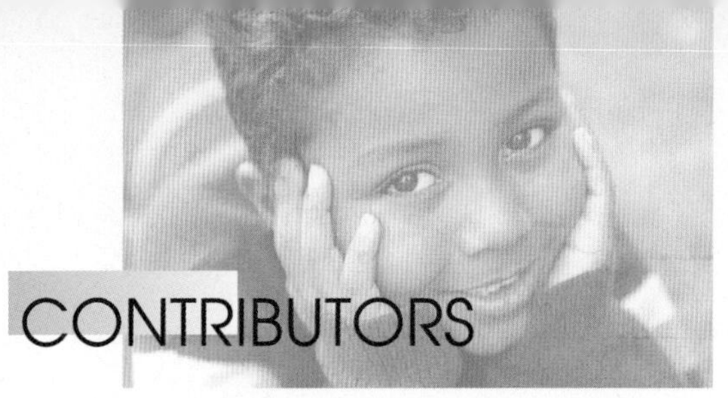

CONTRIBUTORS

Kathie Aduddell, EdD, MSN, RN
Associate Professor
Kennesaw State University, School of Nursing
Kennesaw, Georgia
CHAPTER 1 • Perspectives of Pediatric Nursing
CHAPTER 2 • Factors Influencing Child Health
CHAPTER 11 • Nursing Care of Children During Illness and Hospitalization (co-authored with Kathy Ordelt)
CHAPTER 14 • Medication Administration, Intravenous Therapy, and Nutritional Support
CHAPTER 15 • Pain Management in Children
CHAPTER 20 • Nursing Care of the Child With a Cardiovascular Disorder (co-authored with Carol Holtz)
CHAPTER 28 • Nursing Care of the Child With an Endocrine Disorder

Barbara Browning, RN, MS, CPNP
Clinical Assistant Professor
Georgia State University
Atlanta, Georgia
CHAPTER 8 • Growth and Development of the Adolescent

Susan Carman, BSN, MSN, MBA
Hubertus, Wisconsin
CHAPTER 12 • Nursing Care of the Child in the Community
CHAPTER 16 • Nursing Care of the Child With an Infectious or Communicable Disorder
CHAPTER 30 • Nursing Care of the Child With a Genetic Disorder

Myra Carmon, EdD, CPNP, RN
Director for the Health and Wellness Nursing Collaborative
Georgia State University
Atlanta, Georgia
CHAPTER 7 • Growth and Development of the School-Age Child

Kim Hamilton, RN, BSN
Atlanta, Georgia
CHAPTER 21 • Nursing Care of the Child With a Gastrointestinal Disorder

Carol Holtz, RN, PhD
Professor of Nursing
Kennesaw State University, School of Nursing
Kennesaw, Georgia
CHAPTER 20 • Nursing Care of the Child With a Cardiovascular Disorder (co-authored with Kathie Aduddell)

Maeve Howett, RN, PhD(c), CPNP, IBCLC
Assistant Professor
Emory University
Atlanta, Georgia
CHAPTER 10 • Health Assessment of Children

Randall Johnson, RN, MSN, ARNP
Associate Professor
Florida Hospital College of Health Sciences
Orlando, Florida
CHAPTER 24 • Nursing Care of the Child With a Musculoskeletal Disorder

Kathy Ordelt, RN, CPN, CRRN
Patient and Family Education Coordinator
Children's Healthcare of Atlanta
Atlanta, Georgia
CHAPTER 11 • Nursing Care of Children During Illness and Hospitalization (co-authored with Kathie Aduddell)

Marie Oren-Sosebee, RN, BSN, CWOCN
Wound, Ostomy and Continence Nurse
Children's Healthcare of Atlanta
Atlanta, Georgia
CHAPTER 14 • Medication Administration, Intravenous Therapy, and Nutritional Support

Maggie Payne-Orton, RN, PNP
Clinical Instructor
Emory University
Atlanta, Georgia
CHAPTER 32 • Nursing Care During a Pediatric Emergency

Gayle Wetzel, BSN, MSN, ARNP, CPNP
Professor, Advanced Placement Nursing Program Coordinator
Edison College
Fort Meyers, Florida
CHAPTER 9 • Health Supervision

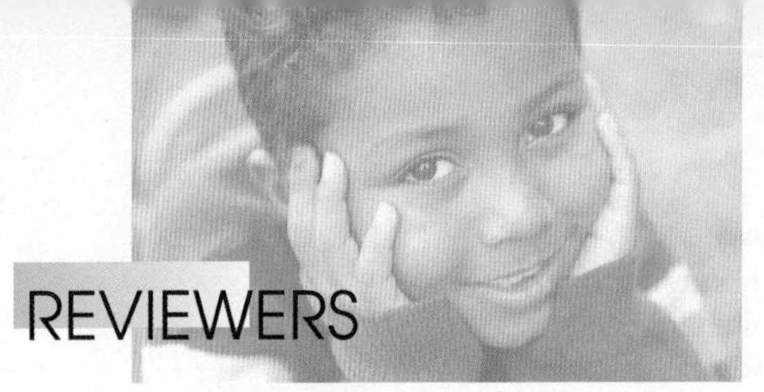

REVIEWERS

Marguerite Aube, BS, MS, CAS
Assistant Professor
University of New England
Portland, Maine

Michele Avila-Emerson, RN, BA, MSN
Fresno City College
Lucille Packard Children's Hospital at Stanford University
Fresno, California

Marty Bachman, RN, PhD
Associate Professor of Nursing
Front Range Community College at Larimer
Fort Collins, Colorado

Vicky Becherer, MSN, RN
Pediatric Clinical Instructor
University of Missouri at St. Louis
St. Louis, Missouri

Jody Bivona, RN, MSN
Nursing Instructor
State University of New York at Ulster
Stone Ridge, New York

Sally Boyster, RN, MS
Professor, Nursing Science Program
Rose State College
Midwest City, Oklahoma

Susan Brillhart, RN, MSN, CPNP
Assistant Professor
Borough of Manhattan Community College
New York, New York

MarJo Bunten, RN, MSN
Assistant Professor
Bradley University
Morton, Illinois

Grace Buttriss, RN, FNP
Nursing Instructor
Queens University of Charlotte
Concord, North Carolina

Karen Carpenter, APRN, BC, FNP, JD
Professor
Quinsigamond Community College
Worcester, Massachusetts

Donna Curry, RN, PhD
Associate Professor
Wright State University
Dayton, Ohio

Dianne DeLong, MSN, RN
Professor, Dean of Professional Accreditation and Curriculum
Lehigh Carbon Community College
Schnecksville, Pennsylvania

Bernadette Dragich, PhD, APRN, BC
Professor
Bluefield State College
Bluefield, West Virginia

Pat Durham-Taylor, RN, PhD
Professor of Nursing
Truckee Meadows Community College
Reno, Nevada

Alison Fisher, RN, MSN, CPN
Instructor
Del Mar College
Corpus Christi, Texas

Lois Griffin, MSN, CFNP
Nursing Instructor
Shelton State Community College
Tuscaloosa, Alabama

Anna Gryczman, MSN, RN, PHN, HNC
Professor
Century College
White Bear Lake, Minnesota

Melanie Hamilton, MSN, BN, RN
Nursing Instructor
Grand Prairie Regional College
Alberta, Canada

Carol Hargate, BS, MPH, CPNP
Assistant Professor
Minnesota State University at Mankato
Mankato, Minnesota

Pat Hendrix, MSN, RN
Director of Nursing
Motlow State Community College
Tullahoma, Tennessee

Jackie Hils-Williams, MSN, RN
Instructor
Golden West College
Huntington Beach, California

Judith Hold, MSN, RN
Nursing Instructor
Chattanooga Technical Institute
Marietta, Georgia

Carol Holtz, RN, PhD
Professor
Kennesaw State University
Kennesaw, Georgia

Carolyn Hulsen, MSN, RN
Professor
Black Hawk College
Eldridge, Iowa

Carrie Huntsman-Jones, MSN, RN, CPN
Assistant Professor
Davis Applied Technical College
Kaysville, Utah

Jean Ivey, DSN, RN, CRNP
Associate Professor
University of Alabama at Birmingham
Birmingham, Alabama

Lynn Jordan, MSN, RN
Professor
Carolinas College of Health Sciences
Charlotte, North Carolina

Katherine Kniest, RN, MSN
Professor
William Rainey Harper College
Palatine, Illinois

Sherry Knoppers, RN, PhDc
Pediatric Nursing Instructor
Grand Rapids Community College
Grand Rapids, Michigan

Penny Leupold, RN, MS
Professor
Joliet Junior College
Joliet, Illinois

Debbie Lewis, RN, MSN, CPN
Instructor
Duquesne University
Pittsburgh, Pennsylvania

Kelli Lewis, BSN, MSN
Practical Nursing Instructor
Rend Lake College
Ina, Illinois

Shirley Mahan, MSN, RN
Assistant Professor
Lincoln Memorial University
Corbin, Kentucky

Larry Manalo, MSN, RN
Director of LVN Program
Allan Hancock College
Santa Maria, California

Barbara Maybury, RN, MsED, MSN
Associate Professor
Northwest Arkansas Community College
Bentonville, Arkansas

Teresa McNabb, RN
Nursing Instructor
South Plains College
Lubbock, Texas

Claire Meggs, MSN, RN
Associate Professor
Lincoln Memorial University
Knoxville, Tennessee

Sandy Olenniczak, RN
Practical Nursing Instructor
Northeast Wisconsin Technical College
Green Bay, Wisconsin

Susan Paterson, RN, MSN
Nursing Instructor
Davenport University Central Region
Midland, Michigan

Lori Peden, MSN, RN, CFNP
Professor
Hocking College
Nelsonville, Ohio

Mary Anne Peters, DNSc, RN
Director of Graduate Nursing Program
LaSalle University
Philadelphia, Pennsylvania

Linda Pina, MSN, RN
Associate Professor
California University of Pennsylvania
California, Pennsylvania

Gena Porter-Lankist, ARNP-C, MSN
Professor
Chipola Junior College
Cottondale, Florida

Susan Reardon, MSN, RN
Nursing Instructor
Allan Hancock College
Lompoc, California

Michelle Renaud, PhD, RN
Associate Professor
Pacific Lutheran University
Tacoma, Washington

Linda Rimer, MSE, RN
Professor
University of Arkansas at Little Rock
Little Rock, Arkansas

Julie Ritland, MSN, ARNP
Assistant Professor
Allen College
Waterloo, Iowa

Melodie Rowbotham, MSN, RN
Clinical Assistant Professor
University of Missouri at St. Louis
O'Fallon, Missouri

Judy Scott, RN
Instructor
Community College of Southern Nevada
North Las Vegas, Nevada

Molly Showalter, BS, RN
Nursing Instructor
North Central Texas College
Gainesville, Texas

Brian Skirvin-Leclair, RN, AS, BSN, MSN
Lecturer in Nursing
Lawrence Memorial, Regis College
Medford, Massachusetts

Bonnie Webster, MS, RN, BC
Nursing Instructor
University of Texas Medical Branch School of Nursing
Galveston, Texas

Patti Witt, MA, CNP
Associate Professor
College of Saint Catherine
Minneapolis, Minnesota

Michele Woodbeck, MS, RN
Assistant Professor
Hudson Valley Community College
Troy, New York

Lisa Woodley, MSN, RN
Clinical Assistant Professor
University of North Carolina School of Nursing
Chapel Hill, North Carolina

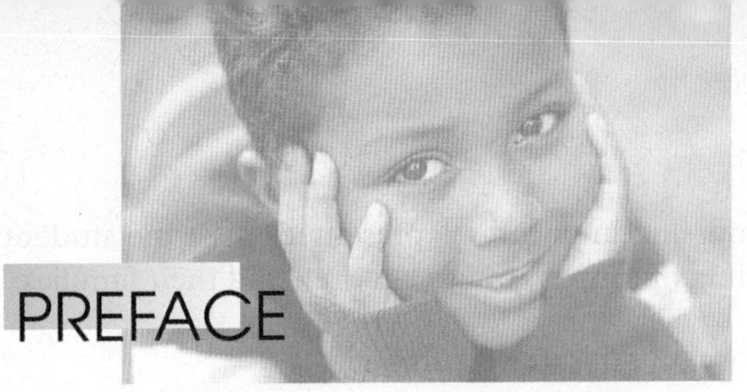

PREFACE

Nursing education is founded upon the principle of mastering simpler concepts first and incorporating those concepts into the student's knowledge base. The student is then able to progress to problem solving in more complex situations. In pediatric nursing, the ability to apply previously learned concepts to new situations is critical. In today's educational climate, with reduced class time being devoted to specialty courses, it is particularly important for nursing educators to focus on key concepts, rather than attempting to cover everything within a specific topic.

The intent of *Essentials of Pediatric Nursing* is to provide the nurse with the basis needed for sound nursing care of children. The main objective is to aid the students in building a strong knowledge base as well as to assist with the development of critical thinking skills. The book covers a broad scope of topics, placing emphasis on common issues and pediatric-specific content. The text presents the important differences when caring for children as compared to caring for adults. Rather than repeating medical-surgical content that the student has already mastered, the text builds upon that knowledge base. A nursing process approach provides relevant information in a concise and non-redundant manner. In Unit IV, specific nursing process content is discussed as appropriate for a given disorder.

Organization

Each chapter of *Essentials of Pediatric Nursing* focuses on a different aspect of pediatric nursing care. The book is divided into four units, beginning with general concepts related to pediatric nursing and followed by normal growth and development and specifics related to caring for children. The fourth unit focuses on nursing management of alterations in children's health.

Unit 1: Introduction to Pediatric Nursing

Unit 1 presents the foundational material the nursing student needs in order to understand how nursing care of the child differs from that of the adult. The unit provides information about general concepts relating to child health. Perspectives on pediatric nursing, the nursing process, factors influencing child health, the family-centered approach, atraumatic care, and communication are key concepts covered in this unit.

Unit 2: Health Promotion for the Growing Child and Family

Unit 2 provides information related to growth and development expectations of the well child from the newborn through adolescence. Though not exhaustive in nature, this unit provides a broad knowledge base related to normal growth and development that the nurse can draw upon in any situation. Common concerns related to growth and development and client/family education are included in each age-specific chapter.

Unit 3: Foundations of Pediatric Nursing

Unit 3 covers broad concepts that provide the foundation for providing nursing care to children. Rather than reiterating all aspects of nursing care, the unit focuses on specific details needed to provide nursing care for children in general. The content remains focused upon differences in caring for children as compared with adults. Topics covered in this unit include anticipatory guidance and routine well-child care (including immunization and safety), health assessment, nursing care of the child in the hospital as well as in the community, concerns common to special-needs children, pediatric variations in nursing procedures, and pain management in children.

Unit 4: Nursing Care of the Child With a Health Disorder

Unit 4 focuses on children's responses to health disorders. This unit provides a comprehensive coverage of illnesses affecting children. It is arranged according to broad topics of disorders organized with a body systems approach and also includes infectious, genetic, and mental health disorders as well as pediatric emergencies. Each chapter follows a similar format in order to facilitate presentation of the information as well as reduce repetition. The chapter begins with a nursing process overview for the particular broad topic, presenting differences in children and how the nursing process applies. The approach provides a general framework for addressing disorders within the chapter. Individual disorders are then addressed with attention to specifics related to pathophysiology, nursing assessment, nursing management, and special considerations. Common pediatric disorders are covered in greater depth than less common disorders. The format of the chapters allows for a strong knowledge base to be built and encourages critical thinking. Additionally, the format is nursing process driven and consistent from chapter to chapter, providing a practical and sensible presentation of the information.

Recurring Features

In order to provide the student and educator with an exciting and user-friendly text, a number of recurring features have been developed.

Key Terms

Each chapter includes a list of key terms that are considered to be vital to understanding the content in the chapter. Each key term appears in boldface, with the definition included in the text. The key terms may also be accessed on thePoint.

Learning Objectives

The provision of learning objectives for each chapter helps to guide the student toward prioritizing information for learning. The objectives also provide a method for the student to evaluate understanding of the presented material.

WOW

Each chapter opens with inspiring Words of Wisdom, which offer helpful, timely, or interesting thoughts. These WOW statements set the stage for the chapter and give the student valuable insight into the nursing care of children and their families.

Case Studies

Real-life scenarios present relevant child and family information that is intended to perfect the student's caregiving skills. Questions about the scenario provide an opportunity for the student to critically evaluate the appropriate course of action.

Watch and Learn Icon

A special icon **WATCH & LEARN** throughout the book directs students to free video clips that highlight growth and development, communicating with children, and providing nursing care to the child in the hospital.

Healthy People 2010

Throughout the textbook, Healthy People 2010 objectives related to children's health and well-being are outlined in box format. Nursing implications or guidance related to working toward achievement of these objectives in provided.

Teaching Guidelines

Teaching Guidelines, presented in most of the chapters, serve as valuable health education tools. The guidelines raise the student's awareness, provide timely and accurate information, and are designed to ensure the student's preparation for educating children and their families about various issues.

Drug Guides

The drug guide tables summarize information about commonly used medications. The actions, indications, and significant nursing implications presented assist the student in providing optimum care to children and their families.

Common Laboratory and Diagnostic Tests

The Common Laboratory and Diagnostic Tests tables in each chapter of Unit 4 provide the student with a general understanding of how a broad range of disorders is diagnosed. Rather than reading the information repeatedly throughout the narrative, the student is then able to refer to the table as needed.

Common Medical Treatments

The Common Medical Treatments tables in each chapter of Unit 4 provide the student with a broad awareness of how a common group of disorders is treated either medically or surgically. The table serves as a reference point for common medical treatments.

Nursing Care Plans

Nursing Care Plans provide concrete examples of each step of the nursing process. Found within the Nursing Process Overview section of each disorder chapter, these nursing care plans summarize issue- or system-related content, thereby minimizing repetition.

Comparison Charts

These charts compare two or more disorders or other easily confused concepts. They serve to provide an explanation that clarifies the concepts for the student.

Nursing Procedures

Step-by-step nursing procedures provide a clear explanation of pediatric variations in order to facilitate competent performance.

Tables, Boxes, Illustrations, and Photographs

Tables and boxes are included throughout the chapters in order to summarize key content areas. Beautiful illustrations and photographs help the student to visualize the content. These features allow the student to quickly and easily access information.

References and Helpful Informational Resources

References and helpful information resources that were used in the development of the text are provided at the end of each chapter. The listings allow the student to further pursue topics of interest. Multiple online sources are also provided as a means for the student to electronically explore relevant content material.

Chapter Worksheets

Chapter worksheets at the end of each chapter assist the student to review essential concepts. Chapter worksheets include:

- **Multiple choice questions**—these questions test the student's ability to apply chapter material. The questions are styled similarly to the national licensing exam (NCLEX-RN).
- **Critical thinking exercises**—these exercises serve to stimulate the student to incorporate the current material with previously learned concepts and reach a satisfactory conclusion. The exercises encourage students to think critically, problem solve, and consider their own perspective on given topics.
- **Study activities**—these activities promote student participation in the learning process. This section encourages increased interaction/learning via clinical, online, and community activities.
- **Answers**—answers to the worksheet are provided on thePoint.

Teaching-Learning Package

Instructor's Resource CD-ROM

This valuable resource for instructors is compatible with WebCT and Blackboard. It includes materials instructors need to teach the pediatric nursing course, including

- **PowerPoint presentations** that correspond to each chapter and serve as a supplement to the instructor's course development
- A **Test Generator** that features hundreds of questions to help instructors create quizzes and tests
- An **Image Bank** that provides access to photographs and illustrations from the text in a convenient, searchable format

Student Resource CD-ROM

The student resource CD-ROM, which is included for free in the front of the book, features video clips highlighting childhood growth and development, communication, and the nursing care provided to a child in the hospital. Pediatric dosage calculation problems, a Spanish-English audio glossary, and an NCLEX Alternate Item Format Tutorial are also included.

ThePoint Solution

ThePoint Solution thePoint (http://thepoint.lww.com), a trademark of Wolters Kluwer Health, is a web-based course and content management system providing every resource that instructors and students need in one easy-to-use site. Advanced technology and superior content combine at thePoint to allow instructors to design and deliver online and off-line courses, maintain grades and class rosters, and communicate with students. Students can visit thePoint to access supplemental multimedia resources, such as Key Concepts, Answers to Worksheets, a Glossary, and NCLEX-style student review questions, to enhance their learning experience. ThePoint Solution package also includes an EBook, so students can search their text electronically, and journal articles to help students understand evidence-based practice. Students can also check the course syllabus, download content, upload assignments, and join an online study group.

For instructors, a wealth of information can be found at thePoint, all designed to make teaching easier. For example:

- **Pre-Lecture Quizzes,** made up of five True/False and five Multiple-Choice questions, are meant to be given at the beginning of class and help evaluate whether students are keeping up with the reading and the material it covers.
- **Assignments,** broken into four types—written, group, clinical, and Web—and organized by learning objective, provide opportunities for in- or after-class activities.
- **Discussion Topics,** also organized by learning objective, allow students to critically think through scenarios and discuss their ideas with other students.
- **Guided Lecture Notes** organize the chapter objective by objective and provide references to appropriate PowerPoint slides and figures from the text.
- **Sample Syllabi** assist instructors with setting up their courses and are provided for four different course lengths: 4, 6, 8, and 10 weeks.

ThePoint . . . where teaching, learning, and technology click!

Online Study Guide to Accompany *Essentials of Pediatric Nursing*

This exciting new resource, built for your WebCT or Blackboard Learning Management System, combines all the helpful activities found in print study guides with additional resources only an online guide can provide. The Online Study Guide is divided into three sections: Assessing Your Understanding, which contains knowledge-based questions, such as Matching, Sequencing, and Fill in the Blank; Applying Your Knowledge, which features application-level questions, including case studies as well as questions based on video vignettes, provided for students within the study guide; and Practicing for NCLEX, which provides NCLEX-style review questions to help students apply and retain the key information from each chapter. The Online Study Guide is a great new way to help assess your students' mastery of information and track their proficiency within the world of pediatric nursing.

Contact your sales representative or visit www.LWW.com/Nursing for more details.

Erickson Stages

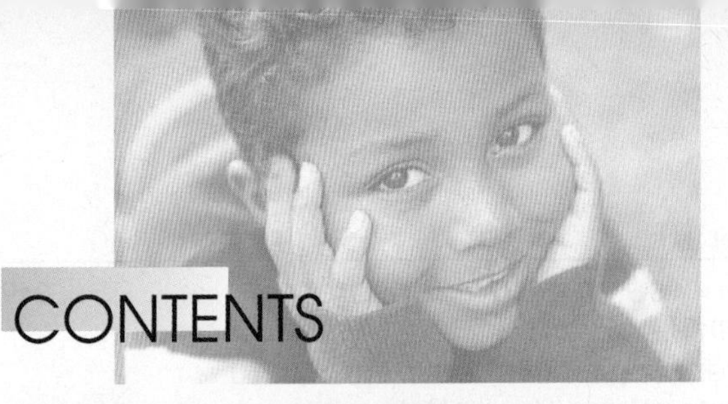

CONTENTS

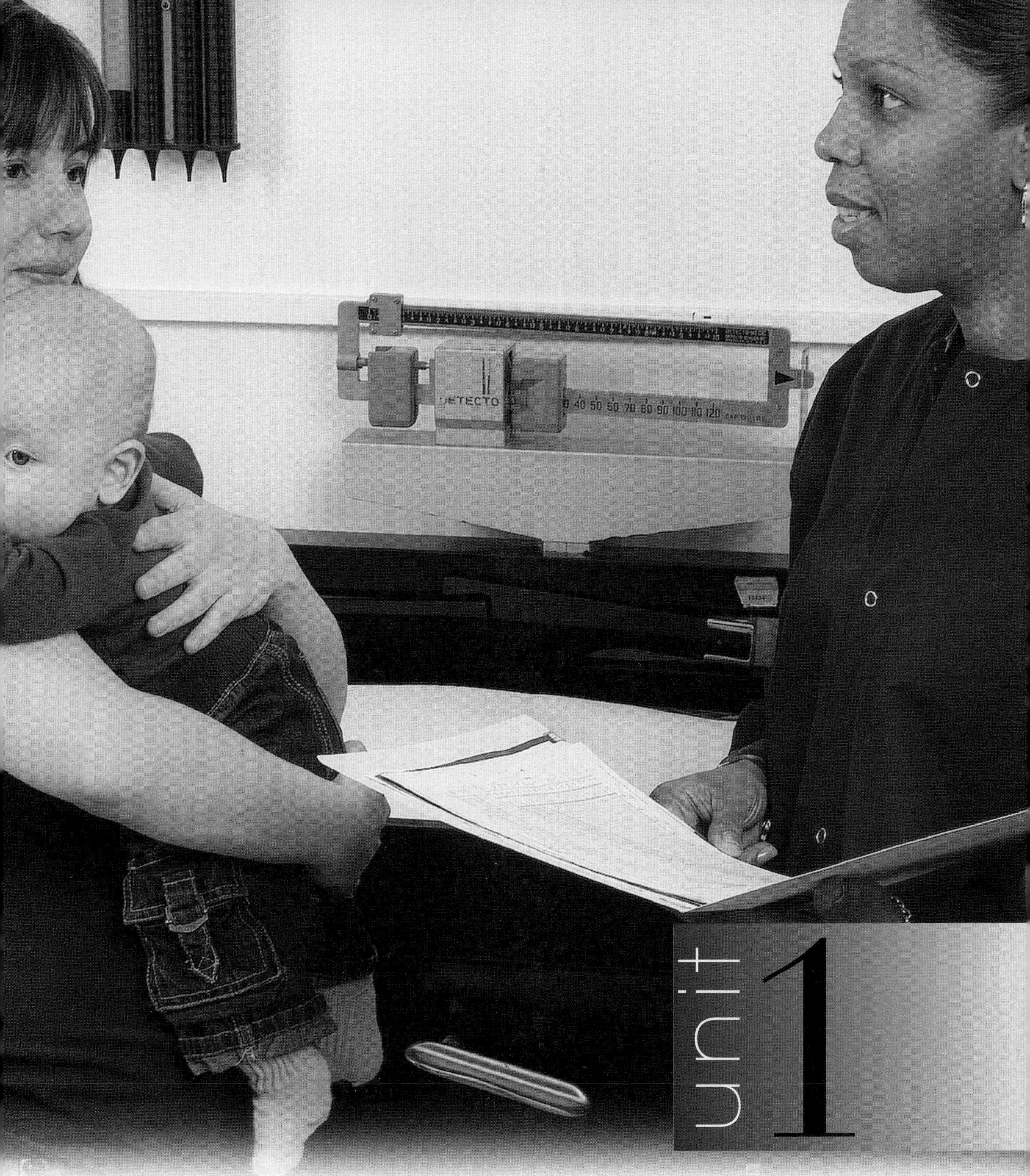

unit 1

Introduction to Pediatric Nursing

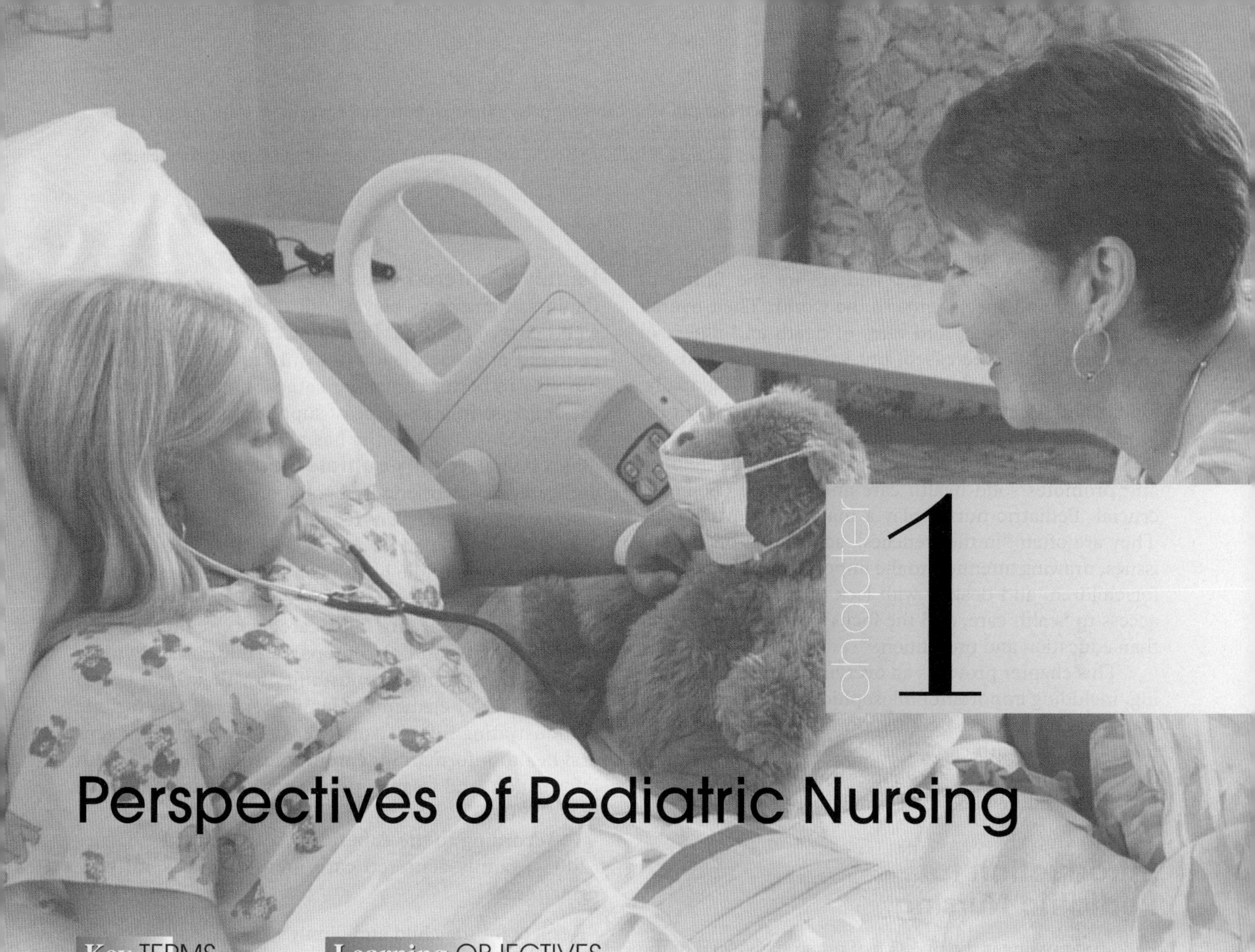

chapter 1

Perspectives of Pediatric Nursing

Key TERMS

advocate
atraumatic care
case management
evidence-based practice
family-centered care
morbidity
mortality
nursing process
standard of care

Learning OBJECTIVES

Upon completion of the chapter, the learner will be able to:

1. Describe the major components, concepts, and influences involved in the nursing practice of children and their families.
2. Identify the key milestones in the evolution of pediatric nursing and child health.
3. Compare the past definitions of health and illness to the current definitions as well as the measurement of health and illness in children.
4. Explain the components of the nursing process as they relate to nursing practice for children and their families.
5. Identify the major roles and functions of pediatric nursing, including the scope of practice and the professional standards for pediatric nurses.

To love children means to see them, respect them, share life with them, but also let them go.

Isabelle Romano is a 6-year-old girl with cerebral palsy. She was born at 28 weeks' gestation and is currently admitted to the hospital due to difficulty breathing secondary to pneumonia. Her parents are very active in her care. Isabelle lives at home with her parents and two brothers, Sergio and Tito. Consider how your role as a nurse can affect this family.

Children are the future of our society and special gifts to the world. Their overall health has improved, and rates of death and illness in some areas have decreased, but we still must focus on children's health both in the United States and globally. Habits and practices established in childhood have profound effects on health and illness throughout life. As a society, creating a population that cares about children and promotes solid health care and lifestyle choices is crucial. Pediatric nurses play a major role in this task. They are often "in the trenches" advocating on various issues, drawing attention to the importance of health care for children, and dealing with lack of resources, lack of access to health care, and the focus on acute care rather than education and prevention.

This chapter provides an overview of pediatric nursing, including important philosophical beliefs, the health status of children, and contemporary issues and trends in children's health care. The chapter concludes with a description of how pediatric nurses use the nursing process to care for children and their families.

Introduction to Pediatric Nursing

Pediatric nursing is the practice of nursing involved in the health care of children from infancy through adolescence. In the United States the number of children under age 18 years is approximately 73.5 million, accounting for 25% of the population (Child Trends, 2006a). The definition of nursing, "the diagnosis and treatment of human responses to actual or potential health problems," also applies to the practice of pediatric nursing (American Nurses Association, 2004). However, the overall goal of pediatric nursing practice is to promote and assist the child in maintaining optimal levels of health while recognizing the influence of the family on the child's well-being. This goal involves the practice of health promotion and disease prevention as well as assisting with care during disease or illness.

Philosophy of Pediatric Nursing Care

Children need accessible, continuous, comprehensive, coordinated, family-centered and compassionate care that focuses on their changing physical and emotional needs (Deal et al., 1998). Pediatric nurses provide this care by focusing on the family, providing atraumatic therapeutic care, and using evidence-based practice. These three concepts represent an overarching philosophy of pediatric nursing care and are integrated throughout the chapters of this text.

Family-Centered Care

Parents or guardians play a critical role in the health and well-being of children. Providing care through a family-centered approach leads not only to better outcomes but also to better consumer satisfaction. The family is the child's primary source of support and strength. The knowledge that the family has about a child's health or illness is vital. **Family-centered care** involves families and caregivers working in a collaborative partnership to determine goals and plans for health care (Woodside et al., 2001). It works well in all arenas of health care, from preventive care of the healthy child to long-term care of the chronically or terminally ill child. Family-centered care enhances parents' and caregivers' confidence in their own skills and also prepares children and young adults for assuming responsibility for their own health care needs. Key elements of family-centered care include demonstrating interpersonal sensitivity, providing general health information, communicating specific health information, and treating people with respect (Woodside et al., 2001).

According to the American Academy of Pediatrics (2003), family-centered care focuses on several core principles:

- Respect for the child and family
- Recognition of the effects of cultural, racial, ethnic, and socioeconomic diversity on the family's health care experience
- Identification of and expansion of the family's strengths
- Support of the family's choices related to the child's health care
- Maintenance of flexibility
- Provision of honest, unbiased information in an affirming and useful approach
- Assistance with the emotional and other support the child and family require
- Collaboration with families
- Empowerment of families

When children's health care is provided through a family-centered approach, many positive outcomes are possible. Anxiety is decreased. Children are calmer and pain management is enhanced. Recovery times are shortened. Families' confidence and problem-solving skills are improved. Communication between the health care team and the family is also improved, leading to greater satisfaction for both health care providers and health care consumers (families). Ways to increase collaboration between the family and the health care team may include a family advisory board, newsletter, or parent resource notebooks. Methods for increasing communication between the health care team and the family may include the use of mailboxes or dry-erase boards for updating the daily plan of care, including the parents' participation in rounds, or through a daily assessment of health status by the child or family.

Vigilant parents are committed to their child's care. They demonstrate resilience in their ability to make it through the emotional upheaval associated with an illness. They may experience changes in their other relationships as well as in the relationships they have with health care providers (Dudley & Carr, 2004). Research has shown that families desire and appreciate nurses' sensitivity to the inconveniences that their child's illness may impose upon the family (Miceli & Clark, 2005). Families want to have their emotional and spiritual needs addressed, their concerns attended to, and their accommodations improved (when the child is hospitalized) (Fig. 1.1). They want to be included and valued in the health care decision-making process (Miceli & Clark, 2005) and to establish rapport with the nurses caring for their child (Espezel & Canam, 2003). Practicing true family-centered care may empower the family, strengthen family resources, and help the child feel more secure throughout the process.

> How could family-centered care help the Romano family described at the beginning of the chapter?

Atraumatic Care

Children may undergo a wide range of interventions, many of which can be traumatic, stressful, and painful. The various settings in which the child receives care can be scary and overwhelming to the child and family, and interacting with various health care personnel in various settings can cause anxiety. Thus, another major component of the pediatric nursing philosophy is providing **atraumatic care**. This is a philosophy of providing therapeutic care through interventions that minimize physical and psychological distress for children and their families. Pediatric nurses must be vigilant for any situation that may cause distress and must be able to identify potential stressors. They take steps to minimize separation of the child from the family, and the nursing care they provide decreases the child's exposure to stressful situations and prevents or minimizes pain and bodily injury. Chapter 3 provides additional information related to atraumatic care.

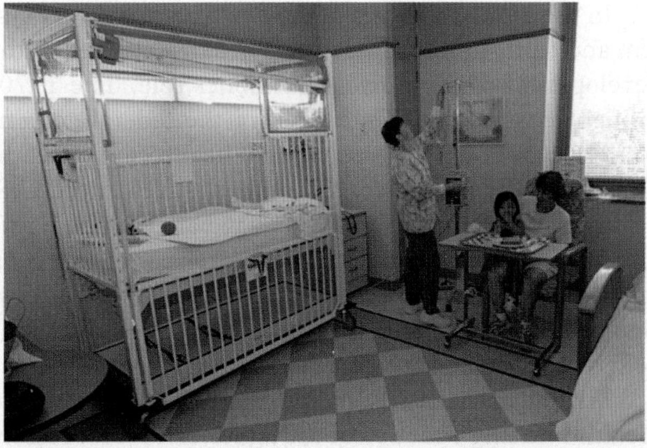

● Figure 1.1 Providing a comfortable area for the parent to rest is an important component of family-centered care.

Evidence-Based, Case Management Care

Modern pediatric health care focuses on an interdisciplinary plan of care designed to meet the child's physical, developmental, educational, spiritual, and psychosocial needs. Nurses coordinate the implementation of this interdisciplinary plan in a collaborative manner to ensure continuity of care that is cost-effective, quality-oriented, and outcome-focused. This type of care is termed **case management**. Box 1.1 highlights the components of case management. When the nurse functions as a case manager, patient and family satisfaction is increased, fragmentation of care is decreased, and outcome measurement for a homogeneous group of patients is possible.

Case management uses a system of plans, often referred to as critical paths, that are derived from standards of care with a multidisciplinary approach that produces clinical practice guidelines. Implementing this philosophy leads to outcomes that are expected as a result of delivery of that care and may lead to future payment tied to the practice guidelines. The Agency for Health Care Policy and Research and the National Guidelines Clearinghouse maintain current clinical practice guidelines. Clinical practice guidelines are rooted in evidence-based practice.

Evidence-based practice involves the use of research findings in establishing a plan of care and implementing that care. Evidence-based practice is a problem-solving approach to making nursing clinical decisions (Newhouse, 2006). This concept of nursing practice includes the use of the best current evidence in making

BOX 1.1

COMPONENTS OF CASE MANAGEMENT

- Collaborative process involving assessment, planning, implementation, coordination, monitoring, and evaluation
- Advocacy, communication, and resource management
- Patient-focused comprehensive care across a continuum
- Coordinated care with an interdisciplinary approach

Commission for Case Management Certification. (n.d.).

decisions about the care of children and their families. Evidence-based practice may lead to a decrease in variations in care while at the same time increasing quality. An example of evidence-based practice is the current pediatric blood pressure measurement recommendations. Due to the difficulty with obtaining consistent and appropriate blood pressure measurements in children, as well as the increase in blood pressure in children over the past several years, the National High Blood Pressure Education Program Working Group published recommendations for routine blood pressure measurement in children. The guidelines address factors affecting the child's blood pressure, use of auscultatory or oscillometric measurement devices, appropriate blood pressure cuff size and application, and site of blood pressure measurement. The goal is to permit early screening and identification of children at risk for hypertension (Schell, 2006). Recent studies provide evidence that nurse-led interventions improve overall health and management of chronic illness.

The Evolution of Pediatric Nursing in Relationship to Child Health

The historical perspective of pediatric nursing includes the devastating epidemics that affected children in the past, societal trends in our country, changes in the health care system, and federal and state regulations. This discussion will provide a brief overview of the evolution of pediatric nursing. By reviewing these historical events, pediatric nurses can gain a better understanding of the current and future status of pediatric nursing.

In past centuries in the United States, the health of the country was poorer than it is today; mortality rates were high and life expectancy was short. When a flood of immigrants from Europe settled in the eastern American cities, infectious diseases were rampant because of the crowded living conditions, inadequate and unsanitary food (e.g., contaminated milk), and harsh working conditions (including child labor). Devastating epidemics of smallpox, diphtheria, scarlet fever, and measles hit children the hardest. During this period, the prevalent view was that children were a commodity; their role was to increase the population and share in the work to be done. This view changed over the years, as public schools were established and the court system began viewing children as minors.

Over time, changes occurred that focused attention on the health of children. In 1870, the first pediatric professorship for a physician was awarded in the United States to Abraham Jacobi, who is known as the father of pediatrics. For the first time, the medical community realized there was a need to provide specialized training and education about children to health care providers. In 1889 Jacobi established milk distribution centers, which provided mothers with uncontaminated milk for their sick infants and also stressed the importance of pasteurization. This one intervention led to a decrease in infant deaths.

In the early 1900s, Lillian Wald established the Henry Street Settlement House in New York City; this was the start of public health nursing. This facility provided medical and other services to poor families. These services included home nurse visits to teach mothers about health care.

Health care personnel were trained to take care of children in hospitals, but parents of hospitalized children were discouraged from visiting to prevent the spread of infection. Restricting parents from being involved in their child's care was also thought to minimize emotional stress.

Nursing in public schools began in 1902 with the appointment of Lina Rogers as a full-time public school nurse in New York. A professional course in pediatric nursing was started in the early 1900s at Teachers' College of Columbia University.

The turn of the 20th century brought new knowledge about nutrition, sanitation, bacteriology, pharmacology, medication, and psychology. Penicillin, corticosteroids, and vaccines, which were developed during this time, assisted with the fight against communicable diseases. By the end of the 20th century, technological advances had significantly affected all aspects of health care. These trends have led to increased survival rates in children. However, many children who survive illnesses that were previously considered fatal are left with chronic disabilities. For example, before the 1960s, extremely premature infants did not survive because of the immaturity of their lungs. Mechanical ventilation and the use of medications to foster lung development have increased survival rates in premature infants, but survivors are often faced with a myriad of chronic illnesses such as bronchopulmonary dysplasia, retinopathy of prematurity, cerebral palsy, or developmental delay. This increased survival has resulted in a significant increase in chronic illness relative to acute illness as a cause of hospitalization and mortality.

In the 1960s, changes in the health care delivery system and shifts in the population's health status led to the development of the nurse practitioner role. The 1970s brought cost-control systems from the federal government because of rapid escalation of health care expenditures. In addition, the considerable changes in the U.S. health care system in the 1980s have affected pediatric nursing and child health care. The emphasis of care is on quality outcomes and cost containment. Some of these changes brought more advanced practice nurses into the field of pediatrics.

Finally, in the 1980s, the Division of Maternal-Child Health Nursing Practice of the American Nurses Association developed maternal-child health standards to provide important guidelines for delivering nursing care.

The Pediatric Nursing Role and Health Care Settings

The professional pediatric registered nurse provides three levels of health care services: primary, secondary, and tertiary. The primary level of service focuses on health promotion and illness prevention and typically occurs in the community. The pediatric nurse may provide this level of service in a variety of settings, including health clinics or offices, schools, homes, daycare centers, and summer camps. The secondary level of service is generally provided in acute treatment centers that focus on the diagnosis and treatment of illness. The pediatric nurse functions at the secondary level when working in settings such as general pediatric hospital units, pediatric intensive care units, emergency departments, ambulatory clinics, surgical centers, and psychiatric centers. The tertiary level of service involves restorative, rehabilitative, or quality-of-life care and takes place in rehabilitation centers or hospice programs or through service with a home health agency.

Although nurses in each setting might have specific roles and responsibilities, they all share universal roles that can be identified as primary and secondary roles, the differentiated practice role, and the advanced practice role. Within all of these roles, the nurse ensures that communication with the child and family is based on the child's age and developmental level.

The primary role of the pediatric nurse is to provide direct nursing care to children and their families, being an **advocate**, educator, and manager. As a child and family advocate, the nurse safeguards and advances the interests of children and their families by knowing their needs and resources, informing them of their rights and options, and assisting them to make informed decisions. In the primary role of educator, the nurse instructs and counsels children and their families about all aspects of health and illness. The pediatric nurse uses and integrates research findings to establish evidence-based practice, managing the delivery of care in a cost-effective manner to promote continuity of care and an optimal outcome for the child and family.

In the secondary role, the pediatric nurse serves as a collaborator, care coordinator, and consultant. Collaborating with the interdisciplinary health care team, the pediatric nurse integrates the child's and family's needs into a coordinated plan of care. In the role of consultant, the pediatric nurse ensures that the child's and family's needs are met through such activities as support group facilitation or working with the school nurse to plan the child's care.

In the differentiated practice role, the nurse's experience, competence, and educational level determine the nurse's role. For example, a clinical coordinator typically holds a baccalaureate degree and fills a leadership role in a variety of settings. The case manager, also usually a baccalaureate-prepared nurse, is responsible for integrating care from before admission to after discharge.

The advanced practice role is an expanded nursing role that requires additional education and skills in the assessment and management of children and their families. The pediatric nurse practitioner (PNP) has a master's degree and national certification in the specialty area. The PNP is an independent and autonomous practitioner, managing children in primary, acute, or intensive care or providing long-term management of the child with a chronic illness. The clinical nurse specialist has a master's degree and provides expertise as an educator, clinician, or researcher, meeting the needs of staff, children, and families.

Various changes in the health care system continue to encourage the development of the advanced practice role for pediatric nursing. Table 1.1 describes the functions of the family nurse practitioner, the neonatal nurse practitioner, and the pediatric nurse practitioner as well as the pediatric clinical specialist and case manager.

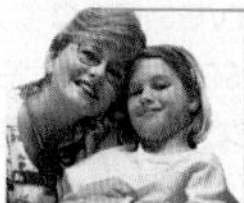

The American Academy of Colleges of Nursing (2005) has recommended that nurse practitioner education be moved from the master's to the doctoral level by the year 2015.

Standards of Care and Performance in Today's Environment

In any role, the professional pediatric nurse is held accountable for nursing actions that adhere to the standards of care. A **standard of care** is a minimally accepted action expected of an individual of a certain skill or knowledge level and reflects what a reasonable and prudent person would do in a similar situation. Professional standards from regulatory agencies, state or federal laws, nurse practice acts, and other specialty groups regulate nursing practice in general. The American Nurses Association (ANA) and the Society of Pediatric Nurses (SPN) have formulated specific standards of care and professional performance for pediatric clinical nursing practice (Table 1.2). These standards are tools that determine if care constitutes adequate, effective, and acceptable nursing practice. They also serve as guides and legal measures for this special area of practice. These standards promote consistency in practice, provide important guidelines for care planning, assist with the development of outcome criteria, and ensure quality nursing care. The ANA-SPN standards specify what is adequate and effective for general pediatric nursing and promote consistency in practice.

Children's Health Status

Since children are a gift to this world, it is society's responsibility to nurture and care for them. Health used to be defined simply as the absence of disease; health was

Table 1.1 Advanced Practice Roles for Pediatric Nurses

Role	Function
Pediatric nurse practitioner (PNP)	• Provides health maintenance care for children (well-child examinations, developmental screening, immunizations, anticipatory guidance, and school physicals) • Diagnoses and treats common childhood illnesses • Provides care to acutely, chronically, or critically ill children (performs in-depth physical assessments and health histories, interprets laboratory and diagnostic tests, prescribes medications, and performs therapeutic treatments) (National Association of Pediatric Nurse Practitioners, 2006)
Family nurse practitioner (FNP)	• Provides health care to individuals throughout the life span • Performs health assessments, orders and interprets diagnostic and laboratory tests, prescribes pharmacologic and nonpharmacologic treatments (American Academy of Nurse Practitioners, 2002)
Neonatal nurse practitioner (NNP)	• Differentiates the nurse practitioner role to the care of the newborn • Functions in similar manner to the PNP or FNP, but within the newborn nursery or neonatal intensive care unit (National Association of Neonatal Nurses, 2002)
Clinical nurse specialist—specialist in specific pediatric areas, such as pediatric oncology clinical nurse specialist	• Serves as a consultant in a particular area of expertise • Researches, educates, and serves as a role model for expert nursing care in specialty field (National Association of Clinical Nurse Specialists, n.d.)
Case manager—specialist in pediatric hospitals and other pediatric health care settings	• Supervises a group of patients from the time they enter a health care setting until they are discharged from the setting • Monitors effectiveness, cost, and patient satisfaction

measured by monitoring the mortality and morbidity of a group. Over the past century, though, the focus of health has shifted to disease prevention, health promotion, and wellness. The World Health Organization (2006) defines health as "a state of complete physical, mental, and social well-being, and not merely the absence of disease or infirmity." Thus, the definition of health is complex; it is not merely the absence of disease or a review of mortality and morbidity statistics.

In 1979, the U.S. Surgeon General's Report, *Healthy People*, presented an agenda for the nation that identified the most significant preventable threats to health. With the series of updates that followed, including the present one, *Healthy People 2010: National Health Promotion and Disease Prevention Objectives*, the country has a comprehensive health promotion and disease prevention agenda that emphasizes children's health (U.S. Department of Health and Human Services, 2000). Major goals are to increase the quality and years of healthy life and to eliminate health disparities between ethnic groups by targeting the lifestyle choices and environmental conditions that cause 70% of premature deaths in the United States. There are 10 specific health indicators, including children's health indicators, that serve as a way to evaluate the progress made in public health; they also serve as focal points to coordinate the national health improvement efforts. For example, one objective under physical activity is to increase the proportion of adolescents who engage in vigorous physical activity three or more days per week for 20 or more minutes per occasion (U.S. Department of Health and Human Services, 2000). Healthy People 2010 1.1 highlights the major health concerns of the 21st century that need to be addressed.

Measurement of Children's Health Status

Measuring a child's health status is not always a simple process. For example, some children with chronic illnesses do not see themselves as "ill" if they can manage their disease. A traditional method of measuring health is to examine mortality and morbidity data. This information is collected and analyzed to provide an objective description of the nation's health.

Mortality

Mortality is the number of individuals who have died over a specific period. This statistic is presented as rates per 100,000 and is calculated from a sample of death certificates. The National Center for Health Statistics, under the Department of Health and Human Services, collects, analyzes, and disseminates these data.

Table 1.2 American Nurses Association/Society of Pediatric Nurses Scope and Standards of Pediatric Nursing Practice

Standard	Description
Standard of care	1. **Assessment:** The pediatric nurse collects health data. 2. **Diagnosis:** The pediatric nurse analyzes the assessment data in determining diagnosis. 3. **Outcome identification:** The pediatric nurse identifies expected outcomes individualized to the client. 4. **Planning:** The pediatric nurse develops a plan of care that prescribes interventions to obtain expected outcomes. 5. **Implementation:** The pediatric nurse implements the interventions identified in the plan of care. 6. **Evaluation:** The pediatric nurse evaluates the child's and family's progress toward attainment of outcomes.
Standards of professional performance	1. **Quality of care:** The pediatric nurse systematically evaluates the quality and effectiveness of pediatric nursing practice. 2. **Performance appraisal:** The pediatric nurse evaluates his or her own nursing practice in relation to professional practice standards and relevant statutes and regulations. 3. **Education:** The pediatric nurse acquires and maintains current knowledge in pediatric nursing practice. 4. **Collegiality:** The pediatric nurse contributes to the professional development of peers, colleagues, and others. 5. **Ethics:** The pediatric nurse's decisions and actions on behalf of children and their families are determined in an ethical manner. 6. **Collaboration:** The pediatric nurse collaborates with the child, family, and health care provider in providing client care. 7. **Research:** The pediatric nurse uses research findings in practice. 8. **Resource utilization:** The pediatric nurse considers factors related to safety, effectiveness, and cost in planning and delivering care.

Neonatal and Infant Mortality

Neonatal mortality is the number of infant deaths occurring in the first 28 days of life per 1,000 live births. The infant mortality rate refers to the number of deaths occurring in the first 12 months of life. It also is documented as the number of deaths in relation to 1,000 live births. The infant mortality rate is used as an index of the general health of a country. Generally, this statistic is one of the most significant measures of children's health. In 2003, the infant mortality rate in the United States was 6.85 per 1,000 live births (Hoyert et al., 2006; Fig. 1.2).

The infant mortality rate varies greatly from state to state as well as between ethnic groups. The United States

HEALTHY PEOPLE 2010

Major health concerns of the 21st century

- Physical activity
- Overweight and obesity
- Tobacco use
- Substance abuse
- Responsible sexual behavior
- Mental health
- Injury and violence
- Environmental quality
- Immunizations
- Access to health care

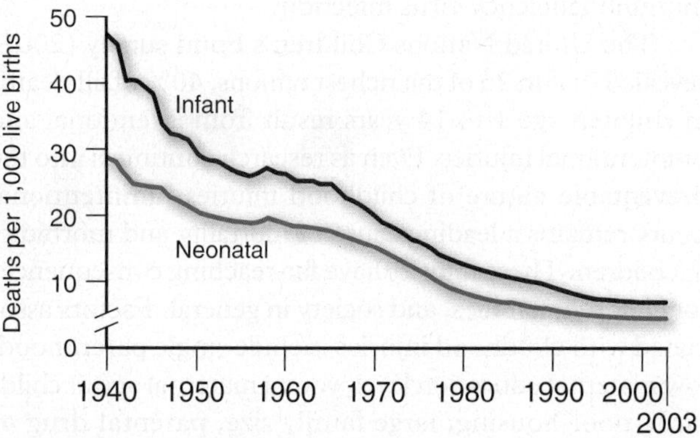

● **Figure 1.2** Infant and neonatal mortality from 1940 to 2003. (Adapted from Hoyert et al., 2006.)

has one of the highest gross national products in the world and is known for its technological capabilities, but it ranked 27th in infant mortality rates among industrialized nations in 2000 (U.S. Department of Health and Human Services, 2006). The main causes of early infant death in this country include problems occurring at birth or shortly thereafter, such as prematurity, low birthweight, congenital anomalies, sudden infant death syndrome, and respiratory distress syndrome.

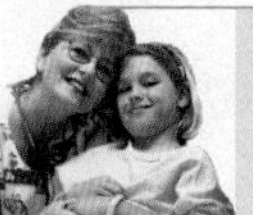

African-Americans and American Indian/Alaskan Native infants have consistently had higher infant mortality rates than other ethnic groups (Federal Interagency Forum on Child and Family Statistics, 2006).

Congenital anomalies remain the leading cause of infant mortality in the United States. Low birthweight and prematurity are major indicators of infant health and significant predictors of infant mortality (Hoyert et al., 2006). The lower the birthweight, the higher the risk of infant mortality; thus, the high incidence of low birthweight (<2,500 g) in the United States plays a factor in the higher infant mortality rate when compared to other countries (Guyer et al., 2000).

Childhood Mortality

Childhood mortality is defined as the number of deaths per 100,000 population in children 1 to 14 years of age. The childhood mortality rate in the United States has decreased by about 50% since 1980. In 2003, the mortality rate for children ages 1 to 4 years was 31 per 100,000 and the rate for children ages 5 to 14 years was 17 per 100,000 (Child Trends, 2006b). The leading cause of death in children is motor vehicle accidents. These deaths can often be prevented through education about the value of using car seats and seat belts, the dangers of driving under the influence of alcohol and other substances, and the importance of pedestrian safety. Other causes of childhood mortality include suicide, homicide, and human immunodeficiency virus infection.

The United Nations Children's Fund survey (2001) revealed that in 26 of the richest nations, 40% of all deaths in children age 1 to 14 years result from intentional and unintentional injuries. Even as research continues into the preventable nature of childhood injuries, unintentional injury remains a leading cause of mortality and morbidity in children. These injuries have far-reaching consequences for children, families, and society in general. Factors associated with childhood injuries include single parenthood, low maternal education level, young maternal age at childbirth, poor housing, large family size, parental drug or alcohol abuse, or low support within the family (United Nations Children's Fund, 2001). One study showed that preschool children who had been injured previously displayed significantly higher numbers of injury behaviors (Bruce et al., 2004). This suggests that screening for injury behaviors can be a useful tool when nurses are providing injury prevention counseling.

Morbidity

Morbidity is the measure of prevalence of a specific illness in a population at a particular time. It is presented in rates per 1,000 population. Morbidity is often difficult to define and record because the definitions used vary widely—for example, visits to the physician or diagnosis for hospital admission. Also, data may be difficult to obtain, such as that gathered by household interviews from research studies. Morbidity statistics are revised less frequently because of the difficulty in defining or obtaining the information.

In general, however, 56% of children enjoyed excellent health and 28% had very good health as reported in a summary of health statistics for children in 2002 (Dey et al., 2004). Factors that may increase morbidity include homelessness, poverty, low birthweight, chronic health disorders, foreign-born adoption, attendance at daycare centers, and barriers to health care. For example, 16% of children live in poverty and have a higher incidence of disease, limited coordination of health services, and limited access to health care, except for visits to the emergency department (Federal Interagency Forum on Child and Family Statistics, 2006). Although the poverty rate declined from 22% in 1993 to 17% in 2004, 47% of African-American children live in poverty; these children are particularly at increased risk for illness (Federal Interagency Forum on Child and Family Statistics, 2006).

The most important aspect of morbidity is the degree of disability it produces, which is identified in children as the number of days missed from school or confined to bed. In 2002, only 25% of children did not miss any school due to illness or injury; however, 6% missed more than 10 days of school because of injury or illness (National Center for Health Statistics, 2004). In the United States during 2002, 3.4 million children (ages 1 to 21 years) were hospitalized (National Center for Health Statistics, 2006). Figure 1.3 shows the major causes of hospitalization by age in the United States.

Common health problems in children include respiratory disorders, such as asthma; gastrointestinal disturbances, which lead to malnutrition and dehydration; and injuries. Twelve percent of children in the United States have asthma, and another 12% of children have respiratory allergies (National Center for Health Statistics, 2004). Diseases of the respiratory system were the major cause of hospitalization for children 1 to 9 years of age

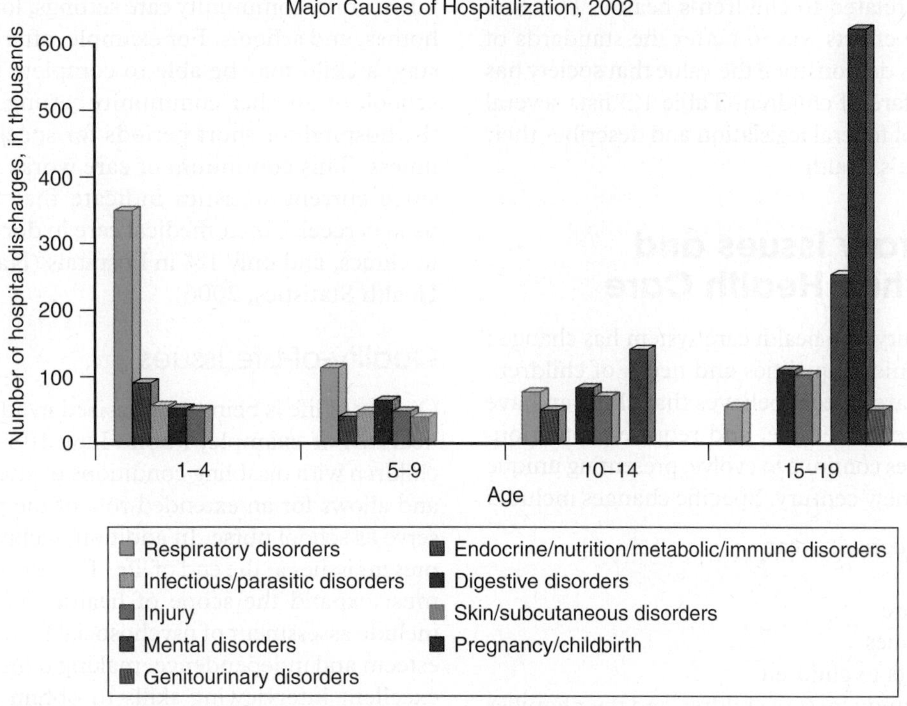

● **Figure 1.3** 2002: causes of hospitalization in children.

(National Center for Health Statistics, 2004). As more immunizations become available, common childhood communicable diseases affect fewer children. The tracking of the leading indicators from *Healthy People 2010* provides some positive information related to improving children's health.

One trend in the United States is the increasing number of children with mental health disorders and related emotional, social, or behavioral problems. The American Academy of Pediatrics (2001) estimates that 13 million children in the United States have mental health–related problems. These problems may limit the child's educational success. They also increase the child's risk for significant mental health problems later in life or emotional problems and possible use of firearms, reckless driving, promiscuous sexual activity, and substance abuse during adolescence. Overall, these behavioral, social, and educational problems can interfere with children's social and academic development.

The incidence of mental health disorders and related emotional, social, or behavioral problems can range from 5% to 30%, depending on how one defines the problems. Some experts include poverty, violence, aggression, noncompliance, school failure, or adjustment issues related to divorce and blended families as part of this group of problems and identify them as a new group of "diseases" of children (Altemeier, 2000). Many times insurance does not reimburse for these problems, leading to additional concerns such as lack of treatment.

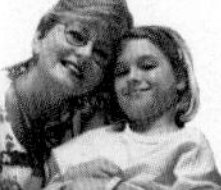

Environmental and psychosocial factors are now an identified area of concern in children. They include academic difficulties, complex psychiatric disorders, self-harm and harm to others, use of firearms, hostility at school, substance abuse, HIV/AIDS, and adverse effects of the media.

Role of the Pediatric Nurse

The nurse's role in relation to morbidity and mortality in children involves educating the family and community regarding the usual causes of deaths, the types of childhood illnesses, and the symptoms that require health care. The goal is to raise awareness and provide guidance and counseling to prevent unnecessary deaths and illnesses in children. The health of children is basic to their well-being and development, and the attention given to children's health in this country has slowly increased over the years. The pediatric nurse is in an excellent position to improve the future health of children.

Federal Legislation Affecting Child Health

Numerous federal programs have had a major impact on child health. President Theodore Roosevelt began the crusade to assist children and their families, especially the poor. The establishment of the Children's Bureau in 1912 began a period of studying economic and social factors related to infant mortality, infant care in rural areas, and other factors related to children's health. The goal of these legislative efforts was to better the standards of care. These actions demonstrate the value that society has placed on the welfare of children. Table 1.3 lists several significant pieces of federal legislation and describes their impact on children's health.

Contemporary Issues and Trends in Child Health Care

Over the past century, the health care system has changed to recognize the unique qualities and needs of children. This new health care system believes that children have a special value, are vulnerable, and require protection. Health care practices continue to evolve, presenting unique challenges for the new century. Specific changes include:

- Health care cost containment
- Preventive care
- Continuum of care
- Quality-of-life issues
- Worldwide threats to children
- Differences and uniqueness of children and their families
- Significant improvements in the diagnosis and treatment of diseases and disorders
- Empowerment of health care consumers
- Reduction in barriers to health care
- Protection of children's rights

Each of these changes will continue to affect children and pediatric nursing practice. Societal needs as well as global needs drive these transformations.

Health Care Cost Containment

A goal of managed care has been to reduce health care costs, and these efforts have shortened hospital stays for children and increased nurses' awareness of the costs of supplies and services. The overall challenge is to maintain the quality of care while reducing its cost.

Preventive Care

Efforts to reduce costs have also led to an increased emphasis on preventive care. Anticipatory guidance is vital during each health contact with children and their families. Education of the family includes everything from keeping the home safe to preventing illness. These are major points of emphasis for pediatric nurses as they deliver care to children and their families.

Continuum of Care

In an effort to become more cost-effective and to provide care more efficiently, the nursing care of children now encompasses a continuum of care that extends from acute care settings such as hospitals to outpatient settings such as ambulatory care clinics, primary care offices, rehabilitative units, community care settings, long-term facilities, homes, and schools. For example, after an acute hospital stay, a child may be able to complete therapy at home, school, or another community setting and can re-enter the hospital for short periods for specific treatments or illness. This continuum of care works well for children, since current statistics indicate that 80% of children usually receive their medical care in doctor's offices, 18% in clinics, and only 1% in hospitals (National Center for Health Statistics, 2006).

Quality-of-Life Issues

Quality of life is being emphasized in addition to physical health. For example, Public Law 108-446 provides for children with disabling conditions to attend regular school and allows for an extended role of the pediatric nurse to serve as school nurse. In addition, technological advances present issues at the end of life. Therefore, pediatric nurses must expand the scope of health care they provide to include assessment of psychosocial factors in areas of self-esteem and independence, making home visits, and using excellent interviewing skills to obtain information that may assist in the care related to these areas.

Concerns Over World Threats and Safety

Disasters such as the terrorist attacks of Sept. 11, 2001, the killings at Columbine High School, or devastating weather events such as Hurricane Katrina can have a significant impact on the well-being of children. The increase in stressors such as war, terrorism, school violence, and natural disasters may reduce children's coping abilities (Ryan-Wenger et al., 2005) and may lead to alterations in growth and development (Crane & Clements, 2005). Children who have experienced these events are at risk for posttraumatic stress disorder, behavioral problems, and depression (Wexler et al., 2006). These disasters may be most difficult for children who have previously gone through a major loss or already suffer from anxiety or depression (Davidhizar & Shearer, 2002). Pediatric nurses must be aware of the effects of world threats on children so that they can assess for alterations and intervene to promote security and stability.

Diverse Patient Populations

The United States is no longer a "melting pot" of various cultures and ethnicities but a society in which each distinct individual brings a diversity and richness that as a whole enriches the country. Today, children do not fit into a set category or group. Children and families vary in terms of culture, family structure, socioeconomic status, background, and circumstances, so each child enters the health care system as a unique individual. Pediatric nurses must have greater sensitivity to the background of

Table 1.3 Milestones in Federal Programs in Support of Children's Health

Date	Action	Impact
1909	First White House Conference on Care of Dependent Children (convened by President Theodore Roosevelt)	Addressed the poor working and living conditions of many children in the United States
1912	U.S. Children's Bureau	Established the first governmental agency to oversee children's health and environmental conditions
1921	Maternity & Infancy (Sheppard-Towner) Act	Provided grants to states to establish maternal and child health divisions in state health departments
1930	White House Conference on Child Welfare Standards and American Academy of Pediatrics	Produced the Children's Charter, documenting the child's need for health, education, welfare, and protection
1935	Title V of the Social Security Act	Established federal–state partnership and provided Aid to Dependent Families and Children (ADFC), maternal-child health services, and child welfare services
1959	14th General Assembly of United Nations	Approved the Declaration of the Rights of the Child
1965	Medicaid Program under Title XIX of Social Security Act; special programs such as Child Health Assessment Program	Provided state block grants to reduce financial barriers to health care for the poor and special services to pregnant women and young children
1966/1974	Women, Infants, Children (WIC) program	Provided nutritional supplementation and education to low-income families; pregnant, postpartum, and lactating women; and infants and children up to age 5
1969	U.S. Children's Bureau moves to Office of Health, Education & Welfare (HEW).	Established greater presence for the programs
1975	Education for All Handicapped Children Act (Public Law 94-142)	Established federally mandated special education in public schools.
	Title XX Social Services	Provided block grants to daycare, emergency shelters, counseling, family planning, and other services for children.
1981	Alcohol, Drug Abuse & Mental Health block grants	Began funding services for children and adolescents with mental health issues
1986	Education of Handicapped Act Amendments (Public Law 99-457)	Established federal funding for states to create statewide, comprehensive, coordinated, and multidisciplinary early-intervention services for handicapped infants and toddlers
1990	Omnibus Budget Reconciliation Act	Extended Medicaid coverage to all children (6 to 18 years) with family income below 133% of poverty level
1993	Family & Medical Leave Act (FMLA)	Allowed eligible employees to take up to 12 weeks of unpaid leave from their jobs every year to care for newborns or newly adopted children or children, parents, or spouses who have a serious health condition; employee can return to previous job or a comparable job with the same conditions

each child and must be able to provide care that addresses the child's uniqueness.

Improvements in Diagnosis and Treatment

Tremendous improvements in technology and biomedicine have created a trend toward earlier diagnosis and treatment of disorders and diseases. Throughout the 1990s remarkable progress was made linking genetics and pathophysiologic processes. For example, female fetuses with congenital adrenal hyperplasia, a genetic disorder resulting in a steroid enzyme deficiency that can lead to disfiguring anatomic abnormalities, are beginning to receive treatment before birth. In addition, many genetic defects are being identified so that counseling and treatment may occur early.

As a result of this improved diagnosis and treatment, the pediatric nurse now cares for children who have survived once-fatal situations, are living well beyond the usual life expectancy for a specific illness, or are functioning and attending school with chronic disabilities. While positive and exciting, these advances and trends pose new challenges for the health care community. For example, as care for premature newborns improves and survival rates have increased, so too has the incidence of long-term chronic conditions such as respiratory airway dysfunction or developmental delays. As a result, pediatric nurses care for children at all stages along the health–illness continuum, from well children, to those who are occasionally ill, to those with chronic, sometimes disabling conditions.

Empowerment of Consumers

Due to the influence of managed care, the focus on prevention, better education, and technological advances, people have taken increased responsibility for their own health. Parents now want information about their child's illness, they want to participate in making decisions about treatment, and they want to accompany their children to all health care situations. As child advocates who value family-centered care, pediatric nurses can provide such empowerment and can address specific issues for children and families. Pediatric nurses must respect the family's views and concerns, address those issues and concerns, regard the parents as important participants in their child's health, and always include the child and family in the decision-making process.

Barriers to Health Care

Even with the federal and state programs available to assist children and families, barriers to appropriate, cost-effective, coordinated, and timely health care remain. Barriers can be financial, sociocultural, or ethnic, or part of the health care system itself.

Financial Barriers

Although the poverty rate is declining in this country, in 2001, 36% of America's households with children had inadequate physical housing, crowded housing, or housing that cost more than 30% of the household income (Federal Interagency Forum on Child and Family Statistics, 2006). In addition, the percentage of children covered by health insurance was 88%, leaving 12% of children uninsured. However, the majority of insurance coverage since 1999 is not from private health insurance but from government-supported plans (Federal Interagency Forum on Child and Family Statistics, 2006). Many children and families do not have insurance, do not have enough insurance to cover services obtained, or cannot pay for services.

Sociocultural and Ethnic Barriers

Sociocultural and ethnic factors also pose barriers. For example, white, non-Hispanic children overall are more likely than African-American and Hispanic children to be in very good or excellent health. The proportion of children ages 6 to 18 who are overweight is increasing, but the largest increase is occurring in African-Americans and Mexican-Americans (Federal Interagency Forum on Child and Family Statistics, 2006). This is just one example of the problems that different ethnic groups face in relation to health.

Lack of transportation, the need for both parents to work, and genetic factors also pose barriers to seeking health care. Knowledge barriers (e.g., lack of understanding of the importance of prenatal care or preventive health care), language barriers (e.g., speaking a different language than the health care providers), or spiritual barriers (e.g., religious beliefs discouraging some forms of treatment) also exist.

Health Care Delivery System Barriers

The health care delivery system itself can create barriers, such as the cost containment movement. Eighty-five percent of employed families with insurance are covered by some type of managed health care plan or health maintenance organization (HMO). This prospective payment system based on diagnosis-related groups (DRGs) limits the amounts of health care the family may receive. This also includes Medicaid reimbursement. As a result, the trend is to discharge patients as soon as possible and deliver care in the home or through community-based services. The overall plan may improve access to preventive services but may limit the access to specialty care, which has a major impact on children with chronic or long-term illnesses.

Protection of Children's Rights

A number of national and international organizations have been formed in recent years to protect children's rights both in the United States and worldwide. These organizations focus on such issues as violence and abuse, child labor and soldiering, juvenile justice, child immigrants and orphaned children, and abandoned or homeless children—all of which can have a negative impact on children's health. A child whose rights are restored and upheld has an improved opportunity for growth, development, education, and health. As advocates for children, nurses support policies that protect children's rights and improve children's health care.

Parents and guardians generally make choices about their child's health and services. As the legal custodians of minor children, they decide what is best for their child. Chapter 3 provides further information pertaining to children's rights in relation to health care decision making.

Confidentiality Issues in Caring for Children

With the establishment of the Health Insurance Portability and Accountability Act of 1996 (HIPAA), confidentiality of health care information is now required. The primary intent of the law was to maintain health insurance coverage for workers and their families when they change or lose jobs. Another aspect of the law requires the Department of Health and Human Services to establish national standards for electronic transactions for health information on individuals. The plan also addresses security and privacy issues involving health information about individuals. For example, no information that clearly identifies a patient can be on public display, including information on a patient's chart. In the pediatric area, information is shared only with the legal parents or guardians or individuals as established in writing by the parents. This law promotes the security and privacy of children's health information.

Computer Privacy

Electronic medical records (EMRs) improve efficiency and accuracy in a variety of clinical settings and may also improve the quality of patient care by simplifying the recording of complete data (Roukema et al., 2006). The EMR allows all health care disciplines to share information about a patient (Adams et al., 2003). The computer can be a powerful tool for improving efficiency and communicating health information in the pediatric arena. In addition to illness data, growth data with appropriate age-based ranges, medication dosages related to weight, and records of immunizations may be communicated across various settings via computer (Hinman et al., 2004). Patient confidentiality and privacy must be maintained as it is with paper documentation. At each point of electronic transmission, patient data must remain secure, and the HIPAA privacy rule applies to electronic patient information (Flores & Dodier, 2005). Nurses can ensure that privacy is maintained when using computerized documentation and an EMR by doing the following:

- Always maintain the security of your personal log-in information; never share it with other health care providers or other persons.
- Always log off when leaving the computer.
- Do not leave patient information visible on a monitor screen when the computer/monitor is unattended.
- Do not use e-mail to communicate confidential patient information.

> Referring back to Isabelle Romano and her family from the beginning of the chapter, what trends in child health care may have affected them?

Use of the Nursing Process in Caring for Children and Their Families

Pediatric nursing involves all the essential components of contemporary nursing practice. The American Nurses Association's (2004) definition of nursing, "the diagnosis and treatment of human responses to actual or potential health problems," also applies to the practice of pediatric nursing. The pediatric nurse makes use of theories and research pertaining specifically to children as well as general nursing concepts and research.

Nurses must know about current trends in health so that they can provide appropriate anticipatory guidance, counseling, and teaching for children and families and can identify high-risk groups so that interventions can be initiated early, before illness or death occurs. The nurse can use the information introduced in the above review of trends to develop and deliver a plan of care that is realistic and relevant to the child's health and welfare. The nurse performs this task using a framework called the **nursing process**.

The nursing process is used to care for the child and family during health promotion, maintenance, restoration, and rehabilitation. It is a problem-solving method based on the scientific method that allows nursing care to be planned and implemented in a thorough, organized manner to ensure quality and consistency of care. The nursing process is applicable to all health care settings and consists of five steps: assessment, nursing diagnosis, outcome identification and planning, implementation, and outcome evaluation.

1. Assessment involves collecting data about the child and family and performing physical assessment during community-based health services, at admission to an acute care setting, at periodic times during the child's hospitalization or care, and during home care visits.

2. The nurse analyzes the data to make judgments about the child's health and developmental status. The nursing diagnoses that result from this judgment process describe health promotion and health patterns that pediatric nurses can manage.
3. The next step in the process involves developing nursing care plans that incorporate goals or expected outcomes that improve the child's dysfunctional health patterns, promote appropriate health patterns, or provide for optimal developmental outcomes. The care plan includes the specific nursing actions that assist in obtaining the outcomes.
4. These interventions are implemented, adapted to the child's developmental level and family status, and modified if the child's response indicates the need. The care plan incorporates the family in addition to the child.
5. The process is continually evaluated and updated during the partnership with the child and family.

Standardized care plans for specific nursing diagnoses and critical pathways for case management are often used in various pediatric settings. In general, care plans and critical pathways are becoming more evidence-based, using a combination of research, group consensus, and past health care decisions to identify the most effective interventions for the child and family. The nurse is responsible for individualizing these standardized care plans based on the data collected during the assessment of the child and family and for evaluating the child's and family's response to the nursing interventions.

The dimensions of pediatric health care are changing. We live in a global community in which distances have been minimized, enabling all of us to learn, share, and exchange information. The pediatric nurse needs to be alert to the wide-ranging developmental and mental health needs of children as well as to the traits and behaviors that may lead to serious health problems. The scope of pediatric health care practice is much broader today, and pediatric nurses must include quality evidence-based interventions when developing the plan of care. In addition, pediatric nurses must incorporate new information about genetics and neurobiology and must continue to keep up with the technology explosion.

In the beginning of the chapter you were introduced to the Romano family. How can you empower this family to help them provide the best care to Isabelle?

References

Books and Journals

Adams, W. G., Mann, A. M., & Bauchner, H. (2003). Use of an electronic medical record improves the quality of urban pediatric primary care. *Pediatrics, 111*(3), 626–632.

Altemeier, W. A. (2000). Prevention of pediatric injuries: so much to do, so little time. *Pediatric Annuals, 29*(6), 324–325.

American Academy of Nurse Practitioners. (2002). *Scope of practice for nurse practitioners.* Retrieved August 23, 2006, from http://www.aanp.org/NR/rdonlyres/edhltucoxqd2xnrfwbve26d-3cowleh5rqqcfmhlcoi3sp7ihpzxry7rdqtkezw5zvpggxsuc7z4iao/scope%2bof%2bpractice%2bv2.pdf.

American Academy of Pediatrics: Committee on Psychosocial Aspects of Child and Family Health. (2001). The new morbidity revisited: A renewed commitment to psychosocial aspects of pediatric care. *Pediatrics, 108,* 1227–1230.

American Academy of Pediatrics, Committee on Hospital Care, Institute for Family-Centered Care. (2003). Policy statement: family-centered care and the pediatrician's role. *Pediatrics, 112*(3), 691–696.

American Association of Colleges of Nursing. (2005). *Commission on collegiate nursing education moves to consider for accreditation only practice doctorates with the DNP degree title.* Retrieved August 23, 2006, from http://www.aacn.nche.edu/Media/NewsReleases/2005/CCNEDNP.htm.

American Nurses Association (2004). *Nursing: Scope and standards of practice.* Silver Spring, MD: American Nurses Association.

American Nurses Association and the Society of Pediatric Nurses. (2003). *Scope and standards of pediatric nursing practice.* Silver Spring, MD: American Nurses Association.

Bruce, B. S., Lake, J. P., Eden, V. A., & Denney, J. C. (2004). Children at risk of injury. *Journal of Pediatric Nursing, 19*(2), 121–127.

Centers for Medicare and Medicaid Services. (2005). *The HIPAA Law and more.* Retrieved August 27, 2006, from http://www.cms.hhs.gov/HIPAAGenInfo/02_TheHIPAALawandMore.asp#TopOfPage.

Child Trends. (2006a). *Child trends data bank.* Retrieved August 30, 2006, from http://www.childtrendsdatabank.org/indicators/53NumberofChildren.cfm.

Child Trends. (2006b). *Infant, child and youth death rates.* Retrieved August 23, 2006, from http://www.childtrendsdatabank.org/indicators/63ChildMortality.cfm.

Commission for Case Management Certification. (n.d.). *Case management practice.* Retrieved August 23, 2006, from http://www.ccmcertification.org/pages/13frame_set1312.html.

Crane, P. A., & Clements, P. T. (2005). Psychological response to disasters: Focus on adolescents. *Journal of Psychosocial Nursing & Mental Health Services, 43*(8), 31–38.

Davidhizar, R., & Shearer, R. (2002). Helping children cope with public disasters: Support given immediately after a traumatic event can counteract or even negate long-term adverse effects. *American Journal of Nursing, 102*(3), 26–33.

Deal, L. W., Shiono, P. H., & Behrman, R. E. (1998). Children and managed health care: analysis and recommendations. *The Future of Children, 8*(2), 4–24.

Dey, A. N., Schiller, J. S., & Tai, D. A. (2004). Summary health statistics for U.S. children: national health interview survey, 2002. *Vital and Health Statistics, 10*(221), 1–78.

Dudley, S. K., & Carr, J. M. (2004). Vigilance: the experience of parents staying at the bedside of hospitalized children. *Journal of Pediatric Nursing, 19*(4), 267–275.

Espezel, H. J. E., & Canam, C. J. (2003). Parent–nurse interactions: Care of hospitalized children. *Journal of Advanced Nursing, 44*(1), 34–41.

Federal Interagency Forum on Child and Family Statistics. (2006). Retrieved September 7, 2006, from: http://childstats.gov/.

Federal Interagency Forum on Child and Family Statistics. (2006). *America's children in brief: Key national indicators of well-being, 2006.* Retrieved August 15, 2006, from http://www.childstats.gov/americaschildren/index.asp.

Flores, J., & Dodier, A. (2005). HIPAA: past, present and future implications for nurses. *Online Journal of Issues in Nursing, 10*(2). Retrieved July 1, 2006, from http://www.nursingworld.org/ojin/topic27/tpc27_4.htm.

Goldrick, B. A. (2004). Vaccine-preventable infections in children: Thwarting pneumococcal infection and pertussis in the very young. *American Journal of Nursing, 104*(2), 34–37.

Guyer, B., Freedman, M. A., Strobino, D. M., & Sondik, E. J. (2000). Annual summary of vital statistics: trends in the health of Americans during the 20th century. *Pediatrics, 106*(6), 1307–1317.

Hinman, A. R., Saarlas, K. N., & Ross, D. A. (2004). A vision for child health information systems: developing child health information systems to meet medical care and public health needs. *Journal of Public Health Management Practice (Suppl.),* S91–S98.

Hoyert, D. L., Heron, M., Kennedy, C., Charlesworth, A., & Chen, J. (2004). Disaster at a distance: Impact of 9.11.01 televised news coverage on mothers' and children's health. *Journal of Pediatric Nursing, 19*(5), 329–339.

Hoyert, D. L., Heron, M., Murphy, S. L., & Kung, H. C. (2006). *Deaths: Final data for 2003.* Health E-Stats. Released January 19, 2006. Retrieved August 27, 2006, from http://www.cdc.gov/nchs/products/pubs/pubd/hestats/finaldeaths03/finaldeaths03.htm#Fig3.

Johnson, J. H., Sabol, B. J., & Baker, E. L. (2006). The crucible of public health practice: Major trends shaping the design of the management academy for public health. *Journal of Public Health Management & Practice, 12*(5), 419–425.

Melnyk, B. M. (2004). Integrating levels of evidence into clinical decision making. *Pediatric Nursing, 30*(4), 323–325.

Miceli, P. J., & Clark, P. A. (2005). Your patient, my child: Seven priorities for improving pediatric care from the parent's perspective. *Journal of Nursing Care Quality, 20*(1), 43–53.

Murphy, S. L., Kung, H., & Division of Vital Statistics. (2006). *Deaths: final data for 2003.* Retrieved August 23, 2006, from http://www.cdc.gov/nchs/products/pubs/pubd/hestats/finaldeaths03/finaldeaths03.htm.

National Association of Clinical Nurse Specialists. (n.d.) *Who we are: clinical nurse specialists.* Retrieved August 23, 2006, from http://www.nacns.org/membership.pdf.

National Association of Neonatal Nurses. (2002). *Education standards for neonatal nurse practitioner programs.* Retrieved August 23, 2006, from http://www.nann.org/files/public/NNP_Standards.pdf.

National Association of Pediatric Nurse Practitioners. (2006). *Scope and standards of practice.* Retrieved August 23, 2006, from http://www.napnap.org/Docs/FinalScope2-25.pdf.

National Association of Pediatric Nurse Practitioners. (2006). *What do PNPs do?* Retrieved August 23, 2006, from http://www.napnap.org/index.cfm?page=15.

National Center for Health Statistics. (2006). *Fast stats A to Z.* Retrieved August 27, 2006, from http://www.cdc.gov/nchs/fastats/default.htm.

Newhouse, R. P. (2006). Examining the support for evidence-based nursing practice. *Journal of Nursing Administration, 36*(7/8), 337–340.

Reasor, J. E., & Farrell, S. P. (2004). Early childhood mental health: Services that can save a life. *Journal of Pediatric Nursing, 19*(2), 140–144.

Roukema, J., Los, R. K., Bleeker, S. E., van Ginneken, A. M., van der Lei, J., & Moll, H. A. (2006). Paper versus computer: feasibility of an electronic medical record in general pediatrics. *Pediatrics, 117*(1), 15–21.

Ryan-Wenger, N. A., Sharrer, V. W., & Campbell, K. K. (2005). Changes in children's stressors over the past 30 years. *Pediatric Nursing, 31*(4), 282–291.

Schell, K. A. (2006). Evidence-based practice: noninvasive blood pressure measurement in children. *Pediatric Nursing, 32*(3), 263–267.

Tiedje, L. B. (2005). Thirty years of maternal-child health policies in the community. *MCN, American Journal of Maternal Child Nursing, 30*(6), 373–379.

United Nations Children's Fund. (2001). A league table of child deaths by injury in rich nations. *Innocenti Report Card, 2.* Retrieved August 24, 2006, from http://www.unicef-icdc.org/siteguide/indexsearch.html.

U.S. Congress. (2004). *Individuals with Disabilities Education Improvement Act of 2004.* Retrieved August 28, 2006, from http://www.ed.gov/policy/speced/guid/idea/idea2004.html#law.

U.S. Department of Health & Human Services. (2000). *Healthy People 2010.* Retrieved August 23, 2006, from http://www.healthypeople.gov/Publications/.

U.S. Department of Health and Human Services. (2006). *Preventing infant mortality.* Retrieved August 23, 2006, from http://www.hhs.gov/news/factsheet/infant.html.

U.S. Department of Health and Human Services, Health Resources and Services Administration, Bureau of Health Professions, Division of Nursing. (2002). *Nurse practitioner primary care competencies in specialty areas: adult, family, gerontological, pediatric, and women's health.* Retrieved August 23, 2006, from http://www.nurse.org/acnp/clinprac/np.comp.spec.areas.pdf.

U.S. Department of Health and Human Services, Health Resources and Services Administration, Maternal and Child Health Bureau. (2004). *Child health USA 2004.* Rockville, MD: U.S. Department of Health and Human Services.

U.S. Department of Health & Human Services, Public Health Service. (1979). *Healthy people: The Surgeon General's report on health promotion and disease prevention* (DHEW publication No. PHS 79-5507). Washington, D.C.: U.S. Government Printing Office.

Wexler, I. D., Branski, D., & Kerem, E. (2006). War and children. *JAMA, 296*(5), 579–581.

Wieck, K. (2000). A vision for nursing: the future revisited. *Nursing Outlook, 48*(1), 7.

Woodside, J. M., Rosenbaum, P. L., King, S. M., & King, G. A. (2001). Family-centered service: developing and validating a self-assessment tool for pediatric service providers. *Children's Health Care, 30*(3), 237–252.

World Health Organization. (2006). *Frequently asked questions.* Retrieved August 30, 2006, from http://www.who.int/suggestions/faq/en/.

Web Sites

www.aahn.org American Association for History of Nursing
www.ahcpr.gov Agency for Healthcare Research and Quality
www.childrensrights.org Children's Rights, Inc.
www.gocrc.com/ Children's Rights Council
www.guidelines.gov National Guidelines Clearinghouse
www.healthypeople.gov; www.health.gov/healthpeople/state/toolkit *Healthy People 2010*
www.hhs.gov U.S. Department of Health & Human Services
http://hrw.org/children Human Rights Watch, Children's Rights
www.odphp.osophs.dhhs.gov Office of Disease Prevention & Health Promotion

Chapter WORKSHEET

MULTIPLE CHOICE QUESTIONS

1. What is the number-one cause for mortality among children?
   a. Human immunodeficiency virus
   b. Congenital anomalies
   c. Motor vehicle accidents
   d. Low birthweight
2. The nurse is assessing the vital signs of a child who is being evaluated in an urgent care center. The child is to be seen by the pediatric nurse practitioner (PNP). The mother asks, "Why is my child seeing the PNP and not the doctor?" What is the best response by the nurse?
   a. "The PNP functions similar to the physician's assistant, so you should be perfectly at ease."
   b. "The child may be seen by the physician instead if you'd like."
   c. "Seeing the PNP is just one more step in having your child evaluated in this setting."
   d. "The PNP is an experienced RN with advanced education in the diagnosis and treatment of children."
3. When caring for children, how does the nurse best incorporate the concept of family-centered care?
   a. Encourages the family to allow the physician to make health care decisions for the child
   b. Uses the concepts of respect, family strengths, diversity, and collaboration with family
   c. Advises the family to choose a pediatric provider who is on the child's health care plan
   d. Recognizes that families undergoing stress related to the child's illness cannot make good decisions
4. In an effort to control health care costs, what is the best recommendation by the nurse?
   a. "Shop around to find the most inexpensive health insurance plan."
   b. "Find a job that provides family health insurance at a minimal cost."
   c. "Stress primary prevention, using the health care system for check-ups."
   d. "Avoid seeing a health care provider until your child becomes ill."
5. The school nurse is planning a screening program. What items should be included to address issues related to the "new morbidity"?
   a. Academic difficulties, violence, and other mental health issues
   b. The number of children with chronic illness at the school
   c. Statistics related to health insurance coverage of the children
   d. HIV infection, asthma and respiratory allergy testing

CRITICAL THINKING EXERCISES

1. Detail how the nursing process fits into the framework of pediatric nursing.
2. Discuss how the role of the pediatric nurse differs from the role of the advanced practice pediatric nurse.

STUDY ACTIVITIES

1. Describe how you will incorporate family-centered care into your nursing care in the pediatric clinical setting.
2. Research a current policy, bill, or issue being debated on the community, state, or national level pertaining to child health or welfare. Summarize the major facts and supporting or opposing issues and present them in a class presentation or paper.
3. Obtain a standardized care plan from the hospital unit. Evaluate whether it is based on evidence-based practice. Develop an individualized care plan for a child you are caring for. Compare and contrast the two types of care plans.
4. The following events were milestones in the support of children's health. Place them in the correct sequence, from oldest to most recent:

   _____ a. Declaration of the Rights of the Child approved
   _____ b. WIC program established
   _____ c. U.S. Children's Bureau established
   _____ d. Sheppard-Towner Act passed
   _____ e. Family and Medical Leave Act passed
   _____ f. Education for all Handicapped Children Act passed.

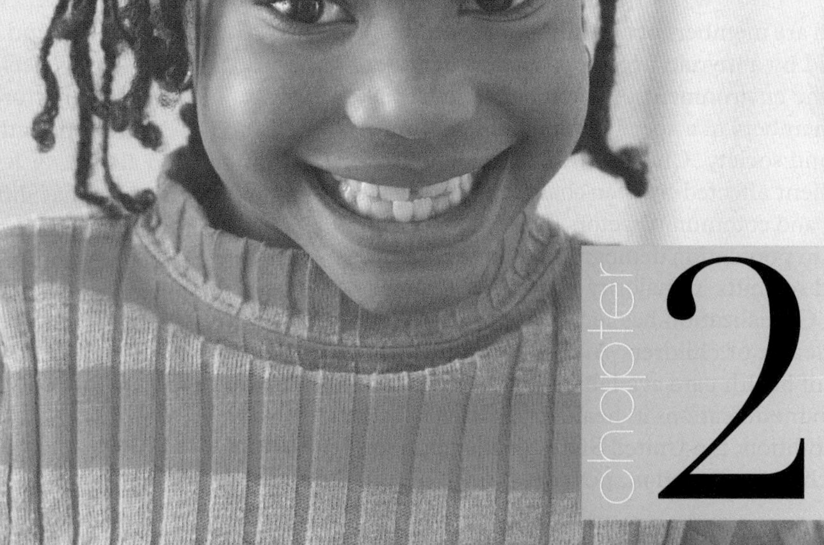

chapter 2

Factors Influencing Child Health

Key TERMS

cultural competence
culture
discipline
enculturation
ethnicity
ethnocentrism
family
family structure
foster care
genetics
heredity
punishment
race
religion
resilience
social capital
spirituality
temperament

Learning OBJECTIVES

Upon completion of the chapter, the learner will be able to:

1. Delineate the structures, functions, and roles of families and the influence on children and their health.
2. Differentiate discipline from punishment.
3. Describe the impact of poverty and homelessness on the health of children.
4. Differentiate between culture, ethnicity, and race.
5. Describe the subcultural and religious influences affecting children and their development.
6. Discuss the sources of violence and how exposure to violence affects children.
7. Compare and contrast the factors associated with health status and lifestyle that affect a child's health.
8. Explain the concept of resiliency as it relates to children and their health status.

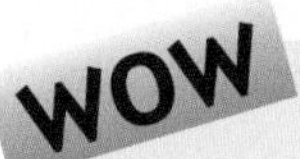

Learning rather than accomplishing should be the focus of raising children.

Miguel Delgado is a 10-month-old boy who is admitted to the pediatric unit for treatment of pneumonia. He is accompanied by his parents and 3-year-old sister, Luisa. Miguel's parents speak Spanish and very little English. The family is Roman Catholic. As the nurse admitting Miguel, how will you facilitate communication? What steps can you take to help ensure ongoing communication with this family despite the language barrier?

When they come into the world, children are members of a family and have already been influenced by a myriad of factors such as heredity, genetics, and the environment. As members of a family, they are also members of a specific population, community, culture, and society. Children live, learn, and grow in an environment affected by ever-changing social, cultural, spiritual, and community factors. For example, dramatic changes in population demographics in the United States have led to shifts in majority and minority population groups. Globalization has led to an international focus on the health of children. Access to health care, and the types of health care available for children, have changed due to modifications in health care delivery and financing. In addition, the United States is still grappling with issues such as immigration, poverty, homelessness, and violence.

Children are on the forefront of many of these trends, often bearing the brunt of the problems and highlighting the changes. The interplay of all these factors creates a situation unique to each child. These factors may affect the child positively, promoting healthy growth and development, or negatively, exposing the child to health risks. To gain the knowledge and skills needed to plan effective care for children, pediatric nurses need to understand how all these factors affect the quality of nursing care and children's health outcomes. By doing so, nurses can create appropriate strategies and plan interventions for achieving the best possible outcomes for children and their families.

This chapter describes the major factors that can influence a child's health and provides information about ways to assist the child and family in achieving their optimal level of health.

Family

The **family** is considered the basic social unit. The U.S. Census Bureau (2007) defines a family as a group of two or more persons related by birth, marriage, or adoption and living together. According to the American Academy of Family Physicians (Ventres & Gobbo, 2005), a family is a group of individuals with a continuing legal, genetic, and/or emotional relationship.

Earlier definitions of family emphasized the legal ties or genetic relationships of people living in the same household with specific roles. Given the diversity of families in today's society, however, some believe that family should be defined as whatever the client says it is (Patterson, 1995) (Fig. 2.1).

The family into which a child is born greatly influences his or her development and health. Children learn health care activities, health beliefs, and health values from their family. The family's structure, the roles assumed by members, and societal changes that affect the family's life can affect the child and his or her health. Children and families are unique: each has different views and requires different methods for support.

Various theories and models have been generated to define a family, to understand its structure and function, and to assess a family's coping and adaptation (Table 2.1).

Family Structure

Family structure is the way that the family is organized and the way that the family members interact with one another on a regular, recurring basis in socially sanctioned ways. Family members can be gained or lost through divorce, marriage, birth, death, abandonment, and incarceration. With these events, the family structure changes and roles are redefined or redistributed.

The traditional nuclear family is no longer considered the dominant family structure. From 1970 to 1996, the percentage of children under age 18 who were living with two married parents decreased steadily from 85% to 68%. In 2005, this percentage was 67% (Child Trends, 2005). Table 2.2 lists some of the family structures found in today's society. Nurses working with children need to understand the child's family structure and any changes that are occurring in it so they can help the family to cope.

Family Roles and Functions

Each family member has a specific position or status and role when interacting with other members of the family. Typical family roles and their functions include:

- Nurturer: the primary caregiver
- Provider: the person who is primarily responsible for generating the family's income
- Decision maker: the person who is responsible for making choices, especially related to lifestyle and leisure time
- Financial manager: the person who handles the money, such as paying bills and saving
- Problem solver: the person to whom other members go for help in solving problems
- Health manager: the person responsible for ensuring that family members maintain their health, such as scheduling doctor visits and ensuring that immunizations are current

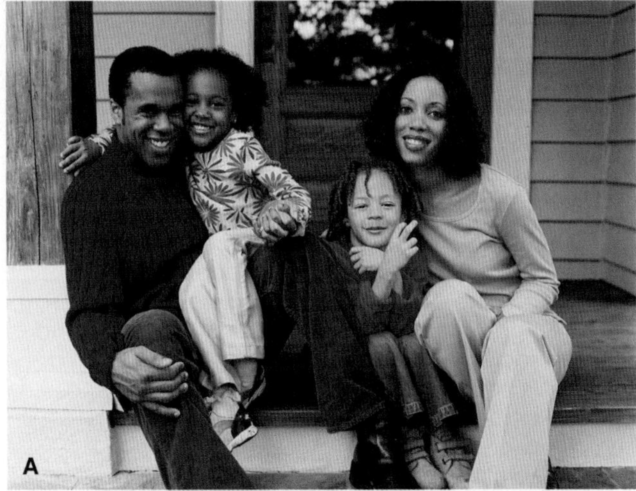

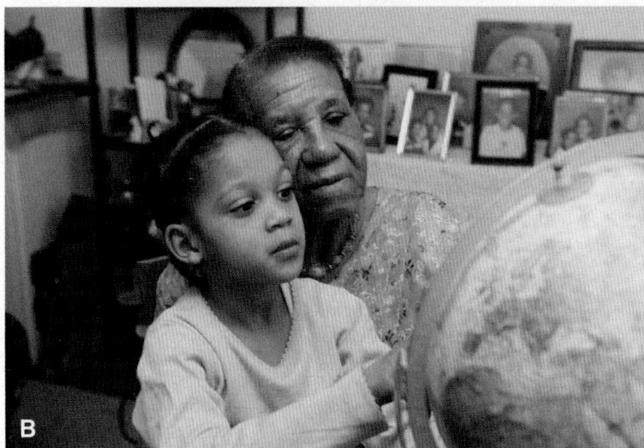

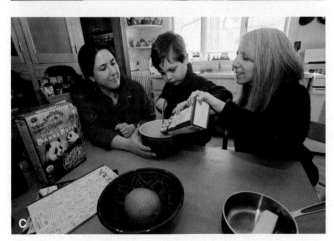

● Figure 2.1 Nurses must recognize family dynamics when providing health care to patients. There are many different family structures, and they influence patient needs. (**A**) The traditional nuclear family is composed of two parents and their biological or adopted children. (**B**) The extended family includes the nuclear family plus other family members, such as grandparents, aunts, uncles, and cousins. (**C**) Gay and lesbian families comprise two people of the same sex sharing a committed relationship, with or without children.

• Gatekeeper: the person who manages information inflow and outflow (Pillitteri, 2007)

Roles and functions are further defined by each family's own traditions and values and the family's set of standards for interaction within and outside the family. For instance, a first-born child may feel that he or she is in a position of power and may attempt to control younger siblings. The youngest child, in response, may learn how to bargain to deal with the situation.

Parental Roles

The caregiver–child interaction is critical to the survival and healthy development of a young child (WHO, 2004). Typically the primary caregivers are the parents. Ideally, parents nurture their children and provide them with an environment in which they can become competent, productive, self-directed members of society. For young children in particular, growth, health, and their very personhood itself depend on the ability of the adults in their life to understand and respond to them (WHO, 2004).

Caregiving includes not only providing physical and emotional care but also imparting the rules and expected behaviors of society. These expected behaviors depend on the culture, values, and beliefs of the family and the child's developmental stage and physical and cognitive abilities.

Parenting Styles

Three major parenting styles seen in this society are authoritarian, authoritative, and permissive. The styles are defined by the amount of control exerted over the child during parenting. Whatever the style, sensitive and responsive caregiving is needed to promote appropriate physical, neurophysiologic, and psychological development (WHO, 2004).

The *authoritarian* parent expects obedience from the child and discourages the child from questioning the family's rules. The rules and standards set forth by the parents are strictly enforced and firm. The parents expect the child to accept the family's beliefs and values and demand respect for these beliefs. The parents are the ultimate authority and allow little, if any, participation by the child in making decisions. Behavior that does not adhere to the family's rules and standards is punished.

The *authoritative* or democratic parent shows some respect for the child's opinions. Although parents still have the ultimate authority and expect the child to adhere to the rules, authoritative parents allow children to be different and believe that each child is an individual. They consistently and firmly enforce the family's rules and standards but do not emphasize punishment.

Permissive or laissez-faire parents have little control over the behavior of their children. Rules or standards

(text continues on page 26)

Table 2.1 Summary of Major Theories Related to Family

Theory	Description	Key Components
Friedman's structural functional theory (Friedman, 1998)	Emphasizes the social system of family, such as the organization or structure of the family and how the structure relates to the function	Identified five functions of families: • Affective function: meeting the love and belonging needs of each member • Socialization and social placement function: teaching children how to function and assume adult roles in society • Reproductive role: continuing the family and society in general • Economic function: ensuring the family has necessary resources with appropriate allocation • Health care function: involving the provision of physical care to keep family healthy
Duvall's developmental theory (Duvall, 1977)	Emphasizes the developmental stages that all families go through, beginning with marriage; the longitudinal career of the family is also known as the family life cycle	Described eight chronological stages with specific predictable tasks that each family completes: • Marriage: beginning of family • Childbearing stage • Family with preschool children • Family with school-aged children • Family with adolescents • Family with young adults • Middle-aged parents • Family in later years
Von Bertalanffy (1968): general system theory applied to families	Emphasizes the family as a system with interdependent, interacting parts that endure over time to ensure the survival, continuity, and growth of its components; the family is not the sum of its parts but is characterized by wholeness and unity	Used to define how families interact with and are influenced by the members of their family and society and how to analyze the interrelationships of the members and the impact that change affecting one member will have on other members
Family stress theory (Boss, 2001)	Addresses the way families respond to stress and how the family copes with the stress as a group and how each individual member copes	Described elements of stress as occurring internally within the family (e.g., values, beliefs, structure) that the family can control or change or externally from outside the family (e.g., culture of the surrounding community, genetics, the family's current time or place) over which the family has no control Mobilization of family resources resulting in either a positive response of constructive coping or negative response of a crisis Identified the main determinant of adequate coping based on the meaning of the stressful event to the family and its individual members
Resiliency model of family stress, adjustment, and adaptation	Addresses the way families adapt to stress and can rebound from adversity	Identified the elements of risks and protective factors that aid a family in achieving positive outcomes

Table 2.2 Types of Family Structures

Structure	Description	Specific Issues
Nuclear family	Husband, wife, and children living in same household	May include natural or adopted children Once considered the traditional family structure; now decreased due to trends in divorce rates or other social situations such as nonmarital childbearing
Binuclear family	Child who is member of two families due to joint custody; parenting is considered a joint venture	Always works better when the interests of the child are put above the parents' needs and desires
Single-parent family	One parent responsible for care of children	May result from death, divorce, desertion, birth outside marriage or adoption Likely to encounter several challenges because of economic, social, and personal restraints; one person as homemaker, caregiver, and financial provider
Commuter family	Adults in the family living and working apart for professional or financial reasons, often leaving the daily care of children to one parent	Similar to single-parent family
Step or blended family	Adults with children from previous marriages or from the new marriage	May lead to family conflict due to different expectations for the child and adults; may have different views and practices related to child care and health
Extended family	Nuclear family and grandparents, cousins, aunts and uncles	Need to determine decision maker as well as primary caretaker of the children May be encouraged and supported by some cultures, such as Hispanic and Asian cultures
Same-sex family (also called homosexual or gay/lesbian family)	Adults of the same sex living together with or without children	May face prejudice against those with different lifestyles
Communal family	Group of people living together to raise children and manage household; unrelated by blood or marriage	May face prejudice against those with different lifestyles Need to determine the decision maker and caretaker of children
Foster family	A temporary family for children who are placed away from their parents to ensure their emotional and physical well-being	May include foster family's children and other foster children in the home Foster children are more likely to have unmet health needs and chronic health problems because they may have been in a variety of settings (American Academy of Pediatrics, 2000).
Grandparents-as-parents families	Grandparents raising their grandchildren if parents are unable to do so	May increase the risk for physical, financial, and emotional stress on older adults May lead to confusion and emotional stress for child if biological parents are in and out of child's life
Adolescent families	Young parents still mastering the developmental tasks of their own childhood	Teenage girls have greater risk for health problems during pregnancy and delivery of premature infants, leading to risk of subsequent health and developmental problems. Probably still need support from their family related to financial, emotional, and school issues

may be inconsistent, unclear, or nonexistent. Permissive parents allow their children to determine their own standards and rules for behavior. Discipline can be lax, inconsistent, or absent.

Discipline

Much of parenting involves increasing desirable behavior and decreasing or eliminating undesirable behavior, a process generally known as **discipline**. There are various opinions in our society about the best or most effective method of discipline. Discipline should be based on expectations that are appropriate for the child's age and should be used to set reasonable, consistent limits while permitting choices among acceptable alternatives (Banks, 2002). Discipline involves teaching and it is ongoing, not something that is done just when the child misbehaves.

The American Academy of Pediatrics (1998) suggests three strategies for effective discipline (Teaching Guideline 2.1):

- Maintaining a positive, supportive, nurturing caregiver–child relationship
- Using positive reinforcement to increase desirable behaviors
- Removing positive reinforcements or using punishment to reduce or eliminate undesirable behaviors

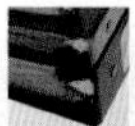

TEACHING GUIDELINE 2.1

Teaching to Promote Effective Discipline

- Set clear, consistent, and developmentally appropriate expected behaviors; offer choices whenever possible.
- Maintain consistency in responding to behaviors; provide encouragement and affection.
- Role-model appropriate behaviors.
- Provide an age-appropriate explanation of the consequence that will occur if the child demonstrates unacceptable behavior.
- Always administer the consequence soon after the unacceptable behavior.
- Keep the consequence appropriate to the age of the child and the situation.
- Stay calm but firm without showing anger when administering the consequence.
- Always praise the child for displaying appropriate behavior.
- Set the environment to assist the child in accomplishing the appropriate behavior; remove temptations that may lead to inappropriate behavior.
- Reinforce that the child's behavior was bad, not that the child was bad.

Attention from parents is one of the most powerful forms of positive reinforcement (Banks, 2002). The key is to focus on the child's appropriate behaviors rather than emphasizing the inappropriate ones. Immediate, consistent, and frequent feedback is crucial. This feedback can be in the form of smiles, praise, special attention, or rewards such as extra privileges or a special token or activity. Providing the feedback immediately is important so that the child learns to associate the feedback with the appropriate behavior, thereby reinforcing the behavior.

Another form of discipline is extinction, which focuses on reducing or eliminating the positive reinforcement for inappropriate behavior. Examples are ignoring the temper tantrums of a toddler, withholding or removing privileges, and requiring "time-out." Withholding or removing privileges such as TV, music, or computer or phone use is most effective for older children and adolescents. The adolescent may be grounded for a short time or not allowed to drive the car. To be effective, the privilege being withheld or removed must be something that the child values.

Time-out is an extinction discipline method that is most effective with toddlers, preschoolers, and early school-aged children. It involves removing the child from the problem area and placing him or her in a neutral, nonthreatening, safe area where no interaction occurs between the child and parents or others for a specifically determined period (Fig. 2.2).

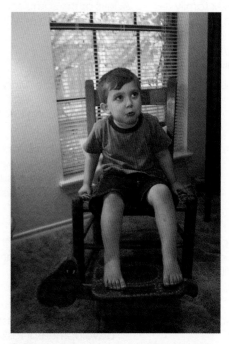

● Figure 2.2 Although he might not like it, quiet solitude helps the child develop inner control.

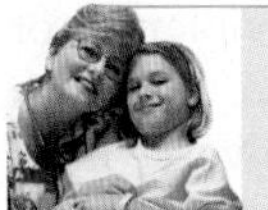

The amount of time that a child spends in time-out is typically 1 minute per year of age; for example, a 3-year-old would spend 3 minutes in time-out. Time-out should not exceed 5 minutes.

Discipline is often confused with **punishment**, but punishment involves a negative or unpleasant experience or consequence for doing or not doing something. Although punishment is sometimes a necessary element of discipline, to be an effective tool it must be coupled with rewards for good behavior (American Academy of Pediatrics, 1998; Banks, 2002).

Punishment may be verbal or corporal. Verbal punishment commonly takes the form of reprimands or scolding (the use of disapproving statements). The statements are intended to change or eliminate the inappropriate behavior.

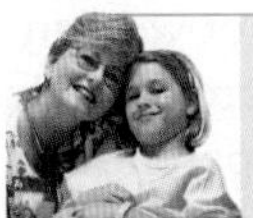

Verbal reprimands can be effective in the short term if they are used sparingly and are focused on the child's specific behavior. If verbal reprimands are used frequently and indiscriminately, they lose their effectiveness, can provoke anxiety in the child, and encourage the child to ignore the parent. Frequent use also may reinforce the behavior by providing the child with attention (American Academy of Pediatrics, 1998; Banks, 2002).

Corporal punishment involves the use of physical pain as a means to decrease inappropriate behavior. The most common form of corporal punishment is spanking (the use of an open hand to the buttocks or an extremity with the intention of modifying behavior without causing injury) (American Academy of Pediatrics, 1998; Banks, 2002). According to the National Survey of Early Childhood Health (Regalado et al., 2004), 29% of parents of children ages 10 to 18 months and 64% of parents of children ages 19 to 35 months spank their children; 11% of parents of children ages 10 to 18 months and 26% of parents of children ages 19 to 35 months reported frequent spanking.

Initially, spanking may be effective because of its sudden and shocking nature. However, over time it loses its effectiveness because its shock value declines. Spanking may stop the negative behavior, but it also increases the chance for physical injury, especially for infants and young children, and may lead to altered caregiver–child relationships. Because the effects of spanking diminish, the intensity of the spanking must be increased to achieve the same effects. Thus, it is important for parents to understand the consequences of its use.

Spanking is a controversial issue. Some argue that it provides children with a model for resolving conflicts using violence, promotes aggressive behavior, and shows children it is acceptable to cause pain in others (Banks, 2002). Various studies have linked spanking in childhood with physical aggression and violence in childhood and persistent anger in adulthood. Because of the negative consequences of spanking and because it has been shown to be no more effective than other methods for managing inappropriate behavior, the American Academy of Pediatrics (1998) recommends that parents use methods other than spanking to respond to inappropriate behavior.

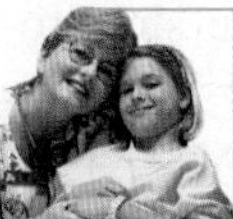

Other forms of discipline, if used incorrectly, can also cause problems for the child and interfere with the caregiver–child relationship. For example, disapproval using tone of voice, facial expression, or gestures can be effective in stopping inappropriate behavior, but if the disapproval comes in the form of verbal statements that attack the child rather than the behavior, negative consequences may occur.

Changes in Parental Roles Over Time

Parental roles evolve due to societal and economic changes as well as individual family changes. Traditionally, the role of provider was assigned to the father. However, with increased numbers of women in the workplace and more households with two parents working, today both parents are often the providers as well as the nurturers to the children. Technological innovations have provided parents with opportunities to work at home, allowing some parents to maintain the provider role while simultaneously fulfilling the nurturer and health manager roles. Fathers also are taking on greater responsibilities related to household management and childcare. The number of children being raised by their fathers alone or their grandparents is increasing. Moreover, as baby boomers age, parents may find themselves caring for both their children and their aging parents.

Temperament

Temperament is the manner in which a child interacts with the environment. The way a child experiences a particular event will be influenced by his or her temperament, and the child's temperament will influence the responses of others, including the parents, to the child. Early on, infants demonstrate differences in their behavior in response to stimuli. These responses are an integral part of the infant's developing personality and individuality. Although a child's temperament is intrinsic, it does change over time. Knowing a child's temperament can help parents understand and accept the characteristics of the child without feeling responsible for having caused them.

The classic theory proposes ten parameters of temperament: activity level, rhythmicity, approach and withdrawal, adaptability, threshold of responsiveness, intensity of reaction, quality of mood, distractibility, attention span, and persistence. This theory seeks to identify behavioral characteristics that lead the child to respond to the world in specific ways.

Using the ten parameters, children's temperaments may be categorized into three major groups—easy (40% of children), difficult (10%), and slow to warm up (15%)—with the remainder categorized as mixed (Behrman et al., 2004). Easy children are even-tempered and have regular biological functions, predictable behavior, and a positive attitude toward new experiences. Difficult children are irritable, highly active, and intense; they react to new experiences by withdrawing. Children in the slow-to-warm-up category are moody and less active and have more irregular reactions; they react to new experiences with mild but passive resistance.

A child's temperament may cause problems if it conflicts with that of the parents (e.g., an active 2-year-old with low-key parents). The "fit" of the parents and children is a powerful predictor of how much conflict there may be in the parent–child relationship (Behrman et al., 2004). If parents want and expect their child to be predictable but that is not the child's style, parents may perceive the child to have problems, and this conflict may affect the child's health. The key is not to label the child but to recognize the strengths and limitations of each group.

Lifestyle

Lifestyle choices affecting health include eating, exercise, use of tobacco, drugs, or alcohol, and methods of coping with stress. Most health problems today are heavily influenced by lifestyle factors. The lifestyle of the parents basically is the lifestyle of the children, so parents who eat poorly and don't exercise have children who also eat poorly and don't exercise. The result is that health problems such as diabetes, obesity, and heart disease are showing up earlier in our society. It is important to maintain a level of physical activity in the child's life through sport activities or hobbies such as dancing.

Special Family Situations

Families face complex challenges as they try to nurture, develop, and socialize their children. When the family structure changes, the effects on children can be life-long. These special situations require astute assessment and proactive intervention to minimize the risk to the child and family.

Divorced Family

Many times divorce is a reason why the family structure changes. Divorce can have a great impact on the child, with chronic and devastating results. According to the American Association of Pediatrics, approximately 40% of children experience the divorce of their parents before their 16th birthday, and parental separation and divorce is as one of the most common and significant risks to the healthy development of children today (Tanner, 2002).

Typically, divorce is not a single event: changes have most likely been occurring in the family for years, and children may have been exposed to turmoil, violence, or changes in structure before the actual divorce. Research has shown that many problems precede the divorce itself and that the effects on the family are often closely related to the level of conflict between the parents (Bryner, 2001). The initial response of children to divorce depends on their age. More than one third of children, however, are still troubled and distressed 5 years after the divorce of their parents, with depression being the most common symptom (Behrman et al., 2004).

Parents need to understand the impact that divorce can have on their children, placing the children's interest in the forefront. Parents can use the rules in Box 2.1 to help reduce tension and conflict, thereby minimizing the impact of separation and divorce on their children.

Single-Parent Families

Single-parent families can result from divorce or separation, death of a spouse, an unmarried woman raising her own child, or adoption by an unmarried man or woman. The U.S. Census Bureau (2004) found that approximately 28% of children under age 18 live with one parent and 68% live with both parents. Of the children under 18 living in single-parent families, 83% lived with the mother and approximately 16.5% lived with the father.

BOX 2.1

10 RULES FOR DIVORCING PARENTS

1. Tell your children about the divorce and the reasons for the divorce in terms that they can understand. Be sure that you and your spouse are present together when telling the children; tell all the children at the same time.
2. Reassure your children that the divorce is not their fault. Repeat this as often as possible and as necessary.
3. Inform the children well in advance of anyone moving out of the house (except when abuse is present or there are concerns for immediate safety).
4. Clearly inform the children about the family structure after the divorce, such as who will live with whom and where; also discuss visitation clearly and honestly.
5. Do not make your children be or act like adults.
6. Do not discuss money or finances with your children.
7. Maintain rules and be consistent in this area.
8. Never force or allow your children to take sides.
9. Avoid belittling your former spouse when the children can hear. However, do not lie to cover up for irresponsible behavior by the other parent.
10. Never put your children in the middle between you and your ex-spouse.

Adapted from Bryner, C. L. (2001). Children of divorce. *Journal of the American Board of Family Practice, 14*(3), 176–183. Accessed 9/21/06. Available at http://www.medscape.com/viewarticle/405852.

Single-parent families have several concerns that can affect the health of the children. Life in a single-parent household can be stressful for the adult and children. The single parent may feel overwhelmed by the responsibility of juggling the care of the children, maintaining a job, and keeping up with the bills and household chores (American Psychological Association, 2004). These issues may be compounded by other pressures, such as custody problems, decreased time available to spend with children, continuing conflicts between parents who are separated or divorced, or changes in relationships with extended family members.

Communication and support are essential to the optimal functioning of the single-parent family. The parent and children need to be able to express their feelings and work through the problems together. Community resources can be helpful. Parents Without Partners, for instance, is an international organization that has over 200 chapters in the United States and Canada. It provides "single parents and their children with an opportunity for enhancing personal growth, self-confidence and sensitivity towards others by offering an environment for support, friendship, and the exchange of parenting techniques" (Parents Without Partners, 2005).

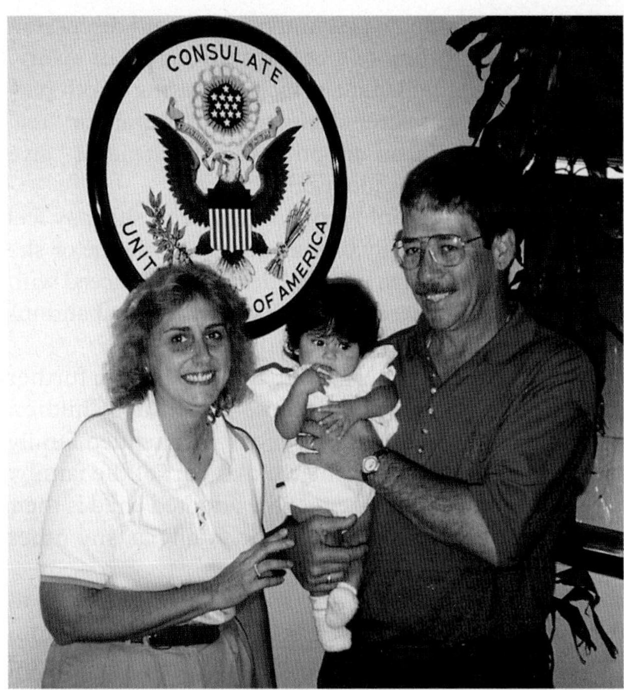

● Figure 2.3 An adopted family in which the child is from a different culture.

Blended Families

Creating a blended family (parents and their stepchildren) can be stressful for the parents and children alike. Although it creates a structure and stability and reduces some of the financial stresses of single parenthood, making the transition to a blended family takes time. Children may feel jealous of the stepparent or feel disloyal toward the previous biological parent. There may be competition or rivalry among the stepchildren. The child may fear that the stepparent is interfering with the child's relationship with the parent or taking away his or her source of love, affection, and attention.

Mutual respect and open, honest communication among all individuals involved are key, and this should include the previous biological parent when possible. Responsibilities for parenting must be shared, including decisions about expectations, limits, and discipline. The continued role of the previous biological parent and the role of the stepparent in the child's life are important to address.

Adopted Families

Adoption can occur domestically (through an agency or intermediary such as an attorney in the family's own area or country), or the family may choose to adopt a child from another country. The child may be of a different culture, race, or ethnicity (Fig. 2.3). An increasing number of single-parent families, blended families, families with gay or lesbian partners, and families with older parents are providing homes to children through adoption (Borchers et al., 2003). Some children are adopted after spending time in foster care.

The amount of contact between the child and the birth mother can vary greatly. In a closed adoption there is no contact between the adoptive parents, the adopted child, and the birth mother. In an open adoption there is as much contact among the individuals as desired.

Regardless of the method used to adopt a child, adoptive families may be faced with unique issues. Some adopted children have complex medical, developmental, behavioral, educational, and psychological issues. They may have been exposed to poverty, neglect, infectious diseases, and lack of adequate food, clothing, shelter, and nurturing, placing them at risk for medical problems, physical growth and development delays or abnormalities, and behavioral, cognitive, and emotional problems. The adoptive parents may know about these problems, but in other situations little if any history may be available.

When should a child be told that he or she was adopted? Most authorities believe that children should be informed at an age young enough so that as they grow older, they do not remember a time when they didn't know they were adopted (Borchers et al., 2003). The timing must be appropriate for the parents as well as the child. As children grow and develop, their understanding of the meaning of adoption changes. Until age 3, most adopted children do not realize there is a difference in the way that they joined their family (Borchers et al., 2003). Usually around this age, children begin to ask questions about being adopted.

Clear, open, honest communication and discussion are essential to promote a healthy, strong relationship. "Positive" adoption language includes saying "birth parent" or "biological parent" instead of "natural" or "real parent" and "make an adoption plan" instead of "give away" or "give up for adoption."

As the adopted child grows older, he or she may feel the loss of a birth family or may question what he or she did that led to the birth parents' decision to proceed with adoption. The adolescent may have issues of abandonment, emotional uncertainty, and identity.

Differences in culture, ethnicity, or race can further influence the adopted child's sense of identity. Children may be subjected to racism or bigotry. Extended family members may not accept the child as part of the family. Parents need to emphasize that the adopted child is their child and is as much a part of the family as any other member.

Adopted adolescents and adults may feel a need to identify their biological parents. Children adopted from other countries may travel to the country of their birth, and children adopted domestically may search for biological relatives. Although this search is an indicator of healthy emotional growth, it can upset the adoptive parents, who may feel rejected. Support, guidance, and open communication are key for all parties involved.

Open acknowledgement of the adoptive relationship helps to nurture a child's self-esteem as he or she learns to understand what it means to join a family through adoption. Effective communication about adoption is important for the long-term mental and physical health and well-being of each child and family (Borchers et al., 2003).

Foster Care Family

Foster care is a situation in which a child is cared for in an alternative living situation apart from his or her parents or legal guardians. The child may be placed in this living situation due to difficulties in the family situation, such as abuse, neglect, abandonment, or the parents' inability to meet the child's needs, due to illness, substance abuse, or death. The child may be sent to live with relatives (kinship care) or foster parents, who are strangers providing protection and shelter in a state-approved foster home.

Over 500,000 children in the United States currently live in some form of foster care, and foster care placements have dramatically increased over the past decade (American Academy of Child and Adolescent Psychiatry [AACAP], 2005). The goal of foster care is to provide temporary services until the child can return home to his or her family or be adopted. Unfortunately, children may remain in foster care for several years or longer and may be moved from one foster family to another.

Many children who are placed in foster care have been the victims of abuse or neglect. Thirty percent of children in foster care have severe emotional, behavioral, or developmental problems (AACAP, 2005). Children who are placed in foster care may experience a wide range of problems, including:

- Physical health problems
- Self-blame and feelings of guilt
- Feelings of being unwanted
- Feelings of helplessness
- Insecurity about the future
- Ambivalent feelings related to foster parents; feelings of being disloyal to birth parents (AACAP, 2005)

Individual attention to the child in foster care is essential. A multidisciplinary approach to care that includes the birth parents, foster parents, child, health care professionals, and support services is important to meet the child's needs for growth and development. Nurses play a key role in advocating for the child.

Genetics

Genetics, the study of heredity and its variations, is a field that has applications to all stages of life and all types of diseases. **Heredity** is the process of transmitting genetic characteristics from parent to offspring. The child's biological traits, including some behavioral traits, gender and race, and certain diseases or illnesses, are directly linked to genetic inheritance. New technologies in molecular biology and biochemistry have led to better understanding of the mechanisms involved in hereditary transmission, including those associated with genetic disorders. These advances are now leading to better diagnostic tests and management options.

Two major areas of study in genetics that are important to pediatrics are cytogenetics and the Human Genome Project. Cytogenetics is the study of genetics at the chromosome level. Chromosomal anomalies occur in 0.4% of all live births and are the prevalent cause of cognitive impairment and congenital anomalies or birth defects (Elias et al., 2007); anomalies are even more common among spontaneous abortions and stillbirths. The Human Genome Project is an international research effort involving the localization, isolation, and characterization of human genes and investigation of the function of the gene products and their interaction with one another. This research project will provide information about genetic diseases to aid in developing new ways to identify, treat, cure, or even prevent them. Chapter 30 offers a more detailed discussion of genetics.

Gender

A child's gender is established when the sex chromosomes join. A child's gender can influence many key aspects, such as physical characteristics and personal attributes. In addition to the development of male or female genitalia, body development, and hair distribution, some diseases or illnesses can be gender-related: for example, scoliosis is more prevalent in females and color blindness is more common in males. An early influence of gender in children involves the survival rate of premature infants: premature girls have a higher survival rate than premature boys.

In addition to the specific biological and physical traits related to gender, there are also social effects. The child develops specific gender attitudes and behaviors that are appropriate in his or her culture, a process called gender identification. Interactions with family members and peers as well as activities and societal values affect how children perceive themselves as a specific gender (Fig. 2.4). If confusion develops with this process, various psychological and social difficulties can arise for the child.

Race

Race indicates membership in a particular group of humans who have biological traits that are transmitted by descent; they may share physical features such as skin color, bone structure, or blood type. Some of the physical variations may be normal in a particular race but may be considered an identifying characteristic of a disorder in other races. For example, epicanthal folds (the vertical folds of skin that partially or completely cover the inner canthi of the eye) are normal in Asian children but may occur with Down syndrome or renal agenesis in other races. In addition, specific malformations and diseases are found in specific races. For example, sickle cell anemia occurs more often in African and Mediterranean groups, and cystic fibrosis is seen more often in individuals from Northwestern Europe.

Society

Society has a major impact on the health of a child. Major components of a society that influence children and their health include social roles, socioeconomic status, the media, and the expanding global nature of society. Each of these areas may influence children's self-concept, the communities they live in, their choice of lifestyle, and their health. Pediatric nurses need to assess these areas and their influence on the child and family so that individualized strategies can be designed and implemented to enhance the positive effects and minimize the negative effects on the child's and family's health.

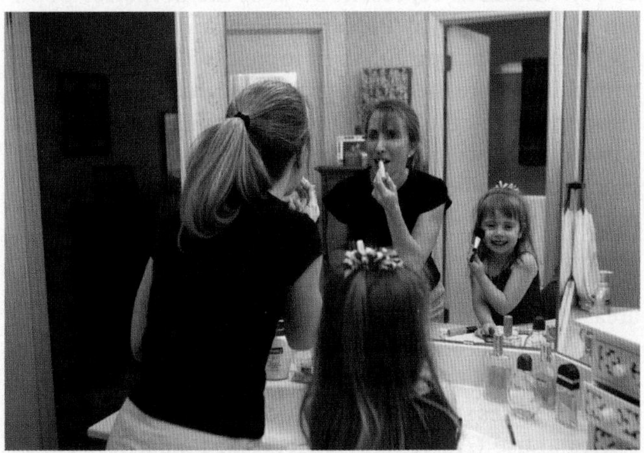

● Figure 2.4 The young child learns to identify with the parent of the same sex.

Social Roles

Society often dictates that specific people behave in specific ways: certain behaviors are permitted and others are prohibited. These patterns are identified as social roles and can be an important factor in the development of self-concept, and a person's self-concept can have a very positive or a very negative influence on his or her health.

For children, social roles influence their ideas about themselves. Box 2.2 lists some typical roles children have in our society. These social roles are generally carried out in groups, such as the family, school, peers, or church or community organizations. At times there may be a conflict in how the different groups expect a child to behave. There also may be conflict for parents related to child-rearing practices. For example, the child's family may believe in creationism, while the school the child attends is teaching evolution. Thus, the child may feel confused as he or she tries to practice the behaviors expected by the different groups.

Socioeconomic Status

An even more important influence on children is the family's socioeconomic status (relative position in society), which takes into account the family's economic, occupational, and educational levels. Children are raised differently by parents of different educational levels, occupations, and incomes. The middle and upper classes often have access to physical and emotional support in the community that is not always available to the lower class (Giger & Davidhizar, 1995). Lower-class parents may need to work long hours to provide basic necessities and have little time or money to enrich the child's life or make healthy lifestyle choices. However, lower-class families may have stronger family relationships if they need to rely

BOX 2.2

EXAMPLES OF SOCIAL ROLES FOR CHILDREN

- Daughter or son
- Brother or sister
- Granddaughter or grandson
- School or daycare roles, such as first-grader, preschooler, honor student
- Ethnic community member
- Church roles, such as acolyte, altar server
- Specialized roles such as developing musician, artist, or athlete

on a family network to meet some of their physical and emotional needs. Lifestyle characteristics, such as cultural norms for health behaviors, may help buffer some lower-class children from health problems (Chen et al., 2006).

Low socioeconomic status can have an adverse influence on children's health. Some families may not be able to afford health insurance or health care. Meals may be unbalanced or irregular. The family's house or apartment may be overcrowded and may have poor sanitation or lead paint. These families may not understand the importance of preventive care or may not be able to afford it, and as a result the children may be inadequately immunized against communicable diseases.

Studies have documented that children who live in low-income neighborhoods, who lack health insurance and whose parents have fewer years of education have increased rates of injury and injury mortality (Marcin et al., 2003). Recently, population-based analysis showed higher rates of injury hospitalization and mortality among children from low-income neighborhoods (Marcin et al., 2003). These children also generally present with more lethal mechanisms of injury, such as pedestrian or firearm injuries.

Poverty

Basic financial stability enhances the general health and well-being of children, and thus an important negative influence on children's health is poverty. Children living in poverty are:

- Two times more likely than other children to die from accidents
- Three times more likely to die from all causes combined
- Four times more likely to die from fires
- Five times more likely to die from infectious diseases and parasites
- Six times more likely to die from other diseases (Children's Defense Fund, 2005)

Children living in poverty are at risk for having difficulty in school, becoming teen parents, and having multiple health problems (Children's Defense Fund, 2005). Overall, they experience diminished health, stunted growth, higher rates of death and illness, and negative effects on their cognitive abilities (Children's Defense Fund, 2005; Behrman, 2004).

The poverty threshold is based on the family's size and income and is used to determine whether a family is living in poverty (Table 2.3). According to the U.S. Census Bureau (2004, 2006a), approximately 12.6% of individuals and 9.9% of families were living below the poverty level. Of the families living below poverty level, 28.7% were single-mother families with no husband present and 13% were single-father families with no wife present. Overall, 17.5% of children under age 18 years were living in poverty. Although the rates have stabilized somewhat after several years of consecutive increases, more children live in poverty than all other Americans, with these rates being highest among minority groups. According to the Children's Defense Fund (2005), 1 in 14 American children lives at less than half the poverty level, and 2,385 babies are born into poverty each day in America.

Table 2.3 U.S. Poverty Thresholds, 2007

Size of Family Unit	Weighted Average Thresholds
1 person	$10,210
2 people	$13,690
3 people	$17,170
4 people	$20,650
5 people	$24,130

Source: National Archives and Records Administration, 2007.

Family structure is an important factor associated with poverty rates for children. The poverty rate for married-couple families is much less than that for families headed by a single parent. Educational level is another important factor: as education increases, unemployment declines and annual income rises. However, a chronic physical or emotional problem in any wage earner may lead to unemployment, and this can cause the family to spiral downward into poverty.

The effects of poverty on children's health can be wide-ranging. The family may be able to afford only substandard housing or a house or apartment in a dangerous neighborhood (e.g., unsanitary conditions, toxins, violence). Poverty may also lead to homelessness.

Homelessness

According to the National Coalition for the Homeless, approximately 1.2 million children are homeless on any given night (National Center on Family Homelessness, 2004). Children represent 39% of the homeless population, with 42% of these children under age 5 years (National Coalition for the Homeless, 2006). Families with children are the fastest-growing segment of the homeless population; the typical homeless family is headed by a woman with two or three children (Bassuk et al., 1998). Homeless families commonly are victims of violence and may have mental health problems.

Homelessness occurs not only in large urban areas but also in midsize cities as well as suburban and rural areas. A family may become homeless due to poverty, lack of affordable housing, decreases in rent subsidies, unemployment, cutbacks in public welfare programs, and personal crises such as divorce, domestic violence, or substance abuse (American Academy of Pediatrics, 2005). Children may choose to run away and become homeless because they have been abused or neglected, lived in foster homes, or are placed in residential treatment or juvenile detention centers (National Association for the Education of Homeless Children, 2007).

Homelessness is not conducive to appropriate growth and development in children, and it damages children's mental health. In homeless children ages 6 to 17 years, the National Mental Health Association (2006) estimates that:

- One in three has at least one major mental health problem interfering with daily activities.
- Approximately one in two experience anxiety, depression, or withdrawal.
- More than one in three exhibit delinquent or aggressive behavior.

In contrast, for school-age children with a home, estimates are approximately one in five or less.

In homeless children, the basic need for a stable shelter goes unmet. They also have a higher incidence of chronic health problems and trauma-related injuries (Bassuk et al., 1998). The most common physical problems are upper respiratory, ear, and skin infections, gastrointestinal disorders such as diarrhea, and infestations such as lice and scabies. They may be exposed to environmental hazards in homeless shelters or overcrowded housing, or, if they live on the street, exposure to the elements, lack of sanitary facilities, and an increased risk of injuries. Homeless children are likely to exhibit poor attention span, trouble sleeping, delayed speech, aggressive behaviors, shyness, and withdrawal (HUD, 1999). Many of these children develop psychological problems such as depression, anxiety disorders, or behavior problems that do not disappear even when the family finds a home. An unbalanced diet may place homeless children at risk for nutritional deficits, which can lead to delayed growth and development. Homeless teens often engage in risky behaviors such as drug use or unprotected sex with multiple partners, so they are more likely to need emergency care, be depressed, and become pregnant (American Academy of Pediatrics, 2005). They may also become teen parents, continuing the cycle of financial instability and homelessness.

Homeless children may have limited access to health care services, especially preventive care such as immunizations, dental care, and well-child services. Lack of immunizations can lead to delayed enrollment in school, and education is vital for these children to help break the cycle of homelessness. When the families do have money, often they need it for food and shelter instead of health care. If they do seek health care, it is generally in an emergency department or a free clinic (Ensign & Santelli, 1998), and such sporadic care is not conducive to the ongoing health needs of a growing child. The family may not follow through with care because they cannot afford it, lack health insurance, or do not have transportation to the clinic or pharmacy.

Some of these children do not go to school or go to various schools because the family moves from place to place. The stress being experienced by the family provides an environment that is not conducive to learning. As a result children present with learning problems, socialization issues, or other behavioral issues.

Media

Today's children are inundated with various forms of media, such as television, video and computer games, movies, magazines, books, and newspapers (Fig. 2.5). Some of the images and information are not always in the best interests of children. Children may identify with and mimic characters who engage in risk-taking behaviors or lifestyles. Sometimes this identification can lead to violence and harm to self and others (Brown & Witherspoon, 2002; Monsen, 2002). Some children may become curious about the substance abuse or sexual activity they see in the media (Strasburger & Donnerstein, 1999). If an image or type of behavior is portrayed as the norm, children may view this as acceptable behavior without examining the potential health risks or other long-term consequences. For example, thinness is portrayed as the body type that is identified with beauty, leading some children to develop unhealthy dieting or other behaviors to develop that body type. For the child who has a body type that does not fit the ideal, depression or self-esteem issues may develop.

Overall, the images children view every day will affect their behavior and possibly their health, and pediatric nurses should take this into account when working with children and their families.

The media's influence relates not only to the content but also to the total viewing time. For example, excessive TV viewing has been linked to obesity and high blood cholesterol levels in children (Andersen et al., 1998). Overuse of computer or video games may lead to poor school performance.

The media can be a positive influence, such as when it offers public service messages on the negative effects

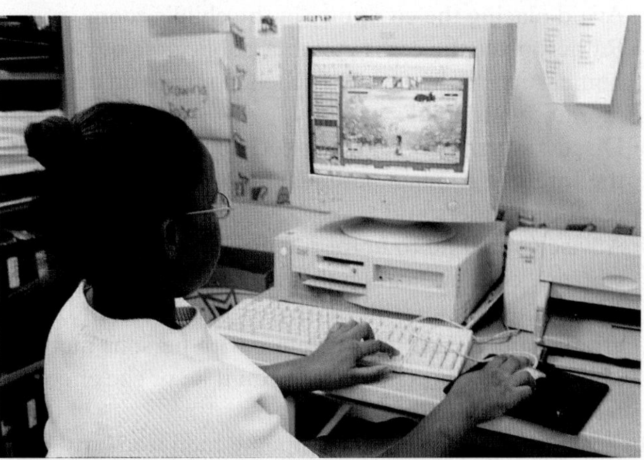

● Figure 2.5 Computer games can be fun and educational, but the child should be monitored while using the computer or other forms of media to minimize negative effects.

of substance abuse, smoking, or gang involvement. Also, public broadcasting networks offer valuable programming.

Widespread access to the Internet has fostered a connection to other areas of the world that would not have been possible in previous years. Children are no longer limited to their immediate surroundings, and they have access to a wealth of information. The Internet can be a valuable resource for parents and children to access information, learn new things, and communicate with friends and family. However, online threats exist that can affect the child's health and safety (American Academy of Pediatrics, 2006), such as sexual predators, pornography, violence, and racism. Parents need to be alert to these hazards and set up safety guidelines (Teaching Guideline 2.2).

Global Society

The world is connected in many ways today: people travel from one nation to another easily, new products and immigrants arrive each day, and the Internet makes worldwide communication simple. The United Nations Children's Fund and the World Health Organization (WHO) lead the world in dealing with the issues for the children of the world. According to these organizations, every year 11 million children die, and over 90% of the children are born into developing or Third World countries. Hundreds of thousands of children born in developing countries are moving to more developed nations such as the United States as refugees, immigrants, or international adoptees. These children become part of this nation.

Pediatric nurses need to be aware of the impact of worldwide events on children. The population explosion and health problems in developing nations and natural and man-made disasters around the world affect the United States and the world in terms of productivity, economics, and politics (WHO, 2004). Children can be displaced by events such as hurricanes or wars, placing them at increased risk for problems such as infectious diseases, malnutrition, and psychological trauma.

According to the United Nations Children's Fund and WHO, young children bear the brunt of the global burden of disease. These organizations have identified six major problems affecting child growth and development and survival:

- Malnutrition, including micronutrient deficiency
- HIV/AIDS
- Acute respiratory infections
- Diarrhea
- Vaccine-preventable diseases such as measles
- Malaria

These organizations work to propose ways to eradicate these conditions by improving the case management skills of providers with adapted guidelines; improving the health systems with good district health planning and management as well as appropriate supplies, medications, information systems, and referral systems; and improving the family and community practices.

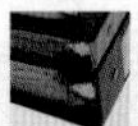

TEACHING GUIDELINE 2.2

Teaching to Promote Safe Internet Use

- Determine a time limit that your child can spend online each day or week and maintain consistency in enforcing this time limit.
- Ensure that use of the Internet does not replace or interfere with homework, friends, or household or school activities.
- Tell your child NEVER to share personal information with anyone online unless you are sure of the person and the child has your permission to do so.
- Urge your child NEVER to share his or her password with anyone, even friends.
- Review Internet sites with your child, and explain which sites are appropriate. Use the safety and parental controls offered by your Internet service provider.
- Avoid placing the computer in the child's room. Rather, place the computer in a public area of your home, such as the den or kitchen, so that you can monitor your child's use.
- Discuss with your child the need for safety while using the Internet. Explain potential hazards in terms the child can understand.
- Advise your child to immediately close any sites or stop any communication that makes him or her confused or uncomfortable. Tell your child NEVER to arrange any face-to-face meeting with persons met online. Urge your child to tell you if he or she encounters such a situation.
- Teach the child NEVER to open e-mail from any unknown senders.
- Be aware of computer use policies in your child's school.

Culture

Culture (the view of the world and a set of traditions that are used by a specific social group and are transmitted to the next generation) plays a critical role in not only the socialization of the child but also the child's experiences related to health and the establishment of specific health practices (Pillitteri, 2003). Culture is a complex phenomenon involving the integration of many components such as beliefs, values, language, time, and personal space that shape a person's actions and behavior. Children learn these patterns of cultural behaviors from their family and community through a process called **enculturation**, which involves acquiring knowledge and internalizing values (Degazon, 1996).

Culture influences every aspect of development and is reflected in childrearing beliefs and practices designed to promote healthy adaptation. Typically, a child begins to understand his or her culture at approximately the age of 5 years. The child's cultural background affects the way that he or she socializes, learns values, and experiences the world. The child's developing beliefs, customs, mode of communication, dress, and actions may all be shaped by his or her culture.

With today's changing demographic patterns, nurses must be able to incorporate cultural knowledge into their interventions so that they can care effectively for culturally diverse children. They must be aware of the wide range of cultural traditions, values, and ethics that exist in the United States today. All nurses must establish **cultural competence**, the ability to apply knowledge about a patient's culture so that health care interventions can be adapted to meet the needs of the patient (Table 2.4). The nurse should know about various culture-based health practices and how they may affect children, as well as the demographics of the local population. The goal is for the nurse to view culture as a point of congruence rather than a potential source of conflict.

> Recall Miguel, the infant described at the beginning of the chapter. Propose appropriate nursing interventions that would assist in providing culturally competent care. How can you best determine the child's and family's cultural preferences?

Cultural Groups

In a society there are typically dominant and minority groups. The dominant group, often the largest group, has the greatest authority to control the values and sanctions of the society (Taylor et al., 2005). As a result, the dominant culture may have the largest impact on the child's health, while minority cultural groups may still maintain some of their own traditions and values.

The relationship of culture to health care can become obscured by the use of broad group titles. In reality, there are many distinct cultural groups, and within a group there may be many subcultures. Geographic differences also can occur. For example, the Latin Americans living in New York may be quite different from the Latin Americans living in Florida. Nurses must be aware of these distinct cultural groups so they can provide culturally competent care.

Nurses should also be aware of the traditional health care values and practices that are passed along from one generation to the next. For example, some cultures believe in consulting folk healers, and this belief may have a major influence on children's health (Table 2.5).

Ethnicity

Ethnicity, a term sometimes used synonymously with culture, involves group membership by virtue of common ancestry. The basic groups are differentiated by their customs, characteristics, language, or similar distinguishing factors. Ethnic groups have their own family structures, languages, food preferences, moral codes, and health care practices. Children learn the accepted mode of behavior by observing and imitating those around them. The influences of culture and ethnicity on children and families are highly variable and dynamic. Probably the most important characteristic of ethnicity is the sense of shared identity felt by members (Davidhizar et al., 1999).

Children who come from a minority group may experience conflict because their native customs are different from those of the dominant culture. Many Americans in the dominant culture do not view themselves as belonging to a specific ethnic group, but many minority groups still identify closely with their ethnicity and emphasize their cultural or racial differences (Davidhizar et al., 1999).

Table 2.4 Components of Cultural Competence

Component	Description
Cultural self-awareness	Exploration of one's own culture and how values, beliefs, and behaviors have influenced personal life Examination of own biases and prejudices Identification of how own background is similar to and different from another's background
Cultural knowledge	Acquisition of information about other cultures from a variety of sources Familiarity with diverse groups and their beliefs, practices, world views, and strategies for decision making
Cultural skills and practices	Incorporation of knowledge of cultural background including specific practices for health Inclusion of family members' roles for decision making
Cultural encounter	Participation in and interaction with persons of diverse cultural backgrounds

Table 2.5 Beliefs and Practices of Selected Cultural Groups

Cultural Group	Beliefs and Practices Affecting Children's Health
African-American	Strong extended family relationships; mother as head of household; elder family members valued and respected Food as a symbol of health and wealth View of health as harmony with nature; illness as disruption in harmony Use of folk healing and home remedies common Belief in illnesses as natural (due to natural forces that the person hasn't protected self against) and unnatural (due to person or spirit) Illness commonly associated with pain Pain and suffering inevitable; relief achieved through prayers and laying on of hands Individuals vulnerable to external forces
Asian-Americans	Strong loyalty to the family Family as the center, with members expected to care for one another Use of complementary modalities with Western health care practices View of life as a cycle, with everything connected to health Pain described by diverse body symptoms Health viewed as a balance between the forces of *yang* and *yin* Respect for authority emphasized
Arab-Americans	Women subordinate to men; young individuals subordinate to older persons Family loyalty is primary Good health associated with eating properly, consuming nutritious foods, and fasting to cure disease Illness due to inadequate diet, shifts in hot and cold, exposure of stomach while sleeping, emotional or spiritual distress, and "evil eye" Little emphasis on preventive care View of pain as unpleasant, requiring immediate control or relief Cleanliness important for prayer
Native Americans	High value on family and tribe; respect for elders Family as an extended network providing care for newborns and children Women as the verbal decision makers Celebrations to mark the stages of growth and development Use of food to celebrate life events and in healing and religious ceremonies Health as harmony with nature; illness due to disharmony, evil spirits Restoration of physical, mental, and spiritual balance through healing ceremonies View of pain as something to be tolerated
Hispanic	Family important; father as the source of strength, wisdom, and self-confidence Mother as the caretaker and decision maker for health View of children as persons to continue the family and culture Use of food for celebrations and socialization Health as God's will maintainable with a balance of hot and cold food intake Freedom from pain indicative of good health; pain tolerated stoically due to belief that it is God's will Folk medicine practices and prayers, herbal teas, and poultices for illness treatment

Stereotyping or labeling can result from **ethnocentrism**, a belief that one's own ethnic group is superior to other ethnic groups. This attitude can lead to a slanted view of the world, and it may hinder the nurse's ability to provide culturally competent care.

Cultural Health Practices

Health practices are often the result of health beliefs derived from a person's culture. For example, do the child and family view health and illness as the result of natural forces, supernatural forces, or the imbalance of forces? Most cultures have remedies that people may use or consider before they seek professional health care. People from some cultures may go to folk healers who they believe can cure certain illnesses. For example, the *curandero* (male) or the *curandera* (female) of the Mexican-American community is believed to have healing powers as a gift from God. Asian-Americans may consult a practitioner who specializes in traditional Asian therapies such as acupuncture, acupressure, and moxibustion. These folk healers are often very powerful in their community, speak the language, and are very familiar with the culture's spiritual or religious aspects.

If the folk remedies or practices of the folk healers are compatible with the health regimen and support appropriate health practices, these practices and beliefs do no harm; in fact, they may even benefit the child and family. However, use of a folk healer can lead to a delay in beneficial treatment or create other problems. Some traditional health practices may be misinterpreted as being harmful, and some actually are harmful. For example, the Vietnamese practice of coining, which involves rubbing the edge of a coin on an oiled symptomatic body area to rid the body of disease, may be misinterpreted as a sign of physical abuse. This practice also can lead to burns, bruising, or welt-like lesions on the child's skin if it is done frequently. *Azarcon* and *greta,* powders containing high amounts of lead, are used as a folk remedy in Mexico to treat digestive problems and can result in lead toxicity. Female circumcision, also called female genital mutilation, can lead initially to hemorrhage and infection and to long-term complications such as cysts, abscesses, urethral damage, and sexual dysfunction

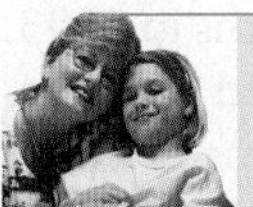

Pediatric nurses can help to shape an individual's lifelong perceptions of health and health services. An understanding of how the child's and family's culture affects their health practices gives the nurse an opportunity to incorporate appropriate and beneficial health practices into the family's cultural milieu, providing sources of strength rather than areas of conflict.

Changing Demographics

Although the proportion of children is decreasing in relationship to the adult population, the racial, ethnic, and cultural diversity among children is significantly increasing in the United States. Thus, the number of culturally diverse children entering the health care system in the United States is increasing. According to the American Community Survey (U.S. Census Bureau, 2005), 75% of the population was white, 12% was Black or African American, and 14.5% was Hispanic. The U.S. Census Bureau reports that the Hispanic population increased by 3.3% from July 1, 2004, to July 1, 2005; this is the fastest-growing population group, accounting for almost half of the total population growth during that time frame. At the same time, non-Hispanic whites accounted for less than one fifth of the total population growth (U.S. Census Bureau, 2006b). In addition, the increasing number of marriages between individuals from different ethnic origins is producing an increasing number of children who have a heritage that represents more than one cultural group.

Immigration

Employment and economic opportunities, expanded human rights, educational opportunities, and other types of freedoms and opportunities encourage many foreigners to move to the United States. Approximately 14 million children in the United States are immigrants or members of an immigrant family (Children's Defense Fund, 2005). Some communities welcome the new members, but others do not. Partly due to fears of terrorism, this country is evaluating, enforcing, and changing many of its immigration laws.

Immigration can affect the health, educational, and social services provided in the United States. It also presents issues related to access to care and the types of care that need to be offered. Immigration imposes unique stresses on children and families, including:

- Depression, grief, or anxiety associated with migration and acculturation
- Separation from support systems
- Inadequate language skills in a society that is not tolerant of linguistic differences
- Disparities in social, professional, and economic status between the country of origin and the United States
- Traumatic events such as war or persecution that may have occurred in their native country (American Academy of Pediatrics, 2005)

Inability to speak English can hinder an immigrant's educational attainment, economic opportunities, and ability to join the mainstream of society. A total of 18% of U.S. children speak a language other than English at home; this number is 72% of children in immigrant families (Hernandez, 2004). Immigrant parents who do not speak English may have trouble enrolling their children in preschool, becoming involved in school activities, helping their children meet college entrance requirements (Hernandez, 2004), and applying for health insurance.

Immigrant children also may arrive in the United States with significant health problems. For example, children from Southeast Asia may have health problems associated with intestinal parasites, poor diets, dental problems, tuberculosis, and hepatitis A and B (Worley et al., 2000).

The health status of immigrant children may be compromised due to the lack of preventive care, immunizations, and dental care. Due to the financial, language, cultural, and other types of barriers immigrant families sometimes face, the children may not receive the necessary preventive care or receive care for minor conditions until they become more serious. Stresses experienced by immigrant children and their families, such as those associated with relocation, separation, and traumatic events, also can have an impact on their psychological health.

Spiritual and Religious Influences

Spirituality is a basic human quality involving the belief in something greater than one's self and a faith that positively affirms life. It is a major influence in many people's lives, providing a meaning or purpose to life and a foundation for and a source of love, relationships, and service. Spirituality is considered a universal human phenomenon with an assumption of the wholeness of individuals and their connectedness to a higher being. During life-changing events and crises, such as a birth of a child with a congenital defect or a serious or terminal illness, families often turn to spirituality for hope, comfort, and relief.

The word "religion" is often used interchangeably with spirituality in our society. However, spirituality is more of a private and individual belief, whereas **religion** is an organized way of sharing beliefs and practicing worship. Over 95% of parents in America believe in God; therefore, spirituality and religion are an important focus when working with children and their families. A person's spiritual and religious beliefs may affect the way in which he or she interprets and responds to illness (Spector, 2000). In some religions, illness is seen as a punishment for sin or wrongdoing. Others religions view illness as a test of strength.

Children view spirituality and religion differently at different developmental stages. Typically, children imitate their parents' rituals when they are toddlers and then develop an increasingly sophisticated understanding of their parents' views during the years up to adolescence. Refer to the chapters on the specific developmental stages for a discussion on how children of different ages view spirituality and religion.

Identifying the child's and family's religious beliefs and customs is important. Families appreciate the recognition of and respect for their beliefs. For example, there may be special dietary restrictions, rituals such as baptism or communion, use of amulets or icons, or practices related to dying that can be incorporated into the child's plan of care. Using open-ended questions and observing for the use of religious articles during assessment can provide clues to the family's beliefs and practices. Visits from spiritual leaders may also be noted. Table 2.6 identifies some of the major religious beliefs that may affect children's health.

> **Recall the Delgado family** described at the beginning of the chapter. What, if any, influence might the family's culture and religious beliefs have on Miguel's care?

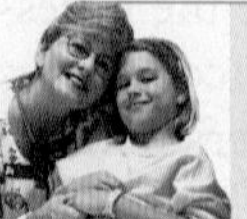

Never make assumptions about a family's religious or spiritual affiliation. Although they may belong to a particular religion, they may not adhere to all of the beliefs or participate in all aspects of the religion. Be alert to clues that would provide insight into their specific beliefs.

Community

Community encompasses a broad range of concepts, from the individual's nation of residence to a particular neighborhood or group. The community surrounding a child affects many aspects of his or her health and general welfare. The child's community consists of the family, school, neighborhood, youth organizations, and other peer groups. All of these groups contribute to the child's experience within any culture and nation (Search Institute, 2007).

The quality of life within the community, positive or negative, has a great influence on a child's ability to achieve developmental tasks and become a functional member of society. The child's school, which is a community by itself, and peer groups are important influences. School programs and community centers can also affect the child's overall health and well-being.

Violence

Although the new century has shown an overall decline in violence by and against children, youth violence is still an important public health problem. Violent crimes include murder, rape, robbery, and aggravated assault. Centers for Disease Control and Prevention (2006) statistics show that for people ages 10 to 24 years:

- Approximately 5,570 individuals were murdered; of those, firearms accounted for 82% of the deaths in 2003.
- More than 750,000 individuals were treated in emergency departments for injuries due to violence in 2004.
- Homicide was the leading cause of death for African-Americans, the second-leading cause of death for Hispanics, and the third-leading cause of death for American Indians, Alaska Natives, and Asian/Pacific Islanders.

In 2003, suicide was the third-leading cause of death in people ages 10 to 24 years. For those ages 10 to 14 years, approximately 30% of suicides were due to firearms; for those 15 to 24 years old, firearms accounted for more than 50% of all suicides (Centers for Disease Control and Prevention, 2006).

Youth violence affects the community as well as the child and family. Studies have shown that youth violence is associated with a disruption in social services, an increase in health care costs, and a decline in property values.

School Violence

In recent years, school violence has received much attention and concern for student safety has increased. As a result, rates of school violence are declining (Children's Defense Fund, 2000). Students are more likely to be victims of violent crimes away from school, but fights, thefts, weapon carrying, teacher victimization, and fear of school environments have increased (Snyder & Sickmund, 1999). The Centers for Disease Control and Prevention (2006) conducted a nationwide survey of high school students about risk behavior and found that approximately 36% of

Table 2.6 Selected Religious Beliefs Affecting Children's Health

Religion	Beliefs about Health and Illness	Dietary Practices	Beliefs About Birth and Death
Buddhist	Illness from karmic causes (ignorant craving) Illness as an opportunity to develop the soul Ultimate goal of achieving nirvana (state of supreme tranquility, purity, and stability)	Generally no special requirements or restrictions Some sects are vegetarian	No baptism Last rite chanting at bedside soon after death
Christian Scientist	Disease viewed as error of human mind that can be dispelled by spiritual truth Health viewed within a spiritual framework; healing through prayer and spiritual regeneration Possible contact of own healing ministry (Christian Science practitioners) if child is hospitalized	No special requirements or restrictions	No baptism or last rites General opposition to human interventions with drugs or other therapies except for legally required immunizations
Hindu	Illness due to sins committed in previous life Acceptance of most medical practice/care Nonviolent approach to life	Meat consumption forbidden Some are strict vegetarians	No baptism View of death as a step in an ongoing cycle to reach nirvana Certain prescribed rites after death, such as washing the body by family and restrictions on who touches the body Cremation common
Islam	Belief that God cures but will accept treatment Compulsory prayers at dawn, noon, afternoon, after sunset, and after nightfall	Ingestion of pork and pork products and alcohol forbidden Fasting (by boys at age 7, girls at age 9, and adults) required during Ramadan (ninth month of Islamic year)	No baptism Special party (*Aqeeqa*) to celebrate birth Specific burial rituals (rinsing and washing, wrapping, special prayers, and burial)
Judaism (orthodox and conservative)	Illness as possible reason for violating some dietary restrictions No treatments or procedures on Sabbath or holy days	Ingestion of blood (such as raw meat) prohibited Kosher dietary laws; highly individualized observance Abstinence from ingestion of pork and predatory fowl and no mixing of milk dishes with meat dishes; ingestion of only fish with fins and scales; no shellfish (strict followers) Fasting during Yom Kippur, and matzo replaces leavened bread during Passover week	No baptism Ritual circumcision of male infants on eighth day of life Ritual of washing body after death; family and close friends remain with the deceased for a period of time No cremation

(continued)

Table 2.6 Selected Religious Beliefs Affecting Children's Health (continued)

Religion	Beliefs about Health and Illness	Dietary Practices	Beliefs About Birth and Death
Mormon (Church of Jesus Christ of Latter-Day Saints)	Belief in divine health via laying on of hands Medical therapy not prohibited Common use of herbal folk remedies	Ingestion of tea, coffee, and alcohol and use of tobacco prohibited Fasting (no food or drink including water) once a month for 24 hours on a designated day	No baptism; infant blessed by church official after the birth Cremation discouraged
Roman Catholic	Care of sick encouraged Misuse of any substance considered harmful to the body and a sin Eucharist as the food of healing and health	Fasting and abstinence from meat and meat products on Ash Wednesday and Good Friday Abstinence on Fridays during Lent	Infant baptism; Sacrament of the Sick if prognosis is poor while child is alive; anointing of the sick Burial and treatment of the body with respect and honor

Sources: Andrews, M. M., & Boyle, J. S. (2003). *Transcultural concepts in nursing care* (4th ed.). Philadelphia: Lippincott Williams & Wilkins; Carson, V. B. (1989). *Spiritual dimensions of nursing practice* (pp. 100–101) Philadelphia: Saunders; Spector, R. E. (2000) *Cultural diversity in health and illness.* Upper Saddle River, NJ: Prentice Hall.

the students reported that they had been involved in a physical altercation at least once in the previous year, and just under one fifth of the students reported carrying a weapon for at least one of the days in the month prior to the survey. Of the students who said they carried a weapon, approximately 5% had carried a gun. The continued coordination among schools, law enforcement, social services, and mental health systems and the development of effective programs will help to reduce these risk behaviors.

Violence in the Home

Violence that occurs in the home, known as domestic violence, affects the lives of many people in America, including children. The U.S. Bureau of Justice estimates that approximately 1 million violent crimes are committed by former spouses, boyfriends, or girlfriends each year, with about 85% of the victims being women (Rennison & Welchans, 2000). This violence is also known as intimate partner abuse, family violence, wife beating, battering, marital abuse, and partner abuse.

Children often witness this violence, and they may be physically, sexually, or emotionally abused themselves (Children's Defense Fund, 2000; DiLauro, 2004). The Federal Child Abuse Prevention and Treatment Act (CAPTA) defines child abuse and neglect as any recent act or failure to act on the part of a parent or caretaker that results in death, serious physical or emotional harm, sexual abuse or exploitation, or an act or failure to act that presents an imminent risk of serious harm to a child (Child Welfare Information Gateway, 2007). Of the number of children identified as being maltreated, 61% were victims of neglect, 19% were victims of physical abuse, 10% were victims of sexual abuse, and 5% were victims of emotional or psychological abuse (Centers for Disease Control and Prevention, 2006b). According to Child Welfare Information Gateway (2006), three children die in America every day as a result of child abuse or neglect. Over 82% of these deaths occur in infants and children younger than 4 years of age.

Children who are exposed to stressors such as domestic violence or who are victims of childhood abuse or neglect (termed adverse childhood experiences) are at high risk for short- and long-term problems. Short-term problems may include sleep disturbances, headaches, stomachaches, depression, asthma, enuresis, aggressive behaviors, decreased social competencies, withdrawal, developmental regression, fears, anxiety, and learning problems (Centers for Disease Control and Prevention, 2006c; Children's Defense Fund, 2000). Long-term problems may include poor school performance, truancy, absenteeism, and difficulty with adult relationships and tasks. There is a strong correlation between the number of exposures to adverse events and negative behaviors such as early initiation of smoking, sexual activity, and illicit drug use, adolescent pregnancies, and suicide attempts (Centers for Disease Control and Prevention, 2006).

Due to the potential impact of violence on children and families, the nurse must perform a thorough assessment to identify violence in the family (Box 2.3). Providing referrals to shelters and child advocacy centers and intervening to assist children in dealing with this issue are key.

BOX 2.3

ASSESSING FOR VIOLENCE

Questions for the Parent

- Do you ever feel afraid in your home?
- What happens when you and ___ (partner's name) argue?
- Do arguments ever become physical (hitting, kicking, pushing, throwing, or punching/breaking objects)?
- Have you ever been threatened with a weapon (gun, knife, other)?
- Have you ever felt trapped or like a prisoner in your own home? Does your partner ever lock you in/out of the house or take your car keys?
- Have your children ever seen or heard violence in the home?
- Have the police ever been involved due to violence in your home?
- Is the violence ever directed at the children? Does __ (partner's name) ever hit, kick, push, or yell at your child when he/she is angry?
- How do you and __ (partner's name) discipline the children?

Questions for the Child

- What happens when Mommy and Daddy (or appropriate partner names) argue/fight? Is there any hitting, pushing, etc.?
- How do you feel when Mommy and Daddy (or appropriate partner names) fight?
- What happens to you when you get in trouble?

If hitting or other physical forms of discipline occur, ask the following:

- What are you hit with? Where on your body? Does it ever leave a mark/bruise?
- Who hits/kicks you? How often does it happen?

Not all children exposed to violence suffer negative consequences. Children have resilience, and preliminary studies have identified protective factors that can help buffer children from the effects of violence and reduce the risk that the child will develop violent behaviors. Examples of protective factors are:

- Strong commitment to school and academic performance
- Involvement in social activities
- Feelings of connectedness to family or other adults outside the family
- Ability to discuss problems with parents or a supportive adult
- Consistent presence of a parent at least once during the day, such as in the morning on awakening, when getting home from school, at dinnertime, or when going to bed.

Thus, interventions need to focus on reducing children's exposure to violence and fostering protective factors.

Schools and Other Community Centers

Children today start school at an earlier age, spend more time in childcare settings, and are involved in various community centers and activities. By age 4, many children are in a preschool setting for several hours a day. Some children spend more time in school and childcare settings than in their family home. Thus, schools have become major influences on children.

Although the primary role of schools has always been academic education, today schools are performing more health-related functions. School also provides a means of socialization. School rules about attendance and authority relationships and the system of sanctions and rewards based on achievement help to teach children behavioral expectations that they will need for future employment and relationships in the adult world. Some consider schools to be a key site for promoting healthy behaviors and teaching about exercise, nutrition, safety, sex, drugs, and behavioral and emotional problems (Hager, 2004). Academic success is linked to healthy behavior, mental health, and avoidance of pregnancy and juvenile justice problems, as well as health, jobs, and self-sufficiency in adult life (Hager, 2004).

Because in many families both parents need to work, many children are enrolled in childcare and after-school programs. Thus, the socialization process begins earlier and involves a larger percentage of the child's waking hours (Fig. 2.6). Community centers and after-school programs can provide support, empowerment, boundaries and expectations, and constructive use of time (Search Institute, 2003).

Children need to feel supported by, cared for, and valued by their community. They need to know what is expected of them and what behaviors are outside the boundaries of the community. They also need to have

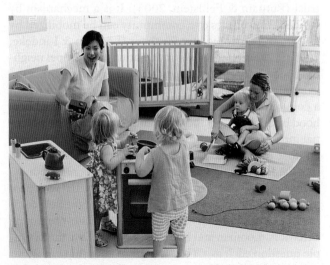

● Figure 2.6 Daycare centers can provide socialization and support for young children.

opportunities that are enriching and constructive. By developing life-long learning skills, positive values, and social competencies, children can feel confidence in their own power, purpose, and worth as well as promise for themselves and their future (Search Institute, 2007).

Peer Groups

A child's friends can have a major influence, positive or negative, on his or her growth and development. Peer group relationships often begin early and are a large part of the child's world, particularly with school-age children and adolescents. This influence starts in play groups in early preschool or elementary school. The child is confronted with a variety of values and belief systems from interactions with his or her friends. To be accepted, the child must conform to the specific values and beliefs of the group. When these values and beliefs differ from those of the adults in the child's world, conflicts can occur, possibly separating children from the adults and strengthening their sense of belonging to the peer group.

When the child's friends are successful in school, sports, or other activities, the growth and development of the child continues in a healthy and positive way. When these groups demonstrate healthy behaviors, the influence is very positive, but peer groups can also exert negative influences on the child. Thus, it is vital to identify the important peer groups in a child's life and the positive or negative behaviors connected with these groups.

Connectedness in Neighborhoods and Communities

Social capital refers to the bonds between individuals that assist communities to achieve a variety of goals, including goals directed at improving children's health. It requires norms of reciprocity, mutual assistance, and trust (Putnam & Feldstein, 2003). It is a mechanism by which the resources of a community can be mobilized by and from the people, not for them (Looman & Lindeke, 2005). Common interests and relationships propel neighborhoods and communities toward engagement. One example is the Neighborhood Watch Program, in which a community invests in the safety of the whole neighborhood by bonding together and sending a message to potential intruders that community members look out for one another (Looman & Lindeke, 2005).

Evidence suggests that the degree of connectedness in neighborhoods and communities is associated with positive health outcomes (Baum, 1999). In connected communities, people find it easy to engage in health-promoting behaviors. Looman and Lindeke (2005) believe that a simple question such as, "How is your relationship with your neighbors?" can help the nurse to understand the patient's social milieu. They suggest three areas to include in nursing interventions and strategies:

- Bringing families together in communities to set the stage for networking
- Disseminating knowledge about what helps create healthy, supported communities
- Thinking of relationships as investments, with social interactions as the processes by which resources for health are exchanged (Looman & Lindeke, 2005)

Health Status and Lifestyle

Obviously, the general health status of a child and specific lifestyles can influence a child's health. Health status may be a factor soon after birth. For example, the incidence of multiple births has been increasing in this country due to the increased use of *in vitro* fertilization and other assisted reproductive technologies (Reynolds et al., 2003). Potential complications of multiple births include intrauterine growth retardation and prematurity (Reynolds et al., 2003), which may lead to chronic health problems in the child. Children with chronic health conditions may also have developmental delays, especially in acquiring skills related to cognition, communication, adaptation, social functioning, and motor functioning. Thus, the beginning health status of a child may affect his or her long-term health and development.

Development and Disease Distribution

The way a child develops is the result of genetics and the environment within the context of a variety of biopsychosocial forces. The biological influences include genetics, *in utero* exposure to teratogens, postpartum illnesses, exposure to hazardous substances, and maturation. Chapters 4 through 8 discuss the forces affecting growth and development for each age group.

Developmental level has a major impact on the health status of children. In general, the distribution of diseases varies with age. For example, certain communicable diseases are more commonly associated with certain age groups. Before the routine use of immunizations, conditions such as measles and mumps were more commonly seen in younger school-age children. The physiologic immaturity of an infant's body systems increases the risk for infection. Ingestion of toxic substances and risk of poisoning are major health concerns for toddlers as they become more mobile and inquisitive. Adolescents are establishing their identity, which may lead them to separate from the family values and traditions for a period of time and attempt to conform with their peers. This journey may lead to risk-taking behaviors, resulting in injuries or other situations that may impair their health.

Nutrition

Adequate nutrition can provide a rich environment for the developing child; conversely, nutritional deprivation can seriously interfere with brain development and other functions. Nutritional requirements change over the child's life and have a great influence on the child's physical growth and intellectual development. Nutrition provides the essentials required to maintain health and prevent illness (Fig. 2.7). Chapters 4 through 8 discuss the specific nutritional requirements and the impact of deficiencies for each developmental stage.

Nutritional deficiencies or excesses, such as iron deficiency anemia and the increasing incidence of childhood obesity, are still common problems in the United States. Some factors contributing to poor nutrition include inadequate food intake, nutritionally unsound social and cultural food practices, the ready availability of processed and nutritionally inadequate foods, lack of nutrition education in homes and schools, and the presence of illness that interferes with ingestion, digestion, and absorption of food. In a growing child, inadequate nutrition is associated with lower cognitive ability, poor emotional and mental health, increased susceptibility to childhood illnesses, and stunted physical growth. "Fast food" or "junk food" diets are one cause of childhood obesity and the recent increases in the number of cases of childhood type 2 diabetes.

Lifestyle Choices

Lifestyle choices that can affect a child's health include patterns of eating, exercise, use of tobacco, drugs, or alcohol, and methods of coping with stress. With the advances in medicine, most health problems today arise due to a person's lifestyle. For children, the lifestyle of the parents basically is the lifestyle of the child. Inactive parents who eat poorly commonly have children with the same habits, resulting in diabetes, obesity, and early heart disease. These typically adult problems are being diagnosed in children and adolescents today. Parents should maintain a level of physical activity in the child's life through sports, hobbies such as dancing, or family activities.

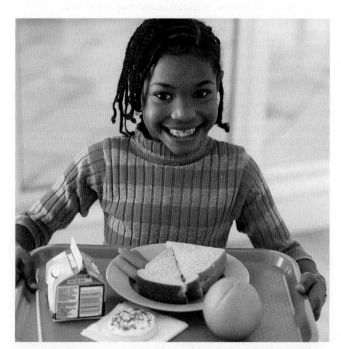

● Figure 2.7 The dietary habits established early in life can have a long-lasting impact on the health of the child and the quality of life.

Environmental Exposure

Some environmental exposures can have a detrimental impact on the child. *In utero,* the child can be affected by poor maternal nutrition or by exposure to the mother's use of alcohol, tobacco, and drugs or infections. It is important for pregnant women to be aware of the risks associated with certain drugs, chemicals, and dietary agents as well as maternal illnesses that may lead to problems for the child. These agents, known as teratogens, may be linked to birth defects in children. Not all drugs or agents are associated with fetal effects, however, and research is ongoing to identify the correlations between teratogens and other variables.

The environment continues to affect a child's health after birth. Exposure to air pollution, tobacco, and water or food contaminants can impair a child's health status. Safety hazards in the home or community can contribute to falls, burns, drowning, or other accidents (statistically, more drownings occur in children in warmer states because more homes have pools). Exposure to second-hand smoke and other pollutants, such as from radiation or chemicals, is a health hazard for children. Because children are smaller and still developing, environmental exposures can cause more health problems for them.

Stress and Coping

Children are exposed to various situations and events that can produce stress. These events can be associated with the normal problems associated with growth and development, such as entering a new classroom, learning a new skill, or being teased by a classmate, or they can be associated with problems such as poverty, divorce, violence, illness, or trauma. Some children can adapt and respond to the stress, while others do not. The term **resilience** refers to the qualities that enable an individual to cope with significant adverse events or stresses and still function competently (Patterson, 2002). Various internal and external protective factors promote resiliency. Internal factors include the person's ability to take control and be proactive, to be responsible for his or her own decisions, to understand and accept his or her own limits and abilities, and to be goal-directed, knowing when to continue or when to stop. External factors include caring relationships with a family member, a positive, safe learning environment at school (including clubs and social organizations), and positive influences in the community (see the discussion earlier in this chapter about protective factors and violence). Promoting the development of resiliency in children aids in the achievement of positive outcomes.

Access to Health Care

The health care system, including the delivery and financing of this system, continues to change and evolve. In the United States, changes in the health care system result from pressures from many directions. These changes reflect shifts in the social and economic realities and results of biomedical and technological progress over the past several decades. The effects are felt by everyone who seeks health care in any form. The method of providing medical care in a high-tech environment has changed to providing health care within a limited-resource environment. Allocating the limited health care resources continues to be the theme.

The U.S. Congress passed legislation in 1997 that led to the creation of the State Children's Health Insurance Program (S-CHIP), and with the development of such public health insurance programs for children, the number of uninsured children declined by over 1.6 million between 1998 and 2001 (Cohen-Ross & Hill, 2003). However, 11.7% of our children still lack health insurance coverage (Cohen-Ross & Hill, 2003). Despite states' efforts to simplify enrollment requirements and support community-based application assistance with grants, contracts, and training, enrollment has not been optimal (Cohen-Ross & Hill, 2003).

It is estimated that more than half of the children who are uninsured are actually eligible for Medicaid or S-CHIP (Institute of Medicine, 2002). Lack of awareness, misconceptions about the application process, discomfort related to receiving governmental assistance, and fear of jeopardizing the family's immigration status are some of the factors that lead to failure to enroll (Cohen-Ross & Hill, 2003). The Future of Children organization recommends strategies such as creating appropriate financing systems, streamlining and coordinating procedures, and providing outreach and public education to make families aware of the opportunities.

Families above the poverty level ("the working poor") may not make enough money to afford to buy health insurance, and many part-time workers do not receive health insurance benefits. Minority children, children in immigrant families, and adolescents are especially hard-hit by the lack of health insurance (Cohen-Ross & Hill, 2003). Typically, individuals without health insurance do not seek health care for maintenance and prevention interventions, a crucial aspect of child health care.

Nursing Management

Nursing care for children and their families involves astute assessment of all of the factors discussed here that may affect the health of children. Nurses play a key role in determining the impact of these factors on children and their families. Pediatric nurses need a sound knowledge base about the family, including the different structures, roles, and functions found in today's society. Knowledge of special situations such as single-parent or adopted families is important to provide individualized care. The nurse should also assess the family's level of stress based on the demands they face and their abilities to meet those demands. Do they have the coping behaviors, patterns, and strategies to have a positive impact on the child's health?

Other assessments need to focus on genetics, social roles, socioeconomic status (e.g., poverty and homelessness), culture and ethnicity, spirituality, and community. Information gathered from these assessments can help the nurse refer the family to community resources that may assist them with stability and health needs. Resources such as state and federal agencies and community agencies such as the United Way or Salvation Army may be of assistance to families.

Nurses work with children and their families in a variety of settings and need to be alert to subtle yet important indicators that may suggest a problem. For example, the child or family may give an inaccurate address or may give as their address a homeless shelter. Parents or children may be embarrassed or ashamed, feeling the stigma of poverty or homelessness. Other clues to problems may include a history of repeated infectious diseases, multiple health problems, or complaints that the child is always hungry. The key is to link children and their families with community resources that will assist with financial stability and meeting the health needs of the children.

Due to changing demographics, immigration, and the global nature of society, nurses must make sure that the care they provide is culturally sensitive. Nursing interventions need to incorporate the family's unique values, beliefs, and actions to ensure that their needs are met.

References

Books and Journals

American Academy of Child and Adolescent Psychiatry. (2005). *Facts for families foster care.* No. 64. Washington, D.C.: Author.

American Academy of Pediatrics (2006). *Setting rules for Internet use.* Accessed 9/26/06. Available at www.aap.org/pubed/ZZZQJ9C0B7C.htm?&sub_cat=17.

American Academy of Pediatrics, Committee on Community Health Services (2005). Providing care for immigrant, homeless, and migrant children. *Pediatrics, 115*(4), 1095–1100.

American Academy of Pediatrics, Committee on Psychosocial Aspects of Child and Family Health. (1998). Guidance for effective discipline. *Pediatrics, 101*(4), 723–728.

American Psychological Association. (2004). *Single parenting and today's family.* Washington, D.C.: Author.

Banks, J. B. (2002). Childhood discipline: Challenges for clinicians and parents. *American Family Physician, 66*(8), 1447–1452.

Bassuk, E. L., & Friedman, S. M. (2005). *Facts on trauma and homeless children.* Los Angeles: National Child Traumatic Stress Network.

Baum, F. (1999). The role of social capital in health promotion: Australian perspectives. *Health Promotion Journal of Australia, 9,* 171–178.

Behrman, R., et al. (2004). *Nelson textbook of pediatrics* (17th ed.). Philadelphia: W. B. Saunders.

Borchers, D. A., Johnson, C., English, K., et al. (2003). Families and adoption: The pediatrician's role in supporting communication. *Pediatrics, 112*(6), 1437–1441.

Boss, P. (2001). *Family stress management.* Newbury Park, CA: Sage.

Brown, J. D., & Witherspoon, E. M. (2002). The mass media and American adolescents' health. *Journal of Adolescent Health, 31*(65), 153–170.

Bryner, C. L. (2001). Children of divorce. *Journal of the American Board of Family Practice, 14*(3), 176–183.

Centers for Disease Control and Prevention (2006a). *Adverse Childhood Experiences Study. Major findings.* Accessed 10/5/06. Available at http://www.cdc.gov/NCCDPHP/ACE/findings.htm.

Centers for Disease Control and Prevention (2006b). *Understanding child maltreatment fact sheet.* Atlanta: Author.

Centers for Disease Control and Prevention (2006c). *Understanding youth violence fact sheet.* Accessed 10/5/06. Available at http://www.cdc.gov/ncipc/factsheets/yvfacts.htm.

Centers for Disease Control and Prevention (2006d). Youth risk behavior surveillance—United States, 2005. *MMWR,* 55(SS-5), 1–112.

Chen, E., Martin, A. D., & Matthews, K. A. (2006). Understanding health disparities: The role of race and socioeconomic status in children's health. *American Journal of Public Health, 96*(4), 702–708.

Children's Defense Fund. (2000). *Fact sheet: Domestic violence and its impact on children.* Accessed 10/16/2005. Available at http://www.childrensdefense.org/childwelfare/domesticviolence/factsheet.aspx.

Children's Defense Fund. (2005). *The state of America's children 2005.* Washington, D.C.: Author.

Child Trends. (2005). *Family structure.* Retrieved May 24, 2007 from http://www.childrensdatabank.org/pdf/59_PDF.pdf

Child Welfare Information Gateway. (2006). *Child abuse and neglect fatalities: Statistics and intervention.* Washington, D.C.: Author.

Child Welfare Information Gateway. (2007). *Definitions in federal law.* Retrieved May 7, 2007 from http://www.childwelfare.gov/can/defining/federal.cfm.

Children's Defense Fund. (2005). *The state of American's children 2005.* Washington, D.C.: Author.

Cohen-Ross, D., & Hill, I. T. (2003). Enrolling eligible children and keeping them enrolled. *Future of Children, 13,* 81–97.

Davidhizar, R., Havens, R., & Bechtel, G. A. (1999). Assessing culturally diverse pediatric clients. *Pediatric Nursing, 25*(4).

Degazon, C. (1996). Cultural diversity and community health nursing practice. In M. Stanhope & J. Lancaster (Eds.), *Community health nursing: Promoting health of aggregates, families and individuals* (pp. 117–134). St. Louis: Mosby Year-Book.

DiLauro, M. D. (2004). Psychosocial factors associated with types of child maltreatment. *Child Welfare, 53,* 69–96.

Duvall, E. (1977). *Marriage and family development* (5th ed.). Philadelphia: J. B. Lippincott.

Elias, E. R., Tsai, A.C., & Manchester, D. K. (2007). Genetics and dysmorphology. In W. W. Hay, M. J. Levin, J. M. Sondheimer, & R. R. Deterding (Eds.), *Current pediatric diagnosis and treatment* (18th ed.). New York: McGraw-Hill.

Friedman, M. M. (1998), *Family nursing: Theory and practice* (4th ed.). Stanford, CT: Appleton & Lange.

Giger, J., & Davidhizar, R. (1995). *Transcultural nursing: Assessment and intervention.* St. Louis: Mosby Year-Book.

Hager, M. (Ed.). (2004). *The future of pediatric education in the 21st century: Proceedings of the conferences chaired by Barry Zuckerman, M.D.* New York: Josiah Macy, Jr. Foundation.

Hernandez, D. J. (2004). Demographic change and the life circumstances of immigrant families. *The Future of Children, 14*(2), 17–47.

Institute of Medicine, Board on Health Care Services. (2002). *Health insurance is a family matter.* Washington, D.C.: The National Academic Press.

Looman, W. S., & Lindeke, L. L. (2005). Health and social context: Social capital's utility as a construct for nursing and health promotion. *Pediatric Health Care, 19*(2), 90–94.

Marcin, J. P., Schembri, M. S., Jingsong, H. E., & Romano, P. S. (2003). A population-based analysis of socioeconomic status and insurance status and their relationship with pediatric trauma hospitalization and mortality rates. *American Journal of Public Health, 93*(3), 461–468.

Monsen, R. B. (2002). Children and the media. *Journal of Pediatric Nursing, 17*(4), 309–310.

National Archives and Records Administration. (2007). 2007 HHS poverty guidelines. *Federal Register, 72*(15), 3147–3148.

National Association for the Education of Homeless Children and Youth and the National Law Center on Homelessness & Poverty. (2004). *The 100 most frequently asked questions on the education rights of children and youth in homeless situations.* Retrieved May 7, 2007 from http://www.naehcy.org/dl/faq.pdf.

National Center for Family Homelessness (2004). *Homeless children: America's new outcasts.* Newton, MA: Author.

National Coalition for the Homeless (2006). *Who is homeless?* Washington, D.C.: Author.

National Mental Health Association (2006). *Children without homes.* Alexandria, VA: Author.

Parents Without Partners (2005). *Mission statement.* Accessed 9/21/06. Available at: http://parentswithoutpartners.org/about.htm.

Patterson, J. (1995). Promoting resilience in families experiencing stress. *Pediatric Clinics of North America, 42*(1), 47–63.

Patterson, J. (2002). Integrating family resilience and family stress theory. *Journal of Marriage and Family, 64*(2), 349–360.

Pillitteri, A. (2007). *Maternal and child health nursing* (5th ed.). Philadelphia: Lippincott Williams & Wilkins.

Putnam, R. D., & Feldstein, L. M. (2003). *Better together: Restoring the American community.* New York: Simon & Schuster.

Regalado, M., Sareen, H., Inkelas, M., Wissow, L. S., & Halfon, N. (2004). Parents' discipline of young children: Results from the National Survey of Early Childhood Health. *Pediatrics, 113*(6.S1), 1952–1958.

Rennison, C. M., & Welchans, S. (2000). *Intimate partner violence, Bureau of Justice Statistics Special Report.* Washington, D.C.: U.S. Department of Justice.

Reynolds, M. A., et al. (2003). Trends in multiple births conceived using assisted reproductive technology, U.S., 1997–2000. *Pediatrics, 111,* 1159.

Search Institute. (2007). *What are developmental assets?* Available at http://www.search-institute.org/assets/.

Snyder, H., & Sickmund, M. (1999). *Juvenile offenders and victims: 1999 national report.* Washington, D.C.: Office of Juvenile Justice and Delinquency Prevention. U.S. Department of Justice.

Spector, R. E. (2000). *Cultural diversity in health and illness* (5th ed.). Upper Saddle River, NJ: Prentice Hall.

Strasburger, V. C., & Donnerstein, E. (1999). Children, adolescents, and the media: Issues and solution. *Pediatrics, 103*(1), 129–139.

Tanner, J. L. (2002). Parental separation and divorce: Can we provide an ounce of prevention? *Pediatrics, 110*(5), 1007–1009.

Taylor, C., Lillis, C., & LeMone, P. (2005). *Fundamentals of nursing* (5th ed.). Philadelphia: Lippincott Williams & Wilkins.

U.S. Census Bureau (2004). *Living arrangements of children under 18 years old: 1960 to present.* Washington, D.C.: Author.

United States Census Bureau. (2005). United States general demographic characteristics: 2005. Retrieved May 7, 2007 from http://factfinder.census.gov/servlet/ADPTable?_bm=y&-geo_id=01000US&-ds_name=ACS_2005_EST_G00_&-_lang=en&_caller=geoselect&-format=.

United States Census Bureau. (2006a). *Income, poverty, and health insurance coverage in the United States: 2005.* Washington, D.C.: Author.

United States Census Bureau (2006b). *Nation's population one third minority.* Washington, D.C.: Author.

United States Census Bureau (2007). *American fact finder.* Retrieved March 22, 2007 from http://finder.census.gov/home/en/epss/glossary_f.html.

Ventres, W., & Gobbo, R. (2005). The A to Z of cross-cultural medicine. *Family Practice Management, 12*(7), 57–58.

Von Bertalanffy, L. (1968). *General systems theory.* London: Penguin Press.

World Health Organization (2004). *Child health in the community.* Geneva, Switzerland: Department of Child and Adolescent Health and Development.

Worley, C., Worley, K., & Kumar, L. (2000). Infectious disease challenges in immigrants from tropical countries. *Pediatrics, 106*(1), e3.

Websites

raisingresilientkids.com Raising Resilient Children Foundation
www.aap.org American Academy of Pediatrics
www.cdc.gov/ncipc Centers for Disease Control, National Center for Injury Prevention and Control
www.childrensdefense.org Children's Defense Fund
www.endabuse.org Family Violence Prevention Fund
www.nationalhomeless.org National Coalition for the Homeless
www.ncadv.org National Coalition Against Domestic Violence
www.nimh.nih.gov National Institute of Mental Health
www.nsc.org National Safety Council
www.unicef.org UNICEF
www.usdoj.gov Office of Juvenile Justice and Delinquency Prevention
www.who.int/child-adolescent-health World Health Organization (WHO)

Chapter WORKSHEET

● MULTIPLE CHOICE QUESTIONS

1. The parents of two school-age children state that they expect their children to adhere to their rules without question and that they make all the decisions. Which type of parenting style does this reflect?

   a. Authoritarian

   b. Democratic

   c. Authoritative

   d. Permissive

2. A single mother asks the nurse for suggestions on disciplining her 2-year-old son. Which suggestion would be most appropriate?

   a. Encourage the mother to emphasize the inappropriate behavior.

   b. Wait an hour or so before enforcing the discipline.

   c. Have the child spend 2 minutes in time-out.

   d. Withhold a privilege from the toddler for a week.

3. The nurse is teaching a group of students about the possible effects of immigration on the health status of children. Which response by the group would indicate the need for additional teaching?

   a. The children of immigrants have better access to preventive care.

   b. The children of immigrants have limited involvement in activities due to the language barrier.

   c. The children of immigrants lack adequate support systems.

   d. The children of immigrants face increased stressors due to relocation.

4. Which would the nurse identify as a protective factor for youth violence?

   a. Exposure to family violence

   b. Limited involvement in social activities

   c. Inconsistency of parental support

   d. Commitment to academic performance

● CRITICAL THINKING EXERCISES

1. A couple has adopted an 11-month-old infant girl from China and have brought her to the health care facility for a check-up. The couple had no contact with the infant's birth parents. The infant spent 7 months in an orphanage before being adopted. Describe the issues that may affect this family.

2. Vanessa Walters brings her 3-year-old son, Tyler, for a well-child visit. Vanessa states, "Tyler is a handful. He always seems to be misbehaving. I just don't know what to do." How should the nurse respond, and what suggestions might be helpful?

3. You've been asked by the local school district to speak to a group of middle school students about Internet safety. Describe the topics that you should address.

● STUDY ACTIVITIES

1. Discuss with fellow students the different types of family structures. Include information about your own family structure. Compare and contrast the roles assumed by each member in the different structures.

2. Create a culture diary or journal for use in clinical practice. Record observations made while caring for children and families of other cultures or ethnicities. Address the preferences that the children and families had relating to food, health care, decision making for the family, view of children, and general health practices.

3. Perform a "spiritual inventory" on yourself. Identify your beliefs about higher authority, life after death, purpose in life, and the value of others who have different beliefs.

4. Search the Internet for sites giving information about violence and its impact on children's health.

5. The nurse is preparing a class for a group of students about homeless children and families. Which of the following factors contribute to homelessness? Select all that apply.

   _____ a. Increase in family income

   _____ b. Job loss

   _____ c. Exposure to abuse or neglect

   _____ d. Cutbacks in public welfare programs

   _____ e. Development of community crisis centers

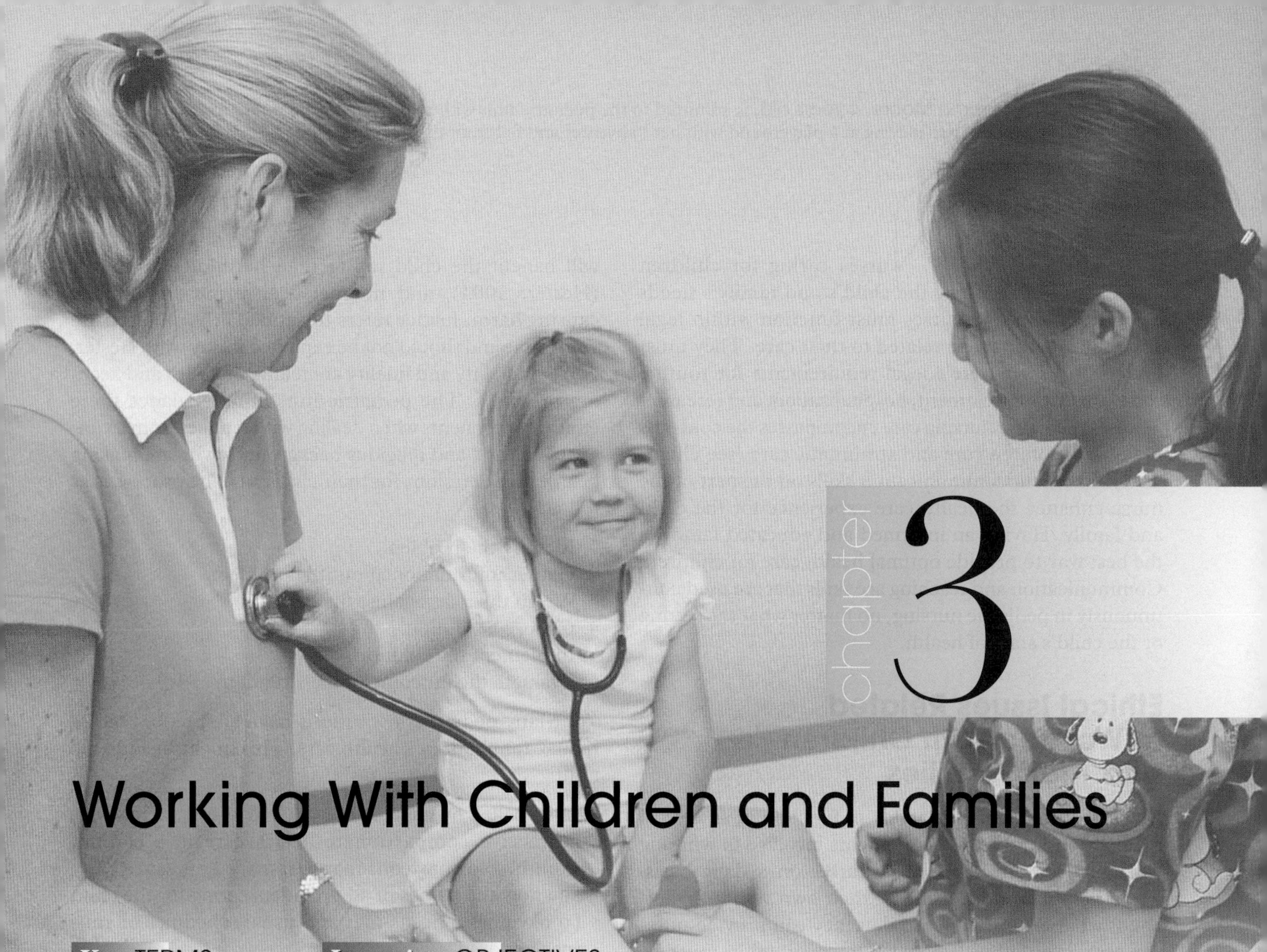

chapter 3

Working With Children and Families

Key TERMS

assent
"do not resuscitate" (DNR) order
emancipated minor
informed consent
mature minor
minor
nonverbal communication
verbal communication

Learning OBJECTIVES

Upon completion of the chapter, the learner will be able to:

1. Identify ethical concepts related to providing nursing care to children and their families.
2. Describe legal issues related to caring for children and their families.
3. Demonstrate the ability to use excellent therapeutic communication skills when interacting with children and their families.
4. Use culturally competent communication when working with children and their families.
5. Describe the process of health teaching as it relates to children and their families.

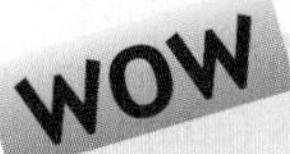

Children need to be seen for who they really are.

Emma Moore, 4 years old, is admitted to the pediatric unit with a suspected head injury from a fall. She was playing at a playground with her babysitter and fell from the top of the slide.

Nurses caring for children and their families make the child's and family's needs a priority. Pediatric nurses must function within legal and ethical boundaries related to their care. They must understand their state's legal requirements for routine care, consent for treatment, hospitalization, and research. The best pediatric nursing care encompasses the concepts of family-centered care and atraumatic care (see Chapter 1). Excellent communication skills on the part of the nurse enhance the health care experience for the child and family. Having an informed and educated family is the best way to provide optimal health care for children. Communication and teaching are skills that are used continuously in pediatric nursing, no matter what the setting or the child's state of health.

Ethical Issues Related to Working With Children and Their Families

Moral development (the ability to function in an ethical manner) and the legal requirements involved in working with children affect pediatric nurses on a daily basis. Pediatric nurses must examine their own values (beliefs about what is important) so that they can provide nursing care in an ethical manner. Each situation must be evaluated individually. The nurse's relationship with the child and family is of prime importance. Every day pediatric nurses are faced with families from a wide variety of religious, cultural, and ethnic backgrounds, and it is critical to treat each family with respect. Family-centered care focuses on the needs of the child and family together and involves ethical treatment of the child. Advances in science and technology have led to an increased number of ethical dilemmas in health care. The parents may refuse treatment for the child, or the child's desires may conflict with the parents' decision, resulting in a powerful ethical dilemma (Linnard-Palmer & Kools, 2004).

Practicing ethically begins with being sensitive to the sanctity and quality of human life. An ethical nurse is accountable and uses sound reasoning to resolve ethical challenges. Ethics includes the basic principles of autonomy, beneficence, nonmaleficence, justice, and veracity. Autonomy refers to self-determination in regard to making health care decisions. Generally, parents have the autonomy to make health care decisions for their child. In certain situations, however, older children have the autonomy to give assent to care (see below), and in special situations, adolescents are granted the autonomy to consent to health care procedures without the parents' knowledge. Beneficence refers to acts of kindness that will benefit the child rather than harming him or her (Hester, 2004), and nonmaleficence means avoiding causing harm. Justice refers to acting fairly; children are vulnerable and should not be exploited in any way (Hester, 2004). Veracity and fidelity are telling the truth and keeping promises. The pediatric nurse must balance these ethical components when dealing with families from a variety of cultural and religious backgrounds who are making health care decisions for their children. The process is as follows:

1. Identify the problem.
2. Gather information about the problem.
3. Weigh the risks against the benefits.
4. Choose a solution.
5. Implement the solution.
6. Evaluate the outcome of the situation.

Many pediatric institutions have adopted a "bill of rights" for children's health care. This might include the right:

- To be called by name
- To receive compassionate health care in a careful, prompt, and courteous manner
- To know the names of all providers caring for the child
- To have basic needs met and usual schedules or routines honored
- To be kept without food or drink when necessary for the shortest time possible
- To be unrestrained if able
- To have parents or other important persons with the child
- To have an interpreter for the child and family when needed
- To object noisily if desired
- To be educated honestly about the child's health care
- To be respected as a person (not having people talk about the child within earshot unless the child knows what is happening)
- For all health care providers to respect the child's confidentiality about his or her illness at all times (adapted from University Children's Hospital, University of California–Irvine, 2006)

Legal Issues Related to Caring for Children

Minors (children less than 18 years of age) generally require adult guardians to act on their behalf. Biological or adoptive parents are usually considered to be the child's legal guardian. When divorce occurs, one or both parents may be granted custody of the child. In certain cases (such as child abuse or neglect, or during foster care), a guardian *ad litem* may be appointed by the courts. This person generally serves to protect the child's best interests (American Bar Association, n.d.). States generally require parental or guardian consent for minors to receive medical treatment, but some exceptions exist (refer to the section on consent below). Confidentiality of patient information should always be maintained within the context of the state law and the institution's policies.

Advance Directives

The Patient Self-Determination Act of 1990 established the concept of advance directives. Advance directives determine the child's and family's wishes should life-sustaining care become necessary. Parents are generally the surrogate decision-makers for children. If the child's interests are not served by prolonged survival, then the physician or advanced practitioner should educate the parents about the extent of the child's illness and potential for ongoing quality of life (Fost, 2006). After discussion with other family members, friends, and spiritual advisors, the parents may make the decision to forego life-sustaining medical treatment, either withdrawing treatment or deciding to withhold certain further treatment or opt not to resuscitate in the event of cardiopulmonary arrest (American Academy of Pediatrics, 1994).

Life-sustaining care may include dialysis, ventilation, cardiopulmonary resuscitation, and artificial nutrition and hydration (Grindel, 2005). Some families may choose to withdraw these treatments if they are already in place or not begin them should the need arise. **"Do not resuscitate (DNR)" orders** are in place for some children, particularly the terminally ill. Some institutions have started using the term AND (Allow Natural Death). No matter what term is used, these orders should include specific instructions regarding the child's and family's wishes (e.g., some families may desire oxygen but not chest compressions or code medications). When the child is hospitalized, the DNR order must be documented in the physician orders and updated according to the facility's policy. DNR orders may also be in place in the home, but only a few states allow emergency medical services to honor a child's DNR order in the home. Children with DNR orders may also still be attending school. In that case, the health care professionals involved should meet with the school officials (the board of education and its legal counsel) to discuss how the DNR request can be upheld in the school setting (American Academy of Pediatrics, 2000).

The U.S. Department of Health and Human Services has published laws related to protecting the welfare of children ("Baby Doe" law). Parents ultimately are the decision-makers for their children. In a situation such as a baby born with brain damage or delivery at an extremely early gestation, parents must be accurately informed about the risks and benefits of treatment before consenting to treatment or deciding to withdraw or forego treatment (Hurst, 2006). Some professionals are recommending the use of prenatal advance directives that would guide care from the time of birth of an extremely premature infant or an otherwise impaired term infant (Catlin, 2005).

The nurse must be knowledgeable about the laws related to health care of children in the state where he or she practices as well as the policies of the health care institution. The nurse must be sensitive to the various ethical situations that he or she may become involved in and should apply knowledge of laws as well as concepts of ethics to provide appropriate care.

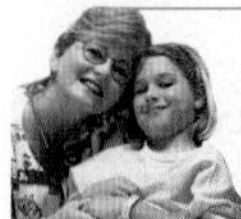

Never assume that the parent accompanying the child is the parent or legal guardian. Always clarify the relationship of the accompanying adult.

Consent

Generally, only persons over the age of majority (18 years of age) can legally provide consent for health care. Since children are minors, the process of consent involves obtaining written permission from a parent or legal guardian. In cases requiring a signature for consent, usually the parent gives consent for care for children less than 18 years of age except in certain situations (see below).

Most care given in a health care setting is covered by the initial consent for treatment signed when the child becomes a patient at that office or clinic or by the consent to treatment signed upon admission to the hospital or other inpatient facility. Certain procedures, however, require a specific process of **informed consent**. Procedures that require informed consent include major and minor surgery; invasive procedures such as lumbar puncture or bone marrow aspiration; treatments placing the child at higher risk, such as chemotherapy or radiation therapy; procedures or treatments involving research; and photography involving children. Applying restraints to children now requires consent.

Informed consent involves disclosure, comprehension, competency, and voluntariness (Taylor et al., 2005). Nurses should involve older children and adolescents in the decision-making process to the extent possible, though the parent is still ultimately responsible for giving consent. Box 3.1 describes the key elements of informed consent, although laws vary from state to state. Nurses must become familiar with state laws as well as the policies and procedures of the health care agency. Treating children without obtaining proper consent may result in charges of assault, and the health care provider and/or facility may be held liable for any damages.

The informed consent process, which must be done before the procedure or specific care, addresses the legal and ethical requirement of informing the child and parent

BOX 3.1
KEY ELEMENTS OF INFORMED CONSENT

- The decision-maker must be of legal age in that state, with full civil rights, and be competent (have the ability to make the decision).
- Present information that is simple, concise, and appropriate to the level of education and language of the individual responsible for making the decision.
- The decision must be voluntary, without coercion, force, or under the influence of duress.
- Have a witness to the process of informed consent.
- Have the witness sign the consent form.

about the procedure. The physician or advanced practitioner is responsible for informing the child and family about the procedure and obtaining consent by providing a detailed description of the procedure or treatment, the potential risks and benefits, and alternative methods available. The nurse's responsibility related to informed consent includes the following:

- Ensuring that the consent form is completed with signatures from the parents or legal guardians
- Serving as a witness to the signature process
- Determining that the parents or legal guardians understand what they are signing by asking them pertinent questions

Special Situations Related to Informed Consent

If the parent is not available, then the person in charge (relative, babysitter, or teacher) may give consent for emergency treatment if that person has a signed form from the parent or legal guardian allowing him or her to do so. During an emergency situation, a verbal consent via the telephone may be obtained. Two witnesses must also be listening simultaneously and will sign the consent form, indicating that consent was received via telephone. Health care providers can provide emergency treatment to a child without consent if they have made reasonable attempts to contact the child's parent or legal guardian (American Academy of Pediatrics, 2003). Table 3.1 gives information about other special situations.

Parental Refusal of Medical Treatment

Parental autonomy (the right to decide for or against medical treatment) is a constitutionally protected right (Linnard-Palmer & Kools, 2004). Ideally, medical care without informed consent should be given only when the child's life is in danger. Parents may refuse treatment when it conflicts with their religious or cultural beliefs,

Table 3.1 Special Considerations Related to Informed Consent

Issue	Definition Average and Good Readers	Nursing Considerations
Child not living with biological or adoptive parents	Child living: • In foster care • With potential adoptive parent • With a relative	Legally appointed guardian must provide consent. Verify authority of legally appointed guardian. Include documentation of who the legal guardian is in the child's medical record (Berger, 2003).
Parent consent after divorce	Ability to give consent for health care rests with parent who has legal custody by divorce degree.	Determine if the parents have joint custody or if there is sole custody by one parent. Even the parent with only physical custody may give consent for emergency care. May need to seek court involvement if there is joint legal custody but parents disagree on care.
Consent for organ donation	For a minor to donate, the parents must be aware of the risks and benefits and must provide emotional support to the child, and there should be a close relationship between the donor and recipient, if living-related donation is occurring.	Potential donors should be referred to local organ procurement organization. Educate family about policies related to organ donation. Legal guardian or parent consents to organ donation (American Academy of Pediatrics, 2002).
Consent for medical experimentation	Requirements include consent of parents, assent of child, and a perceived benefit to the child.	Comply with all federal regulations if federal funds are received. Refer to section on assent.

and the nurse should be aware of some of these common beliefs. Some religions, such as Jehovah's Witnesses, Christian Science, Pentecostal, Faith Assembly, and Evangelical Healers, prefer prayer or faith healing over allopathic medicine (Linnard-Palmer & Kools, 2004). Jehovah's Witnesses refuse blood product administration based on their religious beliefs. The Black Muslim culture advocates vegan diets and refuses pork-based medicines or treatments. Hindus may refuse beef-based foods and medicines. Persons from an Islamic background may refuse the use of any potentially addictive substances such as narcotics or medicines containing alcohol (Linnard-Palmer & Kools, 2004). Sometimes common ground may be reached between the family's religious or cultural beliefs and the health care team's recommendations; communication and education are the keys in this situation.

The health care team must appropriately educate the family and communicate with them on a level that they can understand. The child and family should be informed of what to expect with certain tests or treatments. The health care team should make a clinical assessment of the child's and family's understanding of the situation and note whether there is undue pressure to comply with treatment (Turkoski, 2005). Refusal of medical care may be considered a form of child neglect (Linnard-Palmer & Kools, 2004). If providing medical treatment may save a child's life, health care providers and the judicial system strive to advocate for the child. The state has an overriding interest in the health and welfare of the child and can order that medical treatment proceed without signed informed consent; this is referred to as *parens patriae* (the state has a right and a duty to protect children). In other cases, parents may refuse treatment if they perceive that their child's quality of life may be significantly impaired by the medical care that is offered.

If the parents refuse treatment and the health care team feels the treatment is reasonable and warranted, the case should be referred to the institution's ethics committee. If the issue remains unresolved, then the judicial system becomes involved (Kon, 2006).

Exceptions to Parental Consent Requirement

In some states, a **mature minor** may give consent to certain medical treatment. The health care provider must determine that the adolescent (usually over 14 years of age) is sufficiently mature and intelligent to make the decision for treatment. The provider also considers the complexity of the treatment, its risks and benefits, and whether the treatment is necessary or elective before obtaining consent from a mature minor (American Academy of Pediatrics, 2003).

State laws vary in relation to the definition of an **emancipated minor** and the types of treatment that may be obtained by an emancipated minor (without parental consent). The nurse must be familiar with the particular state's law. Emancipation may be considered in any of the following situations, depending on the state's laws:

- Membership in a branch of the armed services
- Marriage
- Court-determined emancipation
- Financial independence and living apart from parents
- College attendance
- Pregnancy
- Mother less than 18 years of age
- Runaway

The emancipated minor is considered to have the legal capacity of an adult and may make his or her own health care decisions (American Academy of Pediatrics, 2003).

Many states do not require consent or notification of parents or legal guardians when providing specific care to minors. Depending on the state law, health care may be provided to minors for certain conditions, in a confidential manner, without including the parents. These types of care may include pregnancy counseling, prenatal care, contraception, testing for and treatment of sexually transmitted infections and communicable diseases (including HIV), substance abuse and mental illness counseling and treatment, or health care required as a result of a crime-related injury (American Academy of Pediatrics, 2003). These exceptions allow children to seek help in a confidential manner; they might otherwise avoid care if they were required to inform their parents or legal guardian. Again, laws vary by state, so the nurse must be knowledgeable about the laws in the state where he or she is licensed to practice.

There are exceptions to confidential treatment and obtaining consent in children. For example, all states require reporting of suspicion of physical or sexual child abuse and injuries caused by a weapon or criminal act. Abuse cases are reported to the child welfare authorities, criminal acts to the police. The health care provider must also follow public health laws that require reporting certain infectious diseases to the local health department (e.g., tuberculosis, hepatitis, HIV, and other sexually transmitted infections). Finally, there is a duty to warn third parties when a specific threat is made to an identifiable person. Health care providers must strike a balance between confidentiality and required disclosure. If health care information must be disclosed by law, the child or adolescent must be so informed (Feldman-Winter & McAbee, 2002).

Assent

Assent means agreeing to something. In pediatric health care, the term **assent** refers to the child's participation in the decision-making process about health care (McCullough & Stein, 2006). The age of assent depends on the child's developmental level and maturity, though the American Academy of Pediatrics (1995) recommends the age of 7 years (Broome & Richards, 2003). Certainly, the older the child is, the stronger the ethical obligation is to include him or her in the decision-making process (Olechnowicz et al., 2002). The Society of Pediatric Nurses (2006) makes the following recommendations related to research-related assent according to the child's age:

- Child 4 to 6 years of age: Use developmentally appropriate materials to inform the child about the research or treatment.
- Child 7 to 12 years of age: Obtain assent for nontherapeutic research.
- Adolescent 13 to 17 years of age: Obtain assent for therapeutic and nontherapeutic research.

The American Academy of Pediatrics recommends that if a health care provider asks the child's opinion about the direction of treatment or participation in research, then the child's view and desires should be seriously considered.

When obtaining assent, first help the child to understand his or her health condition, depending on the child's developmental level. Next, inform the child of the treatment planned. Then determine what the child understands about the situation and make sure he or she is not being unduly influenced to make a decision one way or another. Lastly, ascertain the child's willingness to participate in the treatment or research (American Academy of Pediatrics, 1995; McCullough & Stein, 2006). Assent should be a process that continues throughout treatment or a research protocol (Miller, 2000).

The converse of assent, dissent (disagreeing with the treatment plan), when given by an adolescent 13 to 17 years of age is considered binding in some states. The Society of Pediatric Nurses (2006) recommends that dissent in the 7- to 12-year-old should also be considered binding. If the decision is made to move forward with treatment despite the child's dissent, then this decision must be explained to the child in developmentally appropriate terms. Research studies involving children must determine whether child assent is necessary, and at what age (Kimberly et al., 2006); researchers must also decide whether a child's objection to participation will be honored (Kon, 2006).

Communication

WATCH & LEARN

Effective communication with children and their parents is critical to quality nursing care. Child- and parent-centered communication increases family satisfaction with nursing care and leads to increased knowledge and health care behaviors on the part of the child and family (Sobo, 2004). Children are often socialized to be passive participants in health care, doing as they are told, with or without protests. "As pediatric nurses, we have an obligation to listen, to hear, and to feel the voices of the children in our care" (McPherson & Thorne, 2000). Children can inform nurses of their experiences in an accurate fashion, and nurses need to be able to discern this information from communication with the child.

Children may be more apt to communicate if they are engaged in another activity. They may use fewer words than adults and tend to rely more on nonverbal communication and silence (Curtin, 2001). Parents more often require neutral communication (i.e., verbal communication that is related to assessing and solving problems), whereas children more often desire affective communication (establishment of rapport and trust, giving comfort). The best communicators in pediatric nursing find a balance between neutral and affective communication (Shin & White-Traut, 2005). Communicating in the pediatric setting can be more difficult than in the adult setting. The pediatric nurse must communicate with different ages of children, as well as on a supportive level with adolescents and parents (Shin & White-Traut, 2005).

Verbal Communication

Communicating through the use of words, either written or spoken, is termed **verbal communication**. Nurses use verbal communication throughout the day when interacting with patients. Good verbal communication skills are necessary when doing nursing assessments and providing child/family teaching. General guidelines for appropriate verbal communication include:

- Use open-ended questions that do not restrict the child's or parent's answers.
- Redirect the conversation to maintain focus.
- Use reflection to clarify the parents' feelings.
- Paraphrase the child's or parent's feelings to demonstrate empathy.
- Acknowledge emotions.
- Demonstrate active listening by using the child's or family's own words.

Remember that most parents are laypersons, so avoid using medical jargon. The abbreviations and shortened terms that health care providers use almost without thinking may sound scary or foreign to children and parents. Avoid using labels; refer to the child by name rather than by a label such as "the boy in the wheelchair" (Fleitas, 2003).

Nonverbal

Nonverbal communication is also referred to as body language. It also includes attending to others and active listening. The nurse should listen to the other person's verbal communication from the beginning of the interaction. When children and parents feel they are being heard, trust and rapport are established. Guidelines for appropriate nonverbal communication include:

- Relax; maintain an open posture, with the arms uncrossed.
- Sit opposite the family and lean forward slightly.
- Maintain eye contact.

- Nod your head to demonstrate interest.
- Note the child's or parent's posture, eye contact, and facial expressions.

Children of all ages want to be listened to without interruption (Deering & Cody, 2002).

Active listening is critical to the communication process. Listening may uncover fears or concerns that the nurse may not have discovered through questioning. Paying attention while children and parents talk is a powerful communication tool. By not listening, the nurse may miss critical information and the family may be reluctant to share further. When interacting with the child and family, determine whether the messages sent by the child's or parent's verbal and nonverbal communication are congruent.

Developmental Techniques for Communicating With Children

Effective communication with children involves a variety of age-appropriate methods. Encouraging children to participate actively gives them some control over the interaction (Shin & White-Traut, 2005). If the child is shy, talk to the parents first to give the child time to "warm up" to you. Use specific and clear phrases in an unhurried, quiet, yet confident manner. Communicate at the child's eye level (Fig. 3.1). Spending time with younger children, even just a few moments, may help them feel more at ease with you (Donat-Bartfield & Passman, 2000). Instead of direct questioning, use dolls, puppets, or stuffed animals with younger children (Fig. 3.2). Metaphors (e.g., referring to white blood cells as "bad guy fighters") help to illustrate concepts to young and school-age children (Fleitas, 2003).

Older children need privacy. Provide the child or adolescent with honest answers at a developmentally appropriate level. Allow children to express their thoughts and feelings. Offer the child choices only when they truly exist (Mandleco, 2005). Box 3.2 lists requirements for communication with children and adolescents.

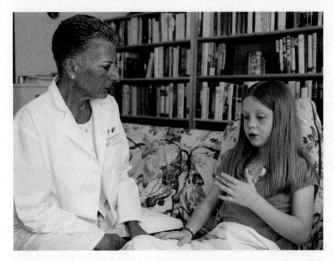

● Figure 3.1 Sitting at the child's level and allowing the child time for self-expression are steps that improve therapeutic communication.

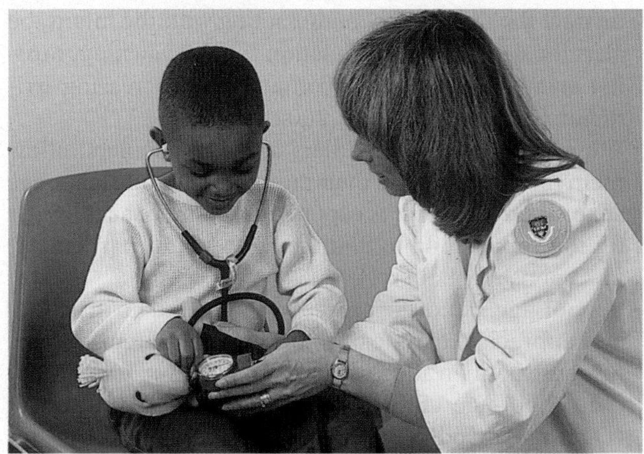

● Figure 3.2 Communication or teaching with dolls may be useful with younger children.

Children feel empowered when health care professionals communicate directly with them. Children may also desire advice about their health care and reassurance about their health status. To be effective when communicating with children of different developmental stages, the nurse must become familiar with how children of different ages communicate and then use age-appropriate techniques for effective communication:

- Infants primarily communicate through touch, sight, and hearing. Communication through play may be helpful in the older infant. Playful persuasion may help to

BOX 3.2

BASICS FOR COMMUNICATING WITH CHILDREN

- Introduce yourself and explain your role.
- Position yourself at the child's level.
- Allow the child to remain near the parent if needed, so the child can remain comfortable and relaxed.
- Smile and make eye contact with the child if culturally appropriate.
- Direct your questions and explanations to the child.
- Listen attentively and pause to allow time for the child to formulate his or her thoughts.
- Use the child's or family's terms for body parts and medical care when possible.
- Speak in a calm, quiet, confident, and unhurried voice.
- Use positive rather than negative statements and directions.
- Encourage the child to express his or her feelings and ask questions.
- Observe for nonverbal cues.
- Ask for permission if you need to approach the child to avoid appearing threatening.

distract the infant. When interacting with the infant, be alert for signs of overstimulation such as yawning, turning away, decreased eye contact, and increasing irritability (Deering & Cody, 2002).

- When working with toddlers and preschoolers, allow them time to complete their thoughts. Though language acquisition at this age is exponential, it often takes longer for the young child to find the right words, particularly in response to a query.
- School-age children are very interested in learning and appreciate simple but honest and straightforward responses. When addressed first and allowed to respond, the school-age child may be eager to communicate (Deering & Cody, 2002).
- Adolescents tend to experience extreme feelings and perceive situations in intense terms. Remain nonjudgmental when communicating with teenagers to avoid alienating them and to keep lines of communication open.

For communication tips related to the child's age, see Table 3.2.

Tips for Communicating With Parents

When communicating with parents, be honest. Parents want to feel valued and should be equal partners in the health care team. Allow the parent to express concerns and ask questions. Explain equipment and procedures thoroughly. Help the parents to understand the long-term as well as short-term effects of the treatment. Teach the parents what the child will feel like and how he or she will look during a procedure. Teach and encourage the parent to perform as much of the child's care as is reasonable and permitted. Ask the parent about his or her perception of the child's progress. Allowing the parents to be involved in the care of their child gives them a sense of control and lets them know they are valued by the health care team. When interacting with families, ask the parents how they are doing and provide positive reinforcement as well as reassurance (Mandleco, 2005).

Communicating Across Cultures

Understanding and respecting the patient's culture helps foster good communication and improves child and family education about health care. Culture, religion, and spirituality are intertwined concepts that affect the child's and family's communication styles, health status, and health beliefs. Nurses must be aware of the family's background, lifestyle, and health care practices to meet their information needs.

Learning about the practices of various cultures is just the beginning; the nurse must assess each family's individ-

Table 3.2 Communicating Effectively With Children

Age	Techniques
Infants	• Respond to crying in a timely fashion. • Allow the infant time to warm up to you. • Use a soothing and calming tone when speaking to the infant. • Talk to the baby directly.
Toddlers	• Approach toddlers carefully; they are often not only fearful but also quite resistant. • Use the toddler's preferred words for objects or actions so he or she is better able to understand. • Toddlers enjoy stories, dolls, and books. • Prepare toddlers for procedures just before they are about to occur.
Preschoolers	• Use play, puppets, or storytelling via a third-party approach. • Speak honestly. • Use simple, concrete terms. • Allow the child to have choices as appropriate. • Prepare preschoolers about 1 hour prior to a procedure.
School-age children	• Use diagrams, illustrations, books, and videos. • Allow the child to honestly express feelings. • Use third-party stories to elicit desired information. • Allow the child to ask questions related to care and treatment. Give the child adequate time for all of the questions to be answered. • Prepare the child a few days in advance for a procedure.
Adolescents	• Always respect the teenager's need for privacy. • Ensure confidentiality. • Use appropriate medical terminology, defining words as necessary. • Use creativity. • Prepare the teen up to 1 week prior to a procedure.

ual beliefs and practices rather than generalizing. The best way to assess the family's cultural practices is to ask and then listen. Determine the language spoken at home and observe the use of eye contact and other physical contact. Demonstrate a caring, nonjudgmental attitude and sensitivity to the child's and family's cultural diversity (McEvoy, 2003).

Working With an Interpreter

Attempting to communicate with a family who does not speak English can be one of the most frustrating situations in which health care providers find themselves. In this situation, interpreters are an invaluable aid and an essential component of patient and family education. Working with an interpreter, whether in person or over the phone, requires coordination of efforts so that both the family and the interpreter understand the information to be communicated. Working as a team, the nurse questions or informs and the interpreter conveys the information completely and accurately (see Healthy People 2010). Table 3.3 presents tips on working with an interpreter to maximize teaching efforts.

Many health care facilities subscribe to Language Line (http://www.languageline.com/), which offers telephone interpreters who speak 150 languages. Additional interpreter resources include:

- Interpreters and translators: American Translators Association (ATA)—www.atanet.org; Center for Applied Linguistics—www.cal.org; Northwest Translators and Interpreters Society—www.notis.net
- Online language resources: Spanish vocabulary—http://www.lingolex.com/spanish.htm; Spanish (pediatric surgery)—http://pedsurgerymex.org/; English-Chinese dictionary—http://www.okdaily.com/go/svc/ecdict.html

HEALTHY PEOPLE 2010

Objective	Significance
Increase the proportion of local health departments that have established culturally appropriate and linguistically competent community health promotion and disease prevention programs.	• Work with professionals and individuals from various cultures to develop materials and programs for health promotion that are culturally competent. • Ensure teaching materials are provided in the appropriate language.

Communicating With Deaf or Hearing-Impaired Children and Families

For hearing-impaired patients and families, determine the method of communication they use (e.g., lip reading, American Sign Language [ASL], or another method or

Table 3.3 Tips on Working With an Interpreter

- **Help the interpreter prepare and understand what needs to be done ahead of time.** A few minutes of preparation may save a lot of time and help communication flow more smoothly in the long run.
- **The interpreter is the "communication bridge," not the "content expert."** The nurse's presence at teaching sessions is vital.
- **The interpreter's timing may not match that of others involved.** It often takes longer to say in some languages what has already been said in English; therefore, plan for more time than you normally would.
- **Speak slowly and clearly.** Avoid jargon. Use short sentences and be concise. Avoid interrupting the interpreter.
- **Pause every few sentences so the interpreter can translate your information.** After 30 seconds of speaking, stop and let the interpreter express the information. Talk directly to the family, not the interpreter.
- **Give the family and the interpreter a break.** Sessions that last longer than 20 or 30 minutes are too long for anyone's attention span and concentration.
- **Express the information in two or three different ways if needed.** There may be cultural barriers as well as language and dialect differences that interfere with understanding. Interpreters may often know the correct communication protocols for the family.
- **Use an interpreter to help ensure the family can read and understand translated written materials.** The interpreter can also help answer questions and evaluate learning.
- **Avoid side conversations during sessions.** These can be uncomfortable for the family and jeopardize patient–provider relationships and trust.
- **Just because someone speaks another language doesn't mean that he or she will make a good interpreter.** An interpreter who has no medical background may not understand or interpret correctly, no matter how good his or her language skills are.
- **Children should not be used as interpreters.** Doing so can affect family relationships, proper understanding, and compliance with health care issues.

Adapted from Weech, W. A. (1999). *Tips for using interpreters.* Foreign Service Institute of the U.S. Department of State.

combination). If the nurse is not proficient in ASL and the child or family uses it, then an ASL interpreter must be available if another adult family member is not present for translation. According to federal law, deaf children and deaf family members must be provided with the ability to communicate effectively with health care providers (Sheehan, 2000).

> In the beginning of the chapter you were introduced to Emma Moore. Discuss ways to facilitate communication with Emma and her family/caregiver.

Atraumatic Care

The health care facility or hospital is an unfamiliar environment for children and parents and may upset or intimidate them. They may feel anxiety, fear, helplessness, anger, or loss of control. Even health care procedures performed in the home or school may be perceived as threatening to children. To minimize the stress experienced by children and their families in relation to health care, pediatric nurses, child life specialists, and other health care professionals recommend the use of atraumatic care. Atraumatic care is defined as therapeutic care that minimizes the psychological and physical distress experienced by children and their families in the health care system (Hockenberry, 2005; Wong, 1989, 2005). This concept is based on the underlying premise of "do no harm." Box 3.3 highlights the major principles of atraumatic care.

Atraumatic care involves guiding children and their families through the health care experience using a family-centered approach by promoting family roles, fostering family support of the child, and providing appropriate information. Help them cope with this experience by using age-appropriate and child-specific interventions. Preparation can help children and their families to adjust to illness and hospitalization. Use appropriate techniques for therapeutic communication (goal-directed, focused, purposeful communication), therapeutic play (type of play that provides an emotional outlet or improves the child's ability to cope with the stress of illness and hospitalization), and patient education to help the child and family understand the reason for the hospitalization and the necessary tests and procedures. In addition, help the family and other health care personnel to obtain the resources and relationships they need for optimal care.

The nurse's greatest ally in the hospital or pediatric specialty clinic in relation to atraumatic care is the child life specialist (CLS). The CLS focuses on the psychosocial care of the child and family (Cole et al., 2001). In addition to preparing children for procedures and providing support, the CLS provides therapeutic play and serves as an advocate for the child and family.

Table 3.4 gives suggestions for incorporating the principles of atraumatic care into nursing care for the child and family.

BOX 3.3

PRINCIPLES OF ATRAUMATIC CARE

- Prevent or minimize physical stressors, including pain, discomfort, immobility, sleep deprivation, inability to eat or drink, and changes in elimination.
  - Avoid or reduce intrusive and painful procedures, such as injections, multiple punctures, urethral catheterization.
  - Avoid or reduce other kinds of physical distress, such as noise, smells, shivering, restraints, skin trauma.
  - Control pain via frequent assessments and use of pharmacologic and nonpharmacologic interventions.
- Prevent or minimize parent–child separation.
  - Promote family-centered care, treating the family as the patient.
  - Use core primary nursing.
  - Consider research findings related to preferences of parents and children and whether or not to be together.
- Promote a sense of control.
  - Elicit the family's knowledge about the child and his or her health condition, promoting partnerships, empowerment, and enabling.
  - Reduce fear of the unknown through education, familiar articles, and decreasing the threat of the environment.
  - Provide opportunities for control, such as participating in care, attempting to normalize daily schedule, and providing direct suggestions.

From Wong, D. (2005). Wong on Web Paper "Beyond First Do No Harm: Principles of Atraumatic Care." Accessed 6/8/2006 from http://www.mosbydrugconsult.com/WOW/op022a.html.

> The physician's orders for Emma include starting intravenous fluids and obtaining blood work upon arrival to the unit. As the admitting nurse, how will you provide atraumatic care?

Teaching Children and Families

Regardless of the type of practice or health care setting, nurses are in a unique position to help families manage the health care needs of their child. Indeed, the family has a right and a responsibility to participate fully in making decisions about health care processes for their child. This is true whether the child is hospitalized with a long-term, devastating illness or needs only health maintenance activities. To accomplish this, families need to be knowledgeable about such things as their child's condition, the health care management plan, and when and how to contact health care providers. With the limited time available in all health care arenas, the pediatric nurse must focus on teaching goals and begin teaching at the earliest opportunity (London, 2004).

Table 3.4 Suggestions for Atraumatic Care

Principle	Suggestions for Nursing Care
Preventing or minimizing physical stressors	• For painful injections, use numbing techniques (see Chapter 14). • During painful or invasive procedures, avoid traditional restraint or "holding down" of the child. Use alternative positioning such as "therapeutic hugging." • If the above-mentioned positions are not an option, have the parent stand near the child's head to provide comfort. • Insert a saline lock if the child will require multiple doses of parenteral medications. • Advocate for minimal laboratory blood draws. • Minimize intramuscular or subcutaneous injections. • Provide appropriate pain management (refer to Chapter 15).
Preventing or minimizing child and family separation	• Promote family-centered care. • In the hospital, provide comfortable accommodations for the parent. • Allow the family the choice about whether to stay for an invasive procedure, and support them in their decision.
Promoting a sense of control	• Maintain child's home routine related to activities of daily living. • In the hospital, use primary nursing. • Encourage the child to have a security item present if desired. • Involve the child and family in planning care from the moment of the first encounter. • Empower the family and child by providing knowledge. • Allow the child and family choices when they are available. • Make the environment more inviting and less intimidating.

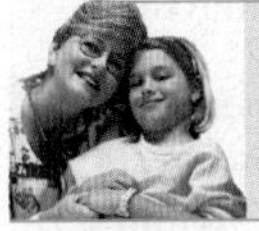

There is no prescription more valuable than knowledge.—C. Everett Koop MD, former Surgeon General of the United States

Patient education occurs when nurses share information, knowledge, and skills with families, thus empowering them to take responsibility for their child's health care. Through patient education, families can overcome feelings of powerlessness and helplessness and gain the confidence and ability to step to the forefront of the health care team. Nurses spend innumerable hours teaching children and families; some days in the hospital, more teaching than nursing care is provided. Given the importance of and the amount of time spent on patient and family education, each nurse should become expert at basic patient education principles. See Healthy People 2010.

Goals of Patient and Family Education

According to the Joint Commission on the Accreditation of Healthcare Organizations (JCAHO) standards, the goal of patient and family education is to:

- Promote interactive communication with providers
- Improve understanding of health status and health care options
- Encourage decision-making about care
- Improve compliance with the plan of care
- Reduce anxiety
- Return a sense of autonomy and control
- Promote healthy lifestyles

Done well, patient education helps to support recovery from illness, enhance return to function, and facilitate patient and family involvement with care and care decisions (JCAHO, 1998–2004). Overall goals for the child and family include allowing families to make informed

HEALTHY PEOPLE 2010

Objective	Significance
Increase the proportion of persons appropriately counseled about health behaviors. (Developmental) Increase the proportion of health care organizations that provide patient and family education; increase the proportion of patients who report that they are satisfied with the patient education they receive from their health care organization.	• Assess health learning needs of children and their families. • Plan health care education in collaboration with children and their families. • Provide health education at each patient encounter.

decisions, ensuring that basic health care skills are present, recognizing when the child has a problem, knowing how to respond to the problem, and having questions answered (London, 2004).

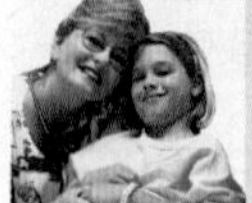

To cope effectively with illness, to understand and participate in decisions about treatment plans, and to maintain and improve health after treatment, patients and their families must have access to the specific knowledge and skills relevant to their conditions (JCAHO, 1996).

Steps of Child and Family Education

The steps of patient and family education are similar to the steps of the nursing process: the nurse must assess, plan, implement, evaluate, and finally document education. Once the nurse reaches a level of comfort and experience with each of these steps, they all blend together into one harmonious whole that becomes an everyday part of nursing practice. Patient education begins with the first patient encounter and proceeds through discharge and beyond. Reassessment after each step or change in the process is critical to success.

Assessing Teaching and Learning Needs

Excellent nursing care begins with a thorough assessment of the patient. In the same way, patient education begins with a learning needs assessment that includes the child's and family's learning needs, learning styles, and potential barriers to learning. Based on the results of the assessment, an individualized plan can be developed to reduce the time and effort required for teaching while maximizing learning for the child and family. Although actual nursing care in pediatrics is given to the child, the educational process is targeted at both the child, when developmentally appropriate, and the adult members of the family. Therefore, it is advisable to conduct a learning needs assessment on both the adult caregivers and the child, when appropriate. Box 3.4 describes the components of a learning needs assessment. This is also a good time to establish rapport with the family, demonstrating your interest in them and your confidence in their ability to learn.

BOX 3.4

COMPONENTS OF LEARNING NEEDS ASSESSMENT

- The child and family's learning needs, including what they want and need to know and what they know already
- Preferred learning style
- Language
- Physical or cognitive limitations and ability to read
- Motivation to learn and emotional concerns
- Social, cultural, and spiritual values

The assessment should be shared with all members of the interdisciplinary team so that the entire team can support the child's and family's learning. Although assessment generally takes place during the first or second meeting with the child and family, it should also occur with each encounter to check for any changes that may occur.

Malcolm Knowles (1990) outlined basic principles to consider when teaching adults. He found that instruction for adults needs to focus more on the process than on the content. Box 3.5 lists four learner-centered principles.

Cultural Impact on Assessment of Learning Needs

In addition to determining the language spoken in the home and use of eye and physical contact, investigate the following during the assessment:

- Who is the person caring for the patient at home?
- Who is the authority figure in the family?
- What is the social support structure?
- Are there any special dietary needs and concerns?
- Are any traditional health practices used (e.g., healers, shamans, talismans, folk remedies and herbs)?

BOX 3.5

SPECIFIC LEARNING PRINCIPLES RELATED TO PARENTS

- **Adults are self-directed.** Adults value independence and want to learn on their own terms. Teaching strategies that include such concepts as role playing, demonstration, and self-evaluation are most helpful. Using this model, nurses can partner with families to ensure that education is interactive and adopt the role of facilitator rather than lecturer.
- **Adults are problem-focused and task-oriented.** Adults learn best when they perceive there is a gap in their knowledge base and want information and skills to fill the gap. Providing a reason to learn can often motivate families that appear slow to comply with their child's care and education.
- **Adults want an immediate need satisfied.** Adults learn best at a time when learning meets an immediate need. Presenting information in an organized, sequential, and timely fashion can often help families understand the importance of learning a particular piece of information or task.
- **Adults value past experiences and beliefs.** Adults bring an accumulated wealth of experiences to each health care encounter; this provides a rich base for new learning. Education should take into account a wide range of backgrounds. Appreciating and using individual differences during teaching encounters can help improve compliance and reduce resistance to educational goals.

Knowles, M. (1990). *The adult learner: A neglected species* (4th ed.). Houston, TX: Gulf Publishing.

- Are any special clothes or other items used to help maintain health?
- What religious beliefs, ceremonies, and spiritual practices are important?

Psychiatrist and anthropologist Arthur Kleinman notes that there is a difference between illness and disease. *Illness* is the personal experience that a sick person has of what is happening to him or her, while *disease* is the health care provider's understanding of the same problem. Kleinman developed a list of eight questions to ask to discover a patient and family's perspective of illness (Rankin & Stallings, 2001):

1. What do you call the problem?
2. What do you think has caused the problem?
3. Why do you think it started as it did?
4. What do you think the sickness does? How does it work?
5. How severe is the sickness? Will it have a short or a long course?
6. What kind of treatment do you think the patient should receive? What are the most important results you hope to receive from the treatment?
7. What are the chief problems the sickness has caused?
8. What do you fear most about the sickness?

Learning needs can then be negotiated with the family and met based on the assessment.

Pediatric issues encountered when teaching immigrant or refugee families might include confusion regarding the use of the English versus the metric scale; preparing formulas and medicines using a "handful" or "pinch" of ingredients rather than specific measurements such as a measuring cup or syringe; access to refrigeration for liquid antibiotics; and breastfeeding practices.

Literacy Issues

Health literacy is the ability to read, understand, and use health care information. The inability to read and comprehend health care information is an enormous problem for many Americans today. Low health literacy affects people of all ages, races, and educational and income levels. Even persons with adequate literacy skills may have difficulty reading and understanding health care information (Fig. 3.3).

Adequate literacy skills are essential for patient and family education, yet many people in America today have marginal reading capabilities. Below are some important facts to consider based on the 1992 National Adult Literacy Survey (Kirsch et al., 1993):

- The average adult in America reads at an eighth-grade level.
- Approximately 1 in 5 (20%) read and understand only information written below a fifth-grade level. This can lead to problems with reading the information on a medication label; reading a bus schedule in order to attend a clinic visit; or reading an appointment card from the physician's office.
- Approximately 1 in 20 (5%) are totally illiterate.
- For the English-speaking Medicaid population, the average reading level is fifth grade; for native Spanish-speaking persons, it is third grade. Immigrants to the United States may be illiterate in their native language (Weiss et al., 1994).

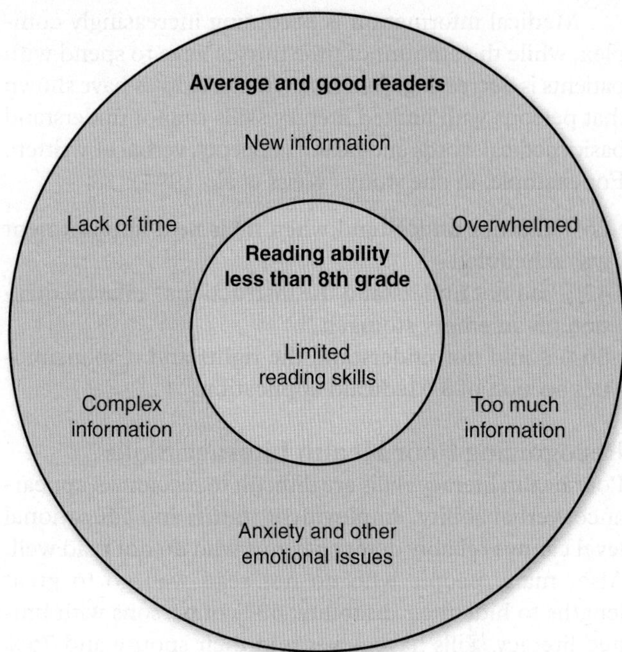

● Figure 3.3 Factors contributing to poor health literacy.

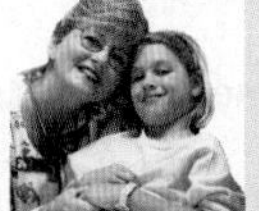

Studies have reported that literacy skills are a stronger predictor of health status than age, income, employment, education, or racial or ethnic group (Weiss, 2003).

Other health literacy studies have suggested that people with inadequate health literacy:

- Have health care needs four times higher than those with higher literacy skills (Weiss et al., 1994)
- Have a 50% higher risk of hospitalization compared to patients with adequate literacy skills (Baker et al., 1998)
- Lack the skills needed to navigate the health care system (Baker et al., 1996; Weiss et al., 1994)

When unfamiliar information is introduced or when emotional distress is present, reading ability and understanding are further reduced. The last grade completed in school does not equate with reading ability: poor readers often read three to five grade levels below the grade they completed. Coupled with the fact that most health care materials are written at a tenth-grade level, it is easy to understand why a disparity exists between health care teaching and patient understanding (Doak et al., 1995).

Medical information is becoming increasingly complex, while the amount of time nurses have to spend with patients is decreasing. As a result, many studies have shown that persons with limited literacy skills cannot understand basic medical words and health concepts, verbal or written. For example, in one study (Weiss et al., 1994):

- 26% did not understand when their next appointment was scheduled.
- 42% did not understand the instructions "take medication on an empty stomach."
- 86% could not understand the rights and responsibilities section of a Medicaid application.

Recognizing Poor Health Literacy Skills

Poor health literacy skills are difficult to recognize: appearance, verbal ability, employment status, and educational level cannot reliably detect persons who do not read well. Also, many people who do not read well go to great lengths to hide their disability; 68% of persons with limited literacy skills have never told their spouse and 75% have never told their health care provider (Weiss, 2003).

Red flags that might indicate poor literacy skills include the following:

- Difficulty filling out registration forms, questionnaires, and consent forms
- Frequently missed appointments
- Noncompliance and lack of follow-up with treatment regimens
- Responses such as, "I forgot my glasses" or "I'll read this when I get home"
- Inability to answer common questions about their treatment or medicines
- Avoiding asking questions for fear of looking "stupid"

Planning Education

Once the assessment is completed, plan mutually agreed-upon, achievable learning goals and objectives. It is important that both the teacher and learner believe the goals can be accomplished. Finding common ground and building a bridge between the child's and family's concerns and what the health care team believes they need to know is a critical part of an education plan. This also is an excellent time to consider which patient education materials and resources can be used to maximize learning and retention.

Planning patient education should involve input from the entire interdisciplinary team when appropriate. Through good communication and collaboration, team members can work together to empower the child and family to become knowledgeable and skillful caregivers. Leaving behind the traditional path of teacher-centered education and providing family-centered education instead requires thought and skill.

To achieve maximum success with education, nurses need to know how people learn. Edgar Dale (1969) suggested that people learn best when they are actively involved in the learning process. Figure 3.4 provides a

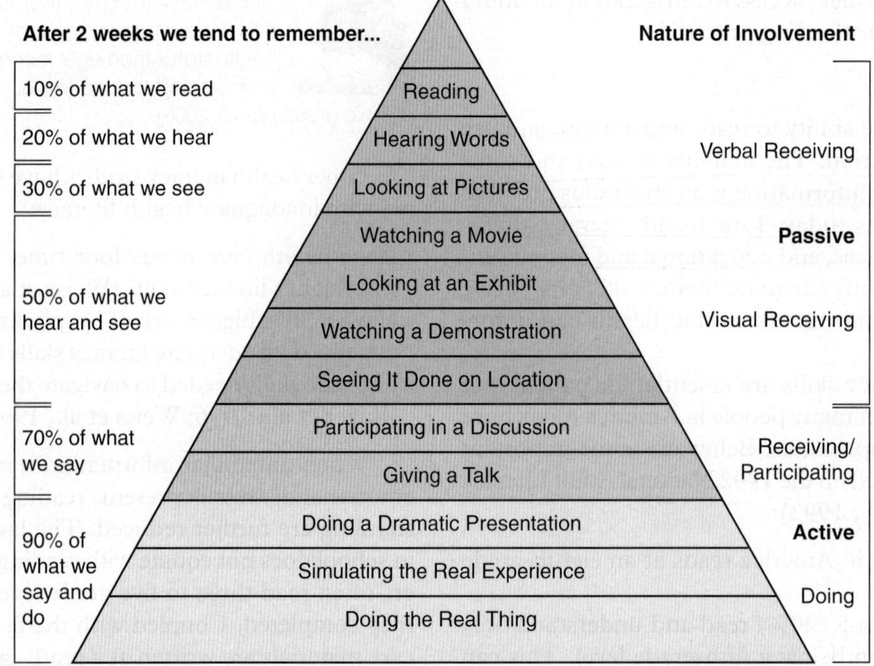

● **Figure 3.4** Cone of Learning. (Adapted from Dale, E. [1969]. *Audio-visual methods in teaching* [3rd ed.]. Austin, TX: Holt, Rinehart, and Winston.)

summary of his principles, known as the "Cone of Learning." The implications for patient education are clear: the more senses used and the more actively involved the learner is, the better he or she will remember what was taught.

Practical Interventions to Enhance Learning

The assessed needs and planned learning objectives lead to good teaching interventions. Evaluate these interventions frequently to ensure that the child and family are learning and meeting agreed-upon goals. Table 3.5 presents six techniques that can help improve learning.

Helping Patients and Families With Poor Health Literacy Skills

Nurses are in an excellent position to create a "blame-free" environment and offer help. It is entirely appropriate to say to the patient, "Many people have a problem reading and remembering the information on this teaching sheet (booklet, manual). Is this ever a problem for you?" For patients with low health literacy, the nurse can adjust oral communication techniques and written materials to assist with learning, and should communicate this need to the entire interdisciplinary health care team.

If literacy problems are known or suspected, the nurse can take several steps to enhance learning, such as:

- Draw pictures or use medical illustrations.
- Use videos.
- Color-code medications or the steps of a procedure.
- Record an audiotape.
- Repeat verbal information often and "chunk" it into small bites.
- Teach a "back-up" family member.

Teaching Children and Adolescents

Teaching children and adolescents is a vital part of pediatric nursing practice. Children and adolescents have a great need for information about their illness as they attempt to master their anxiety and restore feelings of competency, self-confidence, and hope. As with adults, they learn best when their input is valued and they are actively involved in the learning process. The age and developmental level of the child will determine the amount, format, and timing of the information given. Before

Table 3.5 Six Techniques to Improve Learning

Technique	Explanation
Slow down and repeat information often.	Since most of the education in a health care setting is done verbally, repeat important information at least four or five times.
Speak in conversational style using plain, nonmedical language.	When writing directions, write only several words, bullet points, or phrases. Use common, "living-room-type" language containing one or two syllables whenever possible.
"Chunk" information and teach it in small bites using logical steps.	This is especially important when there are large amounts of complex information for the family to learn. Teach for 10 to 15 minutes, give the learner a break, and return later to "chunk" again.
Prioritize information and teach "survival skills" first.	Due to time constraints and multiple demands on the part of staff, coupled with the rapid turn-around times of health care encounters for patients, there never seems to be enough time to teach. Nurses must provide the patient and family with the necessary information to meet their immediate needs. This may include information about: • The child's medical condition • Treatment information • Why the information is important • Possible problems, adverse effects, or concerns • What to do if problems arise • Who to contact for further help, information, or supplies
Use visuals, such as pictures, videos, and models.	Use visual resources to enhance and reinforce learning when available. Drawing simple pictures and charts or using alternative methods such as color-coding often allows learning to occur for families who are having difficulty grasping information or concepts.
Teach using an interactive, "hands-on" approach.	When the learner uses hands-on practice or participates in care, learning occurs more quickly and easily. Learning first on a doll or model can ease anxiety and bolster self-confidence before actually doing care or procedures on the child.

beginning to teach a child, it is important to establish rapport and lay the foundation for good communication. Refer to p. 53 for additional information related to communicating well with children and adolescents.

Teaching Preschool Children

When teaching young children, the nurse or family assumes part or all of the responsibility for what is learned, how it is learned, and when it is learned. Because they have vivid imaginations, young children often attempt to invent pieces of information, or they pick up bits and pieces of misinformation that can lead to false assumptions. Skillfully delivered and timed information can promote trust, calmness, and control in an otherwise apprehensive and uncooperative preschooler. Table 3.6 presents some general guidelines for teaching young children.

Teaching School-Age Children

Unless they are quite ill, school-age children usually want to participate in their care. They have a need to cooperate and achieve. When teaching, speak directly to them and include them in the education plan. Parents can often learn by observing the care being given to their child (Fig. 3.5). Table 3.7 provides some general guidelines to keep in mind when teaching school-age children.

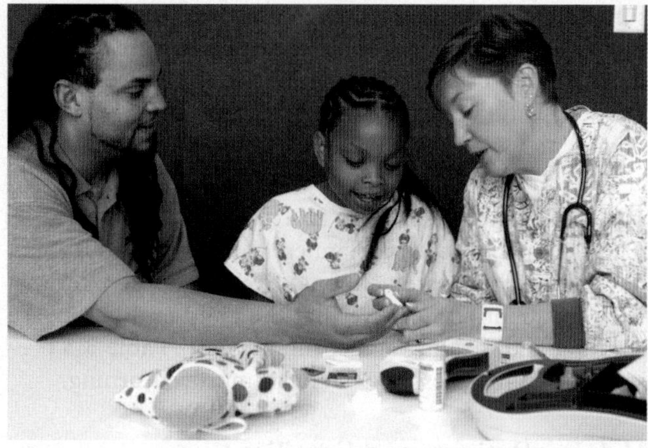

● Figure 3.5 Teach the school-age child and parent together.

Teaching Adolescents

Adolescents are particularly sensitive about maintaining body image and feelings of control and autonomy. This is especially important with health care processes and decisions that affect them. Table 3.8 gives guidelines to use when teaching adolescents.

Table 3.6 General Teaching Tips for Young Children

Teaching Tips	Practical Application
Offer simple, concise, concrete explanations based on the assessed needs, questions, and developmental level of the child.	Use a child's senses and relate what a procedure will look, sound, smell, taste, or feel like ("The MRI machine will sound very loud, like a big train").
Be honest, even when the information you need to convey is not positive. This helps the child to form a bond of trust and confidence with caregivers.	Use the family's words that the child understands; use "soft words" ("This will feel warm" instead of "This will burn").
Time explanations to decrease anxiety and excess worry before the event. Avoid telling unpleasant news close to bedtime.	As a general rule, give toddlers information about procedures, medicines, and other interventions immediately beforehand; give 4- to 7-year-olds information 1 or 2 days in advance.
Parents know their child best. Eliciting information from them about their child's past behaviors and coping skills can often mean the difference between a positive and negative experience for their child.	Teach parents how to coach their child with pain management, visualization, or other methods of distraction when appropriate ("Remember when we went to the beach. . . .").
Provide an active role for the child. This helps to foster a child's sense of self-confidence and control over the situation.	Allow the child to help with simple self-care activities such as holding a dressing or piece of tape. Provide props and dolls to touch and feel as much as possible. ("Your job is to keep your hands still").
Children's wishes must be respected when they verbalize or demonstrate that they do not want more information.	Keep explanations short and simple; know when to stop teaching.
Praise the child and let him or her know how much you appreciate his or her help and cooperation.	Use "please" and "thank you" often ("Thank you. I like the way you held still for me").

Table 3.7 General Guidelines When Teaching School-Age Children

Teaching Tips	Practical Application
Allow the child some control and involvement in the decision-making process.	Offer choices whenever possible (taking the medicine with juice or milk), but don't offer choices when there are no alternatives (taking the medicine).
Children can relate present-day happenings to past experiences.	Use examples and past experiences that are familiar to the child ("Remember when you were first learning to swim . . .").
Achievement and accomplishment are very important to children at this age, so anything they can be actively involved in will help them adjust and learn.	Provide an active role and allow the child to do as much of his or her care as possible. Use props, dolls, games, and computers to enhance learning.
At this age, most children are able to sequence, understand cause-and-effect, and make sense of time.	Teach children the steps involved and how long it will take. ("Today I'm going to teach you how to change your dressing. This will help keep your cut clean. First, wash your hands . . .").
Gaining control over the situation and preparing mentally is important for their self-confidence.	Provide information 3 to 7 days in advance, depending on the child's age and developmental level.
Praise the child and let him or her know how much you appreciate his or her help and cooperation.	Use "please" and "thank you" often ("Thanks! You did a great job using your inhaler").

Evaluating Learning

Teaching, even when done well, does not necessarily mean that learning has occurred. Evaluation of learning is critical to ensure that the patient and family have actually learned what was taught. In a health care setting, evaluation should occur with each educational encounter and goals and interventions should be adjusted accordingly. The nurse, along with the rest of the interdisciplinary team, is responsible for patient and family learning. If they have not learned, the health care team ensures that teaching strategies are adjusted so that the child or family does learn.

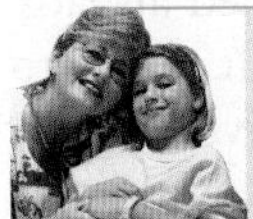

The ultimate goal of education is a change in behavior on the part of the patient and family; this change can occur in their level of knowledge, skill, or both.

Table 3.8 General Guidelines When Teaching Adolescents

Teaching Tips	Practical Application
Allow teens to be in control and involved in the decision-making process.	Speak directly to teens; consider their input in all decisions about their care and education.
Adolescents can process abstract information and understand how their actions affect long-term outcomes.	Provide reasons why something is important and discuss how their lives will be affected by their decision to take care of their health needs ("If you take your asthma medicine, you'll be better able to play tennis").
Adolescents are very concerned about how they look and how they fit in with peers.	Collaborate with the teen to develop acceptable solutions and strategies for dealing with health issues that affect personal appearance and peer acceptance (e.g., wig vs. head scarves for hair loss from chemotherapy).
Adolescents strive for independence and have personal values and ideologies that may conflict with those of parents and the medical community.	Expect some noncompliance with care, despite your best educational efforts. Work together to achieve win–win outcomes of educational goals.

Evaluation can occur in several different ways, depending on the topic and the method of teaching. The child or family may:

- Demonstrate a skill. Learning can quickly and easily be identified using this method.
- Repeat back or teach back the information using their own words.
- Answer open-ended questions. Open-ended questions provide an opportunity to assess for missing or incorrect information. Open-ended questions are those that cannot be answered with a simple "yes" or "no."

Another option to evaluate learning is to provide a "pretend" scenario for the family, mentally placing them in their own home. Have them verbalize all the steps needed to care for their child, from routine care to handling an emergency situation. They will need to convey information accurately and completely as they walk through the steps necessary to provide care for their child independently at home.

Documenting Education for the Child and Family

Documenting patient care and education on the medical record is part of every nurse's professional practice and serves four main purposes. First and foremost, the patient's medical record serves as a communication tool that the entire interdisciplinary team can use to keep track of what the patient and family has learned already and what learning still needs to occur. Next, it serves to testify to the education the family has received if and when legal matters arise. Thirdly, it verifies standards set by the Joint Commission on Accreditation of Healthcare Organizations (JCAHO), Centers for Medicare and Medicaid Services (CMS), and other accrediting bodies that hold health care providers accountable for patient education activities. And lastly, it informs third-party payers of goods and services provided for reimbursement purposes.

Documentation of patient and family education is imperative. It is the only way to ensure that the family's educational plan and objectives have been completed and that the family is ready for discharge. Documentation of patient and family education should include such topics as:

- The learning needs assessment
- Information on the patient's medical condition and plan of care
- Medications, including drug–drug and drug–food interactions
- Modified diets and nutritional needs
- Safe use of medical equipment
- Rehabilitation techniques
- Follow-up care and community resources (JCAHO, 2004)

References

Books and Journals

American Academy of Pediatrics, Committee on Bioethics. (1994). Guidelines on forgoing life-sustaining medical treatment. *Pediatrics, 93*(3), 532–536.

American Academy of Pediatrics, Committee on Bioethics. (1995). Informed consent, parental permission, and assent in pediatric practice. *Pediatrics, 95*(2), 314–317.

American Academy of Pediatrics, Committee on Hospital Care and Section on Surgery. (2002). Pediatric organ donation and transplantation. *Pediatrics, 109*(5), 982–984.

American Academy of Pediatrics, Committee on Pediatric Emergency Medicine. (2003). Consent for emergency medical services for children and adolescents. *Pediatrics, 111*(3), 703–706.

American Academy of Pediatrics, Committee on School Health and Committee on Bioethics. (2000). Policy statement: Do not resuscitate orders in schools. *Pediatrics, 105*(4), 878–879.

American Bar Association. (n.d.). *Facts about children and the law.* Retrieved June 30, 2006, from http://www.abanet.org/media/factbooks/childlaw/pdf.

Baker, D. W., Parker, R. M., Williams, M. V., & Clark, W. S. (1998). Health literacy and the risk of hospital admission. *Journal of General Internal Medicine, 13*(12), 791–798.

Baker, D. W., Parker, R. M., Williams, M. V., Pitkin, K., Parikh, N. S., Coates, W., et al. (1996). The health care experience of patients with low literacy. *Archives of Family Medicine, 5*(6), 329–334.

Bennett, C., & Pflaumer, D. (n.d.). *Positioning & comfort techniques.* Orlando, FL: Florida Children's Hospital.

Berger, J. E. (2003). Consent by proxy for nonurgent pediatric care. *Pediatrics, 112*(5), 1186–1194.

Broome, M. E., & Richards, D. J. (2003). The influence of relationships on children's and adolescents' participation in research. *Nursing Research, 52*(3), 191–197.

Burden-Osmond, C. E. (2002). When children refuse medical treatment: Role of government and assessments. *Defense Counsel Journal, 69*(2), 211–219.

Callister, L. C. (2005). What has the literature taught us about culturally competent care of women and children? *Maternal Child Nursing, 30*(6), 380–388.

Catlin, A. J. (2005). Thinking outside the box: Prenatal care—the call for a prenatal advance directive. *Journal of Perinatal & Neonatal Nursing, 19*(2), 169–176.

Cole, W., Diener, M., Wright, C., & Gaynard, L. (2001). Health care professionals' perceptions of child life specialists. *Children's Health Care, 30*(1), 1–15.

Corjulo, M. T. (2005). Telephone triage for asthma medication refills. *Pediatric Nursing, 31*(2), 116–120, 124.

Curtin, C. (2001). Eliciting children's voices in qualitative research. *American Journal of Occupational Therapy, 55,* 295–302.

Cutilli, C. C. (2005). Do your patients understand? Determining your patients' health literacy skills. *Orthopedic Nursing, 24*(5), 372–377.

Dale, E. (1969). *Audio-visual methods in teaching* (3rd ed.). Austin, TX: Holt, Rinehart, and Winston.

Deering, C. G., & Cody, D. J. (2002). Communicating with children and adolescents. *American Journal of Nursing, 102*(3), 34–41.

Doak, C. C., & Doak, L. G. (eds.). (2004). *Pfizer principles for clear health communication* (2nd ed.). Pfizer Clear Health Communication Initiative. Retrieved June 25, 2006, from http://www.pfizerhealthliteracy.org/pdfs/Pfizers_Principles_for_Clear_Health_Communication.pdf.

Doak, C. C., Doak, L. G., & Root, J. H. (1995). *Teaching patients with low literacy skills* (2nd ed.). Philadelphia: J. B. Lippincott.

Donate-Bartfield, E., & Passman, R. H. (2000). Establishing rapport with preschool-age children: Implications for practitioners. *Children's Health Care, 29*(3), 179–188.

Feldman-Winter, L., & McAbee, G. N. (2002). Legal issues in caring for adolescent patients: Physicians can optimize healthcare delivery to teens. *Postgraduate Medicine, 111*(5), 15. Retrieved from Proquest database June 1, 2006, at http://proquest.umi.com/pqdweb?did=121957428&sid=2&Fmt=3&clientld=2157&RQT=309&VName=PQD.

Figueroa-Altmann, A. R., Bedrossian, L., Steinmiller, E. A., & Wilmot, S. M. (2005). KIDS CARE: Improving Partnerships with children and families: A model from the Children's Hospital of Philadelphia. *American Journal of Nursing, 105*(5), 72A-75A.

Fleitas, J. (2003). The power of words: Examining the linguistic landscape of pediatric nursing. *MCN, 28*(6), 384–390.

Flores, G. (2003). Providing culturally competent pediatric care: Integrating pediatrics, institutions, families, and communities into the process. *Journal of Pediatrics, 143,* 1–2.

Florida Children's Hospital, Child Life Department. (n.d.). *Atraumatic care: an age specific approach.*

Florida Children's Hospital, Child Life Department. (n.d.). *Suggested vocabulary to use with children.*

Fost, N. C. (2006). Ethics of pediatric medicine. In J. A. McMillan (Ed.), *Oski's pediatrics: Principles and practice.* Philadelphia: Lippincott Williams & Wilkins.

Grindel, C. (2005). Advance directives: A call to action. *MEDSURG Nursing, 14*(3), 157, 159.

Hester, C. J. (2004). Adolescent consent: Choosing the right path. *Issues in Comprehensive Pediatric Nursing, 27,* 27–37.

Hockenberry, M. J. (2005). *Wong's essentials of pediatric nursing* (7th ed.). St. Louis: Elsevier Mosby.

Hurst, I. (2006). The legal landscape at the threshold of viability for extremely premature infants: A nursing perspective, part I. *JONA's Healthcare Law, Ethics, and Regulation, 8*(1), 20–28.

Institute for Family-Centered Care. (1999). Family-centered care: Questions and answers. *Advances in Family-Centered Care, 5,* 5.

Institute of Medicine. (2004). *Health literacy.* Washington, D.C.: The National Academies Press.

Joint Commission on Accreditation of Healthcare Organizations. (1996). *Educating hospital patients and their families—examples of compliance.* Oakbrook Terrace, IL: JCAHO.

Joint Commission on Accreditation of Healthcare Organizations. (1998–2004). *Comprehensive accreditation manual for hospitals.* Oakbrook Terrace, IL: JCAHO.

Kimberly, M. B., Hoehn, S. Feudtner, C., Nelson, R. M., & Schreiner, M. (2006). Variations in standards of research compensation and child assent practices: A comparison of 69 institutional review board-approved informed permission and assent forms for 3 multicenter pediatric clinical trials. *Pediatrics, 117*(5), 1706–1711.

Kirsch, I., Jungeblut, A., Jenkins, L., & Kolstad, A. (1993). *Adult literacy in America: A first look at the results of the national adult literacy survey.* Washington, D.C.: National Center for Education Statistics.

Knowles, M. (1990). *The adult learner: A neglected species* (4th ed.). Houston, TX: Gulf Publishing.

Kon, A. A. (2006). Assent in pediatric research. *Pediatrics, 117*(5), 1806–1810.

Kon, A. A. (2006). When parents refuse treatment for their child. *JONA's Healthcare Law, Ethics, and Regulation, 8*(1), 5–9.

Lehna, C. (2005). Interpreter services in pediatric nursing. *Pediatric Nursing, 31*(4), 292–296.

Lindblad, B. M., Rasmussen, B. H., & Sandman, P. O. (2005). Being invigorated in parenthood: Parents' experiences of being supported by professionals when having a disabled child. *Journal of Pediatric Nursing, 20*(4), 288–297.

Linnard-Palmer, L., & Kools, S. (2004). Parents' refusal of medical treatments based on religious and/or cultural beliefs: The law, ethical principles, and clinical implications. *Journal of Pediatric Nursing, 19*(5), 351–356.

London, F. (1990). *No time to teach.* Philadelphia: J. B. Lippincott.

London, F. (2004). How to prepare families for discharge in the limited time available. *Pediatric Nursing, 30*(3), 212–214, 227.

Lustig, J., Gotlieb, E. M., Deutsch, L., Gerstle, R., Lieberthal, A. Shiffman, R., et al. (2001). Special requirements for electronic medical record systems in pediatrics. *Pediatrics, 108*(2), 513–515.

Mandleco, B. (2005). *Pediatric nursing skills and procedures.* Clifton Park, NY: Thomson Delmar.

McCullough, L. B., & Stein, F. (2006). *Pediatric assent and confidentiality in clinical practice.* Retrieved July 5, 2006, from http://www.baylorcme.org/assent/.

McEvoy, M. (2003). Culture and spirituality as integrated concept in pediatric care. *MCN, 28*(1), 39–44.

McPherson, G., & Thorne, S. (2000). Children's voices: Can we hear them? *Journal of Pediatric Nursing, 15*(1), 22–29.

Mika, V. S., Kelly, P. J., Price, M. A., Franquiz, A., & Villarreal, R. (2005). The ABCs of health literacy. *Family and Community Health, 28*(4), 351–357.

Miller, S. (2000). Researching children: Issues arising from a phenomenological study with children who have diabetes mellitus. *Journal of Advanced Nursing, 31*(5), 1228–1234.

Olechnowicz, J. Q., Eder, M., Simon, C., Zyzanski, S., & Kodish, E. (2002). Assent observed: Children's involvement in leukemia treatment and research discussions. *Pediatrics, 109*(5), 806–814.

Purnell, L. D, & Paulanka, B. J. (2003). *Transcultural health care: A culturally competent approach* (2nd ed.). Philadelphia: F. A. Davis Company.

Rankin, S., & Stallings, K. D. (2001). *Patient education: Principles and practice* (4th ed.). Philadelphia: Lippincott Williams & Wilkins.

Schachter, D., Kleinman, I., & Harvey, W. (2005). Informed consent and adolescents. *Canadian Journal of Psychiatry, 50*(9), 534–540.

Schmitt, B. D. (2004). *Pediatric telephone protocols: office version* (10th ed.). Elk Grove, IL: American Academy of Pediatrics.

Sheehan, J. P. (2000). Caring for the deaf: Do you do enough? *RN, 63*(3), 69–70, 72.

Shields, L., & Tanner, A. (2004). Pilot study of a tool to investigate perceptions of family-centered care in different care settings. *Pediatric Nursing, 30*(3), 189–197.

Shin, H., & White-Traut, R. (2005). Nurse-child interaction on an inpatient paediatric unit. *Journal of Advanced Nursing, 52*(1), 56–62.

Simonsen-Anderson, S. (2002). Safe and sound: Telephone triage and home recommendations save lives and money. *Nursing Management, 33*(6), 41–43.

Sobo, E. J. (2004). Pediatric nurses may misjudge parent communication preferences. *Journal of Nursing Care Quality, 19*(3), 253–262.

Society for Pediatric Nurses. (2006). *The role of the staff nurse in protecting children and families involved in research.* Retrieved July 1, 2006, from http://www.pedsnurses.org/pdfs/Protecting%20Children%20and%20Families%20Involved%20in%20Research.pdf.

Staywell Krames. (1999). *A guide to educating patients.* San Bruno, CA: Staywell Company.

Taylor, C., Lillis, C., & LeMone, P. (2005). *Fundamentals of nursing: The art and science of nursing care* (5th ed.). Philadelphia: Lippincott Williams & Wilkins.

Tillett, J. (2005). Adolescents and informed consent: Ethical and legal issues. *Journal of Perinatal and Neonatal Nursing, 19*(2), 112–121.

Titone, J., Cross, R., Sileo, M., & Martin, G. (2004). Taking family-centered care to a higher level on the heart and kidney unit. *Pediatric Nursing, 30*(6), 495–497.

Turkoski, B. B. (2005). When a child's treatment decisions conflict with the parents'. *Home Healthcare Nurse, 23*(5), 123–126.

University Children's Hospital, University of California–Irvine. (2006). *The child's bill of rights.* Retrieved July 2, 2006, from http://ndcweb.hsis.uci.edu/healthcareservices/ChildBillOfRights.htm.

U.S. Congress. (1996). *Public Law 104-191, Health insurance portability and accountability act of 1996.* Retrieved July 1, 2006, from http://aspe.hhs.gov.admnsimp/pl104191.htm.

U.S. Department of Health and Human Services. (2000). Standards for privacy of individually identifiable health information; final rule. *Federal Register, 65*(250), 82461–82829. Retrieved July 1, 2006, from http://frwebgate.access.gpo.gov/cgi-bin/getdoc.cgi?dbname=2000_register&docid=f:28der2.pdf.

U.S. Pharmacopoeia. (2006). *Children and medicines: ten guiding principles for teaching children and adolescents about medicines.* Retrieved July 1, 2006, from http://www.usp.org/audiences/consumers/children/principles/html.

Weech, W. A. (1999). *Tips for using interpreters.* Washington, D.C.: Foreign Service Institute of the U.S. Department of State.

Weiss, B. D. (2003). *Health literacy: A manual for clinicians.* Chicago: American Medical Association Foundation.

Weiss, B. D., Blanchard, J. S., McGee, D. L., Hart, G., Burgoon, W. B., & Smith, K. J. (1994). Illiteracy among Medicaid recipients and its relationship to health care costs. *Journal of Health Care for the Poor & Underserved, 5*(2), 99–111.

Williams, M. V., Davis, T., Parker, R. M., & Weiss, B. D. (2002). The role of health literacy in patient-physician communication. *Family Medicine, 34,* 383–389.

Wong, D. (1989). Principles of atraumatic care. In V. Feeg (Ed.), *Pediatric nursing: Forum on the future:Looking toward the 21st century.* Pitman, NJ: Antony J. Jannetti.

Wong, D. (2005). Wong on Web Paper "Beyond First Do No Harm: Principles of Atraumatic Care." Accessed 6/8/2006 from http://www.mosbydrugconsult.com/WOW/op022a.html.

Wong, D. L. (2002). *Beyond first do no harm: Principles of atraumatic care.* Retrieved June 25, 2006, from http://www3.us.elsevierhealth.com/WOW/op022a.html.

Woodring, B. C. (2004). The role of the staff nurse in protecting children and families involved in research. *Journal of Pediatric Nursing, 19*(4), 311–313.

Websites

www.aap.org American Academy of Pediatrics
www.askme3.org Partnership for Clear Health Communication
www.atanet.org American Translators Association
www.cal.org Center for Applied Linguistics
www.childhealthinfo.com/ Child Health Information Center
www.childrenshealthcare.org/ Children's Healthcare is a Legal Duty
www.diversityrx.org Diversity Rx—issues related to language and culture in health care
www.familycenteredcare.org/ Institute for Family-Centered Care
http://gucchd.georgetown.edu/nccc/ National Center for Cultural Competence
www.hablamosjuntos.org/ Language Policy and Practice in Health Care
www.keepkidshealthy.com/ Guide to Children's Health and Safety
www.languageline.com/ Language Line
www.notis.net Northwest Translators and Interpreters Society
www.omhrc.gov Office of Minority Health, U.S. Department of Health and Human Services
www.tcns.org Transcultural Nursing Society

Chapter WORKSHEET

MULTIPLE CHOICE QUESTIONS

1. When working with children and families, which is a critical strategy for promoting therapeutic communication?
   a. Detailed explanations
   b. Attentive listening
   c. Comforting touch
   d. Closed-ended questions

2. When caring for an adolescent, in which case must the nurse share information with the parents no matter which state the care is provided in?
   a. Pregnancy counseling
   b. Depression
   c. Contraception
   d. Tuberculosis

3. When providing atraumatic care to a child, which action would be most appropriate?
   a. Applying restraints for any procedure that would be uncomfortable
   b. Keeping the lights on in the child's room throughout the day and night
   c. Limiting the use of topical anesthetics for painful injections
   d. Allowing parents and children an informed choice about being together

4. The nurse is caring for a 2-year-old in the hospital, and the mother expresses concern that the toddler will be scared. Which response by the nurse would be most appropriate?
   a. "Don't worry; we practice family-centered and atraumatic care here."
   b. "We will do our best to minimize the stress that your child experiences."
   c. "It will probably be upsetting for you as well, so you should stay home."
   d. "Our practice of atraumatic care will eliminate all pain and stress for your child."

5. When planning patient education for a child and parents, what is the first step the nurse should take?
   a. Decide which procedures and medications the child will be discharged on.
   b. Determine the child's and family's learning needs and styles.
   c. Ask the family if they have ever performed this type of procedure.
   d. Tell the child and family what the goals of the teaching session are.

CRITICAL THINKING EXERCISES

1. A 12-year-old boy is to undergo research treatment for a serious illness. Describe the concept of assent as it relates to this situation.

2. A 3-year-old girl from Saudi Arabia has become seriously ill while visiting the United States. She will require a lengthy hospital stay. Describe the steps the nurse should take to communicate effectively with and provide extensive health care teaching to this child's family.

STUDY ACTIVITIES

1. Develop a teaching plan for one of the families that you care for in the clinical setting. Be sure to follow the appropriate steps for providing education.

2. Interview a child life specialist about the effects that the traditional (not atraumatic) approach to restraining a child for procedures might have on a child of various ages.

3. Research the availability of language interpreters and translators in your local community, compiling a list of the available resources.

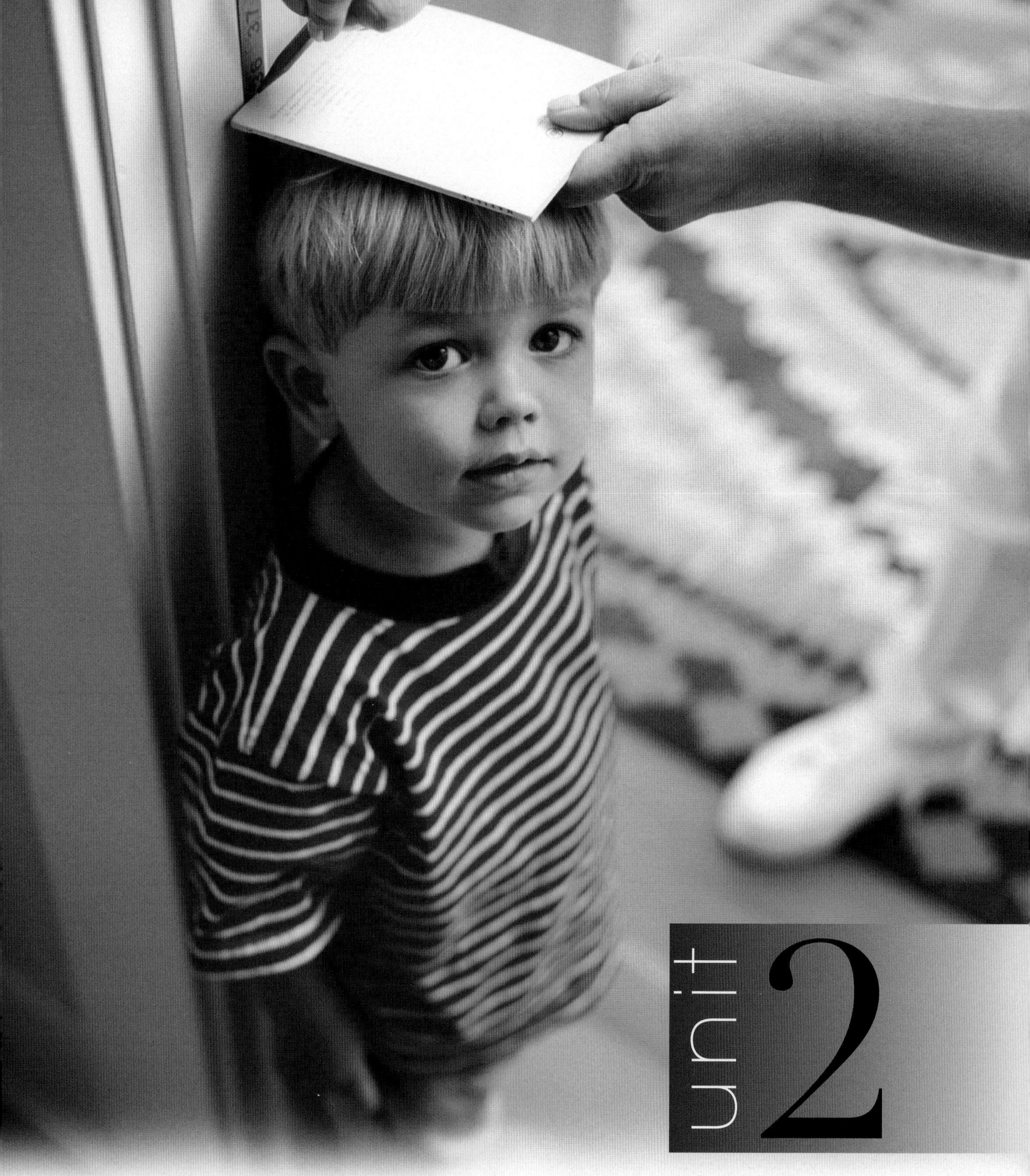

unit 2

Health Promotion for the Growing Child and Family

chapter

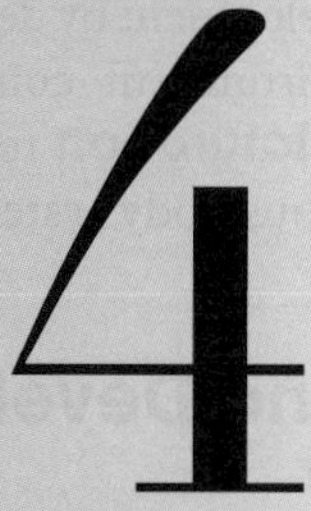

Growth and Development of the Newborn and Infant

Key TERMS

anticipatory guidance
binocularity
cephalocaudal
colic
colostrum
development
discipline
foremilk
growth
hind milk
let-down reflex
maturation
object permanence
prolactin
proximodistal
stranger anxiety
temperament

Learning OBJECTIVES

Upon completion of the chapter, the learner will be able to:

1. Identify normal developmental changes occurring in the newborn and infant.
2. Identify the gross and fine motor milestones of the newborn and infant.
3. Express an understanding of language development in the first year of life.
4. Describe nutritional requirements of the newborn and infant.
5. Develop a nutritional plan for the first year of life.
6. Identify common issues related to growth and development in infancy.
7. Demonstrate knowledge of appropriate anticipatory guidance for common developmental issues.

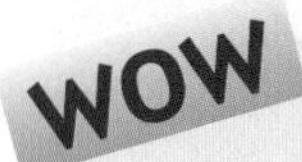

Of all the joys that lighten our hearts, what joy is welcomed like a newborn child?

Allison Johnson is a 6-month-old girl brought to the clinic by her mother and father for her 6-month check-up. As new parents, they have a list of questions and concerns. On assessment you find that Allison's weight is 16 pounds, length 25¾ inches, and head circumference 17 inches. As the nurse caring for her, assess Allison's growth and development, and then teach the parents what changes to expect in Allison over the next few months.

The newborn or neonatal period of infancy is defined as the period from birth until 28 days of age. Infancy is defined as the period from birth to 12 months of age. Growth and development are interrelated, ongoing processes in infancy and childhood. **Growth** refers to an increase in physical size. **Development** is the sequential process by which infants and children gain various skills and functions. Heredity influences growth and development by determining the child's potential, while environment contributes to the degree of achievement. **Maturation** refers to an increase in functionality of various body systems or developmental skills.

Growth and Development Overview

Growth and developmental changes in the first year of life are numerous and dramatic. Physical growth, maturation of body systems, and gross and fine motor skills progress in an orderly and sequential fashion. Though timing may vary from infant to infant, the order in which developmental skills are acquired is consistent. Infants also exhibit vast amounts of learning in the psychosocial and cognitive, language and communication, and social/emotional domains. Adequate growth and development are indicative of health in the infant or young child. Nurses must be familiar with normal developmental milestones so that they can accurately assess the infant's development as well as provide age-appropriate anticipatory guidance to the parents.

Achievement of developmental milestones may be assessed in a variety of ways. While obtaining the health history, the nurse may ask the parent or caregiver if the skill is present and when it was attained. The infant may also demonstrate the skill during the interview or examination, or the nurse may elicit the skill from the infant. A number of screening tools are also used to assess development, such as the Denver II Developmental Screening Test (see Appendix B), Prescreening Developmental Questionnaire (PDQ II), Ages and Stages Questionnaire (ASQ), Infant Toddler Checklist for Language and Communication, and Infant Development Inventory.

Ill or premature infants may exhibit delayed acquisition of physical growth and developmental skills. When assessing the growth and development of a premature infant, use the infant's adjusted age to determine expected outcomes. To determine adjusted age, subtract the number of weeks that the infant was premature from the infant's chronological age. Plot growth parameters and assess developmental milestones based on adjusted age. For example, a 6-month-old boy who was born at 28 weeks' gestation was born 12 weeks early (3 months), so you should subtract 3 months from his chronological age of 6 months to get an adjusted age of 3 months. This infant would demonstrate healthy growth if he were the size of a 3-month-old, and he should be expected to achieve the developmental milestones of a 3-month-old rather than a 6-month-old.

PHYSICAL GROWTH

Ongoing assessments of growth are important so that too-rapid or inadequate growth can be identified early. With early identification, the cause can be diagnosed and the potential for further appropriate growth maximized. Infants grow very rapidly over the first 12 months of life. Weight, length, and head and chest circumference are all indicators of physical growth in the newborn and infant (Table 4.1).

Weight

The average newborn weighs 7 lb 8 oz (3,400 g) at birth. Newborns lose up to 10% of their body weight over the first 5 days of life. The average newborn then gains about 20 to 30 g per day and regains his or her birthweight by 10 to 14 days of age. Most infants double their birthweight by 4 to 6 months of age and triple their birthweight by the time they are 1 year old.

Height

The average newborn is 19 to 21 inches (48 to 53 cm) long at birth. During the first 6 months, length increases

Table 4.1 Average Measurements of Infants at Birth and 6 and 12 Months

Age	Weight	Length	Head Circumference
Birth	7.5 lb (3,400 g)	19–21 in (48–53 cm)	13–14 in (33–35 cm)
6 months	15 lb (6.8 kg)	25–27 in (63.5–68.5 cm)	16.5–17.5 in (42–44.5 cm)
12 months	23 lb (10.5 kg)	28–30 in (71–76 cm)	17.7–18.7 in (45–47.5 cm)

by 1 inch (2.5 cm) per month, then by about a half-inch per month in the second 6 months.

Head and Chest Circumference

Average head circumference of the full-term newborn is 13 to 14 inches (33 to 35 cm). The head circumference is about 1 inch (2 to 3 cm) greater than the chest circumference, which averages 12 to 13 inches (30.5 to 33 cm). The head circumference increases rapidly during the first 6 months: the average increase is about 0.6 inch (1.5 cm) per month. From 6 to 12 months of age, the head circumference increases an average of 0.2 inch (0.5 cm) monthly. The chest circumference is not routinely measured after the newborn period but does increase in size as the child grows.

● ORGAN SYSTEM MATURATION

The newborn and infant's organ systems undergo significant changes as the infant grows. Systems that undergo significant change include the neurologic system, the cardiovascular system, the respiratory system, the gastrointestinal (digestive) system, the renal system, the hematopoietic system, the immunologic system, and the integumentary system.

Neurologic System

The infant experiences tremendous changes in the neurologic system over the first year of life. Critical brain growth and continued myelinization of the spinal cord are occurring. Involuntary movement progresses to voluntary control, and immature vocalizations and crying progress to the ability to speak as a result of maturational changes of the neurologic system.

States of Consciousness

The normal term newborn's ability to move sequentially through states of consciousness reassures parents and health care providers that the neurologic system, though immature, is intact. A normal newborn will ordinarily move through six states of consciousness:

1. Deep sleep: The infant lies quietly without movement.
2. Light sleep: The infant may move a little while sleeping and may startle to noises.
3. Drowsiness: Eyes may close; the infant may be dozing.
4. Quiet alert state: The infant's eyes are open wide and the body is calm.
5. Active alert state: The infant's face and body move actively.
6. Crying: the infant cries or screams and the body moves in a disorganized fashion.

Newborns usually progress through these states slowly, rather than going from deep sleep immediately into outright crying.

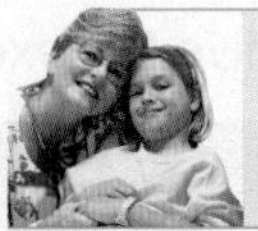

The first period of reactivity (the first 15 minutes after birth) is a quiet alert state and is an opportune time to promote bonding and breastfeeding.

Brain Growth

The nervous system continues to mature throughout infancy, and the increase in head circumference is indicative of brain growth. The brain undergoes tremendous growth during the first 2 years of life. By 6 months of age the infant's brain weighs half that of the adult brain. At age 12 months, the brain has grown considerably, weighing 2½ times what it did at birth. Generally, the anterior fontanel remains open until 12 to 18 months of age to accommodate this rapid brain growth. However, the fontanel may close as early as 9 months of age, and this is not of concern in the infant with age-appropriate growth and development.

In general, the neurologic system matures a significant amount over the first year of life. Myelination of the spinal cord and nerves continues over the first 2 years. Maturation of the nervous system and continued myelination are necessary for the tremendous developmental skills that are achieved in the first 12 months. During the first few months of life, reflexive behavior is replaced with purposeful action.

Reflexes

Primitive reflexes are subcortical and involve a whole-body response. Selected primitive reflexes present at birth include Moro, root, suck, asymmetric tonic neck, plantar and palmar grasp, step, and Babinski. Except for the Babinski, which disappears around 1 year of age, these primitive reflexes diminish over the first few months of life, giving way to protective reflexes. Protective reflexes (also termed postural responses or reflexes) are motor responses related to maintenance of equilibrium. These responses are prerequisites for appropriate motor development and remain throughout life once they are established. The protective reflexes include the righting and parachute reactions. Appropriate presence and disappearance of primitive reflexes, as well as development of protective reflexes, is indicative of a healthy neurologic system. Persistence of primitive reflexes beyond the usual age of disappearance may indicate an abnormality of the neurologic system and should be investigated.

Table 4.2 gives descriptions and illustrations of several primitive and protective reflexes, as well as the timing of appearance and disappearance of these reflexes.

Respiratory System

The respiratory system continues to mature over the first year of life. The respiratory rate slows from an average of 30 to 60 breaths in the newborn to about 20 to 30 in the 12-month-old. The newborn breathes irregularly, with periodic pauses. As the infant matures, the respiratory pattern becomes more regular and rhythmic.

(text continues on page 78)

Table 4.2 Selected Primitive and Protective Reflexes in Infancy

	Description	Age Reflex Appears	Age Reflex Disappears
Primitive Reflexes			
Root	When infant's cheek is stroked, the infant turns to that side, searching with mouth. 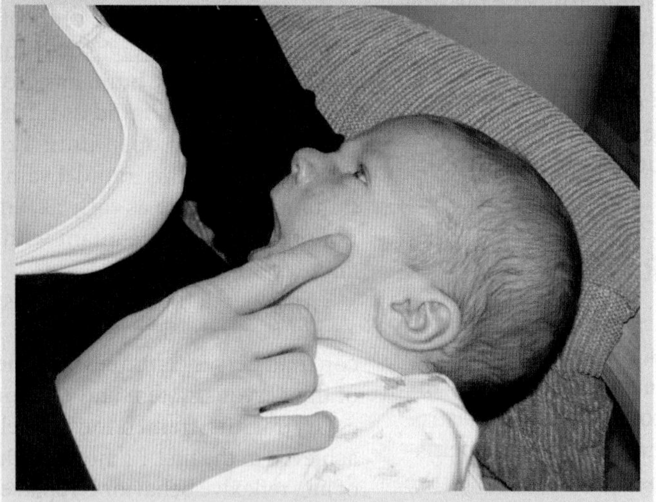	Birth	3 months
Suck	Reflexive sucking when nipple or finger is placed in infant's mouth 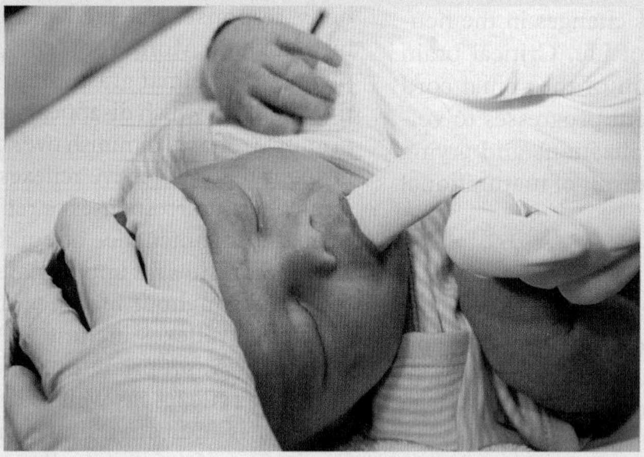	Birth	2–5 months

Table 4.2 Selected Primitive and Protective Reflexes in Infancy (continued)

	Description	Age Reflex Appears	Age Reflex Disappears
Moro	With sudden extension of the head, the arms abduct and move upward and the hands form a "C." 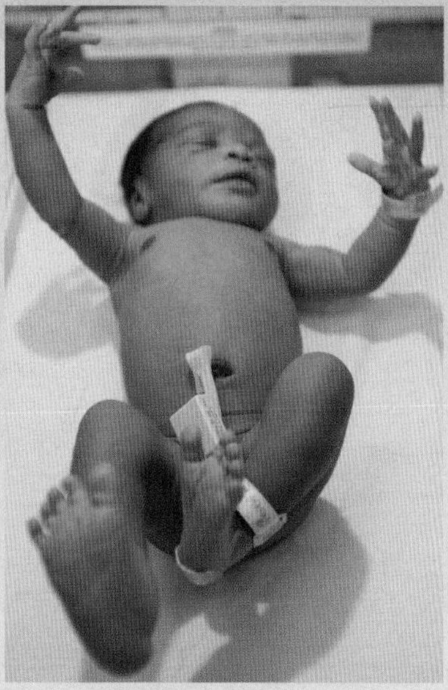	Birth	4 months
Asymmetric tonic neck	While lying supine, extremities are extended on the side of the body to which the head is turned and opposite extremities are flexed (also called the "fencing" position). 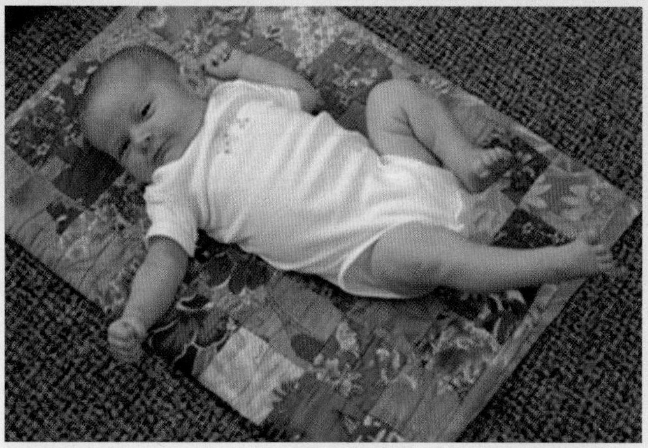	Birth	4 months

(continued)

Table 4.2 Selected Primitive and Protective Reflexes in Infancy (continued)

	Description	Age Reflex Appears	Age Reflex Disappears
Palmar grasp	Infant reflexively grasps when palm is touched. 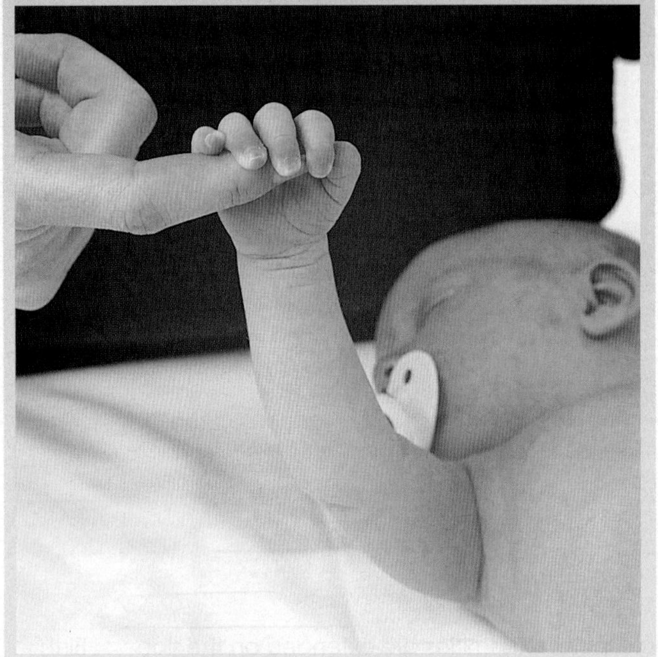	Birth	4–6 months
Plantar grasp	Infant reflexively grasps with bottom of foot when pressure is applied to plantar surface. 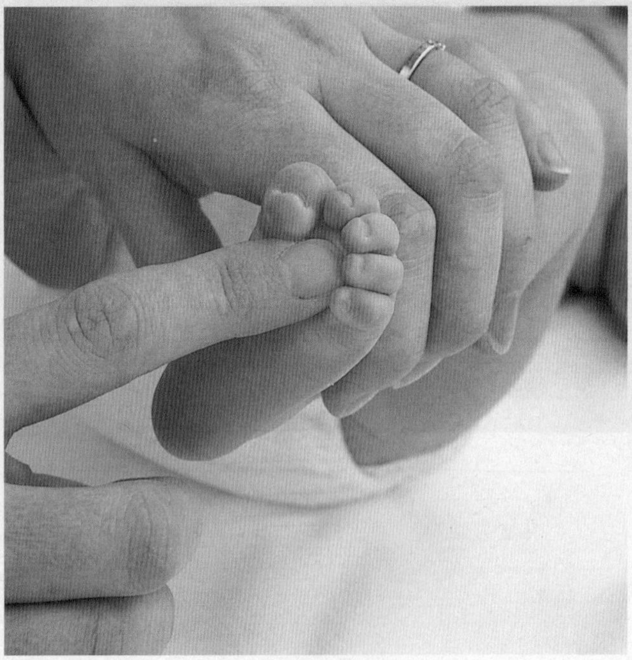	Birth	9 months

Table 4.2 Selected Primitive and Protective Reflexes in Infancy (continued)

	Description	Age Reflex Appears	Age Reflex Disappears
Babinski	Stroking along the lateral aspect of the sole and across the plantar surface results in fanning and hyperextension of the toes. 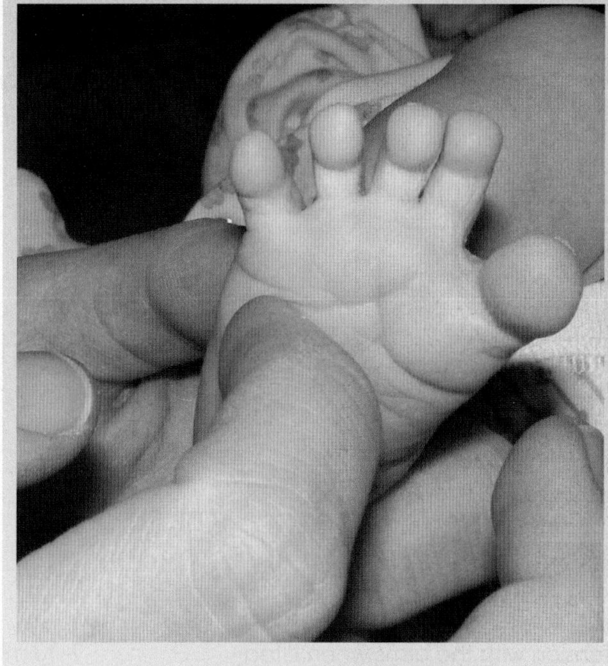	Birth	12 months
Step	With one foot on a flat surface, the infant puts the other foot down as if to "step." 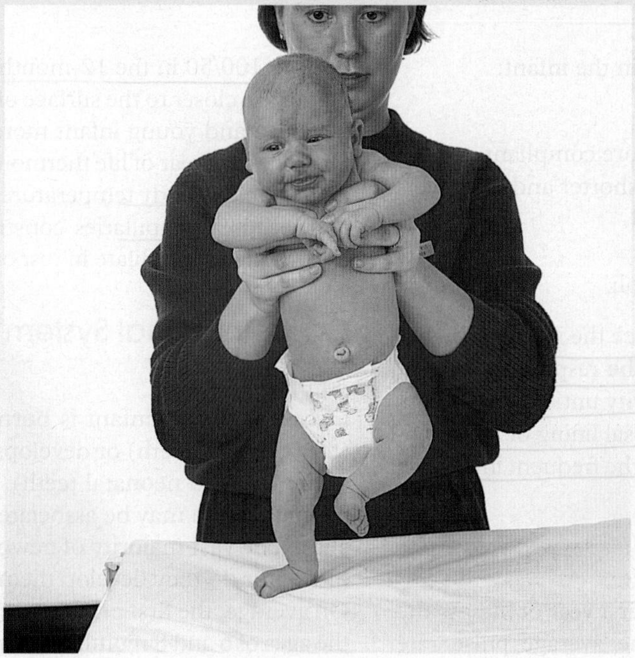	Birth	4–8 weeks

(continued)

Table 4.2 Selected Primitive and Protective Reflexes in Infancy (continued)

	Description	Age Reflex Appears	Age Reflex Disappears
Protective Reflexes			
Neck righting	Neck keeps head in upright position when body is tilted.	4–6 months	Persists
Parachute (sideways)	Protective extension with the arms when tilted to the side in a supported sitting position	6 months	Persists
Parachute (forward)	Protective extension with the arms when held up in the air and moved forward. The infant reflexively reaches forward to catch himself.	6–7 months	Persists
Parachute (backward)	Protective extension with the arms when tilted backward	9–10 months	Persists

In comparison with the adult, in the infant:

- The nasal passages are narrower.
- The trachea and chest wall are more compliant.
- The bronchi and bronchioles are shorter and narrower.
- The larynx is more funnel-shaped.
- The tongue is larger.
- There are significantly fewer alveoli.

These anatomic differences place the infant at higher risk for respiratory compromise. The respiratory system does not reach adult levels of maturity until about 7 years of age. The lack of IgA in the mucosal lining of the upper respiratory tract also contributes to the frequent infections that occur in infancy.

Cardiovascular System

The heart doubles in size over the first year of life. As the cardiovascular system matures, the average pulse rate decreases from 120 to 140 in the newborn to about 100 in the 1-year-old. Blood pressure steadily increases over the first 12 months of life, from an average of 60/40 in the newborn to 100/50 in the 12-month-old. The peripheral capillaries are closer to the surface of the skin, thus making the newborn and young infant more susceptible to heat loss. Over the first year of life thermoregulation (the body's ability to stabilize body temperature) becomes more effective: the peripheral capillaries constrict in response to a cold environment and dilate in response to heat.

Gastrointestinal System

Teeth

Occasionally, an infant is born with one or more teeth (termed natal teeth) or develops teeth in the first 28 days of life (termed neonatal teeth). The presence of natal or neonatal teeth may be associated with other birth anomalies. The vast majority of newborns do not have teeth at birth, nor do they develop them in the first month of life. On average, the first primary teeth begin to erupt between the ages of 6 and 8 months. The primary teeth (also termed deciduous teeth) are lost later in childhood and will be replaced by the permanent teeth. The gums around the emerging tooth often swell. The lower central incisors are usually the first to appear, followed by the upper central incisors (Fig. 4.1). The average 12-month-old has four to eight teeth.

Digestion

The newborn's digestive system is not developed fully. Small amounts of saliva are present for the first 3 months of life and ptyalin is present only in small amounts in the saliva. Gastric digestion occurs as a result of the presence of hydrochloric acid and rennin. The small intestine is about 250 cm long and grows to the adult length over the first few years of life. The stomach capacity is relatively small at birth, holding about one-half to 1 ounce. However, by 1 year of age the stomach can accommodate three full meals and several snacks per day. In the duodenum, three enzymes in particular are important for digestion. Trypsin is available in sufficient quantities for protein digestion after birth. Amylase (needed for complex carbohydrate digestion) and lipase (essential for appropriate fat digestion) are both deficient in the infant and do not reach adult levels until about 5 months of age.

The liver is also immature at birth. The ability to conjugate bilirubin and secrete bile is present after about 2 weeks of age. Conjugation of medications may remain immature over the first year of life. Other functions of the liver, including gluconeogenesis, vitamin storage, and protein metabolism, remain immature during the first year of life.

UPPER
Central incisor
8-12 months
Lateral incisor
9-13 months
Cuspid
16-22 months
First molar
13-19 months
Second molar
25-33 months

LOWER
Second molar
25-33 months
First molar
13-19 months
Cuspid
16-22 months
Lateral incisor
9-13 months
Central incisor
8-12 months

● **Figure 4.1** Sequence and average age of tooth eruption.

Stools

The consistency and frequency of stools change over the first year of life. The newborn's first stools (meconium) are the result of digestion of amniotic fluid swallowed *in utero*. They are dark green to black and sticky (Fig. 4.2). In the first few days of life the stools become yellowish or tan. Generally the formula-fed infant has stools the consistency of peanut butter. Breastfed infants' stools are usually looser in texture and appear seedy. Newborns may have as many as eight to ten stools per day or as few as one stool every day or two. After the newborn period, the number of stools may decrease, and some infants do not have a bowel movement for several days. Infrequent stooling is considered normal if the bowel movement remains soft. Due to the immaturity of the gastrointestinal system, newborns and young infants often grunt, strain, or cry while attempting to have a bowel movement. This is not of concern unless the stool is hard and dry. Stool color and texture may change depending on the foods that the infant is ingesting. Iron supplements may cause the stool to appear black or very dark green.

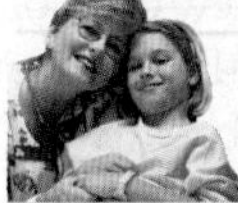

Parents should call the primary care provider if the infant's stools are red, white, or black; mucus-like; frequent and watery; frothy or foul-smelling; hard, dry, formed, or pellet-like; or if the baby is vomiting.

Genitourinary System

In the infant, extracellular fluid (lymph, interstitial fluid, and blood plasma) accounts for about 35% of body weight and intracellular fluid accounts for 40%, compared with the adult quantities of 20% and 40% respectively. Thus, the infant is more susceptible to dehydration. Infants urinate frequently and the urine has a relatively low specific gravity. The renal structures are immature and the glomerular filtration rate, tubular secretion, and reabsorption as well as renal perfusion are all reduced compared with the adult. The glomeruli reach full maturity by 2 years of age.

Integumentary System

In utero the infant is covered with vernix caseosa, which protects the developing infant's skin. At birth, the infant may be covered with vernix (earlier gestational age) or vernix may be found in the folds of the skin, axilla, and groin areas (later gestational age). Production of vernix ceases at birth. Fine downy hair (lanugo) covers the body of many newborns. Often this hair is lost over time and is not replaced. Darker-skinned races tend to have more lanugo present at birth than those with light skin.

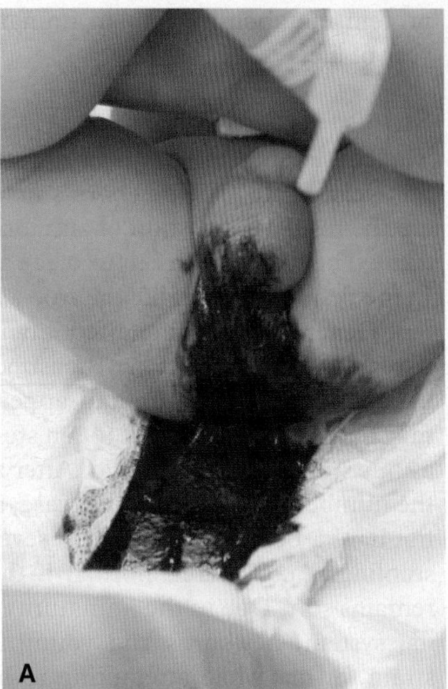

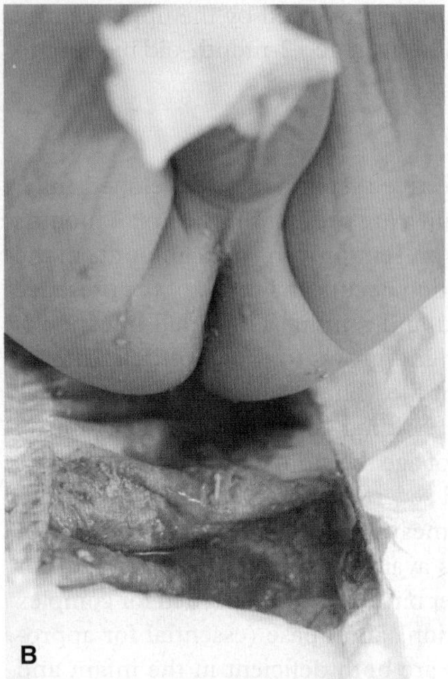

● **Figure 4.2** (**A**) Meconium stool. (**B**) Typical stool after the first few days. Note the yellowish, seedy stool of a breastfed infant.

Acrocyanosis (blueness of the hands and feet) is normal in the newborn; it decreases over the first few days of life (Fig. 4.3). Newborns often experience mottling of the skin (a pink-and-white marbled appearance) because of their immature circulatory system. Mottling decreases over the first few months of life.

The newborn and young infant's skin is relatively thinner than that of the adult, with the peripheral capillaries being closer to the surface. This may cause increased absorption of topical medications.

Hematopoietic System

Significant changes in the hematopoietic system occur over the first year of life. At birth, fetal hemoglobin (HgbF) is present in large amounts. After birth the production of fetal hemoglobin nearly ceases, and adult hemoglobin (HgbA) is produced in steadily increasing amounts throughout the first 6 months. Since HgbF has a shorter lifespan than HgbA, infants may experience physiologic anemia at age 2 to 3 months. During the last 3 months of gestation, maternal iron stores are transferred to the fetus. The newborn typically has 0.3 to 0.5 g of iron stores available. As the high hemoglobin concentration of the newborn decreases over the first 2 to 3 months, iron is reclaimed and stored. These stores may be sufficient for the first 6 to 9 months of life but will become depleted if iron supplementation does not occur. Ongoing iron intake is required throughout the first 15 years of life in order to reach the adult level of 5 g.

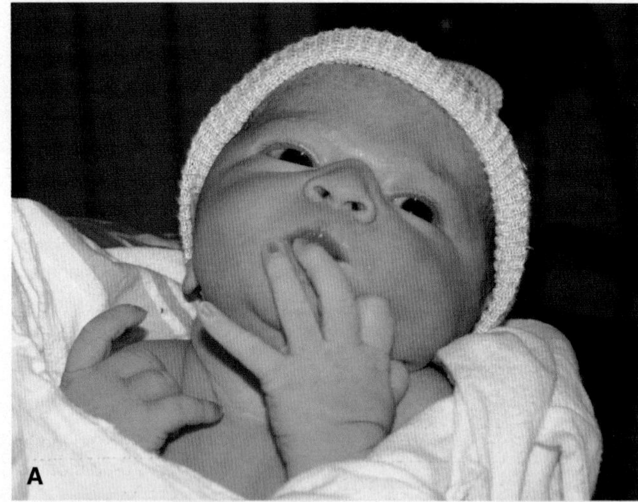

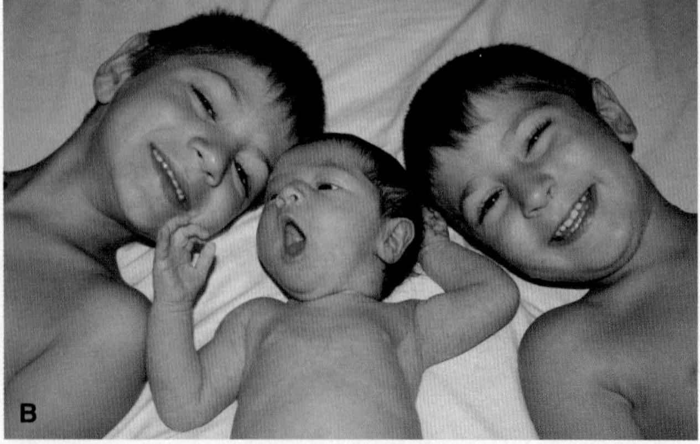

● **Figure 4.3** (**A**) Acrocyanosis. Note blueness of the hands. (**B**) Mottling of the skin in a young infant.

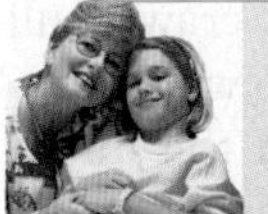

Maternal iron stores are transferred to the fetus throughout the last trimester of pregnancy. Infants born prematurely miss all or at least a portion of this iron store transfer, placing them at increased risk for iron deficiency anemia compared with term infants.

Immunologic System

Newborns receive large amounts of immunoglobulin G (IgG) through the placenta from their mothers. This confers immunity during the first 3 to 6 months of life for antigens to which the mother was previously exposed. Infants then synthesize their own IgG, reaching approximately 40% of adult levels at age 12 months. Immunoglobulin M (IgM) is produced in significant amounts after birth, reaching adult levels by 9 months of age. Immunoglobulin A (IgA), immunoglobulin D (IgD), and immunoglobulin E (IgE) production increases very gradually, maturing in early childhood.

PSYCHOSOCIAL DEVELOPMENT

Erik Erikson (1963) identifies the psychosocial crisis of infancy as Trust versus Mistrust. Development of a sense of trust is crucial in the first year, as it serves as the foundation for later psychosocial tasks. The parent or primary caregiver can have a significant impact on the infant's development of a sense of trust. When the infant's needs are consistently met, the infant develops this sense of trust. But if the parent or caregiver is inconsistent in meeting the infant's needs in a timely manner, then the infant develops a sense of mistrust. Table 4.3 lists activities that promote a sense of trust in infancy.

COGNITIVE DEVELOPMENT

The first stage of Jean Piaget's theory of cognitive development is referred to as the sensorimotor stage (birth to 2 years) (Piaget, 1969). Infants learn about themselves and the world through their developing sensory and motor capacities. Infants' development from birth to1 year of age can be divided into four substages within the sensorimotor stage: reflexes, primary circular reaction, secondary circular reaction, and coordination of secondary schemes. Cause and effect guides most of the cognitive development seen in infancy (see Table 4.3).

The concept of **object permanence** begins to develop between 4 and 7 months of age and is solidified by

Table 4.3 Developmental Theories

Theorist	Stage	Activities
Erikson	Trust vs. Mistrust (birth to 1 year)	Caregivers respond to the infant's basic needs by feeding, changing diapers, and cleaning, touching, holding, and talking to the infant. This creates a sense of trust in the infant. As the nervous system matures, infants realize they are separate beings from their caregivers. Over time the infant learns to tolerate small amounts of frustration and trusts that although gratification may be delayed, it will eventually be provided.
Piaget	• Sensorimotor (birth to 2 years)	• Infant uses senses and motor skills to learn about the world.
	• Substage 1: use of reflexes (birth to 1 month)	• Reflexive sucking brings the pleasure of ingesting nutrition. Infant begins to gain control over reflexes; recognizes familiar objects, odors, and sounds.
	• Substage 2: primary circular reactions (1 to 4 months)	• Thumb-sucking may occur by chance; then the infant repeats it on purpose to bring pleasure. Imitation begins. Object permanence begins. Infant shows affect.
	• Substage 3: secondary circular reactions (4 to 8 months)	• Infant repeats actions to achieve wanted results (e.g., shakes rattle to hear the noise it makes). The infant's actions are purposeful but the infant does not always have an end goal in mind.
	• Substage 4: coordination of secondary schemes (8 to 12 months)	• Infants coordinate previously learned schemes with previously learned behaviors. They may grasp and shake a rattle intentionally or crawl across the room to reach a desired toy. Infant can anticipate events. Object permanence is present at about 8 months of age. The infant begins to associate symbols with events (e.g., waving goodbye means someone is leaving)
Freud	Oral stage (birth to 1 year)	Pleasure is focused on oral activities: feeding and sucking.

about 8 months of age. If an object is hidden from the infant's sight, he or she will search for it in the last place it was seen, knowing it still exists. This development of object permanence is essential for the development of self-image. By age 12 months the infant knows he or she is separate from the parent or caregiver. Self-image is also promoted through the use of mirrors. By 12 months of age, infants can see themselves in the mirror. The 12-month-old will explore objects in different ways, such as throwing, banging, dropping, and shaking. He or she may imitate gestures and knows how to use certain objects correctly (e.g., puts phone to ear, turns up cup to drink, attempts to comb hair).

● MOTOR SKILL DEVELOPMENT

Infants exhibit phenomenal increases in their gross and fine motor skills over the first 12 months of life.

Gross Motor Skills

The term "gross motor skills" refers to those that use the large muscles (e.g., head control, rolling, sitting, and walking). Gross motor skills develop in a **cephalocaudal** fashion (from the head to the tail) (Fig. 4.4). In other words, the baby learns to lift the head before learning to roll over and sit. At birth, babies have poor head control and need to have their necks supported when being held. They can lift their heads only slightly while in a prone position. Over the next several months the infant's motor skills progress at a dramatic rate. First the infant achieves head control, then the ability to roll over, sit, crawl, pull to stand, and, usually around a year of age, to walk independently. Table 4.4 gives details on when the infant develops each specific gross motor skill. Progression of gross motor skills is illustrated in Figures 4.5 through 4.7.

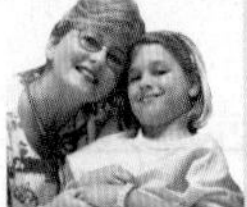

Warning signs that may indicate problems with motor development include the following: arms and legs are stiff or floppy; child cannot support head at 3 to 4 months of age; child reaches with one hand only; child cannot sit with assistance at 6 months of age; child does not crawl by 12 months of age; child cannot stand supported by 12 months of age.

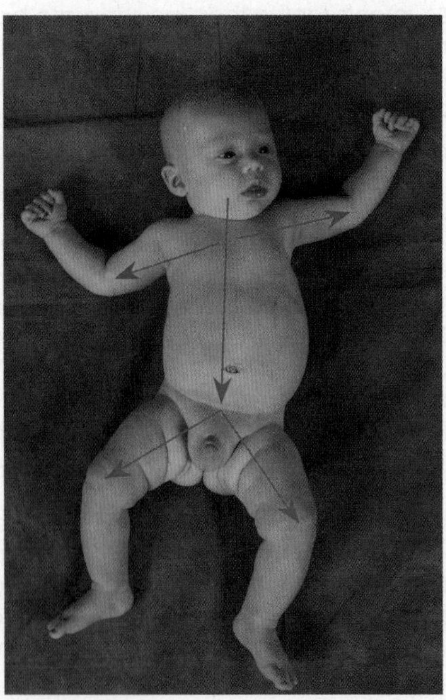

● Figure 4.4 Gross motor skills develop in a cephalocaudal direction, fine motor skills in a proximodistal fashion.

Fine Motor Skills

Fine motor development includes the maturation of hand and finger use. Fine motor skills develop in a **proximodistal** fashion (from the center to the periphery) (see Fig. 4.4). In other words, the infant first bats with the whole hand, eventually progressing to gross grasping, before being capable of fine fingertip grasping (Fig. 4.8). The newborn's hand movements are involuntary in nature, whereas the 12-month-old is capable of feeding himself or herself with a cup and spoon. By 12 months of age the infant should be able to eat with his or her fingers and assist with dressing (e.g., pushing an arm through the sleeve). Table 4.5 gives details on when the infant develops each specific fine motor skill.

● SENSORY DEVELOPMENT

Though hearing should be fully developed at birth, the other senses continue to develop as the infant matures. Though they mature at different rates, sight, smell, taste, and touch all continue to develop after birth.

Sight

The newborn is nearsighted, preferring to view objects at a distance of 8 to 15 inches. Newborns prefer the human face to other objects and may even imitate the facial expressions made by those caring for them. In addition to human faces, newborns show a preference for certain objects, particularly those with contrasts such as black-and-white stripes. The newborn's eyes wander and occasionally cross. At 1 month of age the infant can recognize by sight the people he or she knows best. The infant will study objects within his or her visual range closely. The ability to fuse two ocular images into one cerebral picture (**binocularity**) begins to develop at 6 weeks of age and is well established by 4 months of age. Full color vision develops by 7 months of age, as do distance vision and the ability to track objects.

Hearing

The newborn's hearing is intact at birth and as acute as that of an adult. Newborns prefer the sound of human

Table 4.4 Development of Gross Motor Skills in Infancy

Age	Gross Motor Skills
1 month	Lifts and turns head to side in prone position Head lag when pulled to sit Rounded back in sitting
2 months	Raises head and chest, holds position Improving head control
3 months	Raises head to 45 degrees in prone Slight head lag in pull to sit
4 months	Lifts head and looks around Rolls from prone to supine Head leads body when pulled to sit
5 months	Rolls from supine to prone and back again Sits with back upright when supported
6 months	Tripod sits
7 months	Sits alone with some use of hands for support
8 months	Sits unsupported
9 months	Crawls, abdomen off floor
10 months	Pulls to stand Cruises
12 months	Sits from standing position Walks independently

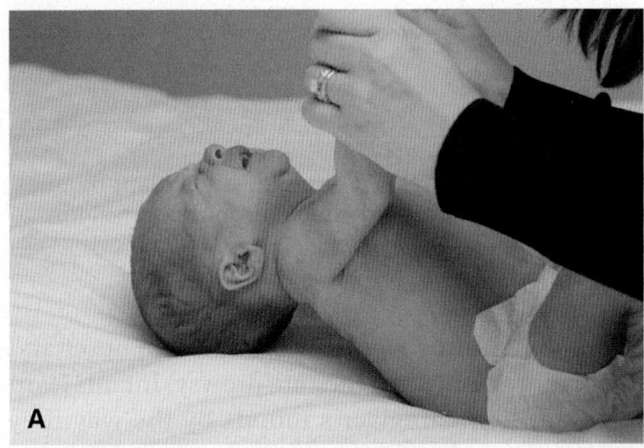

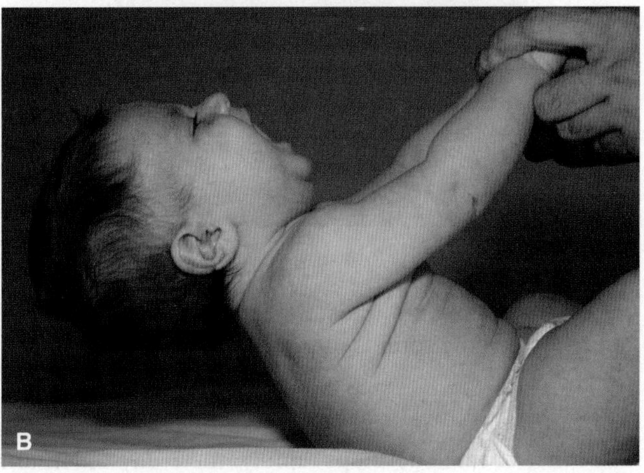

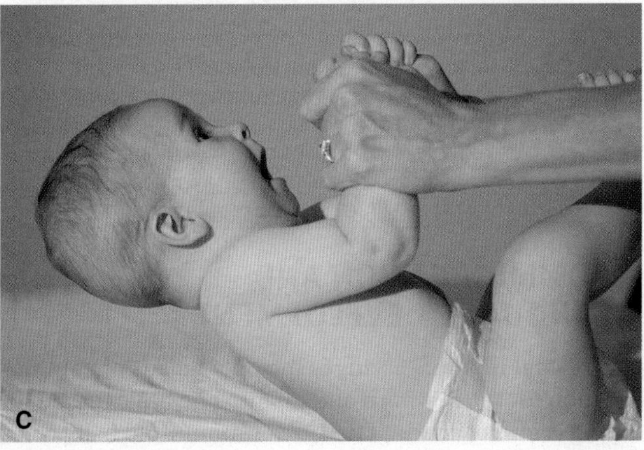

● Figure 4.5 When pulled to sit, an infant shows (**A**) significant head lag (newborn; 2 or 3 weeks old), (**B**) improving head control (2 months old), and (**C**) no head lag (4 months old).

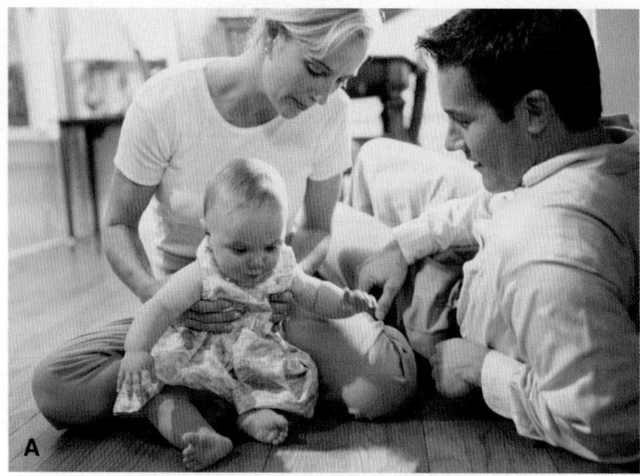

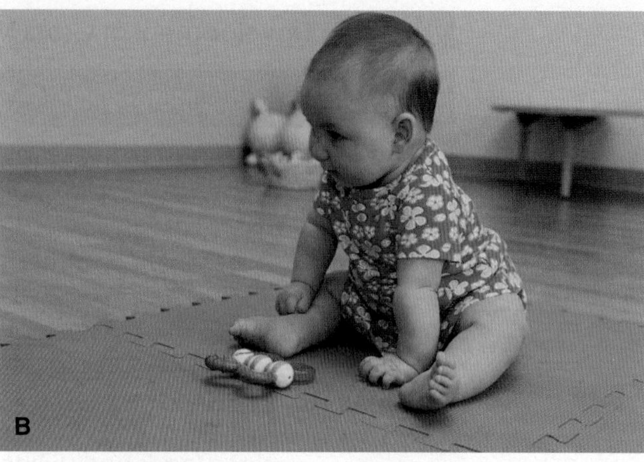

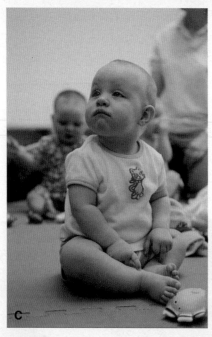

● Figure 4.6 Development of sitting. (**A**) At 4 months, the infant requires significant support. (**B**) The 6-month-old infant sits in tripod fashion. (**C**) The 8-month-old sits alone.

voices to nonhuman sounds. By 1 month of age the infant can recognize the sounds of those he or she knows best.

Smell and Taste

The sense of smell develops rapidly: the 7-day-old infant can differentiate the smell of his or her mother's breast milk from that of another woman and will preferentially turn toward the mother's smell. Newborns prefer sweet tastes to all others. This persists for several months, and eventually the infant will accept non-sweet flavors.

Touch

The sense of touch is perhaps the most important of all the senses for newborn communication. Even the most immature infant responds to soothing stroking. The infant prefers soft sensations to coarse sensations. The infant dislikes rough handling and may cry. Holding, stroking, rocking, and cuddling calms infants when they are upset and makes them more alert when they are drowsy. Infants learn to understand their caregiver's moods by the way they touch them.

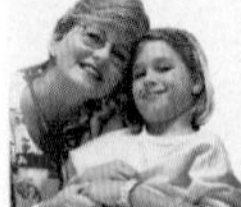

Warning signs that may indicate problems with sensory development include the following: young infant does not respond to loud noises; child does not focus on a near object; infant does not start to make sounds or babble by 4 months of age; infant does not turn to locate sound at age 4 months; infant crosses eyes most of the time at age 6 months.

● COMMUNICATION AND LANGUAGE DEVELOPMENT

For several months, crying is the only means of communication for the newborn and infant. The basic reason for crying is unmet needs. The 1- to-3-month-old baby coos,

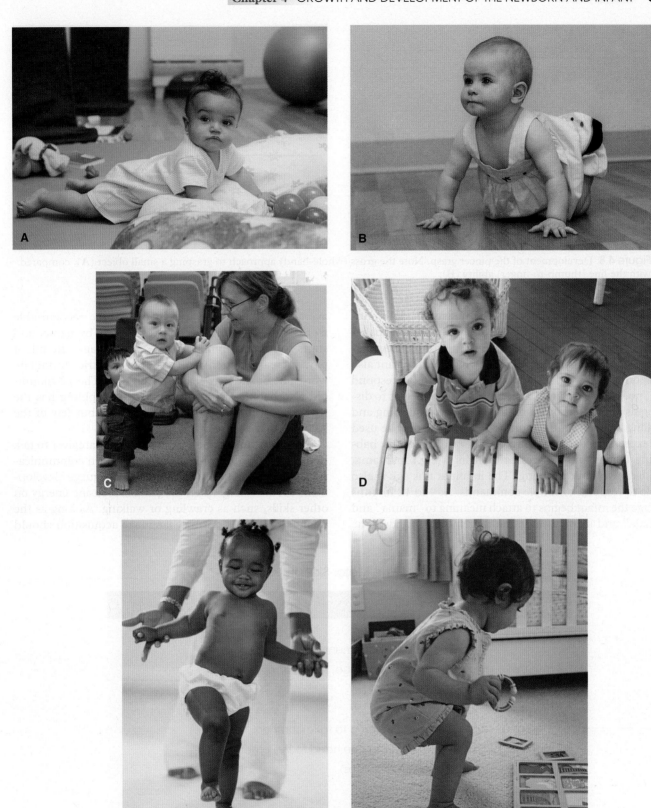

● Figure 4.7 Development of locomotion. (**A**) At 4 months the infant pushes up from a prone position. (**B**) At 8 months, the infant crawls with the abdomen off the floor. (**C**) The infant pulls to stand by 10 months of age. (**D**) The infant cruises along furniture or (**E**) takes steps with assistance at 10 to 11 months of age. (**F**) The infant independently stands from a crouched position and walks around 12 months of age (plus or minus 3 months).

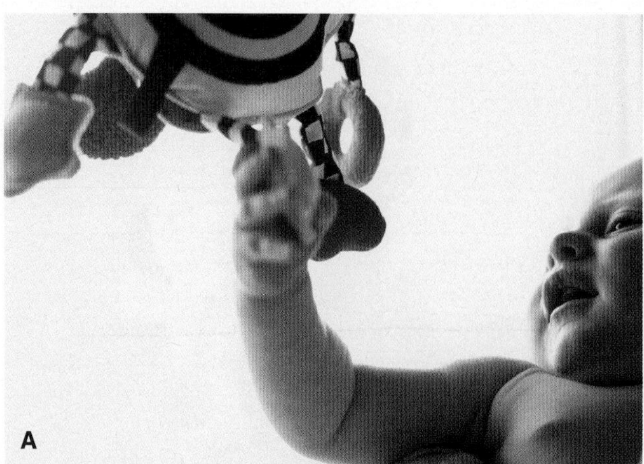

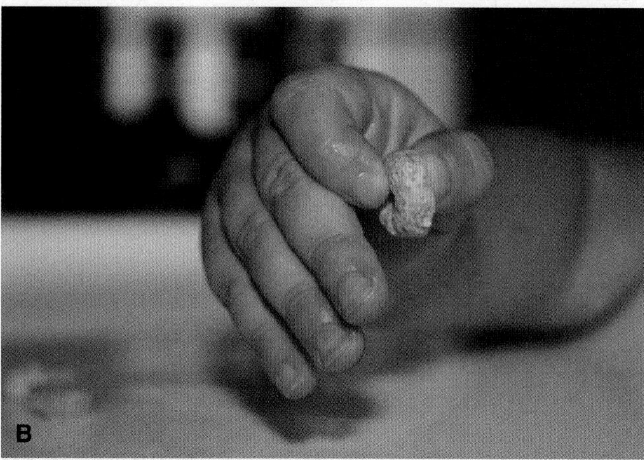

● Figure 4.8 Development of the pincer grasp. Note the gross (whole-hand) approach to grasping a small object (**A**), compared with the fine (thumb-to-finger) ability (**B**).

makes other vocalizations, and demonstrates differentiated crying. At 4 to 5 months of age, the infant makes simple vowel sounds, laughs aloud, performs "raspberries," and vocalizes in response to voices. The infant also responds to his or her own name and begins to respond to "no." Between 4 and 7 months the infant begins to distinguish emotions based on tone of voice. Squealing and yelling begin around 6 months of age; these may be used to express joy or displeasure. At age 7 to 10 months, babbling begins and progresses to strings (e.g., mamama, dadada) without meaning. The infant at this age is also able to respond to simple commands. At 9 to 12 months of age the infant begins to attach meaning to "mama" and "dada" and starts to imitate other speech sounds. The average 12-month-old uses two or three recognizable words with meaning, recognizes objects by name, and starts to imitate animal sounds. At this age, the infant pays increasing attention to speech and tries to imitate words; he or she may also say, "uh-oh." The 12-month-old also babbles with inflection (this babbling has the rhythm and timing of spoken language, but few of the "words" make sense).

It is very important for the parent or caregiver to talk to the infant in order for the infant to learn communication skills. Sometimes regression in language development occurs briefly when the child is focusing energy on other skills, such as crawling or walking. As long as the infant's hearing is normal, language acquisition should

Table 4.5 Development of Fine Motor Skills in Infancy

Age	Fine Motor Skills
1 month	Fists mostly clenched Involuntary hand movements
3 months	Holds hand in front of face, hands open
4 months	Bats at objects
5 months	Grasps rattle
6 months	Releases object in hand to take another
7 months	Transfers object from one hand to the other
8 months	Gross pincer grasp (rakes)
9 months	Bangs objects together
10 months	Fine pincer grasp Puts objects into container and takes them out
11 months	Offers objects to others and releases them
12 months	Feeds self with cup and spoon Makes simple mark on paper Pokes with index finger

continue to progress. Infants in bilingual families may "language mix" (uses some words from each language). This is considered to be a normal progression in language development for these children, but it makes it more difficult for the health care provider to determine delays in communication skills (Fierro-Cobas, 2001).

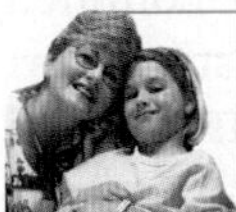

Warning signs that may indicate problems in language development are as follows: infant does not make sounds at 4 months of age; infant does not laugh or squeal by 6 months of age; infant does not babble by 8 months of age; infant does not use single words with meaning at 12 months of age (mama, dada).

SOCIAL AND EMOTIONAL DEVELOPMENT

The newborn spends much of the time sleeping, but by 2 months of age the infant is ready to start socializing. The infant exhibits a first real smile at age 2 months. He or she spends a great deal of time while awake watching and observing what is going on around him or her. By about 3 months of age the infant will start an interaction with a caregiver by smiling widely and possibly gurgling. This prompts the caregiver to smile back and talk to the infant. The infant responds with more smiling, cooing, and gurgles as well as moving the arms and legs. The 3- to 4-month-old will also mimic the parent's facial movements, such as widening the eyes and sticking out the tongue. The baby may hesitate at first, but once the other person responds pleasantly to the infant, the infant engages and gets into the interaction. The infant may cry when the pleasant interaction stops. At 6 to 8 months of age the infant may enjoy socially interactive games such as patty-cake and peek-a-boo.

Stranger Anxiety

Around the age of 8 months the infant may develop **stranger anxiety**. The previously happy and very friendly infant may become clingy and whiny when approached by strangers or people not well known. Stranger anxiety is an indicator that the infant is recognizing himself or herself as separate from others. As the infant becomes more aware of new people and new places, he or she may view an interaction with a stranger as threatening and may start crying, even if the parent is right there. Family members whom the child sees infrequently, as well as others the child does not spend a lot of time with, should approach the infant calmly and slowly, with the parent in sight. Sometimes this will prevent a sudden crying spell.

Separation Anxiety

Separation anxiety may also start in the last few months of infancy. The infant becomes quite distressed when the parent leaves. The infant will eventually calm down and become engaged with the current caregiver. It is not until the infant is older that cognition and memory are sufficient for him or her to understand that the parent will come back.

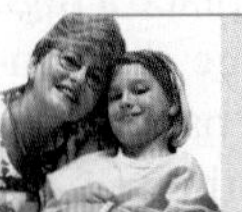

Warning signs of possible problems with social/emotional development include the following: child does not smile at people at 3 months of age; child refuses to cuddle; child does not seem to enjoy people; child shows no interest in peek-a-boo at 8 months of age.

Temperament

Temperament is an individual's nature; it is referred to as the "how" of behavior (Turecki, 2003). Temperament ranges from low or moderately active, regular, and predictable to highly active, more intense, and less adaptable. These are all considered normal along a continuum. An infant's innate temperament affects the way he or she responds to the environment. As parents take note of their infant's usual activity level, how intensely he or she reacts with others and the environment, and how stimulated the baby becomes with interactions, they start to learn about their infant's temperament. The parent should note how adaptable and flexible the infant is as well as how predictable and persistent the baby is.

When parents are familiar with how the baby approaches life on a routine basis, they will be better able to recognize when the baby is not acting like himself or herself. Nurses can help parents interpret observations about their infant's temperament and recommend ways to support the infant's individual behavior. Some infants are slower to warm up than others; those infants should be approached slowly and calmly. Some infants exhibit increased levels of activity compared to quieter, more passive babies; those infants generally require more direct play with the parent or caregiver and will be the type of older infant who is in constant motion. Some infants are loud and some are not. The quiet infant may become overwhelmed with excessive stimulation, whereas the very active baby may need additional stimulation to be satisfied. Becoming familiar with the infant's temperament also helps the parents describe the best approach to the infant by others (e.g., child care workers or health care professionals).

CULTURAL INFLUENCES ON GROWTH AND DEVELOPMENT

Many cultural differences have an impact on growth and development. For instance, certain ethnic groups tend to be shorter than others because of their genetic makeup. These children will not grow to be as tall as those of another ethnic background. Cultural feeding practices in some cultures may lead to overweight in some children. Some cultures and certain religions advocate vegetarianism; those children need nutritional assessment to ensure they are getting enough protein intake for adequate growth.

Parenting styles and health promotion behaviors can also be significantly influenced by culture. Parents and extended family are the most significant influences in an infant's life in most cultures. Certain cultures place a high value upon independence and may encourage their infants to develop quickly, while other cultures "baby" their infants for longer periods. In most cultures the mother takes primary responsibility for caring for the child, but in some cultures, major health-related decisions may be deferred to the father or grandparents.

Health beliefs are often strongly influenced by an individual's religious or spiritual background. Sometimes this creates conflict in the health care setting when the health providers have a different value system than that of the infant's family.

In some cultures infants and children share a bed with their parents. When an infant or child is hospitalized and is accustomed to sleeping with the parents, it may be difficult and distressing for him or her to try to sleep alone.

The nurse should explore the family's cultural practices related to growth and development. Usually these practices are not harmful and can be supported by the health care team, but safety must always be considered. The nurse should not make assumptions about a family's cultural practices based on their skin color, accent, or name; rather, the nurse should perform an adequate assessment.

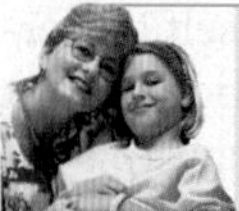

Many communities now include people from a variety of cultures, so it is important for nurses to practice transcultural nursing (nursing care that is directed by cultural aspects and that respects the individual's differences). Many nurse researchers are exploring the cultural aspects of health care and the impact that cultural diversity has upon health.

Refer back to Allison Johnson, who was introduced at the beginning of the chapter. What developmental milestones would you expect Allison to have reached by this age? How would this be different if Allison had been born 6 weeks premature?

The Nurse's Role in Newborn and Infant Growth and Development

WATCH & LEARN

Growth and development affect every aspect of the infant's life. As infants progress through various stages of development, they do so in a predictable fashion. Growth and development are sequential and orderly, though some children develop at faster rates than others. It is important for the nurse to understand growth and development. Health care visits through infancy often focus primarily on **anticipatory guidance** (educating parents and caregivers about what to expect in the next phase of development). The purpose of anticipatory guidance is to give parents the tools they need to support their infant's development in a safe fashion.

Hospital nurses also need to use their knowledge of growth and development when caring for ill infants. Hospitalization often requires the infant to be confined to the crib or the hospital room. Nurses must support growth and development within the constraints imposed by the child's illness.

NURSING PROCESS OVERVIEW

After the infant's current growth and development status has been assessed, problems related to growth and development may be identified. The nurse may then identify one or more nursing diagnoses, including:

- Ineffective breastfeeding
- Risk for disproportionate growth
- Imbalanced nutrition, less than body requirements
- Risk for impaired parent/infant attachment
- Delayed growth and development
- Risk for caregiver role strain

Nursing care planning for the infant with growth and development issues should be individualized based on the infant's and family's needs. The Nursing Care Plan Overview can be used as a guide in planning nursing care for the infant with a growth and development problem. The nurse may choose the appropriate nursing diagnoses from the plan and individualize them as needed. The nursing care plan is intended to serve as a guide, not as an all-inclusive growth and development care plan.

PROMOTING HEALTHY GROWTH AND DEVELOPMENT

Adding a new person to the family produces both excitement and anxiety. Newborns are completely reliant upon their parents or caregivers to fill every need. It is quite a burden and precious responsibility that new parents are taking on. Many parents read the latest books about caring for newborns, while others rely on information received from family and friends. Newborns and their mothers spend only a short time in the hospital after delivery, so it is very important that parents can care for their newborn and know when to call the primary care provider with concerns.

Periodic screening for adequate growth and development is recommended by the American Academy of Pediatrics (AAP) for all infants and children. The prevention of devastating disease is another priority for infants and children. The AAP and the Advisory Committee on

(text continues on page 92)

Nursing Care Plan 4.1

Growth and Development Issues in the Newborn and Infant

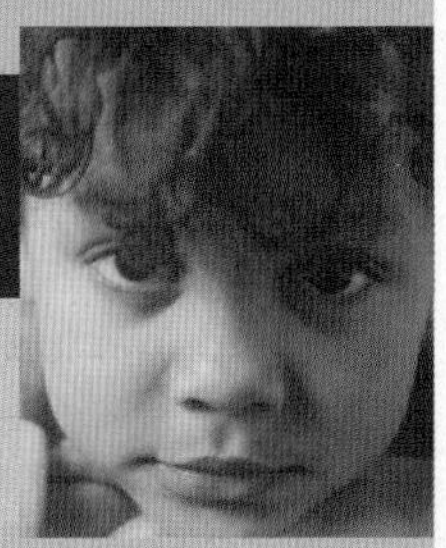

Nursing Diagnosis: Breastfeeding, ineffective, related to lack of exposure, misconceptions, or knowledge deficit as evidenced by first baby, mother's verbalization, or nursing observations

Outcome identification and evaluation

Mother/infant dyad will experience successful breastfeeding: *infant will latch on, suck and swallow at the breast; mother will not experience sore nipples.*

Interventions: promoting effective breastfeeding

- Educate mother on recognition of and response to infant hunger cues *to promote on-cue breastfeeding, which will establish milk supply.*
- Educate mother on appropriate diet and fluid intake *to ensure ability to manufacture adequate supply of breast milk.*
- Demonstrate breastfeeding positions with infant at the breast *(appropriate positioning increases probability of successful latch).*
- Assess infant's latch technique, sucking motion, and audible swallowing *(an appropriately latched infant will take most of the areola in the mouth, suck in spurts, and demonstrate audible swallowing).*
- Assess infant voiding/stool patterns: *at least six voids per day and passage of stool ranging from one or more per day to one every several days is a normal pattern for breastfed infants.*
- Assess infant weight gain: *gain of 15 to 30 g per day after the second week of life indicates infant is receiving appropriate nutrition.*
- Assess mother's nipples for redness or soreness; *if infant appropriately latches on nipples will not become sore.*

Nursing Diagnosis: Risk for altered growth pattern (risk factors: caregiver knowledge deficit, first infant, premature infant, or maladaptive feeding behaviors)

Outcome identification and evaluation

Infant will demonstrate adequate growth and appropriate feeding behaviors: *steady increases in weight, length, and head circumference; infant feeds appropriately for age.*

Interventions: promoting adequate growth

- Observe mother/infant dyad breastfeeding or bottle-feeding *to determine need for further education or identify infant difficulties with feeding.*
- Educate mother about appropriate breastfeeding or bottle-feeding *so that mother is aware of what to expect in normal feeding pattern.*
- When infant is old enough, provide education about addition of solid foods, spoon and cup feeding: *after 6 months of age breast milk or formula needs to be supplemented with a variety of foods.*
- Determine need for additional caloric intake if necessary *(premature infants and infants with chronic illnesses or metabolic disorders often need adjustments in caloric intake to demonstrate adequate or catch-up growth).*
- Obtain daily weights (if hospitalized, weekly if outpatient) and weekly length and head circumference *to determine whether feeding pattern is sufficient to promote adequate growth.*

(continued)

Growth and Development Issues in the Newborn and Infant (continued)

Nursing Diagnosis: Nutrition, altered, less than body requirements, related to possible ineffective feeding pattern or inadequate caloric intake as evidenced by failure to gain weight or by inadequate increases in weight, length, and head circumference over time

Outcome identification and evaluation

Infant will take in adequate nutrients using effective feeding pattern: *Infant will demonstrate adequate weight gain (15 to 30 g per day) and steady increases in length and head circumference.*

Interventions: promoting adequate nutritional intake

- Assess current feeding pattern and daily intake *to determine areas of concern.*
- Increase frequency of breastfeeding or volume of bottle feeding *if needed to meet caloric needs.*
- Introduce solid foods on age-appropriate schedule: *introducing solids at the right time improves the chances that the child will learn to take solid foods.*
- Limit juice intake or discontinue altogether *(juice has little nutritive value and displaces nutrients from breast milk or formula).*
- Use human milk fortifier (if ordered) *to increase caloric density of breast milk.*
- Increase caloric density of formula (if ordered) by mixing to a more concentrated level or with additives (fats or carbohydrates) *to provide increased calories needed to support adequate growth.*
- If infant is taking solids already, choose higher-calorie foods *to maximize nutrient intake.*

Nursing Diagnosis: Parent/infant attachment, altered, risk for (risk factors: premature infant, parental knowledge deficit about normal newborn activity and care, infant with difficult temperament or medical problems)

Outcome identification and evaluation

Parent and infant will demonstrate appropriate attachment via *eye contact, parental response to infant cues, parental verbalization of caring for infant, infant response to parent's caretaking behaviors.*

Interventions: encouraging appropriate parent-infant attachment

- Assess parent's response to infant cues *to determine degree of attachment and level of parent's knowledge about infant care.*
- Assess infant's response to parent's caretaking behaviors *to determine degree of attachment.*
- Determine infant's temperament *to counsel parent effectively about responses appropriate for that type of temperament.*
- Encourage *en face* positioning for holding or feeding the young infant *to encourage give-and-take response between infant and parent.*
- Encourage parent to meet infant's needs promptly and with affection *to promote sense of trust in the infant.*
- Reinforce parent's attempts at improving attachment with infant *(positive reinforcement naturally encourages appropriate behaviors).*

Growth and Development Issues in the Newborn and Infant (continued)

Nursing Diagnosis: Growth and development, altered, related to speech, motor, psychosocial, or cognitive concerns as evidenced by delay in meeting expected milestones

Outcome identification and evaluation

Development will be maximized: *infant will make continued progress toward attainment of developmental milestones.*

Interventions: maximizing development

- Perform developmental evaluation of the infant *to determine infant's current level of functioning.*
- Offer age-appropriate play, activities, and toys *to encourage further development.*
- Carry out interventions as prescribed by developmental specialist, physical therapist, occupational therapist, or speech therapist *(repeated exposure to the activities or exercises is needed to make developmental progress).*
- Provide support to parents of infants with developmental concerns, *as developmental progress can be slow and it is difficult for families to stay motivated and maintain hope.*

Nursing Diagnosis: Caregiver role strain, risk for (risk factors: first baby, knowledge deficit about newborn care, lack of prior exposure, fatigue if premature, ill, or developmentally delayed infant)

Outcome identification and evaluation

Parent will experience competence in role: *will demonstrate appropriate caretaking behaviors and verbalize comfort in new role.*

Interventions: preventing caregiver role strain

- Assess parent's knowledge of newborn/infant care and the issues that arise as a part of normal development *to determine parent's needs.*
- Provide education on normal newborn/infant care *so that parents have the knowledge they need to appropriately care for their new baby.*
- Provide anticipatory guidance related to normal infant development *to prepare parents for what to expect next and how to intervene.*
- Encourage respite for parents *(even a few hours away from the demands of an infant's care can rejuvenate the parents).*

Nursing Diagnosis: Injury, risk for (risk factors: developmental age, infant curiosity, rapidly progressing motor abilities)

Outcome identification and evaluation

Infant safety will be maintained: *infant will remain free from injury.*

Interventions: preventing injury

- Encourage car seat safety *to decrease risk of injury related to motor vehicles.*
- Childproof home: *as infant becomes more mobile, he or she will want to explore everything, increasing risk of injury.*
- Parents should have the poison control center phone number available: *should an accidental ingestion occur, Poison Control can give parents the best advice for appropriate intervention.*
- Never leave an infant unattended in the sink, bathtub, or swimming pool *to prevent drowning.*
- Teach parents first aid measures and infant CPR *to minimize consequences of injury should it occur.*
- Parents should watch the infant at all times *(no amount of childproofing can replace the watchful eye of a caring parent).*

Immunization Practices (ACIP) have made recommendations for immunization schedules. Immunizations are a very important part of the newborn and infant's health visits. Nurses caring for newborns and infants should be familiar with the recommended infant/child periodic screenings (check-ups) as well as the current immunization schedule (see Chapter 9, for further information on immunizations).

Promoting Growth and Development Through Play

Experts in child development and behavior have said repeatedly that play is the work of children. Infants practice their gross and fine motor skills and language through play. Play is a natural way for infants and children to learn. Play is critical to infant development, as it gives infants the opportunity to explore their environment, practice new skills, and solve problems. The newborn prefers interacting with the parent to toys. Parents can talk to and sing to their newborns while participating in the daily activities that infants need, such as feeding, bathing, and changing diapers. Newborns and young infants love to watch people's faces and often appear to mimic the expressions they see.

As infants become older, toys may be geared toward the motor skills or language skills that the child is developing. Parents can promote fine motor development in infants by providing age-appropriate toys. For example, a rattle that a young infant can hold promotes reaching and attaining. The older infant builds fine motor skills by stacking cups or placing smaller toys inside of larger ones. Gross motor skills are reinforced and practiced over and over again when the infant wants to reach something he or she is interested in.

When playing with toys, the infant usually engages in solitary play; he or she does not share with other infants or directly play with other infants. A wide variety of toys are available for infants, but infants often enjoy the most basic ones, such as plastic containers of various shapes and sizes, soft balls, and wooden or plastic spoons.

Books are also very important toys for infants. Reading to all ages of infants is appropriate, and the older infant develops fine motor skills by learning to turn book pages.

Table 4.6 lists age-appropriate toys.

Promoting Early Learning

Research has shown that reading aloud and sharing books during early infancy are critical to the development of neural networks that are important in the later tasks of read-

Table 4.6 Appropriate Toys for Newborns and Infants

Age	Appropriate Toys
Newborn to 1 month	• Mobile with contrasting colors or patterns • Unbreakable mirror • Soft music via tape or music box • Soft, brightly colored toys
1 to 4 months	• Bright mobile • Unbreakable mirror • Rattles • Singing by parent or caregiver, varied music • High-contrast patterns in books or images
4 to 7 months	• Fabric or board books • Different types of music • Easy-to-hold toys that do things or make noise (fancy rattles) • Floating, squirting bath toys • Soft dolls or animals
8 to 12 months	• Plastic cups, bowls, buckets • Unbreakable mirror • Large building blocks • Stacking toys • Busy boxes (with buttons or knobs that make things happen) • Balls • Dolls • Board books with large pictures • Toy telephone • Push–pull toys (older infants)

ing and word recognition. Reading books increases listening comprehension. Infants demonstrate their excitement about picture books by kicking and waving their arms and babbling when looking at them. At 6 to 12 months, the infant reaches for books and brings them to the mouth. Over time, reading leads to acquisition of language skills. Reading picture books and simple stories to infants starts a good habit that should be continued throughout childhood.

Promoting Safety

The most common cause of death in infants between the ages of 6 and 12 months is injury. As infants become more mobile, they risk injury from falls down stairs and off chairs, tables, and other structures. Curiosity leads the infant to explore potentially dangerous items, such as electrical outlets, hot stove or furnace vents, mop buckets, and toilets. Since infants explore so much with their mouths, small objects or hard foods pose a choking hazard. The infant will invariably pick up any accessible object and bring it to the mouth. With increasing dexterity, poisoning from medications, household cleaning products, or other substances also becomes a problem.

Safety in the Car

Motor vehicle accidents are one source of injury, particularly if the infant is improperly restrained. Infants should never be transported in a motor vehicle without proper restraint. Infant car seats should face the rear of the car until the infant is 12 months of age and weighs 20 pounds. The car seat should be secured tightly in the center of the back seat. The infant should never be placed in a front seat that is equipped with an airbag.

Infants should never be left unattended in a motor vehicle. The temperature rises very quickly inside a closed vehicle, and an infant can suffocate from heat in a closed vehicle in the summer. Even during cooler weather, the heat generated within a closed vehicle can reach three to five times the exterior temperature. Kidnapping is also a concern if the baby is left unattended in a vehicle.

Additional information on car safety can be found on www.childsafety.org, www.safekids.org, and www.carseat.org and through the National Highway Traffic Safety Administration at www.nhtsadot.gov.

Safety in the Home

The baby's crib should have a firm mattress that fits snugly in the crib on a secure support. The distance between crib slats should be 2-3/8 inches or less to prevent injury. All crib edges should be smooth. Only well-fitting crib sheets should be used, not sheets intended for large beds. Crib side rails should always be raised when the parent is not right next to the crib. Additional information about crib and playpen safety can be found at www.safekids.org.

Even before the infant can roll over, he or she wiggles and pushes with the feet. The infant can easily fall from a changing table, sofa, or crib with the side rails down, so the infant should never be left unattended on any surface. If infant seats, bouncy seats, or swings are used, the infant should always be restrained in the seat with the appropriate straps.

The AAP does not recommend the use of infant walkers, because the walker may tip over and the baby fall out of it or the infant may fall down the stairs in it. Walkers allow infants access to things they may not otherwise be capable of reaching until they are able to walk alone, such as hot stoves and items on the edge of the countertop.

As the infant becomes more mobile, learning to crawl and walk, new safety issues arise. Safety gates should be used at the tops and bottoms of stairways. Gates may also be used to block curious infants from rooms that may pose physical danger to them because of sharp-edged furniture or decorative objects. Electrical outlets should be covered with approved safety covers. Cabinets and drawers should be secured with child safety latches. Medications, household cleaning supplies, and other potentially hazardous substances should be stored completely out of reach of infants.

Choking is a risk because infants immediately bring small items to the mouth for exploration. To avoid choking, recommend the following to parents:

- Use only toys recommended for children 0 to 12 months of age.
- Avoid stuffed animals with eyes or buttons that can be dislodged by the persistent infant.
- Keep the floor free of small items (accidentally dropped coins, paper clips, straight pins).
- Avoid feeding popcorn, nuts, carrot slices, grapes, and hot dog pieces to infants.

Suffocation is also a risk for infants. Cribs should not have pillows, comforters, stuffed animals, or other soft items in them. Keep plastic bags of any size away from infants. Avoid the risk of strangulation by keeping window blind and drapery cords out of the infant's reach.

Though no safety measure is as effective as close supervision by a watchful parent or caregiver, the above safety measures can be critical to the infant's well-being.

Safety in the Water

Infants can drown in a very small amount of water. Never leave an infant unattended in the sink, a baby bathtub or standard bathtub, a swimming or wading pool, or any other body of water, even if it is quite shallow. The bathroom door should be kept closed and the toilet lid down. Water should be emptied from tubs, pails, or buckets immediately after use. If the family has a swimming pool, a locked fence or locked screen enclosure should surround it. Exterior doors should be kept locked to prevent the older infant from wandering out to the pool. The AAP recommends that parents use caution when enrolling their infant in an aquatic or swim program. The program should be geared toward water survival skills rather than swimming skills, as the infant is not developmentally ready for formal swimming lessons. Completing an aquatic program does not decrease the risk of drowning; vigilant supervision is still always required.

> Remember Allison Johnson, the infant described in the beginning of the chapter? What anticipatory guidance related to safety would you provide to Allison's parents?

Promoting Nutrition

Adequate nutrition is essential for growth and development. Breastfeeding and bottle-feeding of infant formula are both acceptable means of nutrition in the newborn and infant. Breast milk or formula supplies all of the infant's daily nutritional requirements until 4 to 6 months of age, at which time solid foods may be introduced.

Cultural Factors

Many dietary practices are affected by culture, both in the types of food eaten and in the approach to progression of infant feeding. Some ethnic groups tend to be lactose-intolerant (particularly blacks, Native Americans, and Asians); therefore, alternative sources of calcium must be offered. Explore the cultural practices of the family related to infant feeding so that you can support the family's cultural values.

Nutritional Needs

Newborns and infants are experiencing tremendous growth and need diets that support these rapid changes. Table 4.7 compares fluid and caloric needs in the newborn and infant.

Breastfeeding

The National Association of Pediatric Nurse Practitioners (NAPNAP), the AAP, the American College of Obstetrics and Gynecology, the American Dietetic Association, and the U.S. Breastfeeding Committee of the Department of Health and Human Services all recommend breastfeeding as the natural and preferred method of newborn and infant feeding. In their position statement on breastfeeding (2001), NAPNAP identifies "human milk as superior to all substitute feeding methods." Breast milk provides complete infant nutrition.

Breastfeeding or feeding of expressed human milk is recommended for all infants, including sick or premature newborns (with rare exceptions). The exceptions include infants with galactosemia, maternal use of illicit drugs and a few prescription medications, maternal untreated active tuberculosis, and maternal human immunodeficiency virus (HIV) infection in developed countries.

Data from *Healthy People 2010* (2000) indicate that in 1998 64% of U.S. women breastfed in the early postpartum period, 29% of infants were breastfeeding at 6 months of age, and only 16% were still breastfeeding at 1 year of age. Even partial breastfeeding is helpful and offers some of the health benefits of breastfeeding. Pediatric nurses in the community and the hospital are in an excellent position to promote and support breastfeeding, thereby contributing to the *Healthy People 2010* goal of increasing the proportion of mothers who breastfeed their babies.

Breast Milk Composition

Breast milk includes lactose, lipids, polyunsaturated fatty acids, and amino acids. The ratio of whey to casein protein in breast milk makes it readily digestible. The high concentration of fats and the balance of amino acids are believed to contribute to proper myelination of the nervous system. The concentration of iron in breast milk is less than that of formula, but the iron has increased bioavailability and is sufficient to meet the infant's requirements for the first 4 to 6 months of life.

In addition to complete nutrition, immunologic protection is transferred from mother to infant via breast milk and maternal–infant bonding is promoted. The benefits of breastfeeding are listed in Box 4.1.

Breast Milk Supply and Demand

Frequent, on-demand breastfeeding of the newborn is necessary to establish an adequate milk supply. After delivery of the placenta, levels of progesterone drop dra-

Table 4.7 Nutritional Requirements

Nutritional Requirements	Newborn	Infant
Fluid	140–160 mL/kg/day	100 mL/kg/day for first 10 kg, 50 mL/kg/day for next 10 kg
Calories	105–108 kcal/kg/day	1 to 6 months: 108 kcal/kg 6 to 12 months: 98 kcal/kg

HEALTHY PEOPLE 2010

Objective		Significance
Increase the proportion of mothers who breastfeed their babies.		• Encourage breastfeeding in all mothers beginning with the prenatal visit if applicable.
2010 target:		• Provide accurate education related to breastfeeding.
Early postpartum period	75%	• Be available for questions or problems related to initiation and continuation of breastfeeding. Consult lactation consultant as needed or available.
At 6 months	50%	• Encourage pumping of breast milk when mother returns to work in order to continue breastfeeding.
At 1 year	25%	• Refer to local breastfeeding support groups such as La Leche League.

matically, which stimulates the anterior pituitary to produce prolactin. **Prolactin** stimulates the production of milk in the acinar or alveolar cells of the breast. When the infant sucks at the breast, nervous impulses stimulate further production of breast milk.

BOX 4.1

BENEFITS OF BREASTFEEDING

Infant

- Increased bonding with mother
- Immunologic protection
- Breast milk has anti-infective properties
- Decreased incidence and severity of diarrhea
- Decreased incidence of asthma, otitis media, bacterial meningitis, botulism, urinary tract infection
- Possible enhancement of cognitive development
- Decreased incidence of obesity in later childhood

Maternal

- Increased bonding with infant
- Lessens maternal blood loss in the postpartum period
- Decreased risk of ovarian and premenopausal breast cancer
- Reduced incidence of pregnancy-induced, long-term obesity
- Possible delay of return of ovulation in some women
- Always ready; no mixing!
- Economic advantage

The first "milk" to be produced by the breasts is termed **colostrum**. It is produced for the first 2 to 4 days after birth. Colostrum is a thin, watery yellowish fluid that is easy to digest, as it is high in protein and low in sugar and fat. Colostrum is complete nutrition, all that is needed by the newborn for the first 2 to 4 days of life. Transitional breast milk replaces colostrum on day 2 to 4 after birth. By day 10 after birth, mature breast milk is produced. Mature breast milk has a slightly bluish color and appears thin.

The breastfeeding mother produces milk continually. Called **foremilk**, it collects in the lactiferous sinuses, which are small tubules serving as reservoirs for milk located behind the nipples. The **let-down reflex** is responsible for the release of milk from these reservoirs. When the baby sucks at the breast, oxytocin is released from the posterior pituitary, causing the lactiferous sinuses to contract. This allows milk to "let down" into the nipples, and the infant then sucks the milk. The let-down reflex is triggered not only by suckling at the breast but also by thinking of the baby or by the sound of a baby crying. After the foremilk is let down, new, fattier milk is formed. This **hind milk** helps the breastfed infant to grow quickly. Mothers should be informed that the production of oxytocin during suckling may also cause uterine contractions and may cause afterpains during breastfeeding.

Breastfeeding Technique

Before each breastfeeding session, mothers should wash their hands. It is not necessary to wash the breast in most cases. The mother should be positioned comfortably. A number of positions are possible, and they should be varied throughout the day (Fig. 4.9). The mother may hold the breast in a "C" position if that is helpful to her. Stroke the nipple against the baby's cheek (Fig. 4.10). This should stimulate the infant to open the mouth widely. Bring the baby's wide-open mouth to the breast to form a seal around all of the nipple and areola (Fig. 4.11). When the infant is finished feeding, the mother can break the suction by inserting her finger into the baby's mouth, thus releasing the mouth from the nipple (Fig. 4.12). This technique may prevent the infant from pulling on the nipple, which can lead to soreness and cracking.

Watching and listening to the infant feed may assess the adequacy of the baby's latch technique. The infant who is properly latched on to the breast will suck rhythmically, taking most or all of the areola into the mouth. Audible swallowing should be heard as milk is delivered into the infant's mouth. Assess the mother for pain related to breastfeeding. She should not be in pain if the baby is latched on properly.

Establishment of breastfeeding is best achieved if the infant is allowed to feed on demand, whenever he or she is hungry. This may be as often as every 1½ to 3 hours in the neonate. Infants may feed for 10 to 20 minutes on each breast at each feeding, or longer on just one breast, alternating the breast at each feeding. Both methods are acceptable.

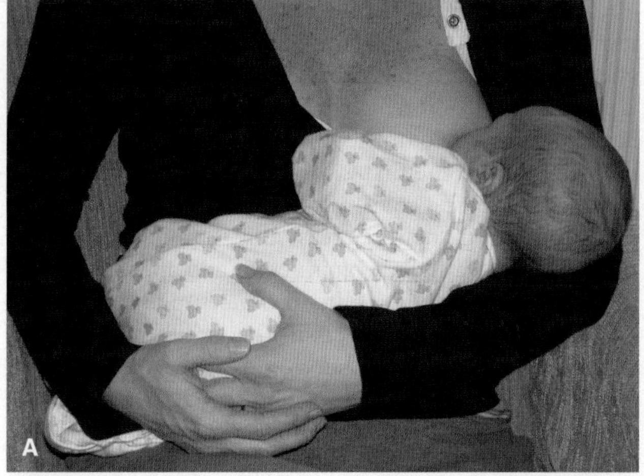

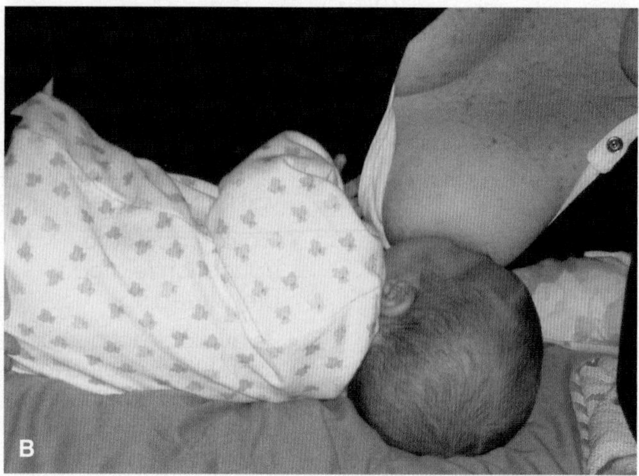

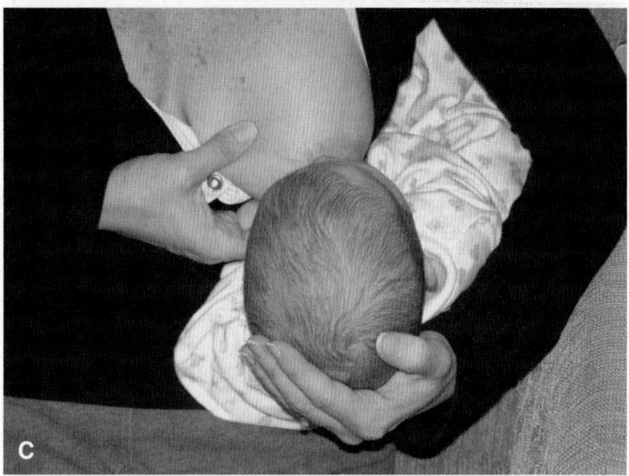

● Figure 4.9 Various positions may be used during breast-feeding: (**A**) cradle hold, (**B**) side-lying, (**C**) football hold.

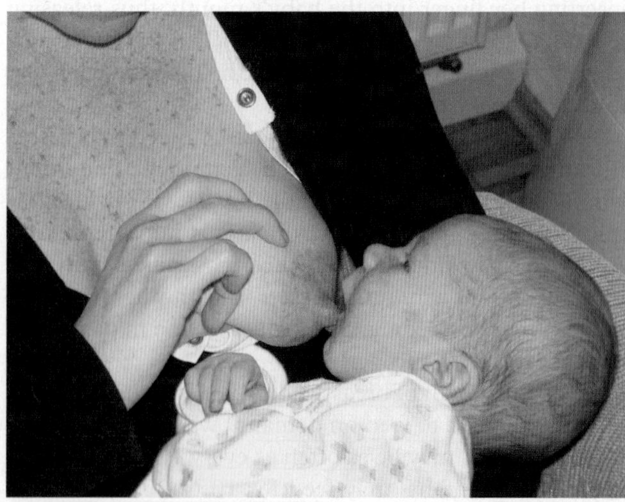

● Figure 4.10 Stroking the infant's cheek with the nipple will elicit the rooting reflex.

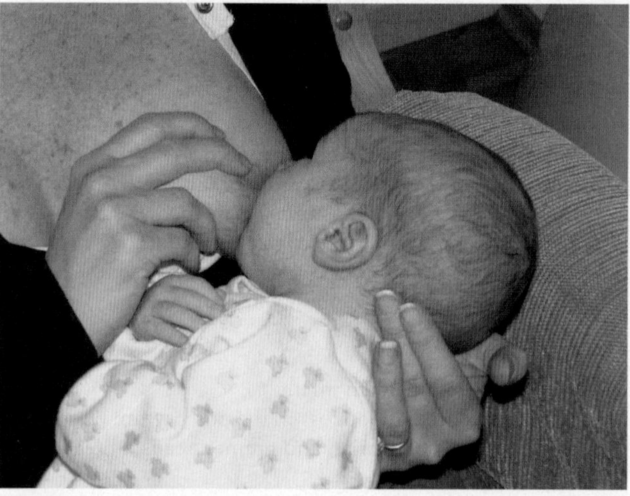

● Figure 4.11 Bringing the infant's open mouth to the breast, rather than bringing the breast to the infant, helps the infant correctly latch on. The infant's mouth forms a seal around all of the nipple and areola. Note the "C" position for holding the breast during latching on.

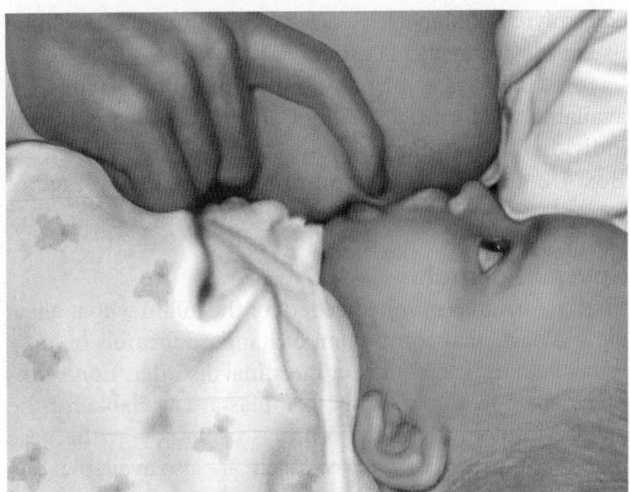

● Figure 4.12 Inserting the little finger between the areola and the infant's mouth helps to break the suction.

The breastfeeding infant does not need supplementation with water or formula even in the first few days of life as long as he or she continues to wet six to eight diapers per day.

Teaching Guideline 4.1 offers solutions for breastfeeding problems. Additional information about breastfeeding may be found on www.aap.org/family/brstguid.htm, www.breastfeeding.com, www.breastfeeding.org, www.lalecheleague.org, www.medela.com, www.promom.org, www.verybestbaby.com, and www.waba.org.br.

Bottle Feeding

For the mother who does not desire to, or cannot, breastfeed, commercially prepared formulas are available for bottle-feeding. These formulas are designed to imitate human milk. Standard infant formulas based on cow's milk provide 20 kcal/ounce and use lactose as a source for carbohydrates. Vegetable oil is used as the source of fat; whey or casein provides protein. Newer cow's milk–based formulas contain long-chain polyunsaturated fatty acids that are thought to improve brain development. Ordinary cow's milk is not recommended for the first year of life.

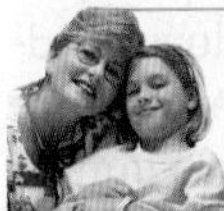

Cow's milk does not provide an adequate balance of nutrients for the growing infant, especially iron. It may also overload the infant's renal system with inappropriate amounts of protein, sodium, and minerals.

Only formulas that are fortified with iron should be used. Iron stores that the infant received prenatally are depleted by 4 to 6 months of age. To prevent iron-deficiency anemia, poor growth patterns, and impaired development, iron-fortified formulas must be used. The AAP recommends that commercial formulas provide 10 to 12 mg of iron per liter (AAP, Committee on Nutrition, 1999). Commercial formulas also provide an adequate blend of essential vitamins and minerals.

Feeding Patterns

Infant feeding is an opportune time to establish good eating behaviors. The infant should always be held while

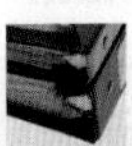

TEACHING GUIDELINE 4.1

Promoting Breastfeeding

Problem	Solutions
Sore nipples	Prevention: encourage appropriate latch on from the beginning. Expose nipples to air between feedings. Allow breast milk to dry on nipples. Aloe vera or vitamin E may help to heal sore nipples. Medical-grade lanolin or preservative-free lanolin (Lansinoh) may be helpful.
Engorgement	Apply warm compresses or encourage the mother to take a warm shower prior to having the baby latch on. Warmth encourages some of the milk to be released, allowing the breast to soften and making it easier for the infant to latch on.
Poor sucking	Feed on cue, not on a schedule. Encourage the sleepy infant by stroking the feet, undressing, and rubbing the head.
Inadequate milk supply	Decrease maternal stress. Encourage adequate maternal diet and fluid intake. Mothers who return to work must pump in order to keep up milk supply when away from infant.
Father feels left out	Encourage father to participate in other aspects of care.
Mother worries about adequacy of breast milk	If infant is voiding six times per day and gaining weight, then he or she is receiving enough milk and appropriate nutrition.

being bottle-fed. Cradling in a semi-upright position allows for additional bonding time, as the infant can see the caregiver's face while feeding (Fig. 4.13). Talking or singing during feeding time also increases bonding. As with breastfed infants, the bottle-fed infant should be fed on cue. Overfeeding with the bottle increases the incidence of gastroesophageal reflux, so families need to learn their baby's cues to hunger and satiety.

It is important to feed the baby when he or she displays signs of hunger. Crying is a late sign of hunger; earlier signs include making sucking motions, sucking on hands, or putting the fist to the chin. The infant should be burped two or three times per feeding, when he or she slows feeding or stops sucking. Newborns may only take a half-ounce to 1 ounce per feeding initially, working up to 2 to 3 ounces in the first few days. They need to feed about six to ten times per day. The infant will gradually be able to ingest more formula per feeding. By 3 to 4 months of age, babies feed four or five times per day and take 6 to 7 ounces per feeding. Most infants will not require specific amounts per feeding; the infant should be fed until full. To prevent overfeeding, healthy bottle-fed infants should be allowed to self-regulate the amount of formula ingested per feeding. When the baby is satiated, he or she might fall asleep, spit out the nipple or formula, play with the nipple, or lie quietly, only sucking once in a while.

Types of Formulas and Bottles

Parents may choose to use commercial formulas that are ready-to-feed or available as a concentrate or as a powder. Parents should follow the instructions for mixing the concentrate or powder to avoid dehydration or fluid and electrolyte imbalances. Ready-to-feed formula should be used as is and never diluted.

A wide variety of baby bottle and nipple types are available for formula feeding, and the choice is purely individual. Few infants require special nipples or bottles. Box 4.2 gives guidelines on preparation and storage of formula and care of bottles.

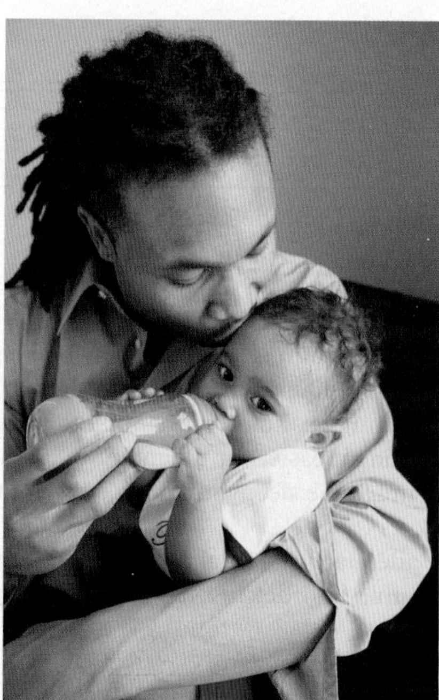

● Figure 4.13 Technique for bottle-feeding the infant.

Special Formulas

Special formulas may be needed for the infant who is allergic to a particular component of standard formula or has a renal, hepatic, metabolic, or intestinal disorder. For example, lactose-free cow's milk formulas are available for the lactose-intolerant child. Formulas using soy as the base ingredient instead of whey or casein are also available. Soy formulas are necessary for infants with a milk allergy, and they may be appealing to the vegetarian family.

These special formulas are designed to meet the nutritional needs of infants, depending on the disorder. Infants who fail to gain weight may be placed on standard infant formula prepared to deliver a higher caloric density per ounce. Preterm infants (those born at less than 34 weeks' gestation) need adequate nutrition to exhibit catch-up growth. Good catch-up growth (quadrupling or even quintupling the birth weight) in the first year or so of life is critical for adequate head growth and avoidance of neurodevelopmental consequences. Premature infant follow-up formulas are designed to provide additional calories, protein, and a particular calcium-to-phosphorus ratio as well as the vitamins and minerals needed for adequate catch-up growth.

Progressing to Solid Foods

After 6 months of age, infants usually require the nutrients available in solid foods in addition to their breast milk or formula. Progressing to feeding solid foods can be exciting and trying. Before solid foods are attempted, the

BOX 4.2

PREPARATION AND STORAGE OF BOTTLES AND FORMULA

- Wash nipples and bottles in hot soapy water and rinse well OR
- Run nipples and bottles through the dishwasher.
- Store tightly covered ready-to-feed formula can after opening in refrigerator for up to 48 hours.
- After mixing concentrate or powdered formula, store tightly covered in refrigerator for up to 48 hours.
- Do not reheat and reuse partially used bottles. Throw away the unused portion after each feeding.
- Do not add cereal to the formula in the bottle.
- Do not sweeten formula with honey.
- Warm formula by placing bottle in a container of hot water.
- Do not microwave formula.

infant should be assessed for readiness to progress. Parents need instruction in choosing appropriate solid foods and support in the progression process.

Assessing Infant Readiness

Several factors contribute to the appropriate timing of solid food introduction. The tongue extrusion reflex is necessary for sucking to be an automatic reaction—that is, when a nipple or other item is placed in the mouth, the tongue extrudes and sucking begins. This reflex disappears at about 4 to 6 months of age. Introducing solid food with a spoon prior to 4 to 6 months of age will result in extrusion of the tongue. The parent may think that the infant does not want the food and is spitting it out intentionally, but this is not the case; the infant simply must be mature enough to eat with a spoon (absence of extrusion reflex).

The ability to swallow solid food does not become completely functional until 4 to 6 months of age. Enzymes to appropriately digest food other than breast milk and formula are also not present in sufficient quantities until the age of 4 to 6 months.

Before the introduction of solid foods and the cup, the infant should be able to sit supported in a high chair. Solids should be fed with a spoon, with the infant in an upright position.

Choosing Appropriate Solid Foods

Iron-fortified rice cereal mixed with a small amount of breast milk or formula is a good choice for the first solid food. The cereal is easily digested and its taste is generally well accepted. The cereal should be quite thin at first; it can be mixed to a thicker consistency as the infant gets older. Once the feeding of cereal with a spoon is successful, other single foods may be introduced. The foods should be puréed to a smooth consistency, whether prepackaged "baby food" or puréed at home.

The introduction of one new food every 4 to 7 days is recommended. This allows for identification of food allergies (Box 4.3). No salt, sugar, or other seasoning should be added to these first foods.

Generally, by 8 months of age the infant is ready for more texture in his or her foods. Soft, smashed table food without large chunks is appropriate. Finger foods such as Cheerios, soft green bean pieces, or soft peas may also be offered. Avoid hard foods that the infant may choke on. Strained, puréed, or mashed meats may be introduced at 10 to 12 months of age.

The cup should be introduced at 6 to 8 months of age. One ounce of breast milk or formula should be placed in the cup while the infant is learning. This will decrease the amount of mess should the cup be spilled. Old-fashioned sippy cups are generally acceptable for use, though older infants quickly learn to drink from an ordinary cup with assistance when they are thirsty. Newer "no-spill" sippy cups are not recommended for general home use. They require sucking much like a bottle and do not really encourage the child to learn cup drinking. They should be reserved for use on long trips in the car or other instances in which spills should be avoided (Rychnovsky, 2000).

Fruit juice is unnecessary and should not be introduced until 6 months of age. If juice is given, it should be limited to 2 to 4 ounces per day. Fruit itself is much more nutritious than fruit juice. If infants are allowed to consume larger quantities of juice, it can displace important nutrients from breast milk or formula.

BOX 4.3

FOODS TO AVOID IN INFANCY

- Honey
- Egg yolks and meats (until 10 months of age)
- Excessive amounts of fruit juice
- Foods likely to cause choking
  - Peanuts
  - Popcorn
  - Other small hard foods (e.g., raw carrot chunks)
  - Grapes and hot dog slices (must be cut in smaller pieces)
- Foods likely to result in allergic reaction
  - Citrus
  - Strawberries
  - Wheat
  - Cow's milk
  - Egg whites
  - Peanut butter

Promoting Healthy Eating Habits

Infants and children learn about food within a social context, so the family plays an important role in creating healthy eating habits. Families "model" eating behaviors; infants and children learn about eating through watching others. Lifelong eating patterns are often established in childhood, so it is important to emphasize healthy eating practices beginning in infancy (Nicklaus & Fisher, 2003). Parents should not let infants eat whatever they want (permissive feeding style); this will lead to fights over eating in the future. Infants may require as many as 20 exposures to a new food before it is accepted. On the other hand, infants should not be coerced into eating all that is provided (authoritarian feeding style). Forcing an infant to eat when he or she is full sets the child up for overeating in the future and may lead to more power struggles. Parents need to find a balance between the permissive and authoritarian feeding styles to establish lifelong healthy eating patterns in their children. By providing education about appropriate diet and feeding behaviors, the nurse can help the family to accomplish this goal.

> **Think back to Allison Johnson.** What questions should you ask Allison's parents related to her nutritional intake? What anticipatory guidance related to nutrition would be appropriate?

Teaching Newborn Care

Educate new parents (and re-educate parents with subsequent additions to the family) about the basics of newborn care. Refer to Teaching Guideline 4.2 for basic newborn care.

Promoting Healthy Sleep and Rest

Newborns sleep about 20 hours a day, waking frequently to feed and quickly returning to sleep. By 3 months of age, most infants sleep 7 to 8 hours per night without waking. They will continue to take about three naps a day. By 4 months of age the infant is more active and alert and may have more trouble going to sleep in the evening. Night waking may occur, but the infant should be capable of sleeping through the night and does not require a night feeding. By 12 months of age infants sleep 8 to 12 hours per night and take two naps per day.

Discuss safe sleeping practices with parents of newborns and infants; the baby should sleep on a firm mattress without pillows or comforters. The baby's bed should be placed away from air conditioner vents, open windows, and open heaters. Sudden infant death syndrome (SIDS) has been associated with prone positioning of newborns and infants, so the infant should be placed to sleep on the back or side. See Healthy People 2010.

In the newborn period, the primary caregiver should try to sleep when the baby is sleeping. Since newborns need to be fed every 1½ to 3 hours around the clock, parents may become exhausted quickly and are often eager for the infant to sleep through the night. Adding rice cereal to the evening bottle has not been proven to discourage night waking and is not recommended. Provide support to parents of newborns and educate them on infant sleeping patterns.

It is important to establish a bedtime routine around 4 months of age due to the infant's increased alertness and activity level. The baby who is 4 months or older needs a time of calming and relaxation before going to sleep. A consistent bedtime routine should be established, perhaps a bath followed by rocking, singing, or reading. The infant should fall asleep in his or her own crib rather than being rocked to sleep or held until sleeping and then put in the crib. After 4 months of age, infants must learn to soothe themselves back to sleep following night waking. Older infants may exhibit head banging as a form of self-soothing and use it to fall asleep at night. Night feedings are unnecessary at this age and will create a routine of further night waking that will be difficult to break. Parents should minimize attention and stimulation provided during a

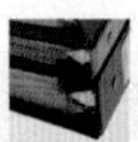

TEACHING GUIDELINE 4.2

Routine Newborn Care

Primary care follow-up	• First visit within first week of life; also see provider if: • Temperature below 98° or above 100.4° F rectally • Poor feeding • "Not acting right" • Excessively sleepy • Vomiting, diarrhea, or difficulty breathing
Weight gain/loss	• Weight loss first 5 to 10 days of life, then should gain weight routinely
Wet diapers	• Minimum of six per day if bottle-feeding or after milk comes in when breastfeeding
Bathing	• Sponge bathe until cord falls off. • Clean the dirty parts daily; full bath every few days. • Do not allow infant to become chilled with the bath.
Umbilical cord care	• Clean base of cord with alcohol. • Dried cord falls off after 1 to 2 weeks. • Call provider if skin is red or cord has drainage, bleeding, or foul odor.
Illness prevention	• Parents and caregivers should practice good hand washing. • Limit exposure to individuals with contagious illness.
Dressing	• Newborns do not usually need additional bundling except in very cold weather. • Dress the infant in the amount of clothing that the parents are comfortable wearing (T-shirt is sufficient in summer, long pants and long-sleeved shirts in winter).
Sleep	• Put the infant to sleep on his or her back or side to decrease the risk for sudden infant death syndrome.

HEALTHY PEOPLE 2010

Objective	Significance
Increase the percentage of healthy full-term infants who are put down to sleep on their backs.	• Begin teaching about "back to sleep" at prenatal or newborn visit. • Use each encounter with the young infant as an opportunity to reinforce the supine position for sleep.

night waking. Briefly checking on the infant to ascertain his or her safety, followed by placing the infant back in a lying position and telling him or her good night, is all that is needed. This may have to be repeated several times before the infant falls back to sleep. It is important to keep interactions brief during the night waking so that the infant learns to fall back to sleep on his or her own. Continued issues with night waking should be discussed with the infant's primary care provider.

> **What anticipatory guidance** should you provide to Allison's parents in relation to sleep?

Promoting Healthy Teeth and Gums

Healthy teeth and gums require proper oral hygiene and appropriate fluoride supplementation. Children over 6 months of age whose drinking water source contains less than 0.3 parts per million may require fluoride supplementation. Excess fluoride ingestion can result in discoloration of the teeth (fluorosis). Early childhood dental caries can result from pooling of milk or juice around teeth and gums.

Before tooth eruption, parents should clean the child's gums after feeding with a damp washcloth. After teeth have erupted, parents can continue to use a soft cloth for tooth cleaning and then eventually use a small soft-bristled toothbrush. Toothpaste is unnecessary in infancy. Infants should not be allowed to take milk or juice bottles to bed, as the high sugar content of the fluid in contact with the teeth all night leads to dental caries (see section on baby bottle mouth below). Weaning from the bottle at age 12 to 15 months may help prevent dental caries. No-spill sippy cups have also been implicated in the development of dental caries and should be avoided. The American Academy of Pediatric Dentistry recommends that infants receive their first dental visit by the age of 1 year.

Promoting Appropriate Discipline

Parenting requires ever-changing adaptations to the developing infant's needs. Unconditional love, patience, and compassion must be balanced with the parents' needs. **Discipline** helps build self-esteem in children as well as setting standards for social interactions. The primary goal of discipline is to teach an infant limits. Discipline should be used to help the infant solve problems. The infant's activities are based on the basic needs of food, security, warmth, love, and comfort (Ateah et al., 2003). Misbehavior is the result of an unmet need, and the parents should respond accordingly.

As the infant is undergoing rapid changes in motor skills, safety needs increase. Nurses should encourage the parents to "childproof" their home so that the infant can develop physical skills without being at risk. In a childproof home, fewer restrictions need to be placed on the infant's behavior, and he or she can explore.

Physical punishment or spanking should never be used in infancy. Infants are at increased risk for physical injury from spanking and cannot make the connection between the spanking and the undesirable behavior (Gottesman, 2000). Providing a safe environment, redirection away from undesirable behaviors, and saying "no" in appropriate instances are far more effective. For example, when the infant is in potential danger (e.g., inserting a key into an electrical outlet, attempting to ingest a poisonous substance, or reaching into the toilet), the parent must use a firm but calm and brisk approach. If the infant knows the parent is serious, he or she will usually comply more quickly.

Remaining calm, firm, and consistent is necessary. Immediacy is also an important component of appropriate discipline. The infant cannot make the connection between a subsequent punishment or discussion of behavior with the earlier event itself. Positive reinforcement should be used to support good behavior.

Addressing Child Care Needs

Many mothers work outside the home, there are many single-parent families, and many families live a distance away from relatives. In all of these circumstances, infants may need to be cared for outside the home, often in child care settings or home day care centers.

Parents contemplating child care must consider a number of factors. Do they want a sitter to come to their home? Will they use a traditional day care center or a home care situation with fewer children? How much can they afford? If families choose to use a freestanding day care center or a home-based day care center, they should make sure that the provider is appropriately licensed. Parents should feel comfortable with the caregiver-to-child ratio. Are the caregivers trained in infant CPR and first aid? Families may need to visit or interview several facilities before finding one that meets their requirements.

When an older infant is attending a child care situation for the first time, it may be helpful to visit the center once or twice beforehand so that the infant can get used to the caregivers from the comfort and security of the parent's lap. Warn parents that separation anxiety in late infancy can cause a disturbing crying episode when the parent leaves. Reassure parents that the infant will not suffer harm due to the separation.

ADDRESSING COMMON DEVELOPMENTAL CONCERNS

Parents commonly have multiple concerns during normal infant growth and development. Although most of these issues are not actual disease states or behavior problems, nurses must be aware of these issues to recognize them and to intervene appropriately.

Colic

Healthy 6-week-old infants cry for a total of about 3 hours every day. Crying and fussing is more prevalent in the evenings. By age 12 weeks, the total amount of crying is about 1 hour per day, and infants are better able to soothe themselves by this age. **Colic** is defined as inconsolable crying that lasts 3 hours or longer per day and for which there is no physical cause. It typically resolves by 3 months of age, coinciding with the age at which infants are better able to soothe themselves (e.g., by finger sucking). The cause of colic is thought to be problems in the gastrointestinal or neurologic system (probably system immaturity), temperament, or parenting style of the mother or father (Nield & Kamat, 2003). Some parents are overly anxious or overly attentive or, at the other extreme, may not give the infant the attention he or she needs. Any of these may contribute to a baby's fussing and crying.

Prolonged crying leads to increased stress among caregivers. Failure to stop the crying leads to frustration, and crying that prevents the parents from sleeping contributes to the exhaustion they are already experiencing.

Educate parents that normal crying increases by the time the infant is 6 weeks old and diminishes by about 12 weeks. When faced with a colicky baby, parents should develop a stepwise approach to checking that all of the infant's basic needs are met. When these needs are met, attempts at soothing the infant may be used. Reducing stimulation may decrease the length of crying. Carrying the infant more may also be helpful. Some infants respond to the motion of an infant swing or a car ride. Vibration, white noise, or swaddling may also help to decrease fussing in some infants. Pacifiers can be soothing to babies who need additional non-nutritive sucking. Parents should try one intervention at a time, taking care not to stimulate the infant excessively in the process of searching for solutions. Nurses should provide ongoing support to the parents of a colicky infant and reassure them that this is a temporary condition that will resolve in time.

Spitting Up

Spitting up (regurgitating small amounts of stomach contents) occurs in all infants. Approximately 50% of normal 2-month-olds spit up at least twice a day (Hobbie et al., 2000). Although spitting up after feeding is normal, it can be a cause of great concern to parents. Overfed babies who feed based on a parent-designed schedule and those who burp poorly are more likely to spit up. For some infants, the amount and frequency of spitting up are significant, and it may indicate gastroesophageal reflux.

Teach parents that feeding smaller amounts on a more frequent basis may help to decrease spitting-up episodes. Always burp the baby at least two or three times per feeding. Keep the baby upright for 30 minutes after feeding and do not lay the infant prone after feeding. Avoid bouncing or excess activity immediately after feeding. Positioning in an infant seat compresses the stomach and is not recommended. When placing the baby in bed, position him or her on the side with the head of the bed slightly elevated.

Reassure parents that if the infant is wetting at least six diapers per 24 hours and gaining weight, the spitting up is normal. If the infant vomits one third or more of most feedings, chokes when vomiting, or experiences forceful emesis, the primary care provider should be notified.

Thumb Sucking, Pacifiers, and Security Items

Infants demonstrate a clear need for non-nutritive sucking: even fetuses can be observed sucking their thumbs or fingers *in utero*. Thumb sucking is a healthy self-comforting activity. Infants who suck their thumbs or pacifiers often are better able to soothe themselves than those who do not. Studies have not shown that sucking either thumbs or pacifiers leads to the need for orthodontic braces unless the sucking continues well beyond the early school-age period. However, pacifier use has been associated with the increased incidence of otitis media (Niemela et al., 2000), and hygiene is always a concern as pacifiers often fall on the floor.

Infants may also become attached to a doll, stuffed animal, or blanket. Just like thumb sucking, the attachment item gives the infant the security to self-soothe when he or she is uncomfortable.

Families need to explore their feelings and cultural preferences about sucking habits and security items. Parents should not try to break the habit during a stressful time for the infant. When the infant is intensely trying to master a new skill such as sitting or walking, he or she may need the sucking or security item to self-soothe. Pacifiers and security items can be physically taken away at some point, but the thumb is attached. The infant who has become attached to thumb sucking should not have additional attention drawn to the issue, as that may prolong thumb sucking.

Families of infants who use pacifiers may want to wean the infant from the pacifier when the child is 6 to 9 months of age. This is the time when the need for additional sucking naturally decreases. Attempts to wean the child from a security blanket or toy should probably be reserved for after infancy.

Teething

Discomfort is common as the tooth breaks through the periodontal membrane. Infants may drool, bite on hard objects, or increase finger sucking. Some infants may become very irritable, refuse to eat, and not sleep well. Fever, vomiting, and diarrhea are generally not considered a sign of teething but rather of illness.

Teething pain results from inflammation. Teach parents that application of cold may be soothing to the gums. The infant may chew on a frozen teething ring, or parents can rub an ice cube wrapped in a washcloth on the gums. Over-the-counter topical anesthetics such as baby Orajel may also be helpful. Parents should apply the ointment correctly to the gums, avoiding the lips, as these ointments cause numbing. Occasionally, oral acetaminophen or ibuprofen may be given to relieve pain.

> **Refer back to 6-month-old Allison Johnson.** List some common developmental concerns of 6-month-old infants. What anticipatory guidance related to these concerns would you provide to her parents?

References

Books and Journals

American Academy of Pediatrics. (1997). Policy statement: Breastfeeding and the use of human milk. *Pediatrics, 100*(6), 1035–1039.

American Academy of Pediatrics. (2000). Policy statement: Changing concepts of sudden infant death syndrome: Implications for infant sleeping environment and sleep position. *Pediatrics, 105*(3), 650–656.

American Academy of Pediatrics. (2000). Policy statement: Swimming programs for infants and toddlers. *Pediatrics, 105*(4), 868–870.

American Academy of Pediatrics. (2001). Policy statement: The use and misuse of fruit juice in pediatrics (RE0047). *Pediatrics, 107*(5), 1201–1213.

American Academy of Pediatrics. (2003). Policy statement: Poison treatment in the home. *Pediatrics, 112*(5), 1182–1185.

American Academy of Pediatrics. (2004). Special challenges in breastfeeding. Accessed 12/20/04 at www.aaporg/healthtopics/breastfeeding.cfm.

American Academy of Pediatrics. (2005). The injury prevention program, age-related safety sheets: Birth to 6 months. Accessed 1/0/05 at www.aap.org/family/birthto6.htm.

American Academy of Pediatrics. (2005). The injury prevention program, age-related safety sheets: 6 to 12 months. Accessed 1/0/05 at www.aap.org/family/6to12mo/htm.

American Academy of Pediatrics, Committee on Nutrition. (1999). Policy statement: Iron fortification of infant formulas (RE9865). *Pediatrics, 104*(1), 119–123.

American College of Obstetrics and Gynecology. (2000). *Breastfeeding: Maternal and infant aspects* (ACOG Educational Bulletin No. 258). Washington, D.C.: American College of Obstetrics and Gynecology.

American Dietetic Association. (2001). Position of the American Dietetic Association: Breaking the barriers to breastfeeding. *Journal of the American Dietetic Association, 101*(10), 1213–1220.

Arias, A., Bennison, J., Justus, K., & Thurman, D. (2001). Educating parents about normal stool pattern changes in infants. *Journal of Pediatric Health Care, 15*(5), 269–274.

Arnold, S., & Bernstein, H. H. (2000). Newborn discharge: A time to be especially thoughtful. *Contemporary Pediatrics, 17*(10), 47–80.

Ateah, C. A., Secco, L., & Woodgate, R. L. (2003). The risks and alternatives to physical punishment use with children. *Journal of Pediatric Health Care, 17*(3), 126–132.

Atkinson, P. M., Parks, D. K., Cooley, S. M., & Sarkis, S. L. (2002). Reach out and read: A pediatric clinic-based approach to early literacy promotion. *Journal of Pediatric Health Care, 16*(1), 10–15.

Blackwell, P. B., & Baker, B. M. (2002). Estimating communication competence of infants and toddlers. *Journal of Pediatric Health Care, 16*(1), 29–35.

Borghese-Lang, T., Morrison, L., Ogle, A., & Wright, A. (2003). Successful bottle feeding of the young infant. *Journal of Pediatric Health Care, 17*(2), 94–101.

Brazelton, T. B. (1983). *Infants and mothers: Differences in development.* New York: Delacourte Press.

Brazelton, T. B. (1992). *Touchpoints, the essential reference: Your child's emotional and behavioral development.* New York: Perseus Books Group.

Brazelton, T. B., & Cramer, B. D. (1990). *The earliest relationship: Parents, infants and the drama of early attachment.* New York: Addison Wesley.

Centers for Disease Control & Prevention. (1998). Recommendations to prevent and control iron deficiency in the United States. *Morbidity and Mortality Weekly Report, 47*(RR-3), 1–36.

Department of Health and Human Services. (2000). *HHS blueprint for action on breastfeeding.* Washington, D.C.: U.S. Department of Health and Human Services.

Erikson, E. H. (1963). *Childhood and society* (2nd ed.). New York: W. W. Norton and Company.

Fierro-Cobas, V. (2001). Language development in bilingual children: A primer for pediatricians. *Contemporary Pediatrics, 18*(7), 79–98.

Fishman, M. A. (1999). Evaluation of the child with neurologic disease. In J. A. McMillan (Ed.), *Oski's pediatrics: Principles and practice.* Philadelphia: Lippincott Williams & Wilkins.

Gabbard, G. O. (2000). Psychoanalysis. In B. J. Sadock & V. A. Sadock (Eds.), *Kaplan and Sadock's comprehensive textbook of psychiatry* (7th ed.). Philadelphia: Lippincott Williams & Wilkins.

Georgieff, M. K. (2001). Taking a rational approach to the choice of formula. *Contemporary Pediatrics, 18*(8), 112–130.

Gilger, M. A. (1999). Normal gastrointestinal function. In J. A. McMillan (Ed.), *Oski's pediatrics: Principles and practice.* Philadelphia: Lippincott Williams & Wilkins.

Gopnik, A. (2003). Crib notes: The innate drive to learn. *Pediatric Basics, 102,* 2–9.

Gottesman, M. M. (2000). Nurturing the social and emotional development of children, a.k.a. discipline. *Journal of Pediatric Health Care, 14*(2), 81–84.

Gottesman, M. M. (2001). Making time for teaching. *Journal of Pediatric Health Care, 15*(2), 94–97.

Green, M. (Ed.) (1998) *Bright futures: Guidelines for health supervision of infants, children and, adolescents* (rev. ed.). Arlington, VA: National Center for Education in Maternal and Child Health.

Harris, J. C. (1999). Developmental perspective. In J. A. McMillan (Ed.), *Oski's pediatrics: Principles and practice.* Philadelphia: Lippincott Williams & Wilkins.

Healthy People 2010. (2000). *Breastfeeding, newborn screening and service systems.* Washington, D.C.: U.S. Department of Health and Human Services. Accessed 10/17/03 at www.healthypeople.gov/Document/HTML/Volume2/16MICH.htm.

Hobbie, C., Baker, S., & Bayerl, C. (2000). Parental understanding of basic infant nutrition: misinformed feeding choices. *Journal of Pediatric Health Care, 14*(1), 26–31.

Kazal, L. A. (2002). Prevention of iron deficiency in infants and toddlers. *American Family Physician, 66*(7), 1217–1224.

Lawrence, R. A., & Lawrence, R. M. (1999). *Breastfeeding: A guide for the medical profession* (5th ed.). St. Louis: Mosby.

Leininger, M. (2001). *Culture, care, diversity and universality: A theory of nursing.* Sudbury, MA: Jones & Bartlett.

National Association of Pediatric Nurse Practitioners. (2001). Position statement: Breastfeeding. *Journal of Pediatric Health Care, 15*(5), 22A.

National Association of Pediatric Nurse Practitioners. (2001). Position statement: Child care. *Journal of Pediatric Health Care, 15*(2), 35A.

National Safe Kids Campaign. *Baby: Crib safety checklist.* Accessed 1/10/05 at http://www.hsca.com/membersonly/USDHHSlink.htm.

Nicklaus, T. A., & Fisher, J. O. (2003). To each his own: Family influences on children's food preferences. *Pediatric Basics, 102,* 13–20.

Nield, L. S., & Kamat, D. (2003). Infant colic: What works, what doesn't? *Consultant for Pediatricians, 2*(6), 230–234.

Niemela, M., Pihakari, O., Pokka, T., & Uhari, M. (2000). Pacifier as a risk factor for acute otitis media: A randomized, controlled trial of parental counseling. *Pediatrics, 106,* 483–488.

Palmer, F. B., & Capute, A. J. (1999). Streams of development: The keys to developmental assessment. In J. A. McMillan (Ed.), *Oski's pediatrics: Principles and practice.* Philadelphia: Lippincott Williams & Wilkins.

Piaget, J. (1969). *The theory of stages in cognitive development.* New York: McGraw-Hill.

Preboth, M. (2002). Physical activity in infants, toddlers, and preschoolers. *American Family Physician, 65*(8), 1694–1696.

Recht, M., & Pearson, H. A. (1999). Diseases of the blood. In J. A. McMillan (Ed.), *Oski's pediatrics: Principles and practice.* Philadelphia: Lippincott Williams & Wilkins.

Record, S., Montgomery, D. R., & Milano, M. (2000). Fluoride supplementation and caries prevention. *Journal of Pediatric Health Care, 14*(5), 247–249.

Rychnovsky, J. D. (2000). No-spill sippy cups. *Journal of Pediatric Health Care, 14*(5), 207–208.

Shelor, S. P. (ed.) (1998). *Caring for your baby and young child: Birth to age 5.* New York: Bantam Books.

Starr, N. B. (2001). Kids and car safety: Beyond car seats and seat belts. *Journal of Pediatric Health Care, 15*(5), 257–259.

Stein, M. T. (2001). Co-sleeping (bedsharing) among infants and toddlers. *Pediatrics 107*(4), 873–877.

Turecki, S. (2003). The behavioral complaint: Symptom of a psychiatric disorder or a matter of temperament? *Contemporary Pediatrics, 20*(8), 111–119.

U.S. Breastfeeding Committee. (2001). Breastfeeding in the United States: A national agenda. Washington, D.C.: U.S. Department of Health and Human Services, Health Resources and Services Administration, Maternal and Child Health Bureau. Accessed 10/17/03 at www.usbreastfeeding.org/USBC-Strategic-Plan-2001.pdf.

Websites

www.aapd.org American Academy of Pediatric Dentistry

www.dbpeds.org recommendations for behavioral and developmental screening in children

www.denverII.com Denver Developmental Screening materials

www.kidshealth.com Nemours Foundation's Center for Child Health Media

www.kidsource.com a parent-supported group for children's health, growth, and development

www.lansinoh.com lanolin for breastfeeding

www.medela.com breastfeeding information from Medela, Inc.

www.orajel.com teething information from Del Pharmaceuticals

www.pediatricinstitute.com Johnson & Johnson Pediatric Institute

www.zerotothree.org The Zero to Three: National Center for Infants, Toddlers and Families

Chapter WORKSHEET

● MULTIPLE CHOICE QUESTIONS

1. The mother of a 3-month-old boy asks the nurse about starting solid foods. What is the most appropriate response by the nurse?
   a. "It's okay to start puréed solids at this age if fed via the bottle."
   b. "Infants don't require solid food until 12 months of age."
   c. "Solid foods should be delayed until age 6 months, when the infant can handle a spoon on his own."
   d. "The tongue extrusion reflex disappears at age 4 to 6 months, making it a good time to start solid foods."

2. The father of a 2-month-old girl is expressing concern that his infant may be getting spoiled. The nurse's best response is:
   a. "She just needs love and attention. Don't worry; she's too young to spoil."
   b. "Consistently meeting the infant's needs helps promote a sense of trust."
   c. "Infants need to be fed and cleaned; if you're sure those needs are met, just let her to cry."
   d. "Consistency in meeting needs is important, but you're right, holding her too much will spoil her."

3. Parents of an 8-month-old girl express concern that she cries when left with the babysitter. How does the nurse best explain this behavior?
   a. Crying when left with the sitter may indicate difficulty with building trust.
   b. Stranger anxiety should not occur until toddlerhood; this concern should be investigated.
   c. Separation anxiety is normal at this age; the infant recognizes parents as separate beings.
   d. Perhaps the sitter doesn't meet the infant's needs; choose a different sitter.

● CRITICAL THINKING EXERCISES

1. The mother of an 11-month-old boy who was born at 24 weeks' gestation is concerned about his size and motor skills. What information should the nurse provide?
2. An infant's mother thinks there may be something wrong with him because "he spits up so much." What further information should the nurse obtain?
3. If you determine that the infant in the question above is experiencing normal spitting up associated with his developmental age, develop a brief teaching plan to review with the mother.

● STUDY ACTIVITIES

1. A mother brings her 9-month-old boy to the clinic for a well-child check-up. She has questions about feeding, speech, and walking. Develop a teaching plan of anticipatory guidance for the 9-month-old infant.
2. Develop a safety plan for the 12-month-old infant.
3. In the clinical setting, observe two infants of the same age, one who is developing appropriately for his or her age and one who is delayed. Note the similarities and differences between the two infants.

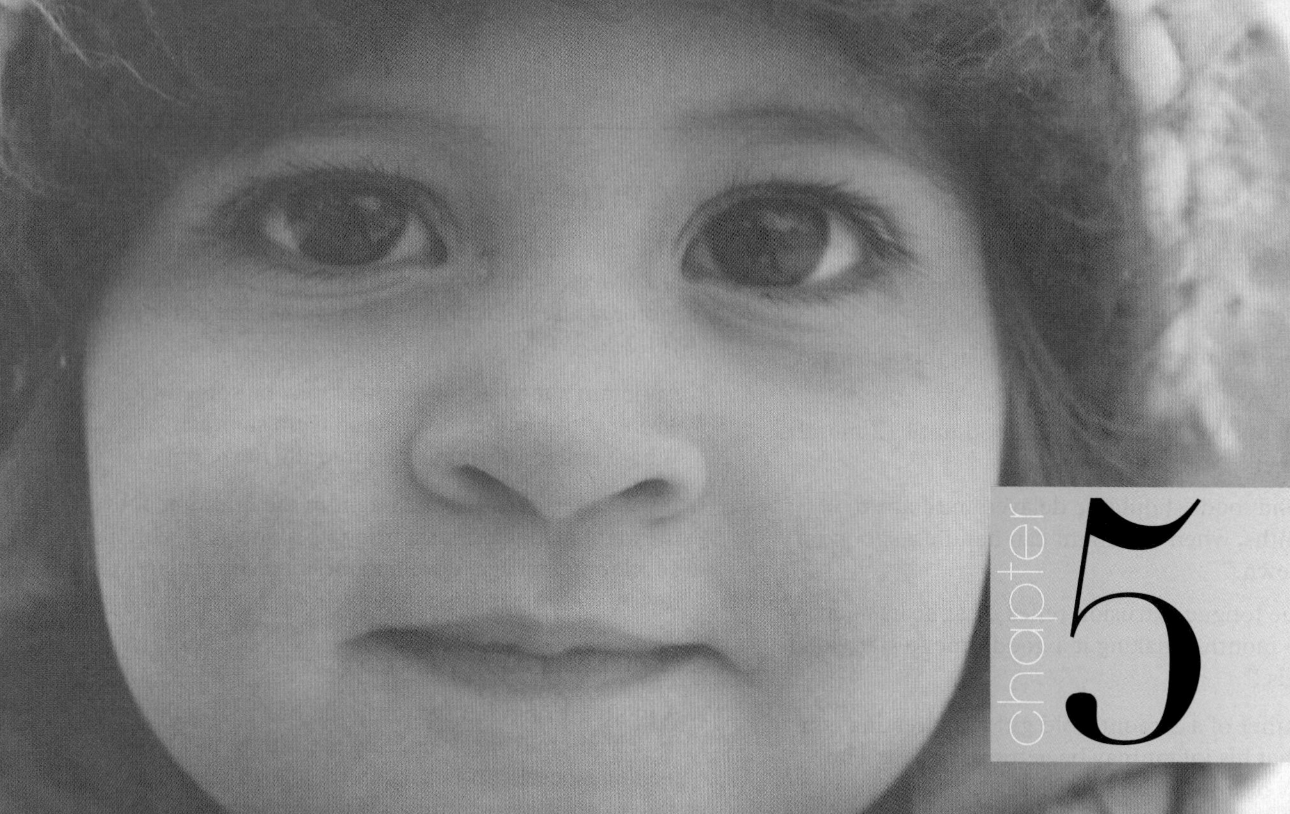

chapter 5

Growth and Development of the Toddler

Key TERMS

animism
echolalia
egocentrism
food jag
individuation
parallel play
physiologic anorexia
regression
ritualism
separation
separation anxiety
sibling rivalry
telegraphic speech

Learning OBJECTIVES

Upon completion of the chapter, the learner will be able to:

1. Explain normal physiologic, psychosocial, and cognitive changes occurring in the toddler.
2. Identify the gross and fine motor milestones of the toddler.
3. Demonstrate an understanding of language development in the toddler years.
4. Discuss sensory development of the toddler.
5. Demonstrate an understanding of emotional/social development and moral/spiritual development during toddlerhood.
6. Implement a nursing care plan to address common issues related to growth and development in toddlerhood.
7. Encourage growth and learning through play.
8. Develop a teaching plan for safety promotion in the toddler period.
9. Demonstrate an understanding of toddler needs related to sleep and rest, as well as dental health.
10. Develop a nutritional plan for the toddler based on average nutritional requirements.
11. Provide appropriate anticipatory guidance for common developmental issues that arise in the toddler period.
12. Demonstrate an understanding of appropriate methods of discipline for use during the toddler years.
13. Identify the role of the parent in the toddler's life and determine ways to support, encourage, and educate the parents about toddler growth, development, and concerns during this period.

WOW *Toddlers will take risks and make many mistakes, but remember that both are an essential part of their growth.*

Jose Gonzales is a 2-year-old boy brought to the clinic by his mother and father for his 2-year-old check-up. During your assessment, you find that his weight is 30 pounds, height 33 inches, and head circumference 19.5 inches. As the nurse caring for him, assess Jose's growth and development, and then provide appropriate anticipatory guidance to the parents.

The toddler period encompasses the second 2 years of life, from age 1 year to age 3 years. This period is a time of significant advancement in growth and development for the child. It can also be quite a challenging time for parents. The theme during the toddler years is one of holding on and letting go. Having learned that parents are predictable and reliable, the toddler is now learning that his or her behavior has a predictable, reliable effect on others. The challenge is to encourage independence and autonomy while keeping the curious toddler safe.

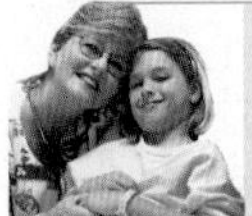

As more grandparents are assuming the primary caregiver role for their grandchildren, nurses should be alert to the possibility of increased stress that is placed upon the older caregiver, particularly during the active and sometimes trying years of toddlerhood.

Growth and Development Overview

Infancy is a time of intense growth and development. Both physical growth and acquisition of new motor skills slow somewhat during the toddler years. Refinement of motor skills, continued cognitive growth, and acquisition of appropriate language skills are of prime importance during the toddler years. The nurse uses the knowledge of normal toddler development as a roadmap for behavioral assessment of the 1- to 3-year-old child.

PHYSICAL GROWTH

The toddler's height and weight continue to increase steadily, though the increase occurs at a slower velocity compared to infancy. Toddler gains in height and weight tend to occur in spurts, rather than in a linear fashion (Fig. 5.1). The average toddler weight gain is 3 to 5 pounds per year. Length/height increases by an average of 3 inches per year. Toddlers generally reach about half of their adult height by 2 years of age. Head circumference increases about 1 inch from when the child is between 1 and 2 years of age, then increases an average of a half-inch per year until age 5. The anterior fontanel should be closed by the time the child is 18 months old. Head size becomes more proportional to the rest of the body near the age of 3 years.

ORGAN SYSTEM MATURATION

Though not as pronounced as the changes occurring during infancy, the toddler's organ systems continue to grow and mature in their functioning. Significant functional changes occur within the neurologic, gastrointestinal, and genitourinary systems. The respiratory and cardiovascular systems undergo changes as well.

Neurologic System

Brain growth continues through toddlerhood, and the brain reaches about 90% of its adult size by 2 years of age. Myelinization of the brain and spinal cord continues to progress and is complete around 24 months of age. Myelinization results in improved coordination and equilibrium as well as the ability to exercise sphincter control, which is important for bowel and bladder training. Integration of the primitive reflexes occurs in infancy, allowing for the emergence of the protective reflexes near the end of infancy or early in toddlerhood. The forward or downward parachute reflex is particularly helpful when the child starts to toddle. Rapid increase in language skills is evidence of continued progression of cognitive development.

Respiratory System

The respiratory structures continue to grow and mature throughout toddlerhood. The alveoli continue to increase

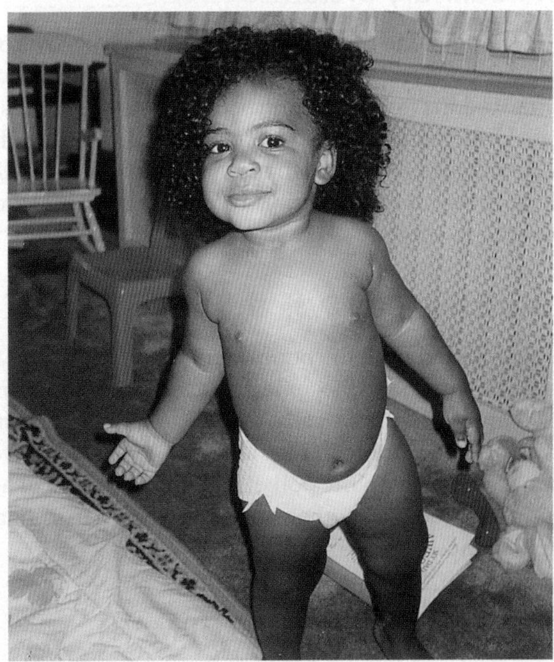

Figure 5.1 The typical toddler appearance is that of a rounded abdomen, a slight swayback, and a wide-based stance.

in number, not reaching the adult number until about 7 years of age. The trachea and lower airways continue to grow but remain small compared with the adult. The tongue is relatively large in comparison to the size of the mouth. Tonsils and adenoids are large and the Eustachian tubes are relatively short and straight.

Cardiovascular System

The heart rate decreases and blood pressure increases in toddlerhood. Blood vessels are close to the skin surface and so are compressed easily when palpated.

Gastrointestinal System

The stomach continues to increase in size, allowing the toddler to consume three regular meals per day. Pepsin production matures by 2 years of age. The small intestine continues to grow in length, though it does not reach the maximum length of 2 to 3 meters until adulthood. Stool passage decreases in frequency to one or two per day, with as many as 25% of toddlers having a bowel movement every other day (Arias, Bennison, Justus, & Thurman, 2001). The color of the stool may change (yellow, orange, brown, or green) depending upon the toddler's diet. Since the toddler's intestines remain somewhat immature, the toddler often passes whole pieces of difficult-to-digest food such as corn kernels. Bowel control is generally achieved by the end of the toddler period.

Genitourinary System

Bladder and kidney function reach adult levels by 16 to 24 months of age. The bladder capacity increases, allowing the toddler to retain urine for increased periods of times. Urine output should be about 1 mL/kg/hour. The urethra remains short in both the male and female toddler, making them more susceptible to urinary tract infections compared to adults.

Musculoskeletal System

During toddlerhood, the bones increase in length and the muscles mature and become stronger. The abdominal musculature is weak in early toddlerhood, resulting in a pot-bellied appearance. The toddler appears to have a swayback along with the potbelly. Around 3 years of age, the musculature strengthens and the abdomen is flatter in appearance.

• PSYCHOSOCIAL DEVELOPMENT

Erikson defines the toddler period as a time of autonomy versus shame and doubt. It is a time of exerting independence. Since the toddler developed a sense of trust in infancy, he or she is ready to give up dependence and to assert his or her sense of control and autonomy (Erikson, 1963). The toddler is struggling for self-mastery, to learn to do for himself or herself what others have been doing for him or her. Toddlers often experience ambivalence about the move from dependence to autonomy, and this results in emotional lability. The toddler may quickly change from happy and pleasant to crying and screaming. Exertion of independence also results in the toddler's favorite response, "no." The toddler will often answer "no" even when he or she really means "yes."

This negativism—always saying "no"—is a normal part of healthy development and is occurring as a result of the toddler's attempt to assert his or her independence. Table 5.1 gives further information related to developing a sense of autonomy.

Cognitive Development

According to Jean Piaget (1969), toddlers move through the last two substages of the first stage of cognitive development, the sensorimotor stage, between 12 and 24 months of age (Table 5.1). Young toddlers engage in tertiary circular reactions and progress to mental combinations. Rather than just repeating a behavior, the toddler is able to experiment with a behavior to see what happens. By 2 years of age, toddlers are capable of using symbols to allow for imitation. With increasing cognitive abilities, toddlers may now engage in delayed imitation. For example, they may imitate a household task that they observed a parent doing several days ago.

Piaget identified the second stage of cognitive development as the preoperational stage. It occurs in children between ages 2 and 7 years. During this stage toddlers begin to become more sophisticated with symbolic thought. The thinking of the older toddler is far more advanced than that of the infant or young toddler, who views the world as a series of objects. During the preoperational stage, objects begin to have characteristics that make them unique from one another. Objects are considered large or small, a particular color or shape, or a unique texture. This moves beyond the connection of sensory information and physical action. Words and images allow the toddler to begin this process of developing symbolic thought by providing a label for the objects' characteristics. Toddlers also use symbols in dramatic play. First they imitate life with appropriate toy objects, and then they are able to substitute objects in their play. A bowl may be used to pretend to eat from, but then later it can be used upside down on the head as a hat (Fig. 5.2). Human feelings and characteristics may also be attributed to objects (**animism**). See Table 5.1 for further explanation of cognitive development in toddlerhood.

Table 5.1 Developmental Theories

Theorist	Stage	Activities
Erikson	Autonomy vs. Shame & Doubt Age 1–3 years	Achieves autonomy and self-control Separates from parent/caregiver Withstands delayed gratification Negativism abounds Imitates adults and playmates Spontaneously shows affection Increasingly enthusiastic about playmates Cannot take turns in games until age 3 years
Piaget	Sensorimotor Substage 5: Tertiary Circular Reactions Age: 12–18 months	• Differentiating self from objects • Increased object permanence (knows that objects that are out of sight still exist (e.g., cookies in the cabinet)) • Uses ALL senses to explore environment • Places items in and out of containers
	Sensorimotor Substage 6: Mental Combinations Age: 18–24 months	• Imitates domestic chores (domestic mimicry) • Imitation is more symbolic • Starting to think before acting • Understands requests and is capable of following simple directions • Has a sense of ownership (my, mine)
	Preoperational Age: 2–7 years	• Time, space, and causality understanding is increasing • Uses mental trial and error rather than physical • Makes mechanical toys work • Plays make-believe with dolls, animals, and people • Increased use of language for mental representation • Understands concept of "two" • Starting to make connections between an experience in the past and a new one that is currently occurring • Sorts objects by shape and color • Completes puzzles with four pieces • Play becomes more complex
Freud	Anal Stage Age: 1–3 years	Focus is on achieving anal sphincter control. Satisfaction and/or frustration may occur as the toddler learns to withhold and expel stool.

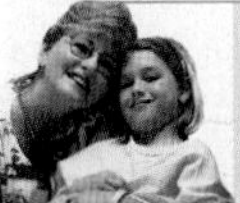

Mothers who are depressed may not be as sensitive to their children as other mothers. For this reason, maternal depression is a risk factor for poor cognitive development. Be alert to the mental status of a toddler's mother so that appropriate referrals can be made if needed.

● MOTOR SKILL DEVELOPMENT

Toddlers continue to gain new motor skills as well as refine others. Walking progresses to running, climbing, and jumping. Pushing or pulling a toy, throwing a ball, and pedaling a tricycle are accomplished in toddlerhood. Fine motor skills progress from holding and pinching to the ability to manage utensils, hold a crayon, string a bead, and use a computer. Development of eye–hand coordination is necessary for the refinement of fine motor skills. These increased abilities of mobility and manipulation help the curious toddler explore and learn more about his or her environment (Fig. 5.3). As the toddler masters a new task, he or she has confidence to conquer the next challenge. Thus, mastery in motor skill development contributes to the toddler's growing sense of self-esteem. The toddler who is eager to face challenges will likely develop more quickly than one who is reluctant. The senses of sight, hearing, and touch are useful in helping to coordinate gross and fine motor movement.

Gross Motor Skills

As gross motor skills are mastered and then used repeatedly, the large muscle groups in the toddler are strengthened. The "toddler gait" is characteristic of new walkers. The toddler does not walk smoothly and maturely. Instead, the legs are planted widely apart, toes are pointed forward, and the toddler seems to sway from side to side while moving forward (Fig. 5.4). Often the toddler seems to speed along, pitching forward, appearing ready to topple over at any moment. The toddler may fall often, but

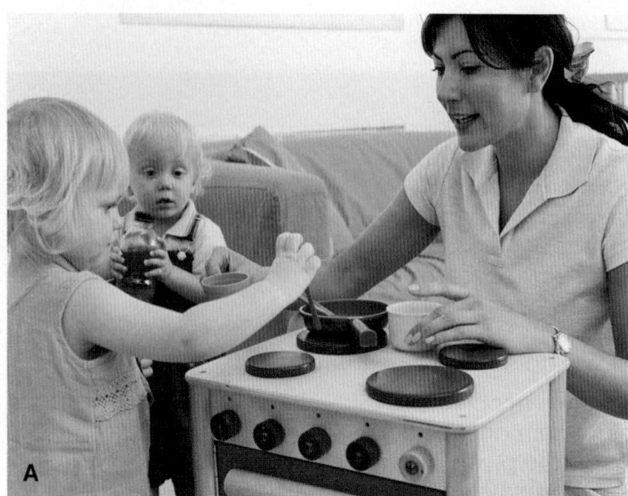
 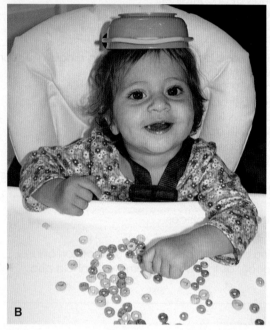

● Figure 5.2 The toddler will (**A**) pretend with items in the way they are intended to be used as well as (**B**) find other creative uses for them.

will use outstretched arms to catch himself or herself (parachute reflex). After about 6 months of practice walking, the toddler's gait is smoother and the feet are closer together. By 3 years of age, the toddler walks in a heel-to-toe fashion similar to that of adults. Toddlers often use physical actions such as running, jumping, and hitting to express their emotions because they are only just learning to express their thoughts and feelings verbally. Table 5.2 lists motor skill expectations in relation to age.

Fine Motor Skills

Fine motor skills in the toddler period are improved and perfected. Holding utensils requires some control and agility, but even more is needed for buttoning and zipping. Adequate vision is necessary for the refinement of

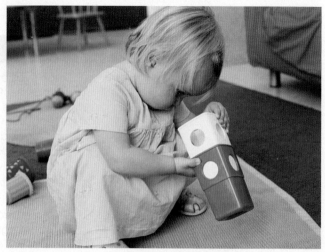

● Figure 5.3 The toddler's curiosity about the world increases, as does her ability to explore it.

fine motor skills because eye–hand coordination is crucial for directing the fingers, hand, and wrist to accomplish small muscle tasks such as fitting a puzzle piece or stringing a bead. See Table 5.2 for age expectations for various motor skills.

● SENSORY DEVELOPMENT

Toddlers use all of their senses to explore the world around them. Toddlers examine new items by feeling them, looking at them, shaking them to hear what sound

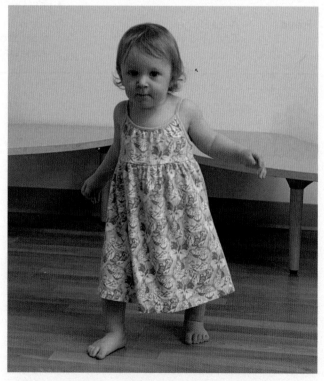

● Figure 5.4 The young toddler (early walker) walks with a wide-based stance, feet pointing forward and arms akimbo.

Table 5.2 Motor Skill Development

Age	Expected Gross Motor Skill	Expected Fine Motor Skills
12–15 months	Walks independently	Feeds self finger foods Uses index finger to point
18 months	Climbs stairs with assistance Pulls toys while walking	Masters reaching, grasping, and releasing: stacks blocks, puts things in slots Turns book pages (singly with board book, multiple if paper) Removes shoes and socks Stacks four cubes
24 months	Runs Kicks ball Can stand on tiptoe Carries several toys, or a large toy while walking Climbs onto and down from furniture without assistance	Builds tower of six or seven cubes Right- or left-handed Imitates circular and vertical strokes Scribbles and paints Starting to turn knobs Puts round pegs into holes
36 months	Climbs well Pedals tricycle Runs easily Walks up and down stairs with alternate feet Bends over easily without falling	Undresses self Copies circle Builds tower of nine or ten cubes Holds a pencil in writing position Screws/unscrews lids, nuts, bolts Turns book pages one at a time

they make, smelling them, and placing them in their mouths. Toddler vision continues to progress and should be 20/50 to 20/40 in both eyes. Depth perception also continues to mature. Hearing should be at the adult level, as infants are ordinarily born with hearing intact. The sense of smell continues to mature, and toddlers may comment if they do not care for the scent of something. Though taste discrimination is not completely developed, toddlers may exhibit preferences for certain flavors of foods. The toddler is more likely to try a new food if its appearance or smell is familiar. Lack of complete taste discrimination places the toddler at risk of accidental ingestion.

• COMMUNICATION AND LANGUAGE DEVELOPMENT

Language development occurs rapidly during the toddler years. The acquisition of language is a dynamic and complex process. The child's age and social interactions and the types of language to which he has been exposed influence language development. Receptive language development (the ability to understand what is being said or asked) is typically far more advanced than expressive language development (the ability to communicate one's desires and feelings). In other words, the toddler understands language and is able to follow commands far sooner than he or she can actually use the words themselves. Language is a very important part of the toddler's ability to organize his or her world and actually make sense of it. Thoughtfully planned use of language can provide behavior guidance and contribute to the avoidance of power struggles. In regard to expressive language development, the young toddler begins to use short sentences and will progress to a vocabulary of 50 words by 2 years of age. **Echolalia** (repetition of words and phrases without understanding) is normally seen in toddlers less than 30 months of age. "Why" and "what" questions dominate the older toddler's language. Telegraphic speech is common in the 3-year-old. **Telegraphic speech** refers to speech that contains only the essential words to get the point across, much like a telegram. Rather than "I want a cookie and milk," the toddler might say, "Want cookie milk." In telegraphic speech the nouns and verbs are present and are verbalized in the appropriate order. Table 5.3 gives an overview of receptive and expressive language development in the toddler.

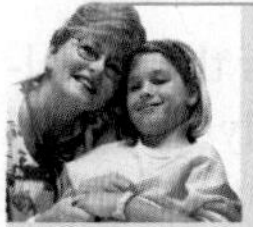

Stuttering usually has its onset at between 2 and 4 years of age. It occurs more often in boys than in girls. About 75% of all cases of stuttering resolve within 1 to 2 years after they start.

Early identification and referral of children with potential speech delays is critical. If a delay is identified, early

Table 5.3 Language Development in Toddlers

Age	Receptive Language	Expressive Language
12 months	Understands common words independent of context Follows a one-step command accompanied by gesture	Uses a finger to point to things Imitates or uses gestures such as waving goodbye Communicates desires with word and gesture combinations Vocal imitation First word
15 months	Looks at adult when communicating Follows a one-step command without gesture Understands 100–150 words	Repeats words that he or she hears Babbles in what sound like sentences
18 months	Understands the word "no" Comprehends 200 words Sometimes answers the question, "What's this?"	Uses at least 5–20 words Uses names of familiar objects
24 months	Points to named body parts Points to pictures in books Enjoys listening to simple stories Names a variety of objects in the environment Beginning to use "my" or "mine"	Vocabulary of 40–50 words Sentences of two or three words (me up, want cookie) Asks questions (what that?) Uses simple phrases Uses descriptive words (hungry, hot) Two thirds of what child says should be understandable Repeats overheard words
30 months	Follows a series of two independent commands	Vocabulary of 150–300 words
36 months	Understands most sentences Understands physical relationships (on, in, under) Participates in short conversations May follow a three-part command	Speech usually understood by those who know the child, about half understood by those outside family Asks "why?" Three- to four-word sentences Talks about something that happened in the past Vocabulary of 1,000 words Can say name, age, and gender Uses pronouns and plurals

intervention may increase the child's potential to acquire age-appropriate receptive and expressive language skills.

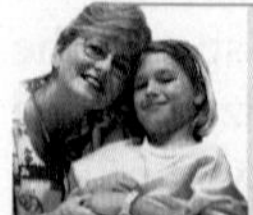

Children with preexisting conditions such as genetic syndromes that are known to have an effect on language development should be referred to a speech–language pathologist as soon as the condition is recognized rather than waiting until the child exhibits a delay.

Of special concern in the toddler years is the development of speech and language in potentially bilingual children. At the age of 1 to 2 years, the potentially bilingual child may blend two languages—that is, parts of the word in both languages are blended into one word. At age 2 to 3 years, the potentially bilingual toddler may mix languages within a sentence. Thus, the assessment of adequate language development is more complicated in bilingual children. Parents of potentially bilingual children may find support and resources at the website www.nethelp.no/cindy/biling-fam.html.

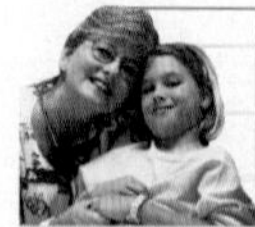

Bilingual children often mix languages, and thus speech delay may be more difficult to assess in this population. The bilingual child should have command of 20 words (between both languages) by 20 months of age and should be making word combinations. If this is not the case, further investigation may be warranted.

● EMOTIONAL AND SOCIAL DEVELOPMENT

Emotional development in the toddler years is focused on **separation** and **individuation**. Seeing oneself as separate from the parent or primary caregiver is accompanied by forming a sense of self and learning to exert control over one's environment. As this need to feel in control of his or her world emerges, the toddler displays **egocentrism** (focus on self). This need for control results in emotional lability: very happy and pleasant one moment, then overreacting to limit setting with a temper tantrum in the next moment. As toddlers identify the boundaries between themselves and the parent or primary caregiver, they learn to negotiate a balance between attachment and independence. Toddlers initially rely on the parents' communication and signals in order to initiate appropriate behavior or inhibit undesirable behavior. They have a difficult time choosing between sets of behaviors as they occur in different situations. Power struggles often occur in this age group, and it is important for parents and caregivers to thoughtfully and intentionally develop the rituals and routines that will provide stability and security for the toddler. Many toddlers rely upon a security item (blanket, doll, or bear) to comfort themselves in stressful situations (Fig. 5.5). This ability to self-soothe is a function of autonomy and is viewed as a sign of a nurturing environment, rather than, as one might suspect, one of neglect.

Children also begin to learn about gender differences in the toddler years. They observe the differences between male and female body parts if they are exposed to them. Toddlers may question parents about these differences and may begin to explore their own genitals. Toddlers also begin to understand and mimic social gender differences. They make observations about gender-specific behavior dependent upon what they are exposed to.

Aggressive behaviors are typically displayed during the toddler years. Toddlers may hit, bite, or push other children and grab toys. Adults can assist the toddler in building empathy by pointing out when someone is hurt and explaining what happened. Toddlers should not be blamed for their impulsive behavior; rather, they should be guided toward socially acceptable actions in order to foster development of appropriate social judgment. It is particularly important for the parent or caregiver to serve as a role model for appropriate behavior, rather than losing his or her own temper, in order for the toddler to be able to learn how to acceptably handle frustrations. Offering limited choices is one way of allowing toddlers some control over their environment and helping them to establish a sense of mastery. Since toddlers naturally have a short attention span, they tend to dawdle. As the toddlers become more self-aware, they start to develop emotions of self-consciousness such as embarrassment and shame.

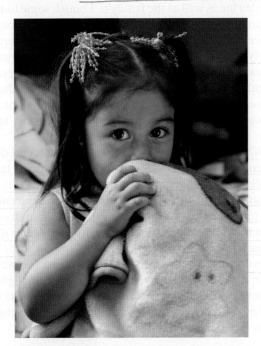

● Figure 5.5 The toddler may be able to self-soothe and produce a sense of comfort during this stage of establishing autonomy by relying upon a security item such as a doll, bear, or blanket.

Though toddlers are becoming more self-aware, they still do not have clear body boundaries. They do not clearly understand the body's functions, though they are beginning to make appropriate connections. Feces may be viewed as a part of the child, and the toddler may become upset at seeing it disappear in the toilet. The toddler will protect his or her body by resisting intrusive procedures such as temperature or blood pressure measurement.

Separation Anxiety

As toddlers become increasingly skilled at mobility, they realize that if they have the capability of leaving, then so does the parent. As self-awareness develops and conflicts over closeness versus exploration occur, **separation anxiety** may reemerge in the 18- to 24-month period. Power struggles may escalate and distress at separating from the parent may increase. Again, a predictable routine with appropriate limit setting may help toddlers to feel safer and more secure during this period. From the age of 24 to 36 months, separation anxiety again eases. The older toddler begins to have a concept of object constancy: he or she has an internal representation of the parent or caregiver and is better able to tolerate separation, knowing that a reunion will occur.

Temperament

Temperament is the biological basis for personality. It is our emotional and motivational core, around which the personality develops over time. Temperament affects how the toddler interacts with the environment. The easygoing toddler may adapt more easily and not mind changes in routine as much as other toddlers. The easygoing toddler usually sleeps and eats well and has more predictable and regular behaviors. However, the toddler may still express frustration by having a temper tantrum. The "difficult" toddler is more likely to have intense reactions, negative or positive, with temper tantrums being more likely, more frequent, and more intense than in other toddlers. The structure and routine that toddlers need to feel secure are essential for the difficult toddler; otherwise, the child feels insecure and as a result is more likely to behave inappropriately. The difficult toddler is also the most active of the three temperament types. The slow-to-warm-up toddler is more of a loner and may be very shy. He or she may experience more difficulty with separation anxiety. The behavior of the slow-to-warm-up toddler is more passive; the toddler may be very watchful and withdrawn and may take longer to mature. Changes in routine usually do not result in as much upset, since the toddler's natural reaction is one of passivity.

Based on the toddler's temperament, make suggestions to the parents for interacting with the toddler in various situations. For example, to avoid temper tantrums in the difficult toddler, suggest that the parent should be especially diligent about maintaining structure and routine as well as avoiding tantrum triggers such as fatigue and hunger. Explain to parents that they may need to exercise additional patience with new activities to which the slow-to-warm-up toddler may need extra time becoming accustomed.

Fears

Common fears of toddlers include loss of parents (which contributes to separation anxiety) and fear of strangers. Some toddlers may be very slow to warm up to people they do not know. The nurse caring for a toddler in the outpatient or hospital setting should take the time to establish a relationship with the toddler in order to allay the toddler's fears. Toddlers may be afraid of loud noises and large or unfamiliar animals. Going to sleep may be a scary time for toddlers as they may be afraid of the dark. A nightlight in the toddler's room may be very helpful.

● MORAL AND SPIRITUAL DEVELOPMENT

During the toddler years, children may feel comfort from the routine of praying, but they do not understand religious beliefs because of their limited cognitive abilities. Reading simple Bible stories can lay a foundation for later religious teachings. Kohlberg's (1984) description of moral development places the older toddler in the preconventional level. The toddler is only just beginning to learn right from wrong and does not understand the larger concept of morality. The toddler will base his or her actions on the avoidance of punishment and the attainment of pleasure. Older toddlers begin to feel empathy for others.

● CULTURAL INFLUENCES ON GROWTH AND DEVELOPMENT

Homelessness or poverty may directly influence the toddler's ability to grow adequately, as resources for the purchase and preparation of appropriate food may be lacking. Appropriate toys (safe ones) may also not be available in those situations. Food customs continue to have an impact on the child's diet and ability to ingest appropriate nutrients. Individual families' value systems have an impact on the toddler's development as well. Some parents desire to keep their child a "baby" for a longer period, thus delaying weaning or continuing to feed the child baby food or puréed food for a longer period. Other families may highly value independence and encourage the toddler to walk everywhere on his or her own rather than carrying the child.

Culture may also affect emotional development. Some families start at a very young age to discourage crying in boys, encouraging them to "act like a big boy" or "be a man." Ridicule for crying at this age may hurt the toddler's self-concept. Educating families about normal growth and development while continuing to value and support cultural practices is important.

> Remember Jose Gonzales, whom you met at the beginning of the chapter? What developmental milestones would you expect him to have reached at his age?

The Nurse's Role in Toddler Growth and Development

WATCH & LEARN

The toddler's growth and development affects his or her everyday life as well as the family's. Though some toddlers may grow more quickly or reach developmental milestones sooner than others, growth and development remains orderly and sequential. Health care visits throughout toddlerhood continue to focus on growth and development. The nurse must have a good understanding of the changes that occur during the toddler years in order to provide appropriate anticipatory guidance and support to the family.

When the toddler is hospitalized, growth and development may be altered. The toddler's primary task is establishing autonomy, and the toddler's focus is mobility and language development. Hospitalization removes most opportunities for the toddler to learn through exploration of the environment. Isolation for contagious illness further constrains the toddler's ability to find some control over the environment. The nurse caring for the hospitalized toddler must use knowledge of normal growth and development to be successful in interactions with the toddler, promote continued development, and recognize delays (see Chapter 11) (Fig. 5.6).

● NURSING PROCESS OVERVIEW

Upon completion of assessment of the toddler's current growth and development status, problems or issues related

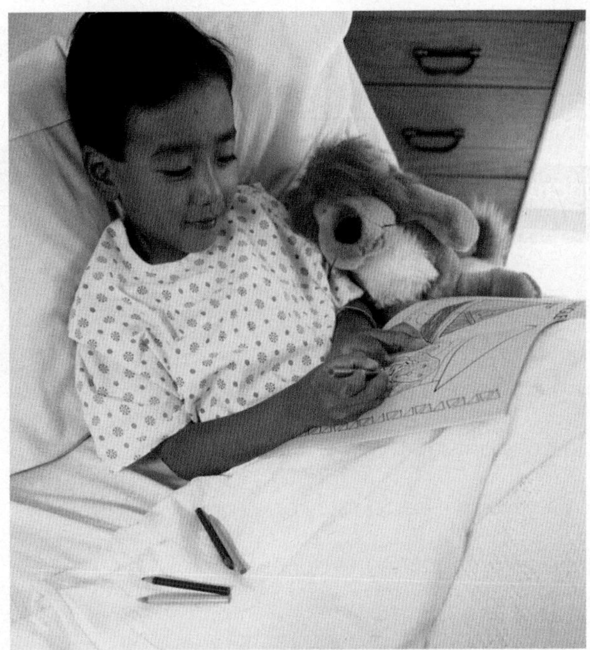

● Figure 5.6 The hospitalized toddler continues to enjoy developmental tasks appropriate for his or her age, such as coloring.

to growth and development may be identified. The nurse may then identify one or more nursing diagnoses, including but not limited to:

- Delayed growth and development
- Imbalanced nutrition, less than body requirements
- Interrupted family processes
- Readiness for enhanced parenting
- Risk for caregiver role strain
- Risk for delayed development
- Risk for disproportionate growth
- Risk for injury

Nursing care planning for the toddler with growth and development issues should be individualized based on the toddler's and family's needs. The nursing care plan may be used as a guide in planning nursing care for the toddler with a growth or developmental concern. The nurse may choose the appropriate nursing diagnoses from the following plan and individualize them as needed. The nursing care plan is intended to serve as a guide only and is not intended to be an inclusive growth and development plan.

● PROMOTING HEALTHY GROWTH AND DEVELOPMENT

Parents who give their toddler love and respect regardless of the child's gender, behavior, or capabilities are helping to lay the foundation for self-esteem. Self-esteem is also built through familiarity with the daily routine. Routine and ritual help toddlers develop a conscience. Making expectations known through everyday routines helps to avoid confrontations. If the toddler knows the routine, he or she knows what to expect and how he or she is expected to act. When routine and limits are absent, the toddler develops feelings of uncertainty and anxiety. Limit setting (and remaining consistent with those limits) helps toddlers master their behavior, develop self-esteem, and become successful participants in the family. Children then are able to learn about cooperation throughout the predictable flow of daily life. Nurses need to be aware of normal developmental expectations in order to determine whether the toddler is progressing appropriately. Table 5.4 lists potential signs of developmental delay. Any toddler with one or more of these concerns should be referred for further developmental evaluation.

Promoting Growth and Development Through Play

Play is the major socializing medium for toddlers. Parents should limit television viewing and encourage creative and physical play instead. Toddlers typically play alongside another child (**parallel play**) rather than cooperatively (Fig. 5.7). The short attention span of the toddler will make him or her often change toys and types of play. It is important to provide a variety of safe toys to allow the toddler many different opportunities for exploring the environment. Toddlers do not need expensive toys; in fact, regular household items sometimes make the most enjoyable toys. Toddlers are egocentric, a normal part of their development. This makes it difficult for them to share. As they are developing a sense of self (who they are as a person), they may see their toys as an extension of themselves. Learning to share occurs in later toddlerhood. Toddlers also like dramatic play and play that recreates familiar activities in the home. Toddlers enjoy introduction to music and musical instruments. They like to listen to music of all kinds and will often dance to whatever they hear on the radio. Toddlers enjoy drums, xylophones, cymbals, and toy pianos. Musical instruments made at home are also enjoyed. A few pebbles or coins inside an empty water bottle with the top tightly secured is a great music maker; an empty butter tub with a lid and a pair of wooden spoons makes a nice drum.

Adequate physical activity is necessary for the development and refinement of movement skills. Toddlers need at least 30 minutes of structured physical activity and anywhere from 1 to several hours of unstructured physical activity per day. Indoor and outdoor play areas should encourage play activities that use the large muscle groups. The activity must occur within a safe environment. Outdoor play structures should be positioned over surfaces that are soft enough to absorb a fall, such as sand, wood chips, or sawdust (Fig. 5.8). Box 5.1 lists recommended age-appropriate toys.

(text continues on page 118)

Nursing Care Plan 5.1

Growth and Development Issues in the Toddler

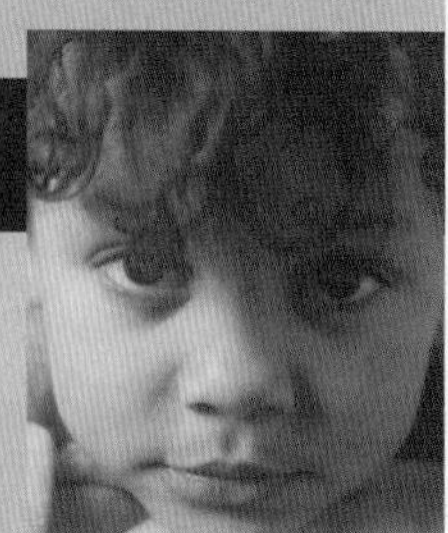

Nursing Diagnosis: Risk for injury related to curiosity, increased mobility, and developmental immaturity

Outcome identification and evaluation

Toddler safety will be maintained: *Toddler will remain free from injury.*

Interventions: preventing injury

- Teach and encourage appropriate use of forward facing car seat *to decrease risk of toddler injury related to motor vehicles.*
- Teach toddlers to stay away from the street and provide constant supervision *to prevent pedestrian injury.*
- Require bicycle helmet use while riding any wheeled toy *to prevent head injury and form habit of helmet use.*
- Childproof the home *to provide a developmentally safe environment for the curious and increasingly mobile toddler.*
- Post poison control center phone number *in case of accidental ingestion.*
- Never leave a toddler unattended in a tub or pool or near any body of water *to prevent drowning.*
- Teach parents first-aid measures and child CPR *to minimize consequences of injury should it occur.*
- Provide close observation and keep side rails up on crib/bed in hospital *because toddlers are at particularly high risk for falling or becoming entangled in tubing as they attempt mobility.*

Nursing Diagnosis: Imbalanced nutrition, less than body requirements, related to inappropriate nutritional intake to sustain growth needs (excess juice or milk intake, inadequate food variety intake) as evidenced by failure to attain adequate increases in height and weight over time

Outcome identification and evaluation

Toddler will consume adequate nutrients while using an appropriate feeding pattern: *Toddler will demonstrate weight gain and increases in height.*

Interventions: promoting appropriate nutrition

- Assess current feeding schedule and usual intake, as well as methods used to feed, *to determine areas of adequacy versus inadequacy.*
- Determine toddler's ability to drink from cup, finger feed, swallow, and consume textures *to determine if additional exposure is needed or if further interventions such as speech or occupational therapy are required.*
- Weigh toddler daily on same scale if hospitalized, weekly on same scale if at home, and plot growth patterns weekly or monthly as appropriate on standardized growth charts *to determine if growth is improving.*
- Wean from bottle by 15 months of age *to discourage excess milk or juice intake in toddler who can carry bottle around.*
- Limit juice to 4 to 6 ounces per day and milk to 16 to 24 ounces per day *to discourage sense of fullness achieved with excess milk or juice intake, thereby increasing appetite for solid foods.*
- Provide three nutrient-dense meals and at least two healthy snacks per day *to encourage adequate nutrient consumption.*
- Feed toddler on a similar schedule daily, without distractions and with the family: *toddlers respond well to routine and structure and may eat better in the social context of meals, and they become distracted easily (TV should be off).*

Growth and Development Issues in the Toddler (continued)

Nursing Diagnosis: Delayed growth and development related to motor, cognitive, language, or psychosocial concerns as evidenced by delay in meeting expected milestones

Outcome identification and evaluation

Development will be enhanced: *Toddler will make continued progress toward realization of expected developmental milestones.*

Interventions: enhancing growth and development

- Screen for developmental capabilities *to determine toddler's current level of functioning.*
- Offer age-appropriate toys, play, and activities (including gross motor) *to encourage further development.*
- Perform interventions as prescribed by physical, occupational, or speech therapist: *participation in those activities helps to promote function and accomplish acquisition of developmental skills.*
- Provide support to families of toddlers with developmental delay *(progress in achieving developmental milestones can be slow and ongoing motivation is needed).*
- Reinforce positive attributes in the toddler *to maintain motivation.*
- Model age-appropriate communication skills *to illustrate suitable means for parenting the toddler.*

Nursing Diagnosis: Risk for disproportionate growth related to excess milk or juice intake, late bottle weaning, and consumption of inappropriate foods or in excess amounts

Outcome identification and evaluation

Toddler will grow appropriately and not become overweight or obese: *Toddler will achieve weight and height within the 5th to 85th percentiles on standardized growth charts.*

Interventions: promoting proportionate growth

- Wean from bottle and discourage use of no-spill sippy cups by 15 months of age *(will keep mobile toddler from carrying around and continually drinking from cup or bottle).*
- Provide juice (4–6 ounces per day) and milk (16–24 ounces per day) from a cup at meal and snack time *to encourage appropriate cup drinking and limit intake of nutrient-poor, high-calorie fluids.*
- Provide only nutrient-rich foods without high sugar content for meals and snacks; *even if the toddler won't eat, it is inappropriate to provide high-calorie junk food just so the toddler eats something.*
- Ensure adequate physical activity *to stimulate development of motor skills and provide appropriate caloric expenditure. This also sets the stage for forming life-long habit of appropriate physical activity.*

Nursing Diagnosis: Interrupted family processes related to issues with toddler development, hospitalization, or situational crisis as evidenced by decreased parental visitation in hospital, parental verbalization of difficulty with current situation, possible crisis related to health of family member other than the toddler

Outcome identification and evaluation

Family will demonstrate adequate functioning: *Family will display coping and psychosocial adjustment.*

Interventions: enhancing family functioning

- Assess the family's level of stress and ability to cope *to determine family's ability to cope with multiple stressors.*
- Engage in family-centered care *to provide a holistic approach to care of the toddler and family.*

(continued)

Growth and Development Issues in the Toddler (continued)

- Encourage the family to verbalize feelings *(verbalization is one method of decreasing anxiety levels)*, and acknowledge feelings and emotions.
- Encourage family visitation and provide for sleeping arrangements for a parent or caregiver to stay in the hospital with the toddler *(contributes to family's sense of control of situation)*.
- Involve family members in toddler's care, *giving them a feeling of control and connectedness.*

Nursing Diagnosis: Readiness for enhanced parenting related to parental desire for increased skills and success with toddler as evidenced by current healthy relationships and verbalization of desire for improved skills

Outcome identification and evaluation

Parent will provide safe and nurturing environment for the toddler.

Interventions: increasing parenting skill set

- Use family-centered care *to provide holistic approach.*
- Educate parent about normal toddler development *to provide basis for understanding the parenting skills needed in this time period.*
- Acknowledge and encourage parent's verbalization of feelings related to chronic illness of child or difficulty with normal toddler behavior *to validate the normalcy of the parent's feelings.*
- Encourage positive parenting with respect to toddlers and their normal development *(helps parents develop approaches to toddlers that can be used in place of anger and frustration).*
- Acknowledge and admire positive parenting skills already present *to contribute to parents' confidence in their abilities to parent.*
- Role model appropriate parenting behaviors related to communicating with and disciplining the toddler *(role modeling actually shows rather than just telling the parent what to do).*

Promoting Early Learning

The parent–child relationship and the interactions between parent and child form the context for the toddler's early learning.

Promoting Language Development

Talking and singing to the toddler during routine activities such as feeding and dressing provides an environment that encourages conversation. Frequent, repetitive naming helps the toddler learn appropriate words for objects. The parent or caregiver should be attentive to what the toddler is saying as well as to his or her moods. Using clarification validates the toddler's emotions and ideas. Parents should listen to and answer the toddler's questions. They should sit down quietly with the toddler and gently repeat what the toddler is saying. Encouragement and elaboration convey confidence and interest to the toddler. The toddler needs time to complete his or her thoughts without being interrupted or rushed because he or she is just starting to be able to make the connections necessary to transfer thoughts and feelings into language.

Parents should not overreact to the child's use of the word "no." They can give the toddler opportunities to use the word "no" appropriately by asking silly questions such as, "Can a cat drive a car?" or "Is a banana purple?" When promoting language development, the parent or primary caregiver should teach the toddler appropriate words for body parts and objects and should help the toddler choose appropriate words to label feelings and emotions. Toddlers' receptive language and interpretation of body language and subtle signs far surpasses their expressive language, especially at a younger age.

Parents should avoid discussing scary or serious topics in the presence of the toddler, since the toddler is very adept at reading emotions.

If the parents speak a foreign language in addition to English, both languages should be used in the home.

Encouraging Reading

Reading to the toddler every day is one of the best ways to promote language and cognitive development (Fig. 5.9). Toddlers particularly enjoy homemade or purchased

Table 5.4 Signs of Developmental Delay

Age or Time Frame	Concern
After independent walking for several months	• Persistent tiptoe walking • Failure to develop a mature walking pattern
By 18 months	• Not walking • Not speaking 15 words • Does not understand function of common household items
By 2 years	• Does not use two-word sentences • Does not imitate actions • Does not follow basic instructions • Cannot push a toy with wheels
By 3 years	• Difficulty with stairs • Frequent falling • Cannot build tower of more than four blocks • Difficulty manipulating small objects • Extreme difficulty in separation from parent or caregiver • Cannot copy a circle • Does not engage in make-believe play • Cannot communicate in short phrases • Does not understand simple instructions • Little interest in other children • Unclear speech, persistent drooling

books about feelings, family, friends, everyday life, animals and nature, and fun and fantasy. Board books have thick pages that are easier for young toddlers to turn; older toddlers can turn paper pages one at a time. The toddler may also enjoy "reading" the story to the parent. Reach Out and Read, a program designed to promote early literacy, offers tips for reading with young children (see Teaching Guideline 5.1).

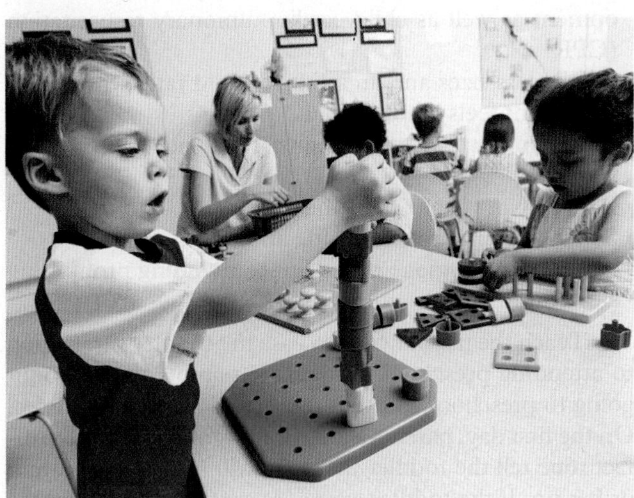

● Figure 5.7 Parallel play. The toddler usually plays alongside another child rather than cooperatively.

Choosing a Preschool

The older toddler may benefit from the structure and socialization provided by attending preschool. Attending preschool will help the toddler become more mature and independent and give the toddler a different source for a sense of accomplishment. At this age, toddlers need

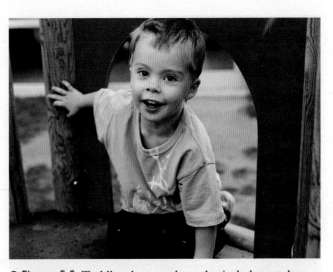

● Figure 5.8 Toddlers love outdoor physical play, such as climbing on playground equipment. An adult should always supervise toddlers when they are playing outdoors.

BOX 5.1

APPROPRIATE TOYS FOR TODDLERS

- Familiar household items such as plastic bowls and cups of various sizes, large plastic serving utensils, pots and pans, wooden spoons, cardboard boxes and tubes (from paper towel rolls), old magazines, baskets, purses, hats
- Child-size household item toys (kitchen, broom, vacuum cleaner, lawnmower, telephone, and so on)
- Blocks, cars and trucks, plastic animals, trains, plastic figures (family, community helpers), simple dolls, stuffed animals, balls, doll beds and carriages
- Manipulative toys with knobs, wind-ups and buttons that make things happen; putting large pegs or shapes into matching holes, stringing large beads on shoelaces, blocks and containers that stack, jigsaw puzzles with large pieces, toys that can be taken apart and put back together again
- Gross motor toys: play gym, push and pull toys, wagons, tricycle or other ride-on toys, tunnels
- Tape or CD players for music, various musical instruments
- Chalk, large crayons, finger paint, Play-Doh, washable markers
- Bucket, plastic shovel and other containers for sand and water play
- Squeaking, floating, squirting toys for the bath

supervised play with some direction that fosters their cognitive development. A strict curriculum is not necessary in this age group. When choosing a preschool, the parent or caregiver should look for an environment that has the following qualities:

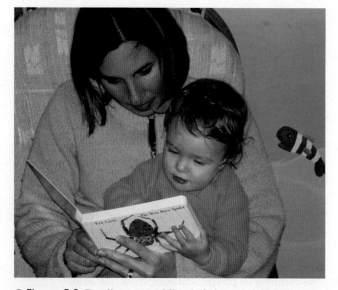

● Figure 5.9 Reading to a toddler daily is one of the best ways to promote language development and school readiness.

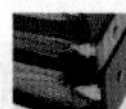

TEACHING GUIDELINE 5.1

Tips for Reading with Young Children

- Make reading part of every day: Read at bedtime or on the bus.
- Have fun: Children who love books learn to read. Books can be part of special time with your child.
- A few minutes is OK: Young children can sit for only a few minutes for a story, but as they grow they will sit longer.
- Talk about the pictures: You do not have to read the book to tell a story.
- Let your child turn the pages: Babies need board books and help to turn pages, but your 3-year-old can do it alone.
- Show your child the cover page: Explain what the story is about.
- Show your child the words: Run your finger along the words as you read them.
- Make the story come alive: Create voices for the story characters and use your body to tell the story.
- Ask questions about the story: What do you think will happen next? What is this?
- Let your child ask questions about the story: Use the story as an opportunity to engage in conversation and to talk about familiar activities and objects.
- Let your child tell the story: Children as young as 3 years old can memorize a story, and many children love an opportunity to express their creativity. (Reach Out and Read, 2003)

- Goals and an overall philosophy with which the parents agree (promotion of independence and self-confidence through structured and free play)
- Teachers and assistants trained in early childhood development as well as child cardiopulmonary resuscitation (CPR)
- Small class sizes and an adult-to-child ratio with which the parent feels comfortable
- Disciplinary procedures consistent with the parents' values
- Parents can visit at any time
- School is childproofed inside and out
- Appropriate hygiene procedures, including prohibiting sick children from attending

Teach the parents how to ease the toddler's transition to attending preschool. Encourage parents to talk about going to preschool and visit the school a couple of times. On the first day, parents should calmly and in a matter-of-fact tone tell the toddler that they will return to pick him or her up. If the toddler expresses separation anxiety, the parent should remain calm and follow through with the plan for school attendance. After a few days of attendance, the toddler will be accustomed to the new routine and crying when parting from the parent should be minimal.

Promoting Safety

Safety is of prime concern throughout the toddler period. Curiosity, mobility, and lack of impulse control all contribute to the incidence of unintentional injury in toddlerhood. Even the most watchful and caring parents have toddlers who run into the street, otherwise disappear from parents, and fall down the stairs. Toddlers require direct observation and cannot be trusted to be left alone. A childproof environment provides a safe place for the toddler to explore and learn. Motor vehicle accidents, drowning, choking, burns, falls, and poisoning are the most common injuries suffered by toddlers. Safety and injury prevention focuses on these categories.

Safety in the Car

The safest place for the toddler to ride is in the back seat of the car. Parents should use the appropriate size and style of car seat for the child's weight and age as required by the state. At a minimum, all children over 20 pounds and up to 40 pounds should be in a forward-facing car seat with harness straps and a clip. A toddler riding in a pickup truck should never ride in the cargo area or truck bed. A full rear seat in the truck is the preferred placement for the toddler car seat. If an appropriate rear seat is unavailable, the air bag should be disarmed and the forward-facing car seat should be secured appropriately in the truck seat. The top tether is additionally required for all forward-facing car seats (American Academy of Pediatrics, Committee on Injury and Poison Prevention, 2000) (Fig. 5.10). Drivers should avoid using the cell phone or attempting to intervene with the children while they are driving. Excellent resources about car seat safety appropriate for both parents and professionals can be found at www.bucklebear.com, www.nhtsa.dot.gov, www.safekids.org, and www.seatcheck.org.

Safety in the Home

Key areas of concern for keeping toddlers safe in the home include avoiding exposure to tobacco smoke, preventing injury, and preventing poisoning.

Avoiding Exposure to Tobacco Smoke

Environmental exposure to tobacco smoke has been associated with increased risk of respiratory disease and infection, decreased lung function, and increased incidence of middle ear effusion and recurrent otitis media. It may also hinder neurodevelopment and may be associated with behavior problems (Brown, 2001). Parents should avoid cigarette smoking entirely to best protect their children. Even smoking outside of the home is suboptimal because smoke lingers on parents' clothing and children who are often carried (such as younger toddlers) face more exposure. Counsel parents to stop smoking (optimal), but if they continue smoking never to smoke inside the home or car with children present.

Preventing Injury

The toddler is able to open drawers and doors, unlock deadbolts, and climb anywhere he or she wants to go. Toddlers have a limited concept of body boundaries and essentially no fear of danger. Toddlers may fall from any height to which they can climb (e.g., play structures, tables, counters). They may also fall from wheeled toys such as tricycles. As toddlers gain additional height and hand dexterity they are able to reach potentially danger-

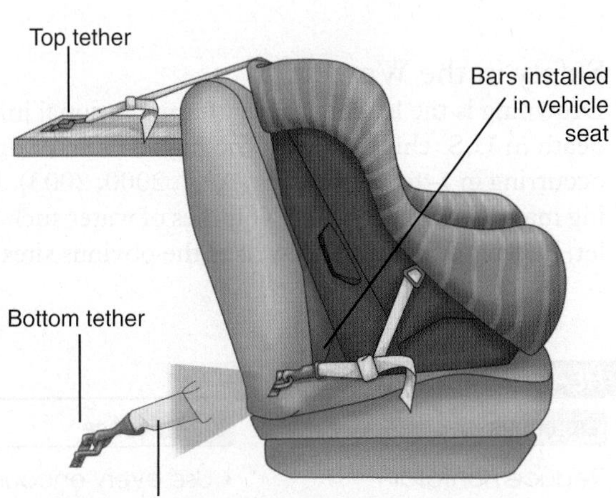

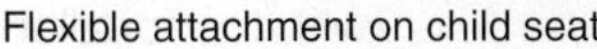

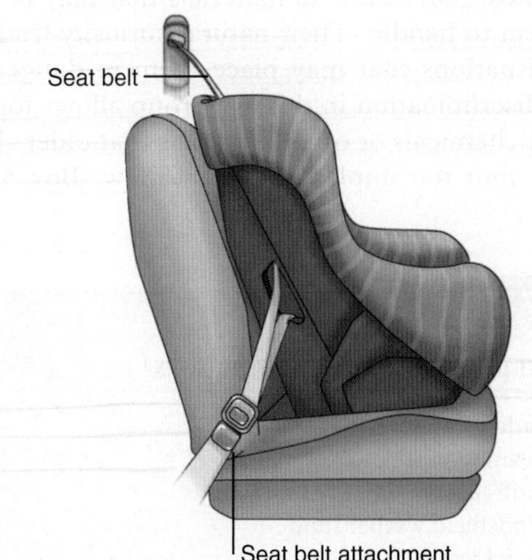

● **Figure 5.10** The top tether further secures the forward-facing car seat. This tether has been a requirement on all forward-facing car seats manufactured since 1999. Also, most vehicles manufactured after 1999 have a specific attachment for the top tether. (U.S. Department of Transportation, National Highway Traffic Safety Administration.)

ous items on the counter or stove, leading to an accidental ingestion, burn, or cut.

To prevent injury in the home, stress the following to parents:

- Never leave a toddler unsupervised out of doors.
- Lock doors to dangerous rooms.
- Install safety gates at the top and bottom of staircases.
- Ensure that window locks are operable; if windows are left opened, then secure all window screens.
- Keep pot handles on the stove turned inward, out of an inquisitive toddler's reach.
- Teach the toddler to avoid the oven, stove, and iron.
- Keep electrical equipment, cords, and matches out of reach.
- Remove firearms from the home, or keep them in a locked cabinet out of the toddler's reach.
- Always require the child to wear a helmet approved by the Consumer Products Safety Commission (CSPC) when riding a wheeled toy. This starts the habit of helmet wearing early, so it can be more easily carried over to the bicycle-riding years of the future.
- Begin teaching the toddler about watching for cars when crossing the street, but always carry or hold the hand of the toddler when crossing the street.
- Teach the toddler to avoid unknown animals.

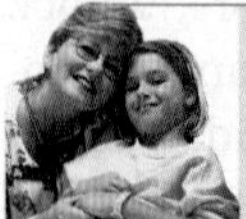

"Bernie Burn," by Sarah Cruz, RN, is a book designed to educate parents and their toddlers about burn prevention while entertaining them. It is endorsed by the American Journal of Nursing and is available from www.littlebootspublishing.com.

Preventing Poisoning

As toddlers become more mobile, they are increasingly able to explore their environment and more easily and efficiently gain access to materials that may be unsafe for them to handle. Their natural curiosity leads them into situations that may place them in danger. Poor taste discrimination in this age group allows for ingestion of chemicals or other materials that older children would find too unpleasant to swallow. Box 5.2 lists most potentially dangerous ingested poisons. Discuss poison prevention in the home at each well-child visit (see Healthy People 2010). The American Academy of Pediatrics recommends that potentially poisonous substances (e.g., medications, cleaners, hair care products, car care products) be stored out of the toddler's teach, out of the toddler's sight, and in a childproof, locked cabinet.

Encourage all families to:

- Store all substances in original containers only.
- Never store any liquid other than soda in a soda pop bottle.
- Do not allow toddlers access to baby powder, lotion, cream, or other toddler hygiene products.
- Ensure all medications have child-safety caps.
- Do not leave within the toddler's reach medications such as lozenges or samples that are not packaged in safety bottles.
- Be very careful with medications that are provided in transdermal patch form.
- Do not refer to medicines as candy, as the toddler many mistake pills for candy and ingest them.
- Do not expose toddlers to hazardous vapors such as paints, cleaners, tobacco smoke, and especially street drugs such as crack and marijuana.
- Keep "button" batteries secured and away from a toddler's reach.
- Keep house plants off the floor, remove them from the home, or hang them or place them on a high shelf.

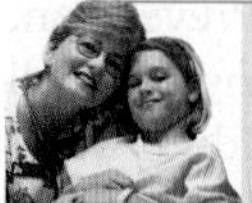

The American Academy of Pediatrics (AAP, 2003a, 2003b) recommends that all families post the Poison Control Center number in a readily accessible place in the home: (800) 222-1222. The AAP discourages the use of syrup of ipecac in the home to induce vomiting after an accidental ingestion.

BOX 5.2

MOST DANGEROUS POTENTIAL POISONS

- Medicines (especially iron)
- Cleaning products
- Antifreeze
- Windshield washer fluid
- Pesticides
- Furniture polish
- Gasoline, kerosene, lamp oil

(AAP, 2003a, b)

Safety in the Water

Drowning is the leading cause of unintentional injury and death in U.S. children, with the highest rate of drowning occurring in 1- to 2-year-olds (AAP, 2000, 2003). Drowning may occur in very small volumes of water such as a toilet, bucket, or bathtub, as well as the obvious sites such as

HEALTHY PEOPLE 2010

Objective	Significance
Reduce nonfatal poisonings	• Use every encounter with the toddler's family as an opportunity to educate about preventing poisonings.

swimming pools and other bodies of water. Toddlers' large heads in relation to their body size place them at risk for toppling over into a body of water that they are inquisitive about. Toddlers should be supervised at all times when in or around the water. In general, most children do not have the physical and cognitive capabilities necessary to truly learn how to swim until 4 years of age. Parents who want to enroll a toddler in a swimming class should be aware that a water safety skills class would be most appropriate. However, even toddlers who have completed a swimming program still need *constant* supervision in the water. Box 5.3 gives recommendations for the prevention of drowning.

Remember Jose Gonzales, the 2-year-old introduced at the beginning of the chapter? What anticipatory guidance related to safety should you provide to his parents?

Promoting Nutrition

The toddler's ability to chew and swallow is improving, and he or she learns to use utensils effectively to feed himself or herself. The early years lay a foundation for the future, and a great deal of parental and societal interest is focused upon nutrition and eating. Forming healthy eating habits has its foundation early in life, and diet has significant influence upon the child's future health status. By establishing healthier food choice patterns early in life, the child is better able to continue these healthy choices later in life. The child less than 2 years of age should not have his or her fat intake restricted, but this does not mean that unhealthy foods such as sweets should be eaten liberally. A diet high in nutrient-rich foods and low in nutrient-poor high-calorie foods such as sweets is appropriate for children of all ages. See Healthy People 2010.

BOX 5.3

PREVENTING DROWNING

- Pools should be fenced with locked gates or screened with locked doors.
- Interior doors should be kept locked.
- Young children should never be left unattended in or near water.
- Water wings or "floaties" are not a substitute for adult supervision or for personal flotation devices.
- U.S. Coast Guard-approved life preservers or personal flotation devices should be available when a young child is in or near a body of water.
- Parents and caregivers should be trained in child cardiopulmonary resuscitation (CPR).

HEALTHY PEOPLE 2010

Objective	Significance
Reduce growth retardation among low-income children under age 5 years.	• Counsel families about the appropriate toddler diet. • Refer eligible families to WIC for grocery supplementation and nutritional counseling.

Weaning

The timing of weaning from breastfeeding is influenced by a number of factors such as cultural beliefs, local and regional ethnic beliefs, the mother's work schedule, desired child spacing, or societal feelings about the nature of the mother–infant relationship. The extent and duration of breastfeeding are inversely related to the development of obesity later in life: children who breastfeed longer are less likely to become obese than those who breastfeed for shorter periods of time. Thus, extending breastfeeding into toddlerhood is believed to be beneficial to the child. Extended breastfeeding provides nutritional, immunologic, and emotional benefits to the child. Contrary to popular belief, it is biologically possible to become pregnant while breastfeeding. Breastfeeding a newborn appropriately can occur while continuing to nurse its older sibling.

Weaning from breastfeeding tends to occur earlier in the United States than in countries around the world, despite recommendations on length of breastfeeding by a number of organizations. Table 5.5 gives recommendations for breastfeeding duration.

Weaning is a highly individualized decision. Educate the mother about the benefits of extended breastfeeding and support her in her decision to wean at a given time.

Weaning from the bottle should occur by 12 to 15 months of age. Prolonged bottle-feeding is associated with the development of dental caries. No-spill "sippy cups" contain a valve that requires sucking by the toddler in order to obtain fluid, thus functioning similar to a baby bottle. Hence, no-spill sippy cups can also be associated with dental caries and are not recommended. Cups with spouts that do not contain valves are acceptable. The 12- to 15-month-old is developmentally capable of consuming adequate fluid amounts using a cup.

Teaching About Nutritional Needs

Adequate calcium intake and appropriate exercise lay the foundation for proper bone mineralization. The toddler requires an average intake of 500 mg calcium per day. Dairy products are considered the primary sources of dietary calcium. One cup of low-fat or whole milk, 8 ounces of low-fat yogurt, and 1½ ounces of cheddar cheese each

Table 5.5 Recommendations for Breastfeeding Duration

Organization	Length of Time
World Health Organization (WHO)	2 years
American Academy of Pediatrics (AAP)	Minimum of 1 year
American Academy of Family Physicians (AAFP)	Minimum of 1 year
American College of Obstetricians and Gynecologists (ACOG)	Minimum of 6 months
National Association of Pediatric Nurse Practitioners (NAPNAP)	Minimum of 1 year
American College of Nurse Midwives (ACNM)	Minimum of 1 year
American Dietetic Association (ADA)	Minimum of 1 year

provide 300 mg of calcium. Broccoli, oranges, sweet potatoes, tofu, and dried beans or legumes are also good sources of calcium (35 to 120 mg calcium per serving).

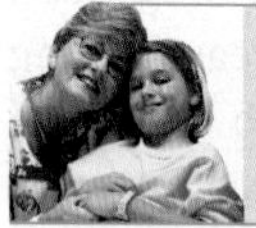

Though a half-cup of cooked spinach contains 120 mg of calcium, it is essentially non-bioavailable, making spinach a poor source of calcium.

Iron-deficiency anemia in the first 2 years of life may be associated with developmental and psychomotor delays. Even after correction of the anemia, the effects can be long-lasting (Eden, 2002). Thus, although it is important for toddlers to consume adequate amounts of iron, they tend to have the lowest daily iron intake of any age group. When breastfeeding or formula feeding ends (most often at 1 year of age), it is often replaced with iron-poor cow's milk. Limiting milk intake to 16 ounces per day, as well as limiting juice intake, can be helpful. Encourage the parents to provide iron-fortified cereals and other foods rich in iron and vitamin C.

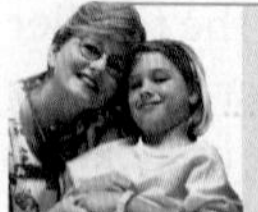

Toddlers who consume a strictly vegan diet (no food from animal sources) are at risk for deficiencies in vitamin D, vitamin B12, and iron. Supplementation with these nutrients should occur to promote adequate nutrition and growth.

Fat or cholesterol intake should not be restricted in children under age 2 years. The first 2 years of life require high energy intake because they are a time of very rapid growth and development. To promote healthy cholesterol levels, children over age 2 years should consume a diet with a total fat content between 20% and 30% of total calories. Saturated fats should account for less than 10% of total calories. Due to daily variations and the pickiness of the toddler, fat intake should be evaluated over a period of several days. The daily recommended intake of fiber for a 1- to 3-year-old is 19 grams. Figure 5.11 gives guidance on serving sizes and daily nutritional needs. Box 5.4 lists common sources of several nutrients.

Parents should encourage toddlers to drink water. Juice intake should be limited to 4 to 6 ounces per day. Milk intake should be limited to 16 to 24 ounces per day. Juice and milk should be served along with meals or snacks. Water should be offered for between-meal drinking. Toddlers should drink from a cup.

Advancing Solid Foods

Parents should offer three full meals and two snacks daily. Portion sizes for toddlers are about one-quarter the size of adult portions. Large portions of a new or different food on the toddler's plate may intimidate the toddler. Normal toddler behaviors of mouthing, handling, tasting, extruding the food from the mouth, and then resampling the food often occur. These behaviors are distasteful to some parents but are a normal part of toddler development. Parents need to understand and tolerate these behaviors rather than scolding the toddler for them. Toddlers are often afraid to try new things anyway, so the parent or caregiver should be flexible with the toddler's acceptance or rejection of new foods. If the toddler refuses healthy food choices at meal or snack time, parents should not substitute high-fat, high-sugar, processed food "just to make sure he's eating something." This sets the stage for future power struggles. The parent decides which foods will be served or offered. The toddler decides how much will be eaten. The toddler self-regulates the amount of food needed to sustain and allow further growth and development. The toddler may not eat well every day but generally, over the course of several days, will consume the foods he or she needs.

Foods should be served near room temperature. Some of the food on the plate should be soft and moist. Food should always be cut into bite-size pieces. Teaching

Food Guide Pyramid For Your Young Child

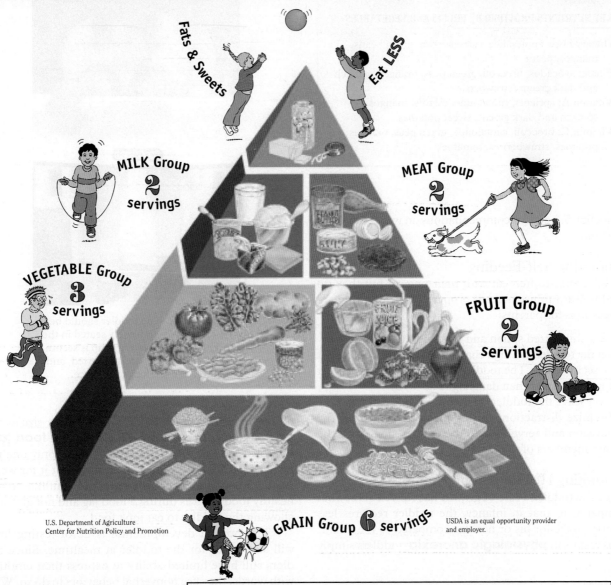

FOOD IS FUN and learning about food is fun, too. Eating foods from the Food Guide Pyramid and being physically active will help you grow healthy and strong.

What Counts As One Serving?

Grain Group
1 slice of bread
½ cup of cooked rice or pasta
½ cup of cooked cereal
1 ounce of ready-to-eat cereal

Vegetable Group
½ cup of chopped raw or cooked vegetables
1 cup of raw leafy vegetables

Fruit Group
1 piece of fruit or melon wedge
¾ cup of juice
½ cup of canned fruit
¼ cup of dried fruit

Milk Group
1 cup of milk or yogurt
2 ounces of cheese

Meat Group
2 to 3 ounces of cooked lean meat, poultry, or fish
½ cup of cooked dry beans, or 1 egg counts as 1 ounce of lean meat.
2 tablespoons of peanut butter count as 1 ounce of meat

Fats and Sweets
Limit calories from these.

Four- to 6-year-olds can eat these serving sizes. Offer 2- to 3-year-olds less, except for milk. Two- to 6-year-old children need a total of 2 servings from the milk group each day.

Provided by ______________________

NIBBLES FOR HEALTH 2 Nutrition Newsletters for Parents of Young Children, USDA, Food and Nutrition Service

● Figure 5.11 The U.S. Department of Agriculture's Young Child Food Pyramid provides a guide for parents and caregivers for determining adequate nutritional intake. (USDA, http://www.fns.usda.gov/tn/Resources/Nibbles/fgp_nibbles.pdf.)

BOX 5.4

KEY NUTRIENTS PROVIDED BY FRUITS AND VEGETABLES

Dietary fiber: applesauce, carrots, corn, green beans, mangos, pears
Folate: avocados, broccoli, green peas, oranges, spinach and dark greens, strawberries
Vitamin A: apricots, cantaloupe, carrots, mangos, spinach and dark greens, sweet potatoes
Vitamin C: broccoli, cantaloupe, green peas, oranges, potatoes, strawberries, tomatoes

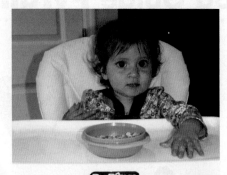

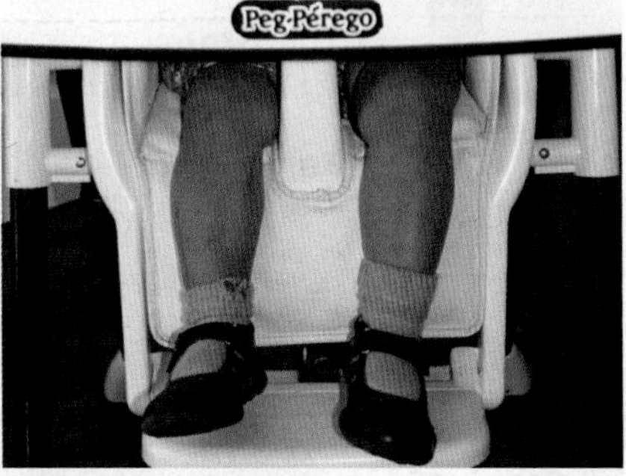

● Figure 5.12 The toddler should be appropriately and safely seated in the high chair. The safety strap is secure, the toddler's feet are supported, and the tray table is locked in place.

Guideline 5.2 gives recommendations on ways to prevent choking.

Promoting Self-Feeding

Toddlers most often eat with their fingers, but they do need to learn to use utensils properly. The following are suggestions for parents:

- Use a child-sized spoon and fork with dull tines.
- Seat the toddler in a high chair or at a comfortable height in a secure chair. The toddler should have his or her feet supported rather than dangling (Fig. 5.12).
- Never leave the toddler unattended while eating.
- Minimize distractions during mealtime. Turn off the television and serve food to the toddler along with the other members of the family.

Promoting Healthy Eating Habits

Since the toddler's rate of growth has slowed somewhat compared to that in infancy, the toddler requires less caloric intake for his or her size compared to the infant. This results in **physiologic anorexia**: toddlers simply do not require as much food intake for their size as they did in infancy. The toddler will also exhibit **food jags**. During a food jag, the toddler may prefer only one particular food for several days, then not want it for weeks. Again, it is important for the parent to continue to offer healthy food choices during a food jag and not give in by allowing the toddler to eat junk food.

The normal developmental issue of testing limits will also occur for the toddler at mealtime. Since toddlers still have limited ability to express their emotions with words, they use nonverbal behaviors to do so. While eating, the toddler may dislike the taste of a particular food or experience a feeling of fullness but will communicate that feeling by screaming or throwing food. When the child exhibits these behaviors, the parent must remain calm and remove the toddler from the situation. Meals should be eaten in a calm and pleasant environment. Parents should serve as role models for appropriate eating habits, but toddlers may also be willing to try more foods if they are exposed to other children who eat those foods. Praise the child for trying a new food, and never punish the toddler for refusing to try something new. A new food may need to be offered many times in a row before the toddler chooses to try it. Parents should be sure to include foods the child is familiar with and likes to eat at the same meal that the new food is being introduced. Teaching Guideline 5.3 lists alternative foods that meet nutritional needs and a list of books for parents of the picky eater.

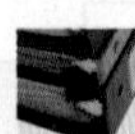

TEACHING GUIDELINE 5.2

Avoiding Choking

- Slowly add foods that are more difficult to chew as the toddler becomes more adept at chewing.
- Cut all foods into bite-sized pieces.
- Avoid foods that are hard to chew and may become lodged in the airway, such as:
  - Nuts
  - Gumdrops or other chewy candies
  - Raw carrots
  - Peanut butter (by itself)
  - Popcorn
- Cut hotdogs and grapes into quarters. Cook carrots until soft; if serving raw, then grate them.
- Always supervise the toddler while he or she is eating.

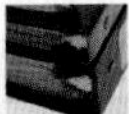

TEACHING GUIDELINE 5.3

Meeting Nutritional Needs of the Picky Eater

Alternative Food Choices for the Picky Eater

- Won't drink milk? Obtain calcium through yogurt (frozen or regular), cheese, pudding, and hot cocoa.
- Poor meat intake? Obtain iron through unsweetened iron-fortified cereals or breakfast bars, raisins; cook with an iron skillet.
- Loves processed white bread? Encourage fiber intake with fresh fruits and vegetables, bran muffins, beans or peas (can be in soup).
- Refuses vegetables? Encourage vitamin A intake with apricots, sweet potatoes, and vegetable juices.

Books for Parents of the Picky Eater

- *Coping with a Picky Eater: A Guide for the Perplexed Parent* by W. Wilkoff. New York: Simon & Schuster, 1998.
- *First Foods* by M. Stoddard. New York: Dorling-Kindersley Publishing, Inc., 1998.
- *How to Get Your Kid to Eat . . . but not too much* by E. Satter. Boulder, CO: Bull Publishing Co., 1987.
- *The "Everything" Baby's First Food Book* by J. Tarlou. Holbrook, MA: Adams Media Corp., 2001.
- *The Family Nutrition Book* by W. Sears & M. Sears. Boston: Little Brown & Co., 1999.
- *The Healthy Baby Meal Planner* by A. Karmel. New York: Simon & Schuster, 2001.

Preventing Overweight and Obesity

In the child younger than 3 years of age, the greatest risk factor for the development of overweight or obesity is having an obese parent. The nurse can screen for overweight in the child over 2 years of age by calculating the body mass index (BMI) and plotting the BMI on the standardized age- and gender-appropriate growth charts (see Appendix A for growth charts, and refer to Chapter 10 for BMI calculation instructions). Trends over time may be predictive of the development of overweight or obesity.

Another factor in development of obesity in young children is juice intake. Since most young children like the sweet taste of juice, they may drink excessive amounts of it. Toddlers who drink excess fruit juice and eat well may develop overweight or obesity because of the high sugar content in the juice. On the other end of the spectrum, some children may actually feel full from juice consumption and decrease their intake of solid foods. These children are at risk for malnutrition. Fruit juice intake should be limited to 4 to 6 ounces per day.

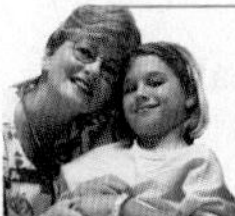

Young children should consume only pasteurized juice, as unpasteurized juice consumption places the toddler at increased risk of *Escherichia coli*, *Salmonella*, and *Cryptosporidium* infection.

> Refer back to Jose Gonzales. What questions should you ask his parents related to his nutritional intake? What anticipatory guidance related to nutrition would be appropriate?

Promoting Healthy Sleep and Rest

The 18-month-old requires 13.5 hours of sleep per day, the 24-month-old 13 hours, and the 3-year-old 12 hours. A typical toddler should sleep through the night and take one daytime nap. Most children discontinue daytime napping at around 3 years of age. The toddler who slept in a crib as an infant will need to move to a youth or toddler bed or even a full-size bed usually sometime in the toddler period. When the crib becomes unsafe (that is, when the toddler becomes physically capable of climbing over the rails), then he or she must make the transition to a bed.

Consistent bedtime rituals help the toddler prepare for sleep. Choose a bedtime and stick to it as much as possible. The nightly routine might include a bath followed by reading a story. The routine should be a calm period with minimal outside distractions. Toddlers often require a security item to help them get to sleep. Older toddlers may be afraid of the dark, so a nightlight is often helpful.

Night waking is a problem for some toddlers. This may occur as a result of change in routine or as a desire for nighttime attention. Attention during night waking should be minimized so that the toddler receives no reward for being awake at night. The book, "Solve Your Child's Sleep Problems," by Dr. Richard Ferber (1986, New York: Fireside Publishing), is an excellent resource for the family with a toddler who resists bedtime or is a persistent night waker. For some toddlers, night waking is caused by nightmares. As the imagination and capacity for make-believe grow, the toddler may not be able to distinguish between reality and pretend. The parent should hold and comfort the toddler after a nightmare. Limiting television viewing (especially shortly before bedtime) may be helpful in limiting nightmares.

Some families practice "co-sleeping" (when children sleep in the parents' bed). Although some professionals believe that co-sleeping may interfere with the toddler's struggle for independence, this theory has not been proven. The nurse should support the family's choice for sleep arrangements unless the co-sleeping is unsafe either physically or psychologically (Stein, 2001).

Provide anticipatory guidance to Jose Gonzales' parents in relation to his sleep.

Promoting Healthy Teeth and Gums

By 30 months of age, the toddler should have a full set of primary ("baby") teeth. Parents may not be aware of the importance of preventing cavities in primary teeth since they will eventually be replaced by the permanent teeth. Poor oral hygiene, prolonged use of a bottle or no-spill sippy cup, lack of fluoride intake, and delayed or absent professional dental care may all contribute to the development of dental caries. Cleaning of the toddler's teeth should progress from brushing with simply water to using a very small amount (pea-sized) of fluoridated toothpaste with brushing beginning at 2 years of age (Fig. 5.13). Weaning from the bottle no later than 15 months of age and severely restricting use of a no-spill sippy cup (the kind that requires sucking for fluid delivery) is recommended.

At age 1 year, the toddler should have his or her first dentist visit to establish current health of the teeth and gums. Eating should be limited to meal and snack times, as "grazing" throughout the day exposes the teeth to food throughout the day. Carbohydrate-containing foods combined with oral bacteria create a decreased oral pH level that is optimal for the development of dental caries (cavities). See Healthy People 2010.

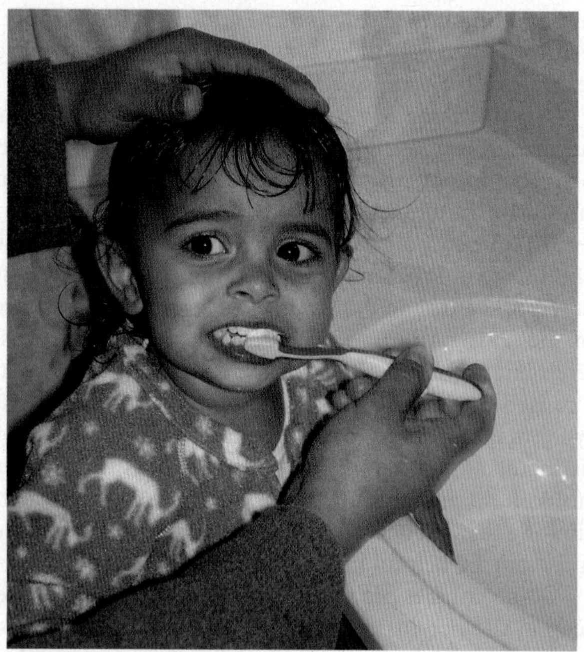

● **Figure 5.13** The parent should brush the toddler's teeth to ensure proper cleaning of the teeth, gums, and tongue. Use only water for brushing before 2 years of age and a pea-sized amount of fluoride-containing toothpaste after age 2 years.

HEALTHY PEOPLE 2010

Objective	Significance
Reduce the proportion of children with untreated dental decay.	• Encourage weaning from bottle by 15 months of age. • Discourage use of no-spill sippy cups. • Refer any toddler with potential or existing caries to pediatric dentist.

Public water fluoridation is a public health initiative that ensures that most children receive adequate fluoride intake to prevent dental caries. Table 5.6 gives recommendations regarding fluoride supplementation. If the water supply contains adequate fluoride, no other supplementation is necessary other than brushing with a small amount of fluoride-containing toothpaste after age 2 years. Excess fluoride ingestion should be avoided, as it contributes to the development of fluorosis (mottling of the enamel). Fluorosis occurs most often in the toddler years. Risk factors for fluorosis development include:

- High fluoride levels in the local water supply
- Use of fluoride-containing toothpaste prior to age 2 years
- Excessive ingestion of fluoride either in toothpaste or foods
  - Fluoride-containing foods: tea, ready-to-eat infant foods containing chicken, white or purple grape juice, and beverages, processed foods and cereals that were manufactured with fluoride-containing water

Promoting Appropriate Discipline

Discipline is a common concern during toddlerhood. The toddler's intense personality and intense emotional reactions can be difficult for parents to understand and cope with. The toddler needs firm, gentle guidance to learn what the expectations are and how to meet them. The parent's love and respect for the toddler teach the toddler to care about himself or herself and for others. Affection is as important as the guidance aspect of discipline. Having realistic expectations of what the toddler is capable of learning and understanding can help the parent in the disciplinary process. The toddler's intense push for autonomy can often test a parent's limits. The easygoing infant usually becomes more challenging in toddlerhood. The toddler's continual quest for new experiences often places the toddler at risk, and his or her negativism very often taxes the parent's patience.

In an effort to prevent the toddler from experiencing harm and in response to his or her continual testing of limits, parents often resort to spanking. Though commonly

Table 5.6 Recommendations for Fluoride Supplementation

	Fluoride Ion Level in Drinking Water (ppm)		
Age	**<0.3 ppm**	**0.3–0.6 ppm**	**>0.6 ppm**
Birth to 6 months	None	None	None
6 months to 3 years	0.25 mg/day	None	None
3–6 years	0.50 mg/day	0.25 mg/day	None
6–16 years	1.0 mg/day	0.50 mg/day	None

ppm: parts per million is equivalent to 1 mg/liter
These recommendations are public domain at www.ada.org and were approved by the American Dental Association, the American Academy of Pediatrics, and the American Academy of Pediatric Dentistry.

accepted, the American Academy of Pediatrics and the National Association of Pediatric Nurse Practitioners recommend against corporal or physical punishment (AAP, Committee on Psychosocial Aspects of Child and Family Health, 1998; NAPNAP, 2002). Recent research points out the dangers inherent in the use of corporal punishment as well as the possibilities for negative effects on the child's future behavior (Box 5.5). Spanking or other forms of corporal punishment lead to a pro-violence attitude, create resentment and anger in some children, and contribute to the cycle of violence (NAPNAP, 2002).

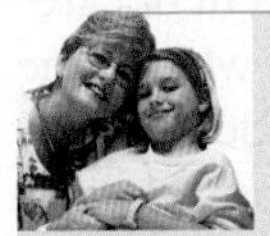

Toddlers less than 18 months of age should NEVER be spanked, as there is an increased possibility of physical injury in this age group. Also, the infant/young toddler is not capable of linking the spanking with the undesired behavior.

Normal toddler development includes natural curiosity, and this curiosity often results in dangerous or problematic activities for the toddler. Toddlers have a difficult time learning the rules and in general do not behave badly intentionally. Providing a childproof environment will allow the toddler to participate in safe exploration, which will meet his or her developmental needs and decrease the frequency of intervention needed on the part of the parents.

Discipline should be focused on limit setting, negotiation, and techniques to assist the toddler to learn problem solving. Parents should provide consistency and commit to the limits that are set.

Offering realistic choices helps give the toddler a sense of mastery. Rules should be simple and limited in number. Maintaining the toddler's schedule of meals and rest/sleep will help to prevent conflicts that occur as a result of hunger or fatigue. Toddlers should not be made to share, as this is a concept they do not understand. Parents should encourage simple activities enjoyed by the children involved and avoid confrontation over toys. Parents should offer toddlers appropriate choices to help them develop autonomy, but should not offer a choice when none exists.

Positive reinforcement should be used as much as possible. "Catching" a child being good helps to reinforce appropriate or desirable behaviors (Gottesman, 2000). When the toddler is displaying appropriate behavior, the parent should reward the child consistently with praise and physical affection.

BOX 5.5

NEGATIVE IMPACT OF PHYSICAL PUNISHMENT

- Spanking is less effective than time-out or other discipline measures to reduce undesired behavior in children.
- The toddler less than 18 months of age:
  - Is not capable of making the appropriate connections between spanking and the undesired behavior
  - Is at increased risk for physical injury from spanking than older children
- Physical punishment:
  - May lead to a pro-violence attitude
  - May create resentment in the toddler
  - Is a poor model for learning effective problem solving
  - May be correlated with antisocial and criminal behavior later in life
  - Leads to increased aggression in preschoolers, school-aged children, and adults
  - When used frequently, may weaken the parent–child relationship
- Childhood corporal punishment increases the probability of depression and substance abuse in adulthood.
- Spanking may lead to more severe forms of punishment and actually to child abuse and maltreatment.
- The more frequently children are hit or spanked, the more likely they are to hit their own children and to be involved in spouse abuse as adults.

(AAP, Committee on Psychosocial Aspects of Child and Family Health, 1998; Ateah et al., 2003; NAPNAP, 2002)

"Time out" can be used effectively at around 2.5 to 3 years of age (refer to Chapter 6 for details). "Extinction" is a particularly useful technique with 2- and 3-year-olds. Extinction involves systematic ignoring of the undesired behavior. Parents sometimes unknowingly contribute to the occurrence of an unwanted behavior simply by the attention they give the toddler (even if is negative in nature, it is still attention). Parents who want to extinguish an annoying (non-dangerous) behavior should resolve to ignore it every time it occurs. When the child withholds the behavior or performs the opposite (appropriate) behavior, they should use compliments and praise. It may be difficult to ignore a difficult behavior, but the results are well worth the effort. Teaching Guideline 5.4 provides tips on avoiding power struggles and offering appropriate guidance to toddlers.

ADDRESSING COMMON DEVELOPMENTAL CONCERNS

Common developmental concerns of the toddler period are toilet teaching, temper tantrums, thumb sucking or pacifier use, sibling rivalry, and regression. An understanding of the normalcy of negativism, temper tantrums, and sibling rivalry will help the family cope with these issues. Prepare parents for these developmental events by giving appropriate anticipatory guidance.

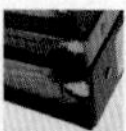

TEACHING GUIDELINE 5.4

Providing Toddlers with Guidance

- When giving the toddler instructions, tell the child what to do, NOT what not to do. This allows for a positive focus. If you must say "no," "don't," or "stop," then follow with a direction of what to do instead.
- Offer limited choices, when a choice is truly available. Say, "Do you want to wear your blue hat or your red hat?" NOT "Do you want to put on your hat?" This gives the toddler some, but not all, control.
- Role model appropriate communication, but don't feel like you have to speak nicely all the time. If the situation warrants, use a firm and even tone to get the point across. Avoid yelling.
- Pay attention to the inflection in your voice. A statement or direction should not end in a questioning tone or with "Okay?" Be clear. Statements should sound like statements, and only questions should end in a questioning tone.
- When a toddler behaves aggressively, label the child's feelings calmly, but be firm and consistent with the expectation. For example, "I know you're mad at your friend, but it is not okay to hit."

Toilet Teaching

When myelinization of the spinal cord is achieved around age 2 years, the toddler is capable of exercising voluntary control over the sphincters. Girls may be ready for toilet teaching earlier than boys. Toddlers are ready for toilet teaching when:

- Bowel movements occur on a fairly regular schedule.
- The toddler expresses knowledge of the need to defecate or urinate. This may be through verbalization, change in activity, or gestures such as:
  - Looks into or grabs diaper
  - Squats
  - Crosses legs
  - Grimaces and/or grunts
  - Hides behind a door or the couch when defecating
- The diaper is not always wet (this indicates the ability to hold the urine for a period of time).
- The toddler is willing to follow instructions.
- The toddler walks well alone and is able to pull down his or her pants.
- The toddler follows caregivers to the bathroom.
- The toddler climbs onto the potty chair or toilet.

Parents should approach toilet teaching with a calm, positive, and nonthreatening manner. Initially it may be helpful to allow the toddler to observe a same-sex family member using the toilet. Start with the toddler fully clothed on the potty chair or toilet while the parent or caregiver talks about what the toilet is used for and when. The toddler will feel most comfortable with a toddler potty chair that sits on the floor (Fig. 5.14). If a potty chair is unavailable, facing toward the toilet tank may make the

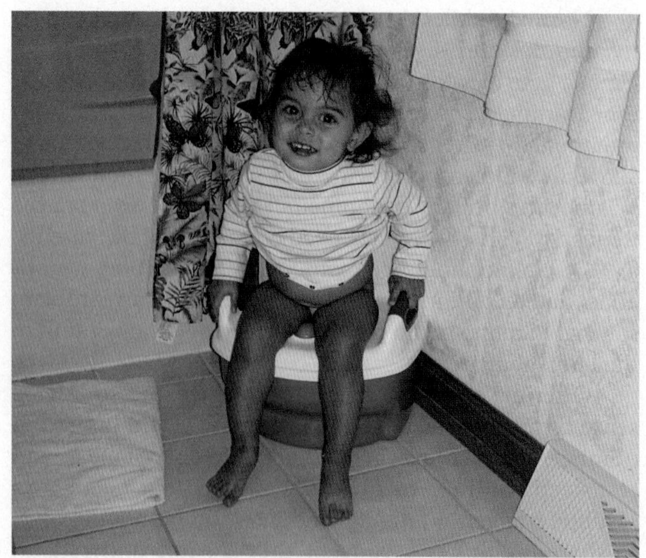

Figure 5.14 The toddler will feel most comfortable with a potty chair that sits on the floor.

toddler feel more secure, as the buttocks remain on the front of the seat rather than sinking through the toilet seat opening. After a week or longer, remove a dirty diaper and place the contents in the toilet. Next try having the toddler sit on the potty chair or toilet without pants or diaper on. The toddler may benefit from watching a caregiver or friend use the toilet. It may also be beneficial to demonstrate using the potty chair with a baby doll that wets.

Parents should always use gentle praise and no reproaches. Usually the best time to achieve success with defecation on the toilet is following a meal. When the toddler has achieved success with bowel control, bladder control will come next. It may be many months before nighttime bladder control is achieved, and the toddler may still require a diaper at night. Parents should use appropriate words for body parts, urination, and defecation, then use those words consistently so the toddler understands what to say and do.

After a couple of weeks of successful toileting, the toddler may start wearing training pants. When toddlers have an accident and don't make it to the toilet, gently remind them about toileting and let them help clean up. Toddlers should never be punished for bowel or bladder "accidents."

With so much attention focused on the genitalia during toilet teaching and the frequency of being without a diaper, it is natural for toddlers to become more focused on their own genitalia. Boys and girls both will explore their genitalia and discover the resulting pleasurable sensation. Masturbation in the toddler often causes a great deal of discomfort in the parent. The parent should not draw attention to the activity, as that may increase its frequency. The parent should calmly explain to the toddler that this is an activity that may only be done in private. If the toddler is masturbating excessively or refuses to stop when in public, then there may be additional stressors in the toddler's life that should be explored.

Negativism

Negativism is common in the toddler period. As the toddler separates from the parent, recognizes his or her own individuality, and exerts autonomy, negativism abounds. Parents should understand that this negativism is a normal developmental occurrence and not necessarily deliberate defiance (though that also occurs). Avoid asking yes-or-no questions, as the toddler's usual response will be "no," whether he or she means it or not. Offering the child simple choices will give the toddler a sense of control. The parent should not ask the toddler if he or she "wants" to do something, if there is actually no choice. "Do you want to use the red cup or the blue cup?" is more appropriate than "Do you want your milk now?" When it is time to go outside, don't ask, "Do you want to put your shoes on?" Instead, state in a matter-of-fact tone that shoes must be worn outside, and give the toddler a choice of type of shoe or color of socks. If the child continues with negative answers, then the parent should remain calm and make the decision for the child.

Temper Tantrums

Even children who displayed an easygoing personality as infants may lose their temper frequently during the toddler years (Fig. 5.15). A toddler who was more intense as an infant may have more temper tantrums. Temper tantrums are a natural result of the frustration that toddlers experience. Toddlers are eager to explore new things, but their efforts are often thwarted (usually for safety reasons). Toddlers do not behave badly on purpose. They need time and maturity to learn the rules and regulations. Some of their frustration may come from lack of language skills to express themselves. Toddlers are just starting to learn how to verbalize feelings and to use alternative actions rather than just "pitching a fit." The temper tantrum may be manifested as a screaming and crying fit or a full-blown episode in which the toddler throws himself or herself on the floor kicking, screaming, and pounding, perhaps even holding the breath. Fatigue or hunger may limit the toddler's coping abilities and promote negative behavior and temper tantrums.

Although tantrums are annoying to parents and caregivers, they are a normal part of the toddler's quest for independence. As toddlers mature, they become better able to express themselves and to understand their environment.

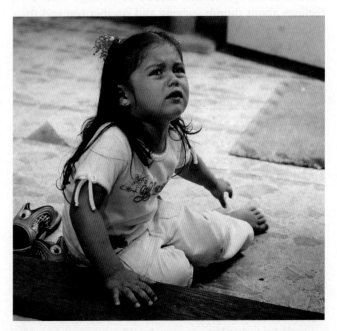

● Figure 5.15 Tantrums are a normal component of toddler development.

Parents need to learn their toddler's behavioral cues in order to limit activity that is frustrating. When the parent notes the beginnings of frustration, a friendly warning might be given. Intervening early with an activity change might prevent a tantrum. Use distraction, refocusing, or removal from the situation.

When a temper tantrum does occur, the best course of action is to ignore the behavior and ensure that the child is safe during the tantrum. Physical punishment will probably just prolong the tantrum and in fact produce more intense negative behavior (Ateah et al., 2003). If the tantrum occurs in public, it may be necessary for the parent to immobilize the child with a big bear hug and use a calm voice to soothe the toddler. It is very important for parents to model self-control. Since toddlers' tantrums most often result from frustration, the role-modeled behavior of self-control helps to teach toddlers to control their temper when they can't get what they want.

Thumb Sucking and Pacifiers

Infants bring their hands to their mouths and begin thumb sucking as a form of self-soothing. This habit may continue into the toddler years and beyond. The pacifier is used for the same reason. Toddlers may calm themselves in a stressful situation by thumb sucking or sucking on a pacifier. Opinions about thumb and finger sucking and pacifier use are significantly affected by family history and culture. For most children there is no need to worry about a sucking habit until it is time for the permanent teeth to erupt. Prolonged and frequent sucking in the withdrawn child is more likely to yield changes to the tooth and jaw structure than sucking that is primarily used for self-soothing. Parents must sort through their own feelings about thumb sucking and pacifier use and then decide how they want to handle the habit.

To ensure safety with pacifier use:

- Use only one-piece pacifiers.
- Replace worn pacifiers with new ones.
- Never tie a pacifier around a toddler's neck.

Parents may want to limit thumb sucking and pacifier use to bedtime, in the car, and in stressful situations. The parent should calmly discuss these limits with the toddler and then remain consistent about enforcing them.

Sibling Rivalry

Many families have subsequent children when their first child is a toddler. The toddler has been accustomed to being the baby and receiving a great deal of attention, both at home and with the extended family. Since toddlers are normally egocentric, bringing a new baby into the home may be quite disruptive. To minimize issues with **sibling rivalry**, parents should attempt to keep the toddler's routine as close to normal as possible. Spend individual time with the toddler on a daily basis. Involve the toddler in the care of the baby. The toddler is capable of fetching a diaper or T-shirt, entertaining the baby with a toy, or helping sing a song to calm the baby. "Helping" the parent care for the baby gives the toddler a sense of importance (Fig. 5.16). The toddler will need significant support while holding the baby.

Regression

Some toddlers experience **regression** during a stressful event (e.g., the birth of a sibling, hospitalization). Stress in a toddler's life affects his or her ability to master new developmental tasks. During regression, the toddler may want to go back to an earlier stage. He or she may desire a bottle or pacifier long ago forgotten. The toddler may stop displaying previously achieved language or motor skills. A significant stress in the toddler's life may also disrupt the toilet teaching process (toilet teaching may not be achieved near the time a sibling is born). When regression occurs, parents should ignore the regressive behavior and offer praise for age-appropriate behavior or attainment of skills.

> **Refer to Jose Gonzales,** the 2-year-old in the case study. List common developmental concerns of the toddler. What anticipatory guidance related to these concerns would the nurse provide to Jose's parents?

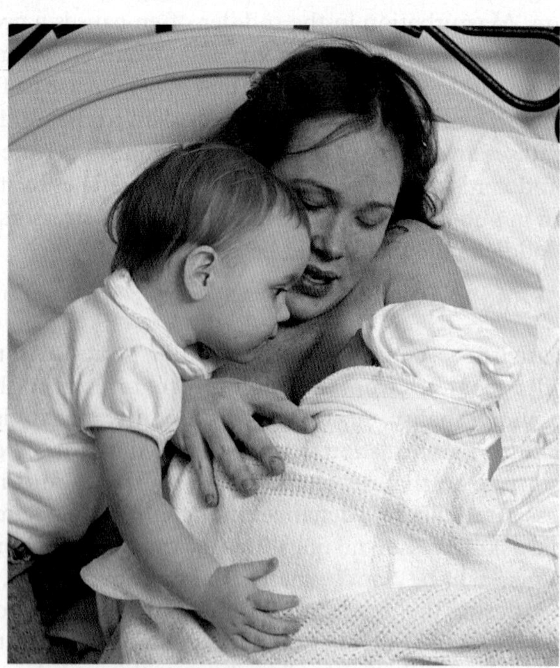

● **Figure 5.16** The toddler may be more likely to accept the new baby in a positive manner if she feels that this is "our baby," not just "mommy's baby." This toddler is meeting her new brother for the first time.

References

Books and Journals

Ackley, B., & Ladwig, G. (2006). *Nursing diagnosis handbook: A guide to planning care* (7th ed.). St. Louis: Mosby.

Adler, M., & Specker, B. (2001). Atypical diets in infancy and childhood. *Pediatric Annals, 30*(11), 630–680.

American Academy of Pediatrics. (2000). Swimming programs for infants and toddlers. *Pediatrics, 105*(4), 868–870.

American Academy of Pediatrics. (2001). Policy Statement: The use and misuse of fruit juice in pediatrics (RE0047). *Pediatrics, 107*(5), 1201–1213.

American Academy of Pediatrics. (2003a). Policy Statement: Poison treatment in the home. *Pediatrics, 112*(5), 1182–1185.

American Academy of Pediatrics. (2003b). Protect your child from poison. Available at www.aap.org/healthtopics/safety.cfm

American Academy of Pediatrics. (2003c). Policy Statement: Prevention of drowning in infants, children and adolescents. *Pediatrics, 112*(2), 437–439.

American Academy of Pediatrics. (2005). The injury prevention program, age-related safety sheets: 2–4 years. Accessed 1/10/05 at www.aap.org/family/2to4yrs.htm

American Academy of Pediatrics, Committee on Injury and Poison Prevention. (2000). Children in pickup trucks. *Pediatrics, 106*(4), 857–859.

American Academy of Pediatrics, Committee on Nutrition. (1998). Cholesterol in childhood. *Pediatrics, 112*(2), 424–430.

American Academy of Pediatrics, Committee on Nutrition. (1999). Calcium requirements of infants, children, and adolescents. *Pediatrics, 104*(5), 1152–1157.

American Academy of Pediatrics, Committee on Nutrition. (2003). Prevention of pediatric overweight and obesity. *Pediatrics, 104*(5), 1152–1157.

American Academy of Pediatrics, Committee on Psychosocial Aspects of Child and Family Health. (1998). Guidelines for effective discipline. *Pediatrics, 101*(4), 723–728.

American Dietetic Association. (2001). Breaking the barriers to breastfeeding: Position of the ADA. *Journal of the American Dietetic Association, 101,* 1213.

American Dietetic Association. (2002). 5 a day for young children up to 2 years of age. Accessed 12/11/03 at http://www.webdietitians.org/Public/NutritionInformation/92_nfs0302.cfm

American Dietetic Association. (2004). Dietary guidance for healthy children aged 2 to 11 years. *Journal of the American Dietetic Association, 104,* 660–677.

Arias, A., Bennison, J., Justus, K., & Thurman, D. (2001). Educating parents about normal stool pattern changes in infants. *Journal of Pediatric Health Care, 15*(5), 269–274.

Ateah, C. A., Secco, L., & Woodgate, R. L. (2003). The risks and alternatives to physical punishment use with children. *Journal of Pediatric Health Care, 17*(3), 126–132.

Atkinson, P. M., Parks, D. K., Cooley, S. M., & Sarkis, S. L. (2002). Reach out and read: A pediatric clinic-based approach to early literacy promotion. *Journal of Pediatric Health Care, 16*(1), 10–15.

Blackwell, P. B., & Baker, B. M. (2002). Estimating communication competence of infants and toddlers. *Journal of Pediatric Health Care, 16*(1), 29–35.

Brazelton, T. B. (1992). *Touchpoints, the essential reference: Your child's emotional and behavioral development.* New York: Perseus Books Group.

Brown, M. L. (2001). The effects of environmental tobacco smoke on children: Information and implications for PNPs. *Journal of Pediatric Health Care, 15*(6), 280–286.

Butler, F. R., & Zakari, N. (2005). Grandparents parenting grandchildren: Assessing health status, parental stress and social supports. *Journal of Gerontological Nursing, 31*(3), 43–54.

Cathey, M., & Gaylord, N. (2004). Picky eating: A toddler's approach to mealtime. *Pediatric Nursing, 30*(2), 101–109.

Centers for Disease Control. (1998). Recommendations to prevent and control iron deficiency in the United States. *Morbidity and Mortality Weekly Report 47(RR-3),* 1–36.

Chan, G. (2001). Calcium needs during childhood. *Pediatric Annals, 30*(11), 666–670.

Cincinnati Children's Hospital Medical Center (2003). Toddler nutrition. Accessed 12/10/03 at http://www.cincinnatichildrens.org/health/info/growth/well/toddler/toddler-nutrition.htm

Deering, C. G., & Cody, D. J. (2002). Communicating with children and adolescents. *American Journal of Nursing, 102*(3), 34–41.

Dettwyler, K. A. (2004). When to wean: Biological versus cultural perspectives. *Clinical Obstetrics and Gynecology, 47*(3), 721–723.

Dowd, M. D., Keenan, H. T., & Bratton, S. L. (2002). Epidemiology and prevention of childhood injuries. *Critical Care Medicine, 30*(11, Suppl.), S385–S392.

Eden, A. (2002). The prevention of iron-deficiency anemia. *Archives of Pediatric and Adolescent Medicine, 156,* 519.

Erikson, E. H. (1963). *Childhood and society* (2nd ed.). New York: W.W. Norton and Company.

Fierro-Cobas, V. (2001). Language development in bilingual children: A primer for pediatricians. *Contemporary Pediatrics, 18*(7), 79–98.

Gabbard, G. O. (2000). Psychoanalysis. In B. J. Sadock & V. A. Sadock (Eds.), *Kaplan and Sadock's comprehensive textbook of psychiatry* (7th ed.). Philadelphia: Lippincott Williams & Wilkins.

Gilger, M. A. (2006). Normal gastrointestinal function. In J. A. McMillan (Ed.), *Oski's pediatrics: Principles and practice* (4th ed.). Philadelphia: Lippincott Williams & Wilkins.

Gottesman, M. M. (2000). Nurturing the social and emotional development of children, a.k.a. discipline. *Journal of Pediatric Health Care, 14*(2), 81–84.

Gottesman, M. M. (2002). Helping toddlers eat well. *Journal of Pediatric Health Care, 16*(2), 92–96.

Green, M., ed. (1998). *Bright futures: Guidelines for health supervision of infants, children and adolescents* (rev. ed.). Arlington, VA: National Center for Education in Maternal and Child Health.

Hogg, T. (2002). *Secrets of the baby whisperer for toddlerhood.* New York: Random House.

Kandarian, P. E. (2001). Tips on getting child's cooperation: You can lead a child to a highchair . . . but will he eat? *ePediatric News, 35*(5). Accessed 9/3/03.

Kazal, L. A. (2002). Prevention of iron deficiency in infants and toddlers. *American Family Physician, 66*(7), 1217–1224.

Kohlberg, L. (1984). *Moral development.* New York: Harper & Row.

Krebs, N. F., Collins, J., & Johnson, S. L. (2004). Screen for and treat overweight in 2 to 5-year-olds? Yes! *Contemporary Pediatrics.* Accessed 11/15/04 at http://www.contemporarypediatrics.com.

LeCuyer-Maus, E. A., & Houck, G. M. (2002). Mother–toddler interaction and the development of self-regulation in a limit-setting context. *Journal of Pediatric Nursing, 17*(3), 184–200.

Lumeng, J. (2005). Is the picky eater a cause for concern? *Contemporary Pediatrics, 22*(3), 71–82.

Mandleco, B. (2004). *Growth and development handbook: Newborn through adolescence.* Clifton Park, NY: Delmar Learning.

National Association of Pediatric Nurse Practitioners. (2001). Position statement: Breastfeeding. [Electronic Version] Available at: http://www.napnap.org/index.cfm?page=10&sec=54&ssec=57

National Association of Pediatric Nurse Practitioners. (2001). Position statement: Child care. *Journal of Pediatric Health Care, 15*(2), 35A.

National Association of Pediatric Nurse Practitioners. (2002). Position statement: Corporal punishment. *Journal of Pediatric Health Care, 16*(3), 34A.

Nicklas, T. A., & Fisher, J. O. (2003). To each his own: Family influences on children's food preferences. *Pediatric Basics, 102,* 13–20.

Niemela, M., Pihakari, O., Pokka, T., & Uhari, M. (2000) Pacifier as a risk factor for acute otitis media: A randomized, controlled trial of parental counseling. *Pediatrics, 106,* 483–488.

Palmer, F. B., & Capute, A. J. (2006). Streams of development: The keys to developmental assessment. In J. A. McMillan (Ed.), *Oski's pediatrics: Principles and practice* (4th ed.). Philadelphia: Lippincott Williams & Wilkins.

Papalia, D. E., Olds, S. W., & Feldman, F. D. (2001). *Human development* (8th ed.). New York: McGraw-Hill.

Piaget, J. (1969). *The theory of stages in cognitive development.* New York: McGraw-Hill.

Preboth, M. (2002). Physical activity in infants, toddlers, and preschoolers. *American Family Physician, 65*(8), 1694–1696.

Record, S., Montgomery, D. R., & Milano, M. (2000). Fluoride supplementation and caries prevention. *Journal of Pediatric Health Care, 14*(5), 247–249.

Rychnovsky, J. D. (2000). No-spill sippy cups. *Journal of Pediatric Health Care, 14*(5), 207–208.

Schmitt, B. D. (2004). Toilet training problems: Underachievers, refusers, and stool holders. *Contemporary Pediatrics, 21*(4), 71–82.

Shelor, S. P. (Ed.). (1998). *Caring for your baby and young child: Birth to age 5.* New York: Bantam Books.

Starr, N. B. (2001). Kids and car safety: Beyond car seats and seat belts. *Journal of Pediatric Health Care, 15*(5), 257–259.

Stein, M. T. (2001). Cosleeping (bedsharing) among infants and toddlers. *Pediatrics 107*(4), 873–877.

Story, M., Holt, K., & Sofka, D. (Eds.). (2002). *Bright futures in practice: Nutrition* (2nd ed.). Arlington, VA: National Center for Education in Maternal and Child Health.

Sullivan, D., & Carlson, S. (2001). Dietary fats for infants and children. *Pediatric Annals, 30*(11), 683–693.

Wacharasin, C., Barnard, K. E., & Spieker, S. (2003). Factors affecting toddler cognitive development in low-income families: Implications for practitioners. *Infants and Young Children, 16*(2), 175–181.

Wilson, M. H., & Levin-Goodman, R. (2006). Injury prevention and control. In J. A. McMillan (Ed.), *Oski's pediatrics: Principles and practice* (4th ed.). Philadelphia: Lippincott Williams & Wilkins.

Zebrowski, P. M. (2003). Developmental stuttering. *Pediatric Annals, 32*(7), 453–465.

Websites

www.aapd.org American Academy of Pediatric Dentistry
www.bucklebear.com information on child passenger safety
www.eatright.org American Dietetic Association
www.5aday.com Produce for Better Health Foundation
www.gerber.com infant and toddler nutrition
www.hanen.org early language intervention programs
www.kidshealth.com the Nemours Foundation's Center for Child Health Media
www.kidsource.com a parent-supported group for children's health, growth, and development
www.littlebootspublishing.com source for burn prevention book "Bernie Burn"
www.nhtsa.dot.gov National Highway Traffic Safety Administration
www.pediatricinstitute.com Johnson & Johnson Pediatric Institute
www.reachoutandread.org early literacy promotion
www.safekids.org National Safe KIDS Campaign
www.seatcheck.org car seat inspection and seat recalls
www.usda.gov/wps/portal/usdahome United States Department of Agriculture; information on young child food guide pyramid
www.zerotothree.org Zero to Three: National Center for Infants, Toddlers and Families

Chapter WORKSHEET

● MULTIPLE CHOICE QUESTIONS

1. The nurse is caring for a hospitalized 30-month-old who is resistant to care, angry, and yells "no" all the time. The nurse identifies this toddler's behavior as

a. Problematic, as it interferes with needed nursing care

b. Normal for this stage of growth and development

c. Normal because the child is hospitalized and out of his routine

2. The mother of a 15-month-old is concerned about a speech delay. She describes her toddler as being able to understand what she says, sometimes following commands, but using only one or two words with any consistency. What is the nurse's best response to this information?

a. The toddler should have a developmental evaluation as soon as possible.

b. If the mother would read to the child, then speech would develop faster.

c. Receptive language normally develops earlier than expressive language.

d. The mother should ask her pediatrician for a speech therapy evaluation.

3. A 2-year-old is having a temper tantrum. What advice should the nurse give the mother?

a. For safety reasons, the toddler should be restrained during the tantrum.

b. Punishment should be initiated, as tantrums should be controlled.

c. The mother should promise the toddler a reward if the tantrum stops.

d. The tantrum should be ignored as long as the toddler is safe.

4. What is the best advice about nutrition for the toddler?

a. Encourage cup drinking and give water between meals and snacks.

b. Encourage unlimited milk intake, because toddlers need the protein for growth.

c. Avoid sugar-sweetened fruit drinks and allow as much natural fruit juice as desired.

d. Allow the toddler unlimited access to the sippy cup to ensure adequate hydration.

● CRITICAL THINKING EXERCISES

1. Develop a teaching plan about safety to present to a toddler-age preschool class.

2. Construct a 3-day menu for a 2-year-old, one that is realistic and will provide the nutrients needed.

3. Develop a plan for educating the parent of a 34-month-old who has been resistant to toilet teaching. Include assessments the nurse will make as well as the plan for teaching.

● STUDY ACTIVITIES

1. Visit a preschool that provides care for special-needs toddlers as well as typical toddlers. Perform a developmental assessment on a typical toddler and one with special needs (both the same age). Compare and contrast your findings.

2. Care for two average 2-year-olds in the clinical setting. Describe each toddler's behavior, response to the parent, and response to the nurse and list strategies used to gain compliance and minimize stress to the toddler.

3. Observe in the toddler classroom of a typical preschool. Choose two toddlers the same age with different temperaments. Record the toddlers' differences and similarities in response to structure and authority, interactions with classmates, attention levels, and language and activity levels.

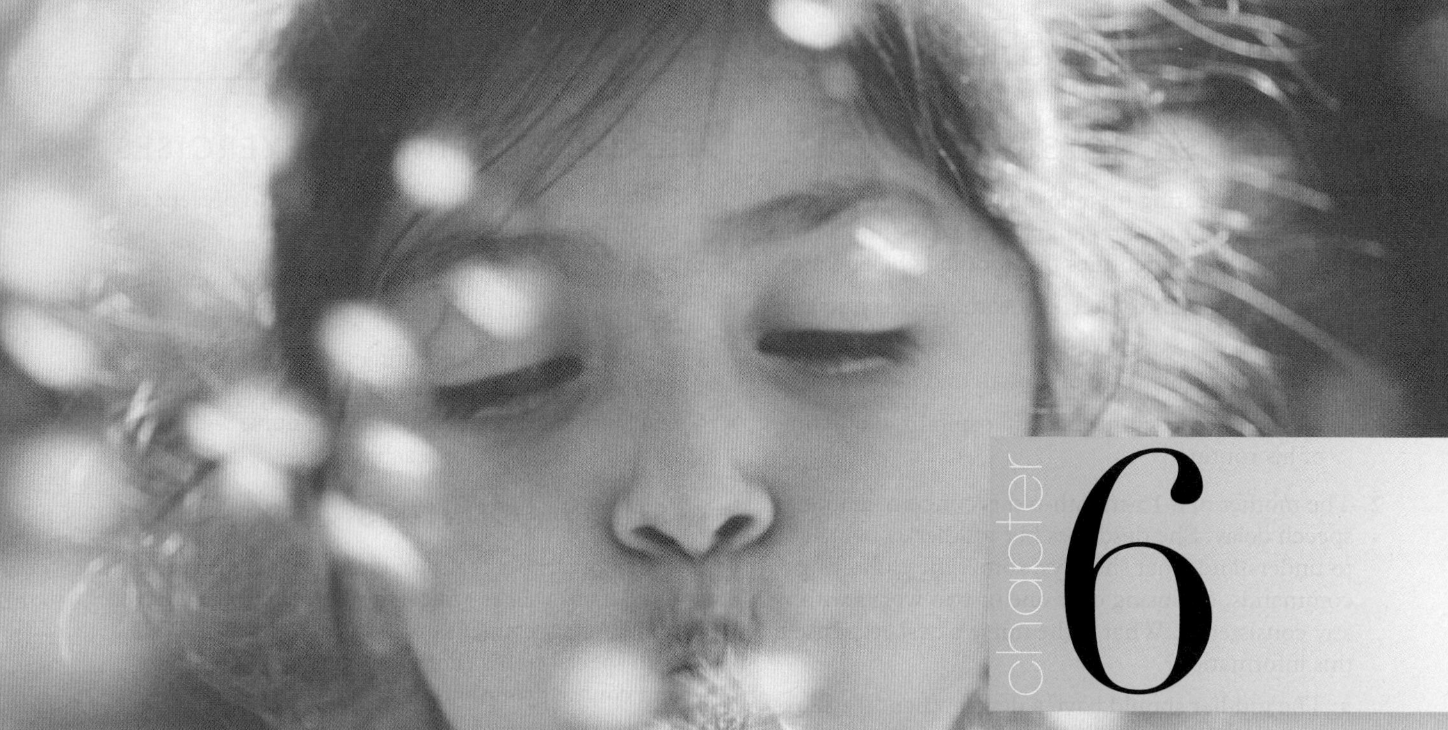

Growth and Development of the Preschooler

Key TERMS

animism
empathy
imaginary friend
magical thinking
preoperational thought
school readiness
telegraphic speech
transduction

Learning OBJECTIVES

Upon completion of the chapter, the learner will be able to:

1. Identify normal physiologic, cognitive, and psychosocial changes occurring in the preschool-aged child.
2. Express an understanding of language development in the preschool years.
3. Implement a nursing care plan that addresses common concerns or delays in the preschooler's development.
4. Integrate knowledge of preschool growth and development with nursing care and health promotion of the preschool-aged child.
5. Develop a nutritional plan for the preschool-aged child.
6. Identify common issues related to growth and development during the preschool years.
7. Demonstrate knowledge of appropriate anticipatory guidance for common developmental issues that arise in the preschool period.

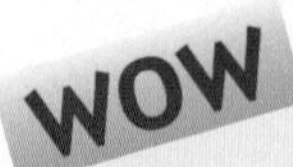

Quality parenting is achieved only by example.

Nila Patel is a 4-year-old girl brought to the clinic by her mother and father for her school check-up. During your assessment you measure her weight to be 44 pounds and her height 40 inches. As the nurse caring for her, assess Nila's growth and development, and then provide appropriate anticipatory guidance to her parents.

The preschool period is the period between 3 and 6 years of age. This is a time of continued growth and development. Physical growth continues much more slowly compared to earlier years. Gains in cognitive, language, and psychosocial development are substantial throughout the preschool period. Many tasks that began during the toddler years are mastered and perfected during the preschool years. The child has learned to tolerate separation from parents, has a longer attention span, and continues to learn skills that will lead to later success in the school-age period. Preparation for success in school occurs during the preschool period because most children enter elementary school by the end of the preschool period.

Growth and Development Overview

The healthy preschooler is slender and agile, with an upright posture. The formerly clumsy toddler becomes more graceful, demonstrating the ability to run more smoothly. Athletic abilities may begin to develop. Major development occurs in the area of fine motor coordination. Psychosocial development is focused on the accomplishment of initiative. Preconceptual thought and intuitiveness dominate cognitive development. The preschooler is an inquisitive learner and absorbs new concepts like a sponge absorbs water.

• PHYSICAL GROWTH

The average preschool age child will grow 2.5 to 3 inches (6.5–7.8 cm) per year. The average 3-year-old is 37 inches tall (96.2 cm), the average 4-year-old is 40.5 inches tall (103.7 cm), and the average 5-year-old is 43 inches tall (118.5 cm). Average weight gain during this time period is about 5 pounds (2.3 kg) per year. The average weight of a 3-year-old is 32 pounds (14.5 kg), increasing to an average weight of 41 pounds (18.6 kg) by age 5. The loss of baby fat and the growth of muscle during the preschool years give the child a stronger and more mature appearance (Fig. 6.1). The length of the skull also increases slightly, with the lower jaw becoming more pronounced. The upper jaw widens through the preschool years in preparation for the emergence of permanent teeth, usually starting around age 6.

• ORGAN SYSTEM MATURATION

Most of the body systems have matured by the preschool years. Myelination of the spinal cord allows for bowel and bladder control to be complete in most children by age 3 years. The respiratory structures are continuing to grow in size, and the number of alveoli continues to increase, reaching the adult number at about 7 years of age. The eustachian tubes remain relatively short and straight. Heart rate decreases and blood pressure increases slightly during the preschool years. An innocent heart murmur may be heard upon auscultation, and splitting of the second heart sound may become evident. The preschooler should have 20 deciduous teeth present.

The small intestine is continuing to grow in length. Stool passage usually occurs once or twice per day in the average preschooler. The 4-year-old generally has adequate bowel control. The urethra remains short in both boys and girls, making them more susceptible to urinary tract infections than adults. Bladder control is usually present in the 4- and 5-year-old child, but an occasional accident may occur, particularly in stressful situations or when the child is absorbed in an interesting activity.

The bones continue to increase in length and the muscles continue to strengthen and mature. However, the musculoskeletal system is still not fully mature, making the preschooler susceptible to injury, particularly with overexertion or excess activity.

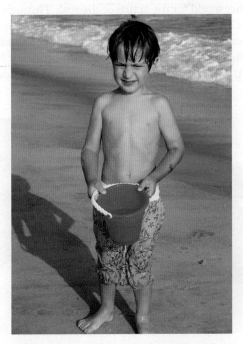

• Figure 6.1 The preschool child has a more slender appearance and erect posture than the toddler.

• PSYCHOSOCIAL DEVELOPMENT

According to Erik Erikson, the psychosocial task of the preschool years is establishing a sense of initiative versus guilt (Erikson, 1963). The preschooler is an inquisitive learner, very enthusiastic about learning new things. Preschoolers feel a sense of accomplishment when succeeding in activities (Fig. 6.2), and feeling pride in one's accomplishment helps the child to use initiative. However, when the child extends himself or herself further than current capabilities allow, he or she may feel a sense of guilt. The superego or conscience development is completed during the preschool period, and this is the basis for moral development (understanding right and wrong). Table 6.1 gives examples illustrating the stage of initiative versus guilt.

• COGNITIVE DEVELOPMENT

According to Jean Piaget's theory, the preschool-age child continues in the preoperational stage. Preoperational thought dominates during this stage and is based on a self-centered understanding of the world. In the preconceptual phase of preoperational thought, the child remains egocentric and is able to approach a problem from a single point of view only. The young preschooler may understand the concept of counting and begins to engage in fantasy play.

Magical thinking is a normal part of preschool development. The preschooler believes that his or her thoughts are all-powerful. The fantasy experienced through magical thinking allows the preschooler to make room in his or her world for the actual or the real. Through make-believe and magical thinking, preschool children satisfy their curiosity about differences in the world around them.

The preschooler often has an **imaginary friend** as well. This friend serves as a creative way for the preschooler to sample different activities and behaviors and practice conversational skills. Despite this imagination, the preschooler is able to switch easily between fantasy and reality throughout the day.

The child in the intuitive phase can count 10 or more objects, correctly name at least four colors, and better understand the concept of time, and he or she knows about things that are used in everyday life, such as appliances, money, and food. The preschooler uses **transduction** when reasoning: he or she extrapolates from a particular situation to another, even though the events may be unrelated. The preschooler also attributes lifelike qualities to inanimate objects (**animism**). Table 6.1 gives further examples illustrating this developmental stage.

The acquisition of language skills in the toddler period is enhanced in the preschool period. The expansion of vocabulary enables the preschooler to progress further with symbolic thought. At this age, children do not completely understand the concept of death or its permanence: they may ask when their grandparent or pet who died is returning.

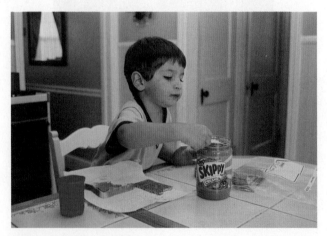

● Figure 6.2 Allowing the preschooler to assist with simple household tasks such as preparing a sandwich encourages the development of initiative.

• MORAL AND SPIRITUAL DEVELOPMENT

The preschool child can understand the concepts of right and wrong and is developing a conscience. That inner voice that warns or threatens is developing in the preschool years. Kohlberg identified this stage (between 4 and 10 years) as the preconventional stage, which is characterized by a punishment-and-obedience orientation. Preschool children see morality as external to themselves; they defer to power (that of the adult). The child's moral standards are those of their parents or other adults who influence them, not necessarily their own. Preschoolers adhere to those standards to gain rewards or avoid punishment. Since the preschool child is facing the psychosocial task of initiative versus guilt, it is natural for the child to experience guilt when something goes wrong. The child may have a strong belief that if someone is ill or dying, then he or she may be at fault and the illness or death is punishment.

As the child's moral development progresses, he or she learns how to deal with angry feelings. Sometimes the way the child chooses to deal with those feelings may be inappropriate, such as fighting and biting. Preschoolers are so involved in imagination and fantasy that lying begins to occur at this age. Preschoolers also use their limited life experiences to make sense of and help them cope with crisis. They need to learn the socially acceptable limits of behavior and are also learning the rewards of manners. The preschool child begins to help out in the family and begins to understand the concept of give-and-take in relationships.

During the preoperational phase of cognitive development, the preschooler's concept of faith is intuitive and

Table 6.1 Developmental Theories

Theorist	Stage	Activities
Erikson	Initiative vs. Guilt Age 3–6 years	• Likes to please parents • Begins to plan activities, make up games • Initiates activities with others • Acts out the roles of other people (real and imaginary) • Develops sexual identity • Develops conscience • May take frustrations out on siblings • Likes exploring new things • Enjoys sports, shopping, cooking, working • Feels remorse when makes wrong choice or behaves badly • Cooperates with other children • Negotiates solutions to conflicts
Piaget	Preoperational substage: Preconceptual phase Age: 2–4 years	• Exhibits egocentric thinking, which lessens as the child approaches age 4 • Short attention span • Learns through observing and imitating • Displays animism • Forms concepts that are not as complete or as logical as the adult's • Able to make simple classifications • By age 4 understands the concept of opposites (hot/cold, soft/hard) • Reasoning is that of specific to specific • Has an active imagination
	Preoperational substage: Intuitive phase Age 4–7 years	• Able to classify and relate objects • Has intuitive thought processes; knows if something is right or wrong, though cannot state why • Tolerates others' differences but doesn't understand them • Very curious about facts • Knows acceptable cultural rules • Uses words appropriately but often without true understanding of their meaning • Has a more realistic sense of causality • May begin to question parents' values
Kohlberg	Punishment–obedience orientation Age 2–4 years (preconventional morality)	• Determines good vs. bad dependent upon associated punishment • Children may learn inappropriate behavior at this stage if parental intervention does not occur (if the child hits, bites, or is verbally disrespectful but is not punished for these activities, the child will view those behaviors as good and continue to participate in them)
Freud	Phallic stage Age 3–7 years	Child's pleasure centers on genitalia and masturbation. Superego is developing and conscience is emerging. Oedipal stage occurs: jealousy and rivalry toward same-sex parent, with love of the opposite-sex parent. This usually resolves by the end of the preschool years, when the child develops a strong identification with the same-sex parent.

projective in nature (Fosarelli, 2003). The preschool child's imagination allows for anything to be possible, so he or she does not have a logical view of the world (as adults do). Preschool children have limited life experiences, so they may project a feeling onto a new person or situation. They may use this projection to help them understand what is going on around them. Preschoolers may project their parents' or caregiver's feelings or characteristics onto "God": if mommy gets angry, then God is probably also angry.

The family's religious beliefs may affect the child's diet, the mode of discipline that parents use, and even how the parents view their children. Knowing about a family's practices of prayer or meditation is helpful to the pediatric nurse, who can help continue the ritual when the child is ill or hospitalized (Fig. 6.3).

MOTOR SKILL DEVELOPMENT

As the preschooler's musculoskeletal system continues to mature, existing motor skills become refined and new ones develop. The preschooler has more voluntary control over his or her movements and is less clumsy than the toddler. Significant refinement in fine motor skills occurs during the preschool period (Table 6.2).

Gross Motor Skills

The preschooler is agile while standing, walking, running, and jumping (Fig. 6.4). He or she can go up and down stairs and walk forward and backward easily. Standing on tiptoes or on one foot still requires extra concentration. The preschooler seems to be in constant motion. He or she also uses the body to understand new concepts (such as using the arms in a "chug-chug" motion when describing how the train wheels work).

Fine Motor Skills

The 3-year-old can move each finger independently and is capable of grasping utensils and crayons in adult fashion, with the thumb on one side and the fingers on the other. He or she can also scribble freely, copy a circle, trace a square, and feed himself or herself without spilling much. These skills become refined over the next 2 years, and by 5 years of age the child can write letters, cut with scissors more accurately, and tie shoelaces (Fig. 6.5).

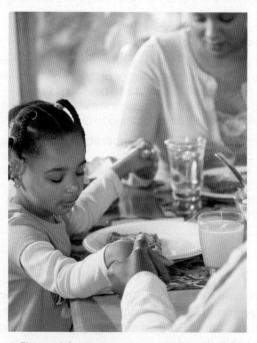

Figure 6.3 The preschool child may participate in religious rituals without having full understanding of their meaning.

SENSORY DEVELOPMENT

Hearing is intact at birth and should remain so throughout the preschool years. The senses of smell and touch continue to develop throughout the preschool years. The young preschooler may have a less discriminating sense of taste than the older child, putting him or her at increased risk for accidental ingestion. Visual acuity continues to progress and should be equal bilaterally. The typical 5-year-old has visual acuity of 20/40 or 20/30. Color vision is intact at this age.

COMMUNICATION AND LANGUAGE DEVELOPMENT

The acquisition of language allows the preschool child to express thoughts and creativity. The preschool years are a time of refinement of language skills. The 3-year-old exhibits **telegraphic speech**, using short sentences that contain only the essential information. Vocabulary at 3 years comprises about 900 words. The preschool child may acquire as many as 10 to 20 new words per day and at age 5 usually has a vocabulary of 2,100 words. By the end of the preschool period, the child is using sentences that are adult-like in structure (Table 6.3).

The 3- to 6-year-old is starting to develop fluency (the ability to smoothly link sounds, syllables, and words when speaking). Initially, the child may exhibit dysfluency or stuttering. Speech may sound choppy, or the child may say repeated consonants or "um." Stuttering usually has its onset between 2 and 4 years of age, and about 75% of children will recover from it without therapy. Parents should slow down their speech and should give the child time to speak without rushing or interrupting. Some sounds remain difficult for the preschooler to enunciate properly: "f," "v," "s," and "z" sounds are usually mastered by age 5 years, but some children do not master the sounds of "sh," "l," "th," and "r" until age 6 or later.

Communication in preschool children is concrete in nature, as they are not yet capable of abstract thought. Despite its concrete nature, the preschooler's communication can be quite elaborate and involved; he or she may talk about dreams and fantasies. In addition to acquiring vocabulary and learning the correct use of grammar, the preschool child's receptive language skills are also becoming refined.

The preschooler is very much in tune with the parent's moods and easily picks up on negative emotions in

Table 6.2 Motor Skill Development

Age	Expected Gross Motor Skills	Expected Fine Motor Skills
4 years	• Throws ball overhand • Kicks ball forward • Catches bounced ball • Hops on one foot • Stands on one foot up to 5 seconds • Alternates feet going up and down steps • Moves backward and forward with agility	• Uses scissors successfully • Copies capital letters • Draws circles and squares • Traces a cross or diamond • Draws a person with two to four body parts • Laces shoes
5 years	• Stands on one foot 10 seconds or longer • Swings and climbs well • May skip • Somersaults • May learn to skate and swim	• Prints some letters • Draws person with body and at least six parts • Dresses/undresses without assistance • Can learn to tie laces • Uses fork, spoon, and knife (supervised) well • Copies triangle and other geometric patterns • Mostly cares for own toileting needs

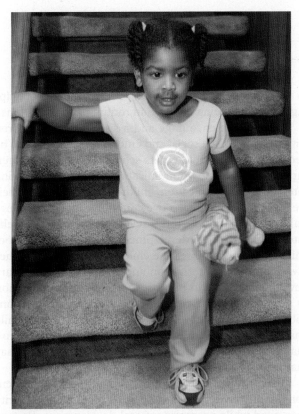

● Figure 6.4 The preschool child is capable of standing on one foot for several seconds and can hop on one foot.

conversations. If the preschooler hears parents discussing things that are frightening to the child, the preschooler's imagination may fuel the development of fears and lead to misinterpretation of what the child has heard.

In the potentially bilingual child, by 4 years of age the child will cease the language mixing exhibited during the toddler years and should be able to use each language as a separate system.

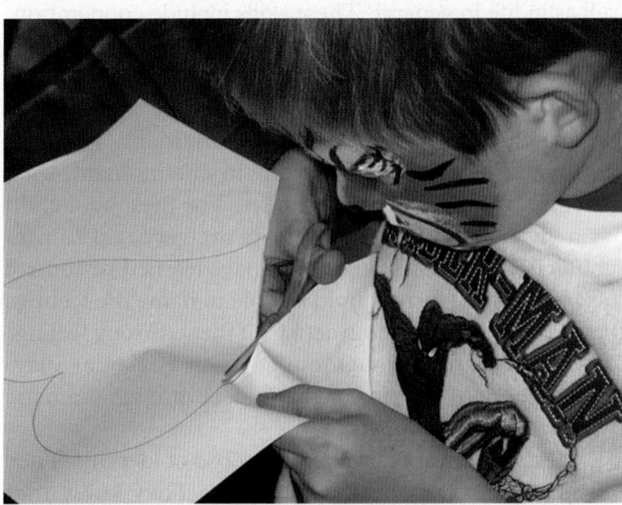

● Figure 6.5 The 5-year-old has the fine motor dexterity to cut well with scissors.

Table 6.3 Communication Skills in the Preschool Child

Age	Communication Abilities
4 years	• Speaks in complete sentences using adult-like grammar • Tells a story that is easy to follow • 75% of speech understood by others outside of family • Asks questions with "who," "how," "how many" • Stays on topic in a conversation • Understands the concepts of "same" and "different" • Asks many questions • Knows names of familiar animals • Names common objects in books and magazines • Knows at least one color • Uses language to engage in make-believe • Follows a three-part command • Can count a few numbers • Vocabulary of 1,500 words
5 years	• Persons outside of the family can understand most of the child's speech • Explains how an item is used • Participates in long, detailed conversations • Talks about past, future, and imaginary events • Answers questions that use "why" and "when" • Can count to 10 • Recalls part of a story • Speech should be completely intelligible, even if the child has articulation difficulties • Speech is generally grammatically correct • Vocabulary of 2,100 words • Says name and address

• EMOTIONAL AND SOCIAL DEVELOPMENT

By the time a child enters kindergarten, he or she should have developed a useful set of social skills that will help him or her have successful experiences in the school setting as well as in life in general. These skills include cooperation, sharing (of things and feelings), kindness, generosity, affection display, conversation, expression of feelings, helping others, and making friends.

Preschoolers tend to have strong emotions. They can be very excited, happy, and giddy in one moment, then extremely disappointed in the next. The preschool child has a vivid imagination, and fears are very real to preschoolers. Most children this age have learned to control their behaviors. They should be able to name the feelings they are having rather than acting on them. Strong feelings may be expressed through outlets such as clay or Play-Doh, water play, drawing or painting, or through dramatic play such as with puppets.

Preschoolers are developing a sense of identity. They recognize that they are boys or girls. They know that they belong to a particular family, community, or culture. They take pride in using self-control rather than giving in to their impulses. The preschool child is capable of helping others and being involved in routines and transitions.

Parents can encourage and assist preschool children with developing the social and emotional skills that will be needed when the child enters school. Preschool children thrive on one-to-one communication with a parent. During interactive communication, children learn to express their feelings and ideas. Interactive communication fosters not only emotional and moral development but also self-esteem and cognitive development. Asking the preschool child questions requires the child to think out his or her own intention or motivation and encourages vocabulary development. Parents may use individual communication as a time to explore right and wrong, thus further contributing to moral development. Being listened to while answering parents' questions gives preschoolers a sense that they are valued, that what they think and have to say matters.

Establishing a few simple rules and enforcing them consistently gives preschoolers the structure and security they need while promoting moral development. Parents or caregivers can help the child give a name to the emotion that is being experienced. Fears are very real to preschoolers because of their active imaginations and may result in a variety of emotions. Parents should validate the feeling or emotion, then discuss with the child alternatives for dealing with the emotion.

Preschoolers are developing their sense of identity, and parents should encourage preschoolers to do simple things for themselves, like dressing and washing their hands and face (Fig. 6.6). Parents should give the child the time he or she needs to complete the task. This helps to establish a sense of accomplishment.

At this age, the child may begin to show an interest in basic sexuality. The preschooler may want to know why boys' and girls' bodies are different, how the reproductive organs function, and where babies come from. The parent should answer the child honestly and directly, using the correct anatomic terms. Long explanations are not necessary, just simple answers. This curiosity is a normal function of the preschool years, and the curiosity may also involve playing with the genitals (see the section on masturbation later in this chapter).

Friendships

Preschoolers need interactions with friends as well. Learning how to make and keep a friend is an important part of social development. Friends may be other children in the neighborhood or those at preschool or day care. A special friend is someone the preschooler can care about, talk to, and play with (Fig. 6.7). The preschooler is more likely to agree to rules and wants to please friends and be like them. The preschooler loves to sing, dance, and act and will enjoy these activities with friends. Disagreements may occur, but the parent can encourage the children to express their views, discuss and resolve conflicts, and continue being friends.

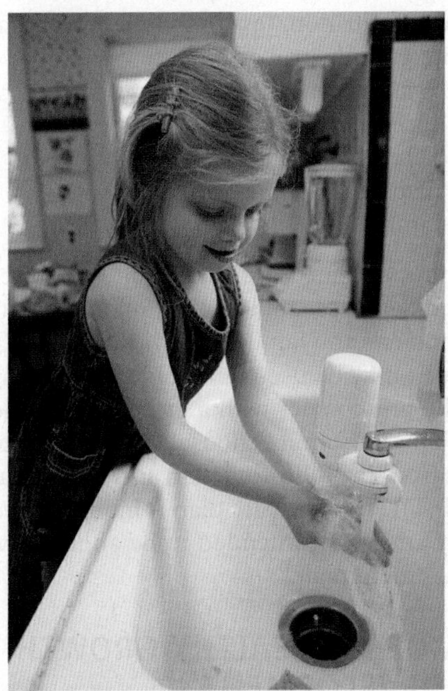

● Figure 6.6 Encouraging the preschooler to complete simple tasks by himself or herself helps to build self-esteem.

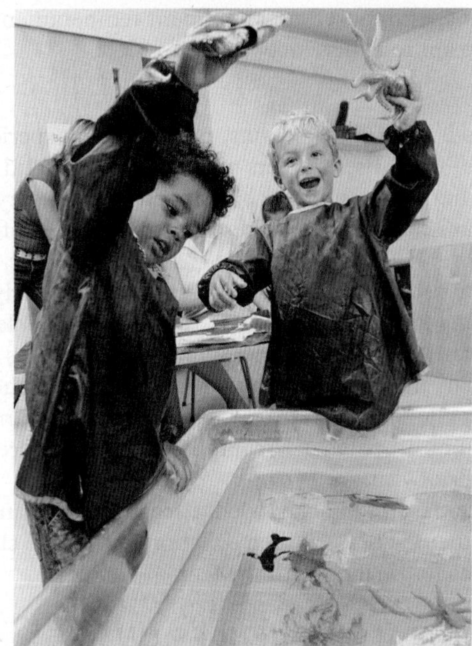

● Figure 6.7 The preschool child begins to develop friendships.

Temperament

By the time children are 3 years old, they recognize that what they do actually matters. It is helpful for the parent to view the child as an active participant in the parent–child relationship. The child's temperament has become a reliable indicator of how a parent might expect the child to react in a certain situation. When the parent is in tune with the preschooler's temperament, it is easier to find ways to ease transitions and changes for that child. In the area of task orientation, temperament may range from the highly attentive and persistent to the more distractible and active.

A child's social flexibility is also evident by this age. A child who is quite adaptable will handle stimuli from the outside world in an approaching rather than a withdrawing manner. Temperament also determines the extent of reactivity (the child's sensory threshold of responsiveness, high versus low). This determines the quality of the child's mood and the intensity of reactions to stimuli, change, or situations. When the parents are familiar with the child's task orientation, social flexibility, and reactivity, they can better structure activities and situations for the child.

The 4-year-old is better at learning self-control and can use setbacks in appropriate behavior as opportunities for growth. Temper tantrums should ease off by this age as the child's language skills are more capable of keeping up with complex ideas. The 4-year-old is able to see the rewards of growing up. This awareness of self-power may, however, lead to additional fears. The 5-year-old who has a more vulnerable type of temperament, as opposed to a confident temperament, may be more apt to experience fears.

Fears

With their vivid imaginations, preschoolers experience a variety of fears. Preschoolers may be scared of loud noises such as fire engine sirens or barking dogs. Imaginary monsters may scare the child. Preschoolers are often afraid of people they do not know as well as strange people (Santa Claus or people who look or dress very differently from what they are accustomed to). Many preschoolers are afraid of the dark. Preschoolers may also fear insects as well as animals they are not familiar with. The preschooler's memory is long enough that he or she may fear returning to the doctor's office when a painful procedure occurred during the prior visit.

Parents should acknowledge fears rather than minimizing them. They can then collaborate with the child on strategies for dealing with the fear.

CULTURAL INFLUENCES ON GROWTH AND DEVELOPMENT

Children may learn prejudice or bias at home before entering school or day care. The ways that families view other races or cultures may be subtly or overtly demonstrated in routine daily activities. The preschool child is developing a conscience, so attitudes of tolerance or bias may influence the child's values. As in the toddler period, the value that the family places on independence will affect the child's development of a healthy self-concept.

Some cultures value reading and education more than others. If reading is not valued in the home, the preschool child's first experience with books may not occur until he or she is in school.

Food served in the home is often very specific to the family's ethnic background. As the preschool child is exposed to persons of other cultures in school, he may or may not like the food that is served. Exploring customs or cultural practices that the family participates in is important so that these practices may be safely incorporated into the child's plan of care.

> Refer back to Nila, who was introduced in the beginning of the chapter. What developmental milestones would you expect Nila to have reached at this age? Nila's mother expresses concerns about her child's imaginary friend, Sasha. How would you respond?

The Nurse's Role in Preschool Growth and Development

WATCH & LEARN

Growth and development in the preschool child remains orderly and sequential. Some preschoolers grow faster than others or reach various developmental milestones sooner than others. Nurses must be aware of the usual growth and development patterns for this age group so that they can assess preschool children appropriately and provide guidance to their families. The changes that the preschool child is experiencing affect not only the child but also the family. Health care visits throughout the preschool period continue to focus on expected growth and development and anticipatory guidance. An additional concern is the preparation for school entry (school readiness).

If the preschooler is hospitalized, growth and development may be altered. Hospitalization hinders the preschool child's ability to explore the environment and engage in make-believe play and thus presents a challenge for the curious and inquisitive child. If the child must be isolated for a contagious illness, the opportunities for exploration and experimentation are further restricted. In addition, a sick preschooler may feel a sense of guilt, worrying that maybe he or she caused the illness by negative thoughts or behaviors.

When caring for the hospitalized preschooler, the nurse must use knowledge of normal growth and development to recognize potential delays, promote continued appropriate growth and development, and interact successfully with the preschooler.

NURSING PROCESS OVERVIEW

Upon completion of assessment of the preschool child's growth and development status, problems or issues related to growth and development may be identified. The nurse may then identify one or more nursing diagnoses, including but not limited to:

- Delayed growth and development
- Imbalanced nutrition, less than body requirements
- Interrupted family processes
- Readiness for enhanced parenting
- Risk for caregiver role strain
- Risk for delayed development
- Risk for disproportionate growth
- Risk for injury

Planning nursing care for the preschool child with growth and development issues should take into account the preschooler's and family's individual needs. The nursing care plan may be used as a guide in planning nursing care for the preschooler with a growth or developmental concern. The nurse may choose the appropriate nursing diagnoses from the following plan and individualize them as needed. The nursing care plan is intended to serve as a guide only and is not intended to be an inclusive growth and development plan.

PROMOTING HEALTHY GROWTH AND DEVELOPMENT

The building of self-esteem continues throughout the preschool period. It is of particular importance during

(text continues on page 147)

Nursing Care Plan 6.1

Growth and Development Issues in the Preschool Child

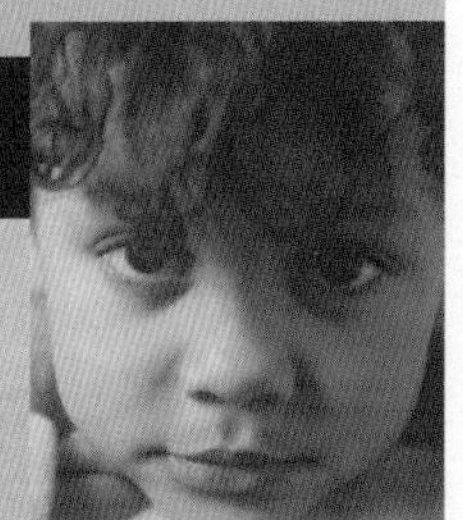

Nursing Diagnosis: Risk for injury related to developmental age, environment, and motor vehicle travel

Outcome identification and evaluation

Child's safety will be maintained: *Child will remain free from injury.*

Interventions: preventing injury

- Teach and encourage appropriate use of forward-facing car seat or booster seat if greater than 40 pounds *to decrease risk of injury related to motor vehicles.*
- Teach preschoolers to stay away from street and to cross the street only when holding the hand of an adult *to prevent pedestrian injury.*
- Require bicycle helmet use while riding any wheeled toy *to prevent head injury and form habit of helmet use.*
- Teach the preschooler appropriate safety rules in the home (avoiding electric outlets, etc.): *the preschooler is able to follow simple directions and carry out directives. Limits help him or her to organize the environment.*
- Post poison control center phone number *(in case of accidental ingestion; the preschool child is very curious).*
- Never leave a preschool child unattended in a tub or pool or near any body of water *to prevent drowning.*
- Provide swimming lessons for children age 4 or 5 *to encourage water safety, but not as a replacement for adult supervision.*
- Teach parents first-aid measures and child CPR *to minimize consequences of injury should it occur.*
- Provide close observation and keep side rails up on bed in hospital *because the preschool child continues to be at risk for falling or injuring self on equipment or tubing (because of curiosity).*

Nursing Diagnosis: Imbalanced nutrition, less than body requirements, related to inappropriate nutritional intake to sustain growth needs (excess juice or milk intake, inadequate food variety intake) as evidenced by failure to attain adequate increases in height and weight over time

Outcome identification and evaluation

Child will consume adequate nutrients: *Child will demonstrate weight gain and increases in height.*

Interventions: promoting appropriate nutrition

- Assess current feeding schedule and usual intake, as well as methods used to feed, *to determine areas of adequacy versus inadequacy.*
- Determine if the preschooler is unable to drink from a cup or does not finger feed or use utensils properly, or if the child has difficulty swallowing or tolerating certain textures of foods *to determine if further interventions such as speech or occupational therapy are required.*
- Weigh child daily on same scale if hospitalized, weekly on same scale if at home, and plot growth patterns weekly or monthly as appropriate on standardized growth charts *to determine if growth is improving.*
- Limit juice to 4 to 6 ounces per day, milk to 16 to 24 ounces per day, *to discourage sense of fullness achieved with excess milk or juice intake, thereby increasing appetite for appropriate solid foods.*
- Provide three nutrient-dense meals and at least two healthy snacks per day *to encourage adequate nutrient consumption.*
- Feed child on a similar schedule daily, without distractions and with the family: *preschool children continue to respond well to routine and structure. They are more interested in the social context of meals and are still apt to become distracted easily, so the TV should be off at mealtimes.*

(continued)

Growth and Development Issues in the Preschool Child (continued)

Nursing Diagnosis: Delayed growth and development related to motor, cognitive, language, or psychosocial concerns as evidenced by delay in meeting expected milestones

Outcome identification and evaluation

Development will be enhanced: *Child will make continued progress toward realization of expected developmental milestones.*

Interventions: enhancing growth and development

- Screen for developmental capabilities *to determine child's current level of functioning.*
- Offer age-appropriate toys, play, and activities (including gross motor) *to encourage further development.*
- Perform interventions as prescribed by physical, occupational, or speech therapist: *participation in those activities helps to promote function and accomplish acquisition of developmental skills.*
- Provide support to families of preschoolers with developmental delay *(progress in achieving developmental milestones can be slow and ongoing motivation is needed).*
- Reinforce positive attributes in the child *to maintain motivation.*
- Model age-appropriate communication skills *to illustrate suitable means for parenting the preschooler.*

Nursing Diagnosis: Risk for disproportionate growth related to excess milk or juice intake, consumption of inappropriate foods or in excess amounts

Outcome identification and evaluation

Child will grow appropriately and not become overweight or obese: *Child will achieve weight and height within the 5th to 85th percentiles on standardized growth charts.*

Interventions:

- Discourage use of no-spill sippy cups *(they contribute to dental caries and allow unlimited access to fluids, possibly decreasing appetite for appropriate solid foods).*
- Provide juice (4–6 ounces per day) and milk (16–24 ounces per day) from a cup at meal and snack time *to encourage appropriate cup drinking and limit intake of nutrient-poor, high-calorie fluids.*
- Provide only nutrient-rich foods without high sugar content for meals and snacks; *even if the preschooler is a picky eater, it is inappropriate to provide high-calorie junk food just so the child eats something.*
- Teach parents to role model appropriate eating (nutrient-rich, varied diet) *to encourage child to try/accept new foods, as well as become familiar with a variety of food.*
- Severely limit the intake of fast foods and foods with high sugar and fat content *to decrease intake of nutrient-poor, high-calorie foods.*
- Ensure adequate physical activity *to stimulate development of motor skills and provide appropriate caloric expenditure. This also sets the stage for forming life-long habit of appropriate physical activity.*
- Teach parents to limit television viewing to 1 to 2 hours per day *to encourage participation in physical activities.*

Nursing Diagnosis: Interrupted family processes related to issues with preschool child's development, hospitalization, or situational crisis as evidenced by decreased parental visitation in hospital, parental verbalization of difficulty with current situation, possible crisis related to health of family member other than the preschool child

Outcome identification and evaluation

Family will demonstrate adequate functioning: *Family will display coping and psychosocial adjustment.*

Growth and Development Issues in the Preschool Child (continued)

Interventions: enhancing family functioning

- Assess the family's level of stress and ability to cope *to determine family's ability to cope with multiple stressors.*
- Engage in family-centered care *to provide a holistic approach to care of the preschooler and family.*
- Encourage the family to verbalize feelings *(verbalization is one method of decreasing anxiety levels)* and acknowledge feelings and emotions.
- Use puppets or dramatic play with the child *to elicit the preschooler's feelings about the current situation.*
- Encourage family visitation and provide for sleeping arrangements for a parent or caregiver to stay in the hospital with the preschooler; *this contributes to family's sense of control in situation.*
- Involve family members in preschooler's care, *giving them a feeling of control and connectedness.*

Nursing Diagnosis: Readiness for enhanced parenting related to parental desire for increased skill level and success with preschool child as evidenced by current healthy relationships and verbalization of desire for improved skills

Outcome identification and evaluation

Parent will provide safe and nurturing environment for the preschool child: *Parents will verbalize new skills they will employ in the family.*

Interventions: increasing parenting skill set

- Use family-centered care *to provide holistic approach.*
- Educate parent about normal preschool development *to provide basis of understanding for parenting skills needed in this time period.*
- Acknowledge and encourage parents' verbalization of feelings related to chronic illness of child or difficulty with normal preschool behavior; *this validates the normalcy of parents' feelings.*
- Encourage positive parenting and respect for preschooler and his/her normal development *(helps parents develop approaches to preschoolers that can be used in place of anger and frustration).*
- Acknowledge and admire positive parenting skills already present *to contribute to parents' confidence in their abilities to parent.*
- Role model appropriate parenting behaviors related to communicating with and disciplining the child *(role modeling actually demonstrates rather than just verbalizes what the parent should strive for).*

these years, as the preschooler's developmental task is focused on the development of initiative rather than guilt. A sense of guilt will contribute to low self-esteem, whereas a child who is rewarded for his or her initiative will have increased self-confidence. The parent who provides a loving and nurturing environment for the preschooler builds upon the earlier foundation.

Routine and ritual continue to be important throughout the preschool years, as they help the child to develop a sense of time as well as provide the structure for the child to feel safe and secure. Daily routine continues to assist with the development of conscience in the preschooler. As in toddlerhood, making expectations known through everyday routines helps to avoid confrontations. The preschooler is developing the maturity to know how to behave in various situations and is capable of learning manners.

Setting limits (and remaining consistent with those limits) continues to be important in the preschool period. Consistent limits provide the preschooler with expectation and guidance. As the preschooler increasingly participates in fantasy and imagination, the limits of routine and structure help guide his or her behavior and ability to distinguish reality.

Nurses caring for preschoolers should have knowledge of normal developmental expectations so they can determine whether the preschool child is progressing appropriately. Table 6.4 lists potential signs of developmental delay. A preschool child with one or more of these concerns should be referred for further developmental evaluation.

Promoting Growth and Development Through Play

Providing sincere encouragement for the preschool child's efforts and accomplishments helps him or her develop a sense of initiative. Giving children opportunities to decide how and with whom they want to play also helps them develop initiative. Preschool children like to write, color, draw, paint with a brush or their fingers, and trace or copy patterns (Fig. 6.8). They may start small collections that may be sorted. They like using toys for their intended purpose as well as for whatever invented purpose they can imagine.

Preschoolers begin to play cooperatively with one another. Play may be focused around a distinct theme. They define roles, make up rules, and assign jobs. They are able to work together toward a common goal such as building a house or fort with discarded boxes. Cooperative play encourages the preschool child to learn to share, take turns and compromise, listen to others' opinions, consider the feelings of others, and use self-control and overcome fears.

Preschoolers have incredible imaginations and love to play "make-believe" (Fig. 6.9). Encouraging pretend play and providing props for dress-up stimulates curiosity and creativity. Fantasy play is usually cooperative in nature. It encourages the preschooler to develop social skills such as taking turns, communication, paying attention, and responding to one another's words and actions. Fantasy play also allows preschoolers to explore complex social ideas such as power, compassion, and cruelty. Through role playing, children begin to develop their sexual identity as well.

Since preschool children have vivid imaginations, it is important to be careful about what television they watch. The preschooler should be limited to 1 to 2 hours per day of quality television. The violence in some television programs may scare the preschool child or inspire him or her to act out violent behavior.

Table 6.4 Signs of Developmental Delay

Age	Concern
4 years	• Cannot jump in place or ride a tricycle • Cannot stack four blocks • Cannot throw ball overhand • Does not grasp crayon with thumb and fingers • Difficulty with scribbling • Cannot copy a circle • Does not use sentences with three or more words • Cannot use the words "me" and "you" appropriately • Ignores other children or does not show interest in interactive games • Will not respond to people outside the family; still clings or cries if parents leave • Resists using toilet, dressing, sleeping • Does not engage in fantasy play
By 5 years	• Unhappy or sad often • Little interest in playing with other children • Unable to separate from parent without major protest • Is extremely aggressive • Is extremely fearful or timid, or unusually passive • Cannot build tower of six to eight blocks • Easily distracted; cannot concentrate on single activity for 5 minutes • Rarely engages in fantasy play • Trouble with eating, sleeping, or using the toilet • Cannot use plurals or past tense • Cannot brush teeth, wash and dry hands, or undress efficiently

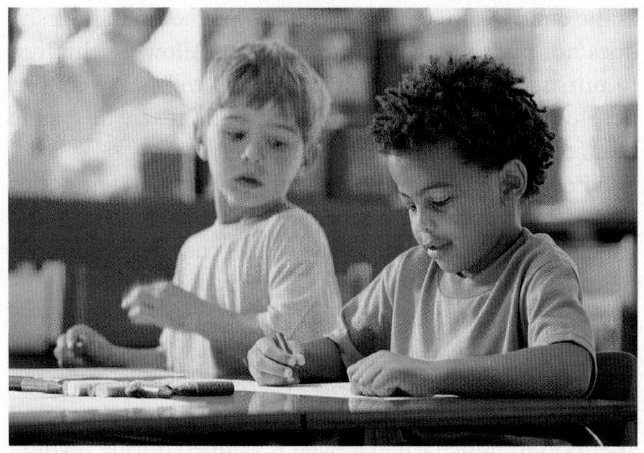

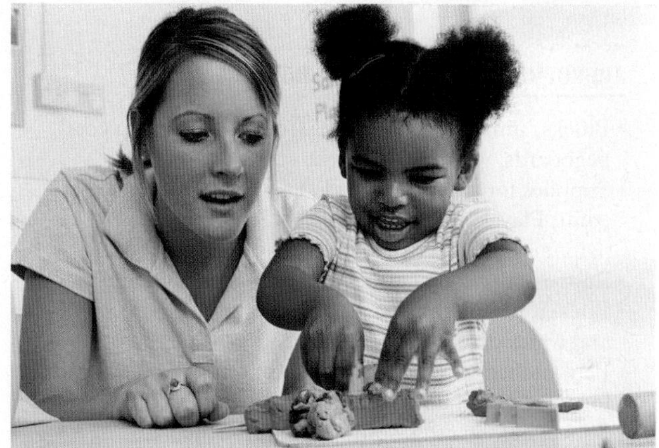

● **Figure 6.8** The preschool child loves to create things, so coloring and molding clay are ideal activities for children this age.

Most preschoolers also engage in dramatic play, fueled by their innate curiosity and vivid imaginations. Three-year-olds may not realize that they are pretending. They run from scary creatures, make plans, and pack their backpacks (never intending to actually leave). Four-year-olds are more sophisticated with dramatic or pretend play: they know they are pretending, and they use dress-up clothes and props to act out more complex roles and scenarios (Fig. 6.10). Five-year-olds are capable of quite complex scenarios. They pretend they are real or fantasy characters. They often use dramatic play to express anxiety, try out negative feelings, or conquer their fears. For example, a child who is afraid of getting a shot at the doctor's office may work through that feeling with pretend play.

Parents should encourage physical activity in the preschool child. Regular physical activity improves gross motor skills, may enhance the child's self-confidence, and allows the child to expend excess energy. Establishing the habit of daily physical activity in the early years is important in the long-term goal of avoiding obesity. The main goal of organized sports at this age should be fun and enjoyment, although of course safety must remain a priority.

Beware of sophisticated toys that claim to teach the young child. These toys are often very expensive and are not necessary. Box 6.1 lists appropriate playthings for the preschool child.

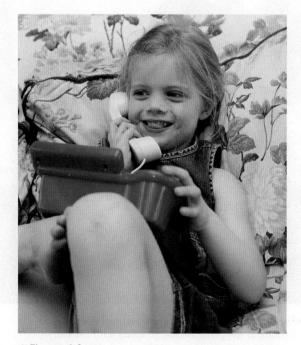

● **Figure 6.9** Preschool children enjoy imitative play.

Promoting Early Learning

The family is the foundation for the child's early growth and development. Parents serve as role models for behav-

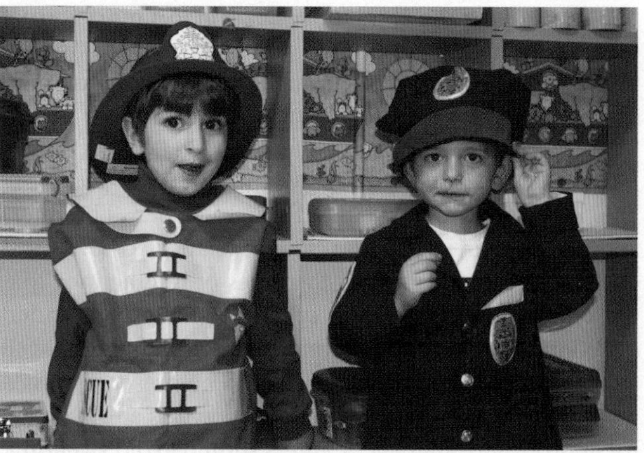

● **Figure 6.10** Preschool children love to dress up and pretend.

BOX 6.1

APPROPRIATE TOYS FOR PRESCHOOLERS

- Blocks, simple jigsaw puzzles (four to six large pieces), pegboards, wooden bead with string
- Supplies for creativity: chalk, large crayons, finger paint, Play-Doh or clay, washable markers, paper, paint and paintbrush, scissors, paste, or glue
- Puppets, dress-up clothes and props for dramatic play
- Bucket, plastic shovel and other containers for sand and water play
- Play kitchen with accessories and pretend food (empty food boxes can be recycled for kitchen play)
- Squeaking, floating, squirting toys for the bath
- Sandbox with shovel and various toys for building
- Dolls that can be dressed and undressed (large buttons, zippers, and snaps), doll care accessories (diapers, bottles, carriage, crib)
- Gross motor toys: tricycle or big wheel (with helmet), jungle gym or swing set (with supervision), hula hoop, tunnel, wagon
- Blocks, Legos, cars and trucks, plastic animals, trains, plastic figures (family, community helpers), stuffed animals, balls, sewing cards
- Tape or CD players for music, various musical instruments
- Simple card and board games (older preschooler)
- Dollhouse with furniture and accessories, people and animals

ior related to education and learning, as well as instilling values in their children. School readiness is a topic that has received a significant amount of national attention in recent years. To succeed in school, children need a safe, responsive home environment that allows them to learn and explore, as well as structure and limits that allow them to learn the socially acceptable behaviors that they will need in school. Language development is critical to the ability to succeed in school and can be encouraged through books and reading. Each of these components is important in readying the child for education in a more formal setting. Promoting language development, choosing a preschool, and making the transition to kindergarten are discussed in more detail below.

Promoting Language Development

The parent serves as the child's first teacher. The interactions between parent and child in relation to books and other play activities model the types of interactions that the child will later have in school. Asking open-ended questions stimulates the development of thinking as well as language in the preschool child. The preschooler is a great imitator, so the parent should serve as a role model for appropriate language. Parents should avoid swearing, as the child is sure to repeat "bad words" even if he or she does not understand what they mean. Allowing children to pursue interests at their own pace will help them to develop the literacy and numeric skills that will enable them to later focus on academic skills.

Preschoolers enjoy books with pictures that tell stories (Fig. 6.11). Stories with repeated phrases help to keep the child's attention. Children like stories that describe experiences similar to their own. The preschool child demonstrates early literacy skills by reciting stories or portions of books. He or she also may retell the story from the book, pretend to read books, and ask questions about the story. The preschool child has enough focus and expanded attention to notice when a page is skipped during reading and will call it to the parent's attention.

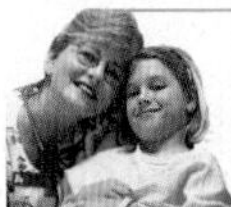

Risk factors for lack of social and emotional readiness for school include insecure attachment in the early years, maternal depression, parental substance abuse, and low socioeconomic status. Nurses should screen for these factors and make referrals if appropriate.

Choosing a Preschool/Starting Kindergarten

Many parents choose to enroll their child in preschool. Preschool should be used primarily as an opportunity to foster the child's social skills and accustom him or her to the group environment. When selecting a preschool

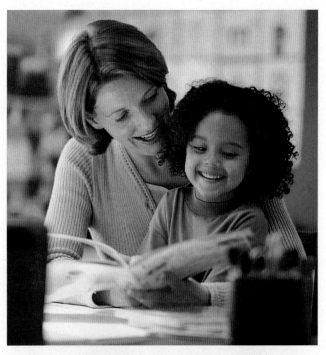

● Figure 6.11 Preschool children enjoy being read to and looking at the pictures that go along with the story.

the parent may want to consider the accreditation of the school, the teachers' qualifications, and recommendations of other parents. The focus of the school environment is also important: What is the daily schedule of activities? Is the school very structured, or does it have a looser environment? The parents must decide how focused on curriculum they want the school to be. The parent should observe the classroom, evaluating the environment, noise level, and sanitary practices as well as how the children interact with each other and how the teachers interact with the children.

The type of discipline used in the school is also an important factor. Parents should not choose a preschool that uses corporal punishment. The American Academy of Pediatrics discourages the use of corporal punishment in the school setting. Corporal punishment may hurt a child's self-esteem as well as his or her ability to achieve in school. It may also lead to disruptive and violent behavior in the classroom. As preschool is the foundation for later education, the child should have the opportunity to build self-esteem and the skills needed for the more formal setting of elementary school.

Whether or not the child attended preschool, kindergarten will be the next big step. Kindergarten hours may be longer than preschool hours, and kindergarten is usually held 5 days per week. This may be a significant change for some children. For most children, the setting and personnel in kindergarten will be new to the child. Rules and expectations are often very different as well. When discussing starting kindergarten with the preschool child, parents should do so in an enthusiastic fashion, keeping the conversation light and positive. Parents should meet with the child's teacher prior to the start of school, if possible, to discuss particular needs or concerns. Parents may want to schedule a tour of the school for the preschooler or attend the school's open house with the child to ease the transition. Practicing the new daily routine prior to the start of school will also be helpful.

Most states require up-to-date immunizations and a health screening of the child before he or she enters kindergarten, so advise parents to plan ahead and schedule these in a timely fashion so that school entrance is not delayed.

Promoting Safety

In the United States, accidental injury remains the leading cause of death for children between the ages of 1 and 14 years. Preschoolers are at an ideal age to be taught about safety and safe behaviors. They are cognitively able to absorb concrete information and they desire to master the situations they are in, but they continue to display poor judgment related to safety issues. Their engagement in fantasy is so strong that it makes it difficult for them to master complicated cause-and-effect relationships. The preschool child is capable of learning safe behaviors but may not always be able to transfer those behaviors to a different situation. Parents must continue to closely supervise preschool children to avoid accidental injury during this period.

Safety in the Car

The young preschooler who weighs less than 40 pounds should use a forward-facing car seat with harness and top tether. The preschooler who weighs between 40 and 80 pounds should ride in a booster seat that uses both the lap and shoulder belts (Fig. 6.12). When the child is large enough to sit up straight with the knees bent at the front edge of the seat, he or she may sit directly on the seat of the car with the lap/shoulder belt securely and appropriately attached. The lap belt should sit low over the hips and upper thighs and the shoulder belt should stay on the shoulder and close to the chest. The back seat of the car is always the safest place for a child to ride. If a child under 12 years of age must sit in the front seat because there are not enough rear seats available, then the front passenger seat air bag should be deactivated. Children should never ride in the cargo area of a pickup truck. See Healthy People 2010.

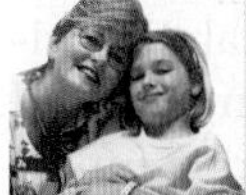

Although motor vehicle accidents remain a major cause of injury and death in the preschool age group, many families do not use appropriate car seat/seat belt safety with their children. Child passenger safety technicians are available to provide proper installation of car seats. To find one in your area, visit www.nhtsa.dot.gov/people/injury/childps/contacts or www.seatcheck.org. The NHTSA Auto Safety Hot Line may be reached at (888) 327-4236.

Safety in the Home

Handguns, matches, bodies of water, bicycle riding, and poisons continue to be sources of potential injury during the preschool years. The majority of injuries in the

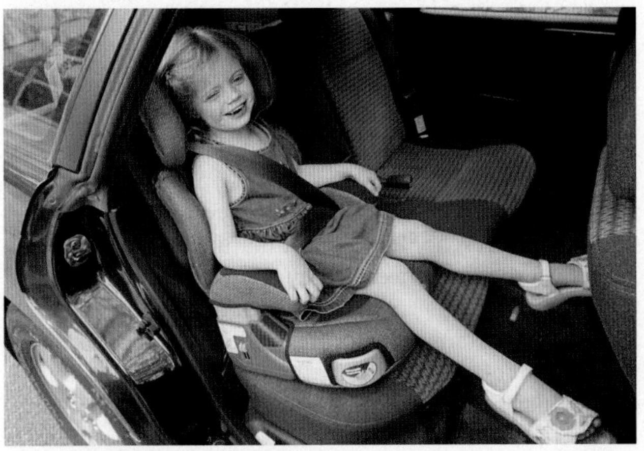

● Figure 6.12 The preschool child who weighs more than 40 pounds should be appropriately secured in an approved booster seat.

HEALTHY PEOPLE 2010

Objective	Significance
Increase use of child restraints.	• Encourage car seat and booster seat use until the child is of the appropriate size and age to progress to seat belts.

preschool years result from motor vehicle accidents, with a significant number of injuries also occurring in or around the home. Bike riders struck by motor vehicles and burns account for a significant percentage of deaths in the preschool age group (Dowd et al., 2002).

Preventing Exposure to Tobacco Smoke

Parents should protect their preschoolers from secondhand tobacco smoke. Exposure to tobacco smoke is associated with an increased incidence of otitis media and respiratory infections, as well as increased symptoms and medication use in children with asthma. Other effects include decreased lung function and behavioral difficulties. The preschool child should never be in an enclosed space (such as a car) where tobacco smoke is present.

Preventing Injury

The preschool child who runs out into the street is at risk for being struck by a car. Teach preschoolers to stop at the curb and never go into the street without a grown-up. The preschooler may learn to ride a bicycle (with or without training wheels). The child must wear an approved bicycle helmet any time he or she rides the bicycle, even if it is just in the driveway. Requiring helmet use in the early years will lead to the habit of helmet use as the child gets older. Allowing the preschooler to choose his or her own helmet may encourage the child to use the helmet.

Bicycles should be safe for this age group. The size must be correct; the balls of the feet should reach both pedals while the child is sitting on the seat and has both hands on the handlebars. Children under 5 years of age have difficulty learning to use hand-operated brakes, so traditional pedal-back brakes are recommended in this age group. Preschoolers are not mature enough to ride a bicycle in the street even if they are riding with adults, so they should always ride on the sidewalk.

It is important to make the inside of the home safe for the preschool child. Parents should install and maintain smoke alarms in the home. Increased physical dexterity and refinement of motor skills enable the preschooler to strike matches or use a lighter and start a fire. The preschool child is capable of washing his or her hands independently, so the water heater should be set at 120 degrees Fahrenheit or below to prevent scalding.

The preschooler's active imagination and desire to play make-believe may result in a firearm injury. The average preschooler is physically capable of handling and firing a gun, particularly a handgun, which is smaller and lighter. If present in the home, firearms should be kept in a locked cabinet with the ammunition stored elsewhere.

Preventing Poisoning

Though taste discrimination is continuing to develop, preschoolers still have unrefined taste discrimination, placing them at risk for accidental ingestion. Parents should never try to coax a child to take a vitamin supplement, tablet, or pill by calling it "candy." Dangerous fluids should be stored in their original containers and should be kept out of reach of preschoolers; they should not be poured into containers that look like ordinary drinking glasses or cups. Potentially dangerous cleaning or personal health and beauty products, gardening and pool chemicals, as well as automotive materials should be kept out of reach of preschoolers and in a locked cabinet if possible. Medications should have childproof caps and should be kept in a locked cabinet. The poison control telephone number should be posted on or near the home phone (1-800-222-1222).

Safety in the Water

Five years of age is an appropriate time for a child to learn to swim. Children at this age are physically capable of this activity and have the cognitive maturity to accomplish the task of swimming and basic water safety. Swimming programs should focus on appropriate swim techniques as well as safety measures. Parents and caregivers should be trained in infant/child CPR. Homes with swimming pools should have lifesaving devices readily accessible. Preschoolers should be taught never to dive into water until an adult has verified its depth. Preschoolers are still too young to be left unattended around any body of water, even if they know how to swim. Preschoolers should never be allowed to swim in a canal or any fast-moving water. Preschoolers who are riding in boats or fishing off riverbanks should wear a personal flotation device. Parents should also be cautioned about close supervision of young children walking, skating, or riding near thin or weak ice. See Healthy People 2010.

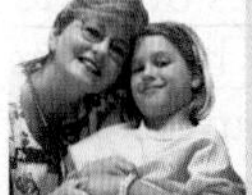

The American Academy of Pediatrics recommends that all swimming pools be secured by a fence that is at least 5 feet high and has a self-latching gate to protect young children from entering a pool area unattended (AAP, 2003).

Recall Nila Patel, the 4-year-old presented at the beginning of the chapter. What anticipatory guidance related to safety should you provide to her parents?

HEALTHY PEOPLE 2010

Objective	Significance
Reduce drownings.	• Never leave a young child unattended in or near the water. • Educate families about water safety. • Remind families that the preschooler's ability to swim does not replace the need for constant supervision while in the pool or other body of water.

Promoting Nutrition

The preschool child has a full set of primary teeth, is able to chew and swallow competently, and has learned to use utensils fairly effectively to feed himself or herself (Fig. 6.13). As in the toddler years, it is important for the preschool child to continue to learn and build upon healthy eating habits. These habits will last throughout the child's life. A diet high in nutrient-rich foods such as whole grains, vegetables, fruits, appropriate dairy foods, and lean meats is appropriate for the preschooler. Nutrient-poor, high-calorie foods such as sweets and typical fast foods should be offered only in limited amounts.

Nutritional Needs

The 3- to 5-year-old requires 500 to 800 mg calcium and 10 mg iron daily. The 3-year-old should consume 19 mg dietary fiber daily, while the 4- to 8-year-old requires 25 mg dietary fiber per day. Box 6.2 lists good calcium and iron

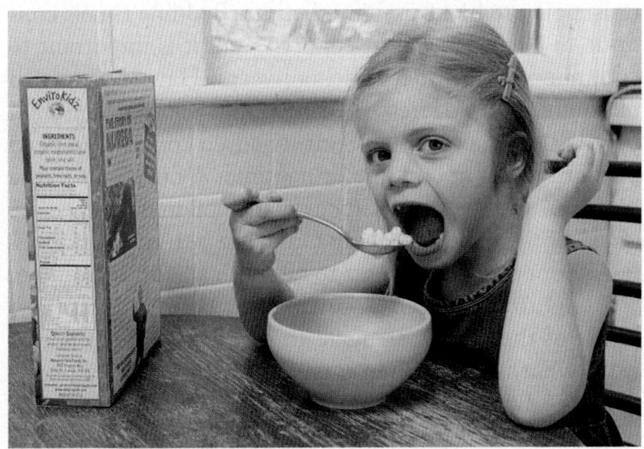

● Figure 6.13 The preschool child has the manual dexterity to handle utensils appropriately and feed himself or herself independently.

BOX 6.2

DAILY CALCIUM AND IRON RECOMMENDATIONS FOR PRESCHOOL CHILDREN

Calcium: 500 mg (3-year-old), 800 mg (4- to 8-year-old)	Iron: 10 mg
Calcium in foods:	**Iron in foods:**
• 8 oz low-fat or whole milk: 300 mg	• ¾ cup 100% fortified prepared cereal: 18 mg
• 8 oz low-fat yogurt: 300 mg	• ¾ cup 50% fortified prepared cereal: 9 mg
• 1½ oz cheddar cheese: 300 mg	• 3 oz beef: 3 mg
• 1 oz dried white beans (cooked): 160 mg	• 3 oz chicken leg: 3 mg
• ¼ cup tofu: 125 mg	• ½ cup cooked lentils: 3 mg
• 1 medium orange: 50 mg	• 3 oz chicken breast: 2 mg
• ½ cup mashed sweet potatoes: 44 mg	• ¼ cup fresh cooked spinach: 1.6 mg
• ½ cup cooked or 1½ cup raw broccoli: 35 mg	• ¼ cup tofu: 0.9 mg
	• 1 slice enriched bread: 0.8 to 0.9 mg
	• ¼ cup frozen spinach, cooked: 0.7 mg

sources. The typical preschooler requires about 85 kcal/kg of body weight. Saturated fats should account for less than 10% of total calories. Preschool children's diets should include a daily total fat intake of no less than 20% and not more than 30% of total calories to promote and maintain healthy cholesterol levels.

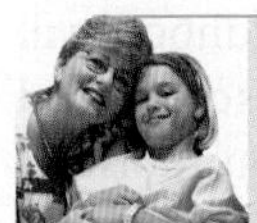

Drinking excess amounts of milk may lead to iron deficiency, as the calcium in milk blocks iron absorption.

Promoting Healthy Eating Habits

Preschool children may be picky eaters. They may eat only a limited variety of foods or foods prepared in certain ways and may not be very willing to try new things. The 3- or 4-year-old may exhibit "food fads," eating only certain foods over a several-day period. As the child gets older, pickiness lessens. By 5 years of age the child is more focused on the social context of eating: table conversation and manners. The 5-year-old is generally more willing to at least try new foods and may like to help with meal preparation and clean-up as appropriate.

If the preschooler is growing well, then the pickiness is not a cause for concern. A larger concern may be the negative relationship that can develop between the parent and child relating to mealtime. The more the parent coaxes, cajoles, bribes, and threatens, the less likely the child is to try new foods or even eat the ones he or she likes that are served. The parent must maintain a positive and patient demeanor at mealtime. The child should be offered a healthy diet, with foods from all groups over the course of the day as recommended by the USDA. The "Food Guide Pyramid for Your Young Child" (from the United States Department of Agriculture) may be used to plan the preschool child's daily diet. See Figure 5.9 in Chapter 5, and note the explanation of serving sizes at the bottom of the chart.

The parent should maintain a matter-of-fact approach, offer the meal or snack, and then allow the child to decide how much of the food, if any, he or she is going to eat. High-fat, nutrient-poor snacks should not be substituted for healthy foods just to coax the child to "eat something." See Healthy People 2010.

Preventing the Development of Overweight and Obesity

Worldwide, over 22 million children under 5 years old are obese. In the past 30 years, the number of U.S. children and adolescents who are overweight has doubled. Eight percent of 4- to 5-year-olds in America are overweight (Williams, 2003). Overweight and obese children are at risk for hypertension, hyperlipidemia, and the development of insulin resistance. Children whose weight is at or above the 95th percentile when 3 to 6 years old have a 50% chance of being obese as adults (Krebs et al., 2004). The risk is increased if one or both parents are overweight. Research has demonstrated that preschool children who are overweight or obese show a preference for higher-fat foods and tend to overeat (Neumark-Sztainer, 2003).

Parents are in an opportune position to exert a positive influence on their preschooler's nutritional intake and activity level. The habits learned in early childhood will likely carry over into the school-age, adolescent, and adult years. Children whose parents take an authoritarian approach to mealtime may learn to overeat, as they are encouraged to finish the entire meal ("Clean your plate!").

HEALTHY PEOPLE 2010

Objective	Significance
Increase the proportion of persons aged 2 years and older who meet dietary recommendations for calcium.	• Screen preschoolers for appropriate dietary intake of calcium. • Educate families about calcium content in foods. • Assist families with choosing a diet that meets calcium needs and is appealing to the young child.

If they are offered appropriate, healthy food choices and access to high-calorie, nutrient-poor food is limited, preschoolers will learn to self-regulate (eat only until full). Food should not be used as either reward or punishment.

Parents should remain positive and patient at mealtime. Mealtimes should continue to be structured. Unstructured meals lead to an increase in fat and calorie consumption. Increased amount of calories as fat has been linked to a higher body mass index (BMI) in preschool children. To limit the chance that overeating will occur, preschoolers should be offered a variety of healthy foods at each meal. This may include one each of a protein source, grain, vegetable, and fruit. The preschool child's serving size is usually one third to one half of the recommended size of an adult serving. The preschool child may imitate the other eaters at the table. Parents have a prime chance to be good role models, setting an example of eating vegetables and fruits.

As with toddlers, fruit juice should be limited to 4 to 6 ounces per day, as excess consumption can lead to excess weight gain. Preschoolers should be encouraged to drink water.

Limiting television viewing and encouraging physical activity are also important strategies for the prevention of overweight and obesity.

> **Refer back to Nila Patel,** the 4-year-old introduced at the beginning of the chapter. What questions should you ask Nila's parents related to nutritional intake? What anticipatory guidance related to nutrition would be appropriate? Nila's mother expresses concerns regarding obesity. How would you address these?

Promoting Healthy Sleep and Rest

The preschool child needs about 12 hours of sleep each day. Some preschool children continue to take a nap during the day. Unless very tired, many preschool children will resist going to bed from time to time. Bedtime rituals continue to be reassuring to children, and it is important to continue them in the preschool years. Having a time of relaxation with a decrease in stimulation will allow the child to fall asleep more easily. Some children continue to need a security item at bedtime or naptime. A nightlight in the bedroom may be necessary, as many children this age are afraid of the dark. Teaching Guideline 6.1 gives information about assisting parents to establish a bedtime routine.

Nightmares often occur in preschool children as a result of the child's struggle to distinguish what is real from what is not. When a child awakens from a nightmare, he or she is often crying and may be able to recount what the dream was about. Parents should validate the child's fear rather than discounting it. Saying, "Yes, I agree, monsters are scary; it's a good thing they aren't real" is more appropriate than, "Don't be silly: monsters

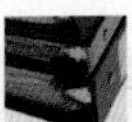

TEACHING GUIDELINE 6.1

Bedtime Routines

- Establish a bedtime as well as morning wake-up time, and enforce them consistently.
- Avoid sugar or caffeine consumption in the evening.
- Avoid stimulating activities such as roughhousing before bedtime.
- Do not allow television watching in bed.
- Make the child's bedroom an inviting and comfortable area of the home.
- Provide a nightlight in the child's bedroom if he or she is afraid of the dark.
- Conform to a nightly routine:
  - Television off at a certain time
  - Bath
  - Quiet game or story reading/telling
  - Bedtime prayer or song
- Maintain quiet in the bedroom and nearby to increase the child's ability to fall asleep.

aren't real." Sometimes children benefit from reading stories about dreams. Recommended books include:

- *Bedtime for Frances* by Russell Hoban
- *Ben's Dream* by Chris van Allsberg
- *In the Night Kitchen* by Maurice Sendak
- *There's a Nightmare in My Closet* by Mercer Mayer

Nightmares should not be confused with night terrors. After a nightmare, the child is aroused and interactive, but night terrors are different: a short time after falling asleep, the child seems to awaken and is screaming. The child usually does not respond much to the parent's soothing, but he or she eventually stops screaming and goes back to sleep. Night terrors are often frightening for parents because the child does not seem to be responding to them. One technique that may help to decrease the incidence of night terrors is to wake the child about 30 to 45 minutes into the sleep cycle. If continued nightly for about a week, the cycle of night terrors may be broken. See Comparison Chart 6.1.

> **Think back to Nila Patel.** What anticipatory guidance would you provide to her parents in relation to sleep during the preschool years?

Promoting Healthy Teeth and Gums

Dental caries prevention continues to be important and can be achieved through daily brushing and flossing. Parents should use only a pea-sized amount of toothpaste to prevent excess fluoride consumption, which can contribute to fluorosis. The preschooler may brush his or her own teeth, but the parent must continue to supervise to ensure adequate brushing. Parents must perform flossing because the preschool child cannot perform this task adequately.

COMPARISON CHART 6.1 Nightmares Versus Night Terrors

	Nightmare	Night Terror
Definition	Scary or bad dream followed by awakening	Partial arousal from deep sleep
When parents become aware	Child awakens parent after episode is over	Screaming and thrashing during the episode awakens the parent
Timing	Usually in the second half of the night	Usually about an hour after falling asleep
Behavior	Crying, may be scared after awakening	Sits up, thrashes, cries, screams, talks, looks wild-eyed. Sweats, may have racing heartbeat.
Responsiveness	Responsive to parent's soothing and reassurances	Child unaware of parent's presence, may scream and thrash more if restrained
Return to sleep	Difficulty going back to sleep if afraid	Rapidly returns to sleep without full awakening
Memory of occurrence	May remember the dream and talk about it later	No memory of event

Information from Ferber, R. (1985). *Solve your child's sleep problems.* New York: Simon & Schuster.

Cariogenic foods should be avoided. If sugary foods are consumed, the mouth should be rinsed with water if it is not possible to brush the teeth immediately. The preschool child should visit the dentist every 6 months.

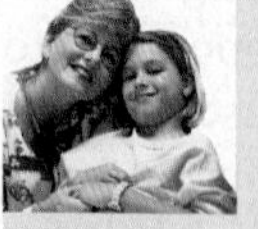

Dental caries prevention is important in the primary teeth, because loss of these teeth to caries may affect the proper formation of permanent teeth as well as the width of the dental arch.

Promoting Appropriate Discipline

Successful discipline results from a loving and nurturing environment in which the preschooler's self-esteem is fostered and where limits are well chosen and enforced consistently. Spanking (striking with the open hand) is the least effective discipline practice and is discouraged by the American Academy of Pediatrics and the National Association of Pediatric Nurse Practitioners. Belts, switches, paddles, or other items should never be used to strike a child. The more the preschool age child is hit, the worse the child's behavior is when assessed 2 years later (Strauss, 1996). The use of physical punishment has been associated with a number of additional problems in adulthood, such as antisocial and criminal behaviors (see Chapter 5).

If parents are consistent with discipline while encouraging the preschooler's normal growth and development of imagination and make-believe, the child will learn to accept that certain things are not allowed. The sense of initiative can be preserved and guilt avoided if the rules are clear and enforced consistently.

Consider THIS!

The more frequently children are hit in the preschool years, the more anger they report as adults (AAP, Committee on Psychosocial Aspects of Child and Family Health, 1998).

Minimize the occurrence of misbehavior by anticipating conditions likely to lead to the undesired or risky action. When the situation becomes difficult, parents should use distraction to changes the preschooler's focus. When discussing the misbehavior, be certain to label the behavior and not the child. This helps to preserve the preschooler's self-esteem. When teaching preschoolers about undesired behavior, be sure they also understand the reason why it is wrong or unacceptable to do it. This helps to encourage the child to use internal controls over behavior. Parents should serve as role models for self-control, including choice of words, the tone they are delivered in, and the actions that accompany them.

Children work harder to obtain praise than to receive punishment, so always reward positive behaviors. Preschool children are becoming capable of understanding the concept of right and wrong. They start to understand each other's feelings (**empathy**) and are cognitively capable of remembering basic rules.

Time-out or time away from the situation can be very effective in this age group. The punishment should be used only for intentional misbehavior (knowing something is forbidden but doing it anyway). It is particularly helpful with dangerous or destructive behavior. The preschooler is given a warning that time-out will occur if the behavior does not stop. The preschooler is removed from the situation and must stay in time-out for a specified period of time. A particular time-out area is helpful; a boring corner of the room without distractions available is a good location. The generally recommended period of time is to require 1 minute of time-out per year of age; thus, a 4-year-old would be in time-out for 4 minutes. Set the timer so the child will know when the time-out is over. If the child gets up before the prescribed time, replace the child in time-out and restart the timer. Time-out works best if used each and every time the undesirable behavior occurs. Also, praise the child when he or she follows the rules and behaves appropriately.

A simple and clear explanation of the misbehavior should be given to the child; parents should also talk about acceptable alternative strategies that the child can use in the future instead of the undesired behavior. Removal of a privilege such as playing with a favorite toy can be as effective as time-out.

Books and other media that are available to help educate parents about appropriate discipline and to help the child learn self-control are listed in Box 6.3.

ADDRESSING COMMON DEVELOPMENTAL CONCERNS

Common developmental concerns of the preschool period include lying, sex education, and masturbation. Parents often express difficulty in dealing with these issues with their preschool children. Offering appropriate anticipatory guidance may give the parents the support and confidence they need to deal with these issues.

Lying

Lying is common in preschool children. It may occur because the child fears punishment, has gotten carried away with imagination, or is imitating what he or she sees the parent do. The parent should ascertain the reason for the lie before punishing the child. If the child has broken a rule and fears punishment, then the parent must determine the truth. The child needs to learn that lying is usually far worse than the misbehavior itself. The punishment for the misbehavior should be lessened if the child admits the truth. The parent should remain calm and serve as

BOX 6.3

SELECTED RESOURCES FOR PARENTS AND PRESCHOOLERS

Books for Parents (about discipline)

- *How to Talk so Kids will Listen and Listen so Kids will Talk* by A. Faber & E. Mazlish (Harper Resource)
- *Kids are Worth It: Giving Your Children the Gift of Inner Discipline* by B. Colorosos (Harper Collins Publishers)
- *Positive Discipline A to Z: 1001 Solutions to Everyday Parenting Problems* by J. Nelson, L. Lott, & S. G. Glenn (Three Rivers Press)
- *Setting Limits with Your Strong-willed Child: Eliminating Conflict by Establishing Clear, Firm and Respectful Boundaries* by R. MacKenzie (Three Rivers Press)
- *The Case Against Spanking: How to Discipline Children without Hitting* by I. A. Hyman (Jossey-Bass)
- *The Nurturing Parent: How to Raise Creative, Loving, Responsible Children* by J. S. Dacey & A. J. Packer (Fireside)
- *Without Spanking or Spoiling: a Practical Approach to Toddler and Preschool Guidance* by E. Crary (Parenting Press)

Books for Preschoolers (about dealing with feelings and learning how to behave):

- *Hands are Not for Hitting* by M. Agassi (Free Spirit Publishing)
- *I Can't Wait* by E. Crary (Parenting Press)
- *I Want It* by E. Crary (Parenting Press)
- *I Want to Play* by E. Crary (Parenting Press)
- *I Was so Mad* by M. Mayer (Golden Books)
- *I Was so Mad* by N. Simon & D. Leder (Albert Whitman & Company)
- *I'm Excited* by E. Crary (Parenting Press)
- *I'm Frustrated* by E. Crary (Parenting Press)
- *I'm Mad* by E. Crary (Parenting Press)
- *I'm Scared* by E. Crary (Parenting Press)
- *Feet are not for Kicking* by E. Verdick (Free Spirit Publishing)
- *Teeth are not for Biting* by E. Verdick (Free Spirit Publishing)
- *When Sophie gets Angry . . . Really, Really Angry* by M. Bang (Blue Sky Press)
- *Words are not for Hurting* by E. Verdick (Free Spirit Publishing)

a role model of an even temper. The next time the misbehavior occurs, the child will be more apt to simply tell the truth.

If the child's lying is really just his or her imagination getting carried away, then the parent should guide the child in distinguishing between myth and reality. The preschooler's imagination is very vivid, and the child needs direction in the use of that faculty. Parents should serve as role models of appropriate behavior for their children to learn it. Children who lie because they hear their parents do it simply must not see or hear their parents do it.

Sex Education

Preschoolers are keen observers but are still not able to interpret all that they see correctly. The child may recognize, but not understand, sexual activity. Preschoolers are very inquisitive and want to learn about everything around them; therefore, they are very likely to ask questions about sex and where babies come from. Before attempting to answer questions, parents should try to find out first what the child is really asking and what the child already thinks about that subject. Then they should provide a simple, direct, and honest answer. The child needs only the information that he or she is requesting. Additional questions will occur in the future and should be addressed as they arise.

Masturbation

The normal curiosity of the preschool years often leads children to explore their own genitals. This behavior may be upsetting to some parents, but masturbation is a healthy and natural part of normal preschool development if it occurs in moderation. If the parent overreacts to this behavior, then it may occur more frequently. Masturbation should be treated in a matter-of-fact way by the parent. The child needs to learn certain rules about this activity: nudity and masturbation are not acceptable in public. The child should also be taught safety: no other person can touch the private parts unless it is the parent, doctor, or nurse checking to see when something is wrong.

Think back to Nila Patel. What are some developmental concerns that are common during the preschool years? What anticipatory guidance related to these concerns would you provide to Nila's parents?

References

Books and Journals

Adler, M., & Specker, B. (2001). Atypical diets in infancy and childhood. *Pediatric Annals, 30*(11), 630–680.

American Academy of Pediatrics. (2000). Swimming programs for infants and toddlers. *Pediatrics, 105*(4), 868–870.

American Academy of Pediatrics. (2001). Policy Statement: The use and misuse of fruit juice in pediatrics (RE0047). *Pediatrics, 107*(5), 1201–1213.

American Academy of Pediatrics. (2003). Policy Statement: Prevention of drowning in infants, children and adolescents. *Pediatrics, 112*(2), 437–439.

American Academy of Pediatrics. (2005). Car safety seats: A guide for families. [Electronic version] Accessed at www.aap.org/family/carseatguide.htm

American Academy of Pediatrics. (2005). The injury prevention program, age-related safety sheets: 5 years. Accessed 1/10/05 at www.aap.org/family/5years.htm

American Academy of Pediatrics, Committee on Injury and Poison Prevention. (2000). Children in pickup trucks. *Pediatrics, 106*(4), 857–859.

American Academy of Pediatrics, Committee on Injury and Poison Prevention. (2003). Poison treatment in the home. *Pediatrics, 112*(5), 1182–1185.

American Academy of Pediatrics, Committee on Nutrition. (1998). Cholesterol in childhood. *Pediatrics, 101*(1), 141–147.

American Academy of Pediatrics, Committee on Nutrition. (1999). Calcium requirements of infants, children, and adolescents. *Pediatrics, 104*(5), 1152–1157.

American Academy of Pediatrics, Committee on Nutrition. (2003). Prevention of pediatric overweight and obesity. *Pediatrics, 104*(5), 1152–1157.

American Academy of Pediatrics, Committee on Psychosocial Aspects of Child and Family Health. (1998). Guidelines for effective discipline. *Pediatrics, 101*(4), 723–728.

American Academy of Pediatrics, Committee on Public Education. (2001). Children, adolescents, and television. *Pediatrics, 107*(2), 423–426.

Ateah, C. A., Secco, L., & Woodgate, R. L. (2003). The risks and alternatives to physical punishment use with children. *Journal of Pediatric Health Care, 17*(3), 126–132.

Atkinson, P. M., Parks, D. K., Cooley, S. M., & Sarkis, S. L. (2002). Reach out and read: A pediatric clinic-based approach to early literacy promotion. *Journal of Pediatric Health Care, 16*(1), 10–15.

Brazelton, T. B. (2001). *Touchpoints three to six: Your child's emotional and behavioral development.* Cambridge, MA: Perseus Publishing Company.

Brown, M. L. (2001). The effects of environmental tobacco smoke on children: Information and implications for PNPs. *Journal of Pediatric Health Care, 15*(6), 280–286.

Chan, G. (2001). Calcium needs during childhood. *Pediatric Annals, 30*(11), 666–670.

Deering, C. G., & Cody, D. J. (2002). Communicating with children and adolescents. *American Journal of Nursing, 102*(3), 34–41.

Dowd, M. D., Keenan, H. T., & Bratton, S. L. (2002). Epidemiology and prevention of childhood injuries. *Critical Care Medicine, 30*(11, Suppl.), S385–S392.

Erikson, E. H. (1963). *Childhood and society* (2nd ed.). New York: W. W. Norton and Company.

Ferber, R. (1985). *Solve your child's sleep problems.* New York: Simon & Schuster.

Fierro-Cobas, V. (2001). Language development in bilingual children: A primer for pediatricians. *Contemporary Pediatrics, 18*(7), 79–98.

Fosarelli, P. (2003). Children and the development of faith: Implications for pediatric practice. *Contemporary Pediatrics, 20*(1), 85–98.

Gabbard, G. O. (2000). Psychoanalysis. In B. J. Sadock & V. A. Sadock (Eds.), *Kaplan and Sadock's comprehensive textbook of psychiatry* (7th ed.). Philadelphia: Lippincott Williams & Wilkins.

Gabriel, J. (2001). Getting ready for school: Pencils, notebook, positive attitude. [electronic article] Available at www.brainconnection.com/topics/?main=fa/emotion-ready

Gottesman, M. M. (2000). Nurturing the social and emotional development of children, a.k.a. discipline. *Journal of Pediatric Health Care, 14*(2), 81–84.

Gottesman, M. M. (2001). Making time for teaching. *Journal of Pediatric Health Care, 15*(2), 94–97.

Kontio, K., Letts, M., & German, A. (2001). Airbags and children: A mixed blessing. *Contemporary Pediatrics, 18*(4), 96–103.

Krebs, N. F., Collins, J., & Johnson, S. L. (2004). Screen for and treat overweight in 2-to 5-year-olds? Yes! *Contemporary Pediatrics.* [Electronic version] Available at www.contemporarypediatrics.com

Leavitt, L. A. (2002). When terrible things happen: A parent's guide to talking with their children. *Journal of Pediatric Health Care, 16*(5), 272–274.

Mandleco, B. (2004). *Growth and development handbook: Newborn through adolescence.* Clifton Park, NY: Delmar Learning.

Martins, Y. (2002). Try it, you'll like it! Early dietary experiences and food acceptance patterns. *Pediatric Basics: The Journal of Pediatric Nutrition and Development, 98,* 12–20.

McEvoy, M. (2000). An added dimension to the pediatric health maintenance visit: The spiritual history. *Journal of Pediatric Health Care, 14*(5), 216–220.

Mobley, C. E., & Evashevski, J. (2000). Evaluating health and safety knowledge of preschoolers: Assessing their early start to being health smart. *Journal of Pediatric Health Care, 14*(4), 160–165.

National Association of Pediatric Nurse Practitioners. (2001). Position statement: Child care. *Journal of Pediatric Health Care, 15*(2), 35A.

National Association of Pediatric Nurse Practitioners. (2002). Position statement: Corporal punishment. *Journal of Pediatric Health Care, 16*(3), 34A.

Nelms, B. C. (2000). Parents are the best toy. *Journal of Pediatric Health Care, 14*(4), 147–148.

Neumark-Sztainer, D. (2003). Childhood and adolescent obesity. *Pediatric Basics: The Journal of Pediatric Nutrition and Development, 101,* 12–20.

Nicklaus, T. A., & Fisher, J. O. (2003). To each his own: Family influences on children's food preferences. *Pediatric Basics: The Journal of Pediatric Nutrition and Development, 102,* 13–20.

Papalia, D. E., Olds, S. W., & Feldman, F. D. (2001). *Human development* (8th ed.). New York: McGraw-Hill.

Passehl, B., McCarroll, C., Buechner, J., Gearring, C., Smith, A. E., & Trowbridge, F. (2004). Preventing childhood obesity: Establishing healthy lifestyle habits in the preschool years. *Journal of Pediatric Healthcare, 18*(6), 315–319.

Piaget, J. (1969). *The theory of stages in cognitive development.* New York: McGraw-Hill.

Record, S., Montgomery, D. R., & Milano, M. (2000). Fluoride supplementation and caries prevention. *Journal of Pediatric Health Care, 14*(5), 247–249.

Shelor, S. P. (ed.). (1998). *Caring for your baby and young child: Birth to age 5.* New York: Bantam Books.

Smith, J., & McSherry, W. (2004). Spirituality and child development: A concept analysis. *Journal of Advanced Nursing, 42*(3), 307–315.

Starr, N. B. (2001). Kids and car safety: Beyond car seats and seat belts. *Journal of Pediatric Health Care, 15*(5), 257–259.

Strauss, M. A. (1996). Spanking and the making of a violent society. *Pediatrics, 98,* 837–842.

Sullivan, D., & Carlson, S. (2001). Dietary fats for infants and children. *Pediatric Annals, 30*(11), 683–693.

Williams, C. L. (2003). Childhood obesity: New epidemic of an old disease. *Pediatric Basics: The Journal of Pediatric Nutrition and Development, 101,* 2–9.

Zebrowski, P. M. (2003). Developmental stuttering. *Pediatric Annals, 32*(7), 453–458.

Websites

www.bcm.tmc.edu/cnrc Children's Nutrition Research Center at Baylor College of Medicine in cooperation with U.S. Department of Agriculture

www.hanen.org early language intervention programs

www.nal.usda.gov/fnic/etext/000008.html Child Nutrition and Health section of the Food and Nutrition Information Center

www.nhtsa.dot.gov National Highway Traffic Safety Administration

www.nutritionforkids.com promotion of nutritional health of children and adolescents

Chapter WORKSHEET

● MULTIPLE CHOICE QUESTIONS

1. The nurse is caring for a hospitalized 4-year-old who insists on having the nurse perform every assessment and intervention on her imaginary friend first. She then agrees to have the assessment or intervention done to herself. The nurse identifies this preschooler's behavior as:

a. Problematic: the child is old enough to begin to have a basis in reality

b. Normal, because the child is hospitalized and out of her routine

c. Normal for this stage of growth and development

d. Problematic, as it interferes with needed nursing care

2. The mother of a 3-year-old is concerned about her child's speech. She describes her preschooler as hesitating at the beginning of sentences and repeating consonant sounds. What is the nurse's best response?

a. Hesitancy and dysfluency are normal during this period of development.

b. Reading to the child will help model appropriate speech.

c. Expressive language concerns warrant a developmental evaluation.

d. The mother should ask her pediatrician for a speech therapy evaluation.

3. The mother of a 4-year-old asks for advice on using time-out for discipline with her child. What advice should the nurse give the mother?

a. If spanking is not working, then time-out is not likely to be helpful either.

b. Place the child in time-out for 4 minutes.

c. Use time-out only if removing privileges is unsuccessful.

d. The child should stay in time-out until crying ceases.

4. A 5-year-old child is not gaining weight appropriately. Organic problems have been ruled out. What is the priority action by the nurse?

a. Allow the child unlimited access to the sippy cup to ensure adequate hydration.

b. Encourage sweets for the extra caloric content.

c. Teach the mother about nutritional needs of the preschooler.

d. Assess the child's usual intake pattern at home.

● CRITICAL THINKING EXERCISES

1. Teach a preschool class about bicycle and street safety. Be certain to design the content at an appropriate developmental level.

2. Construct a 3-day menu for a picky 4-year-old. Include three daily meals and two snacks. Follow the nutritional guidelines recommended by the USDA.

3. Color or draw with a preschool child. Analyze the drawings and interactions or discussions you have with the child, relating them to psychosocial and cognitive development expected at this age.

● STUDY ACTIVITIES

1. Care for two average 3-, 4-, or 5-year old children in the clinical setting (make sure both are the same age). Describe each child's development level, response to hospitalization, and family dynamics.

2. Visit a preschool that provides care for special needs children as well as typically developing children. Perform a development assessment on a typical child and one with special needs (both the same age). Compare and contrast your findings.

3. Observe in a 3-, 4- or 5-year-old classroom of a typical preschool. Choose two children who are the same age with different temperaments. Record the differences and similarities in their response to structure and authority, interactions with classmates, attention levels, and language and activity levels.

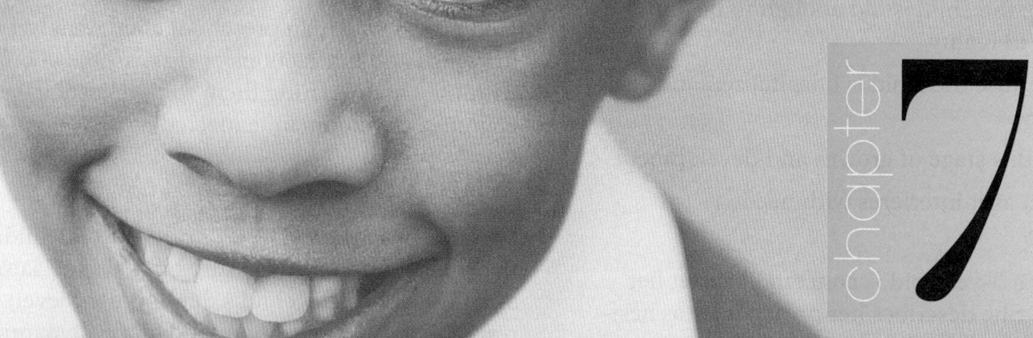

chapter 7

Growth and Development of the School-Age Child

Key TERMS

bruxism
caries
industry
inferiority
malocclusion
prepubescence
principle of conservation
school-age child
school refusal
secondary sexual characteristics
self-esteem

Learning OBJECTIVES

Upon completion of the chapter, the learner will be able to:

1. Identify normal physiologic, cognitive, and moral changes occurring in the school-age child.
2. Describe the role of peers and schools in the development and socialization of the school-age child.
3. Identify the developmental milestones of the school-age child.
4. Identify the role of the nurse in promoting safety for the school-age child.
5. Demonstrate knowledge of the nutritional requirements of the school-age child.
6. Identify common developmental problems in the school-age child.
7. Demonstrate knowledge of the appropriate nursing guidance for common developmental problems.

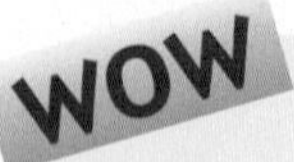

Always give a hundred percent, and you will never doubt your ability to succeed.

Lawrence Jones is a 10-year-old boy brought to the clinic by his mother for his annual school check-up. During your assessment you measure his weight at 62 pounds and his height at 54 inches. As the nurse caring for him, assess Lawrence's growth and development, and then provide appropriate anticipatory guidance to his mother.

School-age children, between the ages of 6 and 12 years, are experiencing a time of slow progressive physical growth, while their social and developmental growth accelerates and increases in complexity. The focus of their world expands from family to teachers, peers, and other outside influences (e.g., coaches, media). The child at this stage becomes increasingly more independent while participating in activities outside the home.

Growth and Development Overview

The school-age years are a time of continued maturation of the child's physical, social, and psychological characteristics. It is during this time that children begin abstract thinking and seek approval of peers, teachers, and parents. Their eye–hand–muscle coordination allows them to participate in organized sports in school or the community. The **school-age child** values school attendance and school activities. The nurse uses knowledge of normal growth and development of the school-age child to assist the child with coping with disruptions and changes during this time period.

● PHYSICAL GROWTH

From 6 to 12 years of age, children grow an average of 2 inches (5 centimeters) per year, increasing their height by 1 to 2 feet. An increase of 4 to 6 pounds (2 to 3 kilograms) per year in weight is expected. In early school-age years, girls and boys are similar in height and weight and appear thinner and more graceful than in previous years. In later school-age years, most girls begin to surpass boys in both height and weight. During this time period there is an approximate 2-year difference between boys and girls. (See Appendix A for growth charts.)

Preadolescent boys and girls do not want to be different from peers of the same sex or the opposite sex, although there are differences in physical and physiologic growth during the school-age years. These differences, especially **secondary sexual characteristics**, are concerning and often a source of embarrassment for both sexes. Girls' early development may be associated with concern about physical appearance and may lead to low **self-esteem**. Boys developing later may have a negative self-concept, which may be linked to risk-taking behaviors such as early sexual activities, substance abuse, or reckless vehicle use.

The differences between girls and boys are more apparent at the end of the middle-school years and may become extreme and a source of emotional problems. These differences in height and weight relationships, and changes in growth patterns, should be explained to parents and children (Fig. 7.1). Physical maturity is not necessarily associated with emotional and social maturity. An 8-year-old who is the size of an 11-year-old will think and act like an 8-year-old. Many times, the expectations placed on these children are unrealistic and can impact the self-esteem and competence of the child.

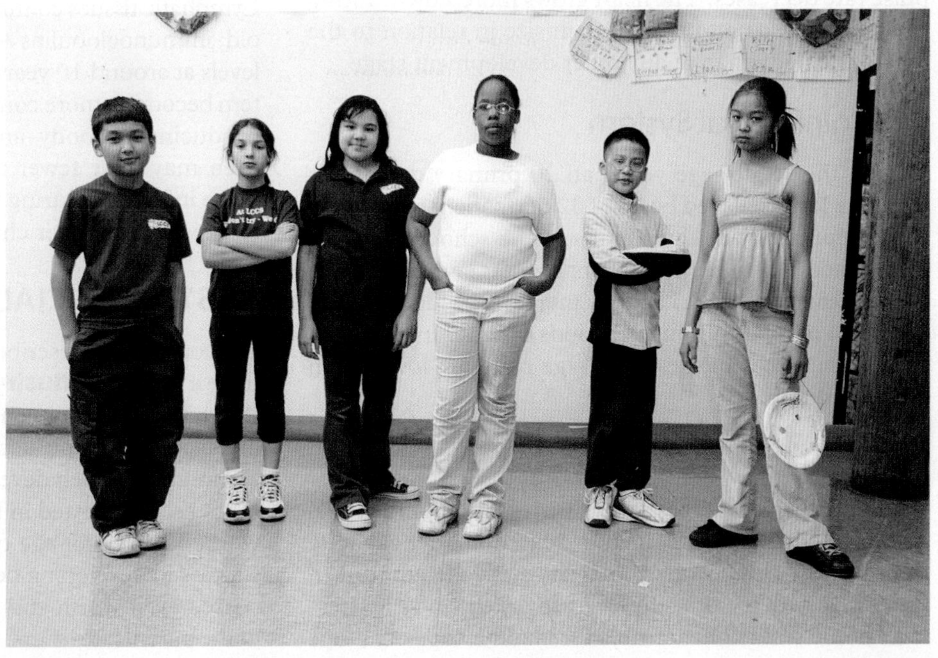

● Figure 7.1 The different growth rates of school-age children are depicted by these same-age school-age children.

This can work in reverse, to similar effect, for an 11-year-old who is the size of an 8-year-old and is therefore treated as such.

ORGAN SYSTEMS MATURATION

Maturation of organs may differ with age or gender. Maturation of organs remains fairly consistent until late school age. In late school-age years (10- to 12-year-olds), boys experience a slowed growth in height and increased weight gain, which may lead to obesity. During this time, girls may begin to have changes in the body that soften body lines. Preadolescence is a period of rapid growth, especially for girls.

Neurologic System

The brain and skull grow very slowly during the school-age years. Brain growth is complete by the time the child is 10 years of age. The shape of the head is longer and the growth of the facial bones changes facial proportions.

Respiratory System

The respiratory system continues to mature with the development of the lungs and alveoli, resulting in fewer respiratory infections. Respiratory rates decrease, abdominal breathing disappears, and respirations become diaphragmatic in nature. The frontal sinuses are developed by 7 years of age. Tonsils decrease in size from the preschool years, but they remain larger than adolescents'. The adenoids and tonsils may appear large normally, even in the absence of infection.

Cardiovascular System

The school-age child's blood pressure increases. Also, the pulse rate decreases. The heart grows more slowly during the middle years and is smaller in size in relation to the rest of the body than at any other development stage.

Gastrointestinal System

During the school-age years, all 20 primary deciduous teeth are lost, replaced by 28 of 32 permanent teeth, with the exception of the third molars. The school-age child experiences fewer gastrointestinal upsets compared with earlier years. Stomach capacity increases, which permits retention of food for longer periods of time. In addition, the caloric needs of the school-age child are lower than in the earlier years.

Genitourinary System

Bladder capacity increases, but varies among individual children. Girls generally have a greater bladder capacity than boys. Urination patterns vary with the amount of fluids ingested, the time they were ingested, and the stress level of the child. The formula for bladder capacity is age in years plus 2 ounces. Therefore, the bladder capacity of the 7-year-old would be 9 ounces. The larger capacity of the bladder allows for the child to experience longer periods between voiding.

Prepubescence

The late school-age years are also referred to as *preadolescence* (the time between middle childhood and the 13th birthday). During preadolescence, **prepubescence** occurs. Prepubescence typically occurs in the 2 years before the beginning of puberty and is characterized by the development of secondary sexual characteristics, a period of rapid growth for girls, and a period of continued growth for boys. There is approximately 2 years' difference in the onset of prepubescence between boys and girls. Sexual development in both boys and girls can lead to a negative perception of physical appearance and lowered self-esteem. Early development in girls can lead to embarrassment, and delayed development in boys can lead to a negative self-concept. Early development may lead to risk-taking behaviors in both boys and girls. It is important for the nurse and parents to educate the late school-age child about body changes to decrease anxiety and promote comfort with these changes in the body.

Musculoskeletal System

Musculoskeletal growth leads to greater coordination and strength, yet the muscles are still immature and can be injured easily. Bones continue to ossify throughout childhood, but mineralization is not complete until maturity; children's bones resist pressure and muscle pull less than mature bones.

Immune System

Lymphatic tissues continue to grow until the child is 9 years old; immunoglobulins A and G (IgA and IgG) reach adult levels at around 10 years of age. Due to the lymphatic system becoming more competent in localizing infections and producing antibody–antigen responses, school-age children may have fewer infections. They may experience more infections during the first 1 to 2 years of school due to exposure to other children who may have infections.

PSYCHOSOCIAL DEVELOPMENT

Erikson (1963) describes the task of the school-age years to be a sense of **industry** vs. **inferiority**. During this time, the child is developing his sense of self-worth by becoming involved in multiple activities at home, school, and in the community, which develops his cognitive and social skills. He is very interested in learning how things are made and work. The school-age child's satisfaction from achieving success in developing new skills leads him to an increased sense of self-worth and level of competence. It is the role of the parents, teachers, coaches, and nurses of the school-age child to identify areas of competency and to build on the child's successful experiences to promote mastery, success, and self-esteem. If the expectations of the parents, teachers, and nurses are set too high, the child will develop a sense of inferiority and incompetence that can affect all aspects of his life. See Table 7.1 for a further explanation of psychosocial development in school-age children.

• COGNITIVE DEVELOPMENT

Piaget's stage of cognitive development for the 7- to 11-year-old is the period of concrete operational thoughts. In developing concrete operations, the child is able to assimilate and coordinate information about her world from different dimensions. She is able to see things from another person's point of view and think through an action, anticipating its consequences and the possibility of having to rethink the action. She is able to use stored memories of past experiences to evaluate and interpret present situations. The school-age child also develops the ability to classify or divide things into different sets and to identify their relationships to each other. The school-age child is able to classify members of four generations on a family tree vertically and horizontally, and at the same time see that one person can be a father, son, uncle, and grandson. It is at this time that the school-age child develops an interest in collecting objects. She starts out collecting multiple objects and becomes more selective as she gets older. Also, during concrete operational thoughts, the school-age child develops an understanding of the **principle of conservation**—that matter does not change when its form changes. For example, if the child pours a half-cup of water into a short, wide glass and into a tall, thin glass, she still only has a half-cup of water despite the fact that it looks like the tall, thin glass has more (Fig. 7.2). She learns about conserving matter in a sequence ranging from the simplest to the more

Table 7.1 Developmental Theories

Theorist	Stage	Activities
Erikson	Industry vs. inferiority	Interested in how things are made and run Success in personal and social tasks Increased activities outside home—clubs, sports Increased interactions with peers Increased interest in knowledge Needs support and encouragement from important people in child's life Needs support when child is not successful Inferiority occurs with repeated failures with little support or trust from those who are important to the child
Piaget	Concrete operational	Learns by manipulating concrete objects Lacks ability to think abstractly Learns that certain characteristics of objects remain constant Understands concepts of time Engages in serial ordering, addition, subtraction Classifies or groups objects by their common elements Understands relationships among objects Starts collections of items Can reverse thought process
Kohlberg	Conventional	
	Stage 3: interpersonal conforming, "good child, bad child"	An act is wrong because it brings punishment Behavior is completely wrong or right Does not understand the reason behind rules If child and adult differ in opinions, the adult is right
	Stage 4: "law and order"	Can put self in another person's position Begins to exercise the "golden rule" Acts are judged in terms of intention, not just punishment
Freud	Latency	A time of tranquility between the Oedipal phase of early childhood and adolescence—focuses on activities that develop social and cognitive skills Develops social skills in relating to same-sex friends through joining clubs like Brownies, Girl Scouts, Boy Scouts

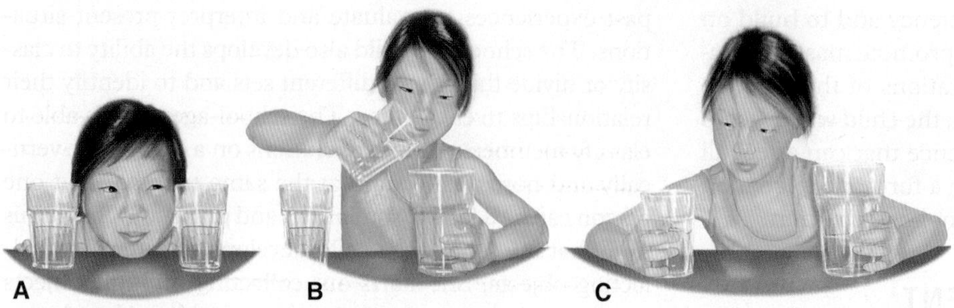

● Figure 7.2 School-age children understand the theory of conservation (**A**). If you pour an equal amount of liquid into two glasses of unequal shape (**B**), the amount of water you have remains the same despite the unequal appearance in the two glasses (**C**).

complex. See Table 7.1 for further information about cognitive development of school-age children.

● MORAL AND SPIRITUAL DEVELOPMENT

During the school-age years, the child's sense of morality is constantly being developed. According to Kohlberg, the school-age child is at the conventional stage of moral development. The 7- to 10-year-old usually follows rules out of a sense of being a "good" person. He wants to be a good person to his parents, friends, and teachers and to himself. The adult is viewed as being right. This is stage 3: interpersonal conformity (good child, bad child), according to Kohlberg. Ten- to 12-year-olds progress to stage 4: the "law and order" stage. At this stage, the child can determine if an action is good or bad based upon the reason for the action, not just on the possible consequences of the action. The older school-age child's behavior is guided by the child's desire to cooperate and by his respect for others. This leads to the school-age child's ability to understand and incorporate into his behavior the concept of the "golden rule." See Table 7.1 for additional information about the moral development of school-age children.

It is during school age that children develop an interest in religion. They are still concrete thinkers and are guided by their family's religious and cultural beliefs. They are comforted by the rituals of their religion, but are just beginning to understand the differences between natural and supernatural. Incorporating religious practices in their lives can assist school-age children in coping with different stressors.

● MOTOR SKILL DEVELOPMENT

Gross and fine motor skills continue to mature throughout the school-age years. Refinement of motor skills occurs, and speed and accuracy increase. To assess the motor skills of school-age children, ask questions about participation in sports and after-school activities, band membership, constructing models, and writing skills.

Gross Motor Skills

During the school-age years, coordination, balance, and rhythm improve, facilitating the opportunity to ride a two-wheel bike, jump rope, dance, and participate in a variety of other sports (Fig. 7.3). Older school-age children may become awkward due to their bodies growing faster than their ability to compensate.

School-age children between the ages of 6 and 8 enjoy gross motor activities such as bicycling, skating, and swimming. They are enthralled with the world and are in constant motion. Sometimes fear is limited due to the strong impulses of exploration. Children between 8 and 10 years of age are less restless, but their energy level continues to be high with activities more subdued and directed. These children exhibit greater rhythm and gracefulness of muscular movements, allowing them to participate in physical activities that require longer and more concentrated attention and effort, such as baseball or soccer.

Between the ages of 10 and 12 years of age (the pubescent years for girls), energy levels remain high but are more controlled and focused. Physical skills in this age group are

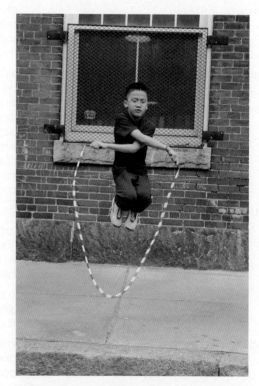

● Figure 7.3 Jumping rope is an example of the increased development of gross motor skills of the school-age child.

similar to adults', with strength and endurance increasing during adolescence.

All school-age children should be encouraged to engage in physical activities and learn physical skills that contribute to their health for the rest of their lives. Cardiovascular fitness, weight control, emotional tension release, and development of leadership and following skills are enhanced though physical activity and team sports.

Fine Motor Skills

Myelinization of the central nervous system is reflected by refinement of fine motor skills. Eye–hand coordination and balance improve with maturity and practice. Hand usage improves, becoming steadier and independent and granting an ease and precision that allows these children to write, print words, sew, or build models or other crafts. The child between 10 and 12 years of age begins to exhibit manipulative skills comparable to adults. School-age children take pride in activities that require dexterity and fine motor skills such as playing musical instruments (Fig. 7.4). Talent and practice become the keys to proficiency.

SENSORY DEVELOPMENT

All senses are mature early in the school-age years. The typical school-age child has 20/20 visual acuity. In addition, ocular muscular control, peripheral vision, and color discrimination are fully developed by the time the child is 7 years of age. Good vision is essential to the physical development and educational progression of school-age children. Vision screening programs conducted by school nurses identify problems with vision and result in appropriate referrals when warranted. Some problems frequently identified include amblyopia, uncorrected refractive errors or other eye defects, and malalignment of the eyes (called *strabismus*). If untreated by age 9 years of age, amblyopia can cause irreversible visual loss. This condition is correctable prior to this time with glasses or patching. Proper screening and referral, as well as notification to parents of the existing condition, are essential to the education and socialization of the school-age child (www.aao.org).

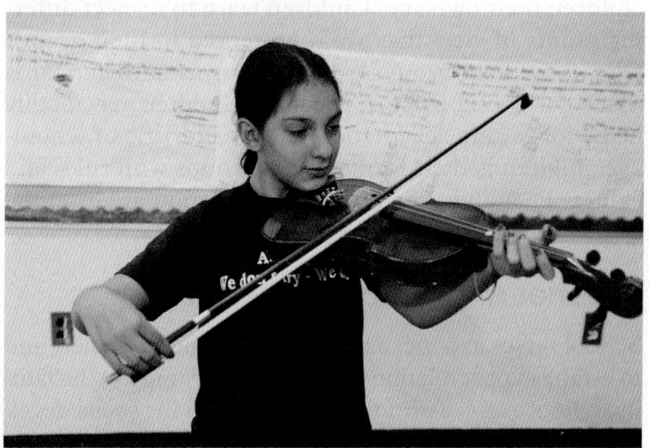

Figure 7.4 School-age children improve their fine motor skills so they can play musical instruments well.

Hearing deficits that are severe are usually diagnosed in infancy, but the less severe may not be diagnosed until the child enters school and has difficulty learning or with speech. It is important to screen children for hearing deficits to ensure proper educational and social progression. With loud music heard over long periods of time each day, there are concerns about these environmental noises affecting hearing in the school-age and adolescent populations.

The sense of smell is mature and can be tested in the school-age child by using scents that children are familiar with, such as chocolate or other familiar odors. In addition, the school-age child may be tested for the sense of touch with objects to discriminate cold from hot, soft from hard, and blunt from sharp.

COMMUNICATION AND LANGUAGE DEVELOPMENT

Language skills continue to accelerate during the school-age years. Vocabulary expands to 8,000 to 14,000 words. Culturally specific words are used, with bilingual children speaking English in school and a second language at home. The school-age child learns to read and reading efficiency improves language skills. Reading skills are improved with increased reading exposure. School-age children begin to use more complex grammatical forms such as plurals and pronouns. Also, they develop metalinguistic awareness—an ability to think about language and comment on its properties. This enables them to enjoy jokes and riddles due to their understanding of double meanings, and play on words and sounds. They are also beginning to understand metaphors such as "a stitch in time saves nine." School-age children may experiment with profanity and dirty jokes if exposed. This age group tends to imitate parents, family members, or others. Therefore, role modeling is very important.

EMOTIONAL AND SOCIAL DEVELOPMENT

Patterns of temperamental traits identified in infancy may continue to influence behavior in the school-age child. Analyzing past situations may provide clues to the way a child may react to new or different situations. Children may react differently over time due to their experiences and abilities. Self-esteem is the child's view of their individual worth. This view is impacted by feedback from family, teachers, and other authority figures.

Temperament

Temperament has been described as the way individuals behave. Some descriptions of temperament are that the child is *easy, slow to warm,* or *difficult.* These behaviors vary from the child who is easy (even-tempered and predictable) to the child labeled as difficult (due to high activity levels, irritability, and moodiness). The child who is easy may adapt to school entry and other experiences smoothly and with little or no stress. The slow-to-warm child may be slow to adapt to changes. The slow-to-warm school-age child may exhibit discomfort when placed in different or new situations such as school. This child may need time to adjust to the new place or situation, and may demonstrate frustration with tears or somatic complaints. The slow-to-warm child should be allowed time to adjust to new situations and people (such as teachers) within his or her own time frame. All of these factors may impact the younger school-age child upon entering the school environment, with changes in authority and the introduction of many peers. The difficult or easily distracted child may benefit from an introduction to the new experience and people by role-playing, by visiting the site and being introduced to the teachers, and by hearing stories or participating in conversations about the upcoming school experience. These children require patience, firmness, and understanding to make the transition into a new situation or experience such as school. The Behavioral Style Questionnaire (BSQ) (McDevitt & Carey, 1978) is a temperament questionnaire for children 3 to 7 years old; the Middle Childhood Temperament Questionnaire is another tool for children 8 to 12 years of age (Hegvik, McDevitt, & Carey, 1982). These tools may be useful for determining type of temperament and guiding interventions.

Self-Esteem Development

Self-esteem mirrors the child's individual self-worth and consists of both positive and negative qualities. Children strive to achieve internalized goals of attainment, although they continually receive feedback from individuals they perceive as authorities (parent or teacher). By the school-age years, children have received feedback related to their performance or tasks. The direction of this feedback influences the child's opinion of self-worth, which influences self-esteem and self-evaluation.

Children face the process of self-evaluation from a framework of either self-confidence or self-doubt. Children who have mastered the earlier developmental task of autonomy and initiative face the world with feelings of pride rather than shame.

If school-age children regard themselves as worthwhile, they have a positive self-concept and high self-esteem. Significant adults in school-age children's lives can manipulate the environment to facilitate success. This success impacts the self-esteem of the child.

Body Image

Body image is how the school-ager perceives his or her body. School-age children are knowledgeable about the human body but may have different perceptions about body parts. School-age children are very interested in peers' views and acceptances of their body, body changes, and clothing. This age group may model themselves after parents, peers, and persons in movies or on television. It is important for late school-agers to feel accepted by peers. If they feel different and are teased, there may be lifelong effects.

School-Age Fears

School-age children are less fearful of harm to their body than in their preschool years, but fear being kidnapped or undergoing surgery. They continue to fear the dark and worry about their past behaviors. They fear death and are fascinated by death and dying. They are less fearful of dogs and noises. The school-age child needs reassurance that his or her fears are normal for this developmental age. Parents, teachers, and other caretakers should discuss the fears and answer questions posed by the child (Hockenberry, Wilson, Winkelstein, & Kline, 2003).

Peer Relationships

The child's concept of self is shaped by relationships with others. Peer relationships influence children's independence from parents. Peers play an important role in the approval and critiquing of skills of school-age children. Previously, only adults such as parents and teachers have been authorities; now, peers influence school-age children's perceptions of themselves. The support of peers helps to support the school-age child by providing enough security to risk the parental conflict brought about when establishing independence. School-age children associate with peers of the same sex most of the time. Although games and other activities are shared by both boys and girls, the child's concept of the appropriate sex role is influenced by his or her relationship with peers.

Continuous peer relationships provide the most important social interaction for school-age children. Valuable lessons are learned from interactions with children their own age. Children learn to respect differing points of view that are represented in their groups (Fig. 7.5). Peer groups establish norms and standards that signify acceptance or rejection. Children may modify behavior to gain acceptance. A characteristic of school-age children is their formation of groups with rules and values. Peer and peer-group identification are essential to the socialization of the school-age child.

Teacher and School Influences

School serves as a means to transmit values of society and to establish peer relationships. Secondary only to the family, school exerts a profound influence on the social development of the child. Often school requires changes for the child and parent. The child enters an environment that requires conforming to group activities that are structured

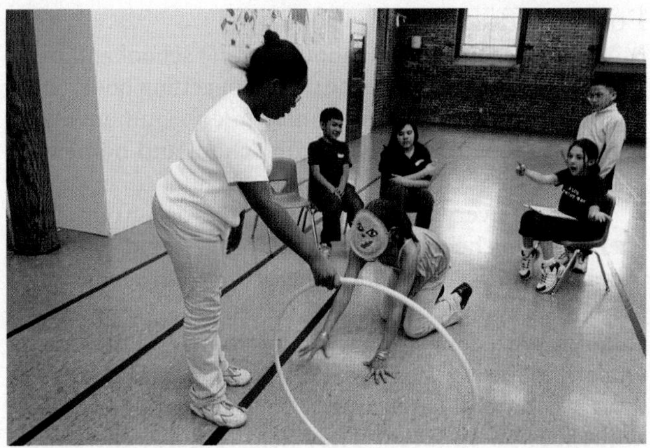

● Figure 7.5 School-age children like to join clubs. These children, in the acting club at school, are rehearsing for a play.

and directed by an adult other than the parent. The parent's attitude and support influences the child's transition into the school setting. Parents that are positive and supportive promote a smooth entry into school. Parents that encourage clinging behaviors may delay a successful transition into school.

To facilitate the transition from home to school, the teacher must have the personality and knowledge of development that will allow him or her to meet the needs of young children. Even though the teacher's responsibilities are primarily to stimulate and guide intellectual development, they must share in shaping the child's attitudes and values. The system of awards and punishment administered by teachers affects the self-concept of children and influences their response to school. Teachers and school are important in shaping the socialization, self-concept, and intellectual development of children.

Family Influences

The school-age years are a time for peer relationships, questioning of parents, and the potential for parental conflict but continued respect for family values. School-age years are the beginning of the time of peer-group influence, with testing of parental and family values. Although the peer group is influential, the family's values usually predominate when parental and peer-group values come into conflict. Even though the school-age child may question the parents' values, the child will usually incorporate the values from parents into his or her values.

Many times in the late school-age and preadolescent period, the child may prefer to be in the company of peers and show a decreased interest in family functions. This may require an adjustment for parents. Parents' awareness of this developmental trend and their continuing support for the child is important while they continue to enforce restrictions and control of behaviors. The school-ager is beginning to strive for independence, but values and parental authority and controls continue to impact choices and values. School-age children continue to need parenting. They do not need parents as pals.

● CULTURAL INFLUENCES ON GROWTH AND DEVELOPMENT

Culture influences habits, beliefs, language, and value. School-age children thrive on learning the music, language, traditions, holidays, games, values, gender roles, and other aspects of culture. Nurses must be aware of the effects on children of various groups' family structures and traditional values. The school-age child's cultural and ethic backgrounds must be considered when assessing growth and development, including differences in growth in children of different racial and cultural backgrounds. Cultural implications must be considered for all children and families in order to provide appropriate care.

> Refer back to Lawrence Jones, who was introduced at the beginning of this chapter. What developmental milestones would you expect him to have reached by this age?

The Nurse's Role in School-Age Growth and Development

WATCH & LEARN

The nurse's role in school-age growth and development includes assessing growth and development, promoting healthy growth and development, and addressing common developmental concerns. The nursing process overview would include an assessment of the individual child and identification of nursing diagnoses needing intervention or referral. The nurse promotes healthy growth and development through anticipatory guidance and goal attainment. Nursing care plans for individual children with common developmental concerns should be individualized considering the needs of the child and the family.

● NURSING PROCESS OVERVIEW

Upon completion of assessment of the school-age child's current growth and development status, problems or issues related to growth and development may be identified. The nurse may then identify one or more nursing diagnoses, including:

- Risk for disproportionate growth
- Imbalanced nutrition: more than body requirements
- Delayed growth and development
- Risk for caregiver role strain
- Risk for injury

Nursing care planning for the school-age child with growth and development issues should be individualized based on the school-age child's and family's needs.

The nursing care plan can be used as a guide in planning nursing care for the school-age child with a growth and development concern. The nurse may choose the appropriate nursing diagnoses from Nursing Care Plan 7.1 and individualize them as needed. The nursing care plan is intended to serve as a guide, not to be an all-inclusive growth and development care plan.

PROMOTING HEALTHY GROWTH AND DEVELOPMENT

The family plays a critical role in promoting healthy growth and development of the school-age child. Respectful interchange of communication between the parent and child will foster self-esteem and self-confidence. This respect will give the child confidence in achieving personal, educational, and social goals appropriate for his or her age. The nurse should observe interactions between parents and school-age children to observe for this respect or lack of respect ("putting the child down"). The nurse can model appropriate behaviors by listening to the child and making appropriate responses. The nurse can be a resource for parents and an advocate for the child in promoting healthy growth and development.

Promoting Growth and Development Through Play

Cooperative play is exhibited by the school-age child. Play for the school-age child includes both organized cooperative activities (such as team sports) and solitary activities. School-age children have the coordination and intellect to participate with other children their age in sports such as soccer, baseball, football, and tennis. The school-age child comprehends that his or her cooperation with others will lead to a unified whole for the team. Additionally, the child learns rules and the value of playing by the rules.

School-age children also enjoy solitary activities including board, card, video, and computer games, and dollhouse and other small-figure play (Fig. 7.6). Many schoolagers start collections of stamps, cars, or other valuable or not-so-valuable items. During the school-age years, children may also begin a scrapbook or keep a diary. They may participate in activities such as dance or karate. Girls and boys may join clubs, gangs, or special interest groups.

Active play has decreased in recent years as television viewing and computer games have increased. This trend has resulted in health risks such as obesity, type 2 diabetes, and cardiovascular problems.

Promoting Learning

School attendance and learning are very important to the school-age child. Parent–child, child–teacher, and child–peer relationships and activities influence the school-age child's learning.

Formal Education

Most children are excited about starting school and making new friends. They like the notion of getting books, having book bags, and having homework assignments. The reality of the work involved with school and homework may decrease the enthusiasm about school.

Peers are very important within this age group. Both peers and teachers influence children. Attending school may be their first experience interacting with a large number of children their own age. Through this interaction, children learn cooperation, competition, and the importance of following the rules. Peer approval and influences grow as the child matures. Teachers have significant influences on children. They help to guide the child's intellectual development by rewarding successes and helping the child deal with failures. The student–teacher relationship is a key to success. Teachers play a role in fostering feelings of industry and preventing feelings of inferiority (Fig. 7.7). School-age children also learn skills, rules, values, and other ways to work with peers and other authority figures.

Parental support is important for school adjustment and achievement. Parents must collaborate with teachers and school personnel to ensure that the child is fulfilling the expectations and requirements for this age group in school. Parents must monitor the child's homework assignments and friends, and observe for any changes in behavior that would indicate school or behavioral problems.

Reading

Encouraging reading is an excellent way to promote learning in the school-age child. Trips to the library and purchasing books help to promote a love of reading. School-age children enjoy being read to as well as reading on their own. Younger school-age children (6 to 8 years) enjoy books that are simple to read with few words on a page, such as the Dr. Seuss books. They enjoy books about animals and trains and simple mysteries. Children 8 to 10 years of age have more advanced reading skills and enjoy those books from early childhood, plus more classic novels and adventures such as the Harry Potter series. Older children enjoy horror stories, mysteries, romances, and adventure stories as well as classic novels. School-age children of all ages benefit from books on topics related to things they may be experiencing, such as a visit to the hospital for a surgical procedure. See Box 7.1 for ideas for parents to promote reading in the school-age child.

Promoting Safety

School-age children become more independent with age. This independence leads to an increased self-confidence and decreased fears, which may contribute to accidents and injuries. School age is a time that the child may walk to school with peers who may influence his or her behavior.

(text continues on page 171)

Nursing Care Plan 7.1

Growth and Development Issues of the School-Age Child

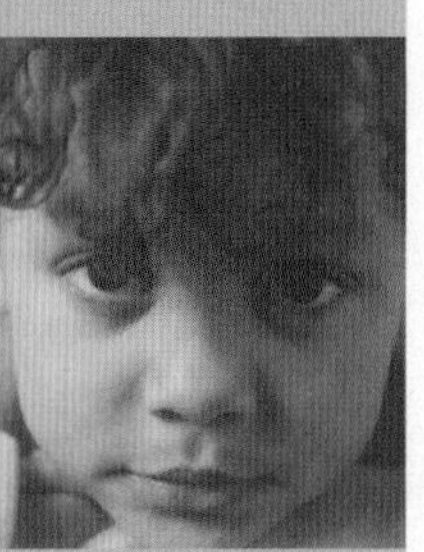

Nursing Diagnosis: Risk for disproportionate growth (risk factors: caregiver knowledge deficit, frequent illnesses)

Outcome identification and evaluation

School-age child will demonstrate adequate growth: *appropriate weight gain for age and sex*

Interventions: promoting proportionate growth

- Assess parent's knowledge of nutritional needs of school-age children *to determine need for further education.*
- Educate mother about appropriate serving sizes and foods *so that mother is aware of what to expect for school-age children.*
- Determine need for additional caloric intake if necessary *(if very active in sports, if have a chronic illness).*
- Plot out height, weight, and body mass index (BMI) *to detect possible pattern.*

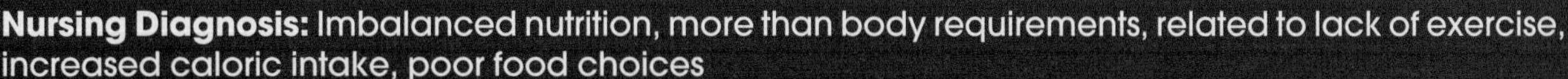

Nursing Diagnosis: Imbalanced nutrition, more than body requirements, related to lack of exercise, increased caloric intake, poor food choices

Outcome identification and evaluation

School-age child will lose weight at an appropriate rate: *increase amount of exercise, make appropriate eating choices, decrease caloric intake to appropriate amount for age and sex*

Interventions: promoting nutrition

- Assess knowledge of parents and child about nutritional needs of school-age children *to determine deficits in knowledge.*
- Have child keep food and exercise diary for 1 week *to determine current patterns of eating and exercise.*
- Interview parents in relationship to their eating habits and exercise habits *to determine where adjustments might need to be made.*
- Analyze preceding data, and base recommendations for changes on these data.
- Discuss ways to decrease temptation to overeat and to make good meal choices (see Teaching Guideline 7.2).
- Have child assist in meal planning and grocery shopping *to allow him some sense of control in process.*
- Incorporate increase in daily exercise, which will stress sense of self-improvement *to increase caloric expenditure and self-esteem.*
- Decrease TV/computer time *to increase caloric expenditure.*
- Develop reward system *to increase self-esteem.*
- Investigate joining weight-loss program for school-age children *to increase self-esteem and to increase awareness that other children have the same problem.*

Nursing Diagnosis: Growth and development, delayed related to speech, motor, psychosocial, or cognitive concerns as evidenced by delay in meeting expected school performances

Outcome identification and evaluation

Development will be maximized: School-age child will make continued progress toward attainment of expected school performances.

Interventions: promoting growth and development

- Perform scheduled evaluation of the school-age child by school and health care provider *to determine current functioning.*
- Develop realistic multidisciplinary plan *to ensure maximizing resources.*
- Carry out interventions as prescribed by developmental specialist, physical therapist, occupational therapist, or speech therapist at home and at school *to maximize benefit of interventions.*
- Have scheduled evaluation meetings *to be able to adapt interventions as soon as possible.*

(continued)

Growth and Development Issues of the School-Age Child (continued)

Nursing Diagnosis: Caregiver role strain, risk for (risk factors: new sibling in household, knowledge deficit about school-age issues, lack of prior exposure, fatigue, ill or developmentally delayed child)

Outcome identification and evaluation

Parent will experience competence in role: will demonstrate appropriate caretaking behaviors and verbalize comfort in caring for a school-age child

Interventions: preventing caregiver role strain

- Assess parent's knowledge of school-age children and the issues that arise as a part of normal development *to determine parent's needs.*
- Provide education on normal issues of school-age children *so that parents are armed with the knowledge they need to appropriately care for their school-age child.*
- Provide anticipatory guidance related to upcoming expected issues related to school-age development *to prepare parents for what to expect next and how to intervene.*

Nursing Diagnosis: Injury, risk for (risk factors: curiosity, increasing cognitive skills and motor abilities)

Outcome identification and evaluation

School-age child's safety will be maintained: *will remain free from injury*

Interventions: preventing injury

- Discuss safety measures needed for the following: bikes, scooters, guns, skateboards, cars, water, and playground *to decrease risk of injury related to those areas.*
- Discuss and develop a fire safety plan *to decrease risk of injury related to fire.*
- Discuss appropriate safety equipment needed for each sport *to decrease risk of injury.*
- Discuss appropriate sports to participate in depending upon age, sex, and maturity of child *to prevent possible injury and to promote child's self-esteem.*
- Parents should have the poison control center phone number available (*in the event of accidental ingestion, poison control can give parents the best advice for appropriate intervention).*
- Teach parents and child first-aid measures and child cardiopulmonary resuscitation (CPR) *to minimize consequences of injury should it occur.*
- Discuss influence of peers on actions of school-age children *to prevent possible injury due to mimicking behavior.*

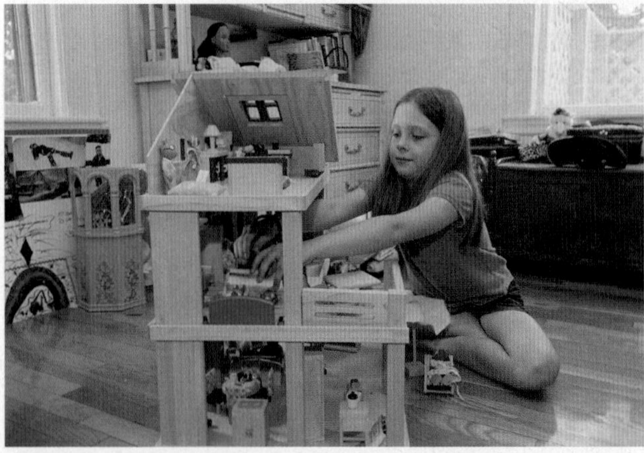

● Figure 7.6 This school-age girl enjoys solitary play with her dollhouse and dolls.

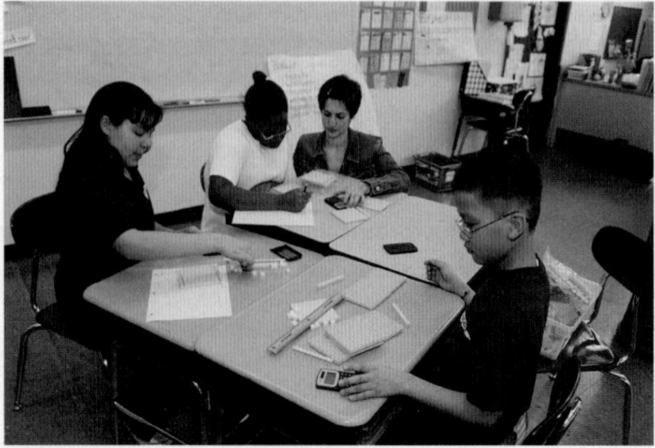

● Figure 7.7 School is important to the school-age child.

BOX 7.1

PROMOTION OF READING IN SCHOOL-AGE CHILDREN

- Parents, read to and with your children.
- Ask teachers and librarians for advice on books appropriate for your child.
- Choose stories that the child can relate to if the child has difficulty reading.
- Choose books with movement if the child has a short attention span.
- Take advantage of all reading opportunities (cereal boxes, road signs).
- Provide choices for the child to select a book of interest.
- Talk about the text and ask questions to improve understanding.
- Keep a record of what the child is reading.
- Visit a library, get a library card, and check out books.
- Parent, demonstrate role modeling through reading books.

Increased independence may also increase exposure to dangerous situations such as the approach of strangers or unsafe streets. Promotion of safe habits during the school-age years is important for parents and nurses. See Teaching Guideline 7.1 for additional information on safety education for nurses and parents.

Unintentional injuries are the leading cause of death in children between 1 and 21 years of age (www.cdc.gov/ncipc). The death rate in children between 5 and 10 years of age is less than for younger children, although the incidence of unintentional injury is higher (Behrman, 1999). Each year, 20% to 25% of all children sustain an injury sufficiently severe to seek medical attention or to miss school (www.cdc.gov). School-age children are very active at home, in the community, and at school. This increased mobility, activity, and time away from parents increases the risk for unintentional injuries. School-age children continue to need supervision and guidance. They need information and rules about car safety, pedestrian safety, bicycle and other sport safety, fire safety, and water safety.

Car Safety

Motor vehicle accidents are a common cause of injury in the school-age child. While traveling in the car, school-age children should always sit in the rear seat. The front seat is dangerous because of passenger-side airbags in most new-model cars. The school-age child should use a three-point restraint system in the rear seat of the car with the shoulder strap and lap belt fitted snugly. In addition, a school-age child over 40 pounds (generally 4 to 8 years of age) should use a belt-positioning, forward-facing booster seat using both lap and shoulder belts. School-age children who outgrow the convertible restraint can sit in a booster seat until their head is higher than the vehicle seat back (usually 4′9″ and taller). Children under 12 years of age should not ride in the front seat of a vehicle with an airbag.

Pedestrian Safety

Children between the ages of 5 and 9 have the highest incidence of pedestrian-related injuries. Young school-age children between 6 and 8 years of age should walk to school or the bus with an older friend, sibling, or parent. Darting out into the street without looking both ways or from between cars is a common occurrence in the school-age years. Teach children safe street and pedestrian practices.

Bicycle and Sport Safety

Bicycling, riding scooters, skateboarding, and inline skating or rollerskating are common activities of school-age children. Laws in most states require helmets for riding bicycles and scooters. In addition, when skating or skateboarding, school-age children should wear a helmet, kneepads, and elbow pads.

Research has shown that head injuries due to bicycle accidents have been reduced by 85% when wearing a well-fitting helmet. National estimates of bicycle helmet ownership in school-age children are 50%, and only approximately 50% of those wear helmets each time they ride their bicycles (see Healthy People 2010). It is important for children to wear helmets that fit and that do not obstruct their vision or hearing. Because school-age children have completed most of their skull growth, a helmet can be worn into adolescence. It is important for the child to have a bicycle that is appropriate for his or her size and age. The child should be able to plant both feet on the ground when sitting on the seat of the bike (Fig. 7.8). It is important to stress to parents the importance of appropriate size and not to get a bike for the child to "grow into." If older school-agers are using the bike for transportation on busy streets, they should be taught to use bike lanes and to give appropriate hand signals for turning. Since the introduction of the scooter in the 1990s, 85% of emergency room visits are attributed to scooter-related injuries (Centers for Disease Control and Prevention, 2000).

Fire Safety

School-age children are eager to help parents with cooking and ironing. They are curious about fire and are drawn to play with fire, matches, and fireworks. Serious burns can occur from any exposure to fire. Educate children about the hazards of fire. In addition, teach children proper behavior around fires at home and outdoors. Always supervise children in the use of matches. In the home setting, parents should develop a fire safety plan with their children, teach children what to do if their clothes catch on fire, and practice evacuating the house in the event of a fire. In the school setting, children should be aware of the appropriate response to fire drills and fire drills should be conducted on a regular basis.

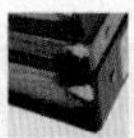

TEACHING GUIDELINE 7.1

Safety Issues and Interventions of the School-Age Child

Safety Issue	Interventions
Car safety	• Should wear seat belt or be in age- and weight-appropriate booster seat at all times. • Fasten seat belt before car is started. • Children under 12 years must sit in back seat. • Utilize childproof locks in back seat. • Establish rules of conduct in car.
Pedestrian safety	• Child should look right, left, then right again before crossing the street. • Cross only at safe crossings. • Older children and adults should provide supervision of younger children. • Should only walk on sidewalks. • Should not dart out between parked cars. • In parking lots, should watch for cars backing up. • If children are playing outside, drivers should be aware of their presence before backing up.
Bike safety: general	• Have a well-maintained and appropriate-size bike for child. • Parents should orient the child to the bike. • Child should demonstrate his or her ability to ride bike safely before being allowed to ride on street. • Safe areas for bike riding should be established as well as routes to and from area of activities. • Should not ride bike barefoot, with someone else on bike, or with clothing that might get entangled in the bike. • Should wear sturdy, well-fitting shoes. • Should wear ANSI-approved helmets. • Bike should be inspected often to ensure it is in proper working order. • A basket should be used to carry heavy objects.
Bike safety in traffic	• All traffic signs and signals must be observed. • If riding at night, the bike should have lights and reflectors and the rider should wear light-colored clothes. • Should ride on the side of the road traveling with traffic. • Should keep close to the side of the road and in single file. • Should watch and listen for cars. • Should not wear headphones while riding a bike. • Never hitch a ride on any vehicles.
Sports safety	• Match sport to child's ability and desire. • Sports program should have warm-up procedure. • Coaches should be trained in cardiopulmonary resuscitation (CPR) and first aid. • Child should wear appropriate protection devices for individual sport.
Skateboarding and inline skating safety	• Should wear helmet, and protective padding on knees, elbows, and wrists • Should not skate in traffic or on streets or highways. • Skating on homemade ramps could be dangerous—should assess ramps for any hazards before skating.
All-terrain vehicle safety	• Should not be operated by children less than 16 years of age. • Should wear helmet and protective coverings. • No nighttime riding. • Should not be used on public roads. • Should not stand up in the vehicle or ride in a person's lap.
Fire safety	• All homes should have working smoke detectors and fire extinguishers. Change the batteries at least twice a year. • Should have fire-escape plan.

(continued)

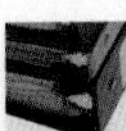

TEACHING GUIDELINE 7.1 (Continued)

Safety Issues and Interventions of the School-Age Child

Safety Issue	Interventions
	• Should practice fire-escape plan routinely. • Nobody should smoke in bed. • Should teach what to do in case of a fire: use fire extinguisher, call 911, and how to put out clothing fire. • Should wear flame-retardant clothing. • Should use stove and other cooking facilities under adult supervision. • All flammable materials and liquids should be stored safely. • Fireplaces should have protective gratings. • Teach children to avoid touching wires they might encounter while playing.
Water safety	• Teach children how to swim. • If swimming skill is limited, must wear life preserver at all times. • Never swim alone—should if at all possible, swim only where there is a life guard. • Should be taught basic CPR. • Should not run or fool around at edge of pool. • Drains in pool should be covered with appropriate cover. • Should wear life jacket when on boat. • Make sure there is enough water to support diving.
Firearm safety	• Should teach never to touch gun—tell adult. • If have guns in household, need to secure them in safe place, use gun safety locks, store bullets in separate place. • Never point a gun at a person.
Toxin safety	• Teach child the hazards of accepting illegal drugs, alcohol, or dangerous drugs. • Store potential dangerous material in safe place.

Water Safety

Teach school-age children swim and water safety. An adult should always supervise children when they are swimming to prevent water-related accidents.

Abuse in Children

Child abuse, including physical abuse and sexual abuse, are common crimes of violence against children. Approximately 10% to 20% of children 3 to 17 years of age are physically abused each year (Murray, Baker, & Lewin, 2000). In 2002, more than 88,000 children were victims

HEALTHY PEOPLE 2010

Objective	Significance
Increase use of helmets by bicyclists.	• Provide education to children and their parents about avoiding head injury through helmet use. • Encourage child to choose a helmet that appeals to him or her (one that looks "cool").

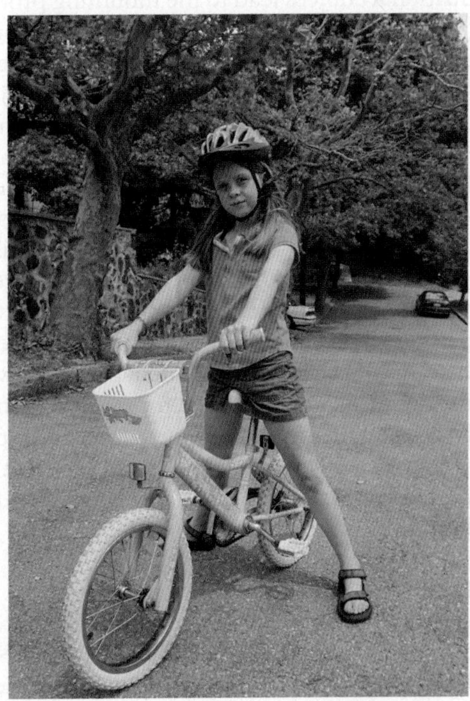

● Figure 7.8 Wearing the appropriate safety equipment and having an appropriately sized bicycle are important to prevent injuries in school-age children.

of sexual abuse (Kellogg & Committee on Child Abuse and Neglect, 2005). The abusers of children are family, friends, and strangers. It is important for parents to teach children the concept of "good touch" vs. "bad touch" prior to school-age years. Whenever the school-age child's behavior yields suspicion of physical or sexual abuse, the nurse should report to the appropriate authorities in his or her state. These topics will be discussed in more depth in Chapter 31.

> **Remember Lawrence Jones,** the 10-year-old presented in the case study? What anticipatory guidance related to safety should you provide to his mother?

Promoting Nutrition

Growth, body composition, and body shape remain constant during late school-age years. Needed calories decrease while the appetite increases. In preparation for adolescence, the body fat composition of school-age children increases. This tendency toward increased body fat occurs earlier in girls than in boys, with the amount of increase greater in girls. Boys have more lean body mass per inch of height than girls.

Diet preferences established in the preschool years continue during the school-age period. As the child grows older, influences of family, media, and peers can impact the eating habits of this age group. Some of these influences are parents' work schedule, outside activities, and exercise level of the child. Decreased exercise levels and poor nutritional choices lead to the mounting problem of obesity seen in this age group. See Box 7.2 for appropriate questions to ask the child and parent regarding nutritional status. Healthy People 2010 provides objectives and actions to improve the nutritional health of children.

Nutritional Needs

School-age children with an average body weight of 20 to 35 kilograms need approximately 70 calories per kilogram daily (1,400 to 2,100 calories per day). The average water requirement per 24 hours ranges from 1,800 to 2,200 milliliters per day. The child needs 28 grams of protein and 800 milligrams of calcium for maintenance of growth and good nutrition. Calcium is needed for the development of strong bones and teeth. Milk, yogurt, and cheese provide protein, vitamins, and minerals and are an excellent source of calcium. Meats, poultry, fish, and eggs provide protein, vitamins, and minerals.

Nutritional Guidelines

School-age children should choose culturally appropriate foods and snacks from the Food Guide Pyramid. School-age children need to limit intake of fat and processed sugars. A prudent diet limits the use of fatty meats, high-fat dairy products, eggs, and hydrogenated shortenings and promotes the consumption of fish and the substitution of polyunsaturated vegetable oils and margarines. The

BOX 7.2

DIETARY QUESTIONS

Dietary Questions

Questions for the Child

- How often do you eat together as a family?
- What are the usual mealtimes?
- How often does the family eat out?
- Do you eat breakfast regularly?
- Where do you eat lunch?
- What do you drink/how much?
- What foods do you eat most often?
- What is your favorite food?
- How often do you eat fast foods?
- What type of exercise do you do?

Questions for the Parents

- How would you describe your child's usual appetite?
- Do you have any special cultural/religious practices regarding food?
- Has your child gained or lost weight recently?
- Do you have any concerns about his or her eating behaviors?
- How does your child exercise? Your family?
- Is there a family history of cancer, hypertension, diabetes, obesity, or heart disease?

HEALTHY PEOPLE 2010

Objective	Significance
Increase the proportion of persons age 2 years and older who consume at least two daily servings of fruit; three daily servings of vegetables, with at least one-third being dark-green or deep-yellow vegetables; and six daily servings of grain products, with at least three being whole grain.	• Educate families about the importance of whole grains, fruits, and vegetables in the diet. • Encourage the child to choose fruits and vegetables that appeal to him or her. • Provide creative suggestions for vegetable preparation to make them more appealing to children.
Increase the proportion of persons age 2 years and older who consume less than 10% of calories from saturated fat, and who consume no more than 30% of calories from fat.	• Educate families about saturated fat-containing foods. • Offer suggestions for alternate sources of protein and fats (chicken or fish, olive oil).

American Heart Association has endorsed a diet for school-age children that includes the recommendations listed in Box 7.3.

> **Regarding Lawrence Jones,** what questions should you ask Lawrence's mother related to nutritional intake? What anticipatory guidance related to nutrition would be appropriate?

Promoting Healthy Sleep and Rest

The number of hours of sleep required for growth and development decreases with age. Children between the ages of 6 and 8 years require about 12 hours of sleep per night. Children between 8 and 10 years of age require 10 to 12 hours of sleep per night, and children between 10 and 12 years of age need 9 to 10 hours of sleep per night. Young school-age children may need an occasional brief nap for an energy boost after being in school for most of the day. Bedtime rituals and consistent schedules continue to be important throughout the school-age years. Parents must facilitate the bedtime schedule and quiet time before bed. Bedtime is a special time for parents and children to read together, listen to stories or soothing music, share events of the day, and exchange expressions of affection. Children should have bedtime expectations as well as wake-up times and methods for waking up (alarm, calling by parent, and so forth).

Night terrors or sleepwalking may occur in 6- to 8-year-olds but should be resolved between the ages of 8 and 10 years. In the older school-age child (11 to 12 years), encourage parents to allow a variation in the sleep schedule on the weekends and a regular schedule on weekdays.

> **Provide anticipatory guidance** to Lawrence Jones's mother in relation to proper sleep for her 10-year-old son.

BOX 7.3

AMERICAN HEART ASSOCIATION'S DIET RECOMMENDATIONS FOR SCHOOL-AGE CHILDREN

- A high-quality protein with every meal
- Milk with added vitamin D and other low-fat dairy products
- Vegetables high in vitamin A
- Fruits high in vitamin C
- Whole-grain or enriched breads or cereals
- Vegetable oils high in polyunsaturated fats
- Meats (4 servings per week of 4 ounces each)
- Fish (1–2 times per week)
- Poultry (1–2 times per week)
- Dark green, leafy, or deep yellow vegetables (at least 4 times per week)
- Eggs (4 times per week)

Promoting Healthy Teeth and Gums

Dental **caries** remains the leading disease in the United States, even though the incidence has been reduced since the introduction of fluoride (www.dentalcare.com). Dental care with emphasis on prevention of caries is important in this age group. Sometimes dental care is not considered to be important by parents of young children because the primary teeth will be replaced by permanent teeth. This perception leads to complications of permanent teeth such as **malocclusion** (see Healthy People 2010).

Proper alignment of teeth is important to tooth formation, speech development, and physical appearance. Many school-age children need braces or other orthodontic devices to correct malocclusion, a condition in which the teeth are crowded, crooked, or misaligned. **Bruxism** or teeth grinding while asleep may continue in the school-age years. Bruxism may result in grinding away of tooth enamel. Teeth grinding may be due to malalignment. A dental evaluation should be scheduled if consistent teeth grinding occurs.

School-age children need to brush their teeth two to three times per day for 3 minutes each time (Fig. 7.9). Parents should replace the toothbrush (soft) every 3 to 4 months. Flossing the teeth at least once daily is recommended by the American Dental Association. Parents must monitor teeth brushing, observe for abnormal alignment of their child's teeth, and schedule regular dental examinations every 6 months to ensure good dental health and prevent dental problems. Children may need help with brushing teeth until they are between 7 and 10 years of age. Dental sealants are recommended for all school-age children. The sealant is a plastic coating applied to biting surfaces to seal out tooth decay on permanent back teeth. In addition, parents should give a fluoride supplement (as directed by the dentist) to their children if fluoride is not in the town's water supply.

HEALTHY PEOPLE 2010

Objective	Significance
Reduce the proportion of children and adolescents who have dental caries in their primary or permanent teeth.	• Encourage appropriate toothbrushing and flossing. • Educate child and family about fluoride use.
Increase the proportion of children who have received dental sealants to their molar teeth.	• Refer school-age children to dentist for molar sealants. • Assist families lacking dental insurance to find resources for the provision of dental care.

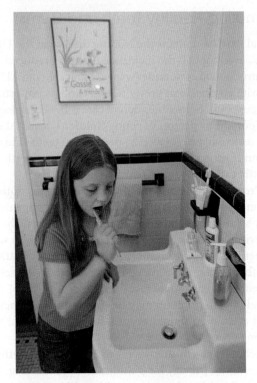

● Figure 7.9 Using correct technique to brush the teeth is important in the prevention of cavities.

Children wearing braces are more prone to cavities; encourage them to brush their teeth after meals and snacks. School nurses can assist these children with brushing after lunch. In addition, the school nurse should promote dental health through education on dental care and gum problems that result from lack of proper dental care. Diet can play a part in dental health. Limiting sticky, high-sugar, and high-carbohydrate foods will decrease the possibility of cavities.

Promoting Appropriate Discipline

Because of the increasing ability of the school-age child to view situations from different angles, the school-age child should be able to see how his actions affect others. Children between 6 and 8 years old are beginning to see the effects of behaviors on others. They are also beginning to realize that their behaviors can have consequences. Children between 8 and 12 years of age are fully aware of the cause and effect of their behaviors. They should be able to express emotions without using violence. Discipline techniques with consequences have both *natural* and *logical* consequences. Natural consequences allow the child to learn the results of their actions. For example, if the child throws a toy out of the window, then he cannot play with the toy anymore. In logical consequences, if the child does not put away her bike, she does not get to ride the bike for the rest of the day.

In disciplining children, parents should teach children the rules established by the family, values, and social rules of conduct. Rules should provide the school-age child with guidelines about behavior that is acceptable and unacceptable. School-age children look to their parents for guidance and as role models. Parents should role model appropriate expressions of feelings and emotions and allow the child to express emotions and feelings. Discuss the effects of the child's temperament on his or her behavior, as well as what constitutes age-appropriate behavior. Include how the parents' temperament can influence the child's temperament.

Effective guidance and discipline focus on the development of the child. They can preserve the child's self-esteem and dignity. Discuss with parents guidelines regarding discipline. Explain to parents that they should never belittle the child. Children may view parents and caretakers negatively if they are consistently belittled or insulted. These negative actions can inhibit learning and teach the child to react unkindly to others. Instead, parents should discipline with praise. Positive acknowledgements of progress are likely to encourage healthy development and appropriate behavior (Barakat & Clark, 2001). Discuss with parents how to be realistic when planning activities so as to not overwhelm the child, resulting in misbehavior. Encourage parents to say "no" only when they mean it, to avoid a negative atmosphere in the home, and to avoid inconsistency.

When misbehaviors occur, the type and amount of discipline is based upon different factors:

- Developmental level of both the child and the parents
- Severity of the misbehavior
- Established rules of the family
- Temperament of the child
- Response of the child to rewards

Keep in mind that school-age children should participate in developing a plan of action for their misbehavior. Whatever methods of discipline are chosen, it is important that parents are consistent in providing discipline in a nurturing environment.

● ADDRESSING COMMON DEVELOPMENTAL CONCERNS

The developmental task (according to Erikson) of the school-age child is industry. They are busy learning, achieving, and exploring. As the school-age child becomes more independent, forces other than the family such as television, video games, and peers influence them. Some of these influences are positive and others are negative. Some of the common developmental concerns for the school-age child are discussed in the following sections. Guidelines to assist the parents and nurses when encountering these concerns are included in Teaching Guideline 7.2.

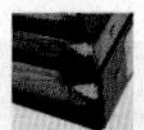

TEACHING GUIDELINE 7.2

Addressing Common Developmental Concerns

Television and Video Games

- Limit television watching and video-game playing to 2 hours per day.
- Monitor television programs.
- Prohibit television or video games with violence.
- Do not put television or video games in children's bedrooms.
- Provide a schedule of accepted television programs for viewing each week.
- Co-view television and video games with the child.
- Encourage sports, interactive play, and reading.

Obesity

- Provide healthy meals and snacks.
- Schedule and encourage daily exercise.
- Encourage involvement in sports.
- Restrict TV and computer-game use.
- Limit the amount of fast-food intake.
- Provide education about healthy nutrition.
- Never use food as a reward.
- Be a good role model.

School Phobia

- Return child to school.
- Investigate cause of the fear.
- Support child.
- Collaborate with teachers.
- Praise success in school attendance.

Latchkey Kids

- Provide rules to follow and expectations, such as
  - Not answering the door or phone
  - No friends in the house when parents are not home
  - No playing with fire
- Teach child to call a trusted neighbor when help is needed and 911 in the event of emergency.
- Post all resource numbers, including after-school help lines if available, in a clearly viewable spot.
- Purchase caller ID for the phone system.
- Enroll the child in an after-school program if available.
- Discuss limitations of outside play.
- Discuss limitations of television viewing and video-game use.
- Make sure the child knows how to contact the parent.
- Set clear homework expectations.
- DO NOT keep guns in the home.

Stealing

- Educate parents about possibility of stealing.
- Discuss ways to teach concept of ownership and property rights.
- Handle situation openly.
- Assist child in developing and enacting a plan to return what was stolen.
- Make sure the punishment is appropriate for the action.

Lying

- Help parents in understanding why the child is lying.
- When the child lies, calmly confront the child and explain why the behavior is not acceptable.
- Educate parents that their behavior should reflect what they teach and expect from their child.
- Educate parents that too-rigid or severe punishments can decrease the child's sense of worth.
- Seek professional help if lying persists in the older school-age child, to rule out underlying problems.

Cheating

- Educate parents that the child must be mature enough to understand the concept of rules.
- Handle cheating situations openly.
- Help parents to understand why their child is cheating and to modify the trigger.
- Develop appropriate punishment; inappropriate punishment could undermine the child.
- Educate parents that their behavior should reflect what they expect from their child.
- Seek professional help if cheating persists in the older school-age child, to rule out underlying problems.

Bullying

The Bullied Child

- Educate parents whose children are at risk for being bullied
  - Children who appear different from the majority
  - Children who act different from the majority
  - Children who have low self-esteem
  - Children with a mental or psychological problem
- Teach parents to role play different scenarios the child may face at school; show the child different ways to react to being bullied.
- Impress upon the child that he or she did not cause the bullying.
- Develop ways to increase the child's self-esteem at home.
- Discuss the situation with the teacher and develop a plan of care.

The Bullying Child

- Educate parents on reasons why it is important to correct the behavior.
- Discuss ways the child can appropriately show his or her anger and feelings.

(continued)

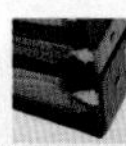

TEACHING GUIDELINE 7.2 (Continued)

Addressing Common Developmental Concerns

- Have parents help the child to see how it feels to be bullied.
- Do not allow fighting at home.
- Reward settling of conflicts without violence.

Tobacco and Alcohol Education

- Inquire about tobacco and alcohol use.
- Discuss the physical and social dangers of tobacco and alcohol use.
- Urge parents to be good role models.
- Limit reading and media materials about alcohol and tobacco use.
- Discuss the influences of tobacco and alcohol use by peers.
- Educate the child on spit tobacco. Let them know it is just as dangerous as smoking tobacco.
- Advocate for a smoke-free environment in the home and other places frequented.
- Avoid having tobacco and alcohol products readily available in the home.

Television and Video Games

The influence of television and video games upon the school-age child is a growing concern for parents and child specialists. Children in the United States spend about 4 hours a day either watching TV or playing video games. During that time, a child will see 8,000 murders by the end of grade school and 40,000 commercials a year. Although a school-age child can determine what is real from what is fantasy, research has shown that this amount of time in front of the TV—watching it or playing video games—can lead to aggressive behavior, less physical activity, and altered body image (see Healthy People 2010).

Although some television shows and video games can have positive influences on children, teach parents guidelines on the use of TV and video games. Parents should set limits on how much TV watching the child can have. The Academy of Pediatrics recommends 2 hours or less of television viewing per day. The parent should establish guidelines on when the child can watch TV, for example, after homework or when chores are completed. Television watching should not be used as a reward. The parents should be aware of what the child is watching. Watch the programs together and use that opportunity to discuss the subject matter with the child. There should be no TV during dinner and no TV in the child's room. The parents need to set an example for the child. Read instead of watching TV or do a physical activity together as a family. If the TV causes fights or arguments, it should be turned off for a period of time.

HEALTHY PEOPLE 2010

Objective	Significance
Increase the proportion of children and adolescents who view television 2 or fewer hours per day.	• Assist families to identify activities other than television for the child to participate in. • Praise craft, music, and sports participation.

Obesity

The Centers for Disease Control and Prevention (CDC) and National Health and Nutrition Examination Survey (NHANES) find that more and more children are overweight. Over the past two decades the number of overweight children and adolescents nearly doubled. The surveys show that 13% of children between 6 and 11 years of age are overweight. Overweight is classified as a body mass index (BMI) greater than 85% and obese is classified as a BMI greater than 95% (see Healthy People 2010).

Obesity occurs when the intake of calories and food exceeds the expenditures. Some factors linked to causing obesity include family role modeling, lack of exercise, and unstructured meals as well as cultural, genetic, environmental, and socioeconomic factors. Some factors that influence lack of exercise include the decreased number of days that school systems offer physical education programs

HEALTHY PEOPLE 2010

Objective	Significance
Reduce the proportion of children and adolescents who are overweight or obese.	• Screen all children for the development of overweight as indicated by an increasing body mass index (BMI) for their age. • Provide accurate diet counseling. • Encourage daily physical activity. • Counsel parents to limit television/computer time daily.

and recess. Also, some children live in unsafe neighborhoods and have no safe place to play outside; therefore they spend time in sedentary activities such as watching TV. Children with low metabolic rates and increased numbers of fat cells tend to gain more weight. Obese children are at risk for cardiovascular diseases, type 2 (non–insulin dependent) diabetes, and orthopedic problems. Also, psychosocial problems and eating disorders are prevalent. When parents do not have knowledge of nutrition, do not monitor snacks or meals, and have unstructured meals, habits are established that lead to obesity. A lack of exercise also contributes to obesity.

Preventing obesity in childhood is important because the fat cells of childhood are carried into adulthood obesity and contribute to disease. Due to the risk of obesity, encourage parents to never use food as a reward. To prevent obesity, establish regular mealtimes and offer healthy foods and snacks. Encourage parents to praise their child's good food choices and to role model appropriate eating and exercise.

School Phobia

School refusal (also called *school phobia* or *school avoidance*) has been defined as frequent absences, dropping out of school, or academic disengagement or disruption (Ruggiero, 1999). School phobia needs to be defined both symptomatically and operationally as the cause for the anxiety. School avoidance occurs in approximately 5% of school-age children. These children may refuse to attend school or create reasons why they cannot go to school.

Some of the fears expressed by school-refusing children include tests, bullying, teacher reprimands, anxieties over toileting in a public bathroom, physical harm, or undressing in the locker room. Due to the emotional distress caused in these children when attending school, they are frequently classified as having school phobia. Young children may complain of stomachache or headache and older children may complain of palpitations or feeling faint.

It is important to investigate specific causes of school refusal/school phobia and take appropriate actions. The physician or nurse practitioner should conduct a physical examination of the child to rule out any physical illness. After these measures are taken, the parent, teacher, school counselor, and school administrator may devise a plan to assist the student to overcome a specific fear. In uncomplicated cases, parents must return the child to school as soon as possible. There may be altered schedules (partial days or decreased hours) to help promote a successful transition back to school. Another idea to help desensitize the child may be to have him or her spend part of the day in the counselor's or school nurse's office.

Latchkey Children

With both parents in the workforce, many children return home alone without adult supervision for a number of hours. These "latchkey kids" are more prone to misbehave and to take risks. The American Academy of Pediatrics recommends that a child come home to a parent, another adult, or a responsible adolescent (www.aap.org).

Most young children are not capable of handling stress or making decisions on their own before 11 or 12 years of age. However, some school-age children are more mature and can be left alone by 8 to 10 years of age; maturity is the key, not the age. Despite the level of maturity, children who are unsupervised are more likely to use alcohol and illegal drugs. In addition, latchkey children may feel isolated from friends because friends may be prohibited from entering the home when parents are not present (Hockenberry et al., 2003).

If children come home to no supervision, they should know the names, addresses, and phone numbers of parents and a neighbor, as well as emergency numbers. They should be given rules about answering the door and the phone. They should tell anyone who comes to the door or who calls that mom is home but busy at this time. Directions as to the handling of the house key and fire safety should be taught and demonstrated (see Teaching Guideline 7.2).

Stealing, Lying, and Cheating

It is during the school-age years that antisocial behaviors can emerge. Children who were previously well behaved may now exhibit behaviors of stealing, lying, and cheating. Parents are usually disturbed by this change in behavior. In turn, they have difficulty in addressing these issues and need help in providing appropriate interventions.

Children between 6 and 8 years old do not fully understand the concept of ownership and property rights. These children may steal things because they like the look of the item. Stealing in the 8- to 10-year-old may occur because the child desires the item or to impress the child's peers. The 10- to 12-year-old child may steal for the same reasons as children between 8 and 10 years of age. In addition, these older children may steal to supplement their perceived inadequate income.

Lying is more common in children between 6 and 8 years old. It is acceptable for these children to tell tall tales, but they should know what truth is and what make-believe is. These younger children typically lie to avoid punishment. However, they do not like others to lie and will tell on them if they lie. Children between 8 and 12 years old typically lie because they are unable to meet expectations of family and peers. They also lie to impress others. If lying persists in older school-age children, parents should discuss the matter with a health care provider because the lying may be evidence of underlying problems.

The concept of cheating is not well understood until the child is 7 years old. Before this age, the desire to "win" is most important and rigid rules are hard to understand. In children between 8 and 12 years old, the concept of cheating is fully understood. It is usually done because of peer pressure, strong pressure placed on the child to succeed by parents, and a sense of low self-esteem. If cheating persists in older school-age children, parents should discuss the matter with a health care provider because the behavior may indicate underlying problems.

In dealing with children who exhibit stealing, lying, or cheating behaviors, parents must first realize the importance of their own behaviors in those areas. Parents are role models to the school-age child. Therefore, when the child sees or hears that parents lie, steal, or cheat (e.g., parents bragging about cheating on their taxes), they think it is all right to mimic those behaviors. Secondly, parents must directly confront any stealing, lying, or cheating behaviors and discuss (and follow through consistently with) the consequences of such behaviors (see Teaching Guideline 7.2).

Bullying

Bullying, defined as inflicting verbal, emotional, or physical abuse upon others, is on the increase during the school-age years. Bullied children are those who report themselves as being lonely and having difficulty in forming friendships. The children who perform the bullying are those children who are reported to have low self-esteem, poor grades, and poor interpersonal skills.

In general, about 10% of all children attending school are frightened and afraid most of the day. Most of the bullying occurs at school. Both boys and girls are bullied; boys usually bully boys and use force more often. Girls can be bullied by both sexes using mainly social alienation and intimidation. Both girls and boys can bully. Girls are usually the bullies in grades 1 through 3, and boys are typically the bullies in grades 4 and above.

Being bullied can have negative results on children throughout life. These children often have increased episodes of common childhood illnesses of headaches, stomachaches, and sleep problems. After the problem of either being bullied or being the bully has been identified, parents must work with the child, the school, and the health care provider to solve the problem (see Teaching Guideline 7.2).

Tobacco and Alcohol Education

School-age children are eager to grow up and be independent. Peers and acceptance are very important at this time. School-age children may be exposed to messages that are in conflict with their parents' values regarding smoking and alcohol. Peers often exert pressure for children to experiment with tobacco and alcohol (see Healthy People 2010).

School-age children are ready to absorb information that deals with drugs and alcohol. Information from parents or other adults who are major influences in the child's life is essential at this time to set clear rules and model behaviors for children to embrace. Discussions with children need to be based on facts and focused on the present. Some topics for discussion include:

- What alcohol and drugs are like and how they harm you
- Differences in medical use vs. illegal use of drugs
- How to think critically to interpret messages seen in advertising, media, sports, and entertainment personalities

See Teaching Guideline 7.2.

HEALTHY PEOPLE 2010

Objective	Significance
Reduce initiation of tobacco use among children and adolescents.	• Educate children and families about the dangers of tobacco use.

Recall Lawrence Jones, the 10-year-old presented at the beginning of the chapter. List potential developmental problems he may experience. What anticipatory guidance related to these concerns should you provide to his mother?

References

Adekoya, N., Thurman, D. J., White, D. D., & Webb, K. W. (2000). Surveillance for traumatic brain injury deaths: United States 1989–1998. *Morbidity and Mortality Weekly Report, 51*(Suppl. 10), 1–16.

American Academy of Pediatrics. (2002). Skateboard and scooter injuries. *Pediatrics, 109*(3), 542–543.

American Academy of Pediatrics, Committee on Nutrition. (2003). Policy statement: prevention of overweight and obesity. *Pediatrics, 112*(2), 424–430. Available at http://aappolicy.aappublications.org/cgi/reprint/pediatrics;112/2/424.pdf.

Barakat, I. S., & Clark, J. A. (2005). *Positive discipline and child guidance.* Retrieved July 9, 2006 from http://muextension.missouri.edu/xplor/hesguide/humanrel/gh6119.htm.

Behrman, R. (1999). When school is out. *The Future of Children, 9*(2), 1–95.

Centers for Disease Control and Prevention. (2000). Unpowered scooter related injuries: United States 1998–2000. *Morbidity and Mortality Weekly Report, 49,* 1108–1110.

Centers for Disease Control and Prevention, National Center for Health Statistics. (2000). *Injury and poisonings episodes and conditions: national health interview survey, 1997.* Retrieved July 10, 2006 from http://www.cdc.gov/nchs/data/series/sr_10/sr10_202.pdf.

Edelman, C. L., & Mandle, C. L. (2002). *Health promotion throughout the lifespan* (5th ed.). St. Louis, MO: Mosby.

Erikson, E. (1963). *Childhood and society* (2nd ed.). New York: Norton.

Fox, J. A. (2002). *Primary health care of infants and children & adolescents.* St. Louis, MO: Mosby.

Green, M., Palfrey, J. S., Clark, E. M., & Anastase, J. M. (Eds.). (2002). *Bright futures: Guidelines for health supervision of infants, children, and adolescents* (2nd ed.). Arlington, VA: National Center for Education in Maternal and Child Health.

Hegvik, R., McDevitt, S., & Carey, W. (1982). The middle childhood temperament questionnaire/develop. *Journal of Developmental and Behavioral Pediatrics, 3*(4), 197–200.

Hockenberry, M., Wilson, D., Winkelstein, M. L., & Kline, N. (2003). *Wong's infant care of infants and children* (7th ed.). St. Louis, MO: Mosby.

Hoekelman, R., Adam, H., Nelson, N., Weitzman, M., & Wilson., M. (2001). *Primary pediatric care.* Philadelphia: Mosby.

James, R. J., Ashwill, J. W., & Droske, S. C. (2002). *Nursing care of children: Principles and practice* (2nd ed.). Philadelphia: Saunders.

Kellogg, N., & Committee on Child Abuse and Neglect. (2005). The evaluation of sexual abuse in children. *Pediatrics, 116*(2), 506–512.

McDevitt, S., & Carey, W. (1978). The measurement of temperament in 3–7 year old children. *Journal of Child Psychology and Psychiatry, 19,* 245–253.

Murray, S. K., Baker, A. W., & Lewin, L. (2000). Screening families with young children for child maltreatment potential. *Pediatric Nursing, 26,* 47–54.

Robinson, T. N. (1999). Reducing children's television viewing to prevent obesity: A randomized controlled trial. *Journal of the American Medical Association, 282*(16), 1561–1567.

Ruggiero, M. (1999). Maladaptation to school. In M. Levine, W. Carey, & A. Croker (Eds.), *Developmental behavioral pediatrics* (pp. 542–550). Philadelphia: Saunders.

Santrock, J. W. (2004). *Life span development.* Boston: McGraw-Hill.

Storey, M., Holt, K., & Sotfka, D. (Eds). (2002). *Bright futures in practice: Nutrition.* Arlington, VA: National Center for Education in Maternal and Child Health.

Web Sites

www.aap.org American Academy of Pediatrics

www.aapd.org American Association of Pediatric Dentistry

www.aao.org American Academy of Ophthalmology

www.americanheartorg/scientific/statements/index.html American Heart Association

www.brightfutures.org Full-text reference to health supervision

www.brightfutures.org/oral health/about.html References on oral health

www.cdc.gov/growthcharts/ Centers for Disease Control and Prevention/National Center for Health Statistics/United States Growth Charts: data files, 2000

www.cdc.gov/mmwr/preview/mmwrhtml/mm4949a2.htm Centers for Disease Control and Prevention/Morbidity and Mortality Weekly Report

www.cdc.gov/nccdphp/dnpa/obesity/consequences.htm Centers for Disease Control and Prevention/National Center for Chronic Disease Prevention and Health Promotion

www.cdc.gov/nchs/about/major/nhanes/growthcharts/datafiles.htm Centers for Disease Control and Prevention/National Center for Health Statistics/National Health and Nutrition Examination Survey/United States Growth Charts: data files, 2002

www.cdc.gov/nchs/releases/01news/overweght99.htm Centers for Disease Control and Prevention/National Center for Health Statistics: prevalence of overweight among children and adolescents, United States, 1999

www.cdc.gov/ncipc/factsheets/childh.htm Centers for Disease Control and Prevention/National Center for Injury Prevention and Control: child health fact sheets

www.dentalcare.com/drn.htm Dental care information

www.eatright.org American Dietetic Association

www.healthypeople.gov/Document/HTML/Volume2/19Nutrition.htm Healthy People 2010 Objectives: leading health indicators

www.healthyschools.org Healthy Schools.org is a nonprofit organization devoted to decreasing environmental exposures in schools.

www.immunize.org Immunization Action Coalition is a nonprofit organization funded by the CDC; a one-stop site for all types of immunization information

www.safekids.com Internet safety for kids

www.sportsparents.com *Sports Illustrated for Kids*–sponsored site with good information for parents and providers of child/adolescent health care

www.taconicnet.com/temperament.htm Taconic Counseling Group, NY. Psychotherapy: Temperament differences in children, 2000

www.tchin.org The Children's Health Network provides this site to offer support to clients, parents, and professionals dealing with heart disease

Chapter WORKSHEET

● MULTIPLE CHOICE QUESTIONS

1. The successful resolution of developmental tasks for the school-age child, according to Erikson, would be identified by:
   a. Learning from repeating tasks
   b. Developing a sense of worth and competence
   c. Using fantasy and magical thinking to cope with problems
   d. Developing a sense of trust
2. Which of the following are reasons that stealing occurs in school-age children? (Choose all that apply)
   a. To escape punishment
   b. High self-esteem
   c. Low expectations of family/peers
   d. Lack of sense of propriety
   e. Strong desire to own something
3. Which of the following will promote weight loss in an obese school-age child? (Choose all that apply)
   a. Unlimited computer and TV time
   b. Role modeling by family
   c. Becoming active in sports
   d. Eating unstructured meals
   e. Involving child in meal planning and grocery shopping
   f. Drinking three glasses of water per day
4. As the school nurse conducting screening for vision in a 6-year-old child, you would refer the child to a specialist if the visual acuity in both eyes is:
   a. 20/20
   b. 20/25
   c. 20/30
   d. 20/50
5. Ms. Jones has two sons, ages 6 and 9, who want to play on the same baseball team. As the school nurse, what advice would you give Ms. Jones?
   a. Having the boys on the same team will make it more convenient for the mother.
   b. Levels of coordination and concentration differ, so the boys need to be on different teams.
   c. Put the boys on the same team because they are both school-age children.
   d. It is best to avoid putting the boys on the same team to prevent sibling rivalry.

● CRITICAL THINKING EXERCISES

1. Ms. Sams brings her 8-year-old son (Frank) to the pediatrician's office for his annual exam. She states that she is concerned about his recent behavior. He went to the grocery store with his friend and his friend's mother and he came home with a Matchbox car. The friend's mother stated she had not purchased the car.
   a. What would be your response to Ms. Sams?
   b. Ms. Sams said she still has the car. What would you advise Ms. Sams to do to make Frank aware of consequences of his actions?
2. Sally's mother is asking the nurse advice about purchasing a 2-wheeled bike for her 7-year-old. What guidance should the nurse offer this parent?
3. Ms. Shaw brings in her 11-year-old daughter for a well-child check. The schoolager says to the nurse, "I look different from my friends. I do not wear bras and my friends are already wearing bras." What would be an appropriate response to this schoolager?
4. Johnny is a 9-year-old whose mother and father both work during the day. He returns home after school. How should the parents prepare Johnny for this experience? What safety rules would be included in the education for Johnny?

● STUDY ACTIVITIES

1. Attend a sporting event (such as soccer or baseball) with school-age teams. Describe the coordination and gross motor functioning of this group.
2. Attend a first-grade class. Observe the behaviors exhibited by the school-age children in this class. How do these behaviors compare with normal values for this age group?

chapter 8

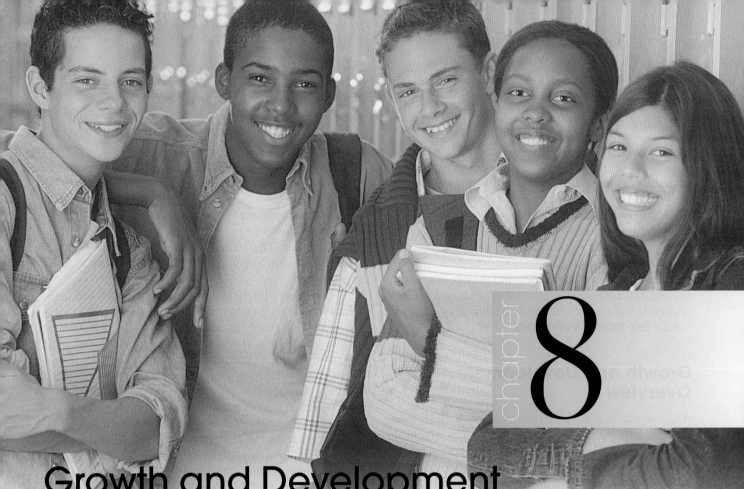

Growth and Development of the Adolescent

Key TERMS

adolescence
adolescent egocentrism
invincibility
menarche
peer groups
puberty
risk-taking behaviors
sexuality

Learning OBJECTIVES

Upon completion of the chapter, the learner will be able to:

1. Identify normal physiologic changes, including puberty, occurring in the adolescent.
2. Discuss psychosocial, cognitive, and moral changes occurring in the adolescent.
3. Identify changes in relationships with peers, family, teachers, and community during adolescence.
4. Describe interventions to promote safety during adolescence.
5. Demonstrate knowledge of the nutritional requirements of the adolescent.
6. Demonstrate knowledge of the development of sexuality and its influence on dating during adolescence.
7. Identify common developmental concerns of the adolescent.
8. Demonstrate knowledge of the appropriate nursing guidance for common developmental concerns.

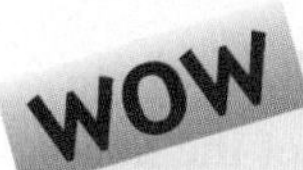

The only way to grow is to let go . . .

Cho Chung is a 15-year-old girl brought to the clinic by her mother for her annual school check-up. During your assessment you measure Cho's weight at 110 pounds and her height at 60 inches. As the nurse caring for her, assess Cho's growth and development, and then provide appropriate anticipatory guidance to her and her mother.

Adolescence spans the years of transition from childhood to adulthood, which is usually between the ages of 11 and 20 years. There is some overlap between late school age and adolescence. The adolescent experiences drastic changes in the physical, cognitive, psychosocial, and psychosexual areas. With this rapid growth during adolescence, the development of secondary sexual characteristics, and interest in the opposite sex, the adolescent needs the support and guidance of parents and nurses to facilitate healthy lifestyles and to reduce **risk-taking behaviors**.

Growth and Development Overview

Adolescence is a time of rapid growth with dramatic changes in body size and proportions. The magnitude of these changes is second only to the growth in infancy. During this time sexual characteristics develop and reproductive maturity is achieved. The age of onset and the duration of the physiologic changes vary form individual to individual. Generally girls enter **puberty** earlier (at 9 to 10 years of age) than boys (at 10 to 11 years). Adolescents will represent varying levels of identity formation and will offer unique challenges to the nurse (Table 8.1).

PHYSIOLOGIC CHANGES ASSOCIATED WITH PUBERTY

The secretion of estrogen in girls and testosterone in boys stimulates the development of breast tissue in girls, pubic hair in both sexes, and changes in male genitalia. These biological changes that occur during adolescence are known as *puberty.* Puberty is the result of triggers among the environment, the central nervous system, the hypothalamus, the pituitary gland, the gonads, and the adrenal glands. Gonadotropin-releasing hormone (GnRH), produced by the hypothalamus, travels though the capillaries to the anterior pituitary gland to stimulate the production and secretion of follicle-stimulating hormone (FSH) and luteinizing hormone (LH). The increased levels of FSH and LH stimulate the gonadal response. LH stimulates ovulation in girls and acts on testicular Leydig cells in boys, prompting maturation of the testicles and testosterone production. FSH with LH stimulates sperm production. Estrogen, progesterone, and testosterone and other androgens are released from the gonads and affect biological changes and changes in various organs, including alterations in muscles, bones, skin, and hair follicles. When serum sex hormones are decreased, the hypothalamus triggers the secretion of GnRH to initiate the proper gonadal responses.

Adolescents experience physical development, hormonal changes, and sexual maturation during puberty that correlate to Freud's genital stage of psychosexual development. The genital stage begins with the production of sex hormones and maturation of the reproductive system.

Girls reach physical maturity before boys and menstruation usually begins between the ages of 9 and 15 years (average 12.8 years). Breast budding (thelarche) occurs at approximately age 9 to 11 years and is followed by the growth of pubic hair. African-American girls reach **menarche** slightly earlier than Caucasian girls (Hoekelman, 2003).

The first sign of pubertal changes in boys is testicular enlargement in response to testosterone secretion, usually occurring in Tanner stage 2 (Fig. 8.1). As testosterone levels increase, the penis and scrotum enlarge, hair distribution increases, and scrotal skin texture changes. During late puberty, boys will typically experience their first ejaculation, which may occur while they are sleeping (nocturnal emissions). Nurses should provide anticipatory guidance to adolescent males regarding involuntary nocturnal emissions (wet dreams) to assure them that this is a normal occurrence.

Tanner stages 3 to 5 usually occur during adolescence. See Figure 8.1 for the increase in breast tissue and pubic hair distribution in girls, and scrotal and penile changes as well as hair distribution changes in boys. The nurse should provide guidance to adolescents about the normalcy of the sexual feelings and evolving body changes that occur during puberty.

PHYSICAL GROWTH

Diet, exercise, and hereditary factors influence the height, weight, and body build of the adolescent. Over the past three decades, adolescents have become taller and heavier than their ancestors and the beginning of puberty is earlier.

The rapid growth during adolescence is secondary only to that of the infant years and is a direct result of the hormonal changes of puberty. Both girls and boys experience changes in appearance and size. Height in girls increases rapidly after menarche and usually ceases 2 to 2½ years after menarche. Boys' growth spurt occurs later than girls' and usually begins between the ages of 10½ and 16 years and ends sometime between the ages of 13½ and 17½ years. Peak height velocity (PHV) occurs at approximately 12 years of age in girls or at about 6 to

Table 8.1 Physiologic Changes of Adolescence

Stage of Adolescence	Puberty Changes in Females	Puberty Changes in Males	Physical Growth in Females	Physical Growth in Males
Early adolescence (11–14 years)	Pubic hair begins to curl and spread over mons pubis; pigmentation increases. Breast bud and areola continue to enlarge; no separation of breast	Pubic hair spreads laterally, begins to curl; pigmentation increases. Growth and enlargement of testes in scrotum (scrotum reddish in color) and continued lengthening of penis	Increase in percentage of body fat Head, neck, hands, and feet reach adult proportions. Senses matured Respiratory rate decreases to 15–20 breaths per minute Heart grows in size and strength, heart rate decreases, blood pressure increases to adult level Full set of permanent teeth with exception of last four molars (wisdom teeth) Liver, kidneys, spleen, and digestive tract mature; enlarge during growth spurt Exocrine and apocrine sweat glands and sebaceous glands become fully functioning.	Increase in percentage of body fat Head, neck, hands, and feet reach adult proportions. Leggy look due to extremities growing faster than the trunk Senses matured Respiratory rate decreases to 15–20 breaths per minute Heart grows in size and strength, heart rate decreases, blood pressure increases Full set of permanent teeth with exception of last four molars (wisdom teeth) Liver, kidneys, spleen, and digestive tract mature; enlarge during growth spurt Exocrine and apocrine sweat glands and sebaceous glands become fully functioning.
Middle adolescence (14–16 years)	Pubic hair becomes coarse in texture and continues to curl; amount of hair increases. Areola and papilla separate from the contour of the breast to form a secondary mound. First menstrual period (average 12.8 years)	Pubic hair becomes coarser in texture and takes on adult distribution. Testes and scrotum continue to grow; scrotal skin darkens; penis grows in width, and glans penis develops. May experience breast enlargement	Reach peak height and weight velocity Muscle mass and strength increase Increase in shoulder, chest, and hip breadth	Voice changes; more masculine due to rapid enlargement of the larynx and pharynx as well as lung changes Growth spurt during this time Muscle mass and strength increase. Increase in shoulder, chest, and hip breadth

(continued)

Table 8.1 Physiologic Changes of Adolescence (continued)

Stage of Adolescence	Puberty Changes in Females	Puberty Changes in Males	Physical Growth in Females	Physical Growth in Males
Late adolescence (17–20 years)	Mature pubic hair distribution and coarseness	Mature pubic hair distribution and coarseness Breast enlargement disappears. Adult size and shape of testes, scrotum, and penis; scrotal skin darkening Ejaculation occurs	Physically mature Ossification of skeletal system complete Eruption of last four molars Basal metabolic rate (BMR) reaches adult levels	Physically mature Ossification of skeletal system complete Eruption of last four molars BMR reaches adult levels

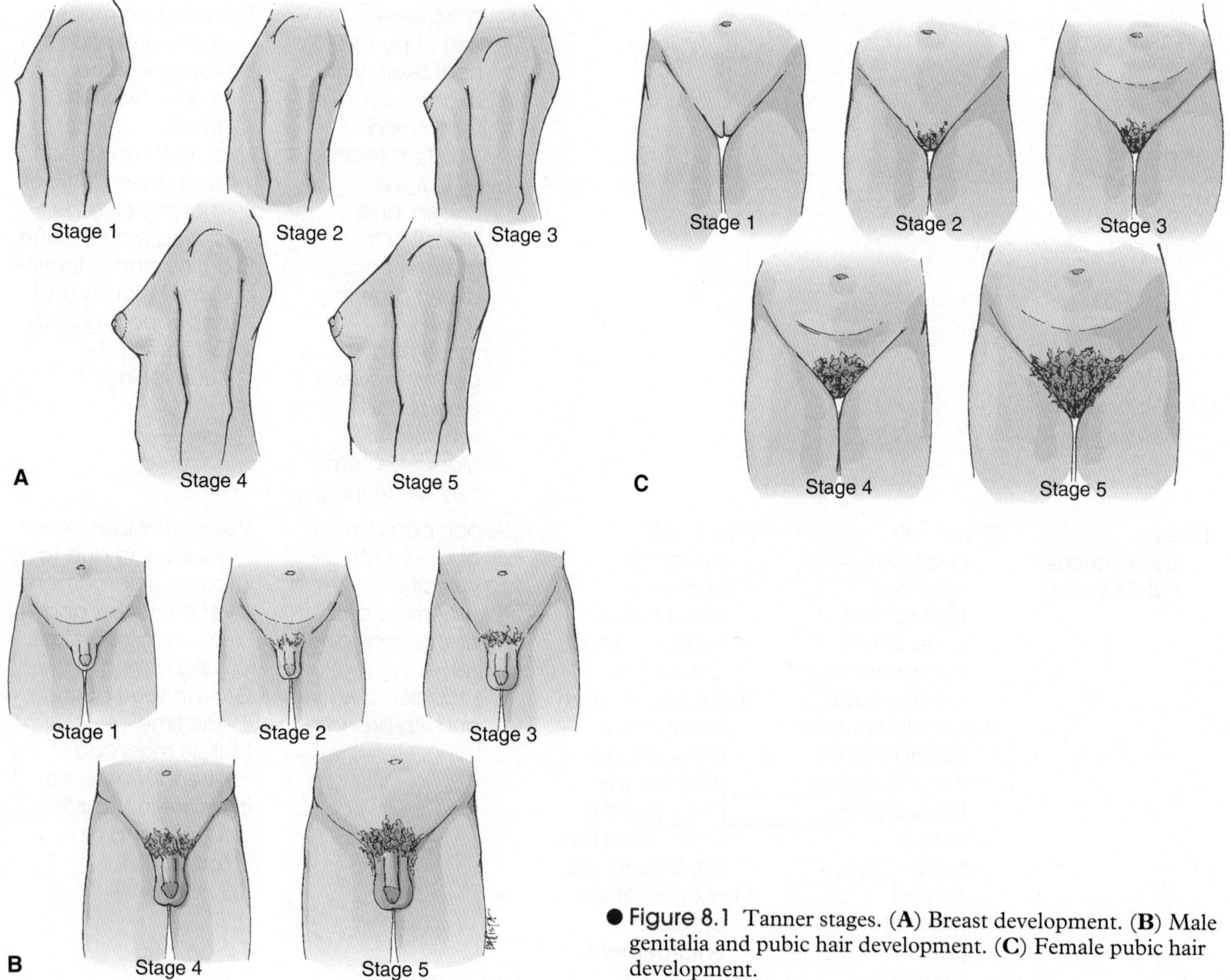

● **Figure 8.1** Tanner stages. (**A**) Breast development. (**B**) Male genitalia and pubic hair development. (**C**) Female pubic hair development.

12 months after menarche. Boys reach PHV at about 14 years of age. Peak weight velocity (PWV) occurs about 6 months after menarche in girls and at about 14 years of age in boys. Muscle mass increases in boys and fat deposits increase in girls (Fig. 8.2).

During early adolescence growth is rapid, but it decreases in middle and late adolescence. Height for adolescent boys who are between the 50th and 95th percentile ranges from 52½ inches (132 centimeters) to 69½ inches (176.8 centimeters). Weight of boys in these percentiles ranges from 77¼ pounds (35.3 kilograms) to 211 pounds (95.76 kilograms). On average, boys will gain 10 to 30 centimeters (4 to 12 inches) in height and 7 to 30 kilograms (15 to 65 pounds) in weight.

Height for girls who are between the 50th and 95th percentile ranges from 57 inches (144.8 centimeters) to 68½ inches (173.6 centimeters), with weight ranging from 60 pounds (27.24 kilograms) to 181 pounds (82.47 kilograms). On average, girls will gain 5 to 20 centimeters (2 to 8 inches) in height and 7 to 25 kg (15 to 55 pounds) in weight during adolescence. See Appendix A for growth charts for this age group. Refer to Chapter 10 for instructions for calculating body mass index (BMI).

ORGAN SYSTEM MATURATION

Adolescence is a time of metabolic slowing and of increasing size of some organs.

Neurologic System

During adolescence there is continued brain growth although the size of the brain does not increase significantly. Neurons do not increase in number, but growth of myelin sheath enables faster neural processing.

Respiratory System

The adolescent years see an increase in diameter and length of the lungs. Respiratory rate decreases and reaches the adult rate. Respiratory volume and vital capacity increase. Volume and capacity are greater in boys than girls, which may be associated with increased chest and shoulder size in boys. The growth of the laryngeal cartilage, larynx, and vocal cords produces the voice changes experienced in adolescence. Deepening of both male and female voices occurs but is more pronounced in boys (Edelman & Mandle, 2002).

Cardiovascular System

There is an increase in size and strength of the heart. Systolic blood pressure increases and heart rate decreases. Blood volume reaches higher levels in boys than girls, which may be due to boys' greater muscle mass.

Gastrointestinal System

The liver, spleen, kidneys, and digestive tract enlarge during the growth spurt in early adolescence, but do not change in function. These systems are mature in early school age.

Musculoskeletal System

The ossification of the skeletal system is incomplete until late adolescence in boys. Ossification is more advanced in girls and occurs at an earlier age. During the growth spurt, muscle mass and strength increase. At similar stages of development, muscle development is generally greater in boys. Estrogen, progesterone, and testosterone (sex steroids) and other androgens are released from the

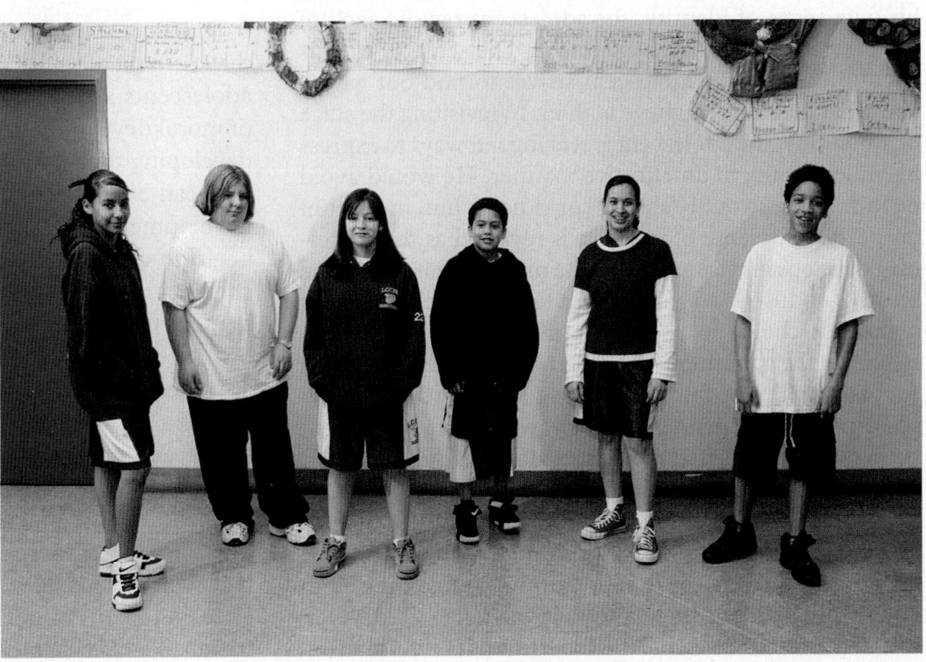

● Figure 8.2 These adolescents reflect the differences in sizes and shapes seen in adolescents of the same age.

gonads and effect changes in the muscles and bones. Low estrogen levels tend to stimulate skeletal growth, while higher levels inhibit growth.

Integumentary System

During adolescence the skin becomes thick and tough. Under the influence of androgens, the sebaceous glands become more active, particularly on the face, back, and genitals. Due to the increased levels of testosterone during Tanner stages 4 and 5 in both boys and girls, both sexes may have increased sebum production, which may lead to the development of acne and oily hair.

The exocrine and apocrine sweat glands function at adult levels during adolescence. The exocrine glands are all over the body and they produce sweat that helps to eliminate body heat through evaporation. The apocrine glands are found in the axillae, genital, and anal areas, and around the breasts. The apocrine sweat glands produce sweat in response to hair follicles. This sweat is produced continuously and is stored and released in response to emotional stimuli.

• PSYCHOSOCIAL DEVELOPMENT

According to Erikson, it is during adolescence that teenagers achieve a sense of identity. As the adolescent is trying out many different roles in regard to his relationships with peers, family, community, and society, he is developing his own individual sense of self. If he is not successful in forming his own sense of self, he develops a sense of role confusion or diffusion. The adolescent culture becomes very important to the teenager. It is through his involvement with teenage groups that the adolescent finds support and help with developing his own identity.

Erikson believed that during the task of developing his own sense of identity, the adolescent revisits each of the previous stages of development. The sense of trust is encountered as the adolescent strives to find out whom and what ideals he can have faith in. In revisiting the stage of autonomy, the adolescent is seeking out ways to express his individuality in an effective manner. He would avoid behaviors that would "shame" or ridicule him in front of his peers. The sense of initiative is revisited as the adolescent develops his vision for what he might become. And the sense of industry is again encountered as the adolescent makes his choice to participate in different activities at school, in the community, at church, and in the work force.

The ability of the adolescent to successfully form a sense of self is dependent upon how well the adolescent successfully completed the former stages of development. Erikson believed that if the adolescent has been successful, he could develop resources during adolescence to overcome any gaps in previous developmental stages. If the adolescent believes that he cannot express himself in any manner due to societal restrictions, he will develop role confusion. See Table 8.2 for additional information.

• COGNITIVE DEVELOPMENT

According to Piaget, the adolescent progresses from a concrete framework of thinking to an abstract one. It is the formal operational period. During this period, the adolescent develops the ability to think outside of the present; that is, she can incorporate into her thinking concepts that do exist as well as concepts that might exist. Her thinking becomes logical, organized, and consistent. She is able to think about a problem from all points of view, ranking the possible solutions while solving the problem. Not all adolescents achieve formal operational reasoning at the same time.

In the early stages of formal operational reasoning, the adolescent's thinking is egocentric. She is very idealistic, constantly challenging the way things are and wondering why things cannot change. These activities lead to the adolescent's feeling of being omnipotent. The adolescent must undergo this way of thinking, even though it can frustrate adults, in her quest to reach formal operational reasoning. As the teenager progresses towards middle adolescence, her thinking becomes very introspective. She assumes others are just as interested in what interests her, which leads her to feel unique, special, and exceptional. That feeling of "being exceptional" leads to the risk-taking behaviors of which teenagers are well known. Also, the teenager feels very committed to her viewpoints. She tries very hard to convince others of her viewpoints and embraces strongly those causes that support her opinions. This idealism can cause the adolescent to reject her family, her culture, her church, and her community beliefs, which can cause conflict with her family, culture, church, and community. See Table 8.2 for additional information.

• MORAL AND SPIRITUAL DEVELOPMENT

It is during the adolescent years that teenagers develop their own set of values and morals. According to Kohlberg, adolescents are experiencing the postconventional stage of moral development. It is only because adolescents are developing their formal operational way of thinking that they can experience the postconventional stage of moral development. At the beginning of this stage, teenagers begin to question the status quo. The majority of their choices are based upon emotions while they are questioning societal standards. As they progress to developing their own set of morals, adolescents realize that moral decisions are based upon rights, values, and principles that are agreeable to a given society. They also realize that those rights, values, and principles can be in conflict with the laws of the given society, but they are able to reconcile the differences. Because adolescents undergo the process of developing their own set of morals at different rates, they might find that their friends view a situation differently. This difference can lead to conflicts and the forming of different friendships. See Table 8.2 for additional information.

Table 8.2 Developmental Theories

Theories	Stages	Activities
Erikson (psychosocial)	Identity vs. role confusion or diffusion Early (11–14 years)	Focuses on bodily changes Experiences frequent mood changes Importance placed upon conformity to peer norms and peer acceptance Strives to master skills within peer groups Defining boundaries with parents and authority figures Early stage of emancipation—struggles to separate from parents while still desiring dependence upon them Identifies with same-sex peers Takes more responsibility for own behaviors
	Middle (14–16 years)	Continues to adjust to changed body image Tries out different roles within peer groups Need for acceptance by peer group at the highest level Interested in attracting opposite gender Time of greatest conflict with parents/authority figures Able to understand implications of behavior and decisions
	Late (17–20 years)	Roles within peer groups established Feels secure with body image Has matured sexual identity Has idealistic career goals Importance of individual friendships emerges Process of emancipation from family almost complete
Piaget (cognitive)	Formal Operations Early (11–14 years)	Limited abstract thought process Egocentrically thinking Eager to apply limited abstract process to different situations and to peer groups
	Middle (14–17 years)	Increased ability to think abstractly or in more idealistic terms Able to solve verbal and mental problems using scientific methods Thinks he or she is invincible—risky behaviors increase Likes making independent decisions Becomes involved/concerned with society, politics
	Late (17–20 years)	Abstract thinking is established Developed critical thinking skills—tests different solutions to problems Less risky behaviors Develops realistic goals and career plans
Kohlberg	Postconventional Level III Early (11–14 years)	Morals based upon peer, family, church, and societal morals Asks broad, usually unanswerable questions about life
	Middle (14–17 years)	Developing own set of morals—evaluate individual morals in relation to peer, family, and societal morals
	Late (17–20 years)	Internalizes own morals and values Continues to compare own morals and values to those of society Evaluates morals of others

Adolescents also begin to question their formal religious practices. As they progress through adolescence, teenagers become more interested in the spiritualism of their religion than in the actual practices of their religion. As teenagers become older, organized religion becomes less important in their lives; rather, their religious beliefs become more personalized.

> **Referring back to Cho Chung,** identify the stage of psychosocial development that she should be in according to Erikson. What approaches for assessment and teaching would be most effective based on the stage you identified?

● MOTOR SKILL DEVELOPMENT

During adolescence, the teenager refines and continues to develop his or her gross and fine motor skills. Because of this period of rapid growth spurts, teenagers may experience times of decreased coordination and have a decreased ability to perform previously learned skills, which can be worrisome for the teenager.

Gross Motor Skills

It is usually during early adolescence that teenagers begin to develop endurance. Their concentration has increased so they can follow complicated instructions. Coordination can be a problem because of the uneven growth spurts. During middle adolescence, speed and accuracy increase while coordination also improves. Teenagers become more competitive with each other (Fig. 8.3). During late adolescence, the teenager usually narrows his or her areas of interest and concentrates on the needed relevant skills.

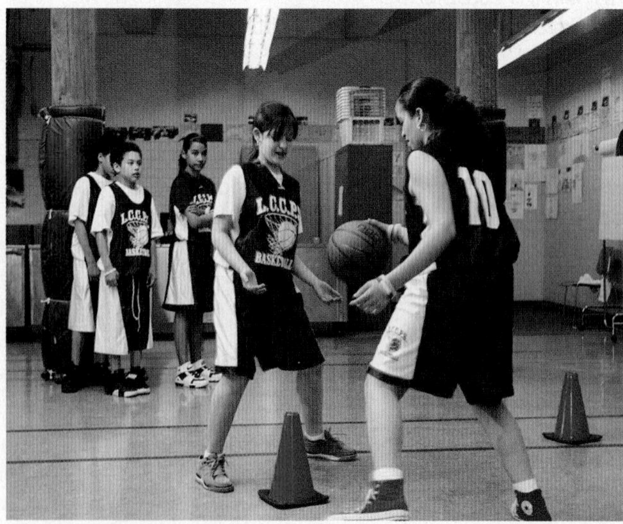

● **Figure 8.3** Adolescents become involved in competitive sports, which draw upon their gross motor skills.

Fine Motor Skills

The use of computers has greatly increased the fine motor skills of teenagers (Fig. 8.4). In the early adolescent years, the teenager increases his ability to manipulate objects. His handwriting is neat and he increases his finger dexterity. The middle adolescent years see the teenager refining his dexterity skills. By late adolescence, the teenager has developed precise eye–hand coordination and finger dexterity.

● COMMUNICATION AND LANGUAGE DEVELOPMENT

Language skills continue to develop and be refined during adolescence. During early adolescence, verbal vocabulary is close to 8,000 words and reading vocabulary is over 50,000 words. Adolescents have improved communication skills, using correct grammar and parts of speech. Vocabulary and communication skills continue to develop during middle adolescence. However, the usage of colloquial speech (slang) increases, causing communication with people other then peers to be difficult at times. By late adolescence, language skills are comparable to those of adults.

● EMOTIONAL AND SOCIAL DEVELOPMENT

Adolescents undergo a great deal of change in the areas of emotional and social development as they grow and mature into adults. Areas that are affected include the adolescent's relationship with parents; self-concept and body image; importance of peers; and **sexuality** and dating.

Relationship With Parents

Families and parents of adolescents experience changes and conflict that require adjustments and the understanding of adolescent development. The adolescent is

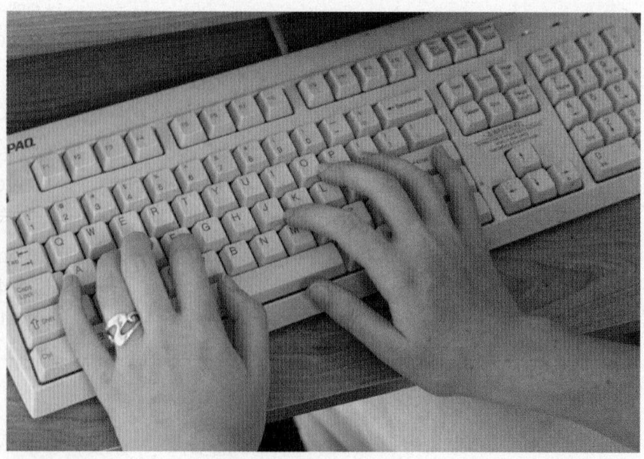

● **Figure 8.4** Using computers has increased the fine motor skills of adolescents.

striving for self-identity and increased independence. She spends more time with peers and less time with family and attending family functions. Parents sense that they have less influence on the adolescent as she spends more time with peers, questions family values, and becomes more mobile. This may lead to a family crisis, and the parents may respond by setting stricter limits or asking questions about the teen's activities and friends. Other parents may drop all rules and assume that the adolescent can manage herself. Both of these responses increase tension in the family. For tips to improve communication with your teenager, see Box 8.1.

With the adolescent attempting to establish some level of independence—and the family learning to let go while focusing on aging parents, their marriage, and other children—a state of disequilibrium occurs. The family may experience more stress than at any other time.

Some families have better outcomes with their adolescents than others. Families who listen to and continue to demonstrate affection for and acceptance of their adolescent have a more positive outcome. This does not mean that the family accepts all of the teen's ideas or actions, but they are willing to listen and attempt to negotiate some limits.

Siblings experience changes in the relationship with the adolescent brother or sister; the older sibling may attempt to parent and the younger sibling may regress in an attempt to avoid the family conflict. Understanding the status of the adolescent–family relationship is essential for the nurse.

Self-Concept and Body Image

Self-concept and self-esteem are tied to body image many times. Adolescents who perceive their body as being different than peers or as less than ideal may view themselves negatively. Adolescent girls often are influenced by peers and the media and want to weigh less and have smaller hips, waist, or thighs. Boys tend to view themselves as being too thin or not muscular enough.

Sexual characteristics are important to the adolescent's self-concept and body image. Boys are concerned about the size of their penis and facial hair while girls are concerned about breast size and the onset of menstruation. Larger breasts are considered more feminine and menstruation is considered the right of passage into adulthood. All of these body changes are important to the adolescent's self-concept.

> **BOX 8.1**
>
> **WAYS TO IMPROVE COMMUNICATION WITH TEENS**
>
> - Set aside appropriate amount of time to discuss subject matter without interruptions.
> - Talk face to face. Be aware of body language.
> - Ask questions to see why he feels that way.
> - Ask her to be patient as you tell your thoughts.
> - Choose words carefully so he understands you.
> - Tell her exactly what you mean.
> - Give praise and approval to your teenager often.
> - Speak to him as an equal—don't talk down to him.
> - Be aware of your tone of voice and body language.
> - Don't pretend you know all the answers.
> - Admit that you do make mistakes.
> - Rules and limits should be set fairly.

Importance of Peers

Peer groups play an essential role in the identity of the adolescent. Adolescent peer relationships are very important in providing opportunities to learn about negotiating differences; for recreation, companionship, and someone to share problems with; for learning peer loyalty; and for creating stability during transitions or times of stress. Learning to work out differences with peers is a skill that is important throughout life. Peers serve as someone safe to discuss family issues with, as the teen emotionally moves away from the family while trying to find his or her identity. Due to changes that have taken place within family systems in society, peer groups play a significant role in the socialization of adolescents (Fig. 8.5).

Peers serve as credible sources of information, role model social behaviors, and act as sources of social reinforcement. Friends provide an opportunity for fun and excitement. Peers impact teens' appearance, dress, social behavior, and language. Peers also can have positive influences on each other, such as promoting college attendance, or negative influences such as involvement with alcohol, drugs, or gangs. Early and middle adolescence are periods when teens are prone to join gangs. Peer role modeling and peer acceptance may lead to the formation of a gang that provides a collective identity and gives a sense of belonging. Peer pressure, companionship, and protection are the most frequent reasons given for joining gangs, particularly those associated with criminal activity.

Parents must know their teen's friends and continue to be aware of potential problems while allowing the teen the independence to become his or her own person. Nurses must remind parents of the importance of peers and the impact they have on the teen's decisions and life choices. The transition to greater peer involvement requires guidance and support. Adolescents who do not have parental or adult supervision and opportunities for conversation with adults may be more susceptible to peer influences and at higher risk for poor peer selections.

Sexuality and Dating

Adolescence is a critical time in the development of sexuality. Sexuality includes the thoughts, feelings, and behaviors related to the adolescent's sexual identity.

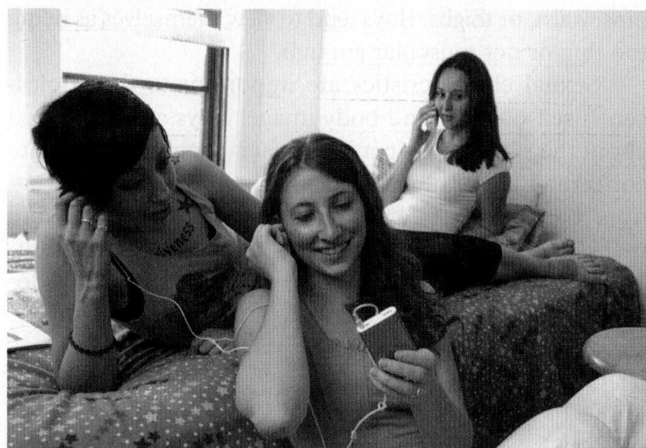

● Figure 8.5 Peers play an important role in shaping the adolescent's identity.

Adolescents usually begin experimentation with heterosexual and homosexual behaviors, although these behaviors may occur earlier in some cultures.

An interest in the opposite sex occurs during adolescence (Fig. 8.6). Some of the reasons cited for this developing interest are physical development and body changes, peer-group pressure, and curiosity. During the past several decades, the age of beginning to date in the United States has dropped. Girls are between 14 and 15 years old, and boys are 15 to 16 years old. Teen dating can range from group dating to single dating to serious relationships. Most early adolescents spend more time in activities with mixed-sex groups, such as dances and parties, than they do dating as a couple. Popular dating activities today include going out to dinner or the movies, "hanging out" at the mall, or visiting each other's home. During this period of early adolescence, teens tend to date for fun and recreation. Also, they may see dating as a way to upgrade social standing by being seen with a popular boy or an attractive girl.

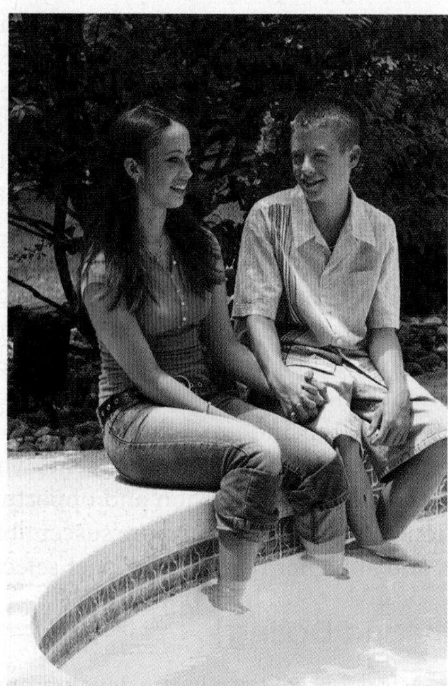

● Figure 8.6 Dating becomes an important aspect of the teenager's life.

Middle and late adolescents have group and single dates. Teens in the 10th through 12th grades are less likely to date at all than a decade ago. Dating or spending time with a potential romantic partner is viewed as a major developmental marker for teens and is one of the most challenging adjustments. Teens who date frequently report more depression and lower levels of autonomy, and experience a higher level of parental conflict even though they have been found to have higher levels of self-esteem and are classified as more popular.

The percentage of teens who date one or more times per week increases with age from 8% among 8th graders, to 15% of 10th grade students, to 29% of 12th grade students (Furman, 2002). Trends in dating are changing, but dating remains a developmental milestone for the adolescent.

Homosexual behavior as a teen does not necessarily indicate that the adolescent will maintain a homosexual orientation. Gay and lesbian adolescents face many challenges due to society's nonacceptance and peer insensitivity. Teens who self-declare as homosexual during high school are at increased risk for such problems as suicide, victimization, risky sexual behaviors, and substance abuse (www.advocatesforyouth.org/glbtq.htm).

Of greatest concern to parents during the adolescent period of developing sexuality and dating are unwanted pregnancy, sexually transmitted infections (STIs), and teen feelings of despair over failed relationships. Many times adolescents are not worried about negative consequences of sexual activity and believe "it will not happen to me."

> **Cho Chung's mother** states that she is concerned about the changes that have occurred in her and Cho's relationship over the past year. Cho seems much more self-centered, always wants to be with her friends, is very critical of her mother and father and seems to be constantly in conflict with them. Based on what you know about this stage of development, what guidance, including approaches and techniques, can you discuss with Mrs. Chung to address her concerns?

● CULTURAL INFLUENCES ON GROWTH AND DEVELOPMENT

Although the adolescent's culture continues to influence the teenager, the desire to be in harmony with peers becomes paramount. That desire can cause conflict with his family and culture. Today's adolescents live in a rapidly changing, increasingly culturally diverse world. They are exposed to many different cultures and ethnic groups. By 2020, about 40% of children and adolescents in the United States will be minorities (Federal Interagency Forum on Child and Family Statistics, 1997).

Attitudes regarding adolescence vary among different cultures. Certain cultures may have more permissive attitudes toward issues facing adolescents, while others are more conservative, for example towards sexuality. Experiencing a rite of passage ceremony to signal the adolescent's movement to adult status varies among cultures. The American culture does not universally have a rite of passage for teenagers. Some religious and social groups do have ceremonies that signal a movement toward the maturity of adulthood, for example, the Jewish bar or bat mitzvah, the Catholic confirmation, and social debuts. In many parts of the world, separate "youth cultures" have developed in an attempt to blend traditional and modern worlds for the adolescent.

It is important for the nurse to recognize the ethnic background of each client. Research has shown that certain ethnic groups are at higher risk for certain diseases. Adolescent African-Americans are at higher risk for developing hypertension. But the major barrier to the adolescent's health and successful achievement of the tasks of adolescence is socioeconomic status. Adolescents at a lower socioeconomic level are at higher risk for developing health care problems and risk-taking behaviors; this may be due to their inability to access health care and to obtain needed services. In caring for adolescents, recognize the influence of their culture, ethnicity, and socioeconomic level upon them.

The Nurse's Role in Adolescent Growth and Development

During adolescence, the teenager faces many challenges. His or her fluctuating relationships with parents and other adult figures may limit him or her from seeking assistance in dealing with the common issues of adolescence. In dealing with adolescents, be aware that they have unpredictable behaviors, are inconsistent with their need for independence, have sensitive feelings, may interpret situations different from what they are, think friends are extremely important, and have a strong desire to belong. The following Nursing Process Overview will address promoting healthy growth and development and dealing with common developmental concerns.

• NURSING PROCESS OVERVIEW

Upon completion of assessment of the adolescent's current growth and development status, problems or issues related to growth and development may be identified. The nurse may then identify one or more nursing diagnoses, including:

- Risk for disproportionate growth
- Imbalanced nutrition: more than body requirements
- Delayed growth and development
- Risk for caregiver role strain
- Risk for injury
- Ineffective coping

Nursing care planning for the adolescent with growth and development issues should be individualized based on the adolescent's and family's needs. Nursing Care Plan 8.1 can be used as a guide in planning nursing care for the adolescent with a growth and development concern. The nurse may choose the appropriate nursing diagnoses from this plan and individualize them as needed. The nursing care plan is intended to serve as a guide, not to be an all-inclusive growth and development care plan.

• PROMOTING HEALTHY GROWTH AND DEVELOPMENT

WATCH & LEARN

It takes multiple groups who address multiple issues to promote healthy growth and development in the adolescent. Some of these groups include sports teams in the school or the community, peers, teachers, band and choir members, and so forth. Also, the family's support and love will influence growth and development.

Promoting Growth and Development Through Sports and Physical Fitness

Many adolescents are involved in team sports that provide avenues for exercise. Adolescents probably spend more time and energy participating in sports than any other age group. Participation in sports contributes to the adolescent's development, educational process, and better health. Sports and games provide an opportunity to interact with peers while enjoying socially accepted stimulation and conflict. Competition in sports activities helps the teenager in processing self-appraisal and in developing self-respect and concern for others. Every sport has some potential for injury. Rapidly growing bones, muscles, joints, and tendons are more vulnerable to unusual strains and fractures. The American Academy of Pediatrics (2006) encourages sports participation by young persons and encourages parents and coaches to be aware of early warning signs of fatigue, dehydration, and injury. See Chapter 24 for a discussion of sports injuries.

Nationwide, approximately two thirds of students participated in physical activities that made them sweat and breathe hard at least 3 out of the past 7 days. Males were

(text continues on page 196)

Nursing Care Plan 8.1

Growth and Development of the Adolescent

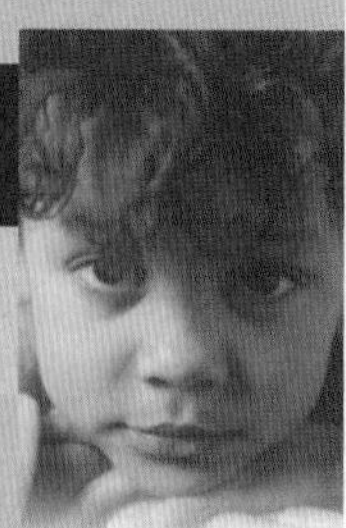

Nursing Diagnosis: Risk for disproportionate growth (risk factors: caregiver and adolescent knowledge deficit, low self-esteem, frequent illnesses)

Outcome identification and evaluation

Adolescent will demonstrate adequate growth: *appropriate weight gain for age and sex*

Intervention: promoting appropriate physical growth

- Assess parents' and adolescent's knowledge of nutritional needs of adolescents *to determine need for further education.*
- Educate parents and adolescent about appropriate serving sizes and foods *so that they are aware of what to expect for adolescents.*
- Determine need for additional caloric intake if necessary *(if very active in sports, if have a chronic illness).*
- Plot out height, weight, and body mass index (BMI) *to detect possible pattern.*
- Assess for risk factors for developing eating disorder *to refer to if needed and plan interventions.*

Nursing Diagnosis: Nutrition, more than body requirements, imbalanced, related to lack of exercise, increased caloric intake, poor food choices, and stresses of adolescence

Outcome identification and evaluation

Adolescent will lose weight at an appropriate rate: *increase amount of exercise, make appropriate eating choices, decrease caloric intake to appropriate amount for age and sex*

Intervention: promoting appropriate nutrition

- Assess knowledge of parents and adolescent about nutritional needs of teenagers *to determine deficits in knowledge.*
- Have adolescent keep a detailed food and exercise diary for 1 week *to determine current patterns of eating and exercise.*
- Interview family in relationship to their eating habits and exercise habits *to determine where adjustments might need to be made.*
- Discuss changes in a positive manner—talk about developing healthy eating habits instead of dieting *to promote compliance.*
- Analyze preceding data, and base recommendations for changes on these data *to promote compliance and to prioritize recommendations.*
- Discuss ways to decrease temptation to overeat, for example, eat slowly, put down the fork between bites, serve food on smaller plates, and count mouthfuls *to allow time to realize that you are full.*
- Have adolescent create meal plans and grocery shop *to allow him or her some sense of control and decision-making.*
- Incorporate increase in daily exercise, which will stress sense of self-improvement to *increase caloric expenditure and self-esteem.*
- Decrease TV/computer time *to increase caloric expenditure.*
- Encourage peer exercise activities *to increase peer interactions and to realize that others are like him or her.*
- Develop reward system *to increase self-esteem.*
- Investigate joining weight loss program for adolescents *to increase self-esteem and to increase awareness that other adolescents have the same problem.*

Growth and Development of the Adolescent (continued)

Nursing Diagnosis: Growth and development, delayed, related to speech, motor, psychosocial, or cognitive concerns as evidenced by delay in meeting expected school performances

Outcome identification and evaluation

Development will be maximized: *Adolescent will make continued progress toward attainment of expected school performance.*

Interventions: promoting growth and development

- Perform scheduled evaluation of the adolescent by school and health care provider *to determine current functioning.*
- Develop realistic multidisciplinary plan *to ensure maximizing resources.*
- Carry out interventions as prescribed by developmental specialist, physical therapist, occupational therapist, or speech therapist at home and at school *to maximize benefit of interventions.*
- Have scheduled evaluation meetings *to be able to adapt interventions as soon as possible.*

Nursing Diagnosis: Caregiver role strain, risk for (risk factors: knowledge deficit about adolescent issues, lack of prior exposure, fatigue, ill or developmentally delayed child)

Outcome identification and evaluation

Parent will experience competence in role: *will demonstrate appropriate caretaking behaviors and verbalize comfort in caring for an adolescent*

Interventions: preventing caregiver role strain

- Assess parent's knowledge of adolescents and the issues that arise as a part of normal development *to determine parent's needs.*
- Provide education on normal issues of adolescence *so that parents are armed with the knowledge they need to appropriately care for their adolescents.*
- Provide anticipatory guidance related to upcoming expected issues related to adolescent development *to prepare parents for what to expect next and how to intervene in an appropriate manner.*

Nursing Diagnosis: Injury, risk for (risk factors: increased motor and cognitive skills and feeling of invincibility)

Outcome identification and evaluation

Adolescent's safety will be maintained: *will remain free from injury*

Interventions: preventing injury

- Discuss safety measures needed for the following: bikes, scooters, guns, skateboards, cars, and water *to decrease risk of injury related to those areas.*
- Discuss and develop a fire safety plan *to decrease risk of injury related to fire.*
- Discuss appropriate safety equipment needed for each sport *to decrease risk of injury.*
- Discuss appropriate sports to participate in depending upon age, sex, and maturity of adolescent *to prevent possible injury.*
- Teach parents and adolescent first-aid measures and cardiopulmonary resuscitation (CPR) *to minimize consequences of injury should it occur.*
- Discuss influence of peers upon actions of adolescents *to prevent possible injury due to mimicking behavior.*

(continued)

Growth and Development of the Adolescent (continued)

Nursing Diagnosis: Coping, ineffective, for coping with normal stress of adolescence (risk factors: low self-esteem, poor relationship with parents and peers, participating in risk-taking behaviors)

Outcome identification and evaluation

Adolescent will demonstrate adequate coping abilities *as evident by management of stress of adolescence and no evidence of participating in risk-taking behaviors.*

Interventions: promoting effective coping

- Assess adolescent's knowledge of normal stress facing teenagers *to determine current knowledge.*
- Assess adolescent's present coping skills *to determine areas for improvement/support.*
- Encourage parents to accept teenager as a unique individual.
- Discuss with parents and adolescent normal developmental issues facing teens *to give them knowledge needed to cope.*
- Provide different situations the teen might be faced with and different solutions.
- Develop with adolescent different solutions to problems.
- Allow for increasing independence and opportunities to solve own problems.
- Encourage development of friends with same values.
- Parents provide unconditional love.
- Assess for any evidence of any risk-taking behaviors (drugs, smoking, suicide).

more likely to participate in vigorous exercises than females (Centers for Disease Control and Prevention [CDC], 20006c). High levels of physical activity may reduce cardiovascular disease risk factors during adolescence.

In relation to youth sports, the role of the nurse is to educate to prevent injuries (Fig. 8.7). This education should include discouraging participation when the teen is tired or has an existing injury.

Adolescence is a good time to develop an exercise program, with aerobic exercise at least 30 minutes per day, four times per week. Nurses should encourage all adolescents to be physically active daily or at least four times per week.

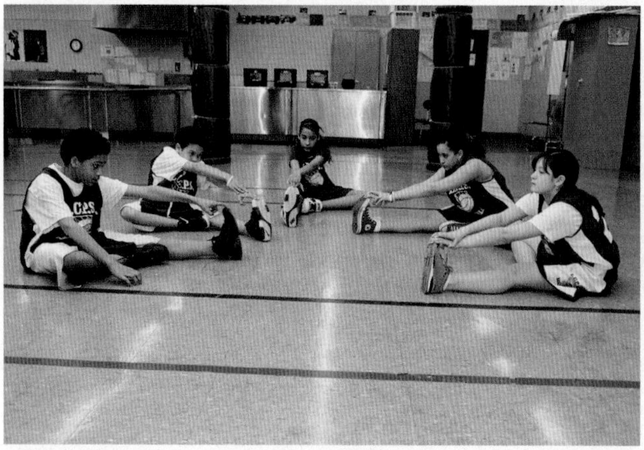

● Figure 8.7 Stretching before exercise is an important part of exercise.

Promoting Learning

School, teachers, family, and peers influence education and learning for the adolescent. Also, activities such athletics and club membership enhance learning through interactions with peers, coaches, club leaders, and others.

School

School plays an essential part in preparing adolescents for the future. Completing school prepares the adolescent for college or employment to make an adequate income. Schools in the United States may not meet the developmental needs of all adolescents. Minority students may not be at the appropriate grade level and the dropout rate may be higher than in nonminority students (Hockenberry, 2004). Dropout rates are highest among Hispanic and American Indian students. Another influencing factor is a lack of parental involvement. Due to single parent families and both parents being in the work force, parents have less time to devote to involvement in their child's school activities.

There is evidence that the transition from elementary school to middle school at age 12 or 13, and then the transition to high school, both occur at the time of physical changes, which may have a negative effect on teens. It is important to observe for transition problems into middle or high school, which may be exhibited by failing grades or behavior problems. Also, students who experience difficulties in school, resulting in negative evaluations and failing grades, may feel alienated from school. Students with failing grades and those repeating grades exhibit more emotional behavior and are more likely to engage in risky behaviors such as tobacco and alcohol use. In 2003, 9% of adolescent boys and 3% of adolescent girls reported carrying a weapon to school (CDC, 2004c). Schools that support peer-group relationships, promote health and fitness, encourage parental involvement, and strengthen community relationships have better student outcomes. Parents, teachers, and health care providers should provide guidance and support.

Other Activities

Adolescents are involved in many other activities that influence learning. Some of these activities include: (1) school activities such as band, choir, or clubs requiring high achievement; (2) athletic activities in the school and community and sometimes in the state or region; (3) art, sewing, and building classes; and (4) work activities when the late adolescent may have a part-time job.

Promoting Safety

Unintentional and intentional injuries are the leading causes of death in persons in the United States under 35 years of age (Minoño, Heron, & Smith, 2006). "At least one adolescent (10 to 19 years of age) dies of an injury every hour of every day," resulting in about 15,000 such deaths each year. Injuries kill more adolescents than all diseases combined. Unintentional injury accounts for about 60% of adolescent injury deaths, while violence (homicide and suicide) accounts for the remaining 40%. Males are more likely than females to die of any type of injury (www.cdc.gov, 2004).

HEALTHY PEOPLE 2010

Objective	Significance
Increase high-school completion.	• Encourage school attendance and completion when encountering teens for well-child or sick visits. • Refer children who have difficulty concentrating or learning for further evaluation. • Praise school accomplishments.

Influencing factors related to the prevalence of adolescent injuries include increased physical growth; insufficient psychomotor coordination for the task; abundance of energy; impulsivity; peer pressure; and inexperience. Impulsivity, inexperience, and peer pressure may place the teen in a vulnerable situation between knowing what is right and wanting to impress peers. On the other hand, teens have a feeling of invulnerability, which may contribute to negative outcomes. Alcohol and other drugs are contributing factors in automobile and firearm accidents among adolescents. Most of the serious or fatal injuries in adolescents are preventable (Fig. 8.8). Nurses must educate parents and adolescents on car, gun, and water safety to prevent unintentional injuries. See Teaching Guideline 8.1 for information on promoting safety.

Motor Vehicle Safety

The largest numbers of adolescent injuries are due to motor vehicle crashes. When the adolescent passes his or her driving test, he or she is able to drive legally. However, driving is complex and requires judgments that the teen is often incapable of exhibiting. Also, the typical adolescent is opposed to authority and is interested in showing peers and others his or her independence. The Youth Risk Behavior Surveillance Survey of high school students found that 16.4% had rarely worn seat belts, and over 33% had ridden with a driver who was drinking alcohol. Adolescents who

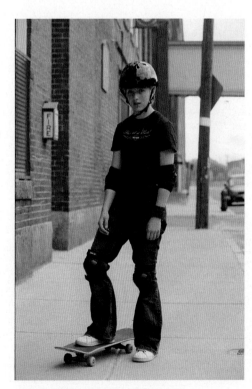

● Figure 8.8 Wearing appropriate safety equipment can prevent injuries.

drive after drinking are more likely than adults to have a crash. Adolescents are also vulnerable to crashes at night. Adolescents do most of their driving at night and have over 50% of their accidents then. Adolescents also cause a disproportionate number of deaths among other passengers and pedestrians (National Highway Traffic Safety Association, n.d.).

It is essential to promote driver education, to teach about the importance of wearing seat belts, and to explain laws about teen driving and curfews (Fig. 8.9). See Teaching Guideline 8.1 for additional information.

Firearm Safety

The risk of dying from a firearm injury among 15- to 19-year-olds has increased by 77% since 1985. In this age group, a firearm causes one in four deaths. Provide education about gun safety. Guns in the home must be kept and locked in a safe location, with ammunition kept separately. Parents must teach adolescents about the dangers of playing with firearms. See Teaching Guideline 8.1 for additional information on gun safety.

Water Safety

Drowning is a needless cause of death in adolescents. Many drownings are a result of risk-taking behaviors. With the independence of the adolescent, many times adult supervision is not prevalent and the teen takes a dare that results in drowning. Provide water safety education and proper supervision to decrease the incidence of risk taking. Teach about swimming lessons for nonswimmers. See Teaching Guideline 8.1 for additional information.

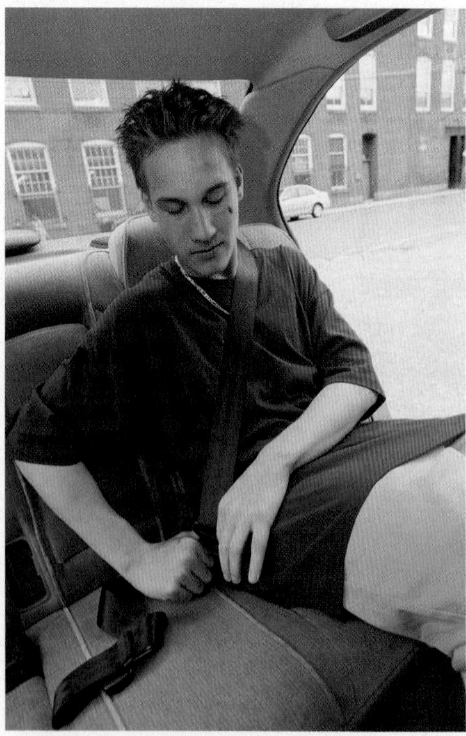

● Figure 8.9 The use of seat belts has led to fewer fatal injuries in car accidents.

Remember Cho Chung, the 15-year-old presented at the beginning of the chapter? What anticipatory guidance related to safety should you provide to Cho and her mother?

Promoting Nutrition

Nutritional needs are increased during adolescence due to accelerated growth and sexual maturation. Adolescents may appear to be hungry constantly and need regular meals and snacks with adequate nutrients to meet the body's anaerobic requirements. Multiple factors influence the adolescent's diet and eating habits (Box 8.2). According to Centers for Disease Control and Prevention (CDC) data, 67% of children between 6 and 19 years of age exceed the dietary guidelines recommended for fat intake; 72% exceed recommendations for saturated fat; and only 21% of high school students eat the five recommended daily servings of fruits and vegetables. Due to this, over 9 million children and adolescents are overweight. In 6- to 11-year-olds, the number of children who are overweight has doubled in the past 20 years. In 12- to 19-year-olds, the obesity rate has tripled over the same period of time (National Center for Health Statistics, 2004).

Nutritional Needs

Teenagers have a need for increased calories, zinc, calcium, and iron for growth. However, the number of calories needed for adolescence depends on the teen's age and activity level as well as growth patterns. Teenage girls who are active require about 2,200 calories per day. Teenage boys who are active require between 2,500 and 3,000 calories per day. Adolescents require about 1,200 to 1,500 milligrams of calcium each day. Adolescents should be made aware of foods high in calcium, including milk, white beans, broccoli, cheese, and yogurt. Adolescent males require 12 milligrams of iron each day and females require 15 milligrams each day. Advise adolescents about foods high in iron (see Box 8.3 and Healthy People 2010). Protein requirements for adolescent girls are 46 grams per day, and 45 to 59 grams for boys. Some foods high in protein are meats, fish, poultry, beans, and dairy products.

Nutritional Assessment

The nurse must understand normal growth and development of the adolescent in order to provide guidance that fits the quest for independence and the need to for teens make their own choices. Assess the eating habits and diet preferences of the adolescent. The assessment should

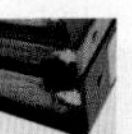

TEACHING GUIDELINE 8.1

Promoting Safety

Safety Issue	Activities
Motor vehicle	• Wear seat belt at all times. • Do not drive with someone who is impaired. • Take driver-education course. • Establish driving rules between parent and adolescent prior to getting license. • Have all passengers wear seat belts. • Do not use cell phone while driving. • Do not drink and drive. • Maintain car in good condition. • Do not drive when tired. • Drive with adult supervision for period of time after receiving license.
Bike: General	• Have a well-maintained and appropriate-size bike for adolescent. • Parents should orient the adolescent to the bike. • Adolescent should demonstrate his or her ability to ride bike safely before being allowed to ride on street. • Safe areas for bike riding should be established as well as routes to and from area of activities. • Should not ride bike barefoot, with someone else on bike, or with clothing that might get entangled in the bike • Should wear sturdy, well-fitting shoes • Should wear ANSI-approved helmets • Bike should be inspected often to ensure it is in proper working order. • A basket should be used to carry heavy objects.
Bike: in traffic	• All traffic signs and signals must be observed. • If riding at night, the bike should have lights and reflectors and the rider should wear light-colored clothes • Should ride on the side of the road traveling with traffic • Should keep close to the side of the road and in single file • Should watch and listen for cars • Should not wear headphones while riding a bike • Never hitch a ride on any vehicles.
All-terrain vehicles	• Should not be operated by adolescent less than 16 years of age • Should wear helmet and protective coverings • No nighttime riding • Should not be used on public roads • Should not stand up in the vehicle or ride in a person's lap • Should not drive if drinking or using drugs
Skateboards/Skates	• Should wear helmet, and protective padding on knees, elbows, and wrists • Should not skate in traffic or on streets or highways • Skating on homemade ramps could be dangerous—should assess ramps for any hazards before skating.
Water safety	• Learn how to swim. • If swimming skill is limited, must wear life preserver at all times • Never swim alone—should if at all possible, swim only where there is a life guard • Should be taught basic cardiopulmonary resuscitation (CPR) • Should not run or fool around at edge of pool • Drains in pool should be covered with appropriate cover. • Should wear life jacket when on boat • Make sure there is enough water to support diving. • Should not swim if drinking alcohol or using drugs

(continued)

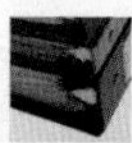

TEACHING GUIDELINE 8.1 (Continued)

Promoting Safety

Safety Issue	Activities
Firearms	• Should never pick up a gun • If guns are in household, should take firearm safety class • If have guns in household, need to secure them in safe place, use gun safety locks, store bullets in separate place • Never point a gun at a person.
Fire safety	• All homes should have working smoke detectors and fire extinguishers. Change the batteries at least twice a year. • Should have fire-escape plan • Should practice fire-escape plan routinely • Nobody should smoke in bed. • Should teach what to do in case of a fire: use fire extinguisher, call 911, and how to put out clothing fire • All flammable materials and liquids should be stored safely. • Fireplaces should have protective gratings. • Avoid touching any downed power lines.
Machinery	• Use safety devices. • Receive training on how to use equipment. • Do not use when alone.
Sports	• Match sport to adolescent's ability and desire. • Sports program should have warm-up procedure and hydration policy. • Should undergo sports physical before start of activity • Coaches should be trained in CPR and first aid. • Should wear appropriate protection devices for individual sport
Sun	• Use of sunscreen with both ultraviolet A (UVA) and ultraviolet B (UVB) protection • Apply sunscreen prior to going out. • Reapply sunscreen often. • Limit sun exposure, especially between 10 a.m. and 2 p.m. • Wear hat when working outside. • Wear sunglasses while outside.
Personal safety	• Never go with a stranger. • Do not enter a car when the driver has been drinking. • Notify adult where you are when out after dark. • Keep cell phone fully charged. • Never give out personal information over the Internet. • Say "no" to drugs, alcohol, smoking, or to being touched when you do not want to be touched.
Toxins	• Teach the hazards of accepting illegal drugs, alcohol, dangerous drugs. • Store potential dangerous material in safe place.

BOX 8.2

FACTORS INFLUENCING THE ADOLESCENT'S DIET

- Peer pressure
- Busy schedules
- Concern about weight control
- Convenience of fast food

include an evaluation of foods from the different food groups that the adolescent eats each day. Also, assess the number of times that fast foods, snacks, and other junk food are eaten per week. This assessment will help the nurse to guide the adolescent in making better food choices at home and in fast-food establishments. Many fast-food restaurants offer baked chicken sandwiches and salads with fewer calories and less fat. Adolescents may be guided in alternating hamburger and fries with more

BOX 8.3

FOODS HIGH IN IRON

- Beef, chicken, fish
- Liver
- Peanut butter
- Nuts and seeds
- Green peas, lima beans
- Spinach
- Strawberries
- Tomato juice
- Whole-grain bread
- Raisins
- Watermelon

nutritious choices. Remember that planning should always include the adolescent.

Nutritional Guidelines

The official U.S. dietary guidelines are based on the Food Guide Pyramid (see Appendix C). This pyramid, designed by the U.S. Department of Agriculture, illustrates a healthy, balanced diet with recommendations for eating foods from the main food groups each day with the exception of fats, oils, and sweets. Table 8.3 outlines daily serving recommendations based on caloric requirements (lower, moderate, or higher). Nurses may use the information in Table 8.3 to help teens plan a healthy diet for themselves. Active teenage girls should eat the number of servings recommended in the "Moderate" column of Table 8.3. Active teenage boys should eat the number of servings recommended in the "Higher" column. Adolescents who are overweight and dieting should base their daily intake on the serving recommendations in the "Lower" column.

What questions should you ask Cho Chung and her mother related to nutritional intake? What anticipatory guidance related to nutrition would be appropriate?

HEALTHY PEOPLE 2010

Objective	Significance
Reduce iron deficiency among young children and females of childbearing age.	• Educate parents and teens about iron-containing foods. • Encourage adolescent females to consume a diet high in iron-rich foods.

Promoting Healthy Sleep and Rest

The average number of hours of sleep that teens require per night is 8. On the weekends, they may sleep 10 to 12 hours per night. Adolescents may stay up later at night and, if they do this during the week, they may have difficulty awakening in the morning. Explain to parents the need to discourage late hours on school nights because it may affect school performance. In this independence-seeking phase of adolescence, the teen may stay up later to do homework or to complete projects. Rapid growth and increased activities may produce fatigue and the need for more rest. Parents may relate that the teen sleeps all the time and never has the time or energy to help with household chores. Provide advice to teens and parents about having realistic expectations; encourage them to agree on a level of normalcy and adequate rest for the teen so that he or she can still fulfill responsibilities in the home.

Provide anticipatory guidance to Cho Chung and her mother in relation to sleep during the adolescent years.

Promoting Healthy Teeth and Gums

Most permanent teeth have erupted with the possible exception of the third molars (wisdom teeth). These molars may become impacted and require surgical removal. The rate of cavities decreases but the need for routine dental visits every 6 months and brushing two to three times per day is very important. Some of the conditions that occur during adolescence include malocclusion, gingivitis, and tooth evulsion. Malocclusion occurs in approximately 50% of adolescents, resulting from facial and mandibular bone growth. The treatment includes braces and other dental devices. Teach the adolescent to brush the teeth more frequently if he or she has braces or other dental devices. Gingivitis is the inflammation of the gums and breakdown of gingival epithelium due to diet and hormonal changes. The use of dental devices/braces makes cleaning more difficult and contributes to gingivitis. Tooth evulsion (knocked-out teeth) may occur during sports and other activities such as falls. The evulsed tooth should be reimplanted as soon as possible. The nurse may see the teen first so it is important that nurses know the proper procedure, which is to reinsert the tooth into its socket if possible or to store it in cool milk or normal saline for transport to the dentist.

Promoting Personal Care

Promotion of personal care during adolescence is an important topic to cover with the adolescent and his or her parents. Topics to discuss include general hygiene tips, caring for body piercings and tattoos, preventing suntanning, and promoting a healthy sexual identity.

Table 8.3 Sample Diet for Three Caloric Levels

Calories for Three Caloric Levels	Lower (About 1,600 Calories)	Moderate (About 2,200 Calories)	Higher (About 2,800 Calories)
Grain group servings	6	9	11
Vegetable group servings	3	4	5
Fruit group servings	2	3	4
Milk group servings	2–3	2–3	2–3
Meat group (ounces)	5	6	7

General Hygiene Tips

Adolescents find that frequent baths and deodorant use are important due to apocrine sweat gland secretory activity. Also, to decrease oily skin due to sexual steroids and hormones, the adolescent should be told to wash his or her face two to three times per day with plain unscented soap. Vigorous scrubbing should be discouraged because it could irritate the skin and lead to follicular rupture. The hair should be shampooed daily to remove excess oil from the hair and scalp. Many over-the-counter medications are available for beginning acne or acne with a few lesions. These preparations may cause drying or redness. Squeezing acne lesions should be discouraged to prevent further irritation and permanent scarring. If the adolescent has severe acne, encourage him or her to ask a parent to make an appointment with a dermatologist.

Caring for Body Piercings and Tattoos

Today, body piercing on the tongue, lip, eyebrow, navel, and nipple is common (Fig. 8.10). Other sites such as the genitals, chin cleft, knuckles, and even the uvula have been used. Generally, body piercing is harmless, but nurses should caution teens about performing these procedures under nonsterile conditions and should educate them about complications. Qualified personnel using sterile needles should perform the procedure. Teach the adolescent to cleanse the pierced area twice a day and more often at some sites.

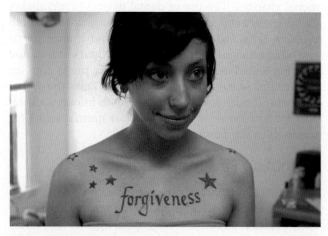

● **Figure 8.10** Having multiple piercings and tattoos can lead to certain health risks.

The complications of body piercing vary by site. Infections from body piercing usually result from unclean tools of the trade. Some of the infections that may occur as a result of unclean tools include hepatitis, tetanus, tuberculosis, and human immunodeficiency virus (HIV). Also, keloid formation and allergies to metal may occur. The navel is an area prone to infection because it is a moist area that endures friction from clothing. After a navel infection occurs, it may take up to a year to heal. Pierced ear cartilage also heals slowly and is prone to infection. Tongue piercings heal very quickly, usually within 4 weeks, probably due to the antiseptic effects of saliva. Other concerns with tongue piercing include tooth damage from biting on the jewelry or partial paralysis if the jewelry pierces a nerve.

Tattoos are becoming more popular among adolescents and are not necessarily a mark of gang membership. Tattoos serve to define one's identity (see Fig. 8.10). Because of the invasiveness of the tattooing procedure, it should be considered a health-risk situation. Like piercings, tattoos are open wounds predisposing to infection (www.cdc.gov/ncidod/diseases/hepatitis/c/tattoo.htm).

Little regulation exists in the tattoo business, and nurses should educate adolescents about the risk of bloodborne infections, skin infections, and allergic reactions to dyes used in the tattoo process. Teach teens to cleanse tattoos with an antibacterial soap and water several times a day and to keep the area moist with an ointment to prevent scab formation. Refer to Box 8.4 for additional information about tattoos.

Preventing Suntanning

Suntanning is popular among adolescents and is influenced by the media, which promotes a link between tan skin and beauty. There is no such thing as a good tan.

BOX 8.4

WHAT ADOLESCENTS NEED TO KNOW ABOUT TATTOOING

- Infections occur as a result of nonsterile equipment used in the procedure.
- Tattoos are open wounds predisposing to infection; sites require proper care with antibacterial soap and water several times per day and application of ointment.
- For most people a tattoo is permanent; new procedures for removal are painful and expensive.

Most exposure to ultraviolet rays occurs during childhood and adolescence, thereby putting people at risk for the development of skin cancer. However, it is difficult to convince adolescents that tanning is harmful to their skin and puts them at risk for skin cancer later in life (see Healthy People 2010).

Educate teens about the benefits and effects of different sun protection products. Explain to them that sun damage and skin cancers can be prevented if sunscreens are used as directed on a regular basis. Encourage sunscreen or sunblock use for water sports, beach activities, and participation in outdoor sports. Also, make adolescents aware of allergies to some sunscreen products. See Teaching Guideline 8.1 for additional information.

Promoting a Healthy Sexual Identity

Encourage parents and teens to have sexuality discussions. In addition, nurses should ensure that adolescents have the knowledge, skills, and opportunities that enable them to make responsible decisions regarding sexual behaviors and sexual orientation. Education for the adolescent should include a discussion about media influences and the use of sexuality to promote products. This discussion should make the adolescent aware of the motives of the media and the need to be an individual and not be influenced by television, magazines, and other forms of advertisement. Encourage parents to be aware of who their adolescents are dating and where they go on their dates. Refer to Teaching Guideline 8.2 for information on counseling related to adolescent sexuality.

Promoting Appropriate Discipline

Adolescents naturally misbehave or do not follow the rules of the house, and parents must determine how to respond. Adolescents need to know the rules and expectations. After rules are established, parents must explain to the adolescent the consequences of breaking the rules.

Offer guidance to parents related to disciplining teens. The parent and the teen should collaborate on what the consequences will be if the rules are broken. Parents must acknowledge and offer reinforcement and support when the teen follows the rules. Consistency and predictability are the cornerstones of discipline, and praise is the most powerful reinforcer of learning.

● ADDRESSING COMMON DEVELOPMENTAL CONCERNS

Adolescence is a time of rapid growth and development with maturation of sexuality. The adolescent period begins with a child and ends with the expectation of adulthood. There are many developmental concerns that present during this period, including obesity, violence, suicide, and homicide. The following is an overview of some of these concerns.

HEALTHY PEOPLE 2010

Objective	Significance
Increase the proportion of persons who use at least one of the following protective measures that may reduce the risk of skin cancer: avoid the sun between 10 a.m. and 4 p.m., wear sun-protective clothing when exposed to sunlight, use sunscreen with a sun protection factor (SPF) of 15 or higher, and avoid artificial sources of ultraviolet light.	• Encourage female teens to use sunscreen-containing makeup. • Discourage teen use of tanning beds. • Remind students to use sunscreen during outdoor organized-sports practice. • Educate teens and families about the risks associated with sun exposure.

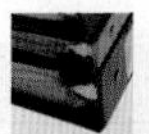

TEACHING GUIDELINE 8.2

Adolescent Sexuality

- It should be your choice to engage in sexual relations. Do not be influenced by peers. When you say "no," be firm and clear about your position.
- Pregnancy, sexually transmitted infections, and human immunodeficiency virus (HIV) infection can occur with any sexual encounter without the use of barrier methods of contraception. Use appropriate contraception if sexually active. Discuss abstinence as a contraceptive method.
- Sexual activity in a mature relationships should be pleasurable to both parties. If your sexual partner is not interested in your pleasure, you need to reconsider the relationship.

Obesity

Over 9 million children and adolescents in the United States are overweight. Over a 20-year time period, from 1980 to 2000, the number of overweight adolescents tripled from 5% to 15%. Although obesity has increased in all segments of the U.S. population, there are differences specific to race, ethnicity, and socioeconomic status. The prevalence of obesity is highest in Hispanic and African-American teens between the ages of 12 and 19 years. Obesity rates are higher in females and in adolescents of lower socioeconomic status.

This increase in obesity in adolescents has led to increases in hypertension, heart disease, and type 2 diabetes. Influential factors causing obesity include food choices, eating practices, and lack of exercise. A study indicated that only 75% to 78% of adolescents ages 11 to 19 eat breakfast. Also, less than 40% of adolescents ages 12 to 19 meet the daily dietary requirement of vegetables and fruits while exceeding the recommendation for saturated fats. Adolescents are busy and eat on the run with many meals from fast-food facilities. In addition, many schools have decreased or discontinued physical education, which has resulted in a more sedentary lifestyle leading to weight gain. Interest in computer games and television watching at home has decreased physical activity and exercise and further contributed to weight gain and obesity (see Healthy People 2010).

Nurses must make parents and adolescents aware of factors leading to obesity. Nurses should recommend:

- Proper nutrition and healthy food choices
- Good eating habits
- Decreased fast-food intake
- Exercising for 30 minutes at least four times per week
- Parents/adolescents exercising more at home
- Decreased computer use and television watching

HEALTHY PEOPLE 2010

Objective	Significance
Increase the proportion of adolescents who engage in moderate physical activity for at least 30 minutes on 5 or more of the previous 7 days, and vigorous physical activity that promotes cardiorespiratory fitness 3 or more days per week for 20 or more minutes per occasion.	• For the nonexercising teen, advise to start slowly by walking. • Work with the teen to identify physical activities that interest the teen. • Praise efforts to participate in a routine exercise plan. • Identify an athletic individual that the teen identifies with and encourage similar activities in the teen.

Violence

The CDC's Injury Center defines violence as threatened or actual physical force or power initiated by an individual that results in physical or psychological injury or death. More than 877,700 adolescents and young adults between 10 and 24 years of age were injured as a result of violence in 2002. Approximately 1 in 13 of these injuries resulted in hospitalization (http://www.cdc.gov/ncipc/factsheets/yvfacts.htm). The issue of youth violence is a growing concern in America's communities. The health and well-being of adolescents and society are threatened by this violence. See Box 8.5 for factors contributing to adolescent violence.

Homicide

Homicide is the fourth leading cause of death in children between 10 and 14 years old, and the second leading cause of death in 15- to 19-year-olds. Most young homicide victims are killed with guns. In 2003, 82% of homicide victims age 10 to 24 years were killed with firearms (CDC, 2006c). Refer to Box 8.5 for factors that contribute to violence among adolescents. In a nationwide survey conducted in 2004, 17% of students reported carrying a weapon on one or more days within the past 30 days (Grunbaum et al., 2004) (see Healthy People 2010).

Suicide

Suicide is the third leading cause of death in adolescents 15 to 19 years of age. In a CDC study in 2001, 19.3% of adolescents surveyed related that they had seriously considered suicide within the past 12 months. The rate of suicide among teens between 15 and 19 years old increased by 11% from 1980 to 1997, and by 10% in 10- to 14-year-olds in the same time period. In 1999, more teenagers and

BOX 8.5

FACTORS CONTRIBUTING TO ADOLESCENT VIOLENCE

- Crowded conditions/housing
- Low socioeconomic status
- Limited parental supervision
- Single parent families/both parents in workforce
- Access to guns or cars
- Drug or alcohol use
- Low self-esteem
- Racism
- Peer or gang pressure
- Aggression

HEALTHY PEOPLE 2010

Objective	Significance
Reduce homicides, physical fighting among adolescents, weapon carrying by adolescents on school property, rate of suicide attempts by adolescents.	• Screen teens at all encounters for indications of violent behaviors. • Provide education related to decreasing school violence at middle and high schools. • Encourage alternate, appropriate methods for dispelling anger. • Screen teens at all encounters for indications of depression.

young adults died from suicide than from cancer, heart disease, acquired immunodeficiency syndrome (AIDS), birth defects, stroke, and chronic lung disease combined (CDC, 2006d). Among adolescents ages 15 to 19, firearm-related suicides accounted for more than 60% of the increase in the overall suicide rate from 1980 to 1997 (see Healthy People 2010).

Dating Violence

Violent behavior that takes place in a context of dating or courtship is not a rare event. Research related to dating violence reveals that its incidence ranges from 9% to 65%. Data from a study of 8th and 9th grade male and female students indicated that 25% had experienced nonsexual dating violence and 8% experienced sexual dating violence. Females are victims of dating violence more often than males and suffer more injuries than males. The likelihood of becoming a victim of dating violence is associated with having female peers who have experienced sexual victimization; lower church attendance; acceptance of dating violence; and personal history of sexual assault (Domestic Violence and Sexual Assault Coalition, 2001).

Gangs

Much of youth violence is a result of the behavior of adolescent gangs. Nationwide there are an estimated 23,388 gangs with 664,906 members; approximately 3% are female. In one study, the risk factors for gang involvement were family, friends, neighborhood, and interpersonal issues. Peers are ranked as being most influential in female gang involvement, followed by neighborhood, family, and self. Gang membership may aid in the formation of identity by providing status and a sense of belonging. Gang membership occurs in cities and in suburban areas, but may differ in composition. The gangs in rural or suburban areas are more diverse racially and include both males and females. All socioeconomic groups are represented in gang membership. Gangs threaten and intimidate with violent behaviors and guns (Walker-Barnes & Arrue, 1998).

Nursing Interventions to Decrease Youth Violence

Nurses working with adolescents should include violence prevention in anticipatory guidance. Violence is a learned behavior. It is often reinforced by the media, television, music, and personal example. Explain to parents, teachers, and peers the importance of being good role models because violence is a learned behavior. Parents should monitor video games, music, television, and other media to decrease exposure to violence. Parents need to know who their adolescent's friends are and monitor for negative behaviors and actions.

The identification of adolescents at risk for suicide is a very important task for the nurse, parents, peers, and counselors. See Box 8.6 for signs of risk factors. The National Center for Injury Prevention and Control (NCIPC) is working to create awareness of suicide as a serious public health problem and is working on strategies to reduce injuries and deaths due to suicide.

Substance Use

Agents commonly abused by children and adolescents include alcohol, hallucinogens, sedatives, analgesics, anxiolytics, steroids, inhalants, and stimulants. The substance abused is related to its availability and cost. Two com-

BOX 8.6

RISK FACTORS FOR SUICIDE IN ADOLESCENTS

- Depression
- Mental health changes
- Poor school performance
- Family disorganization
- Substance abuse
- Homosexuality
- Giving away valued possessions
- Being a loner/having no close friends
- Changes in behavior

mon substances that are more accessible and have the highest incidence of use are tobacco and alcohol. Each day, approximately 4,000 young people under the age of 18 try their first cigarette; 80% of adult smokers started smoking before age 18. It is estimated that 90% of adolescents have tried alcohol by the time they reach adulthood. Research consistently supports the hypothesis that drug use progresses from beer or wine to cigarettes or hard liquor and then to marijuana, followed by illicit drugs.

Some of the long-term effects and consequences of drug and alcohol use include: possibility of overdose and death; unintentional injuries; irrational behaviors; inability to think clearly; unsafe driving and legal consequences; problems with relationships with family and friends; sexual activity and STIs; and health problems such as liver problems (hepatitis) and cardiac problems (sudden death with cocaine). Refer to Table 8.4 for commonly abused drugs and behaviors exhibited (see Healthy People 2010).

HEALTHY PEOPLE 2010

Objective	Significance
Reduce the proportion of adolescents who report that they rode, during the previous 30 days, with a driver who had been drinking alcohol. Reduce steroid use among adolescents. Increase the proportion of adolescents who disapprove of substance abuse and smoking.	• Provide education in the office, hospital, or school related to adverse effects of tobacco, alcohol, and illicit substance use. • Educate families, teens, and coaches about the negative effects of anabolic steroids. • Praise teens for abstaining from the above substances and rising above peer pressure.

Tobacco

Tobacco use remains the leading preventable cause of death in the United States, causing more than 440,000 deaths each year. Long-term consequences of youth smoking are reinforced by the fact that most young people who smoke regularly continue to smoke throughout adulthood. Each day in the United States, about 4,000 12- to 17-year-olds take their first cigarette. More than 6.4 million people will die prematurely because of smoking as adolescents. Although the overall rate of smoking has declined since 1999, rates still remain high: 22% of high-school students report current cigarette use. Seven percent of high-school students use smoke-

Table 8.4 Drugs Commonly Abused

Drug	Manifestations	Considerations
Marijuana	Red eyes, dry mouth, euphoria, relaxation, decreased motivation, loss of inhibition	Considered a gateway drug
Cocaine	Weight loss, euphoria, elation, agitation, pressured speech, tachycardia, hypertension, anorexia, insomnia	Psychotic behavior with large doses; if combined with other drugs can be fatal
Opiates	Elation, euphoria, detachment, drowsiness, constricted pupils, slurred speech, impaired judgment	Self-neglect with malnutrition and dehydration; criminal behaviors to get drugs; infections at injection sites
Amphetamines	Euphoria, agitation, weight loss, insomnia, tachycardia, hypertension	Possible paradoxical effect of depression in children
Hallucinogens	Hallucinations, illusions, depersonalization, heightened awareness, dilated pupils, hypertension, increased salivation, distorted perceptions	Panic flashbacks long after use of drugs; psychotic behaviors
Phencyclidine hydrochloride (PCP)	Euphoria, distorted perceptions, agitation, violence, antisocial behaviors, hypertension, increased salivation, increased pain response	Irrational behaviors, panic, psychosis
Barbiturates	Euphoria followed by depression or hostility; impaired judgment; decreased inhibitions; slurred speech; incoordination	Often used with stimulants; may have a paradoxical effect of hyperactivity in children

less tobacco (CDC, 2004a). Teens who smoke are three times more likely than nonsmokers to use alcohol, eight times more likely to use marijuana, and 22 times more likely to use cocaine. Smoking is associated with a host of other risky behaviors, including fighting and engaging in unprotected sex (www.focusas.com/SubstanceAbuse.html). The short-term health effects of smoking include damage to the respiratory system, addiction to nicotine, and the associated risk of other drug use. Smoking negatively impacts physical fitness and lung growth and increases the potential for addiction in adolescents. Smokeless tobacco may also cause many problems. It can lead to bleeding gums and sores in the mouth that never heal. Smokeless tobacco use leads to discoloration of the teeth and eventually may lead to cancer.

Alcohol

Studies conducted by the National Household Survey on Drug Abuse and the Youth Risk Behavior Survey found that the majority of adolescents under the age of 18 have consumed alcohol, although the legal drinking age is 21. According to the 2004 National Survey of Drug Use and Alcohol, 28.7% of adolescents reported alcohol drinking within the past month, with 20% being binge drinkers and over 6% heavy drinkers. The findings revealed that there were no substantial differences among various sociodemographic subgroups with respect to drinking rates, although alcohol use is lowest in African-Americans and highest in whites. The incidence of alcohol use increases throughout adolescence. Almost two thirds of 12th graders who report consuming alcohol also reported at least one alcohol-related problem. Some of the problems include impaired school performance or work performance; interpersonal problems with friends, family, teachers, and supervisors; physical and psychological impairment; and drunk driving. Alcohol use as an adolescent can lead to prevailing alcohol use as an adult and contribute to physical health problems. Many times alcohol use may precede other drug abuse. Development of more stringent laws and public policies related to curfews and driving help to deter adolescent alcohol use (Johnston, O'Malley, & Bachman, 2002; www.oas.samhsa.gov).

Illicit Drugs

Adolescents may also experiment with or abuse illicit drugs. Substance abuse remains a widespread problem among American adolescents. Although experimentation with marijuana has decreased between 1991 and 2003 among the adolescent population, it still remains the most widely used illicit drug (Eaton et al., 2006). In a 2002 survey, over 53% of adolescents were found to have tried illicit drugs by the time they had finished high school. Thirty-two percent had used inhalants as early as the 8th grade (Johnston et al., 2002).

In 2004, the rates of illicit drug use for adolescents 12 to 17 years of age varied according to race and ethnic groups. American Indian and Alaska Native youths had the highest percentage at 26%. The rate was at 12.2% for youths reporting two or more races. Other racial/ethnic groups were lower, with Asians being the lowest at 6% (www.oas.samhsa.gov).

Data reveal that illicit drug usage for individual drugs reflects rapidly changing determinants specific to that drug. Influencing factors include the psychoactive potential and benefits reported, how risky the drug is to use, how acceptable is it to peer groups, and the accessibility of the drug (Johnston et al., 2002).

Nursing Interventions to Decrease Substance Use Among Teens

Nurses should educate the adolescent on the problems related to alcohol use and abuse. Topics that should be discussed include:

- Short- and long-term effects of alcohol, tobacco, and drugs on health
- Risk factors and implications for unintentional injuries and sexual activity
- Short- and long-term effects of alcohol, tobacco, and drugs on relationships and school performance and progression
- The how and why of chemical dependency
- Impact of substance abuse on society
- Importance of maintaining a healthy lifestyle
- Importance of resisting peer pressure to use drugs and alcohol
- Importance of having confidence in his or her own judgement
- Providing the teen with accurate and up-to-date information (www.coaf.org/family/caregivers/avoid.htm)

Sexually Transmitted Infections and Teen Pregnancy

Most young adolescents have not had intercourse but the likelihood increases with age. The Youth Risk Behavior Surveillance System showed that 6.2% of adolescents had intercourse before 13 years of age, and 47% of all adolescents had been involved in sexual intercourse (CDC, 2006e). This survey found that only about one half of sexually active females used a condom the last time they had intercourse. Adolescence is a time of risk taking, with unprotected sex and multiple sex partners placing adolescents at risk for HIV infection, other STIs, and pregnancy.

Sexually Transmitted Infections

Each year there are four million cases of STIs among teenagers. In the United States, teens who are sexually active experience high rates of STIs. Some groups are at

HEALTHY PEOPLE 2010

Objective	Significance
Increase the proportion of adolescents who have never engaged in sexual intercourse before the age of 15 years. Increase the proportion of adolescents who have never engaged in sexual intercourse.	• Educate teens about the risks of sexually transmitted infections (STIs), human immunodeficiency virus (HIV), and pregnancy associated with sexual intercourse. • Compliment teens for choosing to "wait" to have sex.

higher risk, including African-American youth, abused youth, homeless youth, young men having sex with men (YMSM), and gay, lesbian, bisexual, and transgendered youth. Adolescents and young adults tend to think they are invincible and deny any risks involved in their behavior. This risky behavior exposes them to STIs and HIV/AIDS.

Some of the most prevalent STIs include chlamydia, gonorrhea, human papillomavirus (HPV), and herpes. Chlamydia rates in both males and females have increased over the past decade in 15- to 19-year-olds (Alford, 2003). Gonorrhea rates were higher among females 15 to 19 years old and men 20 to 24 years old. The gonorrhea rates in the United States are 10 times higher than in England and 74 times the rates in France and the Netherlands. Also, there are over one million new cases of genital herpes simplex virus 2 (HSV-2) each year in the United States. Genital HPV is the most common STI in the United States in sexually active youth.

Female adolescents are more susceptible to STIs due to their anatomy. During adolescence and young adulthood, women's columnar epithelial cells are especially sensitive to invasion by sexually transmitted organisms such as chlamydia and gonococcus. These cells extend out over the vaginal surface of the cervix, where they are unprotected by cervical mucus, but recede to a more protected location as women age. STIs will be covered in Chapter 16.

Approximately 25% of cases of STIs reported in the Unites States are among adolescents, which increases the risk of HIV transmission. The effects of HIV and AIDS on adolescents and young adults is of increasing concern, but difficult to get accurate data on, due to the varying ways this population seeks health care services. Some adolescents continue care through pediatricians and adult services, but many are without access to health care. HIV infections are increasing in adolescents and young adults (13 to 24 years). Also, the proportion of adolescents with the diagnosis of AIDS has increased from 3.9% in 1999 to 4.2% in 2004 (National Institute of Allergy and Infectious Diseases, 2006). At least one adolescent in the United States is infected with HIV each hour. Because it takes an average of 10 years for AIDS symptoms to appear when HIV is left untreated, it is obvious that many adults with AIDS were infected during their adolescent years.

Most HIV-infected adolescents are exposed to the virus though sexual intercourse. Recent data suggest that the majority of HIV-infected adolescent males are infected through sex with men. A small number of adolescent males appear to be exposed to the virus through injection of drugs or heterosexual contact. Adolescent females are mostly exposed through heterosexual contact, with a small percentage exposed through injected drug use (www.niaid.nih.gov/factsheets/hivadolescent.htm).

African-American and Hispanic adolescents between the ages of 13 and 19 accounted for 66% and 21%, respectively, of reported adolescent AIDS cases in 2003. Due to adolescents thinking they are invincible, they may delay testing; if they test positive, they may delay or refuse treatment. The inability to trace this population for medical care can lead to increased transmission of HIV. See Chapter 27 for more information on HIV and AIDS.

Health care providers may help these adolescents to understand their situation if:

- Confidentiality is ensured
- Information is explained clearly and at a level the adolescent understands
- Opportunities are provided for the adolescent to ask questions
- Success is emphasized with proper treatment and follow-up

Teen Pregnancy

Each year 860,000 teenage girls become pregnant (March of Dimes, 2006). Despite this incidence, teen births continue to decline, with the sharpest drop in births to African-American teens (CDC, 2003). According to the National Center for Health Statistics, teen births declined by 30% over the past decade and pregnancy in African-American teens was down by 40%. Teenage pregnancy is a source of social, economic, and political concern because of substantial evidence that early childbearing seriously jeopardizes the life chances (such as education, college, career success) of most young parents and their children. Studies suggest that approximately 50% of pregnant teenage girls give birth, 40% have abortions, and the remainder miscarry. Adolescents become pregnant for a variety of reasons (Box 8.7). Adolescents are more likely to produce a low birth weight infant, which increases the incidence of infant mortality, neurologic problems, and childhood illness. Additionally, adolescent mothers often drop

BOX 8.7

PSYCHOLOGICAL REASONS ADOLESCENTS BECOME PREGNANT

- Ambivalence
- 10% want to become pregnant
- 40% did not mind being pregnant
- Escape from home life
- Rite of passage to adulthood
- Peer pressure
- Confrontation of parental authority
- Ignorance

out of school. Over the past two decades, alternative schools with flexible hours and daycare have enabled adolescent parents to obtain an education, overcome economic barriers, and become productive members of society. Adolescents' ability to care for their children has been studied and discussed over the years. The adolescent's lack of experience with caring for children may lead to neglect and even abuse.

Nursing Interventions to Prevent STIs and Teen Pregnancy

Talk to adolescents about sexuality and encourage discussions with parents. Nurses need to be open and respectful of the teen's decision about sexual activity. If adolescents are sexually active, they should be directed to teen clinics and contraceptive options should be explained. In areas where specialized teen clinics are not available, nurses should feel comfortable discussing sexuality, safety, and contraception with teens. The adolescent's lack of abstract thinking may influence contraceptive practices, and feelings of invulnerability may lead to HIV, STIs, or unwanted pregnancies. Nurses in schools and community clinics are in a position to identify teens at risk for HIV, STIs, and pregnancy and to provide guidance, suitable information, and appropriate referrals. Nurses should provide education and information on abstinence, contraception, and the reality of caring for an infant (see Healthy People 2010). Abstinence is the only contraceptive method for complete protection from STIs and pregnancy. Most teens do not seek contraception for 1 year after first intercourse (American Academy of Pediatrics, 1999). Both males and females share the responsibility for birth control. If possible, it is best to meet with both partners when selecting a method of birth control. Refer to Table 8.5 for information about adolescent contraceptive methods. All adolescents require frequent ongoing follow-up to maintain contraception behaviors. If a teen pregnancy does occur, it is important to encourage continued participation in school, sports, and other activities.

> Think back to Cho, who was introduced at the beginning of the chapter. List common developmental concerns of the adolescent. What anticipatory guidance related to these concerns would you provide?

HEALTHY PEOPLE 2010

Objective	Significance
Reduce pregnancies among adolescent females. Increase the proportion of sexually active, unmarried adolescents age 15 to 17 years who use contraception that both effectively prevents pregnancy and provides barrier protection against disease. Increase the proportion of young adults who have received formal instruction before turning 18 years old on reproductive health issues, including all of the following topics: birth control methods, safer sex to prevent human immunodeficiency virus (HIV) infection, prevention of sexually transmitted disease, and abstinence. Reduce acquired immunodeficiency syndrome (AIDS) and the number of HIV infections among adolescents and adults. Reduce the proportion of adolescents and young adults with *Chlamydia trachomatis* infections.	• Provide confidential care to all adolescents. • Build trust to set tone for an accepting educational experience. • Never miss an opportunity to provide appropriate education related to avoidance of sexually transmitted infections (STIs) and HIV. • Provide appropriate education (particularly at well-child visits) about reproductive health. • Encourage condom use in the sexually active adolescent.

Table 8.5 Advantages and Disadvantages of Methods of Adolescent Contraception

Method	Advantages	Disadvantages
Abstinence	No cost Prevention of diseases	May be difficult in teens
Rhythm (no sex during ovulation)	No cost Natural family planning	High failure rate Requires education about fertility times Offers no protection against sexually transmitted infections (STIs)
Condom	Inexpensive/readily available Protects against STIs	Moderate failure rate Requires planning Requires new condom with each intercourse Best used with spermicides
Diaphragm	Some STI prevention Allows for planning after fitting and insertion	Requires consistent use Requires prescription Requires education
Spermicides	Readily available Effective if used with barrier method (condom)	High failure rate Messy Apply with each intercourse
Oral contraception (combination products suppress ovulation, increase thickness of cervical mucus, decrease thickness of uterine lining)	Protection from pregnancy if taken as directed Highly effective Allows for planning	Need prescription and medical visit Expensive for teens Adverse effects of medication include weight gain, bleeding Offers no protection against STIs
Depo-Provera (injectable) Suppresses ovulation for 14–16 weeks	Given every 3 months No estrogen; progestin only Can be used in lactating females	Delay in fertility when discontinued Adverse effects: heavy bleeding and irregular bleeding, weight gain, depression Offers no protection against STIs
Emergency contraceptive pills (combination estrogen and progestin taken within 72 hours and again 12 hours later)	Approximately 85% effective in preventing pregnancy	Should not be used as routine contraception Pregnancy test before and 3 weeks after taking Adverse effect: nausea Offers no protection against STIs

References

Adekoya, N., Thurman, D.J., White, D.D., & Webb, K.W. (2000). Surveillance for traumatic brain injury deaths—United States 1989-1998. *MMWR: Morbidity and Mortality Weekly Report, 51* (SS10), 1–16.

Advocates for Youth. (2001). *Gay, lesbian, bisexual transgender, and questioning (GLBTQ) youth.* Retrieved July 9, 2006 from http://www.advocatesforyouth.org/glbtq.htm.

Advocates for Youth. (2001). *HIV vaccines.* Retrieved July 9, 2006 from http://www.advocatesforyouth.org/hivvaccine.htm.

Alba-Fisch, M. (2000). *Temperament: miss or match.* Retrieved July 9, 2006 from http://www.taconicnet.com/temperament.htm.

Alford, S. (2003). *Adolescents: at risk for sexually transmitted infections.* Retrieved May 7, 2006 from www.advocatesforyouth.org.

American Academy of Pediatrics, Committee on Adolescence. (1999). Contraception and adolescents. *Pediatrics, 104* (5), 1161-1166.

American Academy of Pediatrics, Committee on Nutrition. (2003). Policy statement: prevention of overweight and obesity. *Pediatrics, 112* (2), 424-430.

American Academy of Pediatrics, Council on Sports Medicine and Fitness and Council on School Health. (2006). Active health living: prevention of childhood obesity through increased physical activity. *Pediatrics, 117,* 1834-1842.

Ball, J. W., & Bindler, R.C. (2006). *Child health nursing: Partnering with children and families.* Upper Saddle River, NJ: Prentice Hall.

Barakat, I.S., & Clark, J.A. (2005). *Positive discipline and child guidance.* Retrieved July 9, 2006 from http://muextension.missouri.edu/xplor/hesguide/humanrel/gh6119.htm.

Burstein, G.R., Lowry, R., Klein, J.D., & Santelli, J.S., (2003). Missed opportunities for sexually transmitted diseases, human immunodeficiency virus, and pregnancy prevention services during adolescent health supervision visits. *Pediatrics, 111*(Suppl. 1-1), 996-1001.

Centers for Disease Control and Prevention. (2000). *Unpowered scooter-related injuries: United States, 1998-2000.* Retrieved July 9, 2006 from http://www.cdc.gov/mmwr/preview/mmwrhtml/mm4949a2.htm.

Centers for Disease Control and Prevention. (2004a). Cigarette use among high school students: United States 1991-2003. *Morbidity and Mortality Weekly Report, 53*(52), 499-502.

Centers for Disease Control and Prevention. (2004b). Medical expenditures attributable to injuries in the United States: 2000. *Morbidity and Mortality Weekly Report, 53*(1), 1-4.

Centers for Disease Control and Prevention. (2004c). Violence-related behaviors among high school students: United States, 1991-2003. *Morbidity and Mortality Weekly, 53*(29), 651-655. Retrieved July 9, 2006 from http://www.cdc.gov/mmwr/preview/mmwrhtml/mm5329a1.htm#tab.

Centers for Disease Control and Prevention. (2005). *Physical activity and the health of young people: A report of the surgeon general, Atlanta, GA, DHHS.* Retrieved May 7, 2006 from http://www.cdc.gov/HealthyYouth/PhysicalActivity/.

Centers for Disease Control and Prevention. (2006). *CDC's position on tattooing and HCV infection.* Retrieved July 9, 2006 from http://www.cdc.gov/ncidod/diseases/hepatitis/c/tattoo.htm.

Centers for Disease Control and Prevention. (2006a). *Overweight and obesity: Health consequences.* Retrieved July 9, 2006 from http://www.cdc.gov/nccdphp/dnpa/obesity/consequences.htm.

Centers for Disease Control and Prevention. (2006b). *Tobacco use.* Retrieved July 9, 2006 from http://www.cdc.gov/HealthyYouth/tobacco/index.htm.

Centers for Disease Control and Prevention. (2006c). Youth risk behavior surveillance – United States, 2005. *Morbidity and Mortality Weekly Report, 55* (SS-5). Retrieved July 9, 2006 from http://www.cdc.gov/mmwr/PDF/SS/SS5505.pdf.

Centers for Disease Control and Prevention. National Center for Injury Prevention and Control. (2006d). *Suicide: Fact sheet.* Retrieved July 9, 2006 from http://www.cdc.gov/ncipc/factsheets/suifacts.htm.

Centers for Disease Control and Prevention. (2006e). *Youth online: Comprehensive results.* Retrieved July 9, 2006 from http://apps.nccd.cdc.gov/yrbss/CategoryQuestions.asp?Cat=4&desc=Sexual%20Behavior s.

Centers for Disease Control and Prevention, National Center for Injury Prevention and Control. (2006f). *Youth violence: Fact sheet.* Retrieved July 9, 2006 from http://www.cdc.gov/ncipc/factsheets/yvfacts.htm.

Child Trends. (2003). *Dating.* Retrieved July 9, 2006 from http://www.childtrendsdatabank.org/indicators/73dating.cfm.

Children of Alcoholics Foundation. (n.d.). *How to help kids avoid alcohol and other drugs.* Retrieved July 9, 2006 from http://www.coaf.org/family/caregivers/avoid.htm.

Cool Nurse. (2003). *Dating.* Retrieved July 9, 2006 from http://www.coolnurse.com/dating.htm.

Domestic Violence and Sexual Assault Coalition. (2001). *Facts and statistics on teen dating violence and sexual assault.* Retrieved July 9, 2006 from http://www.dvsac.org/prevparstats.html.

Eaton, D. K., Kann, L., Kinchen, S., Ross, J., et al. (2006). Youth risk behavior surveillance: United States, 2005. *Morbidity and Mortality Weekly, 55* (SS05), 1-108. Retrieved July 9, 2006 from http://www.cdc.gov/mmwr/preview/mmwrhtml/ss5505a1.htm.

Edelman, C.L., & Mandle, C.L. (2002). *Health promotion throughout the lifespan* (5th ed). St. Louis: Mosby.

Erikson, E. (1963). *Childhood and society* (2nd ed.). New York: Norton.

Federal Interagency Forum on Child and Family Statistics. (1997). *America's children: Key national indicators of well-being.* Retrieved July 9, 2006 from http://www.cdc.gov/nchs/data/misc/amchild.pdf.

Fox, J.A. (2002). *Primary health care of infants, children and adolescents* (2nd ed.). St.Louis: Mosby.

Furman, W. (2002). The emerging field of adolescent romantic relationships. *Current Directions in Psychological Science, 11*(5), 177-181.

Green, M., Palfrey, J.S., Clark, E.M., & Anastase, J.M., (Eds.). (2002). *Bright futures: Guidelines for health supervision of infants, children, and adolescents* (2nd ed.). Arlington, VA: National Center for Education in Maternal and Child Health.

Grunbaum, J.A., Kann, L., Kinchen, S., et al. (2004). Youth risk behavior surveillance: United States, 2003 (abridged). *Journal of School Health, 74*(8), 307-324.

Hickman, L.J., Jaycox, L.H. & Aronoff, J. (2004). Dating violence among adolescents: Prevalence, gender distribution, and prevention program effectiveness. *Trauma, Violence & Abuse, 5*(2), 1223-1242.

Hockenberry, M., Wilson, D., Winkelstein, M.L., & Kline, N.E., (2003). *Wong's nursing care of infants and children* (7th ed.). St. Louis: Mosby.

Hoekelman, R., Adam, H., Nelson, N., Weitzman, M., & Wilson, M. (2001). *Primary pediatric care* (4th ed.). St. Louis: Mosby.

Ipp, M. (1997). *Body modification: adolescent piercing and tattooing.* Retrieved July 9, 2006 from http://www.utoronto.ca/kids/bodyprce.html.

James, S., Ashwill, R., & Droske, S. (2002). *Nursing care of children: Principles and practice* (2nd ed.) Philadelphia: W.B.Saunders.

Johnston, L.D., O'Malley, P.M., & Bachman, J.G. (2002). *Monitoring the future: National results on adolescent drug use. National Institute on Drug Abuse.* Bethesda, MD: U.S. Department of Health and Human Services.

Kohlberg, L. (1984). *Essays on moral development.* San Francisco: Harper & Row.

March of Dimes. (2006). *Teenage pregnancy.* Retrieved July 9, 2006 from http://www.marchofdimes.com/professionals/681_1159.asp.

Minono, A.M., Heron, M.P., & Smith, B.L. (2006). Deaths: Preliminary data for 2004. *National Vital Statistics Report, 54*(19). Retrieved July 9, 2006 from http://www.cdc.gov/nchs/data/nvsr/nvsr54/nvsr54_19.pdf.

National Center for Health Statistics. (2004). *NCHS data on overweight and obesity.* Retrieved July 9, 2006 from http://www.cdc.gov/nchs/data/factsheets/overweightobesity.pdf.

National Highway Traffic Safety Association. (n.d.). *Teen Safety.* Retrieved July 9, 2006 from http://www.nhtsa.dot.gov/people/outreach/safesobr/19qp/sect2/page3.html.

National Institute of Allergy and Infectious Diseases, National Institutes of Health. (2006). *HIV infection in adolescents and young adults in the U.S.* Retrieved July 9, 2006 from http://www.niaid.nih.gov/factsheets/hivadolescent.htm.

Palo Alto Medical Foundation. (2004). *Extreme behavior.* Retrieved July 9, 2006 from http://www.pamf.org/teen/life/risktaking/extreme.html.

Piaget, J. (1969). *The theory of stages in cognitive development.* New York: McGraw-Hill.

Robinson, T.N. (1999). Reducing children's television viewing to prevent obesity: A randomized controlled trial. *Journal of the American Medical Association, 282*(16), 1561-1567.

Santrock, J.W. (2004). *Life span development.* Boston: McGraw-Hill.

Storey, M., Holt, K., & Sotfka, D. (Eds.). (2002). *Bright futures in practice: Nutrition.* Arlington, VA: National Center for Education in Maternal and Child Health.

Tanner, J. (1962). *Growth at adolescence* (2nd ed.). Oxford, England: Blackwell Scientific Publications.

United States Department of Health and Human Services. (2000). *Healthy people 2010* (2nd ed., 2 vols.). Washington, DC: U.S. Government Printing Office.

United States Department of Health and Human Services. (2006). *The problem of overweight in children and adolescents.* Retrieved July 9, 2006 from http://www.surgeongeneral.gov/topics/obesity/calltoaction/fact_adolescents.htm.

Walker-Barnes, C.J., & Arrue, R.M. (1998, February). *Girls and gangs: Identifying risk factors for female gang involvement.* Poster presentation, Society for Research on Adolescence.

Websites

www.aap.org American Academy of Pediatrics
www.aapd.org American Academy of Pediatric Dentistry
www.americanheart.org/ American Heart Association
www.brightfutures.org Bright Futures—references for health supervision
www.cdc.gov/ Centers for Disease Control and Prevention

www.cdc.gov/growthcharts/ Growth chart information from the CDC
www.cdc.gov/ncipc/factsheets/children.htm Information about injuries among children and adolescents
www.cdc.gov/powerfulbones/ Powerful Bones. Powerful Girls. The National Bone Health Campaign
www.cdc.gov/tobacco/ CDC's Tobacco Information and Prevention Source (TIPS)
www.coolnurse.com/sex_stuff.htm Sexuality and sexual health information for adolescents
www.dentalcare.com/drn.htm Dental care information from Proctor & Gamble
www.eatright.org American Dietetic Association
www.focusas.com/ Internet clearinghouse of information, resources and support for helping teens
www.healthyschools.org Information on a healthy school environment
www.keepkidshealthy.com/adolescent/adolescentnutrition.html Information on adolescent nutrition
www.obesity.org American Obesity Association
www.safekids.com Internet safety for kids
www.sikids.com/ Sports Illustrated for Kids
www.teenpregnancy.org/ The National Campaign to Prevent Teen Pregnancy
www.taconicnet.com/temperment.htm Taconic Counseling Group, NY. Psychotherapy: Temperament differences in children, 2000
www.tchin.org The Children's Health Network provides this site to offer support to clients, parents, and professionals dealing with heart disease
www.teenpregnancy.org/resources/data/report_summaries/eme National Campaign to Prevent Teen Pregnancy: sex has consequences
www.utoronto.ca/kids/bodyprce.html Body modification: adolescent piercing and tattooing

Chapter WORKSHEET

MULTIPLE CHOICE QUESTIONS

1. When giving parents guidance for the adolescent years, the nurse would advise the parents to: (Choose all that apply)
   a. Accept the adolescent as a unique individual.
   b. Provide strict, inflexible rules.
   c. Listen and try to be open to the adolescent's views.
   d. Screen all of his or her friends.
   e. Respect the adolescent's privacy.
   f. Provide unconditional love.
2. In developing a weight-loss plan for an adolescent, which of the following would you include? (Choose all that apply)
   a. Have parents make all of the meal plans.
   b. Eat slowly and place the fork down between each bite.
   c. Have the family exercise together.
   d. Refer to an adolescent weight-loss program.
   e. Keep a food and exercise diary.
3. Which of the following is associated with early adolescence? (Choose all that apply)
   a. Uses scientific reasoning to solve problems
   b. Still at times wants to be dependent upon parents
   c. Incorporates own set of morals and values
   d. Is influenced by peers and values memberships in cliques
4. Which of the following has the most influence in deterring an adolescent from beginning to drink alcohol?
   a. Drinking habits of parents
   b. Drinking habits of peers
   c. Drinking philosophy of adolescent's culture
   d. Drinking philosophy of adolescent's religion
5. In developing a pregnancy prevention program at school for 15- to 17-year-olds, the school nurse must take into consideration that:
   a. Teenagers think that no harm will come to them.
   b. Teenagers will learn best from their parents.
   c. Teenagers can only think in the here and now.
   d. Teenagers will learn best from professionals.

CRITICAL THINKING EXERCISES

1. During a sports physical examination, Susan, a 16-year-old, tells her health care provider that she is overweight. What additional information would the health care provider obtain?
2. The parents of Joe, a 14-year-old, talk to the school nurse about Joe's behavior at home. He is moody, fights with his younger siblings, only wants to be on his computer, and does not want to go on the family vacation. What advice would give the parents?
3. Jane tells the school nurse that she might be homosexual. What additional information would you obtain?
4. Alicia's parents are worried because all of Alicia's friends wear heavy makeup and have multiple piercings and hair colors. What advice would you give Alicia's parents?

STUDY ACTIVITIES

1. Talk to an early, middle, and late adolescent. Compare and contrast their interactions with you. Identify what psychosocial, cognitive, and moral stage they are in, using examples from their conversations with you.
2. Have an adolescent keep a food and exercise diary for one week. Analyze the information. Develop with the adolescent any interventions needed to promote healthy eating and exercise habits.
3. Plan a class on the dangers of smoking for 15-year-olds.
4. Plan a class for parents on how to keep the lines of communication open for adolescents.

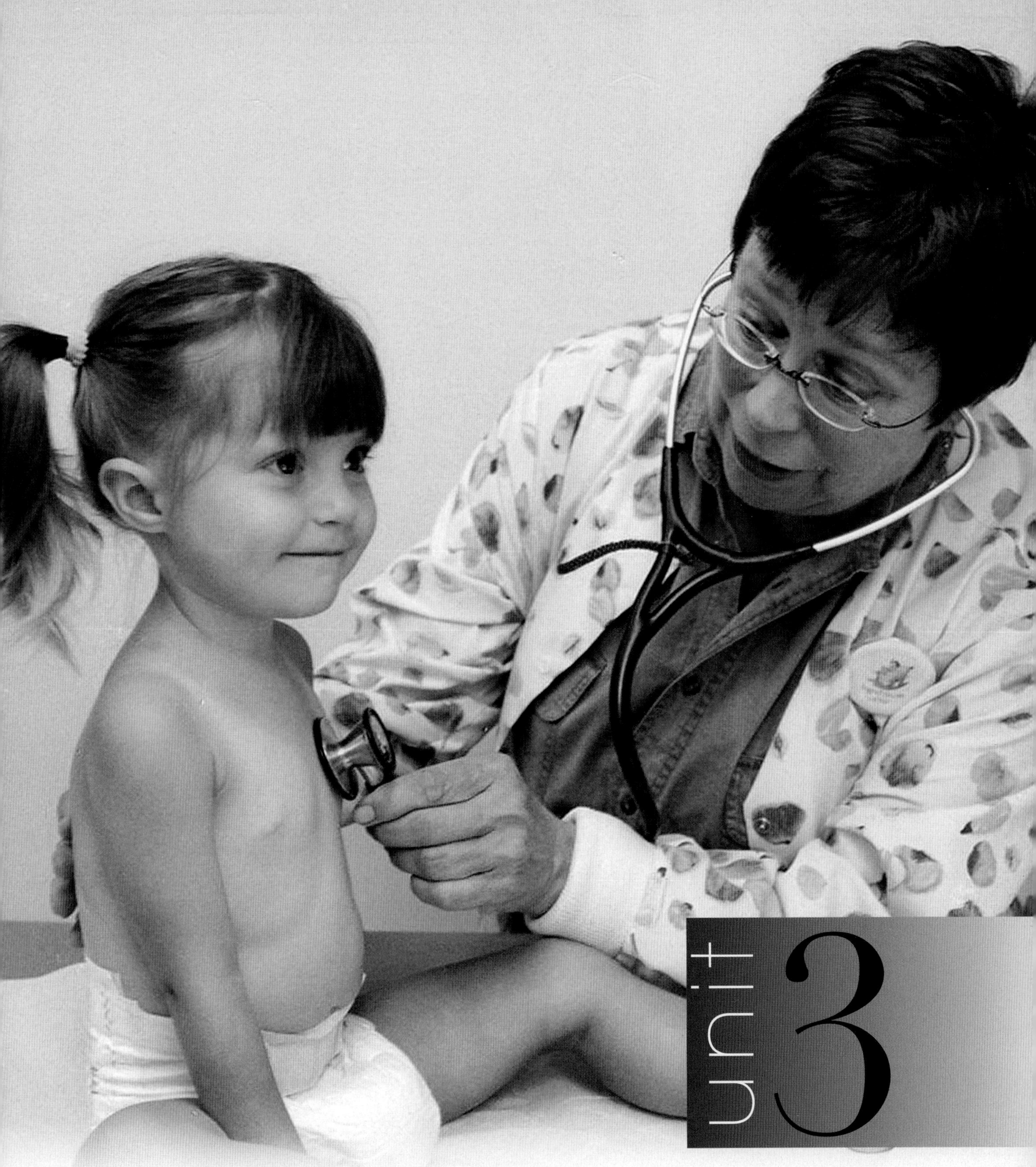

unit 3

Foundations of Pediatric Nursing

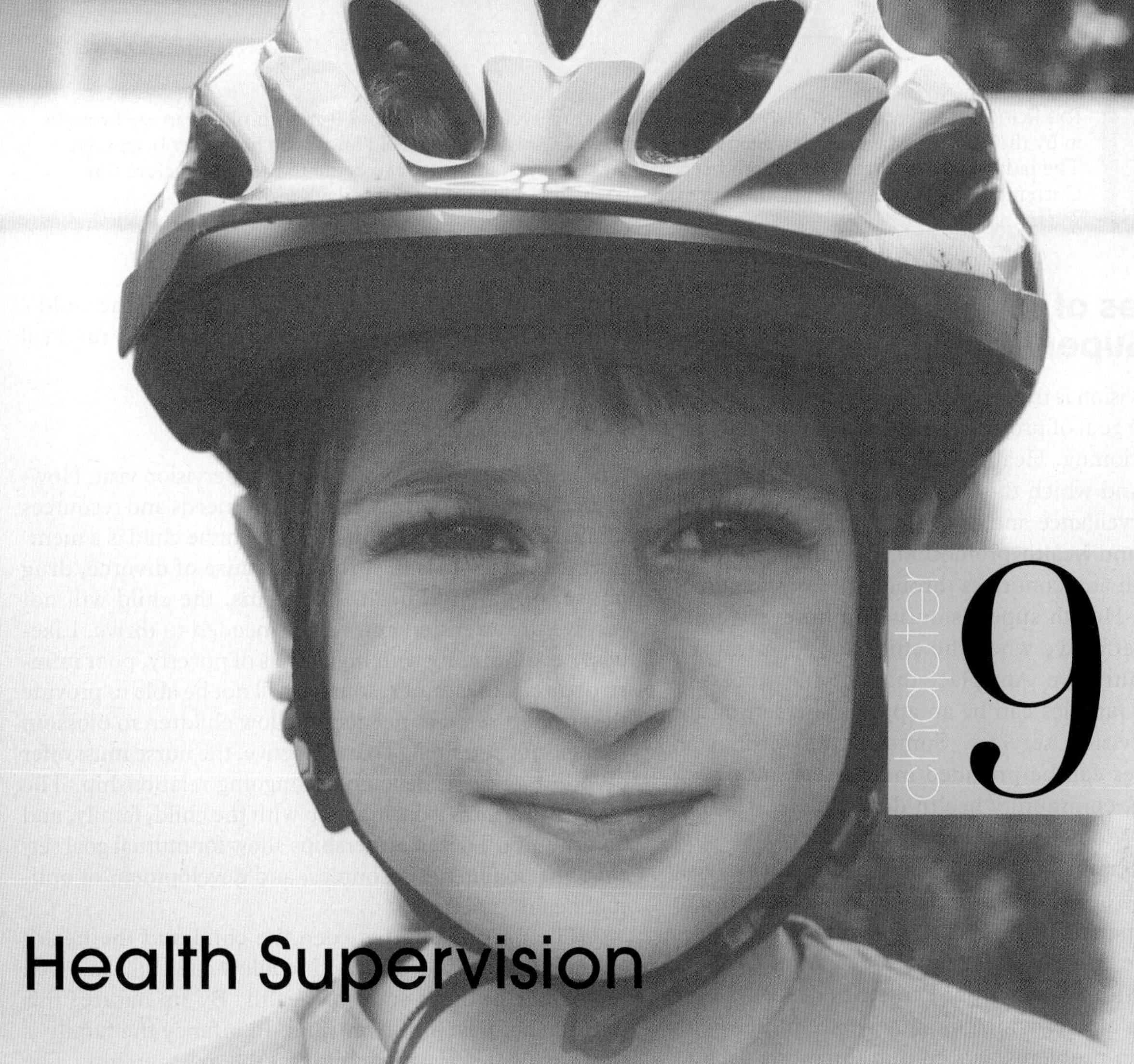

Health Supervision

Key TERMS

active immunity
developmental screenings
developmental surveillance
immunity
medical home
passive immunity
risk assessment
screening tests
selective screening
universal screening

Learning OBJECTIVES

Upon completion of the chapter, the learner will be able to:

1. Describe the principles of health supervision.
2. List the three components of a health supervision visit.
3. Utilize instruments appropriately for developmental and functional testing of children.
4. Demonstrate knowledge of the principles of immunization.
5. Identify barriers to immunization.
6. Identify challenges to health supervision for children with chronic illnesses.

WOW *It is never too late to embrace prevention. It starts with a genuine desire for health improvement.*

The Randall family is seen in the health clinic. Three-year-old Maya and 9-month-old Evan are brought in by their father. Maya was last seen in the clinic when she was 1 year old and Evan has never been seen. The father states that they have both been healthy so they did not need to come to the clinic before this. Currently, Maya is complaining of a sore throat, which is what prompted today's visit.

Principles of Health Supervision

Health supervision is the forward-looking provision of services with the goal of providing the child with an optimal level of functioning. Health supervision has three components around which this chapter is organized: developmental surveillance and screening; injury and disease prevention; and health promotion. Health supervision begins at birth and continues through the completion of adolescence. Health supervision is vital to every child and is most effective when the child has a centralized source of health care. Any place that provides access to children and families can be an appropriate setting for health supervision services. Some of the settings in which services can be provided include private physicians' offices, community health departments, sliding-scale clinics, homeless shelters, daycare centers, and schools. The framework for the health supervision visit is developed from national guidelines available through the U.S. Department of Health and Human Services (DHHS), the American Medical Association (AMA), and the American Academy of Pediatrics (AAP). These organizations also provide guidelines for children with chronic health problems and unique situations such as the internationally adopted child.

Wellness

The focus of pediatric health supervision is wellness. The health supervision visit provides an opportunity to maximize health promotion for the child, family, and community. Nurses have the ability to guide clients to a state of optimal health during these encounters. Health supervision visits must be viewed as a continuum of care and not as isolated episodes of tasks to be accomplished.

Medical Home

A **medical home** is any primary health care provider with a long-term and comprehensive relationship with the family. This continuing relationship fosters the establishment of trust between the provider and the family. In turn, this relationship enhances the probability of comprehensive, coordinated, and cost-effective care. The medical home is the setting that allows the highest level of health supervision. To be effective, the medical home must be accessible, family centered, and community based. It must be integrated into the child's world, not adjacent to it. Characteristics of a medical home are displayed in Box 9.1.

Partnerships

The child is the focus of the health supervision visit. However, the child's health is linked to the needs and resources of the family and community of which the child is a member. If the family is in turmoil because of divorce, drug abuse, or parental health problems, the child will not receive the attention and energy needed to thrive. Likewise, a community with high levels of poverty, poor infrastructure, and lack of resources will not be able to provide the support services needed to allow children to blossom to their full potential. To be effective, the nurse must offer commitment and develop an ongoing relationship. The nurse must form a partnership with the child, family, and community. These partnerships allow for mutual goal setting, marshalling of resources, and development of optimal health practices.

The partnership between the child and the health supervision team is designed to allow the child to reach his or her optimal state of health. By its nature, this partnership develops over time. In infancy the family is the surrogate for the child in the partnership. The child's participation in the partnership increases at a rate that is developmentally appropriate. The partnership increases the child's sense of self-worth and competence. The child's increasing influence in the partnership allows the nurse to tailor health supervision to the

BOX 9.1

MEDICAL HOME CHARACTERISTICS

- Preventive care activities
- Ambulatory and inpatient care available 24 hours a day
- Continuity of care from infancy through adolescence
- Availability of subspecialty consultation and referrals
- Interactive relationships with school and community agencies
- A centralized database containing all pertinent information

Green, M., & Palfrey, J. (Eds.). (2002). *Bright futures: Guidelines for health supervision of infants, children, and adolescents* (2nd ed.). Arlington, VA: National Center for Education in Maternal and Child Health.

child's needs. The partnership allows the child to take increasing responsibility for personal health and optimizes health promotion.

Nurses must validate and enhance the role of family members in the health supervision partnership. The family provides the framework that informs the child's concept of wellness. The health care community must involve the family to have a significant impact on a child's health. The family wants the best possible outcome for their child, and health care decisions are based on the knowledge they possess. When the nurse acknowledges that the family has unique insights to offer on their child's health, a trusting partnership can begin. Nurses can strengthen this partnership by recognizing the family's healthy practices, addressing their health issues, and strengthening their skills. The family's contributions to this partnership enhance the chance of success for health care plans. Families are the ones who must implement any health care strategy and know what expected outcomes are reasonable. They have intimate knowledge of the child's past responses to previous strategies. Their feedback is invaluable to formulating an effective long-term health supervision plan that optimizes their child's wellness.

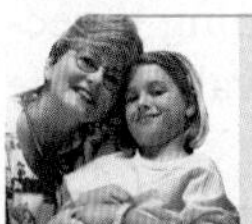

Observe the parent–child interaction during the health supervision visit. The nurse can learn much about the family dynamic by observing the family for behavioral clues:

- Does the parent make eye contact with the infant?
- Does the parent anticipate and respond to the infant's needs?
- Are parents effective when dealing with a toddler's temper tantrum?
- Do the parents' comments increase the school-age child's sense of self-worth?

Behavioral observations are crucial to the proper assessment of the family's needs and issues.

Partnerships between the community and the health promotion team benefit individual clients and the community. When nurses develop partnerships with community agencies such as schools, churches, and ancillary health facilities, barriers to care can be eased. The nurse becomes aware of available resources in the community that will benefit an individual family. With input from community partners, the nurse can perform an assessment of the community's needs. The assessment then provides the foundation for the development of community-based health promotion programs. These programs expand the resources of the community, which in turn enhances the health of its members.

Special Issues in Health Supervision

Special issues in health supervision include cultural influences; community influences; health supervision and the chronically ill child; and health supervision and the internationally adopted child.

Cultural Influences on Health Supervision

A family's definition of health is informed by the culture they inhabit. Successful interactions result when the nurse is aware of the beliefs and interactive styles that are often present in members of a specific culture. If the goals of the health care plan are not consistent with the health belief system of the family, the plan has little chance for success. Optimal wellness for the child requires the nurse and the family to negotiate a mutually acceptable plan of care. A plan must balance the cultural beliefs and practices of the family with those of the health care establishment. The nurse must possess the attributes of cultural competence and sensitivity for the partnership to be successful. Culturally effective care is the result of a dynamic partnership between the nurse and the family.

Most health promotion and disease prevention strategies in the United States have a future-based orientation. They also view the client as an active and controlling agent in his or her own health. This is relevant to the dominant culture; however, the challenge to the nurse is to develop strategies that resonant with clients of alternative cultures. Significant numbers of clients belong to cultures that possess a present-based orientation. For these clients, health promotion activities need shorter-term goals and outcomes to be useful. Clients with a fatalistic worldview will see any actions on their part as ineffective. They feel that a god figure or supernatural forces control their fate and believe that health is gift to be appreciated, not a goal to be pursued. Certain cultures believe health is the result of being in harmony within oneself and the larger universe. From this viewpoint, taking a medication or receiving a treatment is not an effective way to restore health because it does not address the problem of being "out of harmony." An individual's membership in a population does not guarantee that he or she ascribes to all the values of that culture. It is vital for the nurse to explore each client's specific beliefs during the health interview.

Community Influences on Health Supervision

The child is a member of a community as well as a family and a culture. Each community is unique in its strengths, weaknesses, and values. A community can be a contributor to a child's health or be the cause of his or her illnesses. The child's health cannot be totally separated from the health of the surrounding community.

Ideally the child's medical home is within the family's community. Being within the family's community increases access to care. Barriers such as lack of transportation, expense of travel, and time away from the parents' work setting are reduced. The presence of the medical home within the community facilitates the bonds between the health team and schools, churches, and available support services and agencies. Community support and resources are necessary for children with significant problems. A close working relationship between the child's health care provider and community agencies is an enormous benefit to the child (see earlier section, "Partnerships").

The community assessment may reveal problems that are causing or contributing to the child's health deficit. Deteriorating infrastructure can contribute to decreased access to care and increased risk of injury or illness. Poverty has been linked to low birth weight and premature birth. Substandard housing can be directly related to lead poisoning and asthma. Children from communities suffering the large-scale breakdown of family relationships and loss of support systems will be at increased risk for depression; violence and abuse; substance abuse; and human immunodeficiency virus (HIV) infection. A thorough knowledge of the family's community is needed before a health surveillance program can be effective.

Health Supervision and the Child With Chronic Illness

Effective health supervision must be responsive to the individual child's situation. The child with a chronic illness needs to be assessed repeatedly to determine health maintenance needs. These assessments determine the frequency of visits and types of interventions needed. The illness' impact on the functional health patterns of the child determine whether standard health supervision visits need to be augmented.

An effective partnership among the child's medical home, family, and community is vital for a child with a chronic illness. Coordination of medical specialty care, community agencies, and family support networks enhances the quality of life and health of these children. Access to care and services minimizes the risk of injury from the illness. Support groups and community-based resources optimize the family's adaptation to the stressors of chronic illness.

Comprehensive health supervision includes frequent psychosocial assessments. Issues to be covered include:

- Health insurance coverage
- Transportation availability to health care facilities
- Financial stressors
- Family coping effectiveness
- School personnel response to the chronic illness

These are often stressful and emotionally charged issues. The nurse with a trusting and ongoing relationship with the child and family is in the best position to help with these issues. The nurse can assist the family to find financial and medical assistance programs, utilize community resources, and participate in support groups. The nurse can also educate school personnel about the child's illnesses and assist them in maximizing the child's potential for academic success.

Health Supervision and the Child Adopted Internationally

Health supervision of the internationally adopted child must include comprehensive screening for infectious disease. In 2000, nearly 20,000 children were adopted from countries outside the United States. Internationally adopted children typically come from areas with a high prevalence of infectious diseases. China and Russia supply 50% of all international adoptees. Korea, Guatemala, Romania, Vietnam, and the Ukraine account for 32% of internationally adopted children. Proper screening is not only important to the child's health but also to the adopting family and the larger community. Screening is recommended within the first few weeks of arrival into the United States.

Intestinal parasites are a frequently occurring problem. Approximately 25% of international adoptees have one or more pathogens. *Giardia lamblia* is the most common pathogen and is found in 19% of these children. Infected children are frequently symptom free and universal screening is recommended.

Latent tuberculosis is very common, affecting up to 19% of this population. Though active tuberculosis infection has been rarely reported, there was an extensive outbreak of tuberculosis in a North Dakota community in 1998. The index case was an internationally adopted child from the Marshall Islands. Universal screening is recommended for this high-risk population.

Universal screening for hepatitis B, HIV, and syphilis infections is recommended. Due to lack of resources in the home country, screening and treatment for these diseases are sporadic and ineffective. If testing is documented, it is likely to be unreliable. Testing supplies may have been outdated or improperly stored. Also, the test may have been performed before the child's seroconversion occurred.

Components of Health Supervision

Developmental surveillance and screening; injury and disease prevention; and health promotion are the critical components of health supervision for children. Disease prevention and health promotion are concepts well established in adult health supervision. Injury prevention and developmental surveillance/screening are additional components of pediatric health supervision visits that help ensure every child achieves his or her optimum state of wellness.

Developmental Surveillance and Screening

Developmental surveillance is an ongoing collection of skilled observations made over time during health care visits. Components of this surveillance include:

- Noting and addressing parental concerns
- Obtaining a developmental history
- Making accurate observations
- Consulting with relevant professionals

Developmental screenings are brief assessment procedures that identify those children who warrant more intensive assessment and testing. Developmental screening assessments may be observational or by caregiver report (Fig. 9.1).

Development, the emergence of the child's abilities, is a longitudinal process. Within the trust and security of the medical home, family and health providers can share observations and concerns. In collaboration, the family and the health provider observe the child's accomplishments or milestones over time. Data collection for developmental surveillance of infants and young children is performed through developmental questionnaires, health care provider observations, and a thorough physical examination. Reviewing school records and testing can provide academic performance data for the older child. Input from teachers, coaches, and other adults involved with the child can give insight to the child's emotional and social development.

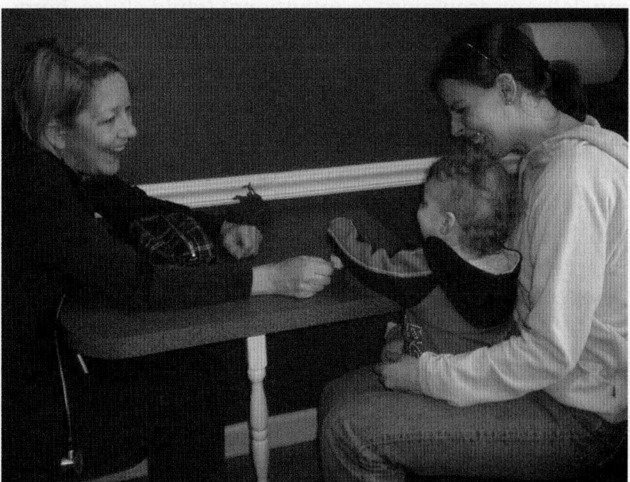

● Figure 9.1 Developmental screening provides the opportunity for the nurse to identify problem areas in the child's development.

When developmental delay is suspected, frequent developmental surveillance is highly warranted. Reemphasizing parental roles and responsibilities fosters cooperation and compliance. It is therefore crucial that parents understand the need for frequent assessments. A pattern of developmental delays warrants a formal evaluation.

It is absolutely critical for the pediatric nurse to understand normal growth and development expectations and become proficient at screening for problems related to development. The historical information obtained from the parent or primary caregiver about developmental milestones may indicate warning signs or identify risk for developmental delay. Refer to Table 9.1 for developmental warning signs and possible deficiency areas. Factors placing the infant or toddler at risk for developmental concerns include:

- Birth weight less than 1,500 grams
- Gestational age less than 33 weeks
- Central nervous system abnormality
- Hypoxic ischemic encephalopathy
- Maternal prenatal alcohol or illicit drug abuse
- Hypertonia
- Hypotonia
- Hyperbilirubinemia requiring exchange transfusion
- Kernicterus
- Congenital malformations
- Symmetric intrauterine growth deficiency
- Perinatal or congenital infection
- Suspected sensory impairment
- Chronic (>3 months) otitis media with effusion
- Inborn error of metabolism
- HIV infection
- Lead level >19 mg/dL
- Parental concern about developmental issues
- Parent with less than high school education
- Single parent
- Sibling with developmental concerns
- Parent with developmental disability or mental illness

Infants or children with any of the above risk factors should be carefully screened for developmental delays. This screening should occur in a prospective manner, with screenings occurring at frequent intervals to identify concerns early.

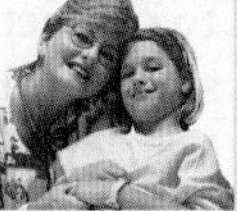

Any child who loses a developmental milestone—for example, the child able to sit without support who now cannot—needs an immediate full evaluation. There is a high likelihood of a significant neurologic problem.

Table 9.1 Infant/Toddler Developmental Warning Signs

Age	Warning Sign	Possible Developmental Concern
Any age	No response to environmental stimulus	Sensory deficit
Any age	Persistently up on toes (longer than 30 seconds) in supported standing position	Cerebral palsy
Before 3 months	Rolls over	Hypertonia
After 2–3 months	Persistent fisting	Neurologic dysfunction
After 4 months	Persistent head lag	Hypotonia
5 months	Not reaching for toys	Motor, visual, or cognitive deficit
6 months	Lack of tripod sitting	Hypotonia
6 months	Not smiling	Visual deficit, attachment issue
6 months	Primitive reflex persistence	Neurologic dysfunction
6 months	Not babbling	Hearing deficit
9 months	No reciprocal vocalizations or facial expressions	Autism spectrum disorders
12 months	No spoon or crayon use	Fine motor delay
15–18 months	Not walking	Gross motor delay
18 months	No imitative play	Autism spectrum disorders
Prior to 18 months	Hand dominance present	Hemiplegia in opposite upper extremity
18 months	No first word	Hearing deficit, expressive language deficit
24 months	Echolalia (repetitive speech) or inability to follow simple commands	Social delay or autism spectrum disorders

A number of developmental screening tools are available to guide the nurse in assessing development. Refer to Table 9.2 for a summary of these assessment tools. The Denver II is a frequently used tool and can be seen in Appendix B. The Denver II should be used for diagnostic purposes only when administered by specifically trained personnel. Nurses not trained in the use of the Denver II should use screening tools based on the Denver II. Many screening methods assist the nurse to identify infants and children who may have developmental delays, thus allowing for prompt identification and referral for more definitive evaluation. The appropriateness of a school-age child's developmental level can be evaluated using additional information. This information can include handwriting samples, ability to draw, school performance, and social skills.

Injury and Disease Prevention

Disease prevention is interventions performed to protect clients from a disease or identify it at early stage and lessen its consequences. These interventions are determined by the results of the nurse's assessment, nationally accepted practice guidelines, and the family's goals. Components of disease prevention include screening tests and immunizations.

Injury prevention is primarily accomplished through education, anticipatory guidance, and physical changes in the environment. Injuries can be unintentional (poisoning, falls, or drowning) or intentional (child abuse, homicide, or suicide). The types of injuries a child is most likely to encounter vary greatly among age groups. Although aggressive public health initiatives have decreased child death rates by injuries significantly in the past 50 years, continued vigilance and innovation are needed. The nurse in partnership with the family and the community can have n enormous impact on child safety. Specific interventions are discussed in Chapters 4, 5, 6, 7, and 8 of this book.

Screening Tests

Screening tests are procedures or laboratory analyses designed to identify those who may have a treatable condition. These tests are designed to assure that no person with the disorder is missed. They have a high sensitivity (a high false-positive rate) and a low specificity (a low false-negative rate). If a screening test result is positive,

Table 9.2 Developmental Screening Tools

Age	Screening Tool	Definition	Nursing Implications
Birth–6 years	Denver II	Assesses personal–social, fine motor–adaptive, language, and gross motor skills	Nurse administered. Requires props (such as ball, crayon, doll) available in the Denver II kit. Simple to learn to administer
Birth–6 years	Denver PRQ	Assesses personal–social, fine motor–adaptive, language, and gross motor skills	Parental report of all items on the Denver II
Birth–6 years	Child Development Inventory (CDI)	Simple questions about infant, toddler, or preschooler behaviors. Measures social, self-help, gross motor, fine motor, expressive language, language comprehension, letters, numbers, and general development as appropriate	A parental-report screening tool
Birth–6 years	Ages and Stages Questionnaire (ASQ)	Assesses communication, gross motor, fine motor, personal–social, and problem-solving skills	A parental-report screening tool, scored by the nurse after completion to determine child's progress in each of the developmental areas
Birth–8 years	Parents' Evaluation of Developmental Status (PEDS)	Screens for a wide range of developmental, behav-ioral, and family issues	A parental-report screening tool that can also be used in nurse interview format. Also available in Spanish
12–96 months	Batelle Developmental Inventory Screening Test	Assesses fine and gross motor, adaptive, personal–social, receptive and expressive language, and cognitive skills	Direct elicitation, parental description, and examiner observation. Requires special training
1–42 months	Bayley Scales of Infant Development II	Provides a mental and motor scale for assessment of cog-nitive, language, personal–social, and fine and gross motor development. A behavior rating scale is obtained during the testing.	Direct elicitation. Thorough. Requires special training
Birth–3 years	Early Language Milestone Scale	Screens for auditory expressive and receptive, visual components of speech	Requires standardized kit
2½–7 years	Denver Articulation Screening	Screens for articulation disorders	5 minutes to administer. Does not evaluate language ability
5–17 years	Goodenough-Harris Drawing Test	A nonverbal screen for mental ability (intelligence)	Child draws a person, which is analyzed for body parts, clothing, proportion, and perspective

follow-up tests with higher specificity are performed. A **risk assessment** is performed by the health care professional in conjunction with the client and includes objective as well as subjective data to determine the likelihood of having a condition. **Universal screening** occurs when an entire population is screened regardless of the client's individual risk. This type of screening is performed when a reliable risk assessment procedure is not available. **Selective screening** is done when a risk assessment indicates the client has one or more risk factors for the disorder.

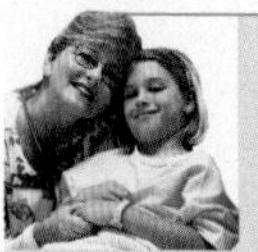

To increase cooperation from young children during screenings, set up a reward system. Easy-to-do rewards include:

- Stamping the back of the child's hand with a "smiley face" icon
- Making an eye cover by placing two stickers back to back over a tongue blade and letting the child keep the cover after the screening
- Copying a design onto a sheet of paper and letting the child take it home to color
- Letting the child play with a simple device such as a penlight or stethoscope

Metabolic Screening

Individual state law determines which metabolic screening tests are mandatory in that state. In some states, mandatory screening is limited to as few as four diseases. The March of Dimes currently recommends universal newborn metabolic screening tests for the following nine diseases:

- Phenylketonuria
- Congenital hypothyroidism
- Galactosemia
- Maple sugar urine disease
- Homocystinuria
- Bionitidase deficiency
- Sickle-cell disease
- Congenital adrenal hyperplasia
- Medium-chain acyl-CoA dehydrogenase deficiency (MCAD)

The nurse needs to confirm that newborn metabolic screening was performed prior to discharge from the birthing unit during any initial health supervision visit. If the test was not performed or was performed at less than 48 hours of age, the screening should be performed at that visit. The metabolic screening results need to be noted in the child's permanent record at the medical home.

Hearing Screening

Universal hearing screening of infants is the guideline established by the AAP. Target screening based on risk factors will only identify 50% of infants with hearing loss. Behavioral observations of the infant's response to sounds, such as a ringing bell, are not sensitive enough to preclude mild to moderate hearing loss. Screening should be done before discharge from the birthing unit; if not, the newborn needs to be screened before 1 month of age. Hearing loss is a common condition in newborns. Even mild hearing loss can cause serious delays in social and emotional development, language acquisition, and cognitive function. Identification of hearing loss by 3 months of age is crucial to prevent or reduce the impact on the child's development. Accepted methodologies for screening newborn hearing are displayed in Table 9.3.

Screening for hearing loss in older children begins with a history from the primary caregivers. If any concerns or problems are noted, objective audiometry should be performed. When the child is capable of following simple commands reliably, the nurse can perform some basic procedures to screen for hearing loss. The whisper test is easy to perform but does require a quiet room that is away from distractions in order to be valid. The Weber's and Rinne tests can be used to screen for sensorineural or conductive hearing loss (Fig. 9.2). Refer to Table 9.3 for additional explanations of hearing screening tests.

Universal hearing screening with objective testing is recommended at ages 4, 5, 6, 8, 10, 12, 15, and 18 years. More frequent screening is recommended if there is any behavior that indicates the child's hearing may be impaired. Repeated hearing screenings are recommended if a child has risk factors for acquired hearing loss such as those listed in Box 9.2; see also Healthy People 2010.

Vision Screening

Newborns with ocular structural abnormalities are at high risk for vision impairment. Ongoing vision screening is performed at every scheduled health supervision visit. The screening procedures for children younger than 3 years of age or any nonverbal child involve evaluating the child's ability to fixate on and follow objects. The neonate should be able to fixate on an object 10 to 12 inches from the face. After fixation, the infant should be able to follow the object to the midline. By 2 months of age, the infant should be able to follow the object 180 degrees. The technique of photoscreening can help identify problems such as ocular malalignment, refractive error, and lens and retinal problems.

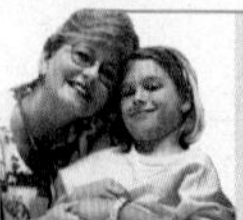

Use objects with black and white patterns when performing vision screening on an infant less than 6 months of age. The infant's vision at this age is more attuned to high-contrast patterns than to colors. Try checkerboard patterns or concentric circles. Animal figures like pandas and dalmatians also work well.

Table 9.3 Hearing Screening Methods

Test Name	Age Group	Characteristics	Nursing Implications
Auditory Brainstem Response (ABR)	Newborn–6 months	Measures electroencephalographic waves Test results may be affected by ear debris	Infant must be quiet (sedation may be needed)
Evoked otoacoustic emissions (EOAE)	Newborn–6 months or developmentally delayed children at the infant's level of functioning	The machine produces clicks that stimulate cilia in the cochlea and measures the response.	Infant must be quiet. Test results may be inaccurate in first 24 hours of life.
Visual reinforcement audiometry (VRA)	6 months–2 years	Visual reward linked to a tone signal Child looks to the visual reward in response to the tone Reward is activated, reinforcing the response	Child must be in an alert and happy state for best results. Schedule for after sleep/rest period. Allow child to sit in parent's lap.
Tympanometry	Over 7 months	Measures tympanic membrane mobility and determines middle ear pressure	The probe must form a seal with the canal. The child must remain still to obtain a valid result.
Conditioned play audiometry (CPA)	2–4 years	Similar to VRA except uses "listening games" Child does listening game at the tone. Receives social reward May be used when developmental age is 2 years	See Nursing Implications for VRA
Pure-tone (conventional) audiometry	4 years and older	Measures hearing acuity through a range of frequencies and intensities Child must wear earphones. Performed in a soundproof room if possible	Teach the child the desired motor response before screening. Administer conditioning trials. Offer two presentations of stimulus to ensure reliability. At a minimum, screen 1,000-, 2,000-, and 4,000-hertz levels at 20 decibels.
Whisper test	4 years and older	One ear is occluded. Examiner stands behind the child and whispers a word. The child must accurately repeat the whispered word.	The child must be in a quiet room and away from distractions. The child should be alert and well rested for accurate results. Consider a reward system to increase compliance.
Weber's test	6 years and older	Place a vibrating tuning fork in the middle of the top of the head. Ask if the sound is in one ear or both ears. The sound should be heard in both ears.	The child must understand the instructions and be able to cooperate.

(continued)

Table 9.3 Hearing Screening Methods (continued)

Test Name	Age Group	Characteristics	Nursing Implications
Rinne test	6 years and older	Place a vibrating tuning fork on the mastoid process to assess bone conduction. The child signals when the sound is gone. Next place a vibrating tuning fork outside the ear to test air conduction. The child signals when the sound is gone. For a passing test, air conduction time should be twice as long as bone conduction time.	The child must understand the instructions and be able to cooperate.

After the age of 3 years. a variety of standardized age-appropriate vision screening charts are available. These charts include the "tumbling E" and Allen figures (Fig. 9.3 A, B). These charts allow for a more precise vision assessment and aid the nurse in identifying preschool children with visual acuity problems. By age 5 or 6, most children know the alphabet well enough to use the traditional Snellen chart for vision screening (Fig. 9.3C). When using any vision-screening chart, several simple steps need to be followed.

- Place the chart at the child's eye level.
- Place a mark on the floor 20 feet from the chart.
- Align the child's heels on the mark.
- The child reads each line with one eye covered and then with the other eye covered (Fig. 9.4).
- The child reads each line with both eyes.

It is important that screenings are performed when children are alert and awake. Fatigue and disinterest can mimic poor vision. In addition to visual acuity screening, children should also be screened for color discrimination. Any child with eye abnormalities or who has failed visual screening needs to be evaluated by a specialist appropriately trained to treat pediatric clients. Refer to Table 9.4 for further information about various vision screening tools; see also Healthy People 2010.

Iron Deficiency Anemia Screening

Iron deficiency is the leading nutritional deficiency in the United States. The increased incidence of iron deficiency anemia is directly associated with periods of

BOX 9.2

RISK FACTORS FOR HEARING IMPAIRMENT

- Family history of hearing loss
- Prenatal infection
- Anomalies of the head, face, or ears
- Low birth weight (less than 1,500 g)
- Hyperbilirubinemia requiring exchange transfusion
- Ototoxic medications
- Low Apgar scores: 4 or less at 1 minute, or 6 or less at 5 minutes
- Mechanical ventilation lasting 5 days
- Syndrome associated with hearing loss
- Bacterial meningitis
- Neurodegenerative disorders
- Persistent pulmonary hypertension
- Otitis media with effusion for 3 months

HEALTHY PEOPLE 2010

Objective	Significance
Increase the proportion of newborns who are screened for hearing loss by age 1 month, have audiologic evaluation by age 3 months, and are enrolled in appropriate intervention services by age 6 months. Increase the proportion of persons who have had a hearing examination on schedule.	• Determine results of newborn hearing screening at first newborn checkup. • Refer any infant with possible hearing deficit for further evaluation. • Insure infants with hearing impairment receive appropriate augmentation (hearing aids). • Insure all children and adolescents receive hearing screenings with well-child checkups as appropriate.

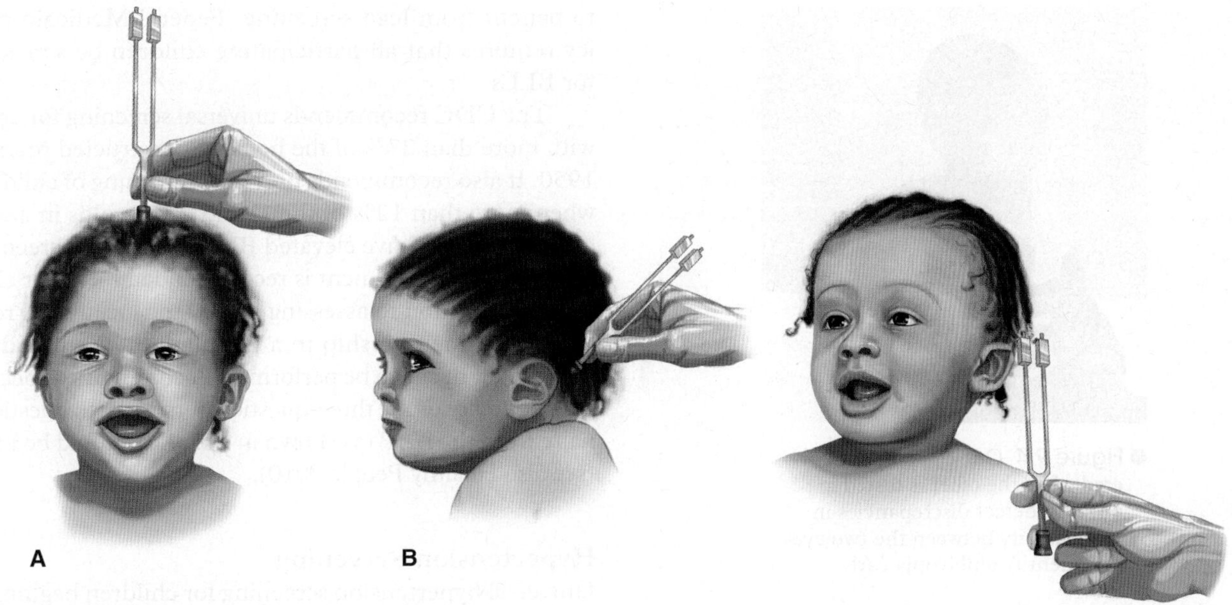

● Figure 9.2 (**A**) Weber's test screens for hearing by assessing sound conducted via bone. (**B**) The Rinne test screens for hearing by comparing sound conduction via bone to sound conduction via air.

diminished iron stores, rapid growth, and high metabolic demands. At 6 months of age, the *in utero* iron stores of a full-term infant are almost depleted. The adolescent growth spurt warrants constant iron replacement. Pregnant adolescents are at even higher risk for iron deficiency, due to the demands of the maternal growth spurt and the needs of the developing fetus. Guidelines for universal iron deficiency anemia screening vary. The Centers for Disease Control and Prevention (CDC) recommend universal screening of high-risk children at various age intervals. The AAP recommends universal screening of all infants at 9 to 12 months;

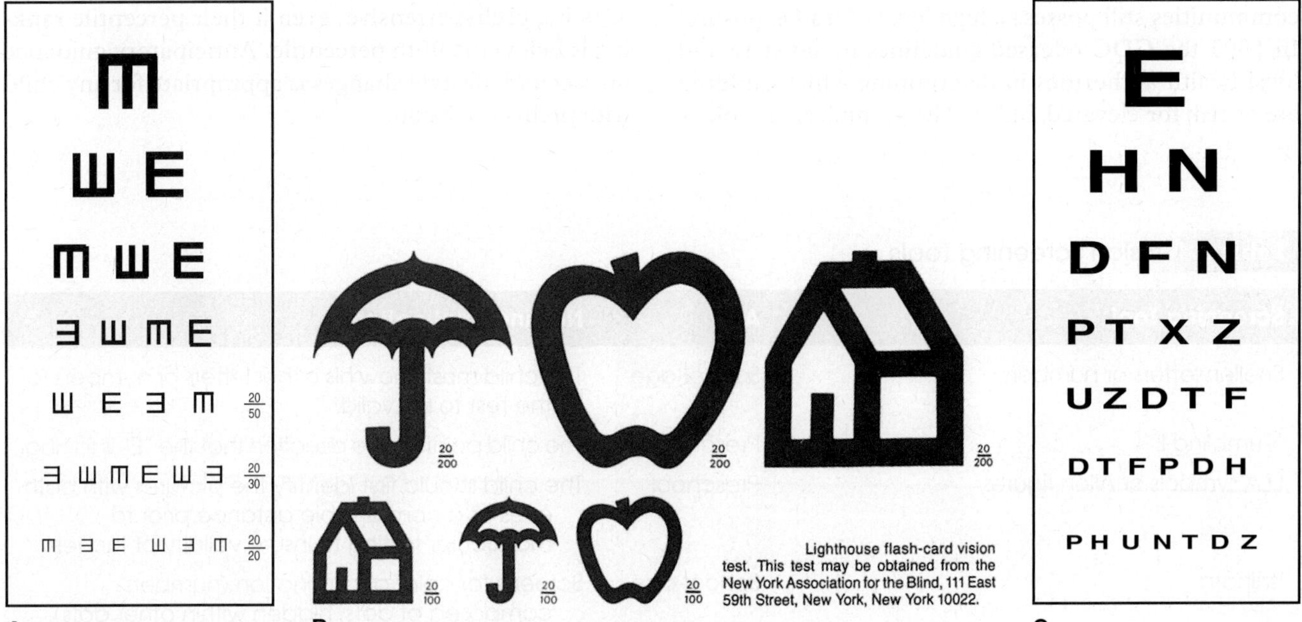
A
B
C
20/50
20/30
20/20
20/200
20/100
E
H N
D F N
P T X Z
U Z D T F
D T F P D H
P H U N T D Z
Lighthouse flash-card vision test. This test may be obtained from the New York Association for the Blind, 111 East 59th Street, New York, New York 10022.

● Figure 9.3 (**A**) The "tumbling E" chart is appropriate for children who do not yet know the alphabet, but who can follow directions to indicate the direction that the arms of the "E" are pointing. (**B**) picture chart similar to the Allen object recognition chart is appropriate for vision screening in the preschool-age child. (**C**) The Snellen eye chart may be used for children age 6 or older who know the alphabet.

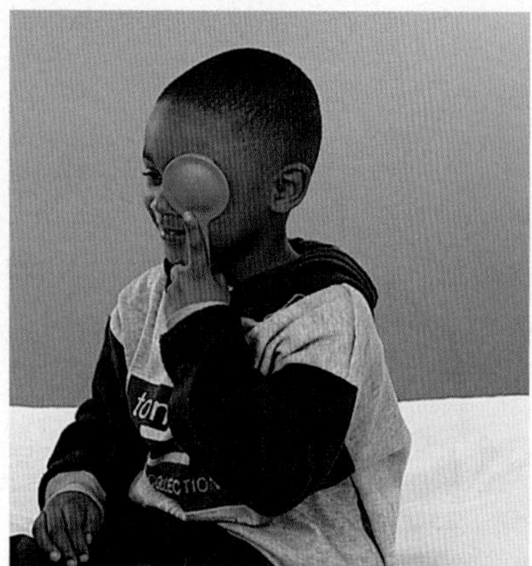

● Figure 9.4 One eye must be covered while the other is tested in order to detect discrepancies in visual acuity between the two eyes and identify amblyopia early.

males at 12 to 18 years; and adolescent females during all routine physical examinations. Both the CDC and the AAP have similar recommendations for selective screening. See Boxes 9.3 and 9.4.

Lead Screening

Elevated blood lead levels (BLLs), 10 micrograms per deciliter or higher, remain a preventable environmental health threat. Although the prevalence of elevated BLLs has declined over the past two decades, certain communities still possess a high level of lead exposure. In 1997 the CDC released guidelines to aid state and local health authorities in determining which children are at risk for elevated BLLs. These children are likely to benefit from lead screening. Federal Medicaid policy requires that all participating children be screened for BLLs.

The CDC recommends universal screening for areas with more than 27% of the housing constructed prior to 1950. It also recommends universal screening of children when more than 12% of the 1- and 2-year-olds in a specific population have elevated BLLs. Targeted screening based on risk assessment is recommended for other children. In addition to assessing risk by the location of residence and membership in a population, an individual assessment needs to be performed. A community-specific questionnaire or the three-question personal risk questionnaire from the AAP (as shown in Box 9.5) should be used (see also Healthy People 2010).

Hypertension Screening

Universal hypertension screening for children beginning at 3 years of age is recommended. If the child has risk factors for systemic hypertension, such as preterm birth and congenital heart disease, then screening begins at the time the risk factor becomes apparent. The prevalence of systemic hypertension in the pediatric population is 1% to 3%.

The guidelines for determining hypertension in children and adolescents mirror the guidelines established for the adult population (Box 9.6). Preadolescent children whose blood pressure is in the 90th to 95th percentile are considered to have prehypertension. Adolescent children whose blood pressure is 120/80 mmHg are categorized as being prehypertensive, even if their percentile ranking is below the 90th percentile. Anticipatory guidance on diet and lifestyle changes is appropriate for any child with prehypertension.

Table 9.4 Vision Screening Tools

Screening Tool	Age	Nursing Implications
Snellen letters or numbers	School-age	The child must know his or her letters or numbers for the test to be valid.
"Tumbling E"	Preschool	The child points in the direction that the "E" is facing.
LEA symbols or Allen figures	Preschool	The child should first identify the pictures with both eyes at a comfortable distance prior to monocular testing to insure validity of the test.
Ishihara	School-age	Screens for color discrimination (numbers composed of dots, hidden within other dots)
Color Vision Testing Made Easy (CVTME)	Preschool	Uses dot pictures like the Ishihara, but instead of numbers has easily identified shapes imbedded in the dots

HEALTHY PEOPLE 2010

Objective	Significance
Increase the proportion of preschool children age 5 years and under who receive vision screening.	• Use preschool-appropriate vision screening tool to assess vision. • Insure screening begins at age 3.

Hyperlipidemia Screening

Hyperlipidemia screening of children can reduce the incidence of adult coronary disease. Atherosclerosis has been documented in children and a link exists between these lesions and high lipid levels. Selectively screening those children at high risk for hyperlipidemia can reduce their lifelong risk of coronary artery disease.

BOX 9.3

COMPARING IRON DEFICIENCY ANEMIA SCREENING GUIDELINES

CDC Recommendations

Universal Screening

- High-risk children only:
  - Ages 9–12 months
  - Repeat 6 months later
  - Ages 2–5 years annually
- Females ages 12–18 years: once every 5–10 years

Selective Screening

Assess infants and children for risk factors at:

- 9–12 months
- 15–18 months
- 2–18 years annually

Screen clients with risk factors.

AAP Recommendations

Universal Screening

- Screen ***all*** infants at 9–12 months.
- Screen males ages 12–18 years at routine physical examinations during their peak growth period.
- Screen adolescent females during all routine physical examinations.

Selective Screening

Assess infants and children for risk factors at:

- 9–12 months
- 15–18 months
- 2–18 years annually

Screen clients with risk factors.

BOX 9.4

RISK FACTORS FOR IRON DEFICIENCY ANEMIA

- Periods of rapid growth
- Low birth weight or preterm infants
- Low dietary intake of meat, fish, poultry, and ascorbic acid
- Macrobiotic diets
- Inappropriate consumption of cow's milk
- Use of infant formula not fortified with iron
- Exclusive breastfeeding after age 6 months without iron-fortified supplemental foods
- Meal skipping, frequent dieting
- Pregnancy or recent pregnancy
- Intensive physical training
- Recent blood loss, heavy/lengthy menstrual periods
- Chronic use of aspirin or nonsteroidal anti-inflammatory drugs
- Parasitic infections

Children at High Risk for Iron Deficiency Anemia

- Low-income families
- Those eligible for the Special Supplemental Nutrition Program for Women, Infants, and Children (WIC)
- Migrants or recently arrived refugees

The risk assessment focuses on the child's family history. Children whose parents or grandparents had premature cardiovascular disease (before 55 years of age) or who have a parent with hypercholesterolemia are screened. If the child's family history is not available, screening is done at the discretion of the health care provider. The nurse also assesses for lifestyle factors that may contribute to hyperlipidemia such as sedentary lifestyle, cigarette smoking, obesity, and high-fat dietary intake. Children with diseases such as diabetes and hypertension are also candidates for hyperlipidemia screening. See Box 9.7 for details.

BOX 9.5

A BASIC PERSONAL-RISK QUESTIONNAIRE FOR LEAD EXPOSURE IN CHILDREN

1. Does your child live in or regularly visit a house or childcare facility that was built before 1950?
2. Does your child live in or regularly visit a house or childcare facility built before 1978 that is being or has recently been renovated or remodeled (within the past 6 months)?
3. Does your child have a sibling or playmate who has or did have lead poisoning?

Remember Maya and Evan, the 3-year-old and 9-month-old from the beginning of the chapter? How would you assess Maya's and Evan's growth and development? Which screening tests are warranted for them and why? What further information would you need to determine which tests should be performed?

HEALTHY PEOPLE 2010

Objective	Significance
Eliminate elevated blood lead levels in children.	• Screen for lead exposure. • Insure that high-risk children have blood lead levels measured.

Immunizations

Immunization is the key activity of disease prevention during health supervision visits. The development of effective vaccines, beginning in the 1940s, revolutionized children's health care in the 20th century. Immunization allowed the focus to shift from disease treatment to disease prevention. The nurse needs to understand the principles of immunizations, the proper use of vaccines, and barriers to immunization. Armed with this knowledge base, the nurse can partner with families to provide the highest level of disease protection to children (Fig. 9.5).

Principles of Immunization

The immune system has the ability to recognize materials present in the body as "self" or "non-self." Foreign materials (non-self) are called *antigens.* When an antigen is recognized by the immune system, the immune system responds by producing antibodies (immunoglobulins) or directing special cells to destroy and remove the antigen.

Immunity is the ability to destroy and remove a specific antigen from the body. The acquisition of immunity can be active or passive. **Passive immunity** is produced when the immunoglobulins of one person are transferred to another. This immunity lasts only weeks or months. Passive immunity can be obtained by injection. It can also be transferred from mothers to infants via colostrum or the placenta. **Active immunity** is acquired when a person's own immune system generates the immune response. Active immunity lasts for many years or for a lifetime. This long-term protection is the result of immunologic memory. After the initial immune response, specialized cells for that antigen continue to exist. When an antigen returns, these memory cells very rapidly produce a fresh supply of antibodies to reestablish protection. This immunity can occur after exposure to natural pathogens or after exposure to vaccines. Vaccines mimic the characteristics of the natural antigen. The immune system mounts a response and establishes an immunologic memory as it would for an infection.

The classification of vaccines is based on the characteristics of the antigen present. The antigen may be viral or bacterial. It may be live attenuated (weakened) or killed. It may be the whole antigen or a portion of it (fractional). Types of vaccines are listed below:

- Live attenuated vaccines are modified living organisms that are weakened. The organism can produce an immune response, but does not produce the complications of the illness.
- Killed vaccines contain whole dead organisms; they are incapable of reproducing but are capable of producing an immune response.
- Toxoid vaccines contain protein products produced by bacteria called *toxins.* The toxin is heat treated to weaken its effect, but it retains its ability to produce an immune response.
- Conjugate vaccines are the result of chemically linking the bacterial cell wall polysaccharide (sugar-based) portions with proteins. This dramatically increases the immune response when compared with presenting the polysaccharide portion alone.

BOX 9.6

PREADOLESCENT CHILDHOOD HYPERTENSION GUIDELINES

Optimal	<90th percentile
Prehypertension	90th to 95th percentile
Stage I	>95th percentile up to 5 mmHg above 99th percentile
Stage II	5 mmHg above 99th percentile, or higher

BOX 9.7

HYPERLIPIDEMIA SCREENING

Screen if parents or grandparents, at <55 years of age, have/had documented:
- Coronary atherosclerosis
- Myocardial infarction
- Angina pectoris
- Peripheral vascular disease
- Cerebrovascular disease
- Sudden cardiac death

Screen if a parent's blood cholesterol level is 240 mg/dL or higher.
Screen at health care provider's discretion:
- Parental history is unobtainable.
- Child has diabetes or hypertension.
- Child has lifestyle risk factors:
  - Cigarette smoking
  - Obesity
  - Sedentary activity pattern
  - High-fat dietary intake

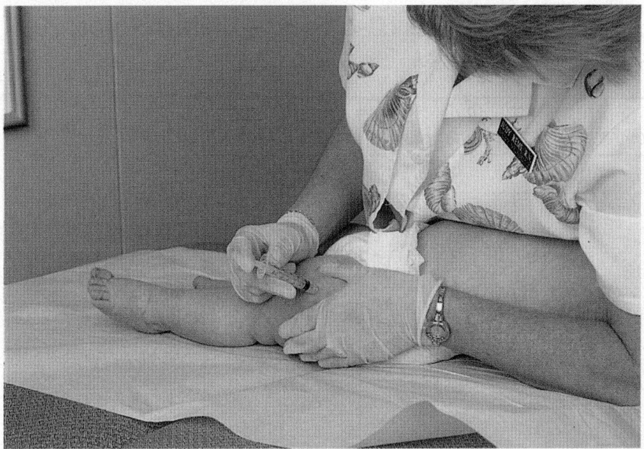

● Figure 9.5 Nurse restraining infant for intramuscular injection into the vastus lateralis.

• Recombinant vaccines use genetically engineered organisms. For example, the hepatitis B vaccine is produced by splicing a gene portion of the virus into a gene of a yeast cell. The yeast cell is then able to produce hepatitis B surface antigen to use for vaccine production.

The safety and efficacy of existing vaccines is constantly being reviewed. Research to improve vaccines is ongoing. The goal is to continue to refine vaccines so that a maximum immune response is produced with the least amount of risk for the client.

Immunization Management

The Advisory Committee on Immunization Practices (ACIP), a branch of the CDC, reviews the recommended immunization schedules at least yearly and updates the schedule to ensure that it accurately reflects current best practices. See Tables 9.5 and 9.6. In addition to the recommended schedule, the ACIP publishes a "catch-up" schedule for children who have not been adequately immunized (Table 9.7). The child's immunization record must be compared with the latest edition of these schedules when assessing the need for immunization.

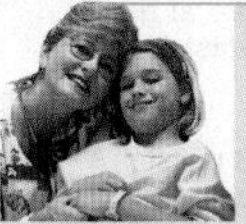

When obtaining an immunization history, ask the question, "When and where did your child receive his (or her) last immunization?" This question allows for more information gathering than the yes–no question, "Are your child's immunizations up-to-date?" The nurse can compare this information with that on the available immunization record; discover in what settings the child is getting health care; and use the information as a starting point in a discussion of any reactions to previous immunizations.

Vaccine storage and administration directly impact the efficacy of a vaccine. Improperly stored or reconstituted vaccines can be rendered ineffective. It is also important to administer the vaccine by the correct route; not all vaccines are given intramuscularly (Box 9.8; Table 9.8). The manufacturer's package insert is the best reference source for any vaccine.

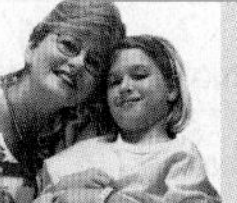

Proper vaccine storage is critical to vaccine efficacy. If you suspect that a vaccine was not maintained at the proper storage temperature, DO NOT USE IT. An ineffective vaccine is of no use in preventing disease.

The Public Health Service Act outlines standards of practice for immunization programs. The act requires that Vaccine Information Statements (VIS; Fig. 9.6) be provided to parents prior to administering an immunization. In accordance with the concept of partnership with the parents, ample time is allowed for reading the VIS and discussing parental concerns. The parents must feel comfortable admitting that they do not understand the information presented. If the parents are illiterate, the nurse presents the information orally and verifies that the parents understand the information. If the information in the VIS is not in the parent's native language, a reliable translator presents the information. At this time the nurse also questions the parents about the child's reactions to previous immunizations and screens for precautions and contraindications for each vaccine to be administered. Parents sign consent forms acknowledging their permission to administer the immunization.

If there is a clinically significant adverse event following an immunization, it should be reported to the Vaccine Adverse Event Reporting System (VAERS). For assistance in obtaining and completing a VAERS form, call 800-822-7967 or visit www.vaers.org.

Proper documentation in the child's permanent record includes the following elements:

- Date vaccine was administered
- Name of vaccine (commonly used abbreviation is acceptable)
- Lot number and expiration date of vaccine
- Manufacturer's name
- Site and route by which vaccine was administered (for example: left deltoid, IM)
- Edition date of VIS given to the parents
- Name and address of the facility administering the vaccine (where the permanent record will be kept)
- Name of person administering the immunization

Families should be provided with a personal record of the child's immunizations. It serves to reinforce the importance of the procedure and acts as a reminder for maintaining the currency of immunizations. Refer to Figure 9.7 for an example of a typical vaccine administration record.

Vaccine Descriptions

This section reviews the most commonly used vaccines. These immunizations are recommended by the ACIP. Each state has laws that determine which immunizations

(text continues on page 235)

Table 9.5 CDC Recommended Immunization Schedule for Persons Aged 0–6 Years—United States, 2007

Vaccine ▼ / Age ►	Birth	1 month	2 months	4 months	6 months	12 months	15 months	18 months	19–23 months	2–3 years	4–6 years
Hepatitis B[1]	HepB	HepB		*See footnote 1*		HepB				HepB Series	
Rotavirus[2]			Rota	Rota	Rota						
Diphtheria, Tetanus, Pertussis[3]			DTaP	DTaP	DTaP		DTaP				DTaP
Haemophilus influenzae type b[4]			Hib	Hib	*Hib*[4]	Hib			Hib		
Pneumococcal[5]			PCV	PCV	PCV	PCV				PCV PPV	
Inactivated Poliovirus			IPV	IPV		IPV					IPV
Influenza[6]								Influenza (Yearly)			
Measles, Mumps, Rubella[7]						MMR					MMR
Varicella[8]						Varicella					Varicella
Hepatitis A[9]							HepA (2 doses)			HepA Series	
Meningococcal[10]										MPSV4	

Range of recommended ages

Catch-up immunization

Certain high-risk groups

This schedule indicates the recommended ages for routine administration of currently licensed childhood vaccines, as of December 1, 2006, for children aged 0–6 years. Additional information is available at http://www.cdc.gov/nip/recs/child-schedule.htm. Any dose not administered at the recommended age should be administered at any subsequent visit, when indicated and feasible. Additional vaccines may be licensed and recommended during the year. Licensed combination vaccines may be used whenever any components of the combination are indicated and other components of the vaccine are not contraindicated and if approved by the Food and Drug Administration for that dose of the series. Providers should consult the respective Advisory Committee on Immunization Practices statement for detailed recommendations. Clinically significant adverse events that follow immunization should be reported to the Vaccine Adverse Event Reporting System (VAERS). Guidance about how to obtain and complete a VAERS form is available at http://www.vaers.hhs.gov or by telephone, 800-822-7967.

1. **Hepatitis B vaccine (HepB).** *(Minimum age: birth)*
   At birth:
   - Administer monovalent HepB to all newborns before hospital discharge.
   - If mother is hepatitis surface antigen (HBsAg)-positive, administer HepB and 0.5 mL of hepatitis B immune globulin (HBIG) within 12 hours of birth.
   - If mother's HBsAg status is unknown, administer HepB within 12 hours of birth. Determine the HBsAg status as soon as possible and if HBsAg-positive, administer HBIG (no later than age 1 week).
   - If mother is HBsAg-negative, the birth dose can only be delayed with physician's order and mothers' negative HBsAg laboratory report documented in the infant's medical record.

   After the birth dose:
   - The HepB series should be completed with either monovalent HepB or a combination vaccine containing HepB. The second dose should be administered at age 1–2 months. The final dose should be administered at age ≥24 weeks. Infants born to HBsAg-positive mothers should be tested for HBsAg and antibody to HBsAg after completion of ≥3 doses of a licensed HepB series, at age 9–18 months (generally at the next well-child visit).

   4-month dose:
   - It is permissible to administer 4 doses of HepB when combination vaccines are administered after the birth dose. If monovalent HepB is used for doses after the birth dose, a dose at age 4 months is not needed.
2. **Rotavirus vaccine (Rota).** *(Minimum age: 6 weeks)*
   - Administer the first dose at age 6–12 weeks. Do not start the series later than age 12 weeks.
   - Administer the final dose in the series by age 32 weeks. Do not administer a dose later than age 32 weeks.
   - Data on safety and efficacy outside of these age ranges are insufficient.
3. **Diphtheria and tetanus toxoids and acellular pertussis vaccine (DTaP).** *(Minimum age: 6 weeks)*
   - The fourth dose of DTaP may be administered as early as age 12 months, provided 6 months have elapsed since the third dose.
   - Administer the final dose in the series at age 4–6 years.
4. ***Haemophilus influenzae* type b conjugate vaccine (Hib).** *(Minimum age: 6 weeks)*
   - If PRP-OMP (PedvaxHIB® or ComVax® [Merck]) is administered at ages 2 and 4 months, a dose at age 6 months is not required.
   - TriHiBit® (DTaP/Hib) combination products should not be used for primary immunization but can be used as boosters following any Hib vaccine in children aged ≥12 months.
5. **Pneumococcal vaccine.** *(Minimum age: 6 weeks for pneumococcal conjugate vaccine [PCV]; 2 years for pneumococcal polysaccharide vaccine [PPV])*
   - Administer PCV at ages 24–59 months in certain high-risk groups. Administer PPV to children aged ≥2 years in certain high-risk groups. See *MMWR* 2000;49(No. RR-9):1–35.
6. **Influenza vaccine.** *(Minimum age: 6 months for trivalent inactivated influenza vaccine [TIV]; 5 years for live, attenuated influenza vaccine [LAIV])*
   - All children aged 6–59 months and close contacts of all children aged 0–59 months are recommended to receive influenza vaccine.
   - Influenza vaccine is recommended annually for children aged ≥59 months with certain risk factors, health-care workers, and other persons (including household members) in close contact with persons in groups at high risk. See *MMWR* 2006;55(No. RR-10):1–41.
   - For healthy persons aged 5–49 years, LAIV may be used as an alternative to TIV.
   - Children receiving TIV should receive 0.25 mL if aged 6–35 months or 0.5 mL if aged ≥3 years.
   - Children aged <9 years who are receiving influenza vaccine for the first time should receive 2 doses (separated by ≥4 weeks for TIV and ≥6 weeks for LAIV).
7. **Measles, mumps, and rubella vaccine (MMR).** *(Minimum age: 12 months)*
   - Administer the second dose of MMR at age 4–6 years. MMR may be administered before age 4–6 years, provided ≥4 weeks have elapsed since the first dose and both doses are administered at age ≥12 months.
8. **Varicella vaccine.** *(Minimum age: 12 months)*
   - Administer the second dose of varicella vaccine at age 4–6 years. Varicella vaccine may be administered before age 4–6 years, provided that ≥3 months have elapsed since the first dose and both doses are administered at age ≥12 months. If second dose was administered ≥28 days following the first dose, the second dose does not need to be repeated.
9. **Hepatitis A vaccine (HepA).** *(Minimum age: 12 months)*
   - HepA is recommended for all children aged 1 year (i.e., aged 12–23 months). The 2 doses in the series should be administered at least 6 months apart.
   - Children not fully vaccinated by age 2 years can be vaccinated at subsequent visits.
   - HepA is recommended for certain other groups of children, including in areas where vaccination programs target older children. See *MMWR* 2006;55(No. RR-7):1–23.
10. **Meningococcal polysaccharide vaccine (MPSV4).** *(Minimum age: 2 years)*
    - Administer MPSV4 to children aged 2–10 years with terminal complement deficiencies or anatomic or functional asplenia and certain other high-risk groups. See *MMWR* 2005;54(No. RR-7):1–21.

The Recommended Immunization Schedules for Persons Aged 0–18 Years are approved by the Advisory Committee on Immunization Practices (http://www.cdc.gov/nip/acip), the American Academy of Pediatrics (http://www.aap.org), and the American Academy of Family Physicians (http://www.aafp.org).

Table 9.6 CDC Recommended Immunization Schedule for Persons Aged 7–18 Years—United States, 2007

Vaccine ▼ / Age ▶	7–10 years	11–12 YEARS	13–14 years	15 years	16–18 years
Tetanus, Diphtheria, Pertussis[1]	*See footnote 1*	Tdap	Tdap		
Human Papillomavirus[2]	*See footnote 2*	HPV (3 doses)	HPV Series		
Meningococcal[3]	MPSV4	MCV4	MCV4	MCV4[3] / MCV4	
Pneumococcal[4]	PPV				
Influenza[5]	Influenza (Yearly)				
Hepatitis A[6]	HepA Series				
Hepatitis B[7]	HepB Series				
Inactivated Poliovirus[8]	IPV Series				
Measles, Mumps, Rubella[9]	MMR Series				
Varicella[10]	Varicella Series				

Range of recommended ages

Catch-up immunization

Certain high-risk groups

This schedule indicates the recommended ages for routine administration of currently licensed childhood vaccines, as of December 1, 2006, for children aged 7–18 years. Additional information is available at http://www.cdc.gov/nip/recs/child-schedule.htm. Any dose not administered at the recommended age should be administered at any subsequent visit, when indicated and feasible. Additional vaccines may be licensed and recommended during the year. Licensed combination vaccines may be used whenever any components of the combination are indicated and other components of the vaccine are not contraindicated and if approved by the Food and Drug Administration for that dose of the series. Providers should consult the respective Advisory Committee on Immunization Practices statement for detailed recommendations. Clinically significant adverse events that follow immunization should be reported to the Vaccine Adverse Event Reporting System (VAERS). Guidance about how to obtain and complete a VAERS form is available at http://www.vaers.hhs.gov or by telephone, 800-822-7967.

1. **Tetanus and diphtheria toxoids and acellular pertussis vaccine (Tdap).** *(Minimum age: 10 years for BOOSTRIX® and 11 years for ADACEL™)*
   - Administer at age 11–12 years for those who have completed the recommended childhood DTP/DTaP vaccination series and have not received a tetanus and diphtheria toxoids vaccine (Td) booster dose.
   - Adolescents aged 13–18 years who missed the 11–12 year Td/Tdap booster dose should also receive a single dose of Tdap if they have completed the recommended childhood DTP/DTaP vaccination series.
2. **Human papillomavirus vaccine (HPV).** *(Minimum age: 9 years)*
   - Administer the first dose of the HPV vaccine series to females at age 11–12 years.
   - Administer the second dose 2 months after the first dose and the third dose 6 months after the first dose.
   - Administer the HPV vaccine series to females at age 13–18 years if not previously vaccinated.
3. **Meningococcal vaccine.** *(Minimum age: 11 years for meningococcal conjugate vaccine [MCV4]; 2 years for meningococcal polysaccharide vaccine [MPSV4])*
   - Administer MCV4 at age 11–12 years and to previously unvaccinated adolescents at high school entry (at approximately age 15 years).
   - Administer MCV4 to previously unvaccinated college freshmen living in dormitories; MPSV4 is an acceptable alternative.
   - Vaccination against invasive meningococcal disease is recommended for children and adolescents aged ≥2 years with terminal complement deficiencies or anatomic or functional asplenia and certain other high-risk groups. See *MMWR* 2005;54(No. RR-7):1–21. Use MPSV4 for children aged 2–10 years and MCV4 or MPSV4 for older children.
4. **Pneumococcal polysaccharide vaccine (PPV).** *(Minimum age: 2 years)*
   - Administer for certain high-risk groups. See *MMWR* 1997;46(No. RR-8):1–24, and *MMWR* 2000;49(No. RR-9):1–35.
5. **Influenza vaccine.** *(Minimum age: 6 months for trivalent inactivated influenza vaccine [TIV]; 5 years for live, attenuated influenza vaccine [LAIV])*
   - Influenza vaccine is recommended annually for persons with certain risk factors, health-care workers, and other persons (including household members) in close contact with persons in groups at high risk. See *MMWR* 2006;55 (No. RR-10):1–41.
   - For healthy persons aged 5–49 years, LAIV may be used as an alternative to TIV.
   - Children aged <9 years who are receiving influenza vaccine for the first time should receive 2 doses (separated by ≥4 weeks for TIV and ≥6 weeks for LAIV).
6. **Hepatitis A vaccine (HepA).** *(Minimum age: 12 months)*
   - The 2 doses in the series should be administered at least 6 months apart.
   - HepA is recommended for certain other groups of children, including in areas where vaccination programs target older children. See *MMWR* 2006;55 (No. RR-7):1–23.
7. **Hepatitis B vaccine (HepB).** *(Minimum age: birth)*
   - Administer the 3-dose series to those who were not previously vaccinated.
   - A 2-dose series of Recombivax HB® is licensed for children aged 11–15 years.
8. **Inactivated poliovirus vaccine (IPV).** *(Minimum age: 6 weeks)*
   - For children who received an all-IPV or all-oral poliovirus (OPV) series, a fourth dose is not necessary if the third dose was administered at age ≥4 years.
   - If both OPV and IPV were administered as part of a series, a total of 4 doses should be administered, regardless of the child's current age.
9. **Measles, mumps, and rubella vaccine (MMR).** *(Minimum age: 12 months)*
   - If not previously vaccinated, administer 2 doses of MMR during any visit, with ≥4 weeks between the doses.
10. **Varicella vaccine.** *(Minimum age: 12 months)*
    - Administer 2 doses of varicella vaccine to persons without evidence of immunity.
    - Administer 2 doses of varicella vaccine to persons aged ≤13 years at least 3 months apart. Do not repeat the second dose, if administered ≥28 days after the first dose.
    - Administer 2 doses of varicella vaccine to persons aged ≥13 years at least 4 weeks apart.

The Recommended Immunization Schedules for Persons Aged 0–18 Years are approved by the Advisory Committee on Immunization Practices (http://www.cdc.gov/nip/acip), the American Academy of Pediatrics (http://www.aap.org), and the American Academy of Family Physicians (http://www.aafp.org).

Table 9.7 Catch-Up Immunization Schedule for Persons Aged 4 Months–18 Years Who Start Late or Who Are ≥1 Month Behind—United States, 2007

The table below provides catch-up schedules and minimum intervals between doses for children whose vaccinations have been delayed. A vaccine series does not need to be restarted, regardless of the time that has elapsed between doses. Use the section appropriate for the child's age.

Vaccine	Minimum age for Dose 1	Minimum interval between doses			
		Dose 1 to Dose 2	Dose 2 to Dose 3	Dose 3 to Dose 4	Dose 4 to Dose 5
CATCH-UP SCHEDULE FOR PERSONS AGED 4 MONTHS–6 YEARS					
Hepatitis B[1]	Birth	4 weeks	8 weeks (and 16 weeks after first dose)		
Rotavirus[2]	6 weeks	4 weeks	4 weeks		
Diphtheria, Tetanus, Pertussis[3]	6 weeks	4 weeks	4 weeks	6 months	6 months[3]
Haemophilus influenzae type b[4]	6 weeks	4 weeks if first dose administered at age <12 months 8 weeks (as final dose) if first dose administered at age 12–14 months No further doses needed if first dose administered at age ≥15 months	4 weeks[4] if current age <12 months 8 weeks (as final dose)[4] if current age ≥12 months and second dose administered at age <15 months No further doses needed if previous dose administered at age ≥15 months	8 weeks (as final dose) This dose only necessary for children aged 12 months–5 years who received 3 doses before age 12 months	
Pneumococcal[5]	6 weeks	4 weeks if first dose administered at age <12 months and current age <24 months 8 weeks (as final dose) if first dose administered at age ≥12 months or current age 24–59 months No further doses needed for healthy children if first dose administered at age ≥24 months	4 weeks if current age <12 months 8 weeks (as final dose) if current age ≥12 months No further doses needed for healthy children if previous dose administered at age ≥24 months	8 weeks (as final dose) This dose only necessary for children aged 12 months–5 years who received 3 doses before age 12 months	
Inactivated Poliovirus[6]	6 weeks	4 weeks	4 weeks	4 weeks[6]	
Measles, Mumps, Rubella[7]	12 months	4 weeks			
Varicella[8]	12 months	3 months			
Hepatitis A[9]	12 months	6 months			
CATCH-UP SCHEDULE FOR PERSONS AGED 7–18 YEARS					
Tetanus, Diphtheria/ Tetanus, Diphtheria, Pertussis[10]	7 years[10]	4 weeks	8 weeks if first dose administered at age <12 months 6 months if first dose administered at age ≥12 months	6 months if first dose administered at age <12 months	
Human Papillomavirus[11]	9 years	4 weeks	12 weeks		
Hepatitis A[9]	12 months	6 months			
Hepatitis B[1]	Birth	4 weeks	8 weeks (and 16 weeks after first dose)		
Inactivated Poliovirus[6]	6 weeks	4 weeks	4 weeks	4 weeks[6]	
Measles, Mumps, Rubella[7]	12 months	4 weeks			
Varicella[8]	12 months	4 weeks if first dose administered at age ≥13 years 3 months if first dose administered at age <13 years			

1. **Hepatitis B vaccine (HepB).** *(Minimum age: birth)*
   - Administer the 3-dose series to those who were not previously vaccinated.
   - A 2-dose series of Recombivax HB® is licensed for children aged 11–15 years.
2. **Rotavirus vaccine (Rota).** *(Minimum age: 6 weeks)*
   - Do not start the series later than age 12 weeks.
   - Administer the final dose in the series by age 32 weeks. Do not administer a dose later than age 32 weeks.
   - Data on safety and efficacy outside of these age ranges are insufficient.
3. **Diphtheria and tetanus toxoids and acellular pertussis vaccine (DTaP).** *(Minimum age: 6 weeks)*
   - The fifth dose is not necessary if the fourth dose was administered at age ≥4 years.
   - DTaP is not indicated for persons aged ≥7 years.
4. ***Haemophilus influenzae* type b conjugate vaccine (Hib).** *(Minimum age: 6 weeks)*
   - Vaccine is not generally recommended for children aged ≥5 years.
   - If current age <12 months and the first 2 doses were PRP-OMP (PedvaxHIB® or ComVax® [Merck]), the third (and final) dose should be administered at age 12–15 months and at least 8 weeks after the second dose.
   - If first dose was administered at age 7–11 months, administer 2 doses separated by 4 weeks plus a booster at age 12–15 months.
5. **Pneumococcal conjugate vaccine (PCV).** *(Minimum age: 6 weeks)*
   - Vaccine is not generally recommended for children aged ≥5 years.
6. **Inactivated poliovirus vaccine (IPV).** *(Minimum age: 6 weeks)*
   - For children who received an all-IPV or all-oral poliovirus (OPV) series, a fourth dose is not necessary if third dose was administered at age ≥4 years.
   - If both OPV and IPV were administered as part of a series, a total of 4 doses should be administered, regardless of the child's current age.
7. **Measles, mumps, and rubella vaccine (MMR).** *(Minimum age: 12 months)*
   - The second dose of MMR is recommended routinely at age 4–6 years but may be administered earlier if desired.
   - If not previously vaccinated, administer 2 doses of MMR during any visit with ≥4 weeks between the doses.
8. **Varicella vaccine.** *(Minimum age: 12 months)*
   - The second dose of varicella vaccine is recommended routinely at age 4–6 years but may be administered earlier if desired.
   - Do not repeat the second dose in persons aged <13 years if administered ≥28 days after the first dose.
9. **Hepatitis A vaccine (HepA).** *(Minimum age: 12 months)*
   - HepA is recommended for certain groups of children, including in areas where vaccination programs target older children. See *MMWR* 2006;55(No. RR-7):1–23.
10. **Tetanus and diphtheria toxoids vaccine (Td) and tetanus and diphtheria toxoids and acellular pertussis vaccine (Tdap).** *(Minimum ages: 7 years for Td, 10 years for BOOSTRIX®, and 11 years for ADACEL™)*
    - Tdap should be substituted for a single dose of Td in the primary catch-up series or as a booster if age appropriate; use Td for other doses.
    - A 5-year interval from the last Td dose is encouraged when Tdap is used as a booster dose. A booster (fourth) dose is needed if any of the previous doses were administered at age <12 months. Refer to ACIP recommendations for further information. See *MMWR* 2006;55(No. RR-3).
11. **Human papillomavirus vaccine (HPV).** *(Minimum age: 9 years)*
    - Administer the HPV vaccine series to females at age 13–18 years if not previously vaccinated.

Information about reporting reactions after immunization is available online at http://www.vaers.hhs.gov or by telephone via the 24-hour national toll-free information line 800-822-7967. Suspected cases of vaccine-preventable diseases should be reported to the state or local health department. Additional information, including precautions and contraindications for immunization, is available from the National Center for Immunization and Respiratory Diseases at http://www.cdc.gov/nip/default.htm or telephone, 800-CDC-INFO (800-232-4636).

BOX 9.8

VACCINE ADMINISTRATION ROUTES

Intramuscular	Subcutaneous
DTaP, DT, Tdap	IPV
Hepatitis B, hepatitis A	MMR
Hib	Varicella
Influenza	MPSV4
Pneumococcal	
HPV	
MCV4	

Modified from Middleton, D., Zimmerman, R., & Mitchell, K. (2005). Childhood vaccine schedules and procedures, 2005 [Special edition]. *Journal of Family Practice,* S16–S25.

are required for school admittance. These requirements can be waived if a contraindication or precaution to the vaccine exists. Contraindications are conditions that justify withholding an immunization either permanently or temporarily. There are only two permanent contraindications: an anaphylactic or systemic allergic reaction to a vaccine component; or with pertussis immunization, encephalopathy without an identified cause within 7 days of the immunization. Temporarily postponing vaccinations is recommended when the child has a severe illness with a high fever, immunosuppression, or has recently received blood products. Postponing vaccination because of a minor respiratory illness or low-grade fever is not appropriate. Precautions are conditions that increase the risk of an adverse reaction or may impair the child's ability to acquire immunity from the vaccine. On an individualized basis, providers must weigh the benefits of immunization against the likelihood of an adverse event. A summary of precautions and contraindications are presented in Table 9.9.

Diphtheria, Pertussis, and Tetanus Vaccines

Immunizations against diphtheria, pertussis, and tetanus diseases is given in combination vaccines. The vaccine currently used for children under age 7 is diphtheria, tetanus, acellular pertussis (DTaP). It contains diphtheria and tetanus toxoids, and pertussis cell wall proteins. The older version of this vaccine—diphtheria, tetanus, pertussis (DPT)—contained killed whole cells of pertussis bacteria and caused more frequent and severe adverse reactions than DTaP. Diphtheria, tetanus (DT) vaccine is used for children under age 7 who have contraindications to pertussis immunization. Full-strength diphtheria toxoid causes significant adverse reactions in people over the age of 7 years. For this group, the TdaP adolescent preparation vaccine is used: It contains tetanus toxoid, reduced diphtheria toxoid, and acellular pertussis vaccine. The lowercase "d" is used to designate the lower dose of diphtheria toxoid. The ACIP recommends that TdaP be used for all tetanus boosters in older children (11 to 12 years) and adolescents, because TdaP provides a boost to diphtheria and pertussis immunization.

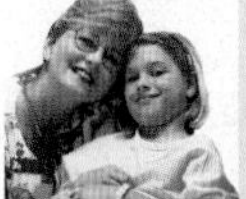

Pertussis cases have steadily risen since the 1970s, with 34% of cases occurring in adolescents. This increase prompted the AAP's recommendation to change the tetanus booster for older children and adolescents from Td to TdaP beginning in 2006, to provide continuing protection against pertussis infection (AAP, 2005).

Haemophilus influenzae *Type B Vaccines*

Haemophilus influenzae type B is a bacterium that causes several life-threatening illnesses in children under 5 years of age. These infections include meningitis, epiglottitis, and septic arthritis. *Haemophilus influenzae* type B conjugate vaccines (Hib) have been extremely effective in cutting the

(text continues on page 240)

Table 9.8 Vaccine Administration: Needle and Site Selection

Client	Needle Size	Needle Length (Inches)	Site
Birth–4 months	25 gauge	5/8	Anterolateral thigh
4–18 months	23–25 gauge	7/8 to 1	Anterolateral thigh
18–36 months	23–25 gauge	7/8 to 1.25	Anterolateral thigh
3–18 years	22–25 gauge	7/8 to 1.5	Deltoid or anterolateral thigh
Male < 120 kg	22–25 gauge	1 to 1.5	Deltoid
Males > 120 kg	22–25 gauge	2	Deltoid
Female < 70 kg	22–25 gauge	1	Deltoid
Female 70–100 kg	22–25 gauge	1.5	Deltoid
Female > 100 kg	22–25 gauge	2	Deltoid
All clients receiving subcutaneous injections	23–25 gauge	5/8 to 3/4	Fat of anterolateral thigh or upper arm

Middleton, D., Zimmerman, R., & Mitchell, K. (2005). Childhood vaccine schedules and procedures, 2005. (Special edition). *Journal of Family Practice,* S16–S25.

DIPHTHERIA TETANUS & PERTUSSIS VACCINES

WHAT YOU NEED TO KNOW

1 Why get vaccinated?

Diphtheria, tetanus, and pertussis are serious diseases caused by bacteria. Diphtheria and pertussis are spread from person to person. Tetanus enters the body through cuts or wounds.

DIPHTHERIA causes a thick covering in the back of the throat.

- It can lead to breathing problems, paralysis, heart failure, and even death.

TETANUS (Lockjaw) causes painful tightening of the muscles, usually all over the body.

- It can lead to "locking" of the jaw so the victim cannot open his mouth or swallow. Tetanus leads to death in about 1 out of 10 cases.

PERTUSSIS (Whooping Cough) causes coughing spells so bad that is hard for infants to eat, drink, or breathe. These spells can last for weeks.

- It can lead to pneumonia, seizures (jerking and staring spells), brain damage, and death.

Diphtheria, tetanus, and pertussis vaccine (DTaP) can help prevent these diseases. Most children who are vaccinated with DTaP will be protected throughout childhood. Many more children would get these diseases if we stopped vaccinating.

DTaP is a safer version of an older vaccine called DTP. DTP is no longer used in the United States.

2 Who should get DTaP vaccine and when?

Children should get 5 doses of DTaP vaccine, one dose at each of the following ages:

✓ 2 months ✓ 4 months ✓ 6 months
✓ 15-18 months ✓ 4-6 years

DTaP may be given at the same time as other vaccines.

3 Some children should not get DTaP vaccine or should wait.

- Children with minor illnesses, such as a cold, may be vaccinated. But children who are moderately or severely ill should usually wait until they recover before getting DTaP vaccine.

- Any child who had a life-threatening allergic reaction after a dose of DTaP should not get another dose.

- Any child who suffered a brain or nervous system disease within 7 days after a dose of DTaP should not get another dose.

- Talk with your doctor if your child:
  - had a seizure or collapsed after a dose of DTaP,
  - cried non-stop for 3 hours or more after a dose of DTaP,
  - had a fever over 105°F after a dose of DTaP.

Ask your health care provider for more information. Some of these children should not get another dose of pertussis vaccine, but may get a vaccine without pertussis, called **DT**.

4 Older children and adults

DTaP should not be given to anyone 7 years of age or older because pertussis vaccine is only licensed for children under 7.

But older children, adolescents, and adults still need protection from tetanus and diphtheria. A booster shot called **Td** is recommended at 11-12 years of age, and then every 10 years. There is a separate Vaccine Information Statement for Td vaccine.

Diphtheria/Tetanus/Pertussis 7/30/2001

● **Figure 9.6** Federal law mandates the use of Vaccine Information Statements (VIS). These should be given to the parent or primary caregiver for each vaccine the child receives. *(continued)*

5 What are the risks from DTaP vaccine?

Getting diphteria, tetanus, or pertussis disease is much riskier than getting DTaP vaccine.

However, a vaccine, like any medicine, is capable of causing serious problems, such as severe allergic reactions. The risk of DTaP vaccine causing serious harm, or death, is extremely small.

Mild Problems (Common)

- Fever (up to about 1 child in 4)
- Redness or swelling where the shot was given (up to about 1 child in 4)
- Soreness or tenderness where the shot was given (up to about 1 child in 4)

These problems occur more often after the 4th and 5th doses of the DTaP series than after earlier doses. Sometimes the 4th or 5th dose of DTaP vaccine is followed by swelling of the entire arm or leg in which the shot was given, lasting 1-7 days (up to about 1 child in 30).

Other mild problems include:

- Fussiness (up to about 1 child in 3)
- Tiredness or poor appetite (up to about 1 child in 10)
- Vomiting (up to about 1 child in 50)

These problems generally occur 1-3 days after the shot.

Moderate Problems (Uncommon)

- Seizure (jerking or staring) (about 1 child out of 14,000)
- Non-stop crying, for 3 hours or more (up to about 1 child out of 1,000)
- High fever, over 105°F (about 1 child out of 16,000)

Severe Problems (Very Rare)

- Serious allergic reaction (less than 1 out of a million doses)
- Several other severe problems have been reported after DTaP vaccine. These include:
  - Long-term seizures, coma, or lowered consciousness
  - Permanent brain damage.

  These are so rare it is hard to tell if they are caused by the vaccine.

Controlling fever is especially important for children who have had seizures, for any reason. It is also important if another family member has had seizures. You can reduce fever and pain by giving your child an *aspirin-free* pain reliever when the shot is given, and for the next 24 hours, following the package instructions.

6 What if there is a moderate or severe reaction?

What should I look for?

Any unusual conditions, such as a serious allergic reaction, high fever or unusual behavior. Serious allergic reactions are extremely rare with any vaccine. If one were to occur, it would most likely be within a few minutes to a few hours after the shot. Signs can include difficulty breathing, hoarseness or wheezing, hives, paleness, weakness, a fast heart beat or dizziness. If a high fever or seizure were to occur, it would usually be within a week after the shot.

What should I do?

- **Call** a doctor, or get the person to a doctor right away.
- **Tell** your doctor what happened, the date and time it happened, and when the vaccination was given.
- **Ask** your doctor, nurse, or health department to report the reaction by filing a Vaccine Adverse Event Reporting System (VAERS) form.

Or you can file this report through the VAERS website at www.vaers.org, or by calling 1-800-822-7967.

VAERS does not provide medical advice.

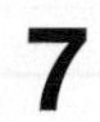

7 The National Vaccine Injury Compensation Program

In the rare event that you or your child has a serious reaction to a vaccine, a federal program has been created to help pay for the care of those who have been harmed.

For details about the National Vaccine Injury Compensation Program, call **1-800-338-2382** or visit the program's website at **www.hrsa.gov/osp/vicp**

8 How can I learn more?

- Ask your health care provider. They can give you the vaccine package insert or suggest other sources of information.
- Call your local or state health department's immunization program.
- Contact the Centers for Disease Control and Prevention (CDC):
  - Call **1-800-232-4636 (1-800-CDC-INFO)**
  - Visit the National Immunization Program's website at **www.cdc.gov/nip**

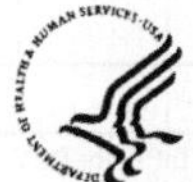

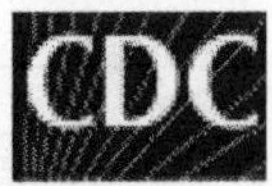

U.S. DEPARTMENT OF HEALTH & HUMAN SERVICES
Centers for Disease Control and Prevention
National Immunization Program

Vaccine Information Statement
DTaP (7/30/01) 42 U.S.C. § 300aa-26

● Figure 9.6 (continued)

Vaccine Administration Record for Children and Teens

Patient name: ____________________

Birthdate: ____________________

Chart number: ____________________

Vaccine	Type of Vaccine[1] (generic abbreviation)	Date given (mo/day/yr)	Source (F,S,P)[2]	Site[3]	Vaccine		Vaccine Information Statement		Signature/ initials of vaccinator
					Lot #	Mfr.	Date on VIS[4]	Date given[4]	
Hepatitis B[5] (e.g., HepB, Hib-HepB, DTaP-HepB-IPV) Give IM.									
Diphtheria, Tetanus, Pertussis[5] (e.g., DTaP, DTaP-Hib, DTaP-HepB-IPV, DT, Tdap, Td) Give IM.									
***Haemophilus influenzae* type b[5]** (e.g., Hib, Hib-HepB, DTaP-Hib) Give IM.									
Polio[5] (e.g., IPV, DTaP-HepB-IPV) Give IPV SC or IM. Give DTaP-HepB-IPV IM.									
Pneumococcal (e.g., PCV, conjugate; PPV, polysaccharide) Give PCV IM. Give PPV SC or IM.									
Rotavirus (Rv) Give oral (po).									
Measles, Mumps, Rubella[5] (e.g., MMR, MMRV) Give SC.									
Varicella[5] (e.g., Var, MMRV) Give SC.									
Hepatitis A (HepA) Give IM.									
Meningococcal (e.g., MCV4; MPSV4) Give MCV4 IM and MPSV4 SC.									
Human papillomavirus (e.g., HPV) Give IM.									
Influenza[5] (e.g., TIV, inactivated; LAIV, live attenuated) Give TIV IM. Give LAIV IN.									
Other									

1. Record the generic abbreviation for the type of vaccine given (e.g., DTaP-Hib, PCV), *not* the trade name.
2. Record the source of the vaccine given as either F (Federally-supported), S (State-supported), or P (supported by Private insurance or other Private funds).
3. Record the site where vaccine was administered as either RA (Right Arm), LA (Left Arm), RT (Right Thigh), LT (Left Thigh), IN (Intranasal), or O (Oral).
4. Record the publication date of each VIS as well as the date it is given to the patient.
5. For combination vaccines, fill in a row for each separate antigen in the combination.

Technical content reviewed by the Centers for Disease Control and Prevention, Nov. 2006.

www.immunize.org/catg.d/p2022b.pdf • Item #P2022 (11/06)

Immunization Action Coalition • 1573 Selby Ave. • St. Paul, MN 55104 • (651) 647-9009 • www.immunize.org • www.vaccineinformation.org

● **Figure 9.7** Sample of a vaccine administration record.

Table 9.9 Contraindications and Precautions for Commonly Used Vaccines

Vaccine	Contraindications	Precautions
Hepatitis A (HepA)	• Standard contraindications* • Infants less than 12 months of age	• Moderate or severe illness
Hepatitis B (HepB)	Standard contraindications*	• Moderate or severe illness with or without acute fever • Infants less than 2,000 grams if mother HBsAg negative
Diphtheria, Tetanus, acellular Pertussis (DTaP) Tetanus, diphtheria, acellular Pertussis (TdaP)	• Standard contraindications* • Previous encephalopathy within 7 days after Diphtheria, Tetanus, Pertussis (DTP) vaccine or DTaP	• Temperature 105 °F (40.5 °C) within 48 hours after previous dose • Continuous crying lasting 3 hours within 48 hours after previous dose • Previous convulsion within 3 days after immunization • Pale or limp episode or collapse within 48 hours after previous dose • Unstable progressive neurologic problem • History of Guillain-Barré syndrome within 6 weeks
Diphtheria, Tetanus (DT)	Standard contraindications*	
Measles, Mumps, Rubella (MMR)	• Standard contraindications*† • Pregnancy or possibility of pregnancy within 4 weeks • Blood products within the past 5 months • Immunocompromised person • If not given same day as varicella and/or yellow fever, hold until spaced 28 days apart	• Thrombocytopenia or history of thrombocytopenic purpura
Varicella	• Standard contraindications*† • Pregnancy or possibility of pregnancy within 4 weeks • Blood products received within the past 5 months • Immunocompromised person • If not given same day as MMR and/or yellow fever, hold until spaced 28 days apart	• Do not give within 24 hours of antiviral medications. • Family history of congenital or hereditary immunodeficiency
Inactivated Polio Virus (IPV)	Standard contraindications*‡	• Moderate or severe acute illness • Pregnancy
Haemophilus Influenza type B (Hib)	Standard contraindications*	• Moderate or severe acute illness
Trivalent Inactivated Influenza Vaccine (TIV)	Standard contraindications*	• History of Guillain-Barré syndrome within 6 weeks
Live Attenuated Influenza Vaccine (LAIV)	Standard contraindications* Client less than 5 years old Client 5 or more years old with chronic illnesses Client with close contact with severely immunosuppressed persons	• Do not give within 48 hours of antiviral medications.
Pneumococcal conjugate vaccine (PCV7) Pneumococcal polysaccharide vaccine (PPV23)	Standard contraindications*	• Moderate or severe acute illness

*1. Do not administer if client has had an anaphylactic reaction to prior dose of vaccine or any of its components. 2. Do not administer if client has a moderate to severe acute illness. Minor illnesses are not a reason to postpone immunization. † Inquire about neomycin or gelatin allergies. ‡ Inquire about neomycin, streptomycin, or polymyxin B allergies.

rates of these diseases in children. There are several different types of Hib conjugate vaccines. HibTITER (HbOC) and ActHib (PRP-T) require three doses for the primary infant series, while PedvaxHIB and Comvax (PRP-OMP) require two doses. These vaccines are interchangeable, but if different brands are administered to a child, then a total of three doses is necessary to complete the primary series in infants. Hib vaccine is not given to children 5 years of age or older.

Polio Vaccine

Inactivated polio vaccine (IPV) is the only polio vaccine currently recommended in the United States. It is a killed virus vaccine that poses no risk for vaccine-acquired disease. Oral polio vaccine (OPV), a live attenuated virus vaccine, was the preferred polio vaccine until 2000. At that time it became apparent that the only victims of poliomyelitis were people who had acquired it from OPV. The ACIP determined that in this country the risks of OPV outweighed the benefits and withdrew its recommendation of OPV.

Measles, Mumps, and Rubella Vaccines

Measles, mumps, rubella (MMR) is a live attenuated virus combination vaccine. It is the one most commonly used in childhood immunizations. MMR can be given the same day as other live attenuated virus vaccines such as varicella vaccine. However, if not given on the same day, the immunizations should be spaced at least 28 days apart. Anaphylactic reactions are believed to be associated with the neomycin or gelatin components of the vaccine, rather than the egg component. The vaccine is not prepared from the allergenic albumen portion of the egg. Egg allergy is no longer a contraindication for measles vaccine. Pregnancy in a child's mother is not a contraindication to the vaccination of the child. Individual measles, mumps, and rubella vaccines are available if needed.

Hepatitis A Vaccine

Hepatitis A vaccine (HepA) is an inactivated whole virus vaccine. The vaccine has been demonstrated to be about 94% effective in preventing hepatitis A infection. Hepatitis A is spread through close physical contact and by eating or drinking contaminated food or water. It is the one of the most frequently reported vaccine-preventable diseases in the United States. Young children are particularly susceptible to hepatitis A because of their close contact with other children, inadequate hygiene practices, and their tendency to place everything in their mouth. Hepatitis A vaccine is recommended to be given to all children at age 12 months, followed by a repeat dose in 6 to 12 months.

Hepatitis B Vaccine

Hepatitis B vaccine (HepB) is a recombinant vaccine. The vaccine is 80% to 90% effective in preventing hepatitis B infection. For infants, the mother's HBsAg status determines when immunization for hepatitis B begins. If the mother's status is positive or unknown, the neonate is immunized within the first 12 hours of life, at 1 to 2 months of age, and at 6 months of age. This is vital, because up to 90% of infected neonates develop chronic carrier status and will be predisposed to cirrhosis and hepatic cancer. If the mother's status is negative, immunizations are done routinely at 2, 4, and 6 months of age. Because hepatitis B is a sexually transmitted infection, it is important to verify the immunization status of all adolescents.

Varicella Vaccine

Varicella vaccine (Var) is a live attenuated virus vaccine. All children age 12 to 15 months who have not had varicella (chickenpox) should be immunized. A second dose is recommended at age 4 to 6 years. The vaccine is an effective varicella postexposure prophylaxis if administered within 3 to 5 days after exposure. Varicella vaccine may be given the same day as other live attenuated virus vaccines. However, if not given on the same day, the immunizations should be spaced at least 28 days apart. Pregnancy in a child's mother is not a contraindication to the vaccination of the child.

Pneumococcal Vaccines

Streptococcus pneumoniae (pneumococcus) is the most common cause of pneumonia, sepsis, and meningitis in children under 2 years of age. The two available pneumococcal vaccines are pneumococcal conjugate vaccine (PCV) and pneumococcal polysaccharide vaccine (PPV). PCV contains seven strains of *Streptococcus pneumoniae.* It does stimulate an immune response in infants and is given at 2 months of age as part of the initial immunization series. PPV contains 23 strains of *Streptococcus pneumoniae.* It does not provoke an immune response in children under 2 years of age. PPV is given to children over 2 years old who are at high risk for pneumococcal sepsis. This group includes children with anatomic/functional asplenia; sickle-sell disease; chronic cardiac, pulmonary, or renal disease; diabetes mellitus; HIV infection; or immunosuppression.

Influenza Vaccines

Influenza immunization is recommended yearly for children between the ages of 6 and 59 months. Children 2 years old or older should be vaccinated if they have chronic health problems. It is also recommended that caregivers and household contacts of these children be immunized. Additionally, the vaccine can be given to anyone wishing to have immunity.

There are two influenza vaccines available, the trivalent inactivated influenza vaccine (TIV) and the live attenuated influenza vaccine (LAIV). LAIV is given intranasally and is indicated for healthy persons between the ages of 5 and 49 years. The virus in LAIV can replicate, and a person who has received LAIV can shed virus for a week. LAIV should not be given to anyone who will be in contact with an immunosuppressed person requiring a protected environment. TIV is suitable for any eligible person age 6 months or older. TIV is not capable of causing disease and is given by intramuscular injection.

Rotavirus Vaccine

Rotavirus is the most common cause of severe gastroenteritis among young children. The virus is shed in the stool and easily spreads via the fecal–oral route. Rotavirus accounts for about 50% of annual hospitalizations for gastroenteritis in children (AAP, 2007a). Severe, watery, crampy diarrhea quickly leads to dehydration in the infected child. The most severe disease occurs in children ages 3 to 35 months (Parashar et al., 2006). The rotavirus vaccine is a live vaccine targeting five strains of rotavirus and is given via the oral route to infants less than 32 weeks of age (CDC, 2006b).

Human Papillomavirus Vaccine

Human papillomavirus (HPV) is a DNA tumor virus transmitted through direct skin-to-skin contact. HPV is contracted most often during vaginal or anal penetrative sexual acts. HPV infection is most common in adolescents and young adults aged 15 to 24 years who are sexually active (CDC, 2006a). HPV causes genital warts and is responsible for the development of cervical cancer. For these reasons, the ACIP and AAP recommended that in 2007, HPV vaccination occur in preadolescent females. The three-vaccine series should begin at age 11 to 12 years. The vaccine is anticipated to prevent most cases of genital warts and cervical cancer (AAP, 2007b).

Meningococcal Vaccine

Meningococcal disease may manifest as meningitis or as a deadly blood infection (meningococcemia). It is caused by the bacterium *Neisseria meningitiditis*, which is spread through direct contact or by air droplets. Since the 1990s, the incidence of meningococcal disease among adolescents and young adults has increased about 60%. About 10% to 12% of infected persons die; of the remaining victims, about 20% suffer severe long-term consequences (NMA, n.d.). For these reasons, the meningococcal vaccine is now recommended for all previously unvaccinated children at age 11 to 12 years. These children should receive the meningococcal conjugated vaccine (MCV4). Certain high-risk groups may be vaccinated at 2 years of age (through age 10) with the meningococcal polysaccharide vaccine (MPSV4) (CDC, 2006b).

> Recall 3-year-old Maya and 9-month-old Evan, introduced at the beginning of the chapter. What immunizations would be appropriate for them to receive? Explain how you would administer the injections and discuss any contraindications or precautions that are necessary.

Barriers to Immunization

A fully immunized child is protected from the discomforts and complications of many infectious diseases. Disease prevention spares the family the emotional and financial burdens that serious illnesses can cause. Effective immunization programs prevent devastating epidemics in a community. Health care dollars not spent treating preventable diseases can be used for other urgent issues. Despite the numerous advantages of an optimal immunization status, many children in this country are not fully immunized.

Many factors to lead to children not being fully immunized. Parental concerns about vaccine safety are a significant cause of inadequate immunization. Misconceptions of what constitutes a contraindication to vaccination and having more than one health care provider are major contributors to inadequate immunization status. The more children in a family, the less likely the children are to be fully vaccinated. The costs for vaccines can also deter families from obtaining immunizations. Parents may want to postpone some of the scheduled immunizations because they are concerned about the effects of multiple injections on their child. Postponing a portion of the immunizations puts the child at risk for contracting disease. Disrupting the optimal spacing of the immunizations can decrease the efficacy of vaccine, further putting the child at risk.

Easing Barriers to Immunization

The AAP recommends the use of manufacturer-produced combination vaccines whenever it will reduce the number of injections at a visit. These combination vaccines have been studied and approved by the U.S. Food and Drug Administration (FDA). The nurse should never mix separate vaccines in the same syringe unless expressly permitted in the product insert for all vaccines involved. Examples of combination vaccines are:

- DTaP: diphtheria, tetanus, acellular pertussis
- MMR: measles, mumps, rubella
- HepB-Hib: hepatitis B virus and *Haemophilus influenzae* type B

The Vaccines for Children (VFC) program was implemented in 1994. Prior to this program, free vaccines were only available to through public health agencies. By providing free vaccines to low-income and uninsured families through their private health care providers, immunization rates have increased tremendously. Additional information on the VFC program is available at http://www.cdc.gov/nip/vfc/provider/provider_home.htm.

Establishing a medical home for every child will help alleviate many of the factors associated with lack of immunization. Parents in a long-term, trust-based relationship with a health care provider are more likely to have their concerns about vaccine safety assuaged. Missed opportunities for immunizations can be reduced by:

- Maintaining a centralized immunization record
- Verifying immunization status at every visit, not just health supervision visits
- Verifying the status of siblings accompanying the child to the appointment
- Providing parents with up-to-date information on vaccines geared to their concerns and needs

An excellent resource for additional information on vaccination recommendations in the United States, the National Immunization Program, may be found at http://www.cdc.gov/nip or by calling 800-235-2522 (National Immunization Hotline) (see Healthy People 2010).

> **Recall Maya and Evan.** Discuss potential barriers to Maya and Evan being fully immunized. As a nurse, how can you help ease these barriers?

Health Promotion

Health promotion focuses on maintaining or enhancing the physical and mental health of clients. The principle components of health promotion are identifying risk factors for a disease, facilitating lifestyle changes to eliminate or reduce those risk factors, and empowering clients at the individual and community level to develop resources to optimize their health. The nurse implements health promotion through education and anticipatory guidance.

Partnership development is the key strategy for success when implementing a health promotion activity. Identifying key stakeholders from the community increases problem solving and provides additional venues for disseminating information. The health promotion message is reinforced at the school; daycare center; Special Supplemental Nutrition Program for Women, Infants, and Children (WIC) office; and church. If families have difficulty accessing health care facilities, the community arenas may be the primary source of health promotion.

Providing Anticipatory Guidance

Anticipatory guidance is primary prevention. The nurse partners with the parents to build a roadmap to optimal health for the child. Healthy People 2010 provides a framework for determining health promotion goals for the client population. *Bright Futures: Guidelines for Health Supervision of Infants, Children, and Adolescents* (2002) is another valuable resource. Although the challenges frequently encountered by most families form the skeleton of the guidance, the nurse fleshes out information provided to parents based on other factors such as results of risk assessments and screening tests, health concerns unique to the child, and the interests and concerns of the parents. Age-related anticipatory guidance information is provided in Chapters 4, 5, 6, 7, and 8 of this book.

> **Provide appropriate** anticipatory guidance for both 3-year-old Maya and 9-month-old Evan.

Promoting Oral Health Care

Effective oral health practices are essential to the overall health of children and adolescents. Dental care is the most prevalent unmet health need among children in the United States. Poor oral health can have significant negative effects on systemic health. Children who suffer from dental caries have increased incidence of pain, decreased appetite, and sleep pattern disturbances. They are at increased risk for abscesses and systemic infections (see Healthy People 2010).

Optimal oral health is not limited to prevention and treatment of dental caries. Oral health includes anticipatory guidance on the topics of nonnutritive sucking habits, injury prevention, oral cancer prevention, and intraoral/perioral piercing. Preventing and treating malocclusion can have significant benefit for children. Comprehensive health care is not possible if oral health is not a priority in the health delivery system.

Optimizing oral health can benefit the community as well as the individual client. There has been a 60% reduction in early childhood caries over the past 50 years since community water supplies were fluoridated at optimal levels. The cost of pediatric oral health care could be reduced 50% with the proper use of fluoride treatments coupled with other preventive measures. These health care dollar savings will benefit community resources.

The dental home enhances the likelihood that the child will obtain appropriate preventive and routine care.

HEALTHY PEOPLE 2010

Objective	Significance
Increase the proportion of young children who receive all vaccines that have been recommended for universal administration for at least 5 years.	• Immunize at every opportunity. If a child is due or past due for vaccinations, provide them at a sick visit if not contraindicated. • Educate families about the benefits and risks of immunization.

HEALTHY PEOPLE 2010

Objective	Significance
Reduce the proportion of children and adolescents who have dental caries in their primary or permanent teeth.	• Teach children and adolescents appropriate toothbrushing and flossing techniques. • Encourage use of fluoride-containing toothpastes. • Encourage routine dental visits.

The American Academy of Pediatric Dentistry (AAPD) adopted the policy of the dental home in 2001. It is modeled on the AAP medical home policy. The dental home provides the same benefits to the child as the medical home. Characteristics of a dental home are listed in Box 9.9. The AAPD recommends that the dental home be established by the infant's first birthday.

Promoting Healthy Weight

Childhood obesity is a growing problem. The number of overweight children has doubled since 1980, while the rate for teens has tripled. The principle causes of this increase in obesity are unhealthy eating habits and decreased physical activity. Research has demonstrated that weight is best managed with a combination of diet and exercise. Nurses will have the maximum effect in promoting healthy weight in children by initiating activities that address both healthy eating patterns and physical fitness. Children, parents, and communities are all targets for healthy weight promotion by nurses.

The focus of healthy weight promotion should be health centered, not weight centered. Emphasizing the benefits of health through an active lifestyle and nutritious eating pattern creates a nurturing environment for the child. This allows the child to maintain self-esteem. Linking success to numbers on a scale increases the possibility of developing eating disorders, nutritional deficiencies, and body hatred. A health-centered orientation also allows the family to develop a lifestyle that respects cultural food patterns and traditions.

The nurse can stress the benefits of the mother's healthy nutritional habits to the fetus at prenatal visits. Parents who have a healthy eating pattern are likely to maintain and encourage those patterns in their children. The nurse provides parents with anticipatory guidance about age-related eating patterns during each health supervision visit. Parents with toddlers and preschoolers may need training in techniques that cope with the child's growing autonomy while providing a variety of nutritious options.

The nurse can begin directly advising children on healthy foods starting at age 3. Information and teaching modalities need to be age appropriate. Using colorful posters and games, the preschool child can learn the difference between healthy and unhealthy food choices. As children enter school age, group and peer-led activities can be very effective. The nurse must gear material toward the teen's growing autonomy in making self-care decisions. Before beginning education to school-age and teenage children, it is important to obtain nutritional histories directly from them. School-agers and teenagers are increasingly eating meals away from the family table. As they spend more time away from their parents, they need to develop the ability to make nutritious choices. The goal is to help older children develop strategies for implementing healthy choices within an increasingly independent lifestyle (see Healthy People 2010). Detailed anticipatory guidance is provided in Teaching Guideline 9.1 and in Chapters 4 to 8.

Healthy physical activity can take many forms. During the preschool years, nurses need to encourage parents to provide a wide variety of physical activities. This exposure to multiple exercise options allows the child to find the one that is most enjoyable and increases the chances of maintaining an active lifestyle. The focus should be on noncompetitive, fun activities such as dance or gymnastics. When the child enters the school-age years, the lure of television and computers can significantly diminish the amount of time spent in physical activity. Parents can influence their children to stay physically active in several ways. They can limit the amount of time spent in sedentary activities and actively encourage the child to pursue any exercise activity that he or she enjoys. In addition to verbal encouragement, parents can stimulate exercise activities by participating in exercise with the child. A simple family walk can increase physical fitness while providing time for increased interaction between parent and child. See Teaching Guideline 9.2 for additional sugges-

BOX 9.9

CHARACTERISTICS OF THE DENTAL HOME

- Preventive health program based on risk assessment
- Anticipatory guidance on oral health developmental issues
- Plans for emergency dental trauma
- Anticipatory guidance on oral hygiene
- Comprehensive dental care
- Referral to specialists for care not available at the dental home

HEALTHY PEOPLE 2010

Objective	Significance
Reduce the proportion of children and adolescents who are overweight or obese.	• Screen all children for the development of overweight as indicated by an increasing body mass index (BMI) for their age. • Provide accurate diet counseling. • Encourage daily physical activity. • Counsel parents to limit television/computer time daily.

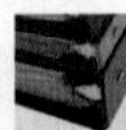

TEACHING GUIDELINE 9.1

Teaching Healthy Eating

Breakfast

1. Don't skip breakfast. You will not have enough energy to play well later in the day. Skipping breakfast can also lower your grades in school.
2. Avoid high-sugar foods at breakfast. They will make you sleepy during the day.
3. Start your breakfast with some fruit. A small glass of juice, berries on your cereal, or a banana are good choices.
4. Protein is important at breakfast. Milk, either in a glass or on cereal, is a good source of protein. So is a serving of yogurt or some peanut butter.

Lunch

1. Check the quality of school-provided lunches. If they are high in fat or sugar, bring your lunch. Many schools publish their daily menus in advance. Check the newspaper or ask the school for a copy.
2. Add a variety of healthy alternatives to your lunches.
   a. Try different types of breads. Pitas, wraps, bagels, and taco shells can be a good change of pace in the sandwich routine.
   b. Freeze fruits before putting them in the lunch box. This will keep the lunch items cool and the fruit fresh tasting. Canned pineapple and grapes freeze well. So do bananas.
   c. Try alternatives to high-fat chips. Dried fruits, baked pretzels, and animal crackers are just a few examples of tasty, healthy treats.
   d. Low-fat chocolate milk is more nutritious than prepackaged juice boxes, which have high sugar concentrations.

Snacks

1. Limit snacks to after school and bedtime. Light snacks such as yogurt or fruit provide good hunger management. A very hungry child will tend to overeat at meals.
2. Children need to learn to eat only when they are hungry. Children often eat out of boredom. Discourage nonstop grazing by planning activities to occupy the child.

Dinner

1. Plan your menu a week ahead. Planning ahead reduces the likelihood of eating out or getting "take-out." Restaurant foods are more likely to be high in fats and carbohydrates.
2. Prepare homemade healthy versions of take-out favorites. Top prepared pizza crust with cooked chicken, vegetables, mushrooms, and cheese. Serve the pizza with a salad for a complete and healthy meal. "Make your own tacos" nights, using lean hamburger and low-fat sour cream, can be a lot of fun for children.
3. Don't turn dinner into a battle zone. Forcing children to eat foods they do not like will only deepen their dislike of them. Give them the healthy foods they do enjoy and eventually they will explore more options.
4. Lead by example. Children eventually adopt the eating patterns of their parents. If they see their parents eat vegetables, they will eventually try them.

TEACHING GUIDELINE 9.2

Teaching Healthy Activity

1. Plan physical activities that your family can do as a group.
2. Write exercise activities on your family's daily schedule.
3. Look for activities that appeal to your child's interest such as dance, team sports, or swimming.
4. Place value on noncompetitive as well as competitive activities.
5. Show your child you believe exercise is important. Exercise daily yourself.
6. Encourage the community to develop safe areas for spontaneous games and activities.

HEALTHY PEOPLE 2010

Objective	Significance
Increase the proportion of adolescents who engage in moderate physical activity for at least 30 minutes on 5 or more of previous 7 days.	• For the nonexercising teen, advise to start slowly by walking. • Work with the teen to identify physical activities that interest the teen. • Praise efforts to participate in a routine exercise plan. • Identify an athletic individual that the teen identifies with and encourage similar activities in the teen.

tions for promoting physical activity; see also Healthy People 2010.

Promoting Personal Hygiene

Hand washing is the first personal hygiene topic that needs to be introduced to children. Hand washing prevents disease by limiting a child's exposure to pathogens. The nurse can introduce the topic to preschool children by the use of cartoons and games. Have the child sing "Twinkle, Twinkle Little Star" while washing his or her hands; this encourages adequate cleansing time. Use soap containers and towels with colorful characters to make the experience more fun. The school-age child can understand the concepts of germs and disease. Slogans such as "Let's drown a germ" can serve as a reminder of the importance of hand washing. The Glo Germ program (www.glogerm.com) is very effective in this age group. A nontoxic substance that shines under a black light is placed on the children's hands. The children can follow how germs travel from object to object. After washing their hands, the children can see if they did a good job. In response to peer pressures, teenagers are usually stringent about personal hygiene. Young teens may need guidance in dealing with pubescent body changes such as adult-type body odor, susceptibility to fungal infections such as tinea pedis (athlete's foot), and acne.

Promoting Safe Sun Exposure

Skin cancers are a significant health problem in the United States. Blistering sunburns in children substantially increase the risk of melanoma and other skin cancers. People with fair skin are at highest risk for skin cancers but anyone can become sunburned and develop skin cancer. When teaching clients about safe sun exposure it is very important to remind them that harmful ultraviolet (UV) rays can reflect off water, snow, sand, and concrete. Being under a shade awning does not guarantee protection. Adequate sun protection requires proper use of sunscreen lotions, avoiding peak sun hours, and wearing proper clothing. See Teaching Guideline 9.3 for more detailed instructions. With proper sun protection starting in infancy, 80% of skin cancers could be prevented.

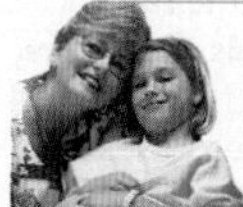

Give children the following physical reference when doing health promotion on safe sun exposure. Tell the child, "Only play outside when your shadow is taller than you are." The child's shadow will be "taller" before 10:00 a.m. and after 2:00 P.M. The nurse can demonstrate this concept by placing a ruler on end and shining a bright light over it. As the nurse moves the light, the child will see the ruler's shadow lengthen.

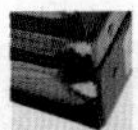

TEACHING GUIDELINE 9.3

Teaching Safe Sun Exposure

Sunscreen

1. Use sunscreen lotions every day. Harmful ultraviolet (UV) rays penetrate clouds and cause damaging sunburns.
2. Use sunscreens with a sun protection factor (SPF) of 15 or higher. An adequate amount for an average-sized child is half an ounce.
3. Apply sunscreens half an hour before sun exposure.
4. Reapply every hour if the child is perspiring heavily.
5. Reapply immediately after swimming.
6. Infants 6 months old or younger should not use sunscreens. Take steps to completely avoid sun exposure with this age group.

Clothing

1. Wear hats. The brim of the hat should be 4 inches or greater and shade the ears. Straw hats need to have a sunproof liner to be effective. Children introduced to hats as young infants usually accept hats as part of the "outfit."
2. Wear UV-blocking sunglasses. The eye is the second most common site for melanoma.
3. Wear long, loose, and lightweight clothing for maximum sun protection.

Lifestyle

1. Avoid sun exposure between 10 A.M. and 4 P.M. This is when UV rays are strongest.
2. Ask your health care provider if your medication will increase your sensitivity to UV rays. If the answer is yes, take extra precautions to reduce sun exposure.
3. Avoid tanning parlors. The devices emit UV rays just like the sun and can cause damage.
4. Check the UV index before going out. The higher the index, the more precautions you should take. UV index figures are available in newspapers, TV, and radio weather reports and on the Internet.
5. Advocate for safe-sun scheduling of recreational activities. Talk to others about scheduling outdoor activities before 10 A.M., after 4 P.M., or in the shade.
6. Consider UV-blocking plastic film for your house and car windows.

References and Helpful Informational Resources

American Academy of Pediatric Dentistry. (2005). Guideline on periodicity of examination, preventive dental services, anticipatory guidance and oral treatment for children. *American Academy of Pediatric Dentistry reference manual 2005–2006.* Retrieved July 9, 2006 from http://www.aapd.org/media/Policies_Guidelines/G_Periodicity.pdf.

American Academy of Pediatric Dentistry. (2004). Policy on the dental home (adopted 2001). *American Academy of Pediatric Dentistry reference manual 2003–2004.* Retrieved June 15, 2004 from http://www.aapd.org/members/referencemanual/pdfs/02-03/P_DentalHome.pdf

American Academy of Pediatric Dentistry. (2004). Policy on use of fluoride (rev. 2003). *American Academy of Pediatric Dentistry reference manual 2003–2004.* Retrieved June 15, 2004 from http://www.aapd.org/members/referencemanual/pdfs/02-03/P_FluorideUses.pdf

American Academy of Pediatrics. (2005). Policy statement. Lead exposure in children: Prevention, detection, and management. *Pediatrics, 116*(4), 1036–1046.

American Academy of Pediatrics, Committee on Children With Disabilities. (2001). Developmental surveillance and screening of infants and young children. *Pediatrics, 108,* 192–196.

American Academy of Pediatrics, Committee on Environmental Health. (1998). Screening for elevated blood lead levels. *Pediatrics, 101,* 1072–1078.

American Academy of Pediatrics, Committee on Infectious Diseases. (1999). Combination vaccines for childhood immunization: Recommendations of the Advisory Committee on Immunization Practices (ACIP), the American Academy of Pediatrics (AAP), and the American Academy of Family Physicians (AAFP). *Pediatrics, 103,* 1064–1077.

American Academy of Pediatrics, Committee on Infectious Diseases. (2005). *Policy statement. Prevention of pertussis among adolescents: Recommendations for use of tetanus toxoid, reduced diphtheria toxoid, and acellular pertussis (Tdp) vaccine.* Retrieved May 8, 2006, from http://www.aap.org/advocacy/releases/Tdap121205.pdf

American Academy of Pediatrics, Committee on Infectious Diseases. (2005). Prevention and control of meningococcal disease: Recommendations for use of meningococcal vaccines in pediatric patients. *Pediatrics, 116*(2), 496–505.

American Academy of Pediatrics, Committee on Infectious Diseases. (2006). Policy statement. Recommended childhood and adolescent immunization schedule: United States, 2006. *Pediatrics, 117*(1), 239–240.

American Academy of Pediatrics, Committee on Infectious Diseases. (2007a). Prevention of rotavirus disease: Guidelines for use of rotavirus vaccine. *Pediatrics, 119*(1), 171–181.

American Academy of Pediatrics, Committee on Infectious Diseases. (2007b). Recommended immunization schedules for children and adolescents—United States, 2007. *Pediatrics, 119*(1), 207–208.

American Academy of Pediatrics, Committee on Nutrition. (1998). Cholesterol in childhood. *Pediatrics, 101,* 141–147.

American Academy of Pediatrics, Committee on Pediatric Work Force. (1999). Culturally effective pediatric care: Education and training issues. *Pediatrics, 103,* 167–170.

American Academy of Pediatrics, Committee on Practice and Ambulatory Medicine, Section on Ophthalmology. (2002). Use of photoscreening for children's vision screening. *Pediatrics, 109,* 524–525.

American Academy of Pediatrics, Committee on Practice and Ambulatory Medicine, Section on Ophthalmology. (2003). Eye examination in infants, children, and young adults by pediatricians. *Pediatrics, 111,* 902–907

American Academy of Pediatrics, Joint Committee on Infant Hearing. (2000). Year 2000 position statement: Principles and guidelines for early hearing detection and intervention programs. *Pediatrics, 106,* 798–817.

Applebaum, E. L. (1999). Detection of hearing loss in children. *Pediatric Annals, 28,* 232–256.

Atkinson, W. L., Pickering, L. K., Schwartz, B., Weniger, B. G., Iskander, J. K., & Watson, J. C. (2002). General recommendations on immunization: Recommendations of the Advisory Committee on Immunization Practices (ACIP) and the American Academy of Family Physicians (AAFP) [Electronic version]. *Morbidity and Mortality Weekly Report, Recommendations and Reports, 51*(RR 2), 1–36. Retrieved May 8, 2006, from http://www.cdc.gov/mmwr/preview/mmwrhtml/rr5102a1.htm

Centers for Disease Control and Prevention. (1998). Recommendations to prevent and control iron deficiency in the United States. *Morbidity and Mortality Weekly Report, Recommendations and Reports, 47*(RR 3), 1–29.

Centers for Disease Control and Prevention. (2002). Contraindications and precautions to routine childhood vaccinations by condition. Retrieved May 8, 2006, from http://www.cdc.gov/nip/publications/pink/Appendices/A/cont_prec.pdf

Center for Disease Control and Prevention. (2006a). *Human papillomavirus: HPV information for clinicians.* Atlanta: Centers for Disease Control and Prevention.

Center for Disease Control and Prevention. (2006b). Recommended immunization schedules for persons aged 0–18 years—United States, 2007. *Morbidity and Mortality Weekly Report, 55*(51 & 52), Q1–Q4.

Centers for Disease Control and Prevention, Advisory Committee on Childhood Lead Poisoning Prevention (ACCLPP). (2000). Recommendations for blood lead screening of young children enrolled in Medicaid: Targeting a group at high risk. *Morbidity and Mortality Weekly Report, Recommendations and Reports, 49*(RR 14), 1–29.

Centers for Disease Control and Prevention, Advisory Committee on Immunization Practice (ACIP). (2000). Preventing pneumococcal disease among infants and children. *Morbidity and Mortality Weekly Report, Recommendations and Reports, 49*(RR 9), 1–38.

Centers for Disease Control and Prevention (ND) Vaccine Information Statements. (n.d.) Retrieved May 8, 2006, from at http://www.cdc.gov/nip/publications/vis

Centers for Disease Control and Prevention's Epidemiology and Prevention of Vaccine-Preventable Diseases. (2004). *Principles of vaccination* (8th ed.). Retrieved July 15, 2004 from http://www.cdc.gov/nip/pink/prinvac.pdf

Centers for Disease Control and Prevention's Epidemiology and Prevention of Vaccine-Preventable Diseases (8th ed.). (2004). *Vaccine administration.* Retrieved July 15, 2004 from http://www.cdc.gov/nip/publications/pink/vacc_admin.pdf

Cincinnati Children's Hospital Medical Center (2005). *Healthy foods and snacking.* Retrieved June 18, 2005, from http://www.cincinnatichildrens.org/health/info/nutrition/eat/food.htm

Colvar, M. R. (2003). Noninvasive hearing testing. *Advance for Nurse Practitioners, 32,* 30–31.

Glo-germ program. (n.d.). Retrieved June 27, 2005, from http://www.glogerm.com

Green, M., & Palfrey, J. (Eds.). (2002). *Bright futures: Guidelines for health supervision of infants, children, and adolescents* (2nd ed.). Arlington, VA: National Center for Education in Maternal and Child Health. Retrieved June 10, 2004, from www.brightfutures.org/bf2/pdf/index.html

Guidelines for childhood obesity prevention programs: Promoting healthy weight in children. (2003). *Journal of Nutrition Education and Behavior, 35*(1), 1–4.

Gust, D., Strine, T., Maurice, E., et al. (2004). Underimmunization among children: Effects of vaccine safety concerns on immunization status. *Pediatrics, 114,* e16–e22. Retrieved July 15, 2004, from http://www.pediatrics.aappublications.org/cgi/content/full/114/1/e16

Holte, L. (2003). Year 2000 position statement: Principles and guidelines for early hearing detection and intervention programs. *Pediatric Annals, 32,* 461–465.

Immunization Action Coalition. (2005). *Summary of rules for childhood and adolescent immunization.* Retrieved June 19, 2005, from 2http://www.immunize.org/nslt.d/n17/rules1.htm

Joint Commission on Infant Hearing. (2000). Position statement: Principles and guidelines for early infant hearing detection and intervention programs. Retrieved July 7, 2003, from www.infanthearing.org/jcih

Killeen, P., & Carlson, L. (2005, March). How to overcome barriers to vaccination: Practical strategies for providers [Special edition]. *Journal of Family Practice,* S26–S29.

March of Dimes. (2004). *State report card on testing for March of Dimes recommended newborn screening conditions.* Retrieved June 30, 2004, from http://www.modimes.org/files/NBS_rc_062404.pdf

Middleton, D., Zimmerman, R., & Mitchell, K. (2005, March). Childhood vaccine schedules and procedures, 2005 [Special edition]. *Journal of Family Practice,* S16–S25.

National High Blood Pressure Education Working Group on High Blood Pressure in Children and Adolescents. (2004). The fourth report on the diagnosis, evaluation and treatment of high blood pressure in children and adolescents. *Pediatrics, 114,* 555–576.

National Meningitis Association. (n.d.) About meningococcal disease. Retrieved January 15, 2007 from http://www.nmaus.org/about_meningitis/

National Partnership for Immunization (ND). *NPI reference guide to vaccines and vaccine safety.* Retrieved July 15, 2004, from http://www.partnersforimmunization.org/pdf/Vaccines.pdf

Newacheck, P., Hughes, D., Hung, Y., et al. (2000). The unmet health needs of America's children. *Pediatrics, 105,* 989–996.

Office of Disease Prevention and Health Promotion, U.S. Department of Health and Human Services. (2000). *Healthy people 2010.* Retrieved June 22, 2005, from http://www.healthypeople.gov

Office of Disease Prevention and Health Promotion, U.S. Department of Health and Human Services. (2000). *Healthy people 2010. Chapter 28: Vision and hearing.* Retrieved July 1, 2003, from http://www.healthypeople.gov/Document/HTML/Volume2/28Vision.htm#_Toc489325915

Parashar, U. D., Alexander, J. P., & Glass, R. I. (2006). Prevention of rotavirus gastroenteritis among infants and children. *Morbidity and Mortality Weekly Report, 55*(RR12), 1–13.

Pickering, L. (Ed.). (2004). *2003 red book: Report of the committee on infectious diseases* (25th ed.). Elk Grove Village, IL: American Academy of Pediatrics.

Ruben, J. R. (2003). *Vision testing in children: An interactive primer.* Retrieved July 6, 2003, from www.aapos.org

Saiman, L., Aronson, J., Gomez-Duarte, C., et al. Prevalence of infectious diseases among internationally adopted children. *Pediatrics, 108,* 608–612.

Simon, J. W., & Daw, P. (2001). Vision screening performed by the pediatrician. *Pediatric Annals, 30,* 446–452.

Staat, M. (2002). Infectious disease issues in internationally adopted children. *Pediatric Infectious Disease Journal, 21,* 257–258.

Story, M., Holt, K., & Sofka, D. (2002). *Bright futures in practice: Nutrition* (2nd ed.). Arlington, VA: National Center for Education in Maternal and Child Health.

University of Iowa, Department of Dermatology. (2002). *Safe sun tips for children.* Retrieved June 18, 2005, from http://www.vh.org/pediatric/patient/dermatology/suntips/index.html

Weber, J., & Kelly, J. (2003). *Health assessment in nursing.* Philadelphia: Lippincott Williams & Wilkins.

Zimmerman, R., Middleton, D., Burns, I., et al. (2005, March). Routine childhood vaccines, 2005 [Special edition]. *Journal of Family Practice,* S3–S15.

Web Sites

www.aap.org American Academy of Pediatrics
www.aapos.org American Association of Pediatric Ophthalmology and Strabismus
www.aoa.org American Optometric Association
www.brightfutures.org Full-text reference to health supervision
www.cdc.gov/ncbddd/child/screen_provider.htm Centers for Disease Control and Prevention/National Center on Birth Defects and Developmental Disabilities: child development
www.cdc.gov/nip Centers for Disease Control and Prevention/National Immunization Program
www.ihsinfo.org International Hearing Society
www.immunizationinfo.org National Network for Immunization Information
www.immunize.org Immunization Action Coalition
www.partnersforimmunization.org National Partnership for immunization: promotes immunization across the lifespan
www.preventblindness.org Prevent Blindness America
www.v2020.org Vision 2020, The Right to Sight
www.vaccinesafety.edu Institute for Vaccine Safety at Johns Hopkins University of Public Health

Chapter WORKSHEET

MULTIPLE CHOICE QUESTIONS

1. During the health interview, the mother of a 4-month-old client makes the statement, "I'm not sure my baby is doing what he should be." What is the nurse's best response?
   a. "I'll be able to tell you more after I do his physical."
   b. "Fill out this developmental screening questionnaire and then I can let you know."
   c. "Tell me more about your concerns."
   d. "All mothers worry about their babies. I'm sure he's doing well."
2. An infant male is at your facility for his initial health supervision visit. He is 2 weeks old and responds to a bell during his examination. You review his all birth records and there is no documentation that a newborn hearing screening was performed. The best action for the nurse to take is:
   a. Do nothing, because responding to the bell proves that the infant does not have a hearing deficit.
   b. Schedule the infant immediately for newborn hearing screening.
   c. Ask the mother to observe for signs that the infant is not hearing well.
   d. Screen again with the bell at the infant's 2-month health supervision visit.
3. A 15-month-old girl is having her first health supervision visit at your facility. Her caregiver has not brought a copy of the child's immunization record, but believes she is fully immunized. The mother states "she had immunizations 3 months ago at the local health department." Which would be the best action by the nurse?
   a. Ask the mother to bring the records at the 18-month health supervision visit.
   b. Start the "catch-up" schedule because there are no immunization records.
   c. Keep the child at the facility while the mother returns home for the records.
   d. Call the local health department and verify the child's immunization status.
4. A 4-year-old child is having a vision screening performed. Which of the following screening charts would be best for determining the child's visual acuity?
   a. Snellen
   b. Ishihara
   c. Allen figures
   d. CVTME
5. Which of the following facilities fulfills the characteristics of a medical home?
   a. An urgent care center
   b. A primary care pediatric practice
   c. A mobile outreach immunization program
   d. A dermatology practice
6. The child's first examination by a dentist should occur:
   a. By the first birthday
   b. By the second birthday
   c. By entry into kindergarten
   d. By entry into first grade

CRITICAL THINKING EXERCISES

1. The client is a 5-year-old boy. During this health supervision visit, his mother states that she has concerns about his hearing. Your facility has been his medical home since birth. He was the product of a normal pregnancy and delivery. He has had frequent ear infections since the age of 8 months. Six months ago he had a ruptured appendix. He was treated with an aminoglycoside. He has been fully recovered for 4 months.
   a. During the health interview, what information does the nurse want to elicit from the mother?
   b. What information does the nurse want to verify from the permanent medical record?
   c. What risk factors for hearing loss does this child have?
   d. What is the best course of action at this time?
2. The nurse must examine a 4-year-old to determine his readiness for school. Describe the developmental, vision, and hearing screening tools that will assist the nurse to identify any problems.

STUDY ACTIVITIES

1. Develop an immunization plan for the following well children: a 2-month-old, an 18-month-old who has never been immunized, and a 5-year-old who was current with all immunizations at age 2.
2. This is the first health supervision visit, since arriving in this country 1 week ago, for a 3-year-old international adoptee from Russia. Develop a health supervision plan for this visit.
3. Develop a healthy weight program for the following: a preschool class, a family in which the parents and the two school-age children are mildly overweight, and a teenage girl who is of normal weight but fears "becoming fat."

chapter 10

Health Assessment of Children

Key TERMS

accommodation
acrocyanosis
auscultation
body mass index (BMI)
cerumen
chief complaint
fontanel
inspection
lanugo
obligate nose breathing
palpation
PERRLA
point of maximal impulse (PMI)
stadiometer
Tanner stages
tympanometer

Learning OBJECTIVES

Upon completion of the chapter, the learner will be able to:

1. Demonstrate an understanding of the appropriate health history to obtain from the child and the parent or primary caregiver.
2. Individualize elements of the health history depending upon the age of the child.
3. Discuss important concepts related to health assessment in children.
4. Describe the appropriate sequence of the physical examination in the context of the child's developmental stage.
5. Perform a health assessment using approaches that relate to the age and developmental stage of the child.
6. Distinguish normal variations in the physical examination from differences that may indicate serious alterations in health status.
7. Determine the sexual maturity of females and males based upon evaluation of the secondary sex characteristics.

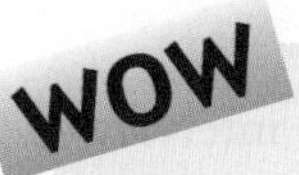

Growth and development is a journey, on which many children venture without a map.

Elliot Simmons, 3 years old, is brought to the clinic for his annual examination. His mother states that he is very fearful and anxious about this visit.

Assessment of the child's health status involves many components: the health interview and history; observation of the parent–child interaction; physical examination; and the child's emotional, physiological, cognitive, and social development. The nurse's skills are vital to the success of the assessment process. The nurse must (Mandleco, 2005):

- Establish rapport and trust
- Demonstrate respect for the child and the parent or caregiver
- Communicate effectively by actively listening, demonstrating empathy, and providing feedback
- Observe systematically
- Obtain accurate data
- Validate and interpret data accurately

The focus of the assessment process depends on the purpose of the visit and the needs of the patient. Assessment is an ongoing process and is repeated to varying degrees at every encounter. Expert nurses are constantly evaluating all of those in their care, whether directly or indirectly as part of conversation and play. Indeed, some of the subtlest developmental signs may express themselves only during relaxed and casual interaction with a child. You can observe gait while watching a child run down the hall; assess fine motor skills and social adaptation while playing a board game; or observe balance and coordination when bouncing a ball. Playful activities such as tickling a child can give the nurse feedback related to upper body strength when the child attempts to push the nurse's arms away. Nurses must also learn to perform a comprehensive and thorough examination of a child in an efficient manner.

A thorough and thoughtful assessment of a child is the foundation upon which a nurse determines the needs of and plan of care for the patient. Nothing can replace it for giving the nurse a snapshot of the life and health of the child. A comprehensive history, a thorough examination, and developmental, functional, or cognitive testing as appropriate will provide practical information about the health of a child and guide the nurse's plan of care. The history and physical examination also provide a time for health education, teaching about expected growth and development, and discussing healthy lifestyle choices. The nurse uses critical thinking skills to analyze the data and establish priorities for nursing intervention or follow-up.

The health assessment may be documented using a number of formats. The information should be easily retrievable and available to all members of the child's health care team.

Health History

The health history provides the nurse with an overall picture of what the child has experienced, highlighting areas of concern such as recurrent upper respiratory infections or headaches. This not only helps the nurse to assess those specific areas more comprehensively but also provides the opportunity to ask focused questions and identify areas where education may be needed. The time used to obtain the health history also gives the nurse an opportunity to interact with the child in a nonthreatening manner, while the child watches the interactions between the nurse and the primary caregiver.

PREPARING FOR THE HEALTH HISTORY

Appropriate materials and a suitable environment are needed when performing a thorough health history. Take into account family roles and values. Consider the age and developmental stage of the child so that you can approach the child appropriately and possibly involve him or her in the health history. Observe the child–parent interaction. Determine the extent of the health history that is needed in a given situation. Being well organized and staying flexible will help ensure success.

Gathering Materials and Preparing Yourself for the Health History

Before you begin, make sure you have materials to record your history data (either a computer or chart paper and a pen), a private space with adequate lighting, chairs for adults and the nurse, and a bed or examination table for the child. The space should be safe for your patient's developmental stage and allow you uninterrupted time for your examination. Sit down for as much of the history taking as possible to demonstrate a relaxed and welcoming manner.

Approaching the Parent or Caregiver

Greet the parent or caregiver by name. While interviewing the parent, provide toys or books to occupy the child, allowing the parent to concentrate on your questions. Use open-ended questions and avoid making judgmental comments. Show respect by remaining approachable. Remember that the structure of the family and its roles and dynamics will affect how the family communicates and how they make decisions about health care. Demonstrate patience and help the parent stay on track when there are several children in the family. Throughout the interview, refer to the child by name and use the correct gender when referring to the child, demonstrating interest and competence.

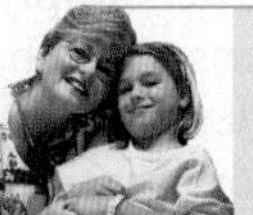

Illness can cause great stress in families and individuals, so nurses must remember to protect themselves from potentially threatening behavior on the part of the family. Sit close to the door, and if you are uncomfortable with a family member, ask for assistance. You may need to keep the door open or have another nurse or security personnel present.

Approaching the Child

Show a professional demeanor while still being warm and friendly to the caregivers and child. A white examination coat or all-white uniform may be frightening to children, who may associate the uniform with painful experiences or find it too unfamiliar. The nurse can wear a variety of professional-looking outfits, whether colorful uniform tops, aprons, or smocks worn over white uniforms, or everyday clothing, depending on the setting of the nurse's practice. Make eye contact if possible and address the child by name. Use slow deliberate gestures rather than very quick or grand ones, which may be frightening to shy children.

Some young children will warm up when given time to be invisible in the room, such as hiding behind a parent before they tentatively appear. Make physical contact with the child in a nonthreatening way at first. Briefly cuddling a newborn before returning it to the caregiver, warmly shaking the hand of older children and teens, and laying your hand on the head or arm of toddlers and preschoolers will convey a gentle demeanor. A joke, a puppet, a silly story, or even a simple magic trick may coax the child into warming up. Being at the same eye level as the child can also be more reassuring than standing over the child. This may require having extra seating for the nurse at the same level as the child and parent/caregiver. Aim to be seen as a trustworthy adult who is the child's partner in feeling better and staying healthy.

Elicit the child's cooperation by allowing him or her control over the pace, the order, or anything else that the child can control while still allowing you to obtain the information you need. All of this establishes a personal relationship with the child and helps gain his or her cooperation.

Communicating With the Child During the Health History

The child should be given opportunities to actively participate in the health history and assessment process. For young children, such as toddlers and preschoolers, ask them to point to where it hurts and allow them to answer questions. Validation of the information by the parent/caregiver is essential because of the limited comprehension and language use of children at these ages. The school-aged child can be more accurate because of his or her increased language skills and maturity level.

Initially, address the child and obtain as much information from him or her as possible. School-aged children should be able to answer questions about interactions with friends and siblings and school and activities they enjoy or are involved in. Ask the parent/caregiver if any additional information or observations should be included.

Adolescents may not feel comfortable addressing health issues, answering questions, or being examined in the presence of the parent/caregiver. The nurse must establish a trusting relationship with the adolescent to provide him or her with optimal health care. Ask adolescents whether they would be more comfortable answering questions alone in the examination area or whether they prefer for their parents to be present. Either way, the parent/caregiver will have an opportunity to talk with the nurse after the health history and assessment are completed.

Demonstrate an interest in the teen by asking questions about school, work, hobbies or activities, and friendships. Begin with these topics to make the teen feel comfortable in communicating with you. Communicate honestly with the adolescent and explain the rationale for various aspects of the health history. Teens are very sensitive to nonverbal communication, so be very aware of your gestures and expressions. Once a rapport has been established, move on to more emotionally charged questions that relate to sexuality, substance use, depression, and suicide.

Always assure the teen that complete confidentiality will be maintained to the extent possible. Current state law will determine the types of information that may be withheld from parents. If the information that the nurse receives indicates that the teen may be in danger, then the nurse must inform the teen that the information will be shared with other providers and/or the parents.

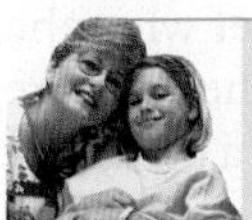

Do not try to become the adolescent's peer. Remain in the role of the health care provider while demonstrating respect and acceptance toward the teen. Clarify the meaning of jargon or slang that the teen uses, but do not use these words yourself, as the teen will simply not accept you as a peer.

Observing the Parent–Child Interaction

Observation of the parent–child interaction begins during the focused conversation of the health interview and continues throughout the physical examination. Explore the family dynamics, not only through questions but also by observing the family for behavioral clues. Does the parent make eye contact with the infant? Does the parent anticipate and respond to the infant's needs? Are the parents ineffective when dealing with a toddler's temper tantrum? The plan of care may need to be adjusted to teach appropriate responses to the infant's needs or toddler's behavior. Do the parents' comments increase the school-age child's sense of self-worth? Behavioral observations are crucial to proper assessment of the family's needs.

Does the parent seem to be coping with the health issue or does he or she appear overwhelmed? Is the parent's/caregiver's behavior appropriate? Does the child look at the parent/caregiver before answering? Does the child seem relaxed and happy with the parent/caregiver, or is the child tense? The infant will appear calm and relaxed if his or her needs are generally met. Crying may occur when the baby is ill or frightened but may also indicate discomfort with the parent or caregiver. Use a calm and comforting voice with the infant. Infants respond well to higher-pitched and soothing voices.

When observing the relationship between the adolescent and the parent/caregiver, does the parent/caregiver allow the adolescent to speak, or does he or she frequently interrupt? Does the parent/caregiver contradict what is being said? Observe the body language of the adolescent. Does the adolescent seem relaxed or tense? Since adolescents are between childhood and adulthood, they have unique needs. They are in a time of multiple physical and emotional changes, many of which they cannot control. They need to know that the nurse is interested in what they have to say. The use of open-ended questions allows the adolescent to talk. "Tell me about your. . . ." or "What have you noticed about. . . ." are comfortable phrases to use to elicit the information needed.

Be aware of your reactions to the adolescent's questions or behaviors, such as your nonverbal and facial expressions. Talk with the adolescent using accurate language that is developmentally and age-appropriate.

Determining the Type of History Needed

The purpose of the examination will determine how comprehensive the history must be. If the health care provider rarely sees the child or if the child is critically ill, a complete and detailed history is in order, no matter what the setting. The child who has received routine health care and presents with a mild illness may need only a problem-focused history. In critical situations, some of the history taking must be delayed until after the child's condition is stabilized. Evaluate the situation to determine the best timing and the extent of the history. Also, be sensitive to repetitive interviews in hospital situations, and collaborate with physicians or other members of the health care team to ensure that a family already under stress does not need to undergo prolonged or repetitive questioning.

Remember Elliot, the 3-year-old being seen for his annual examination? When you enter the room, he is hiding behind his mother's legs. Considering his age and developmental level, how will you proceed with obtaining a health history?

PERFORMING A HEALTH HISTORY

The health interview is the foundation of an accurate health assessment. Information about the child's health will come not only from a physical examination, but also from a careful conversation or interview with the child and/or the caregiver. Depending on the intent of the health assessment, many of the questions will be direct, and many will require the caregiver or child to answer simply "yes" or "no." In other than emergency situations, though, asking open-ended questions offers an excellent opportunity to learn more about the patient's life. For example, "Are you happy at school?" may elicit a brief nod of the head, whereas "Tell me what it's like on your school playground" may result in a story about the child's friends, the kind of activities they enjoy, any bullying that goes on, and so forth. These stories will provide the nurse with clues to the child's stage of physical, emotional, and moral development as well as his or her functional status.

Establish a therapeutic relationship with the child and family. Without the trust that comes from this therapeutic relationship, the family may not reveal vital information due to fear, embarrassment, or mistrust. Use therapeutic communication techniques such as active listening, open-ended questions, and eliminating barriers to communication. Establishing a "medical home" where ongoing health supervision occurs encourages the formation of trust through continuity of care and the family's continuing relationships with health care providers (see Chapter 9).

Components of the Health Interview

The structure of the health interview is determined by the nature of the visit. At an initial visit, large amounts of historical data are collected. Having the family fill out a questionnaire can save time, but a questionnaire is not a substitute for the health interview. The questionnaire may serve as a springboard to begin structured conversations between the family and the nurse. At subsequent visits the health interview can focus on the pertinent issues of that visit as well as any health issues that are being monitored.

The health history includes demographics, chief complaint and history of present illness, past health history, review of systems, family health history, developmental history, functional history, and family composition, resources, and home environment.

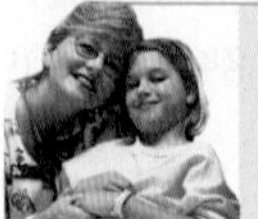

Any questionnaires used in the health care setting must be appropriate to the reading level and primary language of the person filling them out.

Demographics

Questions should start with simple and nonintrusive ones; once a rapport between the nurse and patient has started, sensitive questions can be asked. First obtain data such as the child's name, nickname, birth date, and gender.

Determine the child's race or ethnicity, the language the child understands, and the language the child speaks. Record the child's address and home telephone number and the parent's or caregiver's work telephone number. Identify who the historian is (the child or the parent or caregiver), and note how reliable you consider this source of information to be. Do not assume that an adult with the child is the child's parent. Establish the relationship of the adult to the child, and ask who cares for the child if that person does not. Determine the composition of the household, including other children and other family members or other persons who live there.

Chief Complaint and History of Present Illness

Next, ask about the **chief complaint** (reason for the visit). The reason may not always be apparent to you. A question such as, "What can I help you with today?" or "What did you notice in your baby/child that you wanted to have checked today?" is very welcoming. The response from the child or parent may be a functional problem, a developmental concern, or a disease.

Record the chief complaint in the child's or parent's own words.

Next address the history related to the present illness. For each concern, determine its onset, duration, characteristics and course (location, signs, symptoms, exposures, and so on), previous episodes in patient or family, previous testing or therapies, what makes it better and what makes it worse, and what the concern means to the child and family. Inquire about any exposure to infectious agents.

Past Health History

Ask about the prenatal history (any problems with pregnancy), perinatal history (any problems with labor and delivery), past illnesses, or any other health or developmental problems. Document the child's prior history of illnesses (recurrent, chronic, or serious) and any accidents or injuries in the past. Inquire about any operations or hospitalizations the child has had. Document the child's diet. Note the child's allergies to foods, medications, animals, environmental or contact agents, or latex products. Determine the child's reaction to the allergen as well as its severity. Determine the child's immunization status (refer to Chapter 9 for further information on immunizations). Record any medications the child is taking, the dosage and schedule, as well as when the last dose was given. In preadolescent and adolescent females, determine menstrual history.

Family Health History

Obtaining information about the family's health is a key part of a health interview. Perform a three-generation family health history. This information may be documented in a genogram (Fig. 10.1). Asking about the age and health status of mother, father, siblings, and other family members helps to identify trends and specific health issues. For example, do the grandparents have early-onset coronary artery disease? If they do, the child may benefit from additional health screening. Siblings may exhibit a genetic disease or carry a trait for the disease. This family health information helps to guide future health planning.

Review of Systems

Inquire about current or past history of problems related to:

- Growth and development
- Skin
- Head and neck
- Eyes and vision
- Ears and hearing
- Mouth, teeth, and throat
- Respiratory system and breasts
- Cardiovascular system
- Gastrointestinal system
- Genitourinary system
- Musculoskeletal system
- Neurologic system
- Endocrine system
- Hematologic system

Table 10.1 gives specific questions related to each of these systems.

Developmental History

Determine the age when landmarks in gross motor control were achieved, such as sitting, standing, walking, pedaling, and so on. Ask whether the child has attained fine motor skills such as grasping, releasing, pincer grasp, crayon or utensil use, and handwriting skills. Note the child's age and extent of language acquisition. Document speech

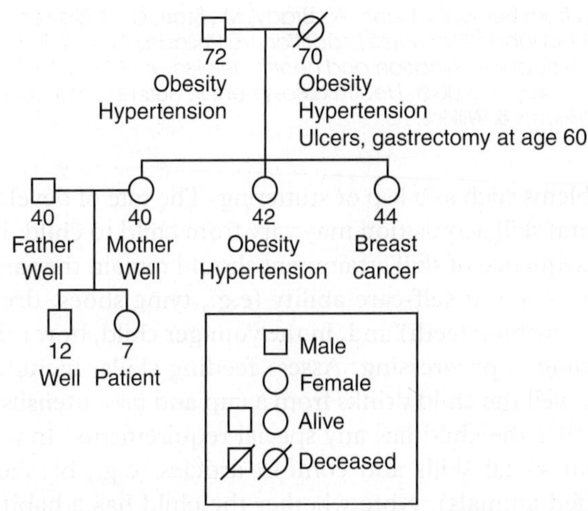

● Figure 10.1 Genogram.

Table 10.1 Questions for the Review of Systems

Systems	Has the Child Experienced:
Growth and development	Weight loss or gain, appropriate energy and activity levels, fatigue, behavioral changes such as irritability, nervousness, anger, or increased crying
Skin	Easy bruising or bleeding, rash, lesion, skin disease, pruritus, birthmarks, or change in mole, pigment, hair, or nails
Head and neck	Head injury, headache, dizziness, syncope
Eyes and vision	Pain, redness, discharge, diplopia, strabismus, cataracts, vision changes, reading difficulties, need to sit close to the board at school or close to the TV at home
Ears and hearing	Earache, recurrent ear infection, tubes in eardrums, discharge, difficulty hearing, ringing, excess cerumen
Mouth, teeth, and throat	Swollen gums, pain with teething, caries, tooth loss, toothache, sores, difficulty with chewing or swallowing, hoarseness, sore throat, mouth breathing, change in voice
Respiratory system and breasts	Nasal congestion or discharge, cough, wheeze, noisy breathing, snoring, shortness of breath or other difficulty breathing, problems with or changes in breasts
Cardiovascular system	Murmur, color change (cyanosis), exertional dyspnea, activity intolerance, palpitations, extremity coldness, high blood pressure, high cholesterol
Gastrointestinal system	Nausea, vomiting, abdominal pain, cramping, diarrhea, constipation, stool-holding, anal pain or itching
Genitourinary system	Dysuria; polyuria; oliguria; narrow urine stream; dark, cloudy, or discolored urine; difficulty with toilet training; bedwetting *Boys:* undescended testicles, pain in penis or scrotum, sores or lesions, discharge, scrotal swelling when crying, changes in scrotum or penis size, addition of pubic hair *Girls:* vaginal discharge, itching rash, problems with menstruation or menstrual cycle
Musculoskeletal system	Joint or bone pain, stiffness, swelling, injury (e.g., broken bones or sprains), movement limitation, decreased strength, altered gait, changes in coordination, back pain, posture changes or spinal curvature
Neurologic system	Numbness, tingling, difficulty learning, altered mood or ability to stay alert, tremors, tics, seizures
Endocrine system	Increased thirst, excessive appetite, delayed or early pubertal changes, problems with growth
Hematologic system	Swelling of lymph nodes, pale color, excessive bruising

Data from Burns, C., Dunn, A., Brady, M., Starr, N., & Blosser, C. (2004). *Pediatric primary care: A handbook for nurse practitioners.* Philadelphia: W. B. Saunders; Jarvis, C. (2004). *Physical examination and health assessment* (4th ed.). St. Louis: Saunders; Weber, J., & Kelley, J. (2003). *Health assessment in nursing* (2nd ed.). Philadelphia: Lippincott Williams & Wilkins.

problems such as a lisp or stuttering. The rate of developmental skill acquisition may vary from child to child, but the sequence of skill attainment should remain the same. Inquire about self-care ability (e.g., tying shoes, dressing, brushing teeth) and, in the younger child, how toilet training is progressing. Assess feeding skills, including how well the child drinks from a cup and uses utensils or whether the child has any special requirements. Inquire about social skills and comfort articles (e.g., blankets, stuffed animals). Note whether the child has a habit of thumb or finger sucking or using a pacifier. Document daycare attendance and preschool or school adjustment and achievements.

Functional History

The functional history should contain information about the child's daily routine. Inquire about:

- Safety measures (e.g., car seats and their placement, use of seat belts, smoke detectors, bike helmets)

- Routine health care and dental care (including dates of dental care and what was done)
- Nutrition, including a 24-hour dietary recall or week-long food diary, use of supplements and vitamins, feeding pattern and satisfaction with diet, amount of "junk food" consumed, food likes and dislikes, and the parent's perception of the child's nutrition (refer to Chapters 4 through 8 for nutritional needs at various ages)
- Physical activity and organized sports, play, and recreation
- Television and computer habits
- Sleep behavior and bedtime
- Elimination patterns and any concerns
- Hearing or vision problems (dates of last screenings and results)
- Relationships with other family members and friends, coping and temperament, discipline strategies, attention or school behavior problems
- Religious involvement and other spiritual practices
- Use of adaptive and assistive devices such as eyeglasses or contact lenses, hearing aids, walker, braces, wheelchair
- Sexual practices

Family Composition, Resources, and Home Environment

Determine the marital status of the parents. Does the child live with the parents, a stepparent, or other family member? Is the child adopted or in foster care? Are the parents the primary caretakers for the child? If not, the primary caretaker should be included in the interview process if possible. Parents may not know some of the child's routines if the child spends much of the time being cared for by someone else. Working parents may learn about a health or behavior issue only after being alerted by the child's daycare center or babysitter. It may be helpful to expand the family history to include the grandparents and their interaction with the child.

Determine the employment status of the parents and their occupations, as this could affect the child's overall well-being; for example, the parents' work schedule may not allow them to spend much time with the child. Assess family income and financial resources, including health insurance and food stamps or other governmental supplemental income. Major family changes can also affect how the parents and child interact, so evaluate for relationship problems or changes.

Ask about the family's home and its age and the home environment. Is there a safe outdoor play area? If there is a pool, are safety features in place? Determine whether the home has electricity and an indoor water supply. Also determine whether the home has heating, air conditioning, and refrigeration. What pets does the family have? How are they housed? Are there infestations of insects or rodents in the home?

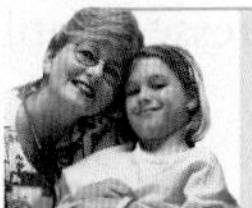

Homes or apartments built prior to 1978 may contain lead-based paint, and children who live there are at an increased risk for the development of lead poisoning.

Performing a Physical Examination

After the history comes the physical examination. It should focus on the chief complaint or any of the systems that engaged the nurse's critical thinking while taking the history. The examination will reflect the nurse's general practice style, the developmental stage and age of the child, the temperament of the child and caregiver, and the health status of the child. A very ill child will not waste energy protesting the examination, so the nurse can move quickly in that situation. A healthy child, however, will express his or her normal developmental stage and will show varying degrees of resistance to the examination.

PREPARING FOR THE PHYSICAL EXAMINATION

When performing the physical examination, being prepared and organized ensures that you will obtain the needed information. The appropriate methods to use and ways to approach the child depend on the child's developmental stage.

Gathering Materials and Preparing for the Examination

The examination area should include an exam table or the child's hospital crib or bed. Appropriate lighting is necessary for adequate observation and inspection. Gather the equipment necessary for the examination such as clean gloves, stethoscope, thermometer, sphygmomanometer, tape measure, reflex hammer, penlight, otoscope/ophthalmoscope, tongue depressor, and cotton ball. An infant or adult scale is needed, as well as a **stadiometer** for children capable of standing independently. Young children may be frightened by seeing a large amount of equipment, so take out one piece of equipment at a time. Some children can be very resistant to what they see as a threat or an invasion of their privacy, so it may help to have washable toys in the examination area to use as distractions during the assessment.

Children and their parents may be able to sense any frustration or anxiety on the part of the examiner, so display a confident and matter-of-fact approach. If the child is not cooperative, do not become discouraged; more time and explanation will usually do the trick.

Regardless of the child's age, if the examination room is cold, the child will be uncomfortable and possibly less cooperative. Provide appropriate covers to ensure the child's comfort, or have the child remain dressed until the time of the examination.

Approaching the Child

Approach the child according to his or her developmental age and stage. Table 10.2 outlines a general approach to the physical examination in each broad developmental category.

If several children are to be seen at the same time, begin with the child who will be most cooperative. If the other children do not see anything scary and realize that their sibling was examined without a problem, it sets the stage for better cooperation from the younger ones.

Newborns and Infants

If the infant is asleep, auscultate the heart, lungs, and abdomen first while the baby is quiet. Count the heart rate and respiratory rate before undressing the baby. Completely undress newborns and infants down to their diaper, removing it just at the end to examine the genitalia, anus, spine, and hips. It is best to examine the infant 1 to 2 hours before a feeding. Having the parent or caregiver hold the child during the examination can help to alleviate fears and anxieties (Fig. 10.2). Allow the parent or caregiver to be a nurturer rather than assisting with painful procedures, unless there are no other choices available.

Perform the assessment in a head-to-toe manner, leaving the most traumatic procedures, such as examination of the ears, nose, mouth, and throat, until last. Also delay eliciting the Moro reflex until the end of the examination, as the startling sensation may make the infant cry. Use firm, gentle handling while examining the infant. Make sure your hands and the stethoscope are warm. Perform the assessment as quickly and completely as possible. Use a soft and crooning voice, smile, and engage the infant in eye contact. If the baby is crying, a pacifier may be useful and brightly colored objects may help distract him or her.

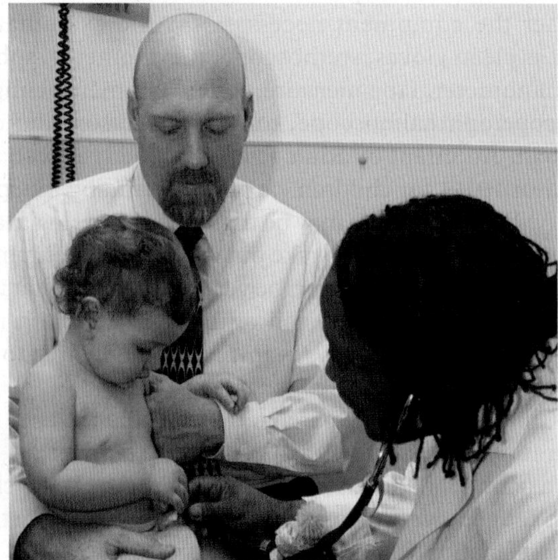

● **Figure 10.2** The infant or toddler may feel more comfortable and secure being examined while sitting in the parent or caregiver's lap.

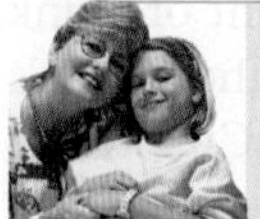

Many older infants demonstrate stranger anxiety as a normal part of development. If the infant is not being held by the parent, make sure the parent is within the infant's view; this will increase the baby's comfort and cooperation.

Toddlers and Preschoolers

Toddlers and preschoolers usually prefer to remove their clothing one item at a time as needed for the examination. After one area is examined, the child may feel more comfortable replacing that item of clothing before removing another one. An examination gown is usually not necessary before school age. Again, make certain the room temperature is comfortable.

When the nurse enters the room, a child of this age is often sitting or standing by the parent. Incorporate play as appropriate during the health assessment. Remember your own facial expressions and tone. Use little touch at the beginning of the encounter with the child and the caregiver.

Introduce the equipment to be used slowly, explaining briefly what is going to happen. Let the child touch and hold the equipment whenever possible, even taking a parent's temperature or putting the blood pressure cuff on a teddy bear (Fig. 10.3). The toddler will prefer to sit on the caregiver's lap. When the toddler must be supine for the abdominal examination, sit in your chair knee-to-knee with the caregiver so the toddler may lie back on the caregiver's and your laps.

Praise the child for being cooperative during the examination. "You did such a good job holding still while I listened to your chest" and similar phrases give positive feedback to the child.

If the child is uncooperative, assess as thoroughly as possible and move on to the next area to be assessed. The caregiver may need to place an arm around the toddler's body to provide restraint for invasive procedures. Use short phrases to tell the toddler what you are going to do, rather than asking if it is OK.

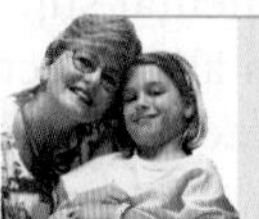

Toddlers are egocentric. Telling a toddler how well another child behaved probably will not be helpful in gaining the young child's cooperation.

The preschooler may fear body invasion and mutilation and will withdraw from any procedure or assessment that is viewed as intrusive. Otherwise, the sense of initiative often leads the preschooler to be cooperative. The preschooler may be willing to undress completely, leaving just the underpants on. Use simple explanations to inform the child about each step of the examination,

Table 10.2 Developmental Considerations for Examination

	Newborn	Infant	Toddler	Preschool	School-age	Early Teen	Late Teen
Place to perform examination	May lie on examination table or in caregiver's lap	In caregiver's lap or on exam table with caregiver right beside infant	Allow some freedom of movement where possible; child may stand between sitting caregiver's legs or sit on the lap.	Some may be willing to sit on exam table with caregiver standing close by with hand on the leg.	Sitting on examination table where they still have eye contact with caregiver	Some may be willing to have their caregiver wait outside the exam room.	Explain to the caregiver that the teen needs privacy and that he or she should wait outside the exam room.
Examination direction	Keep up a running dialog with the caregiver, explaining each step as you do it	Continue to explain each step to the caregiver; address child by name. Perform most invasive parts last.	Introduce yourself to caregiver and child; explain most steps to the child and all steps to caregiver; allow child to handle instruments. Perform most invasive parts last.	Allow child to decide the order of the examination; explain what the instruments do and let the child try them; speak to the caregiver before and after the examination.	Include the child in all parts of the examination; use head-to-toe approach with genital exam last. Speak to the caregiver before and after the examination.	Speak to the child using mature language; appeal to his or her desire for self-care. Use a head-to-toe approach, with genital exam last.	Explain confidentiality to caregiver and teen; allow time talking with them together and separately. Use a head-to-toe approach, with genital exam last.

offering reassurance as appropriate. Allow him or her to "help" by holding the stethoscope or penlight. If choices are available, offer them to the child. Again, always compliment the child on his or her cooperation.

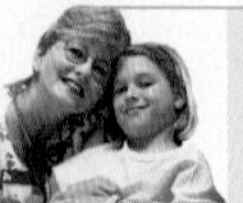

Preschoolers like to play games. To encourage deep breathing during lung auscultation, hold up a finger or a lit penlight and instruct the child to "blow it out."

School-Age Children

The school-age child's thinking is still very concrete, but he or she can be objective and realistic. Avoid using medical jargon and words that may have a double meaning to a young child. Instead of "take your temperature," "take your blood pressure," "hit your knee," or "test," say, "Let's see how warm you are," "I want to listen to you breathe," and other phrases that describe, in words the child can understand, what you are preparing to do. The school-age child may be very interested in how things work and why certain things need to be done and will be responsive to truthful and simple explanations. Instruments that are colorful or look like toys are very helpful until adolescence, when teens are put off by childish things.

Always respect a child's desire to avoid pain and insult. Allow children to wear their underpants under the examination gown to provide a sense of security until the genitalia need to be examined. Allow the child to replace his or her clothing as soon as possible. Privacy and respect for the child's feelings are important to children of this age.

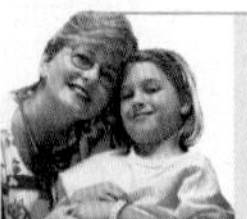

Describing and commenting on your findings during the physical examination is interesting to the school-age child, as children of this age like to learn about how the body works.

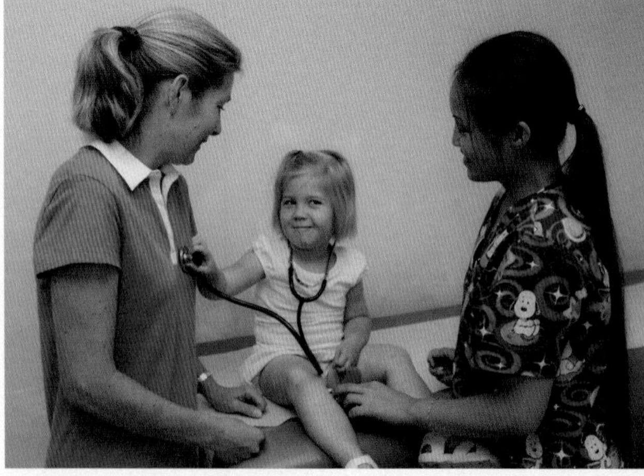

● Figure 10.3 The preschooler enjoys listening to her mother's heart first.

Adolescents

Provide privacy while the adolescent is undressing and putting on a gown. Demonstrate an attitude of respect. Perform the assessment in a head-to-toe manner, exposing only the area to be examined. Provide information about physical changes in a matter-of-fact way, such as, "the hair on your legs is what is expected at this time." This provides information related to sensitive areas that the teen may be reluctant to ask about. It also provides the adolescent with information about the sexual development that is normal and expected. Allow opportunities for the teen to ask questions without the caregiver being present. Assure the adolescent that there are no "dumb questions" about the changes being experienced. Teenage girls should remove their bra so that you can do a breast examination, teach breast self-examination, and check for scoliosis. If the nurse is a male and the patient is an adolescent female, it is appropriate for a female staff member to be present during the breast and genital examination.

Steps of the Physical Examination

The physical examination of children, just as for adults, begins with a systematic **inspection**: checking color, warmth, characteristics, and texture visually and smelling for any odor. **Palpation** follows inspection to validate your observations. Percussion is a useful tool for determining the location, size, and density of organs or masses. Tapping with the reflex hammer elicits deep tendon reflexes. The stethoscope is used to auscultate the heart, lungs, and abdomen.

Performing a Physical Examination

A complete examination includes assessment of the general appearance, vital signs, body measurements, pain assessment, as well as examination of the head, neck, eyes, ears, nose, mouth and throat, skin, thorax and lungs, breasts, heart and peripheral perfusion, abdomen, genitalia and rectum, musculoskeletal system, and neurologic system. The nurse in most settings will not be assessing the breasts, genitalia, or eyes or ears in detail. Be aware of the role of the nurse in different settings and how the nurse can facilitate the assessment process.

General Appearance

Never discount first impressions. As you become more comfortable performing physical examinations, you will develop an ability to describe what you see and hear. Does the child give an impression of being ill or well? What is the child's expression and energy level? Note lethargy, listlessness, excessive activity, or inappropriate attention span for the child's age. Observe the child's state of alertness and whether he or she is responding appropriately to the stress of the situation. Note the child's posture and positioning:

- The newborn's posture is flexed, with arms and legs tucked in.
- The older infant should have improving head and then trunk control.
- The toddler demonstrates lordosis (swayback) and bowlegs, with a relatively large head and protuberant belly.
- The preschooler is more slender and upright in appearance.
- The school-age child and adolescent should demonstrate an upright, straight, and well-balanced posture.

Note whether the child's development appears appropriate. Observing the child initially may yield a wealth of information about the child's development. Is the child active, moving about the room? Does the child's speech seem appropriate for his or her age? Notice whether the family interacts appropriately with one another and the child. Does the child appear clean and well cared for? Does the child appear well nourished or small for age or obese? Do you smell tobacco or alcohol on the family's clothing? Does the child have a toy or transitional object? Is there a baby bottle or pacifier nearby? Do the siblings appear equally well cared for? Is there tension in the room between adults or adolescents? This initial quick assessment of general appearance will serve the nurse well if it is objective; delay your interpretation of what you have assessed until you gather more data.

Measurement of Vital Signs

Measure, document, and interpret the vital signs of children using age-appropriate equipment and approaches. The child's age and size, as well as knowledge of underlying health conditions, will affect your analysis of the vital signs. Vital signs are the temperature, pulse rate, respiratory rate, and blood pressure. In terms of vital signs, there is greater fluctuation in what is considered normal in children compared to adults. Therefore, count the heart rate and respiratory rate for a full minute (this will require comforting an infant or distracting a young child). If possible, perform these measurements when the child is quiet; if the child is crying or otherwise active during the assessment, document this. Many acute care settings require continuous measurement of vital signs using specific monitoring equipment. Also assess the child's pain level when assessing the vital signs.

Temperature

Temperature is measured as it is in adults. Thermometers are available in glass, electronic, and digital types. Use the same type of equipment consistently to allow reliable comparisons to be made and to permit tracking of temperatures during the course of illness. No matter which type of thermometer is used, ensure accuracy by carefully following the manufacturer's instructions.

The routes for taking the child's temperature are tympanic, temporal, oral, axillary, and rectal. Evidence is conflicting as to which method actually correlates best with the child's core, bladder, or arterial temperature, but recent studies support the use of a tympanic temperature as the most accurate, if it is appropriately obtained (El Radhi & Patel, 2006; Nimah et al., 2006). Take the child's temperature using the least invasive method that is best accepted by the child, parent, and health care provider.

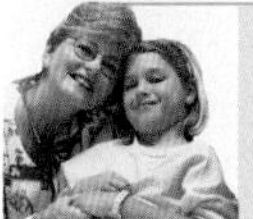

Glass thermometers are rarely used today due to the federal safety recommendations related to glass and mercury.

Choosing a way of measuring temperature depends on what is available at the facility and the child's age and physical condition. Tympanic thermometers measure the temperature within seconds, so this route is ideal for most children. Tympanic temperature reflects the pulmonary artery temperature. Tympanic thermometers are now available with smaller speculums, more appropriate for the infant or young child's ear canal. The accuracy of a tympanic temperature reading depends on the user's technique (Nursing Procedure 10.1). The tympanic method is not affected by the presence of ear wax (Houlder, 2000), but it may be affected by vernix in the newborn's ear.

Temporal scanning is a newer method of temperature measurement that uses infrared scanning on the skin over the temporal artery combined with a mathematical computation to determine the child's arterial temperature. The arterial temperature is considered the most accurate reflection of body temperature. Measure temperature on the exposed side of the head (not the side that has been lying on a pillow or covered by a hat). Slide the sensor tip externally in a horizontal line across the child's forehead, midway between the eyebrows and hairline and ending at the temporal artery. Hold it there until the device registers the temperature reading, which usually requires 1 second. Accuracy may be affected by excessive sweating.

Oral temperature is highly reliable if the child can cooperate. By 4 years of age, the child can hold an electronic oral thermometer in the mouth well enough to obtain a reading. Place the probe under the tongue. The child's mouth remains closed until the device registers the temperature. Have the child sit or lie quietly while the temperature is being taken. Electronic devices provide a

Nursing Procedure 10.1

Tympanic Temperature

1. Note age of child. If younger than 3 years, pull the earlobe back and down.
2. Insert the tympanic thermometer gently into the ear canal with the infrared sensor beam directed toward the center of the tympanic membrane rather than the sides of the ear canal.
3. Push the button to take the temperature and hold until a reading is obtained. The length of time required for the temperature to register varies per manufacturer but is only a few seconds at most.

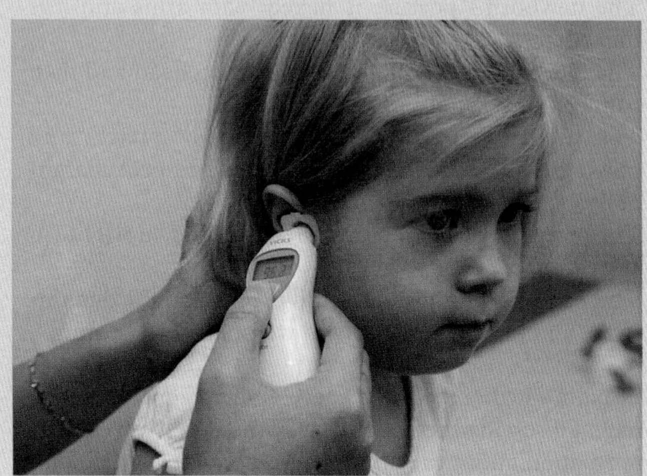

temperature reading in as little as 4 seconds, but again the length of time varies with manufacturer. Oral intake, oxygen administration, and nebulized medications or treatments may affect oral temperature.

The axillary method works well for children who are uncooperative, neurologically impaired, or immunosuppressed or have injuries or surgery to the oral cavity. Place the tip of the electronic or digital thermometer in the axilla to obtain the reading. Make sure the tip is indeed in the axilla and not just between the arm and the child's side. Hold the thermometer parallel rather than perpendicular to the child's side to obtain the most accurate reading. Keep the child's arm pressed down to the side until the thermometer registers, which will be as little as 10 seconds with certain electronic models but 2 or 3 minutes with digital models commonly used at home.

Though long considered to reflect core temperature, the rectal route is invasive, not well accepted by children or parents, and probably unnecessary with the modern alternative methods now available. In addition to its intrusiveness, obtaining the rectal temperature runs the risks of damaging the rectal mucosa and inducing bradycardia in young infants. To take the rectal temperature, position the young infant supine with legs flexed. The older infant or child should be prone or side-lying. Small children may lie across the parent's lap for additional comfort. Apply a water-soluble jelly to the covered probe, insert the thermometer past the anal sphincter no more than 1 inch (2.5 cm), and hold it there until the temperature registers (as little as 15 seconds with certain electronic models but longer with digital models).

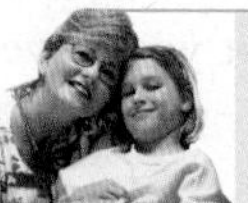

Avoid the rectal route of temperature measurement in the neonate and the immunosuppressed child, as well as the child who has diarrhea, a bleeding disorder, or a history of rectal surgery.

Pulse

Assess the heart rate while the child is resting or sleeping. The heart rate in infants is much faster than in adults. It also varies in infants and children who are anxious, fearful, or crying. As the child grows, the heart rate slows and the range of normal values narrows. Table 10.3 lists heart rate ranges according to the child's age. The radial pulse is difficult to palpate accurately in children less than 2 years of age because the blood vessels lie close to the skin surface and are easily obliterated. For children younger

Table 10.3 Heart Rate and Respiratory Rate Ranges by Age Group

	Newborn	Infant	Toddler	Preschooler	School-age	Adolescent
Heart rate	80–160	80–150	80–140	80–130	75–120	70–100
Respiratory rate	30–70	20–40	20–40	20–30	16–22	15–20

than 2 years of age, auscultate the apical pulse with the stethoscope for a full minute. The **point of maximum intensity (PMI)**, the point on the chest wall where the heartbeat is heard most distinctly, is just above and outside the left nipple of the infant at the third or fourth intercostal space. The PMI moves to a more medial and slightly lower area until 7 years of age, when it is heard best at the fourth or fifth interspace at the midclavicular line (see the section below on chest examination for more information). Apical pulse rate should also be taken if the child has a cardiac problem such as an irregular heart rate or a congenital heart defect, as well as before administration of certain medications such as digoxin. During this procedure with children, allow the young child to examine or handle the stethoscope to become familiar with the equipment. In older children, palpate the radial pulse for a full minute. Note any irregularities in strength or rhythm.

Finally, document the method used to obtain pulse measurement as well as any activity of the child during the assessment and any action taken.

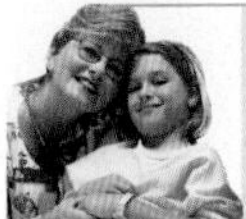

In the infant and young child, the heart rate is often quite elevated due to fear or anxiety when the stethoscope is placed on the chest initially. For an accurate heart rate, wait several seconds until the rate slows, then count for 1 full minute.

Respiratory Rate

Assess respirations when the child is resting or sitting quietly, since respiratory rate often changes when infants or young children cry, feed, or become more active. They also tend to breathe faster when they are anxious or scared. The most accurate respiratory rate is obtained before disturbing the infant or child. This can often be done easily when the parent/caregiver is holding the child before any clothing is removed. Count the respiratory rate for a full minute to ensure accuracy. Infants' respirations are primarily diaphragmatic, so count the abdominal movements. After 1 year of age, count the thoracic movements. Table 10-3 gives ranges of respiratory rate according to the child's age. Document the rate, activity of the child, any deviations from normal, and any action taken.

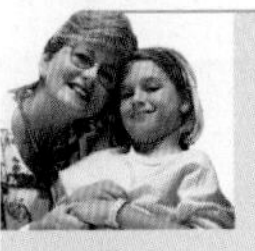

Infants normally display an uneven or irregular breathing pattern, with short pauses between some breaths. This may be accentuated when they are ill.

Measuring Oxygen Saturation

Since the incidence of respiratory dysfunction is high in children who are ill, pulse oximetry is often routinely included in the vital signs assessment. This method is reliable and noninvasive. Pulse oximetry determines the oxygen saturation (SaO_2) in blood by using a sensor that measures the absorption of light waves as they pass through highly perfused areas of the body. The pulse rate on the oximeter should coincide with the apical pulse rate to ensure that the oxygen saturation reading is accurate. Nursing Procedure 10.2 details how to use the pulse oximeter. Identify whether pulse oximetry monitoring will be continuous or intermittent (as with vital signs).

A few guidelines to follow when using pulse oximetry are as follows:

- The probe may be placed on the finger, toe, ear, or foot. Avoid placing the probe on the same extremity with a blood pressure cuff or an intravenous or other type of line.
- Use the physician's orders or health care agency guidelines to set parameters for high and low pulse rate as well as high and low oxygen saturation. Never turn off the alarm settings.
- Ensure that the probe is not applied too tightly, as this will prevent venous flow and cause inaccurate readings.

Potential sources of errors in pulse oximeter readings include abnormal hemoglobin value, hypotension, hypothermia, ambient light interference, motion artifact, and skin breakdown. Falsely low readings may be associated with a nonsecure connection (movement of child's foot or hand), cold extremities/hypothermia, and hypovolemia. Falsely high readings may be associated with carbon monoxide poisoning and anemia.

Blood Pressure

Measure blood pressure yearly at well-child visits. In the hospital or outpatient setting when a child is ill or undergoing surgery or a procedure, the frequency of blood pressure measurement will depend on the child's physical status. Measurement of blood pressure can be frightening to a young child, so include an age-appropriate explanation and perform the procedure after obtaining the pulse rate and respirations. Accuracy of blood pressure measurement depends on the cuff size, as well as the operator's skill (if the heart sounds are auscultated) or accurate calibration of an electronic device. The National Heart, Lung, and Blood Institute (NHLBI) recommends that the cuff bladder width be at least 40% of the circumference of the upper arm at its midpoint. The cuff bladder length should cover 80% to 100% of the circumference of the upper arm. Various pediatric and infant cuffs are available, as well as larger thigh cuffs that may be used on an arm in an obese adolescent.

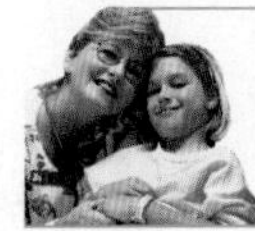

Using an accurate cuff size is important: a wider cuff yields a lower reading and a narrower cuff yields a higher reading.

Measure blood pressure in the upper arm, lower arm, thigh, or calf/ankle. The size of the cuff should match the extremity used. The measurement should be taken in the

Nursing Procedure 10.2

Pulse Oximetry Monitoring

1. Explain the procedure to the child and family (use a penlight to show how the sensor "looks through the skin").
2. Attach the probe to the child and connect to the monitor.
3. Set the parameters for the alarm if monitoring pulse oximetry continuously.
4. Observe and record pulse rate and oxygen saturation.
5. Record the activity level of the child and the percentage of oxygen in use.
6. Check skin condition and rotate sensor position every few hours.

Types of probes

a. infant continuous

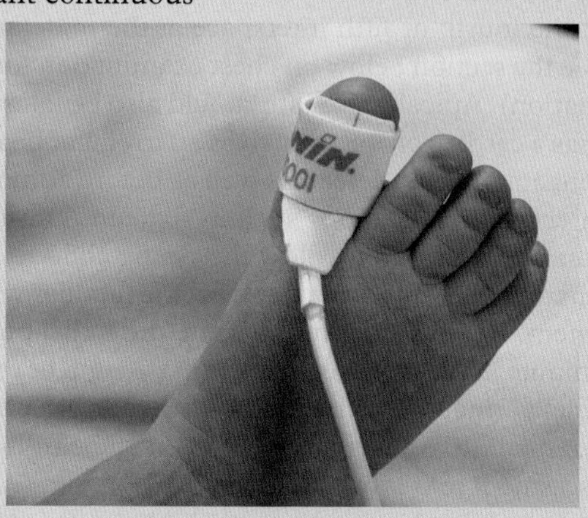

b. finger continuous

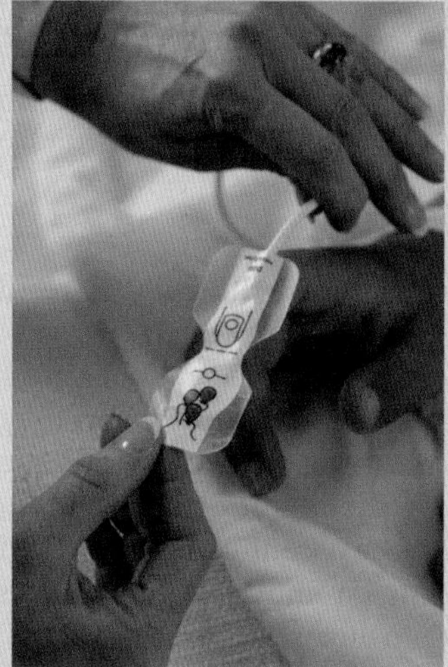

c. finger intermittent

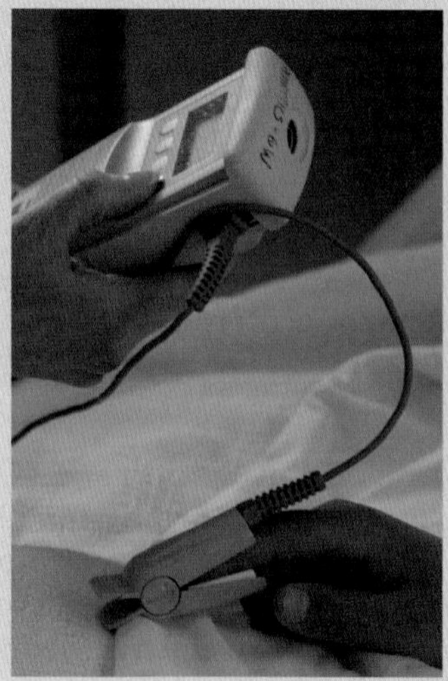

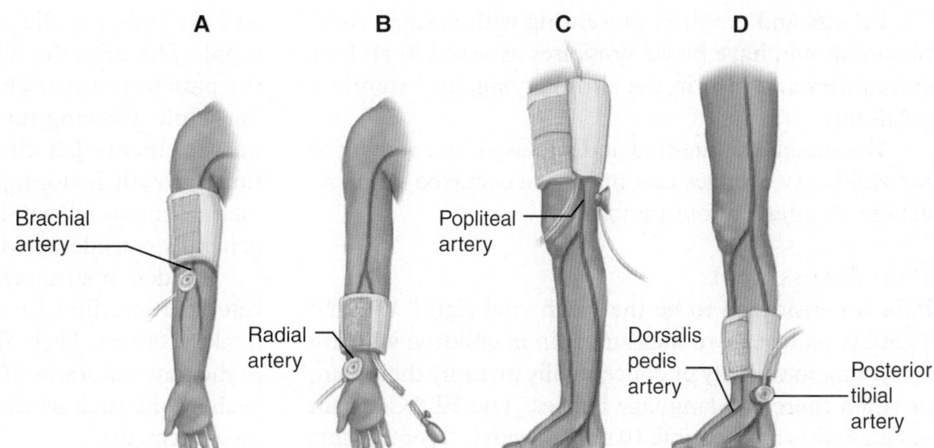

● **Figure 10.4** Various positions of cuff placement and auscultation area for obtaining blood pressure. (**A**) Upper arm. (**B**) Lower arm. (**C**) Thigh. (**D**) Calf/ankle.

same limb, at the same place, and in the same position with each subsequent measurement to ensure consistency in tracking the blood pressure. To measure blood pressure using the upper arm, place the limb at the level of the heart, place the cuff around the upper arm, and auscultate at the brachial artery. When obtaining blood pressure in the lower arm, again, position the limb at the level of the heart, place the cuff above the wrist, and auscultate the radial artery. For measurement in the thigh, place the cuff above the knee and auscultate the popliteal artery. To obtain blood pressure on the calf or ankle, place the cuff above the malleoli or at the midcalf and auscultate the posterior tibial or dorsal pedal artery. Figure 10.4 shows appropriate cuff placement and auscultation points for the various sites.

The NHLBI recommends auscultation as the preferred method of obtaining blood pressure readings in children (Fig. 10.5). Systolic pressure in children is read at the moment you hear the first Korotkoff sound as you lower the manometer pressure (Kay et al., 2001). The point at which the sound disappears is the diastolic pressure. The systolic blood pressure sometimes can be heard

● **Figure 10.5** Auscultation is the preferred method for measuring blood pressure in children.

to a measurement of zero, so document the reading as systolic pressure over "P" for pulse.

Due to the small arm vessels in infants and young children, it may be very difficult to hear the Korotkoff sounds by auscultation. Alternative methods for obtaining blood pressure measurements in children include the use of Doppler or oscillometric (Dinamap) devices. The Doppler ultrasound method uses high-frequency sound waves that bounce off body parts to obtain blood pressure. Apply the gel to the Doppler end and listen with the Doppler device where you would ordinarily auscultate.

With either the Doppler method or auscultation, inflate the cuff 20 mm Hg past the point where the distal pulse disappears. Oscillometric equipment measures the mean arterial pulse and then calculates the systolic and diastolic readings. The accuracy of this method depends heavily on ongoing validation and calibration. Also, the cuff inflates to a preset value often far higher than the infant or child's blood pressure, resulting in a tight, uncomfortable cuff being in place for a longer period of time.

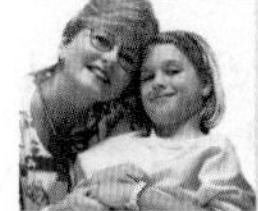

If the oscillometric device yields a blood pressure greater than the 90th percentile for gender and height, repeat the reading using auscultation.

In children older than 1 year, the systolic pressure in the thigh tends to be 10 to 40 mm Hg higher than in the arm; the diastolic pressure remains the same. Refer to Appendix D for the NHLBI blood pressure levels based on gender and height. Systolic blood pressure increases if the child is crying or anxious, so measure the blood pressure with the child quiet and relaxed. If the reading is lower in the leg than in the arm, always consider coarctation of the aorta or interference with circulation to the lower extremities. Also pay attention to the pulse pressure (the difference between the systolic and diastolic readings): unusually wide (more than 50 mm Hg) or narrow (less than 10 mm Hg) pulse pressure readings suggest a congenital heart defect.

Infants and children presenting with cardiac complaints should have blood pressures assessed in all four extremities and also in the sitting, lying, and standing positions.

Document the method and site used, the activity of the child, any changes that may have occurred, and any actions or interventions performed.

Pain Assessment

Pain is considered to be the "fifth vital sign." Use the FLACC pain scale to measure pain in children who are too young to verbally or conceptually quantify their pain, or when there is a language barrier. The FLACC pain scale consists of a possible 10 points, with 0, 1, or 2 points given for each of five clinical signs (see Table 15.7 in Chapter 15).

Children who are older and can express that pain is worsening or improving should use the Pain Faces Scale (see Fig. 15.3 in Chapter 15). Explain that each face represents a person who is happy or sad, depending on how much or how little pain he has: 0 is for a person who is "very happy because he doesn't hurt at all"; 1 means "it hurts just a little bit"; 2, "it hurts a little more"; 3, "it hurts even more"; 4, "it hurts a whole lot"; and 5, "it hurts as much as you can imagine—but you don't have to be crying to feel this bad." Then ask the child to point to the face that best describes the amount of pain being felt.

For additional information related to pain assessment, refer to Chapter 15.

Body Measurements

Appropriate growth in children is usually an indicator of good health. A child who is not growing well may be in poor health, have inappropriate or inadequate dietary intake, or have a chronic disease. Accurate assessment of growth is a critical skill for the pediatric nurse and one that is rarely needed when caring for adults.

Determine the child's height or length, weight, and weight for length or **body mass index (BMI)**. Measure the head circumference for healthy children under age 3. Plot these measurements on a graph so they can be compared with earlier measurements and those of the child's peers. Additional anthropometric measurements used in children may include the chest circumference, mid-upper arm circumference, and skinfold measurement at the triceps, abdomen, or subscapular regions, but these are not performed routinely and are usually used only when a nutritionist consultation is necessary.

The growth chart is a screening tool for nutritional problems as well as a useful screen for chronic illness. Record each measurement in ink with a small dot at the correct location for the child's age and the date of the measurement written above it. Then use a plastic straightedge to connect the previous measurement to the most current one. Children grow at variable rates; in infancy and pre-puberty, the growth velocity is normally more rapid. The growth chart allows the nurse to compare the patient to other children of the same age and gender while allowing for normal genetic variation. When measurements fall close to the same percentiles over time, growth is normal for that child. Children whose measurements fall within the 5th and 95th percentiles are generally considered within the normal growth range.

Sudden or sustained changes in percentile may indicate a chronic disorder, emotional difficulty, or nutritional intake problem. These findings require further assessment of the physical status of the child as well as other types of evaluations such as dietary intake or serum laboratory measurements.

Appendix A gives growth charts for boys and girls, ages birth to 36 months and 2 to 20 years. Special growth charts are available for children with Down syndrome, Turner syndrome, and ethnic groups that are typically smaller in stature as adults. Children may be as much as 10% above or below the predicted measurement and still be normal. Look for a trend over time of healthy growth that is neither too fast nor too slow.

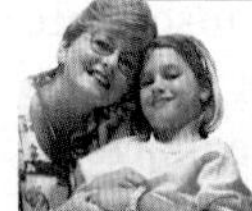

The most valid and reliable growth charts are those supplied by epidemiologists at the Centers for Disease Control and Prevention.

Length or Height

Calculate the length of the infant and toddler in a lying position until the age of 24 months. Use a measuring board (Fig. 10.6) or a cloth or paper measuring tape. Stretch out the legs to get a full extension of the body. Marking the examination paper at the child's head and extended foot is an option. Make sure that the growth chart where the measurement is plotted is marked for

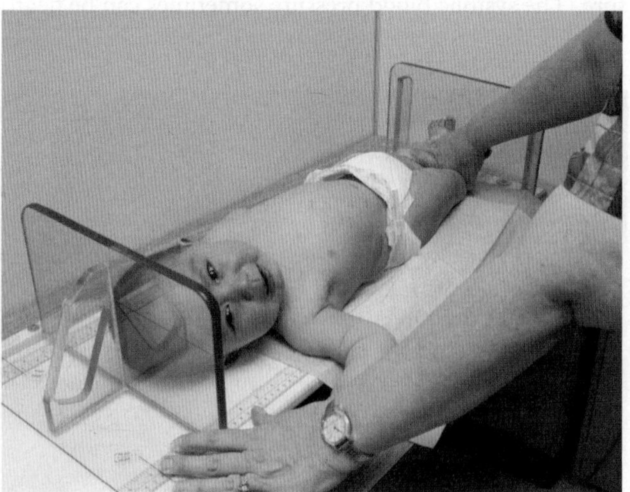

● Figure 10.6 The recumbent measuring board is the most accurate method for obtaining a length measurement in infants and very young children.

length and not height, as the two measurements differ. Document the length in centimeters and inches.

Once the child can cooperate and stand independently, begin measuring the standing height. Using a stadiometer is best (Fig. 10.7), but a cloth or paper tape can be used. Ask the child to remove his or her shoes and check that the back, shoulders, buttocks, and heels are against the wall, with the pelvis tucked as much as possible to correct for lordosis. The chin should be parallel to the floor. Plot this measurement on a growth chart marked for height rather than length. Record the height in centimeters as well as feet and inches.

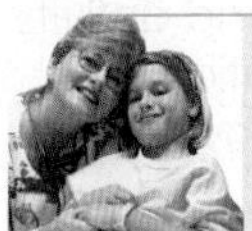

Cloth and paper measuring tapes may stretch over time. Periodically replace or recalibrate all measuring tools.

Weight

Measure weight on a scale that is calibrated between every measurement. Just before placing the child on the electronic scale, press the "zero" or "tare" button and make sure the reading is 0. Calibrate the balance-type scale by setting the weight at zero, observing the beam balance, and making adjustments as necessary. Infants and toddlers should be weighed on a platform-type electronic or balance scale, with examination paper placed between the child and the scale surface. Calibrate the scale with the examination paper in place. Remove the infant's diaper immediately before placing him or her on the scale. Toddlers may sit on the scale with the nurse or caregiver nearby to avoid falls (Fig. 10.8). Weigh older children and adolescents on a standing scale (Fig. 10.9). They may keep their underpants on and wear a lightweight examination gown.

An alternate method for obtaining weight, though much less accurate, is to weigh the caregiver initially and then weigh the caregiver holding the child. The difference between the two weights is the child's weight.

Regardless of the method used, weigh the infant to the nearest 10 g (or half-ounce) and the toddler and older child to the nearest 100 g (or quarter-pound). Record the weight in kilograms and in pounds.

Weight for Length

For children between the ages of newborn and 36 months, plot weight on the growth chart in comparison to the child's length. This allows the nurse to determine whether the child is a healthy weight for how long he or she is. Children placing less than the 5th percentile on the weight-for-length chart are considered underweight. Those placing greater than the 95th percentile are considered to be overweight.

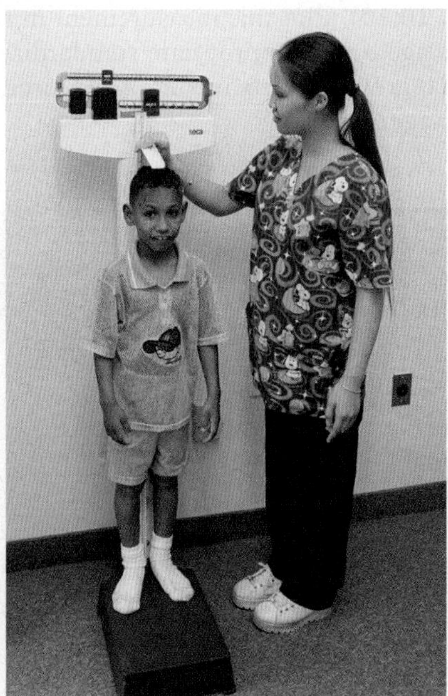

● Figure 10.7 Standing height is most accurately measured with the stadiometer.

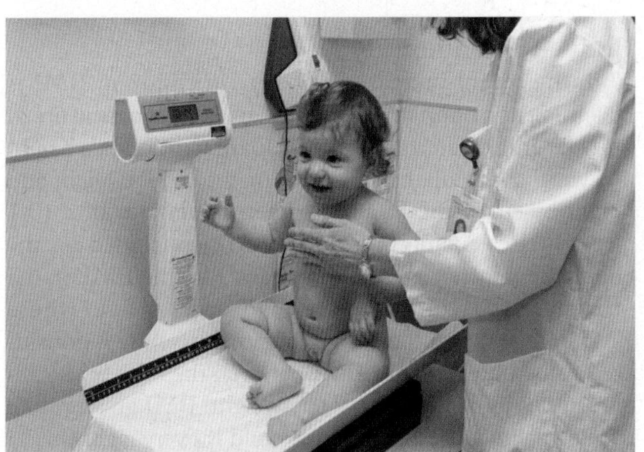

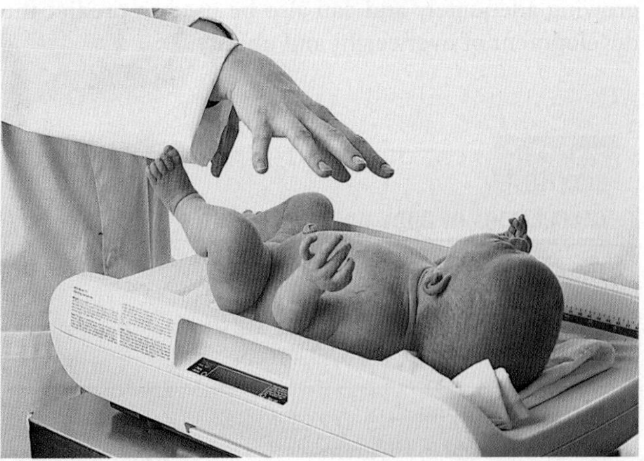

● Figure 10.8 A nurse or caregiver should remain nearby while weighing the infant or toddler.

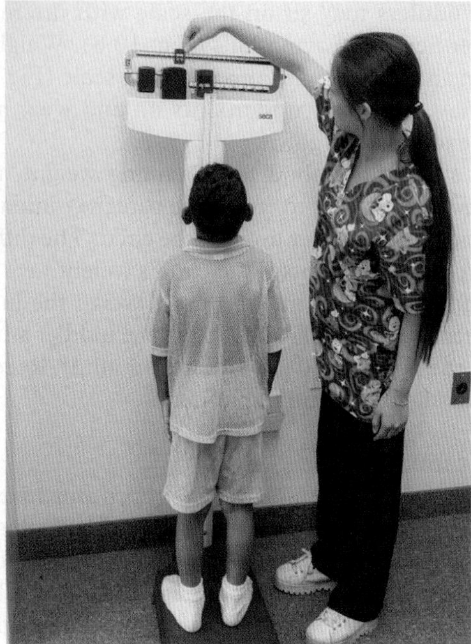

● Figure 10.9 Children who can stand independently can be weighed on a regular standing balance scale.

Body Mass Index

With the recent increase in obesity in children, BMI is becoming an important measurement. BMI is a measure of body fat and is determined by comparing the child's height and weight. Calculate the BMI using the child's weight and height by either the English or metric method. Box 10.1 gives BMI calculation formulas. BMI is included on the charts for children ages 2 to 20 years. Plot the BMI on the growth chart according to the child's age. A child whose BMI for age plots at less than the 5th percentile is considered to be underweight. BMI between the 85th and 95th percentiles indicates risk for overweight. BMI greater than the 95th percentile indicates the child is overweight.

The growth chart can indicate when a child is not growing adequately and can also be used to predict the development of overweight and obesity.

BOX 10.1

CALCULATION OF BODY MASS INDEX (BMI)

English Formula:

$$\frac{\text{weight in pounds}}{(\text{height in inches}) \times (\text{height in inches})} \times 703$$

Metric Formula:

$$\frac{\text{weight in kilograms}}{(\text{height in meters}) \times (\text{height in meters})} \times 10{,}000$$

HEALTHY PEOPLE 2010

Objective	Significance
Reduce the proportion of children and adolescents who are overweight or obese.	• Screen for overweight in all children by plotting weight for length for children less than 36 months and BMI for age for children age 2–20 years. • Assess dietary intake and activity level in all children at risk for or overweight. • Provide diet and activity recommendations to attain a healthy weight or BMI. • Refer significantly overweight children to a pediatric endocrinologist.

Head Circumference

Measure head circumference at well-child visits and upon hospital admission until the third birthday. Then measure it at the annual well-child visit until 6 years old if there are problems such as microcephaly or macrocephaly present at age 3. Measure the largest point across the skull, not including the ears, with a non-stretching cloth or paper tape. Begin at the forehead just above the eyebrows and bring the tape around the head in a taut circle just above the occipital prominence at the back of the head (Fig. 10.10). Plot this measurement in relation to the child's age on the appropriate standardized growth chart (usual growth charts include head circumference only up to age 3 years).

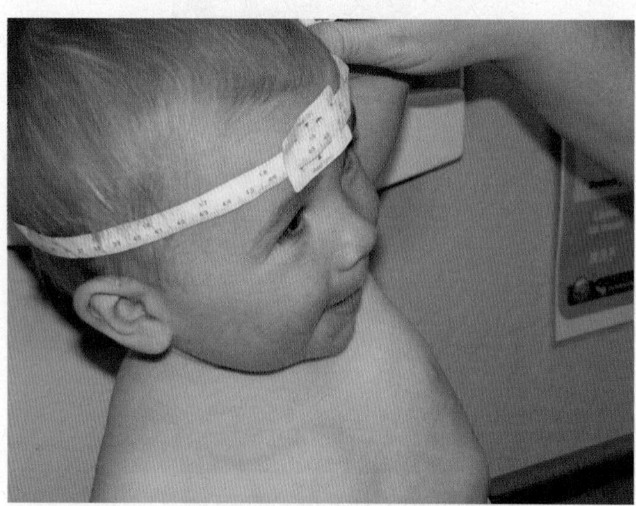

● Figure 10.10 Measure occipito-frontal head circumference at the largest point.

Monitoring Equipment

Sometimes children in acute care settings require continuous monitoring of vital signs. This monitoring could be via an apnea monitor or a cardiopulmonary monitor. The apnea monitor measures abnormal or irregular breathing in infants. The cardiopulmonary monitor generally measures heart rate and respiratory rate. Additional equipment on this monitor also allows for blood pressure and temperature monitoring. Set high and low alarm limits according to the health care facility's policies. Figure 10.11 indicates the placement of electrodes for the apnea and cardiopulmonary monitors. Assess the skin where the electrodes are placed to ensure there is no skin breakdown. If the alarm sounds, immediately check the child to ensure the leads are not disconnected or the child is not in distress.

Skin

The skin is the body's largest organ and reveals information about a child's nutrition, respiratory, cardiac, endocrine, and hydration status all at a glance. A careful skin examination provides an invaluable understanding of a child's health.

Inspection

Inspect the color of the skin. The color should be appropriate to the child's racial or ethnic background, with the nail beds, conjunctivae, soles of the feet, and palms of the hands appearing pink. Normal variations include the following:

- Blueness of the hands and feet, known as **acrocyanosis**, is normal in babies up to several days of age and results from an immature circulatory system completing the switch from fetal to extrauterine life (see Fig. 4.3 in Chapter 4).
- Cooling or warming the newborn and young infant may produce a vasomotor response that causes a mottling of the skin over the trunk and extremities (see Fig. 4.3).
- Babies of darkly pigmented Native American, African, and Asian parents will be paler than their parents for many months until the melanocytes in the epidermis begin production.
- Dark-skinned infants commonly have hyperpigmented areolas, genitals, and linea nigra.

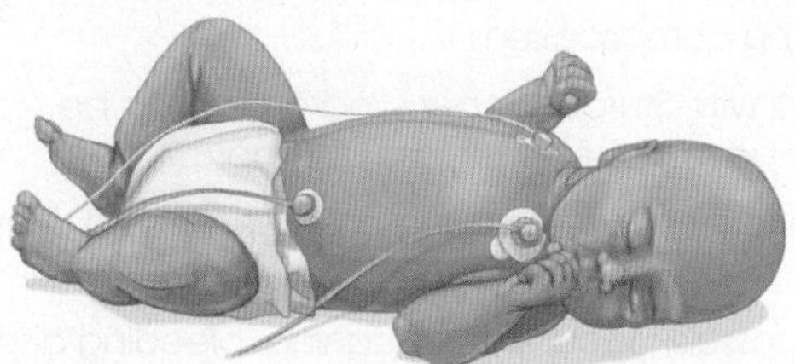

● Figure 10.11 Placement of cardiac apnea monitor leads: white on the right upper chest, black on the left upper chest, red on the abdomen (not over bone).

BOX 10.2

VARIATIONS IN SKIN COLOR AND THEIR CAUSES

- **Pallor** (defined as decreased pinkness in light-skinned patients, ashy-gray in dark-skinned) is caused by anemia, shock, fever, or syncope.
- **Peripheral cyanosis** (blue discoloration) occurs in nails, soles, and palms and may be caused by anxiety or cold; also associated with central cyanosis.
- **Central cyanosis** (blueness of the lips, tongue, oral mucosa, trunk) is caused by hypoxia or circulatory collapse.
- Overall yellow color (**jaundice**) may be physiologic in the newborn or related to liver or hematopoietic disease in any age child.
- **Yellowing** of nose, palms, and soles may result from excess intake of yellow vegetables.
- **Redness** of the skin results from blushing, exposure to cold, hyperthermia, inflammation (localized), or alcohol ingestion.
- **Lack of color** in skin, hair, and eyes is related to albinism.

Other variations related to skin color are discussed in Box 10.2.

Inspect the skin for the presence of **lanugo**. All infants display some degree of lanugo (soft, downy hair on the body, particularly the face and back). Lanugo is more abundant in infants of Hispanic descent and in premature infants and recedes over the first few weeks of life.

Inspect the entire body for nevi and vascular and other lesions. Note their location, size, distribution, characteristics, and color. Pigmented nevi (also termed birthmarks) are indicated by a darker patch of skin and generally do not fade over time. Note the presence of hyperpigmented nevi (formerly called Mongolian spots), which appear as blue or gray, variably and irregularly shaped macules (Fig. 10.12).

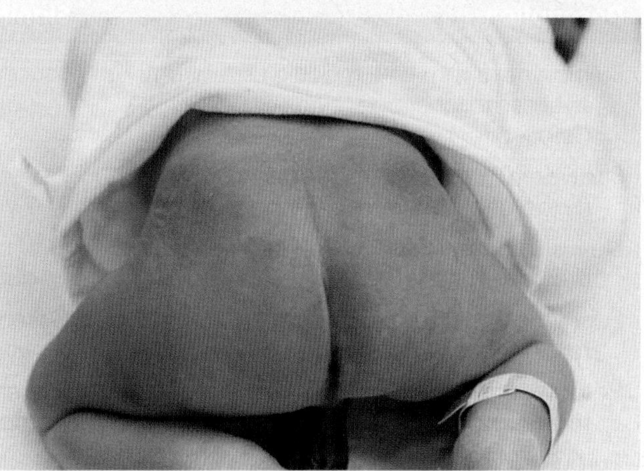

● Figure 10.12 Transient hyperpigmentation most often occurs in darker-skinned infants.

These are a common finding in dark-skinned infants. These nevi fade over months to years as the child's skin pigment darkens. Do not mistake hyperpigmented nevi for bruises. Inspect the skin for vascular lesions. Table 10.4 describes vascular lesions and their significance.

Rashes are common in children and are often associated with communicable diseases. Describe the rash in detail, noting types of lesions, distribution, drying, scabbing, and any drainage. The newborn and young infant may display milia (small white papules) on the forehead, chin, nose, and cheeks. These recede spontaneously. In adolescents the skin examination may reveal open or closed comedones (pimples or blackheads) across the face, chest, and back. Teens may sport tattoos, brandings, or various body piercings; inspect these areas for signs of infection such as erythema or drainage.

Document the presence of any lacerations, abrasions, or burns. Note the distribution of the injury and whether it seems consistent with the mechanism described in the health history. Be alert to the possibility of child abuse if the type or number of burns, lacerations, or bruises seems unusual for the situation.

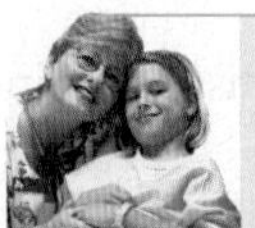

Petechiae or ecchymosis may be found over areas traumatized by the birth process; these may take a few weeks to resolve. Certain cultures use "cupping" or "coining" when a child is ill, and these practices may yield bruises or mild burns.

Palpation

Palpate the skin for temperature, moisture, texture, turgor, and edema. Use the back of your hand to assess the skin's temperature, comparing the right side of the body to the left and the upper body to the lower. The skin should feel uniformly warm. Cool extremities are associated with environmentally cool temperatures as well as impending circulatory collapse and shock. Warm skin may be associated with fever or sunburn, or locally a burn or infectious process. The skin should feel fairly dry, occasionally moister in the creases. Dry, flaking skin may occur in the young infant, particularly if born postmaturely. Overall skin dryness in the well-hydrated child may occur with excess sun exposure, poor nutrition, or overbathing. Moist skin occurs with perspiration, fever resolution, and shock. The infant's and young child's skin is very soft ordinarily. Older children should continue to have a smooth and even skin texture. The preadolescent and adolescent may have oily-feeling skin on the face, shoulders, or back.

Assess skin turgor by elevating the skin on the abdomen in the infant or on the back of hand in the older child or teen. The "pinched-up" skin should quickly return to place. Skin that remains tented is strongly suggestive of moderate to severe dehydration. When edema is present, palpate the edematous area to determine its extent. Palpate any lumps or protrusions to determine firmness or tenderness. Palpate lesions or rashes with a gloved hand to document the size and extent of the lesions.

Hair and Nails

Inspect the hair and scalp, noting distribution of hair as well as color, texture, amount, and quality. The young infant's hair may be absent entirely or quite thick; it will be replaced by hair that is of a texture and color closer to what the child will have throughout childhood. Coarse, dry hair at any age may indicate a thyroid disorder or nutritional deficiency. Inspect the scalp thoroughly; it should be free from lesions and infestations. Note the

Table 10.4 Vascular Lesions and Their Significance

Description	Significance
Salmon nevi: light pink macule usually on eyelids, nasal bridge, back of neck ("stork bite")	Usually fade over time, but may never go away completely. No complications.
Strawberry nevus: raised reddish papule made of blood vessels (hemangiomas)	Present at or develop after birth; recede over time, usually by age 9 years. Usually no complications.
Nevus flammeus: dark purple-red flat patch, grows with the child ("port-wine stain")	May be associated with Sturge-Weber syndrome. May be disfiguring; may be removed with laser therapy.
Ecchymosis: purplish discoloration, changing to blue, brown, black (bruise)	Common on lower extremities in young children. Should correlate with the injury.
Petechiae: pinpoint reddish purple macules that do not blanch when pressed	Broken tiny blood vessels; occur with coughing, bleeding disorders, meningococcemia
Purpura: larger purple macules	Bleeding under the skin; occur with bleeding disorders, meningococcemia

presence of a greasy, scaly plaque on the scalp of infants; termed seborrheic dermatitis or cradle cap, it is benign and easily treated.

Inspect the nails for color, shape, and condition. Full-term infants may have long, papery fingernails that can scratch their skin if not trimmed. Children should have healthy nails. Dry, brittle nails may indicate a nutritional deficiency. Inspect the skin around the nails to ensure that it is intact and without signs of infection. Many children (especially school-age children) have a nervous habit of nail biting or hangnail biting or pulling.

Inspect the school-age child's or adolescent's toenails to ensure they are trimmed in a horizontal fashion. Self-trimming of toenails either too low or in a curved fashion places the child at risk for the development of ingrown nails. Clubbing of the nails indicates chronic hypoxemia related to respiratory or cardiac disease. Nails that curve inward or outward may be hereditary or linked with injury, infection, or iron deficiency anemia.

Head

Examining the head is critical in the newborn and infant periods but should not be overlooked in older children as an opportunity to check for diseases of the scalp and functional and developmental problems that are reflected in poor hygiene of the head and scalp. Note hair distribution and any bald or thinning areas. Use of gloves may be indicated, depending on the overall scalp cleanliness and chance of infestation by head lice (seen as small grayish specks near the base of hair shafts).

Inspection

Examine the head and face for shape and symmetry. In newborns, the head may be temporarily misshapen from uterine positioning or a long vaginal delivery. Some infants have a slight flattening of the back of the head since the recommended sleeping position is supine. Note any irregularities or asymmetry. Observe the infant's head shape by looking down on it from above. Observe whether the head appears centered on the neck or tilts to one side. After 4 months of age, the infant should have achieved enough head control to hold the head erect and in midline when placed in a vertical position. Pull the infant from the supine position into sitting to determine the extent of head lag. To determine the extent of head control in older infants and children, ask the child to turn the head in different directions, either by simple commands or by following a colorful object.

Observe the infant's face when crying, smiling, or babbling for symmetry of muscle movement. In children who are old enough to follow directions, a game of "Simon Says" is a playful way to determine facial symmetry and strength; ask them to puff out their cheeks, make kisses, look surprised, stick out their tongue, and so on (effectively testing function of cranial nerve VII [facial]).

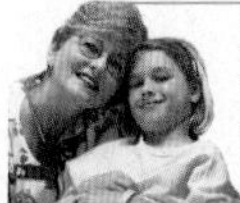

When you note a flattened occiput in an infant, encourage the parent or caregiver to allow the infant "tummy time" while awake and observed and to change the infant's head position frequently when upright in an infant seat.

Palpation

Gently palpate the anterior and posterior **fontanels** (Fig. 10.13), which remain open in infancy to allow for rapid brain growth in the first months of life. Note the size of the fontanels. The anterior fontanel is about the size of a quarter at birth and slowly gets smaller until it can no longer be felt when it is closed by the age of 9 to 18 months. The posterior fontanel is much smaller and may close any time between shortly after birth and approximately 2 months of age. The fontanel should be neither depressed nor taut and bulging, though it is not uncommon to see it pulsate or briefly bulge if the baby cries. In an acutely ill infant, assess the fontanels while obtaining the vital signs. Dehydration can cause the fontanels to be sunken; increased intracranial pressure and overhydration can cause them to bulge. Palpate the skull for asymmetry, overriding or open sutures, and lumps or other deformities. Palpate the jaw joints as the child bites down to assess cranial nerve V (trigeminal). Use the fingertips to palpate for occipital, postauricular, preauricular, submental, and submandibular lymph nodes, noting their size, mobility, and consistency (Fig. 10.14).

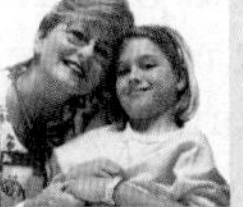

Large fontanels may be associated with Down syndrome or congenital hypothyroidism. A fontanel that becomes larger over time rather than smaller may indicate the development of hydrocephalus, especially if accompanied by an accelerated increase in head circumference.

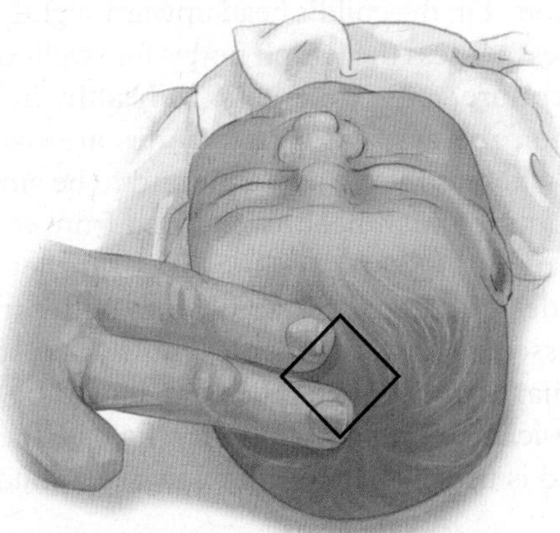

● **Figure 10.13** Note location and size of the anterior and posterior fontanels. The anterior fontanel usually closes between the ages of 9 and 18 months, while the posterior fontanel is usually closed by 2 months of age.

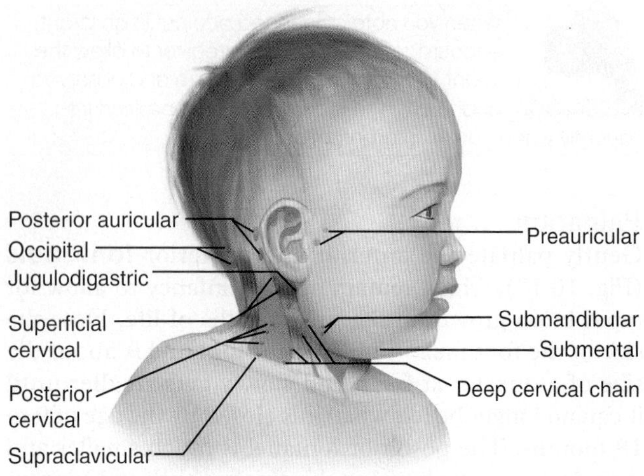

● Figure 10.14 Location of lymph nodes.

Neck

Inspect the neck for symmetry. The infant's neck is short, but by 4 years of age the child's neck should be similar in appearance to the adult's. Webbing or excessive neck skin folds may be associated with Turner syndrome, and lax neck skin may occur with Down syndrome. Assess the flexibility of the neck through a full range of motion. Take younger children through a passive range of motion. Older children will be able to look in all directions on command and stretch their chins to the chests themselves. Test cranial nerve XI (accessory) in the older child by having the child attempt to turn the head against resistance. Assessment of neck mobility is particularly important when infections of the central nervous system are suspected. Pain or resistance to range of motion may indicate meningeal irritation. Do not assess neck mobility in the trauma victim.

Palpate the neck for masses and lymph nodes. Palpate the cervical and clavicular lymph nodes with the distal part of the fingers using gentle but firm pressure in a circular motion. Tilt the child's head upward slightly to allow better access. Assess the lymph nodes for swelling, mobility, temperature, and tenderness. In healthy infants and adolescents, the cervical lymph nodes are usually not palpable, whereas they are often found to be small, nontender, and mobile in healthy children from the ages of 1 year through 11 years (see Fig. 10.14 for locations of lymph nodes). Enlarged cervical lymph nodes frequently occur in association with upper respiratory infections and otitis media. Significant enlargement should be reported to the physician or nurse practitioner. Palpate the trachea; the thyroid is usually palpable only in older children.

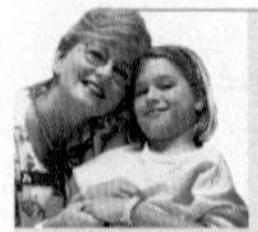

The infant or child who has experienced trauma should have the cervical spine maintained completely immobile until a radiologist has determined that the spinal cord is not damaged.

Eyes

Assessment of the eyes includes evaluation of the external and internal structures as well as screening for visual acuity. Any nurse caring for a child should be adept at examining the external structures. Assessment of the internal structures will also be covered below but is usually performed only by the advanced practitioner. Refer to Chapter 9 for information on vision screening. Determination of visual acuity tests the function of cranial nerve II (optic).

External Structures

Observe the eyes for symmetry and spacing, even distribution of eyelashes and eyelids, and presence of epicanthal folds. Note the child's ability to blink, reporting inability to do so. The eyes should look symmetrical and both should be facing forward in the midline when the child is looking directly ahead. The iris should be perfectly round and the sclerae should be clear. The cornea should be uniformly transparent. Inspect the corners of the eye (medial and lateral canthus) and the conjunctiva (lining of the eyelids). They should be free of discharge, inflammation, or swelling. Epicanthal folds may be present in children of Asian descent, children with genetic abnormalities, or those with fetal alcohol spectrum disorder. Using a small penlight or ophthalmoscope, inspect the function and clarity of the pupil by putting your non-dominant hand on the child's forehead and moving the light toward and away from each eye. This will elicit the blink reflex. Next observe whether the pupil contracts with the light and expands when the light is removed. Make the same motion with a small toy or object and direct the child to look at it. The eyes demonstrate **accommodation**, or focusing at different distances, if the pupil constricts as the object moves closer. If normal findings are present, report **PERRLA** (pupils are equal, round, reactive to light and accommodation) (Fig. 10.15). This is a particularly important assess-

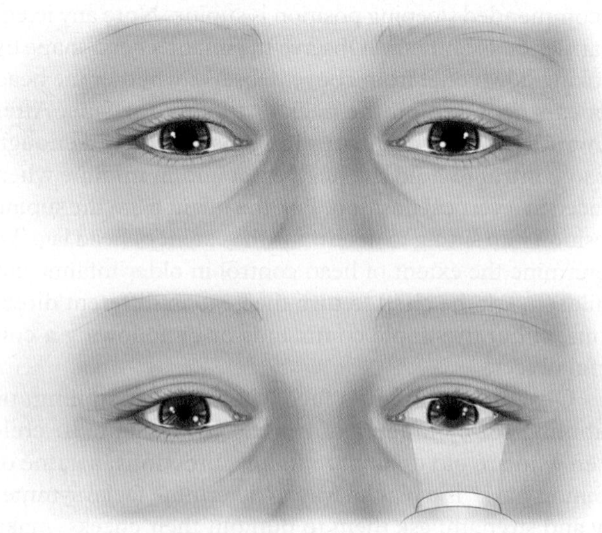

● Figure 10.15 The pupils should be equal, round and reactive to light and accommodation (PERRLA).

ment in head and eye injuries, as well as when other neurologic concerns are present. Absence of pupillary reflexive action after age 3 weeks may indicate blindness.

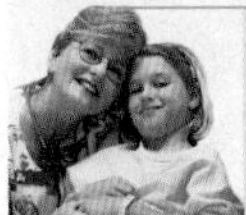

The normal infant may exhibit intermittent strabismus (crossing of the eyes) until about 6 months of age. However, persistent strabismus at any age or intermittent strabismus after 6 months of age should be evaluated by a pediatric ophthalmologist.

Check extraocular muscle motility and function of cranial nerves III and IV (oculomotor and abducens) by instructing the child to follow the light through the six cardinal positions of gaze. Infants and very young children will follow an interesting object. This tests cranial nerve III (oculomotor). Instruct the older child to look downward and inward (testing cranial nerve IV [trochlear]). Assess eye muscle strength using two tests. Using the Hirschberg test, bring the penlight to the middle of your face and direct the child to look at it. The small dot of reflected light seen in the iris should be symmetrically placed in each eye (Fig. 10.16). The cover test also assesses eye muscle strength. Cover one of the child's eyes and instruct the child to focus on an interesting object. The eye should not waver. While the child is still focusing with the first eye, remove the cover from the second. Observe the uncovered eye for movement. Report any movement or drift.

To test peripheral vision, have the child focus on a specific point or object directly in front. Bring a finger or a small object from beyond the range of vision into the area of the peripheral vision. When the child sees the object from the side, while still focusing on the object or point in front, the child should say "stop." This also tests cranial nerve II (optic).

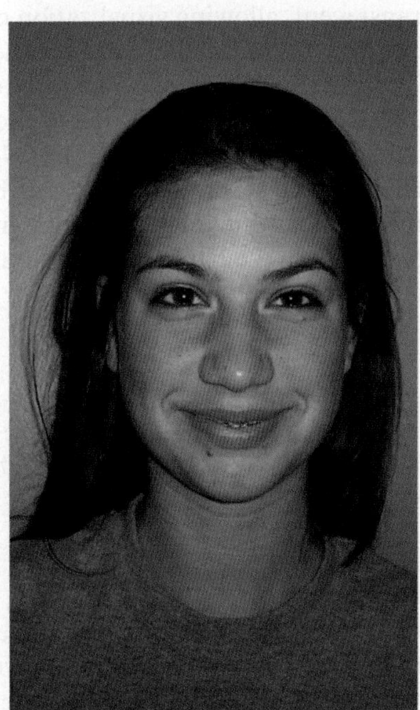

● Figure 10.16 Note reflected light falling symmetrically on each pupil with the Hirschberg test.

Internal Structures

Assessment of the internal structures of the eye is best accomplished by an advanced practitioner with experience in this type of assessment. An adequate assessment requires that the child cooperate. Restraint for eye examination does not usually prove fruitful, as movement and tearing of the eyes interfere with the accuracy of the examination. Use the ophthalmoscope to inspect the internal eye structures. Observe the glow of the pupil, which appears red (creamy-colored in children with very dark eye color). Inspect the optic disk, macula, fovea, and blood vessels. Refer any child with blurring or bulging of the optic disk or hemorrhage of vessels to a pediatric ophthalmologist for further evaluation.

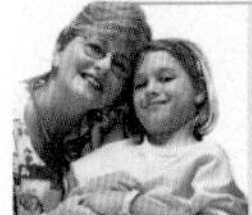

Immediately report absence of the red reflex in one or both eyes, as this may indicate the presence of cataracts.

Ears

Assessment of the ears includes evaluation of the external and internal structures as well as screening for hearing. Any nurse caring for a child should be adept at examining the external structures. Assessment of the internal structures will also be covered below but is usually performed only by the advanced practitioner. Refer to Chapter 9 for information on hearing screening. Testing of hearing also tests the function of cranial nerve VIII (acoustic).

External Structures

Assess the placement of the external ears on the head. They should be symmetrical and placed no lower than the eyes. The pinna should deviate no more than 10 degrees from an imaginary line that is perpendicular to a line drawn between the outer canthus of the eye and the top of the ear. Low-set ears may be associated with genetic abnormalities or syndromes (Fig. 10.17). Note protrusion or flattening of the ears, which may be normal for that child or may indicate inflammation (protrusion) or persistent side-lying (flattening). Note the presence of pits or skin tags in the preauricular area. Observe the exterior ear canal. A waxy **cerumen** that is soft and an orangish-brown color is normally found lubricating and protecting the external ear canal and should be left in place or washed gently away when bathing. Note drainage from the ear canal, which is always considered abnormal. Pull on the auricle and palpate the mastoid process, neither of which should result in pain in the healthy child.

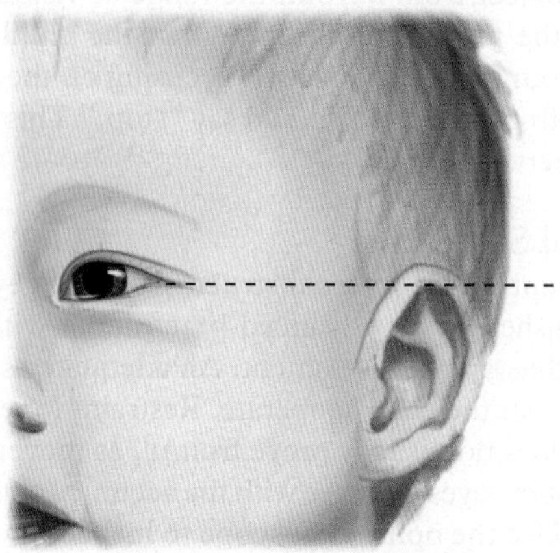

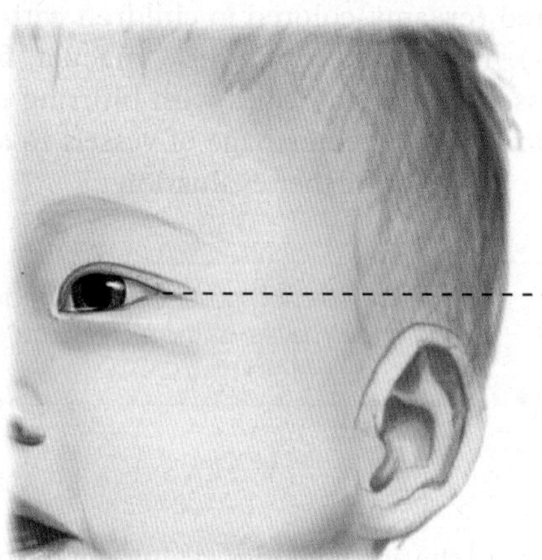

● Figure 10.17 Low-set ears may be associated with chromosomal or other genetic anomalies.

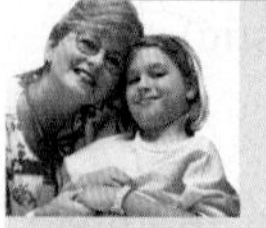

Impacted and dry cerumen can be softened with a few drops of mineral or cooking oil and then gently irrigated from the canal with an ear syringe and warm water.

Internal Structures

Use a **tympanometer** to assess the mobility of the eardrum (tympanic membrane). Gently pull down on the earlobe of infants and toddlers and up on the outer edge of the pinna in older children to straighten the ear canal, and press the tip of the tympanometer over the external canal. A reading of air pressure is recorded by the instrument, and this is useful to assess middle ear disease. Many tympanometers record a wave pattern that may be printed to include in the child's chart.

A nurse practitioner or physician generally performs inspection of the ear canal and tympanic membrane with an otoscope (Fig. 10.18). The otoscopic examination is usually performed near the end of the physical assessment for infants and young children, as they are often quite resistant to this intrusive procedure. The infant or toddler may require restraint in the parent's lap for the otoscopic evaluation. The preschooler may cooperate if the nurse uses a game such as looking for pretend puppies or potatoes in the child's ear. As with the tympanometer, gently pull down on the earlobe of the infant or toddler and up on the outer edge of the pinna in older children to straighten the ear canal. Use an otoscopic speculum appropriate to the size of the child's ear canal. Insert the speculum into the ear canal to visualize the canal and the tympanic membrane. The canal should be pink, should have tiny hairs, and should be free from scratches, drainage, foreign bodies, and edema. The tympanic membrane should appear pearly pink or gray and should be translucent, allowing visualization of the bony landmarks. It may be red if the child has been crying recently. Compress the pneumatic insufflator bulb to provide a puff of air; this causes motion of the tympanic membrane when the middle ear is healthy. Note abnormalities such as a fluid level, bubble or pus behind the tympanic membrane, tympanic membrane immobility, holes or perforations in the tympanic membrane, and the presence of tympanostomy tubes, scarring, or vesicles.

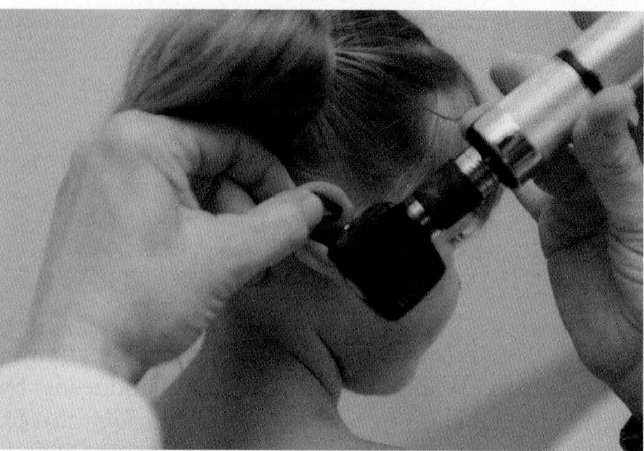

● Figure 10.18 Otoscopic examination allows visualization of the internal structures of the ear.

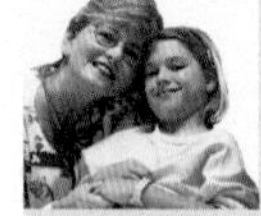

Never attempt to flush a foreign object out with water until it has been identified, because small pieces of sponge, clay, or vegetative material like peas or beans swell with water, further obstructing the ear canal.

Nose and Sinuses

The nose, as with all facial features in a child, should be symmetrical, but it can be displaced temporarily by birth trauma in newborns. Children of Asian or African descent often display a flattened nasal bridge as a normal variation. Ensure that the nares provide unobstructed airflow by alternately occluding one nostril at a time and observing for air movement through the other nostril. If the child is breathing comfortably, there should be little nostril movement visible. Adolescents may have pierced their nose or nasal septum; ensure that the site is free from infection or loose jewelry that could migrate into the sinuses. Ideally the nose should not be draining, though clear mucus may be present if the child has been crying. Assess the amount, color, thickness, and presence of any odor if drainage is present. Inspect the interior of the nose by tilting the child's head backward and pushing the tip of the nose upward. Direct the beam of a penlight in the nostril. The nasal mucosa should be uniformly firm, pink, and free from edema, excoriation, or masses. Test the older child's sense of smell by having the child close the eyes and identify a familiar scent such as peppermint or coffee (cranial nerve I [olfactory]). Palpate the sinuses for tenderness.

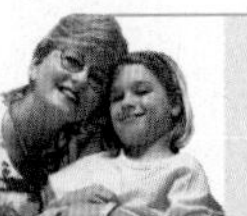

Infants up to 3 to 6 months of age have traditionally been thought to be **obligate nose breathers** because of their long soft palate and relatively large tongue, which allows for swallowing without aspiration during breast or artificial nipple feeding. This lessens with age and as the infant becomes better able to breathe through the mouth when necessary.

Mouth and Throat

Wear a powder-free glove to examine the mouth, teeth, and throat. Inspection of the exterior of the mouth may be done at any point in the examination. Infants and young children may find assessment of the mouth and particularly the pharynx and uvula to be quite intrusive, so delay that part of the assessment until the end of the examination, after otoscopic evaluation. Assess the character and quality of the child's voice and the infant's cry. It should be neither too hoarse nor too shrill.

Inspection of the Mouth

Observe the lips for color, symmetry, and absence of inflammation or edema. Salivation in infants begins at about 3 months of age; drooling occurs because the infant does not learn to swallow saliva until several months later. Next, inspect the interior of the mouth. The mouth is the first part of the digestive system, and a pink, moist, healthy mucosal lining is indicative of a healthy gastrointestinal tract. In infants, the tongue should lie within the mouth at rest and should be capable of extending over the lower gum line to help the baby feed. The tongue extrusion reflex is normal in infants up until the age of 6 months and allows the infant to suckle easily from birth. Observe movement of the tongue when the infant or young child babbles or cries. Ask the older child to touch the tongue to the roof of the mouth and then stick out the tongue and move it from side to side (testing cranial nerve XII [hypoglossal]). Full movement should be present and the tongue should be free from lesions or exudate. Visualize the hard and soft palate (which should be intact) or palpate with the gloved finger.

Most infants have no teeth before the fifth to sixth month. When the teeth begin to erupt, they usually erupt symmetrically at the rate of about one a month, until toddlers have 20 teeth by 30 months of age. The infant may drool for several months before teething. During teething the gums will be swollen at the location of the impending tooth. In older children, the secondary teeth replace the primary teeth much more slowly and with little discomfort from the 5th to the 20th year. Figure 10.19 shows the usual permanent tooth eruption pattern.

Look for dental caries or alignment problems and inspect the gums for signs of infection. Test cranial nerve IX (glossopharyngeal) by having the child identify taste with the posterior portion of the tongue.

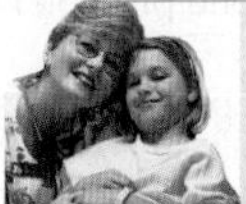

Natal (present at birth) or neonatal (erupting by 30 days of age) teeth should be evaluated by a pediatric dentist for potential extraction, as they may pose an aspiration risk.

Inspection of the Throat

Inspect the tonsils, uvula, and oropharynx. Assess the infant's throat during a yawn or cry, as any forcible attempt to depress the tongue with a tongue depressor produces a strong reflex elevation of the base of the tongue that completely blocks the view of the pharynx. The young child will require restraint so that the nurse can depress the tongue and visualize the back of the mouth without injuring the child (Fig. 10.20). Asking the older child to open wide, stick out the tongue, and say "aaaah" simultaneously will allow for a quick look at the tonsils and pharynx without the need to use a tongue depressor, but the nurse must be very quick because the tongue rises rapidly after those maneuvers are performed.

Tonsils usually cannot be seen in the infant. As the child becomes a toddler, the tonsils become dramatically larger and then begin to decrease in size again by the ninth year. The tonsils should be pink and often have crypts on their surfaces, which are sometimes filled with debris. Is the uvula at midline? Does it rise if the gag reflex is elicited (cranial nerve X [vagus])? Inspect the oropharynx, which should be pink and free from exudate.

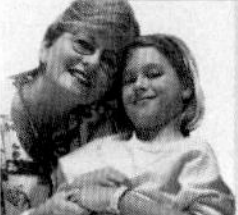

If a gag reflex is inadvertently elicited in the very ill child, the airway may become compromised. Therefore, the pharynx should be examined by asking the child to say "aaah" rather than by depressing the tongue with a tongue depressor.

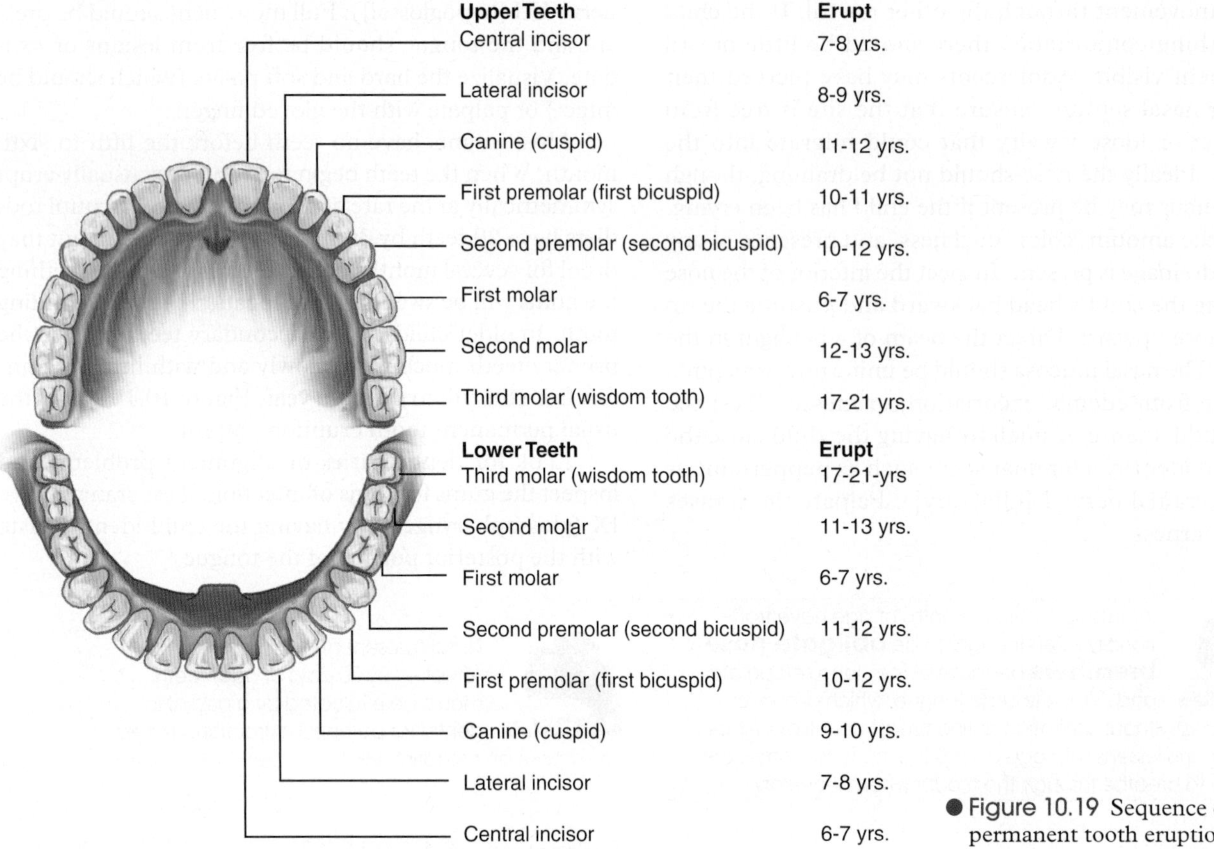

● Figure 10.19 Sequence of permanent tooth eruption.

Thorax and Lungs

Assessment of the thorax and lungs begins by observing the shape and contour of the thorax and determining work of breathing. Accurate auscultation of the lungs is essential, since children often have respiratory infections and disorders and may exhibit alterations in respiratory effort and breath sounds. Note the child's color, which should be pink; cyanosis indicates hypoxia. Listen for audible stridor (inspiratory high-pitched sound), expiratory grunting or snoring, audible wheezing (heard with the naked ear), or cough. Document type and extent of cough. Observe the nail beds for clubbing, which occurs with diseases inducing chronic hypoxic states.

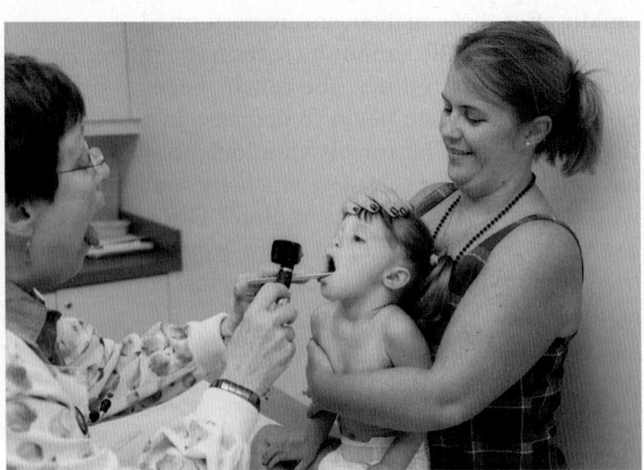

● Figure 10.20 The young child may need to be restrained so that the throat examination can be done safely.

Thorax

Examine the chest with the head in a midline position to determine size and shape as well as symmetry, movement, and bony landmarks. The newborn's chest should be smooth and round, with the transverse diameter nearly equal to the anterior-posterior diameter. The shape of the chest progresses to that of the adult by age 5 to 6 years. At that time the anterior-posterior diameter is about half the transverse diameter (Fig. 10.21). At the point where the xiphoid process and the right and left costal margins meet, the costal angle should measure 90 degrees or less. Inspect for structural deformity such as pectus excavatum (depressed sternum) or pectus carinatum (protuberant sternum) (Fig. 10.22). Note symmetric movement of the chest wall with respiration. Infants and younger children are primarily diaphragmatic breathers, so the abdomen and chest will rise and fall together. Older children, particularly adolescent females, demonstrate thoracic breathing, yet the abdomen and chest should continue to rise and fall together. Asymmetry of chest wall movement is an abnormal finding.

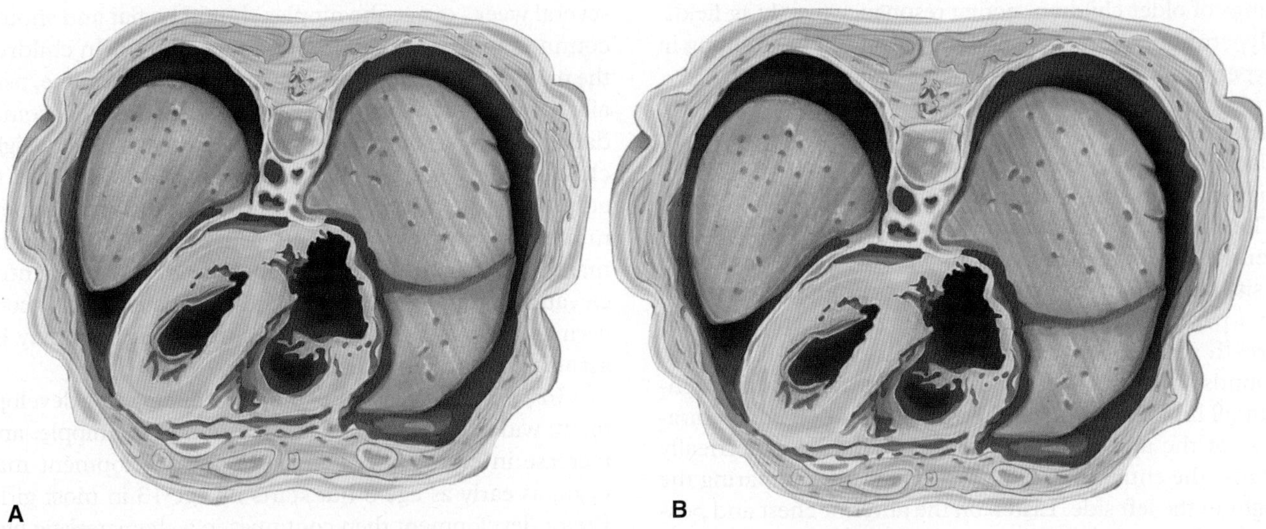

● Figure 10.21 (A) The newborn's chest is round. (B) The adult chest has an anterior-posterior diameter about twice the transverse diameter.

Observe the depth and regularity of respirations, noting the length of the inspiratory and expiratory phases in relation to each other. The newborn and young infant demonstrate an irregular respiratory pattern. Older infants and children should have a more regular respiratory pattern.

Assess the child's respiratory effort by first observing for nasal flaring, which indicates labored breathing. Observe the chest wall and shoulders for accessory muscle use, which normally is not present. If retractions are present, note their location and severity. Typical locations for retraction include the intercostal, subcostal, substernal, suprasternal, and clavicular regions (Fig. 10.23).

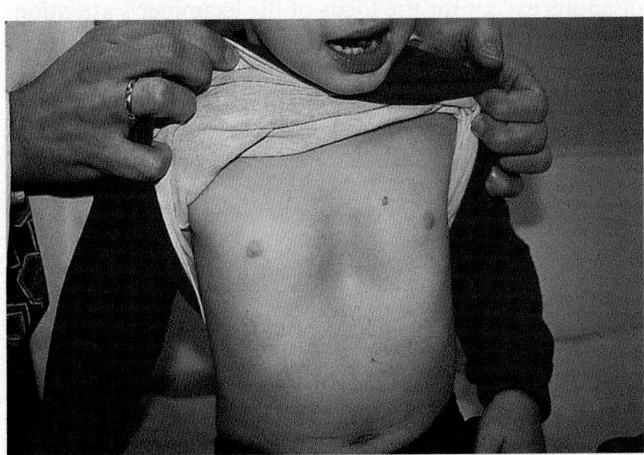

● Figure 10.22 Pectus excavatum: note depression in xiphoid area.

Pay attention to the position the child naturally assumes to breathe comfortably: children in respiratory distress often sit forward and are uncomfortable lying down or talking.

Lungs

Experienced examiners may palpate and percuss the lungs before using **auscultation** to evaluate the breath sounds. Palpate for symmetric respiratory excursion by placing the thumbs and fingers together along the costal margin on the chest or back. Movement should be symmetric with each breath. Palpate for the normal presence of tactile fremitus with the palms or fingertips while the infant is crying or the older child says "99." Indirectly percuss the

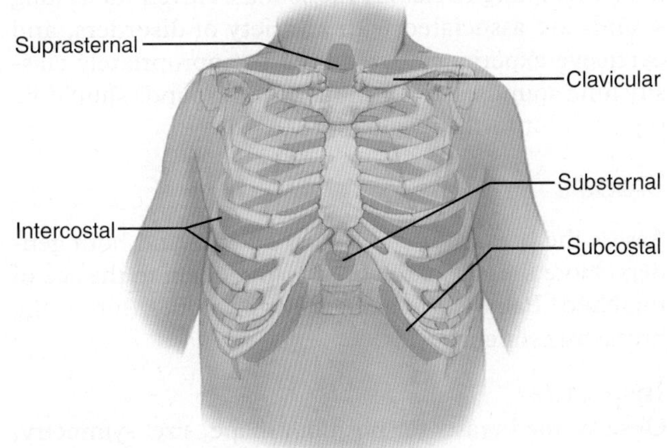

● Figure 10.23 Location of retractions.

lungs of older children, noting resonance over lung fields. Hyperresonance may be present in conditions resulting in hyperaeration of the lungs, such as asthma.

Auscultation

Use the bell of the stethoscope or switch to a small diaphragm to auscultate lung sounds in the infant or child. The adult-sized diaphragm may be used for the adolescent. Auscultate the lung fields with the infant or child in a sitting position, even if that requires propping the infant in a parent's lap. Infants and young children have loud breath sounds because of their thin chest walls. Breath sounds should be clear with adequate aeration throughout all lung fields. Listen to a full inspiration and expiration at the apices of the lungs as well as symmetrically across the entire lung field, systematically comparing the right to the left side. Listen on the anterior chest and posterior chest and in the axillary regions.

Playing games may encourage younger children to cooperate with deep breathing during lung assessment. The child can blow a cotton ball up in the air, blow a pinwheel, or "blow out" the light of the penlight. Older children are capable of deep breathing when instructed to do so.

The child who has a respiratory disorder or who is experiencing respiratory distress may exhibit diminished breath sounds, most often in the lung bases. Diminished breath sounds are softer and quieter than lung sounds demonstrating adequate aeration. In the healthy infant or child, no adventitious sounds should be heard. If noisy breath sounds are heard in the infant or young child, particularly over all lung fields, compare the sound to the noises heard over the trachea or within the nose. Infants and young children with secretions in the nasopharyngeal area may have those sounds transmitted over the lung fields. These sounds usually clear with coughing or airway suctioning; they are not true adventitious sounds. Note adventitious breath sounds such as wheezes or crackles, documenting their location and whether they are present on inspiration, expiration, or both. It is most important to describe the abnormal breath sounds being heard rather than attempting to classify the sounds. Adventitious lung sounds are associated with a variety of disorders, and extensive experience is required to appropriately classify lung sounds. Adventitious breath sounds should be reported for further evaluation.

Breasts

Assess the breasts of children of all ages and both genders. Note the size of the breasts in relation to the age of the child. Palpate the axillary lymph nodes during the breast assessment.

Inspection

Observe the breasts for position, shape, size, symmetry, and color. Newborns of both genders may have swollen nipples from the influence of maternal estrogen, but by several weeks of age the nipples should be flat and should continue to be so in all prepubertal children. In children the nipples are located lateral to the midclavicular line, usually between the fourth and fifth rib. The areola becomes darker in color as the child approaches puberty. Overweight children may appear to have enlarged breasts due to adipose tissue. Note the location of additional (supernumerary) nipples if present (usually located along the mammary ridge); they may appear as darkly pigmented elevated or nipple-like spots. These are usually of no concern as they do not change over time, but they may be associated with renal disorders.

Inspect the breasts for the current stage of development: widening of the areola, elevation of the nipple, and increase in breast size. Female breast development may begin as early as age 8 but starts by age 13 in most girls. Breast development then continues in a characteristic pattern but usually is asymmetric, with one breast larger than the other throughout the lifespan. The sexual maturity rating scale developed by Tanner in 1962 is used to describe breast development (**Tanner stages**; Fig. 10.24). Adolescent boys may develop gynecomastia (enlargement of the breast tissue) due to hormonal pubertal changes. When the hormone levels stabilize, male adolescents then have flat nipples. Occasionally gynecomastia is caused by marijuana use, anabolic steroids, or hormonal dysfunction.

Palpation

Palpate the breasts in a systematic fashion. A tender nodule palpated just under the nipple confirms pubertal changes. This change may be difficult to assess in girls with excessive adipose tissue. Normal breast tissue should feel smooth, firm, and elastic. Note masses or nodules if present. Palpate for axillary lymph nodes with the child's arms relaxed at the side but slightly abducted. Note size and texture of nodes if present.

Heart and Peripheral Perfusion

The examination of the heart in children is identical to that of adults except for the focus of the examiner's attention. Congenital heart defects are the most common cause of heart problems in children, and children with these defects present differently than adults with heart disease.

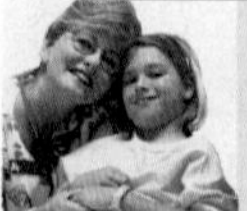

The younger the child, the more responsive the heart rate is to activity changes. It increases with fever, fear, crying, or anxiety and decreases with sleep, sedation, or vagal stimulation.

Inspection

Observe the child's posture. Note the presence of pallor, cyanosis, mottling, or edema, which may indicate a cardiovascular problem. Inspect the anterior chest from the side or at an angle, noting symmetry in shape as well as

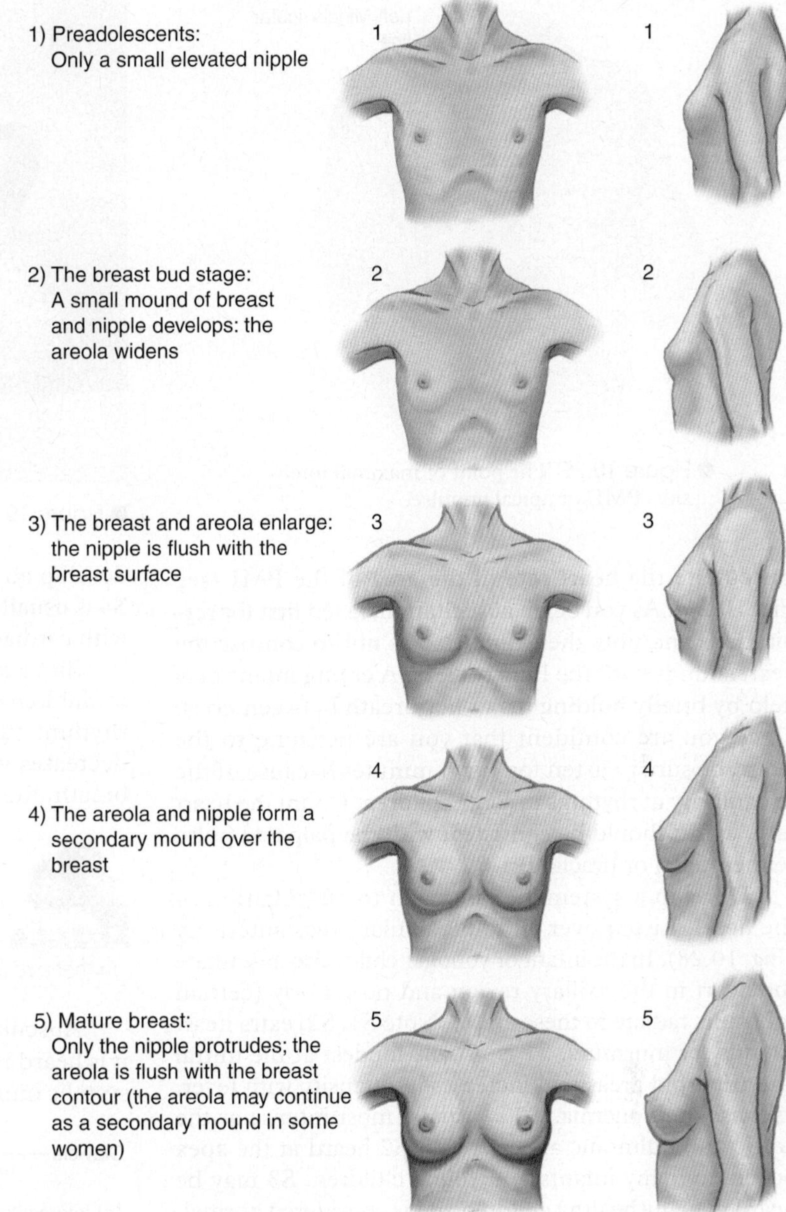

1) Preadolescents:
Only a small elevated nipple
1
1
2) The breast bud stage:
A small mound of breast and nipple develops: the areola widens
2
2
3) The breast and areola enlarge: the nipple is flush with the breast surface
3
3
4) The areola and nipple form a secondary mound over the breast
4
4
5) Mature breast:
Only the nipple protrudes; the areola is flush with the breast contour (the areola may continue as a secondary mound in some women)
5
5

● **Figure 10.24** Tanner sexual maturity rating for breast development.

movement. Observe for the apical impulse, which is visible in about half of children. It occurs at the PMI, which is located at the fourth intercostal space just medial of the child's left midclavicular line until age 4 years, at the fourth intercostal space at the left midclavicular line in children ages 4 to 6 years, and then lateral to the left midclavicular line at the fifth intercostal space in children ages 7 years and older (Fig. 10.25). Note clubbing of the fingertips or distention of neck veins, both of which may be associated with congenital heart disease.

Palpation

Using the fingertips, palpate the chest for lifts and heaves or thrills, which are not normal. Palpate the apical pulse in the area of the PMI (see Fig. 10.25). Check the pulses and compare the upper body to lower body pulses, as well as left versus right, noting strength and quality (Fig. 10.26). The pedal, brachial, and femoral pulses are usually easily palpated. The radial pulse is very difficult to palpate in children less than 2 years of age. Note warmth of the distal extremities. To assess capillary refill time, place slight pressure on the nail beds and quickly release it. Observe the length of time required for refill and return to original color. Compare capillary refill time of the fingers to the toes. A capillary refill time of less than 3 seconds indicates adequacy of perfusion.

Auscultation

Perform auscultation of the heart with the child in two different positions, upright and reclined (Fig. 10.27).

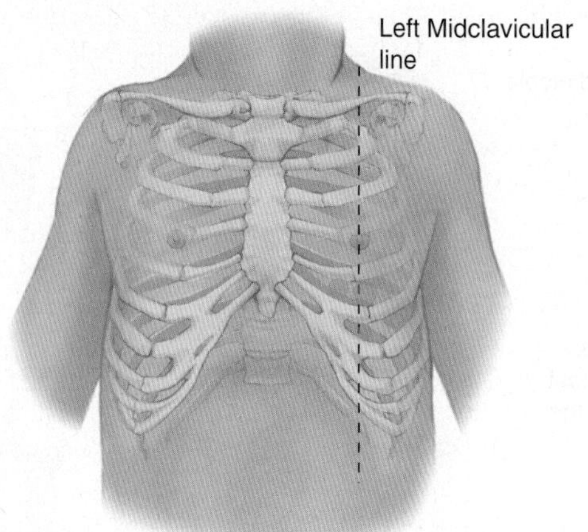

● Figure 10.25 The point of maximal intensity (PMI) or apical impulse.

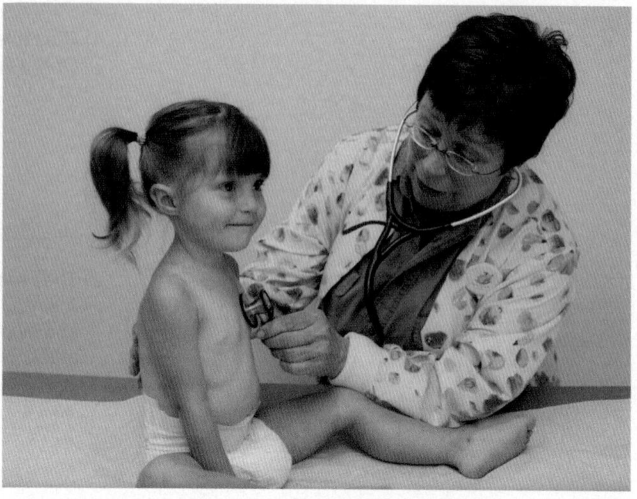

● Figure 10.27 Auscultating the child's heart.

Auscultate the heart rate in the area of the PMI (see Fig. 10.25). As you begin auscultation, listen first for respirations and note their timing so as not to confuse the heart sounds with the lung sounds. A crying infant may help by briefly holding his or her breath between cries. Once you are confident that you are listening to the heart, be sure to listen for 1 to 3 minutes because of the irregularity of rhythms in some children. Count the heart rate, which should be consistent with the palpated pulse (either radial or brachial).

Develop a systematic approach to auscultation of the heart. Listen over all four valvular areas anteriorly (Fig. 10.28). In the infant or younger child, also auscultate the heart in the axillary region and posteriorly (certain murmurs radiate to these areas). Note S1, S2, extra heart sounds, or murmurs. S1 is usually loudest at the mitral and tricuspid areas and increases in intensity with fever, exercise, and anemia. S2 is usually most intense at the aortic and pulmonic areas. A split S2 heard at the apex occurs in many infants and young children. S3 may be heard in many healthy children and is considered normal, though the child with a chronic cardiac condition may develop an S3 when congestive heart failure is present. S4 is usually considered abnormal, most often occurring with cardiac disease.

Sinus arrhythmia is a common and normal finding in children and adolescents. It results in an irregular heart rhythm: the heart rate increases with inhalation and decreases with exhalation. If the child holds his or her breath, the rhythm becomes regular.

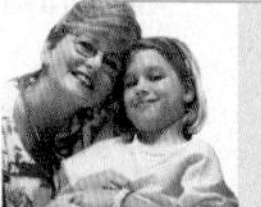

S1 should not vary in intensity at a particular point. If it does, this may indicate a cardiac arrhythmia and the child should be referred for further evaluation.

Auscultate for murmurs. Note the location (where it is heard best or loudest) and timing of the murmur. A systolic murmur occurs in association with S1 (closure of

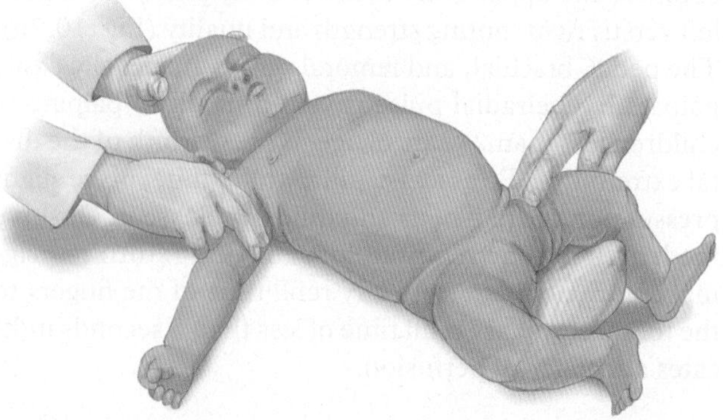

● Figure 10.26 It is important to assess brachial and femoral pulses simultaneously to determine equality or differences in strength and intensity.

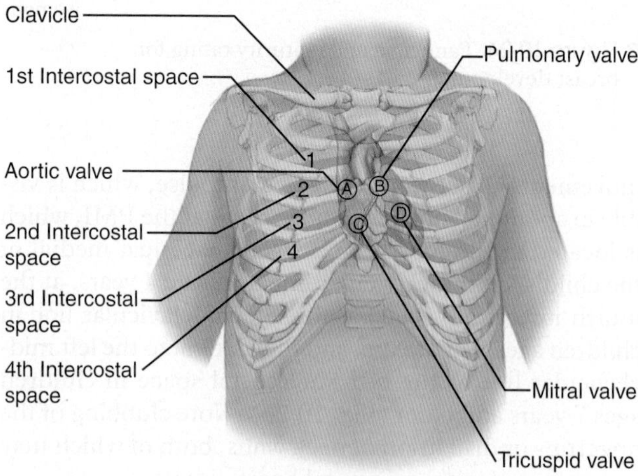

● Figure 10.28 Areas where the sounds of heart valves radiate. A: Aortic valve—second intercostal space, just right of sternum. P: Pulmonic valve—second intercostal space, just left of sternum. T: Tricuspid valve—fourth intercostal space, just right of sternum. M: Mitral valve—fourth intercostal space at left midclavicular line.

the atrioventricular valves), a diastolic murmur in association with S2 (closure of the semilunar valves). Also note the duration of murmur. Does it occur early or late in diastole or systole? Does it occur all the way across systole (holosystolic)? Note the intensity of the murmur. Table 10.5 discusses grading of murmur intensity.

Innocent murmurs occur frequently in children because of the child's more dynamic circulation, thin chest wall, and angulated vessels. An innocent murmur is most often heard at the second or fourth intercostal space, and its timing is systolic. The innocent murmur is usually medium-pitched and musical. Often an innocent murmur disappears when the child changes position. A venous hum that is heard in the supraclavicular area and possibly radiating down the chest is considered an innocent murmur. Refer any child with a murmur to an experienced practitioner for further evaluation.

Abdomen

The abdomen contains organs related to the genitourinary and lymphatic systems, in addition to the gastrointestinal system. These structures lie within the abdomen in approximately the same location as they do in adults. Dividing the abdomen into quadrants simplifies the description of normal organ location and the reporting of abnormalities. Draw an imaginary vertical line from the xiphoid process to the symphysis pubis. Cross this with an imaginary perpendicular line through the umbilicus. The sequence of physical examination is altered for the abdominal assessment: auscultation is done before percussion and palpation because manipulation of the lower abdomen may affect the bowel sounds.

Inspection

Inspect the abdomen for size, shape, and symmetry. The abdomen in the infant and toddler is rounded and protuberant until the abdominal musculature becomes well developed. Though rounded, the abdomen should not be distended (at any age). By adolescence, the stature is more erect and the abdomen begins to appear flat when standing and concave when supine. The thin skin of a young child may allow the visualization of superficial venous circulation across the abdomen. Inspect the abdomen for movement. At eye level with the abdomen, note abdomen and thorax movement occurring simultaneously. Visible peristaltic waves are abnormal and should be reported immediately.

Inspect the newborn's umbilicus for color, bleeding, odor, and drainage. The umbilical stump should slowly dry, become black and hard, and fall away from the cutaneous navel by the end of the second week of life. Note drainage or granulation at the umbilical site indicating delayed drying of the umbilical stump. Inspect the umbilicus in older infants and young children for the presence of umbilical hernia. Because the umbilicus divides the rectus abdominis muscle, it is not uncommon to see an umbilical hernia protrude through and become larger when the infant or toddler strains or cries (Fig. 10.29). This is a benign finding and will usually disappear as the abdomen becomes stronger. Adolescents may have jewelry piercing the umbilicus (Fig. 10.30).

Auscultation

Auscultate the abdomen using the diaphragm or the bell of the stethoscope pressed firmly against the abdomen. Count the bowel sounds in each of the four quadrants for a full minute. Bowel sounds should be present by a few hours after birth and should remain active throughout life. Note whether bowel sounds are normally active, hyperactive, hypoactive, or absent. Normal bowel sounds can be described as growls, gurgles and clicking sounds. Hypoactive bowel sounds may occur postoperatively. Hyperactive bowels sounds are common with diarrhea. Classify bowel sounds as absent after listening for 5 full minutes in each area. Absent bowel sounds may indicate ileus or peritonitis.

Percussion

Indirectly percuss all areas of the abdomen. Normal findings include dullness along the costal margins and tympany

Table 10.5 Grading Heart Murmurs in Children

Grade	Sound
1	Barely audible; sometimes heard, sometimes not. Usually heard only with intense concentration.
2	Quiet, soft; heard each time the chest is auscultated
3	Audible, intermediate intensity
4	Audible, with a palpable thrill
5	Loud, audible with edge of the stethoscope lifted off the chest
6	Very loud, audible with the stethoscope placed near but not touching the chest

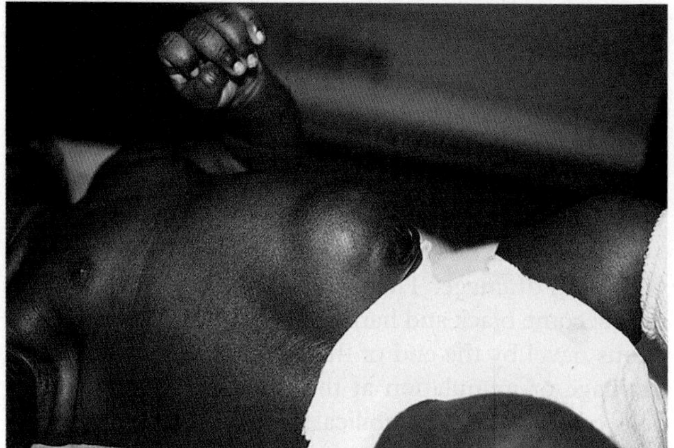

● Figure 10.29 The umbilical hernia may increase in size when the infant cries.

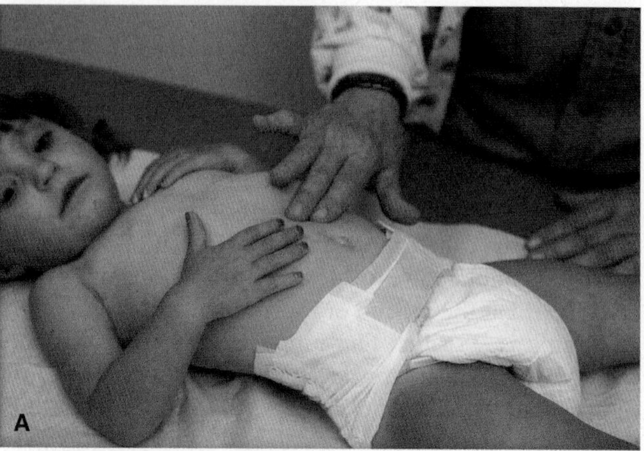

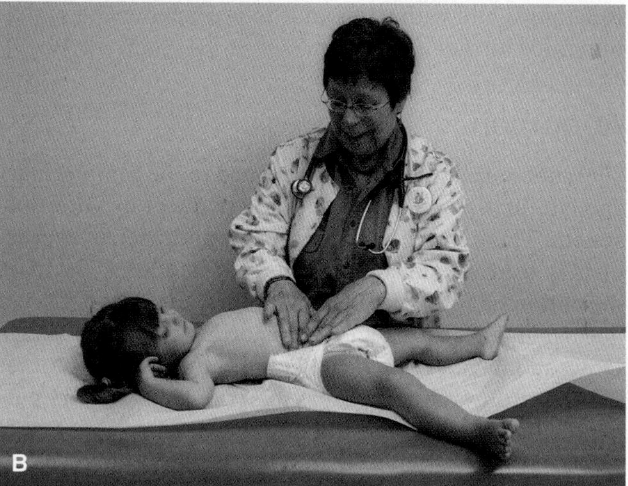

● Figure 10.31 (A) Light and (B) deep palpation of the abdomen.

over the remainder of the abdomen. A full bladder may yield dullness to percussion.

Palpation

Palpate the abdomen with the child in a supine position. If the child's legs are small enough, the knees may be brought up with the nondominant hand to flex the hips and relax the abdomen. Palpate all four quadrants of the abdomen in a systematic fashion, first lightly and then deeply. Apply light pressure with the fingertips to perform light palpation, assessing for tenderness and muscle tone (Fig. 10.31). Note skin turgor by gently elevating a piece of skin and allowing it to fall back into place. Perform deep palpation to assess the organs and any masses. Place one hand on top of the other and palpate from the lower quadrants to the upper (see Fig. 10.31). The edge of the liver may be felt at the right costal margin, and the tip of the spleen can be felt at the left costal margin. The descending colon may be felt in the left lower quadrant as a small column and the bladder as a soft balloon below the umbilicus. The kidneys are rarely palpable. The abdomen should be soft and nontender to palpation. Report firmness, tenderness, or masses. Palpate the inguinal area for the presence of hernia or enlarged lymph nodes.

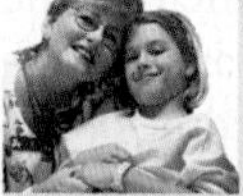

To decrease ticklishness with abdominal palpation, place a flat, warm, still hand on the abdomen while distracting the child before palpation begins. An alternate technique is to first palpate with the child's hand under the examiner's hand.

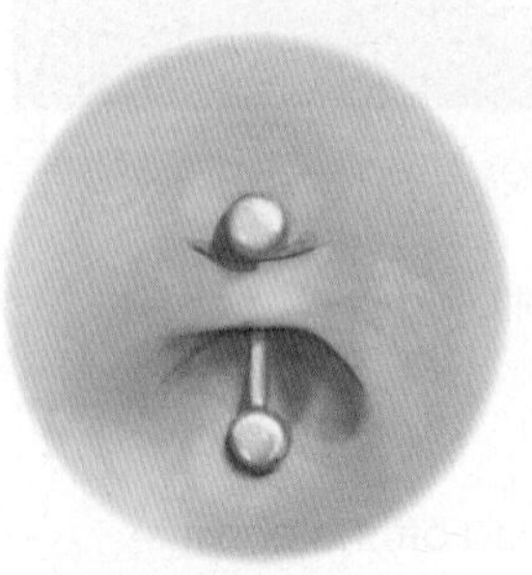

● Figure 10.30 Navel piercing sites should be free from infection.

Genitalia and Anus

Examination of the genitals should immediately follow the abdominal assessment in the younger child and should be reserved for the end of the assessment in the adolescent. Though the anus is part of the gastrointestinal tract, it is best assessed during the genital examination. Ensure privacy for the older child and adolescent. Keep the child covered as much as possible. Use a casual, matter-of-fact approach to place the child or teen at ease. During the genital examination, teach the child or adolescent about normal variations and changes with puberty, as well as issues related to health promotion.

Male

Inspect the penis and scrotum for size, color, skin integrity, and obvious masses. The obese boy's penis may appear small because of additional skin folds. Penis size should correlate with pubertal stage (Fig. 10.32). The penis may have a foreskin that covers the glans, protecting and lubricating it. If present, do not forcibly retract the foreskin. In circumcised males the urinary meatus is exposed and should be at the tip of the glans. Assess the meatus for absence of discharge. If possible, observe the stream of urine for strength of flow and patency of the urethral orifice. Skin lesions may indicate sexually transmitted infection. A foreskin that cannot be retracted in a boy over 3 years of age may indicate phimosis. Report abnormal findings.

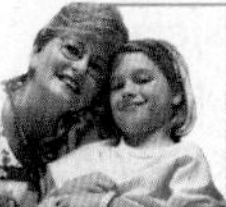

When you first remove a male infant's diaper, this is the ideal time to assess the force of the urine stream and the erection reflex, as the cool air may make the infant void and briefly experience an erection.

Assess the presence and distribution of pubic hair. Inspect the scrotum for size, slight asymmetry, color, and absence of edema. The scrotum may initially be swollen from birth trauma or maternal hormones, but this swelling should decrease in the first few days of life. The scrotum is ordinarily more deeply pigmented than the rest of the boy's skin. Figure 10.32 illustrates scrotal changes that occur with puberty. Assess the testicles by placing one finger over the inguinal canal and palpating the scrotum with the other. This prevents the retractile testes in a young child from slipping back up the inguinal canal. The testicles should be smooth, of similar sizes, and freely moveable. The infant's testicles may be palpated in the scrotum or in the inguinal canal, where they can be easily moved into the scrotum with gentle pressure from the examiner's nondominant hand (Fig. 10.33). Beyond infancy, allow the boy to sit cross-legged to reduce the cremasteric reflex that retracts the testicles during palpation. An adolescent boy may need to stand for the nurse to fully palpate the scrotum. Document the presence of both testicles in the scrotal sac, if they are retractile, or if they are absent. Report undescended testicle or other abnormal findings.

From top to bottom:

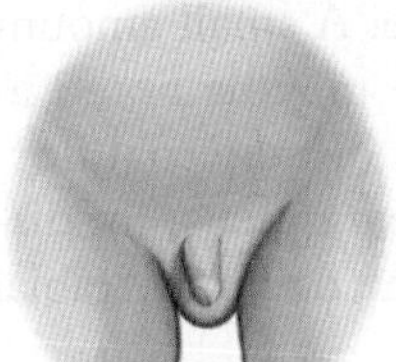

1) No pubic hair and scrotum size and proportion the same as during childhood

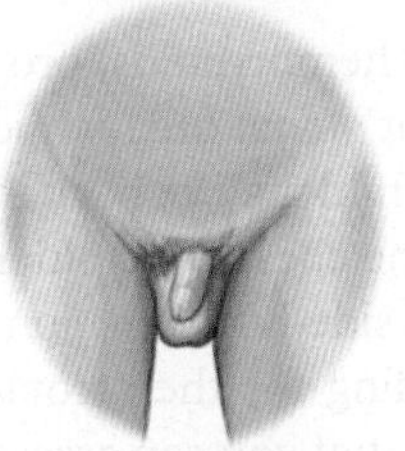

2) Few straight hairs at base of penis, little or no penis enlargement, testes/scrotum begin to enlarge

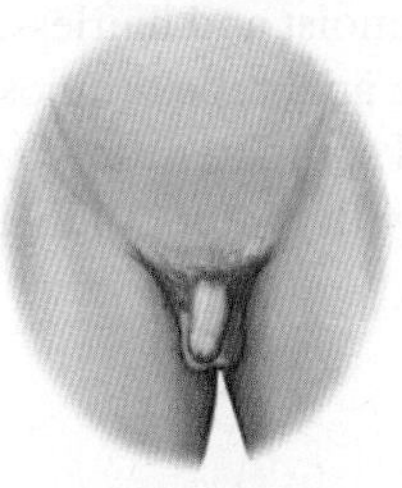

3) Sparse pubic hair growth over entire pubis, penis begins to lengthen, scrotum continues to enlarge

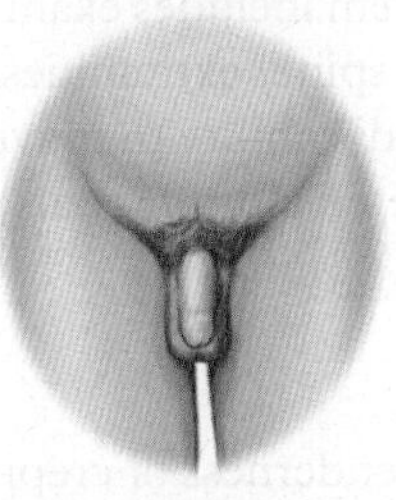

4) Thick pubic hair growth but not on thighs, penis grows in length and diameter, testes almost full grown

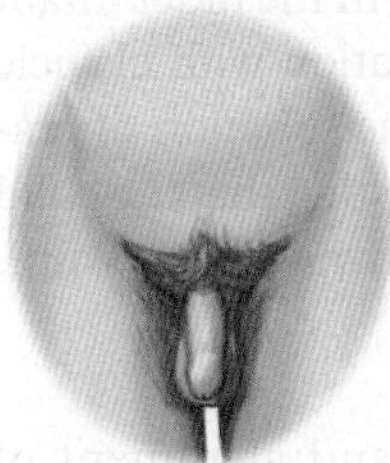

5) Pubic hair growth spread over medial thighs, penis and scrotum are adult size and shape

● **Figure 10.32** Tanner male sexual maturity rating for genitalia and pubic hair.

Female

In most cases, the female genitalia examination is limited to assessment of the external genitalia. Internal examination

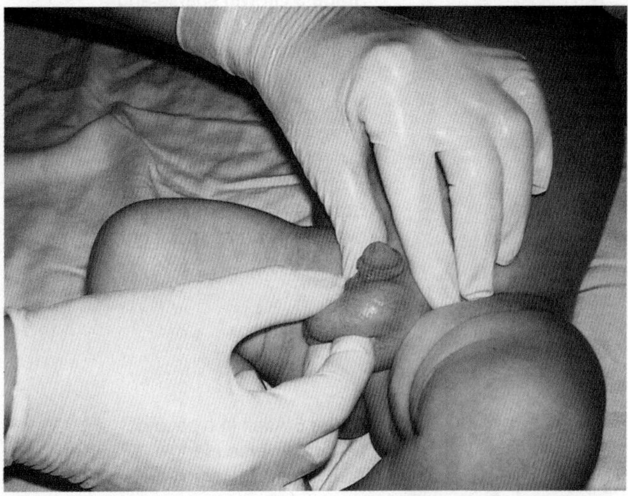

● **Figure 10.33** Placing a digit over the inguinal canal during testicular palpation prevents retraction of the testis into the canal.

is not routinely performed before maturity unless the adolescent anticipates becoming or is sexually active or requests birth control or if pathology is suspected. If an internal examination is needed, refer the child or adolescent to the appropriate advanced practitioner or physician.

Position the infant in the parent's lap or on the examination table or crib. The toddler or preschooler should be examined in the parent's lap, in a frog-legged position. The school-age or adolescent girl should lie on the examination table or bed. Provide for privacy by keeping the genital area covered until it is time for the examination.

Perform the assessment of the external genitalia in a systematic fashion. First, determine the presence and distribution of pubic hair. Infants and young girls (particular those of dark-skinned races) may have a small amount of downy pubic hair. Otherwise, the appearance of pubic hair indicates the onset of pubertal changes, sometimes prior to breast changes. Pubic hair generally begins to appear by age 11 years, with age 13 being the latest. Figure 10.34 illustrates the development of pubic hair through puberty in girls.

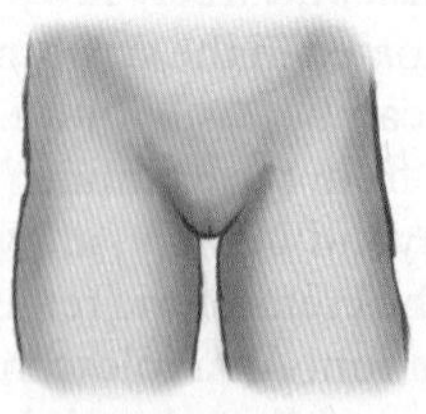

Stage 1 Preadolescents.
No pubic hair. Mons and labia covered with fine vellus hair as on abdomen.

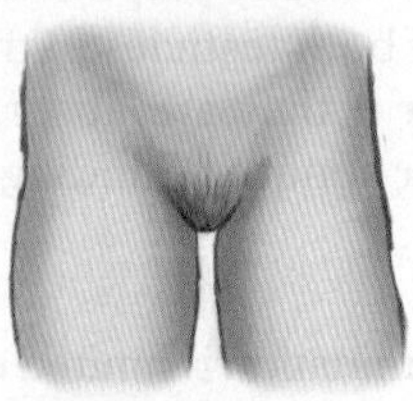

Stage 2 Growth sparse and mostly on labia. Long, downy hair, slightly pigmented, straight or only slightly curly.

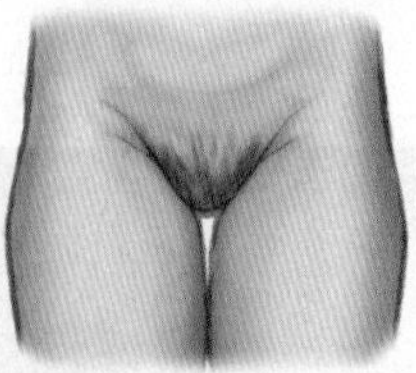

Stage 3 Growth sparse and spreading over mons pubis. Hair darker, coarser, curlier.

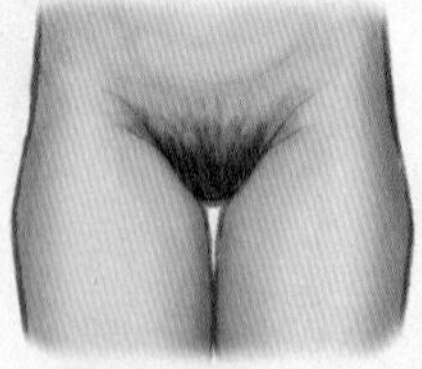

Stage 4 Hair is adult in type but over smaller area; none on medial thigh.

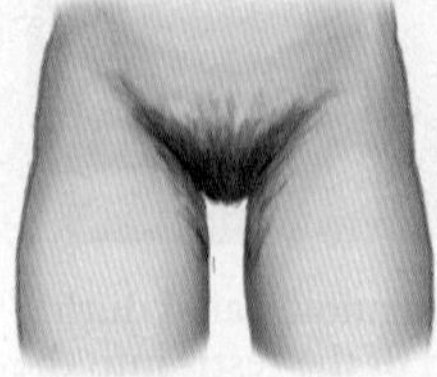

Stage 5 Adult in type and pattern; inverse triangle.
Also on medial thigh surface.

● Figure 10.34 Tanner female sexual maturity rating for pubic hair.

Inspect the labia majora and minora for size, color, and skin integrity. The newborn's labia minora are swollen from the effects of maternal estrogen but will decrease in size and be hidden by the labia majora within the first weeks of life. Redness or swelling of the labia may occur with infection, sexual abuse, or masturbation. Lesions on the external genitalia may indicate sexually transmitted infection. Gently spread the labia to inspect the clitoris, urethral meatus, and vaginal opening. Some girls may prefer to spread the labia themselves. The urinary meatus and vaginal orifice should be visible and not occluded by the hymen. It is not uncommon to see a hymenal tag. Note clitoral size. Inspect the urinary meatus and vaginal opening for edema or redness, which should not be present. Observe for any vaginal discharge. A small amount of blood-tinged or mucoid discharge may be noted in the first few weeks of life as a result of maternal hormone exposure. A small amount of clear mucus-like discharge is normal in all females. If present, document labial adhesion or other abnormal findings.

Anus

Inspect the anal area for fissures, rash, hemorrhoids, prolapse, or skin tags. Examine the infant's anal area while examining the genitalia. The younger child may lie back in the parent's lap and flex the knees to the chest. The older child or adolescent may be prone or in a side-lying position. If the adolescent boy is already standing for the scrotal assessment, have him bend forward so that you can assess the anal area. The anus should appear moist and hairless. Gently stroke the anal area to elicit the anal reflex (quick contraction). If indicated, inspect anal sphincter tone by inserting a gloved finger lubricated with water-soluble jelly just inside the anal sphincter.

Musculoskeletal

Assessment of the musculoskeletal system includes examination of the clavicles and shoulders, spine, extremities, joints, and hips. Determining the child's ability to move all extremities through the full range of motion is also important.

Clavicles and Shoulders

Palpate the clavicles. In the newborn, tenderness or crepitus reveals a fracture sustained at birth. In the older infant or child, a bump indicates callus formation with clavicle fracture. Test shoulder strength and the function of cranial nerve XI in the older child by requesting that the child shrug the shoulders while you apply downward pressure.

Spine

Observe the child's resting posture and alignment of the trunk. The newborn's position will look like the position the baby preferred *in utero* and is one of general flexion. The older infant moves more and can sit unassisted in the second half of the first year. Toddlers stand with a wide-based gait, a slightly swayed back, and the abdomen slightly protruding. The posture straightens in the preschool and school-age years. Adolescents often demonstrate kyphosis as the skeleton and muscles are both growing rapidly (Fig. 10.35).

Inspect the child's spine. The newborn's spine has a single C-shaped curve and remains rounded for the first 3 months of life. The cervical curve begins to develop around 3 to 4 months of age as the baby gains head control. By 12 to 18 months of age, the lumbar curve develops, which corresponds to the onset of walking. The S-shaped spine in older children and adolescents is similar to that of the adult's. The spine should be flexible, with good muscle tone and no rigidity. Assess the back, and hip and shoulder heights for symmetry.

Examine the preadolescent and adolescent for the development of scoliosis. Refer to Chapter 24 for information about scoliosis screening. Scoliosis screening is generally performed during well-child examinations by the physician or nurse practitioner or by the middle or high school nurse on a particular day of the school year.

Note mobility of the vertebral column by having the child bend forward and side to side. Flex the neck and move it from side to side. No resistance or pain should occur. Inspect the back for discoloration, tufts of hair, or dimples. A normal pilonidal dimple is sometimes seen at the base of the spine, but there should be no tuft of hair or nevi along the spine. Document and report abnormal findings.

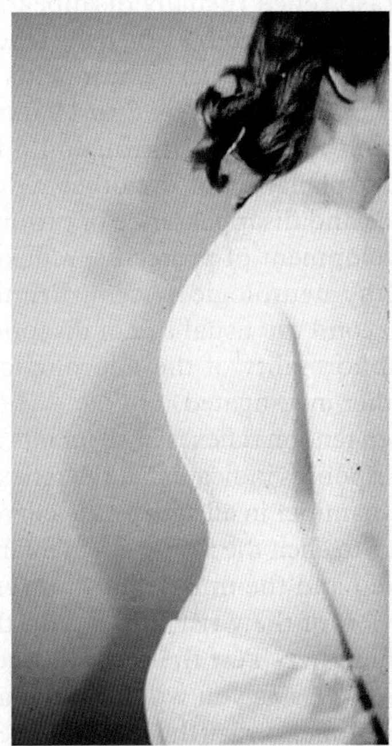

● **Figure 10.35** The teen's posture often demonstrates kyphosis.

Extremities

All children, even newborns, should be able to move all extremities spontaneously. Screen the infant younger than 6 months of age for developmental dysplasia of the hip by performing the Ortolani and Barlow maneuvers (refer to Chapter 24 for additional information). These maneuvers are usually best performed by a proficient examiner. Inspect and palpate the child's upper and lower extremities. Assess for symmetry in size, contour, movement, warmth, and color of the extremities. The infant's feet and legs appear bowed secondary to *in utero* positioning but can be straightened through passive range of motion. Observe the child in a standing position. Bowing of the lower legs (internal tibial torsion) lessens as the toddler begins to bear weight and usually resolves in the second or third year of life as the strength of the muscles and bones increases. When it persists past that time, it is termed genu varum (bow legs). Genu valgum (knock knee) is usually present until the child is 7 years old. Observe the child walking, noting any difficulty with leg position or balance. If the child is reluctant to walk, use play as a way to elicit the behavior. The school-age child should have gait and leg appearance similar to that of the adult.

Note the normal flat foot in the toddler and young child. The arch develops as the child grows and the muscles become less lax, though some children may continue with flexible flat feet; this is considered a normal variation.

Perform passive range of motion of the young infant's extremities. Inability to straighten the foot to midline may indicate clubfoot. Count the fingers and toes, noting abnormalities such as polydactyly (increased number of digits) or syndactyly (webbing of the digits). Palpate the joints for warmth or tenderness. Check the mobility of the joints of the upper and lower extremities by performing range of motion. Determine lower extremity muscle strength by having the child push against the examiner's hands with the soles of the forefoot. Assess upper extremity strength by having the child squeeze the examiner's crossed fingers and/or push up or down against the examiner's outstretched hands.

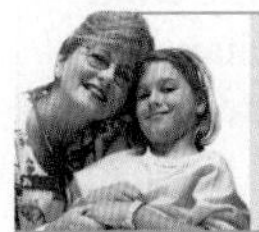

Slight tremors may be noticed in the infant's extremities in the first month of life.

Neurologic

The neurologic examination should include level of consciousness, balance and coordination, sensory function, and reflexes. Motor function is assessed within the musculoskeletal section. Cranial nerve function is generally tested within other portions of the physical assessment as it applies to that section.

Level of Consciousness

Note the state of alertness and attentiveness to parents and the environment in the newborn and infant. Older infants become interactive with other people, as do toddlers and preschoolers. Younger children demonstrate orientation by positive interaction with family members and by crying or fussing when they feel threatened. By school age, the child should be oriented to name and place and a few years later should be able to state the date as well (even if only the day of the week).

Balance and Coordination

Balance and coordination are controlled by the cerebellum. Observe the child's gait to assess balance and coordination. Observe toddlers and older children rising and walking from a seated and supine position. They should be able to stand and balance without straining or holding on to objects. Continue to test cerebellar function by having the younger child skip or hop and requesting that the older child or adolescent walk heel to toe. Further tests of cerebellar function responsible for balance and coordination are discussed in Box 10.3. Demonstrate each test and make sure the child understands your instructions.

BOX 10.3

CEREBELLAR FUNCTION TESTING

- **Romberg:** Ask the school-age or older child to stand still with eyes closed and arms down by the sides. Observe the child for leaning (stand close in case this does occur). This is considered a positive Romberg test, indicating cerebellar dysfunction.

For the following tests, the child should demonstrate accuracy and smoothness:

- **Heel-to-shin:** Have the child lie in a supine position, place one heel on the opposite knee, and run it down the shin.
- **Rapid alternating movements:** The child pats the thighs with the hands, lifts them, turns them over, pats the thighs with the back of the hands, and repeats the process multiple times. An alternate test is for the child to touch the thumb to each finger of the same hand starting at the index finger, then reverse the direction and repeat.
- **Finger-to-finger:** The child's eyes are open. The child touches the examiner's outstretched finger with the index finger, then touches his or her own nose. The examiner moves the finger to a different spot and the child repeats this process several times.
- **Finger-to-nose:** The child's eyes are closed. The child stretches the arm with the index finger extended, then touches his or her nose with that finger, keeping the eyes closed.

Sensory Testing

Portions of sensory testing related to most of the cranial nerves, vision, hearing, taste, and smell have already been incorporated into other sections as appropriate within the physical assessment. Test cranial nerve V (trigeminal) by lightly touching the child's cheek with a cotton ball. The young infant will root toward the side that is touched. With the child's eyes closed, ask the child to identify other locations where he or she is lightly touched (several different ones) to assess sensation. Ask the child to tell you when he or she is touched. Make a game of this activity to encourage cooperation in younger children. In the older child who knows the definition of sharp and dull, test for these sensations with the child's eyes closed. Use the rounded end of a tongue blade for dull and the broken edge of a tongue blade for the sharp sensation. The child should be able to discriminate the sensations of sharp and dull.

Reflexes

Assess the infant's primitive and protective reflexes. The primitive reflexes involve a whole-body response and are subcortical in nature. Selected primitive reflexes present at birth include Moro, root, suck, asymmetric tonic neck, plantar and palmar grasp, step, and Babinski. Most of the primitive reflexes diminish over the first few months of life, giving way to protective or postural reflexes. Protective reflexes are motor responses related to maintenance of equilibrium. They are necessary for appropriate motor development and remain throughout life once they are established. The protective reflexes include the righting and parachute reactions.

Place one finger in each of the infant's hands to elicit the palmar grasp reflex (usually disappears by age 3 to 4 months). Touch the thumb to the ball of the infant's foot to elicit the plantar grasp reflex. The infant's toes will curl down (this reflex disappears by 8 to 10 months). Refer to Table 4.2 and Figures 4.1 through 4.6 in Chapter 4 for additional explanation of the other reflexes. Appropriate presence and disappearance of primitive reflexes, as well as development of protective reflexes, is indicative of a healthy neurologic system. Primitive reflexes that persist beyond the usual age of disappearance may indicate an abnormality of the neurologic system and should be further investigated.

Assess deep tendon reflexes in all infants and children. Appropriate responses indicate that the reflex arc is intact. Use the reflex hammer in all ages or the curved tips of the two first fingers to elicit the responses in infants. The limb must be relaxed and the muscle partly stretched. Use a snapping motion of the wrist to tap with the fingertips or the reflex hammer. Test the biceps, triceps, patellar, and Achilles reflexes as you would in the adult. It may help to place a finger under the infant's knee to encourage relaxation. Young children who tense up when their reflexes are being tested may relax the area if you have them focus on another area, so have the child clasp the hands while testing the Achilles and patellar reflexes. As the child focuses on the hands, the lower extremities relax. Distraction may also be helpful.

Grade the strength of the response using the standard scale from 0 to 4+:

- 0: no response
- 1+: diminished or sluggish
- 2+: average
- 3+: brisker than average
- 4+: very brisk, may involve clonus

The newborn's deep tendon reflexes are normally brisk (3+). They decrease to average (2+), usually by 4 months of age. Healthy children should have reflexes of 2+ if the reflex has been elicited properly. Absent, sluggish, or hyperreactive responses usually indicate disease.

> Refer back to Elliot, the 3-year-old from the beginning of the chapter. What are some important considerations when performing his physical examination?

References

Books and Journals

American Academy of Pediatrics. (2000). Clinical practice guideline: Early detection of developmental dysplasia of the hip (AC0001). *Pediatrics, 105*(4), 896–905.

Anonymous. (n.d.). Points on the pediatric physical exam. Columbia University College of Physicians and Surgeons, Pediatric Clerkship. Available at http://www.columbia.edu/itc/hs/medical/clerkships/peds/Student_Information/Reference_Materials/Pediatric_PE.html#PhysicalExam.

Anonymous. (2002). Pulse oximetry: Update 2002. *Critical Care Nurse, 22*(3), 74–76.

Applebaum, E. L. (1999). Detection of hearing loss in children. *Pediatric Annals, 28*, 352–356.

Barnes, K. (2004). *Paediatrics: A clinical guide for nurse practitioners.* New York: Elsevier.

Barton, S. J., Gaffney, R., Chase, T., Rayens, M. K., & Piyabanditkul, L. (2003). Pediatric temperature measurement and child/parent/nurse preference using three temperature measurement instruments. *Journal of Pediatric Nursing, 18*(1), 314–320.

Benjamin, J. T. (2004). *The continuity clinic notebook: An unfinished story (Department of Pediatrics, Medical College of Georgia).* Retrieved April 20, 2006, from http://www.mcg.edu/pediatrics/CCNotebook/index.htm.

Bergeson, P. S., & Shaw, J. C. (2001). Are infants really obligatory nasal breathers? *Clinical Pediatrics, 40*, 567–569.

Burns, C., Dunn, A., Brady, M., Starr, N., & Blosser, C. (2004). *Pediatric primary care: A handbook for nurse practitioners.* Philadelphia: W. B. Saunders.

Callanan, D. (2003). Detecting fever in young infants: Reliability of perceived, pacifier, and temporal artery temperatures in infants younger than 3 months of age. *Pediatric Emergency Care, 19*(4), 240–243.

Centers for Disease Control and Prevention. (2003). *Using the BMI-for-age growth charts.* Retrieved April 15, 2004, from http://www.cdc.gov/nccdphp/dnpa/growthcharts/training/modules/module1/text/module1print.pdf.

Centers for Disease Control and Prevention. (2004). *CDC growth charts: United States.* Retrieved April 15, 2004, from http://www.cdc.gov/nchs/about/major/nhanes/growthcharts/background.htm.

Centers for Disease Control and Prevention. (2004). *Clinical growth charts.* Retrieved April 15, 2004, from http://www.cdc.gov/nchs/about/major/nhanes/growthcharts/clinical_charts.htm.

El Radhi, A. S., & Barry, W. (2006). Thermometry in paediatric practice. *Archives of Disease in Childhood, 91*, 351–356.

El Radhi, A. S., & Patel, S. (2006). An evaluation of tympanic thermometry in a paediatric emergency department. *Emergency Medicine Journal, 23*(1), 40–41.

Engel, J. K. (2006). *Mosby's pocket guide to pediatric assessment* (5th ed.). St. Louis: Elsevier.

Erickson, B. A. (2003). *Heart sounds and murmurs across the lifespan, with audiotape* (4th ed.). St. Louis: Elsevier.

Exergen Corporation. (2005). Temporal artery thermometer consumer information center. Available at http://www.exergen.com/medical/TAT/tatconsumerpage.htm.

Grap, M. J. (2002). Pulse oximetry. *Critical Care Nurse, 22*(3), 69–74.

Hebbar, K., Fortenberry, J. D., Merritt, R., & Easley, K. (2005). Comparison of temporal artery thermometer to standard temperature measurements in pediatric intensive care unit patients. *Pediatric Critical Care Medicine, 6*(5), 557–561.

Houlder, L. C. (2000). Evidence-based practice: The accuracy and reliability of tympanic thermometry compared to rectal and axillary sites in young children. *Pediatric Nursing, 26*(3), 311–314.

Jarvis, C. (2004). *Physical examination and health assessment* (4th ed.). St. Louis: Saunders.

Jones, H. L., Kleber, C. B., Eckert, G. J., & Mahon, B. E. (2003). Comparison of rectal temperature measured by digital vs. mercury glass thermometer in infants under two months old. *Clinical Pediatrics, 42*(4), 357–359.

Kay, J. D., et al. (2001). Pediatric hypertension. *American Heart Journal, 142*(3), 422–432.

Kiernan, B. (2001). Ask the expert, taking a temperature: Which way is best? *Journal of the Society of Pediatric Nurses, 6*, 192–195.

Killeen, P. (2002). Practical evaluation of pediatric heart murmurs. *Journal of the American Academy of Physician Assistants, 3*, 24–39.

Lanham, D., Walker, B., Klocke, E., & Jennings, M. (1999). Accuracy of tympanic temperature readings in children under 6 years of age. *Pediatric Nursing, 25*(1), 39–42.

Mandleco, B. (2004). *Growth and development handbook: Newborn through adolescence.* Clifton Park, NY: Delmar Learning.

Mandleco, B. (2005). *Pediatric nursing skills and procedures.* Clifton Park, NY: Thomson Delmar.

Mansson, M. E., & Dykes, A. K. (2004). Practices for preparing children for clinical examinations and procedures in Swedish pediatric wards. *Pediatric Nursing, 30*(3), 182–187, 229.

Manworren, R., & Hynan, L. (2003). Clinical validation of FLACC: Preverbal patient pain scale. *Pediatric Nursing, 29*(2), 140–146.

Mau, M. K., Yamasato, K. S., & Yamamoto, L. G. (2005). Normal oxygen saturation values in pediatric patients. *Hawaii Medical Journal, 64*(2), 42, 44–45.

McCaffery, M. (2002). Choosing a faces pain scale. *Nursing '02, 32*(5), 68.

Merkel, S., Voepel-Lewis, T., & Malviya, S. (2002). Pain assessment in infants and young children: The FLACC scale. *American Journal of Nursing, 102*(10), 55–57.

Miller, S. (n.d.). *Introduction to the pediatric physical exam (video).* Columbia University College of Physicians and Surgeons, Pediatric Clerkship. Available at http://www.columbia.edu/itc/hs/medical/clerkships/peds/Student_Information/Reference_Materials/Pediatric_PE.html.

Mintegi, R. S., Gonzalez, B. M., Perez, F. A., Pijoan, Z. J. I., Capape, Z. S., & Benito, F. J. (2005). Infants aged 3–24 months with fever without source in the emergency room: Characteristics, management and outcome. *Annals of Pediatrics, 62*(6), 522–528.

Musumba, C. O., Griffiths, K. L., Ross, A., & Newton, C. R. J. C. (2005). Comparison of axillary, rectal and tympanic temperature measurements in children admitted with malaria. *Journal of Tropical Pediatrics, 51*(4), 242–244.

Nellcor Puritan Bennett, Inc. (2006). *Clinician's guide to Nellcor sensors.* Retrieved 5/1/06 from http://www.nellcor.com/_Catalog/PDF/Product/CliniciansSensorGuide.pdf.

Nimah, M. M., Bshesh, K., Callahan, J. D., & Jacobs, B. R. (2006). Infrared tympanic thermometry in comparison with other temperature measurement techniques in febrile children. *Pediatric Critical Care Medicine, 7*(1), 48–55.

Popovich, D. M., Richiuso, N., & Gale, D. (2004). Pediatric health care providers' knowledge of pulse oximetry. *Pediatric Nursing, 30*(1), 14–20.

Powell, K. R., Smith, K., & Eberly, S. W. (2001). Ear temperature measurements in healthy children using the arterial heat balance method. *Clinical Pediatrics, 40,* 333–336.

Rahi, J. S., & Dezateux, C. (2002). Improving the detection of childhood visual problems and eye disorders. *Lancet, 359,* 1083–1084.

Rideout, M. E., & First, L. R. (2001). Fever: Measuring and managing a sizzling symptom. *Contemporary Pediatrics.* [electronic version]. Available at www.contemporarypediatrics.com.

Roberts, S., & Dallal, G. (2001). The new childhood growth charts. *Nutrition Reviews 59*(2), 31–36.

Rosner, B., Prineas, R., Loggie, J., & Daniels S. R. (1998). Percentiles for body mass index in U.S. children 5 to 17 years of age. *Journal of Pediatrics, 132*(2), 211–222.

Roy, S., Powell, K., & Gerson, L. W. (2003). Temporal artery temperature measurements in healthy infants, children and adolescents. *Clinical Pediatrics, 42*(5), 433–437.

Rubin, S. E. (2001). Management of strabismus in the first year of life. *Pediatric Annals, 30,* 474–480.

Sandlin, D. (2003). New product review: Temporal artery thermometry. *Journal of Perianesthesia Nursing, 18*(6), 419–421.

Sganga, A., et al. (2000). A comparison of four methods of normal newborn temperature measurements. *MCN, 25*(2), 76–79.

Siberry, G. K., Diener-West, M., Schappell, E., & Karron, R. A. (2005). Comparison of temple temperatures with rectal temperatures in children under two years of age. *Clinical Pediatrics, 41*(6), 405–414.

Takayama, J. I., Teng, W., Uyemoto, J., Newman, T. B., & Pantell, R. H. (2000). Body temperature of newborns: What is normal? *Clinical Pediatrics, 39*(9), 503–510.

Tanner, J. M. (1962). *Growth at adolescence.* Oxford, England: Blackwell Scientific Publications.

U.S. Department of Health and Human Services, National Institutes of Health, National Heart, Lung, and Blood Institute. (2005). *The fourth report on the diagnosis, evaluation, and treatment of high blood pressure in children and adolescents* (NIH Publication No. 05-5267). Washington, D.C.: U.S. Department of Health and Human Services.

U.S. Department of Health and Human Services, Substance Abuse and Mental Health Services Administration. (2006). Fetal alcohol spectrum disorder (FASD): The basics. Retrieved March 17, 2006, from http://fascenter.samhsa.gov/educationTraining/fasdBasics.cfm.

Weber, J., & Kelley, J. (2003). *Health assessment in nursing* (2nd ed.). Philadelphia: Lippincott Williams & Wilkins.

Willis, M., Merkel, S., Voepel-Lewis, T., & Malviya, S. (2003). FLACC behavioral pain assessment scale: A comparison with the child's self-report. *Pediatric Nursing, 29*(3), 95–198.

Winch, A. E. (2002). Ask the expert: Obtaining accurate growth measurements in children. *Journal for Specialists in Pediatric Nursing, 7*(4), 166–169.

Wong, D., & Baker, C. (1988). Pain in children: Comparison of assessment scales. *Pediatric Nursing, 14,* 9–17.

Websites

brightfutures.aap.org/web American Academy of Pediatrics, Bright Futures

kidshealth.org/kid Kids' Health for Kids—Nemours Foundation

mchb.hrsa.gov Maternal and Child Health Bureau

www.ahrq.gov/child Agency for Healthcare Research and Quality, Child and Adolescent Health

www.brightfutures.org Bright Futures at Georgetown University

www.cdc.gov/nchs/about/major/nhanes/growthcharts/clinical_charts.htm Centers for Disease Control clinical growth charts

www.childtrendsdatabank.org/indicators/93WellChildVisits.cfm Child Trends Data Bank

www.fda.gov/oc/opacom/kids/default.htm U.S. Food and Drug Administration's Kids' Home Page

www.healthypeople.gov *Healthy People 2010*

www.hhs.gov/kids HHS for Kids (U.S. Department of Health and Human Services)

www.napnap.org National Association of Pediatric Nurse Practitioners

www.pedsnurses.org Society of Pediatric Nurses

Chapter WORKSHEET

MULTIPLE CHOICE QUESTIONS

1. A 5-year-old boy visits the physician's office with an upper respiratory infection. Which approach would give the nurse the most information about the child's developmental level?
   a. Playing a game with the child
   b. Talking with the child about the teddy bear next to him
   c. Using a screening tool during a follow-up office visit
   d. Asking the 10-year-old sibling about the child
2. Which statement indicates the best sequence for the nurse to conduct an assessment in a non-emergency situation?
   a. Introduce yourself, ask about any problems, take a history, do the physical examination.
   b. Perform the physical examination and then ask the family if there are any problems in the child's life.
   c. Do the physical examination while at the same time asking about the child's previous illnesses; then talk about the family's concerns.
   d. Get a complete history of the family's health beliefs and practices, then assess the child.
3. What approach by the nurse would most likely encourage a child to cooperate with an assessment of physical and developmental health?
   a. Explain to the child what's going to happen when the child asks questions.
   b. Explain what is going to happen in words the child can understand.
   c. Force them to cooperate by having a parent hold them down.
   d. Give the child a sticker before beginning the examination.
4. A sleeping 5-month-old girl is being held by the mother when the nurse comes in to do a physical examination. What assessment should be done initially?
   a. Listening to the bowel sounds
   b. Counting the heart rate
   c. Checking the temperature
   d. Looking in the ears
5. Which assessment finding is considered normal in children?
   a. Irregular respiratory rate and rhythm
   b. Split S2 and sinus arrhythmia
   c. Decreased heart rate with crying
   d. Genu varum past the age of 5 years

CRITICAL THINKING EXERCISES

1. A soft and muffled heart murmur is heard in a 4-year-old patient. The mother states that she has never heard that the child has a murmur. What should the nurse do?
2. A nurse is helping a new mother breastfeed her 4-day-old baby. The mother notices that the baby has a bluish cast to the skin on his hands and that sometimes they have a tremor. She asks the nurse if the baby is cold, though the baby is swaddled and comfortably resting against the mother's skin. How might the nurse help teach this mother?
3. Devise a plan for encouraging cooperation of the toddler or preschooler during various parts of the physical examination.

STUDY ACTIVITIES

1. In the clinical setting, obtain a health history on an infant, child, or adolescent.
2. In the clinical setting, compare the approach you use for the physical examination of a toddler versus a school-aged child or adolescent.
3. No matter how thoughtfully and appropriately you plan your assessment, odds are good that you will have difficulty assessing a 2-year-old. Discuss with your classmates the strategies that you have used for success and brainstorm with them about their ideas for assessing a crying or resistant young child.

chapter 11

Nursing Care of Children During Illness and Hospitalization

Key TERMS

child life specialist
denial
magical thinking
regression
sensory deprivation
sensory overload
separation anxiety
therapeutic hugging
therapeutic play

Learning OBJECTIVES

Upon completion of the chapter, the learner will be able to:

1. Identify the major impact and stressors of illness and hospitalization for children in the various developmental stages.
2. Identify the reactions and responses of children and their families during illness and hospitalization.
3. Explain the factors that influence the reactions and responses of children and their families during illness and hospitalization
4. Describe the nursing care that minimizes the stressors of children who are ill or hospitalized.
5. Examine the major components of admission for children to the hospital.
6. Outline the nursing interventions required for children in the specific units or situations in the hospital.
7. Use appropriate safety measures when caring for children of all ages.
8. Describe basic care procedures for children in various health care settings.
9. Review the major components and nursing responsibilities related to patient education and discharge from the hospital.

Sick children need love, hope, faith, and most of all a positive attitude from their nurse.

Jake Jorgenson, 8 years old, was brought to the clinic with a history of headaches, vomiting not related to feeding, and changes in his gait. Initial testing leads to a suspected brain tumor. Jake is to be admitted to the neurologic service at a pediatric hospital for further testing and treatment. Up until this point he has been a healthy child with no previous hospitalizations. He lives at home with his parents and two siblings, Jenny, age 11 and Joshua, age 5. As a nurse on this unit, think of ways you can help prepare Jake and his family for this hospitalization.

Illness, with the occasional consequence of hospitalization, affects children and their families in a variety of ways. Hospitalization is often confusing, complex, and overwhelming for children and their families. Reactions and responses to illness and hospitalization depend on a number of factors, including the unique characteristics and common situations associated with each developmental stage. The result requires nursing strategies that prepare children and their families for this experience while at the same time minimizing negative effects. These strategies include identifying the needs of children and families through astute assessment of nonverbal and verbal behaviors, then validating the information with accurate interpretation and providing appropriate responses and interventions.

Although the nurse implements these strategies throughout the interaction with the child and family, a critical time to ensure the best outcome for the child and family occurs during the admission process. A crucial aspect of these strategies and interventions involves assessing the learning needs and abilities of the child and family. For the interventions to be successful, the nurse must communicate and teach in the most effective method for the individual child and family. The nurse also evaluates the child's and family's competence in performing specific activities prior to discharge.

Hospitalization in Childhood

In today's health care environment, children receive much of their care for illnesses in community health settings such as physician's offices, urgent care settings, or day surgery centers. As a result of this trend, fewer children may actually be admitted to a hospital unit. The children who are hospitalized are generally acutely ill. In addition, hospital stays are often shorter due to economic trends in the health care environment, such as the delivery system of managed care and other factors that attempt to control the escalating cost of health care. Various situations such as acute conditions, trauma, or chronic diseases or illnesses requiring surgical intervention lead to hospitalization for children. According to the Agency for Healthcare Research and Quality (AHRQ, 2000), infections and birth-related problems account for the majority of hospitalizations in children younger than 5 years old, while asthma, injuries, and mental health problems lead to more hospitalizations of older children. Adolescents between 15 and 17 years of age are often hospitalized because of problems related to pregnancy and childbearing (AHRQ, 2000).

Other health problems begin before birth or immediately following birth, such as congenital heart disease or gastrointestinal atresia. Before getting used to the idea of having a new child, the family must now deal with illness and possible extended hospitalizations. Specific genetic or environmental factors also predispose the child to disease and injury, such as the genetic disorder of hemophilia or the environmental factor of homelessness. Many of these factors or situations put the child and family at greater risk for chronic health conditions and long periods of illness, hospitalization, and even death.

Stressors of Hospitalization

In general, children are more vulnerable to the impacts of illness and hospitalization because this is a change from their usual state of health and their routine. They also have limited understanding and coping mechanisms to assist them in relieving the stressors that might occur during this time. As Bricher (2000) states, "Children admitted to the hospital are vulnerable because of their illness, their limitation of understanding, and because they have so little control over what is happening to them." Hospitalization creates a series of traumatic and stressful events that produce uncertainty for all children and their families, whether the hospital stay involves an elective procedure that is planned in advance or is an emergency situation. Specific factors will affect the overall hospital experience as well as the responses and reactions of children and their families.

Besides the physiologic effects of the health problem, the impact of illness and hospitalization on a child include anxiety and fear related to the overall process and the potential for bodily injury and pain. In addition, children are separated from their homes, families, friends, and what is familiar to them, which may result in **separation anxiety** (distress related to removal from family and familiar surroundings). There is a general loss of control over their lives and sometimes their emotions and behaviors. The result may be anger, guilt, **regression** (return to a previous stage of development), acting out, and other types of defense mechanisms to cope with these effects. Children's typical coping strategies are tested during this experience.

Fear and Anxiety

For many children hospitalization is like entering a foreign world, and the result is fear and anxiety. Often anxiety stems from the rapid onset of the illness or injury, particularly when the child has limited experiences with disease or injury. The child hears unfamiliar words and noises, smells unfamiliar odors and eats unfamiliar food, and sees ominous-looking equipment and strangers in unusual attire like surgical caps, masks, or gowns. He or she may hear other children crying. All of these things make hospitalization a difficult experience for children.

Normal fears of childhood include the fear of separation, loss of control, and bodily injury, mutilation, or harm, and all of these are particularly relevant during a hospital stay. Children's fears are similar to adult fears of the unknown, including fear of unfamiliar environments and losing control. Children may be exposed to equipment, people, situations, and procedures that may be new to them and cause them pain (Fig. 11.1). In addition, children of various developmental stages have specific reactions. For example, preschool children have an egocentric view of the environment and events that happen to them and participate in magical, fantasy-type thoughts, both of which may lead to additional fears. Although children are increasingly able to adapt as they grow older, lack of understanding about the need for hospitalization can make such adaptation difficult. Moreover, being hospitalized threatens the sense of control that children are striving for as they develop (Romino et al., 2005).

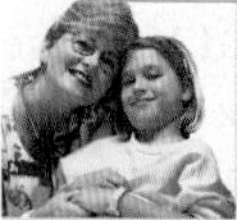

Wollin et al. (2004) interviewed 120 children between the ages of 5 and 12 and their parents to determine preoperative anxiety and fear. Needles, postoperative pain, the unknown, and the presence of many unrecognizable people in the room increased anxiety for children.

Separation Anxiety

Separation anxiety is a major stressor for children of certain ages. It occurs most commonly in children from middle infancy throughout the preschool years, with the peak incidence between the ages of 6 and 30 months. Separation anxiety consists of three stages during which the child exhibits certain behavioral reactions to the stress of the separation. The first phase, protest, occurs when the child is separated from his or her parents or primary caretaker. This phase may last from a few hours to several days. The child reacts aggressively to this separation and exhibits great distress by crying, expressing agitation, and rejecting others who attempt to offer comfort. The child may also exhibit anger and inconsolable grief.

If the parents do not return within a short time, the child exhibits the second phase, despair. The child displays hopelessness by withdrawing from others, becoming quiet without crying, exhibiting apathy, depression, disinterest in play and food, and overall feelings of sadness. Today, health care providers primarily observe the first and second stages because of the shorter hospital stays and the more common use of a family-centered approach to care.

Detachment (also known as **denial**) is the third and final phase of separation anxiety. During this phase the child forms coping mechanisms to protect himself or herself from further emotional pain. This occurs more often during long-term separations. During this stage, the child shows interest in the environment, starts to play again, and forms superficial relationships with the nurses and other children. If the parents return, the child ignores them. A child in this phase of separation anxiety exhibits resignation, not contentment. It is more difficult to reverse this stage, and developmental delays may occur.

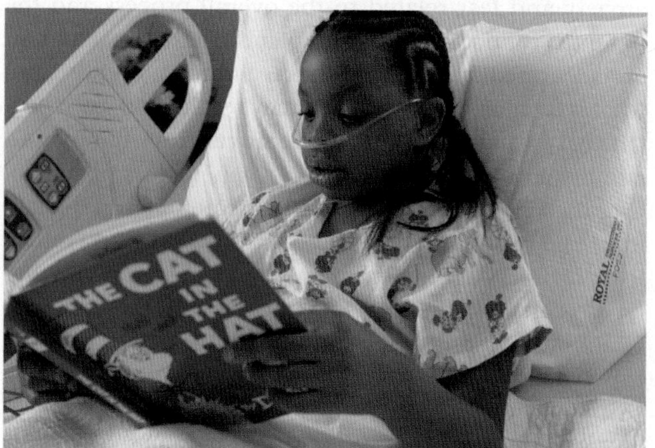

● Figure 11.1 The presence of familiar objects and home routines normalizes the environment and help the child cope with hospitalization. Reading a favorite bedtime story can be comforting.

Loss of Control

When hospitalized, children experience a significant loss of control. This loss of control increases the perception of threat and affects their coping skills. They lose control over routine self-care, their usual tasks, and play as well as decisions related to the care of their own bodies. In the hospital, the child's usual routine is disrupted. He or she cannot choose what to do and at what time. The child can no longer accomplish simple tasks independently as he or she does at home or school. Confinement to the bed or crib worsens this loss of control. For example, if connected to tubes or intravenous lines, the child may not even be able to visit the bathroom alone.

Hospitalization also affects the child's control over decisions related to his or her own body. Many of the procedures and treatments that occur in the hospital are invasive or at least disturbing to children, and much of the time they do not have the option to refuse to undergo them. Adults are presumed to be competent to make health care decisions, but generally children are not (Bricher, 2000). Though parents and nurses of hospitalized children have the children's best interest in mind, children often feel powerless when in the hospital, not having their feelings and wishes respected and having minimal control over events.

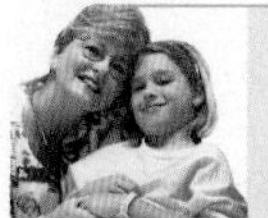

Always ask yourself, "Who speaks for the child?" If you do act as an advocate for a child, make sure you reflect the child's wishes, not what you think his or her wishes might or should be (Bricher, 2000).

Children's Responses to the Stressors of Hospitalization

The stressors that children experience during hospitalization may result in various reactions. Children react to the stresses of hospitalization before admission, during the hospital stay, and after discharge. Defense behaviors such as anger, guilt, regression, and acting out may occur. Many factors influence the amount and degree of reactions the child may experience, and these factors may increase or diminish the child's fears. Children's responses to the stressors of fear, separation anxiety, and loss of control will also vary depending on their age and developmental level. Children with chronic illnesses who have experienced multiple hospitalizations may have different reactions. Chapter 15 gives additional information about the child with a chronic illness.

Infants

Newborns and infants are adapting to life outside the womb with rapid growth and development and establishment of a healthy attachment to parents or primary caregivers. They are dependent on others for nurture and protection. They gain a sense of trust in the world through rhythmic and reciprocal patterns of contact and feeding, resulting in bonding to the primary caregiver. They need a secure pattern of restful sleep, satisfaction of oral and nutritional needs, relaxation of body systems, and spontaneous response to communication and gentle stimuli. The caregiver–infant attachment is critical for psychological health, especially during periods of illness and hospitalization.

Unfortunately, during illness and hospitalization, these critical patterns of feeding, contact, comfort, sleeping, elimination, and stimulation are disrupted, resulting in fear, separation anxiety, and loss of control. By 5 to 6 months of age, infants have developed an awareness of self as separate from mother. As a result, infants of this age are acutely aware of the absence of their primary caregiver and become fearful of unfamiliar persons (Bowlby, 1988). Infants may be separated from their parents when hospitalized if the parents cannot room in because of hospital policy or because the parents must work or care for other children. This results in separation anxiety.

The infant's oral needs, the basic source of infant satisfaction, are often not met in the hospital due to the condition of the child or the procedures that must be performed. The infant is accustomed to having his or her basic needs met by the parent when the infant cries or gestures. The constraints of hospitalization result in loss of control over the environment, leading to additional anxiety in the infant.

Toddlers

Toddlers are more aware of self and can communicate their desires. Because their autonomy is developing, toddlers need to master accomplishments to minimize the development of shame and doubt. Control becomes an issue for toddlers. Toddlers also need opportunities to explore, and they need consistent routines. In addition, toddlers are aware of the need for care and protection of others, so they need familiarity and closeness to the primary caregiver. When the toddler is hospitalized, disruption occurs in this development of autonomy.

Toddlers are often fearful of strangers and can recall traumatic events. Simply walking toward the treatment room where a traumatic procedure previously occurred may result in extreme upset in the toddler. Ordinarily a resurgence in separation anxiety occurs during the toddler years. When the toddler is separated from his or her parents or caregivers in an unfamiliar environment, then separation anxiety is compounded. In response to this anxiety, toddlers may demonstrate behaviors such as pleading with the parents to stay, physically trying to go after the parents, throwing temper tantrums, and refusing to comply with usual routines. Restrictions related to mobility and new skill acquisition result in loss of control. Disruption in usual routines also contributes to loss of control, and the toddler feels insecure. As a result, regression in toilet training and refusal to eat are common reactions in toddlers.

Preschoolers

The preschooler has better verbal and developmental skills to adapt to various situations, but illness and hospitalization can still be stressful. Preschoolers may understand that they are in the hospital because they are sick, but they may not understand the cause of their illness. Preschoolers fear mutilation and are afraid of intrusive procedures since they do not understand the body's integrity. They interpret words literally and have an active imagination. Therefore, when the nurse says, "I need to take some blood," preschoolers' fantasies may run wild. They may not understand the concept of blood and may think everything will come out of their body. They may think that blood is "taken" the same way a child picks up a toy to take it out of the room. Preschoolers' thinking is egocentric; they believe that some personal deed or thought caused their illness, which can lead to guilt and shame. These feelings may be internalized. Overall, preschoolers' concrete, egocentric, and **magical thinking** (type of thinking that allows for fantasies and creativity) limits their ability to understand, so communication and interventions must be on their level.

Separation anxiety may not be as much of an issue as it is in toddlers, since preschoolers may already be spending time away from their parents in preschool. They are, however, still acutely aware of the comfort and security that their family provides for them, so disruptions in these relationships lead to challenges. The preschooler may constantly ask for his or her parents or ask to call the parents. He or she may quietly cry, refuse to eat or take medication, or generally be uncooperative.

In addition, the hospitalized preschooler loses control over the environment. The preschooler is naturally curious about his or her surroundings and learns best by observing and working with objects. This might be limited during hospitalization. Because the preschooler cannot participate in usual activities and explore the environment as usual, the child's normal creative, curious nature may give rise to a variety of fantasies that may present challenges.

School-Age Child

School-age children generally are hospitalized because of long-term illnesses or trauma. The general task of their developmental stage, to develop confidence through a sense of industry, can be disrupted during hospitalization. Even at this time, they generally want to continue to learn and maintain their skills and abilities. The stress of illness or anxiety related to diagnostic tests and therapeutic interventions may lead to inward or outward expressions of distress. If they have learned various coping skills, this distress may be minimized. After 11 years of age there is an increased awareness of physiologic, psychological, and behavioral causes of illness and injury. Typically the school-age child has a more realistic understanding of the reasons for the illness and can better comprehend explanations. School-age children are concerned about disability and death and fear injury and pain. They want to know the reasons why procedures and tests are being performed. They can understand cause-and-effect and how it relates to their illness. They are uncomfortable with any type of sexual examination.

Separation anxiety is not as much of an issue for school-age children. They are accustomed to periods of separation and may already be experiencing some separation anxiety related to being in school. At the same time, they may be missing school and friends as they try to adjust to the unfamiliar environment. They may feel that friends will forget them if they remain in the hospital for a long time. Some school-age children may regress and become needy, demanding their parents' attention or playing with special "comfort toys" they used at a younger age.

Since school-age children are accustomed to controlling self-care and typically are highly social, they like being involved. They are accustomed to making choices about meals and activities and fill their days with activities. Hospitalization presents loss of control by limiting their activities, making them feel helpless and dependent. This may result in feelings of loneliness, boredom, isolation, and depression. The key is to give them opportunities to maintain independence, retain a sense of control, enhance self-esteem, and continue to work toward achieving a sense of industry.

Adolescents

Adolescents fear injury and pain. Since appearance is important to them, they are concerned with how the illness/injury will affect their body image. Anything that changes their perception of themselves has a major impact on their response. Typically, adolescents do not like to be different; they like "being cool," which means being in control and not showing how afraid they may really be. They also may feel ambivalent about wanting their parents to be present. Adolescents typically do not experience separation anxiety related to being away from their parents; instead, their anxiety comes from being separated from friends.

Finally, loss of control is a key factor affecting the behavior of adolescents who are hospitalized. Anger, withdrawal, or general lack of cooperation may occur due to the feelings of loss of control. In addition, their desire to appear confident may lead them to question everything that is being done or that they are asked to do. Their feelings of invincibility may cause them to take risks and be noncompliant with treatment. Overall, adolescents strive for independence, self-assertion, and liberation while developing their identity.

> **Remember Jake,** the 8-year-old with a suspected brain tumor? What responses to hospitalization might you see in him and his family?

Factors Affecting Children's Reaction to Hospitalization

Various factors have a great impact on the ability of children to handle illness and hospitalization, such as the amount of separation from the parents; the age, cognitive level, and developmental level of the child; and any previous experience with illness and hospitalization, which will familiarize the child with the routines and procedures of hospitals. Recent life stresses and changes may also reduce the child's coping abilities and increase his or her vulnerability to anxiety. The child's temperament and coping skills can contribute in a negative or positive way to his or her hospital experience. Finally, the parents' responses to the situation will shape the child's reactions. Because of all of these factors, each child will respond differently and will perceive the hospital experience differently. Box 11.1 lists the factors affecting the child's responses to hospitalization.

Separation from Parents or Primary Caregivers

A widely researched factor associated with children's reactions to hospitalization is the effect of separation from

BOX 11.1

FACTORS AFFECTING A CHILD'S RESPONSE TO ILLNESS AND HOSPITALIZATION

- Developmental age
- Cognitive level
- Previous experience with illness, separation, and hospitalization
- Type and amount of preparation given
- Innate and acquired coping skills
- Seriousness of the diagnosis/onset of illness or injury (e.g., acute or chronic)
- Support systems available, including the family and health professionals
- Cultural background
- Parents' reaction to illness and hospitalization

parents. Over 50 years ago, researchers such as John Bowlby and James Robertson studied the impact that hospitalization has on immediate and long-term emotional distress for the child. Subsequent research led to today's liberal visitation and rooming-in policies of hospitals. These ideas continue to be important components in the care of the ill child and family (Alsop-Shields & Mohay, 2001; Partis, 2000), but today's generally shorter stays in hospitals do not allow time for the various stages of separation anxiety.

Developmental Abilities and Perceptions

The age, cognitive level, and developmental level of children will affect their perceptions of events. This, in turn, will affect their reactions to illness and hospitalization. Younger children, with their limited life experience and immature intellectual capacities, have a more difficult time comprehending what is happening to them. This can be particularly true for toddlers and preschoolers, who perceive the intactness of their bodies to be violated during invasive procedures. In addition, they frequently interpret illness as punishment for wrongdoing or hospital procedures as hostile, mutilating acts. Thus, children below the age of 5 are more vulnerable to emotional distress from hospitalization.

Previous Experiences

In general, children's lack of understanding and minimal experience with illness, hospitalization, and hospital procedures increase their anxiety. However, previous experience with hospitalization and illness can make preparation either easier or more difficult (if the experiences were perceived as negative). For example, if the child associates going to the hospital with the birth of a sibling, he or she may view this experience as positive. However, if the child associates the hospital with the serious illness or death of a relative or close friend, he or she will probably view the experience as negative.

If children have had previous experiences, how the experience unfolded and their response to it determines many of their reactions to the present hospitalization. For example, older children may cling to their parents, kick, or create a scene because of their previous experience. One research study compared the psychological responses of children hospitalized in a pediatric intensive care unit with those hospitalized on a general unit. The children who were younger and more severely ill and who underwent more invasive procedures had significantly more medical fears, a lower sense of control over their health, and ongoing posttraumatic stress responses for 6 months after discharge (Rennick et al., 2002).

Recent Stresses and Changes and Individual Coping Skills

The effects of hospitalization on children are influenced by the nature and severity of the health problem, the condition of the child, and the degree to which activities and routines differ from those of everyday life. A lack of sensory stimulation in the hospital environment produces listlessness, indifference, unhappiness, and even appetite changes. When the child's motor activity is restricted, anger and hyperactivity may result. Play, recreation, and educational opportunities provide an outlet to distract children from the illness, provide them with pleasant experiences, and help them understand their condition.

The ability to work through a situation for children and families will also affect their responses to illness and hospitalization. Of course, this ability depends on the age of child, perceptions of the event, previous situations, encounters with health care personnel, and support from significant others. Table 11.1 lists coping skills used by children and suggestions for promoting positive coping.

Table 11.1 Children and Coping

Behavior/ Methods for Coping	Suggestions to Promote Coping
Ignore or negate the problem Stoicism, passive acceptance Acting out—yelling, kicking, screaming, crying Anger, withdrawal, rejection Intellectualizing	Breathing techniques such as blowing bubbles, pinwheels, or party noise-makers Distraction with books or games Imagery with tapes or scenarios Music Teaching before events or procedures

Parents' Response to Children's Hospitalization

Children sense their parents' anxiety and concern, and even hearing whispers can set off a child's imagination. For example, preschoolers may invent elaborate stories to explain what is happening to them. If parents do not tell the child the truth or do not answer his or her questions, the child will become confused and frightened and the child's trust in the parent may become weakened. It is important for children to believe that someone is in control and that the person can be trusted. Some parents, however, have their own fears and insecurities. Thus, how a child reacts often is shaped by the parents' response to the illness and hospitalization.

The relationship between the family and the hospital staff may also contribute to the stress of the child. These relationships contribute significantly to the quality of the environment. Hospital personnel must assume responsibility for the care of children who are hospitalized by maintaining good partnerships with families.

The Hospitalized Child's Family

Whether planned or unplanned, hospitalization increases the family's stress and anxiety level. The illness or serious injury of one family member affects all members of the family. The process disrupts the family's usual routines and may alter family roles. Parents and siblings have their own reactions to this experience.

Reactions of Parents

Watching a child in pain is difficult, especially when the parent is assisting with the procedure by holding the child. The parent may feel guilty for not seeking care sooner. Parents may also exhibit other feelings such as denial, anger, depression, and confusion. Parents may deny that the child is ill. They may express anger, especially directed at the nursing staff, another family member, or a higher power because of their loss of control in caring for the child. Depression may occur because of exhaustion and the psychological and physical requirements of spending long hours in a hospital caring for a child. Confusion may develop because of dealing with an unfamiliar environment or the loss of a parental role. Finally, the parents' marriage may be strained because of dual roles, long separation, and increased stress.

A recent study indicates that parents have experiences in four categories: facing boundaries, attempting to understand, coping with uncertainty, and seeking reassurance from caregivers (Stratton, 2004). First, parents feel helpless when they play a passive role in their child's care, such as when a medical procedure is required that hurts or traumatizes the child. Then parents attempt to understand by becoming informed and understanding the procedures. Next, they deal with the fear of uncertainty and attempt to promote a sense of comfort by interacting with the hospital staff. They seek reassurance from the caregivers.

Reactions of Siblings

Siblings of children who are hospitalized may experience jealousy, insecurity, resentment, confusion, and anxiety. They may have difficulty understanding why their sibling is ill or getting all the attention, leaving little for them. Certain age groups, such as the preschooler, may feel they caused the illness. Their magical and egocentric thinking combined with little information, contributes to their fears that they may have caused the illness or injury by their thoughts, wishes, or behaviors (Winch, 2001). If the family roles or routines change significantly, the siblings may feel insecure or anxious. They may develop changes in behavior or in school performance during this time.

Four categories of concerns occur for siblings during the hospitalization of a brother or sister:

1. What is wrong? Is my brother/sister going to die? Is he/she going to get better?
2. Is it my fault?
3. Could it happen to me, too?
4. Don't you care about me? (Craft & Wyatt, 1986)

Studies have shown that the level of stress experienced by the siblings was similar to that experienced by the ill child (Simon, 1993).

Factors Influencing Family Reactions

The parenting style and the family–child relationship can influence the hospital experience as well as the family members' coping skills. Cultural, ethnic, and religious variations, values and practices related to illness, general response to stress, and attitudes about the care of a sick child have a significant influence on the family's response and behaviors. For example, religious beliefs can raise problems or can be a source of strength to the family and child. Families already in crisis or without support systems have a more difficult time dealing with the added stress of hospitalization. Chapter 2 gives further explanations of some of these influences on children and their families.

> **Jake's parents are very upset** that he has to be hospitalized. His mother says to you, "I'm worried how Jake is going to react to all of this. What can we do to help him?" How would you address his mother's concerns?

The Nurse's Role in Caring for the Hospitalized Child

In most instances, the nurse is the primary person involved in the care of a hospitalized child. The nurse is probably the first one to see the child and family and will spend more time with them than other health care providers. Nurses are part of a medical community that makes decisions in the child's best interest, but the nurse needs to bear in mind the child's rights and must try to minimize the distress of children so that the hospital stay may be as pleasant an experience as possible (Bricher, 2000). When establishing strategies to care for children in the hospital, nurses should examine the general effects of hospitalization on children in each developmental stage and should strive to understand the factors affecting hospitalization as well as the reactions of the child and family. Nursing Care Plan 11.1 summarizes the nursing care associated with a hospitalized child.

Crole and Smith (2002) divided the nursing care for a hospitalized child into four phases: introduction, building a trusting relationship, making decisions, and providing comfort and reassurance. All of these phases are interconnected. For example, if trust is not established, it becomes difficult to move to the next phase.

The initial contact with children and their families can serve as a foundation for a trusting relationship. Each institution has its own criteria for admission and transfer of pediatric patients, formulated in light of its mission and abilities and limitations (Sigrest et al., 2003). Use favorite toys and common television shows to establish rapport. Allow the child to participate in the conversation without the pressure of having to comply with requests or undergo any procedures. A trusting relationship can be built by using appropriate language, games, and play such as singing a song during a procedure, preparing the child adequately for procedures, and providing explanations and encouragement. Get down to the child's level and play on his or her terms.

The next two phases involve making judgments and providing feedback. Decisions must be made that will affect the trust the child has developed. For example, it is imperative to decide how much control the child will have during treatment, how much information to share with the child about upcoming events, and whether parents should participate. Reinforce the child's use of coping strategies that lead to healthy outcomes by providing options whenever it is safe to do so. Finally, the comfort and reassurance phase uses techniques such as praising the child and providing opportunities to cuddle with a favorite toy.

Preparing Children and Families for Hospitalization

When preparing children for hospitalization, be aware of the situations that may create distress in a child and try to minimize or eliminate them. Even the most minor situations may be frightening to young children. The new experiences associated with hospitalization are often the most stressful for the child and family (Burke et al., 1999). Table 11.2 presents some hospital activities that may seem scary or stressful to a child and gives suggestions for preparing the child and family. Thoughtful preparation for these situations might relieve the stress. Educate children about what to expect so they can cope with their imagination and distinguish reality from fantasy. Describe the intervention and the sequence of steps that will occur, and include sensory information such as how the child will feel.

Good preparation can reduce the child's fears and increase his or her ability to cope with the hospital experience. Preparation should include exploring the child's perceptions, reviewing previous experiences, and identifying coping strategies. Useful techniques include:

- Practicing nursing care on stuffed animals or dolls and allowing the child to do the same
- Avoiding the use of medical terms
- Allowing the child to handle some equipment
- Teaching the child the steps of the procedure or informing him or her exactly what will happen during the hospital stay
- Showing the child the room where he or she will be staying
- Introducing the child to the health care personnel with whom he or she will come in contact
- Explaining the sounds the child may hear
- Letting the child sample the food that they will be served

All techniques used to prepare the child for hospitalization should emphasize the philosophy of atraumatic care. "The main goal of preparation is for the child to participate in a dialogue and a demonstration of the coming procedure so he or she can better understand the situation" (Mansson & Dykes, 2004). Adapt all information to the cognitive and developmental level of the child. Identify what role the child will play in the situation: it is always helpful for children to have something to do, since it shows them that they are included. A rehearsal of what will occur in the hospital allows the child to become comfortable with the situation. If time permits, provide pamphlets that describe the procedure and suggest preparation activities for the child at home before admission.

The child and family may be able to take a tour of the hospital unit or the surgical facility. Videotapes or DVDs, photographs, and books on hospitalization and surgery can serve as resources for the family and child. Many institutions offer programs to familiarize children and families with the hospital experience. For example, one institution uses a "train ride" to help them understand what to expect (Herron, 2005). During the ride, opportunities are provided for role playing, and during stops along the way the child can see, touch, and feel the equipment that may be used (Fig. 11.2).

The American Society of Anesthesiologists has prepared a coloring book entitled "My Trip to the Hospital." This book is designed to alleviate some of the fears that

(text continues on page 299)

Nursing Care Plan 11.1

Overview for the Hospitalized Child and Family

Nursing Diagnosis: Anxiety related to hospital situation, fear of injury or bodily mutilation, separation from family or friends, changes in routine, painful procedures and treatments, and unfamiliar events and surroundings as evidenced by crying, fussing, withdrawal, or resistance

Outcome identification and evaluation:

Child and family will exhibit a decrease in anxiety level as evidenced by positive coping strategies, verbalization or playing out of feelings, appropriate behaviors, positive interactions with staff, child and parent cooperation and participation, and absence of signs and symptoms of increasing anxiety and fear.

Interventions: minimizing anxiety

- Orient child and family to the unit and the child's room *to familiarize them with the facility.*
- Place the child in a room with another child of a similar age, developmental level, and condition severity *to promote sharing.*
- Explain all events, treatments, procedures, and activities to the parents and child (at level the child with understand) in a calm, relaxed manner *to help them prepare for what is to come and decrease fear of the unknown. A calm, relaxed manner helps to establish rapport and instill trust.*
- Encourage parents to room in if possible *to provide the child with support;* if parents cannot stay, encourage them to call *to reduce child's fear of being alone.*
- Urge parents to inform the child when they will be leaving and when they are expected to return *to help child cope with their absence and promote trust.*
- Assess child's usual routine at home and attempt to incorporate aspects of usual routine into hospital routine *to ease the transition to the hospital and promote child participation in routine.*
- Offer comfort measures such as holding, stroking, and rocking *to relieve distress.*
- Provide atraumatic care *to minimize exposure to distress, which would increase anxiety.*
- Encourage the child's participation in play (unstructured and therapeutic play as necessary) *to allow for expression of feelings and fears and promote energy expenditure.*
- Suggest that parents bring in a special toy or object from home *to promote feelings of security.*
- Provide positive reinforcement for participation in care activities *to foster self-esteem.*
- Assess for regression behaviors and inform parents that such behaviors are common *to help alleviate their concerns about this behavior.*
- Provide consistency with care measures *to facilitate trust and acceptance.*

Nursing Diagnosis: Risk for powerlessness related to lack of control over procedures, treatments, and care, and changes in usual routine

Outcome identification and evaluation:

Child and family will demonstrate an increase in control over the situation as evidenced by participation in care activities, identification of needs and choices, and incorporation of appropriate aspects of child's usual routine with that of the hospital.

Interventions: promoting control

- Encourage child and parents to identify areas of concern *to help in determining priority needs.*
- Encourage parent and child to participate in care activities *to promote feelings of control.*
- Incorporate aspects of child's routine at home and use terms similar to those used at home *to foster a sense of normalcy.*

Overview for the Hospitalized Child and Family (continued)

- Offer child choices as much as possible, such as options for foods, drinks, hygiene, activities, or clothing (if appropriate) to *promote feelings of individuality and control.*
- Allow child opportunities for being out of bed or room within limitations as appropriate *to foster independence.*
- Work with child, as age and development allow, and family to set up a schedule to *promote structure and routine.*

Nursing Diagnosis: Deficient diversional activity related to confinement in bed or health care facility, limited mobility, activity restrictions, or equipment as evidenced by verbalization of boredom, lack of participation in play, reading, or schoolwork

Outcome identification and evaluation:

Child will participate in diversional activities as evidenced by engagement in unstructured and therapeutic play that is developmentally appropriate and interaction with family, staff, and other children.

Interventions: promoting adequate diversional activities

- Question child and family about favorite types of activities *to establish a baseline for developing appropriate choices during hospitalization.*
- Assist with planning activities within the limits of the child's condition *to maintain muscle tone and strength without overexerting the child.*
- Spend time with the child *to provide stimulation and foster trust.*
- Enlist the aid of a child life specialist *to provide suggestions for appropriate activities.*
- Encourage interaction with other children *to promote sharing and avoid loneliness.*
- Provide developmentally appropriate opportunities for unstructured and therapeutic play *to facilitate expression of feelings.*
- Encourage short trips to the playroom or activity room *to provide a change of scenery and sensory stimulation.*
- Integrate play activities with nursing care *to achieve therapeutic effect.*

Nursing Diagnosis: Interrupted family processes related to separation from child due to hospitalization, increased demands of caring for an ill child, changes in role function, and effect of hospitalization on other family members such as siblings as evidenced by parental verbalization of issues, parental presence in hospital, or child's hospitalization requiring parent to miss work

Outcome identification and evaluation:

Family will demonstrate positive coping strategies as evidenced by visiting frequently and staying with the child as necessary, sharing of family responsibilities, obtaining assistance for relief or respite, and visiting by other members of the child's family and friends.

Interventions: maximizing family functioning

- Encourage parents and family members to verbalize concerns related to child's illness, diagnosis, and prognosis *to promote family-centered care and identify areas where intervention may be needed.*
- Explain therapies, procedures, child's behaviors, and plan of care to parents to *promote understanding of the child's status and plan of care, which helps to decrease anxiety.*
- Encourage parental involvement in care *to promote feelings of the parents being needed and valued, providing them with a sense of control over their child's health.*
- Identify support system for family and child *to help identify resources available for coping.*
- Educate family and child on additional resources available *to promote a wider base of support to deal with the situation.*
- Suggest ways that parents can divide time between child and other siblings *to prevent feelings of guilt.*

(continued)

Overview for the Hospitalized Child and Family (continued)

- Provide support and positive reinforcement *to promote family coping and foster family strength.*
- Encourage frequent visits by family members, including siblings as appropriate, *to promote ongoing family functioning.*
- Stress the need for adequate rest, sleep, exercise, and nutrition for family members *to promote family health and minimize stress of hospitalization on family.*
- Assist with referrals for resources and help from additional family members and friends as necessary *to allow for respite or relief of care responsibilities.*
- Encourage family to maintain usual routine as much as possible *to minimize the effects of hospitalization on family functioning.*

Nursing Diagnosis: Self-care deficit related to immobility, activity restrictions, regression, or use of equipment, devices, or prescribed treatments as evidenced by inability to feed, bathe or dress self or accomplish other activities of daily living

Outcome identification and evaluation:

Child will participate in self-care within limitations of condition as evidenced by assisting with bathing and hygiene, feeding, toileting, and dressing and grooming.

Interventions: promoting self-care

- Assess child's usual routine for self-care and self-care abilities *to provide a baseline for individualizing interventions.*
- Provide child-sized equipment and devices *to promote child's ability to complete the self-care task.*
- Encourage parents and child to do as much self-are as possible, within limitations of the child's condition and developmental level, *to promote feelings of independence and foster growth and development.*
- Offer praise and encouragement for activities performed *to foster self-esteem, confidence, and competence.*
- Ensure adequate rest periods *to minimize energy expenditure associated with self-care activities.*

Nursing Diagnosis: Risk for delayed growth and development related to stressors associated with hospitalization, current condition or illness, separation from family, and sensory overload or sensory deprivation

Outcome identification and evaluation:

Child will demonstrate developmentally appropriate milestones as evidenced by age-appropriate behaviors and activities.

Interventions: promoting growth and development

- Assess child's developmental stage *to establish a baseline and determine appropriate strategies.*
- Use unstructured and therapeutic play and adaptive toys *to promote developmental functioning.*
- Provide stimulating environment when possible *to maximize potential for growth and development.*
- Praise accomplishments and emphasize child's abilities *to foster self-esteem and encourage feelings of confidence and competence.*
- Include parents in techniques to foster growth and development *to promote feelings of control in their child's care.*

Overview for the Hospitalized Child and Family (continued)

Nursing Diagnosis: Deficient knowledge related to hospitalization, surgery, treatments, procedures, required care, and follow-up as evidenced by questioning and verbalization, lack of prior exposure

Outcome identification and evaluation:

Child and family will demonstrate understanding of all aspects of child's current situation as evidenced by identification of child's and family's needs, verbal statements of understanding and/or need for additional information, return demonstration of procedures and treatments, and verbalization of instructions for follow-up and continued care.

Interventions: providing child and family teaching

- Assess child's and family's willingness to learn *to ensure effective teaching.*
- Provide family with time to adjust to diagnosis *to facilitate their ability to learn and participate in the child's care.*
- Repeat information *to promote multiple opportunities for child and family to learn.*
- Teach in short sessions *to prevent overloading the child and parents with information.*
- Gear teaching to a level of understanding for the child and the family (depends on age of child, physical condition, memory) *to promote learning.*
- Provide reinforcement and rewards *to help facilitate the teaching/learning process.*
- Use multiple modes of learning, such as written information, verbal instruction, demonstrations, and media, when possible *to facilitate learning and retention of information.*
- Provide the child and family with written step-by-step instructions for procedures or care *to allow for reference at a later date.*
- Have child and family provide return demonstrations of care procedures *to ensure effectiveness of teaching.*
- Arrange for trial home care during hospitalization and after discharge as appropriate *to ensure understanding and provide opportunities for additional teaching and learning.*

younger children may have related to the hospital experience. It describes the process from admission (whether it be to the hospital or ambulatory surgery center) through discharge and includes information about preoperative testing, anesthesia, and recovery. The book also includes information for parents. The book is available online at http://www.asahq.org/patientEducation/mytrip.htm.

Parents are instrumental in preparing children by reviewing the materials that are given, answering questions, and being truthful and supportive. Teaching Guideline 11.1 provides suggestions for parents in preparing their child for hospitalization.

Admitting the Child to the Facility

Admitting the child to the facility involves preparing him or her for admission and introducing the child to the unit where he or she will be staying. Use the appropriate hospital forms. Chapter 3 gives general information about communicating with and teaching children and families.

In today's health care environment, the admission process occurs quickly, with little time for extensive preparation; this is why preparation before admission is so important. Of course, the urgency of the child's medical condition also may limit the amount of preparation that can be done in advance.

Types of Admissions and Nursing Care

The hospital units to which a child may be admitted include:

- General inpatient units
- Emergency and urgent care departments
- Pediatric intensive care units
- Outpatient or special procedures unit
- Rehabilitation unit or hospital

Regardless of the site of care, nursing care must begin by establishing a trusting, caring relationship with the child and family. Smile, introduce yourself and give your title. Let the child and family know what will hap-

Table 11.2 Strategies to Reduce Fear of Common Hospitalization Situations

Situation	Strategies to Reduce Fear
Procedure involving intrusion into the body or use of equipment or technology	Describe the procedure and equipment in terms the child can understand. Review the steps of the procedure or steps involved with the use of the equipment. Explain what the child's role will be and what is or isn't allowed. If appropriate, have the child rehearse with the equipment or role play.
Darkness, such as with radiologic examinations or at night	Keep a light on in the examination area. Use a night light in the patient's room. If possible, allow the child to hold the caregiver's or nurse's hand or a favorite toy.
Transport to other areas of the hospital	Allow caregiver to accompany child if possible. Inform the child of where he or she is going, about how long he or she will be there, and approximately when he or she will return. Introduce the child to the person who will be transporting the child.
Numerous personnel in and out of child's room	Identify all staff members working with the child (each shift and each day). Place a small board in the child's room with the name of the nurse caring for the child that shift or day. Inform the child how long the nurse will be caring for the child (adapt this information according to the child's cognitive level; for example, instead of saying that you'll be there for 8 hours, say, "I'll be your nurse until just before dinnertime" or "I'll be your nurse until you go for your test." Say good-bye to the child when leaving for the day; tell the child about his or her new nurse; inform the child of when you will return.

pen and what is expected of them. Ask the family and child what names they prefer to be called by. Maintain eye contact at the appropriate level. With a younger child, start with the family first so the child can see that the family trusts you. Communicate with children at age-appropriate levels.

The next step, as the child's medical condition allows, involves an orientation to the hospital unit. Briefly explain policies and routines and the personnel who will be involved in the care of the child.

During the nursing interview that follows, obtain information about the child's history, routines, and reason for admission. Obtain baseline vital signs, height and weight, and perform a physical assessment. Each health care setting has its own policies and procedures for this. Recognize the needs of the family and child during this

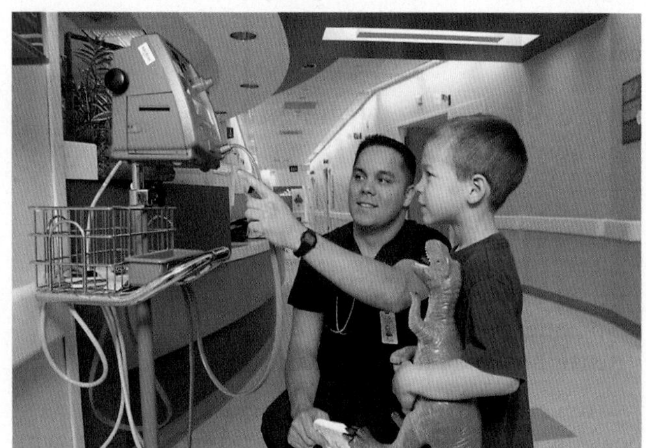

● **Figure 11.2** A child is being prepared for hospitalization by becoming familiar with some of the equipment that might be used.

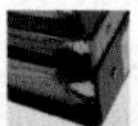

TEACHING GUIDELINE 11.1

Preparing Your Child for Hospitalization

- Read stories about experiences with hospital or surgery.
- Talk about going to the hospital and what it will be like coming home.
- Be honest and encourage child to ask questions.
- Visit the hospital and go through the preadmission tour if time permits.
- Plan support to the child via your presence, telephone calls, and special items brought from home.
- Encourage the child to draw pictures to express how he or she is feeling.
- Include siblings in the preparation.

process. If some of this information already exists, do not ask for it again, except to confirm vital information such as allergies, medications taken at home, and history of the illness. Typically, the information is collected immediately if the child's condition is urgent; otherwise, the information is collected within 8 hours, except for the information that is required for safe care.

General Inpatient Unit Stays

Today, general inpatient unit stays for children are shorter and involve more acute conditions, resulting in little time for admission preparation. Many times the admission procedure and treatment actually occur simultaneously. Sometimes the stay is in a special 23-hour observation unit so the child is in the setting for less than 24 hours. General hospital stays may be in a pediatric hospital, a pediatric unit in a general hospital, or a general unit that occasionally admits children. General units often lack child-oriented services, such as play areas, child-size equipment, and staff familiar with caring for children.

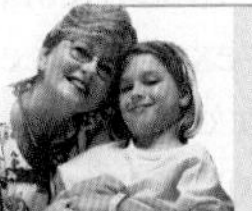

When a child is admitted to a general unit, take extra time to orient and explain the routine and procedures to the child and family. Emphasize that the parents can stay with the child (if institutional policy permits). If possible, place the child in a room close to the nurses' station and order food appropriate for the child's age and developmental level.

Emergency and Urgent Care Departments

The number-one reason for illness and hospitalization in children is injuries from accidents. Many times a family's first experience with the acute care setting is the urgent care or emergency department. Due to the situation, the child and family may experience increased anxiety, and it may become overwhelming as uncertainties develop and critical decisions must be made. The family may be frightened, insecure, and in a state of shock. Procedures and tests are performed quickly, with minimal time for preparation. The family is often ill prepared for the visit, having little money or clothing with them. Siblings may be present if the parents did not have time to get a sitter.

Due to the fast pace of the emergency department, the family may be hesitant to ask questions, so keep the family and child well informed. Allow the family to stay with the child, provide support, and allow the family, and when appropriate the child, to participate in decisions.

Families may have a strong fear of the unknown and may be terrified that the child will die or be permanently disabled. Help the family to identify their concerns and their support systems. Prepare them for what they will experience. Provide comfort such as holding, touching, talking softly, and other appropriate interventions according to age and developmental level.

Pediatric Intensive Care Units

The pediatric intensive care unit (PICU) specializes in caring for children in crisis. The same principles and concepts of general care of children apply to this setting, but everything is intensified. Families will be faced with an unfamiliar, high-tech environment and a large number of staff.

Families must deal with the critical situation that brought them to the PICU. The child will likely experience pain, unusual noises, and increased stimulation and will probably undergo uncomfortable procedures. Parents may face the possibility of losing their child. Sometimes the child cannot talk, eat, or display other appropriate developmental behaviors. **Sensory overload** (increased stimulation) or **sensory deprivation** (lack of stimulation) can affect both child and family.

Welcome families (if institutional policy permits) and encourage them to stay with the child and participate in care. Explain everything to the parents and, when appropriate, to the child. Frequently touch the child and encourage the parents to comfort him or her. Listen for clues about what the child and family need during the PICU stay.

Outpatient or Special Procedure Units

Outpatient or special procedure units are used to keep hospital stays short and decrease the cost of hospitalization. These units may be a part of a general hospital or a freestanding facility. Typically, the child and family arrive in the morning; the child has the procedure, test, or surgery and then goes home later that same day. Examples of surgeries performed in outpatient settings include tympanostomy tube placement, hernia repair, tonsillectomy, cystoscopy, bronchoscopy, and chemotherapy.

This setting minimizes separation of the child from the family. In addition, there is minimal disruption of the family pattern, a decreased risk of infection, and decreased cost. However, these units do not have the equipment for overnight stays, so if complications develop, the child will need to be transported to another facility or another area of the hospital.

Rehabilitation Units

The rehabilitation unit provides care for children beyond the initial period of illness or injury. The care involves an interdisciplinary approach that assists the child to reach his or her fullest potential and achieve developmental skills. For example, rehabilitation units help children regain abilities lost due to neurologic injuries or serious burns. The facilities often resemble a home environment, with special services to help children to relearn activities of daily living and to help them deal with the physical or mental challenges associated with the original illness or injury. Typically, families are encouraged to participate and are given support for their child's eventual return home. There is a balance of nurturing and firm discipline while the child reclaims independence.

Isolation Rooms

Isolation rooms are used for situations involving the risk for infection. When a child is admitted with an infectious disease, or to rule out an infectious disease, or if the child has impaired immune function, isolation will be instituted. Children in this setting may experience sensory deprivation due to the limited contact with others and the use of personal protective equipment such as gloves, masks, and gowns.

Encourage the family to visit often, and help them to understand the reason for the isolation and any special procedures that are required. Introduce yourself before entering the room and allow the child to view your face before applying a mask. Continue to have contact with the child and hold or touch the child often, especially if the parents are not present.

Preparing the Child and Family for Surgery

If the child is to undergo a surgical procedure, whether in the hospital or an outpatient setting, special interventions are necessary. The parents should be allowed to stay with the child until surgery begins. Parents should also be allowed to be with the child when he or she wakes up in the post-anesthesia recovery area. Good preparation provides reassurance and comfort to the child and allows him or her to know what will happen and what is expected of him or her.

Preoperative Care

Preoperative care for the child who is to undergo surgery is similar to that for an adult. The major difference is that the preparation and teaching must be geared to the child's age and developmental level. Many facilities offer special programs to help prepare children and families for the surgical experience. Presurgical preparation programs allow children and their families to experience a "trial run" in a supportive environment to reduce anxiety, increase knowledge, and enhance coping skills (Justus et al., 2006). Books, including the one cited earlier by the American Society of Anesthesiologists, are helpful in preparing the child and family.

Child and family teaching is essential. Like any intervention, adapt the teaching to the child's developmental level. Table 11.3 highlights key teaching strategies based on the child's developmental level. For example, when teaching a toddler or preschooler about breathing exercises, have the child blow a pinwheel or cotton balls across the table through a straw. The child can enjoy the activity while also reaping the respiratory benefits of the activity.

In preparation for surgery, use items such as stuffed animals or dolls to help children understand what is going to happen to them (Fig. 11.3). Allow the child to role-play various experiences with dolls. Dolls designed to simulate surgical experiences have been developed. For example, Shadow Buddies (www.shadowbuddies.org) are custom-made dolls that have the same illness or surgery as the child; the doll may have an ostomy, scar, or catheter. The dolls were developed to help children cope with their illness or disease and send the message that it is okay to be different. These dolls also provide the child with a companion to talk to.

Intraoperative Care

A major controversy is whether parents should be present during anesthesia induction. Proponents argue that the presence of a parent during anesthesia induction is comforting, so the child can remain calm and experience a decreased anxiety level, which in turn decreases catecholamine release and increases oxygenation. As a result, adverse effects such as breath-holding laryngospasm and long-term psychological effects are diminished (Romino, 2005). However, parents must receive thorough preparation; inadequate preparation increases the parents' anxiety, and children experience greater anxiety if accompanied by an anxious parent (Munro & D'Errico, 2000).

Studies have shown that being present at anesthesia induction can also benefit parents. Parents experience high levels of stress when separated from their child during surgery, and allowing parents to be present for anesthesia induction can decrease this stress (Romino, 2005).

Postoperative Care

Postoperative nursing care for a child is similar to that for an adult. However, due to anatomic differences, frequent, astute observation is a must. Assessment of the child's airway, breathing, and circulation is key. The surgical site is inspected and fluids and hydration are administered. If possible, allow parents to be present in the post-anesthesia care unit as soon as possible to provide the child with support and a familiar face.

Pain management is crucial. Use an appropriate pain assessment tool to rate the child's pain. Frequently reassess the child's pain, and use atraumatic care. Expect to administer pharmacologic agents as ordered. Also encourage the use of nonpharmacologic methods. A research study (Huth et al., 2004) showed that distraction techniques such as guided imagery helped children cope with tonsillectomy and adenoidectomy pain. The children who received an educational program about imagery reported less sensory pain, distress, and anxiety while in the outpatient surgery unit, but no differences were found in the reports of pain at home or use of pain medications.

Maintaining Safety During Hospitalization

Safety is a critical aspect of care of the child in the hospital. Due to their age and developmental level, children are vulnerable to harm. Ensure the child has an identification band in place at all times. Sometimes in implementing

Table 11.3 Strategies to Reduce Fear of Common Hospitalization Situations

Developmental Level	Common Fears/Anxieties	Implications for Teaching
Infants and toddlers	Separation	Encourage parents to use a soft tone of voice. Remind parents to use positive facial expressions. Encourage the parent or caregiver to stay with the child as much as possible. Urge the parent or caregiver to use stroking or secure, comfortable holding positions to promote calm. Talk to the child and parents using a soft, comforting tone of voice with the parent or caregiver holding the child. Use terms that the child and parents can understand.
Preschoolers and school-age children	Pain Mutilation Separation Possible punishment for wrongdoings	Provide factual explanations using terms the child and parents can understand. Incorporate pictures and other visual aids in explanation. Allow time for children to play out their concerns and fears. Tailor the timing of education to meet the child's learning needs, allowing enough time for the child to ask questions. For toddlers, provide information as close to the day of surgery as possible to prevent undue anxiety. Some recommend that information be provided no more than 1 week beforehand (Justus et al., 2006).
Adolescents	Loss of independence Effects on body image	Acknowledge the adolescent's right to privacy. Allow as much independence as possible within the constraints of the diagnosis. Provide detailed explanations of the procedure at least 7 to 10 days beforehand. Answer questions honestly, ensuring privacy at all times. Remain available for questions or concerns arising before or after surgery.

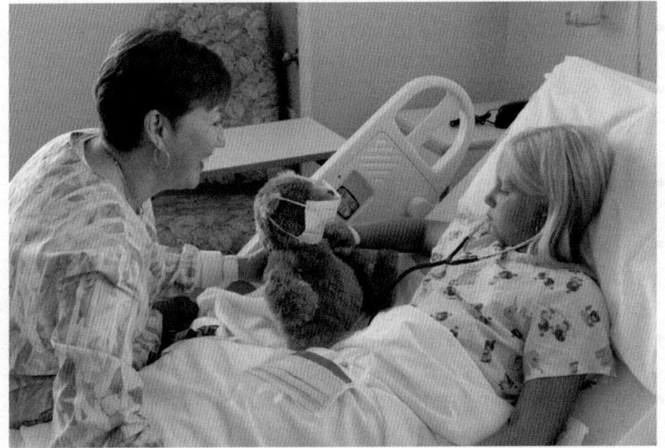

● Figure 11.3 Using a stuffed animal to explain a surgical procedure to the child.

interventions an armband is removed, so make sure it is attached to another extremity. Monitor children closely to avoid accidents such as a child pushing the wrong knob or picking up a piece of equipment or supplies left in the bed or room. Table 11.4 provides nursing goals for ensuring safe, developmentally appropriate care for the hospitalized child.

Use of Restraints

When caring for children, some type of restriction may be necessary. The restriction, often referred to as a restraint, may be needed to ensure the child's safety, allow for a therapeutic or diagnostic procedure to be done, immobilize a body part or limit movement, or prevent disruption of prescribed therapy. However, restraints can be overused and can cause harm to the patient. As a result, the Joint Commission on Accreditation of Healthcare Organizations (JCAHO, 2005) issued standards related to the use of restraints designed to safeguard the patient's physical safety and psychological well-being.

Table 11.4 Nursing Considerations for Providing Safe, Developmentally Appropriate Care

	Ensuring Safety	Promoting Healthy Growth and Development
Infants	• Maintain close supervision of the infant. • Keep one hand on the infant when crib sides are down. • Keep crib rails up all the way when the infant is in the crib. • Avoid leaving small objects that are harmful or that can be swallowed in the crib. • Provide safe and appropriate toys for the infant. • Place infants in rooms close to the nurses' station. • Encourage a family member to stay with the infant at all times.	• Use the *en face* position when holding newborns. • Smile and talk to the infant during bathing, feeding, and other interactions. • Minimize the number of painful or uncomfortable procedures. • Provide comfort during and after procedures by holding or talking, using soothing tones and movements. • When handling the infant, use smooth, continuous movements. • Use gentle stroking and holding, which may reduce stress. • Serve as a role model for first-time parents. • Encourage the family to maintain home routines while in hospital, planning nursing care around the usual feeding and sleep times. • Use the pacifier between feedings to satisfy nonnutritive sucking needs.
Toddlers	• Keep crib side rails up with overhead crib protection intact when the toddler is in the crib. • Never leave toddler alone in the room unless secured in the crib. • Use a bed only for the older toddler who has an adult present in the room at all times. • Avoid leaving small objects than can be swallowed or are harmful in the crib or bed. • Place crib out of reach of cords, equipment, and electrical outlets. • Provide safe and appropriate toys for the toddler. • Always have someone with the toddler when ambulating.	• Encourage the parent to stay with the toddler to decrease separation anxiety. • To promote autonomy, allow the toddler to make appropriate choices, such as which juice to take the medicine with. • Encourage active play in the playroom or with push/pull toys in the hallway (accompanied by an adult). • Expect and plan for regression in areas of toilet training, eating, and other behaviors. • Expect increased temper tantrums in general and intense reactions to intrusive procedures. • Maintain home routine while in hospital, planning nursing care around the usual feeding and sleep times. • Give simple directions with choices appropriate to the hospital situation. • Place toddlers in rooms close to the nurses' station. • Provide close supervision while encouraging independence.
Preschoolers	• Keep bed in low position with the side rails up when the preschooler is in the bed. • Instruct the child to call the nurse or caregiver for help getting out of bed. • Keep harmful objects out of reach of the child.	• Encourage parents to stay with the preschooler in the room as well as other areas of the hospital. • Encourage the preschooler to be involved in care by providing choices and opportunities for the child to help. • Use play as an opportunity to work through the preschooler's fears. • Explain activities in simple, concrete terms, being cautious with language you use because of the preschooler's fantasies and magical thinking. • Expect reactions to pain and bodily injury to be verbally aggressive and specific. • Try to maintain home routines while the child is in the hospital, working them into the plan of care when possible.

Table 11.4 Nursing Considerations for Providing Safe, Developmentally Appropriate Care (continued)

	Ensuring Safety	Promoting Healthy Growth and Development
School-agers	• Keep the bed in the low position with the side rails up while the child is in the bed, explaining that this is a hospital rule, not a punishment.	• Provide opportunities for the child to be involved in care. • Allow children to select their meals, assist with treatments, and keep their rooms neat. • Allow visits with other children if condition allows. • Encourage parents to tell the child when they will return. • Plan care around the child's usual home routines (meals, sleep). • Encourage the child to do schoolwork.
Adolescents	• Be aware of the adolescent's whereabouts. The teen may not wish to stay in the room but may become confused about where the room or unit is located in the hospital.	• Allow teens to interact with others. • Alter hospital routines as possible to allow the teen to sleep in or stay up later at night. • Provide others close to their age as roommates. • Encourage visits from friends. • Provide emotional support for feelings of being alone or away from friends; be alert for regression, which may result in the teen becoming emotional. • Answer questions honestly and with appropriate information. • Give the teen a sense of control by allowing choices. • Be sensitive to concerns about being "different."

According to these standards, hospitals are required to have a policy in place that specifies the following:

- Reason for the restraint
- Patient assessment parameters identifying the need for the restraint
- Use of at least one alternative method for restriction before using a restraint
- Use of the least restrictive type of restraint for the purpose after the decision is made that a restraint is necessary
- Need for a written order by a licensed independent practitioner (LIP) within 1 hour of application of the restraint
- Need for evaluation by LIP within 1 hour of application of the restraint

In addition, the JCAHO standards also identify the need for specific staff training, frequent assessment, and appropriate discontinuation of use.

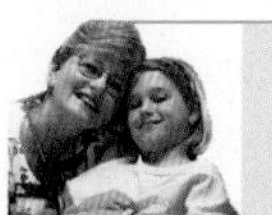

Restraints can promote physical distress in a child. Children also may view restraints as punishment. When determining the need for restraining a child, the nurse needs to consider the child's age, developmental level, mental status, and threat to others and self. Applying the principles of atraumatic care and JCAHO standards, the nurse uses a restraint only when necessary and for the shortest time possible.

Before a restraint is used, other measures need to be tried. Explain why the child should not touch the intravenous site or should maintain a certain position so that the child has a basic understanding of what is necessary. This may be all that is necessary for an older child.

Therapeutic hugging (use of a holding position that promotes close physical contact between the child and a parent or caregiver) may be used for certain procedures or treatments where the child must remain still. For example, the parent can hold the child in his or her lap snugly to prevent the child from moving during an injection or venipuncture. This technique may be used to position a child for intravenous access, injections, an otoscopic examination, or a lumbar puncture. When using this technique, make sure the parent understands his or her role and knows which body parts to hold still in a safe manner.

Alternatively, distraction or stimulation (such as with a toy) can help to gain the child's cooperation. One-to-one supervision and behavior modification techniques may be other alternatives to the use of restraints.

If it is determined that the child requires a restraint, select the most appropriate, least restrictive type of restraint. For example, if the child has an intravenous catheter in the antecubital space that stops flowing when the child bends the arm, an elbow restraint or arm board, rather than a soft wrist restraint or four-point extremity restraint, would be appropriate. With the elbow restraint or arm board, the child's arm flexion is restricted yet he or she can still move the shoulder and hands. A soft wrist restraint would limit the child's ability to move the arm; four-point extremity restraints would restrict the child's ability to move all the extremities. Table 11.5 lists the types of restraints and

Table 11.5 Types of Restraints and Associated Safety Concerns

Type of Restraint	Purpose	Safety Concerns
Clove hitch restraint	Wrist or ankle restraint to prevent range of motion of extremities	Check wrist or ankle for any sign of circulatory, integumentary, or neurologic compromise.
Elbow restraint	Prevents child from flexing and reaching face, head, IV and other tubes	Position the restraint so it does not rub against axilla. Check pulse, temperature, and capillary refill of the extremity.
Mummy restraint	Body restraint using a sheet folded in a square appropriate to size of infant or young child to secure the whole body of the child or every extremity except for one	Ensure that all extremities are secured within the sheet.

Table 11.5 Types of Restraints and Associated Safety Concerns (continued)

Type of Restraint	Purpose	Safety Concerns
Jacket (vest) restraint	Jacket worn by child with ties attached to the child's back and to side of bed. Used to keep children flat in bed, such as after surgery, or safe in chair.	Ensure the child can turn head to side and that the head of the bed is elevated. Place ties in back so child cannot manipulate them.
Crib top bubble restraint	Clear plastic cover over the bed to prevent older infant or young child from falling and climbing out of bed	Ensure that there are no tears or loose plastic.
Specially designed chairs/carts	Chairs/carts with tables or other devices to hold child in specific positions during transport or to prevent child from getting out of device	May need to use a vest or jacket restraints to help keep child in chair/cart. Never leave child unattended. Lock the wheels if the chair/cart is stationary.

the major issues associated with the use of restraints on children.

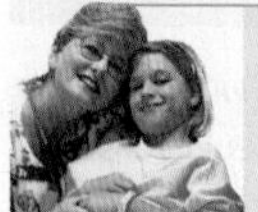

When selecting a restraint, the nurse must choose the least restrictive type of restraint and apply it for the shortest time necessary.

Before applying a restraint, explain the reason for the restraint to the child and the parents. Emphasize that the rationale is to maintain the child's safety; the restraint is not punishment. Having the child and parents state the reason for the restraint demonstrates their understanding.

A written order for the restraint and an evaluation of the child by a LIP must occur within 1 hour of applying the restraint. In addition, the nurse must do the following:

- Ensure that the restraint fits properly.
- Secure the restraints with ties to the bed or crib frame, not the side rails.
- Use a clove-hitch type of knot to secure the restraints with ties (this allows for quick, easy access and release of the restraint).
- Check restraints 15 minutes following initial placement and then every hour for proper placement.
- Assess the temperature of the affected extremities, pulses, and capillary refill, initially after 15 minutes and then every hour after placement.
- Remove the restraint every 2 hours to allow for range of motion and repositioning, with documentation of this process and any findings.
- Encourage parent participation, providing continuous explanations about the reasons for the restraints and tentative time frame for use.
- Offer positive reinforcement to the child and parents.
- Review the criteria for removing the restraints; document removal and continued assessment.

Transport of the Child

Children may need to be transported to other units for diagnostic tests or surgery, to different areas in the same unit, such as the playroom or treatment room, or for discharge. When the child is transported to other areas, specific guidelines need to address safety issues, the age and developmental level of the child, the child's physical condition, and the destination. These factors need to be considered before transport so that the appropriate method can be used with the least amount of risk for the child. Various methods to transport children include carrying the infant and using strollers, wagons, or rolling beds (Fig. 11.4). If possible, the parents should accompany the child to offer support and comfort.

When carrying an infant, good support of the back and head is vital. Rails should be up on all beds and wagons. Use safety belts with strollers and wheelchairs.

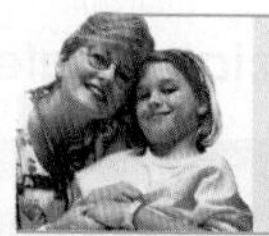

Never leave a child unattended during transport. Keep the child visible at all times during the transport.

Providing Basic Care for the Hospitalized Child

Basic care involves general hygiene measures, including bathing, hair care, oral care, and nutritional care. Young children are dependent on an adult for most, if not all, of their self-care needs. If parents are present, allow them to provide care for the child to decrease the child's stress. Older children may perform hygiene measures themselves but may need some assistance from the nurse.

General Hygiene Measures

General hygiene measures help to maintain healthy skin, hair, and teeth. Skin is a complex structure; its primary function is to protect the tissues that it encloses and to protect itself. Injury to the child's skin may occur when inserting and maintaining an intravenous line, removing a dressing, positioning a child in bed, changing a diaper, using and removing electrode patches, and maintaining restraints. Risk factors for potential problems include impaired mobility, protein malnutrition, edema, incontinence, sensory loss, anemia, and infection. A good time to assess the skin is during bath time.

Bathing

Bathing infants and children is a common daily general hygiene measure in the health care environment. Although the parents or primary caregiver often do this in today's family-centered environment, the nurse is still responsible for ensuring that bathing is done safely and hygienically. Adhere to safety principles to prevent falls, burns, and aspiration of water. Never leave a child alone in a bathtub. Use a gentle, pH-balanced soap with moisturizer if there is a need to rehydrate the skin. Note any condition that might require special considerations or further assessment, such as paralysis, loss of sensation, surgical incisions, skin traction/cast, external lines (intravenous lines, urinary catheters, or feeding tubes), or other alterations in skin integrity. Pay close attention to the ears, between skinfolds, the neck, the back, and the genital area for potential alterations in skin integrity. Table 11.6 highlights specific developmental considerations for bathing.

Before bathing and performing other hygiene measures, assess the family's preferences and home practices for the child, such as time of day, rituals, special equipment, and allergies to products. This is a good time to assess the amount of assistance that might be required by the parents and to address learning needs related to hygiene. Follow general guidelines in bathing any patient with regard to equipment, room temperature, privacy, and use of products such as deodorant and lotion.

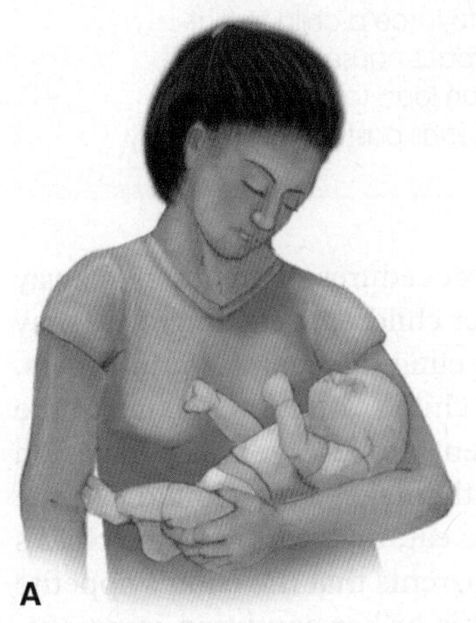

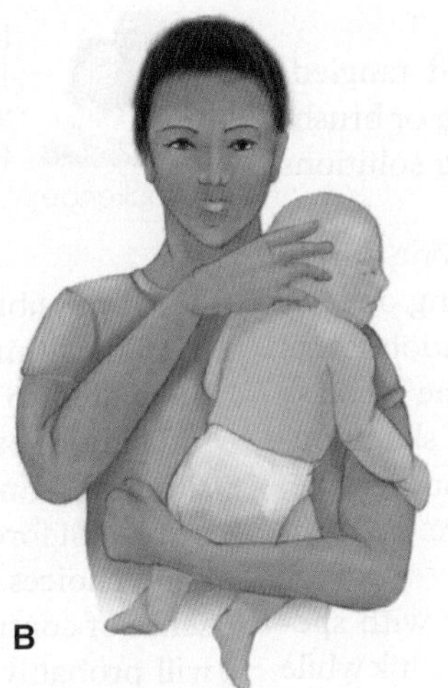

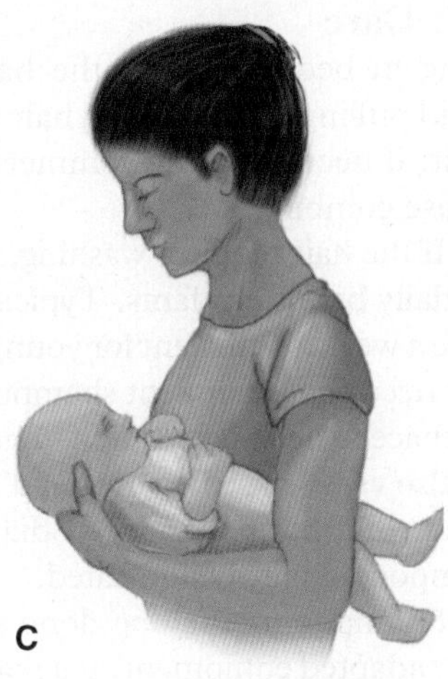

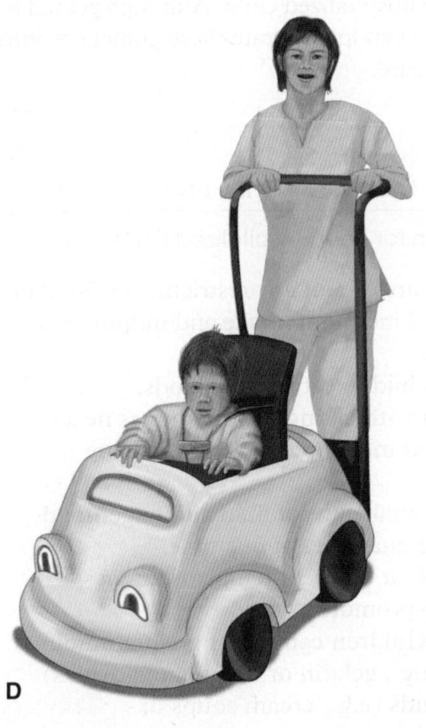

● Figure 11.4 Methods for transporting the infant or child. (**A**) Cradle method for carrying infants up to 3 months of age. One hand grasps the infant's thighs; the other arm supports the infant's head and back. (**B**) The "over-the-shoulder method" for carrying infants up to 7 months of age. Support the head if the infant does not have head control. (**C**) Football method for carrying infants up to 2 months of age. The forearm and hand supports the body and head of the infant. (**D**) A wagon with rails and padding is used to transport small children.

Table 11.6 Developmental Considerations for Bathing

Age of Child	Special Considerations
Infants	Use a sponge bath or tub bath to bathe young infants who cannot sit unaided. Support the infant's body at all times. Ensure appropriate water temperature. Avoid use of talcum powder.
Toddlers	Bathe older infants and toddlers at the bedside or in a regular bathtub, depending on their health condition.
School-age children and adolescents	Older children may prefer a shower if available and acceptable for their health condition. Assess whether a shower would be safe. Provide privacy.

Hair Care

Lying in bed can make the hair matted and tangled. Avoid pulling on the child's hair when combing or brushing it. If necessary, use commercial detangling solutions to ease combing.

If the hair requires washing, this is often done during the daily bath for infants. Typically, shampooing once or twice a week is sufficient for younger children. Adolescents may need more frequent shampooing due to the increase in sebaceous gland secretion. The frequency of shampooing also varies based on the child's condition; for example, if the child has experienced diaphoresis, more frequent shampooing may be indicated.

Shampooing may be done at the bedside with specially adapted equipment, at a readily accessible sink while the child is sitting in a chair or lying on a stretcher, or in a tub or shower. Commercial no-rinse shampoos may be available for use. With these products, the shampoo is applied to the hair and then brushed or combed out.

If the child uses a tub or shower for hair care, monitor the child's safety throughout to ensure that the child does not slip and fall due to the slippery surface or is burned because of improper water temperature.

The child's ethnicity may require special measures for hair care. For example, a child of African-American descent may use a broad-toothed comb for hair care. Ask the child's parents to bring one from home if one is not available. Also ask the child and parents about any products used on the hair to make it easier to handle; the parents can bring some from home. Encourage the parents to help with braiding or plaiting of the hair if desired.

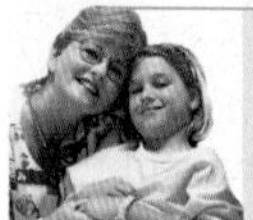

The hair of African-Americans typically is easier to comb when wet, so if possible comb the child's hair soon after shampooing.

Oral Hygiene

Oral hygiene is an important part of basic care. Wipe the infant's gums with a wet cloth after each feeding. Assist children in brushing and flossing their teeth after each feeding or meal and before bedtime. The child who is immunosuppressed needs special attention to oral hygiene, such as using soft toothbrushes and moistened gauze sponges to prevent bleeding and careful inspection of the oral cavity for areas of breakdown.

Nutritional Care

Adequate nutrition is necessary for growth and development and tissue repair, so it is an essential component of care for the ill or hospitalized child.

Frequently, the ill or hospitalized child experiences a loss of appetite, which can affect the child's nutritional status. This may be compounded by other problems such as nausea and vomiting and NPO restrictions for testing or surgery.

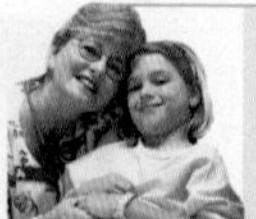

Never attempt to force a child to eat. This can exacerbate nausea and vomiting and can lead to an aversion to food that extends past the hospital stay (Hockenberry, 2004).

If possible, schedule procedures or treatments away from mealtimes. In younger children, refusing to eat may be related to the child's feeling of separation; in others, refusing to eat reflect the child's attempt to control the situation. Encourage parents to use gentle persuasion instead of force to assist with intake. They should give the child choices about what to eat; this reinforces the child's sense of control. Remind parents that the child's appetite will probably improve as his or her condition improves. Teaching Guideline 11.2 provides some tips for promoting nutrition in the hospitalized child. Although geared to parents, nurses also can incorporate these guidelines into the child's plan of care.

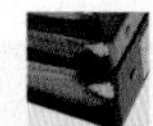

TEACHING GUIDELINE 11.2

Promoting Nutrition for Your Hospitalized Child

- Check with the nurse about any restrictions related to your child's diet. Find out if intake and output are being monitored.
- Encourage your child to eat favorite foods.
- Assist your child with eating or drinking as necessary; be present at mealtimes to help promote socialization.
- Frequently offer small cups of fluid and finger foods; avoid giving large quantities at one time.
- Try offering fluids at different temperatures at different times to promote variety.
- Remember that children can ingest greater amounts of thin liquids (e.g., gelatin or carbonated drinks) than thicker liquids (e.g., cream soups or milkshakes).
- Include ice chips as fluid intake. Ice is approximately equivalent to half the same amount of water (e.g., 1 cup of ice equals a half-cup of water).
- Use straws (unless not allowed) and brightly colored utensils, cups, or dishes to provide contrast and stimulation.
- Offer the child choices; when using a menu, allow the child to choose what he or she wants.
- Avoid spicy or highly seasoned foods.
- Talk with the dietitian to see if any special preferences can be addressed.
- Offer praise to your child for what he or she eats or drinks.
- Never punish the child for not eating or drinking.
- Encourage the older child to help keep track of what he or she eats and drinks.

Addressing the Effects of Hospitalization Developmentally

When addressing the fears, separation anxiety, and loss of control that occur in hospitalized children, the nurse should consider the child's age and cognitive or developmental level. Interventions are then based on how the child experiences these stressors at that age or developmental level. The content, timing, setting, and method of preparation are also based on the child's age and cognitive or developmental level. General guidelines for addressing fear and anxiety, separation anxiety, and loss of control are provided in Box 11.2.

Newborns and Infants

Assess the development or lack of development that is occurring in the infant, and assess the baby's attachment to the parents or primary caregivers. The infant's facial expression is the most consistent indicator of pain or bodily injury. To decrease fear and minimize separation anxiety, avoid separation from the primary caregiver if possible; this will also promote healthy attachment. If the parent or primary caregiver cannot stay with the infant, arrange for volunteers to provide consistent comfort to the baby.

Maintaining the infant's home routine related to sleep and feeding helps decrease feelings of loss of control. Weigh the infant daily, at the same time, on the same scale. Monitor intake and output closely. Be alert to signs of discomfort other than crying, such as a furrowed brow or tense body posture. Additional nursing goals related to promoting growth and development of the infant were presented in Table 11.4 earlier in this chapter.

Toddlers

Key nursing concerns when caring for toddlers center are separation anxiety, adequate growth and development, and autonomy. Establishing a trusting relationship with the toddler through nonthreatening play may decrease the amount of fear the toddler feels. Be alert to subtle, nonverbal indicators of grief or discontent.

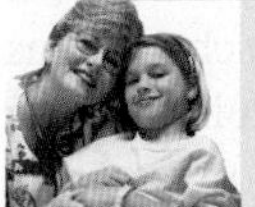

Keep the bed or crib and playroom as "safe" places. Perform invasive procedures such as venipunctures in the treatment room if possible. Never perform any nursing interventions in the playroom, no matter how nonthreatening they may appear to the nurse.

Encourage the parent or primary caregiver to stay with the toddler in the hospital to decrease separation anxiety. Maintaining the home routine related to meals and sleep or a nap provides similar structure and may help decrease the toddler's feelings of loss of control. If indicated, weigh the toddler daily. Closely monitor intake and output. Refer to Table 11.4 for additional nursing considerations related to promoting growth and development in the hospitalized toddler.

Preschoolers

Nursing care for the hospitalized preschooler focuses on their special needs, fears, and fantasies. When working with preschoolers, remember that they use magical thinking and fantasy. Be honest and specific, providing information just prior to the intervention to allay the child's fears. As with toddlers, encouraging parental involvement may decrease the amount of separation anxiety the preschooler experiences while in the hospital. Allowing the preschooler to make simple decisions such as which color bandage to use or whether to take medicine from a cup or syringe helps the child to feel some sense of control. Table 11.4 gives specific nursing considerations related to promoting growth and development for the preschooler in the hospital.

School-Age Children

Provide honest information using concrete, meaningful words to the school-age child to minimize fear of the

BOX 11.2

GUIDELINES TO ADDRESS THE GENERAL EFFECTS OF HOSPITALIZATION

Minimizing Fear and Anxiety	Addressing/Minimizing Separation Anxiety	Addressing Loss of Control
• Know the developmental stages in which magical thinking occurs. • Explain everything to children and their families before it occurs (see Chapter 14). • Use age-appropriate communication techniques. Include the family in this process so they can help the child cope with these fears.	• Know the stages of separation anxiety and be able to recognize them. • Remember that behaviors demonstrated during the first stage do not indicate that the child is "bad." • Encourage the family to stay with the child. • Help the child cope, and intervene before the behaviors of detachment occur. • Try guided imagery, using the child's imagination and enjoyment of play, to help the child relax (Bricher, 2000).	• Minimize physical restrictions, altered routines and rituals, and dependency issues, because they produce loss of control. • Recognize the child's inherent powerlessness in the hospital setting and explore strategies that give children an opportunity to participate in their own health care decisions (Bricher, 2000).

unknown. School-age children are still very attached to their parents, so encouraging parental involvement or rooming-in decreases separation anxiety. Involve the child in making simple decisions and planning the schedule as appropriate to give him or her a sense of control. Nursing considerations when caring for hospitalized school-age children include ensuring safety and promoting growth and development (see Table 11.4 earlier in this chapter).

Adolescents

The adolescent may or may not express fears. Educate the teen honestly: younger teens require more concrete explanations, while older teens can process more abstract concepts. Respect the teen's need for privacy. Encourage visits from the adolescent's friends to minimize anxiety related to separation. Prepare a mutually agreeable schedule with the teen, as appropriate, that includes the teen's preferences while incorporating the required nursing care. Collaborating with the adolescent will provide the teen with increased control. Refer to Table 11.4 earlier in this chapter for additional nursing considerations related to care of the adolescent in the hospital.

> **Think back to Jake,** the 8-year-old from the beginning of the chapter. Discuss nursing care you could provide that will help minimize stressors.

Providing Play, Activities, and Recreation for the Hospitalized Child

Play is an important component in the child's plan of care. Today many health care settings providing care for children have playrooms with age-appropriate toys, equipment, and other creative activities (Fig. 11.5). If the facility is large enough, there may even be a separate area for teens where they can listen to music, play video games, and visit with peers. Obviously, some children will not be able to use these facilities if their activity level is restricted or if isolation is necessary. Children may also play in their rooms. Ensure that opportunities for unstructured play are provided to all children who can engage in play. Therapeutic play may be used to teach children about their health status or to allow them to work through issues in their lives.

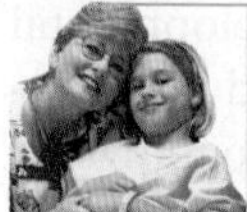

Avoid using the term "playroom" when caring for older school-aged children and adolescents. Instead, call it the "activity room" or "social room." Doing so promotes a greater feeling of maturity and makes it more likely that they will use the area.

Child Life Specialist

The **child life specialist** (CLS) is a specially trained individual who provides programs that prepare children for hospitalization, surgery, and other procedures that could be painful (Child Life Council, 1998–2003). The CLS is a member of the multidisciplinary team and works in conjunction with the health care providers and parents to foster an atmosphere that promotes the child's well-being. Services provided by a CLS include:

- Nonmedical preparation for tests, surgeries, and other medical procedures
- Support during medical procedures
- Therapeutic play
- Activities to support normal growth and development
- Sibling support
- Grief and bereavement support
- Emergency room interventions for children and families
- Hospital preadmission tours and information programs
- Outpatient consultation with families (Child Life Council, 1998–2003; available at http://www.childlife.org/About/what_is_specialist.htm)

Unstructured Play

Unstructured play allows children to control events, ideas, and relationships. Encourage parents to bring small toys

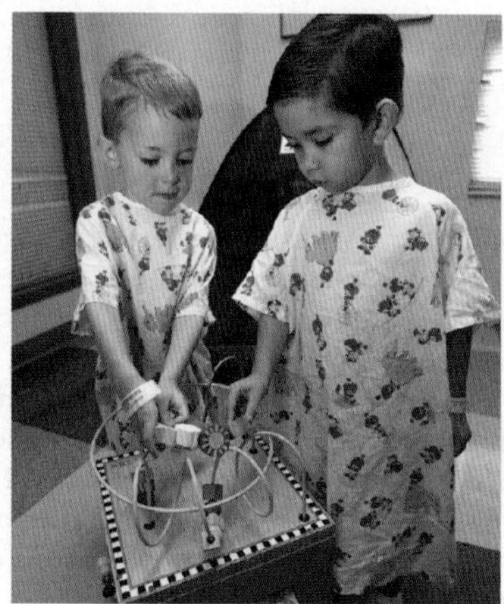

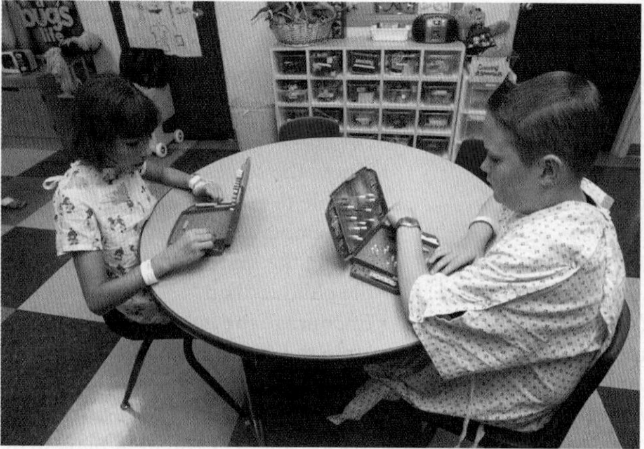

● **Figure 11.5** Children occupied in a hospital playroom. It is important to provide age-appropriate activities for younger and older children alike.

and favorite stuffed animals from home to make the child feel more comfortable in the strange environment of the hospital. Children also enjoy receiving small new toys as surprises when they are hospitalized. Many children enjoy diversional activities such as playing board games or electronic games, reading books, and watching TV, videos, or DVDs. Quiet activities appropriate to the developmental level of the child provide the opportunity for play and encourage the use and development of fine motor skills even if the child is confined to bed. Infants and toddlers enjoy manipulating blocks and playing with stacking toys. The preschooler may enjoy coloring, dollhouses, or playing with plastic building blocks such as Legos. School-age children and adolescents may enjoy playing video games or building a model geared toward their developmental level.

Play as Part of Nursing Care

Play is also an important part of nursing care. Use play as appropriate while providing routine nursing care to the child. An example of the use of play in nursing care involves the school-age child's love of competition and games. To increase range of motion in a school-age child who is hospitalized for traction due to a fracture, have the child throw a soft sponge ball or beanbag ball into hoops, and compete against the child. To increase deep breathing, encourage the child to blow bubbles or blow a whistle. To increase intake of fluids, help the child create a graph to chart the number of glasses of fluids he or she drinks over a period of time. Award the child a sticker, baseball card, special pencil, or other small item if he or she reaches a certain level.

When using play as part of nursing care, it is important to evaluate the outcome of play. Play used in the manner described above should enhance the child's outcome. For example, for the child blowing bubbles, determine whether this activity enhanced coughing and deep breathing.

Therapeutic Play

WATCH & LEARN

Another important aspect of play is **therapeutic play**. Health care professionals use therapeutic play to help the child deal with the physical and psychological challenges associated with illness and hospitalization. Therapeutic play is nondirected and focuses on helping the child cope with his or her feelings and fears. Supervised play with medical equipment in the hospital environment can help children work thorough their feelings about what has happened to them (Fig. 11.6). In a hospital that is large enough or that is a children's hospital, the CLS typically coordinates these activities. Goals include maintaining normal living patterns, minimizing psychological trauma, and promoting optimal development of the child. If a CLS is not available at the facility, the nurse provides this type of activity. There is a greater emphasis on the developmental and psychosocial implications of illness and hospitalization and validation of the child's voice (Bricher, 2000).

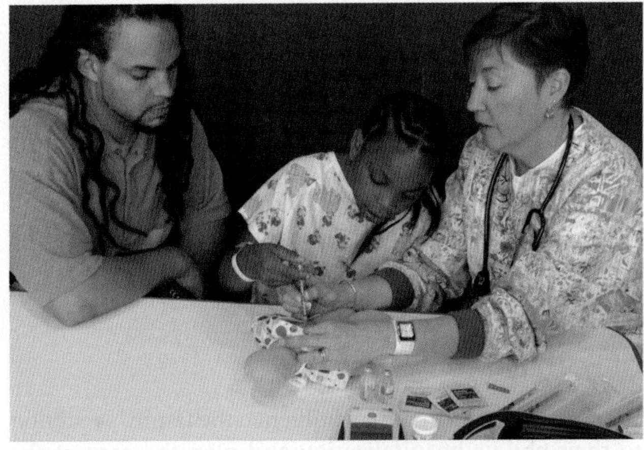

● **Figure 11.6** The nurse supervises play with medical equipment to help the child work through her feelings about being hospitalized.

In emotional outlet play or traumatic play, the child acts out or dramatizes real-life stressors. For example, using a wooden hammer and pegs, a soft sponge ball, or boxing gloves can allow the child to express anger over separation from family and friends. Commercial toys such as anatomically correct dolls and puppets have removable parts so children can see various organs of the body. Sometimes younger children "talk" to puppets and dolls, allowing them to express their feelings to a nonthreatening "person" about a specific situation or what they want from the health care provider. For example, the Shadow Buddies dolls mentioned earlier in the chapter provide a way of coping with a specific condition. For example, there is an ostomy buddy who has a stoma, a cancer buddy with thinning hair and a chest catheter for chemotherapy treatments, and a heart buddy who has a chest incision and a repaired heart. If the child has a dressing, the doll can also get one.

Other types of therapeutic play include drawing and supervised "needle play." Drawing is another method for the child to express his or her thoughts and feelings. Supervised "needle play" assists children who must undergo frequent blood work, injections, or intravenous procedures. A doll can receive an injection as the child works out his or her anger and anxiety. Keep in mind safety and the child's growth and development level before planning this type of directed play; an adult must always be present.

Promoting Schoolwork and Education During Hospitalization

Promote schoolwork and the child's typical activities while he or she is in the hospital. Determine the amount of this schoolwork by assessing the child's condition, the availability of teachers, and the family situation. Many children's hospitals have teachers at the hospitals; there may be classrooms too. These teachers work closely with the child's neighborhood school to continue schoolwork as the child's condition permits. Hospitals without the educational staff will rely on parents to coordinate with the child's school. Parents may bring in schoolbooks and the child's routine work or homework for completion while in the hospital. This connection to the child's school as well as interactions with peers helps maintain normalcy for the child and minimizes the disruption of everyday life.

Addressing the Needs of Family Members

Assess the factors that may influence the family's reaction to their child's hospitalization and plan the care of the child to accommodate some of these issues. Encourage families to have support systems in place before, during, and after hospitalization. Basically, using good communication and tailoring your actions to the family's needs and preferences increase the parents' satisfaction with the health care setting (Marino & Hayes, 2000).

Parents and Caregivers

As stated previously, the anxiety level of caregivers greatly affects the anxiety level of the child. Thus, it is important to help the family work through their feelings. Common sources of parental anger when a child is hospitalized include visiting restrictions, an unexpected change in the child's health status, confusion resulting from conflicting or insufficient information provided by the hospital staff, and feeling undervalued in the care of their child (Griffin, 2003).

The importance of family involvement to the well-being of the child is reflected in the philosophies, policies, procedures, and physical environments where care is delivered. The philosophy of family-centered care places the family at the core of care.

Miles, Carlson, and Brunesen (1999) found four dimensions of support for families:

1. Supportive communication and providing information about the child's illness and treatment plan
2. Parental support focused on respecting, enhancing, and supporting the parental role
3. Emotional support to help parents cope with their emotional responses and needs related to the child's illness
4. Caregiving support, involving the quality of care provided to the child

The family is the primary and continuing provider of the care for the child. Encourage parents to room in with the child throughout the hospital stay, if possible. Facilities can be designed to welcome family participation. For example, having computer ports and fax machines available and providing extra meals and sleeping arrangements for the parents can encourage parents to participate in care. View the parents as vital members of the health care team and partners in the care of the ill child.

Siblings

Family-centered care recognizes the need to treat the child in context of the family, including siblings. Important questions that will affect how siblings deal with the hospitalization of their brother or sister include:

- Was the admission an emergency?
- Were there previous admissions, and how did the siblings perceive those hospitalizations?
- How serious is the illness or trauma?
- Is the prognosis known?

Address the sibling's possible feelings of guilt. Use educational materials, allow time for visits, send photographs back and forth between siblings, and allow siblings to talk on the phone.

Providing Patient Teaching

Not all experiences with hospitalization are negative: in fact, the experience may enhance the child's and family's coping skills, bolster self-esteem, and provide new socialization experiences. It may allow the child to master self-care skills and provides an opportunity for the child and family to learn new information. Parents may learn more about their child's growth and development skills as well as additional parenting or caregiving skills, resulting in improvement in their parenting abilities. In addition, the child's overall health may be improved if because of the hospital stay the child receives current immunizations and the parents learn more about health care practices.

The overall goals of patient and family teaching are to minimize the child's and family's stress, educate them about treatment and nursing care in the hospital, and ensure the family can provide appropriate care at home upon discharge. Providing support before, during, and after hospitalization may minimize stress. Preadmission programs can introduce the child and family to the setting. During the hospital stay, forming partnerships with the child and family, using strategies to promote coping, and providing appropriate preparation for procedures, tests, and surgery serve to decrease stress.

Assess the child's and family's knowledge of the illness and hospital experience. This provides a baseline for teaching. Include hospital rules in child and family teaching. Behavioral changes in hospitalized children often disturb parents or caregivers. Determine the child's usual patterns of behavior and explain to the parents about the child's reaction to hospitalization. Encourage the family to maintain consistent discipline even while in the hospital to provide structure for the child as well as prevent discipline issues after discharge. Also discuss how siblings may react to the hospitalization and provide appropriate teaching to the siblings. Every interaction the nurse has with the child or family provides an opportunity for teaching. Explain the purpose of even simple procedures such as vital signs assessment to the child and family. Provide ongoing information about the child's illness or trauma, treatment plan, and expected outcomes. Chapter 3 gives general principles related to teaching children and their families.

Preparing the Child and Family for Discharge

Discharge planning actually begins upon admission. The nurse assesses the family's resources and knowledge level to determine what education and referrals they may need. Upon discharge, children and their parents or caregivers receive written instructions about home care, and a copy is retained in the medical record. These instructions are individualized for the child. Generally, discharge instructions should include:

- Follow-up appointment information
- Guidelines about when to contact the physician or nurse practitioner (e.g., new or worsening symptoms or indications that the child is not improving)
- Diet
- Activity level allowed
- Medications, including dose, times to be given, route, adverse effects, and special instructions; any prescriptions should be included
- Information on additional treatments the child requires at home.
- Specific dates for when the child may return to school or daycare
- Names and phone numbers of agencies the family has been referred to, such as durable medical equipment providers

Provide and review educational booklets that give basic health information or general care for a child with a particular disease (Fig. 11.7). Videotapes, DVDs, or CD-ROMs may also be used if available. The ability to watch a procedure over and over is helpful to some families. Explain, demonstrate, and request a return demonstration of any treatments or procedures to be done at home. Provide a written schedule if the child is to receive multiple medications, tube feedings, or other medical treatments. For complicated cases, a written teaching plan may be used to provide continuity of child/family education between various nurses. As the family attempts to perform each task, document whether the caregiver continues to require assistance or prompting with the task or whether he or she can perform the task independently.

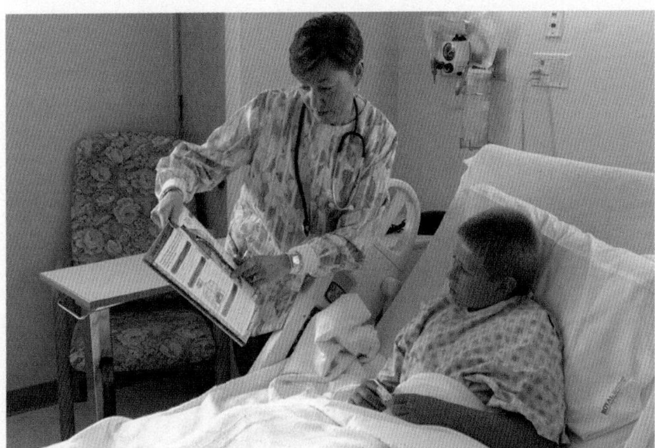

● Figure 11.7 The nurse uses charts with pictures to perform patient teaching before the child goes home.

Parents of children with multiple medical needs may benefit from a trial period of home care. This occurs while the child is still in the hospital, but the parents or caregivers provide all of the care that the child requires. Support the family and praise their accomplishments during this trial period.

References

Books and Journals

AHRQ's Medical Clearinghouse. (1999). Report #00-8014. Annual Report on Access to and Utilization of Health Care for Children and Youth in the United States. Rockville, MD: Author.

Algren, C. L., & Algren, J. T. (1997). Pediatric sedation: Essentials for the perioperative nurse. *Nursing Clinics of North America, 32*(1), 17–30.

Alsop-Shields, L., & Mohay, H. (2001). John Bowlby and James Robertson: Theorists, scientists, and crusaders for improvements in the care of children in hospital. *Journal of Advanced Nursing, 35*(1), 50–58.

Bowlby, J. A. (1988). *A secure base: Parent-child attachment and healthy human development.* New York: Basic Books.

Bricher, G. (2000). Children in the hospital: Issues of power and vulnerability. *Pediatric Nursing, 26*(3), 277.

Burke, S. O., Kauffman, E., Harrison, M. B., & Wiskin, N. (1999). Assessment of stressors in families with a child who has a chronic condition. *MCN: The Journal of Maternal-Child Nursing, 24,* 98–106.

Child Life Council. (1998–2003). What is a child life specialist? Available at: http://www.childlife.org/About/what_is_specialist.htm.

Craft, M. J., & Wyatt, N. (1986). Effect of visitation upon siblings of hospitalized children. *Maternal Child Nursing Journal,* (150), 47–59.

Crole, N., & Smith, L. (2002). Examining the phases of nursing care of the hospitalized child. *Australian Nursing Journal, 9*(8), 30.

Griffin, T. (2003) Facing challenges to family-centered care, II: Anger in the clinical setting. *Pediatric Nursing, 29*(3), 212–214.

Herron, R. (2005). Young patients learn "on tour" with Pediatric Express. *Advance for Nurses, 3*(24), 10.

Hockenberry, M. (2004). *Wong's essentials of pediatric nursing* (7th ed.). St. Louis: Mosby.

Huth, M. M., Broome, M. E., & Good, M. (2004). Imagery reduces children's post-operative pain. *Pain, 110*(1–2), 439–448.

Joint Commission on Accreditation of Healthcare Organizations. (2004). *Setting the standard: The Joint Commission and Health Care Safety and Quality.* Oakbrook Terrace, IL: JCAHO.

JCAHO (2005). Restraint and seclusion. Available at: http://www.jointcommission.org/AccreditationPrograms/Hospitals/Standards/FAQs/Provision+of+Care/Restraint+and+Seclusion/Restraint_Seclusion.htm.

Justus, R., Wyles, D., Wilson, J., et al. (2006). Preparing children and families for surgery: Mount Sinai's multidisciplinary perspective. *Pediatric Nursing, 32*(1), 35–43.

Mansson, M. E., & Dykes, A. (2004). Practices for preparing children for clinical examination and procedures in Swedish pediatric wards. *Pediatric Nursing, 30*(3), 182.

Marino, B. L., Marion, E. K., & Hayes, J. S. (2000). Parents' reports of children's hospital care: What it means for your practice. *Pediatric Nursing, 26*(2), 195–198.

Miles, M. S., Carlson, J., & Brunesen, S. (1999). The nurse-parent support tool. *Journal of Pediatric Nursing, 14,* 44–50.

Munro, H., & D'Errico, F. C. (2000). Parental involvement in perioperative anesthetic management. *Journal of PeriAnesthesia Nursing, 15*(Dec), 397–400.

Partis, M. (2000). Focus: Children. Bowlby's attachment theory: Implications for health visiting. *British Journal of Community Nursing, 5*(10), 499–503.

Pillitteri, A. (2003). *Maternal and child health nursing* (4th ed.). Philadelphia: Lippincott Williams & Wilkins.

Rennick, J. E., Johnston, C. C., Dougerty, G., & Ritchie, J. A. (2002). Children's psychological response after critical illness and exposure to invasive technology. *Journal of Developmental and Behavioral Pediatrics, 23*(3), 133–144.

Romino, S. L., Keatley, V. M., Secrest, J., & Good, K. (2005). Parental presence during anesthesia induction in children. *AORN Journal, 81*(4), 779–792.

Sigrest, T. D., Neff, J. M., Eichner, J. M., & Hardy, D. R. (2003). Facilities and equipment for the care of pediatric patients in a community hospital. *Pediatrics, 111*(5), 1120.

Simon, K. (1993). Perceived stress of nonhospitalized children during the hospitalization of children. *Journal of Pediatric Nursing, 8*(5), 298–304.

Stratton, K. M. (2004). Parents' experiences of their child's care during hospitalization. *Journal of Cultural Diversity, 11*(1), 4.

Weiss, B. D., ed. (1999) *20 common problems in primary care.* New York: McGraw Hill.

Winch, A. (2001). Role play: A nurse's role in helping well children cope with a parent's serious illness and/or hospitalization. *Journal of the Society of Pediatric Nurses, 6*(1), 42–46.

Wollin, S. R., Plummer, J. L., Owen, H., et al. (2004). Anxiety in children having elective surgery. *Journal of Pediatric Nursing, 19*(2), 128–132.

Websites

www.aap.org American Academy of Pediatrics
www.familycentercare.org Institute for Family-Centered Care
www.starbright.org Starbright Foundation

Chapter WORKSHEET

● MULTIPLE CHOICE QUESTIONS

1. The nurse would most likely assess separation anxiety in which child?
   a. A 2-month-old infant
   b. A 15-month-old toddler
   c. A 4-year-old preschooler
   d. An 11-year-old child
2. When developing the preoperative plan of care for an adolescent, the nurse plans interventions to address the adolescent's anxieties and fears related to:
   a. Separation from parents
   b. Punishment for wrongdoings
   c. Changes in body image
   d. Magical thinking
3. The nurse is preparing a 5-year-old boy for surgery on his lower leg. His mother is helping him into the hospital gown and the boy fights removal of his underwear. What is the most appropriate nursing action?
   a. Allow the mother to remove the underwear.
   b. Tell the boy he is acting childishly.
   c. Notify the OR that the underwear is on.
   d. Allow the boy to keep his underwear on.
4. A 6-month-old infant requires restraint to prevent removal of his nasogastric tube. What is the priority nursing intervention?
   a. Tie the restraint loosely to prevent skin breakdown.
   b. Leave the baby unrestrained when directly observed.
   c. Position the restrained infant prone to prevent aspiration.
   d. Place the infant in a room near the nurses' station.
5. A 10-year-old child on a regular diet refuses to eat the food on her meal tray. She requests chicken nuggets, French fries, and ice cream. What is the best nursing action?
   a. Ask that the child's desired foods be sent up from the kitchen.
   b. Negotiate with the child to eat at least part of the food on the tray.
   c. Remove a privilege.
   d. Offer the child cereal and milk from stock on the nursing unit.

● CRITICAL THINKING EXERCISES

1. Becky, an 8-year-old, is admitted to the pediatric unit for an emergency surgery. She is in third grade and very active in after-school programs. Her mother is with her during the admission process but will have to return to work shortly after Becky returns from surgery to the pediatric unit. Would the nurse expect Becky to show separation anxiety? What are the three top nursing diagnoses for Becky?
2. A 6-year-old is admitted to the general pediatric unit after spending several hours in the emergency department with an acute asthma attack. Her mother and two younger siblings are present, but the mother plans to leave shortly to take the siblings home. The father will visit in about 2 hours, after work. What is the overall goal for this child's care? What could the nurse say to promote coping in this child? What would be the best answer if the mother asks if she should stay?

● STUDY ACTIVITIES

1. Shadow a child life specialist in a hospital. Identify his or her role and how he or she works with the nursing staff.
2. Follow a child and family during the admission process, from preadmission to initial time on the unit, to identify the procedures and tasks involved. Examine the response of the child and family and how the nursing staff responds to their needs.
3. Spend a day in the radiology department or the emergency room to learn about the strategies used to prepare children for various procedures.
4. Develop a teaching plan to orient a toddler or preschooler and his or her family to a nursing unit. Include the resources, personnel, and techniques to include in the teaching plan.

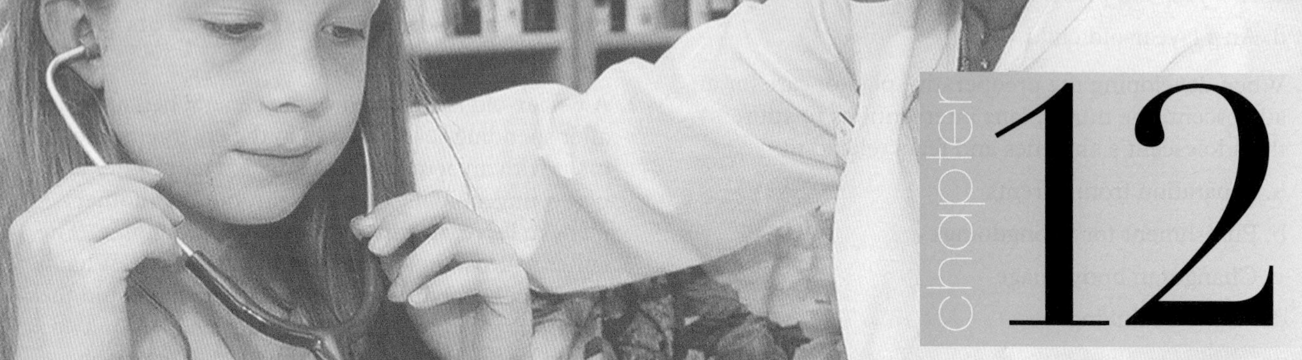

chapter 12

Nursing Care of the Child in the Community

Key TERMS

community
epidemiology
family-centered care
Individualized Health Plan
medically fragile child
outpatient and ambulatory care
technology dependent
triage

Learning OBJECTIVES

Upon completion of the chapter, the learner will be able to:

1. Explain the factors that have created an increased emphasis on community- and home-based nursing care.
2. Describe the various roles of community and home care nurses.
3. Discuss the variety of settings in which community-based care occurs.
4. Examine the major components and key elements of family-centered home health care.
5. Discuss the advantages and disadvantages of home health care.
6. Discuss discharge planning and case management and their role in home care.

WOW *Nurses should leave their "comfort zone" of practice and reach out to patients on their turf to make a difference.*

Jeremy Jacobsen, a 6-year-old boy with cerebral palsy, receives continuous gastrostomy feedings and has frequent respiratory infections. He has been receiving nursing care at home along with therapies for many years but is now ready to make the transition to the local elementary school.

Children receive most of their health care, well and ill care, in the community setting. Nurses play an important role in the health and wellness of a community. They not only meet the health care needs of individuals but go beyond to create interventions that affect the community as a whole. Nurses practice in a variety of settings within a community, such as clinics and physician's offices, schools, shelters, churches, health departments, community health centers, and homes. They promote the health of individuals, families, groups, communities, and populations and promote an environment that supports health.

Community Health Nursing

Nursing in the community is aimed at disease prevention and improvement of the health of populations and communities. Population is defined as "a collection of individuals who have one or more personal or environmental characteristics in common" (Community Health Nurses Association of Canada, 2003, p. 20). **Community** can be defined as a "specific group of people, often living in a defined geographical area, who share a common culture, values, and norms and who are arranged in a social structure according to relationships the community has developed over a period of time" (Community Health Nurses Association of Canada, 2003, p.18). Community health nurses work in geographically and culturally diverse settings. They address current and potential health needs of the population or community. They promote and preserve the health of a population and are not limited to particular age groups or diagnoses. Public health nursing is a specialized area of community health nursing.

Epidemiology can help determine the health and health needs of a population and assist in planning health services. Community health nurses perform epidemiologic investigations in order to help analyze and develop health policy and community health initiatives. Community health initiatives can be focused on the community as a whole or a specific target population with specific needs. *Healthy People 2010* (HP 2010) is an example of national health initiatives developed using the epidemiological process. HP 2010 ensures that health care professionals look at the individual as well as the community. It presumes that there is an unavoidable link between the individual's health and the health of the community (Lurie, 2000). Nurses play a key role in the health of a community and the individuals who reside in it.

HP 2010 is the third edition of national health goals, which were launched in 1979. HP 2010 has two major goals: to increase the quality of life and life expectancy of individuals of all ages and to decrease health disparities among different populations. HP 2010 is a comprehensive health initiatives plan. Nurses can help the nation meet these objectives by educating those in the community on appropriate prevention strategies, such as proper immunization and smoking cessation (see individual chapters for relevant HP objectives and nursing implications). HP 2010 is available online at www.healthypeople.gov.

Community-Based Nursing

In the past the major role of the nurse in the community was that of the community health nurse or public health nurse. This is now a subset of what is considered community-based nursing.

Shifting Responsibilities From Hospital-Based to Community-Based Nursing Care

Over the past 50 years there has been a shift in responsibilities of care for children from the hospital or other institutions to homes and communities (Meleski, 2002). There has been an increase in community-based care due to shorter hospital stays and cost containment. Community care, especially home care, is a rapidly growing service in the United States. Community-based care has been shown to be a cost-effective way to provide care. Increases in disposable income and the longevity of children with chronic and debilitating health conditions have also contributed to the continued shift of health care to the community and home setting. Advances in technology have allowed for improved monitoring of patients in community settings and at home, as well as allowing complicated procedures, such as intravenous administration of antibiotics, to be done at home.

Another major reason for the increase in community care, especially home care, in children is the understanding that an acute care setting is not an appropriate environment for children to grow up in (Hewitt-Taylor, 2005). Caring for children at home not only improves their physical health but also allows for adequate growth and development while keeping them within their family. They are in a familiar environment with the comfort and support of family, which leads to improved care and quality of life.

Role of the Community-Based Nurse

With the shift in responsibilities from hospital care to community care have come changes in nursing care. More opportunities exist for nurses to provide direct care to clients in the community setting, especially the home.

Community-based nursing care differs from nursing care in the acute setting. In the community or home care setting, the nurse provides direct patient care but spends more time in the role of educator, communicator, and manager than the nurse in the acute care setting. In home care the nurse spends a significant amount of time in the supervision or management role. Community-based nursing focuses on the practice of nursing that provides personal care to individuals and families in the community. Community-based nurses focus on promoting and preserving health as well as preventing disease or injury. They are educators, managers of care, and advocates along with being direct providers of care.

Education and Communication

The community-based nurse must use the principles and techniques of interpersonal communication. The nurse must be able to assess the client's and family's learning needs and their readiness to learn. As hospital stays becomes shorter and admissions to the hospital become less frequent, teaching now begins wherever the client or family enters the health care system. Many times initial teaching occurs in the community setting, especially the home. In the community-based setting, client teaching is often focused on assisting the client and family to achieve independence.

Discharge Planning and Case Management

Due to the short length of stays in acute settings and the shift to community settings for children with complex health needs, discharge planning and case management have become an important nursing role. Discharge planning involves the development and implementation of a comprehensive plan for the safe discharge of a client from a health care facility and for continuing safe and effective care in the community and at home. Case management focuses on coordinating health care services while balancing quality and cost outcomes. Often children requiring community-based care, especially home care, have complex medical needs that require an interdisciplinary team to meet the child's physical, psychosocial, medical, nursing, developmental, and education needs. The nurse plays an important role as the link between team members and the client to ensure that the child and family are receiving comprehensive, coordinated care.

Advocacy and Resource Management

Another important role of the community-based nurse is to advocate for the child and family to ensure that their needs are being met and that they have available resources and appropriate health care services. Working in a child and family's home can lead one to become overly involved in the situation. To best serve the child and family, the community-based nurse must be an advocate and educator but avoid becoming a personal friend (Thompson, 2000).

Nurses must have a basic understanding of community, state, and federal resources to ensure they are providing families with the resources they may need. One such resource important in the community-based care of children with complex medical needs is Medicaid and Medicaid waivers. Medicaid is a national program providing medical assistance for children and families with low incomes. It is jointly run by the federal and state governments but is administered state by state; therefore, provisions vary widely. Medical model waivers are state-run programs that use federal and state funds to pay for health care for people with certain medical conditions. Home- and community-based waiver programs, such as the Katie Beckett waiver (also known as the Deeming waiver), allow children and young adults with complex medical needs to be cared for at home and make them eligible for Medicaid based on their own income and assets, regardless of their parents' income. Without medical waiver programs, many children with special needs would either go without health care or would be institutionalized in order to qualify for Medicaid. (Read about Katie Beckett at http://www.partoparvt.org/02sKatie.html.)

Physical Care

The community-based nurse performs less direct physical care than the nurse in the acute care setting. Many times the nurse observes the client or caregiver performing physical care tasks. Excellent assessment skills are especially important in the community care setting. The nurse often functions in a more autonomous role; after data collection, the community-based nurse will often decide whether to initiate, continue, alter, or end physical nursing care. Assessment will go beyond physical assessment of the client to include the environment and the community.

Community-Based Nursing Settings

Community-based nursing takes place in a variety of settings, including physician's offices, clinics, health departments, urgent care centers, hospital outpatient centers, schools, camps, churches, shelters, and clients' homes. Community-based nurses provide well care, episodic ill care. and chronic care. They work to promote, preserve, and improve the health of children and families in these settings.

Outpatient and Ambulatory Care

Outpatient and ambulatory care is health care provided to individuals who do not require care in an acute setting. Due to advances in medical technology, more medical procedures, such as diagnostic tests, treatments, and surgeries, can be administered on an outpatient basis and do not require clients to be hospitalized. Outpatient and ambulatory care delivers convenient and cost-effective health care to children and their families, many times right within their own community. These settings allow for increased independence and permit clients to return to their normal routine as quickly as possible. More and more outpatient and ambulatory care centers are opening; they are being sponsored by health maintenance organizations (HMOs), physician's offices, community agencies and public health departments, and hospitals (Hunt, 2005).

Physician's Office or Clinic, Health Departments, and Urgent Care Centers

Physician's offices, clinics, health departments, and urgent care centers are used by children and their families for well care, episodic ill care, acute care, and care of chronic conditions. For well care and illness or injury, children are often seen by their primary care physician. They may visit a physician's office or clinic or the health department. In more acute situations or for after-hours issues that cannot wait until clinic operating hours, a child may be seen in an urgent care center or may be referred to the emergency department. The American Academy of Pediatrics discourages patients from using urgent care centers or the emergency department for routine care, since it is difficult to provide coordinated, comprehensive family-centered care consistent with a "medical home" concept (see Chapter 9 on medical homes) (Krug et al., 2005).

The nurse's role in these settings includes preparing clients, collecting pertinent health information, performing assessments, assisting the physician with diagnostic testing and procedures, administering injections and medications, changing wound dressings, assisting with minor surgery, helping to maintain records, and educating the child and family about home care and when to call the physician or return to be seen.

An essential component of primary care practice is telephone **triage**. Telephone triage constitutes a large percentage (more than 25%) of pediatric health treatment (Simonsen-Anderson, 2002). Up to 380 calls per week are received in the average pediatric office (Corjulo, 2005). Pediatric office nurses often fill this role. When parents feel comfortable with the providers in their child's medical home office, they often call for advice in order to treat their child at home. A telephone triage nurse needs excellent assessment and critical thinking skills along with solid training and education. The triage nurse needs to assess the patient's entire situation, including current signs and symptoms, history, and home treatment.

Protocols, standardized policies and procedures, and professional judgment guide the triage nurse in the decision-making process. Pediatric telephone protocols are available for purchase through the American Academy of Pediatrics (http://www.aap.org/). The triage nurse needs to determine whether the child requires emergency care, an office visit, or home management. Good listening and the ability to maintain a calm voice when talking to parents are skills necessary for successful telephone triage. The triage nurse should not discourage parents from bringing the child into the office to be seen; triage is not meant to keep children out of the office, and if a parent is very concerned, that is reason enough to be seen.

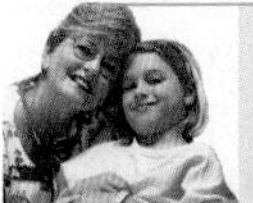

Parents often can pick up on subtle problems in their children. They may not be able to describe accurately signs and symptoms, but they know that their child "isn't acting right." Nurses must listen to parents and act on their concerns.

Outpatient Units

Outpatient units are used to keep hospital stays short and decrease the cost of hospitalization. Outpatient units may be a part of the hospital or a freestanding facility. The child and family arrive in the morning; the child undergoes the procedure, test, or surgery and then goes home in the evening. Examples of surgeries and procedures performed in outpatient settings include tympanostomy tube placement, hernia repair, tonsillectomy, cystoscopy, bronchoscopy, blood transfusions, dialysis, and chemotherapy. The advantages of this environment include minimal separation of the child from the family, minimal disruption of the family pattern, decreased risk of infection, and decreased cost. Disadvantages include that the unit does not have the equipment for overnight stays, so if there are complications the child will need to be transported to the hospital.

Many centers offer preoperative health assessment and teaching sessions. These allow the parent and child to ask questions and resolve them before the procedure. On the day of the procedure, parents should be allowed to be with their child until the procedure begins. Parents should also be allowed to be with their child in the postanesthesia recovery unit as quickly as possible. This provides reassurance and comfort to the child while meeting his or her physical and emotional needs.

The role of the nurse in the outpatient setting includes admission and assessment, preoperative teaching and preparation, client assessment and support, postoperative monitoring, case management, discharge planning, and teaching. Before the procedure the nurse reviews with the family the routine to be followed and any special instructions (such as NPO orders), and familiarizes the child with the setting to help alleviate fears. This may occur during the preoperative health assessment.

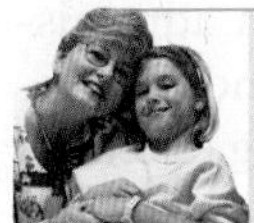

Encourage the parent to bring one of the child's favorite toys, blankets, or games to make the child feel more comfortable.

The nurse performs any surgical preparation and discusses intraoperative procedures as necessary. The nurse provides postoperative care and assessment of the child. Once the child's condition is stable and he or she meets the discharge criteria of the facility, the nurse reviews with the parent postoperative instructions, including pain management, care of the incision if appropriate, diet, activity, including return to school, necessary follow-up, and when to call the physician.

Medically Fragile Daycare Centers

The number of **medically fragile children** (children whose condition is considered medically complex and who require skilled nursing interventions) is growing. Reasons include the increased sophistication of medical technology, the increase in premature deliveries, and the increase in childhood trauma (Cernoch, 1992). It is estimated that 1 million children in the United States have complex, disabling, and costly health conditions (*The Exceptional Parent,* 2000). For many years these children lived in hospitals their entire lives. Due to concerns about the high cost of long-term hospitalization and the diminished quality of life for these children, alternative care settings in the community, such as medically fragile daycare centers, are being developed.

Medically fragile daycare centers are specifically designed to meet the needs of these children. Most centers accept children who have complicated medical needs or are **technology dependent**. Examples include children with multiple congenital anomalies, children who are ventilator dependent, children with respiratory conditions, children with cardiac conditions, and children with cancer. Some centers accept children with less complicated needs, such as cardiorespiratory monitoring or asthma, and some enroll children without health care needs to promote peer relationships and acceptance. Just as at a regular daycare center, the parents or caregivers can drop the child off in the morning and pick the child up in the afternoon. Some centers offer after-school, weekend, or respite services. The centers usually have indoor and outdoor play areas, educational activities, and arts and crafts and provide needed therapies.

Health professionals are present at these centers to provide for the children's medical, emotional, and developmental needs. Nurses trained in pediatric and neonatal care, physical therapists, occupational therapists, speech therapists, child life specialists, and social workers staff the centers; some centers have respiratory therapists on site. Children are able to receive all of their prescribed therapies while at the center. Nursing care includes direct care such as medication administration and dressing changes, assessment and evaluation of the child's overall condition, identifying potential medical emergencies, determining the need for changes in care or treatment and monitoring, and providing frequent treatments or interventions to maintain life and health.

Most centers are located in the community to help ease transportation issues. Some centers provide transportation to and from home or school. Centers are licensed by the state daycare licensing authorities or in some states Physician Prescribed Extended Care (PPEC) agencies. Families may be able to obtain financial assistance from their private insurance or Medicaid. The cost of community-based services, on average, is one third that of inpatient hospitalization (*The Exceptional Parent,* 2000). Other advantages of community-based centers over hospitalization or home care are a decrease in the children's rehospitalization rate and a decrease in family stress (*The Exceptional Parent,* 2000).

Schools

School nursing is a specialized practice of professional nursing and focuses on improving students' health to improve their achievement and success. School nurses work to remove or minimize health barriers to learning to provide students with the best opportunity to achieve academic success. The National Association of School Nurses defines school nursing as "a specialized practice of professional nursing that advances the well-being, academic success, and life-long achievement of students. To that end, school nurses facilitate positive student responses to normal development; promote health and safety; intervene with actual and potential health problems; provide case management services; and actively collaborate with others to build student and family capacity for adaptation, self management, self-advocacy, and learning" (Wolfe & Selekman, 2002, p. 406). See Healthy People 2010.

At the heart of school nursing is the belief that all children have the ability to learn and the right to an education, and that society is best served if all children are educated (Wolfe & Selekman, 2002). School nurses coordinate school health programs and link health service programs within the school and community. School nurses carry out a variety of roles in providing health care to children (Fig. 12.1). Box 12.1 lists some of the activities of the school nurse.

The population of students has changed over the years. Access to public schools for children with disabilities is mandated. Due to improvements in technology, children with chronic conditions or special needs live longer and enter school. There has been an increase in the number of children with psychiatric conditions such as depression, attention-deficit/hyperactivity disorder, and more serious conditions such as bipolar disorder. All have contributed to an increase in the number of children with diverse and sometimes complex health needs in the school system. The essential role of the school nurse has not changed, but the responsibilities and expectations have. School nurses are challenged to meet the growing needs of the changing school population.

HEALTHY PEOPLE 2010

Objective	Significance
Increase the proportion of middle, junior high, and senior high schools that provide school health education to prevent health problems in the following areas: unintentional injury; violence; suicide; tobacco use and addiction; alcohol and other drug use; unintended pregnancy, HIV/AIDS, and STD infection; unhealthy dietary patterns; inadequate physical activity; and environmental health.	• Provide education and training to school staff in health problem areas. • Work with schools to develop appropriate health education with focus on health problem areas. • Provide adequate health care services and health education to students.
Increase the proportion of elementary, middle, and high schools that have a nurse-to-student ratio of at least 1:750.	

Recall Jeremy Jacobsen, the 6-year-old boy with cerebral palsy. In recent years there have been many more children with special needs attending school than ever before. This brings many challenges for the teachers, staff, and school nurses employed by the school district. The principal of Jeremy's elementary school tells the school nurse that many of the teachers and staff have expressed concerns that they do not know anything about the health care needs of these children, including Jeremy. What kinds of interventions might the nurse plan?

Just as nurses in the acute care setting develop nursing care plans, nurses in the school setting develop **Individualized Health Plans** (IHPs). An IHP formalizes the plan of support for a student with complex health care needs. It is a written agreement developed as part of an interdisciplinary collaboration of school staff along with the student, the student's family, and the student's health care provider. The plan describes the student's needs and how the school plans to meet these needs. The nurse plays a critical role in developing these plans. The nurse will use the nursing process and then, based on the nursing assessment and diagnosis, will develop goals and interventions to ensure that the child's needs are being met. Examples of students who may need an IHP are students with asthma, serious allergies, chronic conditions such as type I diabetes, physical disabilities, attention-deficit/hyperactivity disorder, and medication needs. Figure 12.2 gives an example of an IHP for a child with asthma.

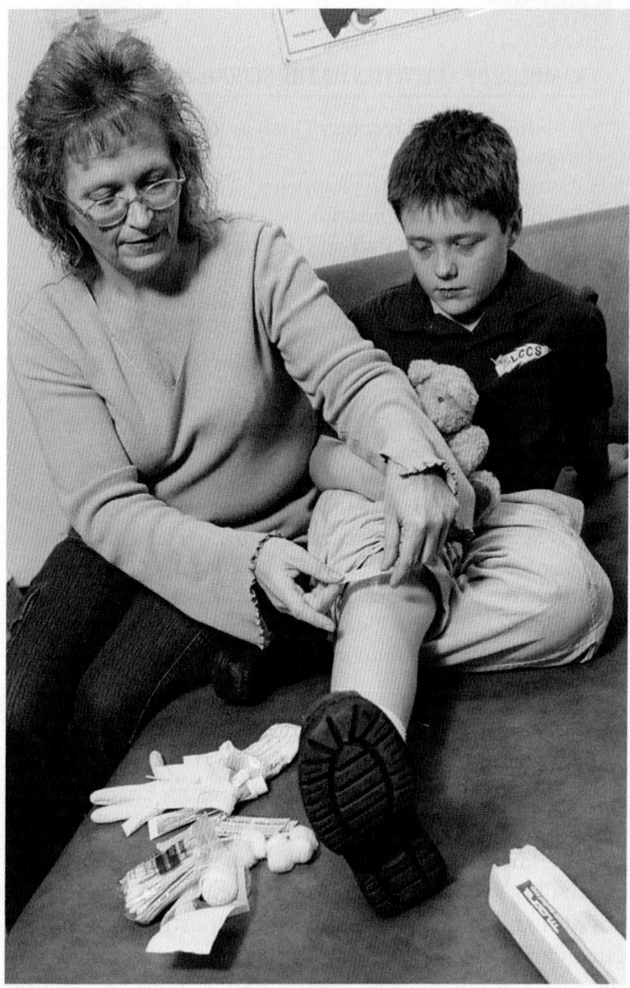

● **Figure 12.1** The school nurse provides nursing assessment as well as health education to students in the school setting.

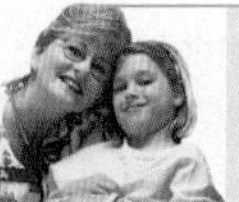

The IHP needs to include directions for care while the child is at school and also must take into account circumstances that may affect the student's health care needs, such as variations in school routine, absence of staff, special outings such as field trips and extracurricular activities, and a plan in case of emergency.

Other Community Settings

Nurses work in a variety of different settings within the community. Their primary focus continues to be on promoting health, preventing disease and injury, and ensuring a safe environment. Nurses play important roles in childcare centers, camps, health department clinics, and shelters. In childcare centers, nurses help address infection control issues and assess for a safe environment. They provide education and training to staff members. A camp nurse ensures a safe environment for all campers and provides first-aid and acute illness care as needed. Camps for children with special needs exist, staffed by specially trained

BOX 12.1
EXAMPLES OF ACTIVITIES OF THE SCHOOL NURSE

- Conduct health screenings (such as vision, hearing, and scoliosis)
- Assess growth and development
- Provide emergency first aid
- Train and educate staff on CPR, first aid, and health issues
- Assess, monitor, and refer students with communicable diseases
- Educate on health promotion and disease prevention (such as immunizations, bike and car safety, decreasing high-risk behaviors, such as smoking, drinking, drug use, and sexual activity)
- Serve as a resource for health issues and education
- Act as a liaison between home, school, and community
- Act as a liaison between health care provider and school
- Reinforce client and family health education (such as discharge instructions, self-care measures)
- Monitor long-term illness in students
- Network with community agencies and make necessary referrals

nurses. These camps cater to children with complex health care needs, such as diabetes, head injuries, and physical disabilities and allow the children the opportunity to experience camp life while providing a safe environment and necessary medical care. Health department and shelter nurses focus on health supervision services and connecting clients to needed community resources.

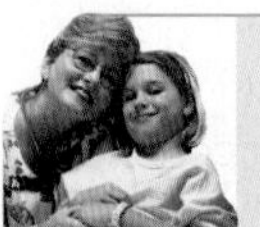

Nurses have a unique opportunity to give back to their community by volunteering their services in various settings, such as shelters and clinics in medically underserved areas.

Home Health Care

Home care provides short- or long-term services for children and their families in the home. It also is used for medically needy and technology-dependent children, such as ventilator-dependent children. Among those who often benefit from home care are children with acute illness, such as a child with osteomyelitis requiring intravenous antibiotics, or chronic health care issues, such as a child with bronchopulmonary dysplasia, that may have required traditional in-hospital care.

Home care is geared toward the needs of the client and family. Private-duty nursing care is used when more extensive care is needed; it may be delivered hourly (several hours per day) or on a full-time, live-in basis. Periodic visiting nurse care is used when the child needs intermittent interventions such as intravenous antibiotic administration, follow-up with patient teaching, and bilirubin monitoring. The goals of nursing care in the home setting include promoting, restoring, and maintaining the health of the child. Home care focuses on minimizing the effects of the illness or disability, along with providing the child or family with the means to care for the illness or disability at home. Nurses in the home care setting are direct providers of care, child and family educators, child and family advocates, and case managers.

There are some disadvantages to home care. The presence of health care professionals in the home can be an intrusion on family privacy. Also, caring for children with complex medical needs can be overwhelming for some families. Financial issues can become a large burden: families may have higher out-of-pocket costs if their insurance does not reimburse for home care. Having one parent at home full time and not earning an income can contribute to increased financial strain, not to mention social isolation of that parent. All of these can lead to increased stress on family members. The advantages of home care usually outweigh the disadvantages, but nurses need to be aware of these potential disadvantages and provide support and resources as necessary.

Family-Centered Home Care

Family-centered care is defined as care that "assures the health and well-being of children and their families through a respectful family–professional partnership. It honors the strengths, cultures, traditions, and expertise that everyone brings to this relationship" (McPherson, 2005). Family-centered care is a challenging pediatric nursing philosophy and is driven by evidence that a nurturing environment improves the chances of positive outcomes for the child. It places the family in a central position relative to the child and to the child's plan of care. The Association for the Care of Children's Health refined key elements of family-centered care in 1994 (Box 12.2).

Family-centered care focuses on increasing support for the emotional and development needs of the child. It encourages families to care for their children at home while health care professionals provide the support, empowerment, education, and expertise in caring for the child that they need. In family-centered care, the family and health care professionals build a partnership of trust to meet the needs of the child. The nurse must value the role of the family and regard family members as the ultimate experts in caring for their child. In home care the family is extensively involved in the child's care, and the home care nurse is there to facilitate this. Family-centered care recognizes that the family is central and constant in the child's life and care, whereas health service systems and support personnel within this system fluctuate (Meleski, 2002).

Any illness, especially a chronic illness, affects the entire family and can disrupt family structure. The parents' role often changes from one of caring for a healthy

Example Individualized Healthcare Plan

Name:	**Birthdate:**
Address:	School:
Home Phone:	Teacher/Counselor:
Parent/Guardian:	Grade:
Day/Work Phone:	IHP Date:
Healthcare Provider:	IEP Date:
Provider's Phone:	Review Dates:
IHP Written by:	ICD-9 Codes:

Assessment Data	Nursing Diagnosis	Student Goals	Interventions	Outcomes
12-year-old diagnosed asthma at age 9 Carries Proventil inhaler at all times	Risk for Ineffective Breathing (NANDA 1.5.1.3) Characterized by shortness of breath, coughing, and/or wheezing related to asthma	Student will demonstrate appropriate use of inhaler at the beginning of school year. Student will initiate treatment when symptoms appear throughout the school year.	**Airway Management (NIC 2K-3140)** **Activities:** Review use of inhaler with student at the beginning of the school year (Nurse). At the beginning of the school year, review with teacher, and other appropriate staff, the signs and symptoms of asthma exacerbation and when student should use inhaler (Nurse).	Symptom Control Behavior (NOC 4Q-1608) Indicators: Recognizes symptom onset **Never** 1 **Rarely** 2 **Sometimes** 3 **Often** 4 **Consistently** 5 Uses preventative measures **Never** 1 **Rarely** 2 **Sometimes** 3 **Often** 4 **Consistently** 5
Independent in identifying symptoms and need for treatment		Student will keep record of peak flow meter readings if required throughout the school year.	Every two months obtain student's record of inhaler use for documentation in health file. Report increased use of inhaler to parents/physician (Nurse).	Uses relief measures **Never** 1 **Rarely** 2 **Sometimes** 3 **Often** 4 **Consistently** 5
M.D. order normal P.E. program		Student will keep record of use of inhaler for health office throughout the school year. Student will avoid having an emergency asthma attack during this school year.	**Emergency plan:** See STUDENT ASTHMA ACTION CARD located in the classroom, locker room, and health office.	Reports controlling symptoms **Never** 1 **Rarely** 2 **Sometimes** 3 **Often** 4 **Consistently** 5

I have read and approve of the above plan for school healthcare:

Parent signature — Date reviewed by the educational team

Nurse signature — Physician signature (optional)

● **Figure 12.2** Example of an individualized health plan. (Adapted from Arnold, M. J. & Silkworth, C. K. [1999]. *The school nurse's source book of individualized healthcare plans: Issues applications in school nursing practice, Vol. II;* and Zentner-Schoessler, S. [1997]. *Computerized version and manual, Vol. I.* North Branch, MN: Sunrise River Press.)

BOX 12.2

KEY ELEMENTS OF FAMILY-CENTERED CARE

- Recognize the concept that the family is the constant in the child's life.
- Share complete and unbiased information with the parents on an ongoing basis.
- Recognize the family's strengths and individuality. Respect different methods of coping.
- Encourage and make referrals to family-to-family support groups.
- Facilitate parent–professional collaboration at all levels of health care.
- Ensure that the design of health care delivery systems is flexible, accessible, and responsive to families.
- Implement appropriate policies that provide emotional and financial support to families.
- Understand and incorporate the developmental needs of children and families into health care delivery systems.

Adapted from Bissell, C. (2006). *Family-centered care.* Obtained from www.communitygateway.org/faq/fcc.htm#key

child to caring for an acutely ill child (Newton, 2000). These role changes can result in stress for the family members and can affect their participation in the child's care. It is important for home care nurses to seek a partnership role with the family regarding care of the child. This can be difficult for both parties. Many times nurses set limits on parental involvement and do not consider the parents' perspective. Many nurses are concerned that the parents may not be able to care for the child safely. It is important for nurses to use self-awareness and reflective practice to help them understand and empower families as well as to develop a partnership for care. A communication framework that can assist nurses in the home care setting is the LEARN framework, which can help create cross-cultural collaboration and communication between nurses and families (Newton, 2000) (Box 12.3).

BOX 12.3

LEARN FRAMEWORK

- L: Listen empathetically and with understanding to the family's perception of the situation.
- E: Explain your perception of the situation.
- A: Acknowledge and discuss the similarities as well as differences between the two perceptions.
- R: Recommend interventions.
- N: Negotiate and agree on the interventions.

Newton, M. S. (2000). Family-centered care: Current realities in parent participation. *Pediatric Nursing, 26*(2), p. 168.

The Nurse's Role in Home Care

Nursing in the home care setting can be challenging. The focus is on meeting the child's physical and psychological needs while involving the family. The nurse uses the nursing process. Assessment in the home is similar to that in the acute care setting but involves obtaining first-hand data about the family and the way it functions. The nurse needs to assess the child's growth and development and thoroughly assess the home environment (refer to Chapter 3 for additional information). The nurse needs to ensure that home offers a safe and nurturing environment for the child.

The nurse needs to assess availability of resources. This includes necessary equipment such as a hospital bed and oxygen, suitable physical and emotional surroundings (are the family members able to deal with the stress of the situation?), ability to contact emergency services, power backup if needed, and ease of evacuation of the child in case of a fire. The nurse needs to assess whether electricity, sanitary conditions, heat, air conditioning, and telephone access are present. If there is no phone in the home, the family needs to have plans for accessing a phone in case of emergency (perhaps a neighbor's phone or a pay phone near the home). The nurse should identify areas of priority and provide appropriate referrals to resources.

During the assessment phase the nurse identifies the person who is the primary caregiver; this may be the mother, father, grandparent, or older sibling. It is essential to include this person when developing the plan of care, as he or she is the expert on the child and family. The primary caregiver can provide insight into direct care and which strategies will be most effective with this child, taking into account the physical layout of the home, the financial ability of the family, and the way the family functions.

The home care nurse must also assess the family's teaching and learning needs. The goals of home care vary. In many situations care must be learned immediately so the child can be cared for at home, such as a child who needs dressing changes four times a day or a child who is ventilator dependent. For example, a child newly diagnosed with diabetes will have some immediate teaching needs, but as the child grows and his or her condition changes, additional care will need to be taught.

Teaching and learning should begin prior to hospital discharge. Early discharge planning, teaching, and case management are keys to promoting a successful transition from the hospital setting to home. The environment differs greatly between the acute setting and home setting. In the acute setting the nurse is in control of the environment; in the home setting, the nurse is a guest in the home. It is important for the nurse to establish a trusting relationship with both the child and family (Fig. 12.3). A trusting therapeutic relationship will make all aspects of care more effective. Box 12.4 gives hints on building this relationship.

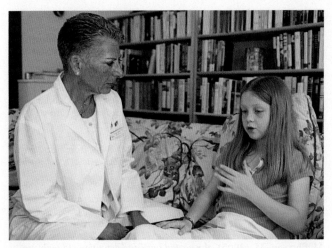

● Figure 12.3 Listening to the child helps to develop a trusting relationship between the home care nurse and the child and her family.

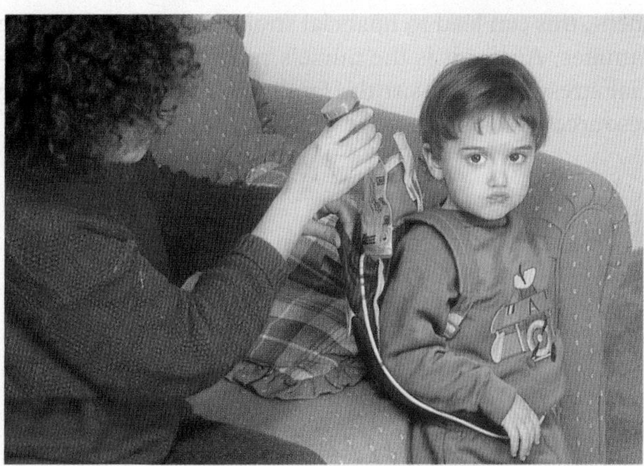

● Figure 12.4 The home care nurse may have to adjust procedures and equipment use to fit the home setting. Placing a feeding pump in a backpack allows this child to receive feedings continuously while at school.

After the assessment is complete, the nurse develops and implements the plan of care. This will include the frequency and duration of the home visits. The nurse will use agency policies, certification standards, and private insurance and/or Medicaid regulations to assist in the development of the plan (Thompson, 2000). The nurse may be the provider of direct care to the child, or the care may be indirect, in which case the nurse plans and supervises the care that is given by others, such as unlicensed personnel and parents.

Nursing care in the home requires excellent assessment and critical thinking skills. The nurse has a great deal of independence since there are no other nurses, supervisors, or physicians on site. When complex care is provided in the home, the nurse may need to adjust procedures to fit the setting. For example, feeding schedules may be adjusted to fit a child's school schedule or equipment may be adjusted to allow a child to receive feedings continuously while at school (Fig. 12.4).

An important role of the home care nurse is empowering children and their families through education (refer to Chapter 3 for further information related to teaching).

BOX 12.4

HINTS TO ESTABLISHING A TRUSTING RELATIONSHIP IN HOME CARE

- Include the child in the conversation and make him or her feel a part of the interaction.
- Address caregivers formally unless otherwise instructed.
- Be friendly. Use a soft, calm voice.
- Be interested in the child's activities.
- Have the primary caregiver present at the initial visit.
- Listen to and show respect to the child and the family.

The nurse assesses the learning needs and provides education that is appropriate to the educational and developmental levels of the child and family. The nurse must encourage the family to participate in the child's care.

Home Care of the Technology-Dependent Child

Due to advances in medicine and technology, a new population of children with chronic disease and disability has emerged. A portion of this population is considered technology dependent, meaning they need medical or technical assistance to remain alive or avoid further disability. To improve the quality of life for these children and to reduce health care costs, more and more family caregivers care for these children at home. These caregivers need to be compassionate and competent and require guidance from health professionals. Meeting the needs of these children usually requires an interdisciplinary team, which may consist of a specialty physician, occupational therapist, speech therapist, physical therapist, nutritionist, special educator, psychologist, social worker, and nurse.

Studies have shown that families of technology-dependent children experience increased emotional, physical, psychological, and financial stress (Fleming, 2004). Due to the intensive, round-the-clock care that many of these children require, physical and emotional exhaustion can occur. To prevent this, respite care is important. It provides support services to temporarily relieve the caregiver of the responsibility for the technology-dependent child. Nurses must assess the need for respite care and assist families in finding appropriate resources (Chapter 13 gives additional information related to respite care).

Home care services have decreased health care costs, but many times the cost to the family is great. The financial burden can increase as one parent has a full-time job at home caring for the technology-dependent child but has no income. Combined with limited third-party reimbursement, this can lead to financial strains and stress for these families. Again, it is the nurse's role to assess for financial stressors and assist the family in finding appropriate resources (refer to above discussion about Medicaid).

As the home care nurse, what can you do to help with Jeremy's transition to school? On your last visit, Jeremy's parents express concerns about this transition and the added stress it is causing the family. They appear tired from the round-the-clock care that Jeremy requires. What suggestions can you make to help ease their stress and fatigue?

References

Books and Journals

Ahmann, E., & Johnson, B. H. (2000). Family-centered care: Facing the new millennium. *Pediatric Nursing, 26*(1), 87–90.

American Academy of Pediatrics, Committee on Pediatric Emergency Medicine. (2005). Pediatric care recommendations for freestanding urgent care facilities. *Pediatrics, 116*(1), 258–260.

Ball, J. W., & Bindler, R. C. (2006). *Child health nursing: Partnering with children and families.* Upper Saddle River, NJ: Prentice Hall.

Bissell, C. (2006). *Family-centered care.* Retrieved July 22, 2006, from http://www.communitygateway.org/faq/fcc.htm#key

Cernoch, J. (1992). Fact sheet number 11: *Respite care for children who are medically fragile.* ARCA National Resource Center for Respite and Crisis Care Services. Obtained on January 20, 2006, at http://www.archrespite.org/archfs11.htm

Community Health Nurses Association of Canada. (2003). *Canadian community health nursing: Standards of practice.* Retrieved July 22, 2006 from http://www.communityhealthnursescanada.org/Standards/Standards%20Practice%20jun04.pdf

Corjulo, M. T. (2005). Telephone triage for asthma medication refills. *Pediatric Nursing, 31*(2), 116–120, 124.

Exceptional Parent (2000). Exceptional professionals: techno-daycare. *The Exceptional Parent, 30*(2), 28–31.

Fleming, J. (2004). *Home health care for children who are technology dependent.* New York: Springer.

Hewitt-Taylor, J. (2005). Children with complex needs: training for care staff. *Journal of Community Nursing, 19*(8). Retrieved July 22, 2006 from http://www.jcn.co.uk/journal.asp?MonthNum=08&YearNum=2005&Type=backissue&ArticleID=831

Hitchcock, J., Schubert, P., & Thomas, S. A. (2003). *Community health nursing: Caring in action* (2nd ed.). New York: Delmar.

Hunt, R. (2005). *Introduction to community-based nursing* (3rd ed.). Philadelphia: Lippincott Williams & Wilkins.

Knopf, A. (2005). Get help—from a telephone triage nurse! *Contemporary Pediatrics.* Retrieved July 22, 2006, from http://www.contemporarypediatrics.com/contpeds/article/articleDetail.jsp?id=174262&pageID=1

Krug, S. E., Bojko, T., Dolan, M. A., et al. (2005). Pediatric care recommendations for freestanding urgent care facilities. *Pediatrics, 116*(1), 258–260.

Lurie, N. (2000). Healthy People 2010: Setting the nation's public health agenda. *Academic Medicine, 75*(1), 12–13.

McPherson, M. (2005). *A new and improved definition of family centered care.* Retrieved July 22, 2006, from http://www.medicalhomeinfo.org/publications/family.html

Meleski, D. D. (2002). Families with chronically ill children [Electronic Version]. *American Journal of Nursing 102* (5), 47–54.

Montagnino, B. A., & Mauricio, R. V. (2004). The child with a tracheostomy and gastrostomy: Parental stress and coping in the home: A pilot study. *Pediatric Nursing, 30*(5), 373–380.

Newton, M. S. (2000). Family-centered care: Current realities in parent participation. *Pediatric Nursing, 26*(2), 164–169.

Simonsen-Anderson, S. (2002). Safe and sound: telephone triage and home recommendations save lives and money. Nursing Management, 33 (6), 41–43.

Thompson, J. M. (2000). Pediatric assessment in the home. *Home Healthcare Nurse, 18*(10), 639–646.

Wanda, M. (1995). Daycare for children who are medically fragile. *The Exceptional Parent, 25*(2), 27–29.

Wolfe, L. C., & Selekman, J. (2002) School nurses: What it was and what it is. *Pediatric Nursing, 28*(4), 403–408.

Websites

www.campnurse.org/ Association of Camp Nurses
www.familycenteredcare.org/ Institute for Family-Centered Care
www.nasn.org National Association of School Nurses

Chapter WORKSHEET

● MULTIPLE CHOICE QUESTIONS

1. The nurse caring for a 5-year-old with diabetes in a family-centered care environment tells the family that there is a support group for parents with children with similar health problems. This discussion is an example of which key element of family-centered care?

   a. The concept that the family is the constant in the child's life

   b. Encourage and make referrals to family-to-family support groups and networks

   c. Recognize family strengths and individuality

   d. Facilitate parent–professional collaboration at all levels of health care

2. The nurse providing home care to a 2-year-old listens to the child's parents talk about how the child and family are adjusting to the child's current illness. Which of the following roles is the nurse participating in?

   a. Case management

   b. Patient and family advocacy

   c. Direct nursing care

   d. Patient and family education

3. A child is to undergo a tympanostomy tube placement in a freestanding outpatient surgery center. What is the major disadvantage associated with this location?

   a. Increased risk for infection

   b. Increased health care costs

   c. Need to be transferred if overnight stay is required

   d. Increased disruption of family functioning

● CRITICAL THINKING EXERCISES

1. A child with cerebral palsy is discharged from the hospital, where he has been receiving treatment for pneumonia. Home health care nurses, through a local agency, are to help the family administer intravenous antibiotic therapy and to monitor the child's health status. As the home health nurse assigned to this child, what should your nursing assessment include?
2. In this situation, what are some nursing interventions that will help ensure family-centered care?
3. When this child is stable and can go back to school, what will be the role of the school nurse in caring for this child?

● STUDY ACTIVITIES

1. Describe health education topics that would be appropriate in an elementary school setting.
2. Shadow a nurse working in a community setting, such as a camp, shelter, or health department. Identify the role the nurse plays in the health of the children and families in the setting and the community.
3. Spend a day in a medically fragile daycare setting. Identify the needs of one child and his or her family, how they may differ from those of a child in a traditional daycare setting, and the role of the nurse in meeting those needs.
4. Develop an IHP for a child with diabetes (use the IHP in Fig. 12.2 as a reference).
5. Shadow a nurse working in a home health care setting. Identify ways he or she helps the family to promote the child's growth and development and to ensure that the child has as normal a childhood as possible. Identify interventions that embody the key concepts of family-centered care.

chapter 13

Nursing Care of the Child With Special Needs

Key TERMS

chronic illness
developmental delay
developmental disability
palliative care
respite care
terminal illness

Learning OBJECTIVES

Upon completion of the chapter, the learner will be able to:

1. Analyze the impact that being a child with special needs has on the child and family.
2. Describe ways that nurses assist children with special needs and their families to obtain optimal functioning.
3. Identify anticipated times when the child and family will require additional support.
4. Plan for transition of the special needs child from the inpatient facility to the home, and from pediatric to adult medical care.
5. Discuss early intervention and public school education for the special needs child.
6. Differentiate developmental responses to death and appropriate interventions.
7. Discuss key elements related to pediatric end-of-life care.

WOW *The touch of a mother's hand and the sound of her voice bring comfort to her special child, and when you bring comfort, you strengthen both of them.*

Preet Singh, a 2-year-old boy who was born at 27 weeks' gestation, is seen in your clinic for the first time. He has a history of hydrocephalus and developmental delay. During the examination, his mother states, "I'm concerned about finding a good, affordable preschool for Preet. His older brother attends public school, but I can't imagine Preet there." After further discussion with Preet's mother, you realize he has not been involved in an early intervention program.

As medicine and scientific technology have advanced, the number of children surviving with health problems that require long-term interventions has increased significantly (Hewitt-Taylor, 2005). Children are now living with conditions that require high-tech treatments for survival. The Maternal Child Health Bureau defines children with special health care needs as those who have or are at risk for a chronic physical, developmental, behavioral, or emotional condition beyond needs generally required by children (Jackson Allen, 2004). According to the Centers for Disease Control and Prevention (CDC)'s National Survey of Children with Special Health Care Needs (2001), about 12.8% of children in the United States have special health care needs (Blumberg, 2003). Of those children with special needs, almost 25% are reported as having conditions that affect their activities usually, always, or a great deal of the time (Blumberg, 2003).

In addition to the direct effects of their special needs, these children and their families are often inadequately insured, have financial needs, have unmet family support needs, or have difficulty obtaining the specialty care that the child requires. Nationwide, 11% report not having a personal doctor or nurse ("medical home") (Blumberg, 2003). Children with special health care needs generally require more intensive and diverse health services, as well as coordination of those services, than do typical children (Child and Adolescent Health Measurement Initiative, 2006). It can be challenging for the family of a child with special needs to navigate the system and obtain all of the services their child requires (Farmer et al., 2003).

Another difficult situation that families may encounter is losing a child to the disease process. A child's chronic illness may progress to the point of becoming terminal. Despite the increased survival rates for children with cancer as a result of improved treatment options and protocols, cancer remains the leading cause of death from disease in all children over the age of 1 year. Less frequently, other diseases also lead to **terminal illness** in children, with congenital defects and traumatic injuries being the more common causes. Caring for the dying child is a family-centered, multidisciplinary process. Nurses must respond to the child's and family's physiologic, emotional, and spiritual needs during this difficult time. Children display differing responses to the dying process and impending death depending on their developmental level. Children and their families need significant amounts of support throughout the process of dying.

For children with special needs, the pediatric nurse fills the critical role of child and family advocate and case manager. When a child is dying, nurses provide physical care of the child and also strive to meet the emotional needs of the child and family. Nurses are in a unique position, both in the inpatient and outpatient setting, to have a significant and positive influence on the lives of these children and their families.

The Medically Fragile Child

When an infant is born very prematurely, when a child is injured and requires long-term rehabilitation and special care, or when a child is diagnosed with a complex chronic health condition, the parents are often devastated initially. The parents of medically fragile children may feel they must adapt to the risk and protect their child. They are interested in preserving their family while compensating for the past, and they cautiously look to the future and become hopeful again. While the infant or child is still in the hospital, nurses can help parents build on their strengths, empowering them to care for their medically fragile infant or special needs child. Education is paramount and should begin as early in the hospitalization as possible. In many situations, particular discharge needs are known early in the course of the infant's or child's hospitalization. Nurses should provide anticipatory guidance about the course of treatment and the expected outcome.

Most children with **chronic illness**, or those who are dependent on technology, progress through stages of growth and development just as typical children do, though possibly at a slower pace. The exception is the child with significant psychomotor retardation, though some developmental progression may occur. Children with special health care needs desire to be treated as normal (Wang & Barnard, 2004), and they want to experience the same events that other children do.

Of particular concern is a growing subset of children with emotional, behavioral, and developmental problems. Children with these needs have even greater difficulty receiving the care and services they require. Many children with emotional, behavioral, or developmental problems also have health problems. Often, these children's problems are not diagnosed early and treatment is difficult. Ongoing counseling and therapy is very difficult for some families to obtain (CDC, 2005). Ultimately, this has a negative impact on the child's physical and mental health and may result in decreased achievement and productivity as the child matures. See Healthy People 2010.

Effect of Special Needs on the Child and Family

The child with special needs and his or her family are both affected by the child's condition and way of living.

HEALTHY PEOPLE 2010

Objective	Significance
Reduce the proportion of children and adolescents with disabilities who are reported to be sad, unhappy, or depressed.	Screen children with special health care needs for depression or sadness. Refer children and their families to mental health providers as needed.

Each member of the family experiences effects related to the child's special needs. Family members' experiences and their responses to the child's illness influence each other directly. They also affect the coping ability of the child with special needs. Children's ability to cope is significantly affected by the family's response to stressors.

Effects on the Child

Children with special health care needs experience differing effects of the chronic illness or disability based on their developmental level, which naturally changes over time for most children.

Infants may fail to develop a sense of trust or attach appropriately with the parents because of frequent hospitalizations, often with multiple caregivers involved, lack of consistency in nurturing, or parental detachment or grieving over the child's condition. The infant's ability to learn through sensorimotor exploration may be impaired due to lack of appropriate stimulation, confinement to a crib, or increased contact with painful experiences.

The toddler may experience difficulty developing autonomy because of increased dependency on the parent or overinvolvement by the parent. Motor and language skill development may be delayed if the toddler is not given adequate opportunities to test his or her limits and abilities.

Limited opportunity also reduces the preschooler's development of a sense of initiative. The preschooler may experience limited opportunities for socialization, causing him or her to withdraw or to feel criticized. Body image development may be hindered due to painful exposures and anxiety. In preschoolers, magical thinking may lead to feelings of guilt for having caused their own disease or condition.

The school-age child may have limited opportunities to achieve a sense of industry because of school absence and inability to participate in activities or competitive events. Lack of socialization limits the school-age child's ability to form peer relationships. The ability to learn via concrete operations is affected by the child's physical limitations or possibly the treatments required.

Adolescents may feel as though they are different from their peers because of their lack of skills/abilities or their appearance. This may hinder the teen's ability to form a sense of personal identity. Since the teen with special health care needs often requires significant amounts of support from the parents, it may be difficult for the adolescent to achieve independence. If the earlier stages of cognitive development have been delayed, then reaching the level of abstract thinking may be blocked.

The child with special health care needs may be able to focus on the positive experiences in his or her life as a method of coping, leading to as much independence as possible. Other children may always feel different from their peers (in a negative sense) and withdraw. Irritability and acting out may also occur. Some children may be compliant and/or seek support for themselves. The child's coping pattern may change over time or with certain situations, such as relapse or worsening of the condition. Children with overprotective parents may display marked dependence and may be very fearful. Children whose parents have been overly indulgent may be more independent and defiant. The nurse must assess the child's individual response to the current health care status and intervene as appropriate.

Effects on the Parents

Raising a child with special needs is generally not the life parents expected to have. Some parents may adapt over time and ultimately accept the child's illness or disability. Others may adapt but do not accept the child's condition and experience the continual fading and re-emergence of chronic sorrow. Denial of their child's problem may prevent parents from progressing through grief, but it also allows them to have hope (Meleski, 2002).

Caring for the special needs child at home (rather than having the child in a facility) may decrease the parents' feelings of anxiety and helplessness (Fig. 13.1). As with

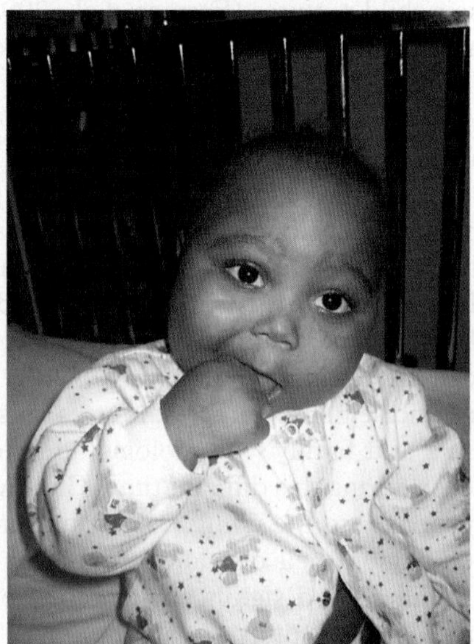

● **Figure 13.1** The special needs child often requires a significant amount of care at home.

typically developing children, parents enjoy witnessing the emotional and social growth of the child (Wang & Barnard, 2004). Parents of special needs children experience a multitude of emotions and changes in their lives; they report that they "live worried" (Coffey, 2006). They feel helpless and overwhelmed at discharge from the hospital. Though willing to carry the burden, they may experience fear, anger, sadness, guilt, frustration, or resentment. Many parents experience grief as a result of losing the "perfect child" they dreamed of.

Stressors of Daily Living

Families with a child who has special health care needs experience life differently than other families. They may have to change their housing situation to accommodate the child's needs. Their sleep is affected. Constant supervision of the technology-dependent child makes it difficult to carry out other basic household activities. In addition to basic childcare and running of the household, medical and technical care must be incorporated into daily life. The family's identity and the parents' employment may be altered radically. Holidays and vacations are affected, as it is difficult to plan activities. Nursing and other health care professional visits are disruptive to family life.

Mothers appear to carry the larger burden of care, though fathers are not unaffected. Somehow, parents eventually take charge, and though they fear failure, they display vigilance, can negotiate and seek information, and become advocates for their child and experts on his or her care. Though parents may feel trapped, isolated, and experience a loss of freedom, their need to survive as a family continues to motivate them. Parents may feel a need to be with their child at all times and experience stress related to coping with the heavy load of caregiving (Case-Smith, 2004).

The extended burden of caregiving can also have adverse health effects on caregivers: only a small percentage of parents of children with special health care needs report that they routinely participate in health-promoting activities for themselves (Kuster et al., 2004). Additionally, parents of children with special health care needs are at increased risk for the development of depression (Wang & Barnard, 2004).

In addition to the caregiving burden, parents experience role conflicts, financial burdens, and the struggle between independence in providing care and the isolation associated with it (Ratliffe et al., 2002). It is very difficult to enjoy spontaneous events outside the home because so much planning is necessary (Case-Smith, 2004; Ratliffe et al., 2002).

The possibility of independence revolves around mobility issues, education, and assistive technology. Though education for all children is federally mandated, parents have anxiety about educational decisions and also find it difficult to obtain the support and educational services the child needs.

Additional stress is associated with transition times in the care of a special needs child. These transition times include:

- Initial diagnosis or change in prognosis
- Increased symptoms
- When the child moves to a new setting (hospital, school)
- During a parent's absence
- During periods of developmental change (Meleski, 2002)

Vulnerable Child Syndrome

"Vulnerable child syndrome" is a clinical state in which the parents' reactions to a serious illness or event in the child's past continue to have long-term psychologically harmful effects on the child and parents for many years. The parents view the child as being at higher risk for medical, developmental, or behavioral problems (Kerruish et al., 2005). Parents exhibit excessive unwarranted concerns and seek health care for their child very frequently. Risk factors for the development of vulnerable child syndrome include preterm birth, congenital anomaly, newborn jaundice, handicapping condition, an accident or illness that the child was not expected to recover from, or crying or feeding problems in the first 5 years of life (Pearson & Boyce, 2004). The parent has difficulty separating from the child, and the child senses that anxiety and then develops symptoms that reinforce the parent's fears. Alternatively (or additionally), the parents may to try to retain control, particularly at times of increasing independence, and fear disciplining the child as they do not want to "upset" the child (O'Connor & Szekely, 2001).

Effects on Siblings

The siblings of children with special health care needs are also affected dramatically. Their relationship with their parents is different than it would have been if they had a typical brother or sister. Parents often need to spend more time with the child with special needs and have less time with their healthy children. Children exhibit emotional and psychological responses to their sibling's long-term needs. Knowledge about the sibling's illness, attitude toward and adjustment to it, the sibling's own self-esteem, how socially supported the sibling is, and the parents' awareness of sibling's feelings are all related to how well the sibling adjusts (Hewitt-Taylor, 2005).

Nursing Management of the Medically Fragile Child

Family-centered care provides the optimal framework for caring for medically fragile children and their families. Family-centered care minimizes the impact of chronic illness and maximizes the child's developmental potential. To provide the best nursing care for these children and the families, the nurse must first develop a trusting relationship with the family.

To ensure optimal functioning, children with special health care needs require comprehensive and coordinated services from multiple professionals. These professionals should work collaboratively to address the child's health, educational, psychological, and social service needs (Farmer et al., 2003). In addition to case management and advocacy, nursing management focuses on screening and ongoing assessment of the child, provision of home care, care of the technology-dependent child, education and support of the child and family, and referral for resources.

Developing a Therapeutic Relationship

Raising children is always challenging, but for the parent of a special needs child it is often overwhelming and exhausting. The parents' needs change continuously, so it is best if the family has a permanent relationship with a health care provider. This promotes trust and a more efficient two-way flow of information (Nuutila & Salanterä, 2006).

Respect the parents' range of emotions and work with them as a team to manage the child's care. Parents need to be recognized for complying with the treatment plan or for other small gains that are made (Jackson Allen, 2004). Empowering the family strengthens them and gives them self-confidence (Lindblad et al., 2005). Feeling supported and invigorated gives parents strength, energy, and hope. Box 13.1 lists principles related to family involvement.

Screening and Ongoing Assessment

Nurses should perform screening to identify children with unmet health care needs (Jackson Allen, 2004). A screening tool developed by the Child and Adolescent Health Measurement Initiative (Fig. 13.2) may help to identify children with special health care needs. Additional information related to the screening tool is available at http://dch.ohsuhealth.com/index.cfm?cfid=6&cftoken=59572841&pageid=458§ionID=133.

Children with special health care needs may attain developmental milestones more slowly than typically developing children. If the Denver II is used for ongoing developmental surveillance of the young child, then the results should be compared from visit to visit to determine progress rather than using it as a screening tool (Ware et al., 2002). Assess special needs children and their families for vulnerable child syndrome.

BOX 13.1

PRINCIPLES RELATED TO FAMILY INVOLVEMENT

Families:

- Define who they are and their culture
- Need to have their basic needs met
- Need to have access to information and training
- Deserve to receive culturally competent care
- Can identify priorities and concerns that lead to policy change
- Know their strengths, limitations, and fears
- Share decision-making power and responsibility for outcomes

Adapted from Federation of Families for Children's Mental Health. (2006). *FFCMH principles for family involvement.*

Promoting Home Care

Home is the most developmentally appropriate environment for all children, even those who are technology dependent. The child's home provides an emotionally nurturing and socially stimulating environment. Children desire to be cared for at home, and those who are cared for at home display an improved physical, emotional, psychological, and social status (Wang & Barnard, 2004).

Technology-dependent children may require supplemental oxygen, assisted ventilation, tracheostomy care, assisted enteral or parenteral feeding, or parenteral medication administration. Traditionally, hospitalization would have been required for these children—in fact, intensive care would have been necessary for children who need assisted ventilation—but with advances in technology, today even children with extensive medical and developmental needs may be cared for at home. Early discharge planning is important, and parents will need detailed instructions and support in caring for the technology-dependent child at home.

Early Discharge Planning

Early discharge planning and ongoing inclusion and education of the family facilitates continuity of care (Swartz, 2005). Box 13.2 provides information about preparing the medically fragile child for discharge.

Caring for the Technology-Dependent Child at Home

Home care nurses are often involved in the care of technology-dependent children. Caring for a technology-dependent child at home is a complex process, yet children thrive in the home care setting with appropriate intervention and care. Many parents feel that rearing a technology-dependent child is different only because of the presence of the equipment. Nurses may tend to think that parents treat the technology-dependent child differently than the other children, while parents value normalization and want to raise and provide discipline to all of their children in the same manner. Parents should tell nurses about their child-rearing expectations, and nurses need to respect the parents' wishes.

Improved collaboration between parents and home care nurses may decrease the parents' stress and maximize opportunities for appropriate growth and development in the technology-dependent child (O'Brien & Wegner, 2002). Thus, a strong relationship, good communication, and negotiation skills are assets to the family and child.

CAHMI Children with Special Health Care Needs (CSHCN) Screening Tool (mail or telephone)

1. Does your child currently need or use **medicine prescribed by a doctor** (other than vitamins)?
   - ☐ Yes ⇐ Go to Question 1a
   - ☐ No ⇐ Go to Question 2

   1a. Is this because of ANY medical, behavioral or other health condition?
   - ☐ Yes ⇐ Go to Question 1b
   - ☐ No ⇐ Go to Question 2

   1b. Is this a condition that has lasted or is expected to last for *at least* 12 months?
   - ☐ Yes
   - ☐ No

2. Does your child need or use more **medical care, mental health or educational services** than is usual for most children of the same age?
   - ☐ Yes ⇐ Go to Question 2a
   - ☐ No ⇐ Go to Question 3

   2a. Is this because of ANY medical, behavioral or other health condition?
   - ☐ Yes ⇐ Go to Question 2b
   - ☐ No ⇐ Go to Question 3

   2b. Is this a condition that has lasted or is expected to last for *at least* 12 months?
   - ☐ Yes
   - ☐ No

3. Is your child **limited or prevented** in any way in his or her ability to do the things most children of the same age can do?
   - ☐ Yes ⇐ Go to Question 3a
   - ☐ No ⇐ Go to Question 4

   3a. Is this because of ANY medical, behavioral or other heath condition?
   - ☐ Yes ⇐ Go to Question 3b
   - ☐ No ⇐ Go to Question 4

   3b. Is this a condition that has lasted or is expected to last for *at least* 12 months?
   - ☐ Yes
   - ☐ No

4. Does your child need or get **special therapy**, such as physical, occupational or speech therapy?
   - ☐ Yes ⇐ Go to Question 4a
   - ☐ No ⇐ Go to Question 5

   4a. Is this because of ANY medical, behavioral or other health condition?
   - ☐ Yes ⇐ Go to Question 4b
   - ☐ No ⇐ Go to Question 5

   4b. Is this a condition that has lasted or is expected to last for *at least* 12 months?
   - ☐ Yes
   - ☐ No

5. Does your child have any kind of emotional, developmental or behavioral problem for which he or she needs or gets **treatment or counseling**?
   - ☐ Yes ⇐ Go to Question 5a
   - ☐ No

   5a. Has this problem lasted or is it expected to last for *at least* 12 months?
   - ☐ Yes
   - ☐ No

● Figure 13.2 The CSHCN Screener. (Reprinted with permission from the Child and Adolescent Health Management Initiative.)

Scoring the Children with Special Health Care Needs (CSHCN©) Screening Tool

Conceptual background

The CSHCN Screener uses consequences-based criteria to screen for children with chronic or special health needs. To qualify as having chronic or special health needs, the following set of conditions must be met:

a) The child currently experiences a specific consequence.
b) The consequence is due to a medical or other health condition.
c) The duration or expected duration of the condition is 12 months or longer.

The first part of each screener question asks whether a child experiences one of five different health consequences:

1) Use or need of prescription medication
2) Above-average use or need of medical, mental health or educational services
3) Functional limitations compared with others of same age
4) Use or need of specialized therapies (OT, PT, speech, etc.)
5) Treatment or counseling for emotional or developmental problems

The second and third parts* of each screener question ask those responding "yes" to the first part of the question whether the consequence is due to any kind of health condition and if so, whether that condition has lasted or is expected to last for at least 12 months.

**NOTE: CSHCN screener question 5 is a two-part question. Both parts must be answered "yes" to qualify.*

All three parts of at least one screener question (or in the case of question 5, the two parts) must be answered "yes" in order for a child to meet CSHCN Screener criteria for having a chronic condition or special health care need.

The CSHCH Screener has three "definitional domains." These are:

1) Dependency on prescription medications
2) Service use above that considered usual or routine
3) Functional limitations

The definitional domains are not mutually exclusive categories. A child meeting the CSHCN Screener© criteria for having a chronic condition may qualify for one or more definitional domains (see diagram below).

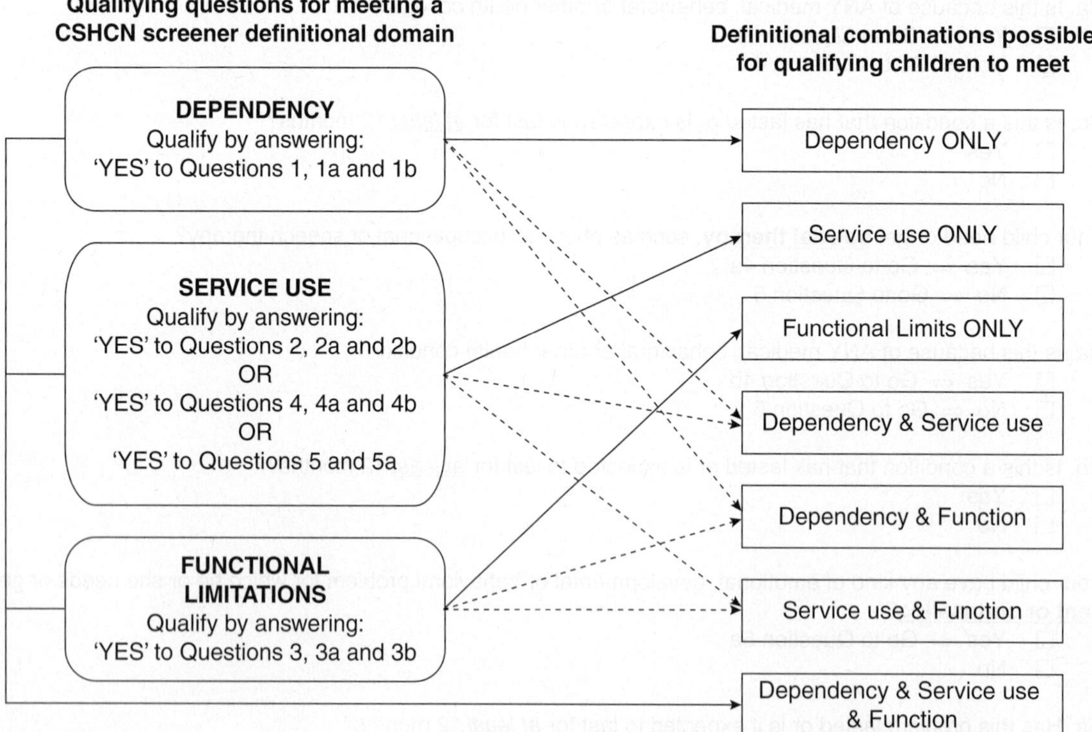

● Figure 13.2 (continued)

BOX 13.2

PREPARING FOR HOME CARE BEFORE DISCHARGE

- Promote liaison with community resources. Develop communication between various services. Plan appointments. Set up home nursing care (either private duty or visits).
- Teach skills, encouraging active caregiving in the hospital setting to increase the parents' self-confidence
- Discuss psychological and emotional issues with parents.
- Obtain/organize equipment and supplies (running out of supplies may cause significant stress on families).
- Refer the family for necessary financial resources.
- Ensure the family's home environment is adequate (enough room for equipment, electricity on, air conditioner for warm weather, heater for cold weather, and refrigeration for food).
- For the baby being discharged from the NICU:
  - Teach the parents about the infant's cues and behaviors and the preemie's different sleep–wake patterns.
  - Encourage kangaroo care and infant massage while in the NICU (as the infant's condition allows).
  - Educate the parents about possible effects on short- and long-term neurodevelopment.
  - Refer to local early intervention program.
  - Assist the family with finding a primary care provider who is experienced in the ongoing follow-up of high-risk infants.

Data from Bakewell-Sachs, S., & Genarro, S. (2004). Parenting the post-NICU premature infant. *MCN, 29*(6), 398–403; and Hewitt-Taylor, J. (2005). Caring for children with complex and continuing health needs. *Nursing Standard, 19*(42), 41–47.

Help the family to incorporate the medical regimen into daily life to minimize the child's self-perception of being "different" (Green & Ray, 2006). Teach families about the technical issues, such as home and travel oxygen therapy, use of the ventilator, suctioning, chest percussion and postural drainage, tube feedings and care of the feeding tube, and medications. Assist parents with the planning and management of routine care, respiratory treatments, nutritional support, and developmental interventions. Reinforce exercises and techniques as prescribed by developmental therapists (Romanko, 2005). Refer to Chapter 12 for additional information about home care nursing.

Providing Care Coordination

Once a child with special health care needs has been identified and has been discharged to the home setting, the nurse plays a vital role in care coordination. Any child with special health care needs benefits from a medical home. The nurse in the medical home is a critical team member, providing ongoing care coordination and follow-up. If such services are available in the local area, refer the child and family with special needs to an integrated health program that provides interdisciplinary, collaborative care for children requiring complex, coordinated care. Box 13.3 lists nursing interventions for families of children with special health care needs.

Providing Ongoing Follow-Up of the Former Premature Infant

Many former premature infants experience a myriad of medical and developmental problems throughout infancy, early childhood, and beyond. Upon or following discharge, many former premature infants display one or many of the following medical or developmental problems:

- Chronic lung disease (bronchopulmonary dysplasia)
- Cardiac changes such as right ventricular hypertrophy and pulmonary artery hypertension
- Growth retardation, poor feeding, anemia of prematurity, other nutrient deficiencies
- Apnea of prematurity, gastroesophageal reflux disease, bradycardia

BOX 13.3

NURSING INTERVENTIONS FOR FAMILIES OF CHILDREN WITH SPECIAL HEALTH CARE NEEDS

- Flag the special needs child's chart.
- Develop written health plans.
- Provide care coordination and collaboration with specialists in other disciplines, early intervention, schools and public agencies.
- Address needs for prior authorization for treatments, medication or specialist referrals; retain copies in the child's chart of authorization forms and approvals.
- Modify office routines to promote family and child comfort.
- Assist parents with childcare decisions. Help parents to understand the child's limits and abilities and the potential health issues (e.g., infections and injuries) associated with childcare.
- Know community resources available to children with special health care needs.
- When the child is hospitalized, encourage high levels of parental participation (if desired by the parent).
- Provide care coordination across multiple health settings.
- Educate childcare providers on child health needs.
- Help parents get involved with parent support networks.

Data from Balling, K., & McCubbin, M. (2001). Hospitalized children with chronic illness: parental caregiving needs and valuing parental expertise. *Journal of Pediatric Nursing, 16*(2), 110–119; Farmer, J. E., Marien, W. E., & Frasier, L. (2003). Quality improvements in primary care for children with special health care needs: Use of a brief screening measure. *Children's Health Care, 32*(4), 273–285; Jackson Allen, P. L. (2004). Children with special health care needs: National survey of prevalence and health care needs. *Pediatric Nursing, 30*(4), 307–314; and Lindeke, L. L., Leonard, B. J., Presler, B., & Garwick, A. (2002). Family-centered care coordination for children with special needs across multiple settings. *Journal of Pediatric Health Care, 16,* 290–297.

- Sudden infant death syndrome (SIDS)
- Rickets (osteopenia) of prematurity
- Hydrocephalus, ventriculomegaly, abnormal head MRI results, ventriculoperitoneal shunt
- Inguinal or umbilical hernias
- Retinopathy of prematurity, strabismus, decreased visual acuity
- Hearing deficits
- Delayed dentition
- Gross motor, fine motor, and language delay, sensory integration issues

Over the long term, former premature infants are at higher risk than typical infants of developing cognitive delay, cerebral palsy, attention-deficit disorder, learning disabilities, difficulties with socialization, and vulnerable child syndrome. Additionally, many former premature infants display alterations in muscle tone at or shortly after discharge from the neonatal intensive care unit (NICU) that require physical therapy intervention.

For these reasons, high-risk infants require special attention and thorough, appropriate assessment to discern subtle changes that may affect their long-term physical, cognitive, emotional, and social outcome. The pediatric nurse should have an understanding of the special concerns that former premature infants and children as well as their families may face.

From the beginning, encourage families to keep a binder that includes all of the infant's pertinent check-up, insurance, and medical and developmental information; this will serve as a resource for the parents, and they will be able to supply complete information when visiting various providers (Kelly, 2006c).

Providing Routine Well-Child Care of the Former Premature Infant

Former premature infants require similar well-child care as typical infants do, with additional visits for management of multiple complex medical issues and developmental screening/intervention. Teach families routine newborn care, including bathing, dressing, and avoidance of passive cigarette smoke. All visits for primary care follow-up will be scheduled based on the infant's chronological age.

Prior to discharge from the NICU, the infant will be tested for oxygen desaturation while seated in the car seat. Clearance will be obtained prior to the infant's discharge. Former preemies require car seat use just as other infants do. Help the parents to find methods of padding the car seat or adding an additional semi-firm cushion inside the seat for the infant to ride in the car safely. Some infants may need to continue cardiac/apnea monitoring while in the car seat.

Since the former premature infant is at increased risk for SIDS compared to the general population, it is critical to teach parents to put the infant on his or her back to sleep (although this is contraindicated with gastroesophageal disease).

Give immunizations according to the current CDC-recommended immunization schedule, based on the infant's chronological age (Kelly, 2006a). All former preemies should receive the flu vaccine as recommended after 6 months chronological age. Respiratory syncytial virus (RSV) prophylaxis is critical for certain groups of premature infants. Administer palivizumab (Synagis) vaccine according to the recommended schedule (refer to Chapter 19 for additional information about RSV prophylaxis) (Kelly, 2006b; Romanko, 2005).

Assessing Growth and Development of the Former Premature Infant

When assessing growth and development of the infant or child who was born prematurely, determine the child's adjusted or corrected age so that you can perform an accurate assessment. The corrected or adjusted age should be used for evaluating progression in growth as well as development. For example, if a 6-month-old infant was born at 28 weeks' gestation (12 weeks or 3 months early), his growth and development expectations are those of a 3-month-old (corrected age). Continue to correct age for growth and development until the child is 3 years old.

Many former premature infants require special diets to foster catch-up growth. Extra calories are needed for increased growth needs. Additional calcium and phosphorus are required for bone mineralization. For these reasons, former preemies should be fed breast milk fortified with additional nutrients or a commercially prepared formula specific for premature infants. When former preemies demonstrate consistent adequate growth (usually by 6 months corrected age), they may be switched to a "term infant formula" such as Similac or Enfamil, concentrated to higher caloric density if needed. Assess the infant's ability to suck efficiently and refer him or her to occupational or speech therapy if the infant is a slow feeder or has difficulty feeding.

All anticipatory guidance related to nutrition is based on the child's corrected age. In other words, begin solids at 6 months corrected age, not chronologic age, and delay the addition of whole milk until 12 months corrected age, rather than 1 year chronologic age. Signs that the former premature infant may be ready to attempt spoon feeding include interest in feeding, decrease in tongue thrust, and adequate head control (Kelly, 2006a).

Early screening and intervention for issues related to development are critical to the attainment of optimal development in the former preemie. The comorbidities that ex-preemies exhibit in the form or prior and current medical problems place these infants at high risk for **developmental delay** (Kelly, 2006b). Even mild developmental delays warrant evaluation and intervention. The Denver II may be used as a screening tool for developmental concerns in the ex-preemie, though it does not always identify children at risk. Parent-report questionnaires demonstrate fairly accurate estimations of developmental problems, and their use is recommended by the American Academy of Pediatrics (AAP, 2001b). Most importantly, assess the child's development based on corrected age until the child is 3 years old. Refer infants and children early if developmental concerns are suspected.

Identifying and Managing Failure to Thrive and Feeding Disorders in Children with Special Needs

Failure to thrive (FTT) is a term used to describe inadequate growth in infants and children. The child fails to demonstrate appropriate weight gain over a prolonged period of time. Length or height velocity and head circumference growth may also be affected. Typical children may experience FTT, but it is much more common in the child with special needs. Adequate nutrition is critical for appropriate brain growth in the first 2 years of life and obviously for growth in general throughout childhood and adolescence. **Developmental disability** may contribute to FTT, as the child's ability to consume adequate nutrition is impaired because of sensory or motor delays, such as with cerebral palsy. Other organic causes of failure to thrive include inability to suck and/or swallow correctly, malabsorption, diarrhea, vomiting, or alterations in metabolism and caloric/nutrient needs associated with a variety of chronic illnesses. Infants and children with cardiac or metabolic disease, chronic lung disease (bronchopulmonary dysplasia), cleft palate, or gastroesophageal reflux disease are at particular risk. Feeding disorders or food refusal may occur in infants or children who have required prolonged mechanical ventilation, long-term enteral tube feedings, or an unpleasant event such as a choking episode. Inorganic causes of FTT include neglect, abuse, behavioral problems, lack of appropriate maternal interaction, poor feeding techniques, lack of parental knowledge, or parental mental illness. Poverty is the single greatest contributing risk factor (Block et al., 2005).

The two categories of causes are not mutually exclusive. Organic causes of FTT may lead to behavioral problems that potentiate problems with adequate growth; hence FTT is thought of as a multifactorial problem.

Screen all children for FTT to identify them early (Locklin, 2005). In addition to poor growth, the infant or child with FTT may present with a history of developmental delay or loss of acquired milestones. Infants or children with feeding problems may display nipple, spoon, or food refusal; difficulty sucking; disinterest in feeding; or difficulty progressing from liquid to puréed to textured food. Perform a detailed dietary history and instruct the parents to complete a 3-day food diary to identify what the child actually eats and drinks. Assess the parent–child interaction, with particular attention to the parent's ability to read and respond to the infant's or child's cues. Observe feeding, noting the child's oral interest or aversion, oral–motor coordination, and swallowing ability, as well as parent–child interactions before, during, and after the feeding (Block et al., 2005). Further aversion to eating may occur as the parent's anxiety over the thought of the child not eating or losing weight leads to attempts to force-feed the child.

Significant FTT may require hospitalization for evaluation and management. Sometimes enteral tube feedings are necessary in order for children with FTT or feeding disorders to demonstrate adequate growth. Box 13.4 lists nursing interventions for the hospitalized child with FTT.

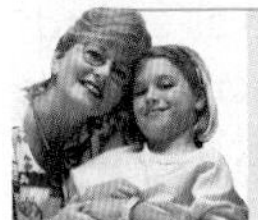

Infants with FTT related to maternal neglect may be less interactive than other infants and avoid eye contact.

Promoting Growth and Development

When caring for the infant with special health care needs in the hospital, provide consistent caregivers to encourage the infant to develop a sense of trust. Allow and encourage the parent to stay with the infant, providing a comfortable place for the parent to sleep. To promote attachment, emphasize the baby's positive qualities. Encourage developmentally appropriate skills and allow the infant to have pleasurable experiences through all of the senses.

For the toddler, begin developmentally appropriate limit-setting and discipline. Encourage independence as the toddler is able. Modify gross motor and sensory activities to accommodate the toddler's limitations. To encourage a sense of control, offer the toddler simple choices. As the preschooler develops, encourage mastery of self-help skills as the child is able. Encourage socialization with same-age peers to develop a sense of friendship. Reinforce to the child that the illness or disability is not a punishment for wrongdoing or the child's fault in any way.

Encourage the school-age child to attend school and make up work that must be missed for medical treatments or appointments. Provide education to the school staff and other students about the child's special needs.

BOX 13.4

NURSING INTERVENTIONS DURING HOSPITALIZATION FOR FAILURE TO THRIVE

- Observe parent/child interactions, especially during feedings.
- Develop an appropriate feeding schedule.
- Provide feedings as prescribed (usually 120 kcal/kg/day is needed to demonstrate proper weight gain).
- Weigh the child daily and maintain strict records of intake and output.
- Educate parents about proper feeding techniques and volumes.
- Provide extensive support to alleviate parental anxiety related to the child's inability to gain weight.

Promote involvement in appropriate sports activities; music, drama, or art activities; and clubs such as Boy Scouts or Girl Scouts. Educate the child about the illness or disability and the course of treatment.

Inform parents of teens that those with chronic illness often participate in the same activities as typical teens, such as risk-taking, rebelling, and trying out different identities. Assist the teen with coping and interpersonal skills. Promote involvement in activities with other teens with special needs as well as typical adolescents. Ensure that the teen participates in rites of passage as able, such as attending the prom or obtaining a driver's license. Discuss future plans with the teen, such as college or vocation, as well as transition to an adult health care provider.

Providing Resources to the Child and Family

Nurses should be familiar with the resources available to children with special health care needs in the community. Educational opportunities for children with special health care needs include early intervention programs and programs offered through the public school system. Financial resources, respite care, and complementary therapies are other areas the nurse should become familiar with.

Educational Opportunities for the Special Needs Child

The foundation for health and development in children is laid during the first years of life. Children with special health care needs often require multiple developmental interventions and special education in the early years in order to reach their developmental potential later in childhood. Children learn best when they are at the stage of maximal readiness, and the early years must not be missed as an opportunity for development. See Healthy People 2010.

Early intervention programs are intended to enhance the development of infants and toddlers with, or at risk for, disabilities, thereby minimizing educational costs and special education. Early intervention is also directed toward enhancing the capacity of families to meet their child's needs as well as to maximize the likelihood of independent living.

HEALTHY PEOPLE 2010

Objective	Significance
Increase the proportion of children and youth with disabilities who spend at least 80 percent of their time in regular education programs.	Ensure that children under age 3 years who may qualify are referred to the local early intervention program. Encourage families to advocate for their child's needs on the individualized education plan.

The Individuals with Disabilities Education Improvement Act (IDEA) of 2004 (formerly called Public Law 99-457) mandates government-funded care coordination and special education for children up to 3 years of age. This early intervention program is administered through each state. Federal law allows each state to define "developmental disability" differently, but in general an evaluation of the child's physical, language, emotional, and social capabilities is performed by qualified personnel to determine eligibility. The law guarantees that eligible children will obtain access to services that will enhance their development. Children who qualify for services receive care coordination, and an individualized family service plan is developed by the service coordinator in conjunction with the family. The service coordinator manages the developmental services and special education that the child requires.

The intent of the program is that the child receives services in a "natural environment," so most services occur in the home or daycare center. Home visits by the service coordinator and maintenance of regular contact with the family ensure the success of the program.

Refer children suspected of developmental delay to the local early intervention program. For children receiving these services, collaborate with the service coordinator on an ongoing basis, with particular involvement at hospital discharge and when transition of services occurs at age 3 years.

> **Think back to Preet,** the 2-year-old boy with a history of hydrocephalus and developmental delay, from the beginning of the chapter. Discuss with his mother the educational opportunities that are available for Preet. Explain what early intervention is and why it is important for Preet.

Schools may have a profound impact on the child's overall health and development. Some children with special needs do not require additional services to succeed in school. For these children, the nurse's role is to assess for school success or failure and determine the effect of the school environment on the child's health. The Individuals with Disabilities Education Act, reauthorized in 2004, provides for the education of children with special needs through the public school system, from age 3 to 21 years. These services are provided within the public school system.

According to the law, each special needs student is entitled to an individualized education program (IEP), which is a written plan designed to meet the preschool, primary, or secondary school student's individual needs. A committee consisting of the child's parent, a regular teacher, a special education teacher, and various other specialists develops the IEP. Nurses may be called to serve upon this committee. The IEP must include measurable short- and long-term goals. Parents are informed of the student's progress routinely and the IEP is reviewed at least annually.

Preschool special education through the local public school system is provided from age 3 to 5 years; access to the curriculum is ensured for all children. A child is eligible for special needs preschool when a significant delay is present in the cognitive, language, adaptive, social-emotional, or motor development domains to the extent that it adversely affects the child's learning ability. The child receives (in the school setting) developmental therapy as needed to augment his or her ability to participate in the education process. The least restrictive environment is preferred, with special needs children participating in classes containing age-appropriate typical peers whenever possible. Special needs preschool services are often offered in the elementary school setting.

Financial and Insurance Resources

Many special needs children whose families demonstrate financial need may be eligible for Supplemental Security Income (SSI). This program was created in 1972 through Public Law 92-603. SSI is a cash assistance program, and monthly benefits vary per individual. SSI qualification also qualifies the child for state-administered Medicaid. Medicaid benefits vary slightly from state to state but generally cover medical visits, medication, hospitalization, and limited adjuvant therapies. The State Children's Health Insurance Program (SCHIP) provides low-cost health insurance to eligible children. Eligibility and the extent of benefits provided by SCHIP vary by state.

Public Law 94-566 provides for state-administered Title V programs under the Maternal and Child Health Bureau Block Grant program. State Title V programs provide community-based, comprehensive service coordination for children with special needs (Mentro, 2003).

Internet Resource for Special Children (www.irsc.org) is an online directory providing a wealth of links to resources for special needs children. Additional online resources include www.childrensdisabilities.info and www.specialchild.com.

Respite Care

Primary caregivers of children with special health care needs must be dedicated, skillful, vigilant, and knowledgeable. Constant care is a stress on the primary caregiver, who needs temporary relief from the daily caregiving demands. **Respite care** provides an opportunity for families to take a break from the daily intensive caregiving responsibilities. Respite care should meet the child's health care needs and offer the child developmental opportunities. Finding and using respite care that the family is comfortable with and trusts may decrease the family's stress and lead to an enhanced quality of life for special needs children and their families. Nurses can facilitate access to respite care, educate respite providers, and ensure quality respite care practices through involvement in community agencies.

Complementary Therapies

Adjuvant therapies are often used by families of children with special health care needs. These may include, among others, homeopathic and herbal medicine, pet therapy, hippotherapy, music, and massage. Many families desire to blend natural or Eastern medicine with traditional allopathic medicine for their special needs child in search of palliation or a cure. When obtaining the health history, ask specifically about homeopathy or herbal medications the child may be taking.

Pet therapy may be used to decrease stress or as a component of psychotherapy.

Hippotherapy is also referred to as horseback riding for the handicapped, therapeutic horseback riding, or equine-facilitated psychotherapy. Individuals with almost any cognitive, physical, or emotional disability may benefit from therapeutic riding or other supervised interaction with horses. The unique movement of the horse under the child helps the child with physical disabilities to achieve increased flexibility, balance, and muscle strength. Children with mental or emotional disabilities may experience increased self-esteem, confidence, and patience as a result of the unique relationship with the horse. A physical therapist or psychotherapist (depending on the situation) generally works very closely with specially trained equine staff. Box 13.5 lists chronic medical conditions for which hippotherapy may be beneficial. Additional information may be obtained through the North American Riding for the Handicapped Association (www.narha.org) or the American Hippotherapy Association (www.americanhippotherapyassociation.org).

BOX 13.5

CONDITIONS BENEFITING FROM HIPPOTHERAPY

- Muscular dystrophy
- Cerebral palsy
- Visual impairment
- Down syndrome
- Mental retardation
- Autism
- Multiple sclerosis
- Emotional disabilities
- Brain injury
- Myelomeningocele
- Spinal cord injury
- Amputation
- Attention-deficit disorder
- Learning disabilities
- Deafness
- Cerebrovascular accident (stroke)

Music may be used to induce positive behavioral changes or various other positive effects (Gasalberti, 2006).

Massage therapy may be beneficial to a wide variety of children. It may be used to reduce pain, promote relaxation, or demonstrate a specific positive effect related to the child's particular medical condition (Gasalberti, 2006).

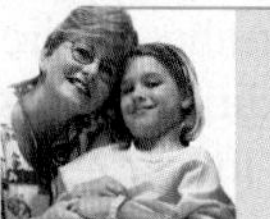

Become familiar with the risks and benefits of homeopathic and herbal medications, as many families use these treatments in an effort to improve their child's quality of life or outcome.

Providing Support and Education

At the time of initial diagnosis, allow and encourage the family to express their feelings. Parents of children with special health care needs require emotional, practical, economic, and social support. Encourage parents to obtain help with daily routines. Encourage stress reduction for the parents through exercise and allowing time for themselves. Be a supportive and encouraging listener, making sure to nurture the whole child, not just his or her special condition (Jackson Allen, 2004).

Parents value peer support groups, sometimes feeling that only other parents of disabled or chronically ill children could understand the heartache, fear, and other emotions they often experience. Pediatric nurses should be proactive in helping families find support systems (Coffey, 2006).

Fathers have the same concerns about their children as mothers do, but they may show this concern differently. It is important for nurses to involve them in the child's care. Teach skills to both parents, and actively involve fathers by asking about their observations and opinions (Ahmann, 2006).

Parents become the experts on their child's needs and care and they should be recognized as such. Parents want to be taken seriously and do not like being ignored (Lindblad et al., 2005). They should be viewed as having reliable and valuable information about their children. By being an active and reflective listener, the nurse can demonstrate to the parents that their opinion is valued, in addition to finding out what the child really needs. Some parents may hesitate to volunteer information, unsure about which information the nurse needs. Show respect for the parents' knowledge of their child's needs by seeking advice on the child's daily care, medical/physical needs, and current developmental level, no matter what the site of care is (Bowie, 2004). See Healthy People 2010.

Families may need additional support from the nurse at times of transition (discussed previously). As the equipment or treatment needs change, adjust the teaching plan. Educate the child and family about the use of adaptive equipment. Ensure that families understand how specific activities must be modified to accommodate the child's needs. Provide anticipatory guidance related to expected developmental changes, including resources and laws related to education. Act as a liaison between the family and the daycare center or school. As the child grows and matures, encourage parents to relinquish caregiving tasks to the child as appropriate to encourage independence and promote self-esteem (Meleski, 2002).

HEALTHY PEOPLE 2010

Objective	Significance
(Developmental) Increase the proportion of children with special health care needs who have access to a medical home.	In the primary care setting, build a relationship with the family to establish a medical home. If available, refer families to multidisciplinary programs for medically complex children.

Assisting the Adolescent With Special Health Needs Making the Transition to Adulthood

Adolescence is a time of physical changes, psychosocial challenges, and initiation of independence from parents. The adolescent with a chronic illness or one who is technology dependent may experience this period differently than other teens. Puberty is often affected by chronic illness (either delayed or earlier). Chronic illness may lead to isolation from peers at a time when peer interaction is the core of psychosocial development. Teens may struggle to fit in with their peers by hiding their illness or health care needs (ignoring them), complying poorly with treatment regimens, or participating in risky behaviors. At a time when the child should be developing independence from the parents, he or she may be experiencing significant dependence related to the special health condition. Adolescents with chronic health disorders demonstrate mental illness at a rate three to four times higher than normally developing adolescents (Burns et al., 2006). For these reasons, the adolescent with special health care needs may require increased amounts of support from the nurse.

With the tremendous increase in technology and health care, about 90% of all children with chronic illness or special health care needs live into adulthood (Lindeke et al., 2001). Making the transition to adult care for a child with special health care needs can be difficult. A written plan for transition to adult care should be initiated in mid-adolescence. Advance planning leads to a smoother transition to adult care. Have ongoing conversations with the teen about this transition. Issues to be resolved prior to the transition include financial resources for medical care, college or vocational school attendance, living arrangements, and caretaking arrangements.

The Adolescent Health Transition Project recommends the following schedule:

- By age 14, ensure that a transition plan is initiated and that the IEP reflects post–high school plans.
- By age 17, explore health care financing for young adults. If needed, notify the local division of vocational rehabilitation by the autumn before the teen is to graduate from high school of the impending transition. Initiate guardianship procedures if appropriate.
- Notify the teen that all rights transfer to him or her at the age of majority. Check the teen's eligibility for SSI the month the child turns 18. Determine if the child is eligible for SSI work incentives.
- If the youth is attending college, contact the college's campus student disability service program.
- By age 21, ensure that the young adult has registered with the Division of Developmental Disabilities for adult services if applicable.

Prior to moving to adult care (with an adult medical specialist), ensure that the adolescent understands the treatment rationale, symptoms of worsening condition, and in particular danger signs. Teach the adolescent about when to seek help from a health professional. Introduce the teen to the medical insurance process. At transition, coordinate a seamless transfer by providing a detailed written plan to the care coordinator or advanced practice nurse (after verbal collaboration).

After the transition, serve as a consultant to the adult office in relation to the teen's needs (Higgins & Tong, 2003). Consult with a transition services coordinator or other service agency as available in the local community (Betz & Redcay, 2002).

The Dying Child

The idea that a child may die is simply unimaginable to most people, yet children die daily. In 2003, a report from the Institute of Medicine stated that about 53,000 children with chronic, life-threatening conditions die each year in the United States (Field & Behrman, 2003). About 28,000 children who die each year are infants (Mellichamp, 2007). Pediatric nurses will inevitably encounter situations in which a child dies. These situations are extremely difficult for all persons involved, and the nurse plays a key role in caring for the dying child and his or her family.

Grieving

Anticipatory grief may be experienced by the family when the diagnosis of terminal illness is made. Families may deny the prognosis, become angry at the health care system or a higher power, or may experience depression. Acute grief is an intense process that occurs around the time of the actual death. Family members may feel short of breath or as though the throat is tight. They may verbalize that the situation is unreal to them or search for reasons why the death was not prevented. Families may also display hostility or restlessness. Each individual will express grief in his or her own manner. Mourning the death of a loved one takes a long time, and families should be supported throughout the process.

Palliative Care of the Dying Child

Appropriate **palliative care** is essential for any child with a life-threatening or progressive incurable condition. Whether palliative care is provided in the home, hospital, or hospice setting, the goal is to provide the best quality of life possible at the end of life while alleviating physical, psychological, emotional, and spiritual suffering. The Last Acts Palliative Care Task Force has established principles on which palliative care of children should be based. These include:

- Respecting patients' goals, preferences, and choices
- Comprehensive caring
- Using the strengths of interdisciplinary resources
- Acknowledging and addressing caregivers' concerns
- Building systems and mechanisms of support (Association of Pediatric Oncology Nurses, 2003)

Hospice Care

Hospice allows for family-centered care in the child's home or a hospice facility. As with adult hospice care, the comfort of the entire family is important. The goals of pediatric hospice care are enhancement of quality of life for the child and family through an individualized plan of care (Children's Hospice International, 2006). The recommended standards for pediatric hospice care do not preclude involvement in ongoing treatment (this is in contrast to adult hospice), but certain eligibility criteria must be met. Parents are educated on ways to comfort and interact with their dying child, such as massage, movement, or singing. Spiritual support is available through a chaplain, social worker, or the family's minister. The nurse not only educates the family about the dying process but also assists them with providing basic care and pain management. The decision to withhold nutrition or hydration may be made in certain instances. Pain management is of utmost importance for the terminally ill child. Ongoing bereavement care is also provided to the family by the hospice after the child's death (Ramer-Chrastek et al., 2002).

Nursing Management of the Dying Child

Though interdisciplinary care is essential for quality care at the end of life, it is the nurse who plays the key role of child/family advocate and who is usually the constant presence throughout the dying process. Nursing management of the dying child focuses on end-of-life decision making, meeting the child's and family's needs, and assisting the family after the child's death. Throughout the process, focus on the family as the unit of care (Malloy et al., 2006).

Assisting the Family With End-of-Life Decision Making

Parents are obligated not only to protect their children from harm but also to do as much good for them as possible, both from an ethical and legal standpoint (Rushton, 2004). When the time comes for end-of-life decision making, parents are often torn about the "right" course of action. Parents may be asked to make decisions about stopping treatment, withdrawing treatment, providing palliative care, or consenting to do not resuscitate (DNR) orders. Patients, parents, and health care providers are generally in agreement that continued suffering is not desired for any child with a terminal illness. When all possible curative attempts have been made, then survival is no longer possible (Hinds et al., 2001).

Nurses involved in this process must examine their own values related to dying and consider the American Nurses Association's code of ethics for nurses as well. The family's feelings must also be acknowledged. During the process of end-of-life decision making, health care providers must assure families that the focus of care is changing and that the child is not being abandoned (Rushton, 2004). Emphasize to parents that no matter what their decision is, the health care team is dedicated to the comfort and expert care of their child.

Ensure that communication is family-centered. Quality of life must be taken into consideration when making decisions to continue or withhold treatment (Jacobs, 2005). Provide parents facing end-of-life decisions with honest information and education from the time of the diagnosis/prognosis forward. Anticipate that parents may vacillate in the decision-making process. Clarify information for them and allow them private time to discuss the options. Do not make judgments about or question the parents' decision. Be sensitive to any ethnic, spiritual, or cultural preferences during the terminal stage of the illness. Encourage parents to interact with other parents who have a child with a terminal illness.

Allowing Natural Death

The decision to institute a DNR order is one of the most difficult decisions a family may ever have to make. DNR refers to withholding cardiopulmonary resuscitation should the child's heart stop beating. Parents may initially feel like this means they are giving up on their child. Nurses must educate families that resuscitation may be inappropriate and lead to more suffering than if death were allowed to occur naturally. The parents need to understand that when a palliative care route is chosen, rather than continuing a curative or treatment route, the focus of the child's care is changing but that the child and family are not being abandoned. Families may wish to specify a certain extent of resuscitation that they feel more comfortable with (e.g., allowing supplemental oxygen but not providing chest compressions). Some institutions are now replacing the DNR terminology with "allow natural death" (AND), which may be more acceptable to families facing the decision to withhold resuscitation (Ramer-Chrastek et al., 2002).

Involving the Dying Child in the Decision-Making Process

End-of-life decision making often involves ethical dilemmas for the patient, family, and health care team. This is particularly true when the parents' wishes conflict with the child's or adolescent's desires. Children should be involved in decision making to the extent that they are able. Discuss intervention within the context of the child's condition and wishes. Children over the age of 7 may "assent" to the continuation or withdrawal of treatment (Hinds et al., 2001). Be available to the older child or adolescent to provide support and information if he or she desires. Talk with the child or adolescent with the parents present, as well as in private. Maintain the child's comfort and dignity. Encourage the child to spend time with other children with a terminal illness. Assure the child that everything will be done to make him or her comfortable.

Consult parents about the timing and depth of end-of-life discussions. Just as parents do, the terminally ill child may vacillate in the decision-making process. Remain sensitive, and respect the child's decisions (Hinds et al., 2001).

Organ or Tissue Donation

With large numbers of organ transplant candidates on waiting lists and the shortage of viable organs, pediatric organ and tissue donation is a priority. For many families, knowing that a child's organs or tissues may save another child's life provides a way to help others despite their own loss. A healthy child who dies unexpectedly is an excellent candidate for organ donation. Many chronic illnesses in children preclude the option of organ or tissue donation, though individual determinations of eligibility should be made.

The discussion of organ donation should be separated from the discussion of impending death or brain death notification. Written consent is necessary for organ donation, so the family must be appropriately informed and educated. Many families who never thought about it before may consider the option of donation if adequately educated about the process. All expenses for organ procurement are borne by the recipient's family, not the donor's. Ask whether the dying child ever expressed a wish to donate organs and whether the parents have considered it.

Families need to know that procurement of the organs does not mar the child's appearance, so that an open casket at the child's funeral is still possible if the family desires. The donating child will not suffer further because of organ donation. The organs or tissues will be harvested in a timely fashion after the declaration of death, so the family need not worry about delay of the wake or funeral. The family's cultural and religious beliefs must be considered, and the team discussing organ donation with the family must do so in a sensitive and ethical manner.

Managing Pain and Discomfort

Pain management is an essential component of care for the child with a terminal illness. Providing for comfort enhances the child's quality of life and minimizes suffering. Assess pain using a developmentally appropriate tool (see Chapter 15 for further information). Provide pain medication around the clock rather than on an "as needed" basis to prevent recurrence or escalation of pain. Determine the child's preferred comfort measures and use them to provide additional relief. Change the child's position frequently but gently to minimize discomfort. Limit nursing care to comfort measures that ease the child's discomfort. Maintain a calm environment, minimizing noise and light.

Easing Anxiety or Fears

Involve the parents and other family members in all phases of the child's care. Explain all aspects of care to the child to minimize anxiety related to nursing interventions. Answer the child's questions honestly. Involve the child in decision making whenever possible. Limit interventions to those related to palliation, rather than treatment, advocating for the child as needed. Remain with the child when a parent or family member is not in the room so the child will not fear dying alone.

Providing Nutrition

Since the body naturally requires less nutrition as the child is dying, do not excessively coax the child to eat or drink. Offer frequent small meals or snacks of the child's choosing. Soups and shakes require less energy to eat and so may be desirable. If the child desires a different food, provide that one. Keep strong odors away from the child to decrease nausea. Administer antiemetics as needed. Provide mouth care and keep the lips lubricated to keep the mouth feeling clean and prevent the discomfort associated with chapped lips. Make sure the environment is a pleasant one for eating.

Supporting the Dying Child and Family

To foster a holistic connection with the child and family, be attuned to the entire family's needs and emotions. Nurses provide physical care through specific tasks and interventions for the dying child, but they also need to be fully present with the child and family. In general, people are uncomfortable with the concept of a dying child. Nurses should work through their own feelings about the situation to be able to be "in the moment" with the child and family. Ask yourself: Can I be fully present with this family? If not, then what can I change to be so?

Families and dying children benefit from the presence of the nurse, not just the interventions he or she performs. Families report that the simple of act of being present with the family is very healing (Mellichamp, 2007). Listen to the child and family; be still and silent for a time to accomplish this. Foster respect for the whole child by attending to him or her as such.

Respect the parents of the dying child by helping them honor the commitments they have made to their child. Acknowledge that parents have diverse needs for information and participation in decision making. Allow and encourage family customs or rituals in relation to death and dying. Families may desire the pastor or priest to be present when the child's death is imminent. Certain rituals may be desired, depending on the family's religious or spiritual background. Ensure that these important events occur, and alter nursing care routines as needed to accommodate them. Respect the family's need to participate in these rituals and customs.

Work collaboratively with the family and health care team to provide for the needs of the child and family (Rushton, 2005). Resources for families of a dying child are listed in Box 13.6. The Make-a-Wish Foundation (www.wish.org) works to grant the wishes of terminally ill children, giving the child and family an experience of hope, strength, and love.

BOX 13.6

RESOURCES FOR FAMILIES OF A DYING CHILD

Websites

- www.joyandhope.org: Project Joy and Hope
- www.chionline.org: Children's Hospice International
- www.compassionatefriends.org: Compassionate Friends

Books

- *Gentle Willow: A Story for Children about Dying* by Joyce Mills
- *35 Ways to Help a Grieving Child* by the Dougy Center for Grieving Children
- *Sad Isn't Bad* by Michaeline Mundy
- *A Child Asks. . . . What Does Dying Mean?* by Lake Pylant Monhollon
- *Talking with Children and Young People about Death and Dying: a Workbook* by Mary Turner
- *The Worst Loss: How Families Heal from the Death of a Child* by Barbara Rosof
- *I Have No Intention of Saying Goodbye: Parents Share Their Stories of Hope and Healing After a Child's Death* by Sandy Fox
- *Stars in the Deepest Night: After the Death of a Child* by Genesse Gentry
- *The Bereaved Parent* by Harriet Schiff
- *You are Special* by Max Lucado

Meeting the Dying Child's Needs According to Developmental Stage

It is important to provide the type of support and education that the dying child needs according to his or her developmental stage. For the infant, unconditional love and trust are of utmost importance. Ensure that the infant's family is available to the child. The toddler, 1 to 3 years old, thrives on familiarity and routine. Maximize the toddler's time with parents, be consistent, provide favorite toys, and ensure physical comfort. Spirituality in the preschool years focuses on the concept of right versus wrong. The 3- to 5-year-old may see death as punishment for wrongdoing; correct this misunderstanding. Use honest and precise language. Help the parents to teach the child that though the family will miss the child, it will continue to function without him or her.

The school-age child has a concrete understanding of death. Children who are 5 to 10 years old need specific, honest details (as desired). Encourage the child to help make decision, and help the child to establish a sense of control.

The young adolescent (10 to 14 years old) will benefit from reinforcement of self-esteem, self-respect, and a sense of worth. Respect the child's need for privacy and time alone as well as time requested with peers. Support the need for independence and encourage the child to participate in decision making. The older teen (14 to 18 years of age) has a more adult-like understanding of death and will need further support through honest, detailed explanations and will want to feel truly involved and listened to.

References

Books and Journals

108th Congress of the United States. (2004). *Individuals with Disabilities Education Improvement Act of 2004.* Retrieved September 3, 2006, from http://frwebgate.access.gpo.gov/cgi-bin/getdoc.cgi?dbname=108_cong_public_laws&docid=f:publ446.108.

Adolescent Health Transition Project. (n.d.) *Transition timeline.* Retrieved September 3, 2006, from http://depts.washington.edu/healthtr/Timeline/timeline.htm.

Ahmann, E. (2006). Supporting fathers' involvement in children's health care. *Pediatric Nursing, 32*(1), 88–90.

American Academy of Pediatrics, Committee on Children with Disabilities. (1995). Guidelines for home care of infants, children, and adolescents with chronic disease. *Pediatrics, 96*(1), 161–164.

American Academy of Pediatrics, Committee on Children with Disabilities. (2001a). Counseling families who choose complementary and alternative medicine for their child with chronic illness or disability. *Pediatrics, 107*(3), 598–601.

American Academy of Pediatrics. (2001b). Policy statement: Developmental surveillance and screening of infants and young children. *Pediatrics, 108,* 192–195.

American Academy of Pediatrics, Committee on Hospital Care and Section on Surgery. (2002). Pediatric organ donation and transplantation. *Pediatrics, 109,* 982–984.

American Academy of Pediatrics, Council on Children with Disabilities. (2005). Policy statement, care coordination in the medical home: Integrating health and related systems of care for children with special health care needs. *Pediatrics, 116*(5), 1238–1244.

American Academy of Pediatrics, Council on Children with Disabilities. (2006). Policy statement: Identifying infants and young children with developmental disorders in the medical home, an algorithm for developmental surveillance and screening. *Pediatrics, 116*(1), 405–420.

American Academy of Pediatrics, Medical Home Initiatives for Children with Special Needs Project Advisory Committee. (2002). Policy statement: The medical home. *Pediatrics, 110*(1), 184–186.

American Nurses Association. (2001). *Code of ethics for nurses with interpretive statements.* Washington, DC: American Nurses Association.

Association of Pediatric Oncology Nurses. (2003). *Precepts of palliative care for children, adolescents and their families.* Retrieved August 1, 2006, from http://www.apon.org/files/public/last_acts_precepts.pdf.

Bakewell-Sachs, S., & Genarro, S. (2004). Parenting the post-NICU premature infant. *MCN, 29*(6), 398–403.

Balling, K., & McCubbin, M. (2001). Hospitalized children with chronic illness: Parental caregiving needs and valuing parental expertise. *Journal of Pediatric Nursing, 16*(2), 110–119.

Baum, L. S. (2004). Internet parent support groups for primary caregivers of a child with special health care needs. *Pediatric Nursing, 30*(5), 381–401.

Bethell, C. D., Read, D., Stein, et al. (2002). Identifying children with special health care needs: Development and evaluation of a short screening instrument. *Ambulatory Pediatrics, 2*(1), 38–48.

Betz, C. L., & Redcay, G. (2002). Lessons learned from providing transition services to adolescents with special health care needs. *Issues in Comprehensive Pediatric Nursing, 25,* 129–149.

Blann, L. E. (2005). Early intervention for children and families with special needs. *MCN, 30*(4), 263–268.

Block, R. W., Krebs, N. F., the Committee on Child Abuse and Neglect, and the Committee on Nutrition. (2005). Failure to thrive as a manifestation of child neglect. *Pediatrics, 116*(5), 1234–1237.

Blumberg, S. J. (2003). *Comparing states using survey data on health care services for children with special health care needs (CSHCN).* Retrieved July 31, 2006, from http://www.cdc.gov/nchs/data/slaits/Comparing_States_CSHCNA.pdf.

Bowie, H. (2004). Mommy first. *Pediatric Nursing, 30*(3), 203–206.

Bratton, S. L., Kolovos, N. S., Roach, E. S., et al. (2006). Pediatric organ transplantation needs: organ donation best practices. *Archives of Pediatrics and Adolescent Medicine, 160*(5), 468–472.

Burns, J. J., Sadof, M., & Kamat, D. (2006). The adolescent with a chronic illness. *Pediatric Annals, 35*(3), 207–216.

Case-Smith, J. (2004). Parenting a child with a chronic medical condition. *American Journal of Occupational Therapy, 58,* 551–560.

Centers for Disease Control and Prevention. (2005). Mental health in the United States: Health care and well being of children with chronic emotional, behavioral, or developmental problems—United States 2001. *Morbidity and Mortality Weekly Report (54),* 985–989.

Child and Adolescent Health Measurement Initiative. (n.d.). *The Children with Special Health Care Needs (CSHCN) Screener.* Retrieved July 31, 2006, from http://www.markle.org/resources/fact/doclibFiles/documentFile_446.pdf.

Child and Adolescent Health Measurement Initiative. (2006). *Approaches to identifying children and adults with special health care needs: A resource manual for state Medicaid agencies and managed care organizations.* Retrieved July 31, 2006, from http://dch.ohsuhealth.com//include/CMS_Manual_revised_apr_06%20compressed.pdf.

Children's Hospice International. (2006). *About children's hospice, palliative and end-of-life care.* Retrieved February 17, 2007, from http://www.chionline.org/resources/about.php.

Coffey, J. S. (2006). Parenting a child with chronic illness: A metasynthesis. *Pediatric Nursing, 32*(1), 51–59.

Farmer, J. E., Marien, W. E., & Frasier, L. (2003). Quality improvements in primary care for children with special health care needs: Use of a brief screening measure. *Children's Health Care, 32*(4), 273–285.

Federation of Families for Children's Mental Health. (2006). *FFCMH principles for family involvement.* Retrieved August 30, 2006, from http://www.ffcmh.org/publication_pdfs/PrinciplesFamilyInvolve.pdf.

Field, M. J., & Behrman, R. E. (eds.). Institute of Medicine, Committee on Palliative and End-of-Life Care for Children and Their Families, Board on Health Sciences Policy. (2003). *When children die: improving palliative and end-of-life care for children and their families.* Washington, DC: The National Academies Press. Retrieved August 1, 2006, from http://www.nap.edu/books/0309084355/html/index.html.

Gance-Cleveland, B. (2006). Family-centered care: Decreasing health disparities. *Journal for Specialists in Pediatric Nursing, 11*(1), 72–76.

Gasalberti, D. (2006). Alternative therapies for children and youth with special health care needs. *Journal of Pediatric Health Care, 20*(2), 133–136.

Green, A., & Ray, T. (2006). Attention to child development: A key piece of family-centered care for cardiac transplant recipients. *Journal for Specialists in Pediatric Nursing, 11*(2), 143–148.

Hack, M. (2001). The outcome of neonatal intensive care. In M. H. Klauss & A. A. Fanaroff, *Care of the high-risk neonate* (pp. 528–535). Philadelphia: W. B. Saunders.

Heilferty, C. M. (2004). Spiritual development and the dying child: the pediatric nurse practitioner's role. *Journal of Pediatric Health Care, 18,* 271–275.

Hewitt-Taylor, J. (2005). Caring for children with complex and continuing health needs. *Nursing Standard, 19*(42), 41–47.

Higgins, S. S., & Tong, E. (2003). Transitioning adolescents with congenital heart disease into adult health care. *Progress in Cardiovascular Nursing, 18*(2), 93–98.

Hinds, P. S., Oakes, L., Furman, W., et al. (2001). End-of-life decision making by adolescents, parents, and healthcare providers in pediatric oncology: Research to evidence-based practice guidelines. *Cancer Nursing, 24*(2), 122–136.

Inkelas, M., & Garro, N. (2005). A picture of needs for children with special health-care needs: What we are learning from the national survey. *Journal of Pediatric Nursing, 20*(3), 207–210.

Jackson Allen, P. L. (2004). Children with special health care needs: National survey of prevalence and health care needs. *Pediatric Nursing, 30*(4), 307–314.

Jacobs, H. H. (2005). Ethics in pediatric end-of-life care: A nursing perspective. *Journal of Pediatric Nursing, 20*(5), 360–369.

Johnson, C. P., Kastner, T. A., & the Committee/Section on Children with Disabilities of the American Academy of Pediatrics. (2005). Helping families raise children with special health care needs at home. *Pediatrics, 115*(2), 507–511.

Kelly, M. M. (2006a). Primary care issues for the healthy premature infant. *Journal of Pediatric Health Care, 20*(5), 293–299.

Kelly, M. M. (2006b). The basics of prematurity. *Journal of Pediatric Health Care, 20*(4), 238–244.

Kelly, M. M. (2006c). The medically complex premature infant in primary care. *Journal of Pediatric Health Care, 20*(6), 367–373.

Kerruish, N. J., Settle, K., Campbell-Stokes, P., & Taylor, B. J. (2005). Vulnerable Baby Scale: Development and piloting of a questionnaire to measure maternal perceptions of their baby's vulnerability. *Journal of Paediatrics and Child Health, 41*(8), 419–423.

Kuster, P. A., Badr, L. K., Chang, B. L., et al. (2004). Factors influencing health-promoting activities of mothers caring for ventilator-assisted children. *Journal of Pediatric Nursing, 19*(4), 276–287.

Lindblad, B., Rasmussen, B. H., & Sandman, P. (2005). Being invigorated in parenthood: Parents' experiences of being supported by professionals when having a disabled child. *Journal of Pediatric Nursing, 20*(4), 288–297.

Lindeke, L. L., Krajicek, M., & Patterson, D. L. (2001). PNP roles and interventions with children with special needs and their families. *Journal of Pediatric Health Care, 15,* 138–143.

Lindeke, L. L., Leonard, B. J., Presler, B., & Garwick, A. (2002). Family-centered care coordination for children with special needs across multiple settings. *Journal of Pediatric Health Care, 16,* 290–297.

Lobar, S. L., Youngblut, J. M., & Brooten, D. (2006). Cross-cultural beliefs, ceremonies, and rituals surrounding death of a loved one. *Pediatric Nursing, 32*(1), 44–50.

Locklin, M. (2005). The redefinition of failure to thrive from a case study perspective. *Pediatric Nursing, 31*(6), 474–479.

Malloy, P., Ferrell, B., Virani, R., et al. (2006). Palliative care education for pediatric nurses. *Pediatric Nursing, 32*(6), 555–561.

Maternal and Child Health Bureau. (2001). *All aboard the 2010 express: A 10-year action plan to achieve community-based service systems for children and youth with special health care needs and their families.* Washington, DC: Department of Health and Human Services.

Meleski, D. D. (2002). Families with chronically ill children: A literature review examines approaches to helping them cope. *AJN, 102*(5), 47–54.

Mellichamp, P. (2007). End-of-life care for infants. *Home Healthcare Nurse, 25*(1), 41–44.

Mentro, A. M. (2003). Health care policy for medically fragile children. *Journal of Pediatric Nursing, 18*(4), 225–232.

Naar-King, S., Siegel, P. T., Smyth, M., & Simpson, P. (2003). An evaluation of an integrated health care program for children with special needs. *Children's Health Care, 32*(3), 233–243.

Neufeld, S. M., Query, B., & Drummond, J. E. (2001). Respite care users who have children with chronic conditions: Are they getting a break? *Journal of Pediatric Nursing, 16*(4), 234–244.

Nuutila, L., & Salanterä, S. (2006). Children with a long-term illness: parents' experiences of care. *Journal of Pediatric Nursing, 21*(2), 153–160.

O'Brien, M. E., & Wegner, C. B. (2002). Rearing the child who is technology dependent: Perceptions of parents and home care nurses. *Journal for Specialists in Pediatric Nursing, 7*(1), 7–15.

O'Connor, M. E., & Szekely, L. J. (2001). Frequent breastfeeding and food refusal associated with failure to thrive: a manifestation of the vulnerable child syndrome. *Clinical Pediatrics, 40*(1), 27–33.

Pearson, S. R., & Boyce, W. T. (2004). The vulnerable child syndrome. *Pediatrics in Review, 25*(10), 345–349.

Ramer-Chrastek, J., Brunnquell, D., & Hasse, S. (2002). Letting nature take its course: One family's choice of hospice home care for their terminally ill infant. *AJN, 102*(10), 24CC-DD, FF, 24II-JJ.

Ratliffe, C. E., Harrigan, R. C., Haley, J., et al. (2002). Stress in families with medically fragile children. *Issues in Comprehensive Pediatric Nursing, 25,* 167–188.

Romanko, E. A. (2005). Caring for children with bronchopulmonary dysplasia in the home setting. *Home Healthcare Nurse, 23*(2), 95–102.

Romesberg, T. (2004). Understanding grief: A component of neonatal palliative care. *Journal of Hospice and Palliative Nursing, 6*(3), 161–170.

Rushton, C. H. (2004). Ethics and palliative care in pediatrics: When should parents agree to withdraw life-sustaining therapy for children? *AJN, 104*(4), 54–63.

Rushton, C. H. (2005). A framework for integrated pediatric palliative care: Being with dying. *Journal of Pediatric Nursing, 20*(5), 311–325.

Schainker, E., & Grant, L. (2003). Medical home meets educational home: How you can make the most of school health services. *Contemporary Pediatrics, 20*(3), 55–81.

Sullivan-Bolyai, S., Sadler, L., Knafl, K. A., & Gilliss, C. L. (2004). Great expectations: A position description for parents as caregivers: Part II. *Pediatric Nursing, 30*(1), 52–56.

Swartz, M. K. (2005). Parenting preterm infants: A meta-synthesis. *MCN, 30*(2), 115–120.

U.S. Department of Health and Human Services, Health Resources and Services Administration, Maternal and Child Health Bureau. (2004). *The national survey of children with special health care needs chartbook 2001.* Rockville, MD: U.S. Department of Health and Human Services.

Verma, R. P., Sridhar, S., & Spitzer, A. R. (2003). Continuing care of NICU graduates. *Clinical Pediatrics, 42*(4), 299–315.

Wang, K. K., & Barnard, A. (2004). Technology-dependent children and their families: A review. *Journal of Advanced Nursing, 45*(1), 36–46.

Ware, C. J., Sloss, C. F., Chugh, C. S., & Budd, K. S. (2002). Adaptations of the Denver II scoring system to assess the developmental status of children with medically complex conditions. *Children's Health Care, 31*(4), 255–272.

Websites

http://depts.washington.edu/healthtr/ Adolescent Health Transition Project

http://genes-r-us.uthscsa.edu National Newborn Screening and Genetics Resource Center
www.aacn.nche.edu/elnec End-of-life Nursing Education Consortium
www.aap.org American Academy of Pediatrics
www.americanhippotherapyassociation.org American Hippotherapy Association
www.cahps.ahrq.gov/default.asp Surveys and tools to advance patient-centered care
www.cdc.gov/ncbddd National Center on Birth Defects and Developmental Disabilities, promoting optimal fetal, infant, and child development; preventing birth defects and developmental disabilities; enhancing quality of life for those with disabilities
www.childrensdisabilities.info/ Articles and resources for families of children with disabilities
www.chionline.org Children's Hospice International
www.dec-sped.org/ Division of Early Childhood, promoting support of families and optimal development of young children with or at risk for developmental delays and disabilities
www.ed.gov/policy/speced/guid/idea/idea2004.html News and information on the Individuals with Disabilities Education Improvement Act of 2004 (IDEA)
www.familiesusa.org Voice for health care consumers, dedicated to achieving high-quality, affordable health care for all Americans
www.familycenteredcare.org/ Institute for Family-Centered Care
www.familyvoices.org A national clearinghouse for information and education related to the health care of children with special health needs
www.fcsn.org Federation for Children with Special Needs
www.ffcmh.org Federation of Families for Children's Mental Health
www.fvkasa.org/ Kids as Self-Advocates
www.infanthearing.org National Center for Hearing Assessment and Management
www.ippcweb.org Initiative for Pediatric Palliative Care
www.irsc.org Internet Resource for Special Children
www.lastacts.org (or www.rwjf.org/newsroom/featureDetail.jsp?featureID=886&type=3) Archive of information from the Last Acts Foundation
www.medicalhomeinfo.org/ American Academy of Pediatrics, National Center of Medical Home Initiatives for Children with Special Needs
www.modimes.org March of Dimes Resource Center, addressing personal and complex problems related to pregnancy and birth defects
www.narha.org North American Riding for the Handicapped Association
www.nectas.unc.edu National Early Childhood Technical Assistance Center
www.nichcy.org/ National Dissemination Center for Children with Disabilities
www.preemie-l.org Parents of Premature Babies, Inc., a nonprofit foundation supporting parents of preterm infants
www.preemies.org Preemies.Org; helps parents of premature infants find other parents using various Internet resources
www.specialchild.com Resources for parents and caregivers of children with special needs
www.ssa.gov Social Security Administration
www.wish.org Make-a-Wish Foundation
www.zerotothree.org Zero to Three, supporting healthy development and well-being of infants and toddlers and their families.

Chapter WORKSHEET

● MULTIPLE CHOICE QUESTIONS

1. The parents of a 5-year-old with special health care needs talk to the parents of a 10-year-old with a similar condition for quite a while each day. What is the nurse's interpretation of this behavior?
   a. The nurse has not provided enough emotional support for the parents.
   b. This relationship between the children's parents is potentially unhealthy.
   c. Support between parents of special children is extremely valuable.
   d. Confidentiality is a pressing issue in this particular situation.
2. The nurse is caring for a child who has received all possible medical care for cancer, yet continues to experience relapse and metastasis. It is time to make the transition from curative care attempts to palliative care. What is the most important nursing consideration at this time?
   a. The health care professionals should make the decision about the child's care.
   b. The family may lose a sense of hope, so cancer treatments should continue.
   c. Involve the family in the decision-making process about the shift to palliative care.
   d. Palliative care can take place only at home, so the child should be discharged.
3. The nurse is caring for a 3-year-old with a gastrostomy tube and tracheostomy who is on supplemental oxygen and multiple medications. The mother is rooming in during this hospitalization. What is the priority nursing action?
   a. Incorporate the mother's assistance in care when convenient.
   b. Recognize the mother as the expert on her child's needs and care.
   c. Recommend that the mother go home to get some rest.
   d. Provide family-centered care since the mother is there.
4. The nurse is caring for a child with a developmental disability who is starting kindergarten this year. The mother is tearful and doesn't want the child to go to school. What is the best response by the nurse?
   a. "Do you need some time alone to collect yourself?"
   b. "You've known for a while this time would come."
   c. "Can I call your husband or a friend for you?"
   d. "It is normal to feel stressed or sad at this time."
5. The parents of a child with a developmental disability ask the nurse for advice about disciplining their child. What is the best response by the nurse?
   a. "You should choose methods that are most congruent with your values about discipline."
   b. "Children like this really can't follow directions, so they may be very hard to discipline."
   c. "Punish your child only for socially unacceptable or offending behaviors."
   d. "Spanking works well for this type of child, as they really don't like pain."

● CRITICAL THINKING EXERCISES

1. A 15-year-old boy is dying of cancer after all medical care options have been exhausted. Describe the plan of care for this child and his family. What strategies should the nurse use to support the child and his family through this difficult process?
2. A 5-month-old infant who was born at 24 weeks' gestation is ready to be discharged from the NICU. She will be going home on oxygen, gastrostomy tube feedings, and eight medications. Develop a teaching plan for the family.

● STUDY ACTIVITIES

1. In the clinical setting, care for a child with a terminal illness. Reflect in your clinical journal about the feelings you had during the care of the child, as well as the feelings and behaviors that you noticed in the child, siblings, parents, and nursing staff.
2. Visit a preschool that provides care for developmentally delayed and typical children. Choose two same-age children, one with a disability or impairment and the other a typical healthy child. Perform a Denver developmental screening or development assessment on each of the two children. Compare and contrast your findings.
3. Spend the day with a home care nurse providing care for a technology-dependent child. What obstacles has the family overcome to have this child at home? What adjustments does the nurse make to provide family-centered care in the home (as compared to the hospital setting)?

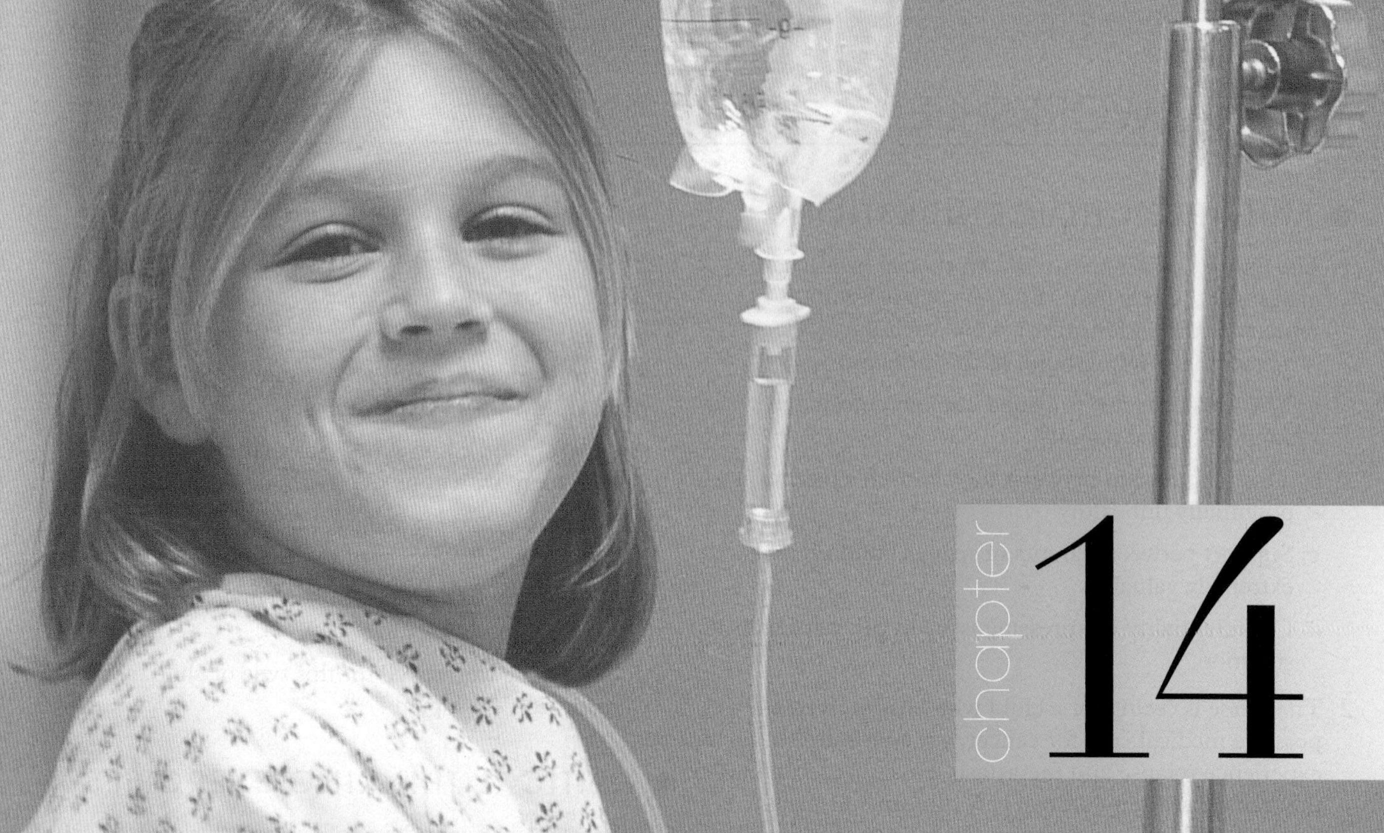

Medication Administration, Intravenous Therapy, and Nutritional Support

Key TERMS

biotransformation
bolus feeding
enteral nutrition
gastrostomy
gavage feedings
infiltration
parenteral nutrition
pharmacodynamics
pharmacokinetics
residual
total parenteral nutrition

Learning OBJECTIVES

Upon completion of this chapter, the learner will be able to:

1. Describe atraumatic methods for preparing children for procedures.
2. Describe the "eight rights" of pediatric medication administration.
3. Explain the physiologic differences in children affecting a medication's pharmacodynamic and pharmacokinetic properties.
4. Accurately determine recommended pediatric medication doses.
5. Demonstrate the proper technique for administering medication to children via the oral, rectal, ophthalmic, otic, intravenous, intramuscular, and subcutaneous routes.
6. Integrate the concepts of atraumatic care in medication administration for children.
7. Identify the preferred sites for peripheral and central intravenous medication administration.
8. Describe nursing management related to maintenance of intravenous infusions in children, as well as prevention of complications.
9. Explain nursing care related to enteral tube feedings.
10. Describe nursing management of the child receiving total parenteral nutrition.

WOW *Parents judge us by our technical abilities and their child's outcome, not by what they believe nurses are capable of doing.*

Lily Kline, a 9-month-old, is admitted to your unit for failure to thrive. The physician has ordered insertion of a nasogastric tube to begin gavage feedings. The parents are very nervous and upset about this. They ask, "What will this tube do for Lily? It sounds very uncomfortable. What do you have to do to insert it? Will it have to stay in all the time? Won't it move?" How would you address their concerns?

The ill child often requires medications, intravenous (IV) therapy, or enteral nutrition to restore health. These procedures occur most often in the inpatient setting, but with today's advanced technology many children may receive treatment in the home, daycare center, school, physician's office, or other community setting.

This chapter begins with an overview of the important aspects of caring for a child who is to undergo a procedure. The key elements of and guidelines for care related to medication administration, IV therapy, and nutritional support in children will be discussed. Child and parent education is emphasized. The chapter will focus on adapting and modifying nursing procedures based on the child's growth and development and providing these treatments using a family-centered, atraumatic approach.

Children and Procedures

Children undergo numerous diagnostic and therapeutic procedures in a wide range of settings during their development. Medication administration, IV therapy, and nutritional support are just three examples. These procedures may be performed in the community or outpatient setting or in a care facility (see Chapters 3 and 11 for additional information). Regardless of the procedure to be performed and the setting, children, like adults, need thorough preparation before the procedure and support during and after the procedure to promote the best outcome.

Before the Procedure

Appropriate preparation for procedures helps to decrease the child's and family's anxiety level, promote the child's cooperation, and support the child's and family's coping skills. Adequate preparation also helps to foster the child's feeling of mastery over a potentially stressful event, as undergoing invasive procedures in particular is extremely distressing for children.

Preparation may include psychological preparation (including explanation and education) as well as preparing the child physically. Employ the concept of atraumatic care when preparing children for a procedure. General guidelines for preparation include the following:

- Provide a description of and the reason for the procedure using age-appropriate language ("the doctor will look at your blood to see why you are sick").
- Describe where the procedure will occur ("the x-ray department has big machines that won't hurt you; it's a little cold there too").
- Introduce strange equipment the child may see ("you will lie on a special bed that moves in the big machine, but you can still see out").
- Describe how long the procedure will last ("you will be in the x-ray department until lunchtime").
- Identify unusual sensations that may occur during the procedure ("you may smell something different" [e.g., alcohol smell], "the MRI machine makes loud noises").
- Inform the child if any pain is involved.
- Identify any special care required after the procedure ("you will need to lie quietly for 15 minutes afterward").

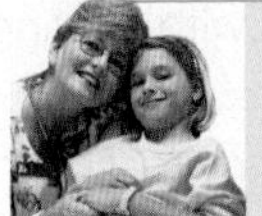

In the hospital, perform all invasive procedures in the treatment room or a room other than the child's room. The child's room should remain a safe and secure area.

A major aspect of preparation involves play. In general, young children respond better to play materials and older children benefit more from viewing peer modeling films. However, consider the child's temperament, coping strategies, and previous experiences as well as developmental needs and cognitive abilities. First, gain trust and provide support. Include the child's parents, because parents are usually the greatest source of comfort for the child. Be short, simple, and appropriate in explaining situations at the child's level of development. Explain what is to be done and what is expected of the child. Avoid terms that have double meanings or might be confusing. Table 14.1 lists alternative words or phrases to use for terms that may be confusing or misunderstood.

During the Procedure

Use a firm, positive, confident approach that provides the child with a sense of security. Encourage cooperation by involving the child in decision making and allowing the child to select from a list or group of appropriate choices. Allow the child to express feelings of anger, anxiety, fear, frustration, or any other emotions. Often this is how a child communicates and copes with the situation. Tell the child that it is okay to scream or cry, but that it is very important to hold still. Use distraction methods such as those listed in Box 14.1.

Toddlers and preschoolers often resist procedures despite preparation for them. Being held down or restrained is often more traumatizing to the young child than the procedure itself. Use alternative methods (positions that provide comfort for the child) to keep the child still during the procedure (Fig. 14.1).

Table 14.1 Alternatives for Confusing or Misunderstood Terms

Term to Avoid	How Children Might Interpret It	Use These Terms Instead
Catheter	Too technical	Tube
Deaden	Kill?	Make sleepy
Dye	"Die"	Special medicine to help the doctor see ______ (part of the body) better
Electrodes	Too technical	Stickers, ticklers, snaps
ICU	"I see you"	Special room with your own nurse
Incision, cut open, make a hole	Too explicit	Special or small opening
Monitor	Too technical	TV screen
Organ	Like a piano?	Special place in the body
Pain	May be too explicit	Child's word for hurt; "boo-boo"
Put to sleep, anesthesia	May confuse with putting a pet to sleep	Special kind of sleep
Shot	Children are scared of shots	Medication under the skin
Stool	Like you sit on?	"Poop" or child's word for it
Stretcher or gurney	"Stretch her"	Rolling bed or special bed on wheels
Take your temperature/BP	Where are you going to "take" them?	See how warm you are/hug your arm
Test	Like at school? (the child will need to perform)	See how your heart is working
Tourniquet	Too technical	Special kind of rubber band
Urine	"You're in?"	"Pee" or child's word for it
X-ray	Don't understand	Picture or big camera to take pictures of the inside of your body

Partially adapted from Florida Children's Hospital, *Suggested vocabulary to use with children.*

After the Procedure

After the procedure, hold and comfort the child. Cuddle and soothe infants. Encourage children to express their feelings through play, such as dramatic play or use of puppets. Gross motor activities such as pounding or throwing are also helpful for children to discharge pent-up feelings and energy. School-age children and adolescents may not outwardly demonstrate behavior indicating the need for comforting; however, provide them with opportunities to express their feelings and be comforted. Remember to praise children for appropriate behavior during the procedure and after all interventions are completed.

BOX 14.1

DISTRACTION METHODS

- Have the child point toes inward and wiggle them.
- Ask the child to squeeze your hand.
- Encourage the child to count aloud.
- Sing a song and have the child sing along.
- Point out the pictures on the ceiling.
- Have the child blow bubbles.
- Play music appealing to the child.

Medication Administration

WATCH & LEARN

At one time or another, every child will need to receive medication. As with adults, pediatric medication administration is a critical component of safe and effective nursing care. However, the need for safety takes on even greater importance due to the physiologic, psychological, and cognitive differences inherent in children. Therefore, the pediatric nurse must adapt administration principles and techniques to meet the child's needs. Medication administration, regardless of the route, requires a solid knowledge base about the drug and its action.

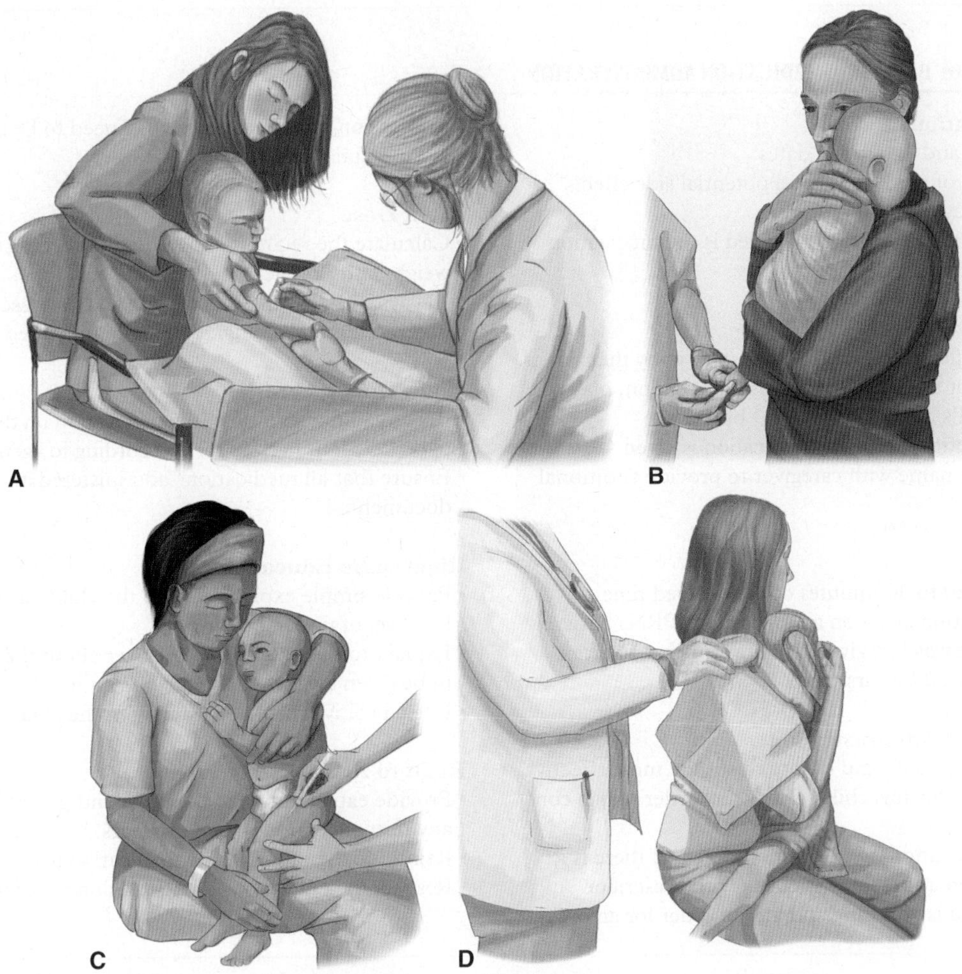

● Figure 14.1 Positioning a child for comfort during a painful procedure. (**A**) Sitting on the parent's lap while undergoing allergy testing provides this toddler with a sense of comfort. (**B**) Position the infant cuddled over the parent's (preferable) or the nurse's shoulder when obtaining a heelstick. (**C**) Use "therapeutic hugging" to maintain a child's position while the child is receiving an IM injection. (**D**) Hold the older child while using a book or story for distraction.

As with medication administration to any patient, the nurse must adhere to the "rights" of medication administration (Box 14.2). Confirming the child's identity and double-checking the dosage before administration of any medication are two critical safeguards that play a major role in preventing medication errors.

Differences in Pharmacodynamics and Pharmacokinetics

Although a drug's mechanism of action is the same in any individual, the physiologic immaturity of some body systems in a child can affect a drug's **pharmacodynamics** (behavior of the medication at the cellular level). As a result, the body may not respond to the drug as intended. The intended effect may be enhanced or diminished, necessitating a change in the dosage to ensure optimal effectiveness without increasing the child's risk for toxicity.

The child's age, weight, body surface area, and body composition also can affect the drug's **pharmacokinetics** (movement of drugs throughout the body via absorption, distribution, metabolism, and excretion). Drugs are administered to children via many of the same routes that are used for adults. However, this similarity ends once the drug is administered.

During the absorption process, drugs move from the administration site into the bloodstream. In infants and young children, the absorption of orally administered medications is affected by slower gastric emptying, increased intestinal motility, a proportionately larger small intestine surface area, higher gastric pH, and decreased lipase and amylase secretion compared with adults. Intramuscular absorption in infants and young children is affected by amount of muscle mass, muscle tone and perfusion, as well as vasomotor instability. Similarly, decreased perfu-

BOX 14.2

EIGHT RIGHTS OF PEDIATRIC MEDICATION ADMINISTRATION

Right Medication
- Check order and expiration dates.
- Know action of medication and potential side effects (use pharmacy, drug formulary).
- Ensure that the medication provided is the medication that is ordered.

Right Patient
- Check identification, since children may deny their identity in attempt to avoid an unpleasant situation, play in another child's bed, or remove ID bracelet.
- Confirm identity each time medication is given.
- Verify child's name with caregiver to provide additional verification.

Right Time
- Give within 20 to 30 minutes of the ordered time.
- For a medication given on an as-needed (PRN) basis, know when it was last given and how much was given during the past 24 hours.

Right Route of Administration
- Check ordered route and ensure this is the most effective and safe route for this child; clarify any order that is confusing or unclear.
- Give the medication by the route ordered. If there is a need to change route, always check with prescriber (e.g., if a child is vomiting and has an order for an oral medication, the medication may need to be given via the IV or rectal route).

Right Dose
- Calculate the recommended dose according to child's weight and double-check your calculations
- Always question the pharmacist and/or prescriber if the ordered dose falls outside the recommended dose range.

Right Documentation
- Record administration of the medication on the appropriate paper or computerized form according to agency policy.
- Ensure that all medications administered and refused are documented.

Right to Be Educated
- Provide simple explanations to the child based on his or her level of understanding.
- Explain to the parents or caregiver about the medication to be given and what to expect from it.
- Use a positive, firm approach with the child.

Right to Refuse
- Provide explanations to the child and parents to clarify any misconceptions or relieve fears.
- Reinforce the rationale for medication use.
- Respect the child's or parents' option to refuse.

sion alters subcutaneous absorption. Absorption by these routes is erratic and may be decreased. In contrast, topical absorption of medications is increased in infants and young children because the stratum corneum is thinner and well hydrated (Lilley et al., 2005; Woo, 2004).

The distribution (movement of a drug from the blood to interstitial spaces and then into cells) of medications is also altered in infants and young children. Medication distribution in children is affected by:

- Higher percentage of body water than adults
- More rapid extracellular fluid exchange
- Decreased body fat
- Liver immaturity, altering first-pass elimination
- Decreased amounts of plasma proteins available for drug binding
- Immature blood–brain barrier, allowing permeation by certain medications (Lilley et al., 2005; Pickar, 2004; Woo, 2004)

Metabolism of medications in children is altered because of differences in hepatic enzyme production and the child's increased metabolic rate. **Biotransformation** (the alteration of chemical structures from their original form, which allows for the eventual excretion of the substance) is affected by the same variations affecting distribution in children. In addition, the immaturity of the kidneys until the age of 1 to 2 years affects renal blood flow, glomerular filtration, and active tubular secretion. This results in a longer half-life and increases the potential for toxicity of drugs primarily excreted by the kidneys (Lilley et al., 2005; Woo, 2004).

Developmental Issues and Concerns

Children are constantly growing and developing. The specific psychosocial, cognitive, physical, and motor developmental levels of children are important. Nurses need a solid understanding of growth and development to ensure safe administration of medications to children. Table 14.2 details some key areas in administering medications to children. Always give developmentally appropriate, truthful explanations before administering medications to children. Include why the drug is needed, what the child will experience, what is expected of the child, and how the parents can participate and

Table 14.2 Growth and Development Issues Related to Pediatric Medication Administration

Stage of Development	Issue/Concern	Nursing Interventions
Infant	Development of trust, which is fostered by consistent care; development of stranger anxiety later in infancy	Involve parents in medication administration to reduce stress for infant. Ensure that parents hold and comfort infant during intervention.
Toddler	Development of autonomy with displays of negativism; rituals, routines, and choices necessary to maintain some sense of control	Follow routines and rituals from home in giving medications if these are safe and positive approaches. Involve parents in medication administration. Offer simple choices (e.g., "Do you want Mom or me to give you your medicine?"). Allow child to touch or handle equipment as appropriate.
Preschooler	Development of initiative, which is fostered when they sense they are helping	Provide an opportunity to play with the equipment and respond positively to explanations and comforting. Provide choices that are possible and keep them simple (e.g., "Do you want juice or water with your medication?" or "Which medication do you want to take first?"). Do not ask, "Will you take your medicine now?" Involve parents in medication administration. Be aware that giving suppositories is particularly upsetting to this age group because of their fears of bodily intrusion and mutilation.
School-aged child	Development of industry, benefiting from being a part of their care; generally very cooperative	Explain to child in simple terms the purpose of the medication. Seek their assistance, such as putting pills in cup or opening the packet, and allow a broader range of choices. Establish a reward system to enhance their cooperation if necessary.
Adolescent	Development of identity, benefiting from much more control over their care	Approach in same manner as adults, with respect and sensitivity to their needs. Maintain the adolescent's privacy as much as possible.

support their child. Refer to Chapters 4 through 8 for further information about growth and developmental issues.

The child's past experiences with taking medications and the approaches that may have been used will often affect how the child reacts. Always approach children positively; let your manner convey the belief that they can accomplish this needed behavior. Never label the child as "bad" if he or she did not fully cooperate in taking medication. When medications must be administered with a needle (intramuscularly or subcutaneously), assure the child that this method is not a consequence of the child's behavior. Help parents to work through the feelings of frustration that may result from the child's refusal to cooperate with medication administration. Provide parents with facts about growth and developmental issues and children's fears and anxiety related to medication administration. Model alternative ways for the parents to deal with undesirable behavior.

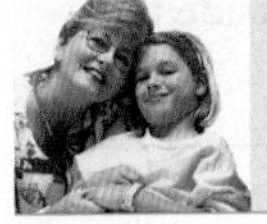

Always administer medications promptly, assist the child in holding still using a comforting position for the child, and reward positive behavior.

Determination of Correct Dose

Administering the correct dose is a key component of medication administration. Many drug references list recommended pediatric dosages, and nurses are responsible for checking doses to ensure that they are appropriate for the child. Two common methods for determining pediatric doses are based on the unit of drug per kilogram of body weight or body surface area (BSA).

Dose Determination by Body Weight

The most common method for calculating pediatric medication doses is based on body weight. The recommended dosage is usually expressed as the amount of drug to be given over a 24-hour period (mg/kg/day) or as a single dose (mg/kg/dose). Differentiate between the 24-hour dosage and the single dose. Use these guidelines to determine the correct dose by body weight:

1. Weigh the child.
2. If the child's weight is in pounds, convert it to kilograms (divide the child's weight in pounds by 2.2).
3. Check a drug reference for the safe dose range (for example, 10 to 20 mg/kg of body weight).
4. Calculate the low safe dose (Box 14.3).
5. Calculate the high safe dose.
6. Determine if the dose ordered is within this range.

The pediatric dosage should not exceed the minimum recommended adult dosage. Generally, once a child or adolescent weighs 50 kg or greater, the adult dose is frequently prescribed. However, always verify that the dose does not exceed the recommended adult dose (Pickar, 2004).

BOX 14.3

DOSAGE CALCULATION USING BODY WEIGHT

After converting the child's weight in pounds to kilograms and checking the safe dose range:

- Calculate the low safe dose range (e.g., 10 to 20 mg/kg and the child weighs 30 kg):
  - Set up a proportion using the low safe dose range $10 \text{ mg}/1 \text{ kg} = x \text{ mg}/30 \text{ kg}$
  - Solve for x by cross-multiplying:
    $1 \times x = 10 \times 30$
    $x = 300$ mg
- Calculate the high safe dose range:
  - Set up a proportion using the high safe dose range $20 \text{ mg}/1 \text{ kg} = x \text{ mg}/30 \text{ kg}$
  - Solve for x by cross-multiplying:
    $1 \times x = 20 \times 30$
    $x = 600$
- Compare the safe dose range (for this example, 300 to 600 mg) with the ordered dose. If the dose falls within the range, the dose is safe. If the dose falls outside the range, notify the prescriber.

Dose Determination by Body Surface Area

Calculating the dosage based on BSA takes into account the child's metabolic rate and growth. It is commonly used for chemotherapeutic agents. Some recommended medication doses may read "mg/BSA/dose." To determine the dose using BSA, you will need to know the child's height and weight, which will be plotted on a nomogram (Fig. 14.2). A nomogram is a graph divided into three columns: height (left column), surface area (middle column), and weight (right column). Use these guidelines to determine BSA:

1. Measure the child's height.
2. Determine the child's weight.
3. Using the nomogram, draw a line to connect the height measurement in the left column and the weight measurement in the right column.
4. Determine the point where this line intersects the line in the surface area column. This is the BSA, expressed in meters squared (m^2).

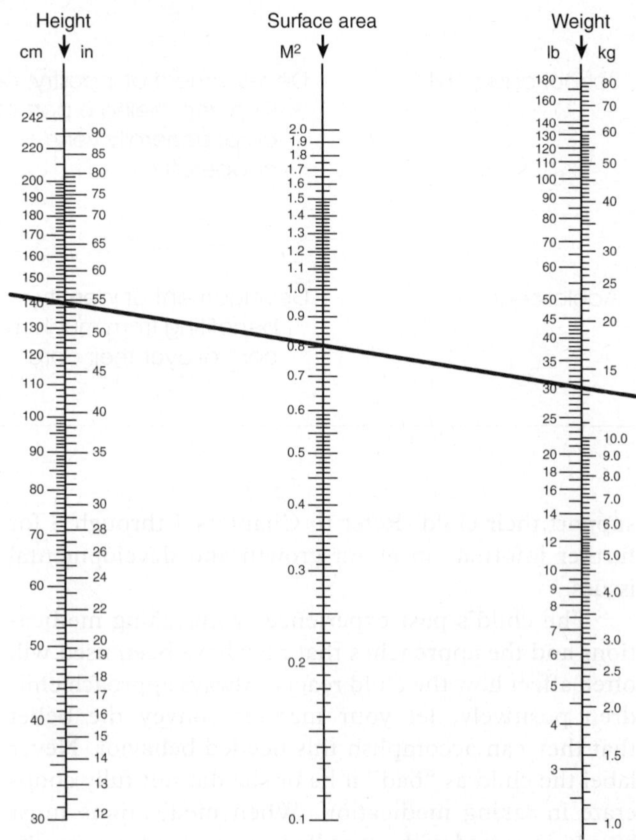

● **Figure 14.2** A nomogram to determine body surface area.

Once you have determined the BSA, use the recommended dosage range to calculate the safe dosage.

Oral Administration

Medications to be given via the oral route are supplied in many forms, such as liquids (elixirs, syrups, or suspensions), powders, tablets, and capsules. Generally, children under the age of 5 to 6 are at risk for aspiration because they have difficulty swallowing tablets or capsules. Therefore, if a tablet or capsule is the only oral form available, it needs to be crushed or opened and mixed with a pleasant-tasting liquid or a small amount (generally no more than a tablespoon) of a nonessential food such as applesauce. However, never crush or open an enteric-coated or time-release tablet or capsule. The crushed tablet or inside of a capsule may taste bitter, so never mix it with formula or other essential foods. Otherwise, the child may associate the bitter taste with the food and later refuse to eat it.

Liquid medications, primarily suspensions, may be less concentrated at the top of the bottle than at the bottom of the bottle. Always shake the liquid to ensure even drug distribution. The key to administering liquid forms of oral medications is to use calibrated equipment such as a medicine cup, spoon, plastic oral syringe, or dropper (Fig. 14.3). If a dropper is packaged with a certain medication, never use it to administer another medication, since the drop size may vary from one dropper to another. If using a syringe for oral administration, only use the type intended for oral medications, not one designed for parenteral administration. When using a dropper or oral syringe (without a needle) for infants or young children, direct the liquid toward the posterior side of the mouth. Give the drug slowly in small amounts (0.2 to 0.5 mL) and allow the child to swallow before more medication is placed in the mouth (Fig. 14.4). A nipple without the bottle attached is sometimes used to administer medication to infants. Place the medication directly in the nipple and keep the nipple filled with medication as the infant sucks so no air is taken in while the infant takes the medication. Always place the infant or young child upright (at least a 45-degree angle) to avoid aspiration. The toddler or young preschooler may enjoy using the oral syringe to squirt the medicine into his or her mouth. Older children can take oral medication from a medicine cup or measured medicine spoon.

As children adapt to swallowing tablets or capsules, administration is similar to that of adults. When helping the younger child learn how to swallow medication, the tablet or capsule can be placed at the back of the tongue or in a small amount of food such as ice cream or applesauce. Always tell children if there is medicine in the food; otherwise they may not trust you.

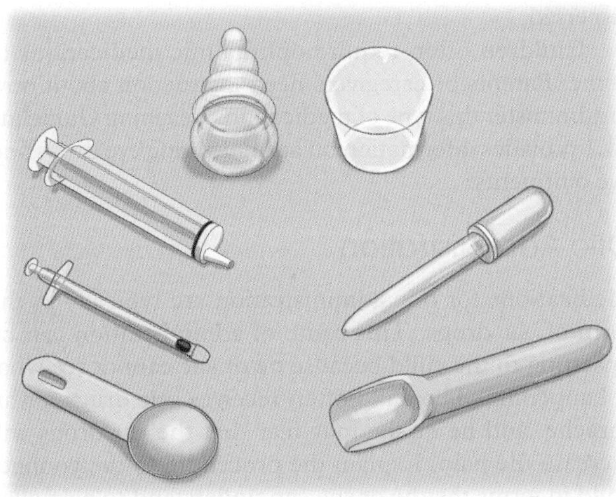

● Figure 14.3 Devices used to administer oral medications to children.

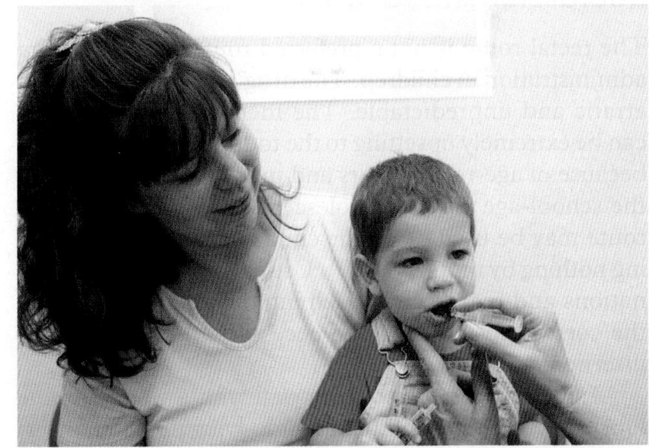

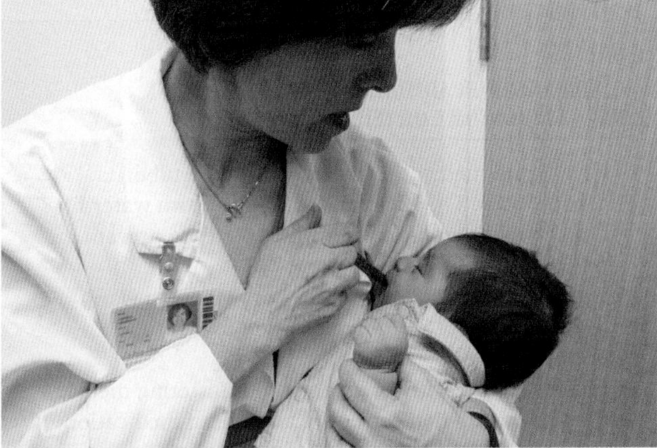

● Figure 14.4 Position the infant or young child for safe medication administration.

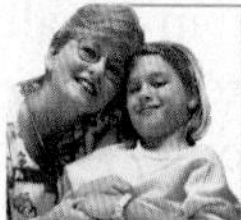

Use the medicine cup or syringe with proper calibration instead of household cups or measuring spoons, since they are not calibrated and may deliver an incorrect dose of medication.

When the child has a nasogastric, orogastric, **gastrostomy** (opening into the stomach), or nasojejunal tube, oral medications may be given via these devices. The tube allows for the medication to be placed directly into the stomach or jejunal area. Medication for administration via a tube must be supplied in a liquid form, or a crushed tablet or opened capsule can be mixed with a liquid (Box 14.4). Always check tube placement prior to administering the medication. After administration, flush the tube to maintain patency.

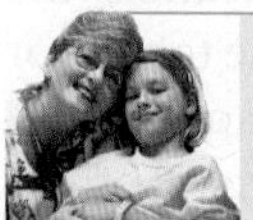

Never force an oral medication into a child's mouth or pinch the child's nose. Doing so increases the risk for aspiration and interferes with the development of a trusting relationship.

Rectal Administration

The rectal route is not a preferred route for medication administration in children. The drug's absorption may be erratic and unpredictable. The method is invasive and can be extremely upsetting to the toddler and preschooler because of age-related fears and may be embarrassing to the school-age child or adolescent. However, the rectal route may be used when the child is vomiting or receiving nothing by mouth (NPO). Use age-appropriate explanations and reassurance. Helping the child to maintain the correct position may be necessary to ensure proper insertion and safety.

Lubricate the suppository well with a water-soluble lubricant. With the child in the side-lying position, insert the suppository into the rectum quickly but gently. Wear gloves or use a finger cot to insert the suppository. Insert the suppository above the anal sphincter. For an infant or child under the age of 3, use the fifth finger for insertion. For an older child, use the index finger. To prevent expulsion of the suppository, hold the buttocks together for several minutes or until the child loses the urge to defecate. If the child has a bowel movement within 10 to 30 minutes after administration of the medication, examine the stool for the presence of the suppository. If it is observed, notify the health care provider to determine if the drug needs to be administered again.

BOX 14.4

GUIDELINES FOR ADMINISTERING MEDICATIONS VIA GASTROSTOMY OR JEJUNOSTOMY TUBES

- Give liquid medications directly into the tube.
- Mix powdered medications well with warm water first.
- Crush tablets and mix with warm water to prevent tube occlusion.
- Open up capsules and mix the contents with warm water to dissolve the contents and prevent tube occlusion.
- Flush the tube with water after administering medications to ensure that the entire amount of medication has been given and to prevent tube occlusion.

Adapted from Children's Healthcare of Atlanta. (2004). *Gastrostomy tube home care manual.*

Ophthalmic Administration

Many children have a fear of having anything placed in their eyes. Provide older children with an age-appropriate explanation to gain their cooperation. Ophthalmic medications are typically supplied in the form of drops or ointment. Ensure that the medication is at room temperature, as chilled medication may be uncomfortable to the child. Proper positioning of the child is necessary to control the child's head, keep the child's hands from interfering, and prevent injury to the eye. Attempt to administer the medication when the child is not crying to ensure that the medication reaches its intended target area.

Place the child in the supine position, slightly hyperextending the neck with the head lower than the body so the medication will be dispersed over the cornea. Rest the heel of your hand on the child's forehead to stabilize it. Retract the lower eyelid and place the medication in the conjunctival sac, being careful not to touch the tip of the tube or dropper to the sac. Wear gloves and maintain sterile technique. For eye drops, place the prescribed number of drops into the lower conjunctival sac (Fig. 14.5). For ointment, apply the medication in a thin ribbon from the inner canthus outward without touching the eye or eyelashes. If the child is old enough to cooperate, instruct the child to gently close the eyes to allow the medication to be dispersed.

Children often require ophthalmic medications at home. Parents or caregivers need instruction about how to administer this type of medication. Teaching Guideline 14.1 provides information on administering eye drops and eye ointments.

Otic Administration

Medications for otic administration are typically in the form of ear drops. This route of administration can be upsetting to the child because he or she cannot see what is happening. The child often receives otic drugs for an earache, and he or she may fear that the ear drops will increase the pain. Explain the procedure to the younger child in terms that he or she can understand to help allay these fears. Gain the older child's cooperation by explaining the purpose of the medication and the procedure for administration.

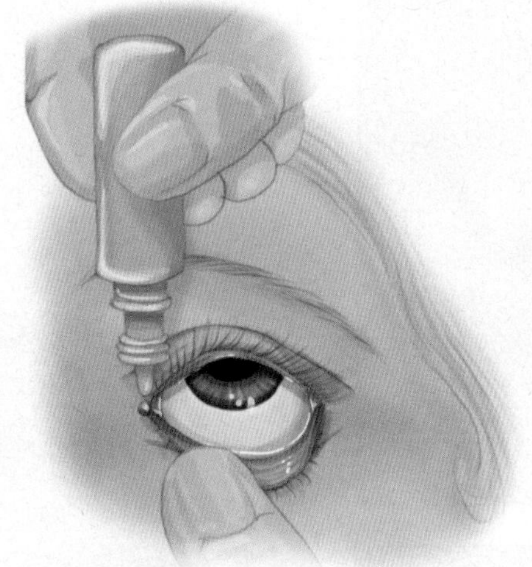
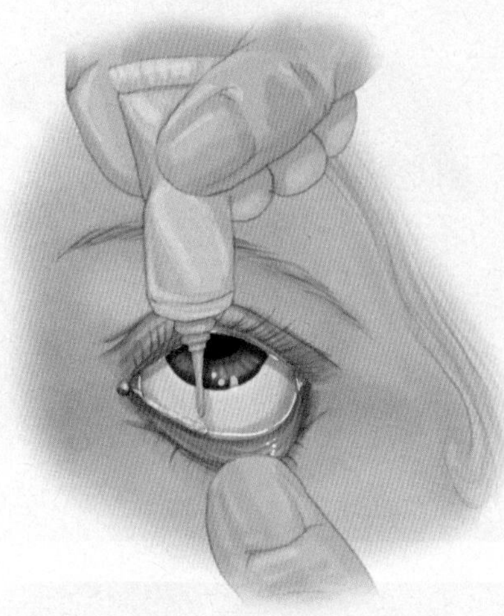

● Figure 14.5 Administering eye drops: gently press the lower lid down and have the child look up as the medication is instilled into the lower conjunctival sac.

Reinforce the need for the child to keep the head still. Younger children may require assistance to do so. Be sure that the ear drops are at room temperature. If necessary, roll the container between the palms of your hands to help warm the drops. Using cold ear drops can cause pain and possibly vertigo when they reach the eardrum.

Place the child in a supine or side-lying position with the affected ear exposed (Fig. 14.6). Pull the pinna downward and back in children under the age of 3 and upward and back in older children. Instill the medication using a dropper. Then have the child remain in the same position for several minutes to ensure that the medication stays in the ear canal. Massage the area anterior to the affected ear to promote passage of the medication into the ear canal. If necessary, place a piece of cotton or a cotton ball loosely in the ear canal to prevent the medication from leaking.

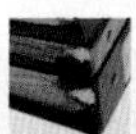

TEACHING GUIDELINE 14.1

Applying Eye Medications

- Wash your hands with soap and water. Dry them thoroughly using paper towels or a clean cloth.
- Allow the eye drops or ointment to come to room temperature (if the medication was stored in the refrigerator). If necessary, warm the eye drops or ointment tube in the palm of your hand. Keep the cap on to avoid any spillage.
- Remove the cap, placing it on a dry, clean surface.
- For young children (3 years or less), obtain assistance to keep their arms and fingers away during the procedure. If doing this procedure alone, wrap the child in a towel or blanket, keeping the arms inside.
- If you are applying eye drops, it may be easiest if you are standing or sitting behind the child, looking over the back of the child's head as he or she reclines. If you are applying an eye ointment, it may be easiest to face the child directly.
- Using one hand, hold the child's forehead in place while raising the eyelid with your thumb.
- With your other hand, hold the eye drop bottle or ointment tube above the eye, using an extended finger against the child's cheek, forehead, or nose to steady your hand.
- Gently squeeze the eye drop bottle, dispensing the proper number of drops, or gently squeeze the ointment tube, dispensing a small trail (about 2 cm) of ointment into the gap between the lower portion of the eye and bottom eyelid.
- Make sure the tip of the bottle or tube does not make contact with the eye or any other surface.
- For eye drops, gently press your finger against the inside corner where the eye meets the nose for about 1 minute, blocking the tears and medication from exiting through the tear duct. This will help the eye retain more of the medication. If your child is old enough, he or she may be able to do this unassisted.
- For ointment, have the child close his or her eye and not rub the area.
- Ask the child not to blink or squeeze the eye shut more than normal, as this may wash away the medication prematurely.
- Gently dab away any tears with a clean tissue.
- If necessary, clean the tip of the bottle or tube with a clean tissue and recap.
- Wash your hands again and dry them thoroughly.

Source: The Pediatric Glaucoma and Cataract Family Association; http://www.pgcfa.org/drops.htm, http://www.pgcfa.org/ointment.htm)

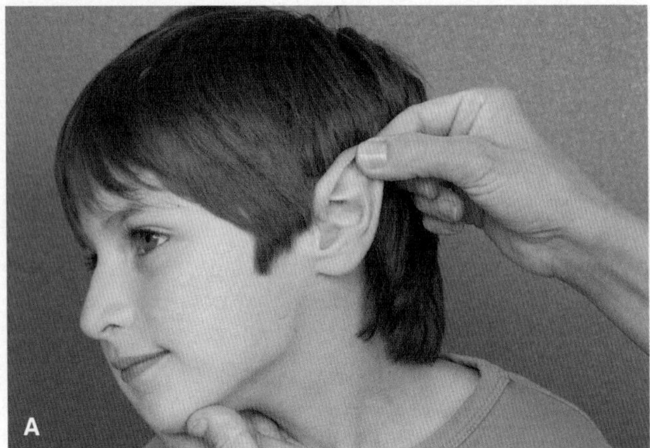

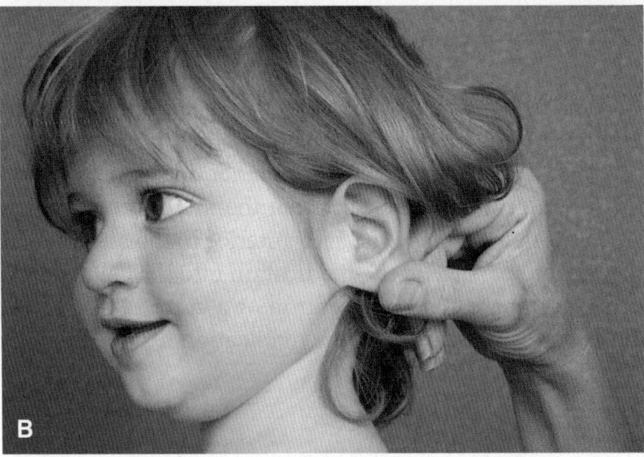

● Figure 14.6 Administering ear drops. (**A**) For a child over age 3 years, the nurse pulls the pinna of the affected ear up and back. (**B**) For the child less than 3 years of age, the nurse pulls the pinna of the ear down and back.

Nasal Administration

Nasally administered medications are typically drops and sprays. Administering nose drops to infants and young children may be difficult, and additional help may be needed to help maintain the child's position. For nose drops, position the child supine with the head hyperextended to ensure that the drops will flow back into the nares. A pillow or folded towel can be used to facilitate this hyperextension. Place the tip of the dropper just at or inside the nasal opening, taking care not to touch the nares with the dropper (Fig. 14.7). Doing so might stimulate the child to sneeze. Although the nasal membranes are not sterile, the drop solution is, and sneezing would contaminate the dropper, leading to contamination of the drop solution when the dropper is returned to the bottle. Once the drops are instilled, maintain the child's head in hyperextension for at least 1 minute to ensure that the drops have come in contact with the nasal membranes.

For nasal sprays, position the child upright and place the tip of the spray bottle just inside the nasal opening and tilted toward the back. Squeeze the container, providing just enough force for the spray to be expelled from the container. Using too great a force can push the spray solution and secretions into the sinuses or Eustachian tube.

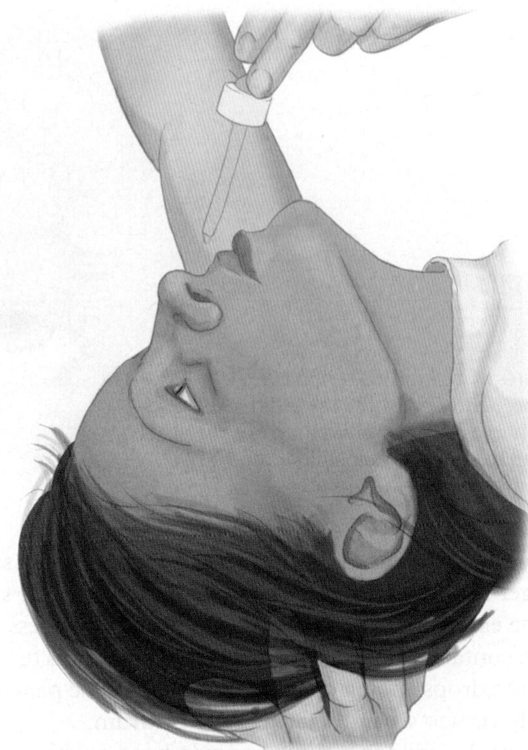

● Figure 14.7 Administering nose drops. Tilt the head down and back to instill nose drops.

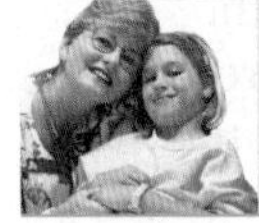

In young infants, instill the medication in one naris at a time, since they are obligate nose breathers.

Intramuscular Administration

Intramuscular (IM) administration delivers medication to the muscle. In children, this method of medication administration is used infrequently because it is painful and children often lack adequate muscle mass for medication absorption. However, IM administration is used to administer certain medications.

Muscle development and the amount of fluid to be injected determine IM injection sites in children. Needle size (gauge and length) is determined by the size of the muscle and the viscosity of the medication. For example, more viscous medications often require a larger-gauge needle. In addition, the needle must be long enough to ensure that the medication reaches the muscle.

The preferred injection site for infants is the vastus lateralis muscle. An alternative site is the rectus femoris muscle. The dorsogluteal site, often used in adults, is not used in children until the child has been walking for at least a year. The muscle has not fully developed and the sciatic nerve occupies a larger portion of this area in the young child. The deltoid muscle, which is a small muscle mass, is used as an IM injection site in children after the age of 4 to 5 years of age due to the small muscle mass. Figure 14.8 illustrates IM injection sites.

Select the needle size and gauge based on the size of the child's muscle. The goal is to use the smallest length and gauge that will deposit the medication in the muscle. Table 14.3 provides general guidelines for solution amount, needle size, and needle gauge when administering IM medications.

Insert the needle into the skin at a 90-degree angle. If the child is a very small infant or has a small muscle mass, use a 45-degree angle.

Subcutaneous and Intradermal Administration

Subcutaneous (SC) administration distributes medication into the fatty layers of the body. It is used primarily for insulin administration. Subcutaneous layers differ among individuals. The preferred sites for SC administration include the anterior thigh, buttocks, upper arms, and abdomen. Use a 3/8- or 5/8-inch needle. Spread the skin tightly or pinch up the skin with the nondominant hand to isolate the tissue from the muscle. Insert the needle at a 45- to 90-degree angle, release the skin if pinched, and inject the medication slowly.

Intradermal (ID) administration deposits medication just under the epidermis. The forearm is the usual site for administration. ID administration is used primarily for tuberculosis screening and allergy testing. A 1-mL syringe with a 5/8-inch, 25- or 27-gauge needle is commonly used to administer the medication. Insert the needle beneath the skin at a 5- to 15-degree angle.

Intravenous Administration

Intravenous (IV) medication administration is commonly used with children, especially when a rapid response to a drug is desired or when absorption via other routes is difficult due to the child's illness or condition. In some cases, the IV route is the only effective method for administering a medication. Use of the IV route requires that the child have an IV device inserted, peripherally or centrally. Although insertion of this device is invasive and traumatic for the child, IV medication administration is considered to be less traumatic when compared to the trauma associated with multiple injections. Unfortunately, the veins of a child are small and easily irritated.

Most medications given by the IV route must be given at a specified rate and diluted properly to prevent overdose or toxicity due to the rapid onset of action that occurs with this route. Therefore, administering medications via the IV route requires knowledge of the drug, the amount of drug to be administered, the minimum dilution of the drug, the type of solution for dilution or infusion, the length of time for infusion, the rate of infusion, the IV tubing volume capacity, and the compatibility of various solutions and medications (Algren & Arnow, 2005). Careful maintenance of the IV site is required to prevent complications.

The primary method for IV medication administration is a syringe pump. This method provides a highly precise rate of infusion. Nursing Procedure 14.1 gives the steps for administering medication via a syringe pump.

If a pump is unavailable, the medication may be administered via a volume control device. The medication is added to the device with a specified amount of compatible fluid and then infused at the ordered rate.

Direct IV push medication typically is reserved for emergency situations and when therapeutic blood levels must be reached quickly to achieve the desired effect (Weinstein, 2006). Direct IV push administration requires that the drug be diluted appropriately and given at a specified rate, such as over 2 to 3 minutes. Care must be taken to prevent fluid overload, which may occur due to flushing needed to maintain IV patency and prevent drug incompatibilities, and from the administration of multiple drug therapies.

Providing Atraumatic Care

When administering any medication, including oral medications, use the principles of atraumatic care (see Chapters 1 and 15 for more information). Children can experience stress and fear or upset when they must take oral medications. The child may become upset or stressed when he or she must be secured snugly or positioned to minimize movement. The child may experience further discomfort if the medication has an unpleasant taste. Encourage the child to participate in care and provide the child with developmentally appropriate options, such as which fluid to drink with the medication or which flavor of ice pop to suck on before or after the administration (see Table 14.2).

To decrease discomfort and pain for the child who is to receive an injection, apply a topical anesthetic such as EMLA cream or vapocoolant spray to the site before injection (see Chapter 15 for additional information). When preparing the site for injection, clean it with alcohol or an antiseptic solution and allow this solution to dry.

Ensuring that the child doesn't move is essential to prevent injury. When administering an injection to a young child, at least two adults should hold him or her; this may also be necessary to help an older child to remain still. Use positions that are comforting to the child, such as those in Figure 14.1. After administration, encourage the parents or caregivers to hold and cuddle the child and offer praise.

Educating the Child and Parents

Teaching the child and parents or caregivers about medication administration is a key component of patient

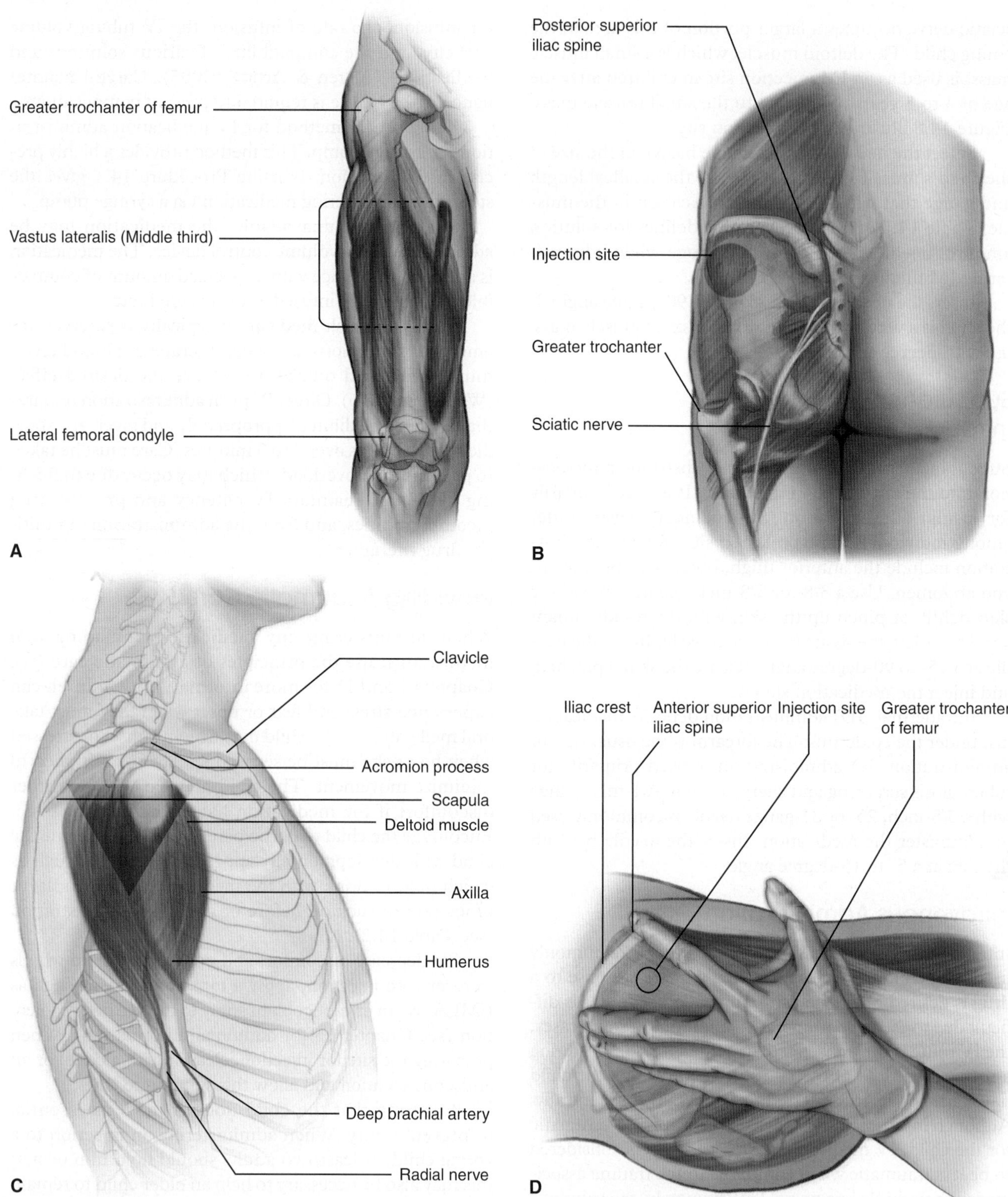

● Figure 14.8 Locating IM injection sites. (**A**) Vastus lateralis: Identify the greater trochanter and the lateral femoral condyle; inject in middle third and anterior lateral aspect. (**B**) Dorsogluteal: Place hand on iliac crest and locate the posterosuperior iliac spine; inject in the outer quadrant formed when an imaginary line is drawn between the trochanter and the iliac spine. (**C**) Deltoid: Locate the lateral side of the humerus, one fingerwidth below the acromion process. (**D**) Ventrogluteal: Place palm of left hand on right greater trochanter so index finger points toward anterosuperior iliac spine, spread middle finger to form a V, and inject in the middle of the V.

Table 14.3 Guidelines for Solution Amount, Needle Length, and Needle Gauge for IM Injections

	Solution Amount					
	Vastus Lateralis	*Dorsogluteal*	*Ventrogluteal*	*Deltoid*	**Needle Length**	**Needle Gauge**
Infant	0.5–1 mL	Not recommended	Not recommended	Not recommended	5/8 inch	25–27
Toddler	1 mL	Not recommended	1 mL	0.5 mL	5/8 to 1 inch	22–23
Preschooler	1.5 mL	1.5 mL	1.5 mL	0.5 mL	5/8 to 1 inch	22–23
School age	1.5–2 mL	1.5–2 mL	1.5–2 mL	0.5 mL	5/8 to 1.5 inch	22–23
Adolescent	2–2.5 mL	2–2.5 mL	2–2.5 mL	1 mL	5/8 to 1.5 inch	22–23

education. Many medications are given in the home, making the parents or caregivers the persons responsible for administration. They need to know what medications they are giving and why, how to give them, and what to expect from the drug, including adverse effects. If the medication is to be given via injection, parents and caregivers need to learn how to administer the injection properly.

Parents and caregivers commonly need suggestions about the best ways to administer the medication to their child. Provide them with tips for administration, such as mixing unpleasant-tasting medications with applesauce or yogurt or offering a favorite liquid as a chaser. Also teach the parents how to measure the amount of drug to be given. Encourage them to use a calibrated device and

Nursing Procedure 14.1

Administering Medication via a Syringe Pump

Purpose: To provide accurate and safe administration of IV medication

1. Verify the medication order.
2. Gather the medication and necessary equipment and supplies.
3. Wash hands and put on gloves.
4. Attach the syringe pump tubing to the medication syringe and purge air from the tubing by gently filling the tubing with medication from the syringe.
5. Insert the syringe into the pump according to the manufacturer's directions.
6. Clean the appropriate port on the child's IV access device or tubing, flush the device or tubing if appropriate (e.g., an intermittent infusion device [saline lock or heparin lock]), and attach the syringe tubing to the IV tubing or device.
7. Set the infusion rate on the pump as ordered.
8. When the medication infusion is completed, flush the syringe pump tubing to deliver any medication remaining in the tubing, according to institution protocol.
9. Document the procedure and the child's response to it.

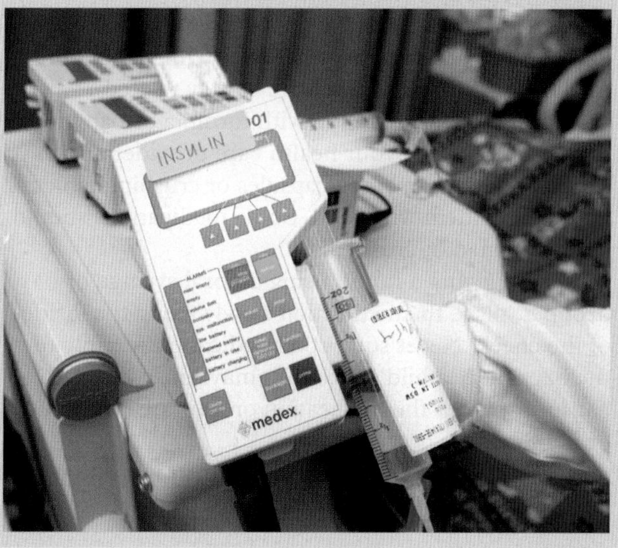

not a typical household spoon, which can vary in the amount that it holds. Teaching Guideline 14.2 gives pointers about oral medication administration.

Intravenous Therapy

IV access provides a route for the administration of medications and fluids. It is commonly used for children because it is the quickest, and often the most effective, method of administration. As with adults, numerous sites and various devices and equipment may be used to provide IV therapy over a short or long period of time. When administering IV therapy, safety is crucial. The nurse must have a solid knowledge base about the fluids or medications to be given as well as a thorough understanding of the child's physical and emotional development. Venipuncture can be a terrifying and painful experience for children and their families. Nurses play a crucial role in providing support and education to the child and family before, during, and after the procedure (refer to p. 57 for additional information related to provision of atraumatic care with procedures).

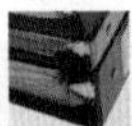

TEACHING GUIDELINE 14.2

Administering Oral Medications

- Be firm when telling your child that it is time for his or her medication. State, "It's time for your medicine" instead of asking, "Will you take your medicine?" or "Can you take your medicine for me?"
- Allow your child to choose an appropriate liquid to help swallow the medication or drink after taking it. Limit the choices to two or three.
- Never bribe or threaten your child to take his or her medication.
- Never refer to the medication as "candy."
- Be honest about the taste of the medication. If necessary, mix it with another food such as applesauce, yogurt, or syrup to help mask the taste.
- If the medication's taste cannot be masked or disguised, have your child hold his or her nose while taking the medication (taste and smell are closely related).
- Do not mix the medication with formula or baby food.
- Always check with your health care provider and pharmacy about opening capsules or crushing tablets and mixing them with food. Some medications should not be opened or crushed.
- If you are giving a liquid using an oral syringe or dropper, place the medication slowly along the inside of the cheek. Never squirt the medication forcibly to the back of the child's throat. It may cause the child to gag and spit out the medication or aspirate it into his or her lungs.
- Always praise the child after taking the medication and provide comfort and cuddling.

Sites

IV therapy may be administered via a peripheral vein or a central vein. Peripheral IV therapy sites commonly include the hands, feet, and forearms (Fig. 14.9). In infants up to about the age of 9 months, the scalp veins may be used. The scalp veins are easily visualized, being covered only by a thin layer of subcutaneous tissue. These veins do not have valves, so the device may be inserted in either direction, although the preference would be in the direction of blood flow. However, use of a scalp vein requires that that area of the infant's head be cleared of hair to enhance visualization. Thus, scalp veins are usually used only if attempts at other sites have been unsuccessful.

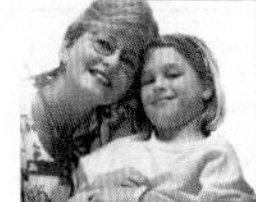

When selecting an IV site in an extremity, always choose the most distal site. Doing so prevents injury to the veins superior to the site and allows additional access sites should complications develop in the most distal site.

Central IV therapy usually is administered through a large vein, such as the subclavian, femoral, or jugular vein or the vena cava. The tip of the device lies in the superior vena cava just at the entrance to the right atrium. The device is inserted surgically or percutaneously and

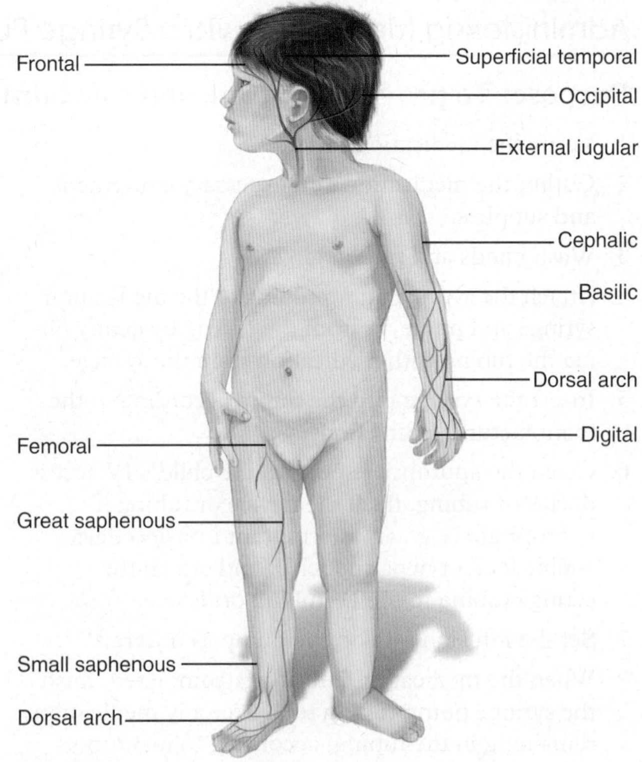

Figure 14.9 Preferred peripheral sites for IV insertion.

exits the body typically in the chest area, just below the clavicle. A device can be inserted via a peripheral vein, such as the median, cephalic, or basilic vein, and then threaded into the superior vena cava.

In the neonate, the umbilical artery or vein may be used as the site for IV therapy. These sites are commonly used during the first few days after birth (Beauman, 2001). The umbilical artery usually is used to administer IV fluids and to obtain arterial blood gases. The umbilical vein is commonly used to infuse IV fluids.

Equipment

The choice of equipment is determined by the solution or medication to be administered, the duration of the therapy, the age and developmental level of the child, the child's status, and the condition of his or her veins. Various types of IV devices are commercially available. In addition, different types of tubing and infusion control devices may be necessary.

Peripheral Access Devices

Devices used for peripheral venous access in a child include over-the-needle catheters or winged-infusion sets, commonly referred to as "butterflies" or scalp vein needles. These devices are inserted into the vein and then connected to the IV solution via tubing to provide a continuous infusion of fluid. These devices can also be inserted for intermittent use if the child does not require a continuous fluid infusion. Typically, the hub of the device is capped or plugged to allow intermittent access, such as for administering medications or obtaining blood specimens. When used in this manner, these devices are termed peripheral intermittent infusion devices or saline or heparin locks.

Needle size on the device also varies. Typically, size ranges from 21 to 25 gauge, depending on the child's size. The rule of thumb is to use the smallest-gauge catheter with the shortest length possible to prevent traumatizing the child's fragile veins.

Central Access Devices

Numerous devices for central venous access are available. The type chosen depends on several factors, including the duration of the therapy, the child's diagnosis, the risks to the child from insertion, and the ability of the child and family to care for the device. The device may have one or multiple lumens. Although central venous access devices can be used short term, the majority are used for moderate- to long-term therapy.

Central venous access devices are indicated when the child lacks suitable peripheral access, requires IV fluid or medication for more than 3 to 5 days, or is to receive specific treatments, such as the administration of highly concentrated solutions or irritating drugs that require rapid dilution. Patient preference is also a consideration. Central venous access is advantageous because it provides vascular access without the need for multiple IV starts, thus decreasing discomfort and fear. However, central venous access devices are associated with complications such as thrombosis due to partial occlusion of the vessel and infection at the site as well as in the blood due to the direct access to the central circulation (de Jonge et al., 2005; Glaser, 2001). Typically, a chest x-ray is performed after a central venous access device is inserted to verify proper placement. No fluids are administered until correct placement is confirmed. Table 14.4 describes the major types of central venous access devices.

Infusion Control Devices

Infants and young children are at increased risk for fluid volume overload compared with adults. Also, malfunction at the IV insertion site, such as infiltration, may result in much greater injury than a similar incident would cause in an adult. Therefore, IV fluids must be carefully administered and monitored. To ensure accurate fluid administration, infusion control devices such as infusion pumps, syringe pumps, and volume control sets may be used.

Infusion pumps used for children are similar to those used for adults. Typically, the IV solution bag is attached to a calibrated volume control set that has been filled with a specified amount of IV solution (Fig. 14.10). The fluid chamber holds a maximum of 100 to 150 mL of fluid that can be infused over a specified period of time as ordered. Usually, a maximum of a 2-hour infusion amount in the chamber avoids accidental fluid overload in the pediatric population. This chamber can be filled every 1 to 2 hours so only small amounts of ordered quantities of fluid can infuse and the child is protected from receiving too much fluid volume.

In addition, syringe pumps may be used to deliver fluid and medications to children. These pumps can be programmed to deliver minute amounts of fluid over controlled periods of time (see discussion on p. 363 for additional information about syringe pumps).

Fluid Administration

Administering IV fluids to an infant or child requires close attention to the child's fluid status. Typically, the amount of fluid to be administered in a day (24 hours) is determined by the child's weight (in kg) using the following formula:

100 mL per kg of body weight for the first 10 kg
50 mL per kg of body weight for the next 10 kg
20 mL per kg of body weight for the remainder of body weight in kg

Table 14.5 gives examples of calculating a child's fluid requirements using body weight. Once the 24-hour total fluid requirement is determined, this amount is divided by 24 hours to arrive at the correct hourly rate of infusion.

Table 14.4 Types of Central Venous Access Devices

Device	Description
Nontunneled central venous catheter (CVC)	Usually used short term One or more lumens Surgical or percutaneous insertion most commonly via the subclavian, internal jugular, or femoral vein with the tip of the catheter at the top of the superior vena cava just above the right atrium Useful for emergency situations Catheter sutured in place at the exit site
Peripherally inserted central catheters (PICC)	Short- to moderate-term therapy Insertion via a peripheral vein such as antecubital, basilic, cephalic, or medial antecubital vein Catheter typically threaded into superior vena cava; distal tip terminates in the superior vena cava, inferior vena cava, or proximal right atrium Insertion via saphenous vein with tip terminating in inferior vena cava above the diaphragm for infants Single or multiple lumens PICC insertion requires additional training and advanced skill.
Tunneled central venous catheter (e.g., Groshong, Hickman/Broviac)	Usually for long-term use Catheter inserted by a physician via small incision in jugular or subclavian vein and tunneled in the subcutaneous tissue under the skin Initially sutured in place to stabilize position; sutures removed after approximately 1 to 2 weeks when cuff on catheter attaches to subcutaneous tissue Single or multiple lumens Some have valves that prevent backflow of blood and air entrance.
Implanted ports (e.g., Port-a-Cath, Infus-a-Port, Mediport)	Surgically inserted by a physician Stainless-steel port with a polyurethane or silicone catheter attached Catheter tip lying in subclavian or jugular vein; port implanted under skin in a subcutaneous pocket, usually on the upper chest wall Port covered completely by skin and visible only as a slight bulging on the chest; possibly more appealing to the older child and adolescent because there are no visible parts or dressings Access to port via a specially angled, non-coring needle (Huber needle) Site preparation and pain relief measures necessary before accessing the port

Inserting Peripheral IV Access Devices

Typically, peripheral IV devices are used for short-term therapy, usually averaging 3 to 5 days. Review the child's diagnosis and medical history for information that may affect therapy, such as site selection or insertion. For example, a child who has a history of chronic illness may have heightened fears and anxieties related to insertion due to his or her previous experiences or difficulty in accessing IV sites. Typically, the nondominant extremity should be used for insertion, but this may not be possible if a right-handed child has a cast on his left arm.

Check the orders for the prescribed therapy. Determine the purpose and length of the IV therapy and the type of fluid or medication that is to be administered. This information aids in selecting the best device and insertion site. For example, the device needs to be of an adequate gauge to allow the solution or medication to infuse into the vein while at the same time allowing

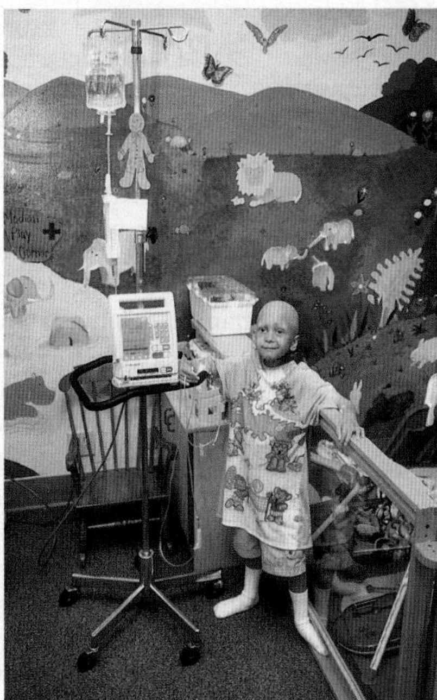

● Figure 14.10 Volume control infusion device.

enough blood flow around the device to promote dilution of the infusion.

Establish rapport with the child and parents. Inform them about IV therapy and what to expect. Be honest with the child. Explain that the venipuncture will hurt but only for a short time. Provide the child with a time frame that he or she can understand, such as the time it takes to brush the teeth or eat a snack. If possible, use therapeutic play to assist the child in coping (see Chapter 11 for more information).

Insertion of an IV therapy device is traumatic. Follow the principles of atraumatic care, including the following:

- Gather all equipment needed before approaching the child.
- If possible, select a site using hand veins rather than wrist or upper arm veins to reduce the risk of phlebitis. Avoid using lower extremity veins if possible because these are associated with an increased risk of infection (CDC, 2002).
- Ensure adequate pain relief using pharmacologic and nonpharmacologic methods prior to insertion of the device (see Chapter 15 for more information about management of pain related to procedures).
- Allow the antiseptic used to prepare the site to dry completely before attempting insertion.
- Use a barrier such as a gauze or washcloth or the sleeve of the child's gown under the tourniquet to avoid pinching or damaging the skin.
- If the child's veins are difficult to locate, use a device to transilluminate the vein (shows the vein's size and direction of travel).
- Make only two attempts to gain access; if you are unsuccessful after two attempts, allow another individual two attempts to access a site. If still unsuccessful, evaluate the need for insertion of another device.
- Encourage parental participation as appropriate in helping to position the child or to provide comfort positioning, such as therapeutic hugging.
- Coordinate care with other departments such as the laboratory for blood specimen collection to minimize the number of venipunctures for the child.
- Secure the IV line using a minimal amount of tape or transparent dressing.

Table 14.5 Intravenous Maintenance Fluid Calculations by Body Weight

<10 kg in weight	100 mL per kg of weight = # mL for 24 hours Example: A child weighs 7.4 kg. 7.4 × 100 = 740 mL (daily requirement) 740/24 = 30.8 or 31 mL/hour
11–20 kg in weight	100 mL per kg of weight for the first 10 kg + 50 mL/kg for the next 10 kg = # mL for 24 hours Example: A child weighs 16 kg. (10 × 100 = 1,000) plus (6 × 50 = 300) Total = 1,300 mL (daily requirement) 1,300/24 = 54 mL/hour
>20 kg in weight	100 mL/kg for the first 10 kg + 50 mL/kg for the next 10 kg + 20 mL/kg for each kg > 20 kg = # mL for 24 hours Example: A child weighs 30 kg. (10 × 100 = 1,000) plus (10 × 50 = 500) plus (10 × 20 = 200) Total = 1,700 mL (daily requirement) 1,700/24 = 70.8 or 71 mL/hr

• Protect the site from bumping by using a security device such as the I.V. House dressing (Fig. 14.11).

Maintaining IV Fluid Therapy

Throughout the course of therapy, monitor the fluid infusion rate and volume closely, as often as every hour. If a volume control set is used to administer the IV infusion, fill the device with the allotted amount of fluid that the child is to receive in 1 hour. Doing so prevents inadvertent administration of too much fluid. Never assume that just because an infusion pump is in use, the infusion is being administered without problems. Pumps can malfunction. The tubing can become blocked, or the IV device can move out of the vein lumen. Not enough fluid, fluid overload, or infiltration of the solution into the tissues can occur.

In addition to monitoring the fluid infusion, closely monitor the child's output. Expected urine output for children and adolescents is 1.0 to 2.0 mL/kg/hour (Weinstein, 2006).

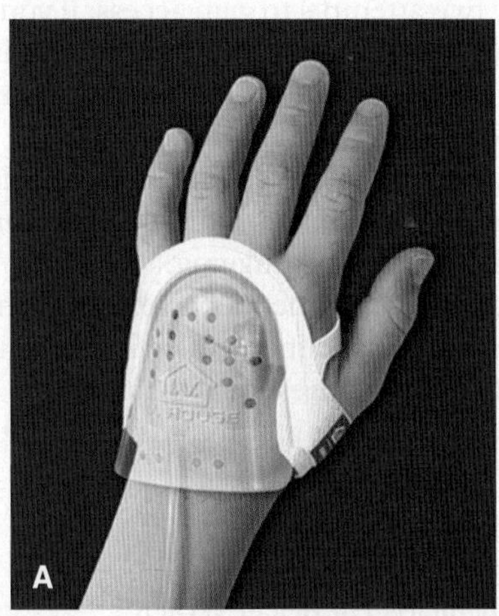

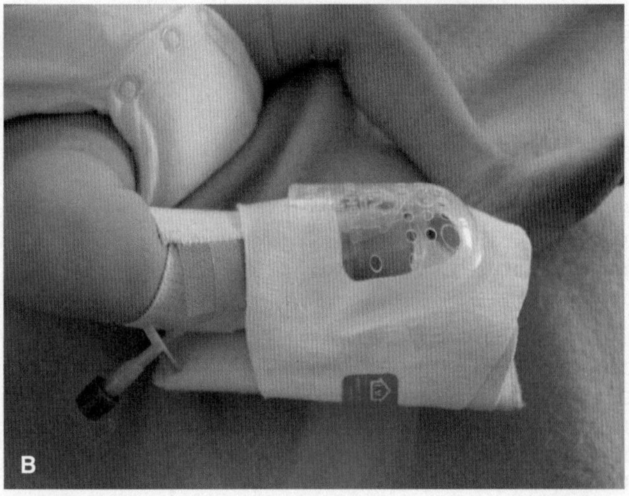

● Figure 14.11 (**A**) IV House over the IV site on a child's hand. (**B**) IV House over the site on an infant's foot.

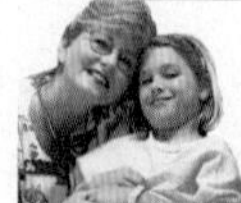

When measuring the output of an infant or child who is not toilet-trained or who is incontinent, weigh the diaper to determine the output. Remember that 1 gram of weight is equal to 1 mL of fluid.

Historically, padded armboards and footboards were used to prevent movement of the IV device, but today these are considered mechanical restraints and as such should be used only as a last resort when no less restrictive method is available or effective. Padded boards also can interfere with inspection of the insertion site. They also restrict movement, increasing the risk of contractures; they may be uncomfortable; and they can irritate the underlying tissue, leading to excoriation and infection. Moreover, research has failed to demonstrate that the use of armboards promotes patency of the IV line (Algren & Arnow, 2005).

Flushing the IV line when the device is used intermittently may be necessary to maintain patency, such as before and/or after medication is administered and after obtaining blood specimens. However, there is much debate as to how often flushing should be done and the best flush solution to use, heparin or saline. Saline has been found to be more compatible with the numerous solutions and medications administered intravenously and less expensive and less irritating to the vein; also, the incidence of pain and phlebitis is less. Heparin is expensive and incompatible with numerous medications and solutions, and it can affect clotting time, depending on the concentration of the flush solution used. Evidence appears to support the use of normal saline flush with catheters larger than 24 gauge, but more studies are needed to determine the effectiveness of normal saline flushes with catheters smaller than 24 gauge. Additional research is also needed to determine the specific frequency interval for flushing and the volume and concentration of the flush solution to use (Knue et al., 2006). Always follow your agency's policy for flushing IV lines.

If the child is receiving IV therapy via a central venous access device, provide site care using sterile technique and flush the device according to agency policy. Note the exit site for the device and inspect it frequently for signs of infection. If the device has multiple lumens, label each lumen with its use (i.e., blood specimen, medication, or fluid). Always check the compatibilities of solutions and medications being given simultaneously.

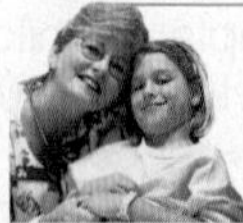

When flushing or administering medications through a peripherally inserted central catheter (PICC) line, use a 5-mL syringe or larger, because PICC lines are fragile. Using a larger-volume syringe exerts less pressure on the PICC, thereby reducing the risk of complications.

Preventing Complications

IV therapy is an invasive procedure that is associated with numerous complications. Strict aseptic technique is necessary when inserting the device and caring for the site. Adherence to standard precautions is key. Inspect the insertion site every 1 to 2 hours for inflammation or **infiltration** (inadvertent infusion of a nonirritant solution or medication into the surrounding tissue) (Weinstein, 2006). Note signs of inflammation such as warmth, redness, induration, or tender skin. Check closely for signs of infiltration such as cool, blanched, or puffy skin. Use of a transparent dressing or IV House dressing provides easy access for assessing the IV insertion site. These types of dressings also help to prevent movement of the catheter hub, thus minimizing the risk of mechanical irritation and complications such as phlebitis or infection.

Typically, an IV site is changed every 72 hours and at any time when the integrity of the system has been compromised or contamination is suspected (Weinstein, 2006). However, with children, the 72-hour time frame may need to be adjusted to minimize the child's exposure to the repeated trauma of insertion. Follow the agency's policies and procedures related to site changes. Consider an alternative route for fluid and medication administration or the insertion of an alternative IV device, such as a PICC line.

Discontinuing the IV Device

Prepare the child for removal of the IV device in much the same manner as for insertion. Many children may fear the removal of the device to the same extent that they feared its insertion. Explain what is to occur and enlist the child's help in the removal. If appropriate, allow the child to assist in removing the tape or dressing. This gives the child a sense of control over the situation and also encourages his or her cooperation. In addition, practice atraumatic care by doing the following:

- Use water or adhesive remover to help loosen the tape.
- If a transparent dressing is in place, gently lift off the dressing by pulling up opposite corners using a motion parallel to the skin surface.
- Avoid using scissors to cut the tape, but if cutting the tape is necessary, be sure that the child's fingers are clear of the tape and scissors.
- Turn off the infusion solution and pump.
- Once all tape and dressings are removed, gently slide the IV device out using a motion opposite to that used for the insertion.
- Apply pressure to the site with a dry gauze dressing and then cover with a small adhesive bandage. If possible, allow the child to choose the bandage.

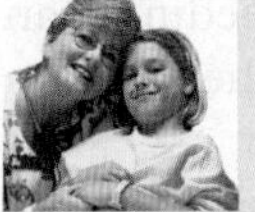

If the IV site was in the arm at or near the antecubital space, do not have the child bend his or her arm after removal of the device. Doing so increases the risk of hematoma formation.

Nutritional Support

Adequate nutrition is important for all individuals but especially for children. The quality of a child's nutrition during the growing years has a major effect on his or her overall health and development (Klossner & Hatfield, 2006). The presence of a chronic illness, disease, or trauma can increase the child's nutritional demands; if the child cannot meet these even with oral supplementation, other measures may be necessary to provide nutritional support. Such measures may include **enteral nutrition** (delivery of nutrition into the gastrointestinal tract via a tube) and **parenteral nutrition** (IV delivery of nutritional substances). The nutritional plan is determined by the child's age, developmental level, and health status.

Enteral Nutrition

Enteral nutrition, commonly called tube feedings, involves the insertion of a tube so that feedings can be delivered directly into the child's gastrointestinal tract. The tube may be inserted via the nose or mouth or through an opening in the abdominal area, with the tube ending in the stomach or jejunum. Nasogastric or orogastric tube feedings are commonly referred to **gavage feedings**. Gastrostomy feedings involve the insertion of a gastrostomy tube through an opening in the abdominal wall and into the stomach. Jejunostomy feedings are similar to gastrostomy feedings except that the tube lies in the jejunum.

Enteral nutrition is indicated for children who have a functioning gastrointestinal tract but cannot ingest enough nutrients orally. The child may be unconscious or have a severely debilitating condition that interferes with his or her ability to consume adequate food and fluids. Other conditions that may warrant the use of enteral nutrition include:

- Failure to thrive
- Inability to suck or tiring easily during sucking
- Abnormalities of the throat or esophagus
- Swallowing difficulties or risk for aspiration
- Respiratory distress
- Metabolic conditions
- Severe gastroesophageal reflux disease (GERD)
- Surgery
- Severe trauma

Enteral feedings may be given via nasogastric, orogastric, gastrostomy, or jejunostomy tubes (Fig. 14.12). Table 14.6 provides additional information about these types of feeding tubes. Enteral feedings are less costly than parenteral feedings; they are considered a safer alternative for nutritional support and are associated with improved outcomes (Westhus, 2004). Tube misplacement is a serious complication of enteral feeding.

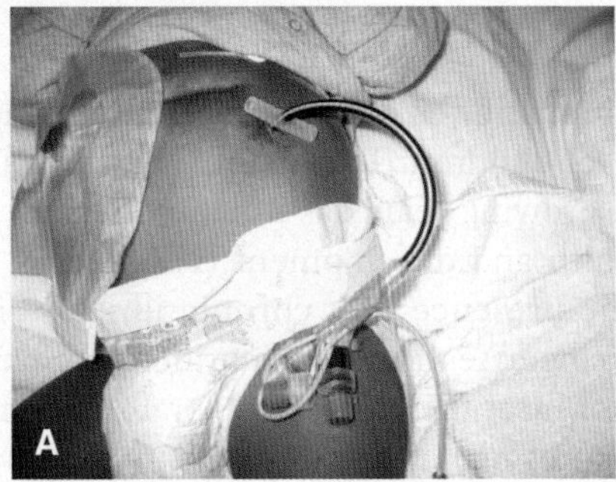

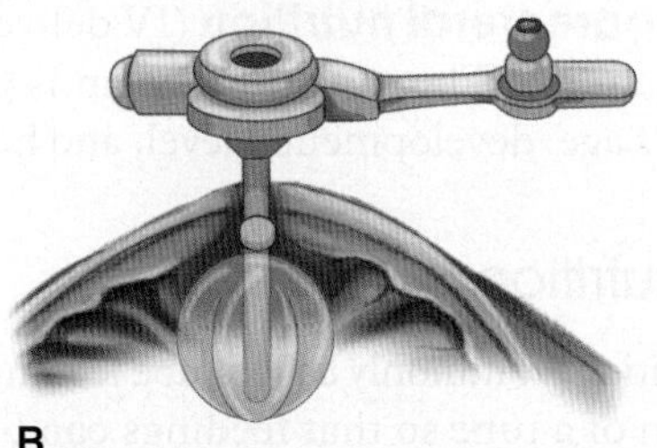

● Figure 14.12 (**A**) Gastrostomy tube. (**B**) Low-profile (button) gastrostomy tube. The filled balloon keeps the tube in place inside the stomach.

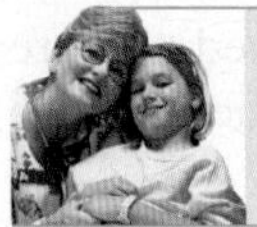

Small-diameter feeding tubes, though more comfortable, may easily become dislodged if the child coughs vigorously.

Inserting a Nasogastric or Orogastric Feeding Tube

Tubes for gavage feeding can be inserted via the nose or mouth. For infants, who are obligate nose breathers, insertion via the mouth may be appropriate. Oral insertion also promotes sucking in the infant. For the older child, nasal insertion is usually the preferred method. If the tube is to remain in place, the nose also is considered to be more comfortable. Nursing Procedure 14.2 gives the steps for inserting a gavage feeding tube.

Once the gavage feeding tube is inserted, checking for placement is essential. Tube placement must be confirmed each time the tube is inserted and prior to each use. Radiologic confirmation of tube placement is considered the most accurate method, but the risks associated with repeated radiation exposure to verify tube placement prohibit its use (Westhus, 2004). Several methods have been proposed as reliable for checking tube placement. Research has shown the following methods to be acceptable:

- Testing the pH of the feeding tube aspirate (pH less than 6 indicates gastric placement; pH over 6 indicates intestinal placement)
- Inspecting the color of the aspirate (clear, tan, or green indicates gastric placement; yellow or bile-stained indicates intestinal placement [Westhus, 2004])

Even with these methods, tube malpositioning can occur. Research also has suggested using measurements of bilirubin, trypsin, and pepsin levels to enhance assessment of tube placement, but no methods are available for bedside testing of these levels (Huffman et al., 2004). Therefore, nurses need to be vigilant in checking for tube placement using the recommended methods and be cautious and proactive if there is any suspicion that the tube may be misplaced.

If the gavage feeding tube is to remain in place, secure it to the child's cheek. Do not tape the tube to the child's forehead because this could lead to irritation and pressure on and possible breakdown of the nasal mucosa. Also measure the length of the tube extending from the nose or mouth to the end and record this information. Double-check this measurement before administering each intermittent tube feeding to verify that the feeding tube is in the proper position. Once the position of the gavage feeding tube is confirmed, the feeding solution or medication can be administered.

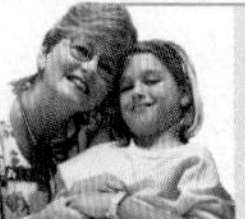

Instilling air into the tube and then auscultating for the sound is no longer considered a viable method for checking tube placement. Air instilled into a tube that is positioned above the gastroesophageal sphincter can still be auscultated as air in the stomach, thereby giving a false-positive result.

Remember Lily, the 9-month-old infant diagnosed with failure to thrive who is to receive gavage feedings with a nasogastric tube? What equipment will be needed, and what steps will you take to complete the procedure?

Administering Enteral Feedings

Enteral feedings can be given continuously or intermittently, regardless of the type of tube used. Intermittent feedings are commonly called **bolus feedings**. With a bolus feeding, a specified amount of feeding solution is given at specific intervals, usually over a short period of time such as 15 to 30 minutes. Given via a syringe, feeding bag, or infusion pump, bolus feedings most closely resemble regular meals. Continuous feedings are given at a slower rate over a longer period of time. In some cases, the feeding may be given during the night so that the child can be free to move about and participate in activities during the day. For continuous feedings, an enteral feeding pump is used to administer the solution at a prescribed rate.

Checking for tube placement is a priority before administering any intermittent tube feeding and periodi-

Table 14.6 Types of Enteral Feeding Tubes

Type of Tube	Indication	Nursing Implications
Nasogastric (inserted via the nose into the stomach) Orogastric (inserted via the mouth into the stomach)	Short-term enteral feeding. Orogastric usually limited to young infants only.	• Long-term use or repeated insertion causes irritation and discomfort. • Silicone and polyurethane tubes are very flexible and more comfortable; they require a stylet or guidewire for insertion. • Length of long-term use varies according to the type of tube used and the institution protocol. Periodically a nasogastric tube is removed and reinserted via the opposite nostril to prevent pressure on the nasal mucosa. • Maintaining orogastric placement between feedings can be difficult due to oral secretions.
Gastrostomy (surgically inserted through the abdominal wall into the stomach) Jejunostomy (surgically inserted through the abdominal wall into the jejunum)	Long-term enteral feeding or when esophageal atresia or stricture is present. Jejunostomy tubes are indicated when gastric feeding is not tolerated.	• The inner section of the tube is below the skin surface with the tip located in the stomach or jejunum (may be balloon, winged, or mushroom-shaped). The outer section appears above the skin surface at the insertion site and has an opening or feeding port to which the feeding solution is attached. • Low-profile gastrostomy device (gastrostomy button) is flush with the abdominal surface. The flip-top opening is anchored by a dome that fits against the stomach wall. Less conspicuous, it allows the child to be more active and mobile. • After initial insertion, the tube length is measured from the insertion site to the far end of the tube and recorded. This measurement is checked at least daily to ensure that the tube has not moved. • For any gastrostomy or jejunostomy tube, the type and size of tube inserted as well as the amount required to fill the balloon if present should be known.

cally during continuous tube feedings, regardless of the type of tube being used. Once placement is confirmed, the feeding can be given. Also, measure the gastric **residual** (the amount remaining in the stomach; indicates gastric emptying time) by aspirating the gastric contents with a syringe, measuring it, and then replacing the contents. Check the residuals periodically, according to the facility's policy, such as every 4 to 6 hours, and before each intermittent feeding. If the residual volume exceeds the amount specified by the physician's order, hold the feeding and notify the physician.

Begin the feeding by placing the child in a supine position with the head and shoulders elevated approximately 30 degrees so that the feeding will remain in the stomach area. Flush the tube with a small amount of water to clear it and prevent occlusion. This is not necessary for a gavage feeding if the tube is being inserted each time a feeding is given. Ensure that the feeding solution is at room temperature. Administer the feeding as per the facility's policy.

Feeding solutions may be placed into the barrel of a syringe or into a feeding bag attached to the feeding tube and allowed to flow by gravity. The rate of flow for gravity-assisted feedings can be increased or decreased by raising or lowering the feeding solution container, respectively. Typically, intermittent feedings last from 15 to 30 minutes. A feeding bag also may be attached to a pump to control the rate of flow. Monitor the child's tolerance to the feeding.

Once the feeding is complete but before the formula completely empties from the container, flush the tube with water. As the water leaves the syringe or tubing, clamp the tube to prevent air from entering the stomach. Then disconnect the syringe or tube-feeding bag from the tube (Children's Healthcare of Atlanta, 2004).

Nursing Procedure 14.2

Inserting a Gavage Feeding Tube

Purpose: To provide a means for delivering nutrition to the child's functioning gastrointestinal tract

1. Verify the order for gavage feeding.
2. Explain the procedure to the child and parents using appropriate language geared to the child's development level.
3. Gather the necessary equipment; remove formula for feeding from refrigerator if appropriate and allow it to come to room temperature.
4. Wash hands and put on gloves.
5. Inspect the child's nose and mouth for deformities that may interfere with passage of the tube.
6. Position the infant supine with the head slightly elevated and with the neck slightly hyperextended so that the nose is pointed upward. If necessary, place a rolled towel or blanket under the neck to help in maintaining this position. Assist the older child to a sitting position if appropriate. Alternatively, have the parent or another person hold the child to promote comfort and reassurance. Enlist the aid of additional persons, such as a parent or other health care team member, to assist in maintaining the child's position.
7. Determine the tubing length for insertion: measure from the tip of the nose to the earlobe to the middle of the area between the xiphoid process and umbilicus. Mark this measurement on the tube with an indelible pen or with a piece of tape.
8. Lubricate the tube with a generous amount of sterile water or water-soluble lubricant to promote passage of the tube and minimize trauma to the child's mucosa.
9. Insert the tube into one of the nares or the mouth. Direct a nasally inserted tube straight back toward the occiput; direct an orally inserted tube toward the back of the throat.
10. Advance the tube slowly to the designated length; encourage the child (if capable) to swallow frequently to assist with advancing the tube.
11. Watch for signs of distress, such as gasping, coughing, or cyanosis, indicating that the tube is in the airway. If these signs develop, withdraw the tube and allow the child to rest before attempting reinsertion.
12. Check for proper placement of the tube by attaching a bulb syringe to the end of the tube and aspirating stomach contents; the pH of the aspirate should be less than 6 (indicating gastric acid) and the color of the aspirate should be clear, tan, or green (indicating gastric secretions); return any aspirated contents to the stomach.
13. Document the type of tube inserted, length of tubing inserted, measurement of external tubing length after insertion, and confirmation of placement.

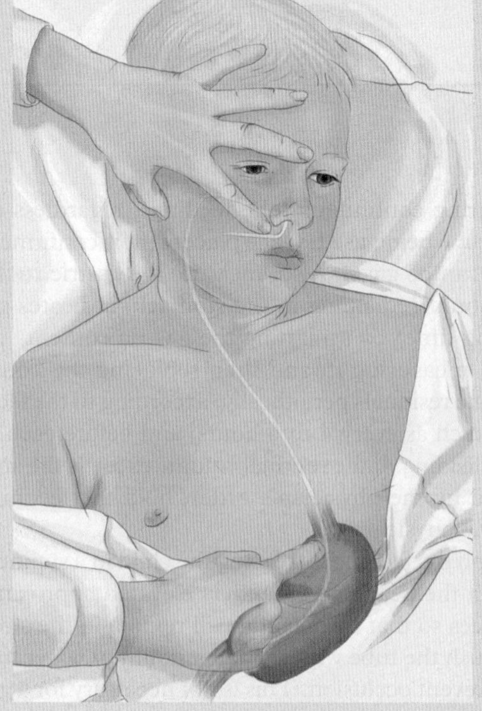

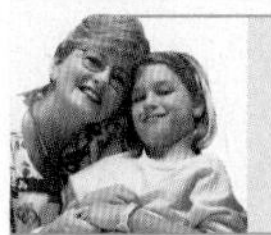

If the child vomits during the feeding, stop the feeding immediately and turn him onto his side or sit him up.

If the child has a gastrostomy button, open the cap and connect an adaptor or insert extension tubing through the one-way valve. This allows access to the gastric conduit. The feeding solution container is connected to the extension tubing or adaptor and the feeding is given as described previously. After the feeding is completed, the extension tubing or adaptor is flushed with water and the flip-top opening is closed.

Burp the infant during and after any type of tube feeding in the same manner as for an infant who is bottle- or breast-fed. Also, position the child on his or her right side with the head slightly elevated, approximately 30 degrees, for about 1 hour after the feeding to facilitate gastric emptying and reduce the risk of aspiration and regurgitation. Weigh the child daily throughout enteral nutrition therapy to determine the effectiveness of the therapy.

Providing Skin and Insertion Site Care

Skin around the insertion gastrostomy or jejunostomy site may become irritated from movement of the tube, moisture, or leakage of stomach or intestinal contents, or due to the adhesive device holding the tube in place. Keeping the skin clean and dry will help prevent most of these problems (Children's Healthcare of Atlanta, 2004). Routine site care includes gentle cleansing with soap and water followed by rinsing or cleaning with water alone.

The skin around a gastrostomy or jejunostomy tube requires cleaning at least once a day. Ordinary soap and water are sufficient to clean about the tube site to prevent buildup. To clean under an external disc or bumper, a cotton-tipped applicator may be used. Diluted hydrogen peroxide is not recommended for cleaning the site because it is irritating and cytotoxic (Burd & Burd, 2003). During insertion site care, rotate the gastrostomy tube or button a quarter-turn to prevent skin adherence and irritation (Children's Healthcare of Atlanta, 2004). Assess the insertion site and condition of the surrounding skin for signs and symptoms of infection, such as erythema, induration, foul drainage, or pain.

Preventing movement of the tube also helps reduce skin irritation. Check the volume of the balloon with a balloon-tipped device about once or twice a week and reinflate the balloon to the initial volume if needed. Measure the external length of a mushroom-tipped device daily and ensure that the tube is stabilized (Burd & Burd, 2003). Tube stabilization methods help prevent the tube from moving around and sliding further into the stomach or jejunum. Stabilize the tube by pulling gently on the tubing and sliding the stabilizer bar or disc snugly against the abdomen. Then, measure and record the length of the tube from the exit site of the abdominal wall to the end of the tube. All future measurements should be the same unless the tube length is changed. For tubes without a stabilizer bar or disc or for additional stabilization needs, several other methods may be used, including nipples, tape, tension loops, and hydroactive dressings (Box 14.5).

Promoting Growth and Development

Some children receive all of their nutritional needs through tube feedings, whereas other children use tube feedings as a supplement to eating by mouth. Feeding time is a special time for infants and children. Occasionally, babies who are fed solely through an enteral feeding tube may forget or lose the desire to eat by mouth. Use a pacifier to help avoid this, allowing the infant to associate the nipple in his or her mouth with a feeding. The sucking motion will also exercise the jaw and promote the flow of the feedings. The saliva produced during sucking aids in digestion. Combined with holding the infant and cuddling, rocking, and talking to him or her, this promotes a more normal feeding time.

Talking with children, playing music, or reading a story promotes an active feeding time. At home, encourage parents to include the feeding as a part of regular family mealtime together to provide socialization for the child. Allow the child to participate in the feedings by gathering supplies and administering the actual feeding so that the child may experience independence and adaptation. If the child also eats food by mouth, feed him or her by mouth first and then administer the tube feeding. During tube feedings in bed, make sure the head of the bed is elevated at least 30 degrees to help prevent vomiting and aspiration.

Children with feeding tubes should be allowed as normal a routine as possible. For example, they can crawl, walk, and jump just like children of the same age and developmental level. However, in some cases, contact sports such as football, hockey, and wrestling should be avoided because of the higher risk of injury. Securing the tubing under the child's clothing will prevent it from becoming accidentally dislodged. Dressing younger children in one-piece outfits helps to prevent them from playing with the gastrostomy or jejunostomy tube and helps to protect the insertion site (Fidanza, 2003).

Educating the Child and Family

Educate children receiving enteral feedings and their parents thoroughly about this method of nutritional support. Reinforce the reason for the therapy and provide the child and parents with opportunities to verbalize their concerns and ask questions. Ensure that the parents understand the risks and benefits of the therapy and the expected duration.

Provide the child, if developmentally appropriate, and parents with opportunities to participate in the feeding sessions. This helps allay some of their fears and anxieties and promotes a sense of control over the situation.

BOX 14.5

METHODS TO STABILIZE A GASTROSTOMY TUBE

Nipple Method

1. Cut a piece of skin protectant (e.g., Stomahesive®) to fit around the G-tube, leaving a small amount of skin showing around the tube.
2. Cut a half-inch from the top of a baby-bottle nipple, just large enough to fit snugly over the tube. Cut three or four holes at the base of the nipple to allow air circulation and site assessment. Slip the nipple over the tube.
3. Secure the tube to the Stomahesive® with four pieces of 1-inch-wide tape around the base of the nipple. Do not cover the holes in the nipple.
4. Gently pull on the tube until slight resistance is felt, anchoring the tube against the stomach or intestinal wall.
5. Place another piece of 1-inch-wide tape where the tube meets the nipple, securing the tube in place.

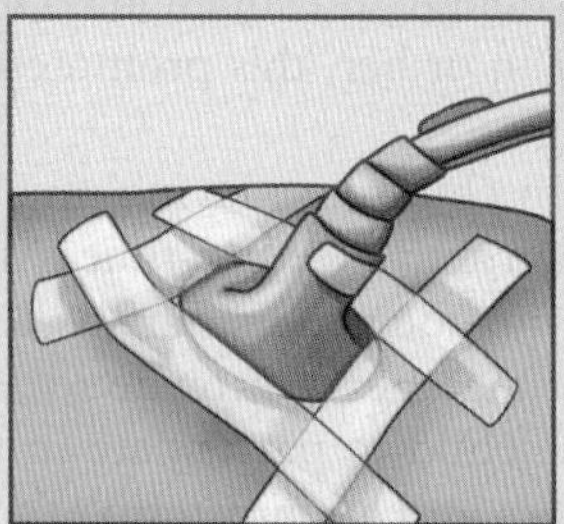

Taping Methods

1. Cut two pieces of 1-inch-wide tape about 4 to 5 inches long.
2. Fold a tab down on each piece of tape.
3. Tape the pieces to the skin and along opposite sides of the tube, sandwiching them together.

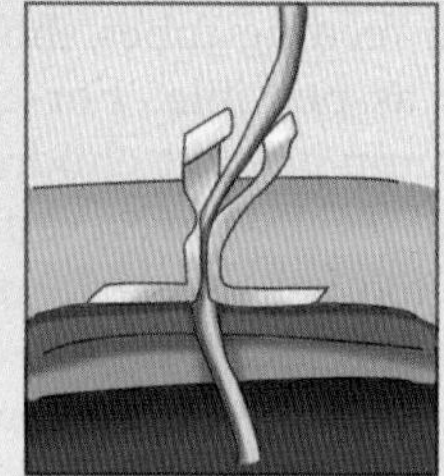

OR

1. Cut two pieces of tape about 6 inches long.
2. Form pieces into two tabs by folding the middle third of each one so it will stick onto itself. Apply these two tabs on either side of the tube directly onto the skin.

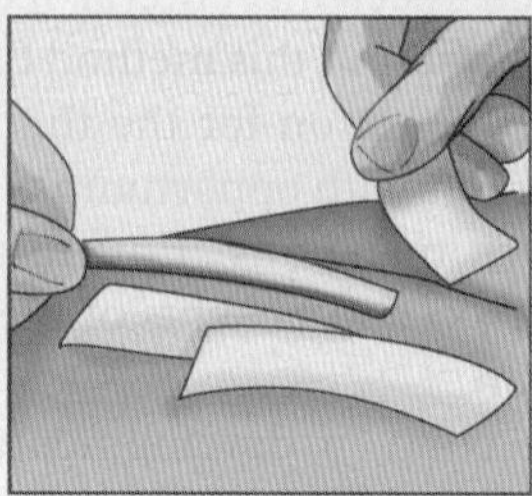

3. Cut a third piece of tape about 8 inches long, using it to go from one tab over the G-tube to the other tab and back again, leaving space at the tube insertion point. This forms an H with the two tabs.

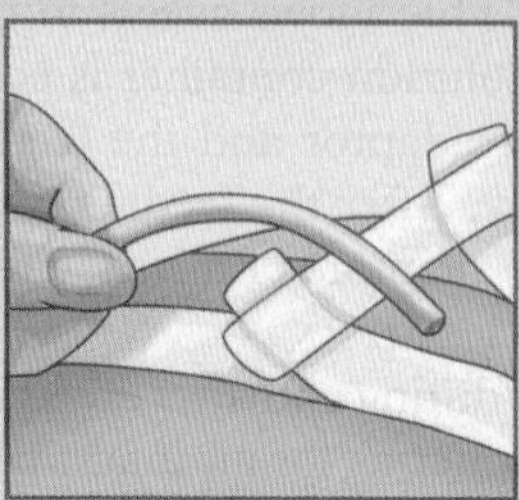

Tension Loop Method

1. Fold the middle third of a piece of tape onto itself. Place the tape onto the skin about 2 to 3 inches from the tube insertion site.
2. Fold each end of a second piece of tape onto itself to make two tabs. Fold this around the tube 3 inches away from the tube insertion site.
3. Tape the two pieces together, keeping the tube at a 90-degree angle from the abdomen.

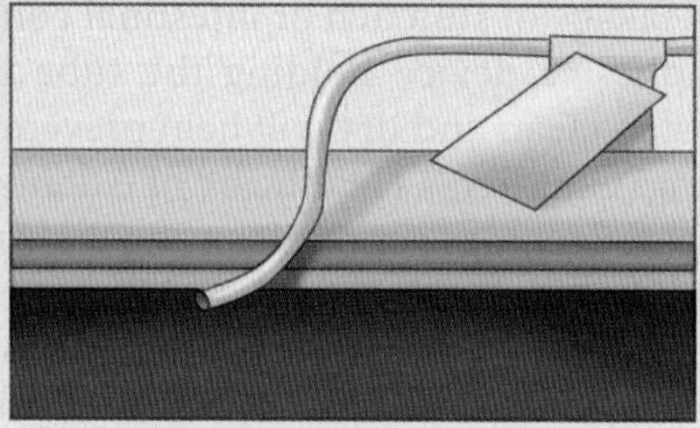

Hydroactive Dressing Method

This method of securing a tube may be used if there is skin breakdown or irritation at the insertion site.

1. Cleanse the skin with soap and water, then rinse. Dry well.
2. Cut a 2-by-3-inch piece of hydroactive dressing material, rounding off the corners. Cut through to the center and then cut a small hole the size of the tube.
3. Remove the paper backing off the hydroactive dressing and apply it to the skin, fitting snugly around the tube.

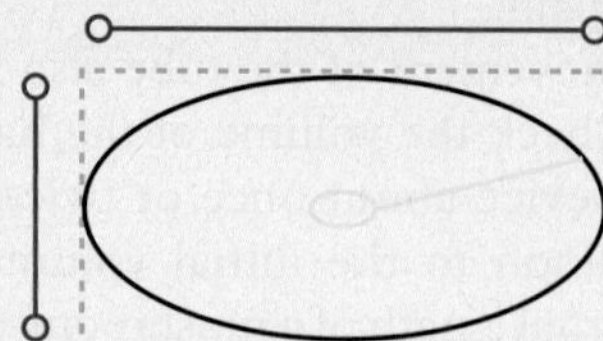

4. Reapply a new dressing every 3 to 5 days or when it becomes wet.

Adapted from Children's Healthcare of Atlanta. (2004). *Gastrostomy tube home care manual.*

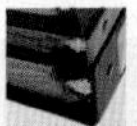

TEACHING GUIDELINE 14.3

Topics to Be Covered for Home Enteral Nutrition

- Type of nutritional support
- Rationale for therapy
- Expected results from therapy
- Duration of therapy
- Frequency of feedings
- Feeding solution and equipment
- Tube insertion technique (if appropriate)
- Methods to check for correct placement
- Steps for administering the feeding (and medication if ordered)
- Procedure for flushing tube
- Frequency of weighing the child
- Signs and symptoms of complications and when to notify health care provider
- Troubleshooting problems, such as clogging of the tube
- Daily tube care (e.g., cleaning the site, rotating tube)
- Site assessment
- Technique for reinsertion/replacement of tube as appropriate
- Equipment suppliers
- Resources for support
- Follow-up visits and referrals

They will also gain valuable practice in learning the skill should the feedings be required at home. Teaching Guideline 14.3 identifies important topics to include in the teaching plan for a child receiving enteral nutrition at home. Education also involves helping the family develop appropriate coping strategies to adapt, solve problems, and negotiate for the support and services they will need after discharge (Burd & Burd, 2003).

> Remember Lily from the beginning of the chapter? She is to be discharged home after having a gastrostomy tube inserted to continue feedings at home.
>
> What teaching is needed for her family prior to discharge?

Parenteral Nutrition

Nutritional support can be administered IV through a peripheral or central venous catheter. The concentration and components of the solution determine the type of parenteral nutrition. Parenteral nutrition given via a central venous access is termed **total parenteral nutrition (TPN)**. Comparison Chart 14.1 gives information about peripheral and central parenteral nutrition.

Administering TPN

Typically, the health care provider determines the concentration and components of the TPN solution based on a thorough assessment of the child's status, including the results of laboratory testing. This information is used as a baseline for evaluating the effectiveness of therapy.

The solution is prepared under sterile conditions in the pharmacy. For TPN, a central venous access device is inserted and secured, if one is not already in place. Use specialized tubing with an in-line filter (0.22 μm) to prevent small microparticles from entering the circulation. If total nutrient admixture (TNA) is being administered, the use of a 1.2-μg filter is recommended.

● **COMPARISON CHART 14.1** Peripheral Parenteral Nutrition vs. Total Parenteral Nutrition

	Peripheral Parenteral Nutrition	Total Parenteral Nutrition
Indications/use	Primarily supplemental Short-term use to supply additional calories and nutrients	Provides all nutrients to meet child's needs Enough calories supplied to maintain a positive nitrogen balance (Weinstein, 2006)
Route	Peripheral vein	Central venous access to allow rapid dilution of hypertonic solution
Child's status	Nutritional status usually within acceptable parameters Oral intake decreased or absent	Child with a nonfunctioning GI tract, such as a congenital or acquired GI disorder Severe failure to thrive Multisystem trauma or organ involvement Preterm newborns
Components	Fluid, electrolytes, and carbohydrates (dextrose); usually no protein or fats Carbohydrate concentration usually limited to 10% (Weinstein, 2006)	Highly concentrated solution of carbohydrates, electrolytes, vitamins, and minerals Lipid emulsion to supply need for essential fatty acids Total nutrient admixture (TNA) with components of TPN plus lipids and other additives in one container

The infusion of the solution is initiated at a slow rate that is gradually increased as ordered based on how the child tolerates the therapy. TPN solutions are highly concentrated glucose solutions that can cause hyperglycemia if given too rapidly. Use of an infusion pump is essential to control the rate of infusion. TPN solutions may be refrigerated until they are to be used. Once started, a single solution of TPN should hang for no longer than 24 hours. Fat emulsions are administered periodically to meet the child's need for essential fatty acids. These solutions are given as a piggyback solution into the TPN line, but below the in-line filter.

Throughout TPN therapy, be vigilant in monitoring the infusion rate, and report any changes in the infusion rate to the health care provider immediately. Adjustments may be made to the rate, but only as ordered by the provider. The infusion rate should never be adjusted more than 10% higher or lower than the current rate (Weinstein, 2006).

Check blood glucose levels frequently, such as every 4 to 6 hours, initially to evaluate for hyperglycemia. These levels can be obtained with a bedside glucose meter. Minimize the trauma and discomfort associated with frequent invasive procedures by using the principles of atraumatic care. If blood glucose levels are elevated, subcutaneous administration of insulin may be needed. Once the child's glucose levels stabilize, the frequency of blood glucose level determinations decreases, such as every 8 to 12 hours, based on the facility's policy.

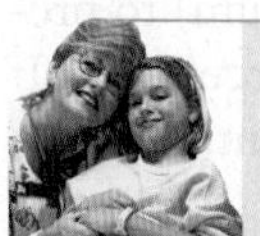

If for any reason the TPN infusion is interrupted or stops, begin an infusion of a 10% dextrose solution at the same infusion rate as the TPN. This helps to prevent rebound hypoglycemia that may occur due to the increased insulin secretion by the child's body in response to the use of the highly concentrated TPN solution.

Perform catheter site care, tubing and filter changes, and dressing changes according to the facility's policy. Inspect the insertion site closely for signs of infection. Also monitor the child's vital signs, daily weights, and intake and output closely for changes. In addition, review laboratory test results, which can aid in early detection of problems, such as infection or electrolyte excesses or deficits.

TPN can be administered continuously over a 24-hour period, or after initiation it may be given on a cyclic basis, such as over a 12-hour period during the night. When administering cycled TPN, the solution is infused at half the prescribed rate for the first and last hour to prevent hyper- and hypoglycemia.

Preventing Complications

Nurses play a key role in minimizing the risk for complications related to use of central venous access devices and TPN. Box 14.6 describes these complications. Key measures to reduce the risk of complications include the following:

BOX 14.6

COMPLICATIONS THAT CAN OCCUR WITH CENTRAL VENOUS ACCESS DEVICES AND TPN

- Air embolism from inadvertent entry of air into the system during tubing or cap changes or accidental disconnection
- Cardiac tamponade due to catheter advancement with movement of the arm, neck, or shoulder
- Catheter occlusion from the development of a fibrin sheath or thrombus at the catheter tip, malpositioning or kinking, or the deposition of precipitates or a blood clot
- Venous thrombosis from injury to the vessel wall during insertion or movement of the catheter after insertion or from chemical irritation due to administration of concentrated solutions, vesicants, and other medications through the catheter
- Hyperglycemia, typically with too rapid an infusion of TPN
- Hypoglycemia, which may occur with rapid cessation
- Dehydration as the child's body attempts to rid itself of excess glucose through renal excretion
- Electrolyte imbalance (particularly potassium, sodium, calcium, magnesium, and phosphorus)
- Infection at the skin insertion site, along the catheter pathway, or in the bloodstream. Organisms can arise from the skin, hands of caregivers, or other areas such as wound drainage, droplets from the lungs, or urine. For example, connection sites can be contaminated during tubing or dressing changes.

- Monitor the child's vital signs closely for changes.
- Adhere to strict aseptic technique when caring for the catheter and administering TPN.
- Ensure that the system remains a closed system at all times. Secure all connections, use occlusive dressings, and clamp the catheter or have the child perform the Valsalva maneuver during tubing and cap changes.
- Adhere to agency policy for flushing of the catheter and maintaining catheter patency.
- Assess intake and output frequently.
- Monitor blood glucose levels and obtain laboratory tests as ordered to evaluate for changes in fluid and electrolytes.

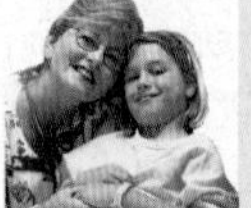

Never administer any medication, blood, or other solution through the TPN lumen. Doing so increases the risk for contamination of the system and subsequent infection.

Promoting Growth and Development

Meals are a time for meeting nutritional needs as well as a time for love, comfort, support, and socialization. TPN meets the child's nutritional needs, but the child's need for love and support also must be met. Implement measures similar to those for children receiving enteral nutrition (see discussion earlier in this chapter). Also provide opportunities for holding and cuddling the child. Allow the older child to participate in activities that can help to occupy the time associated with meals. Encourage the child and parents to participate in the care to promote a sense of independence as well as a sense of control over the situation.

Educating the Child and Family

Children who require long-term TPN therapy may receive TPN in the home. Administering TPN at home requires thorough education of the child and parents. This teaching can occur in the health care agency or in the child's home. The amount of information to be taught can be overwhelming, so ensure that ample time is available. Allow time for questions and concerns. Offer emotional support and guidance whenever necessary.

Provide written and verbal instructions about the care involved. Have the child (if appropriate) and parents demonstrate the care needed, including care of the central venous access device. Review with them the measures for obtaining, storing, and handling the solutions and supplies. Develop plans for troubleshooting problems with devices and equipment, and give instructions on how to recognize and treat complications. Also teach them about danger signs and symptoms that require immediate notification. Be sure they have the name and number of a contact person in case of emergency situations.

Initiate the appropriate referrals for support. Specialized home care infusion services are available for follow-up in the home. In addition, social services can be helpful in providing assistance with finances, health insurance reimbursement, scheduling, transportation, emotional support, and community resources.

References

Books and Journals

Algren, C., & Arnow, D. (2005). Pediatric variations of nursing interventions. In M. J. Hockenberry, *Wong's essentials of pediatric nursing* (7th ed.). St. Louis: Mosby, Inc.

American Academy of Pediatrics, Committee on Hospital Care and Committee on Drugs. (2003). *Prevention of medication errors in the pediatric inpatient setting.* Retrieved December 6, 2006, from http://www.guideline.gov/summary/summary.aspx?ss=15&doc_id=4253&nbr4253.

Association of Operating Room Nurses. (2006). Pediatric medication safety. *AORN Journal, 83*(1), 111–113.

Beauman, S. S. (2001). Didactic components of a comprehensive pediatric competency program. *Journal of Infusion Nursing, 24*(6), 367–374.

Burd, A., & Burd, R. S. (2003). The who, what, why, and how-to guide for gastrostomy tube placement in infants. *Advances in Neonatal Care, 3*(4), 197–205. Available at http://www.medscape.com/viewarticle/462136; accessed 12/28/2006.

Centers for Disease Control & Prevention (2002). Guidelines for prevention of intravascular catheter-related infections. *Morbidity and Mortality Weekly Report, 55*(RR10), 1–26.

Children's Healthcare of Atlanta. (2004). *Gastrostomy tube home care manual.* Atlanta: Children's Healthcare of Atlanta.

de Jonge, R. C., Polderman, K. H., & Gemke, R. J. (2005). Central venous catheter use in the pediatric patient: Mechanical and infectious complications. *Pediatric Critical Care Medicine, 6*(3), 329–339.

Doellman, D. (2003). Pharmacological versus nonpharmacological techniques in reducing venipuncture psychological trauma in pediatric patients. *Journal of Infusion Nursing, 26*(2), 103–109.

Fidanza, S. (2003). *Gastrostomy care.* Broomfield, CO: McKesson Health Solutions LLC.

Florida Children's Hospital, Child Life Department. (n.d.). *Atraumatic care: an age-specific approach.* Orlando, FL: Author.

Florida Children's Hospital, Child Life Department. (n.d.). *Suggested vocabulary to use with children.* Orlando, FL: Author.

Goldberg, E., Kaye, R., Yaworski, J., & Liacouras, C. (2005). Gastrostomy tubes: Facts, fallacies, fistulas, and false tracts. *Gastroenterology Nursing, 28*(6), 485–494.

Huffman, S., Jarczyk, K. S., O'Brien, E., et al. (2004). Methods to confirm feeding tube placement: Application of research in practice. *Pediatric Nursing, 30*(1), 10–13.

Hughes, R. G. (2005). Reducing pediatric medication errors: Children are especially at risk for medication errors. *American Journal of Nursing, 10*(5), 79–84.

Klossner, N. J., & Hatfield, N. (2006). *Introductory maternity and pediatric nursing.* Philadelphia: Lippincott Williams & Wilkins.

Knue, M., Doellman, D., & Jacobs, B. R. (2006). Peripherally inserted central catheters in children. *Journal of Infusion Nursing, 29*(1).

Levine, S. R., Cohen, M. R., Blanchard, N. R., et al. (2001). Guidelines for preventing medication errors in pediatrics. *Journal of Pediatric Pharmacology and Therapeutics, 6,* 426–442.

Lilley, L. L., Harrington, S., Snyder, J. S., & Lake, R. E. (2005). *Pharmacology and the nursing process* (4th ed.). St. Louis: Mosby, Inc.

O'Grady, N. P., Alexander, M., Dellinger, P., et al. (2002). Guidelines for the prevention of intravascular catheter-related infections. *Pediatrics, 110*(51) [electronic version]. Retrieved January 2, 2007, from http://www.pediatrics.org/cgi/content/full/110/5/e51.

Pediatric Glaucoma & Cataract Family Association. (2006). *How to apply eye drops.* Retrieved February 12, 2007, from http://www.pgcfa.org/drops.htm.

Pediatric Glaucoma & Cataract Family Association. (2006). *How to apply eye ointment.* Retrieved February 12, 2007, from http://www.pgcfa.org/ointment.htm.

Phillips, S. K. (2004). Pediatric parenteral nutrition: Differences in practice from adult care. *Journal of Infusion Nursing, 166*(27), 166–170.

Potter, P. A., & Perry, A. G. (2005). *Fundamentals of nursing* (6th ed.). St. Louis: Mosby, Inc.

Stucky, E. R. (2003). Prevention of medication errors in the pediatric inpatient setting. *Pediatrics, 112*(2), 431–436.

Taylor, C., Lillis, C., & Lemone, P. (2005). *Fundamentals of nursing: The art and science of nursing care.* Philadelphia: Lippincott Williams & Wilkins.

Thomas, D. O. (2005). Lessons learned: Basic evidence-based advice for preventing medication errors in children. *Journal of Emergency Nursing, 31*(5), 490–493.

U.S. Pharmacopeia. (2006). *Error-avoidance recommendations for medications used in pediatric populations.* Retrieved December 6, 2006, from www.usp.org/patientSafety/resources/pedRecommnds2003-01-22.html.

Weinstein, S. M. (2006). *Plumer's principles and practice of intravenous therapy* (8th ed.). Philadelphia: Lippincott Williams & Wilkins.

Westhus, N. (2004). Methods to test feeding tube placement in children. *MCN: The American Journal of Maternal Child Nursing, 29*(5), 282–291.

Willock, J., Richardson, J., Brazier, A., et al. (2004). Peripheral venipuncture in infants and children. *Nursing Standard, 18*(27), 43–50, 52, 55.

Woo, T. M. (2004). Pediatric pharmacology update, essentials for prescribing. *Advance for Nurse Practitioners, 12*(6), 22–28.

Websites

http://www.aap.org American Academy of Pediatrics

www.familymanagement.com/childcare/policies/medication.administration.html Medication administration policies

http://www.g-tube.net/spec.spml G-tube Assisted Nutrition

http://www.kidswithtubes.org Kids with Tubes

Chapter WORKSHEET

MULTIPLE CHOICE QUESTIONS

1. A nurse is preparing to administer an intramuscular injection to an infant. What is the most appropriate site for this injection?
   a. Deltoid muscle
   b. Vastus lateralis
   c. Dorsogluteal
   d. Rectus femoris
2. A 3-year-child is to receive a medication that is supplied as an enteric-coated tablet. What is the best nursing action?
   a. Crush the tablet and mix it with applesauce.
   b. Dissolve the medication in the child's milk.
   c. Place a pill in the posterior part of the pharynx and tell the child to swallow.
   d. Check with the prescriber to see if an alternative form can be used.
3. The nurse is caring for an infant who weighs 8.2 kg and is NPO and receiving IV fluid therapy. What rate does the nurse calculate as meeting the child's daily fluid requirements?
   a. 82 mL/hour
   b. 41 mL/hour
   c. 34 mL/hour
   d. 22 mL/hour
4. When administering ear drops to a 2-year-old, which action would be most appropriate?
   a. Tell the child that the drops are to treat his infection.
   b. Pull the pinna of the child's ear down and back.
   c. Have the child turn his head to the opposite side after giving the drops.
   d. Massage the child's forehead to facilitate absorption of the medication.

CRITICAL THINKING EXERCISES

1. When reviewing the medical record of a child, the nurse notes that the ordered dose of medication is different from the recommended dose. How should the nurse proceed?
2. While caring for a 5-year-old child who is receiving IV fluid therapy at a rate of 100 mL/hour, the nurse notes that the infusion is running slowly. The insertion site appears slightly reddened and swollen. What should the nurse do next?
3. A school-aged child is to be discharged, continuing TPN therapy at home. The child lives with his parents and two younger siblings. How would the nurse prepare this child and family for discharge? How could the nurse promote growth and development for this child during TPN therapy?

STUDY ACTIVITIES

1. Review the medical records of several children who are on a pediatric unit in your agency. Note the type of medication, route ordered, and what specific interventions are needed for each child related to the medication administration and developmental age of the child. Compile a list of the most commonly used routes.
2. Interview several parents about their experiences in giving medications to their children. From these interviews, develop a teaching sheet that provides tips to facilitate oral medication administration to children.
3. Create a chart that compares and contrasts the subcutaneous, intramuscular, and intravenous methods of medication administration. Include examples of medications given via these routes, onset of action, appropriate sites, and necessary safety measures for each.
4. An infant is to receive intermittent gavage feedings via a nasogastric tube every 6 hours. The feeding tube was inserted with a previous feeding and remains in place. The nurse is preparing to administer the next scheduled feeding. Place the events in the proper sequence.

   _____ a. Check the placement of the feeding tube.
   _____ b. Position the infant on his right side with the head of the bed slightly elevated.
   _____ c. Allow the feeding to come to room temperature.
   _____ d. Flush the tube with water.
   _____ e. Clamp the tube to prevent air from entering the stomach.
   _____ f. Pour the solution into the barrel of the syringe.

chapter 15

Pain Management in Children

Key TERMS

acute pain
chronic pain
conscious sedation
drug tolerance
epidural
neuromodulators
neuropathic pain
nociceptive pain
nociceptors
pain
pain threshold
patient-controlled analgesia (PCA)
physical dependence
somatic pain
transduction
visceral pain

Learning OBJECTIVES

Upon completion of the chapter, the student will be able to:

1. Identify the major physiologic events associated with the perception of pain.
2. Discuss the factors that influence the pain response.
3. Identify the developmental considerations of the effects and management of pain in the infant, toddler, preschooler, school-age child, and adolescent.
4. Explain the principles of pain assessment as they relate to children.
5. Understand the use of the various pain rating scales and physiologic monitoring for children.
6. Establish a nursing care plan for children related to management of pain, including pharmacologic and nonpharmacologic techniques and strategies.

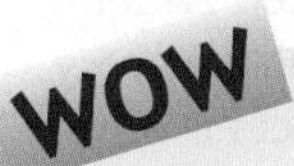

All of our patients in pain deserve as much comfort as we can give.

Aiden Russell is a 6-year-old on the pediatric unit admitted for a wound infection. He requires BID dressing changes. In report you are told that Aiden cries and fights during the dressing change but otherwise seems to be playing and not experiencing much pain. The nurse reporting off states, "Aiden's mother keeps requesting pain medication for Aiden. She states he's complaining of pain most of the time. I'm not sure if I believe her: when I see Aiden, he's playing Nintendo games or watching television and seems to be fine. I've tried to hold off on his pain medication as long as I can."

Pain is a highly individualized, subjective experience that can affect any person of any age. It is a complex phenomenon that involves multiple components and is influenced by a myriad of factors. Pain often has been described as a subjective experience that involves both sensory and emotional factors. **Pain** is defined by the International Association for the Study of Pain as "an unpleasant sensory and emotional experience that is associated with actual or potential tissue damage" (IASP, 2007). The cause of pain is related to the disease process, treatment protocols, surgical interventions, or injury to the child. A definition of pain that is commonly used defines pain as whatever the person says it is, existing whenever the person says it does (McCaffery & Pasero, 1999)—that is, pain is present when the person says that it is. The person experiencing the pain is the only one who can identify pain and know what the pain is like.

Pain is a universal experience. The American Pain Society (1995) has labeled it "the fifth vital sign" to emphasize the importance of assessing pain frequently and providing appropriate treatment. The goal is to encourage health care professionals to assess pain every time that temperature, pulse, respirations, and blood pressure are assessed and to institute measures to manage the pain.

Pain affects adults and children alike, but children may lack the verbal capacity to describe their pain accurately. In addition, many caregivers and health care providers have misconceptions about pain in children, it is difficult to assess the complex nature of the pain experience, and limited resources and research are available related to pain relief strategies for children. All this makes pain management a critical element in the plan of care for children.

Pain is a major source of distress for children and their families as well as health care providers. Pain affects children of all ages, even preterm infants. Various national health associations have issued position papers and guidelines related to the need to treat pain and suffering in children (American Academy of Pediatrics and American Pain Society, 2001). Effective pain management involves initial pain assessment, therapeutic interventions, and reassessment for all children in any health care setting.

Pain in children can result from numerous causes, including procedures, and can lead to serious physical and emotional consequences, such as increased oxygen consumption and alterations in blood glucose metabolism. In addition, the experience of pain early in life may lead to long-term consequences for the child (Howard, 2003). Treating pain reduces anxiety during procedures and decreases the need for physical restraints, reduces anxiety regarding subsequent procedures, and prevents short- and long-term consequences of inadequately treated pain, particularly in newborns.

This chapter describes the pain experience in children, including the types of pain, factors influencing pain, and common fallacies and myths associated with pain in children. The nursing process is applied to provide an overview of the care for a child in pain. Various pain management strategies are described, including nonpharmacologic and pharmacologic interventions and measures to address procedure-related and chronic pain.

Physiology of Pain

The sensation of pain is a complex phenomenon that involves a sequence of physiologic events in the nervous system. These events are transduction, transmission, perception, and modulation.

Transduction

Peripheral nerve fibers extend from the spinal cord to various locations in and throughout the body's tissues, such as skin, joints, bones, and membranes covering the internal organs. At the end of these fibers are specialized receptors, called **nociceptors**, that become activated when they are exposed to noxious stimuli. The noxious stimuli can be mechanical, chemical, or thermal. Mechanical stimuli may include intense pressure to an area, a strong muscular contraction, or extensive pressure due to muscular overstretching. Chemical stimulation may involve the release of mediators, such as histamine, prostaglandins, leukotrienes, or bradykinin, as a response to tissue trauma, ischemia, or inflammation. Thermal stimuli typically involve extremes of heat and cold. This process of nociceptor activation is called **transduction**.

Transmission

When nociceptors are activated by noxious stimuli, the stimuli are converted to electrical impulses that are relayed along the peripheral nerves to the spinal cord and brain. Specialized afferent nerve fibers are responsible for moving the electrical impulse along. Myelinated A-delta fibers are large fibers that conduct the impulse at very rapid rates. The pain transmitted by these fibers is often referred to as fast pain, most commonly associated with mechanical or thermal stimuli (Porth, 2004). Pain also is transmitted by unmyelinated small C fibers. These fibers transmit the impulse slowly and are often activated by chemical stimuli or continued mechanical or thermal stimuli (Porth, 2004). These fibers carry the impulse to the spinal cord via the dorsal horn. Neurotransmitters are released to facilitate the transmission process to the brain.

Several theories have been proposed in an attempt to explain the process of pain transmission. The best known of these is the gate-control theory. According to this theory, the dorsal horn of the spinal cord contains interneuronal or interconnecting fibers. These fibers, when stimulated, close the gate or pathway to the brain, thereby inhibiting or blocking the transmission of the pain impulse. Subsequently, the impulse does not reach the brain where it would be interpreted as pain.

Perception

Once in the dorsal horn of the spinal cord, the nerve fibers divide and then cross to the opposite side and rise upward to the thalamus. The thalamus responds quickly and sends a message to the somatosensory cortex of the brain, where the impulse is interpreted as the physical sensation of pain. The impulses carried by the fast pain A-delta fibers lead to the perception of sharp, stabbing, localized pain that also commonly involves a reflex response to withdraw from the stimulus. The impulses carried by the slow C fibers lead to the perception of diffuse, dull, burning, or aching pain. The point at which the person first feels the lowest intensity of the painful stimulus is termed the **pain threshold** (Fig. 15.1). In addition to sending a message to the cerebral cortex, the thalamus also sends a message to the limbic system, where the sensation is interpreted emotionally, and to the brain stem centers, where autonomic nervous system responses begin.

Modulation

Research has identified substances called **neuromodulators** that appear to modify the pain sensation. These substances have been found to change a person's perception of pain. Examples of these neuromodulators include serotonin, endorphins, enkephalins, and dynorphins.

Pain perception can be modified peripherally or centrally. In the peripheral nerve fibers, chemical substances are released that either stimulate the nerve fibers or sensitize them. Peripheral sensitization allows the nerve fibers to react to a stimulus that is of lower intensity than would be needed to cause pain. As a result, the person perceives more pain. Actions that block or inhibit the release of these substances can lead to a decrease in pain perception.

Modification of pain perception can occur centrally in the spinal cord at the dorsal horn. Substances released by the excited interneurons can potentiate the pain sensation. Other neurochemicals, through their binding to specific receptors, can inhibit the perception of pain.

Types of Pain

Many different systems can be used to classify pain. Most commonly, pain is classified based on its duration, etiology, or source or location.

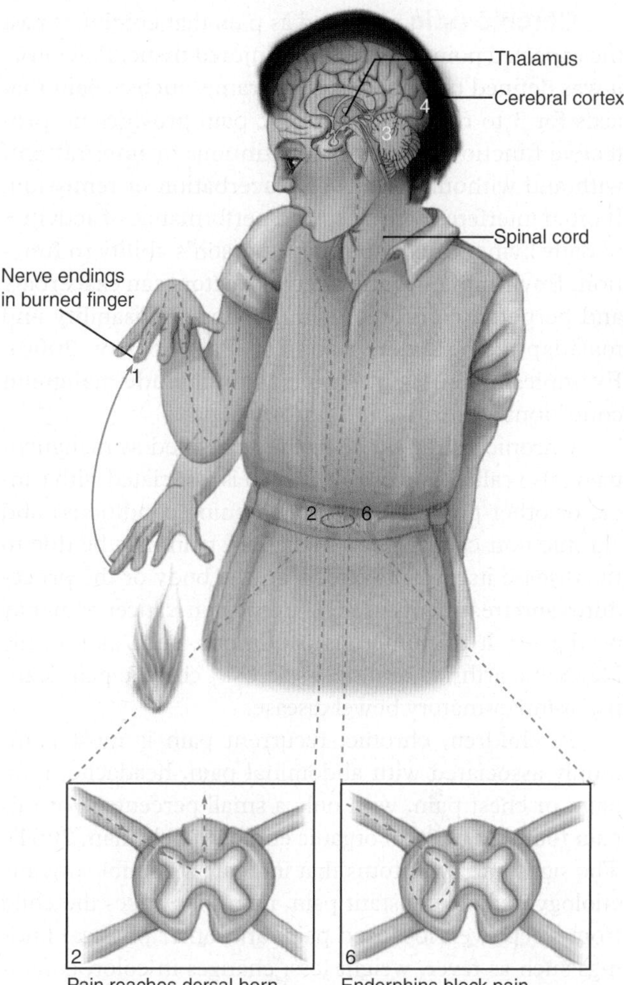

● Figure 15.1 The transmission of pain stimulus.

Classification by Duration

Pain is classified by duration as acute or chronic. **Acute pain** is defined as pain that is associated with a rapid onset of varying intensity. It usually indicates tissue damage and resolves with healing of the injury. Acute pain reflects stimulation of nociceptors and serves a protective function (that is, alerting the person to a problem). Examples of causes of acute pain include trauma, invasive procedures, acute illnesses such as sore throat or appendicitis, and surgery. For example, a child may experience acute pain after operative procedures, trauma, or disease. This type of pain generally last a few days.

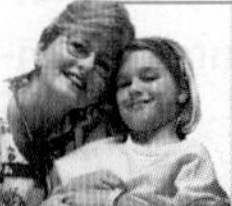

Children often experience pain associated with various procedures done in health care settings. This type of pain is usually short in duration. Preparation of the child and family will help to decrease fears or anxiety. Depending on the type of procedure and the child's age, cognitive level, and temperament, various techniques and methods can be used. Advocating for atraumatic care and adhering to its guidelines will help to minimize procedure-related pain.

Chronic pain is defined as pain that continues past the expected point of healing for injured tissue. Previously it was defined by a specific time frame, such as pain that lasts for 3 to 6 months. Chronic pain provides no protective function. It may be continuous or intermittent, with and without periods of exacerbation or remission. It often interferes with sleep and performance of activities of daily living, thus impairing a person's ability to function. Environmental and affective factors can exacerbate and perpetuate chronic pain, leading to disability and maladaptive behavior (American Pain Society, 2006). Examples of causes of chronic pain include malignant conditions, arthritis, and fibromyalgia.

Chronic pain may be further classified as malignant pain (also called cancer pain, which is associated with cancer or other potentially life-threatening conditions) and chronic non-cancer pain. Malignant pain may be due to the disease itself or its effects on the body or the procedures and treatments used. Chronic non-cancer pain may be the result of numerous conditions, such as juvenile idiopathic arthritis, multiple sclerosis, chronic pancreatitis, or inflammatory bowel disease.

In children, chronic, recurrent pain is most commonly associated with abdominal pain, headache, limb pain, or chest pain, with only a small percentage of this pain found to have an organic etiology (Behrman, 2004). The signs and symptoms that indicate a possible organic etiology include constant pain, pain that wakes the child from sleep, well-localized pain, and other physical findings such as fever, weight loss, changes in color, consistency, or frequency of stools, and urinary tract symptoms (Behrman, 2004). This type of pain lasts for longer periods of time or comes and goes over a period of time.

Classification by Etiology

Pain can be classified by etiology as nociceptive or neuropathic. **Nociceptive pain** reflects pain due to activation of the A-delta fibers and C fibers by noxious stimuli. The pain perceived often correlates closely with the degree or intensity of the stimulus and the extent of real or possible tissue damage (American Pain Society, 2006). With nociceptive pain, nervous system functioning is intact. Reports of nociceptive pain vary depending on the location of the nociceptors being stimulated, ranging from a sharp or burning, to dull, aching, or cramping, to deep aching or sharp stabbing. Examples of conditions that result in nociceptive pain include chemical burns, sunburn, cuts, appendicitis, and bladder distention.

Neuropathic pain is pain due to malfunctioning of the peripheral or central nervous system. It may be continuous or intermittent and is commonly described as burning, tingling, shooting, squeezing, or spasm-like pain. Examples of neuropathic pain include neuropathies, phantom limb pain, and post-stroke pain.

Classification by Source or Location

Pain also may be classified by the source or location of the area involved as somatic pain (superficial and deep) or visceral pain. These classifications typically indicate nociceptive pain. **Somatic pain** refers to pain that develops in the tissues. It can be further divided into two groups: superficial and deep. Superficial somatic pain, often called cutaneous pain, involves stimulation of nociceptors in the skin, subcutaneous tissue, or mucous membranes. Typically the pain is well localized and described as a sharp, pricking, or burning sensation. Superficial somatic pain may be due to external mechanical, chemical, or thermal injury or skin disorders. Tenderness commonly is present. The individual also experiences hyperalgesia (an increased response to noxious stimulus) and allodynia (a painful response to a normally nonpainful or non-noxious stimulus; American Pain Society, 2006).

Deep somatic pain typically involves the muscles, tendons, joints, fasciae, and bones. It can be localized or diffuse and is usually described as dull, aching, or cramping. Deep somatic pain may be due to strain from overuse or direct injury, ischemia, and inflammation. Tenderness and reflex spasm may be present. Additionally, the person may exhibit sympathetic nervous system activation such as tachycardia, hypertension, tachypnea, diaphoresis, pallor, and pupillary dilation.

Visceral pain is pain that develops within organs such as the heart, lungs, gastrointestinal tract, pancreas, liver, gallbladder, kidneys, or bladder. It can be well or poorly localized and is described as a deep ache or sharp stabbing sensation that may be referred to other areas. Visceral pain may be due to distention of the organ, organ muscular spasm or pulling, ischemia, or inflammation. Tenderness, nausea, vomiting, and diaphoresis may be present.

Factors Influencing Pain

Children, like adults, experience neurologic events that result in the perception of pain. However, research has found that environmental and psychological factors may exert a greater influence on the child's perception of pain. Certain factors such as age, gender, cognitive level, temperament, previous pain experiences, and family and cultural background cannot be changed. However, situational factors involving behavioral, cognitive, and emotional aspects can be modified. "Although the causal relationship between an injury and consequent pain seems direct and obvious, what children understand, what they do, and how they feel all affect their pain. Some situational factors can intensify pain and distress, whereas others can eventually trigger pain episodes, prolong pain-related disability, or maintain the repeated pain episodes in recurrent pain syndrome" (McGrath & Hillier, 2003).

Age and Gender

Research has demonstrated that the nervous system structures needed for pain impulse transmission and perception are present by the 24th week of gestation. Therefore, children of any age, including preterm newborns, are capable of experiencing pain. Early on, children can interpret pain as an unpleasant sensation, but this interpretation is based on their comparison with other sensations. As they get older, they learn to use words to describe their pain more fully.

Gender also may play a role in a child's perception of pain, but research has failed to yield concrete evidence supporting it.

Cognitive Level

Cognitive level is a key factor affecting a child's pain perception and response and usually goes hand in hand with the child's age. Cognitive level typically increases with age, thereby influencing the child's understanding of the pain and its impact and his or her choices for coping strategies. In addition, as the child's cognitive level increases, his or her ability to communicate information about pain increases. However, this increased understanding and ability to communicate with advancing age may not apply to the child experiencing developmental delays. For example, a developmentally delayed school-aged child or adolescent may have the cognitive level of a toddler or preschooler. Health care providers need to be cognizant of this difference when caring for the child in pain. Numerous research studies have revealed that young children often describe pain in concrete terms, whereas older children use more abstract terms that involve both physical and psychological components (McGrath & Hillier, 2003).

Temperament

Temperament affects how a child will respond to a situation. Previous experience with a situation or the method used to cope with a new or a threatening or harmful situation along with the child's coping style will affect the child's pain experience. Even mild symptoms of negative mood may affect the perceptions and persistence of pain (Palermo et al., 2005). A child with a "difficult temperament" is more likely to have an increased response to pain.

Previous Pain Experiences

A child identifies pain based on his or her experiences with pain in the past. The number of episodes of pain, the type of pain, the severity or intensity of the previous pain experience, and how the child responded all affect how the child will perceive and respond to the current experience. For example, several research studies have demonstrated that children who had negative experiences with pain involving a routine blood-drawing procedure exhibited an increase in anxiety and stress and greater pain when faced with the procedure again.

Family and Culture

The child's cultural and family background will influence how he or she will express and manage pain. Some cultures transmit the standard of accepting pain stoically; others allow outward expression. The parents have a strong influence on the child's ability to cope. For example, if a parent reacts to the child's pain in a positive manner and offers comfort measures, the child may have an easier time coping. If the parent shows anger or disapproval, the pain experience may be intensified for the child.

Situational Factors

Situational factors involve factors or elements that interact with the child and his or her current situation involving the experience of pain. These factors are highly variable and dependent on the specific situation. Examples of situational factors are highlighted in Table 15.1.

Developmental Considerations

Since children of various developmental ages respond differently to pain and perceive pain in different ways, it is important to review developmental considerations. Refer to Chapters 4 through 8 for a more complete understanding of childhood development. Nurses must understand how children of various ages respond to painful stimuli and what behaviors may be expected based on their developmental level. By understanding these developmental considerations, the nurse can appropriately assess the child's pain and provide effective interventions.

Infants

Research has demonstrated that infants, including preterm infants, experience pain and can distinguish pain from other tactile experiences (McGrath & Hillier, 2003). Much of this research focuses on pain related to invasive procedures, such as heelsticks and intravenous catheter insertion. Research suggests that preterm infants actually experience pain at a greater intensity than their older counterparts. The belief is related to the immaturity of the inhibitory mechanisms that develop higher in the central nervous system at a later time during fetal development. These mechanisms are more complex and do not become functional until later in gestation.

In preterm and term newborns, behavioral and physiologic indicators are used for determining pain. Behavioral indicators include facial expression, body movements, and crying. Physiologic indicators include changes in heart rate, respiratory rate, blood pressure, oxygen saturation levels, vagal tone, palmar sweating, and plasma cortisol or

Table 15.1 Situational Factors Affecting a Child's Pain Experience

Cognitive	Behavioral	Emotional
Information about condition and pain problem, including cause and prognosis	Distress responses; specific behaviors and actions	Anticipatory anxiety
Knowledge about available therapy	Use of therapies	Heightened distress; feelings about scheduled possibly painful treatments
Expectations about the effectiveness of therapy and about the future	Child's or family's response to pain condition	Fear about undiagnosed condition and continuing pain; impact of pain and illness on family
Ability to identify pain triggers	Resolution of stressful situation	Situation-specific stress such as school, sports
Knowledge about stress reduction	Participation in routine activities	Frustration related to interruption in activities
		Underlying anxiety and depression

Adapted from McGrath, P. A., & Hillier, L. M. (2003). Modifying the psychologic factors that intensify children's pain and prolong disability. In N. L. Schecter, C. B. Berde, & M. Yaster, *Pain in infants, children, and adolescents* (2d ed., Fig. 6.1, p. 87). Philadelphia: Lippincott Williams & Wilkins.

catecholamine levels (American Academy of Pediatrics and Canadian Paediatric Society, 2000).

In the younger infant, facial expression is the most common response to pain (Fig. 15.2). The brows may be lowered and drawn together, with the eyes tightly closed. The mouth is open, often forming a square. The body may be stiff, and thrashing may be seen. When the area is stimulated, the infant may demonstrate a generalized reflex withdrawal. The infant may exhibit a high-pitched, shrill cry.

● **Figure 15.2** In the younger infant, facial expression is the most common response to pain.

The older infant often displays similar behavioral manifestations of pain. The older infant may display an angry facial expression, but the eyes are open. He or she often demonstrates a definite withdrawal response when the area is stimulated. The older infant cries loudly and tries to push away the stimulus that is causing the pain. Other manifestations include irritability, restless sleeping, and poor feeding.

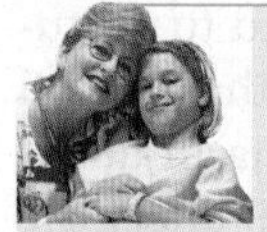

Although an infant usually exhibits typical behaviors indicating pain, absence of these manifestations does not indicate a lack of a pain; the response to pain is highly variable.

Infants are preverbal, so facial expression, diffuse body movements, and other signs, as indicated above, provide helpful feedback that the infant is in pain.

Infants also demonstrate physiologic responses to pain. These may include:

- Increased heart rate, usually averaging approximately 10 beats per minute; possibly bradycardia in preterm newborns
- Decreased vagal tone
- Decreased oxygen saturation
- Palmar or plantar sweating (as measured by skin conductivity testing); not reliable in infants under 37 weeks' gestation

Research has identified some short- and long-term consequences of inadequately treated pain in newborns (Taddio et al., 1997). These include hyperalgesia around a wound from such situations as repeated heelsticks; an increased risk of developing intraventricular hemorrhage with repeated painful stressors; and a change in the pattern of response to subsequent pain. Children's memories of painful experiences can have long-term consequences for their reaction to later painful events and their acceptance of later health care interventions (von Baeyer et al., 2004). Moreover, preterm infants may be at greater risk for experiencing memories of pain due to the often long hospitalizations involving numerous invasive and painful procedures (Johnston et al., 2003).

Toddlers

Toddlers can react to painless procedures as intensely as painful ones, with intense emotional upset and physical resistance or aggression (Hockenberry et al., 2005). They may bite, hit, scream, or kick. Other behaviors may include being very quiet, pointing to where it hurts, or saying such words as "owww." Facial grimacing and teeth clenching may be noted. They may also react with fear and try to hide or leave the room. They often have limited vocabularies, so it may be difficult for them to express pain. Toddlers may demonstrate regressive behaviors, such as clinging to the parent or crying loudly.

Preschoolers

Since preschoolers may differentiate poorly between their self and the external world, the physical and verbal aggression is more goal-directed. They also may become quiet or try to withdraw and hide: the child may say he or she needs to go to the bathroom or needs to get something from another room. Because of their magical type of thinking, preschoolers may believe pain is a punishment for misbehaving or having bad thoughts. Preschoolers may not verbally report their pain, thinking that pain is something to be expected or that the adults are aware of their pain. They can tell someone where it hurts and can use various tools to describe the severity of pain; however, because they may have limited experience with pain, they may have difficulty distinguishing between types of pain (sharp or dull), describing the intensity of the pain, and determining whether the pain is worse or better.

School-Age Children

School-age children can communicate the type, location, and severity of pain. Children over the age of 8 years can use specific words, such as "sharp as a knife," burning, or pulling, to describe their pain. However, they may deny pain in an attempt to appear brave or to avoid further pain related to a procedure or intervention. They may be more concerned with their fear about the illness and its effects rather than the pain. They also may fear being embarrassed by acting-out behaviors. Thus, a typical response might be to withdraw by staring at the television. Other behaviors may include muscular rigidity, such as clenching the fists, stiffening the body, closing the eyes, wrinkling the forehead, or gritting the teeth.

Adolescent

Adolescents are concerned primarily about body image and fear losing control over their behavior. This may result in denial or refusal of medications. Their mood and what they think is expected of them will also affect their response. Adolescents often ask numerous questions and pay close attention to how others respond to them. Fearing that their behavior may be viewed as juvenile, they may attempt to remain stoic, not exhibiting any emotion. Subtle changes such as increased muscle tension with clenched fists and teeth, rapid breathing, and guarding the affected body part may occur. They may also show lack of interest in everyday activities or a decreased ability to concentrate.

Common Fallacies and Myths About Pain in Children

In general, children respond to pain based on the type of pain, the extent of pain, and their age and developmental level. Table 15.2 highlights some common myths and misconceptions related to pain in children. Because of these myths, children have been medicated less than adults with a similar diagnosis, leading to inadequate pain management (Brennan-Hunter, 2001; Fitzgerald & Beggs, 2001).

Nursing Process Overview for the Child in Pain

WATCH & LEARN

Nursing care of the child with pain includes nursing assessment, nursing diagnosis, planning, interventions, and evaluation. Each step of this process must be individualized for each patient. A general understanding of the physiology of pain, factors that influence pain, and effective pain management techniques can help to individualize the child's plan of care.

ASSESSMENT

Assessment of pain in children consists of both subjective and objective data collection. The acronym **QUESTT** is an excellent way to remember the key principles of pain assessment (Baker & Wong, 1987):

- **Question** the child.
- **Use** a reliable and valid pain scale.
- **Evaluate** the child's behavior and physiologic changes to establish a baseline and determine the effectiveness of the intervention. The child's behavior and motor activity may include irritability and protection as well as withdrawal of the affected painful area.

Table 15.2 Myths and Misconceptions About Children and Pain

Myth or Misconception	Fact
Newborns do not feel pain.	Newborns, including preterm newborns, do feel pain. The neurologic and hormonal systems needed for the transmission of painful stimuli are sufficiently developed.
Exposure to pain at an early age has little to no effect on the child. Infants and small children have little memory of pain.	Prolonged or severe pain can lead to increased newborn morbidity. Infants who have experienced pain during the neonatal period respond differently to subsequent painful events (American Academy of Pediatrics and Canadian Paediatric Society, 2000). Repeated exposure to painful procedures and events can have long-term consequences. Memories of pain may be stored in the child's nervous system, influencing later reactions to painful stimuli (Johnston et al., 2003).
The intensity of a child's behavioral reaction indicates the intensity of the child's pain.	Numerous factors affect a child's response to pain. Each child is an individual, with his or her own set of responses.
A child who is sleeping is not in pain.	Sleep may be a coping strategy for the child in pain, or it may reflect exhaustion of the child who is coping with pain.
Children are truthful when they are asked if they are experiencing pain.	Often children deny pain to avoid a painful situation or procedure, embarrassment, or loss of control. Children may assume that others know how they are feeling and thus will not verbalize their complaints.
Children learn to adapt to pain and painful procedures.	Repeated exposure to pain or painful procedures can result in an increase in behavioral manifestations.
Children experience more adverse effects of narcotic analgesics than adults do.	The risk of adverse effects of narcotic analgesics is the same for children as for adults.
Children are more prone to addiction to narcotic analgesics.	Addiction to narcotics when used in children is very rare.

- **Secure** the parent's involvement.
- **Take** the cause of pain into account when intervening.
- **Take** action.

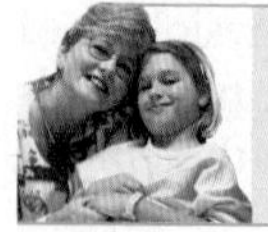

Children do experience pain, and pain management techniques work just as well with children as they do with adults.

Health History

When assessing pain in children, tailor the assessment to the child's developmental level and ask questions geared to the child's cognitive ability. During the health history, determine the child's previous exposure to pain, if any, and how the child responded. This information will provide clues about how the child copes and his or her current response. Attempt to determine what word the child uses to denote pain. Some children may not understand the term "pain" but do understand terms such as "ouchie" or "boo-boo."

The health history also includes questioning the parents about their cultural beliefs related to pain and their child's usual responses. This information aids in planning developmentally and culturally appropriate family-centered care.

Questioning the Child

When questioning the child, phrase the questions in a manner that the child will be able to understand based on his or her developmental level. Some input from the child's family may be helpful in determining where best to focus the questions.

Ask the child what pain means to him or her. Use words that the child may comprehend more easily, such as "hurt," "boo-boo," or "ouch," as appropriate. Inquire about similar experiences in the past and how he or she responded. Determine whether the child let others know that he or she was hurting and how this message was conveyed (e.g., crying, acting out, or pointing to the hurting area).

Review the history of the pain and various influences such as cultural aspects, caregiver attitudes or expectations, previous experiences, and any education or teaching related to pain management. Continue to formulate questions to ascertain the following:

- Location, quality, severity, and onset of the pain, as well as the circumstances in which the child experiences the pain. Have the child point to the area where it hurts or identify the location on a diagram or doll.
- Conditions, if any, that preceded the onset of pain and the conditions that followed the onset of pain
- Any associated symptoms, such as weight loss, fever, vomiting, or diarrhea, which may indicate a current illness
- Any recent trauma, including any interventions that were used in an attempt to relieve the pain

Continue the health history by inquiring about what the child wants others, including the nurse, to do when the child hurts. Conversely, ask the child what he or she doesn't want others to do. Finally, question the child about measures that seem to be most effective in relieving the pain. Ask if there is anything special the child wants to tell the nurse, such as a special pain-relief technique or a specific comfort object.

If the child is experiencing chronic or recurrent pain, suggest the child and family record information in a symptom diary. Explain that this will be helpful in identifying the best ways to manage the pain.

Questioning the Parents

Parents play a key role in assessing pain in children. Often it is the parents who provide information about the child's current and past experiences with pain. In addition, parents can provide information about how the child exhibits and responds to pain. Parents may be aware of subtle changes in the child's behavior that may precede the pain, occur with the pain, or indicate relief of pain. Including the parents in this process helps create a positive experience for all involved and promotes feelings of control over the situation.

The questions posed to the parents are similar in focus to those posed to the child. However, more detailed information may be obtained from the parents because they are usually able to describe events more fully or in greater detail due to their higher cognitive level. Parents typically know their child best.

Parents may assume that nurses have greater expertise when it comes to assessing their child's pain and taking appropriate action. Thus, they may not always report when they notice changes suggesting that their child is uncomfortable. Emphasize the important role that parents play in reporting any changes in their child so that pain relief measures can be instituted as soon as possible.

When questioning the parents, use the following examples as a guide for assessing the child's pain:

- Has your child ever been in pain before? If so, what was the cause of the pain? How long did he or she have the pain? Where was the pain located?
- How did your child react to the pain? What did you do to lessen the pain?
- Did your child let you know that he or she was in pain? Did he or she tell you or did you notice something?
- Are there any special signs that let you know that your child is hurting? If so, what are they?
- Is there anything that your child does or that you do when he or she is hurting that helps relieve the pain?
- Does one thing work better than another when your child is hurting?
- Is there any special information that you want to tell me about your child?

Using Pain Rating Scales

Various pain assessment or pain rating scales are available. These scales allow the child to report his or her pain, and the pain level is quantified. These standardized rating scales provide a greater alignment between the child's pain and the nurse's assessment of the severity of the pain (de Rond et al., 2000).

Many health care facilities have specific policies and procedures related to pain assessment, including the frequency of assessment, the rating tool to use, and nursing interventions to be instituted based on the rating. For example, many facilities require assessment of the child using a specific tool with documentation at least once a shift and 30 minutes to 1 hour after a non-pharmacologic or pharmacologic pain-relief intervention. This process provides a more objective method to determine whether the pain is increasing or decreasing and whether pain-relief methods are effective.

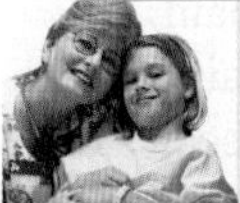

Typically, different pain rating scales are appropriate for different developmental levels. However, children may regress when in pain, so a simpler tool may be needed to make sure that the child understands what is being asked. Regardless of the tool used, nurses need to be consistent in using the same tool so that appropriate comparisons can be made and effective interventions can be planned and implemented. Using the most appropriate tool consistently allows the most accurate assessment of the child's pain.

FACES Pain Rating Scale. The FACES pain rating scale (Fig. 15.3) is a self-report tool that can be used by children as young as 3 years of age. The scale consists of six illustrations of faces arranged horizontally with expressions ranging from smiling (indicating no hurt) to crying

Wong-Baker FACES Pain Rating Scale

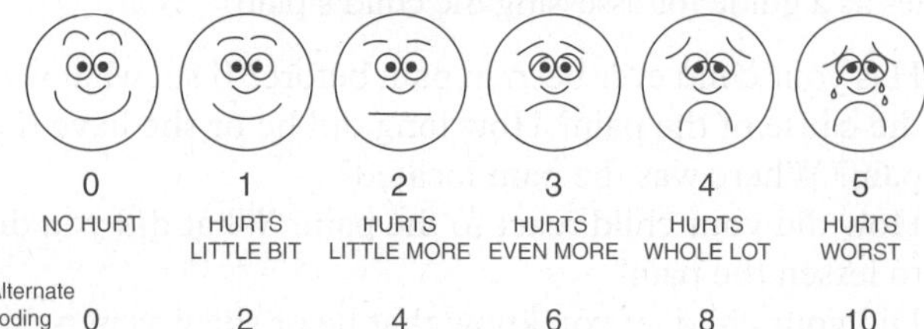

Instructions: Explain to the person that each face is for a person who feels happy because he has no pain (hurt) or sad because he has some or a lot of pain. **Face 0** is very happy because he doesn't hurt at all. **Face 1** hurts just a little bit. **Face 2** hurts a little more. **Face 3** hurts even more. **Face 4** hurts a whole lot. **Face 5** hurts as much as you can imagine, although you don't have to be crying to feel this bad. Ask the person to choose the face that best describes how he is feeling.

● **Figure 15.3** FACES Pain Rating Scale. (From Hockenberry, M. J., Wilson, D., & Winkelstein, M. L. [2005]. *Wong's essentials of pediatric nursing* [7th ed., p. 1259]. St. Louis, MO. Used with permission. Copyright, Mosby.)

with frowning (indicating hurts worst). Under each face is a short description such as "hurts little bit" and a number. The number scale can be 0, 1, 2, 3, 4, and 5 or 0, 2, 4, 6, 8, and 10. The nurse explains the words associated with each face. Then the child is asked to select the facial expression that best describes how he or she is feeling. The nurse then documents the number corresponding to the word description and face.

Oucher Pain Rating Scale. The Oucher pain rating scale is similar to the FACES scale in that it uses facial expressions to indicate increasing degrees of hurt. However, instead of illustrations, six photographs are used: "no hurt" is placed at the bottom of the arrangement and "most hurt" at the top. Alongside the photos is a scale ranging from 0 to 10 that corresponds to the facial expressions in the photographs (Fig. 15.4). After explaining the photos and numeric scale, the child is asked to point to the number that best describes his or her level of pain.

This scale is useful for self-reporting of pain in children from 3 to 13 years of age. Three different scales have been developed for use with Caucasian, Hispanic, and African-American children.

Poker Chip Tool. The poker chip tool is a self-reporting pain assessment tool that uses four red poker chips to quantify the child's level of pain. The chips are arranged in a horizontal line on a surface in front of the child. Starting with the chip closest to the child's left side, the nurse points to the chip and explains that the first chip means a little hurt, the next chip means more hurt, the third chip means more hurt, and the fourth chip means the worst hurt ever. Then the nurse asks the child how many "pieces of hurt" he or she is having (Fig. 15.5). If the child is not experiencing any pain, typically the child will state that he or she isn't having any. When the child identifies the number of

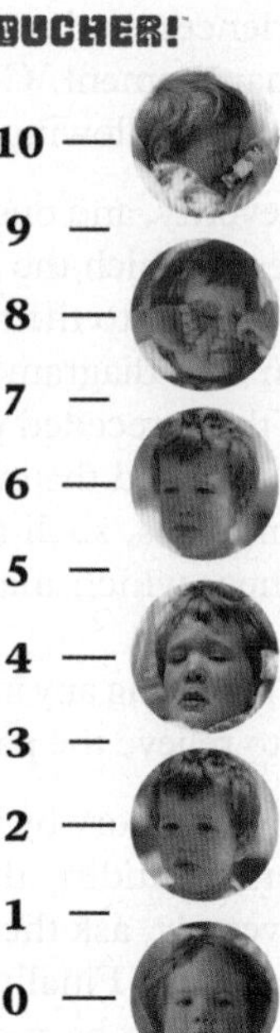

● **Figure 15.4** Oucher Pain Rating Scale.

"pieces of hurt," the nurse follows up by asking the child to tell the nurse more about his or her hurt.

The poker chip tool is useful for assessing pain in children who are 4 years of age or older. Children may view this assessment tool as a game since it involves poker chips. However, the nurse needs to ensure that the child has the cognitive ability to distinguish the numbers.

Word-Graphic Rating Scale. The word-graphic rating scale is a self-reporting scale that consists of a line with

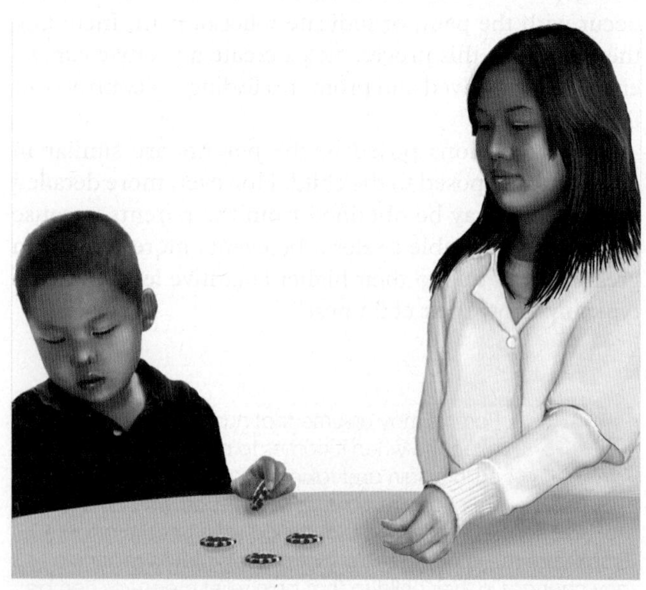

● **Figure 15.5** The poker chip tool. Here the nurse asks the child to identify the number of chips that indicate her degree of "hurt."

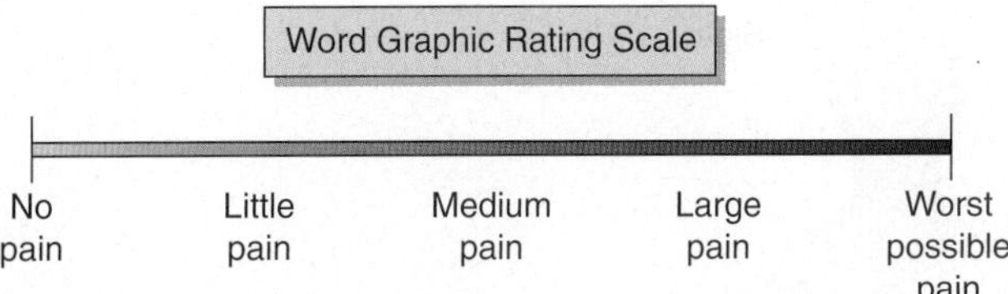

● Figure 15.6 Word-graphic rating scale.

descriptors underneath: no pain, little pain, medium pain, large pain, and worst possible pain (Fig. 15.6). The nurse explains the line and descriptors to the child. Then the child is asked to make a vertical mark on the horizontal line at the point that best describes the child's level of pain. The nurse uses a ruler to measure the distance from the "no pain" starting point to the area marked by the child. This measurement is recorded as the pain score. The word-graphic rating scale is useful for children 4 to 17 years old.

Visual Analog and Numeric Scales. Visual analog and numeric scales involve a horizontal or vertical line with marked endpoints. With a visual analog scale, the end points are identified as no pain and worst pain. A numeric scale typically has endpoints of 0 and 10, reflecting no pain and worst pain, respectively (Fig. 15.7). The nurse explains the scale to the child. With the visual analog scale, the child makes a line that best describes the level of pain. The nurse then measures the distance from the "no pain" endpoint to the child's mark and records this as the pain score. With the numeric scale, the nurse asks the child to pick the number that best describes his or her level of pain.

The numeric scale can be used with children as young as 5 years of age, as long as they can count and understand the concepts related to numeric values. Although research has validated use of the visual analog scale with children as young as 4.7 years of age, the preferred minimum age for using this tool is 7 years (Algren, 2005).

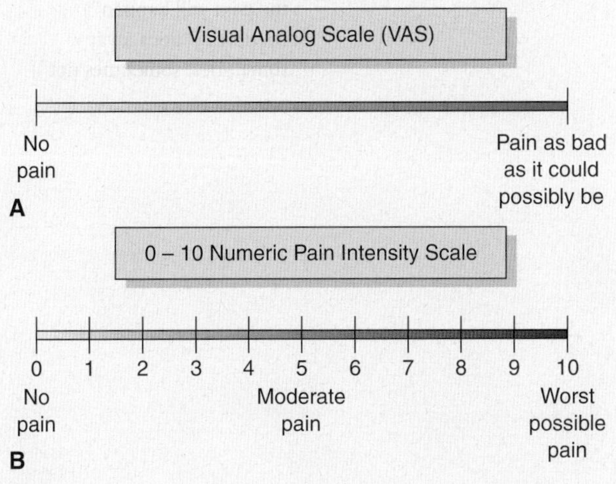

● Figure 15.7 (A) Visual analog scale. (B) Numeric scale.

Adolescent Pediatric Pain Tool. The Adolescent Pediatric Pain Tool is a self-report type of tool useful for older children, usually from ages 8 to 17 years. The tool involves three aspects of assessment. In the first assessment the child identifies the location of the pain on two illustrations of the body, front and back views (Fig. 15.8). The child is instructed to color the areas where he or she is hurting. The child is also instructed to color the area as big or as small as how much he or she is hurting. For example, if the hurt is mild or moderate, the child would color a moderate area of the location; if the pain was severe, he or she would color a much larger area. The second portion of the tool involves a scale that ranges from "no pain" to "worst possible pain"; the child is instructed to identify the severity of his or her pain. The third assessment is a list of words that may be used to describe pain, such as throbbing, pounding, stabbing, or sharp. The child is asked to point to or circle the words that describe the current pain. Children with limited reading skills or vocabulary may have difficulty with some of the words listed to describe pain. Work with the child and encourage the parents to help the child understand the various descriptive words. Parental participation fosters control over the situation and gives the parents some insight into what their child is experiencing.

Physical Examination

Physical examination of the child for pain primarily involves the skills of observation and inspection. These skills are used to assess for physiologic and behavioral changes that indicate pain. Auscultation also may be used to assess for changes in vital signs, specifically heart rate and blood pressure.

Manifestations of Pain

Observe for physical signs and symptoms of pain, keeping in mind the child's developmental level. Look for facial expressions of discomfort, grimacing, or crying. Be alert for movements that may suggest pain. For example, an infant or toddler may pull on the ear when experiencing ear pain. The child may move the head from side to side, suggesting head pain. Typically, children with abdominal pain will lie on one side and draw their knees up to the abdomen. Inspect the child's gait: a limp or avoidance of weight bearing may suggest leg pain. Immobility, guarding of a particular body area, or refusal to move an area may be observed. Inspect the skin for flushing or diaphoresis, possible indicators of pain. Also monitor vital signs for changes. Pulse or heart rate, respiratory rate, and blood pressure may increase. Other physiologic parameters suggesting pain may include elevated intracranial pressure and pulmonary vascular resistance and decreased oxygen saturation levels.

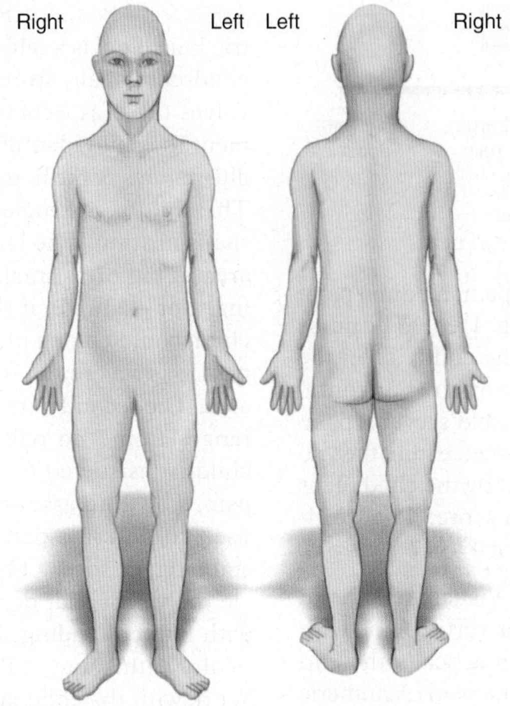

Sensory	Affective	Evaluative	Temporal
Aching ("pain all over")	Awful ("cannot do anything")	Annoying ("cannot sleep")	Always ("pain always there")
Hurting ("pain all over")	Crying ("hurts so bad")	Bad ("cannot stop the hurting")	Comes and goes ("always pain")
Sore ("like a cut")	Frightening ("scared it won't stop")	Miserable ("cannot sleep or do stuff")	Comes on all of a sudden ("no warning")
Beating (procedural pain "spots")	Screaming (afraid of "going to the hospital")	Terrible ("don't like it")	Constant ("never goes away")
Pounding ("gets on your nerves")	Terrifying ("cannot sleep," "really tired," "not going to live")	Uncomfortable ("can't stay in one spot")	Continuous ("pain not going away")
Cutting ("hurts more than a cut")		Uncontrollable ("cannot stop it")	Forever ("never will go away")
Like a sharp knife ("stabbing and sharp")	Dizzy ("don't know where I am")		Once in a while ("in a month sometimes pain; sometimes not")
Sharp (no meaning)			Sneaks up ("don't know when the pain will happen")
Stabbing (no meaning)			Sometimes ("goes away sometimes; sometimes not")
Cramping ("everywhere like a plane crash")			
Crushing (no meaning)			
Pressure ("pushing all over")			
Itching ("all over")			
Scratching ("helps sometimes")			
Shocking (pain "surprises" her)			
Splitting ("splitting in half" her body)			
Numb ("knows pain is there"/procedural pain)			
Stiff ("cannot move")			
Swollen ("meds do not help")			
Tight ("cannot move")			

● **Figure 15.8** Adolescent Pediatric Assessment Tool. (*Top*) Adolescent Pediatric Pain Tool (APPT): Body Outline (Crandall & Savedra, 2005). (*Bottom*) Pain Quality: Words chosen and meaning of words (Crandall & Savedra, 2005).

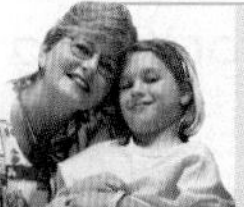

The body responds to acute pain via the sympathetic nervous system, leading to stimulation and subsequently the increase in vital signs. However, if the child has persistent or chronic pain, the body adapts and these changes may be less noticeable; in fact, heart and pulse rate, respiratory rate, and blood pressure may actually decrease.

The child also may exhibit behavioral changes indicating pain. Be alert for irritability and restlessness. Watch for clenching of teeth or fists, body stiffening, or increased muscle tension. Note any changes in the child's behavior—for example, a child who previously was talkative and playful who becomes quiet and almost withdrawn. In addition, pay close attention to the child's cultural background and how these beliefs may be affecting the behavioral response to pain.

Each child is an individual with unique responses to pain, so the nurse must ensure that observations of behavior do indeed reflect the child's pain level. To help ensure the accuracy of observations, several physiologic and behavioral assessment tools have been developed to help quantify the observations.

Physiologic and Behavioral Pain Assessment Tools

Use of physiologic and behavioral pain assessment tools allows measurement of specific parameters and changes that would indicate that the child is experiencing pain. These measurements aid in determining the intensity of the pain experience. Along with the self-report pain-rating scales, measurement of these changes allows the nurse to objectively assess pain and the effectiveness of pain management measures.

Neonatal Infant Pain Scale. The Neonatal Infant Pain Scale (NIPS) is a behavioral assessment tool that is useful for measuring pain in preterm and full-term neonates. Six parameters are measured: facial expression, cry, breathing patterns, arms, legs, and state of arousal (Table 15.3). Each parameter except for cry is scored as a 0 or 1; cry is scored as 0, 1, or 2. The scores are totaled; the maximum score that can be achieved is 7. A higher score indicates increased pain. This tool is not recommended for use in neonates who are too ill to respond or who are receiving paralyzing agents. In these cases, a falsely low score would be produced.

Riley Infant Pain Scale. The Riley Infant Pain Scale (RIPS) is a behavioral assessment tool useful for infants who lack verbal ability. Like NIPS, RIPS measures six parameters: facial expression, body movement, sleep, verbal or vocal ability, consolability, and response to movements and touch (Table 15.4). Each parameter is scored as 0, 1, 2, or 3. The score is totaled; the maximum score that can be achieved is 18. The higher the total score, the more intense the pain.

Pain Observation Scale for Young Children. The Pain Observation Scale for Young Children (POCIS) is a behavioral assessment tool designed for use in children 1 to 4 years of age. This tool measures seven parameters: facial expression, cry, breathing, torso, arms and fingers, legs and toes, and state of arousal (Table 15.5). Each parameter is scored as 0 or 1; the maximum score achievable is 7.

Table 15.3 The Neonatal Infant Pain Scale (NIPS)

Parameter	Finding	Score
Facial expression	Relaxed (restful face; neutral expression)	0
	Grimace (tight facial muscles; furrowed brow, chin, or jaw; negative facial expression)	1
Cry	No cry (quiet; not crying)	0
	Whimper (mild intermittent moaning)	1
	Vigorous crying (loud screaming, shrill, continuous)	2
Breathing patterns	Relaxed	0
	Change in breathing (irregular; faster than usual; gagging; breath holding)	1
Arms	Relaxed (no muscular rigidity; occasional random movements of arm)	0
	Flexed/extended (tense, straight, rigid, or rapid flexion or extension)	1
Legs	Relaxed (no muscular rigidity; occasional random movements of leg)	0
	Flexed/extended (tense, straight, rigid, or rapid flexion or extension)	1
State of arousal	Sleeping/awake (quiet, peaceful; settled)	0
	Fussy (alert, restless, thrashing)	1

From Lawrence, J., Alcock, D., McGrath, P., Kay, J., MacMurray, S. B., & Dulberg, C. (1993). The development of a tool to assess neonatal pain. *Neonatal Network, 12*(6), 59–66.

Table 15.4 The Riley Infant Pain Scale

Parameter	Score
Facial expression	
• Neutral/smiling	0
• Frowning/grimacing	1
• Clenched teeth	2
• Full cry expression	3
Body movement	
• Calm, relaxed	0
• Restless, fidgeting	1
• Moderate agitation or mobility; thrashing, flailing, incessant agitation or strong voluntary mobility	2
• Voluntary immobility	3
Sleep	
• Sleeping quietly with easy respirations	0
• Restless while asleep	1
• Sleeps intermittently (sleep/awake)	2
• Sleeping for prolonged periods of time interrupted by jerky movements or inability to sleep	3
Verbal/vocal	
• No cry	0
• Whimpering, complaining	1
• Pain crying	2
• Screaming, high-pitched cry	3
Consolability	
• Neutral	0
• Easy to console	1
• Not easy to console	2
• Inconsolable	3
Response to movement/touch	
• Moves easily	0
• Winces when touched or moved	1
• Cries out when moved or touched	2
• High-pitched cry or scream when touched or moved	3

From Schade, J. G., Joyce, B. A., Gerkensmeyer, J., & Keck, J. F. (1996). Comparison of three preverbal scales for postoperative pain assessment in a diverse pediatric sample. *Journal of Pain and Symptom Management, 12*(6), 348–359.

The higher the score, the greater the pain being experienced by the child.

CRIES Scale for Neonatal Postoperative Pain Assessment. The CRIES scale is a behavioral assessment tool that also includes measures of physiologic parameters. It was developed to quantify postoperative pain in the newborn. The tool also may be used to monitor the infant's progress over time during recovery or after interventions. The tool assesses five parameters: cry, oxygen required for saturation levels less than 95%, increased vital signs, facial expression, and sleeplessness (Table 15.6). Each parameter is scored as 0, 1, or 2 and then totaled. As with other assessment tools, the higher the score, the greater the infant's pain.

Table 15.5 The Pain Observation Scale for Young Children (POCIS)

Parameter	Finding	Score
Facial expression	Neutral	0
	Grimace (negative)	1
Cry	No cry	0
	Moan, scream	1
Breathing	Relaxed and regular	0
	Irregular and indrawn	1
Torso	At rest, inactive	0
	Tense, shivering	1
Arms and fingers	At rest, inactive	0
	Tense, restless	1
Legs and toes	At rest, inactive	0
	Tense, restless	1
State of arousal	Calm, sleepy	0
	Fussy	1

Reprinted with permission of W. J. C. Boelen-van der Loo, Ph.D.

FLACC Behavioral Scale for Postoperative Pain in Young Children. The FLACC behavioral scale is a behavioral assessment tool that is useful in assessing a child's pain when the child cannot report accurately his or her level of pain. It has been demonstrated to be a reliable tool for children from age 2 months to 7 years of age. This tool measures five parameters: facial expression, legs, activity, cry, and consolability (Table 15.7). Observe the child with the legs and body uncovered. If the child is awake, observe him or her for 2 to 5 minutes; if sleeping, observe the child for 5 minutes or longer. Each parameter is scored as 0, 1, or 2; the scores are totaled, with a maximum achievable score of 10. As with other assessment tools, the higher the score, the greater the pain.

Nursing Diagnoses, Goals, Interventions, and Evaluation

After the assessment is completed, the nurse identifies appropriate nursing diagnoses. The most commonly identified nursing diagnosis would be Acute or Chronic pain. However, the related factors and defining characteristics can vary widely. Nursing diagnoses will focus on the effects of pain on the child—for example, the stress incurred as a result of the pain or the fear or anxiety associated with the pain or events causing the pain. Moreover, pain can affect physiologic functions, such as sleep, nutrition, mobility, and elimination. Examples of common nursing diagnoses may include:

- Acute pain related to repeated need for invasive procedures, surgical experience, recent trauma, or infection

Table 15.6 The CRIES Scale for Neonatal Postoperative Pain Assessment

Assessment	0	1	2
Crying	No	High-pitched, but consolable	High-pitched, inconsolable
Oxygen required for saturation above 95%	No	<30%	>30%
Increased vital signs	Heart rate and blood pressure within 10% of preoperative values	Heart rate or blood pressure 11% to 20% higher than preoperative values	Heart rate or blood pressure 21% or more above preoperative values
Expression	No grimace	Grimace	Grimace with grunt
Sleepless	No	Waking at frequent intervals	Constantly awake
Total infant score			

From Krechel, S. W., & Bildner, J. (1995). CRIES: A new neonatal postoperative pain measurement score. Initial testing of validity and reliability. *Paediatric Anaesthesia, 5,* 53–61.

- Chronic pain related to prolonged illness or injury, effects of cancer on surrounding tissues, or treatment-related effects
- Fear related to the unknown, separation from family, anticipation of invasive procedures, or effects of treatment
- Anxiety related to the stress and uncertainty of the situation
- Deficient knowledge related to current condition and appropriate methods for managing pain
- Disturbed sleep pattern related to inability to manage pain effectively
- Impaired mobility related to increased episodes of pain
- Risk for constipation related to potential adverse effects of narcotic analgesic agents

When caring for a child experiencing pain, the ultimate goal is that the child will be free of pain as evidenced by participation in age-appropriate activities of daily living and vital signs within age-appropriate parameters. However, at times, this may be unrealistic, especially if the child is experiencing chronic pain. Therefore, a more appropriate goal would be that the child reports that his or her pain has decreased to a tolerable level. Pain assessment tools can be used to quantify the amount by which

Table 15.7 FLACC Behavioral Scale

	Scoring		
Category	*0*	*1*	*2*
Face	No particular expression or smile	Occasional grimace or frown, withdrawn, disinterested	Frequent to constant frown, clenched jaw, quivering chin
Legs	Normal position or relaxed	Uneasy, restless, tense	Kicking, or legs drawn up
Activity	Lying quietly, normal position, moves easily	Squirming, shifting back and forth, tense	Arched, rigid, or jerking
Cry	No cry (awake or asleep)	Moans or whimpers, occasional complaint	Crying steadily, screams or sobs, frequent complaints
Consolability	Content, relaxed	Reassured by occasional touching, hugging, or being talked to, distractable	Difficult to console or comfort

Each of the five categories is scored from 0 to 2, which results in a total score between 0 and 10.

the child's pain has decreased. For example, if the child has rated the pain as 7 out of 10, a realistic goal might be that the child reports a pain rating of no more than 4 out of 10. Additional goals would reflect improvement or resolution of the identified problem. For example, a short-term goal for a child experiencing disturbed sleep due to the pain might be that the child sleeps for a minimum of 4 consecutive hours through the night. A long-term goal might be that the child sleeps for 7 to 8 hours undisturbed through the night.

Various interventions can be used for pain management. These interventions include pharmacologic and nonpharmacologic measures. A guiding principle when caring for the child experiencing pain is the provision of atraumatic care (see Chapter 11 for more information). For example, apply a topical anesthetic cream to a site early enough before a venipuncture that it becomes effective. Use an intermittent infusion device to obtain multiple blood specimen samples rather than performing repeated venipunctures. Consider the use of sedation for more painful procedures. In addition to pharmacologic measures, cognitive and behavioral approaches are appropriate for pain management, including pain management related to procedures.

Throughout the child's care, be sure to discuss specific goals and interventions with the child and family as appropriate. Include the family in developing appropriate interventions so they can continue to support the child. Education of the child and family about interventions, including various therapies, is key. Play therapy may be helpful in allowing the child to express his or her feelings and adapt to the stressors of the current situation. Ongoing assessment is needed to determine the effectiveness of the pain relief measures in achieving the desired goals.

Nursing Care Plan 15.1 can be used as a guide in planning nursing care for the child experiencing pain. The nursing care plan should be individualized based on the child's symptoms and needs. Specific information related to pain management and the nurse's role will be discussed later in the chapter.

> When you enter Aiden's room, he is crying and says his leg hurts. What will be your initial action? What will be your plan of care to manage Aiden's pain (refer to QUESTT assessment)? How would you address the statements made by the nurse in report? What approaches can you use to change staff behavior about pain management?

Management of Pain

Three general principles guide pain management in children:

1. Individualize interventions based on the amount of pain experienced during a procedure and the child's personality.
2. Use nonpharmacologic and pharmacologic approaches to ease or eliminate the pain.
3. Use aggressive pharmacologic treatment with the first procedure.

Strategies for pain management include nonpharmacologic interventions such as distraction, relaxation, and guided imagery and pharmacologic interventions such as analgesics, patient-controlled analgesia, local analgesia, epidural analgesia, and conscious sedation.

Nonpharmacologic Management

Various techniques may be available to assist in managing mild pain in children or augment the effectiveness of medications for moderate or severe pain. Many of these nonpharmacologic techniques assist children in coping with pain and give them an opportunity to feel a sense of mastery or control over the situation. Two types of techniques are behavior/cognitive strategies and biophysical strategies. With these techniques as well as administration of medications, parents need to be involved in this process.

Behavioral-Cognitive Strategies

Behavioral-cognitive strategies for pain management involve measures that require the child to focus on a specific area rather than the pain. These strategies help to change the interpretation of the painful stimuli, reducing pain perception or making pain more tolerable. In addition, these strategies help to decrease negative attitudes, thoughts, and anxieties, thereby improving the child's coping mechanisms. Typically, these interventions work well with older children, but some younger children also benefit from these techniques if they are adapted to the child's age and developmental level. Common behavioral-cognitive strategies include relaxation, distraction, imagery, biofeedback, thought stopping, and positive self-talk.

Relaxation

Relaxation aids in reducing muscle tension and anxiety. A wide variety of techniques can be used. Relaxation can be as simple as holding an infant or young child closely while stroking the child or speaking in a soft soothing manner, or having the child inhale and exhale slowly using rhythmically controlled deep breathing. It also can involve more sophisticated techniques such as progressive relaxation. With this technique the child is asked to focus on one area of the body and let that body part go limp. Then in an organized fashion, usually working from the toes to the head or vice versa, the child is asked to focus on another body part, making it go limp. Eventually the exercises work through all body areas, leading to relaxation of the entire body.

Distraction

Distraction involves having the child focus on another stimulus, thereby attempting to shield him or her from

(text continues on page 398)

Nursing Care Plan 15.1

Overview for the Child in Pain

Nursing Diagnosis: Acute pain related to need for invasive procedures, surgery, recent trauma, or infection as evidenced by pain rating scale, facial grimacing, crying, irritability, withdrawal activity, or changes in vital signs

Outcome identification and evaluation

Child will achieve adequate comfort level as evidenced by a decrease in rating number (3 or less) on a pain rating scale, quietness, calm resting behaviors, decrease in crying and irritability, and vital signs within acceptable parameters.

Intervention: promoting pain relief

- Assess pain level using a developmentally appropriate pain rating tool *to establish a baseline.*
- Assess for verbal and nonverbal indicators of pain; question parents about child's typical behaviors and previous experiences with pain *to determine factors that may be influencing child's response to pain.*
- Institute nonpharmacologic methods for pain control based on the child's age and cognitive level; encourage parental participation in use of methods *to provide additional support for the child.*
- Administer pharmacologic agents as ordered using the least traumatic route possible *to alter pain impulse transmission and minimize distress while promoting effective pain relief.*
- Explain the action of the drug and what the child should expect from the medication at a level that the child can understand *to promote trust and reduce fear.*
- Give analgesics around the clock if pain is continuous and can be predicted *to maintain steady blood levels of the drug, thereby maximizing the drug's effect.*
- Perform atraumatic care at all times *to minimize the child's exposure to physical and psychological distress.*
- If a procedure is to be done, explain the purpose of the medication before the procedure and what to expect *to help minimize fear of the unknown.*
- Anticipate timing of procedures or situations that may lead to pain and provide appropriate analgesic therapy as ordered *to ensure that therapy is most effective at the time of the procedure.*
- Ensure that the child's environment is quiet and conducive to rest, dim the lights, close the door or curtain *to reduce sensory overload that would increase the child's pain sensation.*
- Encourage the parents to stroke, touch, caress, and hold the child *to promote feelings of security.*
- Reassess child's pain level after use of nonpharmacologic and pharmacologic methods *to determine effectiveness;* anticipate the need to modify or adapt nonpharmacologic methods or adjust analgesic dosage, route, or frequency *to promote maximum pain relief.*
- Perform nursing care activities after administering analgesic *to prevent exacerbating the child's pain.*
- Use diversional activities, distraction, and play appropriate to the child's age and cognitive level *to promote additional pain relief.*

(continued)

Overview for the Child in Pain (continued)

Nursing Diagnosis: Anxiety related to stress and uncertainty of the situation, unknown cause of pain, lack of familiarity with procedures, testing, and health care facility, and painful procedures, as evidenced by crying, irritability, withdrawal, stoic, or aggressive behaviors

Outcome identification and evaluation

Child and family will demonstrate a decrease in anxiety level as evidenced by age-appropriate positive coping behaviors, verbalization of feelings, playing out of feelings, child and family cooperation with plan of care, and absence of signs and symptoms associated with escalating anxiety.

Intervention: minimizing anxiety

- Assess child's and parents' understanding of the situation, including their understanding of what may be causing the pain and the reasons for the procedures and testing, *to provide baseline information about the child's and parents' knowledge and possible clues to anxiety.*
- Spend time with the child and parents discussing what they think might be happening, encouraging child and parents to talk openly about their feelings, *to facilitate continued expressions and communication.* Allow time for questions and answer questions honestly *to establish rapport and build trust.*
- Approach the child and family in a calm, relaxed manner *to foster trust and communication.*
- Allow the child options related to pharmacologic agent administration as much as possible, such as fluid to drink or snack to eat, extremity to use for venipuncture (right or left), color of bandage, or holding tape or dressing, *to foster feelings of control.*
- Provide atraumatic care *to reduce exposure to distress, which would exacerbate the child's anxiety level.*
- Explain any procedures, tests, activities at a level the child can understand *to reduce fear of the unknown.*
- Incorporate aspects of the child's routine at home as much as possible *to reduce feelings of separation and promote feelings of normalcy.*
- Ensure consistency in care *to facilitate trust and acceptance.*
- Encourage parents in the use of comfort measures such as stroking, cuddling, holding, and rocking *to promote feelings of security and minimize stress.*
- Provide positive reinforcement for choices, participation in activities, and use of appropriate coping methods *to foster self-esteem.*
- Encourage the child's participation in play (unstructured and therapeutic play as needed) *to promote expression of feelings and fears.*

Nursing Diagnosis: Deficient knowledge related to current condition and appropriate methods for managing pain as evidenced by crying, irritability, pushing away, questions and verbalizations about pain and relief methods

Outcome identification and evaluation

Child and parents will demonstrate adequate knowledge about the child's current condition and use of pain relief methods as evidenced by statements about the cause of the child's pain, demonstration of chosen nonpharmacologic relief methods, use of pharmacologic agents, and statements related to signs and symptoms of increased and decreased pain.

Intervention: providing child and family teaching

- Assess child's and parents' knowledge and understanding of child's current condition and current pain level *to establish a baseline for teaching.*

Overview for the Child in Pain (continued)

- Provide time for child and parents to ask questions; answer questions honestly and in terms they can understand *to promote learning.*
- Explain in simplified terms how the child's condition is associated with pain or the rationale for procedures needed that may contribute to pain *to promote understanding and foster trust.*
- Teach in short sessions *to prevent overloading the child and parents with information.*
- Provide reinforcement and rewards *to help facilitate the teaching/learning process.*
- Use multiple modes of learning, such as written information, verbal instruction, demonstrations, and media when possible, *to facilitate learning and retention of information.*
- Instruct parents and child as appropriate in nonpharmacologic methods for pain relief; encourage practice and participation by parents in methods chosen *to foster independence and use of method when necessary.*
- Teach child as appropriate and parents about pharmacologic methods for pain relief; review specific information about drug to be used, including action, duration, administration, possible adverse effects, and care necessary when drug is used, *to promote learning;* have child and parents report back information or demonstrate administration *to evaluate effectiveness of teaching.*
- Provide parents with written information about pain relief methods for use at home if indicated *to allow for reference at a later date.*

Nursing Diagnosis: Disturbed sleep patterns related to inability to manage pain effectively as evidenced by frequent waking by child during night, signs and symptoms of pain including irritability and restlessness, statements about being tired, pain rating scale

Outcome identification and evaluation

Child will exhibit increased ability to sleep during night as evidenced by increasing periods of calm and restfulness (initially starting at 2 hours and gradually increasing to 7 to 8 hours), decreased pain level on pain rating scale, and statements of decreased fatigue.

Intervention: promoting sleep and rest

- Assist child in using nonpharmacologic methods of pain relief, such as imagery, distraction, muscle relaxation, *to promote relaxation.*
- Administer pharmacologic pain relief as ordered *to minimize pain interfering with sleep;* anticipate a change in drug therapy if pain relief is inadequate.
- Cluster nursing care activities *to minimize energy expenditure and disruptions in child's ability to rest.*
- Help child with a nighttime routine similar to one he or she uses at home *to promote feelings of security.*
- Offer child back rub, warm bath, or warm liquids, reading a story, or listening to music *to facilitate relaxation;* provide stroking, hugging, cuddling, rocking, and light touch *to promote a sense of security and calm.*
- Dim the lights and close the curtain or door to the room *to provide a quiet, restful environment.*
- Ensure round-the-clock pain relief for the child through the night *to minimize the risk of pain.*

Nursing Diagnosis: Risk for injury related to possible adverse effects of analgesics

Outcome identification and evaluation

Child will remain free of any injury related to signs and symptoms of adverse effects of analgesic therapy as evidenced by respiratory rate appropriate for age, no complaints of GI upset, dizziness, or sedation or episodes of constipation, nausea, vomiting, or pruritus.

(continued)

Overview for the Child in Pain (continued)

Intervention: promoting safety

- Ensure that the child's call light is within reach *to allow for notification of health care personnel should problems arise.*
- Administer analgesic exactly as prescribed *to reduce the risk of error and development of adverse effects.*
- Assess child's respiratory status closely for changes *to allow for early detection of respiratory depression.*
- If an opioid analgesic is being given, have naloxone readily available *to reverse the action of the narcotic if respiratory depression occurs.*
- Monitor appetite and assess bowel sounds for changes; note any abdominal distention or decreased bowel sounds, *which would suggest decreased peristalsis.*
- Ensure adequate fluid and fiber intake *to reduce risk of constipation.*
- Offer small frequent meals and give medication with food *to minimize risk of GI upset.*
- Assess for nausea and vomiting; if necessary withhold food and fluids *to rest the GI tract* and administer antiemetics until nausea and vomiting resolve.
- Instruct the child to remain in bed after receiving analgesic, raise crib or side rails as appropriate, and instruct the child and parents to have someone accompany the child to the bathroom if allowed *to reduce the risk of falls from sedation.*
- Assess for complaints of itching and observe for rash or reddened areas; if pruritus occurs, urge the child not to scratch and expect to administer antihistamine as ordered *to reduce pruritus.*
- Provide the child with distraction to assist in helping *to reduce effects of pruritus.*

pain. This technique does not eliminate the pain but does help to make it more tolerable. Various methods can be used for distraction, including:

- Counting
- Repetition of specific phrases or words, such as "ouch"
- Listening to music or singing
- Playing games, including computer games
- Blowing bubbles or blowing pinwheels or party favors
- Listening to favorite stories (Fig. 15.9)
- Watching cartoons, television shows, or movies
- Visiting with friends
- Humor

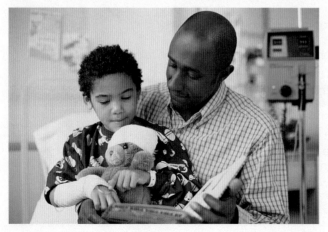

● Figure 15.9 A child using distraction for pain management.

Humor has been demonstrated to be an effective distracting technique for pain management. However, make sure that the technique is age-appropriate and be sure to determine what or who will make the child laugh. If possible, allow the child and his family to choose the materials that they consider humorous.

The type of distraction used depends on the age of the child. For example, a younger child may enjoy blowing pinwheels and blowing bubbles. He or she also will enjoy listening to favorite stories or books. Older children may enjoy computer games, listening to favorite music, or visiting with friends.

Imagery

Imagery involves the use of the imagination to create a mental image. This mental image usually is a positive, pleasurable image, but it need not be real. The child is encouraged to include details and sensations that are associated with the image, such as specific descriptions of the image, colors, sounds, feelings, and smells. In some instances, the child may write down or record the image on a tape or compact disc. When pain occurs, the child is encouraged to create the mental image or read or listen to the description.

Biofeedback

Biofeedback involves having the child gain an awareness of his or her body functions and learn ways to modify them voluntarily. The child usually is taught specific skills about how to modify body functions using an apparatus that measures pain-related changes in muscle tone or physiologic data, such as blood pressure or pulse rate. This teaching usually occurs over several sessions, in advance of the pain experience. With practice, the child learns to control the changes without the apparatus. This technique can be used by older children, such as adolescents, who can concentrate for longer periods of time.

Thought Stopping

Thought stopping involves substituting a pleasurable or positive thought for the painful experience. Examples of positive thoughts might be, "It's only for a short time" or "It's important so I get better." The negative component of the pain is not ignored or suppressed; rather, it is transformed into something positive. Thought stopping also can involve the use of short, positive phrases. For example, the child may repeat "quick stick, feel better, go home soon" when he or she anticipates pain or experiences pain.

Thought stopping is a useful method for reducing anxiety before and during events associated with pain. Children can be taught to use this technique anytime they experience anxiety related to a painful experience. Doing so helps to promote the child's sense of control over the situation.

Positive Self-Talk

Positive self-talk is similar to thought stopping in that it involves the use of positive statements. With positive self-talk the child is taught to say positive statements when he or she is experiencing pain. For example, the child may be taught to say, "I will feel better and be able to go home and play with my friends."

Biophysical Interventions

Biophysical interventions focus on interfering with the transmission of pain impulses reaching the brain. The interventions involve some type of cutaneous stimulation near the site of the pain. This stimulation decreases the ability of the A-delta and C fibers to transmit pain impulses. Examples of biophysical interventions include application of heat and cold, massage and pressure, and transcutaneous electrical nerve stimulation (TENS).

A particular intervention for infants is nonnutritive sucking, which reduces pain behaviors in neonates undergoing painful procedures (Bo & Callaghan, 2000; Morash & Fowler, 2004). Infants derive satisfaction from sucking. In addition, they show reduced pain behaviors after ingestion of sucrose or other sweet-tasting solutions such as glucose, since these substances are mediated through the opioid pathways (Blass & Watt, 1999; Carbajal et al., 1999; Isek et al., 2000; Morash & Fowler, 2004). Nonnutritive sucking is recommended as a technique for providing atraumatic care, but this method must be used with caution in infants with unstable blood glucose levels.

Heat and Cold Applications

Heat and cold applications alter physiologic mechanisms associated with pain. Cold results in vasoconstriction and alters capillary permeability, leading to a decrease in edema at the site of the injury. Due to vasoconstriction, blood flow is reduced and the release of pain-producing substances such as histamine and serotonin also is decreased. Moreover, transmission of painful stimuli via peripheral nerve fibers is decreased.

Heat results in vasodilation and increases blood flow to the area. It also leads to a decrease in nociceptive stimulation and removal of chemical substances that can stimulate nociceptive fibers. The increase in blood flow alters capillary permeability, leading to a reduction in swelling and pressure on nociceptive nerve fibers. Heat may also trigger the release of endogenous opioids, which mediate the pain response.

Massage and Pressure

Massage and pressure, like other biophysical interventions, are believed to inhibit stimulation of the A-delta and C fibers. These methods are helpful in relaxing muscles and reducing tension. In addition, these techniques can aid in distracting the child. Massage can be as simple as rubbing a body part or pressing on an area such as an injection site for about 10 seconds, or it can be more involved, requiring the use of another person to perform the massage. Lotion or ointment can be used during the massage and may provide a comforting effect. Contralateral pressure or massage (i.e., of the opposite area) may be used, especially if the area of pain cannot be accessed or if the affected area is too painful to touch.

A more formal method of pressure application is acupressure. In acupressure the fingertip, thumb, or a blunt instrument is used to apply gentle, firm pressure to specifically designated sites to control pain. The pressure may be applied in one motion followed by releasing, in a circular motion for several minutes and then releasing, or with a vibrating motion using the fingertips. The motion of applying and then releasing pressure is thought to facilitate the release of endogenous endorphins and enkephalins. The techniques of pressure and massage can be taught to children and parents. The techniques are easy to learn and use.

The Nurse's Role in Nonpharmacologic Pain Intervention

The nurse plays a major role in teaching the child and family about nonpharmacologic pain interventions, helping them choose the most appropriate and most effective methods, and ensuring that the child and parents use the method before pain occurs as well as before the pain increases. Teaching Guideline 15.1 lists some helpful instructions for the parents and child about nonpharmacologic pain management.

The nurse also assists the child and parents when using the technique, ensuring that they are using the technique correctly and offering suggestions for modifications or adaptations as necessary.

Parents are important components of the pain management program. Give them the option to stay with the child, or let them know that someone else will support the child if they opt not to stay. Offer simple, concrete ways to assist and help the child to manage pain. Many of the nonpharmacologic techniques can be done by parents, and children may respond better if their parents demonstrate the technique and encourage them to use it. Invite parents to participate in decisions as well as act as a coach to their child during procedures. Prepare the parents and explain the most appropriate pain management approaches and strategies. Discuss the type and amount of pain expected as well as the potential complications associated with pain management approaches. Ask how the parent predicts the child will react to a painful situation. Finally, offer techniques and strategies to the parents as they act as the coach during these situations.

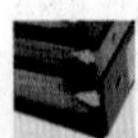

TEACHING GUIDELINE 15.1

Teaching to Manage Pain Without Drugs

- Review the methods available and choose the method(s) that your child and you find best for your situation.
- Learn to identify the ways in which your child shows pain or demonstrates he or she is anxious about the possibility of pain—for example, does he or she get restless, make a face, or get flushed in the face?
- Begin using the technique chosen before your child experiences pain or when your child first indicates he or she is anxious about or beginning to experience pain.
- Practice the technique with your child and encourage the child to use the technique when he or she feels anxious about pain or anticipates that a procedure or experience will be painful.
- Perform the technique with your child; for example, take the deep breath in and out or blow bubbles with him or her; listen to the music or play the computer game with your child.
- Avoid using terms such as "hurt" or "pain" that suggest or cause your child to expect pain.
- Use descriptive terms like pushing, pulling, pinching, or heat.
- Avoid overly descriptive or judgmental statements such as, "this will really hurt a lot" or "this will be terrible."
- Stay with your child as much as possible; speak softly and gently stroke or cuddle your child.
- Offer praise, positive reinforcement, hugs, and support for using the technique even when it was not effective.

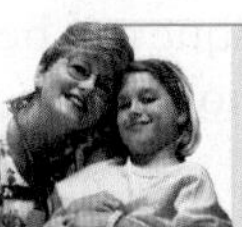

Although parents want to help their children and some are able to act as coaches, the response of the child to pain and stress and to their parents' distraction interventions is highly variable. Some children appear to be soothed by their parents' distraction actions; others appear to become distressed. Be alert to factors that may influence the child's response, including age, sex, diagnosis, ethnicity, previous experience, temperament, anxiety, and coping style. Also be aware of parental factors, including ethnicity, sex, previous experience, belief in the helpfulness of the intervention, parenting style, and parental anxiety (McCarthy & Kleiber, 2006).

Pharmacologic Management

Pharmacologic interventions involve the administration of drugs for pain relief. Administration may occur using a wide variety of methods. The selection of the method is determined by the drug being administered, the child's status, the type, intensity, and location of the pain, and any factors that may be influencing the child's pain. Research overwhelmingly supports the appropriate use of analgesics to reduce pain perception in children (Broome & Huth, 2003).

Medications Used for Pain Management

Analgesics (medications for pain relief) typically fall into one of two categories: nonopioid analgesics and opioid analgesics. Anesthetics also may be used. Drugs such as sedatives and hypnotics also may be used as adjuvant medications to help minimize anxiety or provide or assist with pain relief when typical analgesics are ineffective.

Nonopioid Analgesics

Nonopioid analgesics include acetaminophen and nonsteroidal anti-inflammatory drugs (NSAIDs) such as ibuprofen, ketorolac, naproxen, indomethacin, diclofenac, and piroxicam (Drug Guide 15.1). These agents may be used to treat mild to moderate pain, often for conditions such as arthritis; joint, bone, and muscle pain; headache; dental pain; and menstrual pain. Acetaminophen, probably the most widely known nonopioid analgesic, also is commonly used to treat fever in children, as is ibuprofen.

Drug Guide 15.1 Common Drugs for Pain Management

Drug	Action	Indication	Nursing Implications
Acetaminophen (Tylenol)	Possible inhibition of cyclooxygenase in the central nervous system. Direct action on hypothalamic heat-regulating center.	Mild to moderate pain; arthritis, musculo-skeletal pain, headache	• Administer orally or rectally. Do not exceed five doses of drug in 24 hours. • Caution parents to read labels of other over-the-counter (OTC) drugs carefully; some may contain acetaminophen and if given in conjunction may lead to overdose.
Ibuprofen (Motrin, Advil)	Inhibition of prostaglandin synthesis	Mild to moderate pain, fever	• Administer orally. • Give with food or after meals if GI upset occurs. • Assess for easy bruising, bleeding gums, or frank or occult blood in urine or stool. • Monitor for nausea, vomiting, GI upset, diarrhea or constipation, dizziness or drowsiness. • Caution parents to read labels of OTC medications closely; some may contain ibuprofen or other NSAIDs and if given in conjunction may lead to overdose.
Other NSAIDs: ketorolac (Toradol), diclofenac (Voltaren), indomethacin (Indocin), naproxen (Naprosyn, Aleve)	Inhibition of prostaglandin synthesis	Mild to moderate pain	• Administer oral form with food or after meals if GI upset occurs. • Monitor for headache, dizziness, nausea, vomiting, constipation, or diarrhea. • Assess for signs and symptoms of bleeding, such as bruising, epistaxis, gingival bleeding, or frank or occult blood in urine or stool. • Ketorolac: May also be given IV or IM. In children 2–16 years, recommended as single dose only.

(continued)

Drug Guide 15.1 (continued)

Drug	Action	Indication	Nursing Implications
			• Naproxen: Also available in combination products (caution parents to read OTC labels carefully). • Indomethacin: When administering IV, report oliguria or anuria. • Diclofenac: May also be given rectally.
Opioid agents: morphine, codeine, fentanyl (Sublimaze, Duragesic), hydromorphone (Dilaudid), oxycodone (OxyContin)	Opioid agonist acting primarily at μ-receptor sites (morphine, codeine, fentanyl, hydromorphone, oxycodone)	Moderate to severe acute and chronic pain. Morphine: intractable pain, preoperative sedation. Codeine: also suppresses cough reflex. Fentanyl: pain associated with short procedures such as bone marrow aspiration, fracture reductions, suturing.	• Assess respiratory status frequently, noting any decrease in ventilatory rate or changes in breathing patterns; have naloxone readily available in case of respiratory depression (particularly morphine, fentanyl, hydromorphone). • Monitor for sedation dizziness, lethargy, confusion. • Educate parents and child that the drug may make the child sleepy, drowsy, or lightheaded. • Institute safety measures to prevent injury to the child. • Assess bowel sounds for decreased peristalsis; observe for abdominal distention. • Ensure adequate fiber intake and administer stool softeners as prescribed to minimize risk for constipation. • Monitor urine output for changes and report. • Morphine: May cause itching, particularly facial. • Codeine: May cause nausea, vomiting, abdominal pain. IV administration results in apnea and severe hypotension. Most commonly administered orally in combination with acetaminophen.

Drug Guide 15.1 (continued)

Drug	Action	Indication	Nursing Implications
			• Fentanyl: Observe for chest wall rigidity, which can occur with rapid IV infusion. • Oxycodone is the opioid component of Tylox and Percocet.
Mixed opioid agonist–antagonist: pentazocine (Talwin), butorphanol (Stadol), nalbuphine (Nubain)	Pentazocine: antagonist at μ-receptor sites, agonist at kappa-receptor sites. Butorphanol: high affinity for kappa-receptor sites, minimal affinity for sigma-receptor sites. Nalbuphine: partial agonist at kappa-receptor sites, antagonist at mu-receptor sites.	Moderate to severe pain. Relief of migraine headache (butorphanol). Preoperative analgesia (nalbuphine).	• Monitor the child for sedation. Educate child and parents that the drug may make the child sleepy, drowsy, or lightheaded. • Institute safety measures to prevent injury to the child. • Pentazocine, butorphanol: Monitor for diaphoresis, dizziness. Assess for tachycardia and hypertension. • Butorphanol is given intranasally for migraine headaches.

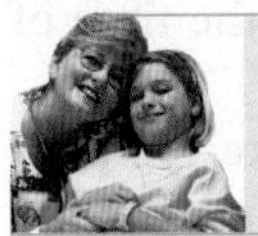

Aspirin should not be used in children for analgesic and antipyretic purposes because of the high risk of Reye's syndrome.

According to the World Health Organization's pain ladder, acetaminophen and NSAIDs are first-line agents for the treatment of pain (WHO, 2006). Although this ladder was developed for the relief of cancer pain, it can be applied to any patient experiencing pain.

Nonopioid agents are typically administered orally or rectally. In some cases, such as with postoperative pain, they may be administered intravenously as a continuous infusion or as bolus doses (Maunuksela & Olkkola, 2003). Administration via intramuscular injection is not recommended because the injection can cause significant pain and the onset of pain relief is not increased.

Adverse effects commonly associated with these agents include gastrointestinal irritation, blood clotting problems, and renal dysfunction. However, research has demonstrated that children experience only mild gastrointestinal upset and negligible effects on a healthy, well-functioning renal system. Blood clotting problems arise primarily when these agents are given perioperatively before primary hemostasis has occurred (Maunuksela & Olkkola, 2003). Nonopioids are relatively safe, have few incompatibilities with other medications, and do not depress the central nervous system. Unfortunately, they exhibit a ceiling effect for analgesia: after a certain level, they do not provide increasing pain relief even when administered at increased doses. As a result, they may be combined with opioids for more effective pain relief.

Opioid Analgesics

Opioid analgesics are typically used for moderate to severe pain. They are classified as either agonists (when they act as the neurotransmitter at the receptor site) or antagonists (when they block the action at the receptor site). Opioid agents that act as agonists include morphine, codeine, fentanyl, meperidine, hydromorphone, oxycodone, and hydrocodone. Opioids that act as mixed agonists–antagonists include pentazocine, butorphanol, and nalbuphine (see Drug Guide 15.1). Opioids can be administered orally, rectally, intramuscularly, or intravenously. In addition, some agents such as fentanyl can be administered transdermally or transmucosally. Morphine is considered the "gold standard" for all opioid agonists; it is the drug to which all other opioids are compared and is usually the drug of choice for severe pain.

Opioid agonists, such as morphine, are associated with numerous adverse effects, resulting primarily from their depressant action on the central nervous system.

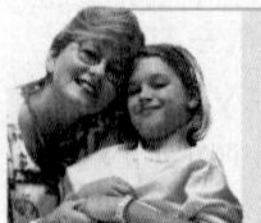

When administering parenteral or epidural opioids, always have naloxone (Narcan) readily available to reverse the opioid's effects should respiratory depression occur.

Opioids stimulate the chemoreceptor trigger zone (CTZ), leading to nausea and vomiting. Moreover, **drug tolerance** (increased dosage required for the same pain relief previously achieved with a lower dose) and **physical dependence** (need for continued administration of the drug to prevent withdrawal symptoms) are commonly noted when opioids are given repeatedly (Yaster et al., 2003). Drug Guide 15.1 gives additional information related to the opioid analgesics.

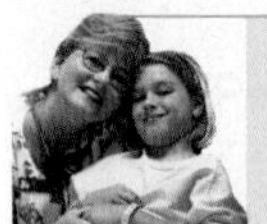

Drug tolerance occurs when increasing doses are required to manage the pain. Physical dependence can occur after as few as 5 days of continuous use of the drug; symptoms of withdrawal begin if it is suddenly stopped. To decrease the risk of withdrawal, the dose can be decreased 10% to 20% per day.

Mixed agonist–antagonists are associated with less respiratory depression than agonists. Unfortunately, like NSAIDs, this group also has a ceiling effect, leading to inadequate effectiveness even with increased dosages. When this occurs, increasing the dosage of the mixed agonist–antagonist or combining it with an agonist provides no additional pain relief.

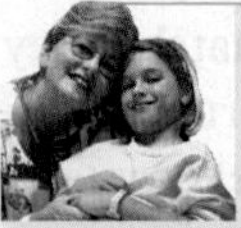

Meperidine, an opioid agonist, is *not* recommended as a first-choice agent for pain relief in children. Meperidine's metabolite, normeperidine, is associated with the development of restlessness, irritability, twitching, agitation, tremors, and most importantly seizures. Normeperidine is a central nervous stimulant and its effects cannot be reversed by an opioid antagonist such as naloxone (American Medical Association, 2006; McCaffrey & Pasero, 1999).

Adjuvant Drugs

Adjuvant drugs are drugs that are used to promote more effective pain relief, either alone or in combination with opioids. These agents are not classified as analgesics. Benzodiazepines, such as diazepam and midazolam, help to relieve anxiety. Midazolam also produces amnesia. Anticonvulsants, such as carbamazepine, and tricyclic antidepressants, such as amitriptyline and nortriptyline, are used to treat neuropathic pain.

Local Anesthetics

Local anesthetics are commonly used to provide analgesia for procedures. They are effective in providing successful pain relief with only minimal risk of systemic adverse effects. However, local anesthetics such as lidocaine historically were not used in children because they need to be injected; the belief was that children feared needles and use of a local anesthetic subjected the child to two needlesticks instead of one. Advances in technology have led to the development of improved methods of delivery such as topical ointments and iontophoresis for administration of local anesthetics, thereby promoting atraumatic care. (For more detailed discussion, see the next section on drug administration methods and later in the chapter on the nurse's role in managing procedure-related pain.)

Drug Administration Methods

With any medication administered for pain management, the timing of administration is vital. Timing depends on the type of pain. For continuous pain, the current recommendation is to administer analgesia around the clock at scheduled intervals to achieve the necessary effect. Scheduled dosing has been associated with decreased pain intensity ratings for children (Paice et al., 2003). As-needed or PRN dosing is not recommended. This method can lead to inadequate pain relief because of the delay before the drug reaches its peak effectiveness, and as a result the child continues to experience pain, possibly necessitating a higher dose of analgesic to achieve relief; this then places the child at risk for overmedication and toxic effects.

For pain that can be predicted or considered temporary, such as with a procedure, analgesia is administered so that the peak action of the drug matches the time of the painful event.

There are various methods for administering pain medications to children. The preferred methods are the oral, rectal, intravenous, topical, or local nerve block routes. Epidural administration and conscious sedation also can be used.

Oral Method

The oral method is often preferred because it is simple, easy, and convenient. The medication may be in the form of a pill, capsule, tablet, syrup, or elixir. Oral administration provides relatively steady blood levels of the drug when administered as a scheduled dose. Effectiveness typically occurs 1 to 2 hours after administration. Higher doses of the medication may be needed to achieve the same effect when switching the child from a parenteral form to an oral form (Hockenberry et al., 2005).

Rectal Method

The rectal method may be used when the child cannot take the medication orally, such as when he or she has difficulty swallowing or is experiencing nausea and vomiting. It is a viable alternative for drug administration. Some analgesics are available in suppository form; for others that are not, the drug can be compounded into a suppository form. The absorption rate varies with rectal administration, and children may find insertion of a suppository uncomfortable and embarrassing.

Intravenous Method

Intravenous analgesia administration is the method of choice in emergency situations and when pain is severe and quick relief is needed. With intravenous administration, the drug usually takes effect within 5 minutes. Intravenous administration can be accomplished with bolus injections or continuous infusions. Continuous infusions may be preferred over bolus doses because steady blood levels are more easily maintained, thereby enhancing the drug's effect in relieving pain. Typically, opioids such as morphine, hydromorphone, and fentanyl are used due to their short half-life and decreased risk for toxicity.

Patient-Controlled Analgesia

In **patient-controlled analgesia (PCA)**, a computerized pump is programmed to deliver an infusion of analgesics via a catheter inserted intravenously, epidurally, or subcutaneously. The analgesic may be given as a continuous infusion, as a continuous infusion supplemented by patient-delivered bolus doses, or as patient-delivered bolus doses only. Typically the child presses a button to administer a bolus dose. The pump has a lockout function that is preset with the dose and time interval: if the child presses the button before the preset time, he or she will not receive an overdose of medication. By delivering small, frequent doses of opioids, the child can experience pain relief without the effects of oversedation. The child also experiences a sense of control over the pain experience.

The child must have the necessary intellect, manual dexterity, and strength to operate the device. This method is usually reserved for use by children 7 years and older, but children as young as 4 years of age have also used this method (Dunbar et al., 1995). With a younger child, a parent or the nurse can press the button.

PCA has been used to control postoperative pain and the pain associated with trauma, cancer, and sickle cell crisis. It can be used in acute care settings or in the home. Most commonly, morphine, hydromorphone, and fentanyl are the drugs used with PCA. The dosage is based on the child's response. Initial bolus doses commonly range from 0.015 to 0.02 mg/kg. Dosages for infusions depend on the child's age, the opioid used, and the type of pain. A commonly used range for morphine infusion to treat postoperative pain ranges from 0.01 to 0.04 mg/kg/hour. Higher dosage ranges have been used to treat the pain associated with sickle cell crisis and cancer (Grandinetti & Buck, 2000).

Local Anesthetic Application

A local anesthetic may sometimes be used to alleviate the pain associated with procedures such as venipuncture, injections, wound repair, lumbar puncture, or accessing of implanted ports. Local anesthesia is a type of regional analgesia that blocks or numbs specific nerves in a region of the body. Medications called local anesthetics include topical forms, such as creams, agents delivered by iontophoresis, and vapocoolants and skin refrigerants, and injectable forms.

Topical Forms

The first choice for the most effective, painless local anesthesia is EMLA (eutectic mixture of local anesthetics [lidocaine and prilocaine]). It achieves anesthesia to a depth of 2 to 4 mm, so it reduces pain of phlebotomy, venous cannulation, and intramuscular injections for up to 24 hours after the injection. However, it requires a 60-minute application time to intact skin using an occlusive dressing for superficial procedures and up to 2 to 3 hours for deeper, more invasive procedures (Box 15.1). Sometimes EMLA

BOX 15.1

APPLYING EMLA

Follow these guidelines when applying EMLA:

- Explain the purpose of the medication to the child and parents, reinforcing that it will help the pain go away.
- Check the scheduled time for the procedure; plan to apply the cream 60 minutes before a superficial procedure such as a heelstick or venipuncture or 2 to 3 hours before a deeper procedure such as a lumbar puncture or bone marrow aspiration.
- Place a thick layer of the cream on the skin at the intended site of the procedure, making sure that the area where the cream is being applied is free of any breaks. Do not rub the cream in once it is applied to the skin.
- Use approximately one third to one half of a 5-g tube for an application.
- Cover the site with a transparent dressing such as Tegaderm or Op-site and secure it so that the dressing is occlusive. Alternatively, use plastic film wrap and tape the edges to secure the dressing.
- Instruct the child not to touch the dressing once it is secured. If necessary, cover the occlusive dressing with a protection device or a loosely applied gauze or elastic bandage.
- After the allotted time, remove the occlusive dressing and wipe the cream from the skin. Inspect the skin for a change in color (blanching or redness), which indicates that the medication has penetrated the skin adequately.
- Verify that sensation is absent by lightly tapping or scratching the area. Use this technique also to demonstrate to the child that the anesthetic is effective. If sensation is present, reapply the cream.
- Prepare the child for the procedure. Assess the child's pain after the procedure to evaluate for pain and to differentiate pain from fear and anxiety.

is not used due to the expense and the time needed to allow the drug to act.

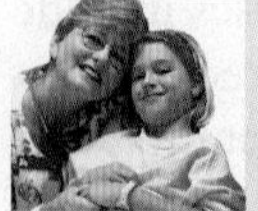

Recommended times for application of EMLA are approximate. Research has shown that children with darker skin may require longer application times (Wong, 2002).

EMLA is available in two forms: a cream and a topical disc. If the disc form is used, an occlusive dressing is not needed. EMLA is approved for use in infants 37 weeks' gestation or older. Maximum dosage and maximum area of application are based on the child's weight. Parents can be taught how to apply the EMLA cream or disc at home in preparation for a procedure (Fig. 15.10).

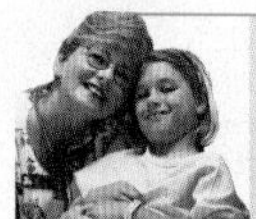

EMLA is contraindicated in children who have congenital or idiopathic methemoglobinemia. It must be used cautiously in those under age 12 months who are receiving methemoglobin-inducing agents, such as sulfonamides, phenytoin, phenobarbital, and acetaminophen. Use of these agents in combination with EMLA increases the child's risk for methemoglobinemia, a condition that could lead to cyanosis and hypoxemia.

TAC (tetracaine, epinephrine, cocaine) and LET (lidocaine, epinephrine, tetracaine) are other examples of topical anesthetics. These are commonly used for lacerations that require suturing. The agent is applied directly to the wound with a cotton ball or swab for 20 to 30 minutes until the area is numb. These methods are not used in patients with known sensitivity to any of these medications.

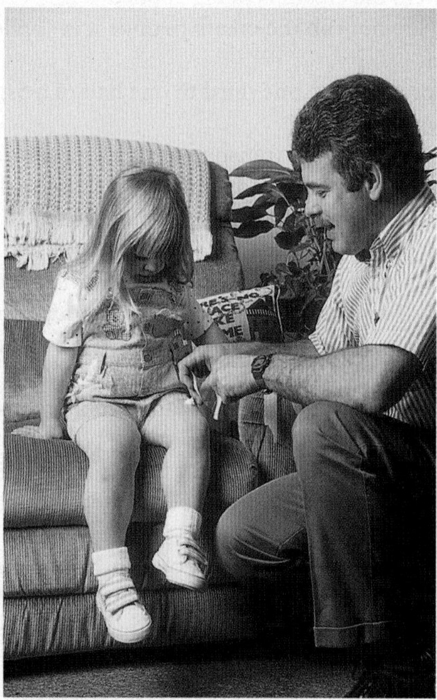

● **Figure 15.10** A parent applies EMLA cream to the child at home in preparation for a procedure.

Researchers have studied LMX4, an over-the-counter topical anesthetic that provides anesthesia to the applied area in 15 to 30 minutes instead of the 60 minutes required by EMLA. The studies showed that an occlusive dressing was not needed when this topical anesthetic was used.

A study published recently in the *Canadian Medical Association Journal* found that a new topical anesthetic containing liposomal lidocaine 4% cream was highly effective in reducing the pain associated with intravenous cannulation. The researchers cited a short onset of action (30 minutes) and minimal vascular effects as benefits. They found that the liposomal encapsulation protects the anesthetic from being metabolized too quickly. Results of this study showed higher intravenous cannulation success rates, less pain, shorter total procedure time, and minor dermal changes among the children (Taddio et al., 2005).

Another choice for local anesthesia is iontophoresis. Iontophoretic lidocaine (Numby Stuff) provides anesthesia to a depth of 8 to 10 mm in approximately 10 minutes and is used over intact skin. A mild electrical current from a small battery-powered generator and two iontophoretic drug-delivery electrodes push drug molecules (lidocaine HCl 2% with epinephrine 1:100,000) into the skin. This type of local anesthesia is not recommended for use in children who have a history of allergy or sensitivity to these drugs; with children who have electrically sensitive equipment such as a pacemaker; or if damaged skin or scar tissue is present. Although children have complained of a tingling or burning sensation from the electric current, recent studies demonstrated this to be a more effective method for pain control than EMLA (Squire et al., 2000).

Vapocoolant spray, another type of local analgesia, can be sprayed onto the skin or administered using a cotton ball soaked in liquid. The depth of anesthesia is not known, but it appears to provide immediate pain control. It is inexpensive and requires no waiting time. The effect lasts for approximately 1 to 2 minutes.

Injectable Forms

Injectable forms of lidocaine or procaine can be administered subcutaneously or intradermally around the procedural area approximately 5 to 10 minutes before the procedure. Common problems with this form of anesthetic include the pain associated with the subcutaneous injection and some burning associated with lidocaine administration, as well as blanching of the skin.

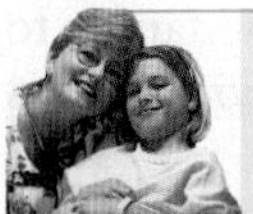

The burning that lidocaine causes on injection may be diminished by buffering lidocaine with sodium bicarbonate, using 10 parts lidocaine and 1 part sodium bicarbonate (1 mL of 1% to 2% lidocaine and 0.1 mL of 8.4% sodium bicarbonate). Then inject 0.1 mL or less of the solution intradermally at the site of venipuncture. Anesthetic action is almost immediate. The solution is stable for only approximately 1 week if not refrigerated.

Epidural Analgesia

For epidural analgesia, a catheter is inserted in the epidural space at L1-2, L3-4, or L4-5. The drug, usually fentanyl or morphine, diffuses into the cerebrospinal fluid and crosses the dura mater to the spinal cord. Then it binds with the opioid receptors located at the dorsal horn. The drugs can be administered as bolus injections (a one-time bolus or on an intermittent schedule), a continuous infusion, or PCA. Usually an opioid, such as morphine, fentanyl, or hydromorphone, is given in conjunction with a long-acting local anesthetic such as bupivacaine.

Epidural analgesia is typically used postoperatively, providing analgesia to the lower body for approximately 12 to 14 hours. The small amount of medication used with this type of analgesia causes less sedation, thereby allowing the child to participate more actively in postoperative care activities. This type of analgesia also is effective for children undergoing upper or lower abdominal surgeries because it controls localized intense pain, somatic pain, and visceral pain.

When epidural analgesia is being administered, additional narcotic analgesics are not given in order to prevent complications such as respiratory depression, pruritus, nausea, vomiting, and urinary retention.

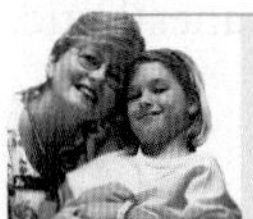

Respiratory depression, although rare when epidural analgesia is used, is always a possibility. When it does occur, it usually occurs gradually over a period of several hours after the medication is initiated. This allows adequate time for early detection and prompt intervention.

Constant assessment is essential because insertion of an epidural catheter and epidural analgesia can lead to infection at the site of the insertion, epidural hematoma, arachnoiditis, neuritis, or spinal headache (rare) due to a cerebrospinal fluid leak. An occlusive dressing is required over the insertion site.

Conscious Sedation

Conscious sedation is a medically controlled state of depressed consciousness that allows protective reflexes to be maintained so the child has the ability to maintain a patent airway and respond to physical or verbal stimulation. This procedure requires adherence to specific protocols as outlined by the Federal Drug Administration Department and Joint Commission on Accreditation of Healthcare Organizations. The depressed state is obtained by using various agents such as morphine, fentanyl, midazolam, or diazepam and other adjuvants such as pentobarbital. Administration of conscious sedation should be atraumatic—that is, by using the oral, topical, or existing intravenous routes (Wong, 2002). Midazolam and fentanyl often are the drugs of choice for conscious sedation because they act quickly, last only a short time, and are available in oral and intravenous formulations (Box 15.2).

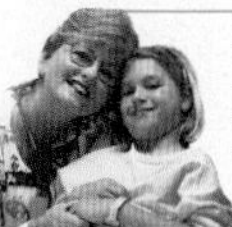

The combination of meperidine (Demerol), promethazine (Phenergan), and chlorpromazine (Thorazine), commonly called DPT, is no longer recommended because it has been shown to cause excessive depression of the central nervous system. In addition, chlorpromazine increases the risk of meperidine toxicity, compounding the risk of severe respiratory depression. Promethazine causes extrapyramidal reactions. The combination also must be administered intramuscularly, which causes the child to experience more pain.

Conscious sedation is used for procedures that are painful and stressful. For example, conscious sedation is suggested instead of restraints, especially for toddlers and preschool children who are undergoing frightening or invasive procedures and who are manifesting extreme

BOX 15.2

ORAL FORMS OF MIDAZOLAM AND FENTANYL

Two of the most commonly used agents for conscious sedation are midazolam and fentanyl. Each of these is available in an oral form, which promotes atraumatic care.

Oral midazolam syrup
- Clear purplish-red cherry-flavored syrup
- Syrup containing 2 mg/mL
- Recommended dosage: 0.25 to 0.5 mg/kg to a maximum dose of 20 mg
- Action usually within 10 to 20 minutes
- Major adverse effects: respiratory depression and arrest

Fentanyl Oralet
- Oral transmucosal formulation
- Candy-type lozenge on a plastic holder
- Available in 200, 300, and 400 mg
- Recommended dose: 5 to 15 mcg/kg
- Not recommended for use in children weighing less than 15 kg
- Onset of action in about 15 minutes of sucking lozenge; duration of action approximately 1 hour

anxiety and behavioral upset (Dresser & Melnyk, 2003). Other indications include situations involving:

- Evidence that the child is experiencing a heightened stress reaction—attempting to flee, crying inconsolably, or flailing
- Verbalization by the child that he or she is frightened and does not want to be touched
- Inability to remain immobilized, such as during laceration repair or computed tomography
- Any procedure that is painful and fear-provoking

Personnel administering conscious sedation must be specially trained, and emergency equipment and medications must be readily available.

The Nurse's Role in Pharmacologic Pain Intervention

The nurse plays a major role in providing pharmacologic pain relief. As with any medication, the nurse is responsible for adhering to the five rights of medication administration: right drug, right dose, right route, right time, and right patient. In addition, the nurse also adheres to three additional rights: the right of the child and parents to be educated; the right of the child to refuse the medication; and the right documentation. The nurse also must have a solid knowledge base about the medications used for pain relief. This knowledge includes information about the drug's pharmacokinetics (absorption, distribution, metabolism, and excretion) and pharmacodynamics (mechanism of action, including adverse effects).

Assessment is crucial when pharmacologic pain interventions are used. An initial assessment of pain provides a baseline from which options for relief can be chosen. Factors that can affect the choice of analgesic, such as the child's age, pain intensity, physiologic status, or previous experiences with pain, also need to be considered. The nurse acts as an advocate for the child and the family to ensure that the most appropriate pharmacologic agent is chosen for the situation.

Assessment is ongoing once the agent is administered. The nurse must monitor physiologic parameters such as level of consciousness, vital signs, oxygen saturation levels, and urinary output for changes that might indicate an adverse reaction to the agent. More intensive monitoring is needed when agents are administered intravenously or epidurally or by conscious sedation. For example, if the child is receiving conscious sedation, interventions include:

- Ensuring that emergency equipment is readily available
- Maintaining a patent airway
- Monitoring the child's level of consciousness and responsiveness
- Assessing the child's vital signs (especially pulse rate, heart rate, blood pressure, and respiratory rate)
- Monitoring oxygen saturation levels

Typically, a specially trained health care provider is specifically designated to perform these activities during the administration of the sedation. Afterwards, the nurse is responsible for ongoing monitoring of the child's status.

Monitor the child closely for evidence of adverse effects. Table 15.8 describes the interventions useful for responding to these adverse effects. Be alert for signs and symptoms of respiratory depression secondary to opioid administration. Have an opioid antagonist such as naloxone (Narcan) and the benzodiazepine antagonist flumazenil (Romazicon) readily available should the child experience respiratory depression.

In addition to assessing physiologic parameters, the nurse must assess the child's and parents' emotional status before and after the agent is administered. For example, increased anxiety and fear may necessitate a change in method of administration, such as topical application instead of an intradermal injection of a local anesthetic.

Table 15.8 Interventions for Common Opioid-Induced Adverse Effects

Adverse Effect	Nursing Interventions
Constipation	Encourage fluid intake unless contraindicated. Ensure intake of high-fiber foods, including fruits, if allowed. Encourage activity, including ambulation if possible. Obtain order for stool softener. Administer laxative as ordered.
Pruritus	Apply cool compresses and lotions. Administer antihistamine as ordered.
Nausea and vomiting	Inform child and parents that these symptoms usually subside in 1 to 2 days. Encourage small frequent meals with bland foods. Administer antiemetic if ordered.

Nonpharmacologic methods may be employed to help lessen anxiety, thereby promoting more effective relief from the drug.

Nurses also are responsible for ensuring that the child and parents are adequately prepared for the use of the pharmacologic agent. The nurse educates the child and parents about the drug, why it is being used, its intended effects, and possible adverse effects, tailoring the teaching to the child's cognitive level. Provide opportunities for the child and parents to ask questions, offering support and guidance throughout the experience. Provide a demonstration or use visual aids so that the child and parents know exactly what to expect. Encourage the use of play to help the child express fears and anxieties related to the administration.

Management of Procedure-Related Pain

One of the most common causes of pain in children is procedure-related pain. The procedure may be minor, such as an intramuscular injection, heelstick, or venipuncture, or it may be more involved, such as lumbar puncture, bone marrow aspiration, or wound care. Regardless, pain is real for children and painful procedures are often extremely distressing to them. Variables that affect pain include the intensity or length of the procedure and the skill of the health care provider performing the procedure.

The Nurse's Role in Managing Procedure-Related Pain

Through the use of behavioral and pharmacologic approaches, nurses can significantly reduce the pain and distress of procedures. The guiding principle is the provision of atraumatic care to the child, which includes the following:

- Using topical EMLA, iontophoretic lidocaine, vapocoolant spray, or buffered lidocaine at the intended site of a skin or vessel puncture
- Incorporating the use of nonpharmacologic strategies for pain relief in conjunction with pharmacologic methods
- Preparing the child and parents ahead of time about the procedure and then keeping all equipment out of site until it is ready to be used
- Using therapeutic hugging (see Chapter 11) to secure the child
- Using the smallest-gauge needle possible or an automated lancet device to puncture the skin
- Using an intermittent infusion device or peripherally inserted central catheter (PICC) if multiple or repeated blood samples are necessary; coordinating care so that several tests can be performed from one sample if possible
- Opting for venipuncture in newborns instead of heelsticks if the amount of blood needed would require much squeezing
- Using kangaroo care (skin-to-skin contact) for newborns before and after heelstick
- Providing nonnutritive sucking with sucrose solution for newborns several minutes before the procedure (Wong, 2002)

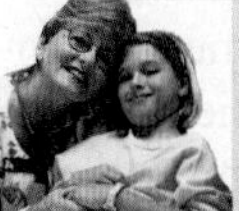

Individualize interventions based on the painfulness of the procedure and the child's developmental age and personality. Use behavioral-cognitive approaches and pharmacologic interventions. For example, encouraging the school-age child to assist during painful procedures in age-appropriate ways may actually help ease some of the pain related to a heightened state of anxiety, or at least assist the child in coping with the situation. Always use appropriate pharmacologic treatment for the first procedure to provide a painless experience for the child.

Nursing care for the child with procedure-related pain includes the child as well as the parents. Be sure to prepare them for the procedure using an appropriate developmental approach. Promote environmental comfort, too. Ensure that the child's privacy is maintained and that the lighting is adequate for the procedure but not so bright as to cause the child discomfort.

Some controversy exists as to whether all procedures should be performed in a treatment room. Research findings suggest that taking a child to a treatment room may be neither feasible nor desirable in all situations and for all procedures. Attention needs to be directed toward the individual needs of the child, the demands of the procedure, and the situational conditions to facilitate the best outcome (Fanurik et al., 2000). The ultimate goal is to do whatever is best for the child.

Unless contraindicated, encourage the parents to be present before, during, and after the procedure to provide comforting support to the child. Also encourage the child and parents to use nonpharmacologic methods to help maximize pain relief and reduce anxiety. For example, nonpharmacologic methods that are helpful for the toddler and preschooler may include positioning the child on the lap and hugging the child, distracting the child with toys or interactive books, and blowing bubbles.

Play therapy can be useful when preparing children for painful procedures. Encourage children to make decisions about their care related to pain management if their condition or procedure allows. It is also helpful to anticipate and recognize painful situations and provide pain medication before the actual procedure to ensure comfort. Many nonpharmacologic strategies can be enhanced and better implemented with the help of the child life specialist or play therapist, who have specialized training in these techniques.

Recall Aiden from the beginning of the chapter. What are some interventions that may be helpful prior to, during, and after his dressing change?

Management of Chronic Pain

Typically, pain in children is acute pain, but chronic pain is a significant problem in the pediatric population, affecting approximately 15% to 20% of children (American Pain Society, 2000). Historically, chronic pain was defined by the duration of the pain, such as longer than 3 to 6 months. However, research has identified elements associated with chronic pain as occurring much earlier in time. Currently, chronic pain is identified as the interplay of biologic, psychological, social, and cultural factors addressed within a developmental framework (American Pain Society, 2000). According to the American Pain Society, children with chronic pain and their families experience significant emotional and social consequences from the pain and disability; also, the experience of chronic pain in childhood may predispose the individual to chronic pain in adulthood.

The Nurse's Role in Managing Chronic Pain

The nurse's role in managing chronic pain in children is similar to that for the child experiencing acute pain or procedure-related pain. Assessment of the child's pain is key and should include a history of the present problem. Questions should focus on the onset of the pain, its intensity, duration, and location, and any factors that alleviate or exacerbate it. In addition, the nurse needs to question the child and parents about the impact of the pain on the child's daily life, such as sleep, play, eating, school, and interactions with peers, other family members, and friends. Impact on the family's life also is addressed.

Another key area of assessment is determining how the pain affects the child's and family's level of stress. Areas to address include the child's and parents' feelings of hopelessness, anxiety, and depression. Also question the child and parents about what they think has caused the pain and how they have coped with it. In addition, ascertain what methods the child and parents have used to alleviate the pain and the success of these methods. Inquire about any home remedies or alternative therapies that may have been used.

Review past physical examination findings for clues to the underlying problem. Observe the child's overall appearance, gait, and posture. Assess the child's cognitive level and emotional response, especially related to the experience of pain. Expect to complete a neurologic examination and observe for muscle spasms, trigger points, and increased sensitivity to light touch. Abnormal body postures assumed by the child due to chronic pain may result in the development of secondary pain in the muscles and fascia. When children tense their muscles due to fear of examination, somatic pain may occur.

Various nonpharmacologic and pharmacologic strategies are used to manage chronic pain. Often multiple strategies are combined to address pain relief as well as the pain's impact on other areas, such as sleep or school functioning. When pharmacologic agents are used, the oral form is the method of choice. As with any pain management strategy, education of the child and family is paramount. A referral to a pediatric pain specialist may be needed if the child's pain is not controlled effectively.

References

Books and Journals

Algren, C. (2005). Family-centered care of the child during illness and hospitalization. In M. Hockenberry, *Wong's essentials of pediatric nursing* (7th ed., pp. 637–705). Philadelphia: Elsevier/Mosby.

American Academy of Pediatrics and American Pain Society (2001). The assessment and management of acute pain in infants, children, and adolescents. *Pediatrics, 108*(3), 793–797.

American Academy of Pediatrics and American Pain Society. (2001). Policy statement: The assessment and management of acute pain in infants, children, and adolescents (0793). *Pediatrics, 105,* 454–461.

American Academy of Pediatrics and Canadian Paediatric Society. (2000). Prevention and management of pain and stress in the neonate. *Pediatrics, 105*(2), 454–461.

American Medical Association. (2006). *AMA pain management: Pediatric pain management (continuing medical education).* Retrieved 9/5/06 from http://www.ama-cmeonline.com/pain_mgmt/module06/01cme/02_01.htm.

American Pain Society (1995). *Pain: The fifth vital sign.* Los Angeles: American Pain Society.

American Pain Society (2000). *Pediatric chronic pain. A position statement.* Available at: http://www.ampainsoc.org/advocacy/pediatric.htm. Accessed 6/6/2006.

American Pain Society (2006). *Pain: Current understanding of assessment, management, and treatments.* APS/National Pharmaceutical Council. Available at http://www.ampainsoc.org/ce/enduring.htm. Accessed 7/6/06.

Baker, C. M. & Wong, D. L. (1987). Q.U.E.S.T.: A process of pain assessment in children. *Orthopaedic Nursing, 6*(1), 11–21.

Beal, J. A. (2005). Evidence for best practices in the neonatal period. *MCN, 30*(6), 397–403.

Behrman, R. E., & Kliegman, R. M. (1998). *Nelson's essentials of pediatrics* (pp. 36–37, 419–420). Philadelphia: W. B. Saunders.

Berde, C. B., & Sethna, N. F. (2002). Analgesics for the treatment of pain in children. *New England Journal of Medicine, 347,* 1094–1103.

Blass, E. M., & Watt, L. B. (1999). Suckling and sucrose-induced analgesia in human newborns. *Pain, 83,* 611–623.

Bo, L. K., & Callaghan, P. (2000). Soothing pain-elicited distress in Chinese neonates. *Pediatrics, 105*(4), e49.

Boelen-van der Loo, W. J. C., Scheffer, E., de Haan, R. J., & de Groot, C. J. (1999). Clinimetric evaluation of the pain observation scale for young children in children aged between 1 and 4 years after ear, nose, and throat surgery. *Developmental and Behavioral Pediatrics, 20*(4), 222–227.

Brennan-Hunter, A. L. (2001). Children's pain: A mandate for change. *Pain, 6,* 29–39.

Broome, M. E., & Huth, M. M. (2003). Nursing management of the child in pain. In N. L. Schecter, C. B. Berde, & M. Yaster, *Pain in infants, children, and adolescents* (2d ed., pp. 417–433). Philadelphia: Lippincott Williams & Wilkins.

Bursch, B. (2000). Pain in infants, children, and adolescents SIG: Policy statement on pediatric chronic pain. *APS Bulletin 10*(3), May/June. Available at: http://www.ampainsoc.org/pub/bulletin/ma00/sig1.htm. Accessed 8/2/06.

Byers, J. F., & Thornley, K. (2004). Cueing in to infant pain. *MCN, 29*(2), 84–91.

Carbajal, R., Chauvet, X., Couderc, S., & Oliver-Martin, M. (1999). Randomized trial of analgesic effects of sucrose, glucose, and pacifiers in term neonates. *British Medical Journal, 319,* 1393–1397.

Crandall, M., & Savedra, M. (2005). Multidimensional assessment using the adolescent pediatric pain tool: A case report. *Journal for Specialists in Pediatric Nursing, 10*(3), 115–123.

De Rond, M. E, de Wit, R., van Dam, F. S., & Muller, M. J. (2000). A pain management program for nurses: Effects on communication, assessment and documentation of patients' pain. *Journal of Pain and Symptom Management, 20,* 424–439.

Dresser, S., & Melnyk, B. M. (2003). The effectiveness of conscious sedation on anxiety, pain, and procedural complications in young children. *Pediatric Nursing, 29*(4), 320–332.

Dunbar, P. J., Buckley, P., Gavrin, J. R., Sanders, J. E., & Chapman, C. R. (1995). Use of patient-controlled analgesia for pain control for children receiving bone marrow transplant. *Journal of Pain and Symptom Management, 10,* 604–611.

Fanurik, D., et al. (2000). Hospital room or treatment room: Where should inpatient pediatric procedures be performed? *Children's Health Care, 29*(2), 103–111.

Fitzgerald, M., & Beggs, S. (2001). The neurobiology of pain: Developmental aspects. *Neuroscientist, 7,* 246–257.

Fratianne, R. B., Prensner, J. D., Huston, M. J., Super, D. M., Yowler, C. J., & Standley, J. M. (2001). The effect of music-based imagery and musical alternate engagement on the burn debridement process. *Journal of Burn Care & Rehabilitation, 22*(1), 47–53.

Grandinetti, C. A., & Buck, M. L. (2000). Patient-controlled analgesia: Guidelines for use in children. *Pediatric Pharmacotherapy, 6*(11). Available at: http://www.medscape.com/viewarticle/410909. Accessed 8/2/06.

Guinsburg, R., Peres, C. A., Almeida, M. F., Balda, R. C., Berenguel, R. C., Tonelotto, J., & Kopelman, B. I. (2000). Differences in pain expression between male and female newborn infants. *Pain, 85,* 127–133.

Hockenberry, M. J., Wilson, D., & Winkelstein, M. L. (2005). *Wong's essentials of pediatric nursing* (7th ed., p. 1259). St. Louis: Mosby.

Howard, R. F. (2003). Current status of pain management in children. *JAMA, 290,* 2464–2469.

International Association for the Study of Pain. (2007). *IASP pain terminology.* Retrieved April 4, 2007 from http://www.iasp-pain.org/AM/Template.cfm?Section=General_Resource_Links&Template=/CM/HTMLDisplay.cfm&ContentID=3058#Pain.

Isek, U., Ozek, E., Bilgen, H., & Ceveci, D. (2000). Comparison of oral glucose and sucrose solutions on pain response in neonates. *Journal of Pain, 1,* 275–278.

Johnston, C. C., Stevens, B. J., Boyer, K., & Porter, F. L. (2003). Development of psychologic responses to pain and assessment of pain in infants and toddlers. In N. L. Schecter, C. B. Berde, & M. Yaster, *Pain in infants, children, and adolescents* (2d ed., pp. 105–127). Philadelphia: Lippincott Williams & Wilkins.

Kaufman, G., Cimo, S., Miller, L., & Blass, E. (2002). An evaluation of the effects of sucrose on neonatal pain with two commonly used circumcision methods. *American Journal of Obstetrics and Gynecology, 186,* 564–568.

Krechel, S. W., & Bildner, J. (1995). CRIES: A new neonatal postoperative pain measurement score. Initial testing of validity and reliability. *Paediatric Anaesthesia, 5,* 53–61.

Lawrence, J., Alcock, D., McGrath, P., Kay, J., MacMurray, S. B., & Dulberg, C. (1993). The development of a tool to assess neonatal pain. *Neonatal Network, 12*(6), 59–66.

Lehr, V. T., & BeVier, P. (2003). Patient-controlled analgesia for the pediatric patient. *Orthopaedic Nursing, 22*(4), 298–304.

Manworren, R. C. B., & Hynan, L. S. (2003). Clinical validation of FLACC: Preverbal patient pain scale. *Pediatric Nursing, 29*(2).

Maunuksela, E., & Olkkola, K. T. (2003). Nonsteroidal anti-inflammatory drugs in pediatric pain management. In N. L. Schecter, C. B. Berde, & M. Yaster, *Pain in infants, children, and adolescents* (2d ed., pp. 171–180). Philadelphia: Lippincott Williams & Wilkins.

McCaffery, M., & Pasero, C. (1999). *Pain: a clinical manual* (2d ed.). St. Louis: Mosby.

McCarthy, A. M., & Kleiber, C. (2006). A conceptual model of factors influencing children's responses to a painful procedure when parents are distraction coaches. *Journal of Pediatric Nursing, 21*(2), 88–98.

McGrath, P. A., & Hillier, L. M. (2003). Modifying the psychologic factors that intensify children's pain and prolong disability. In N. L. Schecter, C. B. Berde, & M. Yaster, *Pain in infants, children, and adolescents* (2d ed., pp. 85–104). Philadelphia: Lippincott Williams & Wilkins.

Merkel, S., Voepel-Lewis, T., & Malviya, S. (2002). Pain assessment in infants and young children: The FLACC scale. *American Journal of Nursing, 102*(10), 54–56, 58.

Merkel, S. I., Voepel-Lewis, T., Shayevitz, J. R., & Malviya, S. (1997). The FLACC: A behavioral scale for scoring postoperative pain in young children. *Pediatric Nursing, 23*(3), 293–297.

Morash, D., & Fowler, K. (2004). An evidence-based approach to changing practice: Using sucrose for infant analgesia. *Journal of Pediatric Nursing, 19*(5), 366–370.

National Association of Neonatal Nurses. (1999). *Position statement #3019: Pain management in infants.* Retrieved 9/1/06 from http://www.nann.org/i4a/pages/index.cfm?pageid=79

National Library of Medicine. (2006). Table 2, pain assessment tools, the word-graphic rating scale. In *Health services/technology assessment text.* Retrieved 9/10/06 from http://www.ncbi.nlm.nih.gov/books/bv.fcgi?rid=hstat6.section.32536.

Oberlander, T. F. (2001). Pain assessment and management in infants and young children with developmental disabilities. *Infants and Young Children, 14*(2), 33–47.

Paice, J. A., Noskin, G. A., Vanagunas, A., & Shott, S. (2003). Efficacy and safety of scheduled dosing of opioid analgesic: A quality improvement study. *Journal of Pain, 6*(10), 639–643.

Palermo, T. M. & Kiska, R. (2005). Subjective sleep disturbances in adolescents with chronic pain: Relationship to daily functioning and quality of life. *Journal of Pain, 6*(3), 201–207.

Porth, C. M. (2004). *Pathophysiology: concepts of altered health states* (7th ed.). Philadelphia: Lippincott Williams & Wilkins.

Puchalski, M., & Hummel, P. (2002). The reality of neonatal pain. *Advances in Neonatal Care, 2,* 233–244.

Razmus, I. S., Daltom, M. E., & Wilson, D. (2004). Pain management for newborn circumcision. *Pediatric Nursing, 30*(5), 414–417, 427.

Schade, J. G., Joyce, B. A., Gerkensmeyer, J., & Keck, J. F. (1996). Comparison of three preverbal scales for postoperative pain assessment in a diverse pediatric sample. *Journal of Pain and Symptom Management, 12*(6), 348–359.

Spagrud, L. J., Piira, T., & von Baeyer, C. L. (2003). Children's self-report of pain intensity. *American Journal of Nursing, 103*(12), 62–64.

Squire, S. J., Kirchhoff, K. T., & Hissong, K. (2000). Comparing two methods of topical anesthesia used before intravenous cannulation in pediatric patients. *Journal of Pediatric Health Care, 14,* 68–72.

Taddio, A. (2001). Pain management for neonatal circumcision. *Pediatric Drugs, 3,* 101–111.

Taddio, A., et al. (1997). Efficacy and safety of EMLA use for pain during circumcision. *New England Journal of Medicine, 336*(17), 1197–1201.

Taddio, A., Soin, H. K., Schuh, S., Koren, G., & Scolnik, D. (2005). Liposomal lidocaine to improve procedural success rates and reduce procedural pain among children: A randomized controlled trial. *Canadian Medical Association Journal, 172*(13), 1691–1695.

Taketokmo, C. K., Hodding, J. H., & Kraus, D. M. (2005). *Lexi-comp's pediatric dosage handbook* (12th ed.). Hudson, OH: Lexi-comp.

Tesler, M. D., Savedra, M. C., Holzemer, W. L., Wilkie, D. J., Ward, J. A., & Paul, S. M. (1991). The word-graphic rating scale as a measure of children's and adolescent's pain intensity. *Research in Nursing and Health, 14*(5), 361–361.

VanHulle, V. C. (2005). Nurses' knowledge, attitudes, & practices regarding children's pain. *American Journal of Maternal Child Nursing, 30,* 177–183.

von Baeyer, C. L., Marche, T. A., Rocha, E. M., & Salmon, K. (2004). Children's memory for pain: Overview and implications for practice. *Journal of Pain, 5*(5), 241–249.

Willis, M. H. W., Merkel, S. I., Voepel-Lewis, T., & Malviya, S. (2002). FLACC behavioral pain assessment scale: A comparison with the child's self-report. *Pediatric Nursing, 29*(3), 195–198.

Wong, D. (2002). *Wong on web paper: Guidelines for atraumatic skin/vessel punctures.* Available at: http://www.mosbydrugconsult.com/WOW/op022aa.html. Accessed 7/9/2006.

Wong, D. (2002). *Wong on web paper: Pediatric conscious sedation.* Available at: http://www.mosbydrugconsult.com/WOW/op042.html. Accessed 7/22/2006.

World Health Organization (2006). WHO's pain ladder. Available at: http://www.who.int/cancer/palliative/painladder/en/. Accessed 7/23/06.

Yaster, M., Kost-Byerly, S., & Maxwell, L. G. (2003). Opioid agonists and antagonists. In N. L. Schecter, C. B. Berde, & M. Yaster, *Pain in infants, children, and adolescents* (2d ed., pp. 181–224). Philadelphia: Lippincott Williams & Wilkins.

Websites

www.ahrq.gov/clinic/ Agency for Healthcare Research and Quality
www.aap.org American Academy of Pediatrics
www.painfoundation.org American Pain Foundation
www.ampainsoc.org American Pain Society
www.canadianpainsociety.ca Canadian Pain Society
www.chionline.org Children's Hospice International
http://www.mayday.coh.org City of Hope Pain/Palliative Care Resource Center
www.iasp-pain.org International Association for the Study of Pain (IASP)
www.kidshealth.org Kids Health
www.napnap.org National Association of Pediatric Nurse Associates and Practitioners
www.childrenshospitals.net National Association of Children's Hospitals and Related Institutions
www.pedsnurses.org Society of Pediatric Nurses
www.virtualpediatrichospital.org Virtual Pediatric Hospital
www.nann.org National Association of Neonatal Nurses

Chapter WORKSHEET

MULTIPLE CHOICE QUESTIONS

1. The nurse is preparing to assess the pain of a 3-year-old child who had surgery the day before. Which pain rating scale would be most appropriate for the nurse to use?
   a. FACES Pain Rating Scale
   b. Poker chip tool
   c. Word-graphic rating scale
   d. Visual analog scale
2. When developing the plan of care for a child in pain, the nurse identifies appropriate strategies aimed at modifying which factors influencing pain?
   a. Gender
   b. Cognitive level
   c. Previous pain experiences
   d. Anticipatory anxiety
3. An adolescent who is a competitive swimmer comes to the emergency department complaining of localized aching pain in his shoulder. He states, "I've been practicing really hard and long to get myself ready for my meet this weekend." The area is tender to the touch. The nurse determines that the adolescent is most likely experiencing which type of pain?
   a. Cutaneous pain
   b. Deep somatic pain
   c. Visceral pain
   d. Neuropathic pain
4. After teaching a child's parents about the different methods of distraction that can be used for pain management, which statement by the parents indicates a need for additional teaching?
   a. "We'll have her focus on her hand and count each finger slowly."
   b. "We'll read some of her favorite stories to her."
   c. "We'll have her imagine that she's at the beach this summer."
   d. "She likes to play video games, so we'll bring in some from home."
5. A child is scheduled for a bone marrow aspiration at 4 p.m. The nurse would plan to apply EMLA cream to the intended site at which time?
   a. 1:30 p.m.
   b. 3:00 p.m.
   c. 3:30 p.m.
   d. 4:00 p.m.

CRITICAL THINKING EXERCISES

1. The nurse asks a 12-year-old girl if she is having pain. She denies pain, even though she is lying on her left side holding her abdomen with her knees flexed up to it. What might be some underlying factors leading the child to deny her pain? How would the nurse go about assessing this child's pain?
2. The nurse comes into the room of a 6-year-old who is sleeping. His mother states, "He's asleep, so he's not in pain." How should the nurse respond?
3. A child who is receiving ibuprofen is experiencing increased pain. The dosage of ibuprofen is increased but is no longer effective in providing adequate pain relief. What is occurring? What would be most likely to happen next?

STUDY ACTIVITIES

1. Interview nurses who work on a pediatric unit about their experiences with managing pain in children. Ask them how they assess pain in children and the major methods they use to assist the children in managing their pain.
2. Interview families of children with chronic illnesses who deal with pain. Ask the parents how they assess their children's pain level and what methods they have used in assisting their children in managing pain.
3. Compare and contrast the drugs fentanyl and midazolam when used for conscious sedation in terms of onset of action, duration, primary effects, and antidotes.
4. A child is receiving epidural analgesia with morphine. The nurse would be alert for which of the following adverse effects? Select all that apply.
   _____ a. Respiratory depression
   _____ b. Pruritus
   _____ c. Constipation
   _____ d. Vomiting
   _____ e. Amnesia
   _____ f. Hematoma

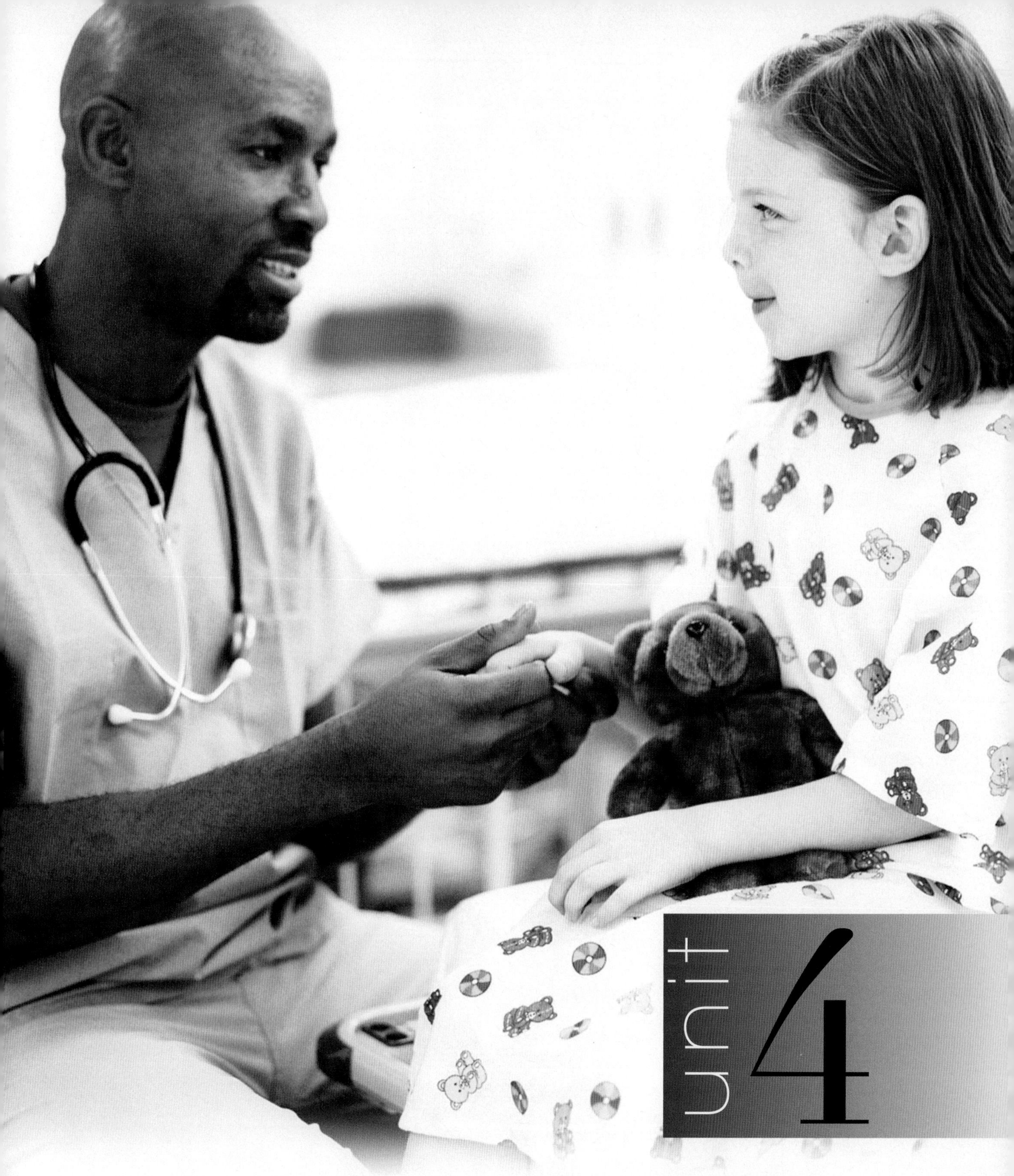

Nursing Care of the Child With a Health Disorder

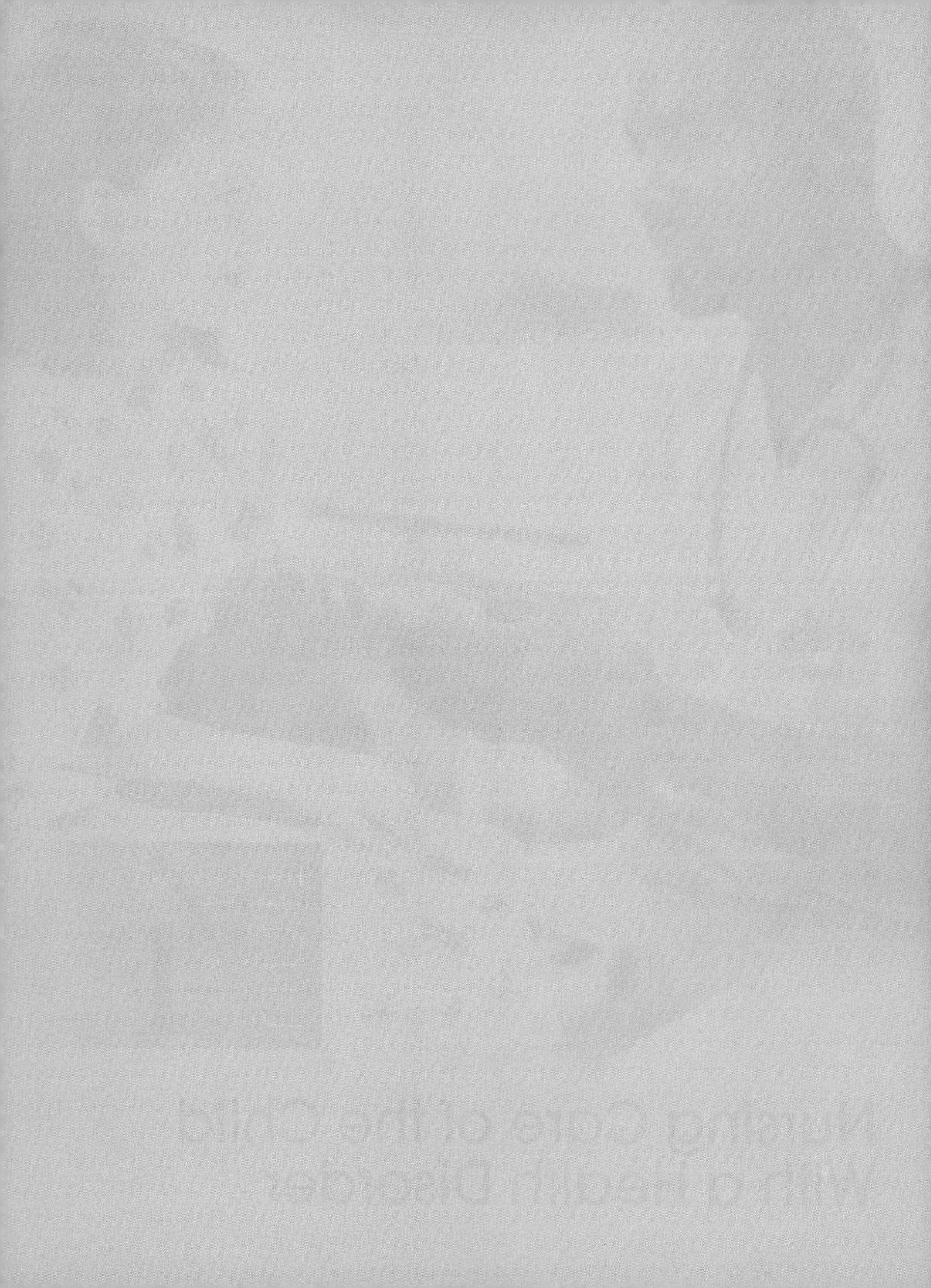

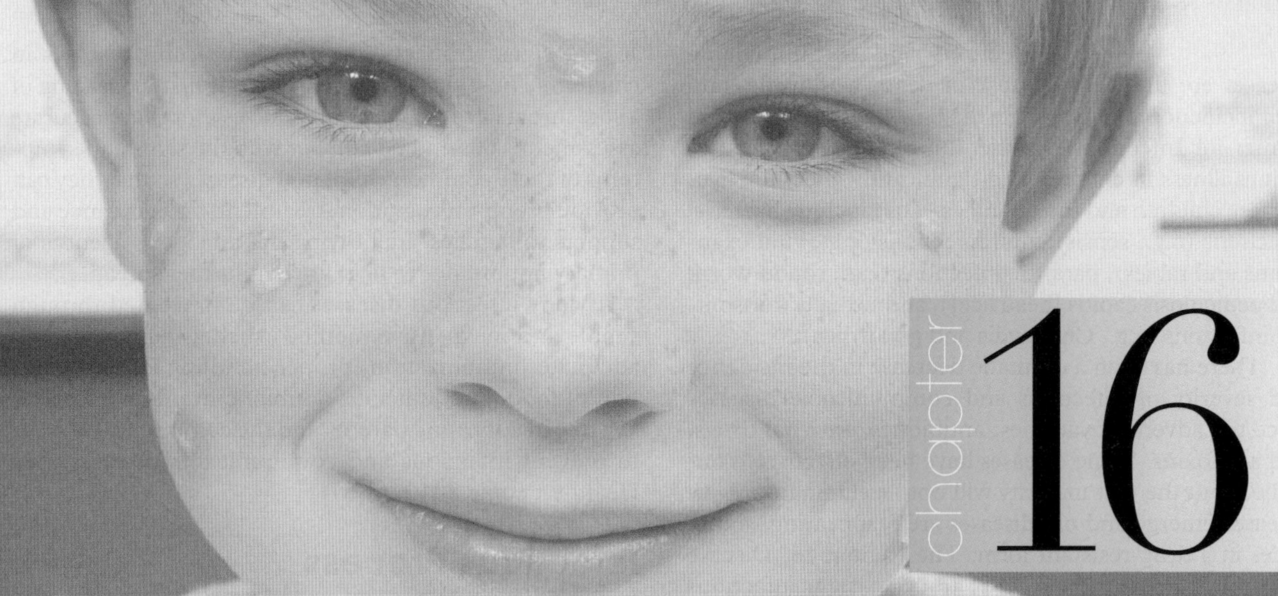

chapter 16

Nursing Care of the Child With an Infectious or Communicable Disorder

Key TERMS

antigen
antibody
chain of infection
communicability
endogenous pyrogens
exanthem
fomites
pathogen
phagocytosis

Learning OBJECTIVES

Upon completion of the chapter, the learner will be able to:

1. Discuss anatomic and physiologic differences in children versus adults in relation to the infectious process.
2. Identify nursing interventions related to common laboratory and diagnostic tests used in the diagnosis and management of infectious conditions.
3. Identify appropriate nursing assessments and interventions related to medications and treatments for childhood infectious and communicable disorders.
4. Distinguish various infectious illnesses occurring in childhood.
5. Devise an individualized nursing care plan for the child with an infectious or communicable disorder.
6. Develop patient/family teaching plans for the child with an infectious or communicable disorder.

WOW *Complete and lasting freedom from infectious disease remains a dream, but one worth fighting a hard battle for.*

Samuel Goldberg, 3 months old, is brought to the clinic by his mother. He presents with a history of fever and nasal congestion. His mother states, "He's been very irritable and crying more than usual."

Infectious and communicable diseases are the leading cause of death worldwide, and their incidence is increasing in the United States (National Center for Infectious Disease, 2003). They can lead to serious illness in children and significantly affect the lives of these children and their families. They include bacterial infections (e.g., sepsis), viral infections (e.g., viral exanthems and rabies), parasitic infections (e.g., round worm and pediculosis capitis [head lice]), and sexually transmitted infections (e.g., Chlamydia and gonorrhea).

There has been a dramatic decrease in the incidence and severity of infections and communicable diseases since the advent of vaccines, antibiotics, antiviral drugs, and antitoxins. Some diseases have been effectively controlled, but the vast majority will not be eliminated. New diseases emerge and old diseases are reappearing, sometimes in a drug-resistant form. The Centers for Disease Control & Prevention (CDC) tracks certain infectious diseases. This list of nationally reportable diseases is revised periodically to add new pathogens or remove diseases as their incidence declines. Reporting by the states to the CDC is voluntary, so slight variations exist from state to state. Box 16.1 lists nationally reportable diseases.

Nurses, particularly those working in schools, childcare centers, and outpatient settings, are often the first to see the signs of infectious or communicable diseases in children. These signs are often vague at first, consisting of a sore throat or rash. Therefore, nurses must have accurate assessment skills and be familiar with the signs and symptoms of these common childhood diseases so that they can provide prompt recognition, treatment, and guidance and support to families. Identifying the infectious agent is of primary importance to help prevent further spread.

Many infectious diseases can be prevented through simple and inexpensive methods such as hand washing, adequate immunization, proper handling and preparation of food, and judicious antibiotic use. Nurses play a key role in educating parents and the community on ways to prevent infectious and communicable diseases. See Healthy People 2010.

Infectious Process

Infection occurs when an organism enters the body and multiplies, causing damage to the tissues and cells. The body's response to this damage due to infection or injury is inflammation. The body delivers fluid, blood, and nutri-

HEALTHY PEOPLE 2010

Objective	Significance
Reduce or eliminate indigenous cases of vaccine-preventable diseases. Congenital rubella syndrome (children under age 1 year); diphtheria (persons under age 35 years); *Haemophilus influenzae* type b (children under age 5 years); hepatitis B (persons aged 2 to 18 years); measles (persons of all ages); mumps (persons of all ages); pertussis (children under age 7 years); polio (wild-type virus) (persons of all ages); rubella (persons of all ages); tetanus (persons under age 35); varicella (persons under age 18).	• Educate children and their families on the importance of proper immunizations. • Assess immunization status at every healthy encounter. • Provide families with a written record of immunizations given.
Achieve and maintain effective vaccination coverage levels for universally recommended vaccines among young children	

BOX 16.1

LIST OF NATIONALLY NOTIFIABLE DISEASES

- Chlamydia
- Diphtheria
- Ehrlichiosis
- Gonorrhea
- Lyme disease
- Malaria
- Measles
- Mumps
- Pertussis
- Poliomyelitis, paralytic
- Q fever
- Rabies
- Rocky Mountain spotted fever
- Rubella
- Streptococcal disease, invasive group A
- Syphilis
- Tetanus
- Varicella (morbidity)
- Varicella (deaths only)

For a complete list of nationally notifiable diseases in the United States, go to www.cdc.gov/epo/dphsi/phs/infdis.htm.

Obtained from the CDC at www.cdc.gov/epo/dphsi/phs/infdis.htm

ents to the area of infection or injury and attempts to eliminate the pathogens and help repair the tissues. The body does this through vascular and cellular reactions. The vascular response is an initial period of vasoconstriction followed by vasodilatation. This vasodilatation allows for the increase of fluids, blood, and nutrients to the area.

The cellular response involves the arrival of white blood cells to the area. White blood cells are the body's defense against infection or injury. The types of white blood cells are neutrophils, lymphocytes, basophils, eosinophils, and monocytes. Elevations in certain portions of the white blood cell count reflect different processes occurring in the body, such as infection, allergic reaction, or leukemia. Table 16.1 gives further explanation of the function of each type of white blood cells. Each type is generally present in a balanced state; the types are reported as a percentage of the total white blood cell count or as the number per certain volume of blood.

The white blood cells use **phagocytosis** to ingest and destroy the **pathogen.** If bacteria escape the action of phagocytosis, they enter the bloodstream and lymph system and the immune system is activated. With activation of the immune system, B lymphocytes (humoral immunity) and T lymphocytes (cell-mediated immunity) are matured and activated. B and T cells recognize and attack infectious pathogens. B cells, which mature in the bone marrow, produce specific antibodies to a specific offending **antigen** (a substance that the body recognizes as foreign). T cells, which mature in the thymus, attack the antigen directly. Once B and T cells have been exposed to an antigen, some cells will remember the antigen: thus, if the particular antigen invades again, the body will act faster.

Infection or inflammation caused by bacteria, viruses, or other pathogens stimulates the release of **endogenous pyrogens** (interleukins, tumor necrosis factor, and interferon) and results in fever. The pyrogens act on the hypothalamus, where they trigger prostaglandin production and increase the body's temperature set point. This triggers the cold response, resulting in shivering, vasoconstriction, and a decrease in peripheral perfusion to help decrease heat loss and allow the body's temperature to rise to the new set point. Fever, defined as a temperature greater than 38° C (100.4° F), then occurs. Box 16.2 gives specific parameters for fever based on the measurement route.

Antipyretics are often used to lower fever and increase the comfort of the patient. They decrease the temperature set point by inhibiting the production of prostaglandins, leading to sweating and vasodilation and therefore heat loss and a drop in temperature.

It is important to distinguish between fever and hyperthermia. Hyperthermia occurs when normal thermoregulation fails, resulting in an unregulated rise in core temperature. Hyperthermia may occur if the central nervous system of the child becomes impaired by disease, drugs, and abnormalities of heat production or thermal stressors, such as being left in a hot automobile or exertional heat stroke. In the absence of hyperthermia and in the normally neurologic child, the body does not allow fever to rise to lethal levels. The body actually produces a natural antipyretic, called cryogen. If there is no hyperthermic insult, it is rare to see a child's temperature rise to greater than 41.4° C (106° F) (Crocetti & Serwint, 2005).

Table 16.1 Function of White Blood Cells by Leukocyte Type

Cell	Cell's Function Is to Combat
Neutrophils (bands and segs)	Pyogenic infection (bacterial)
Eosinophils	Allergic disorders and parasitic infestations
Basophils	Parasitic infections, some allergic disorders
Lymphocytes	Viral infections (measles, rubella, chickenpox, infectious mononucleosis)
Monocytes	Severe infections, by phagocytosis

(Fischbach, 2004; adapted from p. 51)

Stages of Infectious Disease

Infectious diseases follow a similar pattern. They progress through certain stages (Table 16.2) in which **communicability** (ability to spread to others) can be predicted. It is important for nurses to understand these stages to help control and manage infectious diseases.

Chain of Infection

The **chain of infection** is the process by which an organism is spread. Behaviors of infants and young children, mainly pertaining to hygiene, increase their risk for infection by promoting the chain of infection. Poor hygiene habits, including lack of hand washing, placing toys and hands in the mouth, drooling, and leaking diapers, all can contribute to the spread of infection and communicable diseases. Table 16.3 reviews the chain of infection and nursing implications related to it.

BOX 16.2

DEFINITION OF FEVER BY MEASUREMENT ROUTE

- Oral: >37.5° C (99.5° F)
- Rectal: >38° C (100.4° F)
- Axillary: >37.3° C (99.1° F)
- Tympanic: >38° C (100.4° F)

Table 16.2 Stages of Infectious Disease

Stage	Explanation
Incubation	Time of entrance of pathogen into the body and appearance of first symptoms; during this time, pathogens grow and multiply.
Prodrome	Time from onset of nonspecific symptoms such as fever, malaise, and fatigue to more specific symptoms
Illness	Time during which patient demonstrates signs and symptoms specific to an infection type
Convalescence	Time when acute symptoms of illness disappear

Preventing the Spread of Infection

Nurses play a key role in breaking the chain of infection and preventing the spread of diseases. It is very important that nurses not only follow infection control and prevention practices but also educate parents and children on the measures they can take to prevent the spread of infection.

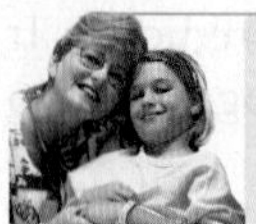

Frequent hand washing is the single most important way to prevent the spread of infection.

Isolation precautions help nurses break the chain of infection and provide strategies to prevent the spread of pathogens among hospitalized patients. Guidelines can be found on the CDC website (www.cdc.gov/ncidod/dhqp/gl_isolation_ptII.html). Additional guidelines are available from various infection control societies and regulatory agencies such as the Occupational Safety and Health Administration. Infection control standards have also been developed by the Joint Commission on Accreditation of Healthcare Organizations. This leads to an array of complex guidelines that all health professionals need to be familiar with.

In 1996, the Hospital Infection Control Practices Advisory Committee (HICPAC) presented guidelines for the hospitalized patient (American Academy of Pediatrics, 2003). It includes two tiers. Tier 1 is standard precautions, which are designed for care of all patients in the hospital regardless of their diagnosis. Tier 2 is transmission-based precautions, designed for patients who are known or suspected to be infected by epidemiologically important pathogens. These pathogens can be spread by airborne, by droplet, or by contact transmission. Box 16.3 gives an overview of standard and transmission-based precautions.

When caring for children, modifications of these guidelines may be appropriate. For instance, diaper changing is routine in the pediatric setting. Since it does not usually soil hands, it is not mandatory to wear gloves (except if gloves are required due to transmission-based precautions). According to the standard precaution guidelines, single rooms are required for those who are incontinent and cannot control bodily excretions. Since the majority of young children are incontinent, obviously this guideline is inappropriate in the pediatric setting. Pediatric units often have common rooms, such as playrooms and schoolrooms. Children placed on transmission-based isolation are not allowed to leave their rooms and therefore are not allowed to use these common rooms.

Variations in Pediatric Anatomy and Physiology

Normal immune function is an amazing protective response by the body. It involves complex responses including phagocytosis, humoral immunity, cellular immunity, and activation of the complement system. Blood and lymph are responsible for transporting the agents of the immune system. Due to the immature responses of the immune system, infants and young children are more susceptible to infection. The newborn displays a decreased inflammatory response to invading organisms, contributing to an increased risk for infection. Cellular immunity is generally functional at birth, and humoral immunity occurs when the body encounters and then develops immunity to new diseases. Since the young infant has had limited exposure to disease and is losing the passive immunity acquired from maternal antibodies, the risk of infection is higher. Young children continue to have an increased risk for infection and communicable disorders because disease protection from immunizations is not complete. (Refer to Chapter 27 for further details.)

Common Medical Treatments

A variety of medications as well as other medical treatments are used to treat infectious disorders in children. Most of these treatments will require a physician's order when the child is in the hospital. The most common treatments and medications are listed in Common Medical Treatments 16.1 and Drug Guide 16.1. The nurse caring for the child with an infectious disorder should be familiar with what the procedures are, how they work, and common nursing implications related to use of these modalities.

Table 16.3 Chain of Infection

Chain Link	Explanation	Nursing Implications
Infectious agent	Any agent capable of causing infection; examples: bacteria, viruses, rickettsiae, protozoa, and fungus	• Control or eliminate infectious agents through: • Hand washing • Wearing gloves • Cleaning, disinfection, or sterilization of equipment
Reservoir	A place where the pathogen can thrive and reproduce; examples: human body, animals, insects, food, water, inanimate objects (e.g., stethoscopes)	• Control or eliminate reservoirs. • Control sources of body fluids, drainage, or solutions that may harbor pathogens. • Follow institution guidelines for disposing of infectious wastes. • Provide proper wound care; change dressings or bandages when soiled. • Assist clients to carry out appropriate skin and oral care. • Keep linens clean and dry.
Portal of exit	A way for the pathogen to exit the reservoir; examples: skin and mucous membranes, respiratory tract, urinary tract gastrointestinal tract, reproductive tract	• Control portals of exit and educate patients and families. • Cover mouth and nose when sneezing or coughing. • Avoid talking, coughing, or sneezing over open wounds or sterile fields. • Use personal protective equipment.
Modes of transmission	Direct transmission: body-to-body contact Indirect transmission: transferred by **fomite** or vector; spread by droplet or airborne transmission	• Wash hands before and after patient contact, invasive procedures, or touching open wounds. • Use personal protective equipment when necessary. • Urge patients and family to wash hands frequently, especially before eating or handling food, after eliminating, and after touching infectious material.
Portal of entry	A way for the pathogen to enter the host; examples: skin and mucous membranes, respiratory tract, urinary tract gastrointestinal tract, reproductive tract	• Use proper sterile technique during invasive procedures. • Provide appropriate wound care. • Dispose of needles and sharps in puncture-resistant containers. • Provide all patients with their own personal care items.
Susceptible host	Any person who cannot resist the pathogen	• Protect susceptible host by promoting normal body defenses against infection. • Maintain integrity of the patient's skin and mucous membranes. • Protect normal defenses by regular bathing and oral care, adequate fluid intake and nutrition, proper immunization.

BOX 16.3

STANDARD PRECAUTIONS AND ISOLATION PRECAUTIONS

Standard Precautions (Tier One)

- Apply to all patients
- Apply to all body fluids, secretions, and excretions except sweat; nonintact skin; and mucous membranes
- Designed to reduce the risk of transmission of microorganisms from recognized and unrecognized sources
- Techniques include:
  - Proper hand hygiene
  - Use of gloves (clean and sterile) when touching blood, body fluids, secretions or excretions, and contaminated items
  - Masks, eye protection, and face shields when patient care may include splashing or sprays of blood, body fluid secretions or excretions
  - Fluid-resistant nonsterile gowns, to protect skin and clothing, when patient care may include splashing or sprays of blood, body fluid secretions or excretions
  - Patient care equipment handled in a manner that prevents skin or mucous membrane exposure and contamination of clothing
  - All used linen is considered contaminated and needs to be handled and disposed of appropriately.
  - Precautions used to prevent injury when using, cleaning, or disposing of needles and sharps
  - Mouthpieces, resuscitation bags, and other ventilation devices should be readily available.

Transmission Based Precautions (Tier Two)

- Designed for patients with known or suspected infection with pathogens for which additional precautions are warranted to interrupt transmission

Airborne

- Designed to reduce the risk of infectious agents transmitted by airborne droplet nuclei or dust particles that may contain the infectious agent
- Examples of such illnesses include measles, varicella, tuberculosis.
- Techniques include standard precautions as well as:
  - Private room (if unavailable, consider cohorting patients with the same disease and consult with an infection control professional)
  - Room with negative air pressure ventilation, with air externally exhausted or high-efficiency particulate air filtered if recirculated
  - If infectious pulmonary tuberculosis is suspected or proven, wear a respiratory protective device, such as N95 respirator, while in the patient's room.
  - Susceptible health care personnel should not enter the room of patients with measles or varicella zoster infections. Those with proven immunity to these viruses need not wear a mask.

Droplet

- Designed to reduce the risk of infectious agents transmitted by contact of the conjunctivae or the mucous membranes of the nose or mouth of a susceptible person with large-particle droplets containing pathogens generated from a person (generally through coughing, sneezing, talking, or procedures such as suctioning) who has a clinical disease or who is a carrier of the disease
- Examples of such illnesses include diphtheria, pertussis, streptococcal group A, influenza, mumps, rubella, scarlet fever.
- Techniques include standard precautions as well as:
- Private room (if unavailable, consider cohorting patients with the same disease. If this is not possible, separation of at least 3 feet between other patients and visitors should be maintained)
- Wear a mask if within 3 feet of the patient.

Contact

- Most important and most common route of transmission of health care–associated infections
- Designed to reduce the risk of infectious agents transmitted by direct or indirect contact. Direct-contact transmission involves skin-to-skin contact and physical transfer of pathogens between a susceptible host and an infected or colonized person. Examples include patient care activities that involve physical contact such as turning and bathing. Direct-contact transmission also can occur between two patients, where one serves as the source of infectious pathogen and the other as a susceptible host. Indirect-contact transmission involves contact of a susceptible host with a contaminated intermediate object, usually inanimate, in the patient's environment.
- Examples of such illnesses include diphtheria*, pediculosis, scabies, multidrug-resistant bacteria.
- Techniques include standard precautions as well as:
  - Private room (if unavailable, consider cohorting patients with the same disease)
  - Gloves (clean or sterile) should be used at all time.
  - Proper hand hygiene after glove removal
  - Use gowns, unless the patient is continent and contact of clothing with patient and patient environmental surfaces is not anticipated. Remove gowns before leaving the patient's room.

Prevention standards are applied in all health care settings and are modified to meet each setting's unique needs. Health care workers must practice within the specific institution's guidelines.

*Certain infections require more than one precaution.

Common Medical Treatments 16.1

Treatment	Explanation	Indication	Nursing Implications
Hydration	Promoting proper fluid balance either orally or intravenously	Child who can't replace insensible loss due to fever, child who is vomiting or has diarrhea	• Encourage oral fluids, if possible. • Offer child fluid he or she prefers; try Popsicles or games to promote fluid intake. • If administering IV fluids, ensure proper fluid and rate per order and assess IV site and fluid intake every hour. • Maintain strict record of intake and output.
Fever reduction	Reducing temperature by use of antipyretics or non-pharmacologic interventions	Febrile child who is uncomfortable or who can't keep up with the increased metabolic demands associated with fever	• Administer antipyretics, such as ibuprofen and acetaminophen. • Avoid aspirin use in children and adolescents. • Use non-pharmacologic interventions such as dressing lightly, removing blankets, use of a fan, tepid bath, and cooling blanket. • Some non-pharmacologic interventions remain controversial. • Make sure that non-pharmacologic measures do not induce shivering or discomfort. If they do, they should be stopped immediately.

Nursing Process Overview for the Child With a Communicable Disorder

Care of the child with an infectious disorder includes assessment, nursing diagnosis, planning, interventions, and evaluation. There are a number of general concepts related to the nursing process that may be applied to the care of children with infectious disorders. From a general understanding of the care involved for a child with an infectious disorder, the nurse can then individualize the care based on the patient's specifics.

> Remember Samuel, the 3-month-old with fever, congestion, and irritability? What additional health history and physical examination assessment information should you obtain?

ASSESSMENT

Assessment of the child with a communicable or infectious disorder includes health history, physical examination, and laboratory and diagnostic testing.

Health History

The health history comprises past medical history, including the mother's pregnancy history, family history, and history of present illness (when the symptoms started and how they have progressed), as well as treatments used at home. The past medical history might be significant for lack of recommended immunizations, prematurity, maternal infection during pregnancy or labor, prolonged difficult delivery, or immunocompromise. Family history might be significant for lack of immunization or recent infectious or communicable disease. When eliciting the history of the present illness, inquire about the following:

- Any known exposure to infectious or communicable disease
- Immunization history
- History of having any common childhood communicable diseases
- Fever
- Sore throat
- Lethargy
- Malaise
- Poor feeding or appetite
- Vomiting

Drug Guide 16.1 Common Drugs for Communicable Disorders

Medication	Action	Indication	Nursing Implications
Antibiotics	Kill and prevent the growth of bacteria	Treatment of bacterial infections such as sepsis	• Check for antibiotic allergies. • Give as prescribed for the length of time prescribed.
Antivirals (e.g., acyclovir)	Kill and prevent the growth of viruses	Treatment of viral infections such as herpes simplex II	• Observe infusion site for signs of tissue damage. • If administering topically, clean and dry area before application and wear gloves. • Give as prescribed for the length of time prescribed.
Antipyretics (acetaminophen, ibuprofen)	Decrease the temperature set point (only in a child with a raised temperature) by inhibiting the production of prostaglandins, leading to heat loss (through vasodilation and sweating) and resulting in a reduction in fever	Febrile child who is uncomfortable or who can't keep up with the increased metabolic demands associated with fever	• Ensure proper dosing, concentration, and dosing interval. • Avoid aspirin use in children and adolescents. • Avoid ibuprofen use in children with a bleeding disorder. • Assess fever and any related symptoms such as tachycardia, shivering, diaphoresis. • Proper education to caregivers on appropriate dosing, concentration, dosing interval, and use of proper measuring device is essential.
Antipruritics (usually antihistamines)	Agents that relieve itching may be given topically or orally.	Relief of discomfort secondary to itching	• When applying topically, wear gloves. • Do not apply to open wounds. • Oral antihistamines may cause drowsiness.

- Diarrhea
- Cough
- Rash (in the older child ask for a description of how it feels; is it painful, does it itch?)

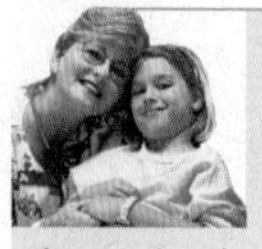

Many childhood infectious and communicable diseases involve a rash. Rashes can be difficult to identify; therefore, a thorough description and history from the caregiver is extremely important.

Physical Examination

Physical examination of the child with an infectious disorder includes inspection, observation, and palpation.

Inspection and Observation

The physical examination should begin with inspection and observation. Assess the child's skin, mouth, throat, and hair for lesions or wounds. Note the color, shape, and distribution of any lesions or wounds. Assess whether there is any exudate from the lesions or wounds. Observe for scratching, restlessness, and avoidance of the use of a body part or guarding of a body part. A thorough and accurate description is important to assist in identifying the rash and causative organism. Observe the child's affect, energy level, and interaction with caregiver. Lethargy can indicate serious infection or sepsis. Observe if there is any discharge from the nose, cough, or respiratory difficulty.

Assess hydration status. Inspect oral mucosa; dry and pale mucous membranes can indicate dehydration. Observe for others signs of dehydration, such as sunken eyes and no tears with crying.

Assessment of vital signs can provide more information about the child's condition. Elevated temperature can indicate infection. Often tachypnea and tachycardia accompany fever. Hypotension may also occur, but it is usually a late sign with sepsis.

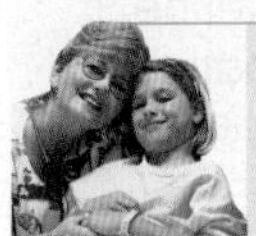

Neonates may not present with fever; some may be hypothermic.

Palpation

Palpate the skin to assess temperature, moisture, texture, and turgor. In a child with an infectious or communicable disease the skin may be warm and moist due to fever. Turgor may be decreased secondary to dehydration. In infants, palpate the fontanels; if sunken, the infant may be dehydrated. Palpate the rash to determine if it is raised or flat. A thorough picture of the presenting rash can help identify the child's illness. Palpate the lymph nodes and note any that are swollen and tender.

Laboratory and Diagnostic Testing

Common Laboratory Diagnostics Tests 16.1 offers an explanation of the laboratory and diagnostic tests used most commonly when considering communicable disorders. The tests can assist the physician in diagnosing the disorder and/or be used as guidelines in determining ongoing treatment. Laboratory or non-nursing personnel obtain some of the tests, while the nurse might obtain others. In either instance the nurse should be familiar with how the tests are obtained, what they are used for, and normal versus abnormal results. This knowledge will also be necessary when providing patient and family education related to the testing.

Performing Venipuncture

Obtaining a blood specimen may be very frightening to children because of the fear of needles, pain, and blood loss. Incorporate the concept of atraumatic care in the performance of all venipunctures or other needlesticks for children. Whether the laboratory technician or the nurse is drawing the blood, the procedure should be performed in an area other than the child's bed, such as the treatment room; the child's bed should be kept as a "safe" area. Provide teaching about the procedure based upon the child's developmental level and readiness to learn. In infants and younger children, additional assistance with positioning and restraint will be needed in perform the procedure safely and to ensure proper collection. Use a topical anesthetic cream or gel, refrigerant spray, or iontophoresis prior to venipuncture. In young infants, administer oral sucrose beginning 1 to 2 minutes prior to the procedure and throughout the course of the venipuncture. Refer to Chapter 14 for additional information related to decreasing the incidence of pain related to venipuncture in infants and children.

The usual sites for obtaining blood specimens via venipuncture are the superficial veins of the dorsal surface of the hand or the antecubital fossa, although other locations may also be used. In specific situations, the jugular or femoral vein may be used and either the physician or advanced practice nurse will perform the venipuncture. Capillary puncture of the child's fingertip, the great toe, or the infant's heel may also be used to obtain blood specimens. Fingertip puncture is similar to that in the adult, directed to the sides of the fingertip. Great toe puncture is performed in the same way. Capillary heel puncture must be performed in the proper location to avoid striking the medial plantar artery or periosteum. Nursing Procedure 16.1 gives instructions related to capillary heel puncture. It is also important to use automatic lancet devices to deliver a more precise puncture depth (Vertanen et al., 2001). The young infant will benefit from the use of oral sucrose via pacifier before and during the capillary puncture.

Performing Arterial Puncture

Occasionally, blood samples may be obtained from an artery rather than a vein or capillary. Blood gases in particular are usually obtained by arterial puncture. Arterial puncture requires additional training and in many institutions is performed only by the respiratory therapist, physician, or nurse practitioner. Children with indwelling venous access devices may be spared the trauma of puncture for blood specimens. Follow your institution's guidelines for withdrawing blood from peripherally inserted venous catheters or central venous catheters. The initial blood will be discarded to prevent contamination with intravenous fluids or medications such as heparin. The discard amount depends on the size of the catheter, the weight of the child, and the institution's guidelines. After aspiration of the specimen, flush the venous access device with normal saline to prevent clogging. The device may then be reconnected to the intravenous fluid or flushed according to the institution's protocol.

NURSING DIAGNOSES, GOALS, INTERVENTIONS, AND EVALUATIONS

Upon completion of a thorough assessment, the nurse might identify several nursing diagnoses, including:

- Altered body temperature: fever
- Impaired comfort

(text continues on page 428)

Common Laboratory and Diagnostic Tests 16.1

Test	Explanation	Indication	Nursing Implications
Complete blood count (CBC)	Evaluate white blood cell count (particularly the percentage of individual white cells)	Detect the presence of inflammation, infection	• Normal values vary according to age and gender. • White blood cell count differential is helpful in evaluating source of infection. • May be affected by myelosuppressive drugs
Erythrocyte sedimentation rate (ESR)	Nonspecific test used in conjunction with other tests to determine presence of infection or inflammation	Detect the presence of inflammation, infection	• Send to laboratory immediately; specimens allowed to stand for longer than 3 hours may produce a falsely low result.
C-reactive protein (CRP)	Nonspecific test that measures a type of protein produced in the liver that is present during episodes of acute inflammation or infection. Usually used to diagnose bacterial infections; does not consistently rise with viral infections.	Detect the presence of infection	• Presence of an intrauterine device may cause positive test results because of tissue inflammation. • Exogenous hormones, such as oral contraceptives, may cause increased levels. • Nonsteroidal anti-inflammatories, salicylates, and steroids may cause decreased levels. • Fasting may be required. • CRP is a more sensitive and rapidly responding indicator than ESR.
Blood culture and sensitivity	Deliberate growing of microorganism in a solid or liquid medium. Once it has grown, it is tested against various antibiotics to determine which antibiotics will kill it.	Detect the presence of bacteria or yeast, which may have spread from a certain site in the body into the bloodstream. Determine which antibiotics the bacteria or yeast is sensitive to.	• Follow aseptic technique and hospital protocol to prevent contamination. • Two cultures obtained from two different sites are preferred. • Ideally obtain before administering antibiotics; if patient is taking antibiotics, notify laboratory and draw specimen shortly before next dose. • Smaller volumes are available for pediatric use. • Deliver to laboratory immediately (within 30 minutes).
Stool culture (including stool for ova and parasites (O&P))	To determine if a bacteria or parasite has infected the intestines	Detect pathogens, including parasites or overgrowth of normal flora in the bowel. Indicated for patients with diarrhea, fever, or abdominal pain.	• Stool must be free of urine, water, and toilet paper. • Do not retrieve out of toilet water. • Deliver to laboratory immediately. • Mineral oil, barium, and bismuth interfere with the detection of parasites; specimen collection should be delayed for 7 to 10 days.

Common Laboratory and Diagnostic Tests 16.1 (continued)

Test	Explanation	Indication	Nursing Implications
			• Often a minimum of three specimens on 3 separate days are required for adequate examination, since many parasites and worm eggs are shed intermittently.
Urine culture	Collection of urine to detect the presence of bacteria in the urine	Detect the presence of bacteria in the urine. Indicated for patients with fever of unknown origin, dysuria, frequency or urgency, or if urinalysis suggests infection.	• Should be obtained by midstream clean-catch, catheterization, or suprapubic aspiration. Avoid contamination with stool, vaginal secretions, hands, or clothing. • Placing bags on the perineum is not acceptable due to high chance of contamination. • Obtain before antibiotics are administered. • Deliver to laboratory immediately or refrigerate.
Genital tract culture	Specimens from the genital tract include urethral, cervical, and anorectal swabs to detect the presence of invasive organisms.	Detect the presence of sexually transmitted infections. Indicated in patients with vaginal discharge, pelvic pain, urethritis, or penile discharge and those at high risk for sexually transmitted infections.	• Menses may alter test. • Female patients should avoid douching or tub bathing 24 hours before a cervical culture (may make fewer organisms available). • Obtain urethral cultures from male patients before voiding, preferably before the first morning void (voiding 1 hour before urethral culture washes secretions out of the urethra). • Fecal material may contaminate a rectal culture. • Transport specimens to laboratory as soon as possible. • Advise patients to avoid intercourse and all other sexual contact until test results are available.
Throat culture	Vigorous swabbing of the tonsillar area and posterior pharynx to detect the presence of invasive organisms	Most reliable method of detecting group A streptococcal pharyngitis. Will also detect *Bordatella pertussis, Corynebacterium diphtheriae.* Also may be used to detect sexually transmitted infections in those who have engaged in oral intercourse. May be performed in those with fever of unknown origin.	• Ensure specimen is of secretions in the pharyngeal or tonsillar area. • When performing on young children, have adult hold child in lap. • Health care worker needs to stabilize head by placing hand on the child's forehead.

Nursing Procedure 16.1

Capillary Heel Puncture

1. Choose the collection site and apply a commercial heel warmer or warm pack for several minutes prior to specimen collection.
2. Assemble equipment:
   - Gloves
   - Automatic lancet
   - Antiseptic wipe
   - Cotton ball or dry gauze
   - Capillary blood collection tube
   - Band-aid
3. Don gloves. Remove the warm pack.
4. Cleanse the site with antiseptic prep pad and allow to dry.
5. Hold the dorsum of the foot with the nondominant hand; with the dominant hand, pierce the heel with the lancet.
6. Wipe away the first drop of blood with the cotton ball or dry gauze.
7. Collect the blood specimen with a capillary specimen collection tube. Avoid squeezing the foot during specimen collection if possible, as it may contribute to hemolysis of the specimen.
8. Hold a dry gauze over the site until bleeding stops, then apply a Band-aid.

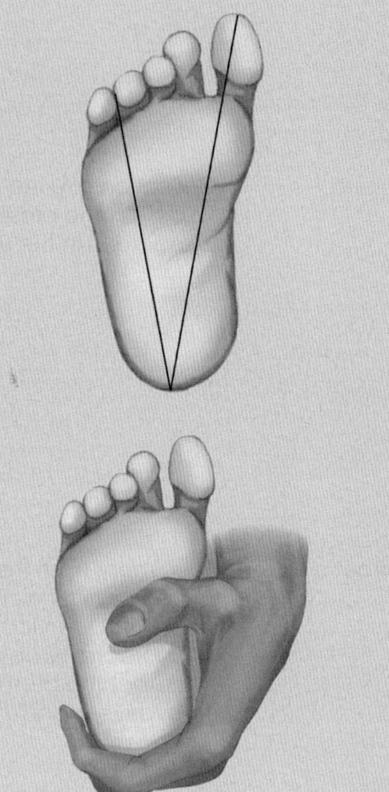

- Impaired skin integrity
- Risk for infection
- Fluid volume deficit
- Social isolation
- Knowledge deficit

> **After completing an assessment of Samuel,** you note the following: rectal temperature of 39° C, poor sucking, and lethargy. Based on these assessment findings, what would your top three nursing diagnoses be for Samuel?

Nursing goals, interventions, and evaluation for the child with a communicable or infectious disorder are based on the nursing diagnoses. Nursing Care Plan Overview 16.1 provides a general guide for planning care for a child with an infectious or communicable disorder. Additional information about nursing management will be included later in the chapter as it relates to specific disorders.

Managing Fever

Fever is one of the most common reasons parents seek medical attention. Most infections or communicable diseases are accompanied by fever. Many parents have great concerns about fever: they fear febrile seizures, neurologic complications, and a potential serious underlying disease. Many health care providers may share these fears. This leads to the common recommendation to intervene and reduce fever. These fears and misconceptions about fever can lead to mismanagement of fever, such as inappropriate dosing of antipyretics or inappropriate use of nonpharmacologic treatments such as sponging the child with alcohol or cold water.

Health care providers need to educate parents that fever is a protective mechanism the body uses to fight infection. Evidence exists that an elevated body temperature actually enhances various components of the immune response. Fever can slow the growth of bacteria and viruses and increase neutrophil production and T-cell proliferation (Corcetti & Serwint, 2005). Studies have shown that the use of antipyretics may prolong illness. Concern also exists that reducing fever may hide signs of serious bacterial illness.

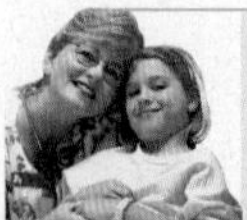

Infants less than 3 months of age with a rectal temperature greater than 38° C should be seen by a physician. They are considered at risk for sepsis until proven otherwise due to their immature immune system and inability to localize or handle infection very well.

(text continues on page 432)

Nursing Care Plan 16.1

Overview for the Child With an Infectious or Communicable Disorder

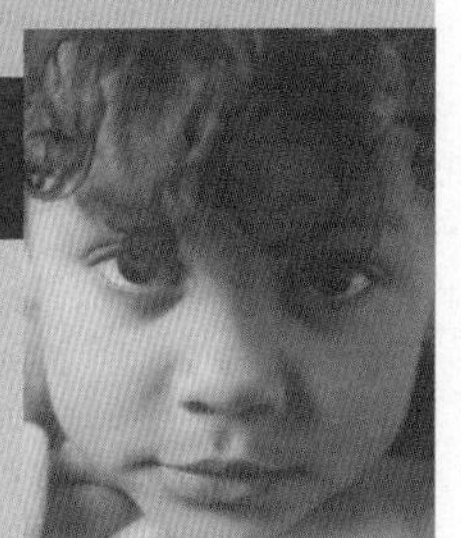

Nursing Diagnosis: Altered body temperature: fever related to infectious disease process as evidenced by rectal temperature greater than 38° C or 100.4° F

Outcome identification and evaluation

Child will maintain temperature within adaptive levels and be comfortable and remain hydrated.

Temperature will be 38° C or 100.4° F or less.

Child will verbalize or exhibit signs of comfort during febrile episode; child will demonstrate adequate signs of hydration.

Interventions: managing fever

- Assess temperature at least every 4 to 6 hours, 30 to 60 minutes after antipyretic is given and with any change in condition; *recognizing the pattern of fever may help identify source.*
- Use same site and device for temperature measurement *to reflect a more accurate trend in temperature, since different sites can result in significant differences in temperature reading.*
- Administer antipyretics per physician order when the child is experiencing discomfort or cannot keep up with the metabolic demands of the fever. *Fever is a protective response of the body to fight infection. Antipyretics provide symptomatic relief but do not change the course of the infection. The major benefits to decreasing fever are increasing comfort in the child and decreasing fluid requirements, helping to prevent dehydration.*
- Notify physician of temperature per institution or specific order guidelines; *increases in temperature may indicate worsening infection and relevant changes in condition.*
- Assess fluid intake and encourage oral intake or administer intravenous fluids per physician order; *increased metabolic rate and diaphoresis related to fever can cause fluid loss and lead to fluid volume deficit.*
- Keep linens and clothing clean and dry; *diaphoresis can leave clothing and linen soaked and increases discomfort for the child.*
- Use of non-pharmacologic measures such as tepid bath and removal of clothing and blankets is controversial. If used, discontinue if shivering begins.

Nursing Diagnosis: Impaired comfort related to infectious and/or inflammatory process as evidenced by hyperthermia, pruritus, rash or skin lesions, sore throat, or joint pain

Outcome identification and evaluation

Pain or discomfort will be reduced to level acceptable to child.

Child will verbalize absence or decrease of pain using a pain scale (FLACC, faces or linear pain scale), will verbalize decrease in uncomfortable sensations such as itching and aches; infants will exhibit decreased crying and ability to rest quietly.

Interventions: improving comfort

- Assess pain and response to interventions frequently with use of pain scales or other pain measurement tools; *provides baseline of pain and allows for evaluation of effectiveness of interventions.*
- Administer analgesics and antipruritics as ordered *to relieve pain via interruption of CNS pathways and to decrease discomfort related to itching.*
- Apply cool compresses to areas of pruritus or provide a cool bath *to decrease inflammation and soothe pruritus.*
- Keep child's fingernails short (use mitts, gloves, or socks over hands if necessary); *short fingernails can help prevent injury to the skin, which leads to increased pain.*

(continued)

Overview for the Child With an Infectious or Communicable Disorder (continued)

- Encourage child to press on rather than scratch the area of pruritus; *pressing on the area that itches can help soothe the itching and prevent scratching, which can lead to injury to the skin.*
- Provide frequent fluids and offer warm fluids such as soup or cold foods such as Popsicles *to help ease the discomfort of a sore throat.*
- Provide cool mist humidification *to help ease the discomfort of a sore throat.*
- Dress the child in light clothing; *restrictive clothing and diaphoresis can lead to increased pruritus.*
- Use diversional activities and distraction appropriate to developmental level: *distraction from pain can reduce the need for pharmacologic agents, and distraction for pruritus can minimize scratching.*

Nursing Diagnosis: Impaired skin integrity related to mechanical trauma secondary to infectious disease process as evidenced by rash, pruritus, and scratching

Outcome identification and evaluation

Child will maintain or regain skin integrity.

Child will not demonstrate increased skin breakdown. Child or parent will be able to describe or demonstrate measures to protect and heal skin and proper care for any lesions.

Interventions: promoting skin integrity

- Monitor skin for color changes, temperature, redness, swelling, warmth, pain or signs of infection, changes in rash lesions, distribution, or size *to help identify problems early and allow for prevention of infection; can also provide information regarding the course of the illness.*
- Encourage fluid intake and proper nutrition *to promote wound healing.*
- Keep child's fingernails short (use mitts, gloves, or socks over hands if necessary); *short fingernails can help prevent injury to the skin, which leads to increased pain.*
- Encourage child to press on rather than scratch the area of pruritus; *pressing on the area that itches can help soothe the itching and prevent scratching, which can lead to injury to the skin.*
- Use antipruritics and topical ointments or creams as ordered *to minimize scratching to prevent injury to skin; can aid in healing.*

Nursing Diagnosis: Risk for infection related to insufficient knowledge regarding measures to avoid exposure to pathogens, increased environmental exposure to pathogens, transmission to others secondary to contagious organism or presence of infectious organisms

Outcome identification and evaluation

Child will exhibit no signs or symptoms of local or systemic infection. Child will not spread infection to others. *Symptoms of infection will decrease over time; others will remain free of infection. Child and family will demonstrate appropriate hygiene measures using proper technique, such as hand washing to prevent the spread of infection.*

Interventions: preventing and controlling infection

- Monitor vital signs; *elevation in temperature may indicate infection.*
- Monitor skin lesions for signs of local infection: *redness, warmth, drainage, swelling, and pain at lesions can indicate infection.*
- Maintain aseptic technique and practice good hand washing *to prevent introduction of further infectious agents and prevent transmission to others.*
- Administer antibiotics as prescribed *to prevent or treat bacterial infection.*

Overview for the Child With an Infectious or Communicable Disorder (continued)

- Encourage nutritious diet and proper hydration according to child's preferences and ability to feed orally *to assist body's natural defenses against infection.*
- Isolate child as required based on transmission-based precautions *to prevent nosocomial spread of infection.*
- Teach child and family preventive measures such as good hand washing, covering mouth and nose with cough or sneeze, and adequate disposal of used tissues *to prevent nosocomial or community spread of infection.*

Nursing Diagnosis: Fluid volume deficit, risk for, related to increased metabolic demands and insensible loss due to fever, vomiting, poor feeding or intake

Outcome identification and evaluation

Fluid volume will be maintained and balanced. *Oral mucosa will remain moist and pink, skin turgor is elastic, urine output is at least 1 to 2 mL/kg/hr.*

Interventions: promoting adequate fluid balance

- Administer IV fluids if ordered *to maintain adequate hydration in children who are NPO, unable to tolerate oral intake, or unable to keep up with fluid losses.*
- When oral intake is allowed and tolerated, encourage oral fluids *to promote intake and maintain hydration.*
- Assess for signs of adequate hydration such as pink and moist oral mucosa, elastic skin turgor, adequate urine output; *discrepancies may identify fluid imbalance.*
- Monitor intake and output *to identify fluid imbalance.*
- Assess urine specific gravity, urine and serum electrolytes, blood urea nitrogen, creatinine, and osmolality and daily weights; *these are reliable indicators of fluid status.*

Nursing Diagnosis: Social isolation related to required isolation from peers secondary to transmission-based precautions, as evidenced by disruption in usual play secondary to inability to leave hospital room, activity intolerance, and fatigue

Outcome identification and evaluation

Child will participate in stimulating activities. *Child is able to verbalize reason for isolation and length of isolation (if developmentally appropriate); child verbalizes interest in activities.*

Interventions: preventing social isolation

- Explain reasons for transmission-based precautions and length of time; *this helps increase understanding and decrease anxiety about isolation. Children sometimes mistake isolation as punishment. Explaining length of time gives child an end point he or she can work toward.*
- Visit child frequently, at least every hour, and try to spend some uninterrupted time to play and allow child time to verbalize feelings about separation from others; *helps establish a therapeutic relationship and demonstrates caring.*
- Let child see caregiver's face before applying mask if appropriate *to help child identify and relate to those caring for him or her and minimize anxiety about strangers and the unknown.*
- Consult child life specialist *to arrange for stimulating activities child enjoys; can help child to better understand reasons for isolation.*
- Contact volunteers to spend time with child, if appropriate: *gives child attention and support, which will assist child with coping and decrease stress.*

(continued)

Overview for the Child With an Infectious or Communicable Disorder (continued)

Nursing Diagnosis: Knowledge deficit related to lack of information regarding medical condition, prognosis, and medical needs as evidenced by verbalization, questions, or actions demonstrating lack of understanding regarding child's condition or care

Outcome identification and evaluation

Child and family will verbalize accurate information and understanding about condition, prognosis and medical needs. *Child and family demonstrate knowledge of condition and prognosis and medical needs, including possible causes, contributing factors, and treatment measures.*

Interventions: providing patient and family teaching

- Assess child's and family's willingness to learn: *child and family must be willing to learn in order for teaching to be effective.*
- Provide family with time to adjust to diagnosis *to help facilitate adjustment and ability to learn and participate in child's care.*
- Repeat information: *allows family and child time to learn and understand.*
- Teach in short sessions; *many short sessions are found to be more helpful than one long session.*
- Gear teaching to level of understanding of the child and family (depends on age of child, physical condition, memory) *to ensure understanding.*
- Provide reinforcement and rewards *to facilitate the teaching/learning process.*
- Use multiple modes of learning involving many senses (provide written, verbal, demonstration and videos) when possible; *the child and family are more likely to retain information when it is presented in different ways using many senses.*

In infants over 3 months of age, fever less than 39° C usually does not require treatment (Behrman et al., 2004). Antipyretics provide symptomatic relief but do not change the course of the infection. The major benefits to decreasing fever are increasing comfort in the child and decreasing fluid requirements, which helps to prevent dehydration. Children with certain underlying conditions, such as cardiovascular disease or pulmonary disease, also benefit from treating fever because such treatment decreases demands on the body.

Home Management of Fever

Management of fever typically occurs at home. Therefore, it is important that guidance and instruction are given at well child visits and reviewed at subsequent visits. Written and video materials related to fever management have been effective in increasing caregivers' knowledge (Broome et al., 2003). Parents can refer to the written instructions when needed (see Teaching Guideline 16.1). The use of acetaminophen and ibuprofen to reduce fever in children has been shown to be safe and effective when the appropriate dose is administered at the appropriate interval (Corcetti & Serwint, 2005). Box 16.4 gives dosing recommendations.

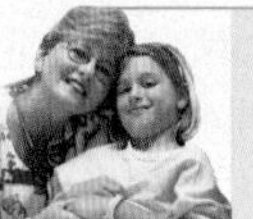

Never give aspirin to children to reduce fever, due to the risk of Reye syndrome.

Acetaminophen Use

Acetaminophen is widely used and accepted, but toxic reactions can be seen in children. Unintentional causes of acetaminophen toxicity include overdosing or incorrect dosing due to failure to read and understand the label instructions, use of an incorrect measuring device or concentration, and co-administration with an over-the-counter fixed-dose combination medication (the parent may not recognize that it has acetaminophen in it). Another factor that may cause acetaminophen toxicity is the controversial but common practice of alternating acetaminophen and ibuprofen to help reduce fever. There is no evidence supporting this practice (American Academy of Pediatrics, 2001), and it can result in overdose or improper administration. It can be hard for parents to keep track of the time each medication is due. Parents may confuse which medication is given every 4 hours and which is given every 6 hours. They may exceed the recommended daily doses or may confuse the strength or dosage of the medicines.

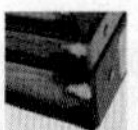

TEACHING GUIDELINE 16.1

Fever Management

- Fever is a sign of illness, not a disease; it is the body's weapon to fight infection.
- Diurnal variation may allow temperature changes as much as 1° C (1.8° F) over a 24-hour period, peaking in the evening.
- In some children fever can be associated with a seizure or dehydration, but this will not lead to brain damage or death. Discuss the facts about febrile seizures (see Chapter 17 for further information on febrile seizures).
- Watch for the signs and symptoms of dehydration; it is important to provide oral rehydration by increasing fluid intake.
- Dress the child lightly and avoid warm, binding clothing or blankets.
- The use of sponging with tepid water is controversial; if used, encourage the parent to give an antipyretic prior to sponging. Ensure the sponging does not produce shivering (which causes the body to produce heat and maintain the elevated set point), and reinforce the importance of using tepid water, not cold water or alcohol. Instruct the parent to stop if the child experiences discomfort.
- Call the physician for:
  - Any child less than 3 months who has a rectal temperature above 38° C (100.4° F)
  - Any child who is lethargic or listless, regardless of temperature
  - Fever lasting more than 3 to 5 days
  - Fever greater than 40.6° C (105° F)
  - Any child who is immunocompromised by illness, such as cancer or HIV, will need further evaluation and treatment.

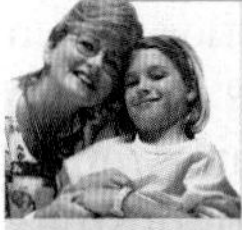

The American Academy of Pediatrics (2001) has stated that due to the lack of evidence supporting the safety or efficacy of alternating acetaminophen with ibuprofen for fever management, extreme discretion should be used when considering this therapy.

BOX 16.4

DOSE RECOMMENDATIONS FOR ACETAMINOPHEN AND IBUPROFEN

Acetaminophen, 10 to 15 mg/kg/dose

- No more than every 4 hours
- No more than 5 doses in a 24-hour period

Ibuprofen, 5 to 10 mg/kg/dose

- Only children greater than 6 months of age
- No more than 4 doses in a 24-hour period

Managing Skin Rashes

Many infectious or communicable diseases are accompanied by skin rashes. These rashes can be very uncomfortable and irritating for the child. Management often occurs at home, so parents need to be educated on ways to relieve the discomfort and protect and maintain skin integrity. Antipruritics, including oral medications or topical creams or ointments, may be prescribed by the physician (see Drug Guide 16.1). Parents need to be instructed on the importance of maintaining skin integrity to prevent infection or scarring. Teach parents to keep their child's fingernails short and hands clean. Explain the importance of discouraging scratching, and discuss distraction techniques they can use with the child. Cool compresses or cool baths can help relieve itching. Encouraging the child to press on rather than scratch the itchy area; this can help relieve discomfort while maintaining skin integrity. Refer to Chapter 25 for more information on managing skin rashes.

Based on your top three nursing diagnoses for Samuel, describe appropriate nursing interventions.

Sepsis

Sepsis is a systemic overresponse to infection resulting from bacteria (most common), fungi, viruses, or parasites. It can lead to septic shock, which results in hypotension, low blood flow, and multisystem organ failure. Septic shock is a medical emergency and patients are usually admitted to an intensive care unit (see Chapter 32). The cause of sepsis may not be known, but common causative organisms in children include *Neisseria meningitidis, Streptococcus pneumoniae,* and *Haemophilus influenzae.* Sepsis can affect any age group but is more common in neonates and young infants. Neonates and young infants have a higher susceptibility due to their immature immune system, inability to localize infections, and lack of IgM immunoglobulin, which is necessary to protect against bacterial infections.

The prognosis for sepsis is variable and depends on the child's age and the cause of the sepsis. Mortality rate may be as high as 40% to 60% for certain types of infections (Behrman et al., 2004). Neonates are at the highest risk, and 50% of neonatal deaths result from serious bacterial infections in the first month of life (Crawford, 2006). Due to this high mortality rate, when a febrile neonate presents, a full work-up is indicated, and usually admission to the hospital to rule out sepsis is the standard of practice.

Pathophysiology

Sepsis results in systemic inflammatory response syndrome (SIRS) due to infection. The pathophysiology of sepsis is complex. It results from the effects of circulating bacterial products or toxins, mediated by cytokine release, occurring as a result of sustained bacteremia. The pathogens cause an overproduction of pro-inflammatory cytokines, previously termed endotoxins, which are responsible for the clinically observable effects of the sepsis. Impaired pulmonary, hepatic, or renal function may result from excessive cytokine release during the septic process.

Therapeutic Management

Therapeutic management of sepsis in infants, especially neonates, is more aggressive than for older children. Neonate and infants with sepsis or even suspected sepsis are treated in the hospital. The infant is admitted for close monitoring along with antibiotic therapy. Intravenous antibiotics are started immediately after the blood, urine, and cerebrospinal fluid cultures have been obtained. The length of therapy and the specific antibiotic used will be determined based on the source of the positive culture and the results of the culture and sensitivity. Common treatment length for positive cultures is 10 to 14 days. If final culture reports are negative and symptoms have subsided, antibiotics may be discontinued (usually after 72 hours of treatment). If the child is not responding to therapy and symptoms worsen, sepsis may be progressing to shock. Management of the child with septic shock is usually done in the intensive care unit.

Nursing Assessment

For a full description of the assessment phase of the nursing process, refer to page 423. Assessment findings pertinent to sepsis are discussed below.

Health History

Elicit a description of the present illness and chief complaint. Signs of sepsis can vary with each child. Some common signs and symptoms reported during the health history might include:

- Child just does not look or act right
- Crying more than usual, inconsolable
- Fever
- Hypothermia (in the neonate and those with severe disease)
- Lethargic and less interactive or playful
- Increased irritability
- Poor feeding or poor suck
- Rash (e.g., petechiae, ecchymosis, diffuse erythema)
- Difficulty breathing
- Nasal congestion
- Diarrhea
- Vomiting
- Decreased urine output
- Hypotonia
- Changes in mental status (confused, anxious, excited)
- Seizures
- Older child may complain of heart racing

Explore the patient's current and past medical history for risk factors such as:

- Prematurity
- Lack of immunizations
- Immunocompromise
- Exposure to communicable pathogens

In neonates and young infants, discuss pregnancy and labor risk factors such as:

- Premature rupture of membranes or prolonged rupture
- Difficult delivery
- Maternal infection or fever, including sexually transmitted infections
- Resuscitation and other invasive procedures
- Positive maternal group beta streptococcal vaginosis

Sepsis may occur in the hospitalized child. Assess for risk factors such as:

- Intensive care unit stay
- Presence of central line or other invasive lines or tubes
- Immunosuppression

Physical Examination

Perform a thorough physical examination of the infant or child with proven or suspected sepsis. Specific findings related to inspection and observation are noted below.

Inspection and Observation

Observe the child's general appearance, color, level of arousal, and hydration status. The child with sepsis may appear lethargic and pale and show signs of dehydration. In neonates and infants, observe the quality of their cry and reaction to parental stimulation, noting weak cry, lack of smile or facial expression, or lack of responsiveness. Inspect the skin for petechiae or other skin lesions. Petechiae may indicate a serious bacterial infection (often *N. meningitidis*), and other skin lesion patterns may help identify the cause of the fever. Observe respiratory effort and rate. The infant or child with sepsis may demonstrate tachypnea and increased work of breathing, such as nasal flaring, grunting, and retractions.

Assess vital signs, noting abnormalities. Note elevation in temperature or hypothermia in the young infant. Note tachypnea or tachycardia in the child or apnea or bradycardia in the infant. Document blood pressure. Hypotension, especially when accompanied by signs of poor perfusion, can be a sign of worsening sepsis with progression to shock (refer to Chapter 32).

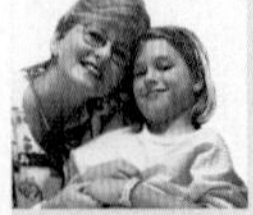

Listen to the parents' descriptions of the neonate's or infant's behavior and appearance, as well as changes they have observed. Many times they are the first to notice when their child is not acting right, even before clinical signs of infection are seen.

Laboratory and Diagnostic Tests

Symptoms of sepsis can be vague in infants. Therefore, laboratory tests play a crucial role in confirming or ruling out sepsis. Common laboratory and diagnostic studies ordered for the assessment of sepsis include:

- Complete blood count: white blood cells will be elevated; in severe cases they may be decreased (this is an ominous sign)
- C-reactive protein: elevated
- Blood culture: positive in septicemia, indicating bacteria is present in the blood
- Urine culture: may be positive, indicating presence of bacteria in the urine
- Cerebrospinal fluid analysis: may reveal increased white blood cells and protein and low glucose
- Stool culture: may be positive for bacteria or other infectious organisms
- Culture of tubes, catheters, or shunts suspected to be infected: the fluid inside those tubes may be tested to detect the presence of bacteria
- Chest x-ray: may reveal signs of pneumonia such as hyperinflation and patchy areas of atelectasis or infiltration

Nursing Management

Monitor the infant or child closely for changes in condition, especially the development of shock. Administer antibiotics as ordered. Refer to the Nursing Care Plan Overview 16.1 for nursing diagnoses and related interventions. In addition to these interventions, reducing risk for infection and providing education to the child and family should be noted.

Preventing Infection

Sepsis is a potentially life-threatening illness, and prevention is important. Hand washing is the most effective intervention against nosocomial infection. Nurses play a key role in minimizing environmental sources through proper cleaning of equipment and disposal of soiled linens and dressings as well as adhering to proper aseptic technique with all invasive procedures. Following your institution's policies and using evidenced-based practice guidelines for interventions such as invasive line dressing changes and intravenous tubing changes can help reduce the risk of infection. Encourage immunization as recommended. To reduce streptococcus group B infection in neonates, screen pregnant woman; if the results are positive, administer intrapartum antibiotics.

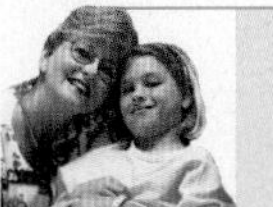

There has been a dramatic reduction in invasive *Haemophilus influenzae* type B diseases since the widespread use of the Hib vaccine. Meningococcal and pneumococcal vaccines also have decreased the incidence of invasive infection, especially in high-risk children.

Educating the Child and Family

Early recognition of the signs of sepsis is essential in preventing morbidity and mortality. Educate parents about the importance of fever, especially in neonates and infants less than 3 months old. Instruct parents to contact their health care provider if their infant or neonate has a fever. A health care provider should see any child with a fever accompanied by lethargy, poor responsiveness, or lack of facial expressions. Signs and symptoms of sepsis can be vague and vary from child to child. Parents need to be encouraged to contact their health care provider if they feel their febrile child is "just not acting right."

Bacterial Infections

Bacteria are one-celled organisms that can live, grow, and reproduce. They exist everywhere. Most are completely harmless and some are very useful. Others can lead to disease either because they are in the wrong place in the body or they are designed to invade and cause disease in humans and animals. Children are at a high risk of developing bacterial infections, which can result in life-threatening illness. Fortunately, many bacterial diseases can be prevented by immunization, such as diphtheria, pertussis, and tetanus (see Chapter 9 for more information related to immunizations).

SCARLET FEVER

Scarlet fever is an infection resulting from a group A streptococcus (GAS). The bacteria produce a toxin that causes a rash. Two children may have a group A streptococcus infection, but both may not get the rash of scarlet fever: only the one who is sensitive to the toxin will develop scarlet fever. It is usually seen in children less than 18 years of age, with the peak incidence between the ages of 4 and 8 years. It is rare in children less than 2 years old. Transmission is airborne and follows contact with respiratory tract secretions. Close contact that occurs in schools and childcare centers facilitates transmission. Foodborne outbreaks have occurred due to human contamination of food. After exposure the incubation period is 2 to 5 days. Communicability is highest during acute infection, and the child is no longer contagious 24 hours after the initiation of appropriate antimicrobial therapy. There has been a dramatic decrease in the mortality from scarlet fever due to antibiotic use, but complications such as rheumatic fever and glomerulonephritis still exist.

Nursing Assessment

Symptoms of scarlet fever begin abruptly. The history may reveal a fever greater than 101° F, chills, body aches, loss of appetite, nausea, and vomiting. Inspect the pharynx, which is usually very red and swollen. The tonsils may have yellow or white specks of pus, and cervical lymph nodes may be swollen. Inspect the skin for the most striking symptom of scarlet fever, which is an erythematous rash appearing on the face, trunk, and extremities. The rash is typically absent from the palms and soles of the feet. It looks like a sunburn but feels like sandpaper (Fig. 16.1). The rash lasts approximately 5 days and is followed by desquamation, typically on the fingers and toes. Early in the illness the tongue develops a thick coat with a strawberry appearance. The tongue will later lose the coating and become bright red (see Fig. 16.1).

Diagnosis is made by identification of GAS on throat culture. Several rapid tests for GAS pharyngitis are available. The accuracy of these tests depends on the quality of the specimen. It is important that the secretions obtained are pharyngeal or tonsillar (refer to Common Medical Treatments 16.1 for more information on throat cultures).

Nursing Management

Care of the child with scarlet fever will usually occur at home. Penicillin V is the antibiotic of choice. In those sensitive to penicillin, erythromycin may be used. Educate the family on the importance of taking the antibiotic as directed and finishing all the medicine.

Encourage fluid intake to maintain adequate hydration due to fever. Teach parents ways to provide comfort for the child. A cool mist humidifier can help soothe the child's sore throat. Soft foods, warm liquids like soup, or cold foods like Popsicles may also be helpful. If the child is hospitalized, droplet precautions, along with standard precautions, are necessary.

CAT SCRATCH DISEASE

Cat scratch disease is a relatively common and occasionally serious disease caused by the bacteria *Bartonella henselae.* It occurs in both children and adults but is more frequent in children under 10 years of age. Cats can carry the bacteria in their saliva, and in 90% of cases the child has had a recent interaction with cats and often kittens (American Academy of Pediatrics, 2003). No evidence exists to support person-to-person transmission. *B. henselae* is transmitted between cats via the cat flea. The incubation period is 7 to 12 days, with lymphadenopathy appearing in 5 to 50 days. Therapeutic management is supportive and is aimed at management of symptoms. The disease itself is usually self-limited, resolving on its own in 2 to 4 months. If lymphadenopathy persists or if the child is immunocompromised, antibiotics may be needed. Painful, swollen nodes may be treated with needle aspiration to provide symptom relief.

Nursing Assessment

Note history of headaches and fatigue. The history may also include interaction or rough play with cats or kittens, resulting in a scratch. Document the temperature, noting fever. Palpate for enlarged lymph nodes, noting their location. A skin papule may be present or reported. Diagnostic tests are available to detect serum antibodies to antigens of *Bartonella* species.

Nursing Management

Administer antibiotics if ordered. No transmission-based isolation is required; standard precautions are sufficient.

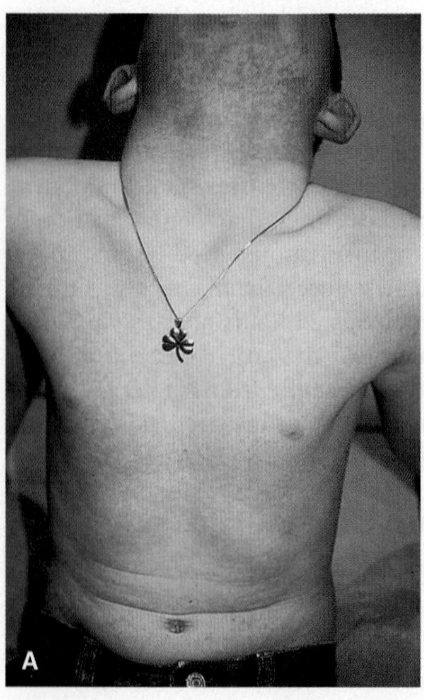

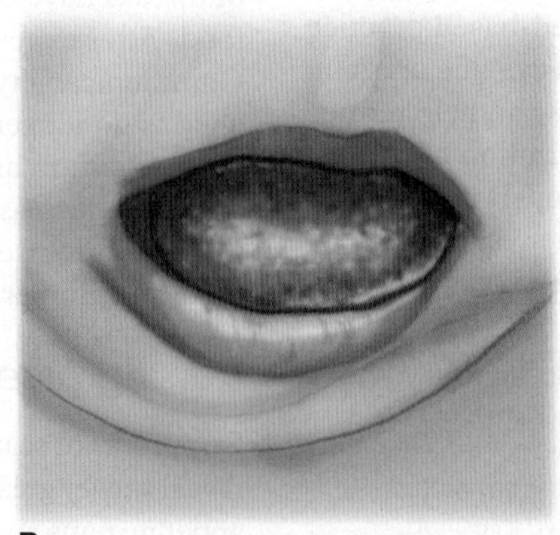

● **Figure 16.1** (**A**) Rash of scarlet fever. (**B**) Strawberry tongue.

Educate the client and family about prevention and control measures. Teach children to avoid rough play with cats and kittens. Teach parents and children to immediately wash any bites or scratches with soap and running water. Explain that cats should never lick open wounds on the child. Control of fleas in cats is important to prevent the spread of *B. henselae*.

● DIPHTHERIA

Diphtheria is caused by infection with *Corynebacterium diphtheriae* and may affect the nose, larynx, tonsils or pharynx. Tonsillar and pharyngeal infections are the most common and will be the focus of this discussion. A pseudomembrane forms over the pharynx, uvula, tonsils, and soft palate (Fig. 16.2). The neck becomes edematous and lymphadenopathy develops. The pseudomembrane causes airway obstruction and suffocation. Diphtheria generally occurs in children less than 15 years old who are unimmunized. Routine infant immunization can prevent the disease from occurring. Therapeutic management involves administration of antibiotics and antitoxin, as well as airway management.

Nursing Assessment

Children at risk for diphtheria are those who are unimmunized. Note history of sore throat and fever, usually less than 38.9° C. As the pseudomembrane forms, swallowing becomes difficult and signs of airway obstruction become apparent. A specimen of the membrane may be cultured for *Corynebacterium diphtheriae*.

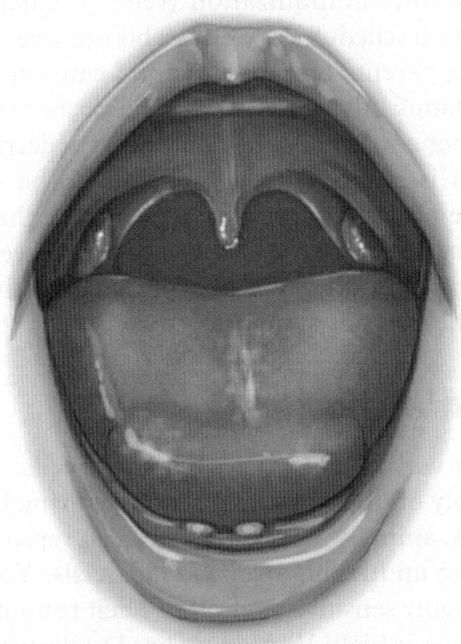

● **Figure 16.2** In diphtheria a pseudomembrane forms over the pharynx, uvula, tonsils, and soft palate.

Nursing Management

Close observation of respiratory status is of utmost importance. Administration of antibiotics and the antitoxin is critical to encourage sloughing of the membrane. The child should remain on strict droplet precautions in addition to standard precautions and should maintain bed rest.

● PERTUSSIS

Pertussis is an acute respiratory disorder characterized by paroxysmal cough (whooping cough) and copious secretions. It primarily occurs in children 4 years and younger and is most severe in children less than 6 months of age. The disease is caused by *Bordatella pertussis*. The incubation period is 6 to 21 days, usually 7 to 10 days. Pertussis usually starts with 7 to 10 days of cold symptoms. The paroxysmal coughing spells then begin and can last 1 to 4 weeks. Convalescence occurs over the course of several weeks to months. Immunization has decreased the incidence of pertussis, but the increasing numbers of unimmunized children, particularly immigrants, contribute to the incidence of the disease. Complications include seizures, pneumonia, encephalopathy, and death.

Therapeutic Management

Therapeutic management of pertussis focuses on eradication of the bacterial infection and respiratory support. CDC guidelines recommend antimicrobial treatment. For infants older than 1 month of age, macrolide drugs, including erythromycin, clarithromycin, and azithromycin, are the drugs of choice. For younger infants, azithromycin should be used and erythromycin and clarithromycin avoided. An alternative to macrolides in children older than 2 months is trimethoprim–sulfamethoxazole (TMP-SMZ).

Nursing Assessment

The most important risk factor for the development of pertussis is the lack of immunization against it. The history may reveal cold and cough symptoms, progressing to paroxysmal coughing spells. During the paroxysms, the child might cough 10 to 30 times in a row, followed by a whooping sound. This might be accompanied by redness in the face, progressive cyanosis, and protrusion of the tongue. Saliva, mucus, and tears flow from the mouth, nose, and eyes. Between the paroxysmal episodes, the child might rest well and appear relatively unaffected. Auscultate the lungs to assess air exchange. The diagnosis may be confirmed by immunofluorescent assay positive for *B. pertussis*.

Nursing Management

Nursing care will focus on providing a high-humidity environment and suctioning frequently to mobilize secretions. Observe for signs of airway obstruction. Encourage fluids to keep secretions thin and maintain adequate hydration. Offer reassurance to the child and family; the coughing episodes can be very frightening. Droplet precautions along with standard precautions are necessary for the hospitalized child.

● TETANUS

Tetanus is an acute, often fatal neurologic disease caused by the toxins produced by *Clostridium tetani.* Tetanus is rare in the United States but continues to be significant worldwide due to lack of routine immunization. It is characterized by increased muscle tone and spasm. *C. tetani* spores can live anywhere but are found most commonly in soil, dust, and feces from human or animals, such as sheep, cattle, chickens, dogs, cats, and rats. The spores can enter the body through a wound that is contaminated, through a burn, or by injecting contaminated street drugs. Once it enters the body, an anaerobic environment allows it to multiply and a poisonous toxin is released.

There are four forms of tetanus. Neonatal tetanus is the most common worldwide, affecting newborns in the first week of life secondary to an infected umbilical stump or unsterile surgical technique during circumcision. Most women in the United States have been immunized and will pass the immunity to their fetus. Along with proper hygiene during delivery and adequate cord care, this makes this type rare in the United States, but in underdeveloped countries it remains a significant problem. The second form is local tetanus. This rare form is characterized by local muscle spasms within the area of the wound. The third type is cephalic tetanus, which is associated with recurrent otitis media or head trauma. It is also rare and affects the cranial nerves, especially facial nerves. Generalized tetanus is the most common form and results in spasms that progress in a descending fashion beginning at the jaw. The most profoundly affected muscles are those of the neck and back. In the United States the fatality rate associated with tetanus has declined and cases are rare, but 3 out of 10 cases will result in death (American Academy of Pediatrics, 2003). The general incubation period is 3 to 21 days; it averages 8 days. Recovery can be long and difficult, and children with tetanus may have to spend several weeks in the hospital in an intensive care setting. It has been suggested that the shorter the incubation period, the higher the risk of more severe illness and poorer prognosis. Complications associated with tetanus include breathing problems, fractures, elevated blood pressure, dysrhythmias, clotting in the blood vessels of the lung, pneumonia, and coma.

Therapeutic management is directed toward supporting respiratory and cardiovascular function. Tetanus immunoglobulin may be given as well as the tetanus vaccine. Removal of the offending organism, by débridement of the wound, may occur, and intravenous antibiotics such as metronidazole may be initiated. In severe cases, the child may require intensive nursing care with mechanical ventilation.

Nursing Assessment

Note history of initial signs such as headache, spasms, crankiness, and cramping of the jaw (lockjaw), which are followed by difficulty swallowing and a stiff neck. Tetanus progresses in a descending fashion to other muscle groups, causing spasms of the neck, arms, legs, and stomach; seizures may result. Document the presence of fever along with an elevated blood pressure and tachycardia. Opisthotonos may be noted due to severe spasms of the neck and back. The spasms or muscle contractions in children may be strong enough to result in fractures. The diagnosis of tetanus is based on the clinical findings of the history and physical examination.

Nursing Management

Nursing management focuses on observing for signs of respiratory distress. Provide a quiet environment with reduced external stimuli to decrease the incidence of spasms. Appropriately manage pain. Encourage adequate nutrition and hydration. Administer sedatives and muscle relaxants as ordered to reduce the pain associated with the muscle spasms and to prevent seizures. Encourage the parents to stay with their child. The child's mental status is unaffected by the disease, and therefore he or she is aware of what is happening. Efforts need to be made to reduce the child's anxiety and to provide reassuring, sympathetic care to the child and family.

Tetanus is a preventable but potentially fatal disease. Education is essential regarding the importance of receiving this routine immunization (refer to Chapter 9 for immunization schedule) as well as a booster every 10 years. Instructing parents on proper wound care can also help prevent tetanus. All wounds should be cleaned thoroughly and a proper antiseptic used. If a wound is deep and contamination is suspected, the child should be seen by a health care professional. If it has been more than 5 years since the last tetanus dose, a booster may be needed. This can help to neutralize the poison and prevent it from entering the nervous system.

Viral Infections

Viruses are very small particles that infect cells. They cannot multiply on their own and require a living host, such as humans, animals, or plants. They can reproduce only by invading and taking over the host cells. Young children are highly sensitive to viruses. Their resistance is low and exposure is high. Viruses are hard to destroy without damaging or killing the living cells they infect. This is why drugs are not used to control them. Many viral diseases can be prevented by immunization such as measles, rubella, varicella, mumps, and poliomyelitis (see Chapter 9 for more information on immunizations).

• VIRAL EXANTHEMS

Many viral infections of the skin in childhood are called viral exanthems. **Exanthem** means rash or skin eruption. Viral exanthems of childhood often present with a distinct rash pattern that assists in the diagnosis of the virus. Table 16.4 discusses common childhood exanthems.

Typically, children with viral exanthems are cared for at home, but there are times when a child may be hospitalized or may develop the disease while being hospitalized. Appropriate transmission-based precautions must be taken.

Immunizations have led to a decrease in the incidence of certain viral exanthems, such as measles, rubella, and varicella (refer to Chapter 9 for immunization information).

Therapeutic management of the viral exanthems focuses on fever management and relief of discomfort.

Nursing Assessment

Obtain the history of the present illness, noting the onset of rash in relation to the onset of fever. Note accompanying symptoms such as respiratory complaints. Document known exposure to childhood diseases. Note immunization status. Inspect the skin for rash, noting the distribution, type, and extent of lesions. Table 16.4 describes the rash as well as accompanying symptoms for each of the viral exanthems.

Nursing Management

Nursing management of viral exanthems focuses on fever reduction, relief of discomfort, and protection of skin integrity. Encourage hydration. Administer antipyretics and antipruritics as needed (refer to Drug Guide 16.1). Nonpharmacologic interventions to reduce fever, such as tepid sponging and cool compresses, may be used. Refer to Nursing Care Plan 16.1 for additional information; care should be individualized based on the child's and family's response to the illness.

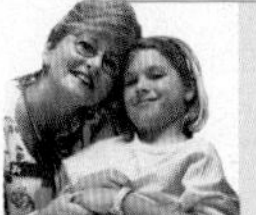

Trim the child's fingernails or cover hands with mitts, gloves, or socks (which work well with younger infants and children) if the rash itches to help prevent breaks in the skin, which can lead to discomfort and infection.

• MUMPS

Mumps, a contagious disease caused by Paramyxovirus, is characterized by fever and parotitis (inflammation and swelling of the parotid gland). Mumps is spread via contact with infected droplets. Infected individuals are contagious for 1 to 7 days prior to onset of symptoms and for 7 to 9 days after parotid swelling begins. The American Academy of Pediatrics recommends immunization against mumps for all children. Mumps occurs most frequently in unimmunized children between 5 and 19 years of age. About one third of all infected prepubertal boys also develop orchitis (inflammation of the testicle). Complications of mumps include meningoencephalitis with seizures and auditory neuritis, which can result in deafness. Therapeutic management is supportive.

Nursing Assessment

Note history of exposure to infected individuals as well as immunization status. Determine history of low-grade fever and onset and progression of parotid swelling. History may also include malaise, anorexia, headache, and abdominal pain. The parotid swelling is easily observed as swelling of the neck either bilaterally or unilaterally (Fig. 16.3). In boys, note orchitis. The diagnosis is usually based on the history and clinical presentation, but serum may be tested for the presence of mumps immunoglobulin G (IgG) or immunoglobulin M (IgM) **antibody.**

Nursing Management

Nursing management of mumps is primarily supportive. Acetaminophen is used for fever management, and occasionally narcotic analgesics may be required for pain management. Oral fluids are encouraged to prevent dehydration. If orchitis is present, ice packs to the testicles and gentle testicular support may be helpful. Hospitalized patients should be confined to respiratory isolation to prevent spread of the disease. Infected children are considered no longer be contagious 9 days following onset of parotid swelling. Current recommendations include first mumps immunization by 15 months of age followed by a second vaccine between 4 and 6 years of age (see Chapter 9 for information related to mumps vaccination).

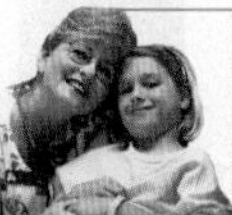

In recent years mumps outbreaks have occurred; mainly they have been seen on college campuses. The mumps vaccine is not 100% effective, and mumps infection can be seen in vaccinated individuals. Per the CDC (2006), one dose of MMR prevents 80% of cases and two doses prevent approximately 90% of cases. During an outbreak it is essential to define the population at risk and transmission setting, identify and isolate suspected cases, and identify and vaccinate susceptible individuals (CDC, 2006).

• POLIOMYELITIS

Poliomyelitis is an infection caused by the highly infectious poliovirus, which is an enterovirus. The virus invades the central nervous system and can progress to total paralysis.

(text continues on page 445)

Table 16.4 Common Viral Exanthems of Childhood

Disease	Causative Organism	Source	Transmission	Incubation Period	Period of Communicability
Rubella (German measles)	Rubella virus	Primarily nasopharyngeal secretions; also present in blood, stool, and urine of infected persons Peak incidence during late winter and early spring	Usually direct or indirect contact with droplets Mother to fetus	14 to 23 days, usually 16 to 18	7 days before to 7 days after onset of rash
Rubeola (measles)	Measles virus	Nasopharyngeal secretions, blood, and urine of infected persons	Highly contagious Usually direct or indirect contact with droplets	10 to 12 days	1 to 2 days before the onset of symptoms (3 to 5 days before onset of rash) to 5 days after rash has appeared
Varicella zoster virus (chickenpox)	Varicella zoster, human herpes virus 3	Nasopharyngeal secretions Peak occurrence late fall, winter, and spring	Highly contagious Direct contact with infected persons or airborne spread, to a lesser degree contact with lesions (scabbed lesions are not infectious) Can be transmitted transplacentally from mother to fetus	14 to 21 days, usually 14 to 16	1 to 2 days before onset of rash until all vesicles have crusted over (about 3 to 7 days after onset of rash)

Exanthem subitum (roseola infantum or sixth disease)	Human herpesvirus 6 (HHV-6); less frequently human herpesvirus 7 (HHV-7)	Unknown, but most adults secrete HHV-6 and HHV-7 in saliva, so may serve as primary source. Usually limited to children <3 years old; peak incidence 6 to 15 months of age	Little is known; suspected to be from saliva of infected person and enters the host through the oral, nasal, or conjunctival mucosa	5 to 15 days, average of 10 days	Unknown, but most likely contagious during fever stage
Erythema infectiosum (fifth disease)	Human parvovirus B19	Infected person Seasonal peaks are in late winter and early spring.	Respiratory route Large droplet spread from nasopharyngeal viral shedding Percutaneous exposure to blood and blood products Mother to fetus	4 to 21 days, average 16 to 17 days	Uncertain, but most children are no longer infectious by the time the rash appears and diagnosis is made. Isolation or exclusion from school, once child is diagnosed, is unnecessary. Those with aplastic crisis may be communicable up to 1 week after onset of symptoms. Those who are immunosuppressed with chronic infection and severe anemia may be communicable for months to years.
Hand, foot and mouth disease, or herpangina (if only mouth) involvement	Coxsackie A viruses (esp. A16)	Spread via fecal–oral route, particularly in children who wear diapers (1- to 4-year-olds) Most common during spring and summer	Direct contact with infected fecal, oral secretions; spread mostly through saliva	3 to 6 days	From time of infection until fever resolves; virus is shed for several weeks after the infection begins

(continued)

Table 16.4 Common Viral Exanthems of Childhood (continued)

Disease	Clinical Manifestations	Management/Complications	Nursing Implications
Rubella (German measles) 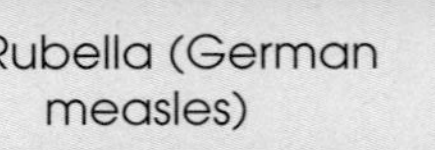 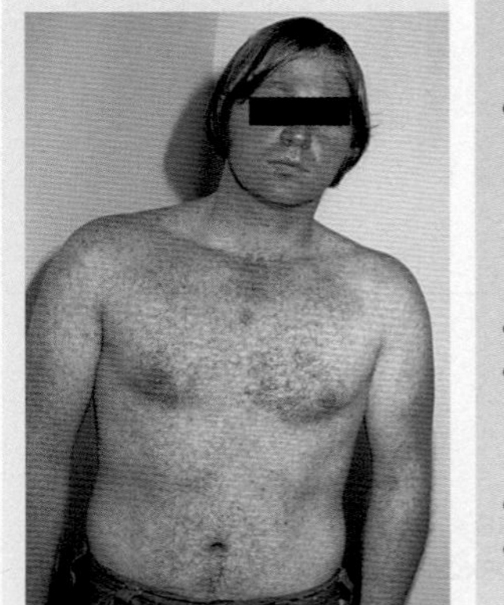	• Characteristic sign is lymphadenopathy (retroauricular, posterior cervical, postoccipital) 24 hours before the onset of the rash; may last up to 1 week. • Rash begins on face and spreads quickly down the neck, trunk, and extremities; on the second day the rash may appear pinpoint and resemble the rash of scarlet fever. • Mild pruritus may occur. • The rash disappears in the same order it spread and is usually cleared by the third day. Desquamation is minimal. • Rubella without a rash has been noted. • Polyarthralgia and polyarthritis are rare in children but common in adolescents.	• Disease is usually mild and self-limiting. • Treatment is mainly supportive. • Complications: Encephalitis and thrombocytopenia are rare. • Maternal rubella during pregnancy can result in miscarriage, fetal death, or congenital malformations.	• Institute comfort measures, such as antipyretics, antipruritics, and analgesics for joint pain. • Contact precautions in addition to standard precautions for the duration of the illness in the hospitalized child • Avoid exposure to pregnant women.
Rubeola (measles) 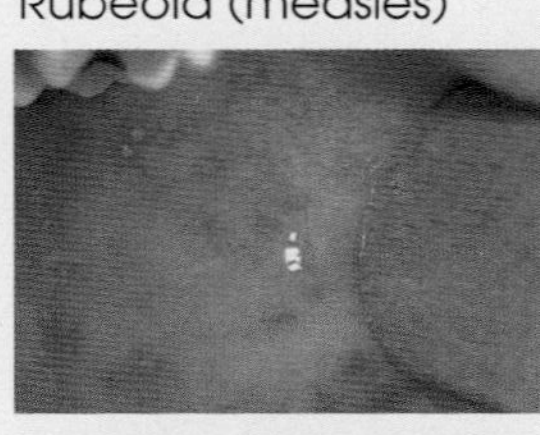 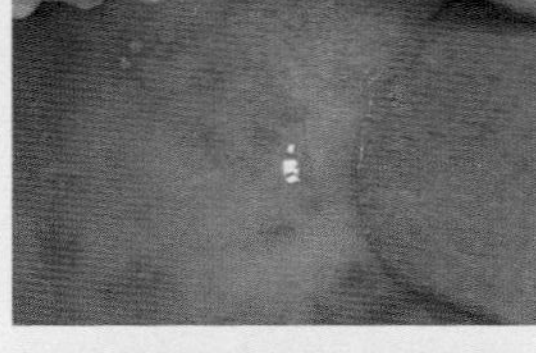	• Prodromal phase: 3 to 5 days, consisting of fever, cough, coryza (inflammation of the mucous membranes lining the nose), conjunctivitis • Followed by Koplik spots • Erythematous maculopapular rash appears 3 to 4 days after the onset of the prodromal phase.	• American Academy of Pediatrics recommends consideration of vitamin A supplementation in children 6 months to 2 years hospitalized for measles or its complications or those with measles and immunodeficiency (Behrman et al., 2004). • In developing countries, treatment with vitamin A can reduce morbidity and mortality. • Treatment is mainly supportive; may include antipyretics, bed rest, maintenance of adequate fluid intake. • Complications: otitis media broncho-pneumonia, laryngotracheobronchitis (croup), and diarrhea common in young children; acute encephalitis	• Institute comfort measures, such as antipyretics and antipruritics. • Provide eye care: clean eyes with warm, moist cloth to remove secretions. • Soothe coryza and cough using cool mist humidification to alleviate symptoms. • Droplet precautions until fifth day of rash in addition to standard precautions

Varicella zoster virus (chickenpox)	• Prodromal symptoms may be present 24 to 48 hours before the onset of the rash, such as fever, malaise, anorexia, headache, and mild abdominal pain. • Lesions often appear first on scalp, face, and trunk; initially intensely pruritic erythematous macules that evolve to papules and then form clear, fluid-filled vesicles • Vesicles eventually erupt, and then lesions scab and crust. • More severe in adolescents and adults than in young children	• Treatment: Antiviral therapy and varicella zoster immune globulin may be used in those considered to be at high risk, such as immuno-compromised, pregnant women, and newborns exposed to maternal varicella • American Academy of Pediatrics does not recommend routine antiviral therapy for the treatment of uncomplicated varicella infection in otherwise healthy children. • In most cases, varicella infection is self-limiting. • Treatment is mainly supportive: fever reduction, antipruritics to relieve itching, and skin care to prevent infection of lesions. • Complications: bacterial superinfection of skin lesions, thrombocytopenia, arthritis, hepatitis, cerebellar ataxia, encephalitis, meningitis, pneumonia, and glomerulonephritis • Congenital infection and life-threatening perinatal infection • Varicella zoster results in a lifelong latent infection. Reactivation results in herpes zoster (shingles), uncommon in childhood.	• Institute comfort measures, such as antipyretics and antipruritics. • Airborne and contact precautions, in addition to standard precautions in the hospitalized child for a minimum of 5 days after onset of rash and as long as vesicular lesions are present • For those with exposure to susceptible persons, airborne and contact precautions, in addition to standard precautions from 8 to 21 days after exposure • Children may return to school or childcare once lesions have crusted.
Exanthem subitum (roseola infantum) 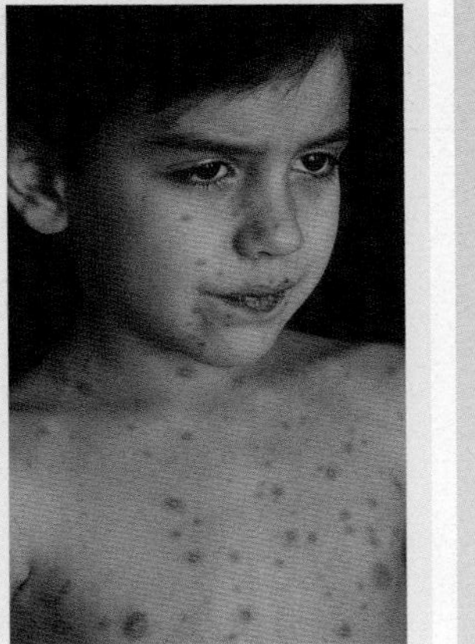	• Prodromal phase: usually asymptomatic but may include upper respiratory signs • Clinical illness: high fever ranging from 37.9° to 40° C (101° to 106° F) for 3 to 5 days; resolves abruptly; rash appears 12 to 24 hours later; rash usually lasts 1 to 3 days	• Generally benign; children generally are quite comfortable • In children who are uncomfortable or irritable or have a history of febrile seizures, antipyretics may be warranted. • Complications: HSV-6 may be responsible for some febrile seizures • Can progress to central nervous system involvement, encephalitis, and meningoencephalitis (rare)	• Institute comfort measures, such as antipyretics, antipruritics. • Standard precautions are sufficient in the hospitalized child.

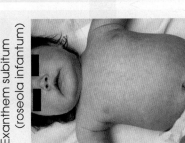

(continued)

Table 16.4 Common Viral Exanthems of Childhood (continued)

Disease	Clinical Manifestations	Management/Complications	Nursing Implications

Erythema infectiosum (fifth disease)	• Prodromal phase: mild symptoms, low-grade fever, headache, mild upper respiratory infection
	• Characteristic rash presents in three stages:
	  • Begins with erythematous flushing and often described as "slapped-cheek" appearance, often with circumoral pallor
	  • Spreads to trunk
	  • Moves peripherally, presenting as a maculopapular, lace-like appearance
	  • Palms and soles are usually spared; rash often is pruritic.
	  • Rash fluctuates in intensity and will disappear and reappear with environmental changes such as exposure to sunlight.
	  • Rash resolves spontaneously over 1 to 3 weeks.
	• Children with preexisting anemias may develop aplastic crisis.
	• In children with aplastic crisis rash is usually absent, but may present with prodromal symptoms of fever, malaise, and myalgia.
		• Disease in usually benign and self-limited.
		• Supportive treatment: antipyretics and antipruritics to improve comfort
		• Children with hemolytic disease, such as sickle cell, or immunodeficiency are at risk for aplastic crisis.
		• Blood transfusion may be necessary in children with aplastic crisis.
		• Complications: arthritis and arthralgia
		• May result in fetal loss if mother is infected during pregnancy (greatest risk seems to be in second trimester). Can also result in congestive heart failure (hydrops fetalis). The risk of transplacental infection is 30% if the woman is infected during pregnancy (Weir, 2005).
			• Institute comfort measures, such as antipyretics, antipruritics.
			• Droplet precautions in addition to standard precautions are required in the hospitalized child.
			• Pregnant women (including health care workers) need to be informed of the potential risks to the fetus and preventive measures to decrease these risks (strict infection control practices, not caring for those likely to be contagious, such as immunocompromised patients with chronic parvovirus infection or patients with parvovirus associated aplastic crisis).
			• The CDCI does not recommended routine exclusion from a workplace where an outbreak is occurring.

Hand foot and mouth disease	• Vesicles on tongue and oral mucosa erode to shallow ulcers; vesicles on hands and feet are football-shaped with erythematous rims. Fever usually occurs first. Extensive mouth lesions may lead to anorexia, dehydration, and drooling.	• Disease is usually mild and self-limiting, resolving within 1 week. • Treatment is mainly supportive. • Dehydration may occur if mouth lesions are significant. Meningitis, encephalitis, and pulmonary edema are rare complications.	• Contact precautions and good hand hygiene are necessary. Encourage oral fluids of preference, Popsicles. Provide analgesics such as acetaminophen as needed.

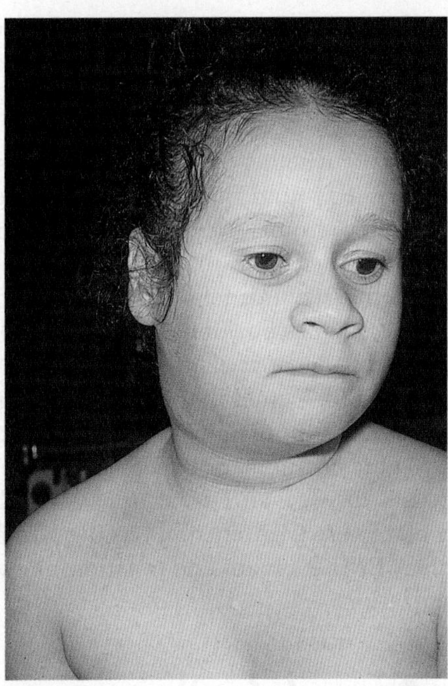

● Figure 16.3 Parotitis associated with mumps.

Transmission occurs through direct or indirect contact. The poliovirus is spread most commonly via the fecal-to-oral route, or by the oral-to-oral route. Polio most commonly occurs in young children and is also referred to as infantile paralysis. This disease is rare due to effective immunization programs but is still seen in developing countries in the eastern Mediterranean region, India, and Africa.

Nursing Assessment

Initial signs and symptoms include fever, fatigue, headache, vomiting, neck stiffness, and limb pain. Symptoms then progress to tremors of the extremities and possible paralysis. Kernig's sign will be positive and deep tendon reflexes will be hyperactive initially and then diminished. Paralysis is asymmetric and generally affects the legs more than the arms. Respiratory problems can occur if the respiratory center of the brain is involved. The poliovirus can be isolated in feces or the pharynx of infected individuals and cerebrospinal fluid evaluation will generally show elevated leukocytes and protein.

Nursing Management

Nursing management is aimed at providing supportive care, focusing on maintaining respiratory status and nutritional status until the illness has run its course. Bed rest will usually be ordered, so skin care is a priority. Maintaining self-care and mobility are also important nursing functions. Long-term care providing therapy and bracing to help strengthen muscles may be needed during and after hospitalization.

No cure for polio exists, but it can be prevented by the polio vaccine, which is routinely administered in developed countries (refer to the immunization schedule in Chapter 9). Oral polio vaccine (OPV) is a live strain, and thus the virus is shed in the stool for up to 6 weeks after immunization, leading to the risk for vaccine-acquired polio in caregivers. For this reason, OPV has been replaced by inactivated polio vaccine (IPV), an injectable form, in the United States. OPV is still used in developing countries, however, so immigrants or travelers whose children were recently immunized in their home country should take precautions if they are immunocompromised or unvaccinated. Areas where polio is endemic, including Afghanistan, Egypt, India, Niger, Nigeria, and Pakistan, agreed to a massive immunization campaign in 2004 and hope to make polio the first eradicated disease of the 21st century (Stephenson, 2004).

● RABIES

Rabies is a preventable viral infection of the central nervous system. It is transmitted to other animals and humans through close contact with the saliva of a rabid animal, usually by a bite. The number of cases of rabies has steadily declined in the United States. It is rare in the United States and Western Europe due to routine vaccination of domestic animals, such as dogs, and the availability of effective postexposure prophylaxis. Now most cases of rabies in these areas are due to wild animals such as raccoons, skunks, bats, and foxes. Rabies continues to be a major health problem in other parts of the world, especially in areas where dogs are not controlled.

Most cases of rabies occur in children less than 15 years of age, and most human deaths occur in developing countries. Children have an increased susceptibility to rabies due to their fearlessness around animals, eagerness to play with animals, shorter stature, and inability to protect themselves. The incubation period for rabies is extremely variable and can range from 20 to 180 days, with the peak at 30 to 60 days (Behrman et al., 2004). The incubation period tends to be shorter in children. Once symptoms of rabies have developed the prognosis is poor: death usually occurs within days of the onset of symptoms. Prevention is paramount and eliminating infection in animal vectors is essential. Successful animal vaccination and animal control campaigns in the United States have led to a very low rate of human rabies cases. Rabies among dogs in the United States has been virtually eliminated. Recently, rabies transmitted from other animals, especially bat bites, has become a cause for concern.

The decision to provide postexposure prophylaxis can be complex. The local health department should be contacted. Several factors need to be considered, such as local epidemiology, type of animal involved, availability of the responsible animal for testing or quarantine, and the circumstances around the exposure, such as a provoked versus unprovoked attack. In the United States, concurrent use of passive and active immunoprophylaxis is recommended. It consists of a regimen of one dose of immune globulin and five doses of human rabies vaccine over a 28-day period. Rabies immune globulin and the first dose of rabies vaccine should be given as soon as possible after exposure, ideally within 24 hours. Additional doses of rabies vaccine should be given on days 3, 7, 14, and 28 after the first vaccination. Rabies immune globulin is infiltrated into and around the wound, with any remaining volume administered intramuscularly at a site distant from the vaccine inoculation. Human rabies vaccine is administered intramuscularly into the anterolateral thigh or deltoid, depending on the age and size of the child. Administration into the gluteus muscle should be avoided, since this site has been associated with vaccine failure (Behrman et al., 2004).

Nursing Assessment

Note history of an animal bite, especially if it was unprovoked, and exposure to bats. Document history of early symptoms of rabies infection, which are nonspecific and flu-like, such as fever, headache, and general malaise. The child may complain of pain, pruritus, and paresthesia at the bite site. As the virus spreads to the central nervous system, encephalitis develops. The disease will have progressive neurologic manifestations, which may include insomnia, confusion, anxiety, changes in behavior, agitation or excitation, hallucinations, hypersalivation, dysphagia, and hydrophobia, which results from aspiration when swallowing liquid or saliva. In some cases progressive paralysis may be present. The client may have periods of lucidity alternating with these neurologic changes.

Laboratory testing may include hair and saliva specimens from which the virus may be isolated. Serum and cerebrospinal fluid can be tested for antibodies to the rabies virus. Direct fluorescent antibody test can be done to diagnose rabies in a suspected animal. The test can only be done postmortem and requires brain tissue from the potentially rabid animal.

Nursing Management

Few patients survive once symptomatic rabies infection develops. Intensive supportive care is required, but recovery is extremely rare. Therefore, it is vital to educate children and families about the importance of seeking medical care after any animal bite to prevent death from rabies infection. Also, teach children to avoid wild animals, stray animals, and any animal with unusual behavior. Teach children not to provoke or attempt to capture wild or stray animals.

Regardless of whether immunoprophylaxis is initiated, appropriate wound management is necessary in all victims of a bite from a potentially rabid animal. This includes a thorough cleansing of all wounds with soap and water. Irrigation of wounds for at least 10 minutes with a virucidal agent, such as povidone–iodine solution, is recommended (Behrman et al., 2004).

When caring for a child requiring postexposure prophylaxis, provide support and education to the child and family. Due to the seriousness and urgency surrounding this disease and treatment, the child and family are often very frightened. Consider comfort measures, such as EMLA cream and positioning, when giving immunization.

Vector-Borne Infections

Children are at a particular risk for contracting vector-borne diseases, which are diseases transmitted by ticks, mosquitoes, or other insect vectors (Table 16.5). Young children are unaware of the health risks around them and cannot take protective measures. Their immature immune system leads to a decreased capacity to resist vector-borne diseases. These diseases can be severe and even fatal, though most are treatable if identified early. Many times the child presents initially with nonspecific symptoms. Coupled with the fact that there are few definitive diagnostic tests available, this can lead to difficulty in promptly recognizing and treating these diseases.

Tick-borne diseases are the most common vector-borne illnesses in the United States. Two of the most common will be covered below.

• LYME DISEASE

Lyme disease, the most common vector-borne disease in the United States, is caused by the spirochete *Borrelia burgdorferi*. It is transmitted to humans via the bite of an infected blacklegged tick. It has been reported in more than 50 countries and is seen in three distinct regions in the United States. Most cases occur in the Northeast, from southern Maine to northern Virginia. Cases have also been reported in the upper Midwest and the West Coast, especially northern California, but with less frequency. Most cases are seen between April and October. Lyme disease can affect any age group, but the reported incidence is highest among children 5 to 10 years of age (Behrman et al., 2004). The prognosis for recovery in children who are treated is excellent.

Table 16.5 Other Vector-Borne Illnesses

Disease	Causative Organism	Geographic Distribution	Vector of Transmission	Manifestations
Mediterranean spotted fever (boutonneuse fever)	*Rickettsia conorii*	Africa, Mediterranean region, India, Middle East	Tick bite	• Fever, headache, maculopapular rash • Eschar may be present at tick bite.
Rickettsialpox	*Rickettsia akari*	Northeastern cities in United States, Europe and Asia, mainly urban settings	Mouse mite bite	• Bite becomes a papule, then pustule, then ulcerates and forms eschar at site. Fever, local adenopathy, headache, myalgia, maculopapular rash that may become vesicular.
Epidemic typhus	*Rickettsia prowazekii*	Africa, South America, Central America, Mexico, Asia; occasional cases seen in United States	Louse feces (typically from the body louse) that are rubbed into broken skin or mucous membranes. Cases in United States associated with louse or flea of flying squirrel.	• Abrupt onset of high fever, chills, and myalgia with severe headache and malaise • Rash appears 4 to 7 days after onset of symptoms, beginning on the trunk and spreading to the extremities. • Maculopapular rash becomes petechial or hemorrhagic, then develops brown pigmented areas. • Changes in mental status may occur. • Flying squirrel–related disease typically presents as a milder illness.
Endemic typhus (murine typhus)	*Rickettsia typhi* and *Rickettsia felis*	Worldwide, especially warm coastal ports. In United States, most prevalent in southern Texas and southern California.	Rat flea or cat flea feces	• Headache, myalgia, and chills that slowly worsen • Fever for 10 to 14 days • Rash appears after 3 to 8 days; it is macular or maculopapular with sparse lesions and no hemorrhage.

(continued)

Table 16.5 Other Vector-Borne Illnesses (continued)

Disease	Causative Organism	Geographic Distribution	Vector of Transmission	Manifestations
Scrub typhus	*Orientia tsutsugamushi*	Southern Asia, Japan, Indonesia, Australia, Korea, Asiatic Russia, India, China	Chigger bite	• Possible necrotic eschar at site of bite, fever, headache, myalgia, cough, and gastrointestinal symptoms • Lymphadenopathy, maculopapular rash on trunk and extremities
Ehrlichioses	3 pathogens: *Ehrlichia chaffeensis, Ehrlichia anaplasma, Ehrlichia ewimgii*	Mostly in southeastern and south-central United States	Tick	• Fever with clinical signs similar to Rocky Mountain spotted fever. Rash is less commonly associated. • May also present with leukopenia, anemia, and hepatitis

Q fever	*Coxiella burnetii*	Worldwide	Inhalation of infected aerosols, ingestion of contaminated dairy products	• Most cases are initially asymptomatic. Occurs in two forms:
				  • Acute: follows initial exposure and presents with abrupt onset of fever, chills, weakness, headache, and loss of appetite
				  • Chronic: occurs years after initial exposure and may present with endocarditis (in patients with underlying heart disease), hepatitis, or fever of unknown origin

Malaria	*Plasmodium* (four species exist that infect humans: *P. falciparum, P. vivax, P. ovale, P. malariae*)	Endemic in tropical areas of the world. Highest risk in sub-Saharan Africa, Papua New Guinea, the Solomon Islands, and Vanuatu. Other areas of risk: Haiti and Indian subcontinent.	Bite of *Anopheles* species of mosquito	• High fever with chills, rigors, sweats, and headache, which may be paroxysmal • Nausea, vomiting, diarrhea, cough, arthralgia, abdominal and back pain may also occur. • Anemia and thrombocytopenia with pallor and jaundice may be seen. • May occur in a cyclic pattern, and depending on the species fever may occur every other day or every third day

Therapeutic Management

In most cases Lyme disease can be cured by antibiotics, especially if they are started early in the illness. Doxycycline is the drug of choice for children older than 8 years. Because it can cause permanent discoloration of the teeth, children less than 8 should be treated with amoxicillin. For patients allergic to penicillin, cefuroxime or erythromycin can be used. Duration of treatment is usually 14 to 21 days.

Nursing Assessment

The clinical signs of Lyme disease are divided into three stages: early localized, early disseminated, and late disease. Untreated patients may progress through the three stages or may present with early disseminated or late disease without having any symptoms of the earlier stages. If children are treated in the early stage, it is uncommon to see them with late disease. Nursing assessment for Lyme disease includes an accurate health history as well as physical examination.

Health History

Explore the health history for a tick bite. Document onset of rash. In early localized disease, the rash usually occurs 7 to 14 days after the tick bite (though it can appear between 3 and 32 days after the bite). In early disseminated disease, the rash usually begins 3 to 5 weeks after the tick bite. Note complaints of fever, malaise, mild neck stiffness, headache, fatigue, myalgia, and arthralgia or pain in the joints. In late disease, note recurrent arthritis of the large joints, such as the knees, beginning weeks to months after the tick bite. The child with late disease may or may not have a history of earlier stages of the disease, including erythema migrans.

Physical Examination

Observe for a rash. Early local disease is characterized by a ring-like rash at the site of the tick bite (erythema migrans) (Fig. 16.4). If untreated, the rash gradually expands and will remain for 1 to 2 weeks. Early disseminated disease should be suspected if multiple areas of erythema migrans are found. The multiple lesions are usually smaller than the primary lesions. Note cranial nerve palsies (especially cranial nerve VII), conjunctivitis, or signs of meningeal irritation, which occur in early disseminated disease.

Laboratory and Diagnostic Testing

Immunoglobulin specific antibody tests may not be positive in the early stage of the disease but may be useful in the later stages. The CDC recommends a two-step test: a sensitive enzyme immunoassay (EIA) or immunofluorescent assay (IFA) followed by a Western immunoblot. If these are negative, no further testing is indicated.

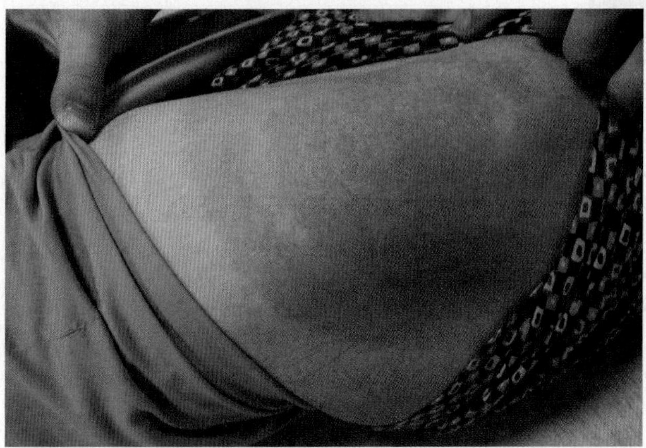

● Figure 16.4 Erythema migrans, a ring-like rash at the site of the tick bite, occurs in Lyme disease.

Nursing Management

Administer antibiotics as ordered. In the hospitalized patient, no transmission-based precautions are necessary. Educate the client and family on the importance of taking the antibiotic as directed and finishing all the medicine. Another important nursing function is educating the client, family, and community on prevention measures (Box 16.5). For infection to occur, the tick must be attached for 24 to 48 hours, so prompt removal of ticks is essential to the prevention of Lyme disease. Teaching Guideline 16.2 gives information on removal of ticks. A vaccine was licensed in 1998 by the U.S. Food and Drug Administration for persons ages 15 to 70, but it has since been withdrawn due to low demand. See Healthy People 2010.

● ROCKY MOUNTAIN SPOTTED FEVER

Rocky Mountain spotted fever (RMSF) is the most severe and frequently reported rickettsial illness in the United States. A rickettsia is a bacteria of the genus Rickettsiae;

> BOX 16.5
>
> **PREVENTION OF TICK-BORNE ILLNESSES**
>
> - Wear appropriate protective clothing when entering tick-infested areas. Clothing should fit tightly around wrists, waists, and ankles. Tuck pants into socks if possible.
> - After leaving the area, check for ticks and remove them promptly.
> - Insect repellent may provide temporary relief but may produce toxicity, especially in children, if used frequently, or in large doses.

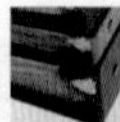

TEACHING GUIDELINE 16.2

Tick Removal

- Use fine-tipped tweezers.
- Protect fingers with a tissue, paper towel, or latex gloves.
- Grasp tick as close to the skin as possible and pull upward with steady, even pressure.
- Do not twist or jerk the tick.
- Once the tick is removed, clean site with soap and water and wash your hands.
- Save the tick for identification in case the child becomes sick. Place in a sealable plastic bag and put it in your freezer. Write date of bite on the bag.

these bacteria are carried as a parasite by many ticks, fleas, and lice and cause disease in humans. RMSF is caused by the bacteria *Rickettsia rickettsii.* The American dog tick and Rocky Mountain wood tick are the primary vectors, although others have been implicated. RMSF can be fatal without prompt and appropriate treatment. Most cases occur between April and September.

RMSF occurs throughout the United States; its name is derived from the fact that it was discovered in the Rocky Mountain region, though few cases are found there today. RMSF is more common in the coastal Atlantic states, with the highest incidence in North Carolina and Oklahoma. It occurs in all age groups but most frequently in children, with the peak incidence in 5- to 9-year-olds (Behrman et al., 2004).

Complications of RMSF include noncardiogenic pulmonary edema, cerebral edema, and multiorgan damage. Long-term neurologic involvement, such as partial paralysis of the lower extremities, hearing loss, loss of bladder and bowel control, movement disorders, and language disorders, may be seen, especially in patients with severe illness who require long hospital stays.

Therapeutic Management

The fatality rate from RMSF has decreased with the widespread use of antimicrobial therapy. However, delays in diagnosis and therapy are significant factors associated with severity of disease and death. In most cases RMSF resolves rapidly with appropriate antibiotic therapy, especially if it is started early. Treatments of choice are tetracyclines, such as doxycycline, and chloramphenicol. Chloramphenicol is the preferred drug in children less than 9 years old due to the risk of teeth staining, though some clinicians use doxycycline to treat children less than 9 because tooth discoloration is dose-dependent and children less than 9 are unlikely to need multiple doses (Behrman et al., 2004). Length of treatment is 5 to 10 days.

Nursing Assessment

Note history of early signs of RMSF, such as sudden onset of fever, headache, malaise, nausea and vomiting, muscle pain, and anorexia. The incubation period varies from 2 to 14 days, with the average being around 7 days after the tick bite. Late signs include a rash, usually seen 2 to 5 days after the onset of the fever, abdominal pain, joint pain, and diarrhea. Inspect the skin for a rash that starts as small, pink, macular, non-itchy, blanchable spots on the wrists, forearms, and ankles. The rash then spreads rapidly over the entire body, including the soles and palms. After several days the rash will appear red, spotted and petechial, or hemorrhagic (Fig. 16.5). Approximately 10% to 15% of patients with RMSF do not have a rash (Behrman et al., 2004). Laboratory findings may include a low leukocyte count, low or decreasing platelet count, and hyponatremia. Biopsy of the rash with immunofluorescent assay and serologic tests may also be used.

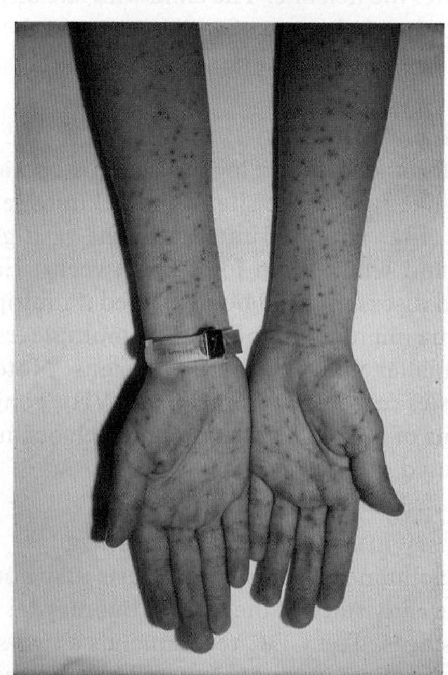

● Figure 16.5 Rash associated with Rocky Mountain spotted fever.

HEALTHY PEOPLE 2010

Objective	Significance
Reduce Lyme disease	• Educate the client, family, and community on prevention measures (refer to Box 16.5).

Nursing Management

Nursing management is similar to that for Lyme disease. Educate the family about completion of the antibiotic course, prevention of tick bites, and appropriate tick removal (refer to Box 16.5 and Teaching Guidelines 16.2).

Parasitic and Helminthic Infections

Parasites are organisms larger than yeast or bacteria that can cause infection. They live in or on a host. Parasites receive nourishment from the host without benefiting or killing the host. Parasites frequently seen in children are scabies and head lice. A helminth is a parasitic intestinal worm. Helminthic infections seen in children include pinworms, roundworms, and hookworms. Children are at an increased risk for parasitic or helminthic infections due to poor hygiene practices: they are typically more careless about hand washing and they tend to put things in their mouths and share toys and objects with other children.

Nursing Assessment and Management

Parents are often embarrassed when they find out that their child has a parasitic or helminthic infection. Reassure them that these infections can occur in any child. Tables 16.6 and 16.7 give nursing assessment and management information related to specific common parasitic and helminthic infections in children.

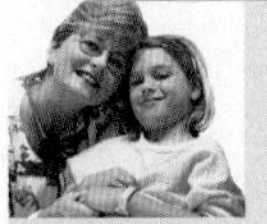

The head louse is becoming increasingly resistant to pediculicides. This may lead parents to resort to home remedies. Parents need to be informed that these remedies are unproven and can be toxic.

As the nurse at a pediatric clinic, you receive a call from a frantic mother. She tells you, "The school sent my daughter home and told me she has lice! We are clean people! I don't understand how this could happen!" How would you address her concerns? Discuss the plan of care for this child. What education and interventions will be necessary to prevent the spread of pediculosis capitis?

Sexually Transmitted Infections

Sexually transmitted infections (STIs), commonly called sexually transmitted diseases, are infectious diseases transmitted through sexual contact, including oral, vaginal, or anal intercourse. Certain infections can be transmitted *in utero* to the fetus or during childbirth to the newborn. Table 16.8 gives information on specific STIs and their effects on the fetus or newborn.

STIs are a major health concern for adolescents. The rates of many STIs are highest in adolescents. It is estimated that before graduating from high school, 25% of adolescents will contract an STI (American Academy of Pediatrics, 2003). Adolescents are at a greater risk for developing STIs for a variety of reasons: they frequently have unprotected intercourse, they are biologically more susceptible to infection, they engage in partnerships of limited duration, and they may have difficulty accessing the health care system.

Detection of STIs also serves as an important warning sign of potential sexual abuse in infants and children. Due to the serious implications that a diagnosis of an STI can have in children, only tests that have high specificities and that can isolate an organism should be used. Also, treatment for the child with a suspected STI may be held until a definitive diagnosis can be made. Chapter 27 provides information related to the human immunodeficiency virus.

Nursing Assessment

Many health care providers fail to assess sexual behavior and STI risks, to screen for asymptomatic infection during clinic visits, or to counsel patients on STI risk reduction. Nurses need to remember that they play a key role in the detection, prevention, and treatment of STIs in adolescents and children. All states allow adolescents to give consent to confidential STI testing and treatment. Table 16.9 discusses common clinical manifestations of the specific STIs in adolescents.

Nursing Management

Encourage the patient to complete the antibiotic prescription. Prevention of STIs among children and adolescents is critical, and health care providers have a unique opportunity to provide counseling and education in this setting. Adapt the style, content, and message to the patient's developmental level. Identify risk factors and risk behaviors and help the patient develop specific individualized actions for prevention. This conversation needs to be direct and nonjudgmental.

Encourage adolescents to postpone sexual intercourse for as long as possible, but explain the need to use barrier methods, such as male and female condoms, if they choose to have sexual intercourse. For teens who have already had sexual intercourse, encourage abstinence at this point and also encourage them to minimize their lifetime number of sexual partners, to use barrier methods consistently and correctly, and to be aware of the connection between drug and alcohol use (see Teaching Guideline 16.3, Table 16.10, and Healthy People 2010).

(text continues on page 463)

Table 16.6 Common Parasitic Infections Seen in Children

Infection	Causative Organism	Transmission	Clinical Manifestations	Diagnosis/Treatment	Isolation/Control Measures
Pediculosis capitis (head lice)	*Pediculus humanus capitis* (head louse)	Direct contact with hair of infested people, less commonly with personal belongings such as combs and hats, of those infested. Incubation period from laying of eggs to hatching of nymph is 6 to 10 days; adult lice will appear 2 to 3 weeks later.	Extreme pruritus is the most common symptom. Adult eggs (nits) or lice may be seen, especially behind the ears and at the nape of the neck.	Diagnosis by identification of eggs, nymph, and lice with the naked eye is possible; adult lice are rarely seen. Treatment: Washing hair with a pediculicide such as permethrin, lindane, malathion. Careful instructions on proper use of any product should be given and strict adherence to application instructions encouraged. Detection of living lice 24 hours after treatment suggests incorrect use, a very heavy infestation, reinfestation, or resistance to treatment. Removal of nits after treatment is not necessary to prevent spread but may be done for aesthetic reasons (American Academy of Pediatrics, 2003).	Contact precautions in addition to standard precautions Control measures: Household and other close contacts should be examined and if infested treated. Bedmates should be treated prophylactically. Children should not be excluded or sent home from school. Importance of environmental measures is controversial. Most children can be treated effectively without treating their clothing and bedding. If needed, dry-cleaning clothing or simply sealing it in a plastic bag for 10 days is effective. Disinfection of headgear, pillowcases, and towels by washing in hot water and drying on the hot cycle may be helpful, even though fomites do not play a role in transmission. Soaking combs and hairbrushes in pediculicide shampoo or hot water can also be done. Temperatures above 53.5 degrees C or 128.3 degrees F are lethal to lice (American Academy of Pediatrics, 2003). Not a sign of poor hygiene; all socioeconomic groups are affected

Pediculosis pubis (pubic lice)	*Phthirus pubis*	Transmission usually occurs through sexual contact; also can be through contaminated items such as towels.	Pruritus of anogenital area; other hairy areas of the body, including eyelashes, eyebrows, axilla, beard, can be affected	Diagnosis by identification of eggs, nymph, and lice with the naked eye is possible; adult lice are rarely seen. Same as treatment with pediculicides to treat head lice. Retreatment is recommended 7 to 10 days later. Petroleum oil is used to treat eyelashes and eyebrows.	Contact precautions in addition to standard precautions All sexual contacts should be treated.
Scabies	*Saracoptes scabiei*	Incubation period from laying of eggs to hatching of nymph is 6 to 10 days; adult lice will appear 2 to 3 weeks later. Transmission usually occurs through prolonged, close personal contact. Incubation period in those without previous exposure is 4 to 6 weeks. People who were previously infested can develop symptoms in 1 to 4 days.	Intense pruritus (especially at night) with presence of erythematous, papular rash with excoriations. The lesions are generally distributed but often are concentrated on the hands and feet and in body folds. May be found on head and neck, which is usually spared in adults. In infants and young children and those who are immunocompromised, the rash may include vesicles, pustules, or nodules.	Diagnosis can be made by a history of itching (especially at night), classic rash, and reports of itching in household or sexual contacts. Mites can be seen on microscopic examination of skin scrapings to confirm diagnosis. Treatment: A scabicide, such as permethrin or lindane, should be applied to the entire body below the head. Treatment of infants and young children should include the head, neck, and body. The cream is left on for a specified time (usually 8 to 14 hours) depending on the type of scabicide. Careful instructions on proper use of any product should be given and strict adherence to application instructions should be urged. Itching may not subside for several weeks, even after successful treatment.	Contact precautions in addition to standard precautions Prophylactic therapy for household members Bedding and clothing worn the 4 days prior to treatment should be laundered in hot water and dried on the hot cycle (mites do not survive more than 3 to 4 days without skin contact). Environmental disinfestation is unnecessary (American Academy of Pediatrics, 2003).

Table 16.7 Common Helminthic Infections in Children

Infection	Causative Organism	Clinical Manifestations	Transmission	Diagnosis/Treatment	Isolation/Control Measures
Roundworm (Ascariasis)	*Ascaris lumbricoides*, common in temperate and tropical areas	Loss of appetite, nausea, vomiting, and abdominal pain may be seen. In significant infestation, partial or complete intestinal obstruction may occur. The more worms, the worse the symptoms.	Human feces are the major source of infected eggs. Hand to mouth is the usual route of transmission. The eggs are swallowed due to unclean hands or contaminated food. They pass into the intestine; larvae then hatch, penetrate the intestinal wall, enter the circulatory system, and migrate to any body tissue.	Diagnosis: Once female worms are in the intestine, eggs can be visualized by microscopic evaluation of the stool. Occasionally a worm may be visualized in vomit or stool. Treatment is with mebendazole, albendazole, or pyrantel pamoate.	• Standard precautions are sufficient. • Sanitary disposal of feces • Proper hand hygiene
Hookworm	*Ancylostoma duodenale* (roundworm) (found mainly in Europe, Africa, China, Japan, India, and the Pacific Islands) and *Necator americanus* (roundworm) (found mainly in the Americas, Caribbean, Africa, Asia, and the Pacific)	Most often people are asymptomatic until significant worms are established. May see pruritic erythematous papular rash at entry site (referred to as ground itch) or pulmonary symptoms as the larvae migrate. One of the greatest concerns in chronic infection is anemia (microcytic hypochromic anemia) secondary to blood loss as the worms suck blood and juices from the intestines. This can lead to hypoproteinemia, edema, pica, and wasting. The infection may result in physical or mental retardation in children.	Hookworms are found in soil and enter the host through pores, hair follicles, and even intact skin (hands and feet are major sites of entry). The maturing larvae travel through the circulatory system into the lungs and then up the bronchial tree and are swallowed with secretions. They then migrate into the intestinal tract and attach to the wall of the small intestines, where they feed and reproduce. Transmission via ingested soil has been seen with *Ancylostoma duodenale* only.	Diagnosis is made through microscopic examination of feces that reveals hookworm eggs. Treatment: Albendazole, mebendazole, and pyrantel pamoate. In children younger than 2 the World Health Organization recommends half the adult dose of albendazole or mebendazole (American Academy of Pediatrics, 2003). Iron supplementation and possible blood transfusion in severe cases.	• Standard precautions are sufficient. • Proper sanitation and disposal of feces • Treatment of all known infested people • Screening of high-risk individuals • Encourage the wearing of shoes and avoiding being barefoot.

Pinworm	*Enterobius vermicularis* (roundworm)	Some people are asymptomatic. May cause anal itching (pruritus ani), especially at night. Other clinical findings may include teeth grinding at night, weight loss, and enuresis.	Fecal–oral route directly, indirectly, or inadvertently by contaminated hands or shared toys, bedding, clothing, toilet seats. Incubation period is 1 to 2 months or longer.	Diagnosis is made when adult worms are visualized in the perianal region; they are best viewed when the child is sleeping. Very few ova are present in stool, so examination of stool is not recommended. Transparent tape pressed to perianal area and then viewed under a microscope may reveal eggs. Three consecutive specimens should be obtained when the child first awakens in the morning. Treatment: Drug of choice is mebendazole, pyrantel pamoate, and albendazole, usually single doses and repeated in 2 weeks. In children less than 2, experience with these drugs is limited; therefore, risks and benefits need to be weighed before administration. All family members should be treated since transmission from person to person is very easy.	Standard precautions are sufficient. Reinfection occurs easily. Infected people should bathe in the morning, which will remove a large portion of the eggs. Frequent changing of underclothes and bedding. Personal hygiene measures such as keeping fingernails short, avoiding scratching of perianal area and nail biting. Good hand hygiene is the most effective preventive measure, especially after using the bathroom and before eating.

Table 16.8 Effects of Sexually Transmitted Infections on the Fetus or Newborn

STI	Effects on Fetus or Newborn
Chlamydia	Newborn can be infected during delivery. Eye infections (neonatal conjunctivitis), pneumonia, low birthweight, preterm birth, stillbirth
Gonorrhea	Newborn can be infected during delivery. Rhinitis, vaginitis, urethritis, inflammation of sites of fetal monitoring. Ophthalmia neonatorum can lead to blindness and sepsis (including arthritis and meningitis).
Herpes type II (genital herpes)	Contamination can occur during birth. Mental retardation, premature birth, low birthweight, death
Syphilis	Can be passed *in utero* Can result in fetal or infant death Congenital syphilis symptoms include skin ulcers, rashes, fever, weakened or hoarse cry, swollen liver and spleen, jaundice and anemia, various deformations.
Trichomoniasis	Fever, irritability, preterm birth, low birthweight
Venereal warts	May develops warts in throat (laryngeal papillomatosis); uncommon but life-threatening

Table 16.9 Sexually Transmitted Infections Common in Adolescents

Disease	Causative Organism	Transmission Mode	Diagnostic Testing	Female Symptoms	Male Symptoms	Treatment
Chlamydia Curable STI Seen frequently among sexually active adolescents and young adults Sexually active adolescents should be screened at least annually.	*Chlamydia trachomatis* (bacteria)	Vaginal, anal, oral sex, and by childbirth	Culture fluid from urethral swabs in males or endocervical swabs for females and conjunctival secretions in neonates	May be asymptomatic Dysuria Vaginal discharge (mucus or pus) Endocervicitis May lead to pelvic inflammatory disease, ectopic pregnancy, infertility Can cause inflammation of the rectum and conjunctiva Can infect the throat from oral sexual contact with an infected partner	May be asymptomatic Dysuria Penile discharge (mucus or pus) Urethral tingling May lead to epididymitis and sterility Can cause inflammation of the rectum and conjunctiva Can infect the throat from oral sexual contact with an infected partner	Azithromycin (Zithromax) Doxycycline (Vibramycin) Erythromycin (EES) Ofloxacin (Floxin) Sexual partners need evaluation, testing, and treatment also.

(continued)

Table 16.9 Sexually Transmitted Infections Common in Adolescents (continued)

Disease	Causative Organism	Transmission Mode	Diagnostic Testing	Female Symptoms	Male Symptoms	Treatment
Gonorrhea Curable STI Patient often coinfected with *Chlamydia trachomatis*	*Neisseria gonorrhoeae* (bacteria)	Vaginal, anal, oral sex, and by childbirth	Staining samples directly for the bacterium, detection of bacterial genes or DNA in urine, and growing the bacteria in laboratory cultures; more than one test may be used	May be asymptomatic or no recognizable symptoms until serious complications such as pelvic inflammatory disease Dysuria Frequency Vaginal discharge (yellow and foul) Dyspareunia Endocervicitis Arthritis May lead to pelvic inflammatory disease, ectopic pregnancy, infertility Symptoms of rectal infection include discharge, anal itching, and occasional painful bowel movements with fresh blood.	Most produce symptoms, but can be asymptomatic Dysuria Penile discharge (pus) Arthritis May lead to epididymitis and sterility Symptoms of rectal infection include discharge, anal itching, and occasional painful bowel movements with fresh blood.	Usually a single dose of one of the following: Cefiximine (Suprax) Ciprofloxacin (Cipro) Ceftriaxone (Rocephin) Ofloxacin (Floxin) Levofloxin (Levaquin) **No Floxin or Cipro if <18 years or pregnant!** Azithromycin (Zithromax) Doxycycline (Vibramycin) Usually will be treated for coinfection with Chlamydia, so a combination is given (such as ceftriaxone and doxycycline). Sexual partners need evaluation, testing, and treatment also.

Herpes type II (genital herpes) Lifelong recurrent viral disease Most people have not been diagnosed. There is no cure.	Herpes simplex virus II (HSV II)	Having sexual contact (vaginal, oral, or anal) with someone who is shedding the herpes virus either during an outbreak or during a period with no symptoms Can be transmitted through close contact such as close skin-to-skin contact	Visual inspection and symptoms or culture Virologic and type-specific serologic tests can tell if herpes simplex virus II is present; does not confirm genital herpes, though most providers will assume a positive HSV II means genital herpes.	Blister-like genital lesions Dysuria Fever, headache, muscle aches	Blister-like genital lesions Dysuria Fever, headache, muscle aches	Acyclovir (Zovirax) Other antivirals Does not cure; just controls symptoms. Sexual partners benefit from evaluation and counseling. If symptomatic, need treatment. If asymptomatic, offer testing and education.
Syphilis	*Treponema pallidum* (spirochete bacteria)	Sexual contact with an infected person	Blood tests Venereal Disease Research Laboratory (VDRL), rapid plasma reagin (RPR), and treponemal tests (e.g., fluorescent treponemal antibody absorbed (FTA-ABS)) can lead to a presumptive diagnosis. Darkfield examination and direct fluorescent antibody tests of lesion exudate or tissue provide definitive diagnosis of early syphilis.	Course of disease divided into four stages **Primary infection:** • Chancre on place of entrance of bacteria (usually vulva or vagina but can develop in other parts of the body) **Secondary infection:** • Maculopapular rash (hands & feet) • Sore throat • Lymphadenopathy • Flu-like symptoms **Latent infection:** • No symptoms • No longer contagious	Course of disease divided into four stages **Primary infection:** • Chancre on place of entrance of bacteria (usually on penis but can develop in other parts of the body) **Secondary, latent, and tertiary infections:** All similar to female symptoms	Penicillin G injection (if penicillin allergy, doxycycline or erythromycin) Sexual partners need evaluation and testing.

(continued)

Table 16.9 Sexually Transmitted Infections Common in Adolescents (continued)

Disease	Causative Organism	Transmission Mode	Diagnostic Testing	Female Symptoms	Male Symptoms	Treatment
				• Many people if not treated will suffer no further signs and symptoms. Some people will go on to develop tertiary or late syphilis. **Tertiary infections:** • Tumors of skin, bones and liver • Central nervous system symptoms • Cardiovascular symptoms • Usually not reversible at this stage		
Trichomoniasis	*Trichomonas vaginalis* (protozoa)	Vaginal intercourse with an infected partner May be picked up from direct genital contact with damp or moist objects, such as towels, wet clothing, or a toilet seat	Microscopic evaluation of vaginal secretions or culture	Many women have symptoms but some may be asymptomatic Dysuria Frequency Vaginal discharge (yellow, green or gray and foul odor) Dyspareunia Irritation or itching of genital area	Most men infected are asymptomatic. Dysuria Penile discharge (watery white)	Metronidazole (Flagyl) Sexual partners need evaluation, testing, and treatment also.

Venereal warts (condylomata acuminata) One of the most common STIs in the United States Could lead to cancers of the cervix, vulva, vagina, anus, or penis No cure; warts can be removed but virus remains	Human papillomavirus	Vaginal, anal, oral sex with an infected partner	Visual inspection Abnormal Pap smear may indicate cervical infection of HPV.	Wart-like lesions that are soft, moist, or flesh colored and appear on the vulva and cervix, and inside and surrounding the vagina and anus. Sometimes appear in clusters that resemble cauliflower-like bumps, and are either raised or flat, small or large.	Wart-like lesions that are soft, moist, or flesh-colored and appear on the scrotum or penis. They sometimes appear in clusters that resemble cauliflower-like bumps, and are either raised or flat, small or large.	May disappear without treatment Treatment is aimed at removing the lesions rather than HPV itself. No optimal treatment has been identified, but several ways to treat depending on size and location. Most methods rely on chemical or physical destruction of the lesion: Imiquimod cream 20% Podophyllin antimitotic solution 0.5% Podofilox solution 5% 5-fluorouracil cream Trichloroacetic acid (TCA) Small warts can be removed by: • Freezing (cryosurgery) • Burning (electrocautery) • Laser treatment Large warts that have not responded to treatment may be removed surgically.

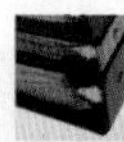

TEACHING GUIDELINE 16.3

Proper Condom Use

- Use latex condoms.
- Use a new condom with each act of sexual intercourse. Never reuse a condom.
- Handle condoms with care to prevent damage from sharp objects such as fingernails and teeth.
- Ensure condom has been stored in a cool, dry place away from direct sunlight. Do not store condoms in wallet or automobile or anywhere they would be exposed to extreme temperatures.
- Do not use a condom if it appears brittle, sticky, or discolored. These are signs of aging.
- Put condom on before any genital contact.
- Put condom on when penis is erect. Ensure it is placed so it will readily unroll.
- Hold the tip of the condom while unrolling. Ensure there is a space at the tip for semen to collect, but make sure no air is trapped in the tip.
- Ensure adequate lubrication during intercourse. If external lubricants are used, use only water-based lubricants such as KY jelly with latex condoms. Oil-based or petroleum-based lubricants, such as body lotion, massage oil, or cooking oil, can weaken latex condoms.
- Withdraw while penis is still erect, and hold condom firmly against base of penis.

Adapted from American Academy of Pediatrics Committee on Infectious Diseases (2003). *Red Book: 2003 Report of the Committee on Infectious Diseases* (26th ed.). Elk Grove Village, IL: American Academy of Pediatrics; and Canadian STD Guidelines (1998 ed., pp. 35–36).

Table 16.10 Barriers to Condom Use and Means to Overcome Them

Perceived Barrier	Intervention Strategy
Decreases sexual pleasure (sensation) Note: Often perceived by those who have never used a condom.	• Encourage patient to try. • Put a drop of water-based lubricant or saliva inside the tip of the condom or on the glans of the penis before putting on the condom. • Try a thinner latex condom or a different brand or more lubrication.
Decreases spontaneity of sexual activity	• Incorporate condom use into foreplay. • Remind patient that peace of mind may enhance pleasure for self and partner.
Embarrassing, juvenile, "unmanly"	• Remind patient that it is "manly" to protect himself and others.
Poor fit (too small or too big, slips off, uncomfortable)	• Smaller and larger condoms are available.
Requires prompt withdrawal after ejaculation	• Reinforce the protective nature of prompt withdrawal and suggest substituting other postcoital sexual activities.
Fear of breakage may lead to less vigorous sexual activity.	• With prolonged intercourse, lubricant wears off and the condom begins to rub. Have a water-soluble lubricant available to reapply.
Non-penetrative sexual activity	• Condoms have been advocated for use during fellatio; unlubricated condoms may prove best for this purpose due to the taste of the lubricant. • Other barriers, such as dental dams or an unlubricated condom, can be cut down the middle to form a barrier; these have been advocated for use during certain forms of non-penetrative sexual activity (e.g., cunnilingus and anolingual sex).
Allergy to latex	• Polyurethane male and female condoms are available. • A natural skin condom can be used together with a latex condom to protect the man or woman from contact with latex.

From the Canadian STD Guidelines (1998 ed., p. 37)

HEALTHY PEOPLE 2010

Objective	Significance
Reduce the proportion of adolescents and young adults with *Chlamydia trachomatis* infections. Reduce gonorrhea. Eliminate sustained domestic transmission of primary and secondary syphilis. (Developmental) Reduce the proportion of persons with human papillomavirus (HPV) infection. Increase the proportion of adolescents who abstain from sexual intercourse or use condoms if currently sexually active. (Developmental) Increase the proportion of all sexually transmitted disease clinic patients who are being treated for bacterial STDs (chlamydia, gonorrhea, and syphilis) and who are offered provider referral services for their sex partners.	• Provide confidential care to all adolescents. • Assess for sexual behaviors and STI risk during clinic visits. Take every opportunity to educate on risks of STIs and risk reduction. • Be direct and nonjudgmental and tailor your approach to the client. • Encourage adolescents to postpone initiation of sexual intercourse for as long as possible. For teens who have already had sexual intercourse, encourage abstinence at this point. • Ensure HPV vaccination in all age-eligible females. • Encourage adolescents to minimize their lifetime number of sexual partners. • Educate about the importance of correct and consistent condom use. • Ensure that up-to-date and complete STI information is included in school-based interventions. • Assist and encourage parents to communicate STI information to their children. • Ensure evaluation and treatment of partners with STI.

References

Books and Journals

Ackley, B. J., & Ladwig, G. B. (2006). *Nursing diagnosis handbook: A guide to planning care* (7th ed.). St. Louis: Mosby.

American Academy of Pediatrics (2001). Policy statement: Acetaminophen toxicity in children. *Pediatrics (108),* 1020–1024.

American Academy of Pediatrics (2003). Tetanus. Retrieved 6/28/04 from http://search.aap.org/aap/CISPframe.html?url=http://www.cispimmunize.org/fam/dtp/tetetill.html.

American Academy of Pediatrics, Committee on Infectious Diseases (2006). *Red book: 2006 report of the committee on infectious diseases* (27th ed.). Elk Grove Village, IL: American Academy of Pediatrics.

Amitai, A., Sinert, R., & Medlin, R. (2006) Tick-borne diseases, Rocky Mountain spotted fever. *Emedicine.* Retrieved 7/22/06 from http://www.emedicine.com/emerg/topic510.htm.

Apolito, K. C. (2006). State of the science: Procedural pain management in the neonate. *Journal of Perinatal and Neonatal Nursing, 20*(1), 56–61.

Barclay, L., & Nghiem, H. T. (2005). CDC revises pertussis guidelines. *Medscape Medical News.* Retrieved 7/22/06 from http://www.medscape.com/viewarticle/519699?src=mp.

Bedford, H. (2003). Measles: The disease and its prevention. *Nursing Standard, 17*(24), 46–52.

Behrman, R. E., Kliegman, R. M., & Jenson, H. B. (2004). *Nelson's textbook of pediatrics* (17th ed.). Philadelphia: Saunders.

Boyer, K. M., & Severin, P. N. (2006). Sepsis and septic shock. In J. A. McMillan (Ed.), *Oski's pediatrics: Principles and practice* (pp. 918–923). Philadelphia: Lippincott Williams & Wilkins.

Bratton, R. L., & Corey, G. R. (2005). Tick-borne diseases. *American Family Physician, 71*(12), 2323–2330.

Broome, M. E., Dokken, D. L. Broome, C. D., Woodring, B., & Stegelman, M. F. (2003). A study of parent/grandparent education for managing a febrile illness using the CALM approach. *Journal of Pediatric Health Care, 17,* 176–183.

Caplan, C. E. (1999). Mumps in the era of vaccines. *Canadian Medical Association Journal, 160,* 865–866.

Carceles, M. D., Alonso, J. M., Garcia-Munoz, M., Najera, M. D., Castano, I., & Vila, N. (2002). Amethocaine-Lidocaine cream, a formulation for preventing venipuncture-induced pain in children. *Regional Anesthesia and Pain Medicine, 27*(3), 289–295.

Carson, S. M. (2003). Alternating acetaminophen and ibuprofen in the febrile child: Examination of the evidence regarding efficacy and safety. *Pediatric Nursing, 29*(5), 379–382.

Centers for Disease Control and Prevention (2005). Nationally notifiable infectious diseases. Accessed 7/22/06 from www.cdc.gov/epo/dphsi/phs/infdis/htm.

Centers for Disease Control and Prevention (2006). *Health advisory: Multistate mumps outbreak.* Accessed 4/25/06 from www.phppo.cdc.gov/HAN/ArchiveSys/ViewMsgV.asp?AlertNum=00243.

Crawford, M. B. (2006). Pediatrics, bacteremia and sepsis. *eMedicine.* Retrieved 7/22/06 from http://www.emedicine.com/EMERG/topic364.htm#section~author_information.

Crocetti, M. T., & Serwint, J. R. (2005). Fever: Separating fact from fiction. *Contemporary Pediatrics.* Retrieved 7/22/06 from www.contemporarypediatrics.com/contpeds/content/content Detail.jsp?id=143315.

Dawson, G. (2005). Chickenpox-related illnesses and deaths are down secondary to varicella vaccination program. *Journal of the National Medical Association, 4,* 453–454.

Eichenfield, L. F., Funk, A., Fallon-Friedlander, S., & Cunningham, B. B. (2002). A clinical study to evaluate the efficacy of ELA-Max (4% liposomal lidocaine) as compared with eutectic mixture of local anesthetics cream for pain reduction of venipuncture in children. *Pediatrics, 109*(6), 1093–1099.

Evans, J. C., McCartney, E. M., Lawhon, G., & Galloway, J. (2005). Longitudinal comparison of preterm pain response to repeated heelsticks. *Pediatric Nursing, 31*(3), 216–221.

Fetzer, S. J. (2002). Reducing venipuncture and intravenous insertion pain with eutectic mixture of local anesthetics: a meta-analysis. *Nursing Research, 51,* 119–124.

Fischbach, F. T. (2004). *A manual of laboratory and diagnostic tests* (7th ed.). Philadelphia: Lippincott Williams & Wilkins.

Flinders, D. C., & De Schweinitz, P. (2004). Pediculosis and scabies. *American Family Physician, 69*(2), 341–348.

Garner, J. S., & the Hospital Infection Control Practices Advisory Committee (1996). Guideline for isolation precautions in hospitals. Retrieved 7/22/06 from http://www.cdc.gov/ncidod/hip/ISOLAT/ISOLAT.HTM.

Garner, J. S., & the Hospital Infection Control Practices Advisory Committee (2005). *Guideline for isolation precautions in hospitals.* Retrieved 7/22/06 from http://www.cdc.gov/ncidod/dhqp/gl_isolation_ptII.html.

Gatti, J. C. (2003). Is oral sucrose an effective analgesic in neonates? *American Family Physician, 67*(8), 1713–1714.

Goldrick, B. A. (2005). Emerging infections: Pertussis on the rise. *American Journal of Nursing, 105*(1), 69–71.

Gradin, M., Eriksson, M., Holmqvist, G., Holstein, A., & Schollin, J. (2002). Pain reduction at venipuncture in newborns: Glucose compared with local anesthetic cream. *Pediatrics, 110*(6), 1053–1057.

Health Canada. (1998). *Canadian STD guidelines.* Retrieved 7/22/06 from www.phac-aspc.gc.ca/publicat/std-mts98/pdf/std98_e.pdf.

Horwitz, N. (2002). Does oral sucrose reduce the pain of neonatal procedures? *Archives of Disease in Childhood, 87*(1), 80–81.

Hotez, P. J., Brooker, S., Bethony, J. M., Bottazzi, M. E., Loukas, A., & Xiao, S. (2004). Current concepts: Hookworm infection. *New England Journal of Medicine, 351*(8), 799–807.

Jain, A., Rutter, N., & Ratnayaka, M. (2001). Topical amethocaine gel for pain relief of heel prick blood sampling: A randomized double-blind controlled trial. *Archives of Disease in Childhood, Fetal and Neonatal Edition, 84,* 56–59.

Kenner, C., & Lott, J. W. (2004). *Neonatal nursing handbook.* St. Louis: Saunders.

Knies, R. C. (2004). Research applied to clinical practice: Sepsis in children. *Emergency Nursing World.* Retrieved 7/22/06 from http://enw.org/Research-SepticKid.htm.

Kucik, C. J., Martin, G. C., & Sortor, B. V. (2004). Common intestinal parasites. *American Family Physician, 69*(5), 1161–1168.

Levin, M. J., & Weinberg, A. (2005). Infections: Viral and rickettsial. In W. W. Hay, M. J. Levin, J. M. Sondheimer, & R. R. Deterding (Eds.), *Current pediatric diagnosis and treatment* (17th ed.) New York: McGraw-Hill.

Lahoti, S., McClain, N., Girardet, R., McNeese, M., & Cheung, K. (2000). Treatment of sexually transmitted diseases part 1: Chlamydia, gonorrhea, and bacterial vaginosis. *Journal of Pediatric Health Care, 14,* 34–36.

McMillan, J. A., & Feigin, R. (2006). Diphtheria. In J. A. McMillan (Ed.), *Oski's pediatrics: Principles and practice* (4th ed., pp. 1059–1062). Philadelphia: Lippincott Williams & Wilkins.

Morash, D., & Fowler, K. (2004). An evidence-based approach to changing practice: Using sucrose for infant analgesia. *Journal of Pediatric Nursing, 19*(5), 366–370.

Moureau, N., & Zonderman, A. (2000). Does it always have to hurt? Premedications for adults and children for use with intravenous therapy. *Journal of IV Nursing, 23*(4), 213–219.

Murray, S. S., & McKinnery, E. S. (2006). *Foundations of maternal-newborn nursing* (4th ed.). St. Louis: Saunders.

National Center for Infectious Diseases. (2003). *About the center.* Retrieved May 19, 2007 from http://www.cdc.gov/ncidod/about.htm.

National Institute of Allergy and Infectious Disease (2004). Human papillomavirus and genital warts. Retrieved 7/22/06 from http://www.niaid.nih.gov/factsheets/stdhpv.htm.

National Institute of Allergy and Infectious Disease (2004). Chlamydia. Retrieved 7/22/06 from http://www.niaid.nih.gov/factsheets/stdclam.htm.

National Institute of Allergy and Infectious Disease (2004). Gonorrhea. Retrieved 7/22/06 from http://www.niaid.nih.gov/factsheets/stdgon.htm.

National Institute of Allergy and Infectious Disease (2005). Syphilis. Retrieved 7/22/06 from http://www.niaid.nih.gov/factsheets/stdsyph.htm.

Niederhauser, V. P. (2006). Pediatric primary care. In S. M. Nettina (Ed.), *Lippincott manual of nursing practice* (8th ed., pp. 1350–1381). Philadelphia: Lippincott Williams & Wilkins.

O'Brien, L., Taddio, A., Ipp, M., Goldbach, M., & Koren, G. (2004). Topical 4% amethocaine gel reduces the pain of subcutaneous measles-mumps-rubella vaccination. *Pediatrics, 114,* e720–724. Retrieved 6/6/06 from www.pediatrics.org/cgi/doi/10.1542/peds.2004-0722.

Ogle, J. W., & Anderson, M. S. (2005). Infections: Bacterial and spirochetal. In W. W. Hay, M. J. Levin, J. M. Sondheimer, & R. R. Deterding (Eds.), *Current pediatric diagnosis and treatment* (17th ed., pp. 1241–1250). New York: McGraw-Hill.

Pagana, K. D., & Pagana, T. J. (2006). *Mosby's manual of diagnostic and laboratory tests* (3rd ed.). St. Louis: Mosby.

Prinzhorn, J., & Churchwell, C. (2004). Fever management in children who are febrile is questionable. *Pediatric Nursing, 30*(4), 322.

Shah, K., & Wolfe, W. (2003). Sepsis. In J. Schaider, S. R. Hayden, S. Wolfe, R. M. Barkin, & P. Rosen (Eds.), *Rosen & Barkin's 5-minute emergency medicine consult.* Philadelphia: Lippincott Williams & Wilkins.

Stephenson, J. (2004). Polio eradication plan. *JAMA, 291*(7), 813. Retrieved 6/18/04 from Proquest database.

Taddio, A., Soin, H. K., Schuh, S., Koren, G., & Scolnik, D. (2005). Liposomal lidocaine to improve procedural success rates and reduce procedural pain among children: A randomized controlled trial. *Canadian Medical Association Journal, 172*(13), 1691–1695.

Takano-Lee, M., Edman, J. D., Mullens, B. A., & Clark, J. M. (2004). Home remedies to control head lice: Assessment of home remedies to control the human head louse, *Pediculus humanus capitis* (Anoplura: Pediculidae). *Journal of Pediatric Nursing, 19*(6), 393–398.

Vertanen, H., Fellman, V., Brommels, M., & Viinikka, L. (2001). An automatic incision device for obtaining blood samples from the heels of the preterm infant causes less damage than a conventional manual lancet. *Archives of Disease in Childhood, Fetal and Neonatal Edition, 84,* 53–55.

Wakim, N., & Henderson, S. (2003). Tetanus. *Topics in Emergency Medicine, 25*(3), 256–262. Retrieved 7/22/06 from Proquest database.

Weir, E. (2005). Parvovirus B19 infection: Fifth disease and more. *Canadian Medical Association Journal, 172*(6), 743.

Weise, K. L., & Nahata, M. C. (2005). EMLA for painful procedures in infants. *Journal of Pediatric Health Care, 19*(1), 42–47.

Workowski, K. A., & William, C. L. (2002). Sexually transmitted diseases treatment guidelines. *MMWR Recommendations Report, 51*(RR06), 1–80. Retrieved 7/22/06 from http://www.cdc.gov/mmwr/preview/mmwrhtml/rr5106a1.htm.

Websites

www.ashastd.org American Social Health Organization

www.cdc.gov/ncidod/about.htm National Center for Infectious Diseases, Centers for Disease Control and Prevention

www.cdc.gov/std Centers for Disease Control and Prevention—Sexually Transmitted Diseases

www.headlice.org National Pediculosis Association

www.lyme.org Lyme Disease Foundation

www.measlesinitiative.org/index3.asp Measles Initiative

www.nfid.org National Foundation for Infectious Diseases

www.teensource.org/RunScript.asp?source=google_grants&Poll_ID=4&p=ASP\Pg0.asp Teen Source (STI information for teens)

Chapter WORKSHEET

● MULTIPLE CHOICE QUESTIONS

1. Compared with adults, why are infants and children at an increased risk for infection and communicable diseases?

a. The infant has had limited exposure to disease and is losing the passive immunity acquired from maternal antibodies.

b. The infant demonstrates an increased inflammatory response.

c. Cellular immunity is not functional at birth.

d. Infants are at an increased risk for infection until they receive their first set of immunizations.

2. A mother calls the clinic because her 2-year-old daughter has a rectal temperature of 37.8° C (100° F). She wonders how high a fever should be before she should give medications to reduce it. What is the best response by the nurse?

a. "All fevers should be treated to prevent seizures."

b. "Antipyretics should be used with any rise in temperature. They can help change the course of the infection."

c. "Give your child aspirin when her fever is above 38° C (100.4° F)."

d. "In a normal healthy child, if your child is not uncomfortable, fevers less than 39° C (102.2° F) do not require medication."

3. A neonate should be evaluated by a physician if which signs and symptoms are present?

a. Acting fussier than normal

b. Refusing the pacifier

c. Rectal temperature above 38° C

d. Mottling is present during bathing

4. As the nurse in a public health department, you have been asked to provide information to local childcare centers on controlling the spread of infectious diseases. What is the best information you can provide?

a. The etiology of common infectious diseases

b. Proper handwashing techniques

c. The physiology of the immune system

d. Why children are at a higher risk of infection than adults

● CRITICAL THINKING EXERCISES

1. A 12-year-old child presents with complaints of a very sore throat and fever. On assessment you find an erythematous rash on his face that feels like sandpaper. You obtain a throat culture that is positive for group A streptococcus. What instructions would you give the parents regarding his care at home?

2. A 1-month-old infant is admitted to the hospital to rule out sepsis. What would be your priority nursing interventions?

3. A 4-year-old child presents with a fever and rash. What three items should the nurse obtain during the health history?

a. Immunization history

b. Any exposure to communicable or infectious diseases

c. Whether the child takes a daily vitamin

d. Thorough description and history of the rash

e. Mother's immunization history

● STUDY ACTIVITIES

1. The 4-year-old presented in question number 3 above was diagnosed with varicella zoster virus. Write a nursing care plan for a child with varicella.

2. You are asked to give a presentation to a group of adolescents on STIs, including transmission, symptoms, treatment, and prevention. What information would you include?

3. A child is brought to the office of the school nurse with intense itching. Upon assessment the nurse finds an erythematous, papular rash with excoriations on the child's hands and feet. As suspected, the diagnosis of scabies is confirmed. What teaching is necessary for the parents, family, and classmates of the child?

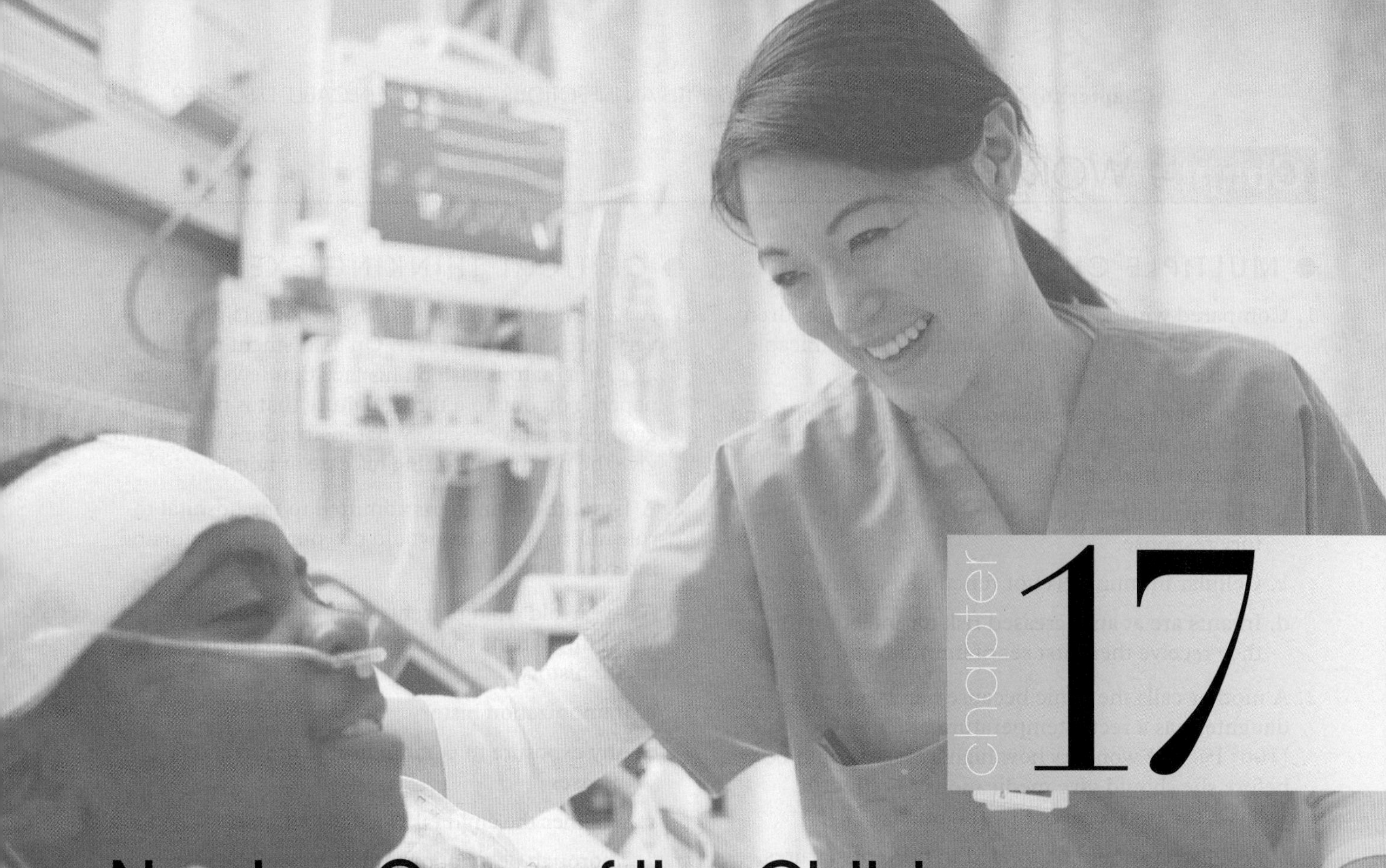

chapter 17

Nursing Care of the Child With a Neurologic Disorder

Key TERMS

automatism
central nervous system (CNS)
cerebrospinal fluid (CSF)
clonic
decorticate posturing
decerebrate posturing
head circumference
intracranial pressure (ICP)
lumbar puncture (LP)
myelinization
myoclonus
neural tube
opisthotonic
postictal
status epilepticus
teratogen
tonic

Learning OBJECTIVES

Upon completion of the chapter, the learner will be able to:

1. Compare how the anatomy and physiology of the neurologic system in children differs from adults.
2. Identify various factors associated with neurologic disease in infants and children.
3. Discuss common laboratory and other diagnostic tests useful in the diagnosis of neurologic conditions.
4. Discuss common medications and other treatments used for treatment and palliation of neurologic conditions.
5. Recognize risk factors associated with various neurologic disorders.
6. Distinguish among different neurologic illnesses based on the signs and symptoms associated with them.
7. Discuss nursing interventions commonly used for neurologic illnesses.
8. Devise an individualized nursing care plan for the child with a neurologic disorder.
9. Develop client and family teaching plans for the child with a neurologic disorder.
10. Describe the psychosocial impact of chronic neurologic disorders on children.

WOW *As long as nurses possess inner integrity, they will be able to handle their patient's life's challenges.*

Antonio Chapman, 3 months old, has had increased irritability, poor sucking and feeding, and a fever for the past 24 hours. Today he is lethargic with a weak cry and is vomiting his feeds.

Neurologic disorders in children often have a devastating and lasting impact. Neurologic disorders can be divided into several categories, including structural disorders, seizure disorders, infectious disorders, trauma to the neurologic system, blood flow disruption disorders, and chronic disorders.

Nurses must be familiar with neurologic conditions affecting children in order to provide prevention, prompt treatment, guidance, and support to families. Neurologic disorders require acute interventions, but many times have long-lasting implications on the child's health and development. Due to the potentially devastating effects that neurologic disorders can have on children and their families, nurses need to be skilled in assessment and interventions in this area and must be able to provide support throughout the course of the illness and beyond.

Variations in Pediatric Anatomy and Physiology

Neurologic disorders can result from congenital problems as well as from infections or traumas. Certain neurologic conditions occur in children more often than adults and will affect their growth and development. Pediatric clients are at an increased risk for different neurologic problems than adults due to anatomic and physiologic differences.

Brain and Spinal Cord Development

Development of the brain and spinal cord occurs early in gestation, in the first 3 to 4 weeks, from the **neural tube**. Infection, trauma, **teratogens**, and malnutrition during this period can result in malformations in brain and spinal cord development and may affect normal **central nervous system (CNS)** development.

At birth, the cranial bones are not well developed and are unfused. Therefore there is an increased risk for fracture. The brain is highly vascular, leading to an increased risk for hemorrhage. Premature infants are at greater risk for brain damage; the more premature the infant, the greater the risk. The premature infant has more capillaries in the periventricular area, which is the brain tissue that lines the outside of the lateral ventricles. These capillaries are fragile and at greater risk for rupture, leading to intracranial bleeding. Also, because the cranium is very soft in the preterm infant, external pressure can change its shape and cause increased pressure in areas of the brain and possible hemorrhage.

The sutures and fontanels present in the newborn help make the skull more flexible and help to accommodate for brain growth that continues after birth. Closure of the fontanels too early or too late can be indicative of problems with brain growth. The child's spine is very mobile, especially the cervical spine region, resulting in a high risk for cervical spine injury.

Nervous System

The development of the nervous system is complete but immature at birth. The infant is born with all the nerve cells that he or she will have throughout life. However, myelinization of these nerves is incomplete. The speed and accuracy of nerve impulses increases as **myelinization** increases. This process accounts for the acquisition of fine and gross motor movements and coordination in early childhood. Myelinization proceeds in the cephalocaudal direction. For example, infants are able to control the head and neck before the trunk and extremities.

The immaturity of the CNS in preterm infants can result in delayed development of motor skills. Premature newborns may have difficulty coordinating sucking and swallowing, leading to feeding and growth issues. Also, episodes of apnea can be problematic in the preterm newborn due to the underdevelopment of the nervous system.

Head Size

The head of the infant and young child is large in proportion to the body. The head of an infant accounts for a quarter of the body height; in adults it accounts for one eighth of the body height (Fig. 17.1). In addition, the infant's and child's neck muscles are not well developed. Both of these differences lead to an increased incidence of head injury from falls. The head is the fastest growing body part during infancy and continues to grow until the child is 5 years old.

Common Medical Treatments

A variety of interventions, including medical treatments and medications, are used to treat neurologic illness in children. Most of these treatments will require a physician's order when the child is hospitalized. The most common treatments and medications used for neurologic disorders are listed in Common Medical Treatments 17.1 and Drug Guide 17.1.

Nursing Process Overview for the Child With a Neurologic Disorder

Care of the child with a neurologic disorder includes assessment, nursing diagnosis, planning, interventions, and evaluation. There are a number of general concepts

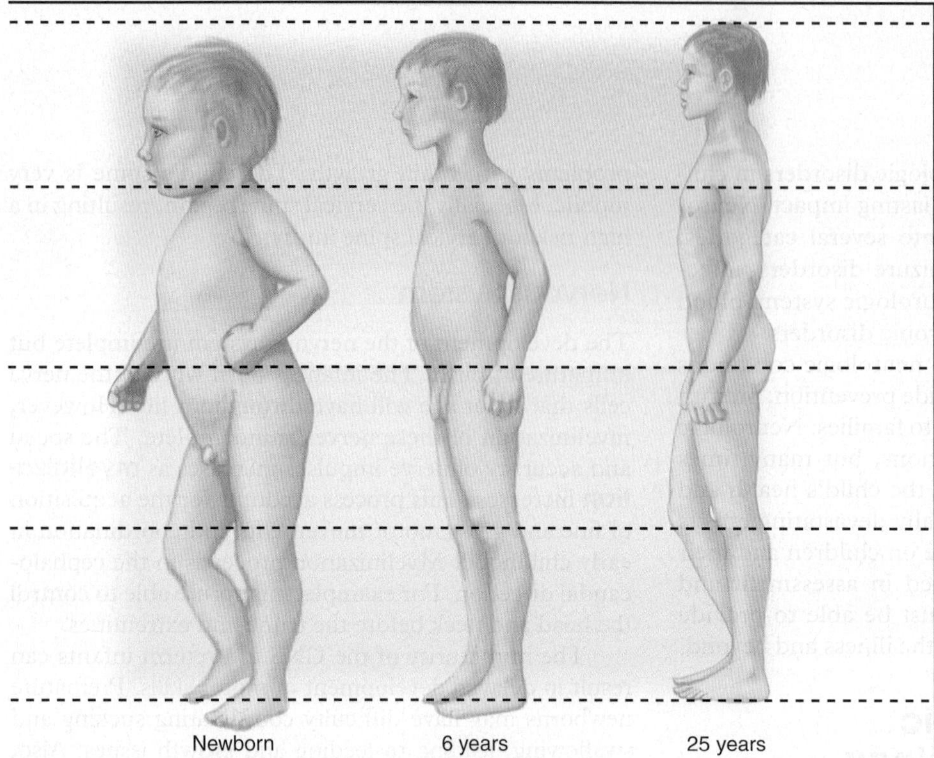

● Figure 17.1 Proportion of head to body height in the newborn, child, and adult.

Common Medical Treatments 17.1

Treatment	Explanation	Indications	Nursing Implications
Shunt placement	A catheter is placed in the ventricle to pass the CSF to the peritoneal cavity, atrium of the heart, or pleural spaces. (Ventriculoperitoneal shunts are commonly used.)	Hydrocephalus, increased ICP	Monitor: • For signs and symptoms of increased ICP • Neurologic status closely • Level of consciousness and vital signs • For signs and symptoms of infection
Ventilation	Hyperventilation to decrease $PaCO_2$, which will result in vasoconstriction and therefore decrease ICP Adequate oxygenation to prevent hypoxia and further damage to the brain	Increased ICP	Monitor: • Arterial blood gases • For signs and symptoms of increased ICP • Pulse oximetry
PT/OT/ST	Therapies are used to improve motor function and ability of clients with neurologic disorders.	Head injury, mental retardation	Ensure adequate communication exists within the interdisciplinary team.

(continued)

Common Medical Treatments 17.1 (continued)

Treatment	Explanation	Indications	Nursing Implications
External ventricular drainage (EVD)	A catheter is temporarily placed in the ventricle and CSF is drained in a closed system to an external reservoir	Most commonly used with shunt infections until CSF is sterile and shunt can be replaced; treats acute-onset hydrocephalus, meningitis, encephalitis, tumors that cause blockage of CSF, closed head injury, subarachnoid hemorrhage, increased ICP; also can be used to monitor ICP	Monitor: • For signs and symptoms of increased ICP • Neurologic status closely • Level of consciousness and vital signs • For signs and symptoms of infection • Level of collection container when drain is unclamped
Ventricular tap	To reduce accumulation of CSF and decrease ICP	Increased ICP	Monitor: • Level of consciousness • Neurologic status
Vagal nerve stimulator	A nerve stimulator is implanted and a lead wire running under the skin is wrapped around the vagus nerve. The stimulator is programmed to provide the appropriate dose of stimulation at preset intervals; additional stimulation can be administered.	Short- and long-term seizure management in children >12 years of age	Monitor: • For signs and symptoms of infection • For seizure activity
Ketogenic diet	Diet involving high intake of fats, adequate protein, and a very low intake of carbohydrates, resulting in a ketosis state. Child is kept in a mild state of dehydration.	Prevention, control, and reduction of seizures, in particular for children with difficult-to-control seizures	Monitor: • Input and output closely • For seizure activity • Growth and nutritional status The diet is time consuming and many clients find it unpalatable; therefore all families and clients do not accept it.

related to the nursing process that can be applied to the management of neurologic disorders. From a general understanding of the care involved for a child with neurologic dysfunction, the nurse can then individualize the care based on client specifics.

Remember Antonio, the 3-month-old with lethargy, a weak cry, and vomiting? What additional health history and physical examination assessment information should the nurse obtain?

ASSESSMENT

Assessment of neurologic dysfunction in children includes health history, physical examination, and laboratory and diagnostic testing.

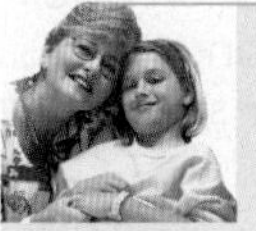

Neurologic assessment should proceed from least invasive to most invasive. The use of toys and familiar objects, as well as incorporating play, will help promote cooperation from the child.

Health History

The health history consists of past medical history, including the mother's pregnancy history, family history, and history of present illness (when the symptoms started and how they have progressed) as well as treatments used at home. The past medical history might be significant for prematurity, difficult birth, infection during pregnancy, nausea, vomiting, headaches, changes in gait, falls,

Drug Guide 17.1

Medication	Action	Indication	Nursing Implications
Antibiotics (oral, parenteral, intrathecal)	Treatment of bacterial meningitis and shunt infections	Meningitis, encephalitis	Check for antibiotic allergies. Monitor serum levels to ensure therapeutic dosing if indicated. Give as prescribed for the length of time prescribed.
Anticonvulsants (oral, parenteral)	Treatment and prevention of seizures. Many are used in combination, but need to be aware of interactions and long-term adverse effects.	Epilepsy, head trauma, neurosurgical procedures	Maintain seizure precautions. Monitor for drug interactions and long-term adverse effects. Monitor and document all seizure activity. Stopping drug abruptly may precipitate seizures or even status epilepticus.
Benzodiazepines Diazepam (oral, rectal, or parenteral) Lorazepam (parenteral or oral)	Anticonvulsant Enhance the inhibition of γ-aminobutyric acid (GABA)	Treatment of status epilepticus	Diazepam is available in rectal form to stop prolonged seizures in children. Useful for home management; nurses must educate family members on administration and when to call MD. Monitor sedation level and for cessation of seizure activity.
Analgesics (acetaminophen, ibuprofen, ketorolac, morphine)	Diminishes pain and provides sedative effect	Used to treat pain in children. Used to help avoid increase in ICP but used cautiously because loss of accurate neurologic evaluation can occur	Monitor for improvements in pain. Monitor sedation and respiratory status with narcotics. Monitor neurologic status closely.
Osmotic diuretics (i.e., mannitol)	Increases plasma osmolality, therefore inducing diffusion back into plasma and extravascular space	Reduces ICP	Monitor electrolytes. Monitor I/O closely. Monitor vital signs. Monitor for signs and symptoms of increased ICP.
Corticosteroids (i.e., dexamethasone)	Suppresses inflammation and normal immune response	Reduces cerebral edema	Give oral doses with food. Dosage must be tapered before discontinuing.

visual disturbances, or recent trauma. Family history might be significant for genetic disorders with neurologic manifestations; seizure disorders; or headaches. When eliciting the history of the present illness, inquire about the following:

- Nausea
- Vomiting
- Changes in gait
- Visual disturbances
- Complaints of headaches

- Recent trauma
- Changes in cognition
- Change in consciousness, including any loss of consciousness
- Poor feeding
- Lethargy
- Increased irritability
- Fever
- Neck pain
- Altered muscle tonicity
- Delays in growth and development
- Ingestion or inhalation of neurotoxic substances or chemicals

Physical Examination

Physical examination of the nervous system consists of inspection and observation; palpation; and auscultation.

Inspection and Observation

Specific areas to inspect and observe include level of consciousness (LOC); vital signs; head, face, and neck; cranial nerve function; motor function; reflexes; sensory function; and **increased intracranial pressure (ICP).**

Level of Consciousness (LOC). Begin the physical examination with inspection and observation. Observe the child's LOC, noting a decrease or significant changes. LOC is the earliest indicator of improvement or deterioration of neurologic status. Extreme irritability or lethargy is considered an abnormal finding. Consciousness consists of alertness, which is a wakeful state and includes the ability to respond to stimuli; and cognition, which includes the ability to process stimuli and demonstrate a verbal or motor response. Five different states constitute the levels of consciousness:

1. *Full consciousness* is defined as a state in which the child is awake and alert; is oriented to time, place, and person; and exhibits age-appropriate behaviors.
2. *Confusion* is defined as a state in which disorientation exists. The child may be alert but responds inappropriately to questions.
3. *Obtunded* is defined as a state in which the child has limited responses to the environment and falls asleep unless stimulation is provided.
4. *Stupor* exists when the child only responds to vigorous stimulation.
5. *Coma* defines a state in which the child cannot be aroused, even with painful stimuli.

The Pediatric Glasgow Coma Scale is a popular scale used to standardize degree of consciousness. It consists of three parts: eye opening, verbal response, and motor response (Fig. 17.2). When assessing LOC in children, consider that the infant or child may not respond to unfamiliar voices in an unfamiliar environment. Therefore it may be helpful to have a parent present to elicit the response.

NEUROLOGIC ASSESSMENT

Pupils	Right	Size	
		Reaction	
	Left	Size	
		Reaction	

++ = Brisk
+ = Sluggish
– = No reaction
C = Eye closed by swelling

GLASGOW COMA SCALE

Eyes open	Spontaneously	4	
	To speech	3	
	To pain	2	
	None	1	
Best motor response	Obeys commands	6	
	Localizes pain	5	
	Flexion withdrawal	4	
	Flexion abnormal	3	
	Extension	2	
	None	1	

Usually record best arm or age-appropriate responses

Pupil scale (mm): 1, 2, 3, 4, 5, 6, 7, 8

	>2 years		<2 years
Best response to auditory and/or visual stimulus	Orientation	5	5 Smiles, listens, follows
	Confused	4	4 Cries, consolable
	Inappropriate words	3	3 Inappropriate persistent cry
	Incomprehensible words	2	2 Agitated, restless
	None	1	1 No response
	Endotracheal tube or trach	T	
COMA SCALE TOTAL			

HAND GRIP: Equal; Unequal; R____L; Weakness

LOC: Alert/oriented × 4; Sleepy; Irritable; Comatose; Disoriented; Combative; Lethargic; Awake; Sleeping; Drowsy; Agitated

MUSCLE TONE: Normal; Arching; Spastic; Flaccid; Weak; Decorticate; Decerebrate; Other ________

EYE MOVEMENT: Normal; Nystagmus; Strabismus; Other ________

FONTANEL/WINDOW: Soft; Flat; Sunken; Tense; Bulging; Closed; Other ________

MOOD/AFFECT: Happy; Content; Quiet; Withdrawn; Sad; Flat; Hostile

● Figure 17.2 Pediatric Glasgow Coma Scale (GCS). The Pediatric GCS provides for developmentally appropriate cues to assess level of consciousness (LOC) in infants and children. Numeric values are assigned to the levels of response and the sum provides an overall picture, as well as an objective measure, of the child's LOC. The lower the score, the less responsive the child.

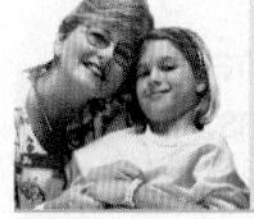

Parents many times will be the first to notice changes in their child's LOC. Listen to parents and respond to their concerns.

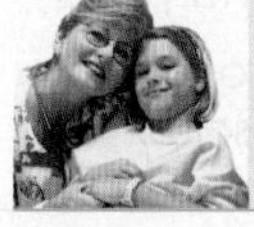

Lack of response to painful stimuli is abnormal and can indicate a life-threatening condition. Report this finding immediately.

Vital Signs. Assessment of vital signs can provide probable underlying causes for altered LOC as well as reveal the adequacy of oxygenation and circulation. Certain neurologic conditions like cerebral infections, increased ICP, coma, brain stem injury, or head injuries can cause alterations in the pediatric client's vital signs.

Head, Face, and Neck. Inspect and observe the head for size and shape. Abnormal skull shape can result from premature closure or widening of sutures. Inspect and observe the face for symmetry. Asymmetry may occur due to paralysis of certain cranial nerves, position *in utero*, or swelling caused by trauma. Assess range of motion of the neck. Alterations in range of motion can indicate CNS infections such as meningitis.

The most dramatic increase in brain volume occurs during the last 3 months of fetal development and the first 2 years of life. The relationship between head and brain growth explains why head circumference is a standard assessment made in children less than 3 years of age. All children less than 3 years old, and any child whose head size is questionable, should have their head circumference measured and plotted on a growth chart (see Appendix A for growth charts). Assessment of the growth trend of the head is important in detecting potential neurologic conditions. Report and investigate any variation in head circumference percentiles over time because variations may indicate abnormal brain or skull growth. A smaller than normal **head circumference** may indicate microcephaly, and a larger than normal head circumference may indicate hydrocephalus.

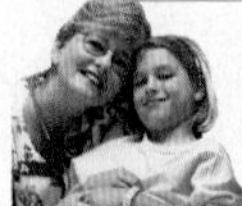

Any assessment that involves movement of the head and neck should not be attempted in cases of trauma or suspected trauma until cervical injury is ruled out. Maintain complete immobilization of the cervical spine until that time.

Cranial Nerve Function. Techniques of assessment of cranial nerve function are similar to techniques for adult assessment. The method of obtaining responses may vary based on age and developmental level of the child. Certain elements of the adult assessment may be omitted. Alterations in cranial nerve function can be the result of compression of a specific nerve, infection, or trauma leading to brain injury. Refer to Table 17.1 for an explanation of cranial nerve assessment in children.

Table 17.1 Assessment of Cranial Nerves in Infants and Children

Cranial Nerve	Function	Assessment Procedure
I (Olfactory)	Sense of smell	Not evaluated in infants and young children. In children, assess child's ability to recognize common smells (i.e., an orange) while eyes are closed.
II (Optic), III (Oculomotor), IV (Trochlear), VI (Abducens)	Vision, motor control and sensation of eye muscles, movement of major eye muscles	Assess oculomotor ability by having child follow object (toy or brightly colored object). Assess vision fields and visual acuity in older child. Assess pupil reaction same as adult. May need to talk to child or have parent in visual field while applying light stimulus
V (Trigeminal)	Mastication muscles and facial sensation	Note strength of infant's suck on pacifier, examiner's thumb, or bottle. In children, assess strength of bite and ability to discern light touch on face.
VII (Facial)	Facial muscles, salivation, and taste	Note symmetry of facial expressions; in infant, monitor during spontaneous cries or smiles. In older child, test as in adults. Assess taste by asking to discern certain common tastes (salt, sugar).
VIII (Acoustic)	Hearing	In infant, note response, to voice. In children, use whisper test or a Weber's or Rinne test.
IX (Glossopharyngeal), X (Vagus)	Motor impulses to heart and other organs, swallowing, and gag reflex	Gag reflex and swallowing tested as in adults. Check time of last feeding, especially in the infant, to avoid vomiting when gag reflex is tested.
XI (Accessory)	Impulses to muscles of shoulders and pharynx	In infants, note symmetry of head position when placed in the sitting position. In children, same as adults
XII (Hypoglossal)	Motor impulses to tongue and skeletal muscles	In infants, note spontaneous tongue movements. In children, same as adults

Use the doll's eyes maneuver to evaluate cranial nerves III, IV, and VI. This maneuver can be helpful when assessing an infant, uncooperative child, or comatose client. It examines horizontal and vertical eye movements by turning the head in one direction and assessing if the eyes move symmetrically in the other direction. For example, if you suddenly turn the child's head to the right, the child's eyes should look to the left symmetrically. Assess vertical eye movements in a similar manner by flexing or extending the neck. Absence of expected eye movements may indicate increased ICP.

When assessing oculomotor function, be sure to note nystagmus or sunset appearance of the eyes. Observe for nystagmus by looking for involuntary, rapid, rhythmic eye movements that may be present at rest or with eye movement. Horizontal nystagmus may occur with lesions in the brainstem and can be the result of certain medications (phenytoin in particular). Vertical nystagmus indicates brainstem dysfunction. *Sunsetting* is when the sclera of the eyes is showing over the top of the iris (Fig. 17.3). Sunset eyes may indicate increased ICP as seen in hydrocephalus. Pupillary response is often abnormal when a neurologic disorder is present. Refer to Figure 17.4 for illustrations of varied pupillary responses.

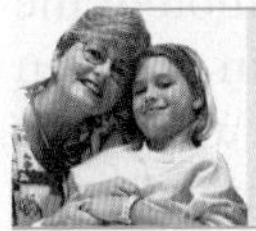

Report immediately the sudden presence of fixed and dilated pupils

Motor Function. Alterations in motor function, like changes in gait, muscle tone, or strength, may indicate certain neurologic problems such as increased ICP, head injury, and cerebral infections. Observe muscle strength, size, and tone in the infant or child. Assess bilaterally and compare. Observe spontaneous activity, posture, and balance and assess for asymmetrical movements. In the infant, observe resting posture, which will normally be a slightly flexed posture. The infant should be able to extend extremities to a normal stretch. Because cortical control of motor function is lost in certain neurologic disorders, postural reflexes reemerge and are directly related to the area of the brain that is damaged. Therefore, it is important to assess for two distinct types of posturing that may occur. **Decorticate posturing** occurs with damage of the cerebral cortex (Fig. 17.5A). **Decerebrate posturing** occurs with damage at the level of the brainstem (Fig. 17.5B).

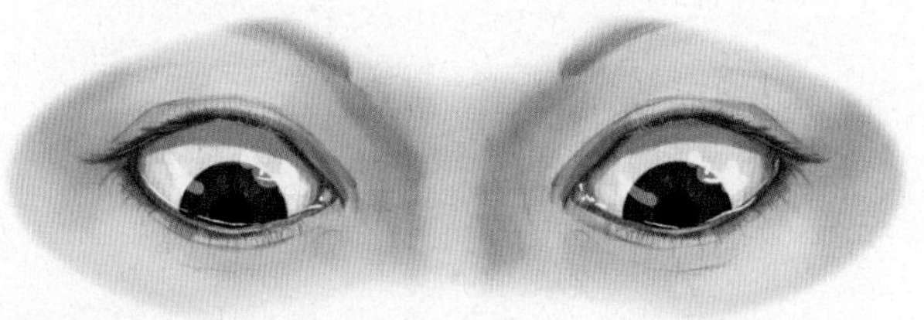

● Figure 17.3 Sunsetting of the eyes is a sign of increased intracranial pressure.

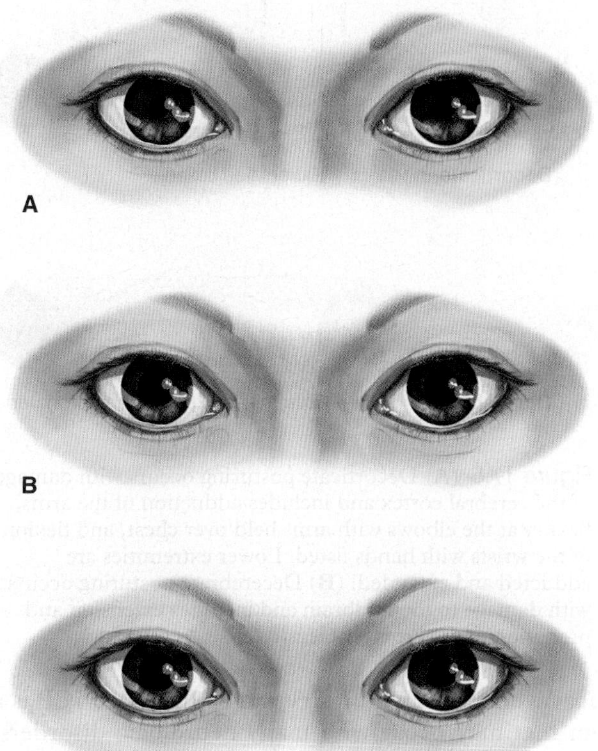

● Figure 17.4 Assessing pupil size and reaction: (**A**) *Pinpoint* is commonly observed in poisonings, brainstem dysfunction, and opiate use. (**B**) *Dilated but reactive* is seen after seizures. *Fixed and dilated* is associated with brainstem herniation secondary to increased intracranial pressure. (**C**) *One dilated but reactive* is associated with intracranial mass.

Both types of posturing are characterized by extremely rigid muscle tone.

Reflexes. Testing of deep-tendon reflexes is part of the neurologic assessment, just as it is in adults. Testing of primitive and protective reflexes in the infant is important because infants cannot perform tasks on command. The Moro's, tonic neck, and withdrawal reflexes are important in assessing neurologic health in infants. Refer to Chapter 4 for a further explanation of primitive and protective reflexes in infants (see Chapter 4, Table 4.2). Absence of certain reflexes, persistence of primitive reflexes after age of normal disappearance, or increases in reflexes may be present in specific neurologic conditions.

Sensory Function. When assessing sensory function, the child should be able to distinguish between light touch, pain, vibration, heat, and cold. When assessing an infant, limit the examination to responses to touch or pain. The normal response in a 4-month-old infant will be movement away from the stimulus. In the child, techniques similar to those used in the adult assessment are followed. Make sure to explain what you are doing to the child, especially before the pin-prick test, to gain continued cooperation. Alterations in sensory function can result from brain or spinal cord lesions.

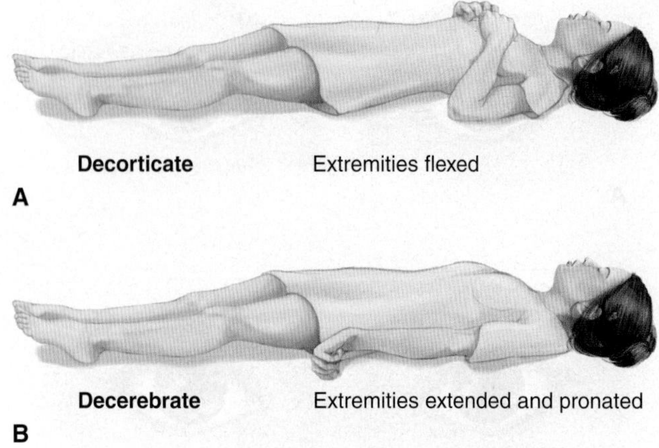

● Figure 17.5 (**A**) Decorticate posturing occurs with damage of the cerebral cortex and includes adduction of the arms, flexion at the elbows with arms held over chest, and flexion of the wrists with hands fisted. Lower extremities are adducted and extended. (**B**) Decerebrate posturing occurs with damage to the midbrain and includes extension and pronation of the arms and legs.

Increased Intracranial Pressure. Increased ICP is a sign that may occur with many neurologic disorders. It may result from head trauma, birth trauma, hydrocephalus, infection, and brain tumors. Observe for signs and symptoms associated with increased ICP while caring for a child with a potential or suspected neurologic disorder. Refer to Comparison Chart 17.1 for early versus late signs and symptoms of increased ICP. As ICP increases, LOC decreases and the signs and symptoms will become more pronounced. It is essential to recognize early signs and symptoms of increased ICP and intervene immediately to prevent long-term damage and possible death.

Palpation

Palpation of the newborn and infant skull and fontanels is an important function of the neurologic examination. Changes in size or fullness of the fontanels may exist in certain neurologic conditions and must be noted. A bulging fontanel can be a sign of increased ICP and is seen in such neurologic disorders as hydrocephalus and head traumas. It is normal for the fontanels to be full or bulging during crying; take this into consideration during assessment.

Note any premature closure of fontanels, which can indicate skull deformities such as craniosynostosis. The posterior fontanel normally closes by 2 months of age and the anterior fontanel normally closes by 12 to 18 months of age. In children with hydrocephalus, widening of the fontanels may be noted, along with a tense appearance and a resulting increase in head circumference.

Auscultation

Advanced practitioners may perform auscultation of the skull. Soft, symmetric bruits may be found in children less than 4 years of age or in children with acute febrile illness. A finding of a loud or localized bruit is usually significant and requires immediate further investigation. Increased ICP, resulting from conditions such as hydrocephalus, tumor, or meningitis, frequently produces

● COMPARISON CHART 17.1 Early vs. Late Signs of Increased Intracranial Pressure

Early Signs	Late Signs
• Headache	• Lowered level of consciousness
• Vomiting, possibly projectile	• Decreased motor and sensory responses
• Blurred vision, double vision (diplopia)	• Bradycardia
• Dizziness	• Irregular respirations
• Decreased pulse and respirations	• Cheyne-Stokes respirations
• Increased blood pressure or pulse pressure	• Decerebrate or decorticate posturing
• Pupil reaction time decreased and unequal	• Fixed and dilated pupils
• Sunset eyes	
• Changes in level of consciousness, irritability	
• Seizure activity	
• In infant will also see:	
• Bulging, tense fontanel	
• Wide sutures and increased head circumference	
• Dilated scalp veins	
• High-pitched cry	

intracranial bruits. Arterial venous malformations may also produce large bruits.

Laboratory and Diagnostic Testing

Common Laboratory and Diagnostic Tests 17.1 offers an explanation of the most commonly used laboratory and diagnostic tests utilized when considering neurologic disorders. The tests can assist the physician in diagnosing the disorder and/or serve as guidelines in determining ongoing treatment. Laboratory or nonnursing personnel obtain some of the tests, while the nurse might obtain others. In either instance, the nurse should be familiar with how the tests are obtained, what they are used for, and normal versus abnormal results. This knowledge will also be necessary when providing client and family education related to the testing. Many of these tests, such as **lumbar puncture** (LP; see Fig. 17.6), can be frightening to parents and the child. Prepare the family and the child and provide support and reassurance during and after the test or procedure.

> After completing an assessment of Antonio, the nurse noted the following: a full anterior fontanel; when being held, Antonio was inconsolable; when lying still, he was calmer and in the opisthotonic position.

NURSING DIAGNOSES AND RELATED INTERVENTIONS

Upon completion of a thorough assessment, the nurse might identify several nursing diagnoses, including:

- Decreased intracranial adaptive capacity
- Ineffective tissue perfusion
- Risk for injury
- Disturbed sensory perception
- Risk for infection
- Pain
- Self-care deficit
- Impaired physical mobility
- Risk for delayed development
- Imbalanced nutrition: less than body requirements
- Risk for deficient fluid volume
- Deficient knowledge
- Interrupted family processes

Nursing goals, interventions, and evaluation for the child with a neurologic disorder are based on the nursing diagnoses.

> Based on the assessment findings, what would be your top three prioritized nursing diagnoses for Antonio?

Nursing Care Plan 17.1 may be used as a guide in planning nursing care for the child with a neurologic disorder. It should be individualized based on the client's symptoms and needs. Additional information will be included later in this chapter related to specific disorders.

> Based on your top three nursing diagnoses for Antonio, describe appropriate nursing interventions.

Seizure Disorders

Seizures occur in approximately 10% of children (Behrman, Kliegman, & Jenson, 2004). Most seizures are caused by disorders that originate outside of the brain such as a high fever, infection, head trauma, hypoxia, toxins, or cardiac arrhythmias. Less than one third of seizures in children are caused by epilepsy (Behrman et al., 2004). Seizure disorders discussed below include epilepsy, febrile seizures, and neonatal seizures.

● EPILEPSY

Epilepsy is a condition in which seizures are triggered recurrently from within the brain. Epilepsy is a common neurologic disorder discovered in childhood, although brain injury or infection can cause epilepsy at any age. Epilepsy is considered present when two or more unprovoked seizures occur more than 24 hours apart. The prognosis for most children with seizures associated with epilepsy is good. Many children will outgrow epilepsy, but some children will have persistent seizures that are difficult to manage and may be unresponsive to pharmacologic interventions. Living with a seizure disorder may have a devastating impact on the quality of life of the child and family.

Pathophysiology

Epilepsy is a complex disorder of the CNS in which brain function is affected. Recurrent or unprovoked seizures are the clinical manifestation of epilepsy and result from a disruption of electrical communication among the neurons of the brain. This disruption results from an imbalance between the excitatory and inhibitory mechanisms in the brain, causing the neurons to either fire when they are not supposed to or not fire when they should. Epilepsy may be acquired and related to brain injury or it may be a familial tendency, but in most cases the cause is unknown.

There are two major categories of seizures: partial and generalized seizures. In partial seizures only one area of the brain is involved, while general seizures involve the entire brain. Partial seizures account for a large portion of childhood seizures and are classified as *simple* or *complex*. Generalized seizures include infantile spasms, absence seizures, tonic-clonic seizures, myoclonic seizures, and atonic seizures. There are many different types of seizures,

(text continues on page 484)

Common Laboratory and Diagnostic Tests 17.1

Test	Explanation	Indications	Nursing Implications
Lumbar puncture (LP)	Withdrawal of CSF from the subarachnoid space for analysis	To diagnose hemorrhage, infection or obstruction Can obtain measurement of spinal fluid pressure	Assist with proper positioning (see Fig. 17.6). Help child maintain position and remain still. Maintain strict asepsis. Assist with collection and transport of specimen. Encourage fluids after procedure if not contraindicated. Keep child flat for 1 hour if ordered. Apply EMLA cream to puncture site 30–60 min before procedure to reduce pain, if ordered.
Head and neck x-ray	Radiographic image of the head and neck will show skull and spine structures	Detects skull and spinal fractures; shows location and course of ventricular catheters; reveals information about increased intracranial pressure (ICP) and skull defects	Children may be afraid. Allow a parent or family member to accompany the child. If the child is unable or unwilling I to stay still for the x-ray, restraint may be necessary. The time of restraint should be limited to the amount of time needed for the x-ray.
Fluoroscopy	Radiographic examination that uses continuous x-rays to show live up-to-date images	Can assess cervical spine for instability during movement	Same as head and neck x-rays. Child will need to cooperate with flexion and extension of neck.
Cerebral angiography	X-ray study of cerebral blood vessels. Involves injection of a contrast medium and use of fluoroscopy	Show vessel defects or space-occupying lesions	Same as head and neck x-rays. Assess for allergy to contrast medium. Push fluids following procedure, if not contraindicated, to help flush out contrast medium.
Ultrasound	Use of sound waves to locate the depth and structure within soft tissues and fluid	Used to assess intracranial hemorrhage in newborns, and ventricular size	Better tolerated by nonsedated children than CT or MRI Can be performed portably at bedside
Computed tomography (CT)	Noninvasive x-ray study that looks at tissue density and structures. Images a "slice" of client's tissue	To diagnose congenital abnormalities, such as neural tube defects, hemorrhage, tumors, fractures	Machine is large and can be frightening to children. Procedure can be lengthy and child must remain still. If unable to do so, sedation may be necessary. Can be performed with or without use of contrast medium; if used, assess for allergy. Encourage fluids postprocedure if not contraindicated.

(continued)

Common Laboratory and Diagnostic Tests 17.1 (continued)

Test	Explanation	Indications	Nursing Implications
Electroencephalogram (EEG)	Measure electrical activity of the brain	To diagnose seizures and brain death	Must remain still. If unable to do so, sedation may be necessary but should be avoided if possible because sedatives can alter the EEG reading. Inform technician of what anticonvulsants the client's taking. Morning anticonvulsants may need to be held.
Magnetic resonance imaging (MRI)	Use of magnetic field to show different tissue compositions	Used to assess tumors and inflammation; used to diagnose congenital abnormalities, such as neural tube defects; shows normal versus abnormal brain tissue	Client may not have any metal devices, internal or external, while undergoing MRI (ensure hospital gown does not have metal snaps). Procedure can be lengthy and child must remain still. Child is placed in long narrow tube and the machine makes a booming noise when it is turned on and off during the procedure; therefore can be difficult to gain cooperation. If the child is unable to remain still, sedation may be necessary. Can be performed with or without use of a contrast medium. If contrast medium is used, assess for allergy. Encourage fluids postprocedure if not contraindicated.
Positron emission tomography (PET)	Similar to CT or MRI but radioisotope is added. Measures physiologic function	Provides information on brain functional development. Can assist in identifying seizure foci. Can assess tumors and brain metabolism	Procedure can be lengthy and child must remain still. If unable to do so, sedation may be necessary. IV access will be needed for the procedure. Encourage fluids postprocedure if not contraindicated, to help body eliminate radioisotopes.
Intracranial pressure (ICP) monitoring (intraventricular catheter, subarachnoid screw or bolt, epidural sensor, anterior fontanel pressure monitor)	A sensing device is placed in the head that monitors the pressure intracranially.	Used to monitor ICP resulting from hydrocephalus, acute head trauma, and brain tumors. Ventricular catheter also allows for draining of CSF to help reduce ICP.	Usually monitored in critical care setting. Monitor for signs and symptoms of increased ICP. Monitor for infection. Keep head of bed elevated 15–30 degrees. Alarms for monitoring device should remain on at all times. Reduce stimulation and avoid interventions that may cause pain or stress and result in an increased ICP.

(continued)

Common Laboratory and Diagnostic Tests 17.1 (continued)

Test	Explanation	Indications	Nursing Implications
Video electroencephalogram (EEG)	Measure electrical activity of the brain continuously along with recorded video of actions and behaviors	Can help determine precise localization of seizure area before surgery. Assists in diagnosis and management of seizures by correlating behaviors with abnormal EEG activity	Ensure that seizure precautions are in place. Parent or caregiver must be with client at all times. Client movements are limited and usually confined to the room. When client changes position, ensure that he or she is still seen by video camera. Boredom can be a problem. Must notify nurse if seizure activity occurs; push the alert button to highlight attack on EEG recoding. Nurse must immediately go to the room, expose as much of the client as possible (remove covers; if at night, turn on light), and avoid blocking the camera. Ask questions (i.e., what is your name, can you raise your left arm, remember the word banana) to help assess responsiveness more accurately. Stay with the client until full recovery has occurred. Ask the client what word you asked them to remember, and document all findings and time of the event.

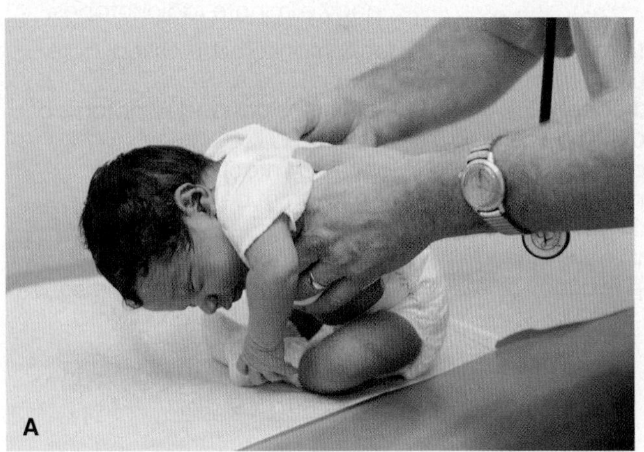

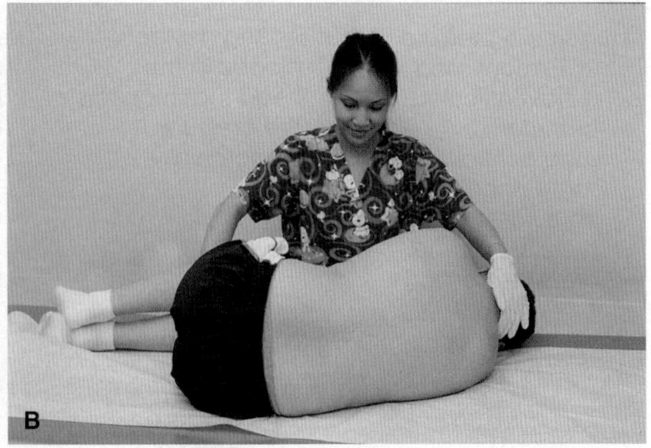

● Figure 17.6 Proper positioning for a lumbar puncture. (**A**) The newborn is positioned upright with head flexed forward. (**B**) Child or older infant is positioned on the side with head flexed forward and knees flexed to abdomen.

Nursing Care Plan 17.1

Overview for the Child with a Neurologic Disorder

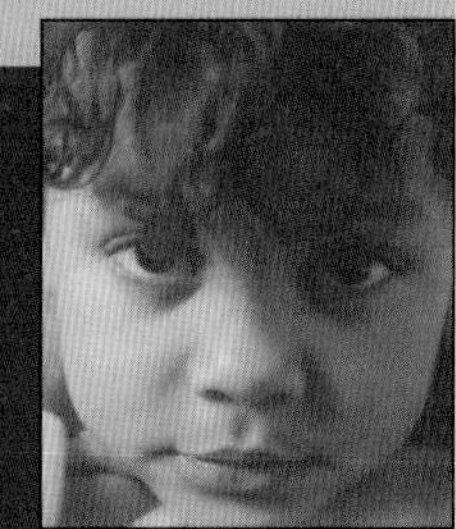

Nursing Diagnosis: Decreased intracranial adaptive capacity related to compression of brain tissue due to increased CSF or cerebral edema secondary to increased. ICP resulting from brain injury, congenital structural defects, brain tumor, decreased reabsorption of CSF, or shunt malfunction as evidenced by vomiting, headache, complaints of visual disturbances, decreased pulse and respirations, elevated blood pressure or pulse pressure, changes in level of consciousness, increased head circumference, or bulging fontanel

Outcome identification and evaluation

Child will remain free of signs and symptoms of increased intracranial pressure as evidenced by *remaining free of headache, vomiting, vision disturbances, vital signs within parameters for age, no signs of altered levels of consciousness, free of excessive irritability or lethargy, head circumference is within parameters for age.*

Interventions: promoting adequate intracranial adaptive capacity

- Assess neurologic status closely, monitor for signs and symptoms of increased ICP: *changes in level of consciousness, signs of irritability or lethargy, changes in pupillary reaction can indicate changes in ICP.*
- Monitor vital signs: *decreased pulse and respiratory rate and increased blood pressure or pulse pressure can indicate increased ICP.*
- Measure head circumference in children <3 years of age: *increases in head circumference outside parameters for age can indicate increased ICP.*
- Elevate head of bed 15–30 degrees to *facilitate venous return and can help to reduce ICP.*
- Minimize environmental stimuli and noise, avoid pain-producing procedures if possible: *all can increase ICP.*
- Have emergency equipment ready and available: *increased ICP can result in respiratory or cardiac failure.*
- Notify MD immediately if changes in assessment are noted: *early intervention is critical to prevent neurologic damage and death.*

Nursing Diagnosis: Risk for ineffective (cerebral) tissue perfusion related to increased ICP, alteration in blood flow secondary to hemorrhage, vessel malformation, cerebral edema

Outcome identification and evaluation

Child will exhibit adequate cerebral tissue perfusion through course of illness and childhood: *Child will remain alert and oriented with no signs of altered level of consciousness; vital signs will be within parameters for age; motor, sensory, and cognitive function will be within parameters for age; head circumference remains within parameters for age.*

Interventions: promoting adequate tissue perfusion

- Assess neurologic status closely, monitor for signs and symptoms of increased ICP: *changes in level of consciousness, signs of irritability or lethargy, changes in pupillary reaction can indicate decreased cerebral tissue perfusion.*
- Monitor vital signs: *decreased pulse and respiratory rate and increased blood pressure or pulse pressure can indicate increased ICP, which can lead to decreased cerebral perfusion.*
- Measure specific gravity of urine: *can detect an oversecretion or undersecretion of antidiuretic hormone*
- Have emergency equipment ready and available: *decreased cerebral perfusion can result in respiratory or cardiac failure.*
- Notify MD immediately if changes in assessment are noted: *early intervention is critical to prevent neurologic damage and death.*

(continued)

Overview for the Child with a Neurologic Disorder (continued)

Nursing Diagnosis: Risk for injury related to altered level of consciousness, weakness, dizziness, ataxia, loss of muscle coordination secondary to seizure activity

Outcome identification and evaluation

Child will remain free of injury as evidenced by *no signs of aspiration or traumatic injury.*

Interventions: preventing injury

- Ensure child has patent airway and adequate oxygenation (have suction, oxygen available at bedside) and place child in side-lying position if possible: *a child with altered level of consciousness may not be able to manage his secretions and is at risk for aspiration and ineffective airway clearance; providing suction and oxygenation can help ensure an open airway and the side-lying position can help secretions drain and prevent obstruction of airway or aspiration.*
- Protect child from hurting self during seizures or changes in level of consciousness by removing environmental obstacles, easing child to lying position, and padding side rails: *helps to keep environment safe*
- Institute seizure precautions for any child at risk for seizure activity (see Box 17.2): *to help prevent injury that can result from acute seizure activity*
- With seizure activity do not insert a tongue blade or restrain child: *can lead to injury to caregiver and child*
- Administer anticonvulsant medications as ordered: *will help to promote cessation and prevention of seizure activity*
- Assist child with ambulation: *help prevent injury in child with weakness, dizziness, ataxia*
- Allow for periods of rest: *to prevent fatigue and decrease risk of injury*

Nursing Diagnosis: Disturbed sensory perception related to presence of neurologic lesion or pressure on sensory or motor nerves secondary to increased ICP, presence of tumor, swelling postoperatively as evidenced by visual disturbances (i.e., reports of double vision), pupillary changes, nystagmus, ataxia, balance disturbances, or loss of response to stimuli

Outcome identification and evaluation

Child will be free of changes in sensory perception or will remain at baseline as evidenced by *no complaints of double vision, PERRLA, no disturbances of gait or balance noted, and no increased in loss of responses to stimuli.*

Interventions: managing disturbed sensory perception

- Assess for changes in sensory perception: *provides baseline data and allows nurse to recognize change in sensory perception early*
- Monitor child for risk of injury secondary to changes in sensory perception: *visual changes, disturbances of gait or balance increase child's risk for injury*
- Notify MD of changes in sensory perception: *can indicate increased ICP and medical emergency*
- Assist child to learn to use adaptive methods to live with permanent changes in sensory perception (i.e., use of eyeglasses) and maximize the use of intact senses: *adaptive devices can enhance sensory input and intact senses can often compensate for impaired senses.*
- Provide familiar sounds (voices, music): *can help relieve anxiety related to changes in sensory perception, especially visual changes*

Overview for the Child with a Neurologic Disorder (continued)

Nursing Diagnosis: Risk for infection related to surgical interventions, presence of foreign body (i.e., shunt), trauma to skull, nutritional deficiencies, stasis of pulmonary secretions and urine, presence of infectious organisms as evidenced by fever, poor feeding, decreased responsiveness and presence of virus or bacteria on laboratory screening

Outcome identification and evaluation

Child will exhibit no signs or symptoms of local or systemic infection and will not spread infection to others: *Symptoms of infection will decrease over time; others will remain free of infection.*

Interventions: preventing infection

- Monitor vital signs: *elevation in temperature can indicate presence of infection.*
- Monitor incision sites for signs of local infection: *redness, warmth, drainage, swelling, pain at incision site can indicate presence of infection.*
- Maintain aseptic technique—practice good hand washing, use proper technique when managing postoperative incisions and external shunts: *to prevent introduction of further infectious agents*
- Administer antibiotics as prescribed: *to prevent or treat bacterial infection*
- Encourage nutritious diet and proper hydration according to child's preferences and ability to feed orally: *to assist body's natural defenses against infection*
- Isolation of child as required: *to prevent nosocomial spread of infection*
- Teach child and family preventive measures such as good hand washing, covering mouth and nose upon cough or sneeze, adequate disposal of used tissues: *to prevent nosocomial or community spread of infection*

Nursing Diagnosis: Self-care deficit related to neuromuscular impairments; cognitive deficits as evidenced by an inability to perform hygiene care and transfer self independently

Outcome identification and evaluation

Child will demonstrate ability to care for self within age parameters and limits of disease: *Child is able to feed, dress, manage elimination within limits of disease and age.*

Interventions: maximizing self-care

- Introduce child and family to self-help methods as soon as possible: *promotes independence from the beginning*
- Encourage family and staff to allow child to do as much as possible: *allows child to gain confidence and independence*
- Teach specific measures for bowel and urinary elimination as needed: *promotes independence, increases self-care abilities and self-esteem*
- Collaborate with physical therapy, occupational therapy, and speech therapy departments to provide child and family with appropriate tools to modify environment and methods to promote transferring and self-care: *allows for maximum functioning*
- Praise accomplishments and emphasize child's abilities: *helps improve self-esteem and encourages feeling of confidence and competence*
- Balance activity with periods to rest: *to reduce fatigue and increase energy for self-care*

Nursing Diagnosis: Impaired physical mobility related to muscle weakness, hypertonicity, impaired coordination, loss of muscle function or control as evidenced by an inability to move extremities, to ambulate without assistance, to move without limitations

Outcome identification and evaluation

Child will be able to engage in activities within age parameters and limits of disease: *Child is able to move extremities, move about environment, and participate in exercise programs within limits of age and disease.*

(continued)

Overview for the Child with a Neurologic Disorder (continued)

Interventions: maximizing physical mobility

- Encourage gross and fine motor activities: *facilitates motor development*
- Collaborate with physical therapy, occupational therapy, and speech therapy departments to strengthen muscles and promote optimal mobility: *facilitates motor development*
- Utilize passive and active ROM and teach child and family how to perform: *prevent contractures, facilitate joint mobility and muscle development (active ROM) to help increase mobility*
- Praise accomplishments and emphasize child's abilities: *helps improve self-esteem and encourages feeling of confidence and competence*

Nursing Diagnosis: Risk for delayed development related to physical disability, cognitive deficits, activity restrictions

Outcome identification and evaluation

Child will demonstrate developmental milestones within age parameters and limits of disease: *Child expresses interest in the environment and people around him or her, and interacts with environment age appropriately.*

Interventions: maximizing development

- Use therapeutic play and adaptive toys: *helps facilitate developmental functioning*
- Provide stimulating environment when possible: *to maximize potential for growth and development*
- Praise accomplishments and emphasize child's abilities: *helps improve self-esteem and encourages feeling of confidence and competence*

Nursing Diagnosis: Nutrition, imbalanced: less than body requirements related to vomiting and difficulty feeding secondary to increased ICP; difficulty sucking, swallowing, or chewing; surgical incision pain or difficulty assuming normal feeding position; inability to feed self as evidenced by decreased oral intake, impaired swallowing, weight loss

Outcome identification and evaluation

Child will exhibit signs of adequate nutrition as evidenced by: *Weight will remain within parameters for age, skin turgor will be good, I/O will be within normal limits, adequate calories will be ingested, vomiting will cease or decrease.*

Interventions: promoting adequate nutrition

- Monitor height and weight: *insufficient intake will lead to impaired growth and weight gain.*
- Monitor hydration status (moist mucous membranes, elastic skin turgor, adequate urine output): *insufficient intake can lead to dehydration.*
- Use techniques to promote caloric and nutritional intake and teach family (i.e., positioning, modified utensils, soft or blended foods, allow extra time): *these techniques can facilitate intake.*
- Assess respiratory system frequently: *to assess for aspiration*
- Monitor for nausea and vomiting and medicate if ordered: *to help reduce vomiting and increase intake*
- Monitor for pain and medicate if ordered: *to help reduce pain related to surgical incisions and trauma, and increase intake*
- Assist family to assume as normal a feeding position as possible: *to help increase oral intake*

Overview for the Child with a Neurologic Disorder (continued)

Nursing Diagnosis: Fluid volume deficit, risk for, related to vomiting, altered level of consciousness, poor feeding or intake, insensible loss due to fever, failure of regulatory mechanisms (as in diabetes insipidus) as evidenced by dry oral mucosa, decreased skin turgor, sudden weight loss, hypotension, and tachycardia

Outcome identification and evaluation

Fluid volume will be maintained and balanced: *oral mucosa moist and pink, skin turgor elastic, urine output at least 1–2 cc/kg/hr*

Interventions: promoting adequate fluid balance

- Administer IV fluids if ordered: *to maintain adequate hydration in children who are NPO or unable to tolerate oral intake*
- When oral intake is allowed and tolerated, encourage PO fluids: *to promote intake and maintain hydration*
- Strict intake and output monitoring: *can help identify fluid imbalance and also detect signs of abnormal pituitary secretions resulting in conditions like syndrome of inappropriate antidiuretic hormone secretion (SIADH) and diabetes insipidus (DI) (see Chapter 28 for further information)*
- Maintain minimum hydration and avoid overhydration in clients where cerebral edema is a concern: *fluid overload can contribute to cerebral edema.*
- Urine specific gravity, urine and serum electrolytes (especially serum sodium), blood urea nitrogen, creatinine and osmolality, and daily weights: *are reliable indicators of fluid status and can also detect signs of abnormal pituitary secretions resulting in conditions like SIADH and DI*

Nursing Diagnosis: Knowledge deficit related to lack of information regarding complex medical condition, prognosis, and medical needs as evidenced by verbalization, questions, or actions demonstrating lack of understanding regarding child's condition or care

Outcome identification and evaluation

Child and family will verbalize accurate information and understanding about condition, prognosis, and medical needs: *Child and family demonstrate knowledge of condition and prognosis and medical needs including possible causes, contributing factors, and treatment measures.*

Interventions: providing client and family teaching

- Assess child's and family's willingness to learn: *child and family must be willing to learn for teaching to be effective.*
- Provide family with time to adjust to diagnosis: *will help facilitate adjustment and ability to learn and participate in child's care*
- Repeat information: *allows family and child time to learn and understand*
- Teach in short sessions: *many short sessions are found to be more helpful than one long session.*
- Gear teaching to a level of understanding of the child and also the family (depends on age of child, physical condition, memory): *to ensure understanding*
- Provide reinforcement and rewards: *help facilitate the teaching–learning process*
- Use multiple modes of learning involving many senses (provide written, verbal, demonstration, and videos) when possible: *child and family more likely to retain information when presented in different ways using many senses*

(continued)

Overview for the Child with a Neurologic Disorder (continued)

Nursing Diagnosis: Family processes, interrupted related to child's illness, hospitalization, diagnosis of chronic illness in child and potential long-term affects of illness as evidenced by family's presence in hospital, missed work, demonstration of inadequate coping

Outcome identification and evaluation

Family will maintain functional system of support and demonstrate adequate coping, adaptation of roles and functions, and decreased anxiety: *Parents are involved in child's care, ask appropriate questions, express fears and concerns, and are able to discuss child's care and condition calmly.*

Interventions: promoting adequate family processes

- Encourage parents and family members to verbalize concerns related to child's illness, diagnosis, and prognosis: *allows the nurse to identify concerns and areas where further education may be needed. Demonstrates family-centered care*
- Explain therapies, procedures, child's behaviors, and plan of care to parents: *understanding the child's current status and plan of care helps decrease anxiety.*
- Encourage parental involvement in care: *allows parents to feel needed and valued with a sense of control over their child's health*
- Identify support system for family and child: *helps nurse identify needs and resources available for coping*
- Educate family and child on additional resources available: *to help them develop a wide base of support*

and the classification of the type of seizure is crucial in assisting with the management and control of seizures. Not all cases are easily classified. The most common seizure types are discussed in Table 17.2.

Therapeutic Management

Management of epilepsy focuses on controlling seizures or reducing their frequency, along with helping the child who has recurrent seizures and his or her family to learn to live with the seizures. The primary mode of treatment is the use of anticonvulsants. There have been significant advances in the treatment of epilepsy due to the many new anticonvulsant medications that have become available in recent years (Table 17.3). Most anticonvulsants are taken orally and are often used in combination. Different medications control different types of seizures, which may be due to individual variation. It can take time to find the right combination to best control an individual's seizures.

If seizures remain uncontrolled, another option for managing them is surgery. Depending on the area of the brain that is affected, it may be possible to remove the area that is responsible for the seizure activity or to interrupt the impulses from spreading and therefore stop or reduce the seizures. The adverse effects range from mild to severe, depending on the area of the brain that is affected. Other nonpharmacologic treatments that may be considered in children with intractable seizures include a ketogenic diet or placement of a vagal nerve stimulator. Refer to Common Medical Treatments 17.1.

Nursing Assessment

For a full description of the assessment phase of the nursing process, refer to page 469. Assessment findings pertinent to epilepsy are discussed below.

Health History

Elicit a description of the present illness and chief complaint, which will usually involve a seizure episode. Gain information to help characterize the episode as a seizure or as a nonepileptic event (see Box 17.1 for a list of nonepileptic events). It is rare to actually observe the child having a seizure; therefore a complete, accurate, and detailed history from a reliable source is essential. *Questions should include:*

- Where did the event occur—while sleeping, eating, playing, or just after waking?
- Description of child's behavior during the event—what types of movements, progression, length, respiratory status, apnea?
- How did the child act after the event?
- Have the episodes been recurrent? If so, how frequent?
- Any precipitating factors such as a fever, fall, activity, anxiety, infection, or exposure to strong stimuli such as flashing lights or loud noises?

Table 17.2 Common Types of Seizures

Type	Description	Characteristics
Infantile spasms	Uncommon type of generalized seizure seen in an epilepsy syndrome of infancy and childhood	Presents as a sudden jerk followed by stiffening May see: • Head flexed, arms extended, and legs drawn up • Arms flung out, knees are pulled up, and the body bends forward (referred to as "jackknife seizures") • Cry may precede or follow Majority of infants have some brain disorder before seizures begin.
	Usually seen between 3–12 months of age and usually stops by 2–4 years of age	The infant seems to stop developing and may lose skills that he or she has already attained after the onset of infantile spasms. Steroid therapy and anticonvulsants are common forms of treatment.
Absence (formerly *petit mal*)	Type of generalized seizure; occurs more frequently in girls than boys Uncommon before age 5	Sudden cessation of motor activity or speech with a blank facial expression or rhythmic twitching of the mouth or blinking of the eyelids Complex absence seizure consists of myoclonic movements of the face, fingers, or extremities and possible loss of body tone. Lasts less than 30 seconds Child may experience countless seizures in a day. Not associated with a post-ictal state May go unrecognized or mistaken for inattentiveness because of subtle change in child's behavior
Tonic-clonic (formerly *grand mal*)	Extremely common generalized seizures. Most dramatic seizure type	Associated with an aura Loss of consciousness occurs and may be preceded by a piercing cry. Presents with entire body experiencing tonic contractions followed by rhythmic clonic contractions alternating with relaxation of all muscle groups Cyanosis may be noted due to apnea. Saliva may collect in the mouth due to inability to swallow. Child may bite tongue. Loss of sphincter control, especially the bladder, is common. Postictal phase: child will be semicomatose or in a deep sleep for approximately 30 minutes to 2 hours; usually responds only to painful stimuli Child will have no memory of the seizure; may complain of headache and feeling fatigue Safety of the child is a primary concern. See Teaching Guideline 17.1.
Myoclonic	Type of generalized seizure that involves the motor cortex of the brain. May occur along with other seizure forms	Sudden, brief, massive muscle jerks that may involve the whole body or one body part Child may or may not lose consciousness.

Table 17.2 Common Types of Seizures (continued)

Type	Description	Characteristics
Atonic	Type of generalized seizure often referred to as "drop attacks." Seen in children with Lennox-Gastaut syndrome	Sudden loss of muscle tone. In children, may only be a sudden drop of the head. Child will regain consciousness within a few seconds to a minute. Can result in injury related to violent fall
Simple partial	Type of partial seizure that occurs in part of the brain. The symptoms seen will depend on which area of the brain is affected.	Motor activity characterized by clonic or tonic movements involving the face, neck, and extremities Can include sensory signs such as numbness, tingling, paresthesia, or pain Usually persists for 10–20 seconds Child remains conscious and may verbalize during the seizure. No post-ictal state
Complex partial	Common type of partial seizure. May begin with a simple partial seizure then progress	May or may not have a preceding aura Consciousness will be impaired. Automatisms and complex purposeful movements are common features in infants and children. Infants will present with behaviors such as lip smacking, chewing, swallowing, and excessive salivation; can be difficult to distinguish from normal infant behavior In older children, will see picking or pulling at bed sheets or clothing, rubbing objects, or running or walking in a nondirective and repetitive fashion These seizures can be difficult to control.
Status epilepticus	Common neurologic emergency in children. Can occur with any seizure activity. Febrile seizures are the most common type. In children with epilepsy, it commonly occurs early in the course of epilepsy. Can be life threatening	Prolonged or clustered seizures where consciousness does not return between seizures. The age of the child, cause of the seizures, and duration of status epilepticus influence prognosis. Prompt medical intervention is essential to reduce morbidity and mortality. Treatment: • Basic life support—ABCs (airway, breathing, circulation) • Administration of anticonvulsants to cease seizures is crucial. Common medications include benzodiazepines such as lorazepam and diazepam, and fosphenytoin. (See Drug Guide 17.1 and Table 17.3) • Blood glucose levels and electrolytes along with evaluation of the underlying cause should be initiated.

Explore the client's current and past medical history for risk factors such as:

- Family history of seizures or epilepsy
- Any complications during the prenatal, perinatal, or postnatal periods
- Changes in developmental status or delays in developmental milestones
- Any recent illness, fever, trauma, or toxin exposure

Children known to have epilepsy are often admitted to the hospital for other health-related issues or complications and treatment of their seizure disorder. The health history should include questions related to:

- Age of onset of seizures
- Seizure control—what medications is the child taking and has he or she been able to take them; when was his or her last seizure?

Table 17.3 Common Anticonvulsant Medications

Medication	Nursing Implications
Phenytoin (IV and PO; IM administration is contraindicated)	Monitor serum levels to ensure therapeutic dosing. Be aware that gingival hyperplasia appears most commonly in children and adolescents. If on prolonged therapy, ensure adequate intake of vitamin D–containing foods. Monitor serum calcium and magnesium levels.
Fosphenytoin (IM or IV only)	Adverse effects are said to be less common than with phenytoin. It does not cause local irritation, but it is a more expensive drug than phenytoin. It is water soluble, therefore allowing faster and easier administration than phenytoin. All dosing is in phenytoin sodium equivalents. It does not precipitate in commonly used IV diluents.
Phenobarbital	Assess for excessive sedation. Monitor serum levels to ensure therapeutic dosing. Monitor for drug interactions. Increase vitamin D–fortified foods or administer supplement if prescribed. Withdrawal symptoms will occur if drug is stopped abruptly. Valproic acid interferes with this drug, causing increased phenobarbital levels.
Felbamate	Monitor for drug interactions, especially if client is taking phenytoin or carbamazepine.
Valproic acid (divalproex sodium, sodium valproate)	Monitor serum levels to ensure therapeutic dosing. Depakote sprinkles are available and useful for children who are unable to tolerate valproate suspension, tablets, or capsules. The contents can be sprinkled on food that does not require chewing.
Carbamazepine	Monitor serum levels to ensure therapeutic dosing; toxicity can occur even with levels slightly above therapeutic range. Plasma concentration decreased by phenytoin, phenobarbital, and valproic acid.
Gabapentin	Do not administer within 2 hours of antacids. Rapidly absorbed in the gastrointestinal tract
Topiramate	Dilantin, tegretol, and valproic acid decrease concentration of topiramate.
Oxcarbazine	Monitor phenytoin levels if administering concurrently.
Zonisamide	Presence of food will delay absorption. Phenytoin, phenobarbital, and carbamazepine all increase the metabolism of this drug.
Lamotrigine	Valproate inhibits metabolism; therefore, monitor serum blood values and decrease the dose if necessary.

IM, intramuscular; IV, intravenous; PO, by mouth.

- Description and classification of seizures—does the child lose consciousness; does the child become apneic?
- Precipitating factors that may contribute to onset of seizures
- Adverse effects related to anticonvulsant medications
- Compliance with medication regimen

BOX 17.1

NONEPILEPTIC EVENTS

- Syncope
- Breath holding
- Jitteriness
- Apnea
- Gastroesophageal reflux
- Cardiac conduction abnormalities
- Migraines
- Tics

Physical Examination

Perform a complete neurologic examination. Careful assessment of the child's mental status, language, learning, behavior, and motor abilities can help provide information about any neurologic deficits. If seizure activity is observed directly, provide a thorough and accurate description of the event. This description needs to include:

- Time of onset and length of seizure activity
- Alterations in behavior such as a cry or changes in facial expression, motor abilities, or sensory alterations prior to the seizure that may indicate an aura
- Precipitating factors such as fever, anxiety, just waking, or eating
- Description of movements and any progression
- Description of respiratory effort and any apnea noted
- Changes in color (pallor or cyanosis) noted
- Position of mouth, any injury to mouth or tongue, inability to swallow, or excessive salivation
- Loss of bladder or bowel control

- State of consciousness during seizure and postictal (after seizure) state—during the seizure the nurse may ask the child to remember a word; after the seizure, assess if child is able to recall it, to help accurately establish current mental state
- Assess: orientation to person, place, and time; motor abilities; speech; behavior; alterations in sensation postictally
- Duration of postictal state

Laboratory and Diagnostic Tests

Laboratory and diagnostic tests are used to evaluate the cause of, and also aid in identifying the type of, seizure activity (refer to Common Laboratory and Diagnostic Tests 17.1). Common laboratory and diagnostic studies ordered for the diagnosis and assessment of epilepsy include:

- Serum glucose, electrolytes, and calcium—to rule out metabolic causes such as hypoglycemia and hypocalcemia
- Lumbar puncture (LP)—to analyze CSF to rule out meningitis or encephalitis
- Skull x-ray examinations—to evaluate for the presence of fracture or trauma
- Computed tomography (CT) and magnetic resonance imaging (MRI) studies—to identify abnormalities and intracranial bleeds and rule out tumors
- Electroencephalographs (EEGs)—EEG findings may be noted with certain seizure types, but a normal EEG does not rule out epilepsy because seizure activity rarely occurs during the actual testing time. EEGs are useful in evaluating seizure type and assisting in medication selection. They can be useful in differentiating seizures from nonepileptic activity.
- Video EEGs—provide the opportunity to see the child's actual behavior on video, accompanied with EEG changes; can improve the chance of catching a seizure because the monitoring is done over a period of time

Nursing Management

Nursing management focuses on preventing injury during seizures; administering appropriate medication and treatments to prevent or reduce seizures; and providing education and support to the child and family to help them cope with the challenges of living with a chronic seizure disorder. See Box 17.2 for a list of basic seizure precautions. In addition to the nursing diagnoses and related interventions discussed in Nursing Care Plan 17.1, interventions common to epilepsy follow.

Relieving Anxiety

Seizures produce fear and anxiety due to their unpredictable nature along with the uncontrolled, forceful, and at times violent appearance. Instruct parents and family members, along with those in the community who may care for the child, on how to respond in case of a seizure (see Teaching Guideline 17.1). This will help to empower the parents, family, and other caregivers, and in turn alleviate some of the anxiety that they may feel.

BOX 17.2

SEIZURE PRECAUTIONS

- Padding of side rails and other hard objects
- Side rails raised on bed at all times when child is in bed
- Oxygen and suction at bedside
- Supervision, especially during bathing, ambulation, or other potentially hazardous activities
- Use of a protective helmet during activity may be appropriate.
- Child should wear a medical alert bracelet.

Managing Treatment

Provide child and family teaching and instruction regarding the administration of anticonvulsant therapy and its importance. Included in this discussion should be common adverse effects, the need to continue the medication unless instructed otherwise by the physician, and the need to call the physician if the child is ill and vomiting and unable to take his or her medication. Encourage parents to discuss unwanted adverse effects with the physician so that they can be addressed and noncompliance with the

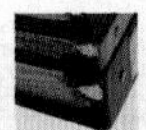

TEACHING GUIDELINE 17.1

How to Respond When Your Child Has a Seizure

Instruct parents and caregivers:

- Remain calm.
- Time seizure episode.
- If child is standing or sitting, ease child to the ground if possible.
- Tight clothing and jewelry around the neck should be loosened if possible.
- Place child on one side and open airway if possible.
- Do not restrain the child.
- Remove hazards in the area.
- Do not forcibly open jaw with a tongue blade or fingers.
- Document length of seizure and movements noted, also cyanosis or loss of bladder or bowel control and any other characteristics.
- Remain with child until fully conscious.
- Call emergency medical services (EMS) if:
  - The child stops breathing
  - Any injury has occurred
  - Seizure lasts for more than 5 minutes
  - This is the child's first seizure
  - Child is unresponsive to painful stimuli after seizure

medication regimen can be reduced. The most common cause of breakthrough seizures is noncompliance.

Providing Family Support and Education

Having a child with a chronic seizure disorder can place stress and anxiety on the family that is often due to fears and misconceptions they may have. An important nursing function is to educate not only the child and family but also the community, including the child's teachers and caregivers, on the reality and facts of the disorder. Encourage parents to be involved in the management of their child's seizures but to allow the child to learn about the disorder and its management as soon as he or she is old enough. Encourage parents to treat the child with epilepsy just as they would a child without this disorder. Children who are brought up no differently than children without epilepsy will be more likely to develop a positive self-image and have increased self-esteem. Any activity restrictions, such as limiting swimming or participation in sports, will be based on the type, frequency, and severity of the seizures the child has. Educate parents and children on any restrictions and encourage parents to place only the necessary restrictions on the child.

The needs of the child and family will change as the child grows and develops. The nurse needs to recognize theses changes and provide appropriate education and support. Referral to support groups is appropriate. The Epilepsy Foundation can be accessed at www.epilepsyfoundation.org. Additional resources can be found at www.paceusa.org and www.epilepsyinstitute.org.

● FEBRILE SEIZURES

Febrile seizures are the most common type of seizure seen during childhood. They usually affect children who are less than 5 years of age, with the peak incidence occurring in children between 18 and 24 months old. It is rare to see febrile seizures in children younger than 6 months and older than 7 years of age. This type of seizure is more commonly seen in boys and there is an increased risk for children who have a family history of febrile seizures. Febrile seizures are associated with a fever, usually related to a viral illness. These seizures are usually benign but can be very frightening for both the child and family. The prognosis is generally excellent for febrile seizures. However, febrile seizures may indicate a serious underlying infectious disease, such as meningitis or sepsis. Though rare, complications associated with febrile seizures include status epilepticus, motor coordination deficits, mental retardation, and behavioral problems.

Therapeutic Management

Treatment includes determination of the cause of the fever and interventions to control the fever. The American Academy of Pediatrics does not recommend long-term or intermittent anticonvulsant therapy for the child who has suffered one or more simple febrile seizures (Shinnar & O'Dell, 2004). Rectal diazepam has been shown to be safe and effective in terminating febrile seizures and may be used in children at high risk for febrile seizures or in children whose parents are extremely anxious. Although anticonvulsant prophylaxis is no longer recommended (Behrman et al., 2004), intermittent use of anticonvulsants at the time of a fever may be used in select groups of children.

Nursing Assessment

A febrile seizure is usually associated with a core temperature that increases rapidly to 39° C or higher. The seizure usually presents as a generalized tonic-clonic seizure that lasts a few seconds to 10 minutes and is followed by a brief postictal period of drowsiness. A simple febrile seizure is defined as a generalized seizure lasting less than 15 minutes that occurs once in a 24-hour period and is accompanied by a fever. It is likely to have stopped by the time a child receives medical attention. Diagnosis is made based on a thorough history and physical examination, accompanied by a determination of the source of the fever. In some cases an LP may be performed to rule out meningitis or encephalitis. This will be based on the age and the clinical presentation of the child.

Risk factors for recurrence of a febrile seizure include young age at first febrile seizure and family history of febrile seizures and high fever. Children who experience one or more febrile seizures are at no greater risk of developing epilepsy than the general population. No evidence exists that febrile seizures cause structural damage or cognitive declines.

Nursing Management

Provide parental support and education regarding febrile seizures. Reassure parents of the benign nature of febrile seizures. Counsel parents on controlling fever; discuss how to keep a child safe during a seizure; and provide instruction and demonstration in the administration of rectal diazepam at the onset of a seizure (if applicable). Instruct parents when to call their physician and when to take their child to the emergency room. Reinforce that any recurrent seizure activity will require prompt medical attention.

● NEONATAL SEIZURES

The incidence of seizures is higher in the neonatal period than in any other age group. The immature brain is more prone to seizure activity. Neonatal seizures are seizures that occur within the first 4 weeks of life and are most commonly seen within the first 10 days. They are different from those in the child or adult because generalized tonic-clonic seizures tend not to occur during the first month of life. Seizures in newborns are associated with underlying conditions such as hypoxic-ischemic encephalopathy, metabolic disorders (hypoglycemia and hypocalcemia), neonatal infection (meningitis and encephalitis), and intracranial hemorrhage. The prognosis depends mainly on the underlying cause of the seizures and the severity of the insult. There is increasing evidence that neonatal seizures have an adverse effect on neurodevelopment and may predispose the infant to cognitive, behavioral, or epileptic complications later in life.

Therapeutic Management

Acute neonatal seizures should be treated aggressively because repeated seizure activity may result in injury to the brain. Treatment focuses on ensuring adequate ventilation; correcting any underlying metabolic disturbance that may exist, such as hypoglycemia; and possibly administering anticonvulsant therapy. Phenobarbital is often used in the initial management of neonatal seizures but efficacy remains uncertain. The dosage of anticonvulsants may be higher in the neonate because neonates metabolize drugs more rapidly than older infants.

Nursing Assessment

Neonatal seizures may be difficult to recognize clinically and may be accompanied by a normal EEG. Several clinical features may help distinguish seizures from nonepileptic activity, such as tremors or jitteriness, in neonates. Autonomic changes such as tachycardia and elevated blood pressure are common with seizures in neonates, but do not occur with nonepileptic events. Also, nonepileptic movements can be suppressed by gently restraining the limb; in true seizures this is not the case. Ocular deviation may be seen with seizure activity but will not be present with nonepileptic activity. The characteristics of seizures seen in the neonatal period differ from those seen in older children. Five major seizure types have been recognized in the neonatal period. See Table 17.4 for information on types of seizures seen in newborn infants.

Laboratory and diagnostic tests including serum testing (e.g., serum glucose, electrolytes, calcium), LP (to analyze CSF), cranial ultrasound, CT, and MRI may be performed to help determine the cause of the seizures. EEGs and video EEGs may assist in the characterization of neonatal seizures and their medical management.

Nursing Management

Nursing management will focus on carrying out interventions to cease seizure activity; monitoring neurologic status closely; recognizing the seizures; preventing injury during seizure activity; and providing support and education to the parents and family.

Structural Defects

Due to the sensitivity of the development of the neurologic system in the first weeks of embryonic life, there exists a potential for defects to occur. These structural defects include neural tube defects, microcephaly, Arnold-Chiari malformation, hydrocephalus, intracranial arteriovenous malformation, and craniosynostosis.

● NEURAL TUBE DEFECTS

Neural tube defects account for the majority of congenital anomalies of the CNS. They are serious birth defects of the spine and the brain and include disorders such as spina bifida occulta, myelomeningocele, meningocele, anencephaly, and encephalocele. The neural tube closes between the third and fourth week *in utero*. The cause of neural tube defects is not known but many factors such as drugs, malnutrition, chemicals, and genetics can adversely affect normal CNS development. Strong evidence exists that maternal preconception supplementation of folic acid

Table 17.4 Types of Seizures Seen in Newborn Infants

Type	Age Affected	Characteristics
Subtle	Preterm and full term	Chewing motions, excessive salivation, alterations in respiratory rate, apnea, blinking, and pedaling movements
Tonic	Preterm	Rigid posturing of the extremities and trunk May be associated with fixed deviation of the eyes
Focal clonic	Full term	Rhythmic twitching of local muscle groups such as the extremities or face
Multifocal clonic	Full term	Similar to focal clonic, except many muscle groups are involved, frequently simultaneously
Myoclonic	Rare in neonatal period	Brief focal jerks, involving one extremity; or multifocal jerks, involving several body parts

can decrease the incidence of neural tube defects in pregnancies at risk by 50% (Behrman et al., 2004). In 1992, the United States Public Health Service recommended that all women of childbearing age who are capable of becoming pregnant take 0.4 mg (400 mcg) of folic acid daily (Merereau et al., 2004). According to the Centers for Disease Control and Prevention (CDC), the number of pregnancies affected by neural tube defects has decreased from 4,000 (1995–1996) to 3,000 (1999–2000) (Merereau et al., 2004). Prenatal screening of maternal serum for alpha-fetoprotein (AFP) and ultrasound examination at 16 to 18 weeks' gestation can help identify fetuses at risk. Anencephaly and encephalocele are discussed below. Refer to Chapter 23 for information on spina bifida occulta, meningocele, and myelomeningocele.

Anencephaly

Anencephaly is a defect in brain development resulting in small or missing brain hemispheres, skull, and scalp. It occurs when the cephalic or upper end of the neural tube fails to close during the third to fourth week of gestation. These infants are born without both a forebrain and a cerebrum, and the condition is incompatible with life. The remaining brain tissue may be exposed. The incidence of anencephaly is 1 in 1,000 live births (Behrman et al., 2004).

Nursing Assessment

Anencephalic infants have a distinctive appearance, with a large defect noted in the vault of the skull (Fig. 17.7). The mother may have had a difficult labor due to the malformation of the head not allowing it to engage in the cervix. The majority of infants will be stillborn. If not, most anencephalic infants die within hours to several days of birth. There have been a few cases in which the infant has lived for several months. The infant is usually blind, deaf, unconscious, and unable to feel pain. Some infants born with anencephaly may be born with a brain stem, but the lack of cerebrum rules out the possibility of gaining consciousness. Reflex actions such as respirations, reactions to sound and touch, and ability to suck may be present.

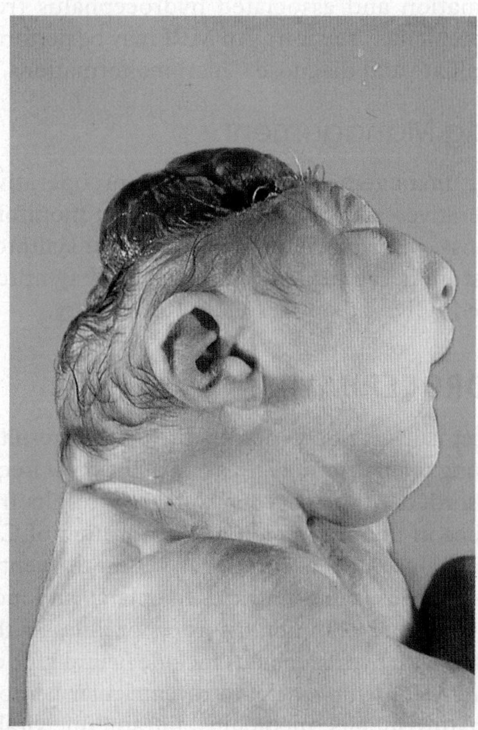

● Figure 17.7 Anencephalic infant.

Nursing Management

The prognosis is extremely poor. Nursing management is supportive in nature and focuses on comfort measures for the dying infant. Some parents may have been aware of the diagnosis prenatally due to screening tests such as AFP and ultrasounds. Parents and family will need support and understanding from all health care professionals during this difficult time. Fear of what the child will look like may be overwhelming. Use of an infant cap can be helpful and allow parents to feel more comfortable holding and comforting their infant. Assisting with anticipatory grieving and decision making related to end-of-life care will also be key nursing interventions.

Encephalocele

Encephalocele is a protrusion of the brain and meninges through a skull defect. It results from failure of the anterior portion of the neural tube to close. Infants born with an encephalocele are at risk for visual problems, microcephaly, mental retardation, and seizures. The prognosis, including the extent of complications and cognitive deficits, will depend on the size and location of the encephalocele and involvement of other brain structures. Encephaloceles are often accompanied by craniofacial and other abnormalities such as hydrocephalus, microcephaly, spastic quadriplegia, ataxia, developmental delay, mental and growth retardation, and seizures. Some children who are affected may display normal intelligence.

Treatment consists of surgical repair, including placement of tissues back into the skull and removal of the sac; possible shunt placement to correct associated hydrocephalus; and corrective repair of any craniofacial abnormalities.

Nursing Assessment

Initial assessment postdelivery will reveal a visible external sac protruding from the skull area. It occurs most commonly in the occipital region but can occur elsewhere, such as frontally or nasofrontally. Generally the lesion is covered by skin, but it may also be open. Therefore, assessment to ensure that the sac covering is intact remains important. Assess neurologic status carefully. Before surgical correction, the infant will be thoroughly examined to determine brain tissue involvement or associated anomalies. Diagnostic procedures such as CT, MRI, and ultrasound may be performed.

Nursing Management

Nursing management will consist of preoperative and postoperative care, along with symptomatic and supportive care. Preoperative and postoperative care will be similar to that for the child with myelomeningocele, with a focus on preventing rupture of the sac, preventing infection, and providing adequate nutrition and hydration. Infants with an encephalocele are at an increased risk for developing hydrocephalus Therefore, monitor for signs and symptoms of increased ICP and head circumference.

● MICROCEPHALY

Microcephaly is defined as a head circumference that is more than three standard deviations below the mean for the age and sex of the infant (Behrman et al., 2004). It may be congenital or it may be acquired and develop in the first few years of life. It generally results in mental retardation due to the lack of functioning brain tissue. There are many causes. Microcephaly can be caused by abnormal development during gestation or follow intrauterine infections such as rubella, toxoplasmosis, and cytomegalovirus. It can also be caused by chromosomal abnormalities or be associated with other syndromes. Acquired microcephaly may occur due to severe malnutrition, perinatal infections, or anoxia in early infancy.

Nursing Assessment

Microcephalic infants will present at birth with a normal or reduced head size. As the child ages, head growth will fail while the face will continue to grow at a normal rate. This results in a small head, a large face, and a loose, often wrinkled scalp. As the child grows older, this smallness of the skull becomes more pronounced. Development of motor functions and speech may be delayed. The degree of mental retardation varies, but it is a common occurrence. Convulsions may be present, and motor deficit ranges from clumsiness to spastic quadriplegia.

Nursing Management

There is no treatment. Nursing care will be supportive and focus on determining the extent of neurologic and cognitive deficits, as well as teaching parents the care of a child with such impairments.

● ARNOLD-CHIARI MALFORMATION

Arnold-Chiari malformation consists of two major subgroups—type I and type II. In type I, symptoms are typically seen in adolescence and adulthood. This type is usually not associated with hydrocephalus and is the more benign form. The deformity is a result of the cerebellar tonsils displacing into the upper cervical canal. The client will usually complain of neck pain, recurrent headaches, lower extremity spasticity, and urinary frequency. Type II is the most common and is usually associated with hydrocephalus and myelomeningocele. The deformity results from the cerebellum, the medulla oblongata, and the fourth ventricle displacing into the cervical canal, resulting in an obstruction of the CSF and causing hydrocephalus. The prognosis depends on the extent of the defect. Symptomatic type II Chiari malformation is the leading cause of death in infants and young children with open neural tube defects (Stevenson, 2004). Treatment of the type II Chiari malformation includes surgical decompression.

Nursing Assessment

Approximately 10% of type II Arnold-Chiari malformations result in symptoms in infancy (Behrman et al., 2004). Symptoms consist of weak cry, stridor, and apnea. These symptoms require prompt medical treatment to reduce mortality. Gastrointestinal disturbances along with a history of chronic aspiration, choking, gagging, prolonged feeding times, and weight loss may also be present. Physical signs include coarse upper airway sounds heard on auscultation and diminished or absent gag reflex. In the older child, signs and symptoms seen are subtler and less frequently life threatening. Upper extremity weakness, spasticity, ataxia, and headaches are frequent signs found. Assessment of shunt function is extremely important in the infant and older child presenting with type II Chiari malformation and associated hydrocephalus (refer to "Hydrocephalus" section). An MRI may be performed to help evaluate and diagnose Chiari malformations.

Nursing Management

Nursing management will focus on preoperative and postoperative care; preventing infection; monitoring of blood loss; improvement of preoperative symptoms in the postoperative period; any signs and symptoms of increased ICP; and any resultant CNS injury.

● HYDROCEPHALUS

Hydrocephalus is not a specific disease, but results from underlying brain disorders. It is one of the most frequently seen disorders of the nervous system. It results from an imbalance in the production and absorption of CSF. In hydrocephalus, CSF accumulates within the ventricular system and causes the ventricles to enlarge and increases in ICP to occur. Common disorders or illnesses that are associated with hydrocephalus include neural tube defects such as myelomeningocele; intraventricular hemorrhage in premature infants; meningitis; intrauterine viral infections; lesions or malformations of the brain such as posterior fossa brain tumors; Chiari malformations; and non-accidental injury. Hydrocephalus may be congenital or acquired. Congenital hydrocephalus is present at birth and is often due to environmental influences during fetal development or a genetic disposition. Causes of congenital hydrocephalus include abnormal intrauterine development, as is the case with myelomeningocele, or intrauterine infections. Acquired hydrocephalus develops at the time of birth or at some point after. It can occur at any age and can result from injury or disease. Acquired hydrocephalus can result from trauma, hemorrhage, neoplasms, or infections.

Hydrocephalus is also classified as obstructive or noncommunicating vs. nonobstructive or communicating. Obstructive or noncommunicating hydrocephalus occurs when CSF is unable to pass between the ventricles and spinal cord. Neural tube defects, neonatal meningitis, trauma, tumors, or Chiari malformations usually result in this type of hydrocephalus. One of the most common causes of obstructive or noncommunicating hydrocephalus in children is aqueductal stenosis, which results from the narrowing of the aqueduct of Sylvius (a passageway between the third and fourth ventricles in the middle brain). Nonobstructive or communicating hydrocephalus occurs when passage of CSF between the ventricles and spinal cord does not occur. Examples include hydrocephalus that results from subarachnoid hemorrhage and intrauterine infections.

Prognosis for the child with hydrocephalus depends mainly on the cause and whether or not brain damage has occurred prior to recognition and treatment. These children are at increased risk for developmental disabilities, visual problems, abnormalities in memory, and reduced intelligence. Long-term follow-up and multidisciplinary care are necessary.

Pathophysiology

CSF is formed primarily in the ventricular system by the choroid plexus. It flows as a result of the pressure gradient that exists between the ventricular system and the venous channels. CSF is absorbed primarily by the arachnoid villi. Hydrocephalus results when there is an obstruction in the ventricular system or obliteration or malfunction of the arachnoid villi. This results in impaired absorption or circulation of the CSF. In rare cases, hydrocephalus can be caused by an overproduction of CSF by the choroid plexus.

Therapeutic Management

Hydrocephalus must be identified early. Treatment needs to be initiated in order to prevent brain tissue damage that can result from the increased ICP that hydrocephalus creates. Specific treatment will depend on the cause. The goals of treatment include relieving hydrocephalus and managing complications associated with the disorder, such as growth and developmental delay. With few exceptions, most cases of hydrocephalus are treated with the surgical placement of an extracranial shunt. Most often a ventriculoperitoneal shunt (VP shunt) is placed. See Figure 17.8 for an illustration of a shunt. The shunt will need to be replaced as the child grows. Therefore, the child will undergo shunt revision surgery at various times during his or her life. It is important for health care professionals and parents to be able to recognize when a shunt needs replacing or when complications are occurring, to decrease the possibility of death or disability that may occur due to increased ICP.

Nursing Assessment

For a full description of the assessment phase of the nursing process, refer to page 469. Assessment findings pertinent to hydrocephalus are discussed below.

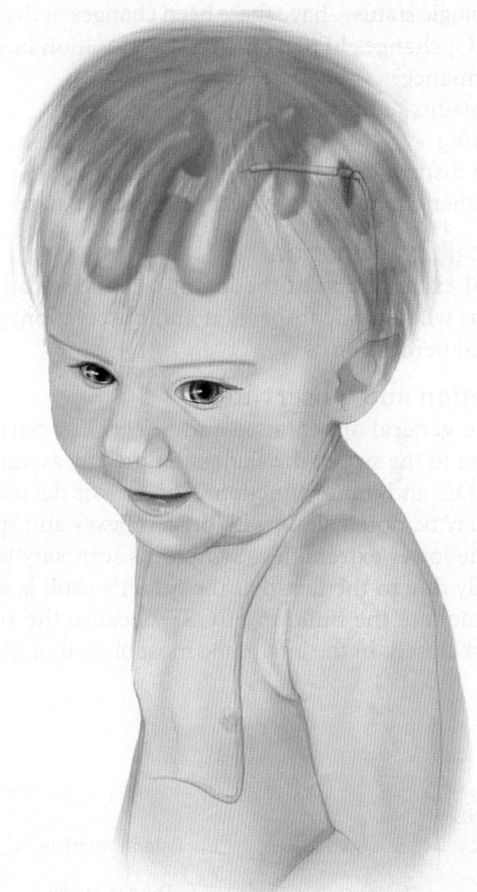

● **Figure 17.8** To treat hydrocephalus, a ventriculoperitoneal (VP) shunt catheter is placed in an enlarged ventricle. The shunt diverts the flow of cerebrospinal fluid (CSF) within the central nervous system to the peritoneum, where CSF is now absorbed across the peritoneal membrane into the body's circulation.

Health History

Explore the pregnancy history and past medical history for:

- Intrauterine infections
- Prematurity with intracranial hemorrhage
- Meningitis
- Mumps encephalitis

Elicit a description of the present illness and chief complaint. Common signs and symptoms reported during the health history of the undiagnosed child might include:

- Irritability
- Lethargy
- Poor feeding
- Vomiting
- Complaints of headache in older children
- Altered, diminished, or changes in LOC

Children known to have hydrocephalus are often admitted to the hospital for shunt malfunctions or other complications of the disease. The health history should include questions related to:

- Neurologic status—have there been changes or decreases in LOC; changes in personality; deterioration in school performance?
- Complaints of headache
- Vomiting
- Visual disturbances
- Any other changes in physical or cognitive state

Physical Examination

Physical examination of the infant or child with hydrocephalus will include inspection and observation; palpation; and percussion.

Inspection and Observation

Observe general appearance and affect. Pay particular attention to the size of the skull and note any asymmetry. Note LOC and motor function. Changes or decreases in LOC may be noted along with brisk reflexes and spasticity of the lower extremities. Symptoms seen vary by age, primarily due to the fact that the infant's skull is able to accommodate the buildup of CSF because the sutures have not closed. In the infant, the most obvious indication is often a rapid increase in head circumference (Fig. 17.9). In the older child, loss of development and changes in personality may be seen. Signs and symptoms associated with increased ICP may be seen (refer to Comparison Chart 17.1).

Palpation

In the infant, palpation of the fontanels may reveal wide-open, bulging fontanels. They will be nonpulsatile and feel tense and very full.

Percussion

Upon percussion of the skull, by advanced practitioners, a positive Macewen's sign may be noted. This is when a "cracked pot" sound is heard during percussion and can indicate separation of the sutures.

Laboratory and Diagnostic Tests

Common laboratory and diagnostic tests ordered for the diagnosis and assessment of hydrocephalus include:

- Skull x-ray studies (may reveal separation of sutures)
- CT
- MRI

CT and MRI are used to evaluate for the presence of hydrocephalus and can also aid in identifying the cause of hydrocephalus. Refer to Common Laboratory and Diagnostic Tests 17.1.

Consider THIS!

Sandra and Michael Graham have brought their 6-month old son, Thomas, to the pediatric unit for observation. Thomas's head circumference has increased from the 25th percentile at the 4-month check-up to the 75th percentile at the 6-month check-up. Upon assessment, the nurse notes a bulging anterior fontanel and persistent primitive reflexes.

What do you think is going on?

Identify early signs.

Identify late signs.

Describe nursing care for Thomas.

What teaching will the nurse do with Sandra and Michael?

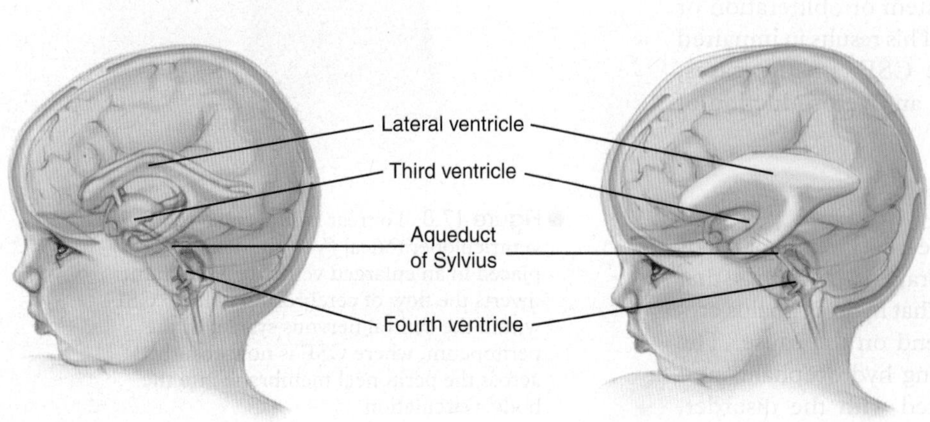

● Figure 17.9 Infant with hydrocephalus. Note broadening of the forehead and large head size.

Nursing Management

Nursing management of the child with hydrocephalus will focus on maintaining cerebral perfusion, minimizing neurologic complications, maintaining adequate nutrition, promoting growth and development, and supporting and educating the child and family. In addition to the nursing diagnoses and related interventions discussed in Nursing Care Plan 17.1, interventions common to hydrocephalus are discussed below.

Preventing and Recognizing Shunt Infection and Malfunction

The major complications associated with shunts are infection and malfunction. Due to the serious nature and potentially devastating affects of shunt infection or malfunction, parents and health professionals need to be aware of the signs and symptoms to provide early recognition and prompt treatment. Signs and symptoms of a shunt infection include elevated vital signs, poor feeding, vomiting, decreased responsiveness, seizure activity, and signs of local inflammation along the shunt tract. Signs and symptoms of shunt malfunction include vomiting, drowsiness, and headache. Signs and symptoms of increased ICP, as listed in Comparison Chart 17.1, can also be indicative of shunt complications.

Infection can occur at any time but is more common 1 to 2 months after placement. Infection is treated with intravenous antibiotics and, if the infection is persistent, the shunt will be removed and an external ventricular drainage (EVD) system will be put into place until the CSF is sterile (refer to Common Medical Treatments 17.1 and Box 17.3).

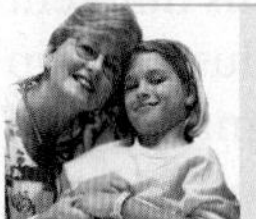

Rapid drainage of CSF, which may occur if the client sits up without the EVD system being clamped, will decrease ICP and can lead to extreme headache, collapse of the ventricles, formation of subdural hematomas, and neurologic deterioration.

A new shunt will be placed after the infection has cleared. Intrathecal administration of antibiotics may be performed by the physician or advanced practitioner. Keeping the peritoneal surgical incision free of feces and urine can help prevent infection. Additionally, inspect surgical incisions after shunt placement for signs and symptoms of infection and any signs of leaking CSF.

Malfunction of the shunt can occur due to kinking, clogging, or separation of the tubing. Blockage is the most common reported complication. A shunt that has been placed within the past year is at higher risk of malfunction. Early recognition and operative intervention are essential to prevent neurologic deficits or possible death from occurring.

BOX 17.3

NURSING MANAGEMENT OF EXTERNAL VENTRICULAR DRAINAGE (EVD) DEVICE

- Ensure all connections are secure and label line as EVD.
- Regularly check that drip chamber of manometer is set at the height prescribed in relation to the client (i.e., zero at clavicle).
- Clamp the drain in the event of client movement or movement anticipated with care. Rezero and open clamps when done.
- Accurately document volume and color of CSF every hour (CSF is normally clear and colorless; cloudiness indicates infection). Notify MD or charge nurse of any significant increase in amount of drainage (if exceeds 10 mL more than previous volumes).
- If minimal or no drainage, check tubing for kinks, blockage, or closed clamps. Check to see if CSF is oscillating in tubing. If blockage is suspected, notify neurosurgery department immediately.
- Entry site into skull should be dressed with a sterile occlusive dressing and should be changed if soiled or nonocclusive.
- Routine CSF samples may be sent for culture and analysis.
- Client may be taking prophylactic antibiotics due to increased risk of infection from the drain.

Supporting and Educating the Child and Family

Hydrocephalus is a serious and chronic illness. It will require lifelong follow-up and regular evaluations. It requires early recognition of complications to prevent neurologic damage. Children will require future surgeries and hospitalizations, which can place a strain on the family and its finances. Potential growth and developmental disabilities are an additional strain. The support of the family in establishing realistic goals and helping the child to achieve his or her developmental and educational potential is important.

The family should be involved in the child's care from the time of diagnosis. Initially parents may be frightened because shunt placement involves entering the brain. Provide parents with accurate information regarding the procedure, and be available to listen to parents' concerns and to answer questions that arise. Ongoing education about the illness and its treatment are important, including signs and symptoms of shunt complications. As the family becomes more comfortable with the diagnosis, treatment, and signs and symptoms of complications, they will become experts on the child's care and will often recognize subtle changes in him or her that may be indicative of shunt complications. Referral to support groups can be helpful for both the family and the child. The National Hydrocephalus Foundation can be accessed at www.nhfonline.org. Additional resources can be found at www.hydroassoc.org and www.hydrocephalus.org.

● INTRACRANIAL ARTERIOVENOUS MALFORMATION (AVM)

Intracranial arteriovenous malformation is a rare congenital disorder. It is caused by an abnormal development of blood vessels and can occur in the brain, brainstem, or spinal cord. AVMs that hemorrhage can lead to serious neurologic deficits and even death. However, some cases of AVMs never cause problems. AVMs account for 30% to 50% of hemorrhagic strokes in children (Ogilvy et al., 2001).

Therapeutic Management

More aggressive treatment strategies are used in children. Treatment options used include surgical excision; endovascular embolization, which involves closing off the vessels of the AVM by injecting glue into them; and radiosurgery, which involves focusing radiation on the AVM. The treatment approach will be based on the age of the client and size and location of the malformation in the brain. The client will usually require at least 24 hours of intensive care monitoring following surgery.

Nursing Assessment

The most common symptoms seen include intracranial hemorrhage (children are more likely to present with hemorrhage than adults), seizures, headaches, and progressive neurologic deficits such as vision problems, loss of speech, problems with memory, and paralysis. In children less than 2 years of age, presentation may include cardiac failure due to arteriovenous shunting in neonates and infants; a large head secondary to hydrocephalus; and seizure activity. Diagnosis is made using diagnostic imaging procedures such as MRI, CT, and arteriography. Due to advances in brain imaging techniques, an increasing number of AVMs are detected before rupture.

Nursing Management

Nursing management for these clients is aimed at supportive care. Monitor for changes in neurologic status, noting any seizure activity, signs or symptoms of increased ICP, or signs and symptoms of intracranial hemorrhage. Hydrocephalus may occur as a result of intracranial hemorrhage secondary to the AVM. An EVD and eventual shunt placement may be necessary (refer to "Hydrocephalus" section).

● CRANIOSYNOSTOSIS

Craniosynostosis is premature closure of the cranial sutures (Fig. 17.10). Complete closure of all sutures does not normally occur until late in childhood. Premature closure can inhibit brain growth and a distorted skull appearance will be evident. In cases where only one suture is fused, neurologic impairments are rarely seen. When two or more sutures are fused, neurologic complications such as hydrocephalus with increased ICP are more likely to occur. The incidence of craniosynostosis is approximately 1 in 2,000 births (Behrman et al., 2004). The cause is unknown, but in 10% to 20% of cases a genetic disorder such as Carpenter's syndrome or Apert's, Crouzon's, or Pfeiffer's disease is present. There are numerous different types of craniosynostosis; they are listed and illustrated in Table 17.5. The prognosis is good for the majority of infants presenting with craniosynostosis, and normal brain development will occur. Exceptions to this are the infant or child who has associated genetic disorders that involve brain function and development.

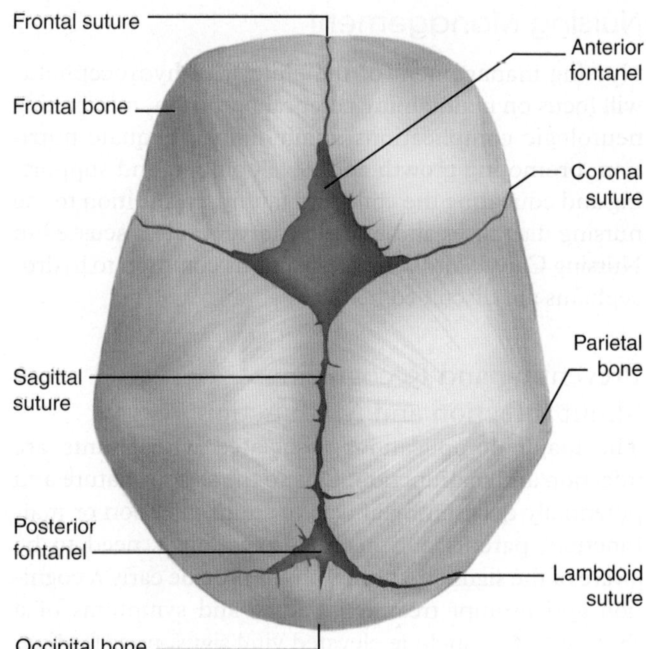

● **Figure 17.10** Skull sutures in the infant.

Surgical correction may be done and allows for normal expansion of the brain and acceptable appearance of the head and skull. If one suture is fused, the surgical intervention is done mainly for cosmetic reasons. If more than one suture is fused, operative intervention is essential to prevent neurologic complications.

Nursing Assessment

Most cases of craniosynostosis are present at birth. Skull deformity is evident as well as a prominent bony ridge that can be palpated. X-ray studies can confirm fusion of the sutures. It is important that craniosynostosis be detected early if it is not evident at birth because premature closure of the suture lines will inhibit brain development.

Table 17.5 Types of Craniosynostosis

Types	Description
Sagittal synostosis (scaphocephaly)	Sagittal suture is closed. Head grows long and narrow in anterior–posterior direction. Broad forehead and a prominent occiput are present. Most common form
Metopic synostosis (trigonocephaly)	Metopic suture is closed Usually a ridge down the forehead can be seen or felt. Triangular-shaped forehead Eyebrows may appear "pinched" on either side. Eyes may also appear close together.
Unilateral coronal synostosis (anterior plagiocephaly)	Early closure of one side of the coronal suture Forehead and orbital rim (eyebrow) have a flattened appearance on that side.
Bicoronal synostosis (brachycephaly)	Very flat, recessed forehead Skull is shortened in the anterior–posterior direction. Commonly seen in Apert's and Crouzon's disease
Lambdoid (posterior plagiocephaly)	Early closure of one lambdoid suture Trapezoid-shaped head in craniosynostosis. Similar to shape found in positional molding or positional plagiocephaly

Therefore, measure head circumference in all children less than 3 years old and compare findings with normal head circumference parameters as well as past measurements of the infant or child.

Nursing Management

Nursing management includes observing hemoglobin and hematocrit levels due to large volumes of blood loss that can occur, and observing for pain, hemorrhage, fever, infection, and swelling. Due to the location of the surgery and incision line, large amounts of facial swelling may be present. This can result in an inability of the child to open his or her eyes for a few days postoperatively. Make sure that parents are aware of this. Encourage the parents to talk to, hold, and comfort their child during this time. Provide support and education to the parents before, during, and after the procedure. Refer families to the Craniosynostosis and Positional Plagiocephaly Support Group, accessible at www.cappskids.org/index.html and 6905 Xanadu Court, Fredericksburg, VA 22407.

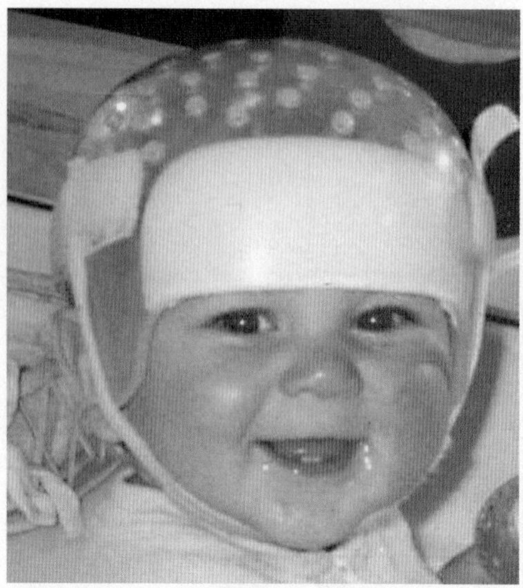

● Figure 17.11 Molding helmet for positional plagiocephaly.

● POSITIONAL PLAGIOCEPHALY

Since the inception of the "back to sleep" program, which recommends placing all infants supine to sleep to decrease the risk of sudden infant death syndrome (SIDS), there has been a dramatic increase in the incidence of positional plagiocephaly. Positional plagiocephaly refers to asymmetry in head shape without fused sutures. It results from gravitational force exertion on the developing cranium. Plagiocephaly in the infant may lead to torticollis.

Medical treatment for positional plagiocephaly is generally conservative, such as changing the infant's position, encouraging "tummy time," and avoiding excessive use of the car seat for infant seating outside of the automobile. Some infants may benefit from the use of a molding helmet (Fig. 17.11).

Nursing Assessment

View the infant's head from the top, noting asymmetry ranging from flattening on one side posteriorly to posterior flattening associated with anterior bulging (Fig. 17.12). Assess neck range of motion to determine if torticollis is also present. Palpate the cranial sutures, which will not feel overlapped as they do when they are fused. Skull x-ray examination or head CT scan will rule out craniosynostosis by demonstrating evidence of open sutures.

Nursing Management

Nursing management is directed toward repositioning the infant to decrease time spent with the flattened area in the dependent position. Position the infant so that turning away from the affected side is necessary for him or her to view objects of interest. Place the infant on the abdomen when awake and supervised. Discourage use of the car seat outside of the automobile. Place a rolled washcloth along the affected side of the head to discourage turning the head in that direction. Following these recommendations may prevent positional plagiocephaly in the infant without congenital torticollis.

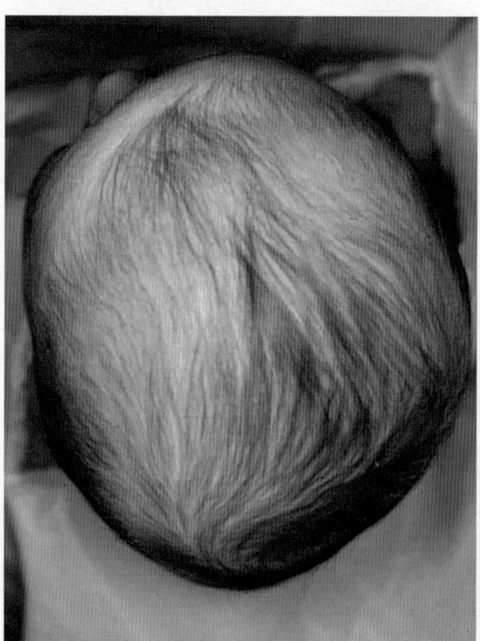

● Figure 17.12 Note flattening of the right posterior parietal and occipital regions of the skull in this infant with positional plagiocephaly.

Infectious Disorders

Infectious disorders of the neurologic system include bacterial meningitis, aseptic meningitis, encephalitis, Reye's syndrome, botulism, and rabies.

● BACTERIAL MENINGITIS

Bacterial meningitis is an infection of the meninges, the lining that surrounds the brain and spinal cord. It is a serious illness in children and can lead to brain damage, nerve damage, deafness, stroke, and even death. It requires rapid assessment and treatment. The leading cause of bacterial meningitis in newborns is group B streptococcus and gram-negative enteric bacilli like *Escherichia coli* (Spiro & Spiro, 2004). In children, the leading causative agents are *Neisseria meningitidis* and *Streptococcus pneumoniae* (Spiro & Spiro, 2004). See Table 17.6 for types of meningitis seen in different age groups. In developed countries, disease resulting from *Haemophilus influenzae* type B, once the most common cause of meningitis in children, has decreased dramatically since the introduction of the Hib vaccine. In less developed countries, infection with *H. influenzae* type B still remains a concern. Most cases of bacterial meningitis occur in the winter and early spring, but it can occur year round (Spiro & Spiro, 2004).

Pathophysiology

Bacterial meningitis causes inflammation, swelling, purulent exudates, and tissue damage to the brain. It can occur as a secondary infection to upper respiratory infections, sinus infections, or ear infections, and can also be the result of direct introduction through LP; skull fracture or severe head injury; neurosurgical intervention; congenital structural abnormalities, like spina bifida; or the presence of foreign bodies, like a ventricular shunt or cochlear implants.

Table 17.6 Common Causes of Meningitis in Different Age Groups

Causative Organism	Age Affected
Escherichia coli	Newborns and infants
Streptococcus group B	Infants less than 1 month old
Haemophilus influenzae type B	1 month–6 years, typically 6–9 months old
Streptococcus pneumoniae	Children older than 3 months of age and adults
Neisseria meningitidis	Children older than 3 months of age and adults

Therapeutic Management

Bacterial meningitis is a medical emergency and requires prompt hospitalization and treatment. Deterioration may be rapid and occur in less than 24 hours, leading to long-term neurologic damage and even death. Intravenous antibiotics will be started immediately after the LP and blood cultures have been obtained if bacterial meningitis is suspected. The length of therapy and specific antibiotic will be determined based on the analysis and the culture and sensitivity of the CSF. Corticosteroids may be ordered to help reduce the inflammatory process. Specific medical treatment varies based on the suspected causative organism and will be determined by the physician.

Nursing Assessment

For a full description of the assessment phase of the nursing process, refer to page 469. Assessment findings pertinent to bacterial meningitis are discussed below.

Health History

Elicit a description of the present illness and chief complaint. Common signs and symptoms reported during the health history might include:

- Sudden onset of symptoms
- Preceding respiratory illness or sore throat
- Presence of fever, chills
- Headache
- Vomiting
- Photophobia
- Stiff neck
- Rash
- Irritability
- Drowsiness
- Lethargy
- Muscle rigidity
- Seizures

Symptoms in infants can be more subtle and atypical, but the history may reveal:

- Poor sucking and feeding
- Weak cry
- Lethargy
- Vomiting

Explore the client's current and past medical history for risk factors such as:

- Young age: 1 month to 5 years, with most cases in children less than 1 year of age and young adults 15 to 24 years of age

- Any fever or illness during pregnancy or around delivery (for infants less than 3 months of age)
- Exposure to ill persons
- Exposure to tuberculosis
- Travel history
- History of maternal illness
- Recent neurosurgical procedure or head trauma
- Presence of a foreign body, such as a shunt or a cochlear implant
- Immunocompromised status
- Close-contact living spaces such as dormitories or military bases
- Daycare attendance

Physical Examination

Observe the general appearance of the client. The infant with bacterial meningitis may rest in the **opisthotonic** position (Fig. 17.13), and the older child may complain of neck pain. In the infant a bulging fontanel may be present, which is often a late sign, and the infant may be consolable when lying still as opposed to being held. Presence of positive Kernig's and Brudzinski's signs can indicate irritation of the meninges (Fig. 17.14). Inspect the client for presence of a rash; a petechial, vesicular, or macular rash may be seen.

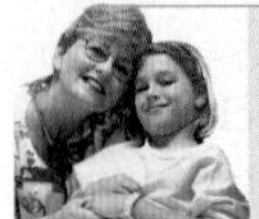

Abrupt eruption of a petechial or purplish rash can be indicative of meningococcemia (infection with N. meningitidis). Immediate medical attention is warranted.

Laboratory and Diagnostic Tests

Common laboratory and diagnostic studies ordered for the assessment of bacterial meningitis include:

- LP—Fluid pressure will be measured and a sample is obtained for analysis and culture. CSF will reveal increased white blood cells (WBCs) and protein and low glucose (the bacteria present feed on the glucose).
- Complete blood count (CBC)—WBCs will be elevated.
- Blood culture—Performed to rule out sepsis. Blood culture will be positive in cases of septicemia.

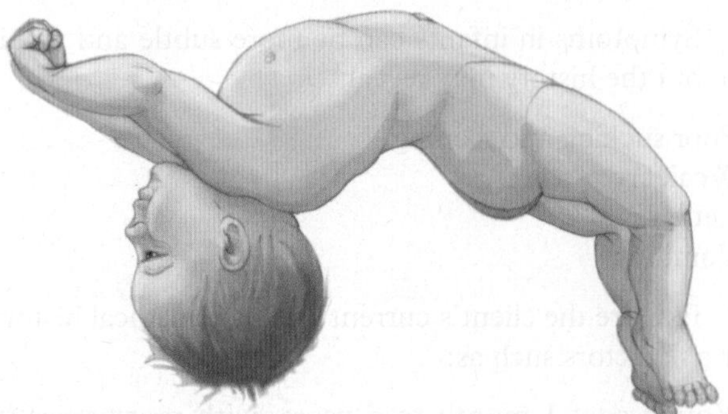

● Figure 17.13 Infant in opisthotonic position: head and neck are hyperextended to relieve discomfort.

Nursing Management

Quickly initiate supportive measures to ensure proper ventilation, reduce the inflammatory response, and help prevent injury to the brain. Interventions are aimed at reducing ICP and maintaining cerebral perfusion along with treating fluid volume deficit, controlling seizures, and preventing injury that may result from altered LOC or seizure activity. Initiate appropriate isolation precautions. In addition to standard precautions, infants and children diagnosed with bacterial meningitis will be placed on droplet isolation until 24 hours of antibiotics have been received to help prevent transmission to others. Refer to Nursing Care Plan 17.1 for nursing diagnoses and related interventions. In addition to those diagnoses and interventions, reducing fever and preventing bacterial meningitis should be noted.

Reducing Fever

Hyperthermia related to infectious process, increased metabolic rate, and dehydration as evidenced by increased body temperature; warm, flushed skin; and tachycardia may be present. Reducing fever is important to help maintain optimal cerebral perfusion by reducing the metabolic needs of the brain. Administer antipyretics such as acetaminophen and NSAIDS such as ibuprofen, per order. Institute nonpharmacologic measures if needed. Reduction of environmental temperature and the use of cooling blankets, fans, cold compresses, and tepid baths may be helpful in reducing fever. Avoid measures that cause shivering because it increases heat production and is therefore counterproductive as well as uncomfortable for the client.

Preventing Bacterial Meningitis

Bacterial meningitis is a serious illness and prevention is important. It is transmitted by direct close contact with respiratory droplets from the nose or throat. Most at risk are those living with the client or anyone with whom the client played or was in close contact. Postexposure prophylaxis and postexposure immunization may be effective. Control measures should be initiated in environments where risk exists. Disinfect toys and other shared objects to decrease transmission of the microorganisms to others.

To reduce group B streptococcus infection in neonates, screen pregnant women; if the screening results are positive, administer intrapartal antibiotics. Vaccines are available for some specific causative organisms, but complete vaccination prevention is not possible at this time. The Hib vaccine is routine starting at 2 months of age and all children should be immunized to continue the reduction of bacterial meningitis caused by *H. influenzae* type B. The pneumococcal vaccine is also routine for all children starting at 2 months of age and should be considered for preschoolers who are at risk. Children at risk

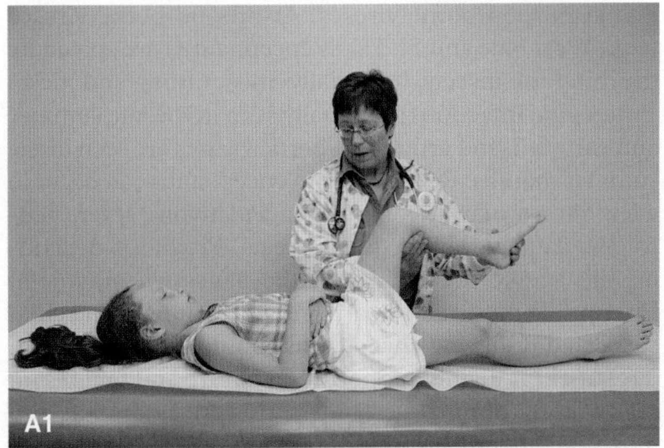

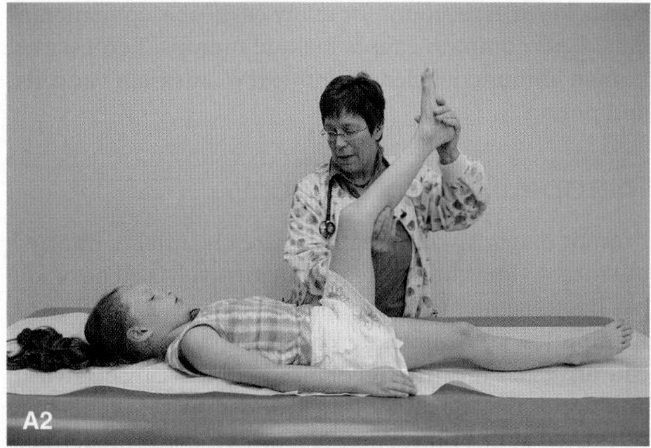

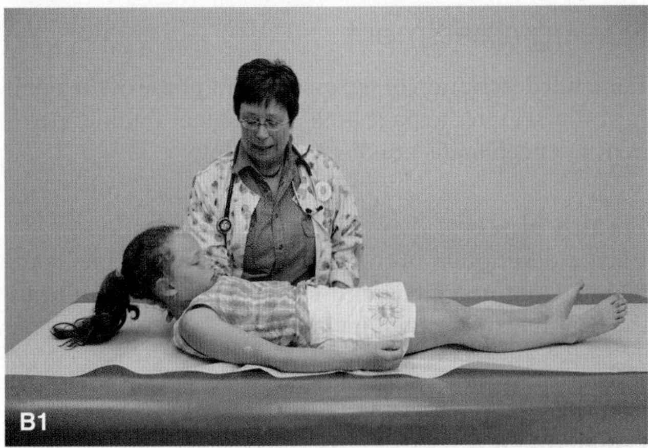

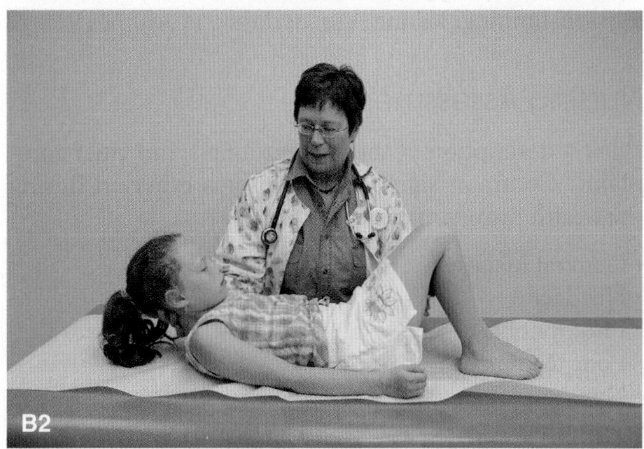

● Figure 17.14 (**A**) Kernig's sign is tested by flexing legs at the hip and knee (**A1**), then extending the knee (**A2**). A positive report of pain along the vertebral column is a positive sign and indicates irritation of meninges. (**B**) Brudzinski's sign is tested by the child lying supine with the neck flexed (**B1**). A positive sign occurs if resistance or pain is met. The child may also passively flex hip and knees in reaction, indicating meningeal irritation (**B2**).

include those with immune deficiency; sickle-cell disease; asplenia; chronic pulmonary, cardiac, or renal disease; diabetes mellitus; cochlear implants; cerebrospinal leaks; and organ transplants.

Meningococcal vaccine is recommended, but not routine, for children age 2 years or older who are at high risk—such as children with chronic conditions or immune suppression or those who travel to high-risk areas or live in crowded conditions. Since the 1990s, a dramatic increase in the incidence of meningococcal meningitis (and the often fatal blood infection meningococcemia) among adolescents and young adults has occurred. Living in close quarters, sleeping less than usual, and sharing personal items such as drinking glasses and lip balm contribute to the increase in disease. For these reasons, current recommendations advise meningococcal vaccination for all children aged 11 to 12 years. Further information and a resource for families can be obtained through the National Meningitis Association, which can be accessed at www.nmaus.org (see Healthy People 2010).

● ASEPTIC MENINGITIS

Aseptic meningitis is the most common type of meningitis, and the majority of children affected are less than 5 years of age. If the causative organism can be identified, it is usually a virus. Enteroviruses, like echovirus and

HEALTHY PEOPLE 2010

Objective	Significance
Reduce bacterial meningitis in young children.	• Encourage appropriate immunization as recommended. • Educate families to complete prescribed courses of antibiotics (to avoid progression of minor bacterial infections to meningitis).

coxsackievirus, account for many cases of aseptic meningitis. Less common causes include mumps, herpesvirus, human immunodeficiency virus (HIV), measles, varicella, and polio.

Therapeutic Management

Prompt diagnosis and treatment are essential to improve outcomes. The child is treated aggressively as if he or she has bacterial meningitis until the diagnosis is confirmed. Antibiotics are administered and continued until the causative organism is recognized. If the cause is viral, antibiotics may be discontinued and antiviral agents may be started at this time. After diagnosis is confirmed, treatment is mainly supportive in nature and the illness is usually self-limiting, lasting 3 to 10 days.

Nursing Assessment

Elicit a description of the present illness and chief complaint. Common signs and symptoms reported during the health history might include:

- General malaise
- Headache
- Photophobia
- Poor feeding
- Nausea
- Vomiting
- Irritability
- Lethargy
- Neck pain
- Positive Kernig's and Brudzinski's signs

The onset of symptoms may be abrupt or gradual. Assessment is similar to that of the child with bacterial meningitis. Signs and symptoms are similar to those seen in bacterial meningitis, but the child is usually less ill.

Nursing Management

Nursing management is similar to the nursing care of the child with bacterial meningitis and will focus on comfort measures to reduce pain and fever. Aseptic meningitis can be managed successfully at home if the child's neurologic status is stable and he or she is tolerating oral intake.

ENCEPHALITIS

Encephalitis is an inflammation of the brain that may also include an inflammation of the meninges. It is a rare complication and can be caused by protozoan, bacterial, fungal, or viral invasion. In children it is most often associated with a viral illness. Most cases of viral encephalitis in children are of unknown cause. In the United States, common causative organisms include the herpes simplex virus; enteroviruses, such as poliovirus and coxsackievirus; and arthropod-borne viruses. Arthropod-borne viruses (e.g., West Nile and St. Louis encephalitis) are spread by the bites of insects, especially mosquitoes and ticks. Enteroviral infections are usually seen in the late summer and early fall, and arthropod-borne viruses are seen in the summer months. Recovery from encephalitis can occur in a few days or may be complicated and involve severe neurologic damage with residual effects. Prognosis depends on the age of the child and the causative organism. Prompt diagnosis and treatment are essential. The child suspected of having encephalitis should be hospitalized. Treatment is mainly supportive in nature and focuses on maintaining optimal cerebral perfusion; hydration and nutrition; and injury prevention.

Nursing Assessment

For a full description of the assessment phase of the nursing process, refer to page 469. Assessment findings pertinent to encephalitis are discussed below.

Health History

Elicit a description of the present illness and chief complaint. Common signs and symptoms reported during the health history might include:

- Fever
- Flu-like symptoms
- Altered LOC
- Headache
- Lethargy
- Drowsiness
- Generalized weakness
- Seizure activity

Explore the client's current history for risk factors such as:

- Recent travel
- Recreational activities, such as hiking and camping
- Animal contacts

Physical Examination

Perform a neurologic examination to distinguish between encephalitis and viral meningitis. In encephalitis, a neurologic examination will reveal changes in sensorium and focal neurologic changes. Neurologic findings vary and reflect the areas of the brain that are involved.

Laboratory and Diagnostic Tests

An LP may be done and the CSF may show an elevated leukocyte count and elevated protein and glucose levels. However, in some cases, levels may be normal. MRI, CT, and EEG procedures may be performed to help identify early changes and provide useful clues in developing a diagnosis.

Nursing Management

Nursing management is similar to nursing care for the child with meningitis. Teach children and their families how to prevent encephalitis. Encephalitis can result from complications of childhood illnesses such as measles, mumps, or chickenpox. Explain the importance of keeping children up-to-date in their immunizations. Effective vaccines are available for a few viral pathogens that cause encephalitis (such as rabies virus and Japanese encephalitis virus), but these vaccines are not routine; they are recommended for those at high risk. For example, postexposure rabies vaccines can be administered to a child who was bitten by a suspected rabid animal. Also, those traveling to areas where Japanese encephalitis is endemic, such as India and China, and planning a prolonged stay or extreme outdoor activity should receive the appropriate vaccine. Vector control and avoiding mosquito and tick bites are the best prevention of arthropod-borne infection. Using insect repellent (repellents containing DEET should be used cautiously in children less than 12 years of age and not at all in children less than 1 year of age); wearing clothing that covers the arms and legs; controlling mosquito populations by eliminating areas of standing water where mosquitoes can breed; and using insect traps and public measures such as sprayed insecticides to reduce the mosquito population can all be helpful in reducing the risk of infection with arthropod-borne viruses. Specific antiviral therapy may be used for diseases caused by the herpes simplex virus.

● REYE'S SYNDROME

Reye's syndrome is a disease that primarily affects children less than 15 years of age who are recovering from a viral illness. The exact cause of Reye's syndrome is unknown. It has been found that Reye's syndrome is a reaction that is triggered by the use of salicylates or salicylate-containing products to treat a viral infection. This reaction causes brain swelling, liver failure, and death in hours if treatment in not initiated. In the 1980s, the adverse effects of salicylates used to treat viral illnesses began to be publicized and the U.S. Food and Drug Administration (FDA) required warning labels to be placed on all salicylate-containing products, such as aspirin. Since then there has been a dramatic decrease in the occurrence of Reye's syndrome.

Nursing Assessment

Elicit a description of the present illness and chief complaint. Common signs and symptoms reported during the health history might include:

- Severe and continual vomiting
- Changes in mental status
- Lethargy
- Irritability
- Confusion
- Hyperreflexia

Explore the client's current and past medical history for risk factors such as:

- A prodromal viral illness, like chickenpox, croup, flu, or an upper respiratory infection
- Ingestion of salicylate-containing products within 3 weeks of the start of the viral illness

Diagnosis can be confirmed by elevated liver function tests and elevated serum ammonia levels.

Nursing Management

Early recognition and treatment are the most important aspects of managing this illness. Nursing management is aimed at maintaining cerebral perfusion, managing and preventing increased ICP, providing safety measures due to changes in LOC and risk for seizures, and monitoring fluid status to prevent dehydration and overhydration.

Education is an important aspect of preventing this disease. Salicylates are found in many products, including many over-the-counter products such as Alka-Seltzer and Pepto-Bismol. For a complete list, go to www.reyessyndrome.org. Recovery from Reye's syndrome is dependent on the severity of swelling of the brain; some children will make a full recovery, while others may suffer long-term neurologic damage.

● BOTULISM

Botulism is a disease that is caused by a toxin produced in the immature intestines of young children resulting from infection with the bacteria *Clostridium botulinum.* It is rare, but can cause serious paralytic illness. Botulism is mainly a food-borne infection but can also be contracted through wound infections or intestinal infections in infants. *C. botulinum* is common in soil and can also be found in a variety of foods, such as improperly preserved home-canned foods. It generally occurs in infants less than 6 months of age. It has been associated with feeding honey and corn syrup to infants; thus these should be avoided in children less than 1 year of age. The disease is not infectious, and the child must ingest the bacterial spores. These spores then multiply in the intestinal tract and produce the toxin, which is absorbed in the immature intestines of the infant. It is generally not a problem for older children because the bacteria do not grow well in mature intestines due to the presence of the normal intestinal flora. Prognosis is good, but if treatment is not initiated, paralysis to the arms, legs, trunk, and respiratory system can develop.

Nursing Assessment

For a full description of the assessment phase of the nursing process, refer to page 469. Assessment findings pertinent to botulism are discussed below.

Health History

Elicit a description of the present illness and chief complaint. Signs and symptoms usually occur soon after ingestion of the bacteria. Common signs and symptoms in infants reported during the health history might include:

- Constipation
- Poor feeding
- Listlessness
- Generalized weakness
- Weak cry

Common signs and symptoms in older children reported during the health history might include:

- Double vision
- Blurred vision
- Drooping eyelids
- Difficulty swallowing
- Slurred speech
- Muscle weakness

Physical Examination and Laboratory and Diagnostic Tests

Assess for a diminished gag reflex, which is indicative of botulism. Diagnostic tests include culturing of stool and serum. Botulism is a rare disease and is difficult to diagnose because symptoms are similar to those seen in other neurologic diseases. Therefore assessment may include diagnostic tests to help rule out other diseases such as Guillain-Barré syndrome, stroke, and myasthenia gravis.

Nursing Management

Treatment is mainly supportive in nature and focuses on maintaining respiratory status and nutritional status. If ordered, administer botulism toxin early in the course of the disease to reduce the severity and progression of the disease.

• RABIES

Rabies is a viral disease that affects both domestic and wild animals. It is transmitted to other animals and humans by means of close contact with the saliva of infected animals, such as through a bite. Most cases of rabies occur in children less than 15 years of age, and most human deaths occur in developing countries.

Nursing Assessment

Rabies infection has a long incubation period. Initial symptoms are fever and pain at the wound site and may include nonspecific symptoms such as headache, vomiting, diarrhea, anorexia, and cough that are seen with many respiratory or gastrointestinal illnesses. As the virus spreads to the CNS, encephalitis develops and signs and symptoms include hyperactivity, disorientation, and changes in behavior. In some cases, progressive paralysis may be present.

Nursing Management

No tests are currently available to detect rabies before the onset of clinical symptoms. Therefore, treatment needs to be initiated promptly for every suspected case of infection with the rabies virus. Immediate therapy is essential. To prevent a fatal outcome, therapy must be started before the virus reaches the CNS and clinical signs appear.

Human deaths can be effectively prevented by vaccination, either preexposure vaccination for those at high risk or as postexposure treatment after any bite from a suspected rabid animal. Vaccination is administered intramuscularly. Therefore, nursing care should include providing information to the child and family regarding the procedure and the use of EMLA cream to decrease discomfort from injection.

Rabies is untreatable, and after symptoms develop it is fatal to both humans and animals. Prevention is paramount and eliminating infection in animal vectors is essential. Successful animal vaccination and animal control campaigns in the United States have led to a very low rate of human rabies cases. Rabies among dogs in the United States has been virtually eliminated. Recently, rabies transmitted from other animal wildlife, especially through bat bites, has emerged as a cause for concern. Educating children and families about the importance of seeking medical care after any animal bite is crucial to preventing death from rabies infection.

Trauma

Trauma or injury is a leading cause of childhood morbidity and mortality in the United States. Injuries from trauma are the number one health risk for children and the leading cause of death in children less than 1 year old (Rowland, 1999). The child faces significant risk of trauma to his or her developing neurologic system, often leading to neurologic disorders with life-threatening and lasting effects. Neurologic trauma may include head trauma, nonaccidental head trauma, birth trauma, and near drowning.

• HEAD TRAUMA

In the United States, injury causes more death in children than disease. Of these injuries, head injury is the most common cause of death and disability in childhood. Common causes of head trauma in children include falls, motor vehicle accidents, pedestrian and bicycle accidents, and child abuse. Many factors make children more susceptible to head trauma than adults. Larger head size in relation to the body, coupled with a higher center of gravity, causes the child to hit his or her head more readily when involved in motor vehicle accidents, bicycle accidents, and falls. Children are also at risk for injury related to psychosocial factors such as their high activity level, curiosity, incomplete motor development, and their lack of knowledge and judgment skills. Also, their dependence on others to care for them places them at a high risk for injuries caused by child abuse. Children younger than 3 years of age have a very mobile spine, especially in the cervical region, along with immature neck muscles. This places them at a higher risk for injury from acceleration/deceleration injuries, which occur when the head receives a blow or is shaken; the sudden acceleration causes deformation of the skull and movement of the brain, allowing brain contents to strike parts of the skull. Bruising of the brain can occur at the point of impact or at that point distant from the impact where the brain collides with the skull. Another result of brain movement is hemorrhages in the brain, which are caused by the shearing forces that may tear small arteries. The child's thin skull places him or her at increased risk for skull fractures and penetrating injuries resulting from head trauma.

Head trauma is a broad term that can include specific patterns of injury. See Table 17.7 for descriptions of common head injuries seen in children. Head trauma in children is serious because it can cause an immediate threat to the child's life as well as a number of complications that can lead to lifelong impairment of an individual's physical, cognitive, and psychosocial functioning. Prognosis for the child who has suffered a head trauma depends on the extent and severity of the injury as well as any complications (see Healthy People 2010).

Nursing Assessment

For a full description of the assessment phase of the nursing process, refer to page 469. Assessment findings pertinent to head trauma are discussed below.

Health History

Take a detailed history, including past medical history along with details of the events surrounding the injury such as mental status at the time of the injury, any loss of consciousness, irritability, lethargy, abnormal behavior, vomiting (if so, how many times), any seizure activity, and any complaints of headache, visual changes, or neck pain.

Physical Examination

Perform a thorough physical examination. Initial physical assessment will focus on the ABCs (airway, breathing, and circulation) (refer to Chapter 32 for further information on emergency management). All children who experience head trauma need an assessment of their neurologic function as soon as they are seen. This includes LOC, pupillary response, and any seizure activity. Fixed and dilated pupils, fixed and constricted pupils, or sluggish pupillary reaction to light will warrant prompt intervention.

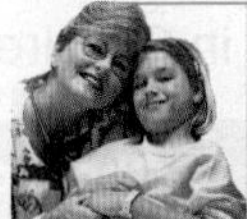

A child's spine must remain stabilized after a head injury until spinal cord injury is ruled out.

Laboratory and Diagnostic Tests

Diagnostic tests that may be utilized include x-ray examinations of the head and neck and CT and MRI scans. These procedures can assist in providing a more definitive diagnosis of the severity and type of trauma.

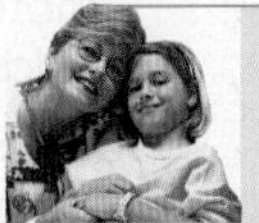

If clear liquid fluid is noted draining from the ears or nose, notification of the physician or advanced practitioner is warranted. If the fluid tests positive for glucose, this is indicative of leaking CSF.

Nursing Management

Nursing management of the child with head trauma depends on the seriousness of the injury. For all head trauma, however, the nurse provides support and education to the family and provides teaching on ways to prevent future head injuries.

Caring for the Child With Mild to Moderate Head Injury

Most children with mild to moderate closed head injury, which refers to brain injury without any penetrating injury to the brain, who suffered no loss of consciousness, no other injury to their head or body, are acting normally after the injury, and were healthy before the injury can be cared for and observed at home. Provide parents and caregivers with clear instructions regarding the care of their child at home. Explain that they must seek medical attention if the child's condition worsens at any time during the first several days after injury. See Teaching Guideline 17.2.

Children with mild closed head injury may exhibit some cognitive and behavioral symptoms, such as difficulty paying attention, problems making sense of what has been seen or heard, and forgetting things, in the early days after the injury. The majority make a full recovery. However, some may experience ongoing cognitive and behavioral difficulties, including slow information processing and attention difficulties.

Caring for the Child With Severe Head Injury

Children with more severe head injury may require intensive care initially until stabilized. Focus will be on maintaining the child's airway; monitoring breathing, circulation, and neurologic status closely; preventing and ceasing any seizure activity; and treating any other injuries that may have occurred as a result of the trauma.

Table 17.7 Common Head Injuries Seen in Children

Types	Description	Characteristics
Skull fractures	A break in the bone surrounding the brain	In the infant and children less than 2 years old, a great deal of force is needed to produce a skull fracture. Due to the flexibility of the immature skull, it is able to withstand a great degree of deformation before a fracture will occur. Can result in little or no brain damage, but may have serious consequences if the underlying brain tissue is injured
Linear skull fracture	A simple break in the skull that follows a relatively straight line	Most common skull fracture. Can result from minor head injuries such as being struck by a rock, stick, or other object; falls; or motor vehicle accidents. Not usually serious unless there is additional injury to the brain
Depressed skull fractures	The bone is locally broken and pushed inward, causing pressure on the brain.	Can result from forceful impact from a blunt object, such as a hammer or another heavy but fairly small object Surgery is often required to elevate the bony pieces and inspect the brain for evidence of injury.
Diastatic skull fracture	A fracture through the skull sutures	Most commonly occurs in the lamboid sutures (refer to Fig. 17.10 for location of sutures) Usually treatment is not required but observation will be necessary.
Compound skull fracture	A laceration of the skin and splintering of the bone	The fracture can be linear or depressed. Generally is the result of blunt force. Usually requires medical intervention and surgery may be necessary.
Basilar skull fracture	A fracture of the bones that form the base of the skull	Can result from severe blunt head trauma with significant force. Due to the proximity to the brainstem, this is a serious head injury. Findings include CSF rhinorrhea and otorrhea, bleeding from the ear, and orbital or postauricular ecchymosis (bruising behind ear is referred to as Battle's sign), and these children are at increased risk for infection because the fracture may allow a portal of entry into the central nervous system.
Concussion	A mild brain injury that is caused by jarring or shaking and results in disruption or malfunction of the electrical activities of the brain	Most common head injury. Results from a blow or jolt to the head caused by sports injuries, motor vehicle accidents, and falls. Confusion and amnesia after the head injury are seen. Loss of consciousness may or may not occur. Noted symptoms may include increased distractibility, and difficulty with concentration. Treatment includes rest and monitoring for neurologic changes that could indicate a more severe injury, such as increased sleepiness, worsening headache, increased vomiting, worsening confusion, difficulty walking or talking, changes in LOC, and seizures.
Contusion	Bruising of cerebral tissue	Results from a blow to the head from incidents such as a motor vehicle accident, falls, or abuse such as shaken baby syndrome. May cause focal disturbances in vision, strength, and sensation. The signs and symptoms will vary based on the extent of vascular injury and can range from mild weakness to prolonged unconsciousness and paralysis. Treatment includes close monitoring for neurologic changes. Surgery is usually not necessary.

(continued)

Table 17.7 Common Head Injuries Seen in Children (continued)

Types	Description	Characteristics
Subdural hematoma	Collection of blood between the dura and cerebrum	Low incidence of fracture. Most common in children less than 2 years old, especially infants. Results from birth trauma, falls, bicycle injuries, and abuse such as shaken baby syndrome. Usually consists of venous bleeding. Symptoms may occur within 3 days of trauma or as late as 20 days. Symptoms include vomiting, failure to thrive, changes in LOC, seizures, and retinal hemorrhage. Treatment depends on clinical symptoms, size of clot, and area of the brain involved. In some cases, the bleed may be closely monitored for resolution. In other cases, treatment may include subdural taps in infants and surgical evacuation in older children. Close monitoring of neurologic status and for signs of increased ICP is indicated.
Epidural hematoma	Collection of blood located outside the dura but within the skull	Relatively uncommon. Often results from skull fracture. Seen when head trauma is severe. Usually arterial bleeding, therefore brain compression occurs rapidly and can result in impairment of the brainstem and respiratory or cardiovascular function. Symptoms include vomiting, headache, and lethargy. Treatment depends on clinical symptoms, the size of the clot, and the area of the brain involved. Treatment includes prompt surgical evacuation and cauterization of the artery. The earlier the bleed is recognized and treated, the more favorable the outcome. Close monitoring of neurologic status is indicated.

Nursing management will continue to focus on evaluation of neurologic status, assessing for changes in LOC and signs and symptoms of increased ICP. Initiate seizure precautions as ordered.

Individualize care to the specific needs of the child. Maintain a quiet environment to help reduce restlessness and irritability. Manage pain and administer sedation as ordered. Observe the level of sedation closely to ensure that LOC will not become altered, which would hinder the ability to assess adequately for neurologic changes. Monitor for the development of complications, which include hemorrhage, infection, cerebral edema, and herniation.

HEALTHY PEOPLE 2010

Objective	Significance
Increase the number of states and the District of Columbia with laws requiring bicycle helmets for bicycle riders.	• Support legislation locally that calls for bicycle helmet laws. • Participate in local "safe kids" activities to demonstrate support for helmet use

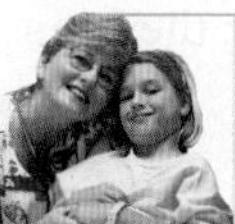

Parents are extremely helpful resources in evaluating a child's behavior for changes or abnormalities. They can provide insight into whether a behavior seen is normal or abnormal for this child. Examples include the ease at which a child is normally aroused, how much the child normally sleeps during the day, and what is the child's normal visual and hearing acuity.

Head injuries can range from a temporary unconsciousness that resolves quickly to children who may remain in a comatose state for a prolonged time. Nursing management of the comatose child is similar to nursing care of the comatose adult.

Providing Support and Education

Provide support and education for the family of a child who has suffered a head trauma. Encourage involvement in the child's care. The extent of residual neurologic damage and recovery may be unclear for the child with a head injury. This can be frustrating and stressful for parents and family. Encourage verbalization of their feelings and concerns. Rehabilitation of the child with permanent brain damage is an essential component of his or her care. It should begin as soon as possible in the hospital setting and may continue for months to years. This can place a strain on the family and its finances. Families need to be involved in the rehabilitation process. The nurse will be a key mem-

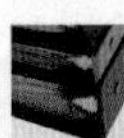

TEACHING GUIDELINE 17.2

Monitoring the Child with Closed Head Injury at Home

Instruct parents and caregivers:

- Stay with the child for the first 24 hours and be ready to take the child to the hospital if necessary.
- Closely observe the child for a few days.
- Wake the child every 2 hours to ensure that he or she moves normally, wakes enough to recognize the caregiver, and responds to the caregiver appropriately.
- Call the medical provider or bring child to the emergency room if the child exhibits any of the following:
  - Constant headache that gets worse
  - Slurred speech
  - Dizziness that does not go away or happens repeatedly
  - Extreme irritability or other abnormal behavior
  - Vomiting more than two times
  - Clumsiness or difficulty walking
  - Oozing blood or watery fluid from ears or nose
  - Difficulty waking up
  - Unequal-sized pupils
  - Unusual paleness that lasts longer than 1 hour
  - Seizures
- Review signs and symptoms of increased intracranial pressure and provide parents with a number they can call if they have questions or concerns.

HEALTHY PEOPLE 2010

Objective	Significance
Reduce hospitalization for nonfatal head injuries.	• Educate children and families about safety such as helmet use when inline skating, skateboarding, bicycling, and playing football or other sports that may result in head injury. • Encourage appropriate child car seat and seat belt use. • Use every encounter with a child and family as an opportunity to provide education related to injury prevention.

ber in ensuring the parents and family are involved with the interdisciplinary team.

Preventing Head Injuries

Prevention of head injuries provides the greatest benefit to children and the community. Nurses play a key role in educating the public on topics such as helmet use with certain sports; bicycle and motorcycle safety; seat belt use; and providing adequate supervision of children to help prevent injuries and accidents—and resultant head trauma—from occurring (see Healthy People 2010).

NONACCIDENTAL HEAD TRAUMA

In the United States, inflicted or nonaccidental head trauma is the leading cause of traumatic death and morbidity during infancy (Hymel, 2002). Causes include violent shaking, referred to as shaken baby syndrome (SBS); blows to the head; and intentional cranial impacts against the wall, furniture, or the floor. The infant's large head size and weak neck muscles place him or her at an increased risk for head trauma due to violent shaking or cranial impacts from adults. The average victim is less than 9 months of age. SBS is a form of child abuse and a significant number of head traumas result from it. It differs from many other forms of child abuse in that frequently there was no intent to harm the child. Shaking happens when the parent or caregiver becomes frustrated or angry because he or she cannot get the baby to stop crying.

The full appearance of neurologic deficits resulting from nonaccidental head trauma may take several years to be identified and recovery can be very slow. Long-term outcomes are not known, but many of these infants and children have poor outcomes and may suffer neurologic defects such as profound mental retardation, spastic quadriplegia, severe motor dysfunction, and blindness. The majority of children with inflicted head injuries have some impairment of motor and cognitive abilities, language, vision, and behavior. These injuries may also contribute to later problems with education and social attainment.

Nursing Assessment

The infant who has been a victim of nonaccidental trauma can present in many ways. Symptoms and physical findings may be similar to those seen in children with accidental head trauma or increased ICP related to infection. Therefore many nonaccidental traumas remain unidentified. Nurses are mandatory reporters of abuse (for further information on this, see Chapter 32), and early recognition of suspected child abuse is essential to prevent death and disability from repetitive inflicted head trauma.

Health History

It is important that health care providers review the child's history closely and pay particular attention to the caregivers' explanation of the child's injury. The health care provider should be alert to any discrepancies between the physical injuries and the history of injury given by the parent, if the stories are conflicting, or if the caregivers are unable to give an explanation for the injury. Also, any previous intracranial or skeletal injuries that cannot be explained should be noted.

In less severe cases, common signs and symptoms may include:

- Poor feeding or sucking
- Vomiting
- Lethargy or irritability
- Failure to thrive
- Increased sleeping
- Difficulty arousing

In more severe cases, the symptoms will be more acute and may consist of:

- Seizure activity
- Apnea
- Bradycardia
- Decreased LOC
- Bulging fontanel

Physical Examination

External bruising of the head and face may be evident in some inflicted head traumas. However, no evidence of external trauma, but the presence of intracranial or intraocular hemorrhages, is the classic presentation of SBS. Retinal hemorrhages are seen in the majority of cases, which is a rare finding in accidental or nontraumatic events.

Laboratory and Diagnostic Tests

Diagnostic tests including CT, MRI, ophthalmologic examination to rule out retinal hemorrhages, and skeletal survey x-rays to rule out or confirm other injuries may be performed to help determine the extent and type of injury.

Nursing Management

Treatment and nursing management will be similar to that for the child with accidental head trauma (see earlier section, "Head Trauma"). Prevention of nonaccidental head trauma, including SBS, is a major concern for all health care professionals. Be aware of risk factors related to the potential for SBS to occur. Recognizing these risk factors will allow appropriate intervention and protection of the child to take place. See Box 17.4 for risk factors related to SBS.

Educating parents and caregivers on appropriate ways to handle stress and ways to cope with a crying infant can help to prevent nonaccidental head trauma (see Teaching Guideline 17.3). Many parents and caregivers may perceive shaking a child as a less violent way to react than other means of enforcing discipline. They need to be aware that shaking a baby, even for only a few seconds, can cause serious brain damage and death. Decreasing mortality and morbidity associated with SBS and nonaccidental injury through early preventive education is an essential nursing concern. Information about the dangers of shaking a baby should be a part of prenatal care and standard discharge teaching on postpartum units. In addition, this information should be

BOX 17.4

RISK FACTORS ASSOCIATED WITH SHAKEN BABY SYNDROME

- Single parent
- Young parent
- Substance abuse by a parent
- Any external factors present such as financial, social, or physical burdens that place stress on the parent
- Premature or sick infant
- Infant with colic

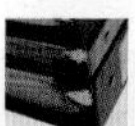

TEACHING GUIDELINE 17.3

Tips to Calm a Crying Baby

Instruct parents and caregivers

- Try to figure out what is upsetting the baby.
  - Is the baby hungry?
  - Is the baby's diaper dry?
  - Is the baby cold or hot?
  - Is the baby overtired or overstimulated?
  - Is the baby in pain?
  - Is the baby sick or running a fever?
- Try to help the baby relax.
  - Turn down the lights.
  - Swaddle the baby.
  - Walk the baby.
  - Rock the baby.
  - Give the baby a breast, bottle, or pacifier.
  - Shhh, talk to, or sing to the baby.
  - Talk the baby for a stroller or car ride.
- Sometimes the baby may continue to cry after all your efforts. If you feel overwhelmed, frustrated, or angry, focus on keeping the baby safe.
  - Stop what you are doing, take a deep breath, and count to 10.
  - Place the baby in a safe place, such as the crib or playpen.
  - Leave the room and shut the door, and find a quiet place for yourself.
  - Check on the baby every 5–15 minutes.
  - Do not be afraid to call for help; call a friend, relative, or neighbor.

provided to the community and in health education classes to reach young potential child care providers.

● BIRTH TRAUMA

Birth traumas are injuries sustained by the newborn during the birthing process. They may result from the pressure of birth, especially from a prolonged or abrupt labor, an abnormal or difficult presentation, cephalopelvic disproportion, or the use of mechanical forces such as forceps or vacuum during delivery. Newborns at risk include multiple deliveries, large-for-date infants, and those with extreme prematurity, a large fetal head, or congenital anomalies. Most injuries are minor and resolve without treatment.

Nursing Assessment

Inspect the head for lumps, bumps, or bruises. Note if swelling or bruising crosses the suture line. See Comparison Chart 17.2 and Figure 17.15 for a comparison of caput succedaneum and cephalohematoma (common types of head trauma resulting from the birth process).

Nursing Management

Nursing management will be mainly supportive and will focus on assessing for resolution of the trauma or any associated complications, along with providing support and education to the parents. Provide parents with explanation and reassurance that these injuries are harmless. It can be very alarming and concerning to parents to see swelling or bruising on their child's head. Provide parents with education regarding the length of time until resolution and when and if they need to seek further medical attention for the condition.

● NEAR DROWNING

Drowning rates have declined, but drowning remains the second leading cause of injury-related death in children between the ages of 1 and 19 years (Bull et al., 2003). Drowning is a preventable problem that is far too prevalent, especially in children. Those at greatest risk of drowning are toddlers and adolescent males.

Near drowning is described as an incident in which a child has suffered a submersion injury and has survived for at least 24 hours. Near-drowning events result in a significant number of injured children and can result in long-term neurologic deficits. In children between the ages of 1 and 4 years, most drowning and near-drowning incidents occur in residential swimming pools. Most incidents are accidental and result from inadequately supervising children who are in or near water; lack of use of personal flotation devices while on recreational water apparatus such as boats; and diving accidents.

Nursing Assessment

Hypoxia is the primary problem resulting from near drowning. Nursing assessment needs to begin with resuscitative measures. The child may be comatose, hypothermic, lack spontaneous respirations, and present with hypoxia and hypercapnea. Gain information about the site of submersion (was it fresh or salt water), the water temperature, the time of submersion, and how long it was until the child received interventions such as

● COMPARISON CHART 17.2 Caput Succedaneum vs. Cephalohematoma

	Caput Succedaneum (see Fig. 17.15a)	Cephalohematoma (see Fig. 17-15b)
Description	An edematous area of the scalp of the newborn	Collection of blood between the skull bone and periosteum
Cause	Pressure from the uterus or vaginal wall during a head-first delivery, also as a result of vacuum extraction	Pressure against the mother's pelvis results in bleeding. Common with forceps births
Characteristics	The swelling may be on any portion of the scalp and may cross the midline and suture lines. Mild discoloration may be present.	Does not cross the midline or suture lines
Treatment	None necessary (only observation)	In most cases only observation is necessary and resolution occurs within 3 to 6 weeks.
Complications	Usually heals spontaneously within a few days and without complication	Anemia; hypotension; underlying skull fracture; rarely leads to an infection such as meningitis. Due to the resolving hematoma, hemolysis of RBCs occurs and the infant may develop hyperbilirubinemia.

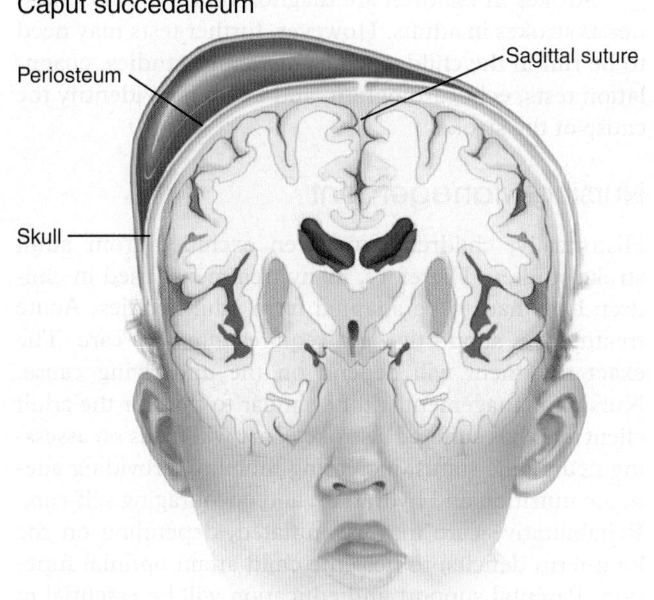

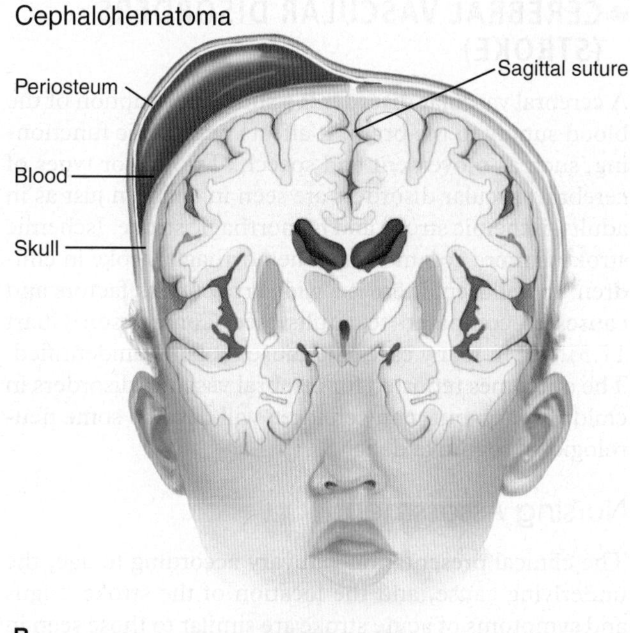

● Figure 17.15 (**A**) Infant with caput succedaneum. Edema is noted at birth and crosses the suture line. (**B**) Infant with cephalohematoma. Bleeding appears within the first 2 to 3 days of birth and does not cross the suture line.

cardiopulmonary resuscitation (CPR) and emergency medical services (EMS).

Nursing Management

Resuscitative measures should be started as soon as the child is pulled from the water, and the child should be transported to a hospital immediately. Management will be based on the degree of cerebral insult that has occurred. The child who has been successfully resuscitated will usually require intensive nursing care and monitoring. Promotion of oxygenation and monitoring for infection related to aspiration of water are primary nursing concerns. Chronic neurologic damage occurs in many near drownings secondary to hypoxia. The child may need rehabilitation and long-term follow-up. Provide parents with support and education relating to their child's condition. Educating children, families, and the community is an important nursing intervention to help prevent drowning (see Teaching Guideline 17.4).

Blood Flow Disruption

Cerebral vascular disorders are among the top ten causes of death in children and occur most frequently in the first year of life (Lynch, Hirtz, DeVeber, & Nelson, 2002). Although they occur less often than in adults, they are still an important cause of mortality and chronic morbidity in children. Many children will develop lifelong cognitive and motor impairments. Improvements in imaging techniques have led to an increase in the reported incidence and prevalence of cerebral vascular disorders in children in recent years. Childhood cerebral vascular disorders (stroke) are usually seen after the first month of life. Periventricular/intraventricular hemorrhage is seen in preterm infants and in infants up to 1 month of age.

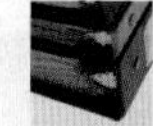

TEACHING GUIDELINE 17.4

Teaching to Prevent Drowning

Instruct parents and caregivers

- Install proper pool fencing.
- Start water safety training at a young age.
- Never leave an infant or young child without adult supervision in or near water (this includes bathtubs).
- Empty water from all containers, such as 5-gallon buckets, immediately after use.
- Use personal flotation devices at all times when near water.
- Learn cardiopulmonary resuscitation (CPR) and keep emergency numbers handy (make sure babysitters are CPR qualified).
- Know the depth of water before permitting a child to jump or dive.

CEREBRAL VASCULAR DISORDERS (STROKE)

A cerebral vascular disorder is a sudden disruption of the blood supply to the brain. It affects neurologic functioning, such as movement and speech. Two major types of cerebral vascular disorders are seen in children just as in adults: ischemic stroke and hemorrhagic stroke. Ischemic stroke is more common than hemorrhagic stroke in children. In children, there is a wide array of risk factors and causes as compared to adults (see Comparison Chart 17.3), but in many cases the cause remains unidentified. The outcomes reported for cerebral vascular disorders in children vary, but many children will develop some neurologic or cognitive deficit.

Nursing Assessment

The clinical presentation will vary according to age, the underlying cause, and the location of the stroke. Signs and symptoms of acute stroke are similar to those seen in the adult and depend on the area of the brain that has been affected. Common signs include:

- Weakness on one side or hemiplegia
- Facial droop
- Slurred speech
- Speech deficits

Strokes in children are diagnosed in the same manner as strokes in adults. However, further tests may need to be run in the child, such as metabolic studies, coagulation tests, echocardiogram, and LP to help identify the cause of the stroke.

Nursing Management

Historically, children have been excluded from adult stroke studies. Therefore, many treatments used in children have had to be adapted from adult studies. Acute treatment is supportive and requires intensive care. The exact treatment will depend on the underlying cause. Nursing management will be similar to that for the adult client who has suffered a stroke. Care will focus on assessing neurologic status, increasing mobility, providing adequate nutrition and hydration, and encouraging self-care. Rehabilitative care may be initiated, depending on the long-term deficits, to help the child attain optimal function. Parental support and education will be essential in helping them care for a child who has new disabilities.

PERIVENTRICULAR/INTRAVENTRICULAR HEMORRHAGE (PVH/IVH)

Intraventricular hemorrhage (IVH), which is bleeding into the ventricles, is the most common intracranial

COMPARISON CHART 17.3 Risk Factors and Causes of Stroke in the Pediatric Client vs. the Adult Client

	Risk Factors and Causes in Children	Risk Factors and Causes in Adults
Ischemic stroke	Cardiac disorders and intracardiac defects (congenital such as ventricular septal defect, atrial septal defect, aortic stenosis or acquired such as rheumatic heart disease) Coagulation abnormalities that lead to thrombosis Sickle-cell disease Infection, such as meningitis Arterial dissection Genetic disorders	Cardiac disease, including atherosclerosis Diabetes mellitus Hyperlipidemia Hypercoagulability states Polycythemia Sickle-cell disease Smoking Increased age Male gender Obesity Excessive alcohol consumption
Hemorrhagic stroke	Vascular malformations such as intracranial arteriovenus malformation (AVM) Aneurysms Warfarin therapy Cavernous malformations Malignancy Trauma Coagulation disorders such as hemophilia Thrombocytopenia Liver failure Leukemia Intracranial tumors such as medulloblastomas	Hypertension Aneurysms Use of anticoagulant medications Smoking Increased age Male gender Obesity Excessive alcohol consumption

bleed seen in preterm infants. Due to the preterm infant's fragile capillaries in the periventricular area, immature cerebral vascular development, and poorly supported vascular bed, these infants are at an increased risk for intracranial bleeds. Causes of rupture of the capillaries leading to IVH vary and include fluctuations in systemic and cerebral blood flow, increases in cerebral blood flow from hypertension, intravenous infusion, seizure activity, increases in cerebral venous pressure due to vaginal delivery, hypoxia, and respiratory distress. The smaller the newborn is, and the more premature, the higher the risk of developing IVH.

Complications of IVH include development of hydrocephalus, periventricular leukomalacia (an ischemic injury resulting from inadequate perfusion of the white matter adjacent to the ventricles), cerebral palsy, and mental retardation. The size and severity of the IVH is measured using a grading system. The system goes from grade I (mild) to grade IV (severe). In some settings, subcategories may be used to further distinguish the severity and extent of bleeding. Infants who experience mild IVH usually suffer no ill effects. Those with more severe grades of IVH are more likely to demonstrate neurologic and cognitive deficits.

Therapeutic Management

Infants with a documented IVH will receive follow-up with scans to monitor the lesion for evidence of progression or resolution. Supportive care includes the correction of underlying medical disturbances that might be related to the development of IVH as well as cardiovascular, respiratory, and neurologic support. Correction of anemia, hypotension, and acidosis along with ventilatory support may be necessary in some cases. If hydrocephalus results, placement of a shunt may be necessary (see "Hydrocephalus" section).

Nursing Assessment

The signs and symptoms seen with IVH vary significantly and there may be no clinical signs evident. Closely monitor newborns who are at an increased risk, such as premature and low-birth-weight newborns. Some symptoms that may be seen include:

- Apnea
- Bradycardia
- Cyanosis
- Weak suck
- Seizure activity
- High-pitched cry
- Bulging fontanel
- Anemia

Premature and low-birth-weight newborns may have a head ultrasonography in the first 10 days of life to assess for the presence of an IVH. Diagnostic tests such as CT and MRI scans also may be performed to document the presence of an IVH and provide more accurate assessment of the severity and size of the bleed.

Nursing Management

Nursing management will include monitoring for signs and symptoms of increased ICP, rapid increases in head circumference, neurologic changes, and delays in attainment of developmental milestones. In addition, provide education and support to the parents.

Chronic Disorders

Chronic disorders in children necessitate multidisciplinary care. Parents and children are in need of a large amount of education and support from the health care team. Chronic neurologic disorders commonly seen in children include headaches and breath holding.

● HEADACHES

Acute and chronic headaches, including migraines, are common reasons why children miss school, visit their primary care physicians, and receive subsequent referrals to neurologists. Children with reports or symptoms of headaches need to be examined thoroughly. Headaches may result from sinusitis or eyestrain or can be indicative of more serious conditions such as brain tumors, acute meningitis, or increased ICP. Migraines are a specific type of headache. They are benign, recurrent, throbbing headaches often accompanied by nausea, vomiting, and photophobia. Acute migraines can occur in children as young as 3 to 4 years old. The cause of migraine headaches is not well understood.

Therapeutic Management

After other acute or chronic conditions are ruled out, management will focus on treating the child's pain. Pharmacologic measures may be utilized in the treatment of chronic headaches and migraines. Medications used in children to treat and prevent headaches are similar to the medications used to treat adults. Recent attention has been paid to headaches caused by medication overuse. The client may have a primary headache disorder that is exacerbated by the frequent use of medications. Although medication overuse headaches are common in children, they are frequently underrecognized and underdiagnosed.

Nursing Assessment

Elicit a description of the present illness and chief complaint. Important health history information to obtain is onset of the pain, aggravating and alleviating factors, frequency and duration of the pain, time of day the pain usually occurs, location of the pain, and quality and intensity of the pain.

In young children, symptoms of headache may be hard to recognize. However, common signs and symptoms may include:

- Irritability
- Lethargy
- Head holding
- Head banging
- Sensitivity to sound or light

Assessment also includes a thorough physical examination to rule out any life-threatening illness, such as a brain tumor or increased ICP. A detailed neurologic exam is warranted. Neuroimaging may be performed based on the child's history and physical exam, if needed, to rule out a brain tumor or mass as the cause of the headaches.

Nursing Management

Nursing measures will focus on support and education. Reassure the child and family that no serious medical or neurologic disease is present. Because headaches are recurring and the cause may be unknown, pain management can be difficult. Provide education to help the child and parents gain control over the headaches. Teach the child and family to a keep very accurate record of headaches and activities surrounding the headaches to help establish a pattern of occurrence and identify triggering factors. Encourage parents and the child to recognize the triggering factors and to avoid them (Box 17.5). Teach the child and family about pain medications and how to use them. Teach other management techniques, which may include exercise, regular attendance at school, use of biofeedback, stress reduction techniques, and possible psychiatric assessment.

BOX 17.5

POTENTIAL HEADACHE TRIGGERS

- Foods, such as chocolate, caffeine, or monosodium glutamate (MSG)-containing foods
- Changes in hormone levels, around menses and ovulation
- Changes in:
  - Weather
  - Season
  - Sleep patterns
  - Meal schedule
- Stress
- Intense activity
- Bright or flickering lights
- Odors, such as strong perfumes

● BREATH HOLDING

Breath holding is a benign behavior of childhood, although it is extremely frightening for parents. It is normally seen in children 1 to 3 years old and typically is outgrown by 5 years of age. It is usually triggered by the child becoming angry or stressed after not getting his or her way. It can also occur as a reflexive response to fear, pain, or being startled. The child stops inhaling and exhaling or hyperventilates, the brain becomes anoxic, and the child becomes cyanotic and then passes out. It usually resolves spontaneously. With the loss of consciousness the child will begin breathing on his or her own and will often begin crying, screaming, and trying to catch his or her breath. The spells usually only last 30 to 60 seconds and, as long as the child does not sustain an injury while falling, have no consequences.

Nursing Assessment

The first time a spell occurs, a doctor should evaluate the child because the event could indicate a seizure. Breath holding also has been shown to be aggravated by iron deficiency anemia and, in rare cases, it could indicate a more serious neurologic condition and therefore warrant a full evaluation. Elicit a full description of the episode and events leading up to it. Also, collect a thorough past medical history and perform a complete physical examination.

Nursing Management

If no underlying condition is found, the child needs no therapy. Nursing management should focus on educating and supporting the parents. Breath holding is a scary event and parents will want information on the effects of the behavior and how to prevent the behavior from recurring. Reassure parents that the child will suffer no ill effects from breath holding and that they should not reinforce the breath holding behavior or give in to the child. Encourage parents to maintain a safe environment when an episode is occurring, but to avoid giving extra attention to the child after the event because this could encourage repetition of the behavior.

References

Amiel-Tison, C., Gosselin, J., & Infante-Rivard, C. (2002). Head growth and cranial assessment at neurologic examination in infancy [Electronic version]. *Developmental Medicine and Child Neurology, 44*(9), 643–649. Retrieved July 9, 2006, from Proquest database.

Anonymous. (2002). Rabies vaccines [Electronic version]. *Weekly Epidemiological Record, 77*(14), 109–120. Retrieved July 9, 2006, from Proquest database.

Anonymous. (2003). Botulism: Information from the World Health Organization [Electronic version]. *Journal of Environmental Health, 65*(9), 51–53. Retrieved July 9, 2006, from Proquest database.

Barnes, N. P., Jones, S. J., Hayward, R. D., Harkness, W. J., & Thompson, D. (2002). Ventriculoperitoneal shunt block: What are the best predictive clinical indicators? [Electronic version]. *Archives of Disease in Childhood, 87*(3), 194–202. Retrieved July 9, 2006, from Proquest database.

Behrman, R. E., Kliegman, R. M., & Jenson, H. B. (2004). *Nelson's textbook of pediatrics* (17th ed.). Philadelphia: Saunders.

Bull, M. J., Agran, P., Dowd, M. D., Garcia, V., et al. (2003). Prevention of drowning in infants, children and adolescents [Electronic version]. *Pediatrics, 112*(2), 437. Retrieved July 9, 2006, from Proquest database.

Cartwright, C. C. (2002). Assessing asymmetrical infant head shapes. *Nurse Practitioner, 27*(8), 33–39.

Castiglia, P. T. (2001). Shaken baby syndrome. *Journal of Pediatric Health Care, 15*(2), 78–80.

Ferguson, L. E., Hormann, M. D., Parks, D. K., & Yetman, R. J. (2002). Neisseria meningitides: Presentation, treatment, and prevention. *Journal of Pediatric Health Care, 16*(3), 119–124.

Fleetwood, I. G., & Steinberg, G. K. (2002). Arteriovenous malformations [Electronic version]. *Lancet, 359*(9309), 863–874. Retrieved July 9, 2006, from Proquest database.

Freeman, J. M. (2003). What every pediatrician should know about the ketogenic diet. *Contemporary Pediatrics, 20*(5), 113–127.

Fulton, D. R. (2000). Shaken baby syndrome [Electronic version]. *Critical Care Nursing Quarterly, 23*(2), 43–51. Retrieved July 9, 2006, from Proquest database.

Halsted, M. J., & Jones, B. V. (2002). Pediatric neuroimaging for the pediatrician. *Pediatric Annals, 31*(10), 661–670.

Hernandez-Diaz, S., Werler, M. M., Walker, A. M., & Mitchell, A. A. (2001). Neural tube defects in relation to use of folic acid antagonists during pregnancy [Electronic version]. *American Journal of Epidemiology, 153*(10), 961. Retrieved July 9, 2006, from Proquest database.

Hobdell, E. (2001). Infant neurologic assessment [Electronic version]. *Journal of Neuroscience Nursing, 33*(4), 190–194. Retrieved July 9, 2006, from Proquest database.

Hymel, K. P. (2002). Inflicted traumatic brain injury in infants and young children [Electronic version]. *Infants and Young Children, 15*(2), 57–66. Retrieved July 9, 2006, from Proquest database.

Jaspreet, G., & Gieron-Korthals, M. (2002). What pediatricians—and parents—need to know about febrile convulsions. *Contemporary Pediatrics, 5*(139).

Jurasek, G. (2001). Options in seizure management [Electronic version]. *Exceptional Parent, 31*(8), 107–113. Retrieved July 9, 2006, from Proquest database.

Kopec, K. (2001). New anticonvulsants for use in pediatric patients (Pt. I). *Journal of Pediatric Health Care, 15*(2), 81–86.

LaRossa, M. M., & Carter, S. L. (2005). Understanding how the brain develops. Retrieved July 9, 2006, from www.pediatrics.emory.edu/neonatology/dpc/brain.htm

Levene, M. (2002). The clinical conundrum of neonatal seizures [Electronic version]. *Archives of Disease in Childhood, 86*(2), F75–F77. Retrieved July 9, 2006, from Proquest database.

Lynch, J. K., Hirtz, D. G., DeVeber, G., & Nelson, K. B. (2002). Report of the National Institute of Neurologic Disorders and Stroke workshop on perinatal and childhood stroke [Electronic version]. *Pediatrics, 109*(1), 116–123. Retrieved July 9, 2006, from Proquest database.

Makaroff, K. L., & Putnam, F. W. (2003). Outcomes of infants and children with inflicted traumatic brain injury [Electronic version]. *Developmental Medicine and Child Neurology, 45*(7), 497. Retrieved July 9, 2006, from Proquest database.

Marthaler, M. T. (2004). Seizures revisited [Electronic version]. *Critical Care, 35*(4), 71–75. Retrieved July 9, 2006, from Proquest database.

Norris, C. M. R., Danis, P. G., & Gardner, T. D. (1999). Aseptic meningitis in the newborn and young infant. *American Family Physician, 59*(10), 2761.

Ogilvy, C. S., Stieg, P. E., Awad, I., Brown, R. D., Jr., et al. (2001). Recommendations for the management of intracranial arteriovenous malformations: A statement for healthcare professionals from a special writing group of the Stroke Council, American Stroke Association [Electronic version]. *Stroke, 32*(6), 1458–1472. Retrieved July 9, 2006, from Proquest database.

Padgett, K., & Boss B. J. (2004). Alterations in neurologic function in children. In S. E. Huether & K. L. Chance (Eds.), *Understanding pathophysiology* (3rd ed., pp. 429–447). St. Louis, MO: Mosby.

Parini, S. M. (2001). 8 Faces of meningitis [Electronic version]. *Nursing, 31*(8), 51–54. Retrieved July 9, 2006, from Proquest database.

Reimschisel, T. (2003). Breaking the cycle of medication overuse headache. *Contemporary Pediatrics, 20*(101). Retrieved July 9, 2006, from www.contemporarypediatrics.com.

Rice, S. (2003). Reye's syndrome isn't just child's play [Electronic version]. *Nursing, 33*(9), 32. Retrieved July 9, 2006, from Proquest database.

Roberts, E. G., & Shulkin, B. L. (2004). Technical issues in performing PET studies in pediatric patients [Electronic version]. *Journal of Nuclear Medicine Technology, 32*(1), 5–13. Retrieved July 9, 2006, from Proquest database.

Rosenblum, R. K., & Fisher, P. G. (2001). A guide to children with acute and chronic headaches. *Journal of Pediatric Health Care, 15*(5), 229–235.

Rowland, R. (1999). Homicide leading cause of injury death in infants [Electronic version]. Retrieved July 9, 2006, from CNN Interactive: www.cnn.com/HEALTH/9905/03/infant.deaths

Saex-Llorens, X., & McCracken, G. H., Jr. (2003). Bacterial meningitis in children [Electronic version]. *Lancet, 361*(9375), 2139. Retrieved July 9, 2006, from Proquest database.

Selekman, J. (2003). Preventing meningitis [Electronic version]. *Pediatric Nursing, 29*(6), 467. Retrieved July 9, 2006, from Proquest database.

Shinnar, S., & O'Dell, C. (2004). Febrile seizures. *Pediatric Annals 33*(6), 395–401.

Simon, N. P. (n.d.). Periventricular/intraventricular hemorrhage (PVH/IVH) in the premature infant. Retrieved July 9, 2006, from www.pediatrics.emory.edu/neonatology/dpc/pvhivh.htm

Spiro, C. S., & Spiro, D. M. (2004). Acute meningitis. *Clinician Reviews, 14*(3), 54–58.

Stevenson, K. L. (2004). Chiari type II malformation: Past, present and future [Electronic version]. *Neurosurgery Focus, 16*(2). Retrieved July 9, 2006, from Proquest database.

Vanore, M. L. (2000). Care of the pediatric patient with brain injury in an adult intensive care unit [Electronic version]. *Critical Care Nursing Quarterly, 23*(3), 38–49. Retrieved July 9, 2006, from Proquest database.

Wheeless, J. W. (2004). Treatment of status epilepticus in children. *Pediatric Annals, 33*(6), 377–383.

Whitley, R. J., & Gnann, J. W. (2002) Viral encephalitis: Familiar infections and emerging pathogens [Electronic version]. *Lancet, 359*(9305), 507–515. Retrieved July 9, 2006, from Proquest database.

Woodward, S., Addison, C. Shah, S., Brennan, F., et al. (2002). Benchmarking best practice for external ventricular drainage [Electronic version]. *British Journal of Nursing, 11*(1), 47–54. Retrieved July 9, 2006, from Proquest database.

Worrall, K. (2004). Use of the Glasgow Coma Scale in infants. *Paediatric Nursing, 16*(4), 45–50.

Web Sites

www.biausa.org/Pages/splash.html Brain Injury Association of America: prevention, research, education, and advocacy

www.cappskids.org/index.html Craniosynostosis and Positional Plagiocephaly Support, Inc.: resources and education for families

www.chasa.org Children's Hemiplegia and Stroke Association: Support for Children with Hemiplegia, Hemiplegic Cerebral Palsy, Infant Stroke, or Childhood Stroke

www.geocities.com/epilepsy911 Epilepsy support group for families

www.hemikids.org Online support group for children with hemiplegia or hemiplegic cerebral palsy

www.hydrocephalus.org Hydrocephalus Foundation

www.pediatricstrokenetwork.com/Pediatric Stroke Network Support group for pediatric stroke

www.pediatricstroke.org A childhood stroke support group

www.safekids.org National Safe Kids Campaign

Chapter WORKSHEET

MULTIPLE CHOICE QUESTIONS

1. When compared with adults, why are infants and children at an increased risk of head trauma?
   a. The head of the infant and young child is large in proportion to the body and the neck muscles are not well developed.
   b. The development of the nervous system is complete at birth but remains immature.
   c. The spine is very immobile in infants and young children.
   d. The skull is more flexible due to the presence of sutures and fontanels.
2. At a well-child visit, hydrocephalus may be suspected in an infant if upon assessment the nurse finds:
   a. Narrow sutures
   b. Sunken fontanels
   c. A rapid increase in head circumference
   d. Increase in weight since last visit
3. A 10-year-old child is admitted to the hospital due to history of seizure activity. As his nurse, you are called into the room by his mother who states he is having a seizure. What would be the priority nursing intervention?
   a. Prevention of injury by removing the child from his bed
   b. Prevention of injury by placing a tongue blade in the child's mouth
   c. Prevention of injury by restraining the child
   d. Prevention of injury by placing the child on his side and opening his airway
4. A 6-month-old infant is admitted to the hospital with suspected bacterial meningitis. She is crying, irritable, and lying in the opisthotonic position. The priority nursing intervention would be:
   a. Educate the family on ways to prevent bacterial meningitis.
   b. Initiate appropriate isolation precautions and begin intravenous antibiotics.
   c. Assess the infant's fontanels.
   d. Encourage the mother to hold the infant and feed her.

CRITICAL THINKING EXERCISES

1. A child is seen in the doctor's office after hitting his head while skateboarding. The child suffered no loss of consciousness, and has no external injuries and no significant past medical history. He is acting appropriately at this time. His only complaint is a dull headache. What instructions would you give the parents regarding his care at home? Include when they should seek further medical care.
2. A 10-year-old child is admitted to the pediatric unit after experiencing a seizure. A complete, accurate, and detailed history from a reliable source is essential. What information would you ask for while obtaining the history?
3. A 6-year-old child is admitted to the hospital because of a possible seizure. The child's mother calls the nurse to the room because the child is "jerking all over" and won't respond when she calls the child's name. List appropriate nursing interventions for this child. Prioritize the list of interventions.
4. Describe the impact of cerebral vascular accident in the child as compared with the adult. How does it affect the child's future? How will the nurse provide care differently for the child stroke victim as compared with the adult?

STUDY ACTIVITIES

1. A 4-month-old child with a history of hydrocephalus has undergone surgery for placement of a VP shunt. What information would you include in the teaching plan?
2. Develop an example of a "headache log" that could be used by the family for chronicling the child's headaches, including triggers, relieving factors, and precipitating events. Ensure that the log is developed at a 6th-grade reading level to make it practical for low literacy parents.
3. In the clinical setting, interview the parent of a child who has suffered significant brain trauma or injury (such as head trauma, IVH, or stroke). Talk with the family about the types of care the child requires. Reflect upon this interview in your clinical journal, and compare how the ongoing care for this child compares with that for a typical child.

chapter 18

Nursing Care of the Child With a Disorder of the Eyes or Ears

Key TERMS

acuity
amblyopia
blindness
conductive hearing loss
deaf
decibel
hearing impairment
nystagmus
pressure-equalizing tubes (PE tubes)
ptosis
sensorineural hearing loss
strabismus
tympanometry
tympanostomy
vision impairment

Learning OBJECTIVES

Upon completion of the chapter, the learner will be able to:

1. Differentiate between the anatomic and physiologic differences of the eyes and ears in children as compared with adults.
2. Identify various factors associated with disorders of the eyes and ears in infants and children.
3. Discuss common laboratory and other diagnostic tests useful in the diagnosis of disorders of the eyes and ears.
4. Discuss common medications and other treatments used for treatment and palliation of conditions affecting the eyes and ears.
5. Recognize risk factors associated with various disorders of the eyes and ears.
6. Distinguish between different disorders of the eyes and ears based on the signs and symptoms associated with them.
7. Discuss nursing interventions commonly used in regard to disorders of the eyes and ears.
8. Devise an individualized nursing care plan for the child with a sensory impairment or other disorder of the eyes or ears.
9. Develop patient/family teaching plans for the child with a disorder of the eyes or ears.
10. Describe the psychosocial impact of sensory impairments on children.

WOW *With the help of a nurse's care and healing, the child's senses provide him or her with an antenna to the universe.*

Enrique Baxter, a 9-month-old, is brought to the clinic by his mother. His mother tells you, "Enrique has been fussy and not eating or sleeping well for the past 2 days."

Children commonly suffer from disorders related to the eyes and ears. Conjunctivitis and otitis media are two very common disorders in childhood. Other inflammatory and infectious conditions also affect the child's eyes or ears. Various alterations such as refractive error, strabismus, and amblyopia affect the development of visual acuity in children. Any alteration in the ear that contributes to hearing loss may have a significant impact on the child's language acquisition. It is important for nurses to be familiar with the most common disorders of the eyes and ears in order to provide appropriate care to these children and to encourage optimal development in all children. In addition, the nurse may be caring for a child with another problem who is also either visually or hearing impaired. The nurse must take these developmental differences into account when planning care for these children.

Variations in Pediatric Anatomy and Physiology

It is important for the nurse to understand the impact of eye and ear disorders on the child's development. Some children may be born with anomalies of the eyes or ears that will have a significant impact on vision and hearing, as well as psychomotor development. On the other hand, disorders affecting the eyes or ears, particularly if chronic or recurrent, can have a significant impact on the development of visual acuity or may cause hearing impairment.

Eyes

Light-skinned children are often born with blue eyes. The iris becomes pigmented over time and eye color is determined by 6 to 12 moths of age. The newborn's sclera may be slightly bluish-tinged but becomes white within weeks. The eyeball of the infant and young child occupies a relatively larger space within the orbit than the adult's does, making it more susceptible to injury (Fig. 18.1).

The spherical shape of the newborn's lens does not allow for distance accommodation, so the newborn sees best at a distance of about 8 to 10 inches. The optic nerve is not completely myelinated, so color discrimination is incomplete. Visual acuity develops over the first few years of the child's life. At birth, acuity ranges from 20/100 to 20/400. By age 2 to 3 years, the visual acuity of most children is 20/50, with 20/20 achieved by age 6 to 7 years. The rectus muscles are uncoordinated at birth and mature over time so that binocular vision (the ability to focus with both eyes simultaneously) may be achieved by 4 months of age. In the very preterm infant, retinal vascularization is incomplete, so visual acuity may be affected.

Ears

Congenital deformities of the ear are often associated with other body system anomalies and genetic syndromes. The presence of ear anomalies may lead to the search for and subsequent diagnosis of the other anomalies or syndromes. The infant's relatively short, wide, and horizontally placed Eustachian tubes allow bacteria and viruses to gain access to the middle ear easily, resulting in increased numbers of ear infections as compared to the adult. As the child matures, the tubes assume a more slanted position, so older children and adults generally have fewer cases of middle ear effusion and infection (Fig. 18.2). Sometimes enlargement of the adenoids contributes to obstruction of the Eustachian tubes, leading to infection.

Common Medical Treatments

A variety of interventions are used to treat disorders of the eyes and ears in children. The treatments listed in Common Medical Treatments 18.1 and Drug Guide 18.1 usually require a physician's order when a child is hospitalized.

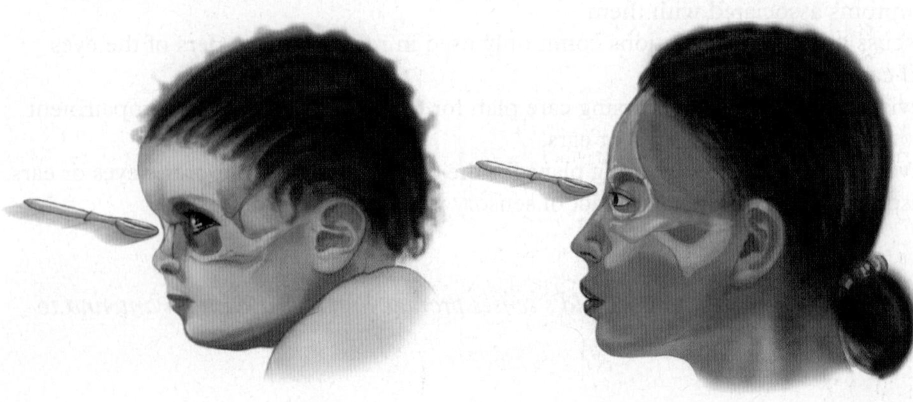

● Figure 18.1 The relatively larger space that the infant's and young child's eyeball occupies within the orbit makes it more susceptible to injury as compared with the adult's eye.

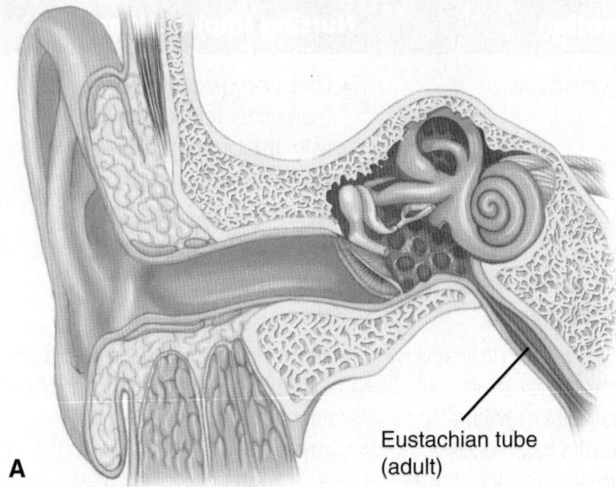

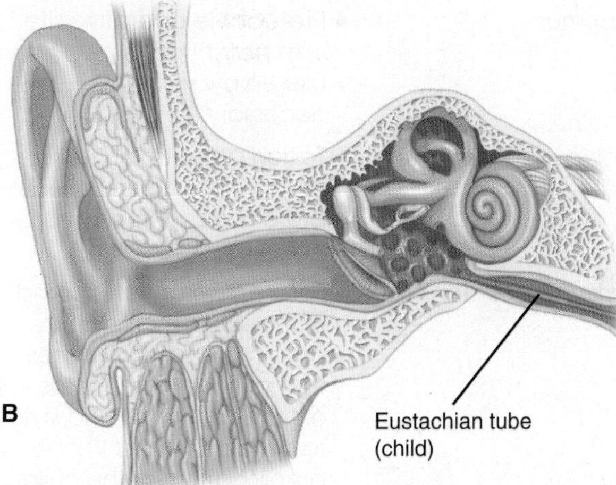

● Figure 18.2 Note the child's relatively shorter, wider Eustachian tubes and their horizontal positioning (**B**) as compared with the adult's (**A**).

> Remember Enrique, the 9-month-old with fussiness and poor feeding who was not sleeping well? What additional health history and physical examination assessment information should you obtain?

Nursing Process Overview for the Child With a Disorder of the Eyes or Ears

Care of the child with a disorder of the eyes and ears includes assessment, nursing diagnosis, planning, interventions, and evaluation. There are a number of general concepts related to the nursing process that can be applied to disorders of the eyes and ears. From a general understanding of the care involved for a child with alterations in the eyes and ears, the nurse can then individualize the care based on client specifics.

ASSESSMENT

Assessment of disorders of the eyes and ears in children includes health history, physical assessment, and laboratory or diagnostic testing.

Health History

The health history comprises past medical history, family history, history of present illness (when the symptoms started and how they have progressed), as well as treatments used at home. The past medical history may be significant for prematurity, genetic defect, eye or ear deformities, visual acuity deficit or blindness, hearing impairment or deafness, recurrent ear infections, or ear surgeries. Family history might be significant for eye or ear deformities or vision or hearing impairment or may reveal contacts for infectious exposure.

When eliciting the history of the present illness, inquire about its onset and progression and the presence of fever, nasal congestion, eye or ear pain, eye rubbing, ear pulling, headache, lethargy, or behavioral changes. Document if the child has corrective lenses or hearing aids prescribed and to what extent these devices are actually used.

Physical Examination

When assessing the eyes and ears, begin with inspection and observation. Palpation is also used when assessing for ear disorders. Testing of visual acuity and hearing is also performed.

Inspection and Observation

The physical examination should begin with inspection or observation. Note whether the child uses eyeglasses, corrective lenses, or a hearing aid. Observe the eyes: note their positioning and symmetry, presence of strabismus, nystagmus, and squinting. The eyelids should open equally (failure to open fully is termed **ptosis**). Note variations in eye slant and the presence of epicanthal folds. Assess the eyes for presence of eyelid edema, sclera color, discharge, tearing, and pupillary equality, as well as size and shape of the pupils. Evert the eyelid to inspect the palpebral conjunctivae for redness. Test for extraocular movements and pupillary light response and accommodation. Note symmetry of corneal light reflex. Note presence of red reflex with an ophthalmoscope. Perform an age-appropriate visual acuity test. Refer to Chapter 9 for more detailed information related to visual acuity testing.

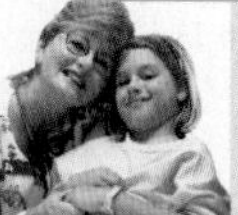
Attempts to inspect the palpebral conjunctivae may be frightening to children. Ask the older, cooperative child to evert the eyelid himself or herself, while the nurse inspects the conjunctivae.

Common Medical Treatments 18.1

Treatment	Explanation	Indication	Nursing Implications
Warm compress	Warm, moist washcloth	Conjunctivitis	• Use very warm water from the tap (to avoid risk of burning, do not microwave).
Corrective lenses	In eyeglass form or as contact lenses	Correction of astigmatism, refractive error, strabismus	• Use a safety strap to help young children wear their eyeglasses.
Patching	An adhesive patch is applied to the healthier eye for several hours each day.	Strabismus, amblyopia, any other eye condition that results in one eye being weaker than the other	• Inform parents that though difficult to obtain, compliance with patching is critical. • A "pirate patch" may coax preschoolers into compliance.
Eye muscle surgery	Surgical alignment of the eyes	Strabismus	• Protect the operative site with patching. • Use elbow restraints if necessary.
Pressure-equalizing (PE) tubes (tympanostomy tubes)	Tiny plastic tubes inserted in the tympanic membrane	Chronic otitis media with effusion	• Teach parents "dry ears" precautions if prescribed or preferred by the surgeon.
Hearing aids	Amplification device worn in the ear	Hearing impairment	• Ensure appropriate fit and adequate amplification. • Direct families to outfitters that provide loaner aids of various brands and styles to determine best fit and amplification for the child.
Cochlear implants	Surgically inserted electronic prosthetic device	Sensorineural hearing loss	• Inform families that the usual minimum age for this procedure is 12 months.

Drug Guide 18.1 Common Drugs for Ear and Eye Disorders

Medication	Action	Indication	Nursing Implications
Antibiotics (oral, otic, ophthalmic)	Treatment of bacterial infections of the eyes and ears	Acute otitis media, otitis externa, conjunctivitis	Teach families to complete the entire course as prescribed. Check for drug allergies prior to administration.
Antihistamines	Block histamine reaction	Allergic conjunctivitis	Topical drops used. Oral agents usually prescribed if allergic rhinitis accompanies the conjunctivitis.
Analgesics	Pain relief	Otitis media, otitis externa, after eye or ear surgery	Narcotic analgesics may be necessary in some instances.

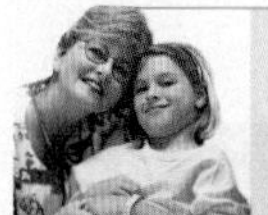

Though the sclerae are bluish in newborns, they become white in the first few weeks of life. Blue sclerae that persist beyond a few weeks of life may be an indicator of osteogenesis imperfecta type I, an inherited connective tissue disorder.

Inspect the ears: note their size and shape, position, and the presence of skin tags, dimples, or other anomalies (Fig. 18.3). Upon otoscopic examination, note presence of cerumen, discharge, inflammation, or a foreign body in the ear canal. Visualize the tympanic membrane and observe its color, landmarks, and light reflex, as well as presence of perforation, scars, bulging, or retraction. Tympanic membrane mobility may be tested with pneumatic otoscopy. Auditory acuity is tested via the whisper test, audiometry, or other age-appropriate test (refer to Chapter 9 for a more detailed explanation of hearing testing).

Palpation

Usually, the eyes are not palpated. In the case of injury the upper eyelid may be everted for examination purposes. Palpate the ear for tenderness over the tragus or pinna. Note the presence of tenderness over the mastoid area (tenderness may be present when otitis media progresses to mastoiditis). Palpate for enlarged cervical lymph nodes (this occurs when the eyes or ears are infected).

Laboratory and Diagnostic Testing

The Common Laboratory and Diagnostic Tests display offers an explanation of the laboratory and diagnostic tests most commonly used for disorders of the eyes and ears. These tests can assist the physician in diagnosing the disorder and/or can be used as guidelines in determining ongoing treatment. Laboratory or non-nursing personnel obtain some of the tests, while the nurse may obtain others. In either instance the nurse should be familiar with how the tests are obtained, what they are used for, and normal versus abnormal results. This knowledge will also be necessary when providing patient and family education related to the testing.

NURSING DIAGNOSES AND RELATED INTERVENTIONS

Upon completion of a thorough assessment, the nurse might identify several nursing diagnoses, including:

- Disturbed sensory perception
- Risk for infection
- Pain
- Delayed growth and development
- Impaired verbal communication
- Deficient knowledge
- Interrupted family processes
- Risk for injury

After completing an assessment of Enrique, the nurse noted the following: fever, tugging at his ears, and increased crying when lying down. Based on the assessment findings, what would your top three nursing diagnoses be for Enrique?

Nursing goals, interventions, and evaluation for the child with an eye or ear disorder are based on the nursing diagnoses. Nursing Care Plan 18.1 may be used as a guide in planning nursing care for the child with an eye or ear disorder, but it should be individualized based on the patient's symptoms and needs. Refer to Chapter 15 for the nursing care plan for pain management. Additional information will be included later in the chapter as it relates to specific disorders.

Based on your top three nursing diagnoses for Enrique, describe appropriate nursing interventions.

(text continues on page 525)

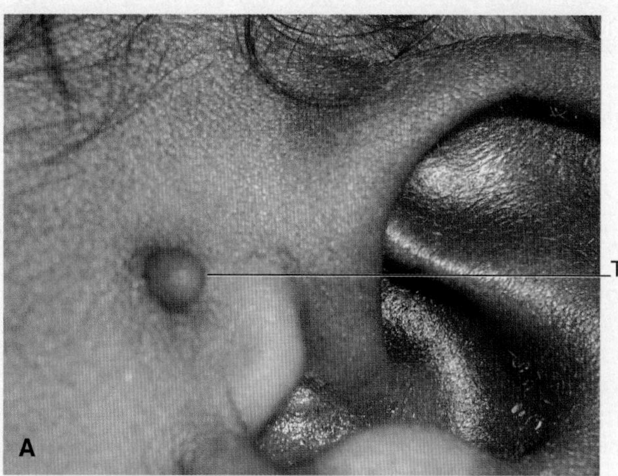

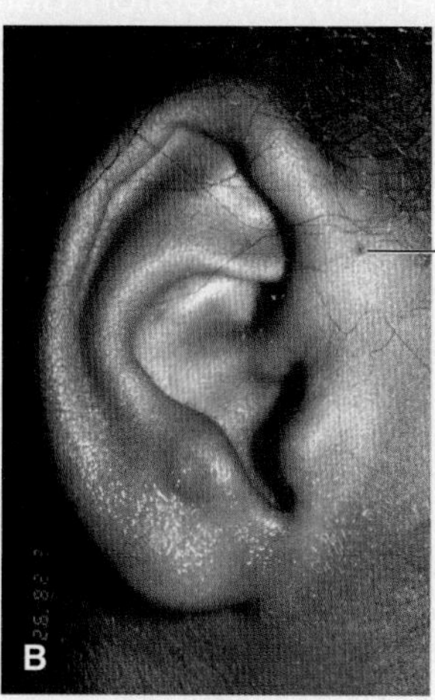

● **Figure 18.3** Note the skin tag (**A**) and preauricular pit (**B**) (in front of the ear).

Common Laboratory and Diagnostic Tests 18.1

Test	Explanation	Indication	Nursing Implications
Culture of eye or ear discharge	Fluid draining from the eye or ear is cultured.	To find appropriate antibiotic coverage for a particular infection	Easy to collect, relatively pain-free. If drainage must be removed from within the ear canal, more likely to be painful.
Tympanic fluid culture	Culture of fluid aspirated from the middle ear	To find appropriate antibiotic coverage for a particular infection	Painful; usually performed only by specially trained physicians
Tympanometry	Probe in ear canal measures movement of the eardrum.	Determines extent of effusion of the middle ear	Quick and easy to perform (seconds). Requires accurate-sized probe for adequate seal of the ear canal.

Nursing Care Plan 18.1

Overview for the Child with a Disorder of Eyes or Ears

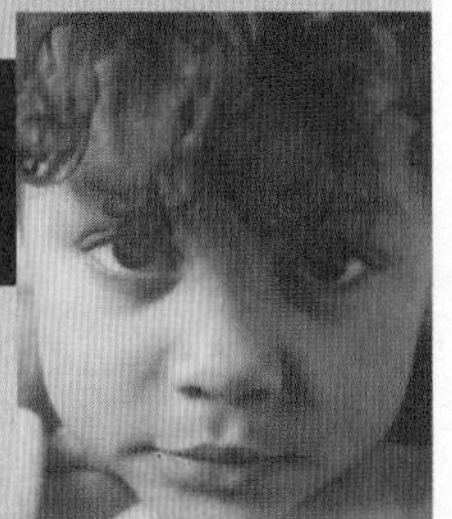

Nursing Diagnosis: Sensory perception, disturbed (visual) related to visual impairment or blindness as evidenced by lack of reaction to visual stimuli, squinting, holding items close

Outcome identification and evaluation

Child will reach maximal vision potential: *Child uses corrective lenses appropriately and is able to participate in play and schoolwork.*

Intervention: improving vision

- Encourage corrective lens use *for enhancement of vision.*
- For the severely impaired or blind child, identify yourself via voice and name items in environment for the child *so that the child is aware of his or her surroundings.*
- Support the family's efforts at vision therapy and other habilitation programs *to promote vision enhancement.*
- Engage the parents in bedside caregiving *because the parents' voice and presence are reassuring to the child.*

Nursing Diagnosis: Sensory perception, disturbed (auditory) related to hearing loss as evidenced by lack of reaction to verbal stimuli, delayed attainment of language milestones

Outcome identification and evaluation

Child will reach maximal hearing and speech potential: *Child uses aids appropriately and communicates effectively.*

Intervention: improving hearing

- Assess hearing ability frequently *because early detection of hearing loss allows for earlier intervention and correction.*
- Assess language development at each visit *to allow for early detection of hearing loss (earlier intervention and correction).*
- Encourage hearing aid use *for amplification of sound.*
- Teach about hearing aid battery safety *to avoid aspiration of battery.*
- Assist child with focusing on sounds in the environment *to encourage listening skills.*
- Refer for and encourage attendance at communication habilitation program *to maximize communication potential.*

Overview for the Child with a Disorder of Eyes or Ears (continued)

Nursing Diagnosis: Risk for infection related to presence of infectious organisms as evidenced by fever, presence of virus or bacteria on laboratory screening.

Outcome identification and evaluation

Child will exhibit no signs of secondary infection and will not spread infection to others: *Symptoms of infection decrease over time, and others remain free from infection.*

Intervention: reducing infection risk

- Maintain aseptic technique and practice good hand washing *to prevent introduction of further infectious agents.*
- Limit number of visitors, screening for recent illness, *to prevent further infection.*
- Administer antibiotics if prescribed *to prevent or treat bacterial infection.*
- Encourage nutritious diet according to child's preferences *to assist body's natural infection-fighting mechanisms.*
- Isolate the child as required *to prevent nosocomial spread of infection.*
- Teach child and family preventive measures such as good hand washing, covering mouth and nose when coughing or sneezing, adequate disposal of used tissues, *to prevent nosocomial or community spread of infection.*

Nursing Diagnosis: Growth and development delay, related to sensory impairment as evidenced by delay in attainment of developmental milestones

Outcome identification and evaluation

Child will achieve optimum independence for age: *Child participates in age-appropriate developmental activities.*

Intervention: encouraging growth and development

- Encourage attainment of developmental milestones with use of assistive devices as needed *for timely developmental achievements.*
- Foster independence in ADLs *to promote sense of accomplishment.*
- Encourage participation in play with another child or within a group *to promote socialization.*
- Assist family to set limits and apply discipline *because structure and routine provide a secure environment in which the developing child can grow.*
- Encourage friendships with other children with a sensory impairment *to promote socialization and let the child know that he or she is not the only one with these challenges.*

Nursing Diagnosis: Impaired verbal communication related to hearing loss as evidenced by lack of or inarticulate speech, lack of alternate communication channel

Outcome identification and evaluation

The child will communicate effectively with the method chosen by the family (this may be sign language, oral/deaf speech, cued speech, or augmentative alternative communication device).

Intervention: improving communication

- Encourage choice of and attendance at communication habilitation program *to promote continued learning.*
- Provide consistency between home and hospital in regard to communication style/devices *to promote continued learning.*
- Support the child's efforts at correct speech to *promote speech development through reinforcement and praise.*
- Encourage family to use spoken language and read books at home *to continue to promote appropriate language development.*

(continued)

Overview for the Child with a Disorder of Eyes or Ears (continued)

Nursing Diagnosis: Deficient knowledge related to sensory impairment (vision or hearing) as evidenced by new diagnosis and parents' questions

Outcome identification and evaluation

Parents express understanding of diagnosis and care of child: *Parents verbalize understanding, demonstrate use of assistive devices, or independently perform medical treatments.*

Intervention: educating the family

- Review diagnosis and plan of care with the parents *to promote understanding of the disease process.*
- Refer family to resources available for sensory impaired children *to provide further education and support to the parents.*
- Demonstrate medical treatments prescribed or use of assistive devices, requiring a return demonstration, *which shows the parents' ability to provide the prescribed care for the child.*
- Encourage exploration of different communication and learning modes available for the sensory impaired child *to allow the child and family to find the right educational and communication style fit.*

Nursing Diagnosis: Family processes, interrupted, related to child's sensory impairment as evidenced by parent verbalization, nonverbal language, altered coping

Outcome identification and evaluation

Parents demonstrate adequate coping and decreased anxiety: *Parents are involved in child's care, ask appropriate questions, and are able to discuss child's care and condition calmly.*

Intervention: encouraging appropriate family interactions

- Encourage parents' verbalization of grief if child is hearing or vision impaired. *Parents must deal with their own feelings of loss to successfully care for the child with an impairment.*
- Encourage parents' verbalization of concerns related to child's illness. *This allows for identification of concerns and demonstrates to the family that the nurse also cares about them, not just the child.*
- Explain therapy, procedures, and child's behavior to parents; *developing an understanding of the child's current status helps decrease anxiety.*
- Encourage parental involvement in care *so that parents may continue to feel needed and valued.*

Nursing Diagnosis: Risk for injury related to vision loss as evidenced by difficulty navigating surroundings

Outcome identification and evaluation

The infant or child will remain free from injury.

Intervention: preventing injury

- Orient the child to hospital surroundings *because awareness is the first step to preventing injury.*
- Encourage parent to be at bedside *so that the child feels more comfortable.*
- Encourage use of assistive devise *to promote safety.*

Infectious and Inflammatory Disorders of the Eyes

Infectious and inflammatory disorders of the eyes include conjunctivitis, nasolacrimal duct obstruction, eyelid lesions, and periorbital cellulitis.

• CONJUNCTIVITIS

Inflammation of the bulbar or palpebral conjunctiva is referred to as conjunctivitis. It can be infectious, allergic, or chemical in nature. Viruses or bacteria may cause infectious conjunctivitis. Adenoviruses and influenza account for the bulk of cases of viral conjunctivitis. The most common bacterial cause is *Staphylococcus aureus,* but many cases are also caused by *Streptococcus pneumoniae, Haemophilus influenzae,* and other bacteria. In the newborn, *Chlamydia trachomatis* and *Neisseria gonorrhoeae* are more common causes. Infectious conjunctivitis is very contagious, so epidemics are common, particularly in young children. Risk factors for acute infectious conjunctivitis include age less than 2 weeks; daycare, preschool, or school attendance; concomitant viral upper respiratory infection; pharyngitis; or otitis media. Concurrent acute otitis media may occur depending upon the bacterial cause (Cook & Walsh, 2005). Complications from simple infectious conjunctivitis are uncommon. Neonates with chlamydial conjunctivitis may be at risk for the development of chlamydial pneumonia.

Allergic conjunctivitis results from exposure to particular allergens. Allergic conjunctivitis may be a seasonal or year-round complaint. A genetic predisposition to allergic conjunctivitis exists, just as it does for asthma, allergic rhinitis, and atopic dermatitis. Allergic conjunctivitis occurs more frequently in school-age children and adolescents than it does in infants and young children because of repeat exposure to allergens over time. In the case of seasonal allergic conjunctivitis, the severity of symptoms and the number of children affected are directly related to the pollen count in the area.

Therapeutic Management

Therapeutic management of conjunctivitis is prescribed depending upon the cause. Bacterial conjunctivitis is generally treated with an ophthalmic antibiotic preparation (drops or ointment). Viral conjunctivitis is a self-limiting disease and does not require topical medication. Eye drops with an antihistamine or mast cell stabilization effect may be helpful in alleviating symptoms of allergic conjunctivitis. If other allergy signs and symptoms are also present, an oral antihistamine may also be prescribed. Table 18.1 compares bacterial, viral, and allergic conjunctivitis.

Pathophysiology

When bacteria or viruses come in contact with the bulbar or palpebral conjunctiva, they are recognized as foreign antigens and an antigen–antibody immune reaction occurs, resulting in inflammation. Allergic conjunctivitis occurs through a different mechanism. Contact with the allergen results in an allergic response (overreaction of the immune response). The mast cell and histamine mediators are then activated, resulting in inflammation.

Nursing Assessment

Nursing assessment of the child with conjunctivitis, regardless of the cause, is similar. It includes health history, physical examination, and in rare instances laboratory testing.

Table 18.1 Types of Conjunctivitis

Type of Conjunctivitis	Conjunctivae	Discharge	Additional Findings	Eyelid Edema	Treatment
Bacterial	Inflamed	Purulent, mucoid	Mild pain	Occasional	Antibiotic drops or ointment
Viral	Inflamed	Watery, mucoid	Lymphadenopathy, photophobia, tearing	Usually present	Symptom relief; antiherpetic agent if cause is herpes
Allergic	Inflamed	Watery or stringy	Itching	Usually present	Antihistamine and/or mast cell stabilizer drops

Health History

Elicit a description of the present illness and chief complaint. Common signs and symptoms reported during the health history might include:

- Redness
- Edema
- Tearing
- Discharge
- Eye pain
- Itching of the eyes (usually with allergic conjunctivitis)

Determine the onset of symptoms and their progression as well as response to treatments used at home. Assess for risk factors for infectious conjunctivitis, such as daycare or school attendance. Note any history of an upper respiratory infection, sore throat, or earache. Question parents about possible infectious exposures. Review the health history for risk factors for allergic conjunctivitis such as a family history and a history of asthma, allergic rhinitis, or atopic dermatitis. Determine seasonality related to the symptoms and whether the symptoms occur after exposure to particular allergens, such as pollen, hay, or animals.

Physical Examination

Observe for eyelid swelling or redness. Inspect the conjunctivae for redness (Fig. 18.4). Note quantity, color, and consistency of discharge. Bacterial infections generally result in a thick, colored discharge, whereas a clear or white discharge is generally seen with viral conjunctivitis. Allergic conjunctivitis often results in a watery discharge, sometimes profuse, which is usually present bilaterally. Contact with an allergen rubbed into one of the eyes may result in unilateral symptoms. Observe the child for other signs of allergic or atopic disease, and document presence of runny nose or cough as well.

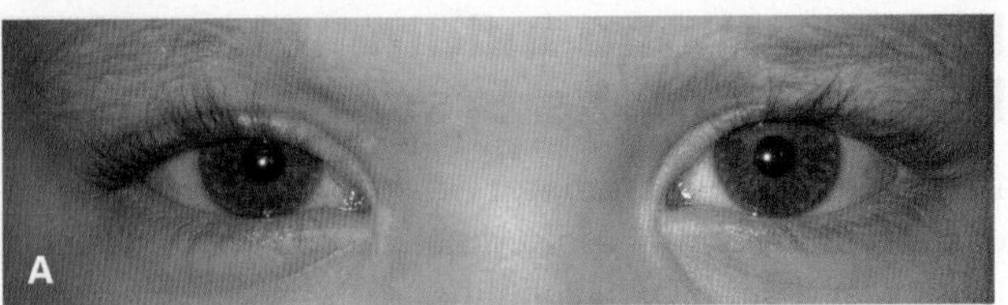

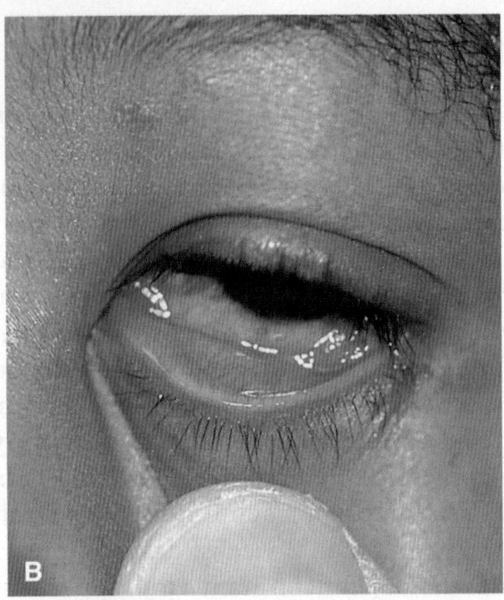

● Figure 18.4 (**A**) Bacterial conjunctivitis: note redness of conjunctiva, copious discolored drainage with matting, and eyelid swelling. (**B**) Allergic conjunctivitis: note redness of conjunctiva, clear watery discharge, rubbing of the eyes.

Laboratory and Diagnostic Tests

Cases of bacterial, viral, and allergic conjunctivitis are generally diagnosed based on history and clinical presentation. Cases of viral and allergic conjunctivitis do not warrant laboratory testing. If bacterial conjunctivitis is suspected, then a bacterial culture of the eye drainage may be performed to determine the exact causative organism, thus allowing the most appropriate antibiotic to be prescribed.

Nursing Management

Nursing management of the various types of conjunctivitis focuses on alleviating symptoms and, for infectious causes, preventing spread.

Alleviating Symptoms

Teach parents how to apply eye drops or ointment (antibiotic for bacterial causes and antihistamine or mast cell stabilizer for allergic). Warm compresses may be used to help loosen the crust that accumulates on the eyelids overnight when drainage is copious, particularly with bacterial conjunctivitis.

The child with allergic conjunctivitis may experience perennial or seasonal allergies (or both). Encourage the child to avoid perennial allergens once the offending allergen is determined (refer to Chapter 19 for additional information related to education about perennial allergen avoidance). Seasonal allergies may include tree pollen in the winter or spring, grass pollen in the summer and ragweed, or flower pollen in the fall.

It is impossible to completely eliminate seasonal allergic responses, partly because it is important for children to participate in physical activity outdoors. Teach families to minimize seasonal allergens on the child's skin and hair. Educate families to:

- Encourage the child not to rub or touch the eyes.
- Rinse the child's eyelids periodically with a clean washcloth and cool water.
- When the child comes in from outdoors, wash the child's face and hands.
- Ensure that the child showers and shampoos before bedtime.

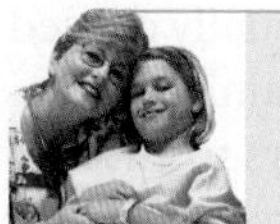

The itching of allergic conjunctivitis may be relieved with cool compresses. An easy way to accomplish this is to have the child hold a tube of yogurt over the affected eye.

Preventing Infectious Spread

Because infectious conjunctivitis is extremely contagious, the parent must wash hands diligently after caring for the child. Teach parents and children about appropriate hand washing, and discourage them from sharing towels and washcloths. Children with viral conjunctivitis may return to school or daycare when symptoms lessen. When mucopurulent drainage is no longer present (usually after 24 to 48 hours of treatment with a topical antibiotic), the child with bacterial conjunctivitis may safely return to daycare or school (Brady, 2005).

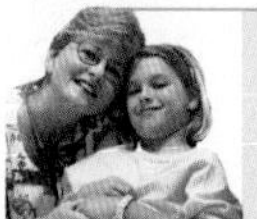

Avoid the use of vasoconstricting eye drops such as Visine to rid the eyes of redness. Rebound vasodilation may occur, and with it the redness returns. This leads to repeated frequent use of the drops to keep the eyes from being red but does not treat the actual cause of the redness.

ConsiderTHIS!

Bryn Carle, a 6-year-old, is brought to the clinic by her mother. She presents with redness of the left eye, edema, and drainage. What other assessment information would be helpful? Based on the history and clinical presentation, Bryn is diagnosed with conjunctivitis. What education will be necessary for the family to assist in alleviating symptoms and preventing infectious spread?

NASOLACRIMAL DUCT OBSTRUCTION

Stenosis or simple obstruction of the nasolacrimal duct is a common disorder of infancy, occurring in about 5% to 20% of the general population (Gross, 2002). It is unilateral in about 65% of cases. Chronic tearing occurs and build-up in the lacrimal sac causes a mucoid or mucopurulent drainage. Over 90% of all cases resolve spontaneously by 1 year of age (American Association for Pediatric Ophthalmology and Strabismus, 2005). No apparent risk factors exist for the development of nasolacrimal duct obstruction or stenosis. Therapeutic management involves a "wait-and-see" approach. Massage may be prescribed, and if secondary bacterial infection is suspected or confirmed, antibiotic ointment or drops may be ordered. If the obstruction does not resolve by 12 months of age, then the pediatric ophthalmologist may probe the duct to relieve the obstruction (a brief outpatient procedure).

Nursing Assessment

Tearing or discharge from one or both eyes is often first noted at the 2-week checkup. Obtain a thorough history about the eye drainage to distinguish it from neonatal conjunctivitis. Determine the onset and progression of symptoms, as well as the newborn's response to any interventions attempted so far. Upon physical examination, note redness of the lower lid of the affected eye. If drainage is present, note its consistency, color, and quantity. Nasolacrimal duct obstruction is usually a diagnosis based upon clinical presentation, but culture of the eye drainage may be used to rule out conjunctivitis or secondary bacterial infection (Fig. 18.5).

Nursing Management

As previously stated, the majority of cases of nasolacrimal duct stenosis resolve spontaneously by 12 months of age. Nevertheless, the continual tearing and discharge is quite upsetting to the parents. Teach parents to clean the eye area frequently with a moist cloth. In addition, teach parents to massage the nasolacrimal duct, which may change the pressure and cause it to open, allowing drainage to occur. Refer to Teaching Guideline 18.1 for appropriate nasolacrimal duct massage technique. Ensure that parents are educated about when and how to administer antibiotic eye drops if ordered.

EYELID DISORDERS

Disorders of the eyelid include hordeolum (stye), chalazion, and blepharitis. Hordeolum is a localized infection

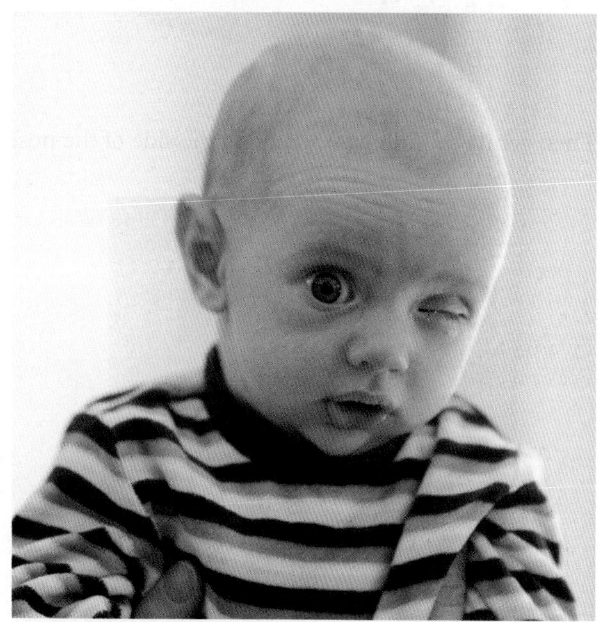

Figure 18.5 Mild eyelid redness and tearing are present in the infant with nasolacrimal duct stenosis. Note the presence of obstruction.

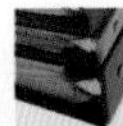

TEACHING GUIDELINE 18.1

Nasolacrimal Duct Massage

- Using the forefinger or little finger, push on top of the bone (the puncta must be blocked).

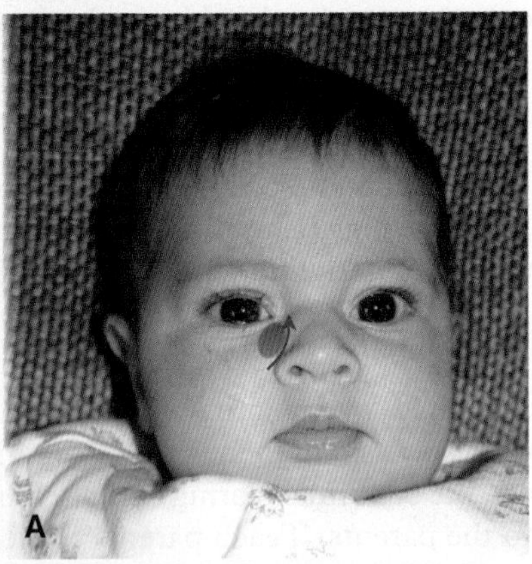

- Gently push in and up.

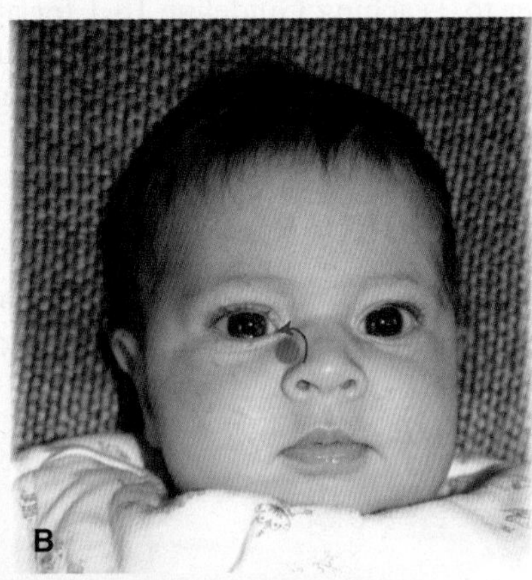

- Then gently push downward along the side of the nose.

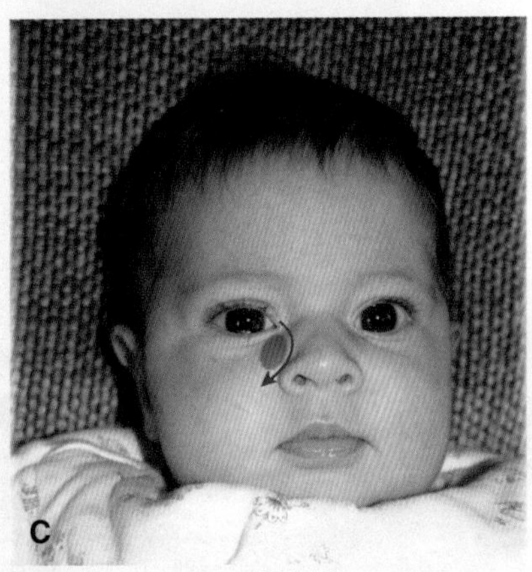

of the sebaceous gland of the eyelid follicle, usually caused by bacterial invasion. Chalazion is a chronic painless infection of the meibomian gland. Blepharitis refers to chronic scaling and discharge along the eyelid margin. Chalazion may resolve spontaneously. Therapeutic management of hordeolum and blepharitis usually involves the use of antibiotic ointment.

Nursing Assessment

Determine the child's health history, noting onset of symptoms, extent and character of eye discharge, and presence of pain (hordeolum is usually painful). Inspect the eyelids, noting redness along the eyelid margin and presence of eyelid edema (hordeolum, blepharitis). Hordeolum may also be quite visible as an enlarged lesion along the lid margin, with purulent drainage present (Fig. 18.6). Chalazion may be visible as a small nodule on the lid margin. The conjunctivae remain clear with all three of these disorders.

Nursing Management

For hordeolum and blepharitis, instruct parents in the administration of antibiotic ointment. Encourage the use of hot, moist compresses. Inform parents that the stye may require several weeks to resolve completely. Also inform parents that chalazion will usually resolve spontaneously; if it does not, it may require minor surgical drainage.

PERIORBITAL CELLULITIS

Periorbital cellulitis is a bacterial infection of the eyelids and tissue surrounding the eye. The bacteria may gain entry to the skin via an abrasion, laceration, insect bite, foreign body, or impetiginous lesion. Periorbital cellulitis may also result from a nearby bacterial infection, such as sinusitis. *Staphylococcus aureus, Streptococcus pyogenes,* and *Streptococcus pneumoniae* are the most commonly implicated bacteria. The bacteria produce either an enzyme or endotoxins that initiate the inflammatory response. Redness, swelling, and infiltration of the skin by the inflammatory mediators occur.

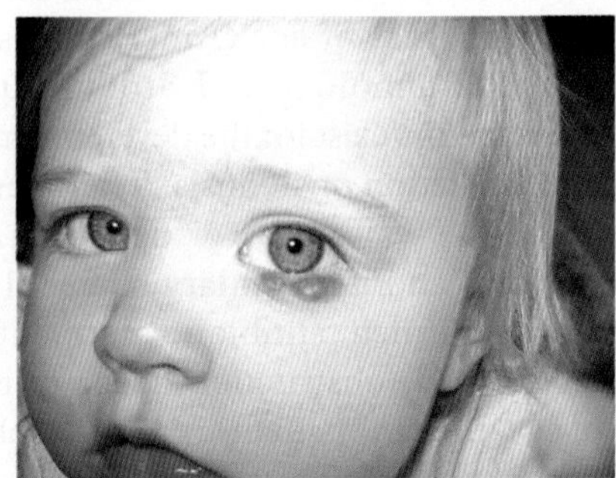

● **Figure 18.6** Hordeolum.

Therapeutic management of periorbital cellulitis focuses on intravenous antibiotic administration during the acute phase followed by completion of the course with oral antibiotics. Complications of periorbital cellulitis include bacteremia and progression to orbital cellulitis, which is a more extensive infection involving the orbit of the eye.

Nursing Assessment

Note the onset and duration of symptoms, as well as any treatment used so far. Document any history of fever. The child may complain of pain around the eye as well as restricted movement of the eye area. Inspect the eye, noting marked eyelid edema as well as a purplish or red color of the eyelid (Fig. 18.7). Usually the conjunctivae are clear and no discharge is present. If the extent of the edema allows the child to open the eye, assess visual acuity, which should be normal.

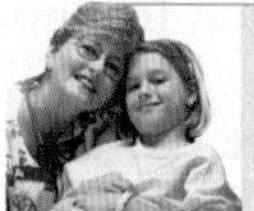

Notify the physician immediately if any of these signs of progression to orbital cellulitis occur: conjunctival redness, change in vision, pain with eye movement, eye muscle weakness or paralysis, or proptosis.

Nursing Management

Apply warm soaks to the eye area for 20 minutes every 2 to 4 hours. Administer intravenous antibiotics as prescribed. Teach families the importance of completing the entire course of oral antibiotic treatment at home. Instruct parents to call the physician or have the child evaluated again if:

- The child is not improving.
- The child reports inability to move the eye.
- Visual acuity changes.
- Proptosis occurs.

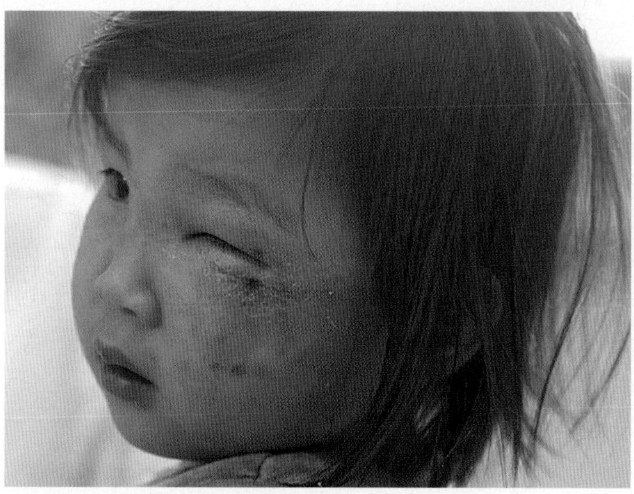

● **Figure 18.7** Periorbital cellulitis.

Eye Injuries

As mentioned earlier, infants and young children are more susceptible to eye injuries than adults since the eyeball is relatively larger in relation to the space within the orbit. Developmental maturity may also play a part in eye injuries. For example, as infants and toddlers learn to walk and run, they do not have the awareness and maturity to avert disaster. Older children involved in sports and school science experiments are also at risk for eye injuries. A few of the more common eye injuries are eyelid injuries, contusion, scleral hemorrhage, corneal abrasion, a foreign body in the eye, and chemical injury.

Therapeutic management depends on the type of injury. Eyelid lacerations may require suturing. Deep lacerations may result in ptosis at a later date, so these patients should be referred to an ophthalmologist. Simple contusions (black eye) usually need only observation, ice, and analgesics. Scleral hemorrhages resolve gradually without intervention over a few weeks. Corneal abrasions may be allowed to self-heal, or antibiotic ointment may be prescribed. Foreign bodies in the eye require removal to prevent further irritation or abrasion. Chemical injuries require irrigation and vision evaluation.

Nursing Assessment

When a child presents with an eye injury, it is very important to obtain an accurate history related to the injury, followed by a focused physical examination, which consists mostly of inspection and observation. The nurse must determine whether an eye injury is non-emergent or emergent in order to provide rapid and appropriate treatment in the case of an emergency so that vision may be preserved.

Health History

Obtain an accurate history. Determine the mechanism of injury and obtain as much detail about the injury as possible. Questions that should be asked during the health history include:

- When did the injury occur?
- What exactly happened?
- Was an object involved? If so, what type of object, and how fast was it going?
- Was it a splash injury?
- Was the child wearing eye protective gear or eyeglasses when the injury occurred?

Determine the extent of pain if present. Document photosensitivity, sensation of a foreign body in the eye, and blurry or lost vision. Inquire about past medical history, including previous eye injury or surgery or vision problems. Determine the child's immunization status.

Physical Examination

Regardless of the type of eye injury, the examination of the child's eye can be quite difficult. The nurse plays an important role in assisting the child and family to cope with the examination. Children with an eye injury often are in acute pain. The area surrounding the eye swells quickly after blunt trauma. The edema and tearing make the eye examination more difficult. Children are very frightened because of the pain and difficulty seeing. Approach the child in a calm and gentle manner. Soothe and coax the child as the eye is examined. Younger children may need to be restrained briefly in order for the examination to proceed safely.

Note the eyelid placement and look for signs of trauma such as bleeding, edema, and eyelid malformation. Evaluate the child's ability to open the eyes. Use a penlight to evaluate the pupils' response to light and accommodation (in the case of non-emergent eye trauma, the pupils should remain equally round and reactive to light and accommodation [PERRLA]). Note redness or irritation of the sclerae and/or conjunctivae. Observe for excessive tearing. Figure 18.8 shows appropriate technique for eversion and examination of the interior of the eyelid.

In a non-emergent situation, evaluate visual acuity via the use of an age-appropriate vision screening tool (refer to Chapter 9 for additional information related to visual acuity screening). Generally, radiologic testing is used only in emergency situations. Table 18.2 gives assessment information specific to eyelid laceration, simple contusion, scleral hemorrhage, corneal abrasion, and foreign body in the eye.

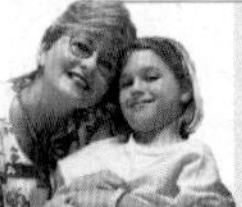

If pupillary reaction is abnormal, vision is affected (decreased acuity from the child's norm, diplopia, or blurriness), or extraocular movements are affected, the child should be immediately referred to an ophthalmologist for further evaluation.

Nursing Management

Children with urgent or emergent conditions must be referred to an ophthalmologist immediately to preserve vision. Urgent and emergent conditions include:

- Traumatic hyphema
- Blowout fracture
- Ruptured globe
- Thermal injury/corneal flash burn
- Extensive animal bite
- Lid laceration with underlying structural involvement
- Corneal abrasion in which corneal penetration is suspected
- Foreign body embedded in the globe

Managing Non-emergent Eye Injuries

Non-emergent eye injuries usually need only simple management. Assist the physician with positioning and distraction of the child for eyelid laceration suturing. The child may require sedation or pain medication for this procedure.

To decrease edema in the child with a black eye (simple contusion), instruct the parent to apply an ice pack to the area for 20 minutes, then remove it for 20 minutes, and continue to repeat the cycle. Tell the parents and child that bruising of the surrounding eye area may take up to 3 weeks to resolve.

The appearance of a scleral hemorrhage may be frightening. Instruct the parents and child about the benign nature of the hemorrhage and its natural history of resolution without intervention over a period of a few weeks.

If the child with a corneal abrasion has pain, analgesics may be helpful. Tell parents that most corneal abrasions heal on their own. If an antibiotic ointment is prescribed,

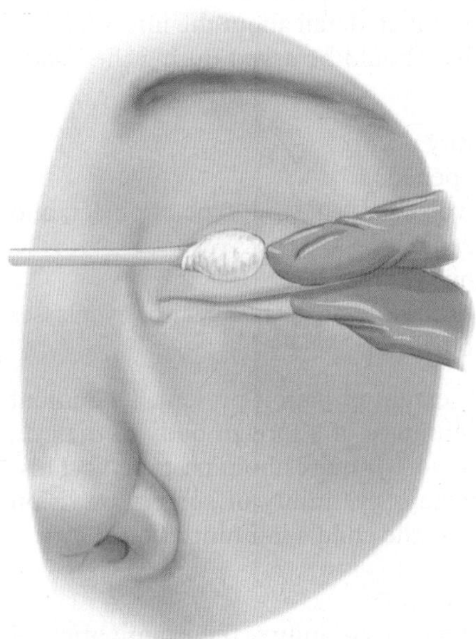

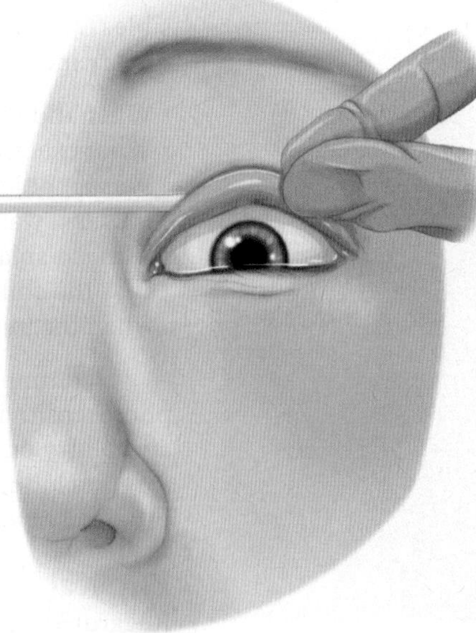

● **Figure 18.8** Eversion of the eyelid for examination. Place a cotton-tipped applicator over the eyelid. Pull the eyelid outward and up over the applicator.

Table 18.2 Assessment of Eye Injuries

Description of Injury	Nursing Assessment
Eyelid injuries: May occur as laceration to the eyelid	• Laceration is noted at any point along the lid. • Vision is unaffected.
Simple Contusion (Black Eye): Occurs as a result of blunt trauma to the eye area	• Bruising and edema of lids or area surrounding eye • PERRLA • Extraocular movements intact • Visual acuity intact • No diplopia or blurred vision • Pain surrounding eye but not within the eye
Scleral Hemorrhage: Caused by blunt trauma or increased pressure such as with coughing	• Painless • Appears as erythema in the sclera; can be quite large initially • Vision unaffected
Corneal Abrasion: Results from foreign body such as sand, grit, or other small object scratching the cornea	• May have tearing • Eye pain • PERRLA • Vision may be blurry. • Photophobia may be present.
Foreign Body: May be dirt, glass, or other small particle	• Tearing • Complaint of "something in the eye" • PERRLA • Vision may be blurry.

instruct the parents in appropriate administration of the ointment.

Foreign bodies may be removed from the eye by gently everting the eyelid and wiping the foreign body away with a sterile cotton-tipped applicator. Irrigation with normal saline may also wash the foreign body away.

For chemical injury, irrigate the eye with copious amounts of water. Consult ophthalmology for further evaluation and management.

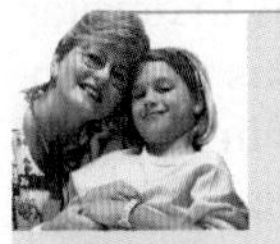

Refer the child with a large foreign body in the eye or one that is imbedded in the globe of the eye to the ophthalmologist for appropriate, safe removal.

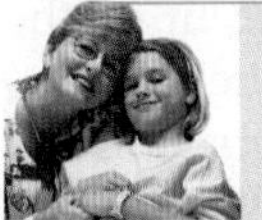

Patching of the eye with a corneal abrasion is no longer recommended, as children are often able to open the eye under the patch, which causes drying of the eye and further irritation, possibly contributing to prolonged recovery from the abrasion.

Eye injuries can be prevented, and nurses play a vital role in educating the public about prevention of eye injuries and use of appropriate safety equipment. See Healthy People 2010.

Visual Disorders

Adequate visual development requires appropriate sensory stimulation to both eyes over the first few years of life. When one or both eyes are deprived of this stimulation, visual development does not progress appropriately, and visual impairment or blindness may result. This may occur when the eyes are not aligned properly, visual acuity between the eyes is disparate, or other problems with the eyes exist. If vision disorders are diagnosed at an early

HEALTHY PEOPLE 2010

Objective	Significance
(Developmental) Increase the proportion of public and private schools that require use of appropriate head, face, eye, and mouth protection for students participating in school-sponsored physical activities; increase the use of appropriate personal protective eyewear in recreational activities and hazardous situations around the home	• Educate the family about appropriate use of eye protective equipment during sports, lawn care, chemical use, and other potentially hazardous activities. • Encourage families to provide appropriate supervision of children (particularly young children) to reduce the risk of injury. • Educate families to teach their children safe practices in and around the home (not running with scissors, etc.).

age and treatment is begun, then vision may progress normally. However, when these disorders go untreated, the young child's developing vision may be significantly reduced. Children must be appropriately screened for these disorders.

Common visual disorders in childhood include refractive errors, astigmatism, strabismus, amblyopia, nystagmus, glaucoma, and cataracts.

REFRACTIVE ERRORS

The most common cause of visual difficulties in children is refractive errors. When the light that enters the lens does not bend appropriately to allow it to fall directly on the retina, then a refractive error occurs. Young children naturally have hyperopia (farsightedness) because the depth of the eye globe is not fully developed until about age 5 years. These children may have blurriness at close range, but by school age this blurriness usually resolves. Childsight.org estimates that about 25% (1.8 million) of all secondary school children living in poverty cannot clearly see in the classroom because of refractive error. Impoverished children often do not have access to appropriate vision care.

When the light entering the eye focuses in front of the retina, it results in myopia (nearsightedness). Children who are nearsighted may see well at close range but have difficulty focusing well on the blackboard or other objects at a distance.

The treatment for both hyperopia and myopia is prescription eyeglasses or contact lenses. Generally, a child 12 years of age can demonstrate the responsibility necessary to wear and care for contact lenses. Contact lenses may be used in younger children but are lost or damaged more readily. Because of the continuing refractive development in the child's vision through adolescence, laser surgery for vision correction is not recommended by the American Academy of Ophthalmology until 18 years of age, though it may be done experimentally in some children (AAO, 2002).

Nursing Assessment

Elicit the health history, noting blurred vision, complaints of eye fatigue with reading, or complaints of eye strain (headache, pulling sensation, or eye burning). Note complaints of difficulty concentrating on or maintaining a clear focus on objects up close, avoidance of up-close work, or poor work performance (hyperopia). Note the risk factor of family history of myopia. Observe for squinting when the child looks at objects at a distance. Observe the hyperopic child for the presence of esotropia. Readily observable physical findings are not noted in the myopic child. Test visual acuity using an age-appropriate screening tool (for more information related to visual acuity screening, refer to Chapter 9). Hyperopia is usually not identified with visual acuity screening alone; it usually requires a retinal examination by an ophthalmologist.

Nursing Management

Nursing management of the child with a refractive error focuses on providing education about corrective lens use and monitoring for the need for new eyeglasses or contact lenses.

Educating About Eyeglass Use

Children may or may not be compliant with wearing eyeglasses. Glasses still carry a stigma, and the child may be teased or bullied. However, many children enjoy the improved vision they achieve when wearing their eyeglasses, and this can help them overcome the teasing they might suffer. Encourage the child with newly prescribed eyeglasses to wear them by having the parent spend "special time" with the child doing an activity that requires the glasses (such as reading or drawing). Teach the parent and child to remove eyeglasses with both hands and to lay them on their side (not directly on the lens on any surface). Instruct the child and family about cleaning the glasses daily with mild soap and water or a commercial cleansing agent provided by the optometrist. Use a soft cloth to clean the glasses, not paper towels, tissues, or toilet paper.

Educating About Contact Lens Use

Teach the older child or adolescent how to care for the contact lenses properly, including lens hygiene and lens insertion and removal. Inform the child and parents that protective eyewear should be worn when the child is participating in contact sports. If the eye becomes inflamed, remove the contact lens and wear eyeglasses until the eye is improved. Consult with the child's eye care provider to determine if medications prescribed for an eye problem can be used while the contact lens is in.

Monitoring for Fit and Visual Correction

Encourage the family to complete visual assessments as scheduled. Since the child's vision is continuing to develop and refraction is not stable, the corrective lens prescription may change more frequently than it does in an adult. As the young child in particular is continuing to grow at a rapid rate, the head size is also changing. Eyeglass frames may hurt or pinch the child as the child's head becomes larger. Teach families to check the fit of the glasses monthly. Monitor for signs of ill fit, such as constant removal of the glasses in an older child or rubbing at the glasses or eyes in the very young child. Monitor for squinting, eye fatigue or strain, and complaints of headache or dizziness, which may indicate the need for a change in the lens prescription. See Healthy People 2010.

ASTIGMATISM

In astigmatism the cornea's curvature is uneven, which results in an irregular quality of vision because the light rays are refracted unevenly. Sometimes the lens is irregularly shaped, having the same result.

HEALTHY PEOPLE 2010

Objective	Significance
(Developmental) Reduce uncorrected visual impairment due to refractive errors; reduce blindness and visual impairment in children and adolescents aged 17 years and under	• Ensure that visual acuity testing begins with an age-appropriate screening tool by 3 years of age and continues yearly throughout childhood and adolescence. • Refer for an eye evaluation any children with complaints of difficulty seeing the front of the classroom or complaints of eye strain or difficulty with close work. • Screen infants and children for asymmetric corneal light reflex for early detection of amblyopia.

Nursing Assessment

Explore the health history for symptoms of astigmatism. Children with astigmatism often have blurry vision and difficulty seeing letters as a whole, so their ability to read is affected. They may have headaches or dizziness. Older children may complain of eye fatigue or strain. Children with astigmatism often learn to tilt their heads slightly so that they can focus more effectively. This may lead to "normal" vision screenings, but the headache and dizziness still warrant further examination by an eye specialist. The diagnosis of astigmatism requires not only a visual acuity test but also a refractive error evaluation by an optometrist or ophthalmologist.

Nursing Management

Corrective lenses can help to, in effect, smooth out the curvature of the cornea, making the light ray refraction occur smoothly. As with refractive errors, encourage the child who requires corrective lenses for astigmatism to wear the eyeglasses or contact lenses regularly.

• STRABISMUS

Strabismus refers to misalignment of the eyes. It is common and occurs in about 4% of children (Optometrists Network, 2006). The most common types of strabismus are exotropia and esotropia. In exotropia the eyes turn outward; in esotropia they turn inward. Because of this unequal alignment, visual development in each eye may proceed at different rates. Diplopia (double vision) may result, so vision in one eye may be "turned off" by the brain to avoid diplopia. Many infants have strabismus intermittently, but this usually resolves by 3 months of age. Intermittent strabismus that persists past 3 months of age or constant strabismus at any age warrants referral to an ophthalmologist for further evaluation.

Therapeutic management of strabismus may include patching of the stronger eye or eye muscle surgery. Corrective lenses are also used for strabismus. Complications of strabismus include amblyopia and visual deficits.

Nursing Assessment

Parents may be the first persons to notice that the child's eyes do not face in the same direction. Question parents about the onset of the problem and whether it is continuous or intermittent. If intermittent, does it occur more often when the child is tired? Elicit the health history, noting complaints of blurred vision, tired eyes, squinting or closing one eye in bright sunlight, tilting the head to focus on an object, or a history of bumping into objects (depth perception may be limited).

Observe the child's eyes for obvious exotropia or esotropia. In the absence of an obvious finding, assessment of the symmetry of the corneal light reflex is extremely helpful (Fig. 18.9). The "cover test" is also a useful tool for the identification of strabismus.

True strabismus should not be confused with pseudostrabismus. In pseudostrabismus, the eyes may appear slightly crossed (as in the child with wide nasal bridge and epicanthal folds), but the corneal light reflex remains symmetric.

Nursing Management

It is extremely important to treat strabismus appropriately in the developing years so that equal visual acuity may be achieved in both eyes. When patching is prescribed, encourage the family to comply with this modality. Encourage eyeglass wearing if prescribed. Provide appropriate postoperative care by protecting the operative site with eye patching.

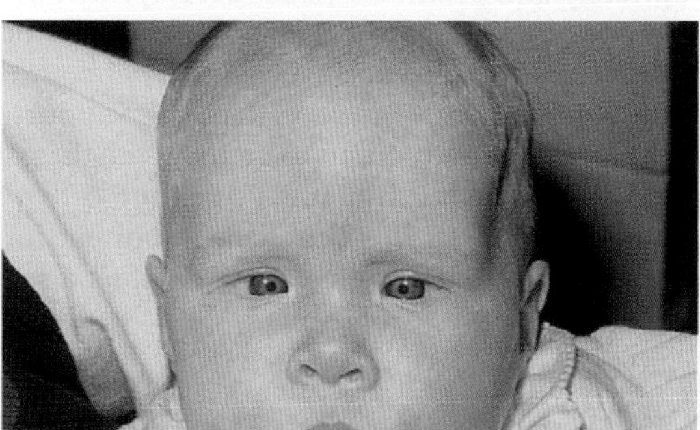

• **Figure 18.9** Esotropia. Test for strabismus by observing symmetry of the corneal light reflex. The reflex falls in the center of one pupil and to the left or right of the pupil of the other eye.

AMBLYOPIA

Amblyopia refers to poor visual development in the otherwise structurally normal eye. It develops within the first decade of life and is more severe the earlier it develops (Bacal & Wilson, 2000). Untreated amblyopia causes more cases of vision loss than all other conditions together in persons younger than 40 years of age. It occurs in about 5% of children (Ruben, 2003). The vision in one eye is reduced because the eye and the brain are not working together properly. While the eyes are fighting to focus differently because of their differences in visual acuity, one eye is stronger than the other. This is why amblyopia is often referred to as "lazy eye."

Amblyopia may be caused by any disorder that affects normal visual development, including strabismus and differences in visual acuity or astigmatism between the two eyes. It may also result from eye trauma, ptosis, or cataract. Children with amblyopia, if untreated, will have worsening of the poorer eye and strain in the better eye, which may also lead to worsening of acuity in that eye. Eventually blindness will result in one or both eyes.

Therapeutic management of amblyopia focuses on strengthening the weaker eye. This may be achieved through patching for several hours per day, using atropine drops in the better eye (once daily), vision therapy, or eye muscle surgery if the cause is strabismus.

Nursing Assessment

One of the most important functions of the nurse is to identify on screening the preschool child with amblyopia. Begin visual acuity testing using an age-appropriate tool by 3 years of age. Observe for asymmetry of the corneal light reflex in the child of any age. This may be the only sign in the preverbal child.

Nursing Management

It is very important for children with amblyopia to receive appropriate treatment during the early years of visual development. Patching the better eye for several hours each day encourages the eye with poorer vision to be used appropriately and promotes visual development in that eye. The once-daily use of atropine drops in the better eye results in blurring in that eye, similarly encouraging use and development of the weaker eye. Support and encourage children and parents to comply with the patching protocol or atropine drop use.

Promoting eye safety is extremely important for the child with amblyopia; if the better eye suffers a serious injury, both eyes may become blind.

NYSTAGMUS

Nystagmus refers to a very rapid, irregular eye movement. It is described by some as "bouncing" of the eyes. It may occur in children with congenital cataracts, but the most common cause is a neurologic problem. It is difficult for the brain and eyes to communicate when the eyes are in continuous motion; thus, visual development may be affected. Children with nystagmus must receive further evaluation by an ophthalmologist and possibly a neurologist.

INFANTILE GLAUCOMA

Infantile glaucoma is an autosomal recessive disorder that is more common in interrelated marriages or relationships. It is often associated with other genetic disorders. It occurs in about 1 of 10,000 live births (www.lighthouse.org). Infantile glaucoma is characterized by obstruction of aqueous humor flow and increased intraocular pressure that results in large, prominent eyes. Vision loss may occur as a result of corneal scarring, optic nerve damage, or, most commonly, amblyopia.

Unlike adult glaucoma, in which medical management is the first step, therapeutic management of infantile glaucoma is focused on surgical intervention. Infantile glaucoma is treated surgically via goniotomy (removal of obstruction of the aqueous humor). Laser surgery is being used as well. Sometimes several surgeries may be necessary to correct the problem. Ongoing medication therapy may also be required.

Nursing Assessment

Note any family history of infantile glaucoma or other genetic disorders. Elicit the health history, noting history of the infant keeping the eyes closed most of the time or rubbing the eyes. Observe the eye for corneal enlargement and clouding; the eye may appear enlarged. Photophobia may occur, so bright light may bother the infant. Tearing or conjunctivitis and eyelid squeezing or spasm may also occur. The pediatric ophthalmologist may use a tonometer to measure the intraocular pressure during the diagnostic phase.

Nursing Management

The main goal of nursing care for the infant with glaucoma is postoperative care. Family education will also be important.

Providing Postoperative Care

Postoperatively the eye will be patched and the child should be maintained on bed rest. Nursing care focuses on protection of the surgical site. Infants and toddlers may require elbow restraints to prevent them from rubbing the affected eye. These children may be quite anxious with one or both eyes patched, since their ability to see will be affected. Use a calm and soothing approach with these children, as well as distraction and developmentally appropriate play activities.

Educating the Family

Instruct parents and children to make sure the child avoids roughhousing and contact sports for at least 2 weeks after surgery. Before the first surgery occurs, prepare parents for the possibility that three or four operations may be necessary. Teach families how to administer postoperative medications. Encourage parents to comply with ongoing recommended visual assessments.

CONGENITAL CATARACT

A congenital cataract is an opacity of the lens of the eye that is present at birth. Sensory amblyopia will result if the infant goes untreated. Complications include visual developmental delay related to amblyopia. In children younger than 5 years of age, congenital cataract causes 16% of the cases of legal blindness (www.lighthouse.org). Bilateral cataracts may be associated with metabolic or genetic syndromes. Surgery to remove the opaque lens can be done as early as 2 weeks of age. The infant is then fitted with a contact lens. Intraocular lens implants are also being used (Watkinson & Graham, 2005). The best visual outcomes occur when cataracts are removed prior to 3 months of age. Glaucoma may occur as a complication after cataract surgery.

Nursing Assessment

Note history of lack of visual awareness. Observe the eyes for apparent cloudiness of the cornea (not always visible). Upon ophthalmoscopic examination, the red reflex will not be observed in the affected eye.

Nursing Management

Postoperative care focuses on protecting the operative site and providing developmentally appropriate activities. Ensure that the protective eye patch is secure. Elbow restraints may be necessary in the older infant to prevent accidental injury to the operative site. Teach families how to administer antibiotic or corticosteroid ophthalmic drops if prescribed for postoperative use. Once the surgical site is healed, the "good" eye may be patched for several hours a day to promote visual development in the eye with the contact or intraocular lens. Regular visual assessments are critical for determining the adequacy of visual development after cataract removal. Instruct parents about the importance of using sunglasses that block ultraviolet rays in the child who has had a lens removed.

HEALTHY PEOPLE 2010

Objective	Significance
(Developmental) Reduce visual impairment due to glaucoma	• Appropriately screen infants and children for glaucoma. • Refer suspected cases to a pediatric ophthalmologist for further evaluation.

HEALTHY PEOPLE 2010

Objective	Significance
(Developmental) Reduce visual impairment due to cataract	• Appropriately screen infants and children for cataract. • Refer suspected cases to a pediatric ophthalmologist for further evaluation.

Retinopathy of Prematurity

Retinopathy of prematurity (ROP) is a disorder characterized by rapid growth of retinal blood vessels in the premature infant. In the fetus, retinal vascularization begins at 4 months and progresses until completion at 9 months or shortly after birth. The premature infant is born with incomplete retinal vascularization, yet new vessels continue to grow between the vascularized and nonvascularized retina. Risk factors include low birthweight, early gestational age, sepsis, high light intensity, and hypothermia. Changes in oxygen tension resulting from hypoxia, oxyhemoglobin dissociation curve changes that occur when adult blood is transfused to the premature infant, and the duration/concentration of supplemental oxygen are thought to play an important role in the development of ROP.

Premature infants should have serial examinations by an ophthalmologist until the ROP has regressed and normal vascularization is seen. If ROP continues to progress, laser surgery may be necessary to prevent blindness (Hack & Klein, 2006). Complications of ROP include myopia, glaucoma, and blindness. Strabismus may occur even in cases of regressed (resolved) ROP. Refractive errors and amblyopia may occur as early as 3 months corrected age. In the first year of life, ophthalmologic examinations may occur frequently so that if corrective lenses are needed, they may be prescribed at the earliest possible time. After 1 year corrected age, former premature infants should continue to have yearly ophthalmologic examinations to detect and treat visual deficits early (Verma, Sridhar, & Spitzer, 2003).

Nursing Assessment

Ensure that all former premature infants are routinely screened for visual deficits. Discuss developmental progress with the parents. Observe for the development of strabismus, manifested by an asymmetric corneal light reflex.

Nursing Management

Nursing management of infants with ROP mainly focuses on ensuring that the family is compliant with the ophthalmologist's follow-up recommendations. Recurrent illness or rehospitalization of premature infants may interfere with scheduled eye follow-up appointments. Ensure that these appointments are rescheduled and that the family understands the importance of them. Many children who have regressed ROP or who require cryotherapy have refractive errors, so even when the ROP is considered resolved, these children should still maintain appropriate ophthalmology follow-up.

Visual Impairment

Vision impairment in children refers to acuity of between 20/60 and 20/200 in the better eye on examination. "Legal blindness" is a term used to refer to vision of less than 20/200 or peripheral vision less than 20 degrees. In most cases, vision may be augmented with corrective lenses. Some blind children can differentiate light versus dark, while others live in total darkness.

Visual impairment in children may result from a number of different causes. In the United States, visual impairment and blindness are most often caused by refractive error, astigmatism, strabismus, amblyopia, nystagmus, infantile glaucoma, congenital cataract, retinopathy of prematurity, and retinoblastoma. Factors that increase the risk for developing visual impairment include: prematurity, developmental delay, genetic syndrome, family history of eye disease, African-American heritage, previous serious eye injury, diabetes, HIV, and chronic corticosteroid use. Trauma is also an important cause of blindness in children.

Children with visual impairments often exhibit motor and cognitive delays as well. With one less sense with which to experience their environment, these children may lag behind in developmental milestones. Visual impairments are associated with many other syndromes. For example, many children with fetal alcohol syndrome have visual impairments, and albinism is associated with blindness.

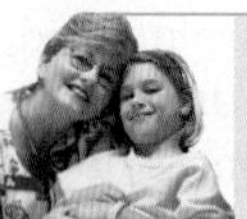

Worldwide, 500,000 children become blind each year. Seventy percent of these cases result from the preventable condition xerophthalmia, caused by vitamin A deficiency. Ten to fifteen percent of cases are caused by trachoma, a treatable infection caused by *Chlamydia trachomatis*.

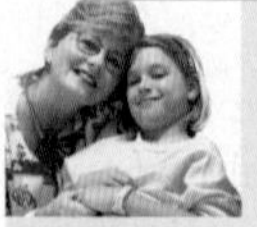

Laser pointers pose a risk of retinal damage in infants and young children. Damage occurs if the child stares at the red light for longer than 10 seconds. They should not be used as toys.

Nursing Assessment

Nursing assessment for visual impairment includes a careful health history, physical examination, and visual acuity testing.

Health History

Parents and nurses alike should be alert to signs of potential visual impairment. One of the most important functions of the nurse is to recognize signs of visual impairment as early as possible. These signs may include:

At any age:
- Dull, vacant stare

Infants:
- Does not "fix and follow"
- Does not make eye contact
- Unaffected by bright light
- Does not imitate facial expression

Toddlers and older children:
- Rubs, shuts, covers eyes
- Squinting
- Frequent blinking
- Holds objects close or sits close to television
- Bumping into objects
- Head tilt, or forward thrust

Physical Examination

Assess for symmetry or asymmetry of corneal light reflex. Perform the "cover test." Use an age-appropriate visual acuity screening tool (refer to Chapter 9 for additional information on visual acuity screening).

Nursing Management

Important nursing functions in relation to visual impairment and blindness are supporting the child and family and promoting socialization, development, and education. In addition, when the child with a visual impairment is hospitalized for any reason, the nurse must plan appropriate care for that child, taking into consideration the child's level of disability. Box 18.1 gives tips on working with the visually impaired child, and these tips should also be taught to families.

Supporting the Child and Family

Provide emotional support to the family with a visually impaired child. Ensure that the child's environment provides familiarity and security. Encourage activities that stimulate development; these activities will vary from child to child depending upon whether the child also demonstrates impairment in other areas, such as hearing or motor skills. The blind infant will not provide the eye contact that parents are looking for, so educate the parents about other indicators that the infant is acknowledging the parents' presence, such as:

- Increased motor activity
- Eyelid movement
- Changes in breathing pattern
- Making sounds

Encourage the family of a visually impaired child to display affection through touch and tone of voice. Refer

BOX 18.1

TIPS FOR INTERACTING WITH THE VISUALLY IMPAIRED CHILD

- Use the child's name to gain attention.
- Identify yourself and let the child know you are there before you touch the child.
- Encourage the child to be independent while maintaining safety.
- Name and describe people/objects to make the child more aware of what is happening.
- Discuss upcoming activities with the child.
- Explain what other children or individuals are doing.
- Make directions simple and specific.
- Allow the child additional time to think about the response to a question or statement.
- Use touch and tone of voice appropriate to the situation.
- Use parts of the child's body as reference points for the location of items.
- Encourage exploration of objects through touch.
- Describe unfamiliar environments and provide reference points.
- Use the sighted-guide technique when walking with a visually impaired child.

Adapted from the Delta Gamma Center for Children with Visual Impairments.

families to support networks and other resources for the blind and visually impaired. Box 18.2 lists some on-line resources for families of children who are visually impaired or blind.

Promoting Socialization, Development, and Education

Blind children, since they lack the visual stimulation that children usually receive, may develop self-stimulatory actions in compensation ("blindisms"). Examples of blindisms are eye pressing, rocking, spinning, bouncing, and head banging. These repetitive behaviors may interfere with the child's ability to socialize. Work with the parents to plan a strategy for the development of alternative behaviors specific to the individual child.

Refer the blind or visually impaired child who is younger than 3 years of age to the local district of Early Intervention to establish case management services for the child's developmental needs. After age 3, state laws provide for public education and related services for children with disabilities. An individualized education plan (IEP) should be developed to maximize the child's learning ability. Nurses may be one of the professionals involved in the development of the IEP.

The severely visually impaired or blind child will need to learn to read Braille and will also need to learn

BOX 18.2

ON-LINE RESOURCES FOR FAMILIES OF CHILDREN WITH VISUAL IMPAIRMENTS

- www.aapos.org: American Association of Pediatric Ophthalmology and Strabismus—Mainly for health care providers, some information and resources for lay persons
- www.acb.org: American Council of the Blind—The nation's leading membership organization of blind and visually impaired people
- www.afb.org: American Foundation for the Blind—Resource for products for people with visual deficits
- www.aoa.org: American Optometric Association—Education and resources for parents
- www.cnib.ca: Canadian National Institute for the Blind—Resources within Canada
- www.helenkeller.org: Helen Keller Services for the Blind—Serves blind, deaf-blind, and visually impaired persons in the New York metropolitan area
- www.icevi.org: International Council for Education of People with Visual Impairment—Promotes equal access to appropriate education for all visually impaired children and youths
- www.lighthouse.org: Lighthouse International—Information on visual disorders, statistics, resources available for families; resource for products for people with visual deficits
- www.napvi.org: National Association for Parents of Children with Visual Impairments—Information, referrals, financial resources; also in Spanish
- www.nei.nih.gov/: National Eye Institute, a division of the National Institutes of Health—Conducts and supports vision research; information for the lay person or health care provider for eye examinations and financial resources
- www.nfb.org: National Federation of the Blind—Information, education, and support for the blind
- www.nichcy.org: National Dissemination Center for Children with Disabilities—Provides information, education, and resources for families and educators; also in Spanish
- www.preventblindness.org: Prevent Blindness America—Resources for lay persons
- www.rfbd.org: Recording for the Blind and Dyslexic—Texts and tapes of books
- www.ropard.org: Association for Retinopathy of Prematurity and Related Diseases—Resources for families and health care providers
- www.sightforstudents.org: Sight for Students—Provides vision examinations and glasses to uninsured children across the country
- www.v2020.org: Vision 2020: The Right to Sight—Information, education, goals for prevention and treatment of blindness worldwide

to navigate the environment with the use of a cane or via another method.

Otitis Media

Otitis media is defined as inflammation of the middle ear with the presence of fluid. It can be subdivided into two categories. Acute otitis media (AOM) refers to an acute infectious process of the middle ear that may produce a rapid onset of ear pain and possibly fever. Otitis media with effusion (OME) refers to a collection of fluid in the middle ear space without signs and symptoms of infection. Chronic otitis media with effusion (chronic OME) is defined as OME lasting longer than 3 months.

ACUTE OTITIS MEDIA

AOM is a common illness in children, resulting from infection (bacterial or viral) of fluid in the middle ear. AOM has a peak incidence in the first 2 years of life, especially between 6 and 12 months of age, though its incidence is increasing in all age groups (Carlson, 2002). Increased susceptibility in infants may be partly explained by the short length and horizontal positioning of the Eustachian tube, limited response to antigens, and lack of previous exposure to common pathogens. AOM occurs mostly in the fall through spring, with the highest incidence in the winter. AOM often recurs in infants and young children when the fluid in the middle ear becomes reinfected. The most significant risk factors for otitis media are Eustachian tube dysfunction and susceptibility to recurrent upper respiratory infections.

Pathophysiology

An upper respiratory infection frequently precedes AOM. Fluid and pathogens travel upward from the nasopharyngeal area, invading the middle ear space. Fluid behind the eardrum has difficulty draining back out toward the nasopharyngeal area because of the horizontal positioning of the Eustachian tube. A viral upper respiratory infection may cause AOM or may place the child at risk for bacterial invasion. Pathogens gain access to the Eustachian tube, where they proliferate and invade the mucosa. Fever and pain occur acutely. Increased pressure behind the tympanic membrane may result in perforation. This may result in decreased pain and yield drainage in the ear canal. Most perforations heal spontaneously and are completely benign.

AOM is most commonly caused by viral pathogens, *Streptococcus pneumoniae, Haemophilus influenzae,* and *Moraxella catarrhalis.* Viral causes of AOM resolve spontaneously.

After clearance of the infection, fluid remains in the middle ear space behind the tympanic membrane, sometimes for several months (otitis media with effusion). This may occur because of the positioning of the Eustachian tubes; which results in difficulty in draining fluid back to the nasopharyngeal area, and/or the high frequency of upper respiratory infections in infants and young children, which again result in back-up of fluid from the nasopharyngeal area.

The most common complications of AOM include:

- Hearing loss
- Expressive speech delay
- Tympanosclerosis (scarring of the tympanic membrane; usually has no effect on hearing)
- Tympanic membrane perforation (acute with resolution or chronic)
- Chronic suppurative otitis media (chronic drainage via perforation or **tympanostomy** tubes)
- Acute mastoiditis (infection of the mastoid process)
- Intracranial infections, including bacterial meningitis and abscesses

Therapeutic Management

Viral causes of AOM usually resolve spontaneously, but bacterial causes may require treatment with an antibiotic. It is unreasonable to obtain a culture of middle ear fluid with every episode of AOM to determine the specific cause. Scientific studies of fluid obtained via tympanostomy in children with AOM have been performed, and clinical decision making is based upon this research. There is great concern in the health care community about the development of antibiotic resistance due to the overuse of antibiotics. For this reason, clinical practice guidelines have been developed for a number of disorders based upon large quantities of research.

Certain diagnosis of AOM is based upon rapid onset of symptoms, signs of fluid in the middle ear, and signs or symptoms of inflammation in the middle ear (complaint of ear pain or visible erythema of the tympanic membrane) (American Academy of Pediatrics & American Academy of Family Physicians, 2004). The choice of antibiotic will depend upon the timing, the child's age, and whether the episode is a first or subsequent infection. The current recommendations by the American Academy of Pediatrics and American Academy of Family Physicians allow for a period of observation or "watchful waiting" in certain children. This allows for natural resolution of AOM related to viral causes and decreases the overuse of antibiotics in the pediatric population.

Recommendations for AOM treatment in previously healthy children are found in Table 18.3. Pain management is also an important component of AOM

Table 18.3 Treatment Recommendations for AOM

Age and Severity of Illness*	Certainty of Diagnosis	Treatment
Less than 6 months old	Certain or possible	Antibiotics
6 months to 2 years	Certain	Antibiotics
6 months to 2 years with severe illness	Possible	Antibiotics
6 months to 2 years with nonsevere illness	Possible	May observe**
Greater than 2 years with severe illness	Certain	Antibiotics
Greater than 2 years with nonsevere illness	Certain	Observe**
Greater than 2 years	Possible	Observe**

*Severe illness is defined as moderate to severe otalgia or fever 39° C or higher. Nonsevere illness is defined as mild otalgia and fever less than 39° C.

**Observation is appropriate only when follow-up can be ensured. If symptoms are persistent or become worse, antibiotics may then be started.

(AAP & AAFP, 2004)

treatment, as is appropriate follow-up to ensure disease resolution.

Nursing Assessment

Nursing assessment of the child with AOM consists of health history and physical examination.

Health History

Elicit a description of the present illness and chief complaint. Note acute, abrupt onset of signs and symptoms. Common signs and symptoms reported during the health history might include:

- Fever (may be low grade or higher)
- Complaints of otalgia (ear pain)
- Fussiness or irritability
- Crying inconsolably, particularly when lying down
- Batting or tugging at the ears (may also occur with teething or OME, or may be a habit)
- Rolling the head from side to side
- Poor feeding or loss of appetite
- Lethargy
- Difficulty sleeping or awakening crying in the night
- Fluid draining from the ear

Determine the child's response to any treatments used thus far. Explore the child's current and past medical history for risk factors such as:

- Young age
- Daycare attendance
- Previous history of AOM or OME
- Antecedent or concurrent upper respiratory infection
- Other risk factors (Box 18.3)

Physical Examination and Diagnostic Testing

The child may complain of pain when the ear is examined. On otoscopic examination, the tympanic membrane will have a dull or opaque appearance and is bulging and/or red (Fig. 18.10). Sometimes pus (greenish or yellowish) may be visible behind the eardrum. Upon pneumatic otoscopy, the eardrum will be immobile. (A physician or nurse practitioner usually performs otoscopic examination.) If

BOX 18.3

RISK FACTORS FOR ACUTE OTITIS MEDIA

- Eustachian tube dysfunction
- Recurrent upper respiratory infection
- First episode of AOM before 3 months of age
- Daycare attendance (increases exposure to viruses causing upper respiratory infections)
- Previous episodes of AOM
- Family history
- Passive smoking
- Crowding in the home or large family size
- Native American, Inuit, or Australian aborigine ethnicity
- Absence of infant breastfeeding
- Immunocompromise
- Poor nutrition
- Craniofacial anomalies
- Presence of allergies (possibly)

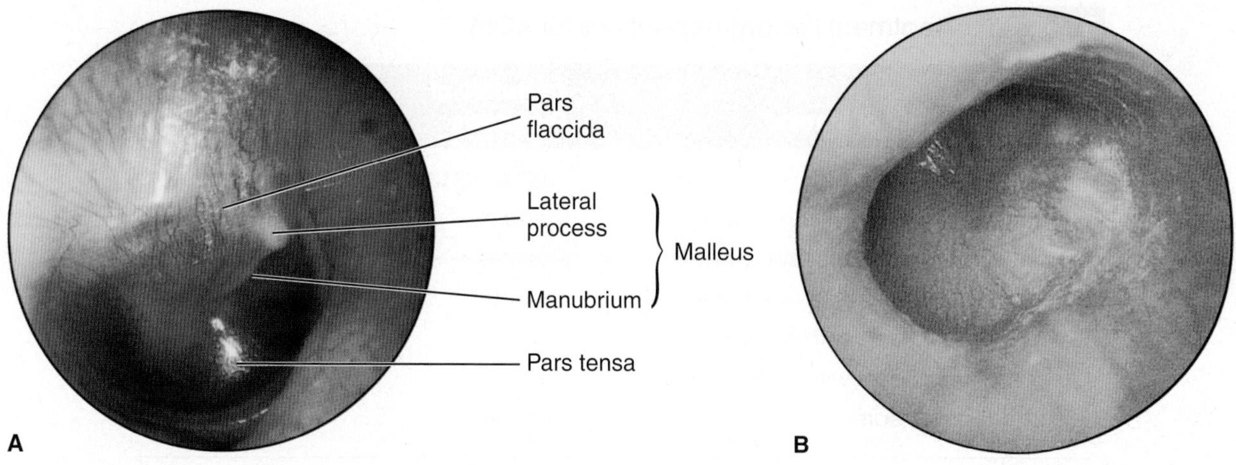

● Figure 18.10 (**A**) Normal tympanic membrane. (**B**) Acute otitis media: note erythema and opacity of the tympanic membrane.

the tympanic membrane has become perforated, drainage may be present in the ear canal, but the canal will otherwise appear normal. Palpate for possible cervical lymphadenopathy. **Tympanometry** is not as useful in the diagnosis of AOM as it is with OME.

Nursing Management

Nursing management of the child with acute otitis media is mainly supportive in nature. It focuses on pain management, family education, and prevention of AOM.

Managing Pain Associated With AOM

Analgesics such as acetaminophen and ibuprofen have been shown to be effective at managing mild to moderate pain associated with AOM. They have the added benefit of reducing fever. Narcotic analgesics such as codeine may be prescribed for severe pain. Application of heat or a cool compress may also be helpful. Instruct the family to have the child lie on the affected side with the heating pad or covered ice pack in place to that ear. Numbing eardrops such as benzocaine (Auralgan) may be helpful in the event of acute, severe pain. They should be used in conjunction with analgesics, though, because of the short duration of action (American Academy of Pediatrics & American Academy of Family Physicians, 2004).

Educating the Family

If the treatment selected for AOM is observation or watchful waiting, explain the rationale for this to the family. Ensure that the family understands the importance of returning for re-evaluation if the child is not improving or if the AOM progresses to severe illness. When antibiotics are prescribed, the family must understand the importance of completing the entire course of antibiotics. Families are tempted to stop giving the antibiotic because the child is usually vastly improved after taking the medication for 24 to 48 hours. Follow-up for resolution of AOM is necessary for all children, and the physician or nurse practitioner will determine the timing of that follow-up. Emphasize the importance of follow-up to the parents, educating them about OME and its potential impact on hearing and speech. See Healthy People 2010.

Preventing AOM

Breastfed infants have a lower incidence of AOM than formula-fed infants, and breast milk's immunologic benefits are well known, so encourage mothers to breastfeed for at least 6 to 12 months. Instruct families to avoid excess exposure to individuals with upper respiratory infections to decrease the incidence of these infections in their child. Infants and children should not be exposed to second-hand smoke. Encourage parents to stop smoking. If quitting smoking is not possible, then instruct parents not to smoke inside the house or automobile. Encourage the parents to have the child immunized with Prevnar and, when appropriate, influenza vaccine.

Though not yet clinically or scientifically proven, Xylitol syrup, a sucrose substitute, may also be protective. Children who are old enough may chew Xylitol-containing gum. Younger children and infants may be given Xylitol syrup. Care should be taken to avoid excessive dosing, as Xylitol can cause diarrhea.

● OTITIS MEDIA WITH EFFUSION

Otitis media with effusion (OME) refers to the presence of fluid within the middle ear space, without signs or symptoms of infection. It may occur independent of AOM or may persist after the infectious process of AOM has resolved. Risk factors for OME include passive smoking, absence of breastfeeding, frequent viral upper respiratory infections, allergy, young age, male sex, adenoid hypertrophy, Eustachian tube dysfunction, and certain congenital disorders. Complications of OME include AOM, hearing loss, and deafness.

HEALTHY PEOPLE 2010

Objective	Significance
Reduce otitis media in children and adolescents	• Teach children and families the importance of hand washing to avoid the common cold (often a precursor to otitis media). • Teach families the importance of appropriate follow-up for eradication of otitis media. • Educate families about the importance of using antibiotics only for true bacterial infections (in order to decrease the development of resistant organisms, many of which cause otitis media).

Nursing Assessment

Nursing assessment of the child with OME includes health history, physical examination, and diagnostic testing.

Health History

Determine the extent of symptoms. Children may be asymptomatic or may experience a popping sensation or fullness behind the eardrum. Explore the health history for risk factors such as passive smoking, absence of breast-feeding, frequent viral upper respiratory infections, allergy, or recent history of AOM.

Physical Examination

Otoscopic examination may reveal a dull, opaque tympanic membrane that may be white, gray, or bluish (Fig. 18.11). If the tympanic membrane is not opaque, a fluid level or air bubble may be visualized. Mobility may be absent or diminished upon pneumatic otoscopy. Tympanometry may be used to confirm the diagnosis of OME.

Nursing Management

OME may take several months to resolve. Nursing management during the resolution phase focuses on education and monitoring for hearing loss.

Educating the Family

Educate the family about the natural history of OME and the anatomical differences in young children that contribute to OME. Inform parents that antihistamines, decongestants, antibiotics, and corticosteroids have not been proven to hasten the resolution of OME and thus are not recommended. OME usually resolves spontaneously, but children should be rechecked every 4 weeks while this resolution is occurring. Teach parents not to feed infants in a supine position and to avoid bottle propping.

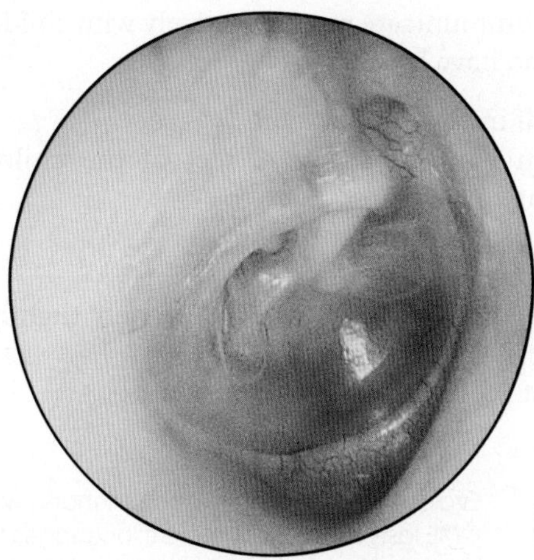

● Figure 18.11 Otitis media with effusion; note dull white tympanic membrane.

Monitoring for Hearing Loss

When OME persists, the primary concern is its effect on hearing. In the infant or toddler who should be experiencing rapid language development, impaired hearing can depress language acquisition significantly. Children with OME who are at risk for speech, language, or learning problems may be referred for evaluation of hearing earlier than a child with OME who isn't at risk (Box 18.4). Children with chronic OME (persistent OME of 3 months' duration or longer) should be referred to a specialist for hearing evaluation. Children who are not already at risk for speech concerns and are not experiencing difficulty with language acquisition may be reassessed every 3 to 6 months as long as hearing loss is not identified. At-risk children may require treatment earlier.

BOX 18.4

CHILDREN AT RISK FOR SPEECH, LANGUAGE, OR LEARNING DIFFICULTIES

- Permanent hearing loss (without OME)
- Speech/language delay (suspected or diagnosed)
- Craniofacial disorder that may interfere with speech
- Any pervasive developmental disorder
- Genetic disorders or syndromes associated with speech or learning problems
- Cleft palate
- Blindness or significant visual impairment

To communicate more effectively with children with OME who have hearing loss:

- Turn off music or television.
- Position yourself within 3 feet of the child before speaking.
- Face the child while speaking.
- Use visual cues.
- Increase the volume of your speech only slightly.
- Speak clearly.
- Request preferential classroom seating.

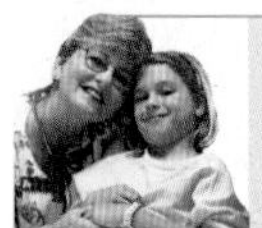

Evaluation of hearing is recommended when OME lasts 3 months or more if language delay, hearing loss, or a learning problem is suspected.

Providing Postoperative Care for the Child With Pressure-Equalizing Tubes

The standard treatment for persistent or problematic OME is surgical insertion of **pressure-equalizing (PE) tubes** into the tympanic membrane (via myringotomy). The tubes stay in place for at least several months usually and generally fall out on their own (Fig. 18.12). The procedure is usually done as an outpatient surgery and the child returns home in the evening. Teach the parents to administer ear drops postoperatively if prescribed. After PE tube placement, the surgeon may recommend avoiding water entry into the ears. If recommended, advise parents to have the child wear ear plugs in the bathtub or while swimming.

Placement of the PE tubes allows for adequate hearing, which in turn encourages appropriate speech development. Placement of PE tubes does not prevent middle ear infection. If the middle ear becomes infected with PE tubes in place, the tubes allow infected fluid to drain from the ear. Tell parents to contact their pediatrician if drainage from the ear is noted. After PE tubes are placed, young children often have rapid increases in language acquisition, and parents should observe for this.

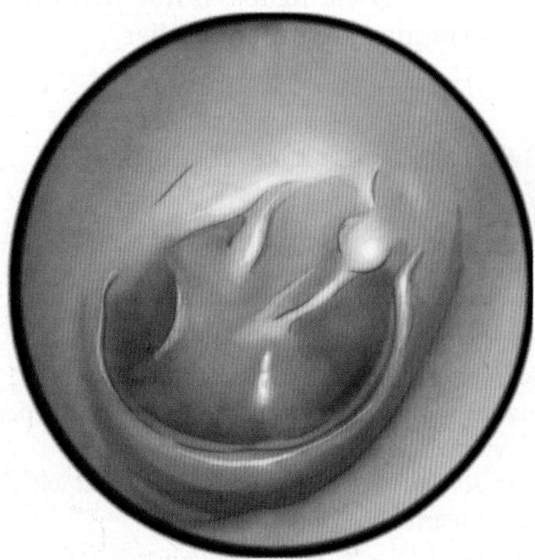

● Figure 18.12 Pressure-equalizing tubes in place in the tympanic membrane.

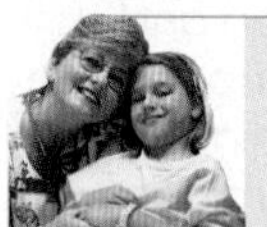

Children with PE tubes who swim in a lake must wear earplugs, as lake water is contaminated with bacteria and entry of that water into the middle ear should be avoided.

● OTITIS EXTERNA

Otitis externa is defined as an infection and inflammation of the skin of the external ear canal. *Pseudomonas aeruginosa* and *Staphylococcus aureus* are typical causative agents, though fungi such as *Aspergillus* and other bacteria also may be implicated. Moisture in the canal contributes to pathogen growth. Otitis externa is commonly known as "swimmer's ear" since it occurs more frequently in those who swim often (and thus have wet ear canals). Changing the pH in the ear canal contributes to the inflammatory process (Zoltan, Taylor, & Achar, 2005).

Nursing Assessment

Nursing assessment of the child with otitis externa focuses on the health history and physical examination.

Health History

Elicit a description of the present illness and chief complaint. Note history of ear itching or pain, ear drainage, or a feeling of fullness in the ear canal, with possible difficulty hearing. Note onset and progression of symptoms, as well as the child's response to treatments. Explore the child's current and past medical history for risk factors such as previous episodes of otitis externa or history of recent swimming in a pool, lake, or ocean.

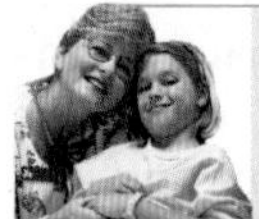

The child with otitis externa usually has significant ear pain. Pressure on the tragus should be avoided, as it can worsen the pain.

Physical Examination

Typically a white or colored discharge can be seen in the ear canal or running from the ear. On otoscopy, the canal is red and edematous, often too swollen for insertion of the speculum and viewing of the tympanic membrane (Fig. 18.13). Diagnosis is based on clinical findings. Occasionally the ear drainage is cultured for bacteria or fungus, particularly if otitis externa is not improving with treatment.

Nursing Management

The primary goals of nursing management are pain relief, treatment of the infection, and prevention of recurrence.

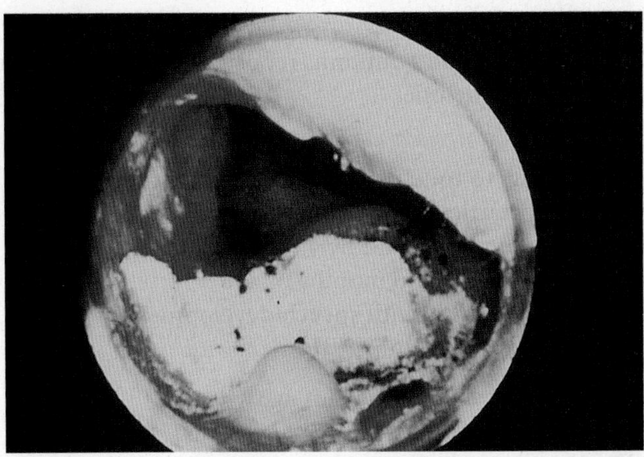

● Figure 18.13 Note edema and erythema of the ear canal as well as purulent discharge in the child with otitis externa.

Managing Pain

Analgesics (often narcotics) may be administered to manage the pain. A warm compress or heating pad to the affected ear is helpful in some children.

Treating the Infection

Antibiotic or antifungal eardrops should be administered as prescribed. In some cases a wick is placed in the ear canal. The wick keeps the antibiotic drops in contact with the skin of the ear canal and promotes healing. Wick insertion can be extremely painful, and younger children will need to be restrained during insertion for their safety.

Preventing Reinfection

Once the infection has resolved, children and their parents should be educated about prevention of further episodes. Since moisture contributes to otitis externa, the ear canals should be kept dry. Encourage the child and parents to use one of the methods described in Teaching Guideline 18.2 after swimming or showering.

Hearing Loss and Deafness

Infants are ordinarily born with the sense of hearing fully developed. Language development in infancy and early childhood is dependent upon adequate hearing, and even the fluctuating hearing loss associated with intermittent bouts of AOM can hinder language development. Hearing loss may be unilateral (involving one ear) or bilateral (involving both ears). The extent of hearing loss is defined based on the softest intensity of sound that is perceived, described in **decibels** (dB). Levels of hearing loss are:

- 0 to 20 dB: normal
- 20 to 40 dB: mild loss
- 40 to 60 dB: moderate loss
- 60 to 80 dB: severe loss
- Greater than 80 dB: profound loss (ASHA, 2007)

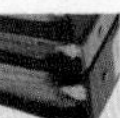

TEACHING GUIDELINE 18.2

Preventing Otitis Externa

1. Avoid the use of cotton swabs, headphones, and earphones.
2. Wear earplugs when swimming.
3. Promote ear canal dryness and alternate pH. Use one or more of the following methods:
   - Dry the ear canals using a hair dryer set on a lower setting.
   - Administer solutions that have a drying effect on the auditory canal skin and change the pH of the canal to discourage organism growth in susceptible children. The following solutions can be used:
     - A few drops of Domeboro solution can be placed in the canal, and then allowed to run out.
     - A mixture of half rubbing alcohol and half vinegar (squirted into the canal and then allowed to run out). The alcohol solution should be used only when the ear canals are healthy. Using it while the canals are inflamed will cause stinging and increased pain.

Hearing loss may be congenital or of delayed onset. Congenital hearing loss affects about 2 to 3 infants per 1,000 live births in the United States (Holte, 2003). About 10% of all newborns have at least one risk factor for hearing impairment (Verma et al., 2003). Most congenital hearing loss is inherited through a recessive gene, with only about 20% of cases resulting from an autosomal dominant trait (Applebaum, 1999). Congenital hearing loss accounts for about one half of all the cases of hearing impairment; the remainder are acquired. Premature infants and those with persistent pulmonary hypertension of the newborn are at increased risk for hearing loss compared with other infants (Verma et al., 2003). Hearing loss commonly occurs with a large number of congenital or genetic syndromes, as well as in association with anomalies of the head and face. As of 2005, a variety of newborn universal hearing screening mandates have been passed by legislation in 37 states, thus allowing for earlier identification of infants with congenital hearing loss (National Center for Hearing Assessment and Management, 2005). See Healthy People 2010.

Delayed-onset hearing loss may be conductive, sensorineural, or mixed. **Conductive hearing loss** results when transmission of sound through the middle ear is disrupted, as in the case of OME. When fluid fills the middle ear, the tympanic membrane is unable to move properly, and partial or complete hearing loss occurs. **Sensorineural hearing loss** is caused by damage to the hair cells in the cochlea or along the auditory pathway. This may result from kernicterus, use of ototoxic medication, intrauterine infection with cytomegalovirus

HEALTHY PEOPLE 2010

Objective	Significance
(Developmental) Increase the proportion of newborns who are screened for hearing loss by age 1 month, have audiologic evaluation by age 3 months, and are enrolled in appropriate intervention services by age 6 months	• Encourage appropriate hearing assessments. • Refer children who are diagnosed with a hearing deficit to local services for the deaf or hearing impaired.

or rubella, neonatal or postnatal infection such as meningitis, severe neonatal respiratory depression, or exposure to excess noise. Mixed hearing loss occurs when the cause may be attributed to both conductive and sensorineural problems. See Healthy People 2010.

Regardless of the cause of hearing loss, early intervention can make a difference in the child's ability to communicate. Once the hearing loss has been determined, intervention can begin. Hearing aids, cochlear implants, communication devices, and speech education may enable these children to communicate verbally. Improved communication beginning in infancy and early childhood may also improve the child's school achievement.

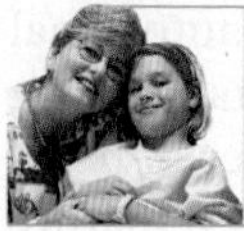

The ear plugs or covers used to block ambient noise in premature infants in the NICU may decrease the preemie's risk for hearing loss.

Nursing Assessment

Nursing assessment of the child with hearing loss or impairment focuses on the health history, physical examination, and hearing testing.

HEALTHY PEOPLE 2010

Objective	Significance
(Developmental) Increase the use of appropriate ear protection devices, equipment, and practices. Reduce noise-induced hearing loss in children and adolescents aged 17 years and under.	• Educate children and families about the dangers of excess noise and its potential for damaging hearing. • Encourage appropriate use of ear protection devices.

Health History

Common signs and symptoms reported during the health history might include:

Infant:
- Wakes only to touch, not environmental noises
- Does not startle to loud noises
- Does not turn to sound by 4 months of age
- Does not babble at 6 months of age
- Does not progress with speech development

Young child:
- Does not speak by 2 years of age
- Communicates needs through gestures
- Does not speak distinctly, as appropriate for his or her age
- Displays developmental (cognitive) delays
- Prefers solitary play
- Displays immature emotional behavior
- Does not respond to ringing of the telephone or doorbell
- Focuses on facial expressions when communicating

Older child:
- Often asks for statements to be repeated
- Is inattentive or daydreams
- Performs poorly at school
- Displays monotone or other abnormal speech
- Gives inappropriate answers to questions except when able to view face of speaker

At any age:
- Speaks loudly
- Sits very close to TV or radio, or turns volume to loud
- Responds only to moderate or loud voices

Signs of hearing loss should be investigated as early as possible in order for appropriate communication intervention to begin.

Explore the child's current and past medical history for risk factors such as congenital anomalies, genetic syndrome, infection, family history, kernicterus, neonatal ventilator use, ototoxic medication, or exposure to excess noise. Note whether newborn hearing screening was done, along with the results.

Physical Examination and Laboratory and Diagnostic Tests

Determine the child's level of interaction with the environment. For preschoolers and older children, administer the whisper test, keeping in mind that this is a gross screening test only. Perform the Weber and Rinne tests (refer to Chapter 10 for further explanation). If further evaluation is needed, the nurse may be responsible for administering an otoacoustic emissions test or auditory brain stem evoked response test, either in the hospital or outpatient office.

Nursing Management

The primary goal of nursing care for the child with a hearing impairment is to provide education and support to the family and child. Individualize care for the child with a hearing impairment and the family based on their specific responses to the hearing impairment.

Augmenting Hearing

Compliance with hearing aids and communication curriculums is critical so that the child can develop hearing and speech. Hearing aids should be cleaned daily with a damp cloth. Batteries are usually changed weekly. When inserting the aid, the volume should be turned down, then adjusted to the appropriate level after insertion. As the infant or child grows, the hearing aid will need to be reassessed for proper fit. Many deaf schools and other organizations provide loaner hearing aids so that the best fit and amplification may be determined prior to purchase. Assist the family to explore this type of option in the local community. See Healthy People 2010.

When cochlear implants are used, the nurse focuses on postoperative care of the incision site and pain management.

Promoting Communication and Education

Families and children need to learn how to communicate effectively with one another. If the child learns American Sign Language, for instance, the parents and siblings should as well. Table 18.4 gives information on communication options for hearing-impaired children and their families. Communication may also be enhanced by the use of text telephone service in the home and closed-caption television. Bells and alarms in the home may use lights rather than sound to alert the child. Provide a sign language interpreter for the child at health care visits if the parent is not present for interpretation.

Encouraging Education

Refer the child less than 3 years of age to the local district of Early Intervention for case management of developmental needs. At 3 years of age and beyond, state laws provide for public education and related services for children with disabilities. An IEP should be developed to maximize

HEALTHY PEOPLE 2010

Objective	Significance
(Developmental) Increase access by persons who have hearing impairments to hearing rehabilitative services and adaptive devices, including hearing aids, cochlear implants, or tactile or other assistive or augmentative devices	• Know resources available in the local area for the deaf and hearing impaired. • Refer children with hearing deficits to these resources and to service providers for augmentative devices.

Table 18.4 Comparing Communication Options for the Hearing Impaired

Spoken Language	
Oral deaf education (auditory-verbal therapy)	Uses technology to boost auditory potential; teaches children to notice sound and give it meaning. Develops oral speech.
Cued speech	A system using hand signs to clarify lip-reading; gives the person clues about the sounds the speaker is making
Signed Language	
American Sign Language (ASL)	Entirely communicated through hand signs, gestures, and facial expressions. Has its own grammar and syntax.
Combination: Total Communication	Combines auditory training and teaching of spoken language with SEE ("signing exact English"; corresponds to the words and syntax of English)
Augmentative and Alternative Communication (AAC)	
May use gestural communication	Can also include physical devices such as notebooks, communication boards, charts, or computers. Ranges from very low-tech to technologically complex.

BOX 18.5

ON-LINE RESOURCES FOR FAMILIES OF CHILDREN WITH HEARING IMPAIRMENTS

- www.agbell.org: Alexander Graham Bell Association for the Deaf and Hard of Hearing—Wide range of programs and services, advocating independence through listening and talking
- www.asha.org: American Speech-Language-Hearing Association (ASHA)—Information, education, referrals, and resources for the hearing impaired
- www.audiology.org: American Academy of Audiology (AAA)—Education, referrals for audiologists, resources
- www.auditory-verbal.org: Auditory-Verbal International (AVI)—Advocates for listening, amplification of hearing, and learned speech
- www.chs.ca: Canadian Hearing Society—Resources within Canada
- www.cici.org: Cochlear Implant Association—Support, information, advocacy for rights and services
- www.cuedspeech.org: National Cued Speech Association—Promotes and supports the effective use of cued speech
- www.entnet.org: American Academy of Otolaryngology–Head and Neck Surgery—Education and resources
- www.ihsinfo.org: International Hearing Society—Education, referrals, information on hearing aids
- www.jtc.org: John Tracy Clinic—Worldwide free service for families of preschool children with hearing loss
- www.lhh.org: League for the Hard of Hearing—Hearing rehabilitation and human services agency
- www.oraldeafed.org: Oral Deaf Education—Promotes spoken language use in the hearing impaired for effective communication

the child's learning ability. Nurses may be involved in the development of the IEP.

Some children attend schools specifically geared toward deaf students. The choice of school will depend upon the family's preferences and resources.

Providing Support

The diagnosis of a significant disability can be extremely stressful for the family. Encourage families to express their feelings and provide emotional support. Ensure that the needs of any siblings are also attended to. When the family is ready, encourage them to network with other families who have children with similar needs. Educate the family about the child's prescribed plan of care. Refer families to resources and support groups (Box 18.5).

References

Books and Journals

Abelson, M. (2001). Tackling pediatric infectious conjunctivitis. *Review of Ophthalmology, 8*(1), 70–72.

Altemeier, W. A. (1999). A trip through the ear in search of deafness. *Pediatric Annals, 28,* 342–344.

American Academy of Family Physicians, American Academy of Otolaryngology–Head and Neck Surgery, and American Academy of Pediatrics Subcommittee on Otitis Media With Effusion. (2004). Clinical practice guideline: Otitis media with effusion. *Pediatrics, 113,* 1412–1429.

American Academy of Ophthalmology. (2002). *Summary recommendations for LASIK.* [electronic version] available at www.aao.org/.

American Academy of Pediatrics. (2001). Screening examination of premature infants for retinopathy of prematurity. *Pediatrics, 108,* 809–811.

American Academy of Pediatrics. (2002). Use of photoscreening for children's vision screening. *Pediatrics, 109,* 524–525.

American Academy of Pediatrics. (2003). Eye examination in infants, children and young adults by pediatricians. *Pediatrics, 111,* 902–907.

American Academy of Pediatrics. (2003). Hearing assessment in infants and children: Recommendations beyond neonatal screening. *Pediatrics, 111,* 436–440.

American Academy of Pediatrics and American Academy of Family Physicians, Subcommittee on Management of Acute Otitis Media. (2004). Clinical practice guidelines: Diagnosis and management of acute otitis media. *Pediatrics, 113,* 1451–1465.

American Association for Pediatric Ophthalmology and Strabismus (AAPOS). (2005). *Congenital nasolacrimal duct obstruction.* [electronic version] available at www.aapos.org.

American Speech-Language-Hearing Association. (2007). *Type, degree and configuration of hearing loss.* Retrieved March 28, 2007 from http://www.asha.org/public/hearing/disorders/types.htm.

Applebaum, E. L. (1999). Detection of hearing loss in children. *Pediatric Annals, 28,* 352–356.

Bacal, D. A., & Wilson, M. C. (2000). Strabismus: Getting it straight. *Contemporary Pediatrics, 17*(2), 49–60.

Balkany, T. J., Hodges, A. V., Eshraghi, A. A., Butts, S., Bricker, K., Lingval, J., Polak, M., & King, J. (2002). Cochlear implants in children: A review. *Acta Otolaryngology, 122,* 356–362.

Belkengren, R., & Sapala, S. (2003). Pediatric management problems. *Pediatric Nursing, 29*(1), 38.

Block, S. (2005). Diagnosing acute otitis media: It's what you see, not what you hear. *Contemporary Pediatrics, suppl,* 3–8.

Brady, M. T. (2005). Infectious disease in pediatric out-of-home child care. *American Journal of Infection Control, 33*(5), 276–285.

Brophy, M., Sinclair, S. A., Hostetler, G., & Xiang, H. (2006). Pediatric eye injury-related hospitalizations in the United States. *Pediatrics, 117* (6), 2267.

Brown, M. L. (2001). The effects of environmental tobacco smoke on children: Information and implications for PNPs. *Journal of Pediatric Health Care, 15,* 280–286.

Brunnell, P. A., Abelson, M. B., D'Arienzo, P. A., Friedman, F. N., Granet, D. B., Lanier, B. Q., & Spangler, D. L. (2001). The diagnosis and management of red eye. *Infectious Disease in Children (Suppl.),* 2–15.

Brunnell, P. A., Wagner, R. S., Cuming, G. S., Dorfman, M. S., & Murphey, D. K. (2006). Bacterial conjunctivitis in children: Containing the infection. *Infectious Diseases in Children (Suppl.),* 2–19.

Byers, J. F. (2003). Developmental care and the evidence for their use in the NICU. *Maternal Child Nursing, 28*(3), 174–182.

Carlson, L. (2002). Update on otitis media. *American Journal for Nurse Practitioners, 6*(10), 9–16.

Carlson, L. H. (2005). Otitis media: New information on an old disease. *Nurse Practitioner, 30*(3), 31–41.

Casey, J. R. (2005). Treatment of AOM post-PCV7: Judicious antibiotic therapy. *Contemporary Pediatrics (Suppl.),* 16–23.

Celeste, M. (2002). A survey of motor development for infants and young children with visual impairments. *Journal of Visual Impairment & Blindness, 96*(3), 169–174.

Centers for Disease Control. (2003). Pneumococcal conjunctivitis at an elementary school—Maine, Sept. 20 to Dec. 6, 2002. *MMWR, 52*(4), 64–66.

Chentsova, E. V., & Petriaslivili, G. G. (2004). *Moscow Helmholtz Eye Research Institute,* http://pdm.medicine.wisc.edu/chentsova.htm. Accessed October 26, 2005.

Coody, D., Banks, J., Yetman, R., et al. (1997). Eye trauma in children: Epidemiology, management, and prevention. *Journal of Pediatric Healthcare, 11,* 182–188.

Cook, K. A., & Walsh, M. (2005). *Otitis media.* [electronic version] Available at http://www.emedicine.com/emerg/topic351.htm.

DeRespinis, P. A. (2001). Eyeglasses: Why and when do children need them? *Pediatric Annals, 30,* 455–461.

Downey, D., & Hurtig, R. (2003). Augmentative and alternative communication. *Pediatric Annals, 32,* 467–474.

Effron, D. (2003). Acute diagnosis: What cause of sudden illness? *Consultant for Pediatricians, 2,* 41–43.

Forbes, B. J. R. (2001). Management of corneal abrasions and ocular trauma in children. *Pediatric Annals, 30,* 465–472.

Granet, D. B. (2002). Acute bacterial conjunctivitis: Common and manageable. *Contemporary Pediatric (Suppl.),* 13–15.

Gross, R. D. (2002). Case study: Nasolacrimal-duct obstruction. *Infectious Diseases in Children (Suppl.),* 18–19.

Hack, M., & Klein, N. (2006). Young adult attainments of premature infants. *Journal of the American Medical Association, 295*(6), 695–696.

Harrison, C. J. (2004). How will the new guideline for managing otitis media work for your practice? *Contemporary Pediatrics, 21*(6), 24–40.

Harrison, C. J. (2005). The microbiology of acute otitis media: Past, present, and future. *Contemporary Pediatrics (Suppl.),* 8–16.

Hoberman, A., & Paradise, J. L. (2000). Acute otitis media: Diagnosis and management in the year 2000. *Pediatric Annals, 29,* 609–620.

Hoffman, R. (1997). Evaluating and treating eye injuries. *Contemporary Pediatrics, 14*(4), 74–98.

Holte, L. (2003). Early childhood hearing loss: A frequently overlooked cause of speech and language delay. *Pediatric Annals, 32,* 461–465.

Joint Commission on Infant Hearing (2000). *Position statement: Principles and guidelines for early infant hearing detection and intervention programs.* www.infanthearing.org/jcih. Accessed July 7, 2003.

Kemper, K. J. (2002). Otitis media: When parents don't want antibiotics or tubes. *Contemporary Pediatrics, 19,* 47–58.

Michel, F. K., & Sulewski, M. E. (2000). Focused assessment of the patient with eye trauma: The essentials. *Topics in Emergency Medicine, 22*(4), 1–8.

Montgomery, D. (2005). A new approach to treating acute otitis media. *Journal of Pediatric Health Care, 19*(1), 50–52.

National Center for Hearing Assessment and Management. (2005). Legislative activities. Available at www.infanthearing.org.

National Institutes of Health. Chapter 28: Vision and hearing. *Healthy People 2010.* http://www.healthypeople.gov/Document/HTML/Volume2/28Vision.htm#_Toc489325915, accessed July 1, 2003.

Optometrists Network. (2006). *Strabismus.* Retrieved March 28, 2007 from http://www.strabismus.org/.

Rahi, J. S., & Dezateux, C. (2002). Improving the detection of childhood visual problems and eye disorders. *Lancet, 359,* 1083–1084.

Rahi, J. S., Logan, S., Timms, C., Russell-Eggitt, I., & Taylor, D. (2002). Risk, causes, and outcomes of visual impairment after loss of vision in the non-amblyopic eye: A population-based study. *Lancet, 360,* 597–602.

Ramsey, A. M. (2002). Diagnosis and treatment of the child with a draining ear. *Journal of Pediatric Health Care, 16,* 161–169.

Randleman, J. B., & Sachdeva, D. (2005). *Chemical eye burns.* Retrieved October 24 2005 from http://www.emedicinehealth.com/chemical_eye_burns/article_em.htm.

Roddey, O. F., & Hoover, H. A. (2000). Otitis media with effusion in children: A pediatric office perspective. *Pediatric Annals, 29,* 623–629.

Rosenthal, M. (2005). Achieve eradication, rather than clinical cure when treating AOM. *Infectious Diseases in Children, 18*(11), 57–58.

Ruben, J. R. (2003). Vision testing in children: An interactive primer. *American Academy of Pediatric Ophthalmology and Strabismus.* Retrieved from www.aapos.org on July 6, 2003.

Rubin, S. E. (2001). Management of strabismus in the first year of life. *Pediatric Annals, 30,* 474–480.

Sadovsky, R. (2003). Distinguishing periorbital from orbital cellulitis. *American Family Physician, 67*(6), 1349, 1353.

Sagraves, R. (2002). Increasing antibiotic resistance: Its effect on the therapy for otitis media. *Journal of Pediatric Health Care, 16,* 79–85.

Sander, R. (2001). Otitis externa: A practical guide to treatment and prevention. *American Family Physician, 63,* 927–937.

Shields, J. A., & Shields, C. L. (2001). Pediatric ocular and periocular tumors. *Pediatric Annals, 30,* 491–501.

Simon, J. W., & Kaw, P. (2001). Vision screening performed by the pediatrician. *Pediatric Annals, 30,* 446–452.

Slattery, W. H., & Fayad, J. N. (1999). Cochlear implants in children with sensorineural inner ear hearing loss. *Pediatric Annals, 28,* 359–363.

St. Lukes Cataract and Laser Institute. (2006). *Eye conditions: do you know how to treat a chemical burn?* Retrieved June 24, 2006 from http://www.stlukeseye.com/conditions/chemicalburn.asp.

Verma, R. P., Sridhar, S., & Spitzer, A. R. (2003). Continuing care of NICU graduates. *Clinical Pediatrics, 42*(4), 299–315.

Wagner, R. S. (2001). Management of congenital nasolacrimal duct obstruction. *Pediatric Annals, 30,* 481–488.

Wagner, R. S. (2005). Treating pediatric conjunctivitis: A pediatric ophthalmologist's perspective. *Infectious Diseases in Children, 18*(10), 5.

Wagner, R. S., Alcorn, D., Gigliotti, F., & Rabinowitz, R. (2000). Management of conjunctivitis part 2: mimics and nonbacterial disease. *Contemporary Pediatrics (Suppl.),* 3–14.

Walling, A. D. (2005). Selecting a topical treatment for seasonal allergic conjunctivitis. *American Family Physician, 71*(7), 1409.

Watkinson, S., & Graham, S. (2005). Visual impairment in children. *Nursing Standard, 19*(51), 58–65.

Wetmore, R. F. (2000). Complications of otitis media. *Pediatric Annals, 29,* 637–646.

Zoltan, T. B., Taylor, K. S., & Achar, S. A. (2005). Health issues for surfers. *American Family Physician, 71*(12), 2313–2317.

Websites

www.aapos.org American Association of Pediatric Ophthalmology and Strabismus.

www.acb.org American Council of the Blind (goal is to improve the well-being of all blind and visually impaired people)

www.agbell.org Alexander Graham Bell Association for the Deaf and Hard of Hearing

www.aoa.org American Optometric Association.

www.asha.org American Speech-Language-Hearing Association (ASHA)

www.audiology.com American Academy of Audiology (AAA)

www.auditory-verbal.org Auditory-Verbal International, Inc. (AVI)

www.childsight.org A division of Helen Keller Worldwide

www.chs.ca Canadian Hearing Society

www.cici.org Cochlear Implant Association

www.cnib.ca Canadian National Institute

www.colorado.edu/slhs/mdnc Marion Downs National Center for Infant Hearing

www.dgckids.org Delta Gamma Center for Children with Visual Impairments

www.entnet.org American Academy of Otolaryngology–Head and Neck Surgery

www.helenkeller.org Helen Keller Services for the Blind (helping blind and visually impaired persons to develop independence)

www.hkworld.org Helen Keller Worldwide

www.icevi.org International Council for Education of People with Visual Impairments

www.ihsinfo.org International Hearing Society

www.infanthearing.org National Center for Hearing Assessment and Management

www.ingenweb.com/cuedspeech National Cued Speech Association

www.jewishbraille.org/ Jewish Braille International (provides a wide variety of Braille books and magazines)

www.johntracyclinic.org John Tracy Clinic

www.lhh.org League for the Hard of Hearing

www.lighthouse.org Lighthouse International

www.napvi.org National Association for Parents of Children with Visual Impairments

www.nei.nih.gov/ National Eye Institute, a division of the National Institutes of Health

www.nfb.org National Federation of the Blind

www.nichcy.org National Information Center for Children and Youth with Disabilities

www.nystagmus.org/ American Nystagmus Network, Inc.

www.oraldeafed.org Oral Deaf Education

www.pgcfa.org/ Pediatric Glaucoma and Cataract Family Association (Canada)

www.preventblindness.org Prevent Blindness America

www.ropard.org Association for Retinopathy of Prematurity and Related Diseases

www.rpbusa.org Research to Prevent Blindness

www.spedex.com/vapvi National Association for Parents of Children with Visual Impairments

www.v2020.org Vision 2020, The Right to Sight

Chapter WORKSHEET

● MULTIPLE CHOICE QUESTIONS

1. Which situation would cause the nurse to become concerned about possible hearing loss?
   a. A 12-month-old who babbles incessantly, making no sense
   b. An 8-month-old who says only "da"
   c. A 3-month-old who startles easily to sound
   d. A 3-year-old who drops the letter "s"
2. A 4-year-old complains of extreme pain when the tragus is touched. Though not diagnostic, this sign is most indicative of which disorder?
   a. Acute otitis media
   b. Acute tympanic effusion
   c. Otitis interna
   d. Otitis externa
3. The nurse is caring for an infant who has undergone surgery for infantile glaucoma. What is the priority nursing intervention?
   a. Place the child prone postoperatively for comfort.
   b. Teach the family use of the contact lens.
   c. Place elbow restraints on the infant.
   d. Provide a mobile for optical stimulation.
4. A 2-year-old has been prescribed eye patching for strabismus 6 hours per day. What teaching does the nurse provide for the mother?
   a. Try to patch 6 hours per day, but if you miss some it is OK.
   b. Patching is necessary to strengthen vision in the weaker eye.
   c. Patching will keep the eye from turning in.
   d. Since the child is so young, patching can be delayed until school age.

● CRITICAL THINKING EXERCISES

1. A 16-month-old toddler is being seen for his sixth ear infection. What particular information about his growth and development must the nurse ask about? Be specific about the questions you would ask.
2. How would you distinguish allergic conjunctivitis from acute bacterial conjunctivitis?
3. A 13-month-old has been diagnosed with severe visual impairment. Develop a list of sample nursing diagnoses for this situation.

● STUDY ACTIVITIES

1. Develop a sample plan for teaching a low-literacy parent about the etiology, treatment, and complications of recurrent acute otitis media.
2. While in the pediatric clinical setting, compare the play styles of a sighted child with those of a visually impaired child.
3. Research hearing and vision resources in your local community.

chapter 19

Nursing Care of the Child With a Respiratory Disorder

Key TERMS

atelectasis
atopy
clubbing
coryza
cyanosis
expiration
hypoxemia
hypoxia
infiltrate
inspiration
laryngitis
oxygenation
pharyngitis
pulmonary
pulse oximetry
rales
retractions
rhinitis
rhinorrhea
stridor
subglottic stenosis
suctioning
tachypnea
tracheostomy
ventilation
wheeze
work of breathing

Learning OBJECTIVES

Upon completion of the chapter, the learner will be able to:

1. Compare how the anatomy and physiology of the respiratory system in children differs from that of adults.
2. Identify various factors associated with respiratory illness in infants and children.
3. Discuss common laboratory and other diagnostic tests useful in the diagnosis of respiratory conditions.
4. Discuss common medications and other treatments used for treatment and palliation of respiratory conditions.
5. Recognize risk factors associated with various respiratory disorders.
6. Distinguish different respiratory illnesses based on the signs and symptoms associated with them.
7. Discuss nursing interventions commonly used for respiratory illnesses.
8. Devise an individualized nursing care plan for the child with a respiratory disorder.
9. Develop patient/family teaching plans for the child with a respiratory disorder.
10. Describe the psychosocial impact of chronic respiratory disorders on children.

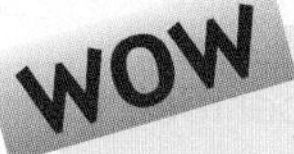

Restoring a full breath allows a child to participate fully in life's adventures.

Alexander Roberts, 4 months old, is brought to the clinic by his mother. He presents with a cold and has been coughing a great deal for 2 days. Today he has had difficulty taking the bottle and is breathing very quickly. Mrs. Roberts says he seems tired.

Respiratory disorders are the most common causes of illness and hospitalization in children. These illnesses range from mild, non-acute disorders (such as the common cold or sore throat), to acute disorders (such as bronchiolitis), to chronic conditions (such as asthma), to serious life-threatening conditions (such as epiglottitis). Chronic disorders, such as allergic rhinitis, can affect quality of life, but frequent acute or recurrent infections also can interfere significantly with quality of life for some children.

Respiratory infections account for the majority of acute illness in children. The child's age and living conditions and the season of the year can influence the etiology of respiratory disorders as well as the course of illness. For example, younger children and infants are more likely to deteriorate quickly. Lower socioeconomic status places children at higher risk for increased severity or increased frequency of disease. Certain viruses are more prevalent in the winter, whereas allergen-related respiratory diseases are more prevalent in the spring and fall. Children with chronic illness such as diabetes, congenital heart disease, sickle cell anemia, and cystic fibrosis and children with developmental disorders such as cerebral palsy tend to be more severely affected with respiratory disorders. Parents might have difficulty in determining the severity of their child's condition and might either seek care very early in the course of the illness (when it is still very mild) or wait and present to the health care setting when the child is very ill.

Nurses must be familiar with respiratory conditions affecting children in order to provide guidance and support to families. When children become ill, families often encounter nurses in outpatient settings first. Nurses must be able to ask questions that can help determine the severity of the child's illness and determine whether they must seek care at a health facility. Since respiratory illness accounts for the majority of pediatric admissions to general hospitals, nurses caring for children require expert assessment and intervention skills in this area. Detection of worsening respiratory status early in the course of deterioration allows for timely treatment and the possibility of preventing a minor problem from becoming a critical illness. Difficulty with breathing can be very frightening for both the child and parents. The child and the family need the nurse's support throughout the course of a respiratory illness.

Nurses are also in the unique position of being able to have a significant impact upon the burden of respiratory illness in children by the appropriate identification of, education about, and encouragement of prevention of respiratory illnesses. See Healthy People 2010.

Variations in Pediatric Anatomy and Physiology

Respiratory conditions often affect both the upper and lower respiratory tract, though some affect primarily one or the other. Respiratory dysfunction in children tends to be more severe than in adults. Several differences in the infant's or child's respiratory system account for the increased severity of these diseases in children compared with adults.

Nose

Newborns are obligatory nose breathers until at least 4 weeks of age. The young infant cannot automatically open his or her mouth to breathe if the nose is obstructed. The nares must be patent for breathing to be successful while feeding. Newborns breathe through their mouths only while crying.

The upper respiratory mucus serves as a cleansing agent, yet newborns produce very little mucus, making them more susceptible to infection. However, the newborn and young infant may have very small nasal passages, so when excess mucus *is* present, airway obstruction is more likely.

Infants are born with maxillary and ethmoid sinuses present. The frontal sinuses (most often associated with sinus infection) and the sphenoid sinuses develop by age 6 to 8 years, so younger children are less apt to acquire sinus infections than are adults.

Throat

The tongue of the infant relative to the oropharynx is larger than in adults. Posterior displacement of the tongue can quickly lead to severe airway obstruction. Through early school age, children tend to have enlarged tonsillar and

HEALTHY PEOPLE 2010

Objective	Significance
Reduce hospitalization rates for three ambulatory-care-sensitive conditions: pediatric asthma and immunization-preventable pneumonia and influenza.	• Appropriately educate children with asthma and their families about the ongoing management of asthma. • Encourage pneumococcal and influenza vaccinations per recommendations.

adenoidal tissue even in the absence of illness. This can contribute to an increased incidence of airway obstruction.

Trachea

The airway lumen is smaller in infants and children than in adults. The infant's trachea is approximately 4 mm wide compared with the adult width of 20 mm. When edema, mucus, or bronchospasm is present, the capacity for air passage is greatly diminished. A small reduction in the diameter of the pediatric airway can significantly increase resistance to airflow, leading to increased **work of breathing** (Fig. 19.1).

In teenagers and adults the larynx is cylindrical and fairly uniform in width. In infants and children less than 10 years old, the cricoid cartilage is underdeveloped, resulting in laryngeal narrowing. Thus, in infants and children, the larynx is funnel-shaped. When any portion of the airway is narrowed, further narrowing from mucus or edema will result in an exponential increase in resistance to airflow and work of breathing. In infants and children, the larynx and glottis are placed higher in the neck, increasing the chance of aspiration of foreign material into the lower airways. Congenital laryngomalacia occurs in some infants and results in the laryngeal structure being weaker than normal, yielding greater collapse on **inspiration**. Box 19.1 gives details related to congenital laryngomalacia.

The child's airway is highly compliant, making it quite susceptible to dynamic collapse in the presence of airway obstruction. The muscles supporting the airway are less functional than those in the adult. Children have a large amount of soft tissue surrounding the trachea, and the mucous membranes lining the airway are less securely attached compared with adults. This increases the risk for airway edema and obstruction. Upper airway obstruction resulting from a foreign body, croup, or epiglottitis can result in tracheal collapse during inspiration.

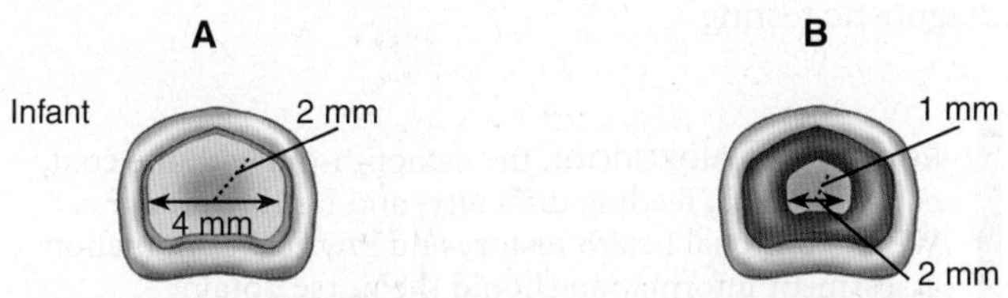

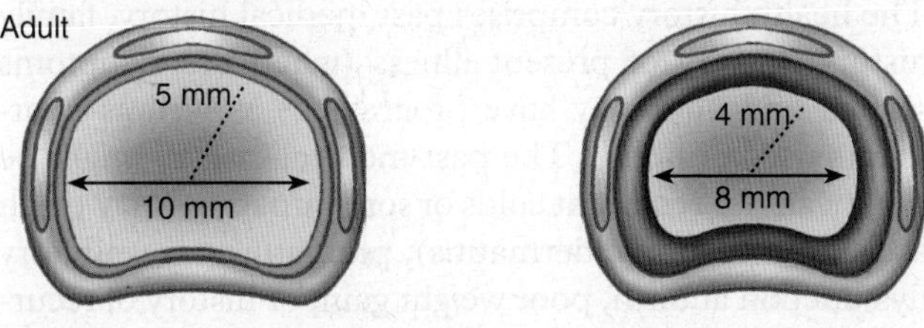

● Figure 19.1 (**A**) Note the smaller diameter of the child's airway under normal circumstances. (**B**) With 1 cm of edema present, note the exponential decrease in airway lumen diameter as compared with the adult.

> BOX 19.1
> **CONGENITAL LARYNGOMALACIA**
> - Inspiratory stridor is present and is intensified with certain positions.
> - Suprasternal retractions may be present, but the infant exhibits no other signs of respiratory distress.
> - Congenital laryngomalacia is generally a benign condition that improves as the cartilage in the larynx matures. It usually disappears by age 1 year.
> - The crowing noise heard with breathing can make parents very anxious. Reassure parents that the condition will improve with time.
> - Parents become very familiar with the "normal" sound their infant makes and are often able to identify intensification or change in the stridor. Airway obstruction may occur earlier in infants with this condition, so intensification of stridor or symptoms of respiratory illness should be evaluated early by the primary care provider.

Lower Respiratory Structures

The bifurcation of the trachea occurs at the level of the third thoracic vertebra in children, compared to the level of the sixth thoracic vertebra in adults. This anatomic difference is important when suctioning children and when endotracheal intubation is required (see Chapter 32 for further discussion). This difference in placement also contributes to risk for aspiration. The bronchi and bronchioles of infants and children are also narrower in diameter than the adult's, placing them at increased risk for lower airway obstruction (see Fig. 19.1). Lower airway obstruction during exhalation often results from bronchiolitis or asthma or is caused by foreign body aspiration into the lower airway.

Alveoli develop at approximately 24 weeks' gestation. Term infants are born with about 50 million alveoli. After birth, alveolar growth slows until 3 months of age and then progresses until the child reaches 7 or 8 years of age, at which time the alveoli reach the adult number of around 300 million. Alveoli make up most of the lung tissue and are the major sites for gas exchange. Oxygen moves from the alveolar air to the blood, while carbon dioxide moves from the blood into the alveolar air. Smaller numbers of alveoli, particularly in the premature and/or young infant, place the child at a higher risk of **hypoxemia** and carbon dioxide retention.

Chest Wall

In older children and adults the ribs and sternum support the lungs and help keep them well expanded. The movement of the diaphragm and intercostal muscles alters volume and pressure within the chest cavity, resulting in air movement into the lungs. Infants' chest walls are highly compliant (pliable) and fail to support the lungs adequately. Functional residual capacity can be greatly reduced if respiratory effort is diminished. This lack of lung support also makes the tidal volume of infants and toddlers almost completely dependent upon movement of the diaphragm. If diaphragm movement is impaired (as in states of hyperinflation such as asthma), the intercostal muscles cannot lift the chest wall and respiration is further compromised.

Metabolic Rate and Oxygen Need

Children have a significantly higher metabolic rate than adults. Their resting respiratory rates are faster and their demand for oxygen is higher. Adult oxygen consumption is 3 to 4 liters per minute, while infants consume 6 to 8 liters per minute. In any situation of respiratory distress, infants and children will develop hypoxemia more rapidly than adults. This may be attributed not only to the child's increased oxygen requirement but also to the effect that certain conditions have on the oxyhemoglobin dissociation curve.

Normal oxygen transport relies upon binding of oxygen to hemoglobin in areas of high pO_2 (pulmonary arterial beds) and release of oxygen from hemoglobin when the pO_2 is low (peripheral tissues). Normally, a pO_2 of 95 mm Hg results in an oxygen saturation of 97%. A decrease in oxygen saturation results in a disproportionate (much larger) decrease in pO_2 (Fig. 19.2). Thus, a small decrease in oxygen saturation is reflective of a larger decrease in pO_2. Conditions such as alkalosis, hypothermia, hypocarbia, anemia, and fetal hemoglobin cause oxygen to become more tightly bound to hemoglobin, resulting in the curve shifting to the left. Conditions common to pediatric respiratory disorders such as acidosis, hyperthermia, and hypercarbia cause hemoglobin to decrease its affinity for oxygen, further shifting the curve to the right.

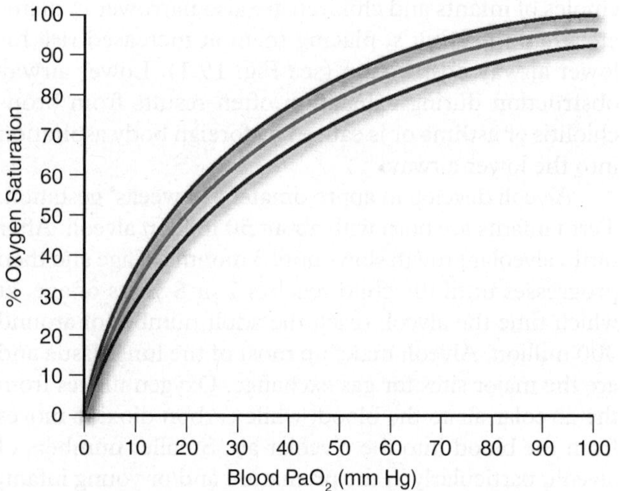

● **Figure 19.2** Normal hemoglobin dissociation curve (*green*), shift to the right (*red*), and shift to the left (*black*).

Common Medical Treatments

A variety of interventions are used to treat respiratory illness in children. The treatments listed in Common Medical Treatments 19.1 and Drug Guide 19.1 usually require a physician's order when a child is hospitalized.

Nursing Process Overview for the Child with a Respiratory Disorder

Care of the child with a respiratory disorder includes assessment, nursing diagnosis, planning, interventions, and evaluation. There are a number of general concepts related to the nursing process that can be applied to respiratory disorders. From a general understanding of the care involved for a child with respiratory dysfunction, the nurse can then individualize the care based on client specifics.

ASSESSMENT

Assessment of respiratory dysfunction in children includes health history, physical examination, and laboratory or diagnostic testing.

> Remember Alexander, the 4-month-old with the cold, cough, fatigue, feeding difficulty, and fast breathing? What additional health history and physical examination assessment information should the nurse obtain?

Health History

The health history comprises past medical history, family history, history of present illness (when the symptoms started and how they have progressed) as well as treatments used at home. The past medical history might be significant for recurrent colds or sore throats, **atopy** (such as asthma or atopic dermatitis), prematurity, respiratory dysfunction at birth, poor weight gain, or history of recurrent respiratory illnesses or chronic lung disease. Family history might be significant for chronic respiratory disorders such as asthma or might reveal contacts for infectious exposure. When eliciting the history of the present illness, inquire about onset and progression, fever, nasal congestion, noisy breathing, presence and description of cough,

(text continues on page 556)

Common Medical Treatments 19.1 Respiratory Disorders

Treatment	Explanation	Indication	Nursing Implications
Oxygen	Supplemented via mask, nasal cannula, hood, or tent or via endotracheal or nasotracheal tube	Hypoxemia, respiratory distress	Monitor response via work of breathing and pulse oximetry.
High humidity	Addition of moisture to inspired air	Common cold, croup, tonsillectomy	Infant may require extra blankets with cool mist, and frequent changes of bedclothes under oxygen hood or tent as they become damp.
Suctioning	Removal of secretions via bulb syringe or suction catheter	Excessive airway secretions (common cold, flu, bronchiolitis, pertussis)	Should be done carefully and only as far as recommended for age or tracheostomy tube size, or until cough or gag occurs
Chest physiotherapy (CPT) and postural drainage	Promotes mucus clearance by mobilizing secretions with the assistance of percussion or vibration accompanied by postural drainage (see Chapter 14 for more information about CPT and postural drainage)	Bronchiolitis, pneumonia, cystic fibrosis, or other conditions resulting in increased mucus production. Not effective in inflammatory conditions without increased mucus.	May be performed by respiratory therapist in some institutions, by nurses in others. In either case, nurses must be familiar with the technique and able to educate families on its use.
Saline gargles	Relieves throat pain via salt water gargle	Pharyngitis, tonsillitis	Recommended for children old enough to understand the concept of gargling (to avoid choking)
Saline lavage	Normal saline introduced into the airway, followed by suctioning	Common cold, flu, bronchiolitis, any condition resulting in increased mucus production in the upper airway	Very helpful for loosening thick mucus; child may need to be in semi-upright position to avoid aspiration
Chest tube	Insertion of a drainage tube into the pleural cavity to facilitate removal of air or fluid and allow full lung expansion	Pneumothorax, empyema	Should tube become dislodged from container, the chest tube must be clamped immediately to avoid further air entry in to the chest cavity.
Bronchoscopy	Introduction of a bronchoscope into the bronchial tree for diagnostic purposes. Also allows for bronchiolar lavage.	Removal of foreign body, cleansing of bronchial tree	Watch for postprocedure airway swelling, complaints of sore throat.

Drug Guide 19.1 Common Drugs for Respiratory Disorders

Medication	Action	Indication	Nursing Implications
Expectorant (guaifenesin)	Reduces viscosity of thickened secretions by increasing respiratory tract fluid	Common cold, pneumonia, other conditions requiring mobilization and subsequent expectoration of mucus	Encourage deep breathing before coughing in order to mobilize secretions. Maintain adequate fluid intake. Assess breath sounds frequently.
Cough suppressants (dextromethorphan, codeine, hydrocodone)	Relieves irritating, non-productive cough by direct effect on the cough center in the medulla, which sup-presses the cough reflex	Common cold, sinusitis, pneumonia, bronchitis	Should be used only with nonproductive coughs in the absence of wheezing
Antihistamines	Treatment of allergic conditions	Allergic rhinitis, asthma	May cause drowsiness or dry mouth
Antibiotics (oral, parenteral)	Treatment of bacterial infections of the respiratory tract	Pharyngitis, tonsillitis, sinusitis, bacterial pneumonia, cystic fibrosis, empyema, abscess, tuberculosis	Check for antibiotic allergies. Should be given as prescribed for the length of time prescribed.
Antibiotics (inhaled)	Treatment of bacterial infections of the respiratory tract	Used in cystic fibrosis	Can be given via nebulizer
Beta$_2$ adrenergic agonists (short-acting) (i.e., albuterol, levalbuterol)	May be administered orally or via inhalation. Relax airway smooth muscle, resulting in bronchodilation. Inhaled agents result in fewer systemic side effects.	Acute and chronic treat-ment of wheezing and bronchospasm in asthma, bronchiolitis, cystic fibrosis, chronic lung disease. Prevention of wheezing in exercise-induced asthma.	Can be used for acute relief of bronchospasm. May cause nervousness, tachycardia and jitteriness.
Beta$_2$ adrenergic agonists (long-acting) (i.e., salmeterol)	Administered via inhalation Long-acting bronchodilator does not produce an acute effect so should not be used for an asthma attack.	Long-term control in chronic asthma. Prevention of exercise-induced asthma.	Used only for long-term control or for exercise-induced asthma. Not for relief of bronchospasm in an acute wheezing episode.
Racemic epinephrine	Produces bronchodilation	Croup	Assess lung sounds and work of breathing. Observe for rebound bronchospasm.
Anticholinergic (ipratropium)	Administered via inhala-tion to produce bronchodilation without systemic effects	Chronic or acute treat-ment of wheezing in asthma and chronic lung disease	In children, generally used as an adjunct to beta$_2$ adrenergic agonists for treatment of bronchospasm

Drug Guide 19.1 Common Drugs for Respiratory Disorders (continued)

Medication	Action	Indication	Nursing Implications
Antiviral agents (amantadine, rimantidine, zanamivir, oseltamivir)	Treatment and prevention of influenza A	Influenza A	Amantadine, rimantidine: Monitor for confusion, nervousness, and jitteriness. Zanamivir, oseltamivir: Well tolerated but expensive
Virazole (Ribavirin)	Treatment of severe lower respiratory tract infection with RSV	Usually reserved for treatment of RSV in the ventilated client. Has not been shown to significantly reduce length of stay, morbidity, or mortality.	Administer via aerosol with the small-particle aerosol generator (SPAG). Suction patients on assisted ventilation every 2 hours; monitor pulmonary pressures every 2 to 4 hours. May cause blurred vision and photosensitivity.
Corticosteroids (inhaled)	Exert a potent, locally acting anti-inflammatory effect to decrease the frequency and severity of asthma attacks. May also delay pulmonary damage that occurs with chronic asthma.	Maintenance program for asthma, chronic lung disease. Acute treatment of croup syndromes.	Not for treatment of acute wheezing. Rinse mouth after inhalation to decrease incidence of fungal infections, dry mouth, and hoarseness. Minimal systemic absorption makes inhaled steroids the treatment of choice for asthma maintenance program.
Corticosteroids (oral, parenteral)	Suppress inflammation and normal immune response. Very effective, but long-term or chronic use can result in peptic ulceration, altered growth, and numerous other side effects.	Treatment of acute exacerbations of asthma or wheezing with chronic lung disease. Acute treatment of severe croup.	May cause hyperglycemia. May suppress reaction to allergy tests. Consult physician if vaccinations are ordered during course of systemic corticosteroid therapy. Short courses of therapy are generally safe. Children on long-term dosing should have growth assessed.
Decongestants (e.g., pseudephedrine)	Treatment of runny or stuffy nose	Common cold, limited but possible usefulness in sinusitis and allergic rhinitis	Assess child periodically for nasal congestion. Some children react to decongestants with excessive sleepiness or increased activity.
Leukotriene receptor antagonists (montelukast, zafirlukast, zileuton)	Decrease inflammatory response by antagonizing the effects of leukotrienes (which mediate the effects of airway edema, smooth muscle constriction, altered cellular activity)	Long-term control of asthma in children age 1 year and older. Montelukast: for allergic rhinitis in children 6 months and older.	Given once daily, in the evening. Not for relief of bronchospasm during an acute wheezing episode, but may be continued during the episode.

(continued)

Drug Guide 19.1 Common Drugs for Respiratory Disorders (continued)

Medication	Action	Indication	Nursing Implications
Mast-cell stabilizers (cromolyn, nedocromil)	Administered via inhalation. Prevent release of histamine from sensitized mast cells, resulting in decreased frequency and intensity of allergic reactions.	Maintenance program for asthma and chronic lung disease, pre-exposure treatment for allergens	For prophylactic use, not to relieve bronchospasm during an acute wheezing episode. Can be used 10 to 15 minutes prior to exposure to allergen, to decrease reaction to allergen.
Methylxanthines (theophylline, aminophylline)	Administered orally or intravenously. To provide for continuous airway relaxation. Sustained-release oral preparation can be used to prevent nocturnal symptoms. Requires serum level monitoring.	Used late in the course of treatment for moderate or severe asthma in order to achieve long-term control. Also indicated for apnea of prematurity (see "Caffeine").	Monitor drug levels routinely. Report signs of toxicity immediately: tachycardia, nausea, vomiting, diarrhea, stomach cramps, anorexia, confusion, headache, restlessness, flushing, increased urination, seizures, arrhythmias, insomnia.
Caffeine	Stimulates the respiratory center	Apnea of prematurity	See "Methylxanthines."
Pulmozyme (dornase alfa)	Enzyme that hydrolyzes the DNA in sputum, reducing sputum viscosity.	Cystic fibrosis	Monitor for dysphonia and pharyngitis.
Synagis (palivizumab)	Monoclonal antibody used to prevent serious lower respiratory RSV disease	For certain high-risk groups of children	Should be administered monthly during the RSV season. Given intramuscularly only.

rapid respirations, increased work of breathing, ear, nose, sinus, or throat pain, ear pulling, headache, vomiting with coughing, poor feeding, and lethargy. Also inquire about exposure to second-hand smoke. Children exposed to environmental smoke have an increased incidence of respiratory illnesses such as asthma, bronchitis, and pneumonia (Sheahan & Free, 2005). See Healthy People 2010.

HEALTHY PEOPLE 2010

Objective	Significance
Reduce the proportion of children who are regularly exposed to tobacco smoke at home.	• Educate the family about the effects that passive smoking has on children. • Encourage families to join smoking cessation programs.

Physical Examination

Physical examination of the respiratory system includes inspection and observation, auscultation, percussion, and palpation.

Inspection and Observation

Color. Observe the child's color, noting pallor or cyanosis (circumoral or central). Pallor (pale appearance) occurs as a result of peripheral vasoconstriction in an effort to conserve oxygen for vital functions. **Cyanosis** (a bluish tinge to the skin) occurs as a result of **hypoxia**. It might first present circumorally (just around the mouth) and progress to central cyanosis. Newborns might have blue hands and feet (acrocyanosis), a normal finding. The infant might have pale hands and feet when cold or when ill, as peripheral circulation is not well developed in early infancy. It is important, then, to note if the cyanosis is central (involving the midline), as this is a true sign of hypoxia. Children with low red blood cell counts might not demonstrate cyanosis as early in the course of hypoxemia as children with normal hemoglobin levels. Therefore, absence of cyanosis or the degree of cyanosis present is not always an accurate indication of the severity of respiratory involvement.

Note the rate and depth of respiration as well as work of breathing. Often the first sign of respiratory illness in infants and children is **tachypnea.**

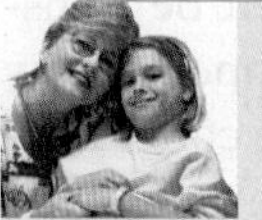

A slow or irregular respiratory rate in an acutely ill infant or child is an ominous sign. See Chapter 32: Nursing Care of the Child During a Pediatric Emergency.

Nose and Oral Cavity. Inspect the nose and oral cavity. Note nasal drainage and redness or swelling in the nose. Note the color of the pharynx, presence of exudates, tonsil size and status, and presence of lesions anywhere within the oral cavity.

Cough and Other Airway Noises. Note the sound of the cough (is it wet, productive, dry and hacking, tight?). If noises associated with breathing are present (grunting, stridor, or audible wheeze) these should also be noted. Grunting occurs on **expiration** and is produced by premature glottic closure. It is an attempt to preserve or increase functional residual capacity. Grunting might occur with alveolar collapse or loss of lung volume, such as in atelectasis, pneumonia, and pulmonary edema. **Stridor,** a high-pitched, readily audible inspiratory noise, is a sign of upper airway obstruction. Sometimes wheezes can be heard with the naked ear; these are referred to as audible wheezes.

Respiratory Effort. Assess respiratory effort for depth and quality. Is breathing labored? Infants and children with significant nasal congestion may have tachypnea, which usually resolves when the nose is cleared of mucus. Mouth breathing also may occur when a large amount of nasal congestion is present. Increased work of breathing, particularly if associated with restlessness and anxiety, usually indicates lower respiratory involvement. Assess for the presence of nasal flaring, retractions, or head bobbing. Nasal flaring can occur early in the course of respiratory illness and is an effort to inhale greater amounts of oxygen.

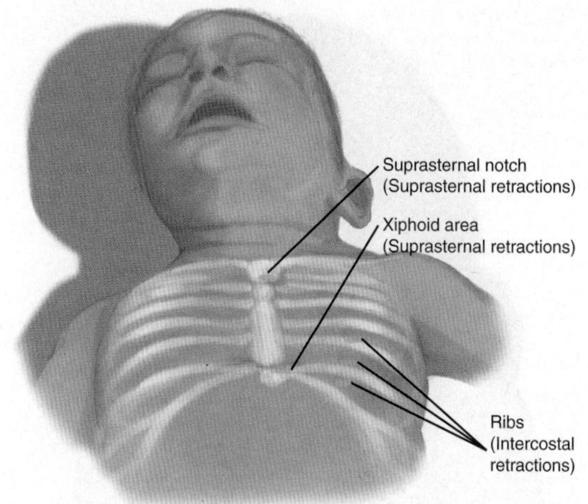

● Figure 19.3 Location of retractions.

Retractions (the inward pulling of soft tissues with respiration) can occur in the intercostal, subcostal, substernal, supraclavicular, or suprasternal regions (Fig. 19.3). Document the severity of the retractions: mild, moderate, or severe. Also note the use of accessory neck muscles. Note the presence of paradoxical breathing (lack of simultaneous chest and abdominal rise with the inspiratory phase; Fig. 19.4). Bobbing of the head with each breath is also a sign of increased respiratory effort.

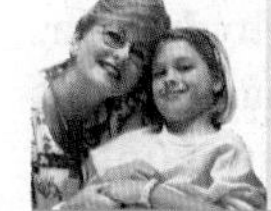

Seesaw (or paradoxical) respirations are very ineffective for ventilation and oxygenation. The chest falls on inspiration and rises on expiration.

Anxiety and Restlessness. Is the child anxious or restless? Restlessness, irritability, and anxiety result from difficulty in securing adequate oxygen. These might be very early signs of respiratory distress, especially if accompanied by tachypnea. Restlessness might progress to listlessness and lethargy if the respiratory dysfunction is not corrected (Fig. 19.5).

Clubbing. Inspect the fingertips for the presence of **clubbing,** an enlargement of the terminal phalanx of the finger, resulting in a change in the angle of the nail to the fingertip (Fig. 19.6). Clubbing might occur in children

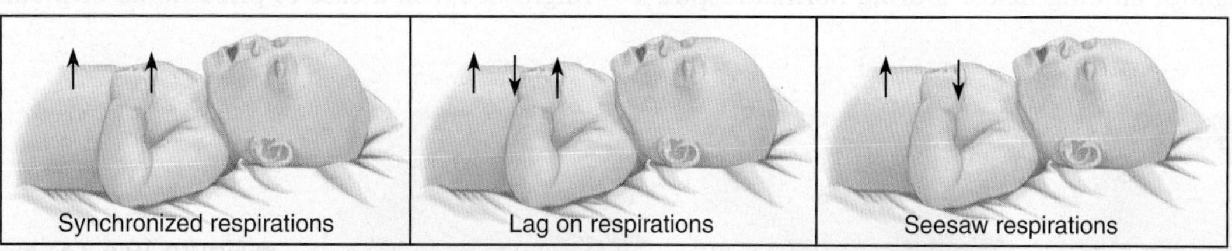

● Figure 19.4 Seesaw respirations.

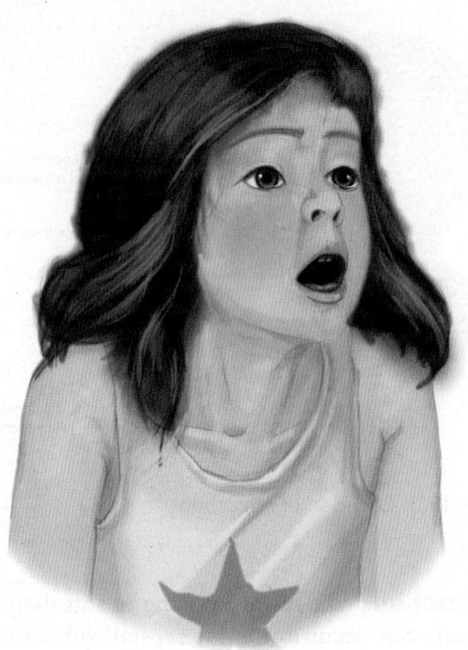

● Figure 19.5 Hypoxia and respiratory distress lead to anxiety and air hunger.

with a chronic respiratory illness. It is the result of increased capillary growth as the body attempts to supply more oxygen to distal body cells.

Hydration Status. Note the child's hydration status. The child with a respiratory illness is at risk for dehydration. Pain related to sore throat or mouth lesions may prevent the child from drinking properly. Nasal congestion interferes with the infant's ability to suck effectively at the breast or bottle. Tachypnea and increased work of breathing interfere with the ability to safely ingest fluids.

Assess the oral mucosa for color and moisture. Note skin turgor, presence of tears, and adequacy of urine output.

Auscultation

Assess lung sounds via auscultation. Evaluate breath sounds over the anterior and posterior chest, as well as in the axillary areas. Note the adequacy of aeration. Breath sounds should be equal bilaterally. The intensity and pitch should be equal throughout the lungs; document diminished breath sounds. In the absence of concurrent lower respiratory illness, the breath sounds should be clear throughout all lung fields. During normal respiration, the inspiratory phase is usually softer and longer than the expiratory phase.

Prolonged expiration is a sign of bronchial or bronchiolar obstruction. Bronchiolitis, asthma, pulmonary edema, and an intrathoracic foreign body can cause prolonged expiratory phases.

Infants and young children have thin chest walls. When the upper airway is congested (as in a severe cold), the noise produced in the upper airway might be transmitted throughout the lung fields. When upper airway congestion is transmitted to the lung fields, the congested-sounding noise heard over the trachea is the same type of noise heard over the lungs but is much louder and more intense. To ascertain if these sounds are truly adventitious lung sounds or if they are transmitted from the upper airway, auscultate again after the child coughs or his or her nose has been suctioned. Another way to discern the difference is to compare auscultatory findings over the trachea to the lung fields to determine if the abnormal sound is truly from within the lung or is actually a sound transmitted from the upper airway.

Note adventitious sounds heard on auscultation. Wheezing, a high-pitched sound that usually occurs on expiration, results from obstruction in the lower trachea or bronchioles. Wheezing that clears with coughing is most likely a result of secretions in the lower trachea. Wheezing resulting from obstruction of the bronchioles, as in bronchiolitis, asthma, chronic lung disease, or cystic fibrosis, that does not clear with coughing. **Rales** (crackling sounds) result when the alveoli become fluid-filled, such as in pneumonia. Note the location of the adventitious sounds as well as the timing (on inspiration, expiration, or both). Tachycardia might also be present. An increase in heart rate often initially accompanies hypoxemia.

Percussion

When percussing, note sounds that are not resonant in nature. Flat or dull sounds might be percussed over partially consolidated lung tissue, as in pneumonia. Tympany might be percussed with a pneumothorax. Note the presence of hyperresonance (as might be apparent with asthma).

Palpation

Palpate the sinuses for tenderness in the older child. Assess for enlargement or tenderness of the lymph nodes of the head and neck. Document alterations in tactile fremitus detected on palpation. Increased tactile fremitus might occur in a case of pneumonia or pleural effusion.

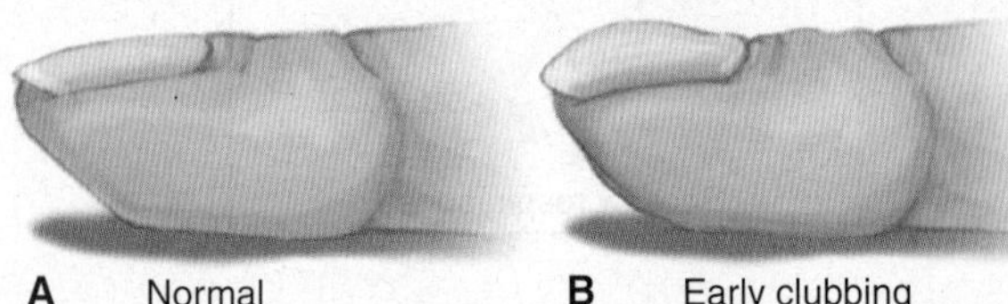

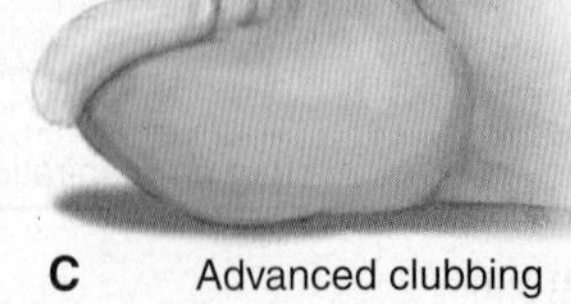

● Figure 19.6 (A) Normal fingertip. (B) Clubbing.

Fremitus might be decreased in the case of barrel chest, as with cystic fibrosis. Absent fremitus might be noted with pneumothorax or atelectasis.

Compare central and peripheral pulses. Note the quality of the pulse as well as the rate. With significant respiratory distress, perfusion often becomes compromised. Poor perfusion might be reflected in weaker peripheral pulses (radial, pedal) when compared to central pulses.

Laboratory and Diagnostic Testing

Common Laboratory and Diagnostic Tests 19.1 explains the laboratory and diagnostic tests most commonly used for a child with a respiratory disorder. The tests can assist the physician in diagnosing the disorder and/or be used as guidelines in determining ongoing treatment. Laboratory or non-nursing personnel obtain some of the tests, while the nurse might obtain others. In either instance the nurse should be familiar with how the tests are obtained, what they are used for, and normal versus abnormal results. This knowledge will also be necessary when providing patient and family education related to the testing.

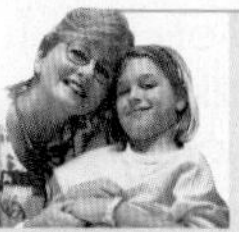

Ambient light may interfere with pulse oximetry readings. When the pulse oximeter probe is placed on the infant's foot or young child's toe, covering the probe and foot with a sock may help to ensure an accurate measurement.

Common Laboratory and Diagnostic Tests 19.1 Respiratory Disorders

Test	Explanation	Indication	Nursing Implications
Allergy skin testing	Suggested allergen is applied to skin via scratch, pin or prick. A wheal response indicates allergy to the substance. Carries risk of anaphylaxis. (Nursing note: Antihistamines must be discontinued before testing, as they inhibit the test.)	Allergic rhinitis, asthma	Close observation for anaphylaxis is necessary. Epinephrine and emergency equipment should be readily available. Some children react to the skin test almost immediately; others take several minutes.
Arterial blood gases	Invasive method (requires blood sampling) of measuring arterial pH, partial pressure of oxygen and carbon dioxide, and base excess in blood	Usually reserved for severe illness, the intubated child, or suspected carbon dioxide retention	Hold pressure for several minutes after a peripheral arterial stick to avoid bleeding. Radial arterial sticks are common and can be very painful. Note if the child is crying excessively during the blood draw, as this affects the carbon dioxide level.
Chest x-ray	Radiographic image of the expanded lungs: can show hyperinflation, atelectasis, pneumonia, foreign body, pleural effusion, abnormal heart or lung size	Bronchiolitis, pneumonia, tuberculosis, asthma, cystic fibrosis, bronchopulmonary dysplasia	Children may be afraid of the x-ray equipment. If a parent or familiar adult can accompany the child, often the child is less afraid. If the child is unable or unwilling to hold still for the x-ray, restraint may be necessary. Restraint should be limited to the amount of time needed for the x-ray.
Fluorescent antibody testing	Determines presence of respiratory syncytial virus (RSV), adenovirus, influenza, parainfluenza or *Chlamydia* in nasopharyngeal secretions	Bronchiolitis, pneumonia	To obtain a nasopharyngeal specimen instill 1 to 3 mL of sterile normal saline into one nostril, aspirate the contents using a small sterile bulb syringe, place the contents in sterile container, and immediately send them to the lab.

(continued)

Common Laboratory and Diagnostic Tests 19.1 Respiratory Disorders (continued)

Test	Explanation	Indication	Nursing Implications
Fluoroscopy	Radiographic examination that uses a fluorescent screen—"real-time" imaging	Identification of masses, abscesses	Requires the child to lay still. Equipment can be frightening. Children may respond to presence of parent or familiar adult.
Gastric washings for AFB	Determines presence of AFB (acid-fast bacilli) in stomach (children often swallow sputum)	Tuberculosis	Nasogastric tube is inserted and saline is instilled and suctioned out of the stomach for the specimen.
Peak expiratory flow	Measures the maximum flow of air that can be forcefully exhaled in 1 second. Measured in liters per second.	Daily use can indicate adequacy of asthma control.	It is important to establish the child's "personal best" by taking twice-daily readings over a 2-week period while well. The average of these is termed "personal best." Charts based on height and age are also available to determine expected peak expiratory flow.
Pulmonary function tests	Measures respiratory flow and lung volumes	Asthma, cystic fibrosis, chronic lung disease	Usually performed by a respiratory therapist trained to do the full spectrum of tests. Spirometry can be obtained by the trained nurse in the outpatient setting.
Pulse oximetry	Noninvasive method of continuously (or intermittently) measuring oxygen saturation	Can be useful in any situation in which a child is experiencing respiratory distress	Probe must be applied correctly to finger, toe, foot, hand, or ear in order for the machine to appropriately pick up the pulse and oxygen saturation.
Rapid flu test	Rapid test for detection of influenza A or B	Influenza	Should be done in first 24 hours of illness so that medication administration can begin. Have the child gargle with sterile normal saline and then spit into a sterile container. Send immediately to the lab.
Rapid strep test	Instant test for presence of strep A antibody in pharyngeal secretions	Pharyngitis, tonsillitis	Results in 5 to 10 minutes. Negative tests should be backed up with throat culture.
RAST (radioallergosorbent test)	Measures minute quantities of immunoglobulin E in the blood. Carries no risk of anaphylaxis but is not as sensitive as skin testing.	Asthma (food allergies)	Blood test that is usually sent out to a reference laboratory
Sinus x-rays, computed tomography (CT), or magnetic resonance imaging (MRI)	Radiologic tests that may show sinus involvement	Sinusitis, recurrent colds	X-ray results are usually received more quickly than CT or MRI results.

Common Laboratory and Diagnostic Tests 19.1 Respiratory Disorders (continued)

Test	Explanation	Indication	Nursing Implications
Sputum culture	Bacterial culture of invasive organisms in the sputum	Pneumonia, cystic fibrosis, tuberculosis	Must be true sputum, not mucus from the mouth or nose. Child can deep breathe, cough, and spit, or specimen may be obtained via suctioning of the artificial airway.
Sweat chloride test	Collection of sweat on filter paper after stimulation of skin with pilocarpine. Measures concentration of chloride in the sweat.	Cystic fibrosis	May be difficult to obtain sweat in a young infant
Throat culture	Bacterial culture (minimum of 24 to 48 hours required) to determine presence of streptococcus A or other bacteria	Pharyngitis, tonsillitis	Can be obtained on separate swab at same time as rapid strep test to decrease trauma to the child (swab both applicators at once). Do not perform immediately after the child has had medication or something to eat or drink.
Tuberculin skin test	Mantoux test (intradermal injection of purified protein derivative)	Tuberculosis, chronic cough	Must be given intradermally; not a valid test if injected incorrectly

NURSING DIAGNOSES, GOALS, INTERVENTIONS, AND EVALUATION

Upon completion of a thorough assessment, the nurse might identify several nursing diagnoses, including:

- Ineffective airway clearance
- Ineffective breathing pattern
- Impaired gas exchange
- Risk for infection
- Pain
- Risk for fluid volume deficit
- Altered nutrition, less than body requirements
- Activity intolerance
- Fear
- Altered family processes
- Pain

> After completing an assessment of Alexander, the nurse notes the following: lots of clear secretions in the airway, child appears pale, respiratory rate 68, retractions, nasal flaring, wheezing, and diminished breath sounds. Based on these assessment findings, what would your top three nursing diagnoses be for Alexander?

Nursing goals, interventions, and evaluation for the child with a respiratory disorder are based on the nursing diagnoses. Nursing Care Plan 19.1 can be used as a guide in planning nursing care for the child with a respiratory disorder. The nursing care plan should be individualized based on the patient's symptoms and needs; refer to Chap. 15 for detailed information on pain management. Additional information will be included later in the chapter as it relates to specific disorders.

> Based on your top three nursing diagnoses for Alexander, describe appropriate nursing interventions.

Oxygen Supplementation

Oxygen may be delivered to the child by a variety of methods (Fig. 19.7). Since oxygen administration is considered a drug, it requires a physician's order, except when following emergency protocols outlined in a health care facility's policies and procedures. Many health care settings develop specific guidelines for oxygen administration that are often coordinated by respiratory therapists, yet the nurse still remains responsible for ensuring that oxygen is administered properly.

Oxygen sources include wall-mounted systems as well as cylinders. The supply of oxygen available from a wall-mounted source is limitless, but use of a wall-mounted source restricts the child to the hospital room. Cylinders are portable oxygen tanks; the D-cylinder holds a little less

(text continues on page 565)

Nursing Care Plan 19.1

Overview for the Child with a Respiratory Disorder

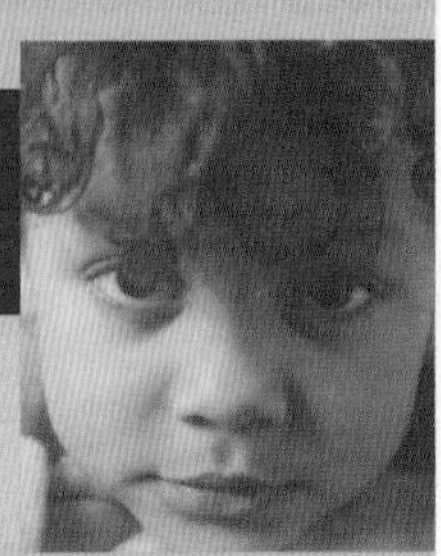

Nursing Diagnosis: Ineffective airway clearance related to inflammation, increased secretions, mechanical obstruction, or pain as evidenced by presence of secretions, productive cough, tachypnea, and increased work of breathing

Outcome identification and evaluation

Child will maintain patent airway, *free from secretions or obstruction, easy work of breathing, respiratory rate within parameters for age.*

Interventions: maintaining a patent airway

- Position with airway open (sniffing position if supine): *open airway allows adequate ventilation.*
- Humidify oxygen or room air and ensure adequate fluid intake (intravenous or oral) *to help liquefy secretions for ease in clearance.*
- Suction with bulb syringe or via nasopharyngeal catheter as needed, particularly prior to bottle-feeding *to promote clearance of secretions.*
- If tachypneic, maintain NPO status *to avoid risk of aspiration.*
- In older child, encourage expectoration of sputum with coughing *to promote airway clearance.*
- Perform chest physiotherapy if ordered *to mobilize secretions.*
- Ensure emergency equipment is readily available *to avoid delay should airway become unmaintainable.*

Nursing Diagnosis: Ineffective breathing pattern related to inflammatory or infectious process as evidenced by tachypnea, increased work of breathing, nasal flaring, retractions, diminished breath sounds

Outcome identification and evaluation

Child will exhibit adequate ventilation: *respiratory rate within parameters for age, easy work of breathing (absence of retractions, accessory muscle use, grunting), clear breath sounds with adequate aeration, oxygen saturation >94% or within prescribed parameters.*

Interventions: promoting effective breathing patterns

- Assess respiratory rate, breath sounds, and work of breathing frequently *to ensure progress with treatment and so that deterioration can be noted early.*
- Use pulse oximetry to monitor oxygen saturation in the least invasive manner *to note adequacy of oxygenation and ensure early detection of hypoxemia.*
- Position for comfort with open airway and room for lung expansion and use pillows or padding if necessary to maintain position *to ensure optimal ventilation via maximum lung expansion.*
- Administer supplemental oxygen and/or humidity as ordered *to improve oxygenation.*
- Allow for adequate sleep and rest periods *to conserve energy.*
- Administer antibiotics as ordered: *may be indicated in the case of bacterial respiratory infection.*
- Encourage incentive spirometry and coughing with deep breathing (can be accomplished through play) *to maximize ventilation (play enhances the child's participation).*

Overview for the Child with a Respiratory Disorder (continued)

Nursing Diagnosis: Gas exchange, impaired, related to airway plugging, hyperinflation, atelectasis as evidenced by cyanosis, decreased oxygen saturation, and alterations in arterial blood gases

Outcome identification and evaluation

Gas exchange will be adequate: *Pulse oximetry reading on room air is within normal parameters for age, blood gases within normal limits, absence of cyanosis.*

Interventions: promoting adequate gas exchange

- Administer oxygen as ordered *to improve oxygenation.*
- Monitor oxygen saturation via pulse oximetry *to detect alterations in oxygenation.*
- Encourage clearance of secretions via coughing, expectoration, chest physiotherapy, and suctioning: *mobilization of secretions may improve gas exchange.*
- Administer bronchodilators if ordered (albuterol, levalbuterol, and racemic epinephrine) *to treat bronchospasm and improve gas exchange.*
- Provide frequent contact and support to the child and family *to decrease anxiety, which increases the child's oxygen demands.*
- Assess and monitor mental status (confusion, lethargy, restlessness, combativeness): *hypoxemia can lead to changes in mental status.*

Nursing Diagnosis: Risk for infection related to presence of infectious organisms as evidenced by fever or presence of virus or bacteria on laboratory screening

Outcome identification and evaluation

Child will exhibit no signs of secondary infection and will not spread infection to others: *symptoms of infection decrease over time; others remain free from infection.*

Interventions: preventing infection

- Maintain aseptic technique, practice good hand washing, and use disposable suction catheters *to prevent introduction of further infectious agents.*
- Limit number of visitors and screen them for recent illness *to prevent further infection.*
- Administer antibiotics if prescribed *to prevent or treat bacterial infection.*
- Encourage nutritious diet according to child's preferences and ability to feed orally *to assist body's natural infection-fighting mechanisms.*
- Isolate the child as required *to prevent nosocomial spread of infection*
- Teach child and family preventive measures such as good hand washing, covering mouth and nose when coughing or sneezing, adequate disposal of used tissues *to prevent nosocomial or community spread of infection.*

Nursing Diagnosis: Fluid volume deficit, risk for, related to decreased oral intake, insensible losses via fever, tachypnea, or diaphoresis

Outcome identification and evaluation

Fluid volume will be maintained: *Oral mucosa moist and pink, skin turgor elastic, urine output at least 1 to 2 mL/kg/hr.*

Interventions: maintaining adequate fluid volume

- Administer intravenous fluids if ordered *to maintain adequate hydration in NPO state.*
- When allowed oral intake, encourage oral fluids. Popsicles, favorite fluids, and games can be used *to promote intake.*
- Assess for signs of adequate hydration (elastic skin turgor, moist mucosa, adequate urine output).
- Strict intake and output monitoring *can help identify fluid imbalance.*
- Urine specific gravity, urine and serum electrolytes, blood urea nitrogen, creatinine, and osmolality *are reliable indicators of fluid status.*

(continued)

Overview for the Child with a Respiratory Disorder (continued)

Nursing Diagnosis: Nutrition, altered: less than body requirements related to difficulty feeding as evidenced by poor oral intake, tiring with feeding

Outcome identification and evaluation

Child will maintain adequate nutritional intake: *Weight gain or maintenance occurs. Child consumes adequate diet for age.*

Interventions: promoting adequate nutritional intake

- Weigh on same scale at same time daily: *weight gain or maintenance can indicate adequate nutritional intake.*
- Calorie counts over a 3-day period *are helpful in determining if caloric intake is sufficient.*
- Assist family and child to choose higher-calorie, protein-rich foods *to optimize growth potential.*
- Coax young children to eat better by playing games and offering favorite foods *resulting in improved intake.*

Nursing Diagnosis: Activity intolerance related to high respiratory demand as evidenced by increased work of breathing and requirement for frequent rest when playing

Outcome identification and evaluation

Child will resume normal activity level: *Activity is tolerated without difficulty breathing. Pulse oximetry readings and vital signs within parameters for age and activity level.*

Interventions: increasing activity tolerance

- Provide rest periods balanced with periods of activity. Group nursing activities and visits to allow for sufficient rest. *Activity increases myocardial oxygen demand so must be balanced with rest.*
- Provide small, frequent meals to prevent overtiring (*energy is expended while eating*).
- Encourage quiet activities that do not require exertion *to prevent boredom.*
- Allow gradual increase in activity as tolerated, keeping pulse oximetry reading within normal parameters, *to minimize risk for further respiratory compromise.*

Nursing Diagnosis: Fear related to difficulty breathing, unfamiliar personnel, procedures, and environment (hospital) as evidenced by clinging, crying, fussing, verbalization, or lack of cooperation

Outcome identification and evaluation

Fear/anxiety will be reduced: *decreased episodes of crying or fussing, happy and playful at times.*

Interventions: relieving fear

- Establish trusting relationship with child and family *to decrease anxiety and fear.*
- Explain procedures to child at developmentally appropriate level *to decrease fear of unknown.*
- Provide favorite blanket or bear to patient, as well as comfort measures preferred by client such as rocking or music *for added security.*
- Involve parents in care *to give child reassurance and decrease fear.*

Overview for the Child with a Respiratory Disorder (continued)

Nursing Diagnosis: Family processes, altered, related to child's illness or hospitalization as evidenced by family's presence in hospital, missed work, demonstration of inadequate coping

Outcome identification and evaluation

Parents demonstrate adequate coping and decreased anxiety: *Parents are involved in child's care, ask appropriate questions and are able to discuss child's care and condition calmly.*

Interventions: promoting adequate family processes

- Encourage parents' verbalization of concerns related to child's illness: *allows for identification of concerns and demonstrates to the family that the nurse also cares about them, not just the child.*
- Explain therapy, procedures, and child's behavior to parents; *developing an understanding of the child's current status helps decrease anxiety.*
- Encourage parental involvement in care *so that parents may continue to feel needed and valued.*

than 400 liters of oxygen and the E-cylinder holds about 650 liters of oxygen. Cylinders turn on with a metal key that is kept with the tank. The tank empties relatively quickly if the child requires a high flow of oxygen, so this is not the best oxygen source in an emergency. The cylinder is useful for the child on low-flow oxygen because it allows mobility.

Respiratory therapists usually maintain the respiratory equipment that is found in the emergency room or hospital. However, in an outpatient setting the nurse may be responsible for maintaining respiratory equipment and checking the level of oxygen in the office's oxygen tanks each day.

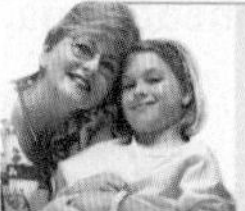

Oxygen is highly flammable, so use safety precautions. Post signs ("Oxygen in Use"); inform the family to avoid matches, lighters, and flammable or volatile materials; and use only facility-approved equipment.

The efficiency of oxygen delivery systems is affected by several variables, including the child's respiratory effort, the liter flow of oxygen delivered, and whether the equipment

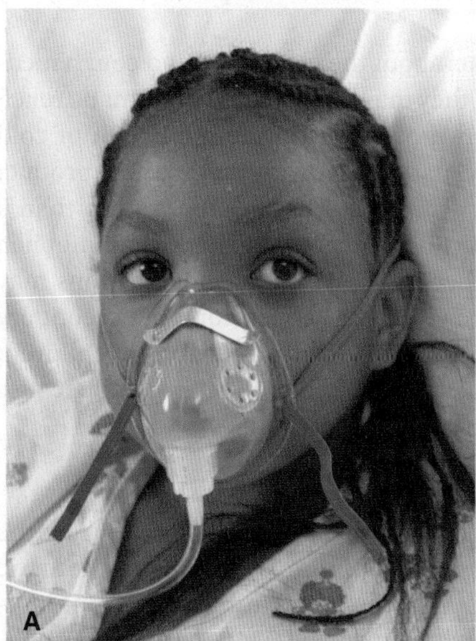

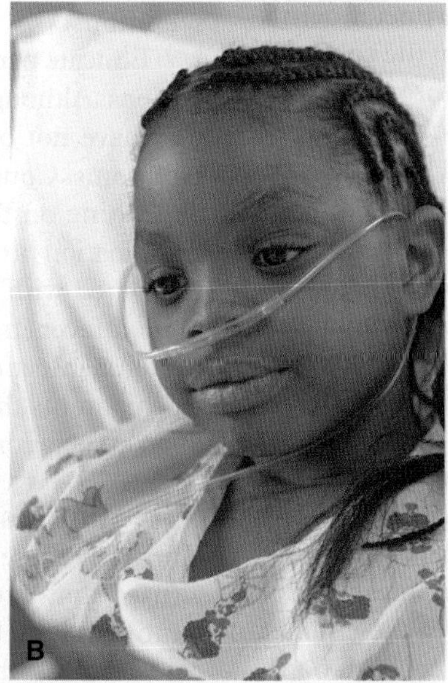

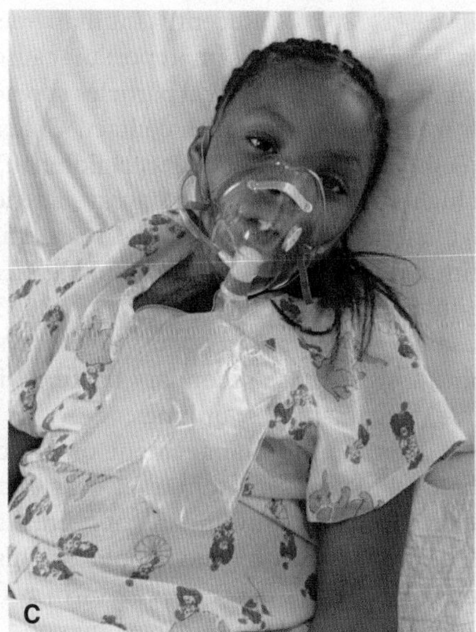

● **Figure 19.7** (**A**) Simple oxygen mask provides about 40% oxygen. (**B**) The nasal cannula provides an additional 4% oxygen per 1 L of oxygen flow (i.e., 1 L will deliver 25% oxygen). (**C**) The nonrebreather mask provides 80%–100% oxygen.

is being used appropriately. In general, oxygen facemasks come in infant, child, and adult sizes. Select the mask that best fits the child. In addition, ensure that the mask is sealed properly to decrease the amount of oxygen that escapes from the mask. Ensure that the liter flow is set according to the manufacturer's recommendations for use with that particular delivery method. The oxygen flow rate or concentration is usually determined by the physician's order. Whichever method of delivery is used, provide humidification during oxygen delivery to prevent drying of nasal passages and to assist with liquefying secretions. Table 19.1 gives details on oxygen delivery methods.

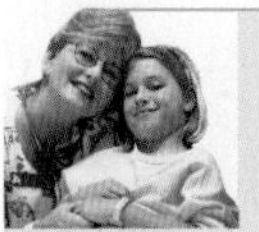

Monitor vital signs, color, respiratory effort, pulse oximetry, and level of consciousness before, during, and after oxygen therapy to evaluate its effectiveness.

Acute Infectious Disorders

Acute infectious disorders include the common cold, sinusitis, influenza, pharyngitis, tonsillitis, laryngitis, croup syndromes, respiratory syncytial virus (RSV), pneumonia, and bronchitis.

• COMMON COLD

The common cold is also referred to as a viral upper respiratory infection (URI) or nasopharyngitis. Colds can be caused by a number of different viruses, including rhinoviruses, parainfluenza, RSV, enteroviruses, and adenoviruses (National Institute of Allergy and Infectious Diseases, 2004). Recently, human meta-pneumovirus has been identified as an important cause of the common cold (Burke, 2004). Viral particles spread through the air or from person-to-person contact. Colds occur more frequently in winter. They affect children of all ages and have a higher incidence among daycare attendees and school-age children. It is not unusual for a child to have six to nine colds per year. Passive smoking increases the risk of catching colds (Johannsson et al., 2003). Spontaneous resolution occurs after about 7 to 10 days. Potential complications include secondary bacterial infections of the ears, throat, sinuses, or lungs.

Therapeutic management of the common cold is directed toward symptom relief. Nasal congestion may be relieved via humidity and use of normal saline nasal wash or spray followed by suctioning. Antihistamines are not indicated, as they dry secretions further. Over-the-counter cold preparations are available singly and in combinations. These preparations have not been proven to reduce the length or severity of the cold but may offer symptomatic relief in some children.

Nursing Assessment

The child may have either a stuffy or runny nose. Nasal discharge is usually thin and watery at first but may become thicker and discolored. The color of nasal discharge is *not* an accurate indicator of viral versus bacterial infection. The child may be hoarse and complain of a sore throat. Cough usually produces very little sputum. Fever, fatigue, watery eyes, and appetite loss may also occur. Symptoms are generally at their worst over the first few days and then decrease over the course of the illness.

Assess for risk factors such as daycare or school attendance. Inspect for edema and vasodilation of the mucosa. Diagnosis is based on clinical presentation rather than lab or x-ray studies. Comparison Chart 19.1 differentiates causes of nasal congestion.

Nursing Management

Nursing management of the child with a common cold consists of promoting comfort, providing family education, and preventing spread of the cold.

Promoting Comfort

Nursing care of the common cold is aimed at supportive measures. Nasal congestion may be relieved with the use of normal saline nose drops, followed by bulb syringe suctioning in infants and toddlers. Older children may use a normal saline nose spray to mobilize secretions. A cool mist humidifier also helps with nasal congestion. Generally, other over-the-counter nose sprays are not recommended for use in children, but they are sometimes prescribed for very short-term use. Promotion of adequate oral fluid intake is important to liquefy secretions.

Educate parents about the use of cold and cough medications. Although they may offer some symptomatic relief, they have not been proven to shorten the length of cold symptoms. Counsel parents to use the appropriate product depending on the symptom relief desired, rather than a combination product. Products containing acetaminophen combined with other "cold symptom" medications may mask a fever in the child who is developing a secondary bacterial infection. As with all viral infections in children, teach parents that aspirin use should be avoided because of its association with Reye syndrome.

Providing Family Education

Currently there are no medications available to treat the viruses that cause the common cold, so symptomatic treatment is all that is necessary. Antibiotics are not indicated unless the child also has a bacterial infection. Explain to parents the importance of reserving antibiotic use for appropriate illnesses. Provide education about the use of normal saline nose drops and bulb suctioning

Table 19.1 Oxygen Delivery Methods

Delivery Method	Description	Nursing Implications
Simple mask	Provides 35% to 60% oxygen with a flow rate of 6 to 10 L/minute. Oxygen delivery percentage affected by respiratory rate, inspiratory flow, and adequacy of mask fit.	• Must maintain oxygen flow rate of at least 6 L/minute to maintain inspired oxygen concentration and prevent rebreathing of carbon dioxide • Mask must fit snugly to be effective but should not be so tight as to irritate the face.
Venturi mask	Provides 24% to 50% oxygen by using a special gauge at the base of the mask that allows mixing of room air with oxygen flow	• Set oxygen flow rate according to percentage of oxygen desired as indicated on the gauge/dial. • As with simple mask, must fit snugly
Nasal cannula	Provides low oxygen concentration (22% to 44%) but needs patent nasal passages	• Must be used with humidification to prevent drying and irritation of airways • Can provide very small amounts of oxygen (as low as 25 cc/minute) • Maximum recommended liter flow in children is 4 L/minute. • Children can eat or talk while on oxygen. • Inspired oxygen concentration affected by mouth breathing • Requires patent nasal passages
Oxygen tent	Provides high-humidity environment with up to 50% oxygen concentration	• Oxygen level drops when tent is opened. • Must change linen frequently as it becomes damp from the humidity • Secure edges of tent with blankets or by tucking edges under mattress. • Young children may be fearful and resistant. • Mist may interfere with visualization of child inside tent.
Oxygen hood	Provides high concentration (up to 80% to 90%) for infants only. Allows easy access to chest and lower body.	• Liter flow must be set at 10 to 15 L/minute. • Good method for infant but need to remove for feeding • Can and should be humidified
Partial rebreathing mask	Simple facemask with an oxygen reservoir bag. Provides 50% to 60% oxygen concentration.	• Must set liter flow rate at 10 to 12 L/min to prevent rebreathing of carbon dioxide • The reservoir bag does not completely empty when child inspires if flow rate is set properly.
Nonrebreathing mask	Simple facemask with valves at the exhalation ports and an oxygen reservoir bag with a valve to prevent exhaled air from entering the reservoir. Provides 95% oxygen concentration.	• Must set liter flow rate at 10 to 12 L/min to prevent rebreathing of carbon dioxide • The reservoir bag does not completely empty when child inspires if flow rate is set properly.

COMPARISON CHART 19.1 Causes of Nasal Congestion

Sign or Symptom	Allergic Rhinitis	Common Cold	Sinusitis
Length of illness	Varies, may have year-round symptoms	10 days or less	Longer than 10 to 14 days
Nasal discharge	Thin, watery, clear	Thick, white, yellow, or green; can be thin	Thick, yellow or green
Nasal congestion	Varies	Present	Present
Sneezing	Varies	Present	Absent
Cough	Varies	Present	Varies
Headache	Varies	Varies	Varies
Fever	Absent	Varies	Varies
Bad breath	Absent	Absent	Varies

to clear the infant's nose of secretions. Normal saline nasal wash using a bulb syringe to instill the solution is also helpful for children of all ages with nasal congestion. Though normal saline for nasal administration is available commercially, parents can also make it at home (Box 19.2). Teaching Guideline 19.1 gives instructions on use of the bulb syringe.

Counsel parents about symptoms of complications of the common cold. These include:

- Prolonged fever
- Increased throat pain or enlarged, painful lymph nodes
- Increased or worsening cough, cough lasting longer than 10 days, chest pain, difficulty breathing
- Earache, headache, tooth or sinus pain
- Unusual irritability or lethargy
- Skin rash

If complications do occur, tell parents to notify the health care provider for further instruction or reassessment.

Preventing the Common Cold

Teaching about ways to prevent the common cold is a vital nursing intervention. Explain that frequent hand washing helps to decrease the spread of viruses that cause the common cold. Teach parents and family to avoid second-hand smoke as well as crowded places, especially during the winter. Avoid close contact with individuals known to have a cold. Encourage parents and families to consume a healthy diet and get enough rest (Torpy, 2003). See Healthy People 2010.

BOX 19.2

HOMEMADE SALT WATER NOSE DROPS

Mix 8 oz distilled water, a half-teaspoon sea salt, and a quarter-teaspoon baking soda. Keeps for 24 hours in the refrigerator, but should be allowed to come to room temperature prior to use.

Consider THIS!

Corey Davis, a 3-year-old, is brought to the clinic by her mother. She presents with a runny nose, congestion, and a nonproductive cough. Her mother says, "She is miserable."

What other assessment information would be helpful?

Based on the history and clinical presentation, Corey is diagnosed with a common cold. What education would be helpful for this family? Include ways to improve Corey's comfort and ways to prevent the common cold.

SINUSITIS

Sinusitis (also called rhinosinusitis) generally refers to a bacterial infection of the paranasal sinuses. The disease may be either acute or chronic in nature, with the treatment approach varying with chronicity. Approximately 5% of upper respiratory infections are complicated with acute sinusitis. In young children the maxillary and ethmoid sinuses are the main sites of infection. After age 10 years, the frontal sinuses may be more commonly involved. Mucosal swelling, decreased ciliary movement, and thickened nasal discharge all contribute to bacterial invasion of the nose. Nasal polyps also place the child at risk for bacterial sinusitis. Complications include orbital cellulitis and intracranial infections such as subdural empyemas.

Symptoms lasting less than 30 days generally indicate acute sinusitis, whereas symptoms persisting longer than 4 to 6 weeks usually indicate chronic sinusitis. Sinusitis is managed with antibiotic treatment. The course of treatment is a minimum of 10 days. The current American

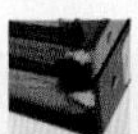

TEACHING GUIDELINE 19.1

Using the Bulb Syringe to Suction Nasal Secretions

- Hold the infant on your lap or on the bed with head tilted slightly back.

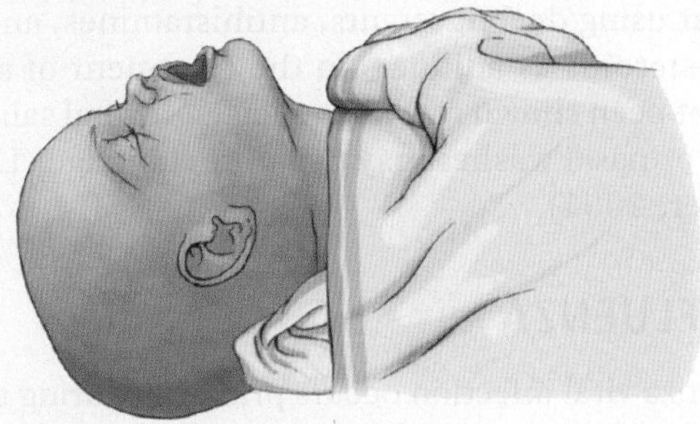

- (If using saline) Instill several drops of saline solution in one of infant's nostrils.

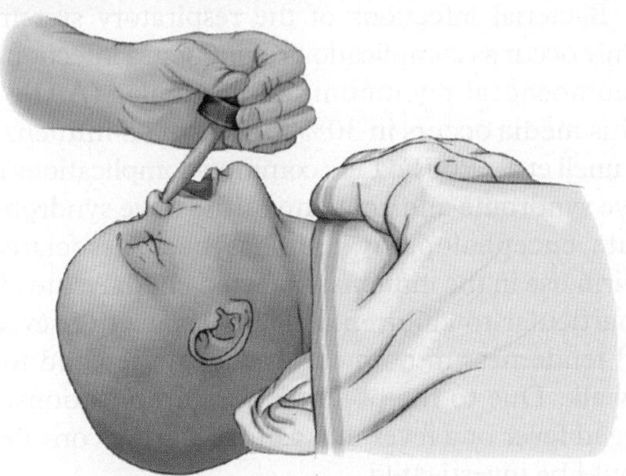

- Compress the sides of the bulb syringe completely. Use only a rubber-tipped bulb syringe.

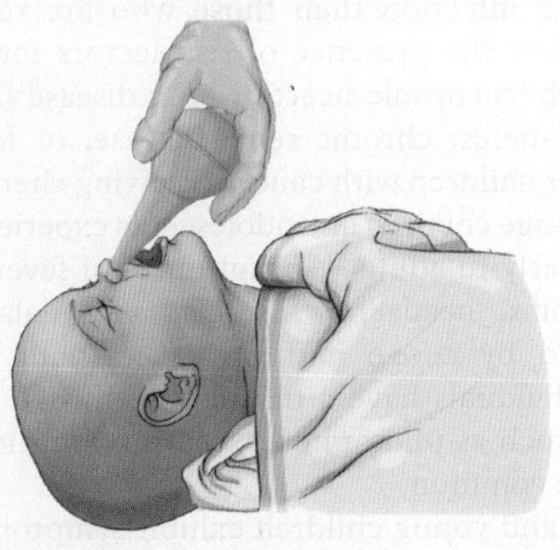

- Place rubber tip in infant's nose and release pressure on the bulb.

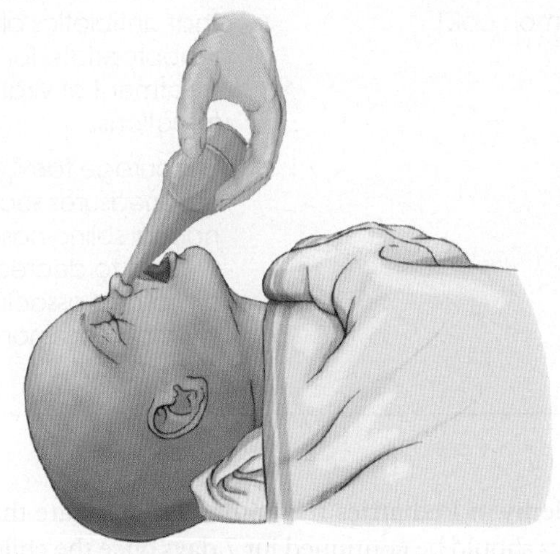

- Remove the syringe and squeeze bulb over tissue or the sink to empty it of secretions.

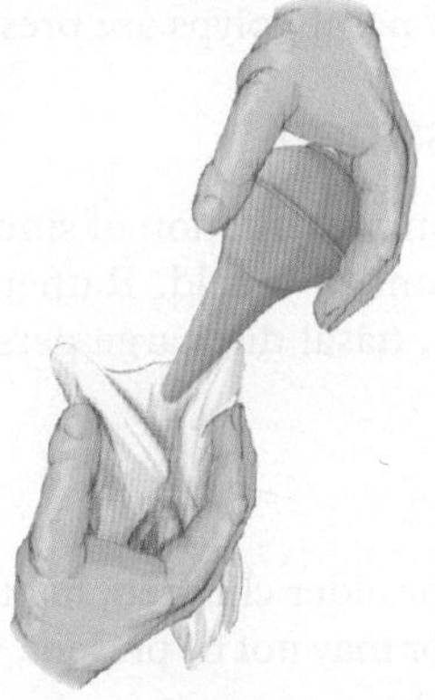

- Repeat on alternate nostril if necessary. Using a bulb syringe prior to bottle-feeding or breastfeeding may relieve congestion enough to allow the infant to suck more efficiently.
- Clean the bulb syringe thoroughly with warm water after each use and allow to air dry.

HEALTHY PEOPLE 2010

Objective	Significance
Reduce the number of courses of antibiotics prescribed for the sole diagnosis of the common cold.	• Appropriately educate families that the cause of the common cold is a number of viruses and that antibiotics are inappropriate for the treatment of viral infections. • Encourage families to use measures such as normal saline nasal washes to decrease symptoms associated with the common cold more quickly.

Academy of Pediatrics recommendations state that antibiotics should be continued for 7 days once the child is free from symptoms to eradicate the infection (AAP, 2001). Naturally, chronic sinusitis requires a longer course of treatment than acute sinusitis. Surgical therapy may be indicated for children with chronic sinusitis, particularly if it is recurrent or if nasal polyps are present.

Nursing Assessment

The most common presentation of sinusitis is persistent signs and symptoms of a cold. Rather than improving after 7 to 10 days, nasal discharge persists. Explore the history for:

- Cough
- Fever
- In preschoolers or older children, halitosis (bad breath)
- Facial pain may or may not be present, so is not a reliable indicator of disease.
- Eyelid edema (in the case of ethmoid sinus involvement)
- Irritability
- Poor appetite

Cold symptoms that are severe and not improving over time may also indicate sinusitis (Leung & Kellner, 2004). Assess for risk factors such as a history of recurrent cold symptoms or a history of nasal polyps.

On physical examination, note eyelid swelling, extent of nasal drainage, and halitosis. Inspect the throat for evidence of postnasal drainage. Inspect the nasal mucosa for erythema. Palpate the sinuses, noting pain with mild pressure. The diagnosis may be made based on the history and clinical presentation, augmented by x-ray, computed tomography scan, or magnetic resonance imaging findings in some cases (Leung & Kellner, 2004). (Refer to Comparison Chart 19.1, which differentiates the causes of nasal congestion.)

Nursing Management

Normal saline nose drops or spray, cool mist humidifiers, and adequate oral fluid intake are recommended for children with sinusitis. Teach families the importance of continuing the full course of antibiotics to eradicate the cause of infection. Also educate the family that using decongestants, antihistamines, and intranasal steroids as adjuncts in the treatment of sinusitis has not been shown to be beneficial. Normal saline nose spray or nasal washes may promote drainage (Leung & Kellner, 2004).

INFLUENZA

Influenza viral infection occurs primarily during the winter. "The flu" is spread through inhalation of droplets or contact with fine-particle aerosols. Infected children shed the virus for 1 to 2 days before symptoms begin. Average annual infection rates in children range from 35% to 50% (Brunell et al., 2001). Influenza viruses primarily affect the upper respiratory epithelium but can cause systemic effects as well. Children with chronic heart or lung conditions, diabetes, chronic renal disease, or immune deficiency are at higher risk than other children for more severe influenza infection.

Bacterial infections of the respiratory system commonly occur as complications of influenza infection, severe pneumococcal pneumonia in particular (AAP, 2002). Otitis media occurs in 30% to 50% of all influenza cases (Brunell et al., 2001). Less common complications include Reye syndrome and acute myositis. Reye syndrome is an acute encephalopathy that has been associated with aspirin use in the influenza-infected child. Acute myositis is particular to children. A sudden onset of severe pain and tenderness in both calves causes the child to refuse to walk. Due to the potential for complications, a prolonged fever or a fever that returns during convalescence should be investigated.

Nursing Assessment

Children who attend daycare or school are at higher risk for influenza infection than those who are routinely at home. Note the presence of risk factors for severe disease, such as chronic heart or lung disease (such as asthma), diabetes, chronic renal disease, or immune deficiency or children with cancer receiving chemotherapy. School-age children and adolescents experience the illness similarly to adults. Abrupt onset of fever, facial flushing, chills, headache, myalgia, and malaise are accompanied by cough and **coryza**. About half of infected individuals have a dry or sore throat. Ocular symptoms such as photophobia, tearing, burning, and eye pain are common.

Infants and young children exhibit symptoms similar to other respiratory illnesses. Fever greater than

39.5° C is common. Infants may be mildly toxic in appearance and irritable and have a cough, coryza, and pharyngitis. Wheezing may occur, as influenza also can cause bronchiolitis. An erythematous rash may be present, and diarrhea may also occur. Diagnosis may be confirmed by a rapid assay test.

Nursing Management

Nursing management of influenza is mainly supportive. Symptomatic treatment of cough and fever and maintenance of hydration are the focus of care. Amantadine hydrochloride (Symmetrel) and other newer antiviral drugs can be effective in reducing symptoms associated with influenza if started within the first 24 to 48 hours of the illness.

Preventing Influenza Infection

Yearly vaccination against influenza is recommended for high-risk groups. Children who are 6 months or older considered high risk are those who:

- Have chronic heart or lung conditions
- Have sickle cell anemia or other hemoglobinopathy
- Are under medical care for diabetes, chronic renal disease, or immune deficiency
- Are on long-term aspirin therapy (risk of developing Reye syndrome after the flu)

Among otherwise healthy children, infants and toddlers are at highest risk for developing severe disease. All healthy children between the ages of 6 and 59 months should also be immunized. Refer to Chapter 9 for more information on immunizations.

● PHARYNGITIS

Inflammation of the throat mucosa (pharynx) is referred to as **pharyngitis**. A sore throat may accompany nasal congestion and is often viral in nature. A bacterial sore throat most often occurs without nasal symptoms. Group A streptococci account for 15% to 30% of cases, with the remainder being caused by other viruses or bacteria (Bisno, 2001).

Complications of group A streptococcal infection include acute rheumatic fever (see Chapter 20) and acute glomerulonephritis (see Chapter 22). An additional complication of streptococcal pharyngitis is peritonsillar abscess; this may be noted by asymmetric swelling of the tonsils, shift of the uvula to one side, and palatal edema. Retropharyngeal abscess may also follow pharyngitis and is most common in young children (Ebell et al., 2000). It can progress to the point of airway obstruction and requires careful evaluation and appropriate treatment.

Viral pharyngitis is usually self-limited and does not require therapy beyond symptomatic relief. Group A streptococcal pharyngitis requires antibiotic therapy. If either the rapid diagnostic test or throat culture (described below) is positive for group A streptococci, penicillin is generally prescribed. Appropriate alternative antibiotics include amoxicillin and, for those allergic to penicillin, macrolides and cephalosporins (Hayes & Williamson, 2001).

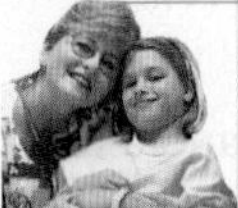

A "strep carrier" is a child who has a positive throat culture for streptococci when asymptomatic. Strep carriers are not at risk for complications from streptococci as are those who are acutely infected with streptococci and are symptomatic.

Nursing Assessment

Onset of the illness is often quite abrupt. The history may include a fever, sore throat and difficulty swallowing, headache, and abdominal pain, which are quite common. Inquire about recent incidence of viral or strep throat in the family, daycare, or school setting.

Inspect the pharynx and tonsils, which may demonstrate varying degrees of inflammation (Fig. 19.8). Exudate may be present but is not diagnostic of bacterial infection. Note the presence of petechiae on the palate. Inspect the tongue for a strawberry appearance. Palpate for enlargement and tenderness of the anterior cervical nodes. Inspect the skin for the presence of a fine, red, sandpaper-like rash (called scarlatiniform), particularly on the trunk or abdomen, a common finding with streptococcus A infection.

The nurse may obtain a throat swab for rapid diagnostic testing and throat culture. If both tests are being obtained, the applicators may be swabbed simultaneously to decrease perceived trauma to the child. The rapid strep test is a sensitive and reliable measure rarely

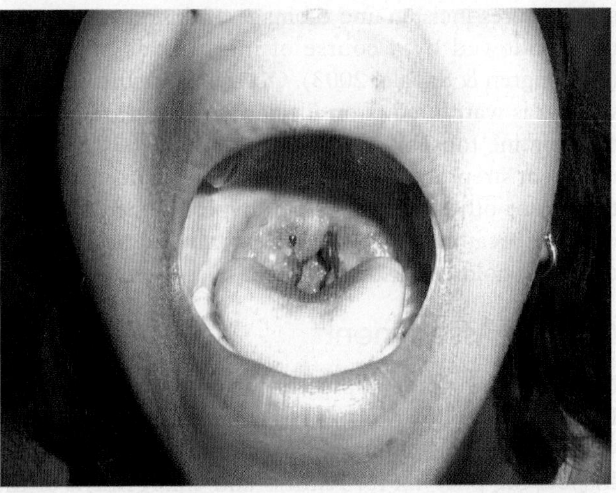

● Figure 19.8 Note the red color of the pharynx, as well as redness and significant enlargement of the tonsils.

resulting in false-positive readings (Farrar-Simpson et al., 2005). If the rapid strep test is negative, the second swab may be sent for a throat culture.

Nursing Management

Nursing management of the child with pharyngitis focuses on promoting comfort and providing family education.

Promoting Comfort

Saline gargles (made with 8 oz of warm water and a half-teaspoon of table salt) are soothing for children old enough to cooperate. Analgesics such as acetaminophen and ibuprofen may ease fever and pain. Sucking on throat lozenges or hard candy may also ease pain. Cool mist humidity helps to keep the mucosa moist in the event of mouth breathing. Encourage the child to ingest Popsicles, cool liquids, and ice chips to maintain hydration.

Providing Family Education

Parents may be accustomed to "sore throats" being treated with antibiotics, but in the case of a viral cause antibiotics will not be necessary and the pharyngitis will resolve in a few days. For the child with streptococcal pharyngitis, urge parents to have the child complete the entire prescribed course of antibiotics (Parmet, 2004). After 24 hours of antibiotic therapy, instruct the parents to discard the child's toothbrush to avoid reinfection. Children may return to day care or school after they have been receiving antibiotics for 24 hours, as they are considered noncontagious at that point.

TONSILLITIS

Inflammation of the tonsils often occurs with pharyngitis and thus may also be viral or bacterial in nature. Viral infections require only symptomatic treatment. Treatment for bacterial tonsillitis is the same as for bacterial pharyngitis. Peritonsillar abscess may follow a bout of tonsillitis and requires incision and drainage of the pus-containing mass followed by a course of intravenous antibiotics (Belkengren & Sapala, 2003). Occasionally surgical intervention is warranted. Tonsillectomy (surgical removal of the palatine tonsils) may be indicated for the child with recurrent streptococcal tonsillitis, massive tonsillar hypertrophy, or other reasons. When hypertrophied adenoids obstruct breathing, then adenoidectomy (surgical removal of the adenoids) may be indicated.

Nursing Assessment

Note whether fever is present currently or by history. Inquire about the history of recurrent pharyngitis or tonsillitis. Note if the child's voice sounds muffled or hoarse. Inspect the pharynx for redness and enlargement of the tonsils. As the tonsils enlarge, the child may experience difficulty breathing and swallowing. When tonsils touch at the midline ("kissing tonsils" or 4+ in size), the airway may become obstructed (see Fig. 19.8). Also, if the adenoids are enlarged, the posterior nares become obstructed. The child may breathe through the mouth and may snore. Palpate the anterior cervical nodes for enlargement and tenderness. Rapid test or culture may be positive for streptococcus A (Johansson & Mannson, 2003).

Nursing Management

Tonsillitis that is medically treated requires the same nursing management as pharyngitis. Nursing care for the child after tonsillectomy is described below.

Promoting Airway Clearance

Until fully awake, place the child in a side-lying or prone position to facilitate safe drainage of secretions. Once alert, he or she may prefer to sit up or have the head of the bed elevated. Suctioning, if necessary, should be done carefully to avoid trauma to the surgical site. Dried blood may be present on the teeth and the nares, with old blood present in emesis. Since the presence of blood can be very frightening to parents, alert them to this possibility.

Maintaining Fluid Volume

Hemorrhage is unusual postoperatively but may occur any time from the immediate postoperative period to as late as 10 days after surgery (Peterson & Losek, 2004). Inspect the throat for bleeding. Mucus tinged with blood may be expected, but fresh blood in the secretions indicates bleeding. Early bleeding may be identified by continuous swallowing of small amounts of blood while awake or sleeping. Other signs of hemorrhage include tachycardia, pallor, restlessness, frequent throat clearing, and emesis of bright red blood.

To avoid trauma to the surgical site, discourage the child from coughing, clearing the throat, blowing the nose, and using straws. Upon discharge, instruct the parents to immediately report any sign of bleeding to the physician. To maintain fluid volume postoperatively, encourage children to take any fluids they desire; Popsicles and ice chips are particularly soothing. Citrus juice and brown or red fluids should be avoided: the acid in citrus juice may irritate the throat, and red or brown fluids may be confused with blood if vomiting occurs.

Relieving Pain

For the first 24 hours after surgery, the throat is very sore. Adequate pain relief is essential to establish adequate oral fluid intake. An ice collar may be prescribed, as well as analgesics with or without narcotics. Counsel parents to maintain pain control upon discharge from the facility, not only for the child's sake but also to enable the child to continue to drink fluids (Louloudes, 2006).

INFECTIOUS MONONUCLEOSIS

Infectious mononucleosis is a self-limited illness caused by the Epstein-Barr virus. It is characterized by fever, malaise, sore throat, and lymphadenopathy. Mononucleosis is commonly called the "kissing disease" since it is transmitted by oropharyngeal secretions. It can occur at any age but is most often diagnosed in adolescents and young adults. Some infected individuals may have concomitant streptococcal pharyngitis. Complications include splenic rupture, Guillain-Barré syndrome, and aseptic meningitis (Jensen, 2004).

Nursing Assessment

Note any history of exposure to infected individuals. Determine history of fever and onset and progression of sore throat, malaise, and other complaints. Observe for periorbital edema. Inspect the pharynx and tonsils for inflammation and the presence of patches of gray exudate. Petechiae may be present on the palate. Palpate for bilateral nontender enlargement of the posterior cervical lymph nodes. After 3 to 5 days of illness, the pharynx may become edematous and the tonsillar exudate more extensive. Lymphadenopathy may progress to include the anterior cervical nodes, which may become tender. Palpate the abdomen for the presence of splenomegaly or hepatomegaly. An erythematous maculopapular rash may appear as the illness progresses. Definitive diagnosis may be made by Monospot or Epstein-Barr virus titers.

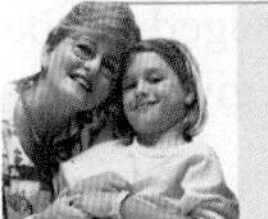

The Monospot is usually negative if obtained within the first 7 to 10 days of illness with infectious mononucleosis. Epstein-Barr virus titer is reliable at any point in the illness.

Nursing Management

Nursing management of mononucleosis is primarily symptomatic. The throat may be very sore, so analgesics and salt-water gargles are recommended. Bed rest should be encouraged while the child is febrile. Frequent rest periods may be necessary for several weeks after the onset of illness, as fatigue may persist as long as 6 weeks. During the acute phase, if tonsillar or pharyngeal edema threatens to obstruct the airway, then corticosteroids may be given to decrease the inflammation. In the presence of splenomegaly or hepatomegaly, strenuous activity and contact sports should be avoided. Appearance of rash or jaundice should be reported to the physician.

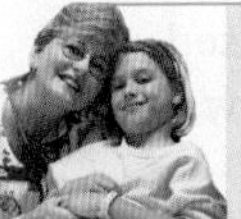

Concomitant strep throat in the presence of infectious mononucleosis should be treated with an antibiotic other than ampicillin, as it may cause an allergic-type rash if used in the presence of mononucleosis.

LARYNGITIS

Inflammation of the larynx is termed **laryngitis**. It may occur alone or in conjunction with other respiratory symptoms. It is characterized by a hoarse voice or loss of the voice (so soft as to make it difficult to hear). Oral fluids might offer relief, but resting the voice for 24 hours will allow the inflammation to subside. Laryngitis alone requires no further intervention.

CROUP

Children between 3 months and 3 years of age are the most frequently affected with croup, though croup may affect any child. Croup is also referred to as laryngotracheobronchitis because inflammation and edema of the larynx, trachea, and bronchi occur as a result of viral infection. Parainfluenza is responsible for the majority of cases of croup. Other causes include adenovirus, influenza virus A and B, RSV, and rarely measles virus or *Mycoplasma pneumoniae* (Bjornson et al., 2004). The inflammation and edema obstruct the airway, resulting in symptoms. Mucus production also occurs, further contributing to obstruction of the airway. Narrowing of the subglottic area of the trachea results in audible inspiratory stridor. Edema of the larynx causes hoarseness. Inflammation in the larynx and trachea causes the characteristic barking cough of croup. Symptoms occur most often at night, and croup is usually self-limited, lasting only about 3 to 5 days (Leung et al., 2004).

Croup often presents suddenly at night, with resolution of symptoms in the morning. Complications of croup are rare but may include worsening respiratory distress, hypoxia, or bacterial superinfection (as in the case of bacterial tracheitis). Croup is usually managed on an outpatient basis, with only 1% to 2% of cases requiring hospitalization (Leung et al., 2004).

Corticosteroids (usually a single dose) are used to decrease inflammation and racemic epinephrine aerosols demonstrate the alpha-adrenergic effect of mucosal vasoconstriction, helping to decrease edema (Bjornson et al., 2004; Schooff, 2005). Children with croup may be hospitalized if they have significant stridor at rest or severe retractions after a several-hour period of observation. Comparison Chart 19.2 gives information comparing croup to epiglottis.

Nursing Assessment

Note the age of the child; children between 3 months and 3 years of age are most likely to present with viral croup (laryngotracheobronchitis). History may reveal a cough that developed during the night (most common presentation) and that sounds like barking (or a seal). Inspect for presence of mild URI symptoms. Temperature may be normal or elevated mildly. Listen for inspiratory stridor and observe for suprasternal retractions. Auscultate

COMPARISON CHART 19.2 Croup vs. Epiglottitis

	Spasmodic Croup	Epiglottitis
Preceding illness	None or minimal coryza	None or mild upper respiratory infection
Usually affects age:	3 months to 3 years	1 to 8 years
Onset	Usually sudden, often at night	Rapid (within hours)
Fever	Variable	High
Barking cough, hoarseness	Yes	No
Dysphagia	No	Yes
Toxic appearance	No	Yes
Cause	Viral	*Haemophilus influenzae* type B

the lungs for adequacy of breath sounds. Various scales are available for scoring croup severity, though these are of limited value in the clinical assessment and treatment of croup (Leung et al., 2004). Croup is usually diagnosed based on history and clinical presentation, but a lateral neck x-ray may be obtained to rule out epiglottitis.

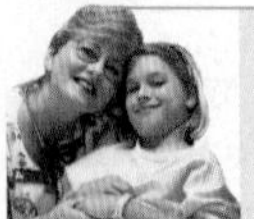

The child with fever, a toxic appearance, and increasing respiratory distress despite appropriate croup treatment may have bacterial tracheitis (Orenstein, 2004). Notify the physician of these findings in a child with croup.

Nursing Management

If the child's care is being managed at home, advise parents about the symptoms of respiratory distress and instruct them to seek treatment if the child's respiratory condition worsens. Teach parents to expose their child to humidified air (via a cool mist humidifier or steamy bathroom). Though never clinically proven, use of humidified air has long been recommended for alleviating coughing jags and anecdotally reported as helpful. Administer dexamethasone if ordered or teach parents about home administration. Explain to parents that the effects of racemic epinephrine last about 2 hours and the child must be observed closely as occasionally a child will worsen again, requiring another aerosol. Teaching Guideline 19.2 gives information about home care of croup.

EPIGLOTTITIS

Epiglottitis (inflammation and swelling of the epiglottis) is most often caused by *Haemophilus influenzae* type b. Extensive use of the Hib vaccine since the 1980s has resulted in a significant decrease in the incidence of epiglottitis. Epiglottitis usually occurs in children between the ages of 2 and 7 years and can be life threatening (Leung et al., 2004). Respiratory arrest and death may occur if the airway becomes completely occluded. Additional complications include pneumothorax and pulmonary edema. Therapeutic management focuses on airway maintenance and support. Intravenous antibiotic therapy is necessary (Tanner et al., 2002). The child will be managed in the intensive care unit. Comparison Chart 19.2 gives information comparing croup to epiglottitis.

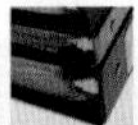

TEACHING GUIDELINE 19.2

Home Care of Croup

- Keep the child quiet and discourage crying.
- Allow the child to sit up (in your arms).
- Encourage rest and fluid intake.
- If stridor occurs, take the child into a steamy bathroom for 10 minutes.
- Administer medication (corticosteroid) as directed.
- Watch the child closely. Call the physician if:
  - The child breathes faster, has retractions, or has any other difficulty breathing
  - The nostrils flare or the lips or nails have a bluish tint
  - The cough or stridor does not improve with exposure to moist air
  - Restlessness increases or the child is confused
  - The child begins to drool or cannot swallow

Adapted from Knutson, 2004.

Nursing Assessment

Carefully assess the child with suspected epiglottitis. Note sudden onset of symptoms and high fever. The child has an overall toxic appearance. He or she may refuse to speak or may speak only with a very soft voice. The child may refuse to lie down and may assume the characteristic position, sitting forward with the neck extended. Drooling may be present. Note anxiety or a frightened appearance. Note the child's color. Cough is usually absent. A lateral neck x-ray may be performed to determine the presence of epiglottitis. This is done cautiously, so as not to induce airway obstruction with changes in position of the child's neck (Bjornson et al., 2004; Tanner et al., 2002).

Nursing Management

Do not leave the child unattended. Keep the child and parents as calm as possible. Allow the child to assume a position of comfort. *Do not* place the child in a supine position, as airway occlusion may occur. Provide 100% oxygen in the least invasive manner that is most acceptable to the child. Do not under any circumstance attempt to visualize the throat: reflex laryngospasm may occur, precipitating immediate airway occlusion. If the child with epiglottitis experiences complete airway occlusion, an emergency tracheostomy may be necessary. Ensure that emergency equipment is available and that personnel specifically trained in intubation of the pediatric occluded airway and percutaneous tracheostomy are notified of the child's presence in the facility (Bjornson et al., 2004; Tanner et al., 2002).

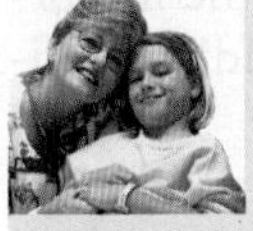

Epiglottitis is characterized by dysphagia, drooling, anxiety, irritability, and significant respiratory distress. Prepare for the event of sudden airway occlusion.

● BRONCHIOLITIS (RSV)

Bronchiolitis is an acute inflammatory process of the bronchioles and small bronchi. Nearly always caused by a viral pathogen, RSV accounts for the majority of cases of bronchiolitis, with adenovirus, parainfluenza, and human meta-pneumovirus also being important causative agents. This discussion will focus on RSV bronchiolitis.

The peak incidence of bronchiolitis is in the winter and spring, coinciding with RSV season. RSV season in the United States and Canada generally begins in September or October and continues through April or May. Virtually all children will contract RSV infection within the first few years of life. RSV bronchiolitis occurs most often in infants and toddlers, with a peak incidence around 6 months of age. The severity of disease is related inversely to the age of the child, with the most severe cases occurring between 1 and 3 months of age (Weisman & Groothius, 2000). The frequency and severity of RSV infection decrease with age. Repeated RSV infections occur throughout life but are usually localized to the upper respiratory tract after toddlerhood.

Therapeutic Management

Management of RSV focuses on supportive treatment. Supplemental oxygen, nasal and/or nasopharyngeal suctioning, oral or intravenous hydration, and inhaled bronchodilator therapy are used. Many infants are managed at home with close observation and adequate hydration. Hospitalization is required for children with more severe disease. The infant with tachypnea, significant retractions, poor oral intake, or lethargy can deteriorate quickly, to the point of requiring ventilatory support, and thus warrants hospital admission.

Pathophysiology

RSV is a highly contagious virus and may be contracted through direct contact with respiratory secretions or from particles on objects contaminated with the virus (Lauts, 2005). RSV invades the nasopharynx, where it replicates and then spreads down to the lower airway via aspiration of upper airway secretions. RSV infection causes necrosis of the respiratory epithelium of small airways, peribronchiolar mononuclear infiltration, and plugging of the lumens with mucus and exudate. The small airways become variably obstructed; this allows adequate inspiratory volume but prevents full expiration. This leads to hyperinflation and atelectasis (Cooper et al., 2003) (Fig. 19.9). Serious alterations in gas exchange occur,

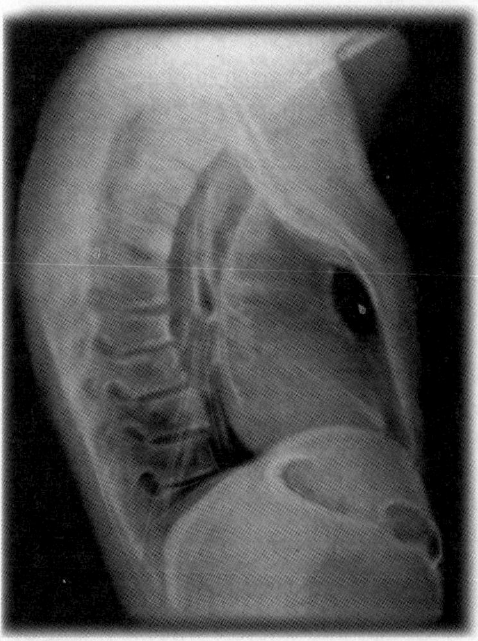

● Figure 19.9 Hyperinflation with atelectasis is noted upon chest x-ray.

with arterial hypoxemia and carbon dioxide retention resulting from mismatching of pulmonary ventilation and perfusion. Hypoventilation occurs secondary to markedly increased work of breathing.

Nursing Assessment

For a full description of the assessment phase of the nursing process, refer to page 552. Assessment findings pertinent to bronchiolitis are discussed below.

Health History

Elicit a description of the present illness and chief complaint. Common signs and symptoms reported during the health history might include:

- Onset of illness with a clear runny nose (sometimes profuse)
- Pharyngitis
- Low-grade fever
- Development of cough 1 to 3 days into the illness, followed by a wheeze shortly thereafter
- Poor feeding

Explore the child's current and past medical history for risk factors such as:

- Young age (less than 2 years old), more severe disease in a child less than 6 months old
- Prematurity
- Multiple births
- Birth during April to September
- History of chronic lung disease (bronchopulmonary disease)
- Cyanotic or complicated congenital heart disease
- Immunocompromise
- Male gender
- Exposure to passive tobacco smoke
- Crowded living conditions
- Daycare attendance
- School-age siblings
- Low socioeconomic status
- Lack of breastfeeding

Physical Examination

Examination of the child with RSV involves inspection, observation, and auscultation.

Inspection and Observation

Observe the child's general appearance and color (centrally and peripherally). The infant with RSV bronchiolitis might appear air-hungry, exhibiting various degrees of cyanosis and respiratory distress, including tachypnea, retractions, accessory muscle use, grunting, and periods of apnea. Cough and audible wheeze might be heard. The infant might appear listless and disinterested in feeding, surroundings, or parents.

Auscultation

Auscultate the lungs, noting adventitious sounds and determining the quality of aeration of the lung fields. Earlier in the illness, wheezes might be heard scattered throughout the lung fields. In more serious cases, the chest might sound quiet and without wheeze. This is attributed to significant hyperexpansion with very poor air exchange.

Laboratory and Diagnostic Tests

Common laboratory and diagnostic studies ordered for the assessment of RSV bronchiolitis include:

- Pulse oximetry: oxygen saturation might be significantly decreased
- Chest x-ray: might reveal hyperinflation and patchy areas of atelectasis or infiltration
- Blood gases: might show carbon dioxide retention and hypoxemia
- Nasal-pharyngeal washings: positive identification of RSV can be made via enzyme-linked immunosorbent assay (ELISA) or immunofluorescent antibody (IFA) testing

Nursing Management

RSV infection is usually self-limited, and nursing diagnoses, goals, and interventions for the child with bronchiolitis are aimed at supportive care. Children with less severe disease might require only antipyretics, adequate hydration, and close observation. They can often be successfully managed at home, provided the primary caregiver is reliable and comfortable with close observation. Parents or caregivers should be educated to watch for signs of worsening and must understand the importance of seeking care quickly should the child's condition deteriorate.

Hospitalization is required for children with more severe disease, and children admitted with RSV bronchiolitis warrant close observation. In addition to the nursing diagnoses and related interventions discussed in the Nursing Care Plan for respiratory disorders, interventions common to bronchiolitis follow.

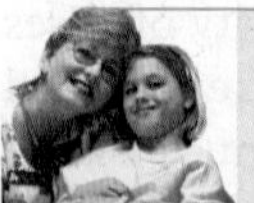

Currently no safe and effective antiviral drug is available for definitive treatment of RSV. Aerosolized ribavirin is recommended only for the highest-risk, most severely ill patients (Lauts, 2005). Routine antibiotic use is discouraged in RSV bronchiolitis treatment because the secondary bacterial infection rate of the lower airway is very low.

Maintaining Patent Airway

Infants and young children with RSV tend to have copious secretions. Position the child with the head of the bed elevated to facilitate an open airway. These children often require frequent assessment and suctioning to maintain a patent airway (Lauts, 2005). Use a Yankauer or tonsil-tip suction catheter to suction the mouth or pharynx of older infants or children, rinsing the catheter after each suctioning. Nasal bulb suctioning may be sufficient to clear the airway in some infants, while others will require nasopharyngeal suctioning with a suction catheter. Nursing Procedure 19.1 gives further information. The routine use of sterile normal saline is not indicated in all children, as its use has been demonstrated to result in decreased oxygen saturations for up to 2 minutes after suctioning is complete (Ridling et al., 2003). Adjust the pressure ranges for suctioning infants and children between 60 and 100 mm Hg, 40 and 60 mm Hg for premature infants.

Promoting Adequate Gas Exchange

Infants and children with bronchiolitis might deteriorate quickly as the disease progresses. In the child ill enough to require oxygen, the risk is even greater. Assessment should include work of breathing, respiratory rate, and oxygen saturation. The percentage of inspired oxygen (FiO_2) should be adjusted as needed to maintain oxygen saturation within the desired range. Positioning the infant with the head of the bed elevated may also improve gas exchange. Frequent assessment is necessary for the hospitalized child with bronchiolitis (Cooper et al., 2003; Steiner, 2004).

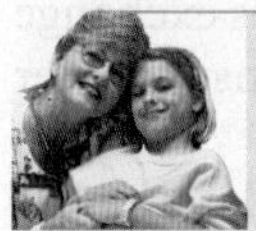

In the tachypneic infant, slowing of the respiratory rate does not necessarily indicate improvement: often, a slower respiratory rate is an indication of tiring, and carbon dioxide retention may soon be followed by apnea.

Reducing Risk for Infection

Since RSV is easily spread through contact with droplets, inpatients should be isolated according to hospital policy to decrease the risk of nosocomial spread to other patients. Patients with RSV can be safely cohorted. Attention to hand washing is necessary, as droplets might enter the eyes, nose, or mouth via the hands.

Providing Family Education

Educate parents to recognize signs of worsening distress. Tell parents to call their physician or nurse practitioner if the breathing is rapid or becomes more difficult or if the child cannot eat secondary to tachypnea. Children who are less than 1 year of age or who are at higher risk (those who were born prematurely or who have chronic heart or lung conditions) might have a longer course of illness. Instruct parents that cough can persist for several days to weeks after resolution of the disease, but infants usually act well otherwise.

Preventing RSV Disease

Strict adherence to hand-washing policies in daycare centers and when exposed to individuals with cold symptoms is important for all groups. Though generally benign in healthy older children, RSV can be devastating in young infants or children with pre-existing risk factors. Palivizumab (Synagis) is a monoclonal antibody effective in the prevention of severe RSV disease in those who are most susceptible. It is given as an intramuscular injection once a month throughout the RSV season. Though quite costly, it is covered by most insurance policies and Medicaid for those who qualify. It is generally indicated for use in certain children less than 2 years of age. Qualifying factors include:

- Prematurity
- Chronic lung disease (bronchopulmonary dysplasia) requiring medication or oxygen
- Certain congenital heart diseases
- Immunocompromise (AAP, 2003)

Nursing Procedure 19.1

Nasopharyngeal or Artificial Airway Suction Technique

1. Check to ensure the suction equipment works properly before starting.
2. After washing your hands, assemble the equipment needed:
   - Appropriate-size sterile suction catheter
   - Sterile gloves
   - Supplemental oxygen
   - Sterile water-based lubricant
   - Sterile normal saline if indicated
3. Don sterile gloves, keeping dominant hand sterile and nondominant hand clean.
4. Preoxygenate the infant or child if indicated.
5. Apply lubricant to the end of the suction catheter.
6. If indicated for loosening of secretions, instill sterile saline.
7. Maintaining sterile technique, insert the suction catheter into the child's nostril or airway.
   - Insert only to the point of gagging if inserting via the nostril.
   - Insert only 0.5 cm further than the length of the artificial airway.
8. Intermittently apply suction for no longer than 10 seconds, while twisting and removing the catheter.
9. Supplement with oxygen after suctioning.

More information related to recommendations for Synagis use can be found at http://aappolicy.aappublications.org/cgi/reprint/pediatrics;112/6/1442.pdf.

● PNEUMONIA

Pneumonia is an inflammation of the lung parenchyma. It can be caused by a virus, bacteria, mycoplasma, or fungus. It may also result from aspiration of foreign material into the lower respiratory tract (aspiration pneumonia). Pneumonia occurs more often in winter and early spring. It is common in children but is seen most frequently in infants and young toddlers. Viruses are the most common cause of pneumonia in younger children and the least common cause in older children (Table 19.2). Viral pneumonia is usually better tolerated in children of all ages. Children with bacterial pneumonia are more apt to present with a toxic appearance, but rapid recovery generally occurs if appropriate antibiotic treatment is instituted early.

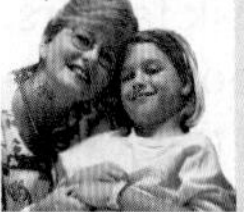

Community-acquired pneumonia (CAP) refers to pneumonia in a previously healthy person that is contracted outside of the hospital setting. CAP is a common cause of lower respiratory infection in North America (Ostapchuk et al., 2004).

Pneumonia is usually a self-limited disease. A child who presents with recurrent pneumonia should be evaluated for chronic lung disease such as asthma or cystic fibrosis. Potential complications of pneumonia include bacteremia, pleural effusion, empyema, lung abscess, and pneumothorax (Nield et al., 2005). Excluding bacteremia, these are often treated with thoracentesis and/or chest tubes as well as antibiotics if appropriate. Pneumatoceles (thin-walled cavities developing in the lung) might occur with certain bacterial pneumonias and usually resolve spontaneously over time.

Therapeutic management of children with less severe disease includes antipyretics, adequate hydration, and close observation. Even bacterial pneumonia can be successfully managed at home if the work of breathing is not severe and oxygen saturation is within normal limits. However, hospitalization is required for children with more severe disease. The child with tachypnea, significant retractions, poor oral intake, or lethargy might require hospital admission for the administration of supplemental oxygen, intravenous hydration, and antibiotics.

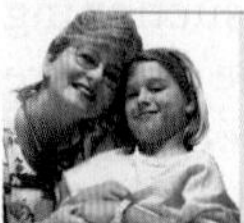

Haemophilus influenzae type B has been nearly eliminated as a cause of pneumonia in the United States and other developed countries as a result of universal immunization with Hib vaccine.

Pathophysiology

Pneumonia occurs as a result of the spread of infectious organisms to the lower respiratory tract from either the upper respiratory tract or the bloodstream. In bacterial pneumonia, mucus stasis occurs as a result of vascular engorgement. Cellular debris (erythrocytes, neutrophils, and fibrin) accumulates in the alveolar space. Relative hyperexpansion with air trapping follows. Inflammation of the alveoli results in atelectasis. **Atelectasis** is defined as a collapsed or airless portion of the lung, so gas exchange becomes impaired. The inflammatory response further impairs gas exchange (Nield et al., 2005).

Viral pneumonia usually results in an inflammatory reaction limited to the alveolar wall. Aspiration of food, fluids, or other substances into the bronchial tree can result in aspiration pneumonia. Aspiration is the most common cause of recurrent pneumonia in children and often occurs as a result of gastroesophageal reflux disease (Turcios & Patel, 2003). Secondary bacterial infection often occurs following viral or aspiration pneumonia and requires antibiotic treatment.

Nursing Assessment

For a full description of the assessment phase of the nursing process, refer to page 552. Assessment findings pertinent to pneumonia are discussed below.

Table 19.2 Common Causes of Pneumonia According to Age

Age Group	Most Common Causative Agents
1 to 3 months	RSV, other respiratory viruses (parainfluenza, influenza, adenovirus); *Streptococcus pneumoniae, Chlamydia trachomatis*
4 months to 5 years	Respiratory viruses, *Streptococcus pneumoniae, Chlamydia pneumoniae, Mycoplasma pneumoniae*
5 to 18 years	*Mycoplasma pneumoniae, Chlamydia pneumoniae, Streptococcus pneumoniae*

(Nield et al., 2005; Ostapchuk, 2004)

Health History

Elicit a description of the present illness and chief complaint. Note onset and progression of symptoms. Common signs and symptoms reported during the health history include:

- Antecedent viral URI
- Fever
- Cough (note type and whether productive or not)
- Increased respiratory rate
- History of lethargy, poor feeding, vomiting, or diarrhea in infants
- Chills, headache, dyspnea, chest pain, abdominal pain, and nausea or vomiting in older children

Explore the child's past and current medical history for risk factors known to be associated with an increase in the severity of pneumonia, such as:

- Prematurity
- Malnutrition
- Passive smoke exposure
- Low socioeconomic status
- Daycare attendance
- Underlying cardiopulmonary, immune, or nervous system disease

Physical Examination

Physical examination consists of inspection, auscultation, percussion, and palpation.

Inspection

Observe the child's general appearance and color (centrally and peripherally). Cyanosis might accompany coughing spells. The child with bacterial pneumonia may appear ill. Assess work of breathing. Children with pneumonia might exhibit substernal, subcostal, or intercostal retractions. Tachypnea and nasal flaring may be present. Describe cough and quality of sputum if produced.

Auscultation

Auscultation of the lungs might reveal wheezes or rales in the younger child. Local or diffuse rales may be present in the older child. Document diminished breath sounds.

Percussion and Palpation

In the older child, percussion might yield local dullness over a consolidated area. Percussion is much less valuable in the infant or younger child. Tactile fremitus felt upon palpation may be increased with pneumonia.

Laboratory and Diagnostic Tests

Common laboratory and diagnostic studies ordered for the assessment of pneumonia include:

- Pulse oximetry: oxygen saturation might be significantly decreased or within normal range
- Chest x-ray: varies according to patient age and causative agent. In infants and young children, bilateral air trapping and perihilar **infiltrates** are the most common findings. Patchy areas of consolidation might also be present. In older children, lobar consolidation is seen more frequently.
- Sputum culture: possibly useful in determining causative bacteria in older children and adolescents
- White blood cell count: might be elevated in the case of bacterial pneumonia

Nursing Management

Nursing diagnoses, goals, and interventions for the child with pneumonia are primarily aimed at providing supportive care and education about the illness and its treatment. Prevention of pneumococcal infection is also important. Children with more severe disease will require hospitalization. Refer to the Nursing Care Plan on page 562 for nursing diagnoses and related interventions. In addition to the interventions listed in the Nursing Care Plan, the following should be noted.

Providing Supportive Care

Ensure adequate hydration and assist in thinning of secretions by encouraging oral fluid intake in the child whose respiratory status is stable. In children with increased work of breathing, intravenous fluids may be necessary to maintain hydration. Allow and encourage the child to assume a position of comfort, usually with the head of the bed elevated to promote aeration of the lungs. If pain due to coughing or pneumonia itself is severe, administer analgesics as prescribed. Provide supplemental oxygen to the child with respiratory distress or hypoxia as needed.

Providing Family Education

Educate the family about the importance of adherence to the prescribed antibiotic regimen. Antibiotics may be given intravenously if the child is hospitalized, but upon discharge or if the child is managed on an outpatient basis, oral antibiotics will be used.

Teach the parents of a child with bacterial pneumonia to expect that following resolution of the acute illness, for 1 to 2 weeks, the child might continue to tire easily and the infant might continue to need small, frequent feedings. Cough may also persist after the acute recovery period but should lessen over time.

If the child is diagnosed with viral pneumonia, parents might not understand that their child does not require an antibiotic. Pneumonia is often perceived by the public as a bacterial infection, so most parents will need an explanation related to treatment of viral infections. As with bacterial pneumonia, the child may experience a week or two of weakness or fatigue following resolution of the acute illness.

The young child is at risk for the development of aspiration pneumonia. Parents need to understand that the child might be at risk for injury related to his or her age and developmental stage. To prevent recurrent or further aspiration, teach the parents the safety measures in Teaching Guideline 19.3.

Preventing Pneumococcal Infection

Children at high risk for severe pneumococcal infection should be immunized against it. This includes all children between 0 and 23 months of age, as well as children between 24 and 59 months of age with certain conditions such as immune deficiency, sickle cell disease, asplenia, chronic cardiac conditions, chronic lung problems, cerebrospinal fluid leaks, chronic renal insufficiency, diabetes mellitus, and organ transplants. For additional information refer to Chapter 9. See Healthy People 2010.

HEALTHY PEOPLE 2010

Objective	Significance
Reduce invasive pneumococcal infections.	• Provide accurate information to families about pneumococcal disease. • Encourage pneumococcal immunization per recommendations.

BRONCHITIS

Bronchitis is an inflammation of the trachea and major bronchi. It is often associated with a URI. Bronchitis is usually viral in nature, though *Mycoplasma pneumoniae* is also an important causative agent in children over 6 years of age. Recovery usually occurs within 5 to 10 days. Therapeutic management involves mainly supportive care. Expectorant administration and adequate hydration are important. If *Mycoplasma* is the cause, antibiotics are indicated (Orenstein, 2004).

Nursing Assessment

The illness might begin with a mild URI. Fever develops, followed by a dry, hacking cough that might become productive in older children. The cough might wake the child at night. Auscultation of the lungs might reveal coarse rales. Respirations remain unlabored. The chest x-ray might show diffuse alveolar hyperinflation and perihilar markings.

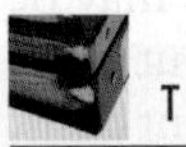

TEACHING GUIDELINE 19.3

Preventing Aspiration

- Keep toxic substances such as lighter fluid, solvents, and hydrocarbons out of reach of young children. Toddlers and preschoolers cannot distinguish safe from unsafe fluids due to their developmental stage.
- Avoid oily nose drops and oil-based vitamins or home remedies to avoid lipid aspiration into the lungs.
- Avoid oral feedings if the infant's respiratory rate is 60 or greater to minimize the risk of aspiration of the feeding.
- Discourage parents from "force-feeding" in the event of poor oral intake or severe illness to minimize the risk of aspiration of the feeding.
- Position infants and ill children on their right side after feeding to minimize the possibility of aspirating emesis or regurgitated feeding.

Nursing Management

Nursing management is aimed at providing supportive care. Teach parents that expectorants will help loosen secretions and antipyretics will help reduce the fever, making the child more comfortable. Encourage adequate hydration. Antibiotics are prescribed only in cases believed to be bacterial in nature. Discourage the use of cough suppressants: it is important for accumulated sputum to be raised.

TUBERCULOSIS

Tuberculosis is a highly contagious disease caused by inhalation of droplets of *Mycobacterium tuberculosis* or *Mycobacterium bovis*. Children usually contract the disease from an immediate household member. Annually about 1,000 U.S. children contract active tuberculosis disease (Reznik & Ozuah, 2005). Nonwhite children and children with chronic illness or malnutrition are more susceptible to infection. After exposure to an infected individual, the incubation period is 2 to 10 weeks. The inhaled tubercle bacilli multiply in the alveoli and alveolar ducts, forming an inflammatory exudate. The bacilli are spread by the bloodstream and lymphatic system to various parts of the body. Though pulmonary tuberculosis is the most common, children may also have infection in other parts of the body, such as the gastrointestinal tract or central nervous system (Starke & Munoz, 2004). See Healthy People 2010.

In the case of drug-sensitive tuberculosis, the American Academy of Pediatrics recommends a 6-month course of oral therapy. The first two months consist of isoniazid, rifampin, and pyrazinamide given daily. This is followed by twice-weekly isoniazid and rifampin; administration must be observed directly (usually by a public health nurse). In the case of multidrug-resistant tuberculosis, ethambutol or streptomycin is given via intramuscular injection (AAP, 2003).

HEALTHY PEOPLE 2010

Objective	Significance
Reduce tuberculosis. Increase the proportion of all tuberculosis patients who complete curative therapy within 12 months. Increase the proportion of contacts and other high-risk persons with latent tuberculosis infection who complete a course of treatment.	• Assess the health history of all infants, children, and adolescents for risk factors for tuberculosis infection. • Provide tuberculosis screening as recommended. • Refer all tuberculosis infections to the local public health department. • Educate families about the importance of completing medication therapy as prescribed for active and latent tuberculosis, and the need for appropriate follow-up and retesting for tuberculosis infection.

Nursing Assessment

Routine screening for tuberculosis infection is not recommended for low-risk individuals, but children considered to be at high risk for contracting tuberculosis should be screened using the Mantoux test. Children considered to be at high risk are those who:

- Are infected with HIV
- Are incarcerated or institutionalized
- Have a positive recent history of latent tuberculosis infection
- Are immigrants from or have a history of travel to endemic countries
- Are exposed at home to HIV-infected or homeless persons, illicit drug users, migrant farm workers, or nursing home residents

Children with chronic illnesses (except HIV infection) are not more likely to become infected with tuberculosis but should receive special consideration and be screened prior to initiation of immunosuppressant therapies (Reznik & Ozuah, 2005).

The presentation of tuberculosis in children is quite varied. Children can be asymptomatic or exhibit a broad range of symptoms. Symptoms may include fever, malaise, weight loss, anorexia, pain and tightness in the chest, and rarely hemoptysis. Cough might or might not be present and usually progresses slowly over several weeks to months. As tuberculosis progresses, the respiratory rate increases and the lung on the affected side is poorly expanded. Dullness to percussion might be present, as well as diminished breath sounds and crackles. Fever persists and pallor, anemia, weakness, and weight loss are present. Diagnosis is confirmed with a positive Mantoux test, positive gastric washings for acid-fast bacillus, and/or a chest x-ray consistent with tuberculosis (Reznik & Ozuah, 2005).

Nursing Management

Hospitalization of children with tuberculosis is necessary only for the most serious cases. Nursing management is aimed at providing supportive care and encouraging adherence to the treatment regimen. Most nursing care for childhood tuberculosis is provided in outpatient clinics, schools, or a public health setting. Supportive care includes ensuring adequate nutrition and adequate rest, providing comfort measures such as fever reduction, preventing exposure to other infectious diseases, and preventing reinfection.

Providing Care for the Child with Latent Tuberculosis Infection

Children who test positive for tuberculosis but who do not have symptoms or radiographic/laboratory evidence of disease are considered to have latent infection. These children should be treated with isoniazid for 9 months to prevent progression to active disease. Follow-up and appropriate monitoring can be achieved via the child's primary care provider or local health department.

Preventing Infection

Tuberculosis infection is prevented by avoiding contact with the tubercle bacillus. Thus, hospitalized children with tuberculosis must be isolated according to hospital policy to prevent nosocomial spread of tuberculosis infection. Promotion of natural resistance through nutrition, rest, and avoidance of serious infections does not prevent infection. Pasteurization of milk has helped to decrease the transmission of *Mycobacterium bovis.* Administration of bacille Calmette-Guérin (BCG) vaccine can provide incomplete protection against tuberculosis and is not widely used in the United States.

Acute Noninfectious Disorders

Acute noninfectious disorders include epistaxis, foreign body aspiration, respiratory distress syndrome, acute respiratory distress syndrome, and pneumothorax.

● EPISTAXIS

Epistaxis (a nosebleed) occurs most frequently in children younger than adolescent age. Bleeding of the nasal mucosa occurs most often from the anterior portion of the septum. Epistaxis may be recurrent and idiopathic (meaning there is no cause). The majority of cases are benign, but in children with bleeding disorders or other hematologic concerns, epistaxis should be further investigated and treated.

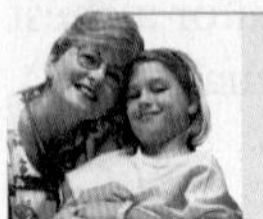

The child with recurrent epistaxis or epistaxis that is difficult to control should be further evaluated for underlying bleeding or platelet concerns.

Nursing Assessment

Explore the child's history for initiating factors such as local inflammation, mucosal drying, or local trauma (usually nose picking). Inspect the nasal cavity for blood.

Nursing Management

The presence of blood often frightens children and their parents. The nurse and parents should remain calm. The child should sit up and lean forward (lying down may allow aspiration of the blood). Apply continuous pressure to the anterior portion of the nose by pinching it closed. Encourage the child to breathe through the mouth during this portion of the treatment. Ice or a cold cloth applied to the bridge of the nose may also be helpful. The bleeding usually stops within 10 to 15 minutes. Apply petroleum jelly or water-soluble gel to the nasal mucosa with a cotton-tipped applicator to moisten the mucosa and prevent recurrence.

• FOREIGN BODY ASPIRATION

Foreign body aspiration occurs when any solid or liquid substance is inhaled into the respiratory tract. It is common in infants and young children and can present in a life-threatening manner (Qureshi & Mink, 2003). The object may lodge in the upper or lower airway, causing varying degrees of respiratory difficulty. Small, smooth objects such as peanuts are the most frequently aspirated, but any small toy, article, or piece of food smaller than the diameter of the young child's airway can potentially be aspirated: popcorn, vegetables, hot dogs, fruit snacks, coins, latex balloon pieces, pins, and pen caps are commonly seen (Qureshi & Mink, 2003).

Foreign body aspiration occurs most frequently in children ages 6 months to 5 years. Children this age are growing and developing rapidly. They tend to explore things with their mouths and can easily aspirate small items.

The child often coughs out foreign bodies from the upper airway. If the foreign body reaches the bronchus, then it may need to be surgically removed via bronchoscopy. Postoperative antibiotics are used if an infection is also present. Complications of foreign body aspiration include pneumonia or abscess formation, hypoxia, respiratory failure, and death (Orenstein, 2004).

Nursing Assessment

The infant or young child might present with a history of sudden onset of cough, wheeze, or stridor. Stridor suggests that the foreign body is lodged in the upper airway. Sometimes the onset of respiratory symptoms is much more gradual. When the item has traveled down one of the bronchi, then wheezing, rhonchi, and decreased aeration can be heard on the affected side. A chest x-ray will demonstrate the foreign body only if it is radiopaque (Fig. 19.10).

Nursing Management

The most important nursing intervention related to foreign body aspiration is prevention. Anticipatory guidance for families with 6-month-olds should include a discussion of aspiration avoidance. This information should be reiterated at each subsequent well-child visit through age 5. Tell parents to avoid letting their child play with toys with small parts and to keep coins and other small objects out of the reach of children. Teach parents not to feed peanuts and popcorn to their child until he or she is at least 3 years old. When children progress to table food, teach parents to chop all foods so that they are small enough to pass down the trachea should the child neglect to chew them up thoroughly. Carrots, grapes, and hot dogs should be cut into small pieces. Harmful liquids should be kept out of the reach of children.

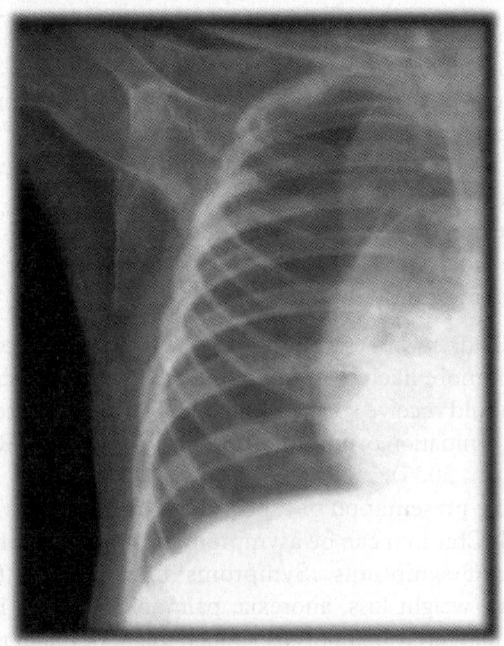

● **Figure 19.10** Foreign body is noted in the bronchus upon chest x-ray.

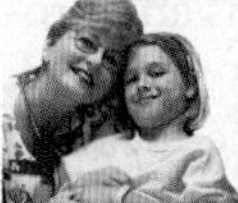

Items smaller than 1.25 inches (3.2 cm) can be aspirated easily. A simple way for parents to estimate the safe size of a small item or toy piece is to gauge its size against a standard toilet paper roll, which is generally about 1.5 inches in diameter.

● RESPIRATORY DISTRESS SYNDROME

Respiratory distress syndrome (RDS) is a respiratory disorder that is specific to neonates. It results from lung immaturity and a deficiency in surfactant, so it is seen most often in premature infants. Other infants who might experience RDS include infants of diabetic mothers, those delivered via cesarean section without preceding labor, and those experiencing perinatal asphyxia. It is believed that each of these conditions has an impact on surfactant production, thus resulting in RDS in the term infant (Stoll & Kliegman, 2004).

The administration of surfactant via endotracheal tube shortly after delivery helps to decrease the incidence and severity of RDS. Management of RDS focuses on intensive respiratory care, usually with mechanical ventilation. Newer techniques for ventilatory support are also available (Table 19.3).

Pathophysiology

The lack of surfactant in the affected newborn's lungs results in stiff, poorly compliant lungs with poor gas exchange. Right-to-left shunting and hypoxemia result. As the disease progresses, fluid and fibrin leak from the pulmonary capillaries, causing hyaline membrane to form in the bronchioles, alveolar ducts, and alveoli. Presence of the membrane further decreases gas exchange. Complications of RDS include air leak syndrome, bronchopulmonary dysplasia, patent ductus arteriosus and congestive heart failure, intraventricular hemorrhage, retinopathy of prematurity, necrotizing enterocolitis, complications resulting from intravenous catheter use (infection, thrombus formation), and developmental delay or disability (Stoll & Kliegman, 2004).

Nursing Assessment

The onset of RDS is usually within several hours of birth. The newborn exhibits signs of respiratory distress, including tachypnea, retractions, nasal flaring, grunting, and varying degrees of cyanosis. Auscultation reveals fine rales and diminished breath sounds. If untreated, RDS progresses to seesaw respirations, respiratory failure, and shock.

Nursing Management

Rarely, mucus plugging can occur in the neonate placed on a ventilator after surfactant administration. Therefore, close observation and assessment for adequate lung expansion are critical. In addition to expert respiratory intervention, other crucial nursing goals include maintenance of normothermia, prevention of infection, maintenance of fluid and electrolyte balance, and promotion of adequate nutrition (parenterally or via gavage feeding). Nursing care of the infant with RDS generally occurs in the intensive care unit.

● ACUTE RESPIRATORY DISTRESS SYNDROME

Acute respiratory distress syndrome (ARDS) occurs following a primary insult such as sepsis, viral pneumonia,

Table 19.3 Alternatives to Traditional Mechanical Ventilation

Mode	Description	Additional Information
High-frequency ventilators (high frequency, oscillating, or jet)	Provide very high respiratory rates (up to 1,200 breaths per minute) and very low tidal volumes	May decrease risk of barotrauma associated with ventilator pressures
Nitric oxide	Causes pulmonary vasodilation, helping to increase blood flow to alveoli	Safe; no long-term developmental risks
Liquid ventilation	Perfluorocarbon liquid acts as a surfactant. Provides an effective medium for gas exchange and increases pulmonary function.	Virtually no reported physiologic sequelae
Extracorporeal membrane oxygenation (ECMO)	Blood is removed from body via catheter, warmed and oxygenated in the ECMO machine, and then returned to infant.	Labor-intensive. Risk of bleeding is great.

smoke inhalation, or near-drowning. Acute onset of respiratory distress and hypoxemia occur within 72 hours of the insult in infants and children with previously healthy lungs. The alveolar–capillary membrane becomes more permeable and pulmonary edema develops. Hyaline membrane formation over the alveolar surfaces and decreased surfactant production cause lung stiffness. Mucosal swelling and cellular debris lead to atelectasis. Gas diffusion is impaired significantly. ARDS can progress to respiratory failure and death, though some individuals recover completely or have residual lung disease.

Medical treatment is aimed at improving **oxygenation** and **ventilation**. Mechanical ventilation is used with special attention to lung volumes and positive end-expiratory pressure (PEEP). Newer treatment modalities show promise for improving outcomes of ARDS.

Nursing Assessment

Tachycardia and tachypnea occur over the first few hours of the illness. Significantly increased work of breathing with nasal flaring and retractions develops. Auscultate for breath sounds, which might range from normal to high-pitched crackles throughout the lung fields. Hypoxemia develops. Bilateral infiltrates can be seen on a chest x-ray.

Nursing Management

Nursing care of the child with ARDS is mainly supportive and occurs in the intensive care unit. Closely monitor respiratory and cardiovascular status. Comfort measures such as hygiene and positioning as well as pain and anxiety management, maintenance of nutrition, and prevention of infection are also key nursing interventions. The acute phase of worsening respiratory distress can be frightening for a child of any age, and the nurse can be instrumental in soothing the child's fears. As the disease worsens and progresses, especially when ventilatory support is required, psychological support of the family as well as education about the intensive care unit procedures will be especially important.

PNEUMOTHORAX

A collection of air in the pleural space is called a pneumothorax. It can occur spontaneously in an otherwise healthy child, or as a result of chronic lung disease, cardiopulmonary resuscitation, surgery, or trauma. Trapped air consumes space within the pleural cavity, and the affected lung suffers at least partial collapse. Needle aspiration and/or placement of a chest tube is used to evacuate the air from the chest. Some small pneumothoraces resolve independently, without intervention (Cunnington, 2002).

Nursing Assessment

Primary pneumothorax (spontaneous) occurs most often in adolescence. The infant or child with a pneumothorax might have a sudden or gradual onset of symptoms. Chest pain might be present as well as signs of respiratory distress such as tachypnea, retractions, nasal flaring, or grunting. Assess potential risk factors for acquiring a pneumothorax, including chest trauma or surgery, intubation and mechanical ventilation, or a history of chronic lung disease such as cystic fibrosis. Inspect the child for a pale or cyanotic appearance. Auscultate for increased heart rate (tachycardia) and absent or diminished breath sounds on the affected side. The x-ray reveals air within the thoracic cavity (Fig. 19.11).

Nursing Management

The child with a pneumothorax requires frequent respiratory assessments. Pulse oximetry might be used as an

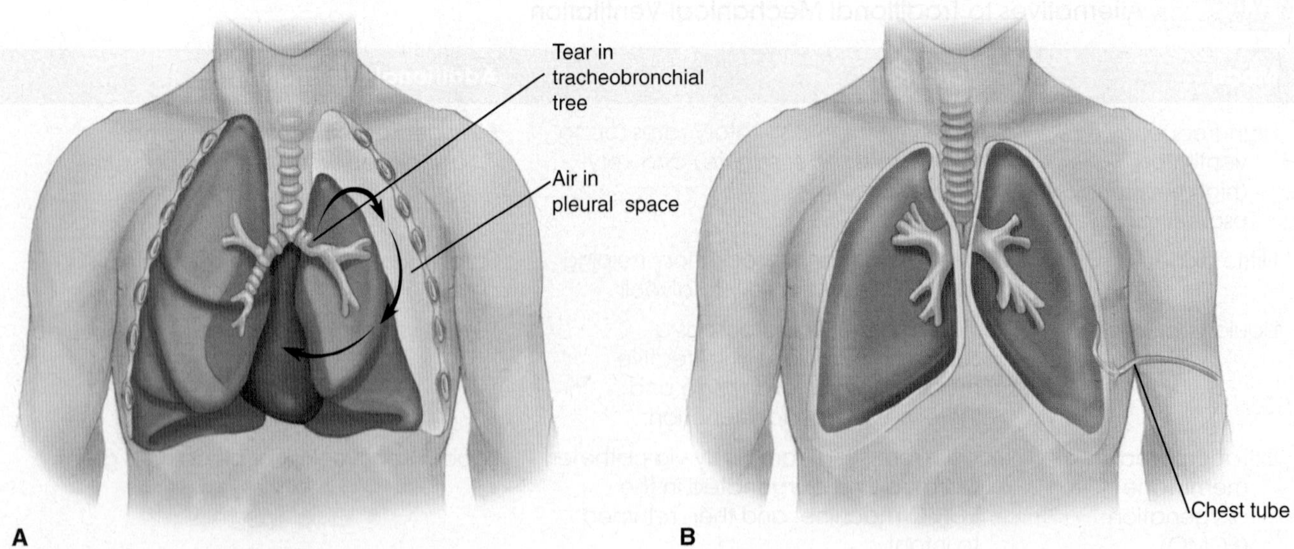

● Figure 19.11 Pneumothorax.

adjunct, but clinical evaluation of respiratory status is most useful. In some cases, administration of 100% oxygen hastens the reabsorption of air, but it is generally used only for a few hours. If a chest tube connected to a water seal or suction is present, provide care of the drainage apparatus as appropriate (Fig. 19.12). A pair of hemostats should be kept at the bedside to clamp the tube should it become dislodged from the drainage container. The dressing around the chest tube is occlusive and is not routinely changed. If the tube becomes dislodged from the child's chest, apply Vaseline gauze and an occlusive dressing, immediately perform appropriate respiratory assessment, and notify the physician.

Chronic Diseases

Chronic respiratory disorders include allergic rhinitis, asthma, chronic lung disease (bronchopulmonary dysplasia), cystic fibrosis, and apnea.

● ALLERGIC RHINITIS

Allergic **rhinitis** is a common chronic condition in childhood, affecting up to 40% of children (Hagemann, 2005). Allergic rhinitis is associated with atopic dermatitis and asthma, with as many as 80% of asthmatic children also suffering from allergic rhinitis (Corren, 2000). Perennial allergic rhinitis occurs year-round and is associated with indoor environments. Allergens commonly implicated in perennial allergic rhinitis include dust mites, pet dander, cockroach antigens, and molds. Seasonal allergic rhinitis is caused by elevations in outdoor levels of allergens. It is typically caused by certain pollens, trees, weeds, fungi, and molds. Complications from allergic rhinitis include exacerbation of asthma symptoms, recurrent sinusitis and otitis media, and dental malocclusion.

Pathophysiology

Allergic rhinitis is an intermittent or persistent inflammatory state that is mediated by immunoglobulin E (IgE). In response to contact with an airborne allergen protein, the nasal mucosa mounts an immune response. The antigen (from the allergen) binds to a specific IgE on the surface of mast cells, releasing the chemical mediators of histamine and leukotrienes. The release of mediators results in acute tissue edema and mucous production (Banasiak & Meadows-Oliver, 2005). Late-phase mediators are released and more inflammation results. IgE binds to receptors on the surfaces of mast cells and basophils, creating the sensitization memory that causes the reaction with subsequent allergen exposures. Allergen exposure then results in mast cell degranulation and release of histamine and other chemotactic factors. Histamine and other factors cause nasal vasodilation, watery rhinorrhea, and nasal congestion. Irritation of local nerve endings by histamine produces pruritus and sneezing (Hagemann, 2005). Treatment of allergic rhinitis is aimed at decreasing response to these allergic mediators as well as treating inflammation.

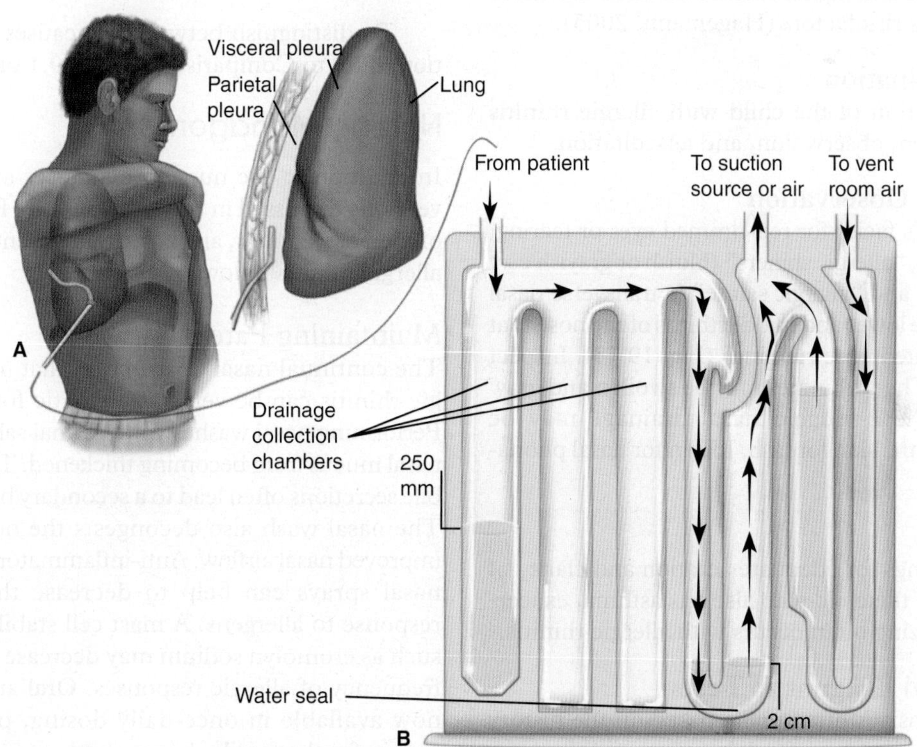

● Figure 19.12 The chest tube is connected to suction or water seal via a drainage container.

Nursing Assessment

For a full description of the assessment phase of the nursing process, refer to page 552. Assessment findings pertinent to allergic rhinitis are discussed below.

Health History

Elicit a description of the present illness and chief complaint. Common signs and symptoms reported during the health history might include:

- Mild, intermittent to chronic nasal stuffiness
- Thin, runny nasal discharge
- Sneezing
- Itching of nose, eyes, palate
- Mouth breathing and snoring

Determine the seasonality of symptoms. Are they perennial (year-round) or do they occur during certain seasons? What types of medications or other treatments have been used, and what was the child's response?

Explore the history for the presence of risk factors such as:

- Family history of atopic disease (asthma, allergic rhinitis, or atopic dermatitis)
- Known allergy to dust mites, pet dander, cockroach antigens, pollens, or molds
- Early childhood exposure to indoor allergens
- Early introduction to foods or formula in infancy
- Exposure to tobacco smoke
- Environmental air pollution
- Recurrent viral infections

Nonwhite race and higher socioeconomic status have also been noted as risk factors (Hagemann, 2005).

Physical Examination

Physical examination of the child with allergic rhinitis includes inspection, observation, and auscultation.

Inspection and Observation

Observe the child's facies for red-rimmed eyes or tearing, mild eyelid edema, "allergic shiners" (bluish or grayish cast beneath the eyes), and "allergic salute" (a transverse nasal crease between the lower and middle thirds of the nose that results from repeated nose rubbing) (Fig. 19.13). Inspect the nasal cavity. The turbinates may be swollen and gray/blue in color. Clear mucoid nasal drainage may be observed. Inspect the skin for rash. Listen for nasal phonation with speech.

Auscultation

Auscultate the lungs for adequate aeration and clarity of breath sounds. In the child who also has asthma, exacerbation with wheezing often occurs with allergic rhinitis.

Laboratory and Diagnostic Tests

The initial diagnosis is often made based on the history and clinical findings. Common laboratory and diagnostic studies ordered for the assessment of allergic rhinitis may include:

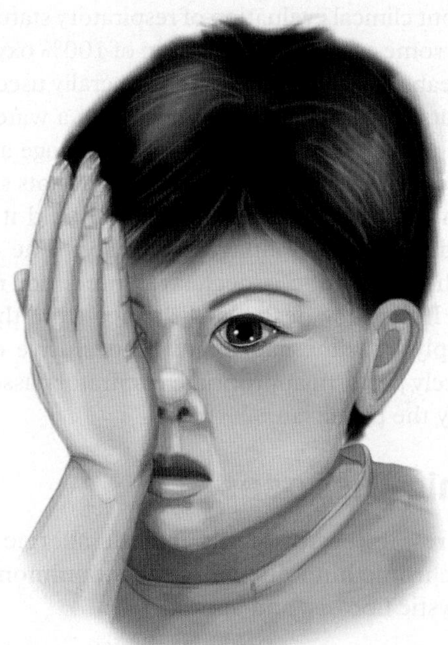

● **Figure 19.13** Allergic shiners beneath the eyes and allergic salute across the nose.

- Nasal smear (positive for eosinophilia)
- Positive allergy skin test
- Positive RAST

To distinguish between the causes of nasal congestion, refer to Comparison Chart 19.1 on page 568.

Nursing Management

In addition to the nursing diagnoses and related interventions discussed in the Nursing Care Plan for disorders of the nose, mouth, and throat, interventions common to allergic rhinitis follow.

Maintaining Patent Airway

The continual nasal obstruction that occurs with allergic rhinitis can be very problematic for some children. Performing nasal washes with normal saline may keep the nasal mucus from becoming thickened. Thickened, immobile secretions often lead to a secondary bacterial infection. The nasal wash also decongests the nose, allowing for improved nasal airflow. Anti-inflammatory (corticosteroid) nasal sprays can help to decrease the inflammatory response to allergens. A mast cell stabilizing nasal spray such as cromolyn sodium may decrease the intensity and frequency of allergic responses. Oral antihistamines are now available in once-daily dosing, providing convenience for the family. Some children may benefit from a combined antihistamine/nasal decongestant if nasal congestion is significant. Leukotriene modifiers such as montelukast may also be beneficial for some children (Banasiak & Meadows-Oliver, 2005).

Providing Family Education

One of the most important tools in the treatment of allergic rhinitis is learning to avoid known allergens. Teaching Guideline 19.4 gives information on educating families about avoidance of allergens. Children may be referred to a specialist for allergen desensitization (allergy shots). Products helpful with control of allergies are available from a number of vendors, such as www.onlineallergyrelief.com.

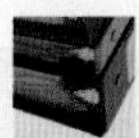

TEACHING GUIDELINE 19.4

Controlling Exposure to Allergens

Tobacco

- Avoid all exposure to tobacco smoke (this includes self-smoking).
- If parents cannot quit, they must not smoke inside the home or car.

Dust Mites

- Use pillow and mattress covers.
- Wash sheets, pillowcases, and comforters once a week in 130 degree F water.
- Use blinds rather than curtains in bedroom.
- Remove stuffed animals from bedroom.
- Reduce indoor humidity to <50%.
- Remove carpet from bedroom.
- Clean solid surface floors with wet mop each week.

Pet Dander

- Remove pets from home permanently.
- If unable to remove them, keep them out of bedroom and off carpet and upholstered furniture.

Cockroaches

- Keep kitchen very clean.
- Avoiding leaving out food or drinks.
- Use pesticides if necessary, but ensure that the asthmatic child is not insidc the home when it is sprayed.

Indoor Molds

- Repair water leaks.
- Use dehumidifier to keep basement dry.
- Reduce indoor humidity to <50%.

Outdoor Molds, Pollen, and Air Pollution

- Avoid going outdoors when mold and pollen counts are high.
- Avoid outdoor activity when pollution levels are high.

● ASTHMA

Asthma is a chronic inflammatory airway disorder characterized by airway hyperresponsiveness, airway edema, and mucus production. Airway obstruction resulting from asthma might be partially or completely reversed. Severity ranges from long periods of control with infrequent acute exacerbations in some children to the presence of persistent daily symptoms in others (Kieckhefer & Ratcliffe, 2004). It is the most common chronic illness of childhood and affects about 9 million American children (Kumar et al., 2005). A small percentage of children with asthma account for a large percentage of health care use and expense (Wakefield et al., 2005). Asthma accounts for about 12 million lost school days per year and a significant number of lost workdays on the part of parents (Lara et al., 2002). The incidence and severity of asthma are increasing; this might be attributed to increased urbanization, increased air pollution, and more accurate diagnosis.

Severity ranges from symptoms associated only with vigorous activity (exercise-induced bronchospasm) to daily symptoms that interfere with quality of life. Though uncommon, childhood death related to asthma is also on the rise worldwide. Air pollution, allergens, family history, and viral infections might all play a role in asthma. Many children with asthma also have gastroesophageal disease, though the relationship between the two diseases is not clearly understood.

Complications of asthma include chronic airway remodeling, status asthmaticus, and respiratory failure. Children with asthma are also more susceptible to serious bacterial and viral respiratory infections.

Current goals of medical therapy are avoidance of asthma triggers and reduction or control of inflammatory episodes. Current recommendations by the National Asthma Education and Prevention Program suggest a stepwise approach to management as well as avoidance of allergens. The stepwise approach involves increasing treatment as the child's condition worsens, then backing off treatment as he or she improves (Table 19.4). Leukotriene modifiers have been found to be effective in the short-term management of chronic asthma (Berkhof et al., 2003). Long-term prevention usually involves inhaled steroids. Bronchodilators may be used in the acute treatment of bronchoconstriction or in the long-acting form to prevent bronchospasm. Exercise-induced bronchospasm may occur in any child with asthma or as the only symptom in the child with mild intermittent asthma. Most children may avoid exercise-induced bronchospasm by using a longer warm-up period prior to vigorous exercise and, if necessary, inhaling a short-acting bronchodilator just prior to exercise. See Healthy People 2010.

Table 19.4 Asthma Severity Classification and Treatment Approach

Classification & Referral	Symptoms	Lung Function	Long-Term Control	Quick Relief
Step 1: Mild intermittent	• One or two times a week • No symptoms and normal PEFR between exacerbations • Intensity of exacerbations varies, though usually brief in length. • Nighttime symptoms one or two times a month	PEFR 80% or more of predicted, variability <20%	No daily medication needed	Short-acting bronchodilator PRN symptoms
Step 2: Mild persistent (referral to asthma specialist should be considered)	• Symptoms more than twice a week but less than once a day • Exacerbations may affect activity level. • Nighttime symptoms <2 times a month	PEFR 80% or more of predicted, with 20% to 30% variability	Daily anti-inflammatory medication (low-dose inhaled corticosteroid) (preferred) OR cromolyn OR leukotriene modifier	Short-acting bronchodilator PRN symptoms
Step 3: Moderate persistent (referral to asthma specialist recommended)	• Daily symptoms • Daily use of inhaled short-acting beta$_2$-agonist • Exacerbations affect activity. • Exacerbations 2 or more times a week; may last days • Nighttime symptoms >1 time a week	PEFR 60% to 80% of predicted, with variability >30%	Daily anti-inflammatory medication (medium-dose inhaled corticosteroid OR low-dose inhaled corticosteroid AND long-acting bronchodilator)	Short-acting bronchodilator PRN symptoms up to TID
Step 4: Severe persistent (referral to asthma specialist recommended)	• Continual symptoms • Limited physical activity • Frequent exacerbations • Frequent nighttime symptoms	PEFR 60% or less of predicted, with variability >30%	Daily anti-inflammatory medicine (high-dose inhaled corticosteroid) and long-acting bronchodilator. May need systemic corticosteroids.	Short-acting bronchodilator PRN symptoms up to TID

PEFR, peak expiratory flow rate.

Adapted from National Asthma Education and Prevention Program. (1997, July). *Expert panel report 2: Guidelines for the diagnosis and management of asthma* (NIH Publication No. 97-4051) and (2002). *Update on selected topics.* (Publication No. 02-5075). Bethesda, MD: National Institutes of Health, National Heart, Lung and Blood Institute. These recommendations are intended to be used as a guide in individualized asthma care.

HEALTHY PEOPLE 2010

Objective	Significance
Reduce asthma deaths, hospitalizations for asthma, and hospital emergency department visits for asthma.	• Provide appropriate education and triage to families of children with asthma, particularly when the child is experiencing symptoms or a decreased peak flow rate.

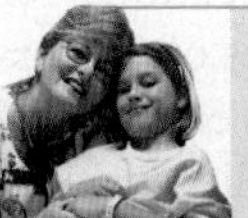

Currently many manufacturers use chlorofluorocarbon (CFC) as the propellant in metered-dose inhalers. In 2005, the U.S. Food and Drug Administration announced that these types of inhaler would be phased out of the market by the end of 2008. Environmentally friendly formulations of hydrofluoroalkane (HFA) will be used in all metered-dose inhalers by that time (Bederka, 2006).

Pathophysiology

In asthma, the inflammatory process contributes to increased airway activity. Thus, control or prevention of inflammation is the core of asthma management. Asthma results from a complex variety of responses in relation to a trigger. When the process begins, mast cells, T lymphocytes, macrophages, and epithelial cells are involved in the release of inflammatory mediators. Eosinophils and neutrophils migrate to the airway, causing injury. Chemical mediators such as leukotrienes, bradykinin, histamine, and platelet-activating factor also contribute to the inflammatory response. The presence of leukotrienes contributes to prolonged airway constriction (Banasiak & Meadows-Oliver, 2005). Autonomic neural control of airway tone is affected, airway mucus secretion is increased, mucociliary function changes, and airway smooth muscle responsiveness increases (Kiecheter & Ratcliffe, 2004). As a result, acute bronchoconstriction, airway edema, and mucus plugging occur (Fig. 19.14).

In most children, this process is considered reversible and until recently it was not considered to have long-standing effects on lung function. Current research and scientific thought, however, recognize the concept of airway remodeling. Airway remodeling occurs as a result of chronic inflammation of the airway. Following the acute response to a trigger, continued allergen response results in a chronic phase. During this phase, the epithelial cells are denuded and the influx of inflammatory cells into the airway continues. This results in structural changes of the airway that are irreversible, and further loss of pulmonary function might occur (Kiecheter & Ratcliffe, 2004).

Nursing Assessment

For a full description of the assessment phase of the nursing process, refer to page 552. Assessment findings pertinent to asthma are discussed below.

Health History

Elicit a description of the present illness and chief complaint. Common signs and symptoms reported during the health history might include:

- Cough, particularly at night: hacking type of cough that is initially nonproductive, becoming productive of frothy sputum
- Difficulty breathing: shortness of breath, chest tightness or pain, dyspnea with exercise
- Wheezing

Explore the child's current and past medical history for risk factors such as:

- History of allergic rhinitis or atopic dermatitis
- Family history of atopy (asthma, allergic rhinitis, atopic dermatitis)

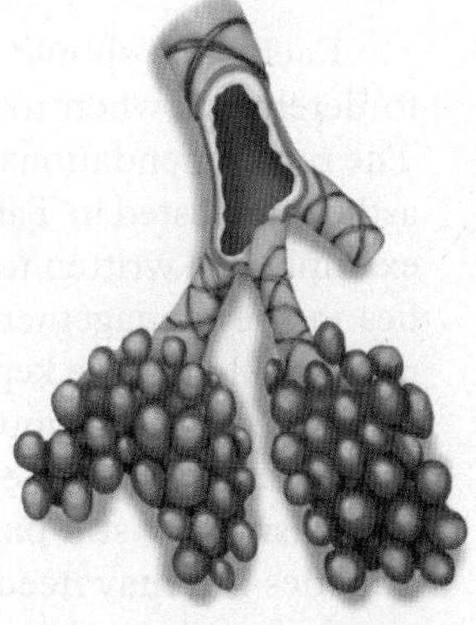

Normal airway

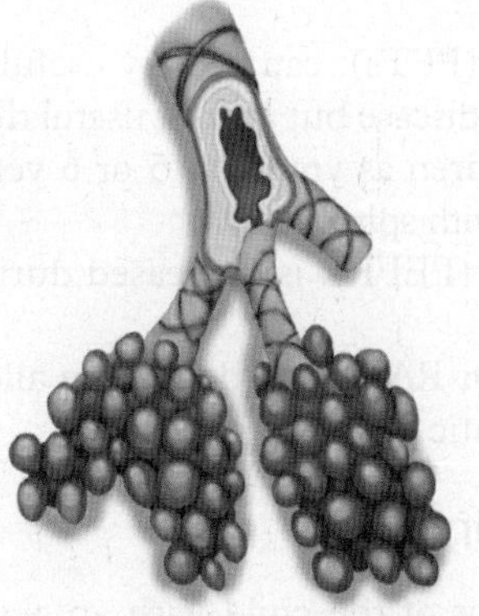

Airway with inflammation

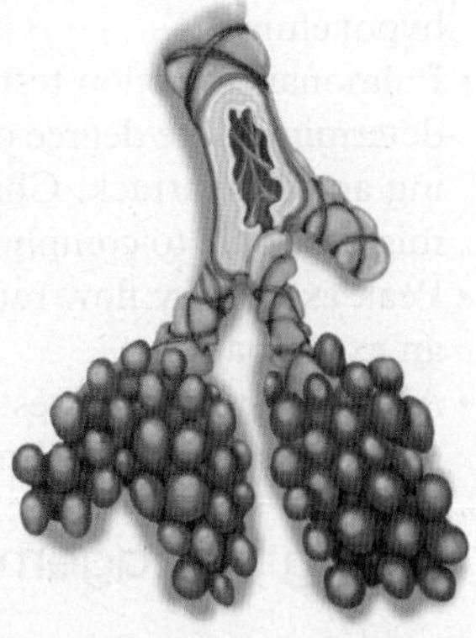

Airway with inflammation, bronchospasm, and mucus production

● Figure 19.14 Note airway edema, mucus production, and bronchospasm occurring with asthma.

- Recurrent episodes diagnosed as wheezing, bronchiolitis, or bronchitis
- Known allergies
- Seasonal response to environmental pollen
- Tobacco smoke exposure (passive or self-smoking)
- Poverty

Physical Examination

Physical examination of the child with asthma includes inspection, auscultation, and percussion.

Inspection

Observe the patient's general appearance and color. During mild exacerbations, the child's color might remain pink, but as the child worsens, cyanosis might result. Work of breathing is variable. Some children present with mild retractions, while others demonstrate significant accessory muscle use and eventually head-bobbing if not effectively treated. The child may appear anxious and fearful or be lethargic and irritable. An audible wheeze might be present. Children with persistent severe asthma may have a barrel chest and routinely demonstrate mildly increased work of breathing.

Auscultation and Percussion

A thorough assessment of lung fields is necessary. Wheezing is the hallmark of airway obstruction and might vary throughout the lung fields. Coarseness might also be present. Assess the adequacy of aeration. Breath sounds might be diminished in the bases or throughout. A quiet chest in an asthmatic child can be an ominous sign. With severe airway obstruction, air movement can be so poor that wheezes might not be heard upon auscultation. Percussion may yield hyperresonance.

Laboratory and Diagnostic Tests

Laboratory and diagnostic studies commonly ordered for the assessment of asthma include:

- Pulse oximetry: oxygen saturation may be significantly decreased or normal during a mild exacerbation
- Chest x-ray: usually reveals hyperinflation
- Blood gases: might show carbon dioxide retention and hypoxemia
- Pulmonary function tests (PFTs): can be very useful in determining the degree of disease but are not useful during an acute attack. Children as young as 5 or 6 years might be able to comply with spirometry.
- Peak expiratory flow rate (PEFR): is decreased during an exacerbation
- Allergy testing: skin test or RAST can determine allergic triggers for the asthmatic child

Nursing Management

Initial nursing management of the child with an acute exacerbation of asthma is aimed at restoring a clear airway and effective breathing pattern as well as promoting adequate oxygenation and ventilation (gas exchange). Refer to the Nursing Care Plan on page 562. Additional considerations are reviewed below.

Educating the Child and Family

Asthma is a chronic illness and needs to be understood as such. Figure 19.15 displays the "Kids with Asthma Bill of Rights" developed by the American Lung Association. Teach families of children with asthma, and the children themselves, how to care for the disease. Symptom-free periods (often very long) are interspersed with episodes of exacerbation. Parents and children often do not understand the importance of maintenance medications for long-term control. They may view the episodes of exacerbation (sometimes requiring hospitalization or emergency room visits) as an acute illness and are simply relieved when they are over. Frequently during the periods between acute episodes, children are viewed as disease-free and long-term maintenance schedules are abandoned. The prolonged inflammatory process occurring in the absence of symptoms, primarily in children with moderate to severe asthma, can lead to airway remodeling and eventual irreversible disease.

To provide appropriate education to the child and family, determine the severity of the asthma as outlined in the NAEPP Expert Panel Report: Guidelines for the Diagnosis and Management of Asthma (Kumar et al., 2005). Stress the concept of maintenance medications for the prevention of future serious disease in addition to controlling or preventing current symptoms.

Educate families and children on the appropriate use of nebulizers, metered-dose inhalers, spacers, dry-powder inhalers, and Diskus, as well as the purposes, functions, and side effects of the medications they deliver. Require return demonstration of equipment use to ensure that children and families can use the equipment properly (Teaching Guideline 19.5).

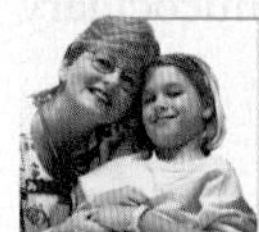

The NAEPP recommends use of a spacer or holding chamber with metered-dose inhalers to increase the bioavailability of medication in the lungs.

Each child should have a management plan in place to determine when to step up or step down treatment. The recommendations for treatment based on severity of asthma are listed in Table 19.4. Figure 19.16 provides an example of a written format that may be helpful to families in the management of asthma. This written action plan should also be kept on file at the child's school, and relief medication should be available to the child at all times. Children who experience exercise-induced bronchospasm may still participate in physical education or athletics but may need to be allowed to use their medicine before the activity.

(text continues on page 594)

KIDS WITH ASTHMA

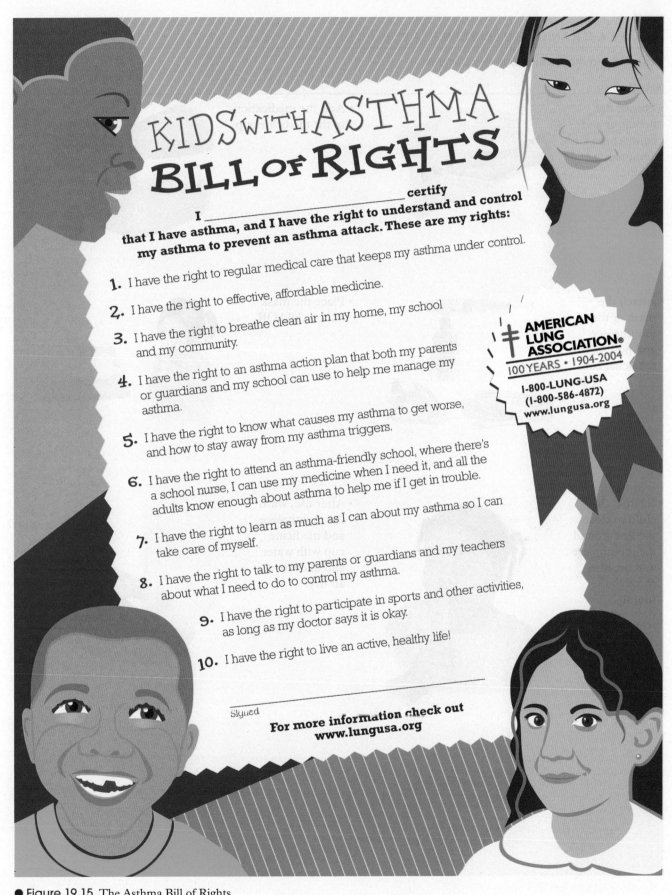

I ______________________ certify
that I have asthma, and I have the right to understand and control
my asthma to prevent an asthma attack. These are my rights:
1. I have the right to regular medical care that keeps my asthma under control.
2. I have the right to effective, affordable medicine.
3. I have the right to breathe clean air in my home, my school and my community.
4. I have the right to an asthma action plan that both my parents or guardians and my school can use to help me manage my asthma.
5. I have the right to know what causes my asthma to get worse, and how to stay away from my asthma triggers.
6. I have the right to attend an asthma-friendly school, where there's a school nurse, I can use my medicine when I need it, and all the adults know enough about asthma to help me if I get in trouble.
7. I have the right to learn as much as I can about my asthma so I can take care of myself.
8. I have the right to talk to my parents or guardians and my teachers about what I need to do to control my asthma.
9. I have the right to participate in sports and other activities, as long as my doctor says it is okay.
10. I have the right to live an active, healthy life!
Signed
For more information check out
www.lungusa.org
AMERICAN
LUNG
ASSOCIATION®
100 YEARS • 1904-2004
1-800-LUNG-USA
(1-800-586-4872)
www.lungusa.org

● Figure 19.15 The Asthma Bill of Rights.

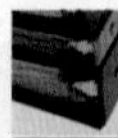

TEACHING GUIDELINE 19.5

Using Asthma Medication Delivery Devices

Nebulizer

- Plug in the nebulizer and connect the air compressor tubing.

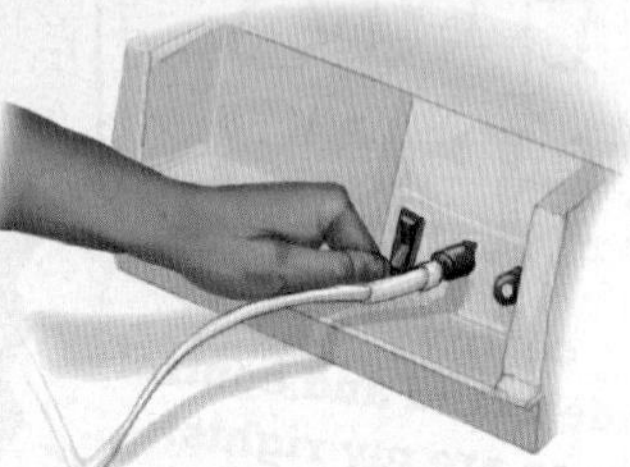

- Add the medication to the medicine cup.

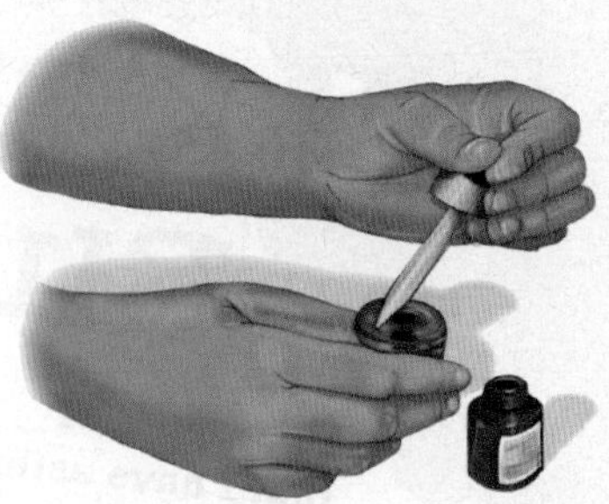

- Attach the mask or the mouthpiece and hose to the medicine cup.

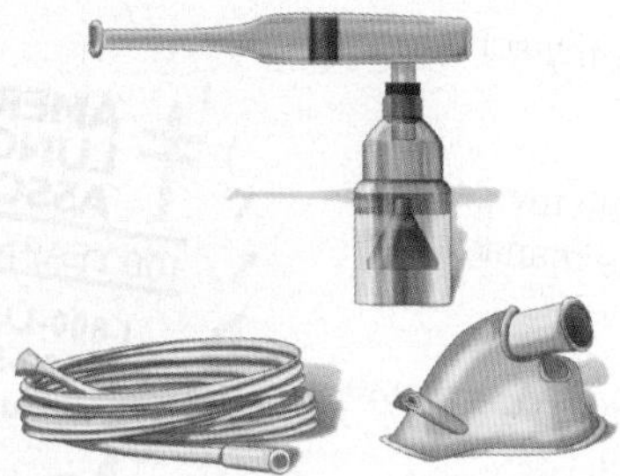

- Place the mask on the child OR

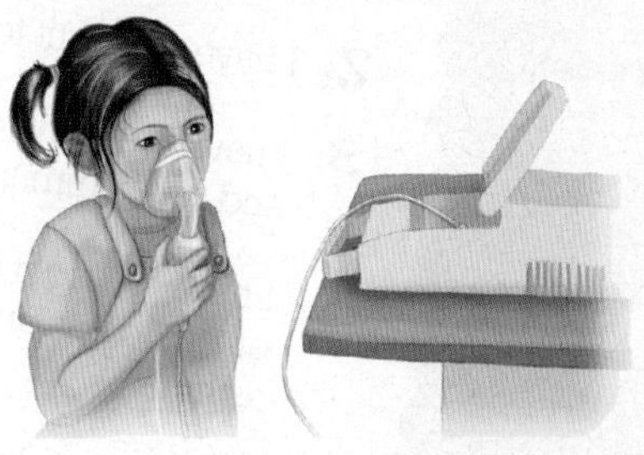

- Instruct the child to close the lips around the mouthpiece and breathe through the mouth.

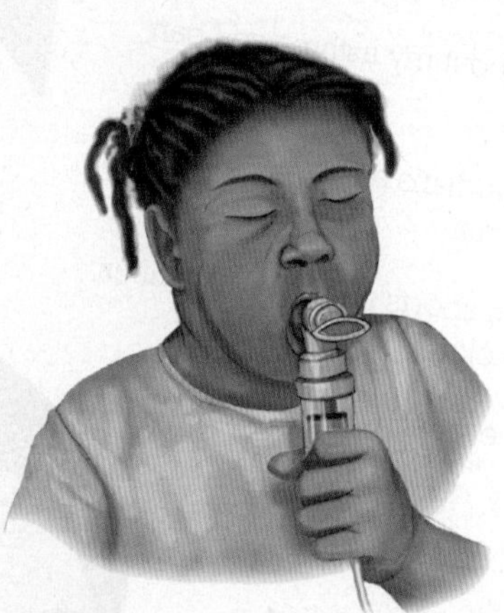

- After use, wash the mouthpiece and medicine cup with water and allow to air dry.

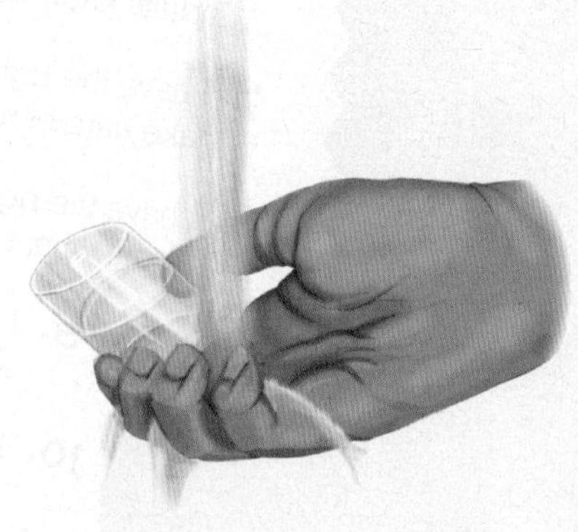

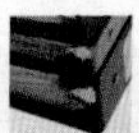

TEACHING GUIDELINE 19.5 (Continued)

Using Asthma Medication Delivery Devices

Metered-Dose Inhaler

- Shake the inhaler and take off the cap.

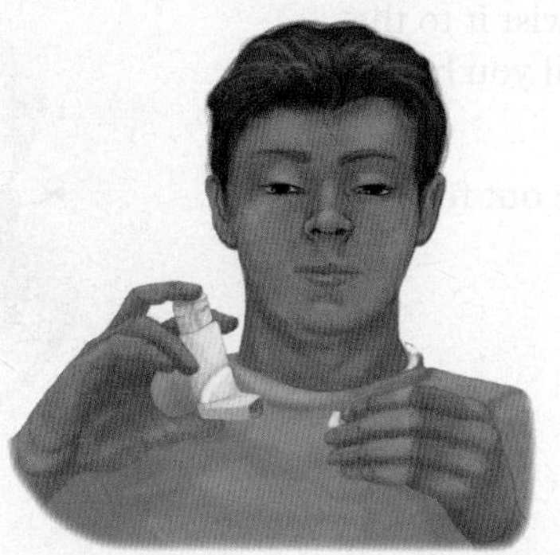

- Attach the inhaler to the spacer or holding chamber.
- Breathe out completely.

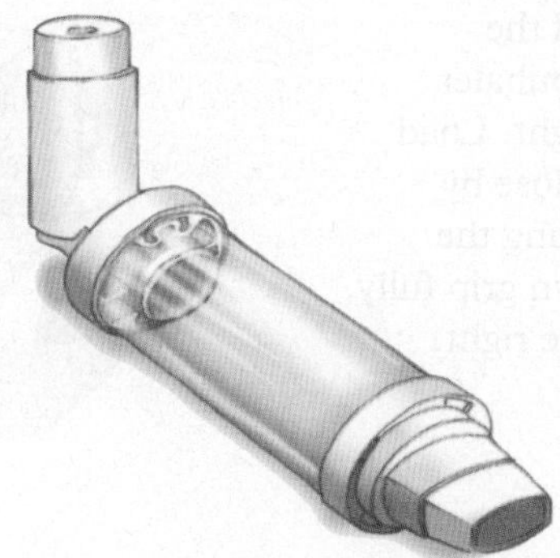

- Put the spacer mouthpiece in the mouth (or place the mask over the child's nose and mouth, ensuring a good seal).

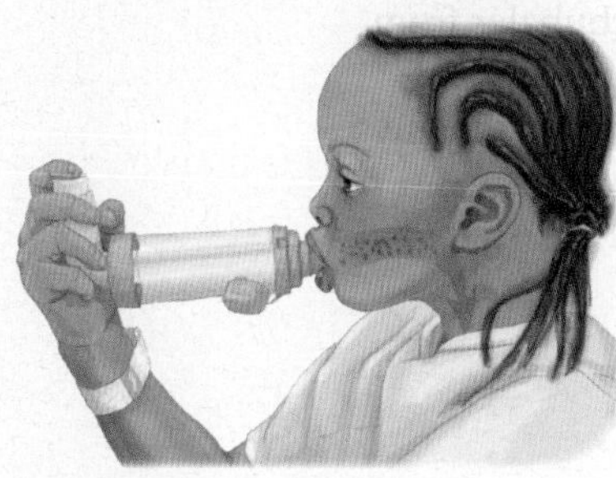

- Compress the inhaler and inhale slowly and deeply. Hold the breath for a count of 10.

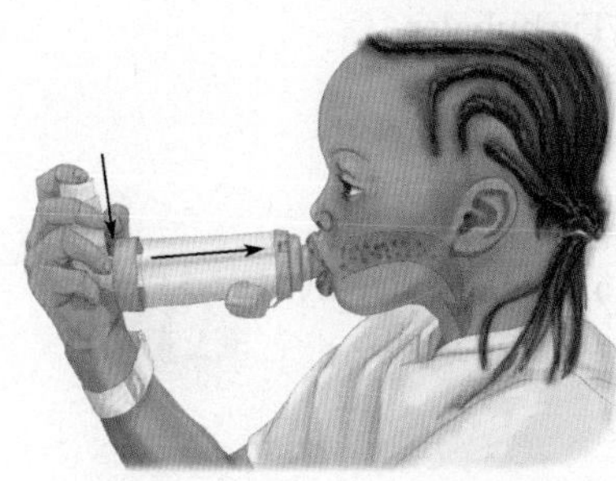

Diskus

- Hold the Diskus in a horizontal position in one hand and push the thumbgrip with the thumb of your other hand away from you until mouthpiece is exposed.

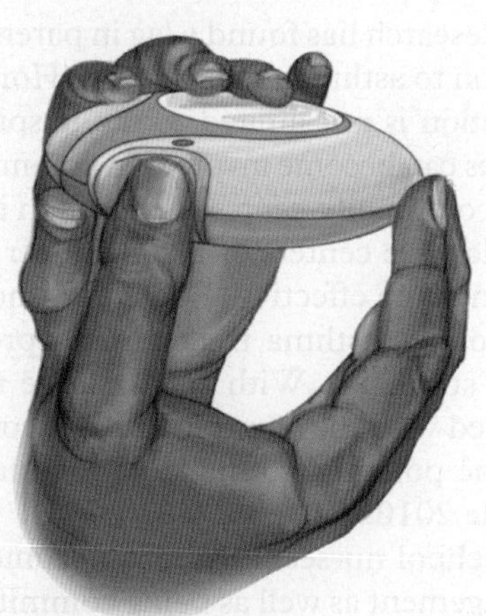

- Push the lever until it clicks (the dose is now loaded).
- Breathe out fully.

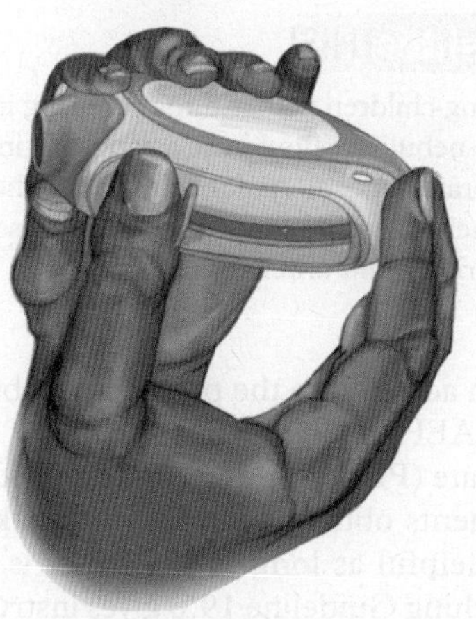

- Place your mouth securely around the mouthpiece and breathe in fully and quickly through your mouth.

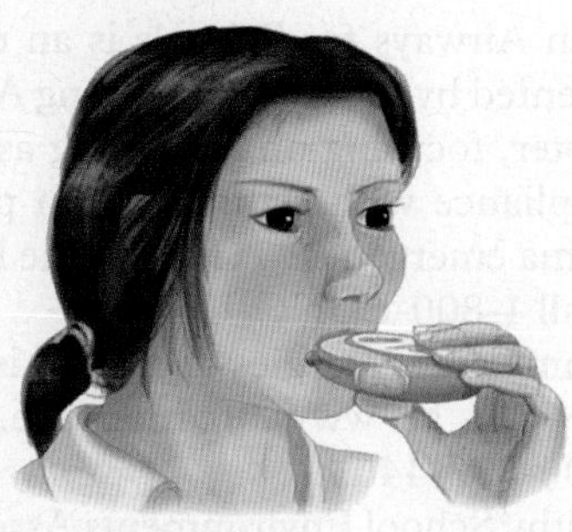

- Remove the Diskus, hold the breath for 10 seconds, and then breathe out.

(continued)

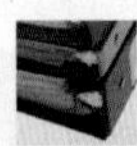

TEACHING GUIDELINE 19.5 (Continued)

Using Asthma Medication Delivery Devices

Turbuhaler

- Hold the Turbuhaler upright. Load the dose by twisting the brown grip fully to the right.

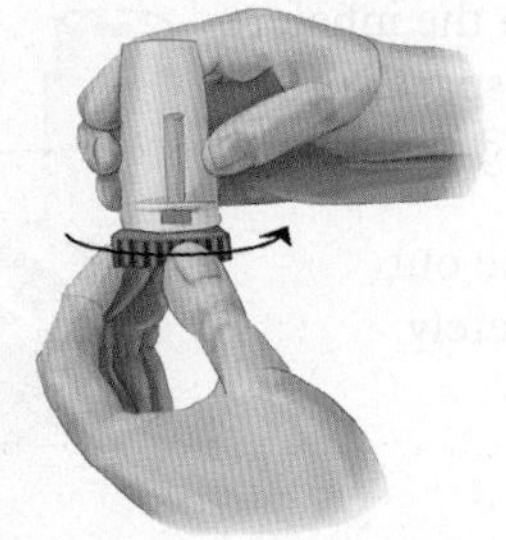

- Then twist it to the left until you hear it click.
- Breathe out fully.

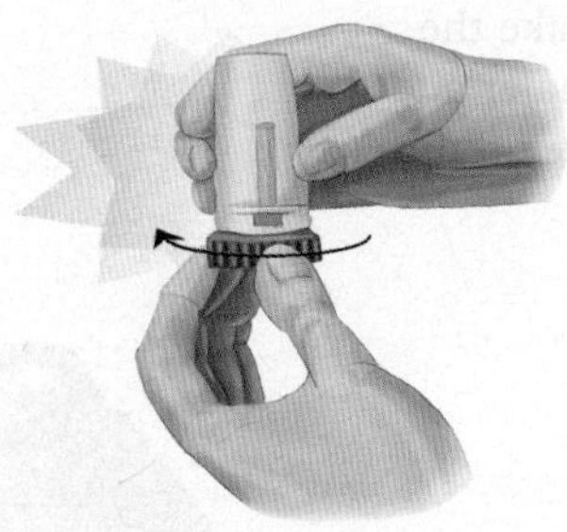

- Holding the Turbuhaler horizontally, place the mouth firmly around the mouthpiece and inhale deeply and forcefully.

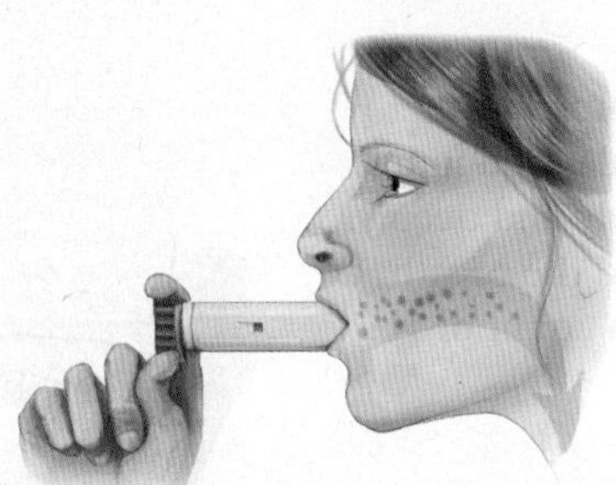

- Remove the Turbuhaler from the mouth and then breathe out.

Consider THIS!

Young children with asthma receiving inhaled medications via a nebulizer should use a snugly fitting mask to ensure accurate deposition of medication to the lungs. "Blow-by" via nebulizer should be discouraged, as medication delivery is variable and unreliable.

In addition to the presence or absence of symptoms, the NAEPP recommends the use of the peak expiratory flow rate (PEFR) to determine daily control. PEFR measurements obtained via a home peak flow meter can be very helpful as long as the meter is used appropriately (Teaching Guideline 19.6 gives instructions on peak flow meter use). The child's "personal best" is determined collaboratively with the health care practitioner during a symptom-free period. PEFR is measured daily at home using the peak flow meter. The asthma management plan then gives specific instructions based on the PEFR measurement (Table 19.5).

Avoidance of allergens is another key component of asthma management. Avoiding known triggers helps to prevent exacerbations as well as long-term inflammatory changes. This can be a difficult task for most families, particularly if the affected child suffers from several allergies. Teaching Guideline 19-4 outlines strategies for allergen avoidance.

Research has found a lag in parent/child education in relation to asthma management (Horner, 2004). Asthma education is not limited to the hospital or clinic setting. Nurses can become involved in community asthma education: community-centered education in schools, churches, and daycare centers or through peer educators has been shown to be effective. Education should include pathophysiology, asthma triggers, and prevention and treatment strategies. With such a large number of children affected with this chronic disease, community education has the potential to make a broad impact. See Healthy People 2010.

School nurses must also become experts in asthma management as well as being committed to ongoing education of the child and family (Sander, 2002). Resources for schools include:

- Open Airways for Schools is an educational program presented by the American Lung Association or its local chapter, focusing on increasing asthma awareness and compliance with asthma action plans and decreasing asthma emergencies. Contact the local lung association or call 1-800-LUNG-USA.
- Asthma and Allergies at School is a kit available from AANMA at www.breatherville.org/schoolhouse or 1-800-878-4403.
- Healthy School Environments Assessment Tool is available at http://www.epa.gov/schools/.

Asthma Action Plan

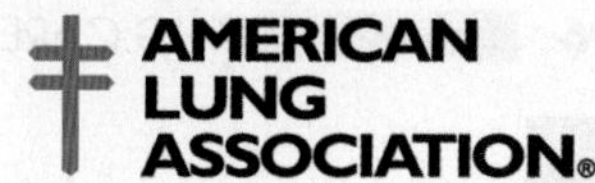

General Information:

- Name ______
- Emergency contact ______ Phone numbers ______
- Physician/Health Care Provider ______ Phone numbers ______
- Physician Signature ______ Date ______

Severity Classification	Triggers	Exercise
○ Mild Intermittent ○ Moderate Persistent ○ Mild Persistent ○ Severe Persistent	○ Colds ○ Smoke ○ Weather ○ Exercise ○ Dust ○ Air pollution ○ Animals ○ Food ○ Other ______	1. Pre-medication (how much and when) ______ 2. Exercise modifications ______

Green Zone: Doing Well

Peak Flow Meter Personal Best = ______

Symptoms

- Breathing is good
- No cough or wheeze
- Can work and play
- Sleeps all night

Peak Flow Meter

More than 80% of personal best or ______

Control Medications

Medicine	How Much to Take	When To Take It

Yellow Zone: Getting Worse

Contact Physician if using quick relief more than 2 times per week.

Symptoms

- Some problems breathing
- Cough, wheeze or chest tight
- Problems working or playing
- Wake at night

Peak Flow Meter

Between 50 to 80% of personal best or ______ to ______

Continue control medicines and add:

Medicine	How Much to Take	When To Take It

IF your symptoms (and peak flow, if used) return to Green Zone after one hour of the quick relief treatment, THEN

- ○ Take quick-relief medication every 4 hours for 1 to 2 days
- ○ Change your long-term control medicines by ______
- ○ Contact your physician for follow-up care

IF your symptoms (and peak flow, if used) DO NOT return to the GREEN ZONE after 1 hour of the quick relief treatment, THEN

- ○ Take quick-relief treatment again
- ○ Change your long-term control medicines by ______
- ○ Call your physician/Health Care Provider within ______ hours of modifying your medication routine

Red Zone: Medical Alert

Ambulance/Emergency Phone Number: ______

Symptoms

- Lots of problems breathing
- Cannot work or play
- Getting worse instead of better
- Medicine is not helping

Peak Flow Meter

Between 0 to 50% of personal best or ______ to ______

Continue control medicines and add:

Medicine	How Much to Take	When To Take It

Go to the hospital or call for an ambulance if

- ○ Still in the red zone after 15 minutes
- ○ If you have not been able to reach your physician/health care provider for help
- ○ ______

Call an ambulance immediately if the following danger signs are present

- ○ Trouble walking/talking due to shortness of breath
- ○ Lips or fingernails are blue

● Figure 19.16 Asthma Action Plan.

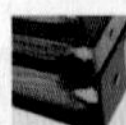

TEACHING GUIDELINE 19.6

Using a Peak Flow Meter

- Slide the arrow down to "zero."
- Stand up straight.
- Take a deep breath and close the lips tightly around the mouthpiece.
- Blow out hard and fast.
- Note the number the arrow moves to.
- Repeat three times and record the highest reading.
- Keep a record of daily readings, being sure to measure peak flow at the same time each day.

Data from the American Lung Association.

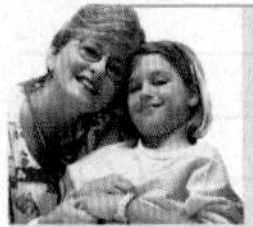

Exposure to second-hand smoke increases the need for medications in children with asthma as well as the frequency of asthma exacerbations. Both indoor air quality and environmental pollution contribute to asthma in children.

HEALTHY PEOPLE 2010

Objective	Significance
Reduce activity limitations among persons with asthma. (Developmental) Reduce the number of school or workdays missed by persons with asthma. Increase the proportion of persons with asthma who receive formal patient education, including information about community and self-help resources, as an essential part of the management of their condition.	• Encourage appropriate physical activity in children with asthma. • Provide extensive education to children and families about peak flow meter use and its meaning, maintenance and rescue medications, symptoms of asthma exacerbation, and a written plan for how to "step up" and "step down" asthma management. • Refer children and their families to local asthma or Internet resources and support groups. • Refer families to formal classes on asthma education.

Promoting the Child's Self-Esteem

Fear of an exacerbation and feeling "different" from other children can harm a child's self-esteem. In qualitative research studies, children have made such statements as "my body shuts down" and "I feel like I'm going to die" (Yoos et al., 2005). The fatigue and fear associated with chronic asthma may reduce the child's confidence and sense of control over his or her body and life. In addition to coping with a chronic illness, the asthmatic child often also has to cope with school-related issues. Moodiness, acting out, and withdrawal correlate with increases in school absence, which can contribute to poor school performance. To live in fear of an exacerbation or to be unable to participate in activities affects the child's self-esteem.

Through education and support, the child can gain a sense of control. Children need to learn to master their disease. Accurate evaluation of asthma symptoms and

Table 19.5 Assessment of Peak Expiratory Flow Rate (PEFR)

Zone*	PEFR	Symptoms	Action
Green: Good control	>80% personal best	None	Take usual medications.
Yellow: Caution	50% to 80% personal best	Possibly present	Take short-acting inhaled beta$_2$-agonist right away. Talk to your health care provider.
Red: Medical alert	<50% personal best	Usually present	Take short-acting inhaled beta$_2$-agonist right away. Go to office or emergency department.

*The National Asthma Education and Prevention Program recommended the "traffic light" approach for educating individuals on PEFRs and management plans.

improvement of self-esteem may help the child to experience less panic with an acute episode. Improved self-esteem might also help the child cope with the disease in general and with being different from his or her peers. The school-age child has the cognitive ability to begin taking responsibility for asthma management, with continued involvement on the part of the parents. Transferring control of asthma care to the child is an important developmental process that will contribute to the child's feeling of control over the illness (Buford, 2004).

Promoting Family Coping

Parent denial is an issue in many families. The family, through education and encouragement, can become the experts on the child's illness as well as advocates for the child's well-being. The resilient child is better able to cope with difficulties presented to him or her, including asthma. Cohesiveness and warmth in the family environment can improve a child's resiliency as well as contribute to family hardiness. Parents need to be allowed to ask questions and voice their concerns. A nurse who understands the family's issues and concerns is better able to plan for support and education. Provide culturally sensitive education and interventions that focus on increasing the family's commitment to and control of asthma management. As the child and parents become confident in their ability to recognize asthma symptoms and cope with asthma and its periodic episodes, the family's ability to cope will improve (Svavarsdottir & Rayens, 2005).

CHRONIC LUNG DISEASE

Chronic lung disease (formerly termed bronchopulmonary dysplasia [BPD]) is often diagnosed in infants who have experienced RDS and continue to require oxygen at 28 days of age. It is a chronic respiratory condition seen most commonly in premature infants. It results from a variety of factors, including pulmonary immaturity, acute lung injury, barotrauma, inflammatory mediators, and volutrauma. Epithelial stretching, macrophage and polymorphonuclear cell invasion, and airway edema affect the growth and development of lung structures. Cilia loss and airway lining denudation reduce the normal cleansing abilities of the lung. The number of normal alveoli is reduced by one third to one half. Lower birthweights, white race, and male gender pose increased risk for development of chronic lung disease. Complications include pulmonary artery hypertension, cor pulmonale, congestive heart failure, and severe bacterial or viral pneumonia. (Harvey, 2004; Stoll & Kliegman, 2004).

Anti-inflammatory inhaled medications are used for maintenance, and short-acting bronchodilators are used as needed for wheezing episodes. Supplemental long-term oxygen therapy may be required in some infants.

Nursing Assessment

Tachypnea and increased work of breathing are characteristic of chronic lung disease. After discharge from the NICU, these symptoms can continue. Exertion such as activity or oral feeding can cause dyspnea to worsen. Failure to thrive might also be evident. Auscultation might reveal breath sounds that are diminished in the bases. These infants have reactive airway episodes, so wheezing might be present during times of exacerbation. If fluid overload develops, rales may be heard.

Nursing Management

If the infant is oxygen dependent, provide education to the parents about oxygen tanks, nasal cannula use, pulse oximetry use, and nebulizer treatments. Often these children require increased-calorie formulas to grow adequately. Fluid restrictions and/or diuretics are necessary in some infants. Follow-up echocardiograms might be used to determine resolution of pulmonary artery hypertension prior to weaning from oxygen. Encourage developmentally appropriate activities. It might be difficult for the oxygen-dependent infant or toddler to reach gross motor milestones or explore the environment because the length of his oxygen tubing limits him or her.

Parental support is also a key nursing intervention. After a long and trying period of ups and downs with their newborn in the intensive care unit, parents find themselves exhausted caring for their medically fragile infant at home.

CYSTIC FIBROSIS

Cystic fibrosis is an autosomal recessive disorder that occurs about once in every 3,300 live white births and about once in every 16,000 live black births (Boat, 2004). A deletion occurring on the long arm of chromosome 7 at the cystic fibrosis transmembrane regulator (CFTR) is the responsible gene mutation. DNA testing can be used prenatally and in newborns to identify the presence of the mutation. The American College of Obstetrics and Gynecology currently recommends screening for cystic fibrosis to any person seeking preconception or prenatal care. At present, 11 states include testing for cystic fibrosis as part of newborn screening (Gross, 2004).

Cystic fibrosis is the most common debilitating disease of childhood among those of European descent. Medical advances in recent years have greatly increased the length and quality of life for affected children: about 50% now live past the age of 30 years (Boat, 2004), and many live a high-quality life into their 40s (Carpenter & Narsavage, 2004). Complications include hemoptysis, pneumothorax, bacterial colonization, cor pulmonale, volvulus, intussusception, intestinal obstruction, rectal prolapse, gastroesophageal reflux disease, diabetes, portal hypertension, liver failure, gallstones, and decreased fertility.

Therapeutic Management

Therapeutic management of cystic fibrosis is aimed toward minimizing pulmonary complications, maximizing lung function, preventing infection, and facilitating growth. All children with cystic fibrosis who have pulmonary involvement require chest physiotherapy with postural drainage several times daily to mobilize secretions from the lungs. Physical exercise is encouraged. Recombinant human DNase (Pulmozyme) is given daily using a nebulizer to decrease sputum viscosity and help clear secretions. Inhaled bronchodilators and anti-inflammatory agents are prescribed for some children. Aerosolized antibiotics are often prescribed and may be given at home as well as in the hospital. Choice of antibiotic is determined by sputum culture and sensitivity results. Pancreatic enzymes and supplemental fat-soluble vitamins are prescribed to promote adequate digestion and absorption of nutrients and optimize nutritional status. Increased-calorie, high-protein diets are recommended, and sometimes supplemental high-calorie formula, either orally or via feeding tube, is needed. Some children require total parenteral nutrition to maintain or gain weight (McMullen, 2004). Lung transplantation has been successful in some children with cystic fibrosis.

Pathophysiology

In cystic fibrosis, the CFTR mutation causes alterations in epithelial ion transport on mucosal surfaces, resulting in generalized dysfunction of the exocrine glands. The epithelial cells fail to conduct chloride, and water transport abnormalities occur. This results in thickened, tenacious secretions in the sweat glands, gastrointestinal tract, pancreas, respiratory tract, and other exocrine tissues. The increased viscosity of these secretions makes them difficult to clear. The sweat glands produce a larger amount of chloride, leading to a salty taste of the skin and alterations in electrolyte balance and dehydration. The pancreas, intrahepatic bile ducts, intestinal glands, gallbladder, and submaxillary glands become obstructed by viscous mucus and eosinophilic material. Pancreatic enzyme activity is lost and malabsorption of fats, proteins, and carbohydrates occurs, resulting in poor growth and large, malodorous stools. Excess mucus is produced by the tracheobronchial glands. Abnormally thick mucus plugs the small airways, and then bronchiolitis and further plugging of the airways occur. Secondary bacterial infection with *Staphylococcus aureus*, *Pseudomonas aeruginosa*, and *Burkholderia cepacia* often occurs. This contributes to obstruction and inflammation, leading to chronic infection, tissue damage, and respiratory failure. Nasal polyps and recurrent sinusitis are common. Boys have tenacious seminal fluid and experience blocking of the vas deferens, often making them infertile. In girls, thick cervical secretions might limit penetration of sperm (Boat, 2004; Simpson & Ivey, 2005). Table 19.6 gives further details of the pathophysiology and resulting respiratory and gastrointestinal clinical manifestations of cystic fibrosis.

Nursing Assessment

For a full description of the assessment phase of the nursing process, refer to page 552. Assessment findings pertinent to cystic fibrosis are discussed below.

Health History

Elicit a description of the present illness and chief complaint. Common signs and symptoms reported during the health history in the undiagnosed child might include:

- A salty taste to the child's skin (resulting from excess chloride loss via perspiration)
- Meconium ileus or late, difficult passage of meconium stool in the newborn period
- Abdominal pain or difficulty passing stool (infants or toddlers might present with intestinal obstruction or intussusception at the time of diagnosis)
- Bulky, greasy stools
- Poor weight gain and growth despite good appetite
- Chronic or recurrent cough and/or upper or lower respiratory infections

Children known to have cystic fibrosis are often admitted to the hospital for pulmonary exacerbations or other complications of the disease. The health history should include questions related to:

- Respiratory status: has cough, sputum production, or work of breathing increased?
- Appetite and weight gain
- Activity tolerance
- Increased need for pulmonary or pancreatic medications
- Presence of fever
- Presence of bone pain
- Any other changes in physical state or medication regimen

Physical Examination

The physical examination includes inspection, auscultation, percussion, and palpation.

Inspection

Observe the child's general appearance and color. Check the nasal passages for polyps. Note respiratory rate, work of breathing, use of accessory muscles, position of comfort, frequency and severity of cough, and quality and quantity of sputum produced. The child with cystic fibrosis often has a barrel chest (anterior–posterior diameter approximates transverse diameter) (Fig. 19.17). Clubbing of the nail beds might also be present. Note whether rectal prolapse is present. Does the child appear small or thin for his or her age? The child might have a protuberant abdomen and thin extremities, with decreased amounts of subcutaneous fat present. Observe for the presence of edema (sign of cardiac or liver failure). Note distended neck veins or the presence of a heave (signs of cor pulmonale).

Table 19.6 Pathophysiology of Cystic Fibrosis and Resultant Respiratory and Gastrointestinal Clinical Manifestations

Defect in the CFTR Gene Affects	Pathophysiology	Clinical Manifestations
Respiratory tract	• Infection leads to neutrophilic inflammation. • Cleavage of complement receptors and immunoglobin G leads to opsonophagocytosis failure. • Chemoattractant interleukin-8 and elastin degradase contribute to inflammatory response. • Thick, tenacious sputum that is chronically colonized with bacteria results. • Air trapping related to airway obstruction • Pulmonary parenchyma is eventually destroyed.	• Airway obstruction • Difficulty clearing secretions • Respiratory distress and impaired gas exchange • Chronic cough • Barrel-shaped chest • Decreased pulmonary function • Clubbing • Recurrent pneumonia • Hemoptysis • Pneumothorax • Chronic sinusitis • Nasal polyps • Cor pulmonale (right-sided heart failure)
Gastrointestinal tract	• Decreased chloride and water secretion into the intestine (causing dehydration of the intestinal material) and into the bile ducts (causing increased bile viscosity) • Reduced pancreatic bicarbonate secretion • Hypersecretion of gastric acid • Insufficiency of pancreatic enzymes necessary for digestion and absorption • Pancreas secretes thick mucus.	• Meconium ileus • Retention of fecal matter in distal intestine, resulting in vomiting, abdominal distention and cramping, anorexia, right lower quadrant pain • Sludging of intestinal contents may lead to fecal impaction, rectal prolapse, bowel obstruction, intussusception. • Obstructive cirrhosis with esophageal varices, and splenomegaly • Gallstones • Gastroesophageal reflux disease (compounded by postural drainage with chest physiotherapy) • Inadequate protein absorption • Altered absorption of iron and vitamins A, D, E, and K • Failure to thrive • Hyperglycemia and development of diabetes later in life

Auscultation

Auscultation may reveal a variety of adventitious breath sounds. Fine or coarse crackles and scattered or localized wheezing might be present. With progressive obstructive pulmonary involvement, breath sounds might be diminished. Tachycardia might be present. Note the presence of a gallop (might occur with cor pulmonale). Note the adequacy of bowel sounds.

Percussion

Percussion over the lung fields usually yields hyperresonance due to air trapping. Diaphragmatic excursion might be decreased. Percussion of the abdomen might reveal dullness over an enlarged liver or mass related to intestinal obstruction.

Palpation

Palpation might yield a finding of asymmetric chest excursion if atelectasis is present. Tactile fremitus may be decreased over areas of atelectasis. Note if tenderness is present over the liver (might be an early sign of cor pulmonale).

Laboratory and Diagnostic Tests

Common laboratory and diagnostic studies ordered for the diagnosis and assessment of cystic fibrosis include:

- Sweat chloride test: considered suspicious if the level of chloride in collected sweat is above 50 mEq/L and diagnostic if the level is above 60 mEq/L (Fig. 19.18)
- Pulse oximetry: oxygen saturation might be decreased, particularly during a pulmonary exacerbation

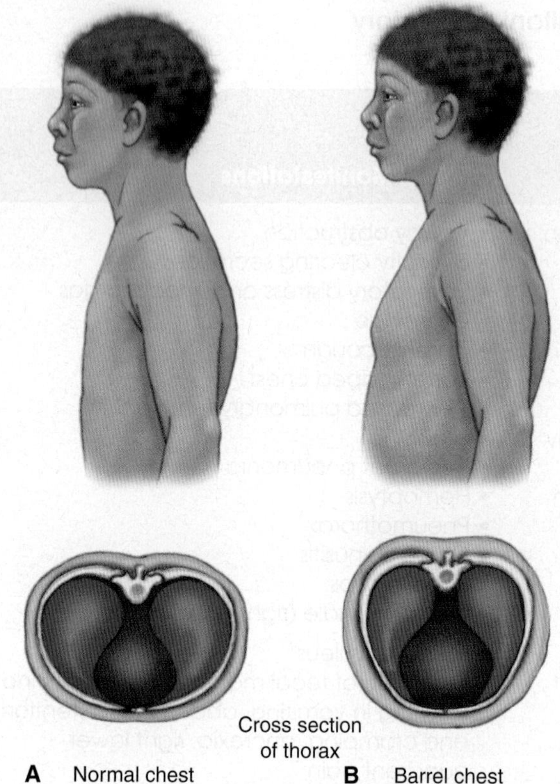

● Figure 19.17 (A) Normal chest shape—transverse diameter > anterior-posterior diameter. (B) Barrel chest—transverse diameter = anterior-posterior diameter.

- Chest x-ray: may reveal hyperinflation, bronchial wall thickening, atelectasis, or infiltration
- Pulmonary function tests: might reveal a decrease in forced vital capacity and forced expiratory volume, with increases in residual volume (Boat, 2004; McMullen, 2004)

Nursing Management

Management of cystic fibrosis focuses on minimizing pulmonary complications, promoting growth and development, and facilitating coping and adjustment of the child and family. In addition to the nursing diagnoses and related interventions discussed in the Nursing Care Plan Overview for respiratory disorders, interventions common to cystic fibrosis follow.

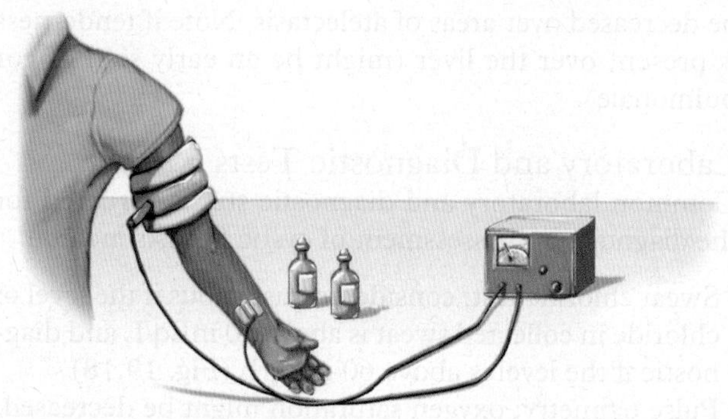

● Figure 19.18 Sweat chloride test.

Maintaining Patent Airway

Chest physiotherapy is often used as an adjunct therapy in respiratory illnesses, but for children with cystic fibrosis it is a critical intervention. Chest physiotherapy involves percussion, vibration, and postural drainage, and either it or another bronchial hygiene therapy must be performed several times a day to assist with mobilization of secretions. Nursing Procedure 19.2 gives instructions on the chest physiotherapy technique.

For older children and adolescents, the flutter-valve device, positive expiratory pressure therapy, or a high-frequency chest compression vest may also be used. The flutter valve device provides high-frequency oscillation to the airway as the child exhales into a mouthpiece that contains a steel ball. Positive expiratory pressure therapy involves exhaling through a flow resistor, which creates positive expiratory pressure. The cycles of exhalation are repeated until coughing yields expectoration of secretions. The vest airway clearance system provides high-frequency chest wall oscillation to increase airflow velocity to create repetitive cough-like shear forces and to decrease the viscosity of secretions (Goodfellow & Jones, 2002). Breathing exercises are also helpful in promoting mucus clearance. Encourage physical exercise, as it helps to promote mucus secretion as well as providing cardiopulmonary conditioning. Ensure that Pulmozyme is administered, as well as inhaled bronchodilators and anti-inflammatory agents if prescribed.

Preventing Infection

Vigorous pulmonary hygiene for mobilization of secretions is critical to prevent infection. Aerosolized antibiotics can be given at home as well as in the hospital. Children with frequent or severe respiratory exacerbations might require lengthy courses of intravenous antibiotics.

Maintaining Growth

Pancreatic enzymes must be administered with all meals and snacks to promote adequate digestion and absorption of nutrients. The number of capsules required depends on the extent of pancreatic insufficiency and the amount of food being ingested. The dosage can be adjusted until an adequate growth pattern is established and the number of stools is consistent at one or two per day. Children will need additional enzyme capsules when high-fat foods are being eaten. In the infant or young child, the enzyme capsule can be opened and sprinkled on cereal or applesauce. A well-balanced, high-calorie, high-protein diet is necessary to ensure adequate growth. Some children require up to 1.5 times the recommended daily allowance of calories for children their age. A number of commercially available nutritional formulas and shakes are available for diet supplementation.

Nursing Procedure 19.2

Performing Chest Physiotherapy

1. Provide percussion via a cupped hand or an infant percussion device. Appropriate percussion yields a hollow sound (not a slapping sound).

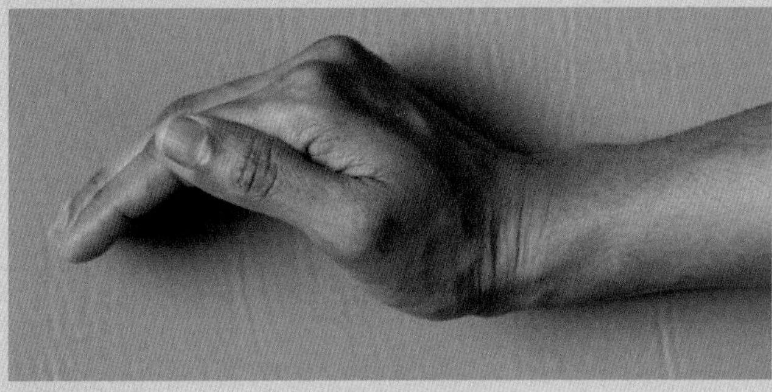

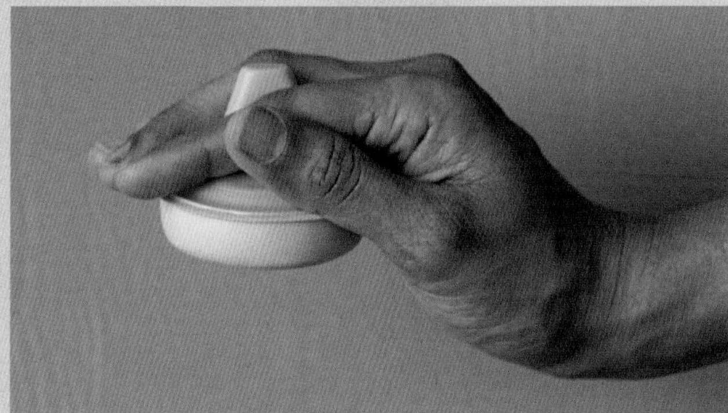

2. Percuss each segment of the lung for 1 to 2 minutes.

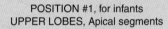

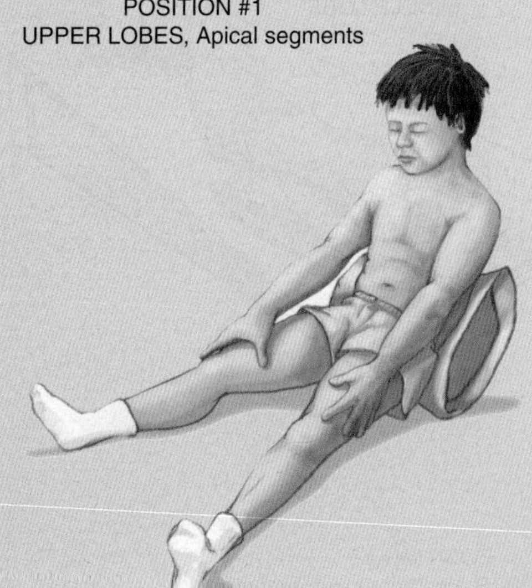

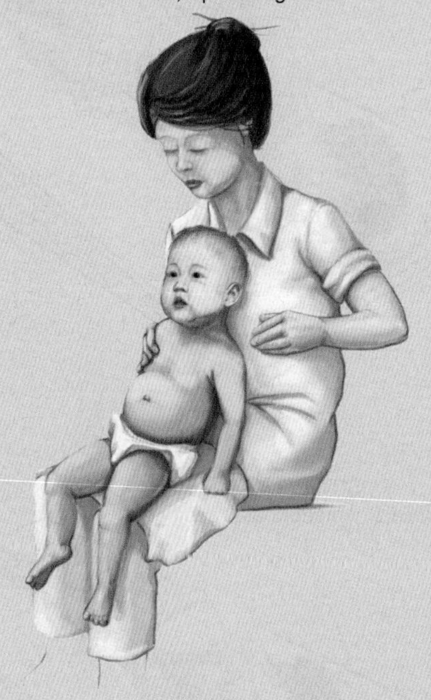

(continued)

Nursing Procedure 19.2

Performing Chest Physiotherapy (continued)

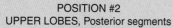

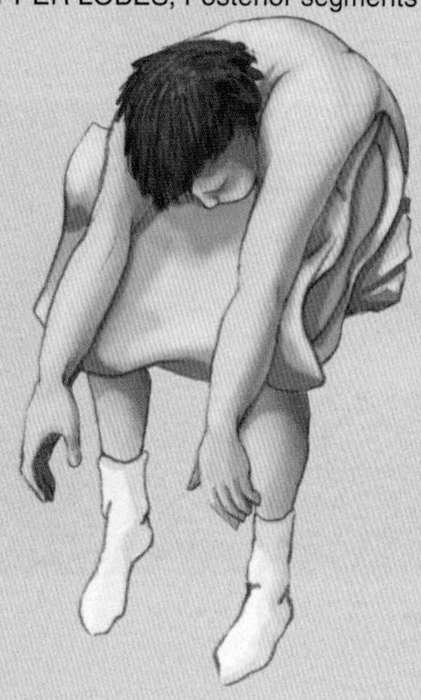

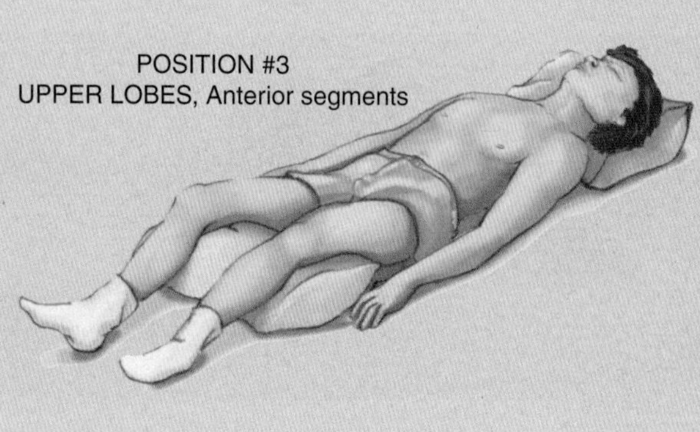

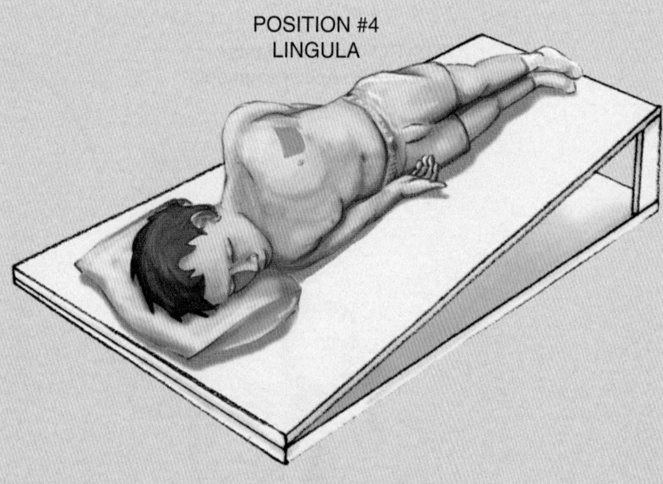

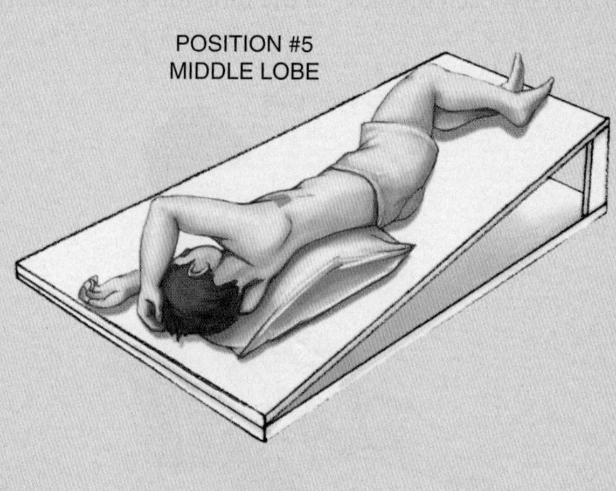

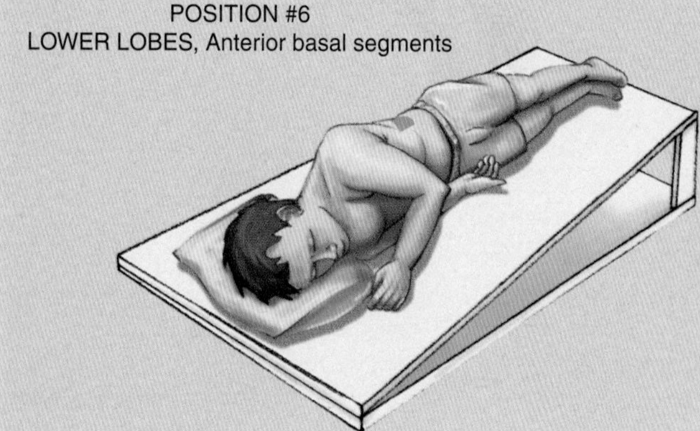

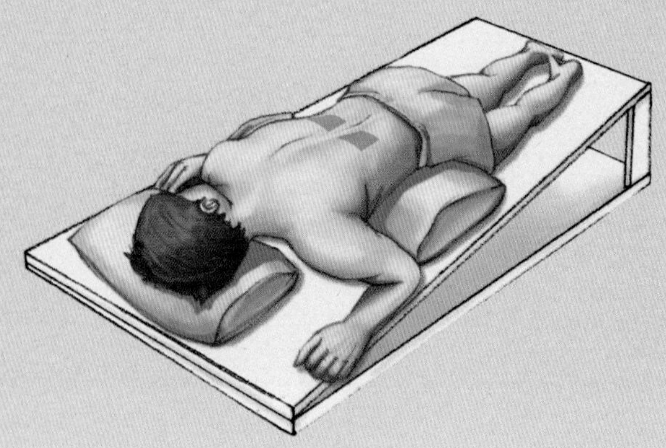

Nursing Procedure 19.2

Performing Chest Physiotherapy (continued)

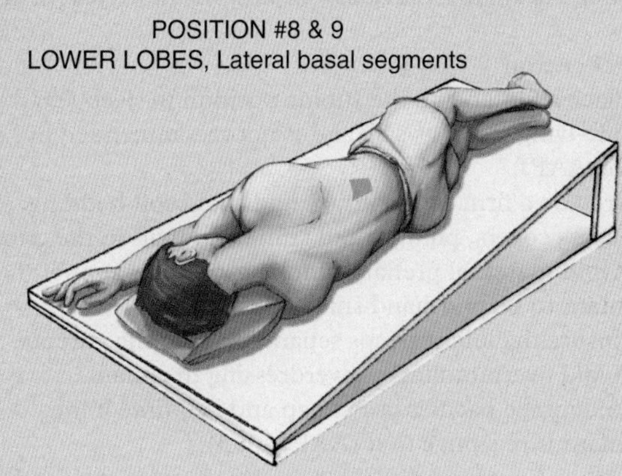

POSITION #10
LOWER LOBES, Superior segments

3. Place the ball of the hand on the lung segment, keeping the arm and shoulder straight. Vibrate by tensing and relaxing your arms during the child's exhalation. Vibrate each lung segment for at least five exhalations.
4. Encourage the child to deep breathe and cough.
5. Change drainage positions and repeat percussion and vibration.

In infants, breastfeeding should be continued with enzyme administration. Some infants will require fortification of breast milk or supplementation with high-calorie formulas. Commercially available infant formulas can continue to be used for the formula-fed infant and can be mixed to provide a larger amount of calories if necessary. Supplementation with vitamins A, D, E, and K is necessary. Administer gavage feedings or total parenteral nutrition as prescribed to provide for adequate growth.

Promoting Family Coping

Cystic fibrosis is a serious chronic illness that requires intervention on a daily basis. It can be hard to maintain a schedule that requires pulmonary hygiene several times daily as well as close attention to appropriate diet and enzyme supplementation. Adjusting to the demands that the illness places on the child and family is difficult. Continual ongoing adjustments within the family must occur. Children are frequently hospitalized, and this may place an additional strain on the family and its finances. Children with cystic fibrosis may express fear or feelings of isolation, and siblings may be worried or jealous (Carpenter & Narsavage, 2004). The family should be encouraged to lead a normal life through involvement in activities and school attendance during periods of wellness.

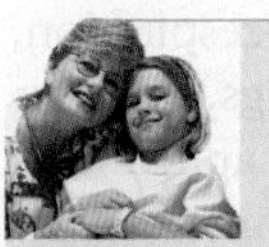

Massage therapy performed by the parent, nurse, or licensed massage therapist may help to decrease anxiety in the child with cystic fibrosis. It may have the added benefit of improving respiratory status, but it does not replace chest physiotherapy (Huth et al., 2005).

Starting at the time of diagnosis, families often demonstrate significant stress as the severity of the diagnosis and the significance of disease chronicity become real for them. The family should be involved in the child's care from the time of diagnosis, whether in the outpatient setting or in the hospital. Ongoing education about the illness and its treatments is necessary. Once the initial shock of diagnosis has passed and the family has adjusted to initial care, the family usually learns how to manage the requirements of care. Powerlessness gives way to adaptation. As family members become more comfortable with their understanding of the illness and the required treatments, they will eventually become the experts on the child's care. It is important for the nurse to recognize and respect the family's changing needs over time.

Providing daily intense care can be tiring, and noncompliance on the part of the family or child might occur as a result of this fatigue. Overvigilance may also occur as a result of the need for control over the difficult situation as well as a desire to protect the child. Families welcome support and encouragement. Most families will eventually progress past the stages of fear, guilt, and powerlessness. They move beyond those feelings to a way of living that is different than what they anticipated but is something that they can manage.

Refer parents to a local support group for families of children with cystic fibrosis. The Cystic Fibrosis Foundation has chapters throughout the United States and can be accessed at www.cff.org. Additional resources can be found at www.cysticfibrosis.com, www.cfri.org, and www.cfww.org.

Parents of children with a terminal illness might face the death of their child at an earlier age than expected.

Assisting with anticipatory grieving and making decisions related to end-of-life care are other important nursing interventions.

Preparing the Child and Family for Adulthood With Cystic Fibrosis

With current technological and medication advances, many more children with cystic fibrosis are surviving to adulthood and into their 30s and 40s. Lung transplantation is now being used in some patients with success, thus prolonging life expectancy (barring transplant complications). Children should have the goal of independent living as an adult, as other children do. Making the transition from a pediatric medical home to an adult medical home should be viewed as a rite of passage (Madge & Byron, 2005). Pediatric clinics are focused on family-centered care that heavily involves the child's parents, but adults with cystic fibrosis need a different focus, one that views them as independent adults.

Adults with cystic fibrosis can make the transition from pediatric to adult care with thoughtful preparation and coordination. They desire and deserve a smooth transition in care that will result in appropriate ongoing medical management of cystic fibrosis provided in an environment that is geared toward adults rather than children.

Adults with cystic fibrosis are able to find rewarding work and pursue relationships. Most men with cystic fibrosis are capable of sexual intercourse, though unable to reproduce. Females might have difficulty conceiving, and when they do they should be cautioned about the additional respiratory strain that pregnancy causes. All children of parents with cystic fibrosis will be carriers of the gene.

APNEA

Apnea is defined as absence of breathing for longer than 20 seconds; it might be accompanied by bradycardia. Sometimes apnea presents in the form of an acute life-threatening event (ALTE), an event in which the infant or child exhibits some combination of apnea, color change, muscle tone alteration, coughing, or gagging. Apnea may also occur acutely at any age as a result of respiratory distress. This discussion will focus on apnea that is chronic or recurrent in nature or that occurs as part of an ALTE.

Apnea in infants may be central (unrelated to any other cause) or occur with other illnesses such as sepsis and respiratory infection. Apnea in newborns might be associated with hypothermia, hypoglycemia, infection, or hyperbilirubinemia. Apnea of prematurity occurs secondary to an immature respiratory system. Apnea should not be considered as a predecessor to sudden infant death syndrome (SIDS). Current research has not proven this theory, and SIDS generally occurs in otherwise healthy young infants (AAP, Task Force on Sudden Infant Death Syndrome, 2005; Ramanathan et al., 2001). Box 19.3 gives more information about SIDS and its prevention.

BOX 19.3

SUDDEN INFANT DEATH SYNDROME (SIDS)

Definition

Sudden death of a previously healthy infant <1 year of age

Prevention

- Place all infants in the supine position to sleep (even side-lying is not as safe and is not recommended by the AAP).
- Provide a firm sleep surface and avoid soft bedding, excess covers, pillows, and stuffed animals in the crib.
- Avoid maternal prenatal smoking and exposure of the infant to second-hand smoke.
- Ensure the infant sleeps separately from the parents.
- Avoid overbundling or overdressing the infant.
- Encourage pacifier use at nap and bed time if the infant is receptive to it (AAP, 2005).

Support and Information

- www.sidsalliance.org: SIDS alliance
- www.sidscenter.org: National SIDS/Infant Death Resource Center
- www.asip1.org: Association for SIDS and Infant Mortality Program
- sids-network.org/: Sudden Infant Death Syndrome Network, Inc.

Therapeutic management of apnea varies depending upon the cause. When apnea occurs as a result of another disorder or infection, treatment is directed toward that cause. In the event of apnea, stimulation may trigger the infant to take a breath. If breathing does not resume, rescue breathing or bag-valve-mask ventilation is necessary. Infants and children who have experienced an ALTE or who have chronic apnea may require ongoing cardiac/apnea monitoring. Caffeine or theophylline is sometimes administered, primarily in premature infants, to stimulate respirations.

Nursing Assessment

Question the parents about the infant's position and activities preceding the apneic episode. Did the infant experience a color change? Did the infant self-stimulate (breathe again on his or her own), or did he or she require stimulation from the caretaker? Assess risk factors for apnea, which may include prematurity, anemia, and history of metabolic disorders. Apnea may occur in association with cardiac or neurologic disturbances, respiratory infection, sepsis, child abuse, or poisoning.

In the hospitalized infant, note absence of respiration, position, color, and other associated findings, such as emesis on the bedclothes. If an infant who is apneic fails to be stimulated and does not breathe again, pulselessness will result.

Nursing Management

When an infant is noted to be apneic, gently stimulate him or her to take a breath again. If gentle stimulation is unsuccessful, then rescue breathing or bag-valve-mask ventilation must be started.

To avoid apnea in the newborn, maintain a neutral thermal environment. Avoid excessive vagal stimulation and taking rectal temperatures (the vagal response can cause bradycardia, resulting in apnea). Administer caffeine or theophylline if prescribed and teach families about the use of these medications.

Infants with recurrent apnea or ALTE may be discharged on a home apnea monitor (Fig. 19.19). Provide education on use of the monitor, guidance for when to notify the physician or monitor service about alarms, and training in infant CPR. The monitor is usually discontinued after 3 months without a significant event of apnea or bradycardia. In some ways the monitor gives parents peace of mind, but in others it can make them more nervous about the well-being of their child. Also, the alarm on home monitors is extremely loud and parents often go for months with inadequate sleep. Providing appropriate education to the parents about the nature of the child's disorder as well as action to take in the event of apnea may give the family a sense of mastery over the situation, thus decreasing their level of anxiety. Refer families to local area support groups such as those offered by Parent to Parent and Parents Helping Parents.

Tracheostomy

A **tracheostomy** is an artificial opening in the airway; usually a plastic tracheostomy tube is in place to form a patent airway. Tracheostomies are performed to relieve airway obstruction, such as with **subglottic stenosis** (narrowing of the airway sometimes resulting from long-term intubation). They are also used for pulmonary toilet and in the child who requires chronic mechanical ventilation. The tracheostomy facilitates secretion removal, reduces work of breathing, and increases patient comfort. In some cases the tracheostomy facilitates mechanical ventilation weaning. It may be permanent or temporary depending on the condition that leads to the tracheostomy. The tracheostomy tube varies in size and type depending on the child's airway size and health and the length of time the child will require the tracheostomy. Silastic tracheostomy tubes are soft and flexible; they are available with a single lumen or may have an outer and inner lumen. Both types have an obturator (the guide used during tube changes). Typically, the tubes with inner cannulas are used with older children and in children with increased mucus production. Cuffed tracheostomy tubes are generally used in older children also. The cuff is used to prevent air from leaking around the tube. The funnel-shaped airway in younger children acts a physiological cuff and prevents air leak. Figure 19.20 shows various types of tracheostomy tubes.

Complications immediately postoperatively include hemorrhage, air entry, pulmonary edema, anatomic damage, and respiratory arrest. At any point in time the tracheostomy tube may become occluded and ventilation compromised. Complications of chronic tracheostomy include infection, cellulitis, and formation of granulation tissue around the insertion site (Russell, 2005).

Nursing Assessment

When obtaining the history for a child with a tracheostomy, note the reason for the tracheostomy, as well as the size and type of tracheostomy tube. Inspect the site. The stoma should appear pink and without bleeding or drainage. The tube itself should be clean and free from secretions. The tracheostomy ties should fit securely, allowing one finger to slide beneath the ties (Fig. 19.21). Inspect the skin under the ties for rash or redness. Observe work of breathing.

When caring for the infant or child with a tracheostomy, whether in the intensive care unit, the patient floor, or the home, a thorough respiratory assessment is necessary. Note presence of secretions and their color, thickness, and amount. Auscultate for breath sounds, which should be clear and equal throughout all lung fields. Pulse oximetry may also be measured. When infection is suspected or secretions are discolored or have a foul odor, a sputum culture may be obtained.

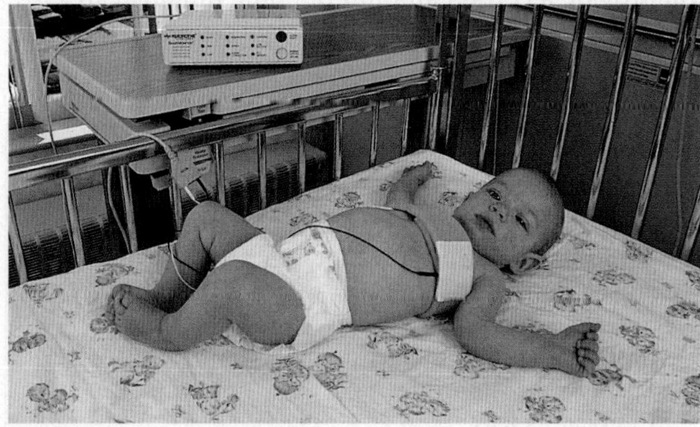

● Figure 19.19 The home apnea monitor uses a soft belt with Velcro attachment to hold two leads in the appropriate position on the chest.

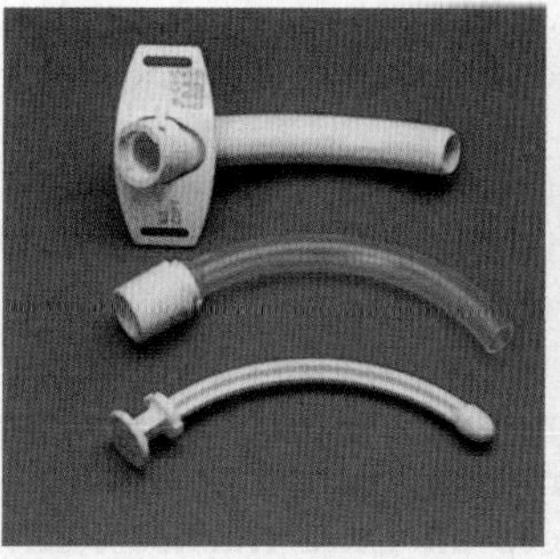

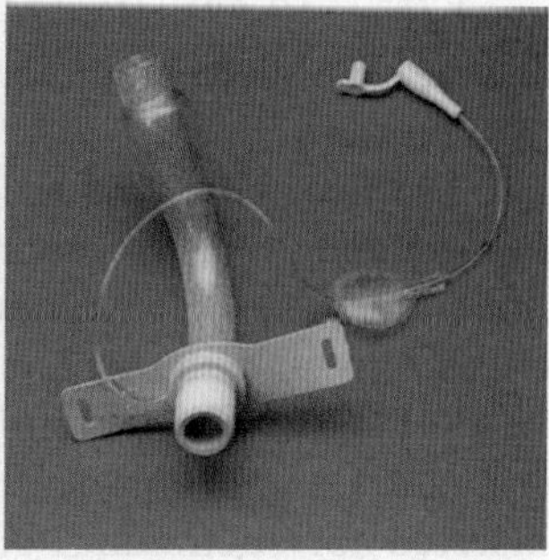

● Figure 19.20 Note smaller size and absence of inner cannula on particular brands of pediatric tracheostomy tubes.

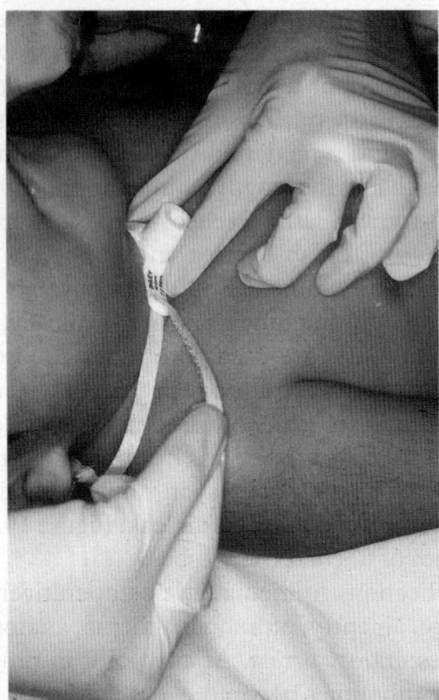

● Figure 19.21 Properly fitting trach ties. One finger width fits between the ties and the child's neck.

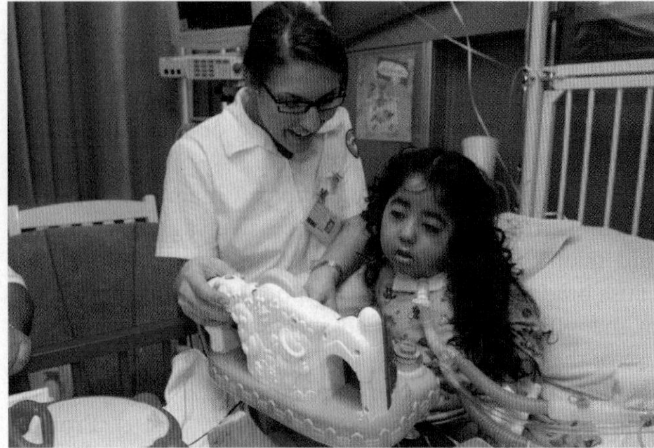

● Figure 19.22 The trach collar allows for humidification of inspired air or supplemental oxygen.

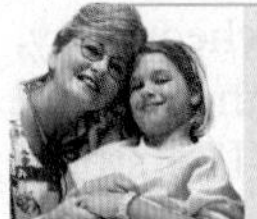

Keep small toys (risk of aspiration), plastic bibs or bedding (risk of airway occlusion), and talcum powder (risk of inhalation injury) out of reach of the child with a tracheostomy.

Nursing Management

In the immediate postoperative period the infant or child may require restraints to avoid accidental dislodgment of the tracheostomy tube. Infants and children who have had a tracheostomy for a period of time become accustomed to it and usually do not attempt to remove the tube. Since air inspired via the tracheostomy tube bypasses the upper airway, it lacks humidification, and this lack of humidity can lead to a mucus plug in the tracheostomy and hypoxia. Provide humidity to either room air or oxygen via a tracheostomy collar or ventilator, depending upon the child's need (Fig. 19.22). Box 19.4 lists the equipment that should be available at the bedside of any child who has a tracheostomy.

Tracheostomies require frequent suctioning to maintain patency. The appropriate length for insertion of the suction catheter depends on the size of the tracheostomy and the child's needs. Place a sign at the head of the child's bed indicating the suction catheter size and length (in centimeters) that it should be inserted for suctioning. Keep an extra tracheostomy tube of the same size and one size smaller at the bedside in the event of an emergency.

Many pediatric tracheostomy tubes do not have an inner cannula that requires periodic removal and cleaning, so periodic removal and replacement of the chronic tracheostomy tube is required. Clean the removed tracheostomy tube with half-strength hydrogen peroxide and pipe cleaners. Rinse with distilled water and allow it to dry. The tracheostomy tube can be reused many times if adequately cleaned between uses.

Perform tracheostomy care every 8 hours or per institution protocol. Change the tracheostomy tube only as needed or per institution protocol. Nursing Procedure 19.3 gives information about tracheostomy care.

If the older child or teen has a tracheostomy tube with an inner cannula, provide care of the inner cannula similar to that of an adult. Involve parents in care of the tracheostomy and begin education about caring for the tracheostomy tube at home as soon as the child is stable. Refer the family to local support groups or to www.tracheostomy.com, which offers many resources for a family whose child has a tracheostomy. The child with a tracheostomy often qualifies for a Medicaid waiver that will provide a certain amount of home nursing care.

BOX 19.4

EMERGENCY EQUIPMENT (AVAILABLE AT BEDSIDE)

- Two spare tracheostomy tubes (one the same size and one a size smaller)
- Suction equipment
- Stitch cutter (new tracheostomy)
- Spare tracheostomy ties
- Lubricating jelly
- Bag-valve-mask device
- Call bell within child's/parent's reach

Nursing Procedure 19.3

Tracheostomy Care

1. Gather the necessary equipment:
   - Cleaning solution
   - Gloves
   - Precut gauze pad
   - Cotton-tipped applicators
   - Clean tracheostomy ties
   - Scissors
   - Extra tracheostomy tube in case of accidental dislodgement
2. Position the infant/child supine with a blanket or towel roll to extend the neck.
3. Open all packaging and cut tracheostomy ties to appropriate length if necessary.
4. Cleanse around the tracheostomy site with prescribed solution (half-strength hydrogen peroxide or acetic acid, normal saline or soap and water if at home) and cotton-tipped applicators working from just around the tracheostomy tube outward.
5. Rinse with sterile water and cotton-tipped applicator in similar fashion.
6. Place the precut sterile gauze under the tracheostomy tube.
7. With the assistant holding the tube in place, cut the ties and remove from the tube.
8. Attach the clean ties to the tube and tie or secure in place with Velcro.

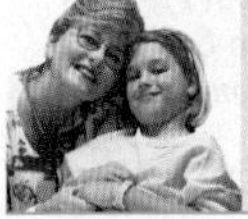

Always change tracheostomy ties with an assistant to avoid the tube being accidentally dislodged.

References

Ackley, B. J., & Ladwig, G. B. (2006). *Nursing diagnosis handbook: A guide to planning care* (7th ed). St. Louis: Mosby.

Advanced Respiratory. (2002). *Chest physiotherapy: the gold standard?* Retrieved May 13, 2006, from www.thevest.com/research/whitepapers/1101AACPTGoldStandard.pdf

American Academy of Pediatrics. (2001). Clinical practice guidelines: Management of sinusitis. *Pediatrics*, 108, 798–808.

American Academy of Pediatrics (2002). Policy statement: Reduction of the influenza burden in children. *Pediatrics, 110,* 1246–1252.

American Academy of Pediatrics. (2003). Tuberculosis. In L. K. Pickering (ed.), *Red Book: 2003 report of the committee on infectious diseases.* Elk Grove Village, IL: American Academy of Pediatrics.

American Academy of Pediatrics, Committee on Infectious Disease and Committee on Fetus and Newborn. (2003). Revised indications for the use of palivizumab and respiratory syncytial virus immune globulin intravenous for the prevention of respiratory syncytial virus infections. *Pediatrics, 112*(6), 1442–1446.

American Academy of Pediatrics, Task Force on Sudden Infant Death Syndrome. (2005). Policy Statement: The changing concept of sudden infant death syndrome: Diagnostic coding shifts, controversies regarding the sleeping environment, and new variables to consider in reducing risk. *Pediatrics, 116*(5), 1245–1255.

American Academy of Pediatrics & American Heart Association (2002). Airway and ventilation. In L. Chameides & M. F. Hazinski (eds.), *Pediatric advanced life support.* Dallas: American Heart Association.

American Association of Respiratory Care. (2004). AARC clinical practice guideline: nasotracheal suctioning—2004 revision & update. *Respiratory Care, 49*(9), 1080–1084.

American Heart Association. (2002). *PALS provider manual.* Dallas: American Heart Association.

American Thoracic Society (2000). Targeted tuberculin testing and treatment of latent tuberculosis infection. *American Journal of Respiratory and Critical Care Medicine, 161,* S221–S247.

Anonymous. (2005). Montelukast sodium for young children. *Nurse Practitioner, 30*(11), 76.

Auwaerter, P. G. (2002). Infectious mononucleosis in active patients. *Physician & Sports Medicine, 30*(11), 43–46.

Balinsky, W., & Zhu, C. W. (2004). Pediatric cystic fibrosis: Evaluating costs and genetic testing. *Journal of Pediatric Health Care, 18,* 30–34.

Banasiak, N. C., & Meadows-Oliver, M. (2005). Leukotrienes: Their role in the treatment of asthma and seasonal allergic rhinitis. *Pediatric Nursing, 31*(1), 35–38.

Bederka, M. (2006). Asthma studies you shouldn't miss: A look back at important research developments from 2004–2005. *Advance for Nurse Practitioners.* [electronic version] http://nurse-practitioners.advanceweb.com/.

Belkengren, R., & Sapala, S. (2003). Pediatric management problems. *Pediatric Nursing, 29*(2), 133–134.

Berkhof, J., Parker, K., & Melnyk, B. M. (2003). The effectiveness of anti-leukotriene agents in childhood asthma: Evidence to guide clinical practice. *Pediatric Nursing, 29*(1), 60–62.

Bisno, A. L. (2001). Acute pharyngitis. *New England Journal of Medicine, 344*(3), 205.

Bjornson, C. L., Klassen, T. P., Williamson, J., Brant, R., Mitton, C., Plint, A., Bulloch, B., Evered, L., & Johnson, D. W. (2004). A randomized trial of a single dose of oral dexamethasone for mild croup. *New England Journal of Medicine, 351,* 1306–1313.

Boat, T. F. (2004). Cystic fibrosis. In R. E. Behrman, R. M. Kliegman, & H. B. Jenson. *Nelson textbook of pediatrics* (17th ed.). Philadelphia: W. B. Saunders.

Brown, M. L. (2001). The effects of environmental tobacco smoke on children: information and implications for PNPs. *Journal of Pediatric Health Care, 15,* 280–286.

Buchfa, V. L., & Fries, C. M. (2004). Respiratory care. In E. J. Mills (Ed.), *Nursing procedures.* Philadelphia: Lippincott Williams & Wilkins.

Buford, T. A. (2004). Transfer of asthma management responsibility from parents to their school-age children. *Journal of Pediatric Nursing, 19*(1), 3–12.

Burke, M. G. (2004). Human metapneumovirus: Newly recognized villain. *Contemporary Pediatrics.* [electronic version] available www.contemporarypediatrics.com.

Carpenter, D. R., & Narsavage, G. L. (2004). One breath at a time: Living with cystic fibrosis. *Journal of Pediatric Nursing, 19*(1), 25–32.

Celik, S. A., & Kanan, N. (2006). A current conflict: use of isotonic sodium chloride solution on endotracheal suctioning in critically ill patients. *Dimensions of Critical Care Nursing, 25*(1), 11–14.

Cincinnati Children's Hospital Medical Center, (2000). Evidence-based clinical practice guideline of community-acquired pneumonia in children 60 days to 17 years of age. [Online]. www.guidelines.gov

Cooper, A. C., Banasiak, N. C., & Allen, P. J. (2003). Management and prevention strategies for respiratory syncytial virus (RSV) bronchiolitis in infants and young children: A review of evidence-based practice interventions. *Pediatric Nursing, 29*(6), 452–456.

Corren, J. (2000). The association between allergic rhinitis and asthma in children and adolescents: Epidemiologic considerations. *Pediatric Annals, 29,* 400–402.

Cunnington, J. (2002). Spontaneous pneumothorax. In S. Barton (Ed.), *Clinical evidence concise.* United Kingdom: BMJ Publishing Group.

Donahue, M. (2002). "Spare the cough, spoil the child:" Back to the basics of airway clearance. *Pediatric Nursing, 28,* 107–111.

Edgtton-Winn, M., & Wright, K. (2005). Tracheostomy: a guide to nursing care. *Australian Nursing Journal, 13*(5), S1–S4.

Farrar-Simpson, M. A., Gaffney, K. F., & Deleon, E. E. (2005). School-age girl with sore throat. *Pediatric Nursing, 31*(4), 341–344.

Flume, P. A., Strange, C., Ye, X., Ebeling, M., Hulsey, T., & Clark, L. L. (2005). Pneumothorax in cystic fibrosis. *Chest, 128*(2), 720–728.

Galley, R. (2005). Understanding pulse oximetry. *Clinician Reviews, 15*(10), 32–36.

German, J. A., & Harper, M. B. (2002). Environmental control of allergic disease. *American Family Physician, 66,* 3, 421–426, 429.

Goodfellow, L. T., & Jones, M. (2002). Bronchial hygiene therapy. *American Journal of Nursing 102*(1), 37–43.

Gross, S. D., Boyle, C. A., Botkin, J. R., Comeau, A. M., Kharrazi, M., Rosenfeld, M., & Wilfond, B. S. (2004). Newborn screening for cystic fibrosis: Evaluation of benefits and risks and recommendations for state newborn screening programs. *Morbidity and Mortality Weekly Report, 53*(RR12), 1–36.

Grossman, S., & Grossman, L. C. (2005). Pathophysiology of cystic fibrosis: Implications for critical care nurses. *Critical Care Nurse, 25*(4), 46–51.

Hagemann, T. M. (2005). Pediatric allergic rhinitis drug therapy. *Journal of Pediatric Health Care, 19,* 238–244.

Hall, K. L., & Zalman, B. (2005). Evaluation and management of apparent life-threatening events in children. *American Family Physician, 71*(12), 2301–2308.

Harvey, K. (2004). Bronchopulmonary dysplasia. In P. L. Jackson & J. A. Vessey (Eds.), *Primary care of the child with a chronic condition.* St. Louis: Mosby.

Hamilton, C., Steinlechner, B., Gruber, E., Simon, P., & Wollenek, G. (2004). The oxygen dissociation curve: quantifying the shift. *Perfusion, 19,* 141–144.

Hayes, C. S., & Williamson, H. (2001). Management of group A beta hemolytic streptococcal pharyngitis. *American Family Physician, 63,* 1557–1565.

Hayes, J. S., Ladebauche, P., Saucedo, K., Volicer, B., Richards, T., Nicolosi, R., & Reece, S. (2001). Asthma in Head Start children: Prevalence, risk factors, and health care utilization. *Pediatric Nursing, 27,* 396–399.

Horner, S. D. (2004). Effect of education on school-age children's and parents' asthma management. *Journal for Specialists in Pediatric Nursing, 9*(3), 95–102.

Horner, S. D., & Fouladi, R. T. (2003). Home asthma management for rural families. *Journal for Specialists in Pediatric Nursing, 8*(2), 52–61.

Hsiao, G., Black-Payne, C., & Campbell, G. D. (2001). Pneumonia, part 1: Making the diagnosis. *Journal of Respiratory Diseases for Pediatricians, 3,* 69–79.

Huth, M. M., Zink, K. A., & Van Horn, N. R. (2005). The effects of massage therapy in improving outcomes for youth with cystic fibrosis: An evidence review. *Pediatric Nursing, 31*(4), 328–332.

Jensen, H. B. (2004). Epstein-Barr virus. In R. E. Behrman, R. M. Kliegman, & H. B. Jenson (Eds.), *Nelson textbook of pediatrics* (17th ed.). Philadelphia: W. B. Saunders.

Johannsson, A., Halling, A., & Hermansson, G. (2003). Indoor and outdoor smoking. *European Journal of Public Health, 13*(1), 61–66.

Johansson, L., & Mansson, N. (2003). Rapid test, throat culture and clinical assessment in the diagnosis of tonsillitis. *Family Practice, 20*(2), 108–111.

Kieckhefer, G., & Ratcliffe, M. (2004). Asthma. In P. L. Jackson & J. A. Vessey (Eds.), *Primary care of the child with a chronic condition.* St. Louis: Mosby.

Knutson, D., & Aring, A. (2004). Information from your family doctor: What should I know about croup? *American Family Physician, 69*(3), 541–542.

Kumar, C. Edelman, M., & Ficorelli, C. (2005). Children with asthma: A concern for the family. *Maternal Child Nursing, 306*(30), 306–311.

Lara, M., Rosenbaum, S., Rachelefsky, G., Nicholas, W., Morton, S. C., Emont, S., Branch, M., Genovese, B., Vaiana, M. E., Smith, V., Wheeler, L., Platts-Mills, T., Clark, N., Lurie, N., & Weiss, K. B. (2002). Improving childhood asthma outcomes in the United States: A blueprint for policy action. *Pediatrics, 109*(5), 919–930.

Lauts, N. M. (2005). RSV: Protecting the littlest patients. *RN, 68*(12), 47–51.

Lemanske, R. F. (2002). Inflammation in childhood asthma and other wheezing disorders. *Pediatrics, 109*(2), 368–372.

Leung, A. K. C., & Kellner, J. D. (2004). Acute sinusitis in children: Diagnosis and management. *Journal of Pediatric Health Care, 18,* 72–76.

Leung, A. K. C., Kellner J. D., & Johnson, D. W. (2004). Viral croup: A current perspective. *Journal of Pediatric Health Care, 18,* 297–301.

Lieberman, P. (2000). A pathophysiologic link between allergic rhinitis and asthma. *Pediatric Annals, 29,* 405–410.

Louloudes, A. P. (2006). Pediatric respiratory disorders. In S. M. Nettina (Ed.), *Lippincott manual of nursing practice.* Philadelphia: Lippincott Williams & Wilkins.

Madge, S., & Bryon, M. (2002). A model for transition from pediatric to adult care in cystic fibrosis. *Journal of Pediatric Nursing, 17*(4), 283–288.

McCool, F. D., & Rosen, M. J. (2006). Nonpharmacologic airway clearance therapies: AACP evidence-based clinical practice guidelines. *Chest, 129*(1), 250S–259S.

McGarry, G. (2002). Recurrent idiopathic epistaxis (nosebleeds). *Clinical evidence concise, 7,* 59.

McMillan, J. A., Abramson, J. S., Katz, S. L., & Offit, P. A. (2005). Reducing the risk of influenza: Prevention strategies to help both the young and the old. *Contemporary Pediatrics supplement, 22*(1), 1–8.

McMullen, A. H. (2004). Cystic fibrosis. In P. L. Jackson & J. A. Vessey (Eds.), *Primary care of the child with a chronic condition* (4th ed.). St. Louis: Mosby.

Meissner, H. C. (2005). Prepare your patients for the RSV season. *Infectious Diseases in Children, 18*(11), 6, 9.

Moore, T. (2003). Suctioning techniques for the removal of respiratory secretions. *Nursing Standard, 18*(9), 47–55.

Myers, T. R. (2005). AARC clinical practice guideline: selection of an oxygen delivery device for neonatal and pediatric patients. *Respiratory Care, 47*(6), 707–716.

National Asthma Education and Prevention Program. (1997). *Expert panel report 2: Guidelines for the diagnosis and management of asthma* (NIH Publication No. 97-4051). Bethesda, MD: National Institutes of Health, National Heart, Lung and Blood Institute.

National Asthma Education and Prevention Program. (2002). *Expert panel report 2: Guidelines for the diagnosis and management of asthma—update on selected topics 2002* (NIH Publication No. 02-5074). National Institutes of Health, National Heart, Lung and Blood Institute.

National Institute of Allergy and Infectious Diseases. (2004). The common cold. [electronic version] available at www.niaid.nih.gov/factsheets/cold.htm.

Nield, L. S., Mahajan, P., & Kamat, D. M. (2005). Pneumonia: Update on causes and treatment options. *Consultant for Pediatricians, 4*(8), 365–370.

Orenstein, D. M. (2004). Bacterial tracheitis. In R. E. Behrman, R. M. Kliegman, & H. B. Jenson (Eds.), *Nelson textbook of pediatrics* (17th ed.). Philadelphia: W. B. Saunders.

Orenstein, D. M. (2004). Bronchiolitis. In R. E. Behrman, R. M. Kliegman, & H. B. Jenson (Eds.), *Nelson textbook of pediatrics* (17th ed.). Philadelphia: W. B. Saunders.

Orenstein, D. M. (2004). Bronchitis. In R. E. Behrman, R. M. Kliegman, & H. B. Jenson (Eds.), *Nelson textbook of pediatrics* (17th ed.). Philadelphia: W. B. Saunders.

Orenstein, D. M. (2004). Foreign bodies in the larynx, trachea and bronchi. In R. E. Behrman, R. M. Kliegman, & H. B. Jenson (Eds.), *Nelson textbook of pediatrics* (17th ed.). Philadelphia: W. B. Saunders.

Ostapchuk, M., Roberts, D. M., & Haddy, R. (2004). Community-acquired pneumonia in infants and children. *American Family Physician, 70*(5), 899–908.

Pagana, K. D., & Pagana, T. J. (2006). *Mosby's manual of diagnostic and laboratory tests* (3rd ed.). St. Louis: Mosby.

Parmet, S. (2004). Sore throat. *Journal of the American Medical Association, 291*(13), 1664.

Peterson, J., & Losek, J. D. (2004). Post-tonsillectomy hemorrhage and pediatric emergency care. *Clinical Pediatrics, 43,* 445–448.

Popovich, D. M., Richiuso, N., & Danek, G. (2004). Pediatric health care providers' knowledge of pulse oximetry. *Pediatric Nursing, 30*(1), 14–20.

Prober, C. G. (2004). Pneumonia. In R. E. Behrman, R. M. Kliegman, & H. B. Jenson (Eds.), *Nelson textbook of pediatrics* (17th ed.). Philadelphia: W. B. Saunders.

Pruitt, W. C., & Jacobs, M. (2003). Basics of oxygen therapy. *Nursing, 33*(10), 43–45.

Qureshi, S., & Mink, R. (2003). Aspiration of fruit gel snacks. *Pediatrics, 111*(3), 687–689.

Ramanathan, R., Corwin, M. J., Hunt, C. E., Lister, G., Tinsley, L. R., Baird, T., Silvestri, J. M., Crowell, D. H., Hufford, D., Martin, R. J., Neuman, M. R., Weese-Mayer, D. E., Cupples, L. A., Peucker, M., Willinger, M., & Keens, T. G. (The Collaborative Home Infant Monitoring Evaluation [CHIME] Study Group). (2001). Cardiorespiratory events recorded on home monitors: Comparison of healthy infants with those at increased risk for SIDS. *Journal of the American Medical Association, 285*(17), 2199–2207.

Reznik, M., & Ozuah, P. O. (2005). A prudent approach to screening for and treating tuberculosis. *Contemporary Pediatrics, 22*(11), 73–88.

Ridling, D. A., Martin, L. D., & Bratton, S. L. (2003). Endotracheal suctioning with or without instillation of isotonic sodium chloride solution in critically ill children. *American Journal of Critical Care, 12*(3), 212–219.

Robertson, J., & Shilkofski, N. (2005). *The Harriet Lane handbook: a manual for pediatric house officers* (17th ed.). St. Louis: Mosby.

Roman, M. (2005). Tracheostomy care. *MedSurg Nursing, 14*(2), 143–145.

Russell, C. (2005). Providing the nurse with a guide to tracheostomy care and management. *British Journal of Nursing, 14*(8), 428–433.

Sagraves, R. (2002). Increasing antibiotic resistance: Its effect on the therapy for otitis media. *Journal of Pediatric Health Care, 16,* 79–85.

Sander, N. (2002). Making the grade with asthma, allergies, and anaphylaxis. *Pediatric Nursing, 28*(6), 593–598.

Schneiderman, J. (2002). Ethmoid and maxillary sinusitis. *Consultant for Pediatricians, 1*(4), 131–134.

Schooff, M. (2005). Glucocorticoids for treatment of croup. *American Family Physician, 71*(1), 66.

Sharma, G. (2005). Cystic fibrosis. On emedicine.com, available at www.emedicine.com/cgi-bin/foxweb.exe/checkreg@/em/checkreg?http://www.emedicine.com/ped/topic535.htm.

Sheahan, S. L., & Free, T. A. (2005). Counseling parents to quit smoking. *Pediatric Nursing, 31*(2), 98–109.

Simpson, T., & Ivey, J. (2005). Toddler with a chronic cough. *Pediatric Nursing, 31*(1), 48–49.

Skoner, D. P. (2001). Why we must do a better job of controlling asthma. *Contemporary Pediatrics, 18*(8), 49–62.

Stadtler, A. C., Tronick, E. Z., & Brazelton, T. B. (2001). The Touchpoints Pediatric Asthma Program. *Pediatric Nursing, 27,* 459–461.

Starke, J. R., & Munoz, F. (2004). Tuberculosis. In R. E. Behrman, R. M. Kliegman, & H. B. Jenson (Eds.), *Nelson textbook of pediatrics* (17th ed.). Philadelphia: W. B. Saunders.

Steiner, R. W. P. (2004). Treating acute bronchiolitis associated with RSV. *American Family Physician, 69*(2), 325–330.

Steyer, T. (2002). Peritonsillar abscess: Diagnosis and treatment. *American Family Physician, 65,* 93–96.

Stoll, B. J., & Kliegman, R. M. (2004). Hyaline membrane disease (respiratory distress syndrome). In R. E. Behrman, R. M. Kliegman, & H. B. Jenson (Eds.), *Nelson textbook of pediatrics* (17th ed.). Philadelphia: W. B. Saunders.

Strunk, R. (2002). Defining asthma in the preschool age child. *Pediatrics, 109,* 357–361.

Suddaby, B., & Mowery, B. (2002). Tracheostomy troubles. *Pediatric Nursing, 28,* 162.

Svavarsdottir, E. K., & Rayens, M. K. (2005). Hardiness in families of young children with asthma. *Journal of Advanced Nursing, 50*(4), 381–390.

Taketokmo, C. K., Hodding, J. H., & Kraus, D. M. (2005). *Lexi-comp's pediatric dosage handbook (12th ed.).* Hudson, Ohio: Lexi-comp.

Tanner, K., Fitzsimmons, G., Carrol, E. D., Flood, T. J., & Clark, J. E. (2002). *Haemophilus influenzae* type b epiglottitis as a cause of acute upper airways obstruction. *British Medical Journal, 325,* 1099–1100.

Taylor, Z., Nolan, C. M., & Blumberg, H. M. (2005). Controlling tuberculosis in the United States: Recommendations from the American Thoracic Society, CDC, and the Infectious Diseases Society of America. *Morbidity and Mortality Weekly Report, 54*(RR12), 1–81.

Torpy, J. (2003). Coughs, colds and antibiotics. *Journal of the American Medical Association, 289*(20), 2750.

Turcios, N., & Patel, P. (2003). Pneumonia that recurs: Your diagnostic challenge. *Contemporary Pediatrics 3,* 82.

U.S. Department of Health and Human Services. (2000). *Healthy people 2010: Understanding and improving health.* Washington, D.C.: Department of Health and Human Services.

Vinson, J. A. (2002). Children with asthma: Initial development of a child resilience model. *Pediatric Nursing, 28*(2), 149–158.

Wachter, K. (2005). Many children manage own asthma medications. *Pediatric News, 39*(7), 38.

Wakefield, P. L., Sockrider, M. M., & White, L. (2005). A new approach to wheezing in infants and preschoolers: Shedding light on a difficult diagnosis. *Contemporary Pediatrics, 22*(3), 54–61.

Wakefield, P. L., Sockrider, M. M., & White, L. (2005). A new approach to wheezing in infants and preschoolers: Toward more effective treatment. *Contemporary Pediatrics, 22*(3), 63–68.

Weisman, L. E., & Groothius, J. R. (2000). *Contemporary diagnosis and management of respiratory syncytial virus.* Newtown, PA: Handbooks in Health Care Co.

Yoos, H. L., Kitzman, H., McMullen, A., Sidora-Arcoleo, K., & Anson, E. (2005). The language of breathlessness: Do families and health care providers speak the same language when describing asthma symptoms? *Journal of Pediatric Health Care, 19*(4), 197–205.

Websites

asthmatrack.org/ Ed's Asthma Track—for parents of children with asthma

www.aaaai.org American Academy of Allergy, Asthma, and Immunology

www.aafa.org Asthma and Allergy Foundation of America

www.aanma.org/ Allergy & Asthma Network Mothers of Asthmatics—offers extensive resources for families with children who have asthma

www.acaai.org/ American College of Allergy, Asthma, and Immunology

www.adcouncil.org/issues/Childhood_Asthma/ childhood asthma attack prevention

www.asthma-carenet.org/ The Childhood Asthma Research and Education (CARE) network founded by the National Heart, Lung and Blood Institute

www.asthmaandchildren.com/ information about asthma and children (supported by AstraZeneca)

www.asthmabusters.org/ online club for kids with asthma

www.asthmacamps.org/asthmacamps/ consortium on children's asthma camps

www.cff.org Cystic Fibrosis Foundation

www.cfri.org Cystic Fibrosis Research, Inc.

www.cfww.org Cystic Fibrosis Worldwide

www.childasthma.com/ Childhood Asthma Foundation

www.cysticfibrosis.com support forum for the cystic fibrosis community

www.guideline.com National Guideline Clearinghouse

www.jcaai.org Joint Council of Allergy, Asthma, and Immunology

www.lungusa.org/site/pp.asp?c=dvLUK9O0E&b=22691 American Lung Association, section on children and asthma

www.niaid.nih.gov National Institute of Allergy and Infectious Disease

www.noattacks.org site provides education about asthma, section for children, also available in Spanish

www.tracheostomy.com Aaron's Tracheostomy Site

Chapter WORKSHEET

● MULTIPLE CHOICE QUESTIONS

1. A 5-month-old infant with RSV bronchiolitis is in respiratory distress. The baby has copious secretions, increased work of breathing, cyanosis, and a respiratory rate of 78. What is the most appropriate *initial* nursing intervention?
   a. Attempt to calm the infant by placing him in his mother's lap and offering him a bottle.
   b. Alert the physician to the situation and ask for an order for a stat chest x-ray.
   c. Suction secretions, provide 100% oxygen via mask, and anticipate respiratory failure.
   d. Bring the emergency equipment to the room and begin bag-valve-mask ventilation.

2. A toddler has moderate respiratory distress, is mildly cyanotic, and has increased work of breathing, with a respiratory rate of 40. What is the priority nursing intervention?
   a. Airway maintenance and 100% oxygen by mask
   b. 100% oxygen and pulse oximetry monitoring
   c. Airway maintenance and continued reassessment
   d. 100% oxygen and provision of comfort

3. The nurse is caring for a child with cystic fibrosis who receives pancreatic enzymes. The nurse realizes that the child's mother understands the instructions related to giving the enzymes when the mother makes which of the following statements?
   a. "I will stop the enzymes if my child is receiving antibiotics."
   b. "I will decrease the dose by half if my child is having frequent, bulky stools."
   c. "Between meals is the best time for me to give the enzymes."
   d. "The enzymes should be given at the beginning of each meal and snack."

4. Which of these factors contributes to infants' and children's increased risk for upper airway obstruction as compared with adults?
   a. Underdeveloped cricoid cartilage and narrow nasal passages
   b. Small tonsils and narrow nasal passages
   c. Cylinder-shaped larynx and underdeveloped sinuses
   d. Underdeveloped cricoid cartilage and smaller tongue

5. Which is the most appropriate treatment for epistaxis?
   a. With the child lying down and breathing through the mouth, apply pressure to the bridge of the nose.
   b. With the child lying down and breathing through the mouth, pinch the lower third of the nose closed.
   c. With the child sitting up and leaning forward, apply pressure to the bridge of the nose.
   d. With the child sitting up and leaning forward, pinch the lower third of the nose closed.

● CRITICAL THINKING EXERCISES

1. A 10-month-old girl is admitted to the pediatric unit with a history of recurrent pneumonia and failure to thrive. Her sweat chloride test confirms the diagnosis of cystic fibrosis. She is a frail-appearing infant with thin extremities and a slightly protuberant abdomen. She is tachypneic, has retractions, and coughs frequently. Based on the limited information given here and your knowledge of cystic fibrosis, choose three of the categories below as priorities to focus on when planning her care:
   a. Prevention of bronchospasm
   b. Promotion of adequate nutrition
   c. Education of the child and family
   d. Prevention of pulmonary infection
   e. Balancing fluid and electrolytes
   f. Management of excess weight gain
   g. Prevention of spread of infection
   h. Promoting adequate sleep and rest

2. A child with asthma is admitted to the pediatric unit for the fourth time this year. The mother expresses frustration that the child is getting sick so often. Besides information about onset of symptoms and events leading up to this present episode, what other types of information would you ask for while obtaining the history?

3. The mother of the child in the previous question tells you that she smokes (but never around the child), the family has a cat that comes inside sometimes, and she always gives her child the medication prescribed. She gives salmeterol and budesonide as soon as the child starts to cough. When he is not having an episode, she gives him albuterol before his baseball games. Diphenhydramine helps his runny nose in the springtime. Based on this new information, what advice/instructions would you give the mother?

4. A 7-year-old presents with a history of recurrent nasal discharge. He sneezes every time he visits his cousins, who have pets. He lives in an older home that is carpeted. Tobacco smokers live in the home. His mother reports that he snores and is a mouth breather. She says he has symptoms nearly year-round, but they are worse in the fall and the spring. She reports that diphenhydramine is somewhat helpful with his symptoms, but she doesn't like to give it to him on school days because it makes him drowsy. Based on the history above, develop a teaching plan for this child.

5. The nurse is caring for a 4-year-old girl who returned from the recovery room after a tonsillectomy 3 hours ago. She has cried off and on in the past 2 hours and is now sleeping. What areas in particular should the nurse assess and focus on for this patient?

● STUDY ACTIVITIES

1. While caring for children in the pediatric setting, compare the signs and symptoms of a child with asthma to those of an infant with bronchiolitis. What are the most notable differences? How does the history of the two children differ?

2. The nurse is caring for a child with asthma. The child has been prescribed Advair (fluticasone and salmeterol), albuterol, and prednisone. Develop a sample teaching plan for the child and family. Include appropriate use of the devices used to deliver the medications, as well as important information about the medications (uses and side effects).

3. While caring for children in the pediatric setting, compare the signs and symptoms and presentation of a child with the common cold to those of a child with either sinusitis or allergic rhinitis.

4. While caring for children in the pediatric setting, review the census of clients and identify those at risk for severe influenza and thus those who would benefit from annual influenza vaccination.

5. Compare the differences in oxygen administration between a young infant and an older child.

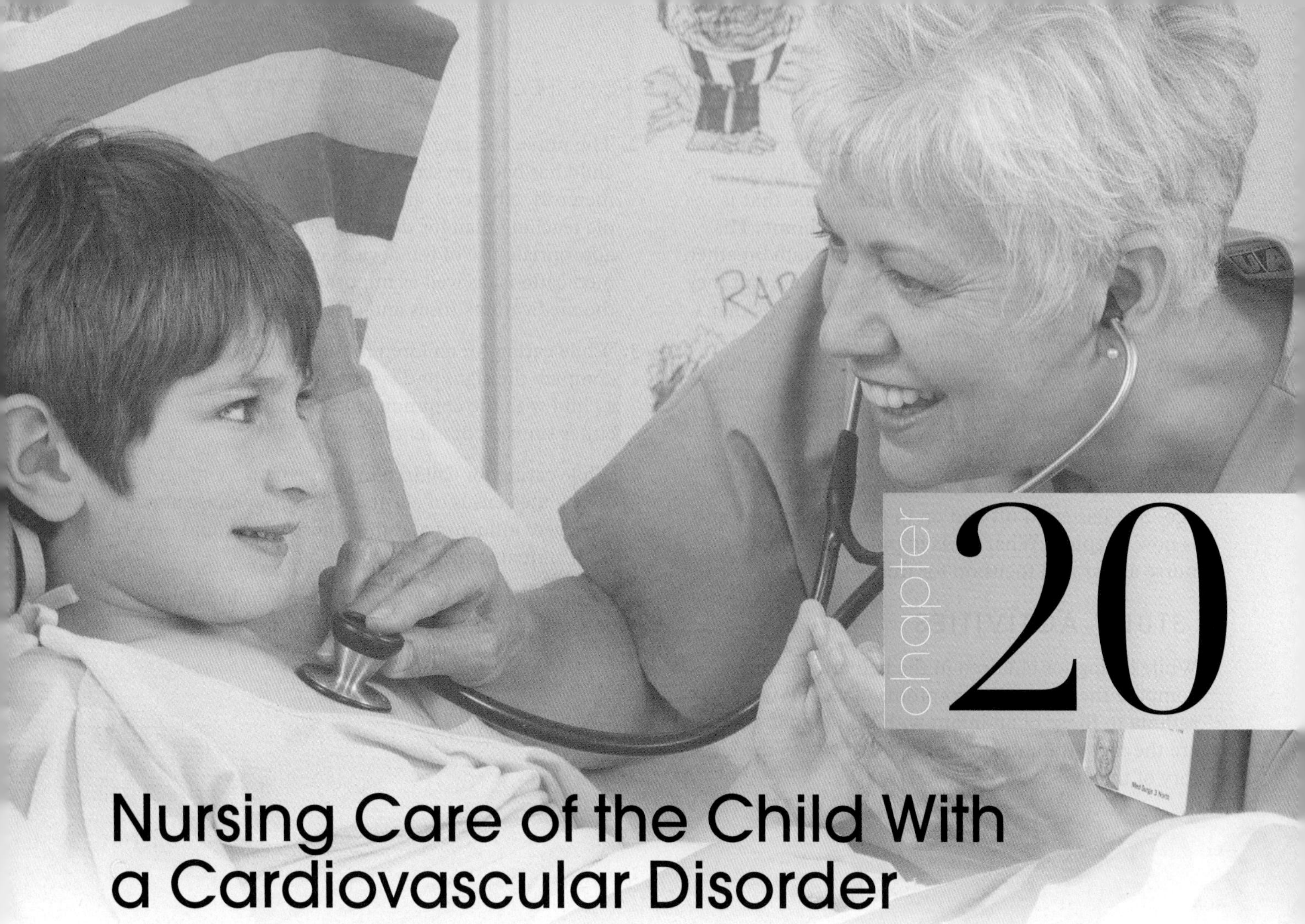

chapter 20

Nursing Care of the Child With a Cardiovascular Disorder

Key TERMS

arrhythmia
cardiac monitoring
cardiac output
cardiomegaly
clubbing
congenital heart defect
echocardiography
electrocardiogram (ECG, EKG)
heart failure
orthotopic
polycythemia
sinus bradycardia
sinus tachycardia
tetralogy of Fallot

Learning OBJECTIVES

Upon completion of the chapter, the learner will be able to:

1. Compare anatomic and physiologic differences of the cardiovascular system in infants and children versus adults.
2. Describe nursing care related to common laboratory and diagnostic tests used in the medical diagnosis of pediatric cardiovascular conditions.
3. Distinguish cardiovascular disorders common in infants, children, and adolescents.
4. Identify appropriate nursing assessments and interventions related to medications and treatments for pediatric cardiovascular disorders.
5. Develop an individualized nursing care plan for the child with a cardiovascular disorder.
6. Describe the psychosocial impact of chronic cardiovascular disorders on children.
7. Devise a nutrition plan for the child with renal insufficiency.
8. Develop patient/family teaching plans for the child with a cardiovascular disorder.

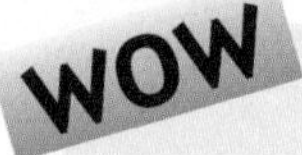

The heart of the matter is healing the child's heart so he or she can embrace life to its fullest.

Logan Bernstein, 6 weeks old, is brought to the clinic by his mother. He presents with poor feeding. His mother states, "Logan falls asleep while feeding, and he's always very sweaty during feedings."

Cardiovascular disease is a significant cause of chronic illness and death in children. Typically cardiovascular disorders in children are divided into two major categories: congenital heart disease (CHD) and acquired heart disease. Congenital heart disease is defined as structural anomalies that are present at birth, though they are often not diagnosed until later in life. CHD accounts for the largest percentage of birth defects, and about 40,000 babies are born annually with a **congenital heart defect** (American Heart Association [AHA], 2006c). Acquired heart disease includes disorders that occur after birth. These disorders develop from a wide range of causes, or they can occur as a complication or long-term effect of CHD. Over 100 genes have been identified that may be involved in the development of CHD (Cunningham et al., 2005). Additional noncardiac anomalies occur in about 28% of children with CHD. CHD is also commonly associated with chromosomal abnormalities and occurs at a rate of about 3% in children with first-degree relatives who have CHD (Fixler, 2006). Many congenital heart defects result in heart failure and chronic cyanosis, leading to failure to thrive.

The diagnosis of a cardiovascular disorder in any person can be extremely frightening and overwhelming. This is even truer for the child and his or her parents. Early on, children learn that the heart is necessary for life, so knowing that there is a heart problem can promote feelings of dread. These feelings are compounded by the child's age, the view of the child as being vulnerable and defenseless, and the stressors associated with the disorder itself. The child and parents need much support and reassurance.

Nurses need to have a sound knowledge base about cardiovascular conditions affecting children so that they can provide appropriate assessment, intervention, guidance, and support to the child and family. Cardiovascular disorders require acute interventions that often have long-term implications for the child's health and growth and development. Due to the potentially overwhelming and devastating effects that cardiovascular disorders can have on children and their families, nurses need to be skilled in assessment and interventions in this area and able to provide support throughout the course of the illness and beyond. This chapter describes the nursing management of children with congenital and acquired cardiovascular disorders, highlighting the common procedures used for treatment.

Variations in Pediatric Anatomy and Physiology

The cardiovascular system undergoes numerous changes at birth. Structures that were vital to the fetus are no longer needed. Circulation via the umbilical arteries and vein is replaced with the child's own closed independent circulation. Changes in the size of the heart, pulse rate, and blood pressure also occur.

Circulatory Changes From Gestation to Birth

The fetal heart is developed within the first 21 days of gestation, with the development of the heart rate and fetal blood circulation. The four chambers of the heart and arteries are formed during gestational months 2 through 8. During fetal development, oxygenation of the fetus occurs via the placenta; the lungs, though perfused, do not perform oxygenation and ventilation. The foramen ovale, an opening between the atria, allows blood flow from the right to the left atrium. The ductus arteriosus allows blood flow between the pulmonary artery and the aorta, shunting blood away from the pulmonary circulation (Molczan, 2006; Valente et al., 2006). Figure 20.1 illustrates fetal circulation.

With the first breath, several changes occur in the cardiopulmonary system that enable the newborn to make the transition from fetal circulation to normal circulation. As the newborn breathes for the first time, the lungs inflate, reducing pulmonary vascular resistance to blood flow. As a result, pulmonary artery pressure drops. Subsequently, pressure in the right atrium decreases. Blood flow to the left side of the heart increases the pressure in the left atrium. This change in pressure leads to closure of the foramen ovale. The drop in pressure of the pulmonary artery promotes closure of the ductus arteriosus, which is located between the aorta and pulmonary artery. The ductus venosus, located between the left umbilical vein and the inferior vena cava, closes because of a lack of blood flow and vasoconstriction. The closed ductus arteriosus and ductus venosus eventually become ligaments. With the lack of blood flow to the umbilical arteries and vein, these structures atrophy.

Structural and Functional Differences

The structure and function of the infant's and child's cardiovascular system differ from those of adults, depending on age. In infants and children under 7, the heart lies more horizontally. As a result, the apex lies higher, below the fourth intercostal space. In the infant, the heart lies higher in the chest and occupies over half of the chest width. As the lungs grow over time, the heart is displaced downward. The toddler/preschooler (between 1 and 6 years) has a heart four times the birth size. By school age (between 6 and 12 years) the child's heart is 10 times the

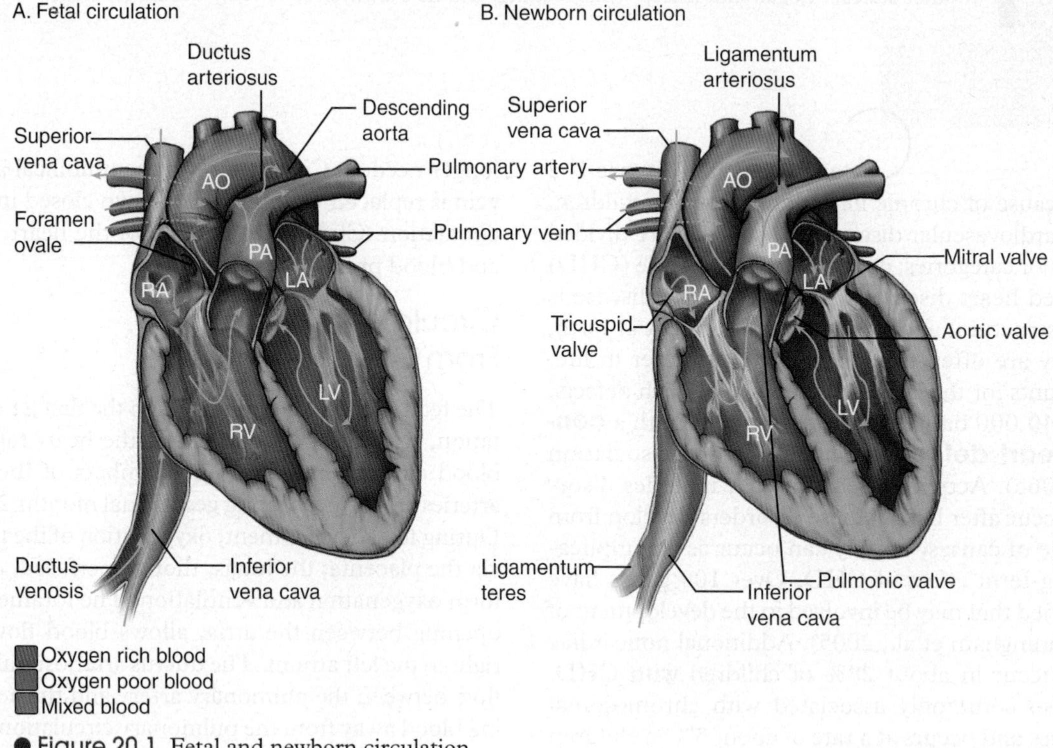

● **Figure 20.1** Fetal and newborn circulation.

size it was at birth. However, the heart is smaller proportionally at this time than at any other stage in life. During the school-age years, the heart grows more vertically within the thoracic cavity. During adolescence, the heart continues to grow in relation to the teen's rapid growth.

At birth, the ventricle walls are similar in thickness, but with time the left ventricular wall thickens. The immature myocytes of the infant's heart are thinner and less compliant than those of the adult. Right ventricular function dominates at birth, and over the first few months of life, left ventricular function becomes dominant. The infant's heart at rest exhibits a greater resting tension than the adult's, so volume loading or increased stretch may actually lead to decreased **cardiac output**. The infant's sarcoplasmic reticulum is less well organized than the adult's, making the infant dependent on serum calcium for contraction. Inotropic response to calcium in the actin and myosin (contractile proteins) increases with age (Craig et al., 2001).

The normal heart rate is higher in infancy than in adulthood, limiting the infant's ability to increase cardiac output by increasing the heart rate. The heart's efficiency increases as the child ages and the heart rate drops over time. The normal infant heart rate averages 120 to 130 beats per minute (bpm), the toddler's or preschooler's is 80 to 105 bpm, the school-age child's is 70 to 80 bpm, and the adolescent's averages 60 to 68 bpm. Innocent murmurs and physiologic splitting of heart sounds may be noted in infancy or childhood. These findings are related to the change in the size of the heart in relation to the thoracic cavity. The infant's and child's blood vessels widen and increase in length over time. The normal infant's blood pressure (BP) is about 80/40 mm Hg. The BP increases over time to the adult level. The toddler or preschooler's BP averages 80 to 100/64 mm Hg, the school-age child's 94 to 112/56 to 60 mm Hg, and the adolescent's 100 to 120/50 to 70 mm Hg (Frietas-Nichols, 2004; Luxner, 2005; Muscari, 2004).

Common Medical Treatments

A variety of medications as well as other medical treatments and surgical procedures are used to treat cardiovascular problems in children. Most of these treatments will require a physician's order when the child is in the hospital. The most common treatments and medications are listed in Common Medical Treatments 20.1 and Drug Guide 20.1. The nurse caring for the child with a cardiovascular disorder should be familiar with what the procedures and medications are and how they work as well as common nursing implications related to use of these modalities.

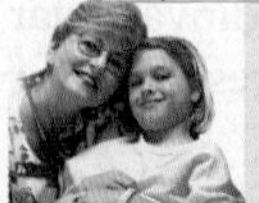

Give digoxin at regular intervals, every 12 hours, such as at 8 a.m. and 8 p.m., 1 hour before or 2 hours after a feeding. If a digoxin dose is missed and more than 4 hours have elapsed, withhold the dose and give the dose at the regular time; if less than 4 hours have elapsed, give the missed dose. If the child vomits digoxin, **do not** give a second dose. Monitor potassium levels, as a decrease enhances the effects of digitalis, causing toxicity.

(text continues on page 618)

Common Medical Treatments 20.1

Treatment	Explanation	Indication	Nursing Implications
Oxygen	Supplemented via mask, nasal cannula, hood, and tent or via endotracheal/ nasotracheal tube	Hypoxemia, respiratory distress, heart failure	Monitor response via work of breathing and pulse oximetry.
Chest physiotherapy (CPT) and postural drainage	Promotes mucus clearance by mobilizing secretions with the assistance of percussion or vibration accompanied by postural drainage (refer to Chapter 14 for additional information related to CPT and postural drainage)	Mobilization of secretions, particularly in postoperative period or with heart failure	May be performed by respiratory therapist in some institutions, by nurses in others. In either case, nurses must be familiar with the technique and able to educate families on its use.
Chest tube	Drainage tube is inserted into the pleural cavity to facilitate removal of air or fluid and allow full lung expansion.	After open heart surgery, pneumothorax	If tube becomes dislodged from container, the chest tube must be clamped immediately to avoid further air entry into the chest cavity.
Pacing	External wiring connected to a small generator used to electrophysiologically correct cardiac arrhythmias or heart block (temporary). Permanent pacing achieved with an implantable internal pacemaker.	Bradyarrhythmias, heart block, cardiomyopathy, sinoatrial or atrioventricular node malfunction	Provide close observation of the child, pacing unit, and ECG. Maintain asepsis at pacing lead insertion site. Explain to child and family that the permanent pacemaker may be felt under the skin. Advise against participation in contact sports.

Drug Guide 20.1

Medication	Action	Indication	Nursing Implications
Alprostadil (Prostin VR: prostaglandin E_1)	Direct vasodilation of the ductus arteriosus smooth muscle	Temporary maintenance of ductus arteriosus patency in infants with ductal-dependent congenital heart defects	• Apnea occurs in 10% to 20% of neonates within first hour of infusion. • Monitor arterial BP, respiratory rate, heart rate, ECG, temperature, pO_2; watch for abdominal distention. • Fresh IV solution required every 24 hours • Reposition catheter if facial or arm flushing occurs. • Use with caution in neonate with bleeding tendency. • Contraindicated in respiratory distress syndrome or persistent fetal circulation
Digoxin (Lanoxin)	To increase contractility of the heart muscle by decreasing conduction and increasing force	Heart failure, atrial fibrillation, atrial flutter, supraventricular tachycardia	• Prior to administering each dose, count apical pulse for 1 full minute, noting rate, rhythm, and quality. Withhold if apical pulse is <60 in an adolescent, <90 in an infant.

Drug Guide 20.1 (continued)

Medication	Action	Indication	Nursing Implications
			• Avoid giving oral form with meals, as altered absorption may occur. • Monitor serum digoxin levels (therapeutic range: 0.8–2 ng/mL). • Notes signs of toxicity: nausea, vomiting, diarrhea, lethargy, bradycardia. • Ginseng, hawthorn, and licorice intake increases risk for drug toxicity. • Note contraindications (ventricular fibrillation and hypersensitivity to digitalis). • Avoid rapid IV administration, as this may lead to systemic and coronary artery vasoconstriction.
Furosemide (Lasix)	Inhibits resorption of sodium and chloride in ascending loop of Henle	Management of edema associated with heart failure, or management of hypertension in combination with antihypertensives	• Administer with food or milk to decrease GI upset. • Monitor BP, renal function, electrolytes (particularly potassium), and hearing. • May cause photosensitivity.
Heparin	Interferes with conversion of prothrombin to thrombin, preventing clot formation	Prophylaxis and treatment of thromboembolic disorders, especially after cardiac surgery	• Administer SQ, not IM. • Dose is adjusted according to coagulation test results. • Monitor for signs of bleeding, platelet counts. • Ensure that the antidote, protamine sulfate, is available. • Do not administer with uncontrolled bleeding or if subacute bacterial endocarditis is suspected.
Indomethacin (Indocin)	Inhibits prostaglandin synthesis	To close patent ductus arteriosus	• Monitor heart rate, BP, ECG, urine output; monitor for murmur. • Monitor serum sodium, glucose, platelet count, BUN, creatinine, potassium, and liver enzymes. • May mask signs of infection • Note development of edema.
Spironolactone (Aldactone)	Competes with aldosterone to result in increased water and sodium excretion (spares potassium)	Management of edema due to heart failure, treatment of hypertension	• Administer with food. • Monitor serum potassium, sodium, and renal function. • May cause drowsiness, headache, arrhythmia. • May cause false elevations in digitalis level. • Teach patients to avoid high-potassium diets, salt substitutes, and natural licorice. • Contraindicated in hyperkalemia, renal failure, and anuria.

Drug Guide 20.1 (continued)

Medication	Action	Indication	Nursing Implications
Antibiotics			
Penicillin G benzathine (PCN-G) Penicillin V potassium (Pen-VK)	Inhibits bacterial wall synthesis in susceptible gram-positive organisms, such as streptococci, pneumococci, and staphylococci	Mild to moderate infections, prophylaxis of endocarditis and rheumatic fever	• Contraindications include hypersensitivity to penicillins. • Report hypersensitivity reactions (chills, fever, wheezing, pruritus, anaphylaxis) immediately. • PCN-G: administer IM. • Pen-VK: administer orally on empty stomach 1 hour prior to or 2 hours after a meal.
Erythromycin	Inhibits RNA transcription in susceptible organisms, such as streptococci, pneumococci, and staphylococci	Children with penicillin allergy, mild to moderate infections, endocarditis, and rheumatic fever prophylaxis	• Contraindicated in preexisting liver disease. • IV administration may result in CV abnormalities. • Abdominal distress common with oral use. • Fever, dizziness, rash may occur.
Antihypertensive Drugs			
Angiotensin-converting enzyme (ACE) inhibitors (captopril (Capoten), enalapril (Vasotec))	Competitive inhibition of ACE	Management of hypertension. Heart failure management in conjunction with digitalis and diuretics.	• Monitor BP, renal function, WBC count, serum potassium. • Discontinue if angioedema occurs. • Captopril: administer orally on empty stomach 1 hour before or 2 hours after meals. • Enalapril: may administer orally without regard to food.
Beta-adrenergic blockers (propranolol (Inderal), atenolol (Tenormin), sotalol (Betaspace))	Competitively blocks response to $beta_1$- and $beta_2$-adrenergic stimulation (propranolol, sotalol), $beta_1$ only (atenolol), decreasing heart rate and force of contraction	Management of hypertension, arrhythmias; prevention of myocardial infarction (propranolol, atenolol). Arrhythmia management (sotalol).	• Monitor ECG and BP. • Propranolol: administer with food. • Atenolol, sotalol: administer without regard to food. Do not stop drug abruptly. • May result in bradycardia, dizziness, nausea and vomiting, dyspnea, hypoglycemia (propranolol). • Contraindications: heart block, uncompensated heart failure, cardiogenic shock, asthma, or hypersensitivity.
Hydralazine (Apresoline)	Direct vasodilation of arterioles	Management of moderate to severe hypertension, heart failure	• Monitor heart rate, BP. • Closely monitor BP with IV use. • Administer oral dose with food. • May cause palpitations, flushing, tachycardia, dizziness, nausea and vomiting. • Notify physician if flu-like symptoms occur. • Contraindicated in rheumatic valvular disease.

Nursing Process Overview for the Child With a Cardiovascular Disorder

Care of the child with a cardiovascular disorder includes all of the typical steps of the nursing process: assessment, nursing diagnosis, planning, interventions, and evaluation. There are a number of general concepts related to the nursing process that may be applied to any child with a cardiovascular disorder. The nurse should be knowledgeable about the procedures, treatments, and medication as well as familiar with the nursing implications related to these interventions. With an understanding of these concepts, the nurse can individualize the care based on the patient's and family's needs.

> **Remember Logan, the 6-week-old** with poor feeding? What additional health history and physical examination assessment information should the nurse obtain?

ASSESSMENT

When assessing a child with a cardiovascular disorder, expect to obtain a health history, perform a physical examination, and prepare the child for laboratory and diagnostic testing.

Health History

The health history comprises a history of the present illness, past medical history, and family history. Depending on his or her age, the child should be included in the health history interview; the child's age will determine the degree of involvement and the terminology used. Table 20.1 gives examples of typical questions that can be used when obtaining the child's health history.

History of Present Illness

Elicit the history of the present illness, which addresses when the symptoms started and how they have progressed. Inquire about any treatments and medications used at home. Ask parents about history of orthopnea, dyspnea, easy fatigability, growth delays, squatting, edema, dizziness, and/or frequent occurrences of pneumonia, which can be significant signs of pediatric heart disease (Muscari, 2004). The history of present illness may reveal a history of poor feeding, including fatigue, lethargy, and/or vomiting, or failure to thrive, even with adequate caloric intake. The parents may report diaphoresis, which is often seen in early heart failure. Delays in gross motor development, cyanosis (possibly reported by the parents as more of a gray

Table 20.1 Examples of Questions for Obtaining a Child's Health History

Questions	Provides Information About:
• What types and amounts (dosages) of medications has the child received? What were they used for? • Who prescribed them? • Were they effective? Did the child experience any adverse effects?	• Possible underlying conditions that may be related to the child's current status • Other health care personnel involved in the child's care as well as the parents' health care beliefs and patterns • How the medications may be affecting the child's health
• To whom does the child go for medical evaluation? How often? Were the visits for regular health check-ups or for situational problems? Were there previous hospitalizations? What for?	• The child's health status and the parents' health care knowledge, practices, and beliefs
• Has the child experienced any growth delay? Does the child have any problems with activity and coordination?	• Problems that may result from impaired cardiac output, adequacy of tissue oxygenation, and concomitant disorders associated with heart disease
• Does the child's skin color change when crying? If so, what color do you see?	• Effectiveness of tissue oxygenation. A blue or gray skin color may be due to cyanosis.
• Does the child stop frequently during play to sit or squat?	• The child's exercise tolerance and tissue oxygenation
• Does the child have feeding difficulty? Does the child tire easily or sleep excessively?	• The child's energy expenditure, ability to tolerate activity, and tissue oxygenation
• Does the child frequently develop strep throat?	• Child's risk for developing rheumatic fever and heart disease

color than blue), and tachypnea (indicative of heart failure) may also be reported by the parent or caregiver.

Past Medical History

The past medical history includes information about the child as well as the mother's pregnancy history. Assess the child's past medical history for:

- Problems occurring after birth (history of the child's condition after birth may reveal evidence of an associated congenital malformation or other disorder)
- Frequent infections
- Chromosomal abnormalities
- Prematurity
- Autoimmune disorders
- Use of medications, such as corticosteroids

Assess the mother's pregnancy, labor, and delivery history. Be sure to include information about the status of the neonate at birth. Also inquire about maternal use of medications, including illicit or over-the-counter drugs and alcohol; exposure to radiation; presence of hypertension; and maternal viral illnesses such as coxsackievirus, cytomegalovirus, influenza, mumps, or rubella. A history of significant problems related to labor and delivery is also important: stress or asphyxia at birth may be related to cardiac dysfunction and pulmonary hypertension in the newborn.

Assess for additional risk factors such as:

- Family history of heart disease or CHD (investigate the history further if heart disease occurred in a first-degree relative)
- Hyperlipidemia
- Diabetes mellitus
- Obesity
- Inactivity
- Stress
- High-cholesterol diet (Freitas-Nichols, 2004; Muscari, 2004)

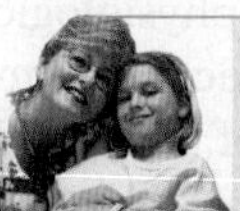

Medications taken by pregnant women such as isotretinoin (Accutane) for acne, lithium, and some antiseizure medications may be linked to the development of congenital heart defects. In addition, smoking during pregnancy, febrile illness in the first trimester, rubella infection during pregnancy, exposure of the pregnant woman to strong cleaning products, repeated x-rays, and any harmful or poisonous material can increase the risk of CHD.

Physical Examination

Physical examination of the child with a cardiovascular condition consists of inspection, palpation, and auscultation. In addition, obtain the child's vital signs and measure the child's height and weight. Plot this information on a standard growth chart to evaluate nutritional status and growth. If the child is less than 3 years of age, measure and plot the head circumference also.

Inspection

Assess the child's overall appearance. Inspect the color of the skin, noting cyanosis. Inspect the skin for edema. In infants, peripheral edema occurs first in the face, then the presacral region, and then the extremities. Edema of the lower extremities is characteristic of right ventricular heart failure in older children.

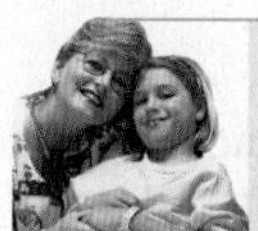

CHD should be suspected in the cyanotic newborn who does not improve with oxygen administration.

Inspect the fingers and toes for **clubbing**. Clubbing (which usually does not appear until after 1 year of age) implies severe congenital heart disease due to chronic hypoxia. The first sign of clubbing is softening of the nail beds, followed by rounding of the fingernails, followed by shininess and thickening of the nail ends (see Fig. 19.6 in Chapter 19).

Obtain the child's temperature; fever would suggest infection. Assess respirations, including rate, rhythm, and effort. Note location and severity of retractions if present. Inspect the chest configuration, noting any prominence of the precordial chest wall, which is often seen in infants and children with **cardiomegaly**. Note visible pulsations, which may indicate increased heart activity. Also inspect the neck veins for engorgement or abnormal pulsations. Note abdominal distention (Frietas-Nichols, 2004; Muscari, 2004; Valente et al., 2006).

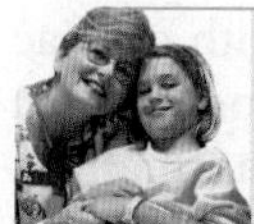

Children with cardiac conditions resulting in cyanosis will often have baseline oxygen saturations that are relatively low because of the mixing of oxygenated with deoxygenated blood.

Palpation

Palpate the right and left radial or brachial pulse to assess cardiac rate and rhythm. Throughout infancy and childhood, the rate may vary. Palpate the femoral pulse; it should be readily palpable and equal in amplitude and strength to the brachial or radial pulse. A femoral pulse that is weak or absent in comparison to the brachial pulse is associated with coarctation of the aorta. Palpate apical pulses for rate, rhythm, and quality. Significant variations in pulse occur with activity, so the most accurate heart rate may be determined during sleep. In older children, exercise and emotional factors may influence the heart rate. A bounding pulse is characteristic of patent ductus arteriosus or aortic regurgitation. Narrow or thready pulses may occur in children with heart failure or severe aortic stenosis. Note **tachycardia**, **bradycardia**, irregularities in rhythm, diminished peripheral pulses, or thready pulse. Palpate the child's abdomen for hepatomegaly, a sign of right-sided heart failure in the infant and child.

Auscultation

Auscultate the apical pulse for a full minute to determine heart rate and rhythm. Note irregularities in rhythm, tachycardia or bradycardia. Auscultate the heart for murmurs. Many children have functional or innocent murmurs, but all murmurs must be evaluated on the basis of the following characteristics:

- Location
- Relation to the heart cycle and duration
- Intensity: grade I, soft and hard to hear; grade II, soft and easily heard; grade III, loud without thrill; grade IV, loud with a precordial thrill; grade IV, loud, audible with a precordial thrill; grade V, loud, audible with a stethoscope; grade VI, very loud, and audible with a stethoscope or with the naked ear
- Quality: harsh, musical, or rough; high, medium, or low pitch
- Variation with position (sitting, lying, standing) (Freitas-Nichols, 2004; Muscari, 2004; Valente et al., 2006)

Auscultate for the character of heart sounds. Note distinct, muffled, or distant heart sounds. Abnormal splitting or intensifying of S2 sounds occurs in children with major heart problems. Ejection clicks, which are high-pitched, are related to problems with dilated vessels and/or valve abnormalities. Heard throughout systole, they can be early, moderate, or late. Clicks on the upper left sternal border are related to the pulmonary area. Aortic clicks are best heard at the apex and can be mitral or aortic in origin. A mild to late ejection click at the apex is typical of a mitral valve prolapse. The S3 heart sound may be heard in children and is associated with cardiac abnormalities. The S4 heart sound is not normally heard and is always associated with cardiac abnormalities (Driscoll, 2006; Muscari, 2004).

Auscultate the BP in the upper extremities and lower extremities and compare the findings; there should be no major differences between the upper and lower extremities. Determine the pulse pressure by subtracting the diastolic pressure from the systolic pressure. The pulse pressure is less than 50 Hg, or less than half the systolic pressure. A widened pulse pressure, which usually is accompanied by a bounding pulse, is associated with patent ductus arteriosus, aortic insufficiency, fever, anemia, or complete heart block. A narrowed pulse pressure is associated with aortic stenosis. Note hypotension or hypertension.

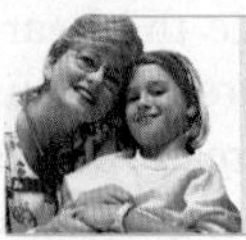

Children and parents must be alerted if a heart murmur is detected, even if it is benign.

Laboratory and Diagnostic Testing

Common Laboratory and Diagnostic Tests 20.1 explains the laboratory and diagnostic tests most commonly used when considering cardiovascular disorders in children. The tests can assist the physician in diagnosing the disorder or can be used as guidelines in determining ongoing treatment. Laboratory or non-nursing personnel obtain some of the tests, while the nurse might obtain others. In either instance the nurse should be familiar with how the tests are obtained, what they are used for, and normal versus abnormal results. This knowledge will also be necessary when providing patient and family education related to the testing.

Cardiac Catheterization

Cardiac catheterization is the definitive study for infants and children with cardiac disease and thus deserves special attention in this section on assessment of cardiovascular disorders. Cardiac catheterization has become almost a routine diagnostic procedure and may be performed on an outpatient basis. However, it is highly invasive and not without risks, especially in sick infants and children. Indications for cardiac catheterization include:

- Cardiovascular disease causing cyanosis in infants: these infants need to be catheterized as soon as they are in a reasonably stable condition
- Severe heart failure or progressive problems such as pulmonary edema
- Questionable anatomic or physiologic abnormalities
- Planned cardiac surgery
- Progressive monitoring related to pulmonary hypertension
- Periodic assessment after repair of a cardiac defect
- Therapeutic interventions such as septostomy or balloon valvotomy

Cardiac catheterization may be categorized as diagnostic, interventional, or electrophysiologic. Diagnostic cardiac catheterization typically is used to identify structural defects. Interventional cardiac catheterization is used as a treatment measure to dilate occluded or stenotic structures or vessels or close some defects. Electrophysiologic cardiac catheterization involves the use of electrodes to identify abnormal rhythms and destroy sites of abnormal electrical conduction. The type of catheterization performed varies based on the individual needs of the patient. The procedure lasts from 1 to 3 hours (Driscoll, 2006; Mullins, 2006b; Muscari, 2004).

Performing Cardiac Catheterization

In cardiac catheterization, a radiopaque catheter is inserted into a blood vessel and is then guided through the vessel to the heart with the aid of fluoroscopy. For a right-sided catheterization, the catheter is threaded to the right atrium via a major vein such as the femoral vein. With a left-sided catheterization, the catheter is threaded to the aorta and heart via an artery. Once the tip of the catheter is in the heart, contrast material is injected via the catheter and radiographic images are taken.

Common Laboratory and Diagnostic Tests 20.1

Test	Explanation	Indication	Nursing Implications
Arteriogram (angiogram: visualization of arteries or veins)	Radiopaque contrast solution is injected through a catheter and into the circulation. X-rays are then taken to visualize the structure of the heart and blood vessels.	To observe blood flow to parts of body and detect lesions; to confirm a diagnosis. Catheters can be used to remove plaques.	• Make sure the parent signs a consent form. • Administer premedication as ordered. • Obtain child's weight to determine amount of dye needed. • Keep the child NPO before the procedure according to institutional protocol. • After the procedure, maintain the child on bed rest. • Observe the puncture site for bleeding. • Monitor vital signs frequently and check the pulse distal to the site.
Ambulatory electrocardiographic monitoring (Holter)	Monitoring of the heart's electrical patterns for 24 hours using a portable compact unit	To identify and quantify arrhythmias in a 24-hour period during normal daily activities	• Instruct the child and parent to push the "event button" whenever chest pain, syncope, or palpitations occur. • Normal daily activities should be carried out during the testing period. • Having the child wear a snug undershirt over the leads helps to keep them in place.
Chest x-ray	A radiographic film of the chest area; will determine size of the heart and its chambers and pulmonary blood flow	Serves as a baseline for comparison with films taken after surgery; used to identify abnormalities of the lungs, heart, and other structures in the chest	• Instruct patient not to wear jewelry or any metal around neck or on the hospital gown. • Explain to the child and family that no pain or discomfort should result. • If a portable x-ray at bedside is done, remove electrodes temporarily.
Echocardiogram	Noninvasive ultrasound procedure used to assess heart wall thickness, size of heart chambers, motion of valves and septa, and relationship of great vessels to other cardiac structures	Specific diagnosis of structural defects; determines hemodynamics and detects valvular defects	• Assure the child that the echo does not hurt. • Instruct the child about ECG lead placement and use of gel on the scope's wand during the procedure. • Encourage the child to lie still throughout the test.

Common Laboratory and Diagnostic Tests 20.1 (continued)

Test	Explanation	Indication	Nursing Implications
Electrocardiogram (ECG, EKG)	A graphic record produced by an electrocardiograph (device used to record the electrical activity of the myocardium to detect transmission of the cardiac impulse through the conductive tissues of the muscle). Facilitates evaluation of the heart rate, rhythm, conduction, and musculature.	To detect heart rhythm and chamber overload; also serves as a baseline for measuring postoperative complications	• Assure the child that monitoring is a painless procedure. • Place electrodes in the appropriate location. • The child must lie still during the ECG recording period (usually about 5 minutes). • Wipe electrode paste or jelly off after procedure.
Exercise stress test	Monitoring of heart rate, blood pressure, ECG, and oxygen consumption at rest and during exercise	Quantifies exercise tolerance; can be used to provoke symptoms or arrhythmias	• Child should be NPO for 4 hours prior to test. • Obtain baseline ECG and vital signs. • Instruct child to verbalize symptoms during testing. • Usually takes about 54 minutes.
Hemoglobin (Hgb) and hematocrit (Hct)	Measures the total amount of hemoglobin in the blood and indirectly measures the red blood cell number and volume	To detect anemia or polycythemia (may occur with CHD resulting in cyanosis)	• False elevations occur with dehydration. • May be obtained quickly via capillary puncture. • Normal values vary with age.
Partial pressure of oxygen (pO_2)	Measures the amount of oxygen in the blood	To determine the presence and degree of hypoxia	• Most accurate result is with arterial specimen (venous and capillary specimens demonstrate lower levels). • Observe child for cyanosis. • Supplement with oxygen per protocol.

While the catheter is in the heart, several procedures can be performed. The blood pressures, changes in cardiac output or stroke volume, and oxygen saturation in each heart chamber and major blood vessels are recorded. With the injection of contrast material, information is revealed about the heart anatomy, ventricular wall motion and ejection fraction, intracardiac pressures and hemodynamic parameters, cardiac valve function, and structural abnormalities. The movement of the contrast material is filmed so that the details of the cardiac procedure are recorded. Samples of heart tissue to evaluate for infection, muscular dysfunction, or rejection after a transplant may also be obtained.

Nursing Management

Although cardiac catheterization may be considered nearly routine, for the child and parents or guardians, the procedure can be a source of much anxiety. Therefore, the nurse needs to educate the parents and, if appropriate for age, the child about all aspects of the procedure. The procedure is commonly performed on an outpatient basis, but some health care providers require the child be admitted for an overnight stay for observation. Nursing management of the child undergoing cardiac catheterization includes preprocedure nursing assessment and preparation of the child and family, postprocedural nursing care, and discharge teaching.

Before the Procedure. A thorough history and physical examination are necessary to establish a baseline. Obtain vital signs. Note fever or other signs and symptoms of infection, which may necessitate rescheduling the procedure. Obtain the child's height and weight to aid in determining medication dosages. Assess the child for any allergies, especially to iodine and shellfish, because some contrast materials contain iodine as a base. Review the child's medications: medications such as anticoagulants are typically withheld for several days or longer prior to the procedure to reduce the child's risk for bleeding. Check the results of any laboratory tests, such as hemoglobin and hematocrit levels.

Perform a complete physical examination. Pay particular attention to assessing the child's peripheral pulses, including pedal pulses. Use an indelible pen to mark the location of the child's pedal pulses so they can be easily assessed after the procedure. Document the location and quality in the child's medical record.

Teach the parents and child, if appropriate, about the procedure, including what the procedure involves, how long it will take, and any special instructions from the health care provider. Use a variety of teaching methods as appropriate, such as videotapes, books, and pamphlets. Adapt these teaching methods to the child's developmental stage. For example, introduce the younger child to equipment through play therapy. For school-age and older children and their parents, offer a tour of the cardiac catheterization laboratory. Mention sounds and sights they may experience during the procedure. Explain the use of intravenous fluid therapy, sedation, and, if ordered, anesthesia to the child and parents. Tell the child that he or she may feel a sensation of the heart racing when the catheter is inserted. Also warn the older child that he or she may experience a feeling of warmth or stinging when the contrast material is injected. Encourage the child to use familiar ways to help him or her relax. If necessary, teach the child simple relaxation measures.

Typically, food and fluid are withheld for 4 to 6 hours before the procedure. Prescribed medications may be taken with a sip of water. On the day of the procedure, check to ensure that a signed informed consent form is on the child's medical record and that all necessary assessment data have been included. Just before the procedure, ask the child to void and administer a sedative, as ordered. If appropriate and permitted, allow the parents to accompany the child to the catheterization area.

Teach the child and family what to expect after the procedure is completed. Inform the parents of the possible complications that might occur, such as bleeding, low-grade fever, loss of pulse in the extremity used for the catheterization, and arrhythmias. Explain to the child that he or she will have a dressing over the catheter site and that he or she will need to keep the leg straight for several hours after the procedure. Teach the child and parent that frequent monitoring will be required after the procedure.

After the Procedure. Throughout the postprocedure period, closely monitor the child for complications of bleeding, **arrhythmia**, hematoma and thrombus formation, and infection. After the procedure, evaluate the child's vital signs, the neurovascular status of the lower extremities, and the pressure dressing over the catheterization site every 15 minutes for the first hour and then every 30 minutes for 1 hour. Vital signs should remain within acceptable parameters. Hypotension may signify hemorrhage due to perforation of the heart muscle or bleeding from the insertion site. Expect to monitor cardiac rhythm and oxygen saturation levels via pulse oximetry for the first few hours after the procedure to help identify possible complications.

Assess the child's distal pulses bilaterally for presence and quality. The pulse of the affected extremity may be slightly less than that of the other extremity in the initial postprocedure period, but it should gradually return to baseline. Also assess the color and temperature of the extremity; pallor or blanching would indicate an obstruction in blood flow. Check capillary refill and sensation to evaluate blood flow to the area.

Maintain bed rest in the immediate postprocedure period. Ensure that the child maintains the extremity in a straight position for approximately 4 to 8 hours, depending on the approach used and the facility's policy. Some facilities require straight positioning for 4 to 6 hours after a right-sided catheterization and for 6 to 8 hours after a left-sided catheterization to ensure healing of the vessel. Inspect the pressure dressing frequently. Check to make sure that it is dry and intact, without evidence of bleeding. Reinforce the dressing as necessary and report any evidence of drainage on the dressing. If there is a risk of the dressing becoming soiled or wet, cover it with plastic.

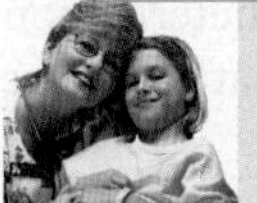

If bleeding occurs after a cardiac catheterization, apply pressure 1 inch above the site to create pressure over the vessel, thereby reducing the blood flow to the area.

Monitor the child's intake and output closely to ensure adequate hydration. The contrast material has a diuretic effect, so assess the child for signs and symptoms of dehydration and hypovolemia. Typically, the child resumes oral intake as tolerated, beginning with sips of clear liquids and progressing to his or her preprocedure diet. Continue intravenous fluids as ordered and encourage oral fluid intake as allowed and ordered to promote elimination of the contrast material.

Allow the child to talk about the experience and how and what he or she felt. Provide positive reinforcement for the child's actions.

Provide patient and family education before the child is discharged home (Teaching Guideline 20.1). Areas to address include site care, signs and symptoms of complica-

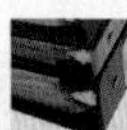

TEACHING GUIDELINE 20.1

Providing Care After a Cardiac Catheterization

- Change the pressure dressing on the day after the procedure. Apply a dry sterile dressing or adhesive bandage for the next several days. Keep the dressing dry; cover it with plastic if there is a chance that the dressing could become wet or soiled.
- When changing the dressing, inspect the insertion site for redness, irritation, swelling, drainage, and bleeding. Report any of these to the health care provider.
- Check the temperature, color, sensation, and pulses on the child's extremities and compare. Report any changes to the health care provider.
- Resume the child's usual diet after the procedure; report any nausea or vomiting.
- Check the child's temperature at least once a day for approximately 3 days after the procedure. Report any temperature elevation of 100.4° F or greater.
- Avoid giving the child a tub bath for approximately 3 days after the procedure; use sponge baths or showers instead.
- Discourage strenuous exercise or activity for approximately 3 days after the procedure.
- Watch for changes in the child's appearance, such as changes in skin color, reports of the heart "fluttering" or "skipping a beat," fever, or difficulty breathing.
- Give acetaminophen (Tylenol) or ibuprofen (Motrin) for complaints of pain.
- Schedule a follow-up appointment with the health care provider in the time specified.

tions (especially within 24 hours after the catheterization, such as fever, bleeding or bruising at the catheterization site, or changes in color, temperature, or sensation in the extremity used), diet, and activity level.

NURSING DIAGNOSES AND RELATED INTERVENTIONS

Upon completion of a thorough assessment, the nurse might identify several nursing diagnoses. These may include but are not limited to:

- Decreased cardiac output related to structural defect, congenital anomaly, or ineffective heart pumping
- Ineffective tissue perfusion related to inadequate cardiac function or cardiac surgery
- Imbalanced nutrition, less than body requirements, related to increased energy expenditure and fatigue
- Risk for delayed growth and development related to effects of cardiac disease and treatments, inadequate nutrition, or frequent separation from caregivers secondary to illness
- Risk for infection related to need for multiple invasive procedures or cardiac surgery
- Excess fluid volume related to ineffective cardiac muscle function
- Interrupted family process related to crisis associated with heart disease, frequent need for testing and hospitalizations, or stresses associated with care demands
- Activity intolerance related to ineffective cardiac muscle function, increased energy expenditure, or inability to meet increased oxygen or metabolic demands
- Pain

After completing Logan's assessment, the nurse noted the following: poor weight gain, tachypnea with occasional nasal flaring, crackles heard on auscultation, and edema noted in the face, presacral area and extremities. Based on these assessment findings, what would your top three nursing diagnoses be for Logan?

Nursing goals, interventions, and evaluation for the child with a cardiovascular disorder are based on the nursing diagnoses. Nursing Care Plan 20.1 can be used as a guide in planning nursing care for the child with a cardiovascular disorder. The nursing care plan overview should be individualized based on the patient's symptoms and needs. Refer to Chapter 15 for detailed information about pain assessment and management. Additional information will be included later in the chapter as it relates to specific disorders.

Based on your top three nursing diagnoses for Logan, describe appropriate nursing interventions.

Congenital Heart Disease

In North America, more than 1% of newborn infants have CHD resulting from numerous causes. The prevalence of CHD is about 8 per 1,000 live births; premature infants have a higher rate (Fixler, 2006). Many chromosome defects are associated with CHD, including Down syndrome, velocardiofacial syndrome, Turner syndrome, trisomy 13, trisomy 18, Williams syndrome, Prader-Willi syndrome, and cri-du-chat (Marian et al., 2004). About one third of infants with CHD will have disease serious enough to result in death or will require cardiac catheterization or cardiac surgery within the first year of life. Complications of CHD include heart failure, hypoxemia, growth retardation, developmental delay, and pulmonary vascular disease. As many as 13% of children with CHD experience severe failure to thrive (Chen et al., 2004).

With advances in palliative and corrective surgery in the past 20 years, many more children are now able to survive into adulthood (Fulton & Freed, 2004). As many as 70% to 85% of children with CHD grow to be adults, yet many have problems related to education, insurance,

(text continues on page 628)

Nursing Care Plan 20.1

Overview for the Child With a Cardiovascular Disorder

Nursing Diagnosis: Decreased cardiac output related to structural defect, congenital anomaly, or ineffective heart pumping as evidenced by arrhythmias, edema, murmur, abnormal heart rate, or abnormal heart sounds

Outcome identification and evaluation

Child or infant will demonstrate adequate cardiac output; *will have elastic skin turgor, brisk capillary refill, demonstrate pink color, pulse and blood pressure within normal limits for age, regular heart rhythm, adequate urinary output.*

Interventions: increasing cardiac output

- Monitor vital signs closely, especially BP and heart rate, *to detect increases or decreases.*
- Monitor cardiac rhythm via cardiac monitor *to detect arrhythmias quickly.*
- Observe for signs of hypoxia such as tachypnea, cyanosis, tachycardia, bradycardia, dizziness, and/or restlessness *to identify this change early.*
- Administer oxygen as needed *to correct hypoxia.*
- Place child in knee-to-chest or squatting position as needed *to increase systemic vascular resistance.*
- Administer antiarrhythmics, vasopressors, ACE inhibitors, beta blockers, corticosteroids, or diuretics as prescribed *to improve cardiac output.*
- Monitor for signs of thrombosis such as restlessness, seizure, coma, oliguria, anuria, edema, hematuria, or paralysis *to identify this condition early.*
- Administer adequate hydration *to decrease possibility of thrombosis formation.*
- Cluster nursing care and other activities *to allow adequate periods of rest.*
- Anticipate child's needs *to decrease the child's stress, thereby decreasing oxygen consumption requirement.*

Nursing Diagnosis: Excess fluid volume related to ineffective cardiac muscle function as evidenced by weight gain, edema, jugular vein distention, dyspnea, shortness of breath, abnormal breath sounds, or pulmonary congestion

Outcome identification and evaluation

Child will attain appropriate fluid balance, *will lose weight (fluid), edema or bloating will decrease, lung sounds will be clear and heart sounds normal.*

Interventions: encouraging fluid loss

- Weigh daily on same scale in similar amount of clothing; *in children weight is the best indicator of changes in fluid status.*
- Monitor location and extent of edema (measure abdominal girth daily if ascites is present); *decrease in edema indicates positive increase in oncotic pressure.*
- Protect edematous areas from skin breakdown: *edema leads to increased risk for alterations in skin integrity.*
- Auscultate lungs carefully to identify crackles *(indicating pulmonary edema).*
- Assess work of breathing and respiratory rate *(increased work of breathing is associated with pulmonary edema).*
- Assess heart sounds for gallop *(presence of S3 may indicate fluid overload).*
- Maintain fluid restriction as ordered *to decrease intravascular volume and workload on the heart.*
- Strictly monitor intake and output *to quickly note discrepancies and provide intervention.*
- Provide sodium-restricted diet as ordered *(restricting sodium intake allows better renal excretion of extra fluid).*
- Administer diuretics as ordered and monitor for adverse effects. *Diuretics encourage excretion of fluid, elimination of edema, reduce cardiac filling pressures, and increase renal blood flow. Adverse effects include electrolyte imbalance as well as orthostatic hypotension.*

(continued)

Overview for the Child With a Cardiovascular Disorder (continued)

Nursing Diagnosis: Imbalanced nutrition, less than body requirements, related to increased energy expenditure and fatigue as evidenced by weight loss or height and weight below accepted standards

Outcome identification and evaluation

Child will improve nutritional intake resulting in *steady increase in weight and length/height, will feed without tiring easily.*

Interventions: promoting adequate nutrition

- Determine body weight and length/height norm for age *to determine goal to work toward.*
- Assess child for food preferences that fall within dietary restrictions: *child will be more likely to consume adequate amounts of foods that he or she likes.*
- Weigh child daily or weekly (according to physician order or institutional standard) and measure length/height weekly *to monitor for increased growth.*
- Offer highest-calorie meals at the time of day when the child's appetite is the greatest *(to increase likelihood of increased caloric intake).*
- Provide increased-calorie shakes or puddings within diet restriction *(high-calorie foods increase weight gain).*
- Consult with the pediatric dietician *to provide optimal caloric intake within dietary restrictions.*
- Provide small, frequent feedings *to discourage tiring with feeding.*
- Feed infants with special nipple as needed *to decrease amount of energy expended for sucking.*
- Administer vitamin and mineral supplements as prescribed *to attain/maintain vitamin and mineral balance in the body.*

Nursing Diagnosis: Ineffective tissue perfusion related to inadequate cardiac function or cardiac surgery as evidenced by pallor, cyanosis, edema, changes in mental status, prolonged capillary refill, clubbing, or diminished pulses

Outcome identification and evaluation

Child will demonstrate adequate tissue perfusion: *Child will be alert, not restless or lethargic, will have pink color, decrease in edema, normal perfusion and strong pulses.*

Interventions: promoting tissue perfusion

- Assess level of consciousness, pulse, BP, peripheral perfusion, and skin color frequently *to determine baseline and ongoing improvement.*
- Administer cardiac glycosides or vasodilators as ordered *to promote cardiac output necessary for proper perfusion.*
- Monitor pulse oximetry and arterial blood gas results *to assess ability to appropriately oxygenate.*
- Supplement oxygen as needed *to provide oxygen to organs for proper functioning.*
- Monitor hemoglobin and hematocrit *to identify blood loss.*
- Strictly assess intake and output *to determine adequacy of renal perfusion.*
- Position with head of bed elevated *to decrease blood volume returning to heart.*
- Change position every 2 to 4 hours *to promote circulation and avoid skin breakdown in areas of poor perfusion.*

Overview for the Child With a Cardiovascular Disorder (continued)

Nursing Diagnosis: Risk for delayed growth and development related to effects of cardiac disease and necessary treatments, inadequate nutrition, or frequent separation from caregivers secondary to illness

Outcome identification and evaluation

Child will display development appropriate for age, *will display evidence of cognitive and motor function within normal limits (individualized for each child).*

Interventions: promoting appropriate development

- Promote adequate caloric intake *to stimulate growth and provide adequate energy.*
- Provide age-appropriate developmental activities *to stimulate development.*
- Consult with the physical or occupational therapist or child life specialist *to determine activities most appropriate for the child within the constraints of the child's illness.*
- Schedule daily activities to allow for essential rest periods *for energy conservation.*
- Encourage parents, teachers, and playmates to be sensitive to child's self-image, using positive comments, *to improve the child's self-concept.*
- As energy allows, encourage participation in all activities as feasible *to allow the child to feel normal.*

Nursing Diagnosis: Risk for infection related to need for multiple invasive procedures or cardiac surgery as evidenced by break in skin integrity, decreased hemoglobin, or inadequate nutritional intake

Outcome identification and evaluation

Child will remain free from infection: *vital signs will be within normal limits, white blood cell count normal, cultures negative. Child will exhibit no signs or symptoms of infection.*

Interventions: preventing infection

- Maintain strict hand hygiene *to prevent spread of infectious organisms to the child.*
- Assess temperature *to detect elevation early in course of infection.*
- Avoid contact with persons with known infections *to prevent risk of becoming ill.*
- Ensure appropriate immunization, including pneumococcal and influenza vaccinations, *to prevent development of common childhood illness.*
- Administer prophylactic antibiotics prior to all dental procedures, surgery, and many invasive procedures *to prevent subacute bacterial endocarditis.*
- Encourage good dental hygiene *to reduce the risk of endocarditis.*

Nursing Diagnosis: Interrupted family processes related to crisis associated with heart disease, frequent need for testing and hospitalizations, or stresses associated with care demands, as evidenced by inadequate parental coping, frequent separations of parent and child, or inadequate support

Outcome identification and evaluation

Family will maintain functional system of support and will demonstrate adequate coping, adaptation of roles and functions, and decreased anxiety: *Parents are involved in child's care, ask appropriate questions, express fears and concerns, and can discuss child's care and condition calmly.*

Interventions: promoting family processes

- Provide ongoing support to the child and family *to help them cope.*
- Encourage parents and family members to verbalize concerns related to child's illness, diagnosis, and prognosis: *allows the nurse to identify concerns and areas where further education may be needed. Demonstrates family-centered care.*

(continued)

Overview for the Child With a Cardiovascular Disorder (continued)

- Allow families to grieve over the loss of a "perfect" child: *parents must work through those grief feelings so they can be fully "present" for this chronically ill child.*
- Explain therapies, procedures, child's behaviors, and plan of care to parents: *Understanding the child's current status and plan of care helps decrease anxiety.*
- Encourage parents to be involved in care: *allows parents to feel needed and valued and gives them a sense of control over their child's health.*
- Identify support system for family and child: *helps nurse identify needs and resources available for coping.*
- Educate family and child on additional resources available *to help them develop a wide base of support.*
- Encourage parents to seek genetic counseling *to provide them with the information required to make an informed decision about having another child.*

Nursing Diagnosis: Activity intolerance related to ineffective cardiac muscle function, increased energy expenditure, or inability to meet increased oxygen or metabolic demands as evidenced by squatting positions, shortness of breath, cyanosis, or fatigue

Outcome identification and evaluation

Child will increase activity level as tolerated: *child participates in play and activities (specify particular activities and level as individualized for each child).*

Interventions: promoting activity

- Assess level of fatigue and activity tolerance *to determine baseline for comparison.*
- Note extent of dyspnea, oxygen requirement, or color change with exertion *to provide baseline for comparison.*
- Cluster care activities, allowing rest periods in between, *to conserve child's energy.*
- Work with the parent and child to determine a mutually satisfactory daily schedule *to allow adequate rest and energy conservation.*
- Instruct family and child in prescribed activity restrictions *to prevent fatigue while allowing some activity.*
- In the infant, avoid long periods of crying or prolonged nipple feeding *(expends excessive calories).*
- Provide neutral thermal environment *to avoid increased oxygen and energy needs associated with excessive heat or cold.*

and employment (Doroshow, 2001). Hypothermia and cardiopulmonary bypass required during cardiac surgery for CHD may have a long-term impact on the child's cognitive ability and academic function (Griffin et al., 2003; Mahle et al., 2000, 2006). Due to the potential long-term effects that CHD may have on these children, nurses must be expertly equipped to care for them.

Pathophysiology

The exact cause of CHD is unknown. However, the belief is that it results from an interplay of several factors, including genetics (e.g., chromosomal alterations) and maternal exposure to environmental factors (e.g., toxins, infections, chronic illnesses, and alcohol).

Congenital heart defects result from some interference in the development of the heart structure during fetal life. Subsequently, the septal walls or valves may fail to develop completely, or vessels or valves may be stenotic, narrowed, or transposed. Structures that formed to allow fetal circulation may fail to close after birth, altering the pressures necessary to maintain adequate blood flow.

After birth, with the change from fetal to newborn circulation, pressures within the chambers of the right side of the heart are less than those of the left side and pulmonary vascular resistance is less than that for the systemic circulation. These normal pressure gradients are necessary for adequate circulation to the lungs and the rest of the body. However, these pressure gradients become disrupted if a structure has failed to develop, a fetal structure has failed to close, or a narrowing, stenosis, or transposition of a vessel has occurred. For example, blood typically flows from an area of higher pressure to lower pressure. If the ductus arteriosus fails to close, blood will move from the aorta to the pulmonary artery, ultimately increasing right atrial pressure. With this shunting of blood, highly oxygenated blood can mix with less oxygenated blood, interfering with the amount available to the tissues via the systemic circulation. Some of the defects may result in significant hypoxemia, the sequelae of which include clubbing, polycythemia, exercise intolerance, hypercyanotic spells, brain abscess, and cerebrovascular accident (Fulton & Freed, 2004).

The traditional approach to categorizing CHD has been in terms of whether the child exhibits cyanosis as a clinical manifestation—cyanotic versus acyanotic defects. However, children with acyanotic defects may exhibit cyanosis, and children with cyanotic defects may not demonstrate cyanosis unless they are seriously ill. Many children with congenital heart defects shift between cyanotic and acyanotic states depending on their hemodynamic status (Suddaby, 2001). Therefore, this chapter will categorize the disorders based on hemodynamic characteristics (blood flow patterns in the heart):

- Disorders with decreased pulmonary blood flow: tetralogy of Fallot, tricuspid atresia
- Disorders with increased pulmonary blood flow: patent ductus arteriosus (PDA), atrial septal defect (ASD), ventricular septal defect (VSD)
- Obstructive disorders: coarctation of the aorta, aortic stenosis, pulmonary stenosis
- Mixed disorders: transposition of the great vessels (TGV), total anomalous pulmonary venous return (TAPVR), truncus arteriosus, and hypoplastic left heart syndrome (Suddaby, 2001)

Therapeutic Management

Prenatal education about avoiding certain substances or infection is essential to promote optimal outcomes for the fetus. Parents of children with CHD are encouraged to receive genetic counseling because of the probability of having subsequent children with a congenital heart defect. Children with small septal defects are urged to lead a normal life and often require no medical intervention. Therapeutic management of other forms of CHD focuses on palliative care or a surgical corrective approach necessary for most of the defects. In newborns and very young infants with severe cyanosis (tricuspid atresia, TGV), a prostaglandin infusion will maintain patency of the ductus arteriosus, improving pulmonary blood flow. Definitive correction of structural disorders requires surgical intervention. Table 20.2 describes the surgical procedures used for the various congenital heart defects and the relevant nursing measures. Nursing management for the child with CHD will be provided following the disorders section.

• DISORDERS WITH DECREASED PULMONARY BLOOD FLOW

Defects involving decreased pulmonary blood flow occur when there is some obstruction of blood flow to the lungs. As a result of the obstruction, pressure in the right side of the heart increases and becomes greater than that of the left side of the heart. Blood from the higher-pressure right side of the heart then shunts to the lower-pressure left side through a structural defect. Subsequently, deoxygenated blood mixes with oxygenated blood on the left side of the heart. This mixed blood, which is low in oxygen, is pumped via the systemic circulation to the body tissues.

Defects with decreased pulmonary blood flow are characterized by mild to severe oxygen desaturation. Typically, the child exhibits oxygen saturation levels ranging from 50% to 90%, which can produce severe cyanosis. To compensate for low blood oxygen levels, the kidneys produce the hormone erythropoietin to stimulate the bone marrow to produce more red blood cells (RBCs). This increase in RBCs is called **polycythemia**. Polycythemia can lead to an increase in blood volume and possibly blood viscosity, further taxing the workload of the heart. Although the number of RBCs increases, there is no change in the amount of blood that reaches the lungs for oxygenation (Chamberlain, 2006; Driscoll, 2006a; Suddaby, 2001). Disorders within this classification include tetralogy of Fallot and tricuspid atresia.

Tetralogy of Fallot

Tetralogy of Fallot is a congenital heart defect that actually comprises four heart defects: pulmonary stenosis (a narrowing of the pulmonary valve and outflow tract, creating an obstruction of blood flow from the right ventricle to the pulmonary artery), VSD, overriding aorta (enlargement of the aortic valve to the extent that it appears to arise from the right and left ventricles rather than the anatomically correct left ventricle), and right ventricular hypertrophy (the muscle walls of the right ventricle increase in size due to continued overuse as the right ventricle attempts to overcome a high pressure gradient). Surgical intervention is usually required during the first year of life. The rate for survival into adulthood with a good functional long-term result is greater than 90% (Neches et al., 2006a).

Pathophysiology

With pulmonary stenosis, the blood flow from the right ventricle is obstructed and slowed, resulting in a decrease in blood flow to the lungs for oxygenation and a decrease in the amount of oxygenated blood returning to the left atrium from the lungs. The obstructed flow also increases the pressure in the right ventricle. This blood, which is poorly oxygenated, is then shunted across the VSD into the left atrium. Poorly oxygenated blood also travels through the overriding aorta (if it extends to both ventricles). In some cases when the VSD is large, the pressure in the right ventricle may be equal to that of the left ventricle. In this case, the path of blood shunting depends on which circulation is exerting the higher pressure, pulmonary or systemic.

Table 20.2 Common Surgical Procedures and Nursing Measures for Congenital Heart Defects

Disorder	Surgical Procedure	Nursing Measures
Tetralogy of Fallot	Palliation with systemic-to-pulmonary anastomoses: • Blalock-Taussig shunt: an end-to-side anastomosis (or connection with a small Gore-tex tube) of the subclavian artery and the pulmonary artery • Waterston shunt: anastomosis of the ascending aorta and the pulmonary artery • Definitive correction involves patch closure of the ventricular septal defect and repair of the pulmonary valve and right ventricular outflow tract.	• Avoid BP measurements and venipunctures in the affected arm after a Blalock-Taussig shunt. Pulse will not be palpable in that arm because of use of the subclavian artery for the shunt. • Monitor for ventricular arrhythmias after corrective repair.
Tricuspid atresia	• Palliation with Blalock-Taussig shunt or pulmonary artery banding may be performed. • At 3 to 6 months of age, the superior vena cava is detached from the heart and connected to the pulmonary artery (Glenn procedure). • By age 2 to 5 years, a modified Fontan procedure may be performed. Systemic venous return is redirected to the pulmonary artery directly.	• Monitor for atrial arrhythmias, left ventricular dysfunction, and protein-losing enteropathy. • Some children may eventually require a pacemaker.
Atrial septal defect	• If small, the defect may be sutured closed. Larger defects may require a patch of pericardium or synthetic material. • Ostium secundum ASD may be repaired percutaneously via cardiac catheterization with an Amplatzer septal occluder (other brands are also available).	• Monitor for atrial arrhythmias (lifelong) after surgical closure. • With the Amplatzer device, strenuous activity should be avoided for 1 month after the procedure.
Ventricular septal defect	• If surgical closure is required, it should be performed before permanent pulmonary vascular changes develop. • Surgical closure may be in the form of suture closure of the VSD, transcatheter placement of a device in the defect, or Dacron patch closure.	• Monitor for ventricular dysrhythmias or AV block. • With the clamshell occluding or Amplatzer device, strenuous activity should be avoided for 1 month after the procedure.
Atrioventricular canal defect	• Pulmonary artery banding as palliation in very young infants • Surgical correction by 3 to 18 months of age • Patch closure of the septal defects and suturing of the valve leaflets or valve reconstruction are performed.	• Monitor for complete heart block postoperatively. • Teach parents that mitral regurgitation is a long-term complication and may require valve replacement.
Patent ductus arteriosus	• PDA is closed by coil embolization or device via cardiac catheterization. • May also be surgically ligated	• Monitor for bleeding and laryngeal nerve damage.

Table 20.2 Common Surgical Procedures and Nursing Measures for Congenital Heart Defects (continued)

Disorder	Surgical Procedure	Nursing Measures
Coarctation of the aorta	• Balloon angioplasty via cardiac catheterization is possible in some children. • Most common surgical repair is resection of the narrowed portion of the aorta, followed by end-to-end reanastomosis.	• Preoperatively, administer prostaglandin medications as ordered to relax the ductal tissue. • Postoperatively, measure and compare BP in all four extremities and quality of upper vs. lower pulses.
Aortic stenosis	• Balloon dilatation is accomplished via the umbilical artery in the newborn or the femoral artery via cardiac catheterization in the older child.	• Provide routine post-catheterization care. • Teach parents that long-term aortic regurgitation requiring valve replacement may occur.
Pulmonary stenosis	• Balloon dilation valvuloplasty is performed via cardiac catheterization to dilate the valve. This is effective in all but the most severe of cases, which will require surgical valvotomy.	• Provide routine post-catheterization care for balloon dilation. • Explain to parents that prognosis is excellent.
Transposition of the great vessels (arteries)	• Balloon atrial septotomy is usually done as soon as the diagnosis is made. A balloon-tipped catheter is passed through the atrial septum to enlarge the atrial septum. • Surgical correction involves switching the arteries into their normal anatomic positions.	• Administer prostaglandin to maintain the open state of the ductus arteriosus, which will allow the mixing of poorly oxygenated blood with well-oxygenated blood. • Monitor for rapid respirations and cyanosis. • Administer oxygen as needed preoperatively.
Total anomalous pulmonary venous return	The pulmonary vein is repositioned to the back of the left atrium and the ASD is closed.	• Monitor for dysrhythmias, heart block, and persistent heart failure.
Truncus arteriosus	VSD repair, separation of the pulmonary arteries from the aorta, with subsequent connection to the right ventricle with a valve conduit	• Preoperatively, administer prostaglandin infusion to prevent closing of the ductus arteriosus.
Hypoplastic left heart syndrome	• Heart transplantation is the treatment of choice. • Palliative staged treatment. First: Norwood procedure, reconstruction of the aorta and pulmonary arteries includes a cardiac transplant. Second: bidirectional Glenn procedure, connection of the superior vena cava to the right pulmonary artery to increase the blood flow to the lungs. Third: modified Fontan procedure.	• Preoperatively, administer prostaglandin infusion to prevent closing of the ductus arteriosus. • After palliative repairs, monitor for dysrhythmias or worsening ventricular function.
Valve disorders	• The incompetent valve is replaced with a valve prosthesis.	• Lifelong anticoagulation therapy is necessary with prosthetic valves. • Monitor prothrombin times. • Monitor heart sounds for alterations.

Regardless of which way shunting occurs, a mixing of oxygenated and poorly oxygenated blood occurs, with this blood ultimately being pumped into the systemic circulation. The oxygen saturation of the blood in the systemic circulation is reduced, leading to cyanosis. The degree of cyanosis depends on the extent of the pulmonary stenosis, the size of the VSD, and the vascular resistance of the pulmonary and systemic circulations. In some children, cyanosis is so severe that it leads to severe hypoxia, dysrhythmias, and sudden death (Betz & Sowden, 2005).

Tetralogy of Fallot is usually diagnosed during the first weeks of life due to the presence of a murmur and/or cyanosis. Some newborns may be acutely cyanotic, while others may exhibit only mild cyanosis that gradually becomes more severe, particularly during times of stress as the child grows older. Most often, infants with tetralogy of Fallot have a PDA at birth, providing additional pulmonary blood flow and thereby decreasing the severity of the initial cyanosis. Later, as the ductus arteriosus closes, such as within the first days of life, more severe cyanosis can occur (Fig. 20.2).

Nursing Assessment

Nursing assessment consists of health history, physical examination, and laboratory and diagnostic tests.

Health History and Physical Examination

Obtain the health history, noting a history of color changes associated with feeding, activity, or crying. Determine if the infant or child is demonstrating hypercyanotic spells. Hypercyanosis develops suddenly and is manifested as increased cyanosis, hypoxemia, dyspnea, and agitation. If the infant's oxygen demand is greater than the supply, such as with crying or during feeding, then the spell progresses to anoxia. When the degree of cyanosis is severe and persistent, the infant may become unresponsive. As the infant gets older, he or she may use specific postures, such as bending at the knees or assuming the fetal position, to relieve a hypercyanotic spell. The walking infant or toddler may squat periodically. These positions improve pulmonary blood flow by increasing systemic vascular resistance. Ask the parents if they have noticed any of these unusual positions (Driscoll, 2006a). Note history of irritability, sleepiness, or difficulty breathing.

During the physical examination, observe the skin color and note any evidence of cyanosis. Also observe for changes in skin color with positional changes, and inspect the fingers for clubbing. Note if the child has a hypercyanotic spell during the assessment. Count the child's respiratory rate and observe work of breathing, noting retractions, shortness of breath, or noisy breathing. Document oxygen saturation via pulse oximetry; it will likely be decreased. Auscultate the chest for adventitious breath sounds, which may suggest the development of heart failure. Auscultate the heart, noting a loud, harsh murmur characteristic of this disorder.

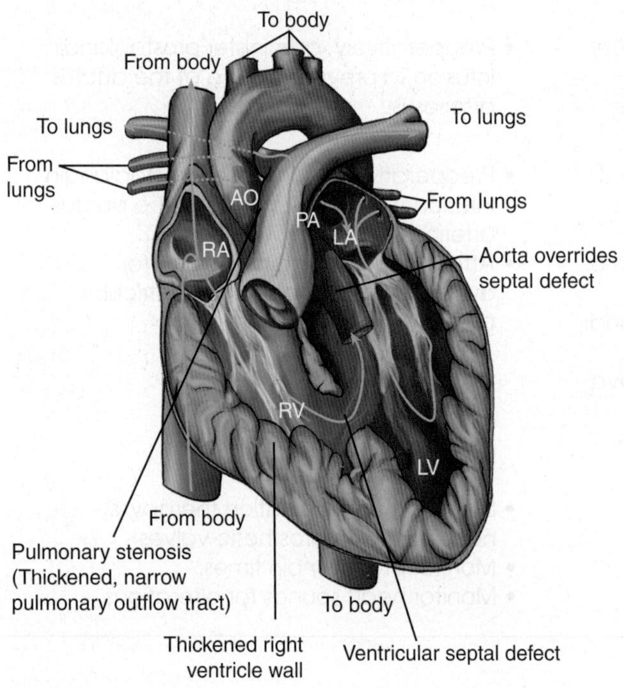

● Figure 20.2 Tetralogy of Fallot.

Laboratory and Diagnostic Tests

Note increased hematocrit, hemoglobin, and RBC count associated with polycythemia. Additional testing may include:

- Echocardiography, possibly revealing right ventricular hypertrophy, decreased pulmonary blood flow, and reduced size of the pulmonary artery
- ECG, indicating right ventricular hypertrophy
- Cardiac catheterization and angiography, which reveal the extent of the structural defects

Consider THIS!

Ava Gardener, 2 weeks old, is brought to the clinic by her mother. She presents with trouble feeding. Her mother states, "When Ava eats, she seems to have trouble breathing, and recently I've noticed a bluish color around her lips." What other assessment information would you obtain?

Ava is to be admitted to the hospital secondary to suspected tetralogy of Fallot. What education and interventions may be necessary for this child and family? How can you assist the family to cope?

Tricuspid Atresia

Tricuspid atresia is a congenital heart defect in which the valve between the right atrium and right ventricle fails to develop. As a result, there is no opening to allow blood to flow from the right atrium to the right ventricle and subsequently through the pulmonary artery into the lungs.

Pathophysiology

In tricuspid atresia, blood returning from the systemic circulation to the right atrium cannot directly enter the right ventricle due to agenesis of the tricuspid valve. Subsequently, deoxygenated blood then passes through an opening in the atrial septum (either an ASD or through a patent foramen ovale) into the left atrium, never entering the pulmonary vasculature. Thus, deoxygenated blood mixes with oxygenated blood in the left atrium. The blood then travels to the lungs through a PDA. The foramen ovale and ductus arteriosus must remain open for the newborn to maintain minimally adequate oxygenation (Fig. 20.3).

Nursing Assessment

Nursing assessment consists of health history, physical examination, and laboratory and diagnostic tests.

Health History and Physical Examination

Note the infant's history since birth. Document history of cyanosis either at birth or a few days later when the ductus arteriosus closed. Note history of rapid respirations and difficulty with feeding. Inspect the skin for cyanosis or a pale gray color. Observe the apical impulse, noting overactivity. Evaluate the baby's sucking strength (will usually have a weak or poor suck). Count the respiratory rate, noting tachypnea. Note increased work of breathing. Auscultate the lungs, noting crackles or wheezes if heart failure is beginning to develop. Auscultate the heart, noting a murmur. Palpate the skin, noting coolness and clamminess of the extremities. Document the presence of clubbing in the older infant or child.

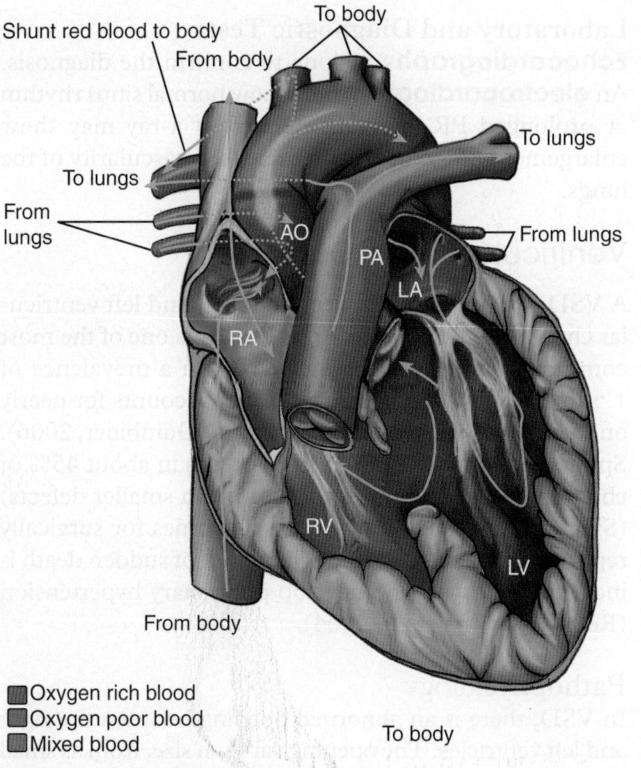

● **Figure 20.3** Tricuspid atresia.

Laboratory and Diagnostic Testing

Laboratory and diagnostic testing is similar to that for tetralogy of Fallot. A complete blood count (CBC) is needed to assess compensatory increases in hematocrit, hemoglobin, and erythrocyte count (RBC) indicating the development of polycythemia. Oxygen saturation levels (typically reduced) may be determined by pulse oximetry or arterial blood gases. Additional testing may include:

- Echocardiography, revealing absence of tricuspid valve, underdeveloped right ventricle
- ECG, indicating possible heart failure
- Cardiac catheterization and angiography, which reveal the extent of the structural defects

● DISORDERS WITH INCREASED PULMONARY FLOW

Most congenital heart defects involve increased pulmonary blood flow. Normally, the left side of the heart has a higher pressure than the right side. Defects with connections involving the left and right sides will shunt blood from the higher-pressure left side to the lower-pressure right side. Even a small pressure gradient such as a 1- to 3-mm difference between the left and right sides will produce a movement of blood from the left to the right. In turn, the increase of blood on the right side of the heart will cause a greater amount of blood to move through the heart. If the amount of blood flowing to the lungs is large, the child may develop **heart failure** early in life. In addition, right ventricular hypertrophy may result. Sometimes with ventricular hypertrophy the right side of the heart pumps so forcefully that left-to-right shunting is reversed to right-to-left shunting. If this occurs, deoxygenated blood mixes with oxygenated blood, thereby lowering the overall blood oxygen saturation level.

Excessive blood flow to the lungs can produce a compensatory response such as tachypnea or tachycardia. Tachypnea increases caloric expenditure; poor cellular nutrition from decreased peripheral blood flow leads to feeding problems. Subsequently, the infant experiences poor weight gain, which retards overall growth and development. Increased pulmonary blood flow results in decreased systemic blood flow, so sodium and fluid retention may occur. Increased pulmonary blood flow also places the child at higher risk for pulmonary infections. As the child grows, the continuous increased pulmonary blood flow will cause vasoconstriction of the pulmonary vessels, actually decreasing the pulmonary blood flow. This may lead to pulmonary hypertension. Therefore, preventing the development of pulmonary disease via early surgical correction is essential.

For children with congenital defects with increased pulmonary blood flow, oxygen supplementation is not helpful. Oxygen acts as a pulmonary vasodilator. If pulmonary dilation occurs, pulmonary blood flow is even greater, causing tachypnea, increasing lung fluid retention, and eventually causing a much greater problem with oxygenation. Over time, continuous increased pulmonary blood flow may cause pulmonary vasoconstriction and pulmonary hypertension. Surgical correction is essential before pulmonary disease develops (Driscoll, 2006a; Gumbiner, 2006; Mullins, 2006a; Suddaby, 2001; Vick & Bezold, 2006). Examples of defects with increased pulmonary blood flow are ASD, VSD, atrioventricular canal defect, and PDA.

Atrial Septal Defect

An ASD is a passageway or hole in the wall (septum) that divides the right atrium from the left atrium (Fig. 20.4). Three types of ASDs are identified based on the location of the opening:

- Ostium primum (ASD1): the opening is at the lower portion of the septum
- Ostium secundum (ASD2): the opening is near the center of the septum

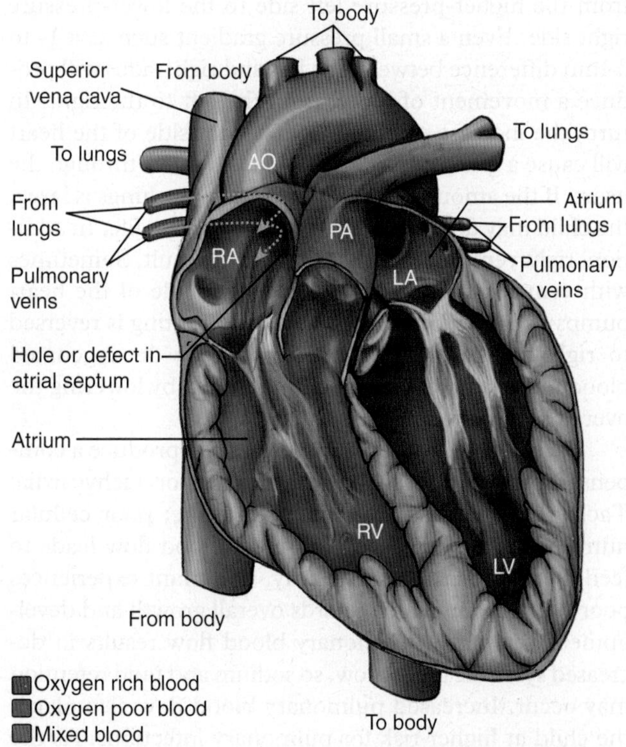

● **Figure 20.4** Atrial septal defect; note the opening between the two atria.

- Sinus venosus defect: the opening is near the junction of the superior vena cava and the right atrium

When the ASD is small, as many as 80% of infants may have a spontaneous closure within the first 18 months of life. If not spontaneously closed by age 3, the child will most likely need corrective surgery.

Pathophysiology

With ASD, blood flows between the opening from the left atrium to the right atrium due to pressure differences. The shunting increases the blood volume entering the right atrium. This, in turn, leads to increased blood flow into the lungs. The defect if untreated can cause problems such as pulmonary hypertension, heart failure, atrial arrhythmias, or stroke (Driscoll, 2006a; Vick & Bezold, 2006).

Nursing Assessment

Most children with ASDs are asymptomatic. However, a very large defect can cause increased blood flow, leading to heart failure, which results in shortness of breath, easy fatigability, or poor growth.

Health History and Physical Examination

Obtain the health history, noting poor feeding as an infant, decreased ability to keep up with peers, or history of difficulty growing. Observe the child's chest, noting a hyperdynamic precordium. Auscultate the heart, noting a fixed split second heart sound and a systolic ejection murmur, best heard in the pulmonic valve area. Palpate along the left sternal border for a right ventricular heave.

Laboratory and Diagnostic Tests

Echocardiography is done to confirm the diagnosis. An **electrocardiogram** may show normal sinus rhythm or prolonged PR intervals. The chest x-ray may show enlargement of the heart and increased vascularity of the lungs.

Ventricular Septal Defect

A VSD is an opening between the right and left ventricular chambers of the heart (Fig. 20.5). It is one of the most common congenital heart defects, with a prevalence of 1.5 to 2.5 per 1,000 live births. VSD accounts for nearly one third of all congenital heart defects (Gumbiner, 2006). Spontaneous closure of the VSD occurs in about 45% of children by age 3 years (most often with smaller defects) (Singh et al., 2004). Long-term outcomes for surgically repaired VSD are good, though the risk of sudden death is increased in those who develop pulmonary hypertension (Roos-Hesselink et al., 2004).

Pathophysiology

In VSD, there is an abnormal opening between the right and left ventricles. The opening varies in size, from as small as a pinhole to a complete opening between the ventricles

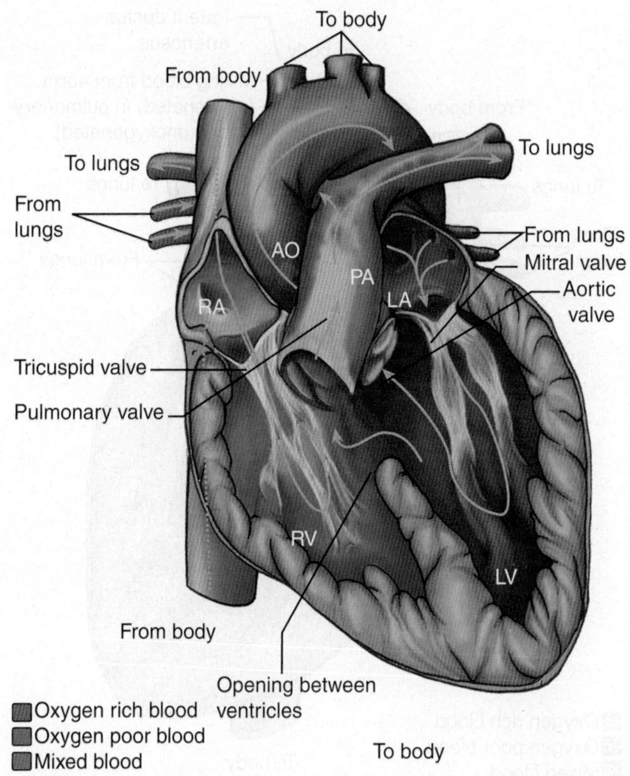

● **Figure 20.5** Ventricular septal defect; note the opening between the ventricles.

so that the right and left sides are as one. Children with small VSDs may remain asymptomatic. In other children, blood shunts across the opening in the septum. Pulmonary vascular resistance and systemic vascular resistance determine the direction of blood flow. A left-to-right shunt results when pulmonary vascular resistance is low. Increased amounts of blood flowing into the right ventricle are then pumped to the pulmonary circulation, eventually causing an increase in pulmonary vascular resistance. Increased pulmonary vascular resistance leads to increased pulmonary artery pressure (pulmonary hypertension) and right ventricular hypertrophy. When the pulmonary vascular resistance exceeds the systemic vascular resistance, right-to-left shunting of blood across the VSD occurs, resulting in Eisenmenger syndrome (pulmonary hypertension and cyanosis). Heart failure commonly occurs in children with moderate to severe VSD. Children with VSD are also at risk for the development of aortic valve regurgitation as well as infective endocarditis.

Nursing Assessment

Initially, the newborn may not exhibit any signs and symptoms at birth because left-to-right shunting is most likely minimal due to the high pulmonary resistance common after birth.

Health History and Physical Examination

Determine the health history, which commonly reveals signs of heart failure around 4 to 8 weeks of age. Note history of tiring easily, particularly with exertion or feeding. Document the child's growth history, noting difficulty thriving. Ask the parent about color change or diaphoresis with nipple feeding in the infant. Note history of frequent pulmonary infections, shortness of breath, and possibly edema. Inspect the extremities for edema, noting whether pitting is present. Note mild tachypnea.

Auscultate the heart, noting a characteristic holosystolic harsh murmur along the left sternal border. In some instances, a murmur may be noted only with excessive blood flow across the opening. Adventitious lung sounds may be auscultated if the child is experiencing heart failure. Palpate the chest for a thrill.

Laboratory and Diagnostic Tests

Magnetic resonance imaging (MRI) or echocardiogram with color flow Doppler may reveal the opening as well as the extent of left-to-right shunting. These studies also may identify right ventricular hypertrophy and dilation of the pulmonary artery resulting from the increased blood flow. Cardiac catheterization may be used to evaluate the extent of blood flow being pumped to the pulmonary circulation and to evaluate hemodynamic pressures.

Atrioventricular Canal Defect

Atrioventricular canal defect (atrioventricular septal defect [AVSD], AV canal, or endocardial cushion defect) accounts for 4% to 5% of congenital heart disease and occurs in 2 of every 10,000 live births. Forty percent of children with Down syndrome and CHD have this defect (Driscoll, 2006a).

Pathophysiology

AV canal defect occurs as a result of failure of the endocardial cushions to fuse (Fig. 20.6). These cushions are needed to separate the central parts of the heart near the tricuspid and mitral (AV) valves. The complete AV canal defect involves atrial and ventricular septal defects as well as a common AV orifice and a common AV valve. Partial and transitional forms of AV canal defect also occur, involving variations of the complete form.

The complete AV canal defect permits oxygenated blood from the lungs to enter the left atrium and ventricle, crossing over the atrial or ventricular septum and returning to the lungs via the pulmonary artery. This recirculation problem, which typically involves a left-to-right shunt, is inefficient because the left ventricle must pump blood back to the lungs and also meet the body's peripheral demand for oxygenated blood. Subsequently, the left ventricle must pump two to three times more blood than in a normal heart. Therefore, this specific type of cardiac defect causes a large left-to-right shunt; an increased workload of the left ventricle; and high pulmonary arterial pressure, resulting in an increased amount of blood in the lungs and causing pulmonary edema (Driscoll, 2006a; Vick & Bezold, 2006).

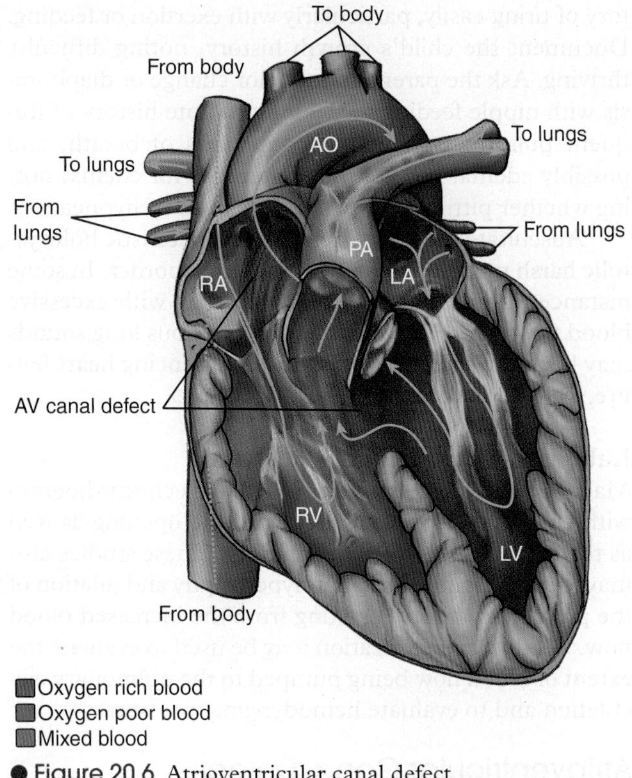

● Figure 20.6 Atrioventricular canal defect.

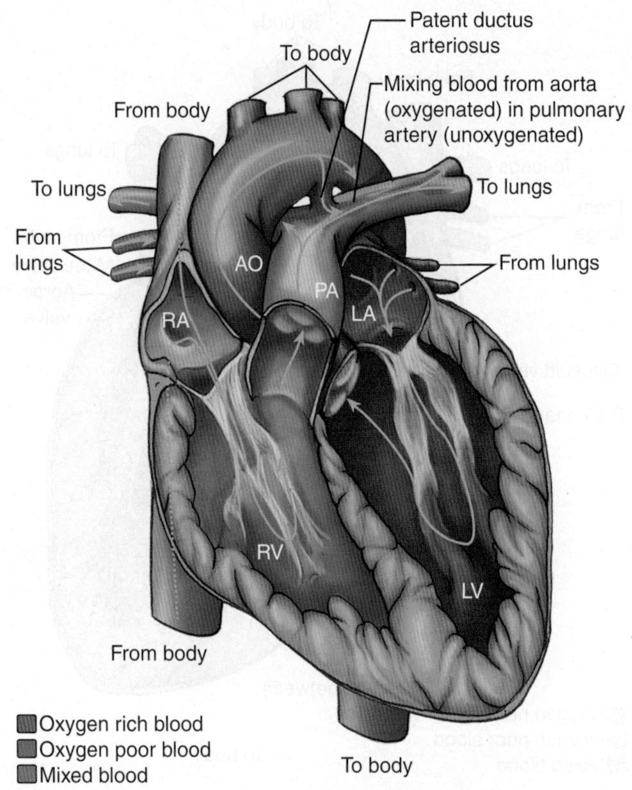

● Figure 20.7 Patent ductus arteriosus.

Nursing Assessment

The infant with a complete AV canal defect commonly exhibits moderate to severe signs and symptoms of heart failure. However, for infants with partial or transitional AV canal defects, the signs and symptoms will be more subtle.

Health History and Physical Examination

Obtain the health history, noting frequent respiratory infections and difficulty gaining weight. Ask the parent if the infant has been experiencing difficulty feeding or increased work of breathing.

Inspect the skin, fingernails, and lips for cyanosis. Observe for retractions, tachypnea, and nasal flaring. Auscultate the lungs and heart, noting rales and a loud murmur. The murmur is commonly noted within the first 2 weeks of life. Infants with partial or transitional AV canal defect may display more subtle signs.

Laboratory and Diagnostic Tests

Echocardiography will reveal the extent of the defect and shunting as well as right ventricular hypertrophy. Electrocardiogram may indicate right ventricular hypertrophy and possible first-degree heart block due to impulse blocking before reaching the AV node.

Patent Ductus Arteriosus

PDA is failure of the ductus arteriosus, a fetal circulatory structure, to close within the first weeks of life (Fig. 20.7). As a result, there is a connection between the aorta and pulmonary artery. PDA is the second most common congenital heart defect and accounts for 10% of CHD cases (Mullins, 2006a). PDA occurs much more frequently in premature than in term infants: 45% of infants less than 1,750 g at birth and 80% of infants less than 1,200 g will display a PDA. PDA occurs 30 times more often in infants born at high altitudes compared with those born at sea level (Driscoll, 2006a). Infants with other congenital heart defects that result in right-to-left shunting of blood and cyanosis may additionally display a PDA. In these infants, the PDA allows for some level of oxygenated blood to reach the systemic circulation.

Pathophysiology

Failure of the ductus arteriosus to close leads to continued blood flow from the aorta to the pulmonary artery. Blood returning to the left atrium passes to the left ventricle, enters the aorta, and then travels to the pulmonary artery via the PDA instead of entering the systemic circulation. This altered blood flow pattern increases the workload of the left side of heart. Pulmonary vascular congestion occurs, causing an increase in pressure. Right ventricular pressure increases in an attempt to overcome this increase in pulmonary pressure. Eventually, right ventricular hypertrophy occurs.

Nursing Assessment

The symptoms of PDA depend on the size of the ductus arteriosus and the amount of blood flow it carries. If it is small, the infant may be asymptomatic. Some infants demonstrate signs and symptoms of heart failure.

Health History and Physical Examination

Determine the health history, which may reveal frequent respiratory infections, fatigue, and poor growth and development. On physical examination, note tachycardia, tachypnea, bounding peripheral pulses, and a widened pulse pressure. The diastolic blood pressure typically is low due to the shunting. Auscultate the lungs and heart, noting rales if heart failure is present. Note a harsh, continuous, machine-like murmur, usually loudest under the left clavicle at the first and second intercostal spaces.

Laboratory and Diagnostic Tests

Echocardiogram reveals the extent of the defective opening and confirms the diagnosis. Electrocardiogram may be normal or it may indicate ventricular hypertrophy, especially if the defect is large. Chest x-ray demonstrates cardiomegaly.

● OBSTRUCTIVE DISORDERS

Another group of congenital heart defects is classified as obstructive disorders. These disorders involve some type of narrowing of a major vessel, interfering with the ability of the blood to flow freely through the vessel. As a result, peripheral circulation or blood flow to the lungs is affected. Increased pressure backing up toward the heart causes an increased workload on the heart. Examples of defects in this group include coarctation of the aorta, aortic stenosis, and pulmonic stenosis.

Coarctation of the Aorta

Coarctation of the aorta is narrowing of the aorta, the major blood vessel carrying highly oxygenated blood from the left ventricle of the heart to the rest of the body (Fig. 20.8). It is the third most common congenital heart defect. Coarctation occurs more than twice as often in males as in females (Morriss, 2006).

Pathophysiology

Coarctation of the aorta occurs most often in the area near the ductus arteriosus. The narrowing can be preductal (between the subclavian artery and ductus arteriosus) or postductal (after the ductus arteriosus). As a result of the narrowing, blood flow is impeded, causing pressure to increase in the area proximal to the defect and to decrease in the area distal to it. Thus, blood pressure is increased in the heart and upper portions of the body and decreased in the lower portions of the body. Left ventricular afterload is increased, and in some children this may lead to heart failure. Collateral circulation also may develop as the body attempts to ensure adequate blood flow to the descending aorta. Due to the elevation in blood pressure, the child is also at risk for aortic rupture, aortic aneurysm, and cerebrovascular accident (CVA).

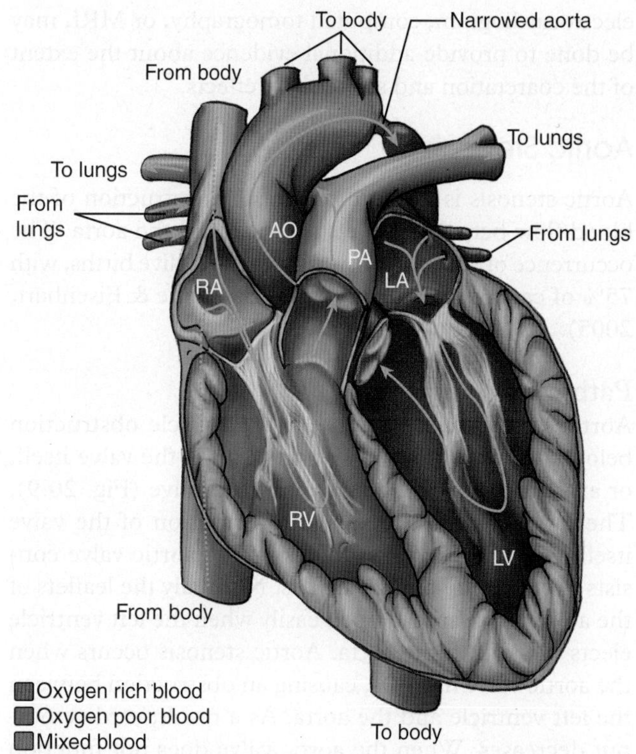

● Figure 20.8 Coarctation of the aorta.

Nursing Assessment

The extent of the symptoms depends on the severity of the coarctation. Some children with coarctation of the aorta grow well into the school-age years before the defect is discovered.

Health History and Physical Examination

Determine the health history, noting problems with irritability and frequent epistaxis. In older children, there also may be reports of leg pain with activity, dizziness, fainting, and headaches. Assess pulses throughout, noting full, bounding pulses in the upper extremities with weak or absent pulses in the lower extremities. Determine BP in all four extremities. BP in the upper extremities may be 20 mm Hg or higher than that in the lower extremities. Inspect the school-age child's chest, noting notching of the ribs. Auscultate the heart for a soft or moderately loud systolic murmur, most often heard at the base of the heart.

Laboratory and Diagnostic Tests

Diagnosis of coarctation of the aorta is based primarily on the history and physical examination. In addition, an echocardiogram may disclose the extent of narrowing and evidence of collateral circulation. Chest x-ray may reveal left-sided cardiac enlargement and rib notching indicative of collateral arterial enlargement. Other tests, such as electrocardiogram, computed tomography, or MRI, may be done to provide additional evidence about the extent of the coarctation and subsequent effects.

Aortic Stenosis

Aortic stenosis is a condition causing obstruction of the blood flow between the left ventricle and the aorta. The occurrence of aortic stenosis is 4 per 1,000 live births, with 75% of cases occurring in males (Balentine & Eisenhart, 2005).

Pathophysiology

Aortic stenosis can be caused by a muscle obstruction below the aortic valve, an obstruction at the valve itself, or an aortic narrowing just above the valve (Fig. 20.9). The most common type is an obstruction of the valve itself, called aortic valve stenosis. The aortic valve consists of three very pliable leaflets. Normally the leaflets of the aortic valve spread open easily when the left ventricle ejects blood into the aorta. Aortic stenosis occurs when the aortic valve narrows, causing an obstruction between the left ventricle and the aorta. As a result, cardiac output decreases. When the aortic valve does not function properly, the left ventricle must work harder to pump blood into the aorta. Because of the increased workload, the left ventricular muscle hypertrophies. If this continues, left ventricular failure can occur, leading to a backup of pressure in the pulmonary circulation and pulmonary edema. Heart failure may occur, but this is more commonly seen in the infant (Driscoll, 2006a).

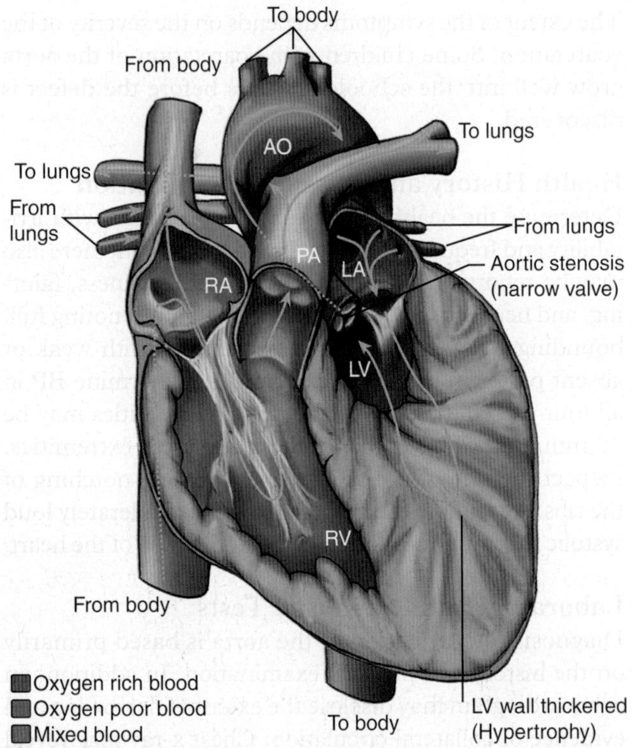

● **Figure 20.9** Aortic stenosis.

Nursing Assessment

Typically, the child with aortic stenosis is asymptomatic. However, it is important to obtain an accurate health history and perform a physical examination.

Health History and Physical Examination

Obtain the child's health history, noting easy fatigability or complaints of chest pain similar to anginal pain when active. Dizziness with prolonged standing also may be reported. In the infant, note difficulty with feeding. Palpate the child's pulse; if aortic stenosis is severe, the pulses may be faint. Palpate the child's chest, noting a thrill at the base of the heart. Auscultate the heart, noting a systolic murmur best heard along the left sternal border with radiation to the right upper sternal border.

Laboratory and Diagnostic Tests

The echocardiogram is the most important noninvasive test to identify aortic stenosis. An electrocardiogram may be normal in children with mild to moderate forms of aortic stenosis. For children with severe aortic stenosis, left ventricular hypertrophy may be determined from the electrocardiogram. For children experiencing easy fatigability and chest pain, an exercise stress test may be done to evaluate the degree of cardiac compromise.

Pulmonary Stenosis

Pulmonary stenosis is a condition that causes an obstruction in blood flow between the right ventricle and the pulmonary arteries. Pulmonary stenosis occurs in 7% to 12% of all cases of CHD (Cheatham, 2006). It is often associated with various genetic syndromes. Children may be asymptomatic, although some children with severe stenosis may exhibit dyspnea and fatigue with exertion (demonstrating hypercyanotic spells similar to those in children with tetralogy of Fallot).

Pathophysiology

Pulmonary stenosis may occur as a muscular obstruction below the pulmonary valve, an obstruction at the valve, or a narrowing of the pulmonary artery above the valve (Fig. 20.10). Valve obstruction is the most common form of pulmonary stenosis. Normally the pulmonary valve is constructed with three thin and pliable valve leaflets; they spread apart easily, allowing the right ventricle to eject blood freely into the pulmonary artery. The most common problem causing pulmonary stenosis is that the pulmonary valve leaflets are thickened and fused together along their separation lines, causing the obstruction to blood flow. The right ventricle has an additional workload, causing the muscle to thicken, resulting in right ventricular hypertrophy and decreased pulmonary blood flow. When the pulmonary valve is severely obstructed, the right ventricle cannot eject sufficient blood into the

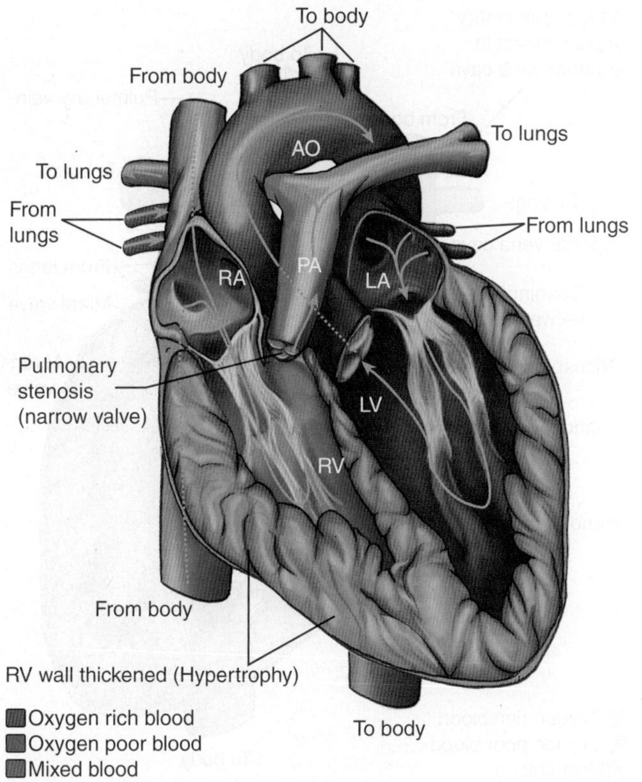

● Figure 20.10 Pulmonary stenosis.

pulmonary artery. As a result, pressure in the right atrium increases, which could lead to a reopening of the foramen ovale. If this occurs, deoxygenated blood would pass through the foramen ovale into the left side of the heart and would then be pumped to the systemic circulation. In some cases, a PDA may be present, thus allowing for some compensation by shunting blood from the aorta to the pulmonary circulation for oxygenation.

Nursing Assessment

The child with pulmonary stenosis may be asymptomatic or may exhibit signs and symptoms of mild heart failure. If the stenosis is severe, the child may demonstrate cyanosis. Therefore, it is important for the nurse to obtain an accurate health history and physical examination.

Health History and Physical Examination

Elicit the health history, noting mild dyspnea or cyanosis with exertion. Document the child's growth history, which is typically normal. Carefully palpate the sternal border for a thrill (not always present). Auscultate the heart, noting a high-pitched click following the second heart sound and a systolic ejection murmur loudest at the upper left sternal border.

Laboratory and Diagnostic Tests

An echocardiogram reveals the extent of obstruction present at the valve, as well as right ventricular hypertrophy. An electrocardiogram also helps to detect right ventricular hypertrophy.

● MIXED DEFECTS

Mixed defects are congenital heart defects that involve a mixing of well-oxygenated blood with poorly oxygenated blood. As a result, systemic blood flow contains a lower oxygen content. Cardiac output is decreased, and heart failure occurs. Examples of mixed defects include transposition of the great vessels, total anomalous pulmonary venous connection, truncus arteriosus, and hypoplastic left heart syndrome.

Transposition of the Great Vessels (Arteries)

Transposition of the great vessels (TGV) is a congenital heart defect in which the pulmonary artery and the aorta arise from the ventricle opposite that from which they normally arise. Thus, the vessels are transposed from their normal positions. The aorta arises from the right ventricle instead of the left ventricle and the pulmonary artery arises from the left ventricle instead of the right ventricle. Transposition of the great vessels accounts for approximately 5% of all CHD cases. It is most often diagnosed in the first few days of life when the child manifests cyanosis, which indicates decreased oxygenation. As the ductus arteriosus closes, the symptoms will worsen. Heart failure may also be present in the first weeks to months of life. If untreated, 50% of affected infants will die in the first month of life and 90% in the first year.

Pathophysiology

In TGV there is no connection or communication between the pulmonary and systemic circulations (Fig. 20.11). TGV creates a situation in which poorly oxygenated blood returning to the right atrium and ventricle is then pumped out to the aorta and back to the body. Oxygenated blood returning from the lungs to the left atrium and ventricle is then sent back to the lungs through the pulmonary artery. Unless there is a connection somewhere in the circulation where the oxygen-rich and oxygen-poor blood can mix, all the organs of the body will be poorly oxygenated. Often the ductus arteriosus remains patent, allowing for some mixing of blood. Similarly, if a VSD is also present, mixing of blood may occur and cyanosis will be delayed. However, these associated defects can lead to increased pulmonary blood flow that increases pressure in the pulmonary circulation. This predisposes the child to heart failure.

Nursing Assessment

Significant cyanosis without a murmur in the newborn period is highly indicative of TGV. In about 10% of infants, cyanosis will not develop until several days of age as the PDA closes (Molczan, 2006). In infants with septal defects, cyanosis may be further delayed.

Health History and Physical Examination

Elicit the health history, noting onset of cyanosis with feeding or crying. Observe the infant for cyanosis while active

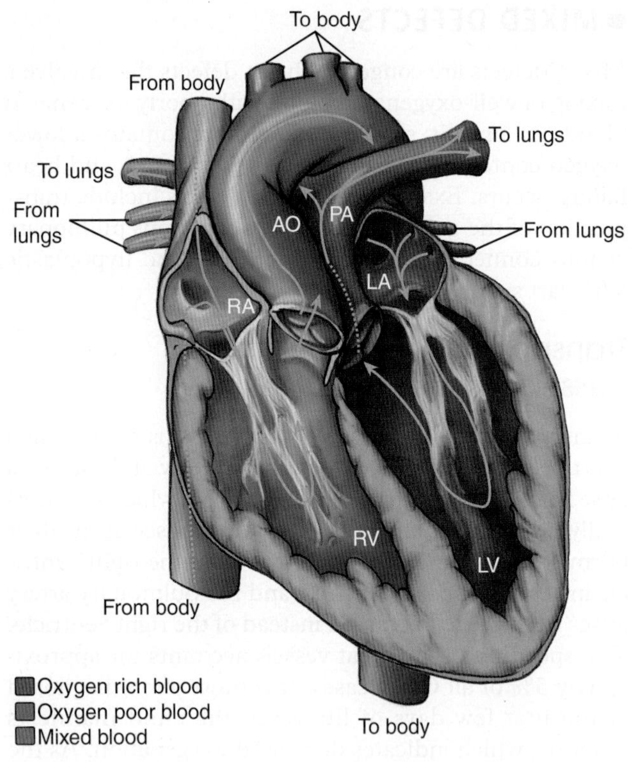

● Figure 20.11 Transposition of the great vessels.

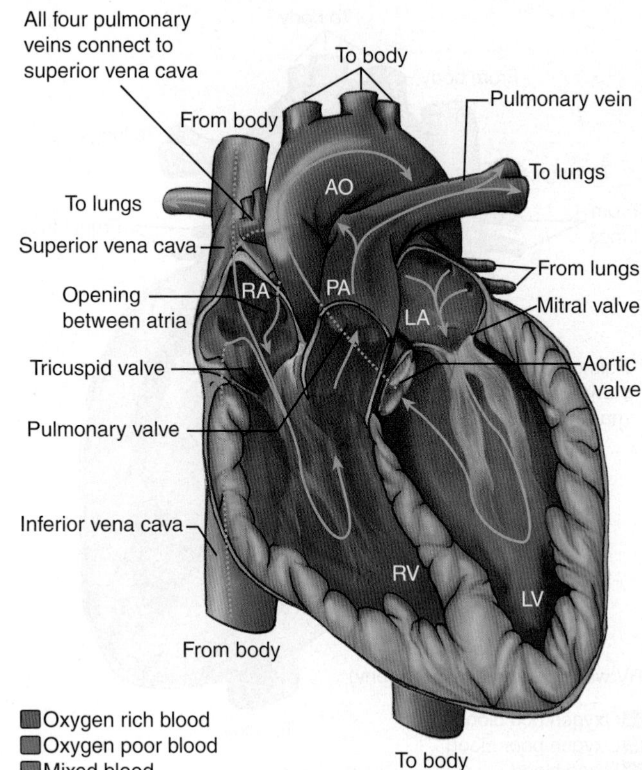

● Figure 20.12 Total anomalous pulmonary venous connection.

and at rest. Observe the chest, noting a prominent ventricular impulse. Auscultate the heart, noting a loud second heart sound. A murmur may be heard if the ductus remains open or a septal defect is present. If heart failure is present, note edema, tachypnea, and adventitious lung sounds.

Laboratory and Diagnostic Tests

Echocardiography clearly reveals evidence of the transposition. Cardiac catheterization may be performed, determining low oxygen saturation levels due to the mixing of the blood.

Total Anomalous Pulmonary Venous Connection

Total anomalous pulmonary venous connection (TAPVC) is a rare congenital heart defect in which the pulmonary veins do not connect normally to the left atrium; instead, they connect to the right atrium, often by way of the superior vena cava. Males exhibit this disorder three times more often than females (Ward, 2006).

Pathophysiology

Oxygenated blood that would normally enter the left atrium now enters the right atrium and passes to the right ventricle. As a result, the pressure on the right side of the heart increases, leading to hypertrophy. TAPVC is incompatible with life unless there is an associated defect present that allows for shunting of blood from the highly pressured right side of the heart. A patent foramen ovale or an ASD is usually present. Since none of the pulmonary veins connect normally to the left atrium, the only source of blood to the left atrium is blood that is shunted from the right atrium across the defect to the left side of the heart (Fig. 20.12). The highly oxygenated blood from the lungs completely mixes with the poorly oxygenated blood returning from the systemic circulation. This causes an overload of the right atrium and right ventricle. The increased blood volume going into the lungs can lead to pulmonary hypertension and pulmonary edema.

Nursing Assessment

The degree of cyanosis present with TAPVC depends on the extent of the associated defects. For example, if the foramen ovale closes or the ASD is small, significant cyanosis will be present. The physical examination findings will vary depending on the type of TAPVC the infant has, whether obstruction is present, and which other associated cardiac anomalies are present.

Health History and Physical Examination

Note history of cyanosis, tiring easily, and difficulty feeding. Observe the chest for prominence of the right ventricular impulse and retractions with tachypnea. Auscultate the heart, noting fixed splitting of the second heart sound and a murmur. Palpate the abdomen for hepatomegaly.

Laboratory and Diagnostic Tests

An echocardiogram will reveal the abnormal connection of the pulmonary veins, enlargement of the right atrium and right ventricle, and an ASD if present. The chest x-ray will demonstrate an enlarged heart and pulmonary edema. Cardiac catheterization can also be useful to visualize the abnormal connection of the pulmonary veins, particularly if an obstruction is present.

Truncus Arteriosus

Truncus arteriosus is a congenital heart defect in which only one major artery leaves the heart and supplies blood to the pulmonary and systemic circulations. It affects males and females equally and accounts for 1% to 4% of all CHD cases (Slesnick & Kovalchin, 2006). A VSD may also be present.

Pathophysiology

The one great vessel contains one valve which comprises two to five leaflets and is positioned over both the left and right ventricles (Fig. 20.13). Due to the location, blood from the left ventricle mixes with blood from the right ventricle. Pressure in the pulmonary circulation typically is less than that of the systemic circulation, leading to increased blood flow to the lungs. As a result, systemic blood flow is decreased. Over time, the increased pulmonary blood flow can lead to pulmonary vascular disease.

Nursing Assessment

Typically, the infant demonstrates cyanosis in varying degrees depending on the extent of compromise in the systemic circulation. Obtain an accurate health history and perform a physical examination.

Health History and Physical Examination

Elicit the health history, noting history of cyanosis that increases with periods of activity such as feeding. Also note history of tiring easily, difficulty in feeding, and poor growth. Count the respiratory rate, which may be elevated. Observe for nasal flaring, grunting or noisy breathing, retractions, and restlessness. Auscultate the lungs, noting adventitious breath sounds, and the heart, noting a murmur associated with a VSD.

Laboratory and Diagnostic Tests

An echocardiogram will confirm the presence of truncus arteriosus as the anatomy of the great vessels, the single truncal valve, and the VSD will be seen. On rare occasions a cardiac catheterization may be done to determine pressures in the pulmonary arteries.

Hypoplastic Left Heart Syndrome

Hypoplastic left heart syndrome (HLHS) is a congenital heart defect in which all of the structures on the left side of the heart are severely underdeveloped (Fig. 20.14). The mitral and aortic valves are completely closed or very small. The left ventricle is nonfunctional. Thus, the left side of the heart is completely unable to supply blood to the systemic circulation. HLHS is the fourth most com-

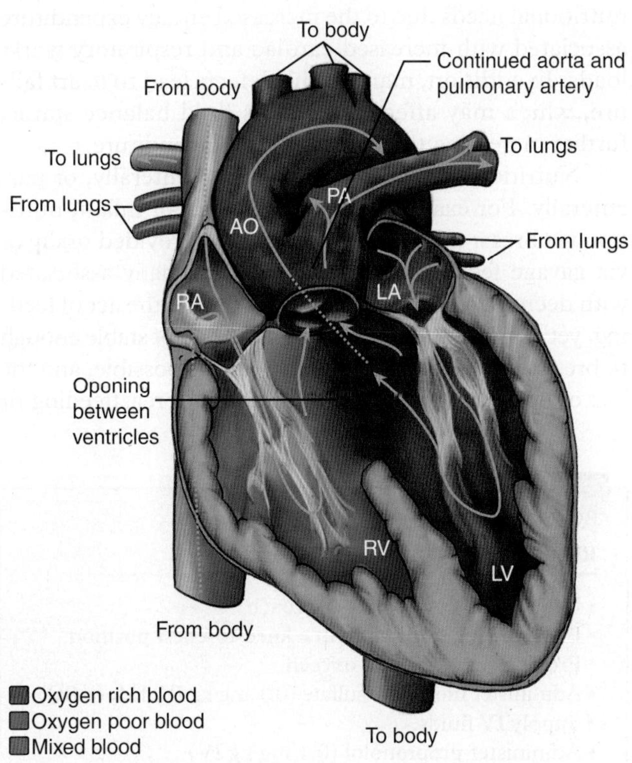

● Figure 20.13 Truncus arteriosus.

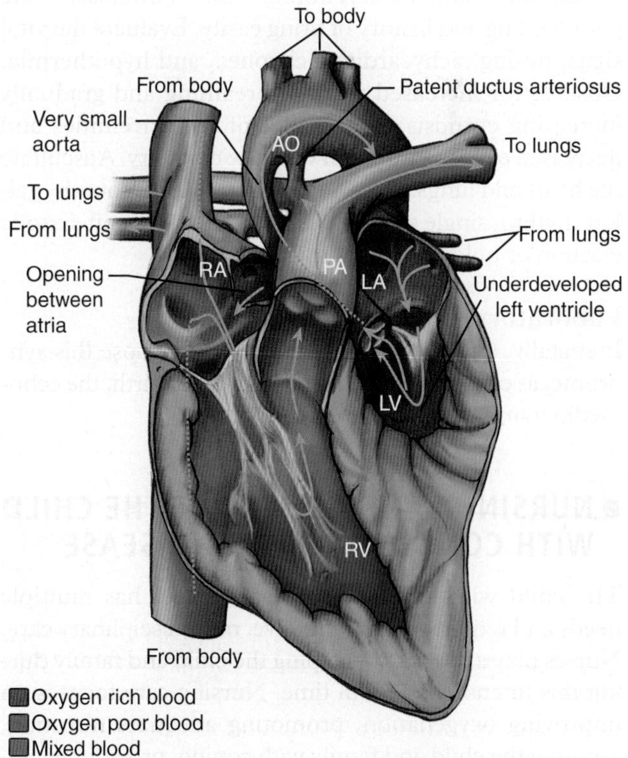

● Figure 20.14 Hypoplastic left heart syndrome.

mon congenital heart defect. It appears to have a multifactorial and autosomal recessive inheritance pattern. Almost 30% of infants with HLHS also have a definable genetic or other congenital anomaly in addition to the heart defect (Eidem, 2006). The options for treatment include palliative care, cardiac transplantation within the first few weeks of life, or palliative reconstructive surgery consisting of three stages, beginning within days to weeks of birth (Ziegler, 2003).

Pathophysiology

With HLHS, the right side of the heart is the main working part of the heart. Blood returning from the lungs into the left atrium must pass through an ASD to the right side of the heart. The right ventricle must then pump blood to the lungs and also to the systemic circulation through the PDA. A few days after birth, when the ductus arteriosus closes, the heart cannot pump blood into the systemic circulation, causing poor perfusion of the vital organs and shock. Death will occur rapidly without intervention.

Nursing Assessment

Initially after birth, the newborn may be asymptomatic because the ductus arteriosus is still patent. However, as the ductus begins to close at a few days of age, the newborn will begin to exhibit cyanosis. Some infants may present with circulatory collapse (shock) and must be resuscitated emergently.

Health History and Physical Examination

Obtain the health history, noting onset of cyanosis. Note poor feeding and history of tiring easily. Evaluate the vital signs, noting tachycardia, tachypnea, and hypothermia. Observe for increased work of breathing and gradually increasing cyanosis. Note pallor of the extremities and decreased oxygen saturation via pulse oximetry. Auscultate the heart and lungs. Note adventitious breath sounds, gallop rhythm, single second heart sound, and a soft systolic ejection or holosystolic murmur.

Laboratory and Diagnostic Tests

Prenatally, a fetal echocardiogram can diagnose this syndrome, as can a maternal ultrasound. After birth, the echocardiogram illustrates the defect.

NURSING MANAGEMENT OF THE CHILD WITH CONGENITAL HEART DISEASE

The child with a congenital heart defect has multiple needs and requires comprehensive, multidisciplinary care. Nurses play a key role in helping the child and family during this intensely stressful time. Nursing care focuses on improving oxygenation, promoting adequate nutrition, assisting the child and family with coping, providing postoperative nursing care, preventing infection, and providing patient and family education. An important component of education involves preparing the child and parents for discharge. In addition to the nursing management presented below, refer to Nursing Care Plan 20.1 for additional interventions appropriate for the child with CHD. Individualize nursing care specific to the child's needs.

Improving Oxygenation

Due to the hemodynamic changes accompanying the underlying structural defect, oxygenation is key. Provide frequent ongoing assessment of the child's cardiopulmonary status. Assess airway patency and suction as needed. Position the child in Fowler's or semi-Fowler's position to facilitate lung expansion. Monitor vital signs, especially heart and respiratory rates. Monitor the child's color and oxygen saturation levels closely, using these to guide oxygen administration. Observe for tachypnea and other signs of respiratory distress, such as nasal flaring, grunting, and retractions. Auscultate the lungs for adventitious sounds. Provide humidified supplemental oxygen as ordered, warming it to prevent wide temperature fluctuations. Anticipate the need for assisted ventilation if the child has difficulty maintaining the airway or experiences deterioration in oxygenation capacity. Box 20.1 lists interventions related to relief of hypercyanotic spells.

Promoting Adequate Nutrition

Adequate nutrition is critical to foster growth and development as well as to reduce the risk for infection. Children with congenital heart defects typically have increased nutritional needs due to the increased energy expenditure associated with increased cardiac and respiratory workloads. In addition, many of the defects lead to heart failure, which may affect the child's fluid balance status, further increasing the child's energy expenditure.

Nutrition may be provided orally, enterally, or parenterally. For example, for the newborn or infant, nutrition via breast milk or formula may be provided orally or via gavage feedings. Breastfeeding is usually associated with decreased energy expenditure during the act of feeding, yet some infants in intensive care are not stable enough to breastfeed. Gavage with breast milk is possible, and the use of human milk fortifier (either with breastfeeding or

BOX 20.1

RELIEVING HYPERCYANOTIC SPELLS

- Use a calm, comforting approach.
- Place the infant or child in a knee-to-chest position.
- Provide supplemental oxygen.
- Administer morphine sulfate (0.1 mg/kg IV, IM, or SQ).
- Supply IV fluids.
- Administer propranolol (0.1 mg/kg IV).

added to the gavage feed) adds additional calories that the infant requires. Formula-fed infants may also require increased-calorie formula, which may be achieved by more concentrated mixing of the formula or through the use of additives such as Polycose or vegetable oil. Consult the nutritionist to determine the individual infant's caloric needs and prescription of appropriate feeding.

Cutting a large hole in the nipple or "cross-cutting" the nipple decreases the work of feeding for some infants. Generally, nipple feedings should be limited to a 20-minute duration, as feeding for longer periods results in excess caloric expenditure. Many infants may feed orally for 20 minutes, receiving the remainder of that feeding via orogastric or nasogastric tube. Offer older children small, frequent feedings to reduce the amount of energy required to feed or eat and to prevent overtiring the child. When needed, administer and monitor total parenteral nutrition as prescribed.

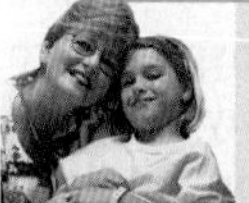

Breastfeeding a child before and after cardiac surgery may boost the infant's immune system, which can help fight postoperative infection. If breastfeeding is not possible, mothers can pump milk and the breast milk may be given via bottle, dropper, or gavage feeding.

Assisting the Child and Family to Cope

The diagnosis of CHD is especially overwhelming for the child and the parents. The numerous examinations, diagnostic tests, and procedures are sources of stress for the infant or child regardless of age and for the parents. The parents may fear long-term disability or death or may worry that allowing the child to engage in any activity will worsen his or her status. Thus, the parents may tend to overprotect the child. It is important for the parents to continue parenting the child, even when the child requires extended hospitalizations or intensive care (Fernandes, 2005). Explain all that is happening with the child, using language the parents and child can understand. Allow the parents and child to voice their feelings, concerns, or questions. Provide ample time to address these questions and concerns. Encourage the parents, and the child as developmentally appropriate, to participate in the child's care.

If the child is a newborn or infant, encourage attachment and bonding. Emphasize the child's positive attributes, including the normal aspects of the infant. Help the parents to experience the joy of a new infant, seeing the beauty of the child, no matter how ill the infant is (Fernandes, 2005). Urge the parents to touch, stroke, pat, and talk to the infant. Encourage them to hold the infant close, using kangaroo care as appropriate. If the child is older, offer suggestions as to how the parents can meet the child's emotional needs. For example, encourage them to bring a favorite toy or object from home while the child is hospitalized.

Provide developmentally appropriate explanations to the child. Encourage play therapy to help the child understand what is happening.

Preventing Infection

Teach parents proper hand hygiene. Provide appropriate dental care. Make sure the child receives prophylaxis for infective endocarditis as needed. Ensure that children 24 months or younger who have hemodynamically significant heart defects receive respiratory syncytial virus (RSV) prophylaxis as recommended during RSV season (Ressel, 2004).

Providing Care for the Child Undergoing Cardiac Surgery

Cardiac surgery may be necessary to correct a congenital defect or to provide symptomatic relief. The surgery may be planned as an elective procedure or done as an emergency. Open-heart surgery involves an incision of the heart muscle to repair the internal structures. This may require cardiopulmonary bypass. Closed-heart surgery involves structures related to the heart but not the heart muscle itself and may be performed with or without cardiopulmonary bypass (Kopf & Mello, 2006; Muscari, 2004).

Providing Preoperative Care

The preoperative nursing assessment complements the history and physical examination and provides important baseline information for comparison during the postoperative period. Establish a relationship with the child and parents. Identify problems that may require particular nursing interventions during the postoperative period. Before cardiac surgery, interview the parents and, if age-appropriate, the child. Focus the interview on the history of the present illness, cardiac risk factors, the child's present physical and functional status, additional medical problems, current medications and drug allergies, the child's and family's understanding of the illness and planned procedure, and the family support system.

The preoperative physical assessment includes:

- Temperature and weight measurements
- Examination of extremities for peripheral edema, clubbing, and evaluation of peripheral pulses
- Auscultation of the heart (rate, rhythm, heart sounds, murmurs, clicks, and rubs)
- Respiratory assessment, including respiratory rate, work of breathing, and auscultation of the lungs for breath sounds

Obtain any necessary laboratory and diagnostic tests to establish a baseline. In addition, review the results of any tests done previously. Testing may include CBC, electrolyte levels, clotting studies, urinalysis, cultures of blood and other body secretions, renal and hepatic function tests, chest x-ray, electrocardiogram, echocardiogram, and cardiac catheterization.

In most nonemergent cases, preoperative assessment is performed in an outpatient setting and the patient is admitted to the hospital on the day of surgery. Nursing care during this phase focuses on thorough patient and parent education. If the surgery is an emergency, patient teaching must be done quickly, emphasizing the most important elements of the child's care.

Child and parent education typically includes the following topics:

- Heart anatomy and its function, including what area is involved with the defect that is to be corrected
- Events before surgery, including any testing or preparation such as a skin scrub
- Location of the child after surgery, such as a pediatric intensive care unit, which may include a visit to the unit if appropriate and explanation of the sights and sounds that may be present
- Appearance of the child after surgery (equipment or devices used for monitoring, such as oxygen administration, electrocardiogram leads, pulse oximeter, chest tubes, mechanical ventilation, or intravenous lines)
- Approximate location of the incision and coverage with dressings
- Postoperative activity level, including measures to reduce the risk of complications, such as coughing and deep-breathing exercises, incentive spirometry, early ambulation, and leg exercises
- Nutritional restrictions, such as nothing by mouth for a specified time before surgery and use of intravenous fluids
- Medications, such as anesthesia, sedation, and analgesics as well as medications the child is taking now that need to be continued or withheld

Prepare and educate the child at an age- and developmentally appropriate level. Advise parents to read books with their child about CHD and hospitalization such as:

- "Clifford Visits the Hospital" by N. Bridwell, 2000 (Scholastic Inc.)
- "Franklin Goes to the Hospital" by P. Bourgeois, 2000 (Scholastic Paperbacks)
- "Pump the Bear" by G. O. Whittingon, 2000 (Brown Books)
- "Blue Lewis and Sasha the Great" by C. D. Newell, 2005 (Cally Press)
- "Cardiac Kids: A Book for Families Who Have a Child with Heart Disease" by V. Elder, 1994 (Dayton Area Heart and Cancer Association)
- "When Molly Was in the Hospital: A Book for Brothers and Sisters of Hospitalized Children" by D. Duncan, 1994 (Rayve Productions) (siblings)
- "A Night Without Stars" by J. Howe, 1993 (Camelot) (older children)

Additionally, parents may order "It's My Heart", a parent resource book, free of charge from the Children's Heart Foundation at http://www.childrensheartfoundation.org/its_my_heart.htm.

Parents may also help their child by buying a small thrift-store suitcase, spray-painting it, and allowing the child to decorate it with his or her name, pictures of family, stickers, or favorite story characters. This will be the child's "hospital suitcase" that the child may pack with toys and videos to bring to the hospital. Hospital tours are appropriate for school-age children, and older children and teens may benefit from an intensive care unit tour before surgery.

Instruct parents to stop food and liquids at the designated time, depending on the child's age, and to give all medications as directed. Some medications may be withheld before surgery. If the child's nutritional status is poor or questionable, nutritional supplementation may be ordered for a period of time preoperatively to ensure that the child has the best possible nutritional status before surgery. When it is time for the child to be transported to the surgical area, allow the parents to accompany the child as far as possible, depending on the institution's policy. Also reinforce with the child that the parents will be present at the bedside when he or she awakens from surgery.

Providing Postoperative Care

The child will usually be transported from the operating room to the intensive care unit. Depending on the age, postoperative stability, and type of surgery, the child may stay in the intensive care unit for several hours up to several days. Vigilant nursing care aids in the transition of the child and parents after surgery and reduces the risk of complications.

During the postoperative period the nurse should do the following:

- Assess vital signs frequently, as often as every 1 hour, until stable.
- Assess the color of the skin and mucous membranes, check capillary refill, and palpate peripheral pulses.
- Observe cardiac rate and rhythm via electronic monitoring and auscultate heart rate, rhythm, and sounds frequently.
- Monitor hemodynamic status via arterial and/or central venous lines (left and right atrial, and pulmonary artery pressures, pulmonary artery oxygen saturation).
- Provide site care and tubing changes according to the institution's policy.
- Auscultate lungs for adventitious, diminished, or absent breath sounds.
- Assess oxygen saturation levels via pulse oximetry and arterial blood gases as well as work of breathing and level of consciousness frequently.
- Administer supplemental oxygen as needed.
- Monitor mechanical ventilation and suction as ordered.

- Inspect chest tube functioning, noting amount, color, and character of drainage.
- Inspect the dressing (incision and chest tube) for drainage and intactness. Reinforce or change the dressing as ordered.
- Assess the incision for redness, irritation, drainage, or separation.
- Monitor intake and output hourly.
- Maintain accurate intravenous infusion rate; restrict fluids as ordered to prevent hypervolemia.
- Assess for changes in level of consciousness. Report restlessness, irritability, or seizures.
- Obtain ordered laboratory tests, such as CBC, coagulation studies, cardiac enzyme levels, and electrolyte levels. Report abnormal results.
- Administer medications, such as digoxin or inotropic or vasopressor agents, as ordered, watching the child closely for possible adverse effects.
- Encourage the child to turn, cough, deep breathe, use the incentive spirometer, and splint the incisional area with pillows.
- Assess the child's pain level and administer analgesics as ordered. Allow time for the child to rest and sleep.
- Assist the child to get out of bed as soon as possible and as ordered.
- Assess daily weights.
- Administer small, frequent feedings or meals when oral intake is allowed.
- Position the child in a comfortable position, one that maximizes chest expansion. Change position frequently.
- Assess the child for complications (Box 20.2).
- Provide emotional and physical support to the child and family, making appropriate referrals such as to social services for assistance.
- Prepare the patient and family for discharge (Beke et al., 2005).

BOX 20.2

POSSIBLE COMPLICATIONS AFTER CARDIAC SURGERY

- Atelectasis
- Bacterial endocarditis
- Cardiac arrhythmias
- Cardiac tamponade
- Cerebrovascular accident
- Heart failure
- Hemorrhage
- Pleural effusion
- Pneumonia
- Pneumothorax
- Postperfusion syndrome
- Postcardiac surgery syndrome
- Pulmonary edema
- Seizures
- Wound infection

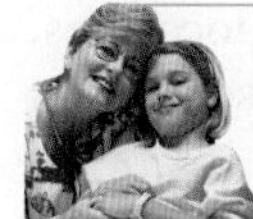

Abrupt cessation of chest tube output accompanied by an increase in heart rate and increased filling pressure (right atrial) may indicate cardiac tamponade (Beke et al., 2005).

Providing Patient and Family Education

Provide patient and family education throughout the child's stay. Initially, teaching focuses on the underlying defect and measures to treat or control the problem. If the child requires surgery, teaching shifts to preoperative and postoperative events. Emphasize discharge teaching for each admission. Teaching Guideline 20.2 highlights the major areas to be addressed in patient and family education.

Acquired Cardiovascular Disorders

Acquired cardiovascular disorders occur in children as a result of an underlying cardiovascular problem or may refer to other cardiac disorders that are not congenital. The most common type of acquired cardiovascular disorder in children is heart failure. Other acquired disorders include

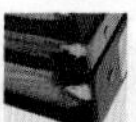

TEACHING GUIDELINE 20.2

Caring for the Child With a Congenital Heart Disease

- Give medications, if ordered, exactly as prescribed.
- Weigh the child at least once a week or as ordered, at approximately the same time of the day with the same scale, and wearing the same amount of clothing.
- Allow the child to engage in activity as directed. Provide time for the child to rest frequently throughout the day to prevent overexertion.
- Provide a nutritious diet, taking into account any restrictions for fluids or foods.
- Use measures to prevent infection, such as frequent handwashing, prophylactic antibiotics, and skin care.
- Adhere to schedule for follow-up diagnostic tests and procedures.
- Support the child's growth and development needs.
- Use available community support services.
- Notify the primary care provider if the child has increasing episodes of respiratory distress, cyanosis, or difficulty breathing; fever; increased edema of the hands, feet, or face; decreased urinary output; weight loss or difficulty eating or drinking; increased fatigue or irritability; decreased level of alertness; or vomiting or diarrhea.

rheumatic fever, cardiomyopathy, infective endocarditis, hyperlipidemia, hypertension, and Kawasaki disease.

● HEART FAILURE

Heart failure occurs most often in children with CHD and is the most common reason for admission to the hospital for children with CHD. Eighty percent of all cases of heart failure in children with CHD occur by the age of 1 year (Freitas-Nichols, 2004). Heart failure also occurs secondary to other conditions such as myocardial dysfunction following surgical intervention for CHD, cardiomyopathy, myocarditis, fluid volume overload, hypertension, anemia, or sepsis or as a toxic effect of certain chemotherapeutic agents used in the treatment of cancer. Heart failure refers to a set of clinical signs and symptoms that reflect the heart's inability to pump effectively to provide adequate blood, oxygen, and nutrients to the body organs and tissues.

The child experiencing heart failure requires a multidisciplinary approach to care. Collaboration is necessary to achieve improved cardiac function, restored fluid balance, decreased cardiac workload, and improved oxygen delivery to the tissues.

Pathophysiology

Cardiac output is controlled by preload (diastolic volume), afterload (ventricular wall tension), myocardial contractility (inotropic state), and heart rate. Protracted alterations in any of these factors may lead to heart failure. In the event of reduced cardiac output, multiple compensatory mechanisms are activated. When the ventricular contraction is impaired (systolic dysfunction), reduced ejection of blood occurs, and therefore cardiac output is reduced. Diminished ability to receive venous return (diastolic dysfunction) occurs when high venous pressures are required to support ventricular function. As a result of decreased cardiac output, the renin-angiotensin-aldosterone system is activated as a compensatory mechanism. Fluid and sodium retention as well as improved contractility and vasoconstriction then occur. Initially blood pressure is supported and organ perfusion is maintained, but increased afterload worsens systolic dysfunction. As the heart chambers dilate, myocardial oxygen consumption increases and cardiac output is limited by excessive wall stretch. Over time, the capacity of the heart to respond to these compensatory mechanisms fails, and cardiac output is further decreased (Craig et al., 2001; Talner & Carboni, 2003). Figure 20.15 shows the clinical manifestations that occur related to the mechanisms of heart failure.

Therapeutic Management

Management of heart failure is supportive. Promotion of oxygenation and ventilation is of utmost importance. Digitalis, diuretics, inotropic agents, vasodilators, antiarrhythmics, and antithrombotics have been widely used in children for palliation of symptoms (Kay et al., 2001a; Rosenthal et al., 2004). Many children with heart failure require management in the intensive care unit until they are stabilized. Augmenting nutrition and ensuring adequate rest are also key components of management.

Nursing Assessment

For a full description of the assessment phase of the nursing process, refer to page 618. Specific assessment findings related to heart failure are discussed below.

Health History

When obtaining the health history, elicit a description of the present illness and chief complaint. Common complaints reported during the health history might include:

- Failure to gain weight or rapid weight gain
- Failure to thrive
- Difficulty feeding
- Fatigue
- Dizziness, irritability
- Exercise intolerance
- Shortness of breath
- Sucking and then tiring quickly
- Syncope
- Decreased number of wet diapers

Infants with heart failure often display subtle signs such as difficulty feeding and tiring easily. Pay close attention for reports of these problems from the parents. Also be alert for statements such as "the baby drinks a small amount of breast milk (or formula) and stops, but then wants to eat again very soon afterwards"; "the baby seems to perspire a lot during feedings"; or "the baby seems to be more comfortable when he's sitting up or on my shoulder than when he's lying flat." In addition, the parents may report episodes of rapid breathing and grunting.

The child's current and past medical history also provides additional clues. Question the parents about any history of congenital heart defects and treatments such as surgery to repair the defect. Determine the current medication regimen. Also ask about any recent or past infections, such as streptococcal infections or fever.

Physical Examination

Weigh the child and note recent rapid weight gain or lack of weight gain. Obtain the child's vital signs, noting tachycardia or tachypnea. These findings are often the first indicators of heart failure in an infant or older child. Measure the BP in the upper and lower extremities, comparing the findings for differences. Note decreased BP, which may be due to impaired cardiac muscle function. Inspect the skin color, noting pallor or cyanosis. Also observe for diaphoresis (profuse sweating). Inspect the face, hands, and lower extremities for edema. Observe for increased work

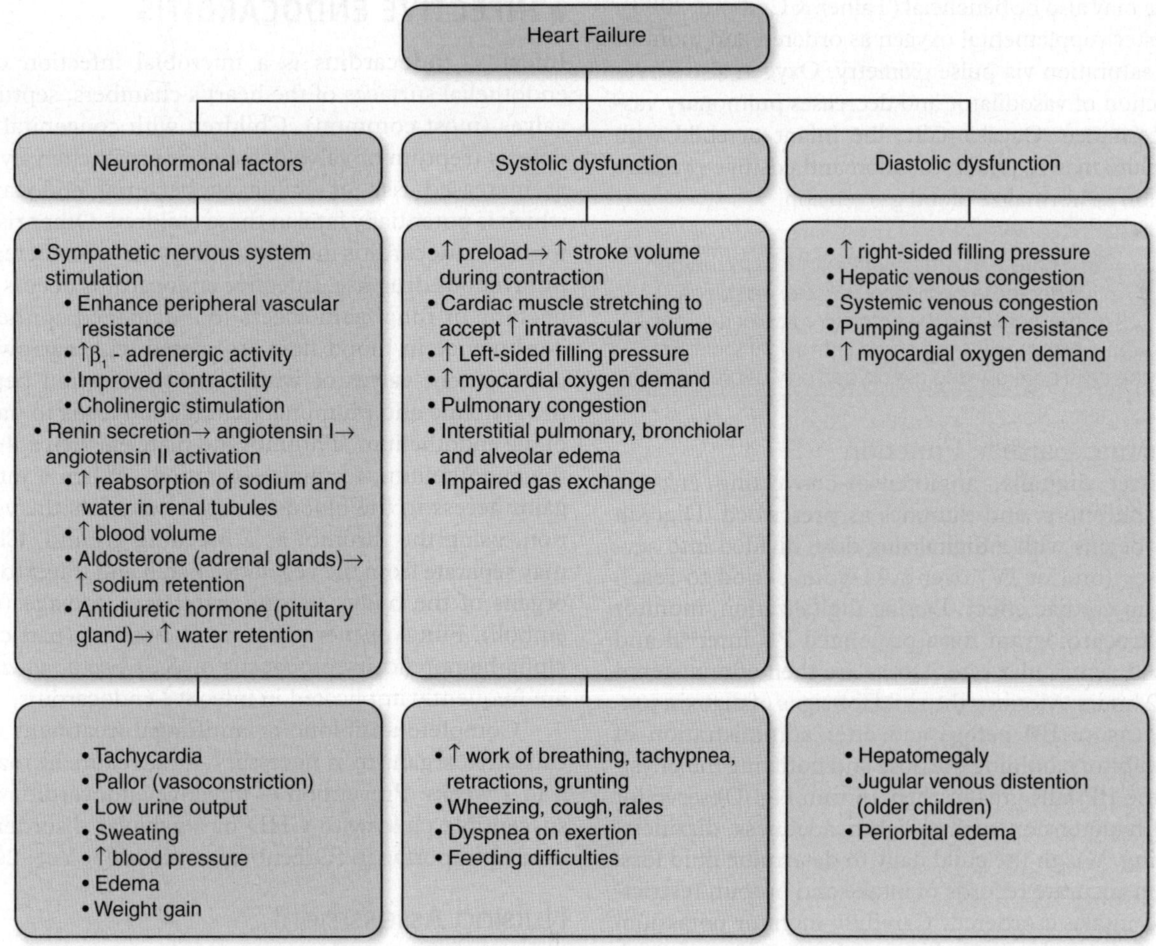

Heart Failure
Neurohormonal factors
Systolic dysfunction
Diastolic dysfunction
• Sympathetic nervous system stimulation
• Enhance peripheral vascular resistance
• ↑β1 - adrenergic activity
• Improved contractility
• Cholinergic stimulation
• Renin secretion→ angiotensin I→ angiotensin II activation
• ↑ reabsorption of sodium and water in renal tubules
• ↑ blood volume
• Aldosterone (adrenal glands)→ ↑ sodium retention
• Antidiuretic hormone (pituitary gland)→ ↑ water retention
• ↑ preload→ ↑ stroke volume during contraction
• Cardiac muscle stretching to accept ↑ intravascular volume
• ↑ Left-sided filling pressure
• ↑ myocardial oxygen demand
• Pulmonary congestion
• Interstitial pulmonary, bronchiolar and alveolar edema
• Impaired gas exchange
• ↑ right-sided filling pressure
• Hepatic venous congestion
• Systemic venous congestion
• Pumping against ↑ resistance
• ↑ myocardial oxygen demand
• Tachycardia
• Pallor (vasoconstriction)
• Low urine output
• Sweating
• ↑ blood pressure
• Edema
• Weight gain
• ↑ work of breathing, tachypnea, retractions, grunting
• Wheezing, cough, rales
• Dyspnea on exertion
• Feeding difficulties
• Hepatomegaly
• Jugular venous distention (older children)
• Periorbital edema

● Figure 20.15 Pathophysiology of heart failure. (From Kay et al., 2001a; Talner et al., 2003.)

of breathing, such as nasal flaring or retractions. Note the presence of a cough, which may be productive with bloody sputum. Auscultate the apical pulse, noting its location and character. Listen for a murmur, which may suggest a congenital heart defect, a gallop rhythm, or an accentuated third heart sound, suggesting sudden ventricular distention. Auscultate the lungs, noting crackles or wheezes suggestive of pulmonary congestion. Palpate the peripheral pulses, noting weak or thready pulses. Note the temperature and color of the extremities; they may be cool, clammy, and pale.

Assess the child's abdomen, looking for distention indicative of ascites. Gently palpate the abdomen to identify hepatomegaly or splenomegaly.

Laboratory and Diagnostic Tests

The diagnosis of heart failure is based on the child's signs and symptoms and is confirmed with several laboratory and diagnostic tests. These include:

- Chest x-ray, revealing an enlarged heart and/or pulmonary edema
- Electrocardiogram, indicating ventricular hypertrophy
- Echocardiogram, revealing the underlying cause of heart failure, such as a congenital heart defect

Other tests may be done to support the diagnosis. For example, the CBC may show evidence of anemia or infection. Electrolyte levels may reveal hyponatremia secondary to fluid retention and hyperkalemia secondary to tissue destruction or impaired renal function. Arterial blood gas results may demonstrate respiratory alkalosis in mild heart failure or metabolic acidosis. Tissue hypoxia may be evidenced by increased lactic acid and decreased bicarbonate levels.

Nursing Management

Nursing management of the child with heart failure focuses on promoting oxygenation, supporting cardiac function, providing adequate nutrition, and promoting rest.

Promoting Oxygenation

Position the infant or child in a semi-upright position to decrease work of breathing and lessen pulmonary congestion. Suction as needed. Chest physiotherapy and postural drainage may also be beneficial (Talner & Carboni, 2003). Administer supplemental oxygen as ordered and monitor oxygen saturation via pulse oximetry. Oxygen also serves the function of vasodilator and decreases pulmonary vascular resistance. Occasionally, the infant or child with heart failure may require intubation and positive-pressure ventilation to normalize blood gas tension.

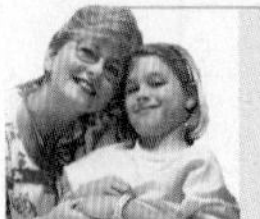

In a child with a large left-to-right shunt, oxygen will decrease pulmonary vascular resistance while increasing the systemic vascular resistance, which leads to increased left-to-right shunting. Monitor the child carefully and use oxygen only as prescribed.

Supporting Cardiac Function

Administer digitalis, angiotensin-converting enzyme (ACE) inhibitors, and diuretics as prescribed. Digoxin therapy begins with a digitalizing dose divided into several doses (oral or IV) over a 24-hour period to reach maximum cardiac effect. During digitalization, monitor the electrocardiogram for a prolonged PR interval and decreased ventricular rate. Doses are then administered every 12 hours. Monitor the child for signs of digoxin toxicity. Measure BP before and after administration of ACE inhibitors, holding the dose and notifying the physician if the BP falls greater then 15 mm Hg. Observe for signs of hypotension such as lightheadedness, dizziness, or fainting. Weigh the child daily to determine fluid loss. Maintain accurate records of intake and output, restricting fluid intake if ordered. Carefully monitor potassium levels, administering potassium supplements if prescribed. Sodium intake is not usually restricted in the child with heart failure (Rosenthal et al., 2004).

Providing Adequate Nutrition

Due to the increased metabolic rate associated with heart failure, the infant may require as much as 150 calories/kg/day. Older children will also require higher caloric intake than typical children. Offer small, frequent feedings if the child can tolerate them. During the acute phase of heart failure, many infants in particular will require continuous or intermittent gavage feeding to maintain or gain weight. Concentrate infant formula to 24 to 28 calories/ounce as instructed by the nutritionist (Talner & Carboni, 2003).

Promoting Rest

Minimize metabolic needs to decrease cardiac demand. The infant or older child with heart failure will usually limit activities based upon energy level. Ensure adequate time for sleep, and attempt to limit disturbing interventions. Provide age-appropriate activities that can be performed quietly or in bed, such as books, drawing, and video or board games. The older child or adolescent with significant heart failure may require home schooling. As the child improves, a rehabilitation program may be helpful for maximizing activity within the child's cardiovascular status limits (Talner & Carboni, 2003).

INFECTIVE ENDOCARDITIS

Infective endocarditis is a microbial infection of the endothelial surfaces of the heart's chambers, septum, or valves (most common). Children with congenital heart defects (septum or valve defects) or prosthetic valves are at increased risk of acquiring bacterial endocarditis, which is potentially fatal in these children. Other risk factors for endocarditis include central venous catheters and intravenous drug use. Infective endocarditis occurs when bacteria or fungi gain access to a damaged epithelium. Turbulence in blood flow associated with narrowed or incompetent valves or with a communication between the systemic and pulmonary circulation leads to damage of the endothelium. Thrombi and platelets then adhere to the endothelium, forming vegetations. When a microbe gains access to the bloodstream, it colonizes the vegetation, using the thrombi as a breeding ground. Clumps may separate from the vegetative patch and travel to other organs of the body, causing significant damage (septic emboli). Fungi or more commonly bacteria (particularly alpha-hemolytic streptococcus or *Staphylococcus aureus*) are frequently implicated in infective endocarditis.

Complete antibiotic or antifungal treatment of the causative organism is necessary, and treatment may last 4 to 7 weeks. Prevention of infective endocarditis in the susceptible child with CHD or a valvular disorder is of utmost importance (Greenberg et al, 2005; Yee, 2005).

Nursing Assessment

For a full description of the assessment phase of the nursing process, refer to page 618. Assessment findings related to endocarditis are discussed below.

Health History

Obtain the health history, noting intermittent, unexplained low-grade fever. Document history of fatigue, anorexia, weight loss, or flu-like symptoms (arthralgia, myalgia, chills, night sweats). Note history of CHD, valve disorder, or heart failure.

Physical Examination

Measure the child's temperature, noting low-grade fever. Observe for edema if heart failure is also present. Note petechiae on the palpebral conjunctiva, the oral mucosa, or the extremities. Inspect for signs of extracardiac emboli:

- Roth's spots: splinter hemorrhages with pale centers on sclerae, palate, buccal mucosa, chest, fingers, or toes
- Janeway lesions: painless flat red or blue hemorrhagic lesions on the palms or the soles
- Osler's nodes: small, tender nodules on the pads of the toes or fingers
- Black lines (splinter hemorrhages) under the nails

Evaluate the electrocardiogram for a prolonged PR interval or dysrhythmias. Auscultate the heart for a new or changing murmur. Auscultate the lungs for adventitious breath sounds. Palpate the abdomen for splenomegaly (Greenberg et al., 2005; Yee, 2005).

Laboratory and Diagnostic Tests

Diagnosis is usually based on the clinical presentation. Laboratory tests may reveal:

- Blood culture: bacteria or fungus
- CBC: anemia, leukocytosis
- Urinalysis: microscopic hematuria
- Echocardiogram: cardiomegaly, abnormal valve function, area of vegetation

Nursing Management

Nursing management focuses on maintaining IV access for at least 4 weeks to appropriately administer the antibiotic or antifungal course of therapy. Monitor the child's temperature and subsequent blood culture results.

Ideally, infective endocarditis in children should be prevented. Children at increased risk for the development of infective endocarditis include those with:

- Valvular dysfunction or prosthetic valves
- Mitral valve prolapse with regurgitation
- Most congenital heart defects (certain simple septal defects are excluded)
- Surgically constructed systemic-to-pulmonary shunts
- Hypertrophic cardiomyopathy

Children, at high risk should practice good oral hygiene, including regular tooth brushing and flossing. Instruct parents or the older child to carry emergency medical identification at all times. A wallet card is available from the American Heart Association at http://www.americanheart.org/downloadable/heart/1023826501754walletcard.pdf. The card may be presented to any health care provider and includes the recommended antibiotic prophylactic regimen. Instruct the parents to notify the primary care provider or cardiologist if the child develops flu-like symptoms or a fever.

High-risk children (as noted above) who are undergoing procedures that increase the risk for the introduction of the types of bacteria responsible for endocarditis should receive prophylaxis as recommended by the American Heart Association. Usual antibiotics for prophylaxis may include ampicillin, amoxicillin, gentamicin, or vancomycin. Box 20.3 lists procedures for which antibiotic prophylaxis in high-risk children is recommended.

BOX 20.3

PROCEDURES FOR WHICH INFECTIVE ENDOCARDITIS PROPHYLAXIS IS RECOMMENDED

Dental Procedures

- Tooth extractions
- Periodontal procedures
- Dental implant placement
- Replacement of avulsed tooth
- Root canal or surgery
- Intraligamentary local anesthetic injections
- Any prophylactic dental procedure during which bleeding is anticipated

Respiratory Tract Procedures

- Tonsillectomy, adenoidectomy
- Rigid bronchoscopy
- Surgery involving the respiratory mucosa

Gastrointestinal Tract Procedures

- Esophageal varices sclerotherapy
- Dilation of esophageal stricture
- Endoscopic retrograde cholangiography for biliary obstruction
- Other biliary tract surgery
- Surgery involving the gastrointestinal mucosa

Genitourinary Tract Procedures

- Cystoscopy
- Urethral dilation
- Surgery involving the prostate

Data from American Heart Association. (2006a). *Bacterial endocarditis.* Retrieved 11/29/06 from http://www.americanheart.org/presenter.jhtml?identifier=4436; American Heart Association. (2006b). *Bacterial endocarditis wallet card.* Retrieved 11/29/06 from http://www.americanheart.org/downloadable/heart/102382650175 4walletcard.pdf; Greenberg, J. D., Bonwit, A. M., & Roddy, M. G. (2005). Subacute bacterial endocarditis prophylaxis: A succinct review for pediatric emergency physicians and nurses. *Clinical Pediatric Emergency Medicine, 6*(4), 266–272; and Yee, C. A. (2005). Endocarditis: The infected heart. *Nursing Management, 36*(2), 25–30.

● ACUTE RHEUMATIC FEVER

Acute rheumatic fever (ARF) is a delayed sequela of group A streptococcal pharyngeal infection. In the United States this disease occurs more often in school-age children between 5 and 15 years of age in areas where streptococcal pharyngitis is more prevalent, especially during the colder months. It usually develops 2 to 3 weeks after the initial streptococcal infection. Current understanding of the disease process of ARF is that the child develops an antibody response to surface proteins of the bacteria. The antibodies then cross-react with antigens in cardiac muscle and neuronal and synovial tissues, causing carditis, arthritis, and chorea (involuntary random, jerking movements). ARF affects the joints, central nervous system, skin, and subcutaneous tissue and causes chronic, progressive damage to the heart and valves. Most attacks of ARF last 6 to 12 weeks and then are resolved, but rheumatic fever may recur with subsequent streptococcal infections.

Diagnosis of ARF is based on the modified Jones' criteria (Box 20.4). Therapeutic management is directed

BOX 20.4

MODIFIED JONES CRITERIA (AMERICAN HEART ASSOCIATION)

Diagnosis of acute rheumatic fever requires the presence of either two major criteria or one major plus two minor criteria.

Major Criteria
- Carditis
- Migratory polyarthritis
- Subcutaneous nodules
- Erythema marginatum
- Sydenham chorea

Minor Criteria
- Arthralgia
- Fever
- Elevated erythrocyte sedimentation rate or C-reactive protein
- Prolonged PR interval

Data from Jaggi, P., & Shulman, S. T. (2006). Group A streptococcal infections. *Pediatrics in Review, 27,* 99–105; and Parrillo, S. J., & Parrillo, C. V. (2006). *Rheumatic fever.* Retrieved 11/13/06 from http://www.emedicine.com/emerg/topic509.htm.

toward managing inflammation and fever, eradicating the bacteria, preventing permanent heart damage, and preventing recurrences. A full 10-day course of penicillin therapy (or equivalent) as well as corticosteroids and nonsteroidal anti-inflammatory drugs is used. Continuous prophylaxis with monthly intramuscular injections of penicillin G benzathine or daily oral doses of penicillin or erythromycin following the initial illness is recommended to prevent a new streptococcal infection and recurrent ARF. Prophylaxis is continued until adulthood (no valvular disease) or age 40 years (with valvular disease) (Martin & Green, 2006).

Nursing Assessment

Elicit a description of the present illness and chief complaint, noting fever and joint pain. Explore the patient's recent medical history for risk factors such as documented streptococcal infection or sore throat within the past 2 to 3 weeks, or for past history of ARF. Observe the child for Sydenham chorea, a movement disorder of the face and upper extremities. Inspect the skin for evidence of the classic rash, erythema marginatum, a maculopapular red rash with central clearing and elevated edges. Auscultate the heart, noting a murmur. Palpate the surfaces of the wrist, elbows, and knees for firm, painless, subcutaneous nodules. Note prolonged PR interval on the electrocardiogram. Throat culture will provide definitive diagnosis of current streptococcal infection, while streptococcal antibody tests may yield evidence of recent infection. Echocardiogram is required to determine if carditis if present.

Nursing Management

Nursing management of the child with ARF focuses on ensuring compliance with the acute course of antibiotics as well as prophylaxis following initial recovery from ARF. Allow the child to verbalize the frustration he or she may be feeling in relation to chorea symptoms. Offer support for dealing with the abnormal movements. Educate the child and others that the sudden jerky movements of chorea will eventually disappear, though they may last as long as several months. Some children may require a neuroleptic agent such as haloperidol (Haldol) for management of chorea. Administer corticosteroids or nonsteroidal anti-inflammatory agents for control of joint pain and swelling.

● CARDIOMYOPATHY

Cardiomyopathy is a condition in which the myocardium cannot contract properly. The incidence of cardiomyopathy among children is increasing; it occurs at a rate of 1.13 per 100,000 (AHA, 2006d). Cardiomyopathy may occur in children with genetic disorders or congenital heart defects, as a result of an inflammatory or infectious process or hypertension, or after cardiac transplantation or surgery, but most commonly it is idiopathic. Cardiomyopathy clusters in infancy and adolescence. Three types of cardiomyopathy exist. Restrictive cardiomyopathy is rare in children and results in atrial relaxation. Dilated cardiomyopathy is the most common type in childhood and may result in heart failure because of ventricular dilatation with decreased contractility. There is some familial tendency toward dilated cardiomyopathy, and it is also associated with Duchenne and Becker muscular dystrophy (Marian et al., 2004). Children with dilated cardiomyopathy may present with heart failure. Hypertrophic cardiomyopathy is more common in adolescence and results in hypertrophy of the heart muscle, particularly the left ventricle, affecting the heart's ability to fill. About two thirds of all cases of hypertrophic cardiomyopathy are familial, with some inherited in an autosomal dominant fashion (Marian et al., 2004; Maron, 2004).

There is no cure for cardiomyopathy, meaning that currently heart muscle function cannot be restored. Therapeutic management is directed toward improving heart function and blood pressure. Mechanical ventilation and vasoactive medications are needed in many children. ACE inhibitors, beta blockers, or calcium channel blockers may be used. Pacemakers or surgery are helpful in some children. Nearly 40% of children with cardiomyopathy either die or require heart transplantation (Strauss & Lock, 2003).

Nursing Assessment

Explore the health history for risk factors such as:

- Congenital heart defect, cardiac transplantation or surgery
- Duchenne or Becker muscular dystrophy
- History of myocarditis, HIV infection, or Kawasaki disease
- Hypertension
- Drugs, alcohol, or radiation exposure
- Connective tissue, autoimmune, or endocrine disease
- Maternal diabetes
- Familial history of sudden death

Inquire about a history of respiratory distress, fatigue, or poor growth (dilated) or chest pain, dizziness, or syncope (hypertrophic). Observe the child for extremity edema and abdominal distention. Note increased work of breathing. Auscultate the heart, noting tachycardia and irregular rhythm. Evaluate heart rhythm via electrocardiogram, noting dysrhythmias or indications of left ventricular hypertrophy.

Chest x-ray may reveal cardiomegaly or congested lungs. Echocardiogram demonstrates increased heart size, poor contractility, decreased ejection fraction, or asymmetric septal hypertrophy. Cardiac catheterization is usually performed to aid in the diagnosis.

Nursing Management

Many children with cardiomyopathy require intensive care initially. Monitor for complications such as blood clots or arrhythmias, which could lead to cardiac arrest. Refer to the prior section on heart failure for nursing interventions related to heart failure, which may be present with dilated cardiomyopathy. Administer vasoactive and other medications as prescribed, monitoring the child closely for response to these therapies as well as for complications. Support the child in choosing activities that fit within the prescribed restrictions. Provide extensive emotional support to the child and family, who may experience significant stress as they realize the severity of this illness.

HYPERTENSION

Hypertension affects only 1% to 3% of children and adolescents but often leads to long-term health consequences such as cardiovascular disease and left ventricular hypertrophy (Cromwell et al., 2005a). In children, acceptable BP values are based on gender, age, and height. Hypertension is defined as BP persistently greater than the 95th percentile for gender, age, and height. Prehypertension refers to BP that is persistently between the 90th and 95th percentiles. BP is considered normal when the systolic and diastolic values are less than the 90th percentile for gender, age, and height (USDHHS, NHLBI, 2005).

Childhood hypertension may be further defined as primary or secondary. Primary hypertension in children is rare, but its incidence increases with age, so it is more common in adolescence than in early childhood. Hypertension in children most frequently occurs secondary to an underlying medical problem (most often renal disease). Mild to moderate hypertension in childhood is usually asymptomatic and usually is determined only upon BP screening during a well-child visit or during follow-up for known risk factors.

Therapeutic management depends on the extent of the hypertension and the length of time it has existed. Weight reduction, appropriate diet, and increased physical activity are important components of management of prehypertensive and asymptomatic hypertensive children. Some children are candidates for and require antihypertensive medications or diuretics.

Pathophysiology

The balance between cardiac output and vascular resistance determines the BP. An increase in either of these variables, in the absence of a compensatory decrease in the other, increases the mean BP. Factors regulating cardiac output and vascular resistance include changes in electrolyte balance, particularly sodium, calcium, and potassium.

Nursing Assessment

Elicit the health history, determining the presence of risk factors for hypertension such as:

- Family history
- Obesity
- Hyperlipidemia
- Renal disease (including frequent urinary tract infections)
- Systemic lupus erythematosus
- Congenital heart disease
- Neurofibromatosis, Turner syndrome, and other genetic disorders
- Prematurity
- Prolonged neonatal ventilation
- Umbilical artery catheterization
- Diabetes mellitus
- Increased intracranial pressure
- Malignancy
- Solid organ transplant
- Medications known to raise BP

Signs and symptoms reported during the health history might include growth retardation (with certain chronic medical conditions), obesity, and, particularly in older children, headache, subtle behavioral or school performance changes, fatigue, blurred vision, nosebleed, or Bell's palsy.

Determine the child's weight and height/length. Plot these growth parameters on the gender-appropriate chart for the child's age. Note the percentile for height/length, as it will be used to determine the BP percentile (see Appendix A). Measure the BP in all four extremities (to rule out coarctation of the aorta). Ensure that the child is relaxed and sitting or reclined. Refer to Chapter 10 for specific information related to accurate BP measurement in children.

Physical Examination

Inspect the skin for:

- Acne, hirsutism, or striae (associated with anabolic steroid use)
- Café-au-lait spots (associated with neurofibromatosis)
- Malar rash (associated with lupus)
- Pallor, diaphoresis, or flushing (associated with pheochromocytoma)

Observe the extremities for edema (renal disease) or joint swelling (lupus). Inspect the chest for apical heave (ventricular hypertrophy) or wide-spaced nipples (Turner syndrome). Auscultate heart sounds, noting tachycardia (associated with primary hypertension) or murmur (associated with coarctation of the aorta). Palpate the abdomen for a mass or enlarged kidney (Flynn, 2001).

Laboratory and Diagnostic Testing

Though diagnosis of hypertension is based upon BP measurements, additional laboratory or diagnostic tests may be used to evaluate the underlying cause of secondary hypertension, including:

- Urinalysis, blood urea nitrogen, and serum creatinine: may determine presence of renal disease
- Renal ultrasound or angiography: may reveal kidney or genitourinary tract abnormalities
- Echocardiogram: may show left ventricular hypertrophy
- Lipid profile: determines the presence of hyperlipidemia (USDHHS, NHLBI, 2005)

Nursing Management

Salt restriction and potassium or calcium supplements have not been scientifically shown to decrease BP in children (Kay et al., 2001b). However, certain children may benefit from salt restriction, as some children seem to be sensitive to salt intake (Flynn, 2001). Assist the child and family to develop a plan for weight reduction if the child is overweight or obese. Encourage the child and family to control portion sizes, decrease the intake of sugary beverages and snacks, eat more fresh fruits and vegetables, and eat a healthy breakfast (USDHHS, NHLBI, 2005). Consult the nutritionist for additional assistance with meal planning. To increase physical activity, the child should find a sport or type of exercise in which he or she is interested. Aerobic activities involving running, walking, or cycling are particularly helpful. When a child requires antihypertensive therapy, teach the child and family how to administer the medication. Caution the parents about side effects related to antihypertensives. Teach the parent to measure the child's BP as determined by the primary care physician or specialist, as well as to keep appointments for BP follow-up. See Healthy People 2010.

HEALTHY PEOPLE 2010

Objective	Significance
Increase the proportion of persons appropriately counseled about health behaviors	• To prevent development of hypertension, encourage children to maintain a healthy weight and participate in regular exercise.

• KAWASAKI DISEASE

Kawasaki disease is an acute systemic vasculitis occurring mostly in infants and young children. It is the leading cause of acquired heart disease among children and occurs more frequently in the winter and spring (Newburger et al., 2004). Over 4,000 children are hospitalized annually in the United States with Kawasaki disease, and though it affects all ethnic groups, it occurs more frequently in those of Asian or Pacific descent (Newburger et al., 2004). It is a self-limited syndrome but causes serious cardiovascular sequelae in up to 25% of affected children (Newburger et al., 2004). Coronary artery aneurysm results in myocardial infarction and death in some children (Driscoll, 2006a). Therapeutic management of acute Kawasaki disease focuses on reducing inflammation in the walls of the coronary arteries and preventing coronary thrombosis. Chronic management of children developing aneurysms during the initial phase is directed toward preventing myocardial ischemia (Newburger et al., 2004). In the acute phase, high-dose aspirin in four divided doses daily and a single infusion of intravenous immunoglobulin (IVIG) are used. Children whose fever persists longer than 48 hours after initiation of aspirin therapy may receive a second dose of IVIG. Pulsed-dose corticosteroid therapy may also be used to prevent or halt coronary dilatation and inhibit progression to aneurysm (Dummer & Newburger, 2004).

Pathophysiology

Though the etiology is still unknown, Kawasaki disease may result from an infectious cause. Current thought is that some infectious organism (as yet unidentified) causes disease in genetically susceptible people. Kawasaki disease appears to be an autoimmune response mediated by cytokine-induced endothelial cell surface antigens that leads to vasculitis. Neutrophils, followed by mononuclear cells, T lymphocytes, and immunoglobulin A–producing plasma cells, infiltrate the vessels. Inflammation then occurs in all three layers of the small and medium-sized blood vessels. Edema and smooth muscle necrosis occur in the vessel wall media in severe cases. Generalized systemic vasculitis occurs in the blood vessels throughout the body due to the inflammation and edema. As elastin and collagen fibers fragment, the structural integrity of the vessel wall is impaired. This mechanism leads to coronary dilatation (ectasia) or aneurysm. Some children never develop coronary artery changes, while others develop an aneurysm in either the acute phase or as a long-term sequela. Infants are at the highest risk for coronary aneurysm or ectasia (Newburger et al., 2004).

Nursing Assessment

Nursing assessment consists of determining the health history, physical examination, and laboratory and diagnostic testing.

Health History

Elicit the health history, noting any of the following:

- Fever
- Chills
- Headache
- Malaise
- Extreme irritability
- Vomiting
- Diarrhea
- Abdominal pain
- Joint pain

Of particular note is a history of high fever (39.9° C) of at least 5 days' duration that is unresponsive to antibiotics.

Physical Examination

Observe for significant bilateral conjunctivitis without exudate. Inspect the mouth and throat for dry, fissured lips, strawberry (cracked and reddened) tongue, and pharyngeal and oral mucosa erythema. Note hyperdynamic precordium. Evaluate the skin for:

- Diffuse, erythematous, polymorphous rash
- Edema of the hands and feet
- Erythema and painful induration of the palms and soles
- Desquamation (peeling) of the perineal region, fingers, and toes, extending to the palms and soles
- Possible jaundice

Palpate the neck for cervical lymphadenopathy (usually unilateral) and the joints for tenderness. Palpate the abdomen for liver enlargement. Auscultate the heart, noting tachycardia, gallop, or murmur (Newburger et al., 2004; Rowley, 2004).

Laboratory and Diagnostic Testing

The CBC may reveal mild to moderate anemia, an elevated white blood cell count during the acute phase, and significant thrombocytosis (elevated platelet count [500,000 to 1 million]) in the later phase. The erythrocyte sedimentation rate (ESR) and the C-reactive protein (CRP) level are elevated. Echocardiogram is performed as soon as possible after the diagnosis is confirmed to provide a baseline of a healthy heart or to evaluate for coronary artery involvement. Echocardiograms may be repeated during the illness and as part of long-term follow-up. Occasionally cardiac involvement warrants cardiac catheterization.

Nursing Management

In addition to the administration of aspirin and immunoglobulin, nursing management of the child with Kawasaki disease focuses on monitoring cardiac status, promoting comfort, and providing family education.

Monitoring Cardiac Status

Administer intravenous and oral fluids as ordered, evaluating intake and output carefully. Prepare the child for the echocardiogram. Assess frequently for signs of developing heart failure such as tachycardia, gallop, decreased urine output, or respiratory distress. Evaluate quality and strength of pulses. Provide cardiac monitoring as ordered, reporting arrhythmias.

Promoting Comfort

Provide acetaminophen for fever management and apply cool cloths as tolerated. Keep the environment quiet and cluster nursing care activities to decrease stimulation and hence irritability. Teach parents that irritability is a prominent feature of Kawasaki disease, and support their efforts to console the child. Apply petrolatum jelly or another lubricating ointment to the lips. Encourage the older child to suck on ice chips; the younger child may suck on a cool, moist washcloth. Popsicles are also soothing. Provide comfortable positioning, particularly if the child has joint pain or arthritis.

Providing Patient and Family Education

Teach parents to continue to monitor the child's temperature after discharge until the child has been afebrile for several days. Children with prolonged or recurrent fever may require a second dose of IVIG. Inform parents that irritability may last for up to 2 months after initial diagnosis with Kawasaki disease. Toxic effects of aspirin therapy such as headache, confusion, dizziness, or tinnitus should be reported to the primary care provider. Nonsteroidal anti-inflammatory agents should be avoided while aspirin therapy is ongoing. For children with continued arthritis (which resolves in several weeks), range-of-motion exercises with a morning bath may help to decrease stiffness.

Instruct parents to avoid measles and varicella vaccination for 11 months after high-dose IVIG administration (Newburger et al., 2004). It is critical that the family comply with regularly scheduled cardiology follow-up appointments to determine development or progression of coronary artery ectasia or aneurysm. If the child has severe cardiac involvement, teach the parents about infant and/or child cardiopulmonary resuscitation before discharge from the hospital.

● HYPERLIPIDEMIA

Hyperlipidemia refers to high levels of lipids (fats/cholesterol) in the blood. High lipid levels are a risk factor for the development of atherosclerosis, which can result in coronary artery disease, a serious cardiovascular disorder occurring in adults. Children with high lipid levels, though remaining asymptomatic, are likely to have high levels as adults, which increases their risk for coronary artery disease. Therefore, detection, screening, and early intervention are important, especially if there is a family tendency toward heart disease (Labarthe et al., 2003).

Pathophysiology

Cholesterol is a building block for hormones and cell membranes. It occurs naturally in foods derived from animals such as eggs, dairy products, meat, poultry, and seafood. Cholesterol is also manufactured in the body. Together, cholesterol and triglycerides are known as lipids. Very-low-density lipoprotein (VLDL) is a lipoprotein composed mainly of triglycerides with only small amounts of cholesterol, phospholipid, and protein. VLDLs are easily converted to low-density lipoproteins (LDLs). Cholesterol is expressed in terms of LDL cholesterol or high-density lipoprotein (HDL) cholesterol. LDLs contain relatively more cholesterol and triglycerides than they do protein. HDLs contain about 50% protein, with the rest being cholesterol, triglyceride, and phospholipid. High levels of cholesterol and triglycerides place a person at risk for atherosclerosis. Elevated VLDL and LDL levels and decreased HDL levels produce a particular increase in the risk for atherosclerosis.

Therapeutic Management

Screening children for hyperlipidemia is of prime importance for early detection, intervention, and subsequent prevention of adult atherosclerosis. The National Cholesterol Education Program recommends screening for hyperlipidemia in children over 2 years of age if:

- The parent has a total cholesterol level above 240 mg/dL
- There is a family history of cardiovascular disease in a parent or grandparent before age 55 years
- If the family history is unavailable

All children should eat a diet with the appropriate amount of fats (see the section on nursing management below) and should participate in physical activity. When diet and exercise are not enough to lower cholesterol to appropriate levels, medications such as resins, fibric acid derivatives, statins, or niacin may be used.

Nursing Assessment

Elicit the health history, noting risk factors such as family history of hyperlipidemia, early heart disease, hypertension, diabetes or other endocrine abnormality, cerebral vascular accident, or sudden death. Note prior lipid levels if available. Measure the child's height and weight, plotting them on standardized growth charts. Note overweight or obesity, as these are risk factors associated with hyperlipidemia. Typically, there are no other particular physical findings associated with hyperlipidemia. Table 20.3 gives details about the interpretation of cholesterol levels.

Nursing Management

Instruct families that the child must fast for 12 hours before lipid screening (initially and on follow-up samples). Dietary management is the first step in the prevention and management of hyperlipidemia in children over 2 years of age. The diet should consist primarily of fruits, vegetables, low-fat dairy products, whole grains, beans, lean meat and poultry, and fish. As in adults, fat should account for no more than 30% of daily caloric intake. Fat intake may vary over a period of days, as many young children are picky eaters. Limit saturated fats by choosing lean meats, removing skin from poultry before cooking, and avoiding palm, palm kernel, and coconut oils as well as hydrogenated fats. Teach families to read nutrition labels to determine the content of the food. Limit intake of processed or refined foods as well as high-sugar drinks; these products provide minimal nutrition and significant calories. Children over 2 years of age should have 60 minutes per day of vigorous play or physical activity. Refer parents to "Healthy Habits for Healthy Kids—A Nutrition and Activity Guide for Parents" published by the American Dietetic Association, available at http://www.wellpoint.com/healthy_parenting/index.html.

Table 20.3 Interpretation of Cholesterol Levels for Children Age 2 to 19 Years

Total Cholesterol (mg/dL)	LDL Cholesterol (mg/dL)	Interpretation
<170	<100	Normal
170–200	100–130	Borderline
>200	>130	High

Starc, T. J. (2001). Management of hyperlipidemia in children. *Progress in Pediatric Cardiology, 12*(2), 205–213.

If medications are required, teach the child and family about the dose, administration, and possible adverse effects. Assist the family to develop a medication dosing plan that is compatible with school and work schedules to increase compliance.

Heart Transplantation

Heart transplantation is indicated in children with end-stage heart disease related to cardiomyopathy or inoperable CHD. Candidates for heart transplantation are infants and children whose medical and surgical options have been exhausted and who have a 12- to 24-month life expectancy (Gabrys, 2005). Between 350 and 390 children have received a heart transplant each year since 1991 (Boucek et al., 2006). The 5-year survival rate is 75% and the 10-year rate is 65% (Gabrys, 2005).

A comprehensive evaluation is performed to determine whether the child is a candidate for heart transplant. The evaluation includes:

- Chest x-ray, electrocardiogram, echocardiogram, exercise stress test, cardiac catheterization, pulmonary function tests
- CBC with differential, prothrombin and partial thromboplastin time, serum chemistries and electrolytes, blood urea nitrogen, and creatinine
- Urinalysis and urine creatinine clearance
- Blood, throat, urine, stool, and sputum cultures for bacteria, viruses, fungi, and parasites
- Epstein-Barr virus, cytomegalovirus, varicella, herpes, hepatitis, and HIV titers
- HLA typing and panel reactive antibody typing and titer
- Computed tomography or MRI scan, electroencephalogram
- Consults with neurology, psychology, genetics, social work, nutritionist, physical and occupational therapy, and financial coordinator or case manager

Children with irreversible lung, liver, kidney, or central nervous system disease, recent malignancy (past 5 years), or chronic viral infection may be excluded as candidates.

Once candidacy is determined, the transplant center registers the child as a potential recipient with the United Network for Organ Sharing (UNOS). Blood type, body size, length of time on the waiting list, and medical urgency are used to evaluate compatibility. Children awaiting transplantation may need continuous or intermittent hospitalization. Coordination of organ procurement and the transplantation procedure is essential (Canter, 2000; Gabrys, 2005).

Surgical Procedure and Postoperative Therapeutic Management

Most transplantation procedures are **orthotopic**, which means that the recipient's heart is removed and the donor heart is implanted in its place in the normal anatomic position (del Rio, 2000). Cardiopulmonary bypass and hypothermia are used to maintain circulation, protect the brain, and oxygenate the recipient during the procedure. Postoperatively, the child may have near-normal heart function and capacity for exercise and may be able to return to school.

Immunosuppressive therapy is necessary for the rest of the child's life to avoid rejection of the transplanted heart. Usually a three-drug regimen is used that includes calcineurin inhibitors (cyclosporine, tacrolimus), cell toxins (mycophenolate mofetil, azathioprine), and corticosteroids. Ongoing follow-up is provided by the cardiologist and transplant surgeon. Complications of heart transplantation include bacterial, fungal, and viral infection and heart rejection. Neoplasm may occur as a result of chronic immunosuppression.

Nursing Management

Preoperative nursing care for the child undergoing a heart transplant is similar for children undergoing other types of heart surgery. In addition, the nurse should assist with the comprehensive pretransplant evaluation. Care for the child in the post-transplant period is intense and complex. Evaluate the family's ability to perform the tasks that will be necessary. Teach families about the evaluation and transplantation process, as well as the waiting period. In the immediate preoperative period, perform a thorough history and physical examination and obtain last-minute blood work. Provide preoperative teaching similar to other cardiac surgeries. Older children, adolescents, and parents may enjoy the book *Future Conditional* by J. Hatton (1996, Yorkshire Art Circus), which was written by one of the first heart transplant survivors.

Postoperatively, provide frequent assessments and routine care for cardiac surgery patients. In addition, monitor the child closely for infection or signs of rejection. Acute rejection may be indicated by low-grade fever, fatigue, tachycardia, nausea, vomiting, abdominal pain, and decreased activity tolerance, though some children will be asymptomatic. Maintain strict handwashing techniques and isolate the child from other children with infections. Though live vaccines are contraindicated in immunosuppressed children, inactivated vaccines should be given as recommended (Centers for Disease Control and Prevention, 2006). Teach children and families that the child may return to school and usual activities about 3 months after the transplant. Provide emotional support to the child related to body image changes such as hair growth, gum hyperplasia, weight gain, moon facies, acne, and rashes that occur due to long-term immunosuppressive therapy.

References

Books and Journals

Abdallah, H. (2006). *Pediatric cardiac testing.* Retrieved 10/3/06 from http://www.childrenheartinstitute.org/testing/testhome.htm.

Ackley, B. J., & Ladwig, G. B. (2006). *Nursing diagnosis handbook: A guide to planning care* (7th ed.). St. Louis: Mosby.

AGA Medical Corporation. (2006). *Amplatzer™ septal occluder (ASD).* Retrieved 11/19/06 from http://www.amplatzer.com/us/medical_professionals/aso.html.

Al-Karaawi, Z. M., Lucas, V. S., Gelbier, M., & Roberts, G. J. (2001). Dental procedures in children with severe congenital heart disease: A theoretical analysis of prophylaxis and non-prophylaxis procedures. *Heart, 85,* 66–68.

American Academy of Pediatrics, National High Blood Pressure Education Program, Working Group on High Blood Pressure in Children and Adolescents. (2004). The fourth report on the diagnosis, evaluation, and treatment of high blood pressure in children and adolescents. *Pediatrics, 114*(2), 555–576.

American Heart Association. (2006a). *Bacterial endocarditis.* Retrieved 11/29/06 from http://www.americanheart.org/presenter.jhtml?identifier=4436.

American Heart Association. (2006b). *Bacterial endocarditis wallet card.* Retrieved 11/29/06 from http://www.americanheart.org/downloadable/heart/1023826501754walletcard.pdf.

American Heart Association. (2006c). *Diseases, conditions and treatments.* Retrieved 11/18/06 from http://www.americanheart.org/presenter.jhtml?identifier=3028667.

American Heart Association. (2006d). *Youth and cardiovascular diseases—statistics.* Retrieved 11/13/06 from http://www.americanheart.org/downloadable/heart/1136818182083Youth06.pdf

Balentine, J., & Eisenhart, A. (2005). *Aortic stenosis.* Retrieved 11/19/06 from http://www.emedicine.com/emerg/topic40.htm.

Barbas, K. H., & Kelleher, D. K. (2004). Breastfeeding success among infants with congenital heart disease. *Pediatric Nursing, 30*(4), 285–289.

Beke, D. M., Braudis, N. J., & Lincoln, P. (2005). Management of the pediatric postoperative cardiac surgery patient. *Critical Care Nursing Clinics of North America, 17*(4), 405–416.

Betz, C. L., & Sowden, L. A. (2005). *Mosby pediatric nursing reference* (5th ed.). St. Louis: Mosby.

Bezold, L. I. (2006). Cardiovascular embryology. In J. A. McMillan (Ed.), *Oski's pediatrics: Principles and practice.* Philadelphia: Lippincott Williams & Wilkins.

Boucek, M. M., Waltz, D. A., Edwards, L. B., et al. (2006). Registry of the International Society for Heart and Lung Transplantation: Ninth official pediatric heart transplantation report, 2006. *Journal of Heart and Lung Transplantation, 25,* 893–903.

Bricker, J. T. (2006). Hypertension. In J. A. McMillan (Ed.), *Oski's pediatrics: Principles and practice.* Philadelphia: Lippincott Williams & Wilkins.

Broyles, B. (2006). *Case studies in pediatrics.* Clifton Park, NY: Thomson Delmar Learning.

Brumund, M., & Strong, W. (2002). Murmurs, fainting, chest pain: Time for a cardiology referral? *Contemporary Pediatrics, 2,* 155. Retrieved 11/22/06 from http://www.contemporarypediatrics.com/contpeds/article/articleDetail.jsp?id=126596&searchString=congenital%20heart%20disease.

Cannon, B. C. (2006). Abnormalities in rate and rhythm. In J. A. McMillan (Ed.), *Oski's pediatrics: Principles and practice.* Philadelphia: Lippincott Williams & Wilkins.

Canter, C. E. (2000). Preoperative assessment and management of pediatric heart transplantation. *Progress in Pediatric Cardiology, 11*(2), 91–97.

Carpenito-Moyet, L. J. (2004). *Nursing care plans & documentation: Nursing diagnoses and collaborative problems.* Philadelphia: Lippincott Williams & Wilkins.

Centers for Disease Control and Prevention, National Immunization Program. (2006). *General recommendations on immunization: epidemiology and prevention of vaccine-preventable diseases.* Retrieved 12/20/06 from http://www.cdc.gov/nip/ed/vpd2006/Slides/chap02-genrecs9.ppt#324,1,Slide 1.

Chamberlain, R. S. (2006). Pediatric cardiovascular disorders. In S. M. Nettina (Ed.), *Lippincott manual of nursing practice.* Philadelphia: Lippincott Williams & Wilkins.

Chang, R. R., Chen, A. Y., & Klitzner, T. S. (2000). Factors associated with age and operation for children with congenital heart disease. *Pediatrics, 105,* 1073–1081.

Cheatham, J. P. (2006). Pulmonary stenosis. In J. A. McMillan (Ed.), *Oski's pediatrics: Principles and practice.* Philadelphia: Lippincott Williams & Wilkins.

Chen, C.-W., Li, C.-Y., & Wang, J.-K. (2004). Growth and development of children with congenital heart disease. *Journal of Advanced Nursing, 47*(3), 260–269.

Chen, C.-W., Li, C.-Y., & Wang, J.-K. (2005). Self-concept: Comparison between school-aged children with congenital heart disease and normal school-aged children. *Journal of Clinical Nursing, 14,* 394–402.

Christensen, D. D., Vincente, R. N., & Campbell, R. M. (2005). Presentation of atrial septal defect in the pediatric population. *Pediatric Cardiology, 26*(6), 812–814.

Coleman, K. B. (2002). Genetic counseling in congenital heart disease. *Critical Care Nursing Quarterly, 25*(3), 8–16.

Connor, J. A. (2003). Initial outcome for infants born with hypoplastic left heart syndrome. *Dissertation Abstracts International* (UMI No. 3088310).

Connor, J. A., Arons, R. R., Figueroa, M., & Gebbie, K. M. (2004). Clinical outcomes and secondary diagnoses for infants born with hypoplastic left heart syndrome. *Pediatrics, 114*(2), e160–165. Retrieved 11/18/06 from http://www.pediatrics.org/cgi/content/full/114/2/e160.

Couch, S. C., Daniels, S. R., & Deckelbaum, R. J. (2003). Current concepts of diet therapy for children with hypercholesterolemia. *Progress in Pediatric Cardiology, 17*(2), 179–186.

Craig, J., Fineman, L. D., Moynihan, P., & Baker, A. L. (2001). Cardiovascular critical care problems. In M. A. Q. Curley & P. A. Moloney-Harmon (Eds.), *Critical care nursing of infants and children* (2nd ed.). Philadelphia: W. B. Saunders Company.

Cromwell, P. F., Munn, N., & Zolkowski-Wynne, J. (2005a). Evaluation and management of hypertension in children and adolescents (part 1): Diagnosis. *Journal of Pediatric Health Care, 19*(3), 172–175.

Cromwell, P. F., Munn, N., & Zolkowski-Wynne, J. (2005b). Evaluation and management of hypertension in children and adolescents (part 2): Evaluation and management. *Journal of Pediatric Health Care, 19*(5), 309–313.

Cunningham, F. G., Leveno, K. L., Bloom, S. L., et al. (2005). *Williams obstetrics* (22nd ed.). New York: McGraw-Hill Companies.

Daniels, S. R. (2001). Obesity in the pediatric patient: Cardiovascular complications. *Progress in Pediatric Cardiology, 12*(2), 161–167.

del Rio, M. J. (2000). Transplantation in complex congenital heart disease. *Progress in Pediatric Cardiology, 11*(2), 107–113.

Dooley, K. J., & Bishop, L. (2002). Medical management of the cardiac infant and child after surgical discharge. *Critical Care Nursing Quarterly, 25*(3), 98–104.

Doroshow, R. W. (2001). The adolescent with simple or corrected congenital heart disease. *Adolescent Medicine, 12*(1), 1–23.

Driscoll, D. J. (2006a). *Fundamentals of pediatric cardiology.* Philadelphia: Lippincott Williams & Wilkins.

Driscoll, D. J. (2006b). Tricuspid atresia. In J. A. McMillan (Ed.), *Oski's pediatrics: Principles and practice.* Philadelphia: Lippincott Williams & Wilkins.

Du, Z., & Hijazi, Z. M. (2001). *Transcatheter closure of ventricular septal defect.* Retrieved 11/19/06 from http://www.fac.org.ar/scvc/llave/pediat/hijazi/hijazii.htm.

Dummer, K. B., & Newburger, J. W. (2004). Acute management of Kawasaki disease. *Progress in Pediatric Cardiology, 19*(2), 129–135.

Eidem, B. W. (2006). Hypoplastic left heart syndrome. In J. A. McMillan (Ed.), *Oski's pediatrics: Principles and practice.* Philadelphia: Lippincott Williams & Wilkins.

Einarson, K. D., & Arthur, H. M. (2003). Predictors of oral feeding difficulty in cardiac surgical infants. *Pediatric Nursing, 29*(4), 315–319.

El-Said, G. M., Baghdady, Y. M. K., & El-Said, H. G. (2006). Rheumatic fever. In J. A. McMillan (Ed.), *Oski's pediatrics: Principles and practice.* Philadelphia: Lippincott Williams & Wilkins.

El-Said, G. M., Baghdady, Y. M. K., & El-Said, H. G. (2006). Rheumatic heart disease. In J. A. McMillan (Ed.), *Oski's pediatrics: Principles and practice.* Philadelphia: Lippincott Williams & Wilkins.

Evangelista, J. K., Parsons, M., & Renneburg, A. K. (2000). Chest pain in children: Diagnosis through history and physical examination. *Journal of Pediatric Health Care, 14*(1), 3–8.

Fernandes, J. R. H. (2005). The experience of a broken heart. *Critical Care Nursing Clinics of North America, 17*(4), 319–327.

Ferrieri, P., & the Jones Criteria Working Group. (2002). Proceedings of the Jones criteria workshop. *Circulation, 106,* 2521. Retrieved 11/29/06 from http://circ.ahajournals.org/cgi/content/full/106/19/2521?ck=nck#top.

Fixler, D. E. (2006). Epidemiology of congenital heart disease. In J. A. McMillan (Ed.), *Oski's pediatrics: Principles and practice.* Philadelphia: Lippincott Williams & Wilkins.

Flynn, J. T. (2001). Evaluation and management of hypertension in childhood. *Progress in Pediatric Cardiology, 12*(2), 177–188.

Flynn, J. (2003). Recognizing and managing the hypertensive child. *Contemporary Pediatrics, 20,* 38. Retrieved 11/22/06 from http://www.contemporarypediatrics.com/contpeds/article/articleDetail.jsp?id=111767&searchString=hypertension.

Friedman, R. A., & Starke, J. R. (2006). Infective endocarditis. In J. A. McMillan (Ed.), *Oski's pediatrics: Principles and practice.* Philadelphia: Lippincott Williams & Wilkins.

Freitas-Nichols, J. (2004). Cardiovascular disorders. In C. E. Burns et al., *Pediatric primary care: A handbook for nurse practitioners* (3rd ed.). Philadelphia: W. B. Saunders.

Fulton, D. R., & Freed, M. D. (2004). The pathology, pathophysiology, recognition, and treatment of congenital heart disease. In V. Fuster, R. W. Alexander, & R. A. O'Rourke (Eds.), *Hurst's the heart* (11th ed., pp. 1785–1850). New York: McGraw-Hill Companies.

Fyfe, D. A., & Parks, W. J. (2002). Noninvasive diagnostics in congenital heart disease: Echocardiography and magnetic resonance imaging. *Critical Care Nursing Quarterly, 25*(3), 26–36.

Gabrys, C. A. (2005). Pediatric cardiac transplants: A clinical update. *Journal of Pediatric Nursing, 20*(2), 139–143.

Gidding, S. S., Dennison, B. A., Birch, L. L., et al. (2006). Dietary recommendations for children and adolescents: A guide for practitioners. *Pediatrics, 117,* 544–559.

Green, A. (2004). Outcomes of congenital heart disease: A review. *Pediatric Nursing, 30*(4), 280–284.

Greenberg, J. D., Bonwit, A. M., & Roddy, M. G. (2005). Subacute bacterial endocarditis prophylaxis: A succinct review for pediatric emergency physicians and nurses. *Clinical Pediatric Emergency Medicine, 6*(4), 266–272.

Griffin, K. J., Elkin, T. D., & Smith, C. J. (2003). Academic outcomes in children with congenital heart disease. *Clinical Pediatrics, 42*(5), 401–409.

Gumbiner, C. H. (2006). Ventricular septal defect. In J. A. McMillan (Ed.), *Oski's pediatrics:Principles and practice.* Philadelphia: Lippincott Williams & Wilkins.

Hagler, D. J. (2001). Palliated congenital heart disease. *Adolescent Medicine, 12*(1), 23–35.

Hershberger, R. E. (2005). Familial dilated cardiomyopathy. *Progress in Pediatric Cardiology, 20*(2), 161–168.

Huhta, J. C. (2006). Echocardiography and electrocardiography. In J. A. McMillan (Ed.), *Oski's pediatrics: Principles and practice.* Philadelphia: Lippincott Williams & Wilkins.

Jaggi, P., & Shulman, S. T. (2006). Group A streptococcal infections. *Pediatrics in Review, 27,* 99–105.

Karch, A. M. (2007). *Lippincott's nursing drug guide.* Philadelphia: Lippincott Williams & Wilkins.

Kay, J. D., Colan, S. D., & Graham, T. P. (2001a). Congestive heart failure in pediatric patients. *American Heart Journal, 142*(5), 923–928.

Kay, J. D., Sinaiko, A. R., & Daniels, S. R. (2001b). Pediatric hypertension. *American Heart Journal, 142*(3), 422–432.

Kopf, G. S., & Mello, D. M. (2006). Cardiovascular surgery in the newborn. In J. A. McMillan (Ed.), *Oski's pediatrics: Principles and practice.* Philadelphia: Lippincott Williams & Wilkins.

Koppel, R. I., Druschel, C. M., Carter, T., et al. (2003). Effectiveness of pulse oximetry screening for congenital heart disease in asymptomatic newborns. *Pediatrics, 111*(3), 451–455.

Labarthe, D. R., Dai, S., & Fulton, J. E. (2003). Cholesterol screening in children: Insights from Project HeartBeat! and NHANES III. *Progress in Pediatric Cardiology, 17*(2), 169–178.

Lawoko, S., & Soares, J. J. F. (2006). Psychosocial morbidity among parents of children with congenital heart disease: A prospective longitudinal study. *Heart & Lung, 35*(5), 310–314.

Luxner, K. L. (2005). *Delmar's pediatric nursing care plans.* Clifton Park, NY: Thomson Delmar Learning.

Mahle, W. T., Clancy, R. R., Moss, E. M., et al. (2000). Neurodevelopmental outcome and lifestyle assessment in school-aged and adolescent children with hypoplastic left heart syndrome. *Pediatrics, 100*(5), 1082–1089.

Mahle, W. T., Visconti, K. J., Freier, M. C., et al. (2006). Relationship of surgical approach to neurodevelopmental outcomes in hypoplastic left heart syndrome. *Pediatrics, 117*(1), e90–97.

Marian, A. J., Brugada, R., & Roberts, R. (2004). Cardiovascular disease due to genetic abnormalities. In V. Fuster, R. W. Alexander, & R. A. O'Rourke (Eds.), *Hurst's the heart* (11th ed., pp. 1747–1733). New York: McGraw-Hill Companies.

Marino, B. S., & Fine, K. S. (2007). *Blueprints: Pediatrics* (4th ed.). Philadelphia: Lippincott Williams & Wilkins.

Maron, B. J. (2004). Hypertrophic cardiomyopathy in childhood. *Pediatric Clinics of North America, 51*(5), 1305–1346.

Martin, J. M., & Green, M. (2006). Group A streptococcus. *Seminars in Pediatric Infectious Diseases, 17*(3), 140–148.

McConnell, M. E., & Elixson, E. M. (2002). The neonate with suspected congenital heart disease. *Critical Care Nursing Quarterly, 25*(3), 17–25.

McCrindle, B. W. (2003). Drug therapy of hyperlipidemia. *Progress in Pediatric Cardiology, 17*(2), 141–150.

Milan, C., & Chandran, L. (2006). What's new in Kawasaki disease? *Contemporary Pediatrics.* Retrieved 11/22/06 from http://www.contemporarypediatrics.com/contpeds/article/articleDetail.jsp?id=356254&sk=&date=&pageID=7.

Miller-Hoover, S. (2003). Pediatric and neonatal cardiovascular pharmacology. *Pediatric Nursing, 29*(2), 105–115.

Molczan, K. (2006). Cardiac anomalies in the neonate: High index of suspicion important. *Journal of Emergency Nursing, 32,* 94–97.

Moran, A. M., Newburger, J. W., Sanders, S. P., et al. (2000). Abnormal myocardial mechanics in Kawasaki disease: Rapid response to gammaglobulin. *American Heart Journal, 139*(2), 217–223.

Morelius, E., Lundh, U., & Nelson, N. (2002). Parental stress in relation to the severity of congenital heart disease in the offspring. *Pediatric Nursing, 28*(1), 28–34.

Morriss, M. J. H. (2006). Coarctation of the aorta. In J. A. McMillan (Ed.), *Oski's pediatrics: Principles and practice.* Philadelphia: Lippincott Williams & Wilkins.

Mullins, C. E. (2006a). Patent ductus arteriosus. In J. A. McMillan (Ed.), *Oski's pediatrics: Principles and practice.* Philadelphia: Lippincott Williams & Wilkins.

Mullins, C. E. (2006b). Therapeutic cardiac catheterization. In J. A. McMillan (Ed.), *Oski's pediatrics: Principles and practice.* Philadelphia: Lippincott Williams & Wilkins.

Muscari, M. E. (2004). *Lippincott's review series: Pediatric nursing.* Philadelphia: Lippincott Williams & Wilkins.

Neches, W. H., Park, S. C., & Ettedgui, J. A. (2006a). Tetralogy of Fallot. In J. A. McMillan (Ed.), *Oski's pediatrics: Principles and practice.* Philadelphia: Lippincott Williams & Wilkins.

Neches, W. H., Park, S. C., & Ettedgui, J. A. (2006b). Transposition of the great arteries. In J. A. McMillan (Ed.), *Oski's pediatrics: Principles and practice.* Philadelphia: Lippincott Williams & Wilkins.

Neilson, D., & Robin, N. (2002). Advances in the genetics of pediatric heart disease. *Contemporary Pediatrics, 1,* 85. Retrieved 11/22/06 from http://www.contemporarypediatrics.com/contpeds/article/articleDetail.jsp?id=126571&searchString=congenital%20heart%20disease.

Newburger, J. W., Takahashi, M., Gerber, M. A., et al. (2004). Diagnosis, treatment and long-term management of Kawasaki disease: A statement for health professionals from the Committee on Rheumatic Fever, Endocarditis, and Kawasaki Disease, Council on Cardiovascular Disease in the Young, American Heart Association. *Pediatrics, 114*(6), 1708–1733.

Pagana, K. D., & Pagana, T. J. (2006). *Mosby's manual of diagnostic and laboratory tests* (3rd ed.). St. Louis: Mosby.

Park, M. K., Menard S. W., & Schoolfield, J. (2005). Oscillometric blood pressure standards for children. *Pediatric Cardiology, 26*(5), 601–607.

Parrillo, S. J., & Parrillo, C. V. (2006). *Rheumatic fever.* Retrieved 11/13/06 from http://www.emedicine.com/emerg/topic509.htm.

Penny, D. J., & Shekerdemian, L. S. (2001). Management of the neonate with symptomatic congenital heart disease. *Archives of Disease in Childhood, 84*(3), F141–F145.

Phend, C. (Nov. 15, 2006). AHA: Pregnant smokers increase baby's heart defect risk. *Medpage Today.* Retrieved 11/15/06 from http://www.medpagetoday.com/MeetingCoverage/AHAMeeting/tb/4527.

Ressel, G. W. (2004). AAP releases policy statement on the prevention of RSV infections. *American Family Physician, 69*(4), 993–994.

Rhodes, J., Curran, T. J., Camil, L., et al. (2005). Impact of cardiac rehabilitation on the exercise function of children with serious congenital heart disease. *Pediatrics, 116*(6), 1339–1345.

Roodpeyma, S., Karmali, Z., Afshar, F., & Naraghi, S. (2002). Risk factors in congenital heart disease. *Clinical Pediatrics, 41*(9), 653–658.

Roos-Hesselink, J. W., Meijboom, F. J., Spitaels, S. E. C., et al. (2004). Outcome of patients after surgical closure of ventricular septal defect at young age: Longitudinal follow-up of 22–34 years. *European Heart Journal, 25*, 1057–1062.

Rosenthal, D., Chrisant, M. R., Edens, E., et al. (2004). International Society for Heart and Lung Transplantation: practice guidelines for management of heart failure in children. *Journal of Heart and Lung Transplantation, 23*, 1313–1333.

Rowley, A. H. (2004). The etiology of Kawasaki disease: A conventional infectious agent. *Progress in Pediatric Cardiology, 19*(2), 109–113.

Singh, V. N., Sharma, R. K., Reddy, H. K., & Nanda, N. C. (2004). *Ventricular septal defect.* Retrieved 12/3/06 from http://www.emedicine.com/radio/topic740.htm.

Slesnick, T. C., & Kovalchin, J. P. (2006). Truncus arteriosus. In J. A. McMillan (Ed.), *Oski's pediatrics: Principles and practice.* Philadelphia: Lippincott Williams & Wilkins.

Starc, T. J. (2001). Management of hyperlipidemia in children. *Progress in Pediatric Cardiology, 12*(2), 205–213.

Stauffer, N. R., & Murphy, K. (2002). Prenatal diagnosis of congenital heart disease: The beginning. *Critical Care Nursing Quarterly, 25*(3), 1–7.

Strauss, A., & Lock, J. E. (2003). Pediatric cardiomyopathy—a long way to go. *New England Journal of Medicine, 348*(17), 1703–1705.

Suddaby, B., & Mowery, B. (2002). Progression of congenital heart disease. *Pediatric Nursing, 28*(1), 69.

Suddaby, E. C. (2001). Contemporary thinking for congenital heart disease. *Pediatric Nursing, 27*(3), 233–238, 270.

Taketokmo, C. K., Hodding, J. H., & Kraus, D. M. (2005). *Lexi-comp's pediatric dosage handbook* (12th ed.). Hudson, OH: Lexi-comp.

Talner, N. S., & Carboni, M. P. (2003). Congestive heart failure. In C. D. Rudolph, A. M. Rudolph, M. K. Hostetter, et al., *Rudolph's pediatrics* (21st ed.). New York: McGraw-Hill.

Tani, L. Y., Veasy, L. G., Minich, L. L., & Shaddy, R. E. (2003). Rheumatic fever in children younger than 5 years: Is the presentation different? *Pediatrics, 112*(5), 1065–1068.

Taylor, M. L. (2005). Coarctation of the aorta: A critical catch for newborn well-being. *Nurse Practitioner, 30*(12), 34–44.

Towbin, J. A., & Bowles, N. E. (2006). Cardiomyopathy. In J. A. McMillan (Ed.), *Oski's pediatrics: Principles and practice.* Philadelphia: Lippincott Williams & Wilkins.

Towbin, J. A., Lowe, A. M., Colan, S. D., et al. (2006). Incidence, causes, and outcomes of dilated cardiomyopathy in children. *JAMA, 296*(15), 1867–1876.

U.S. Department of Health and Human Services. (2000). *Healthy people 2010: Understanding and improving health.* Washington, D.C.: Department of Health and Human Services.

U.S. Department of Health and Human Services, National Institutes of Health, National Heart, Lung, and Blood Institute. (2005). *The fourth report on the diagnosis, evaluation, and treatment of high blood pressure in children and adolescents (NIH Publication No. 05-5267).* Washington, D.C.: U.S. Department of Health and Human Services.

Uzark, K., & Jones, K. (2003). Parenting stress and children with heart disease. *Journal of Pediatric Health Care, 17*(4), 163–168.

Valente, A. M., Fleishman, C. E., & Talner, N. S. (2006). Cardiovascular disease in the newborn. In J. A. McMillan (Ed.), *Oski's pediatrics: Principles and practice.* Philadelphia: Lippincott Williams & Wilkins.

Vick, G. W., & Bezold, L. I. (2006). Defects of the atrial septum, including the atrioventricular canal. In J. A. McMillan (ed.), *Oski's pediatrics: Principles and practice.* Philadelphia: Lippincott Williams & Wilkins.

Ward, K. E. (2006). Anomalous pulmonary venous connections. In J. A. McMillan (Ed.), *Oski's pediatrics: Principles and practice.* Philadelphia: Lippincott Williams & Wilkins.

Watt, R. H. (2004). Congenital heart disease: an overview of the condition and treatment options. *Lippincott's Case Management, 9*(4), 205–208.

Webb, G. D., Smallhorn, J. F., Therrien, J., & Redington, A. N. (2005). Congenital heart disease. In D. P. Zipes, P. Libby, R. O. Bonow, & E. Braunwald. *Braunwald's heart disease: A textbook of cardiovascular medicine* (7th ed.). St. Louis: Elsevier.

Yee, C. A. (2005). Endocarditis: The infected heart. *Nursing Management, 36*(2), 25–30.

Ziegler, V. L. (2003). Ethical principles and parental choice: Treatment options for neonates with hypoplastic left heart syndrome. *Pediatric Nursing, 29*(1) 65–69.

Websites

http://hp2010.nhlbihin.net/ncep.htm National Cholesterol Education Program

www.childrensheartfoundation.org Children's Heart Foundation (awareness, education, and research for children's heart disease)

www.childrenheartinstitute.org Children's Heart Institute (helps children and parents to understand the defects)

www.childrenscardiomyopathy.org Children's Cardiomyopathy Foundation (focused on broadening the understanding of pediatric cardiomyopathy)

http://chin.org/ Congenital Heart Information Network

www.pcmregistry.org/index.htm Pediatric Cardiomyopathy Registry

www.spcnonline.com Society of Pediatric Cardiovascular Nurses

www.unos.org United Network for Organ Sharing

www.wellpoint.com/healthy_parenting/index.html "Healthy Habits for Healthy Kids—A Nutrition and Activity Guide for Parents"

Chapter WORKSHEET

MULTIPLE CHOICE QUESTIONS

1. The nurse is caring for a 5-year-old child with a congenital heart anomaly causing chronic cyanosis. When performing the history and physical examination, what is the nurse least likely to assess?

a. Obesity from overeating

b. Clubbing of the nail beds

c. Squatting during play activities

d. Exercise intolerance

2. A 2-day-old infant was just diagnosed with aortic stenosis. What is the most likely nursing assessment finding?

a. Gallop and rales

b. Blood pressure discrepancies in the extremities

c. Right ventricular hypertrophy on ECG

d. Heart murmur

3. Sam, age 11, has a diagnosis of rheumatic fever and has missed school for a week. What is the most likely cause of this problem?

a. Previous streptococcal throat infection

b. History of open heart surgery at 5 years of age

c. Playing too much soccer and not getting enough rest

d. Exposure to a sibling with pneumonia

4. The nurse is caring for a child after a cardiac catheterization. What is the nursing priority?

a. Allow early ambulation to encourage activity participation.

b. Check pulses above the catheter insertion site for strength and quality.

c. Assess extremity distal to the insertion site for temperature and color.

d. Change the dressing to evaluate the site for infection.

5. While assessing a 4-month-old infant, the nurse notes that the baby experiences a hypercyanotic spell. What is the priority nursing action?

a. Provide supplemental oxygen by face mask.

b. Administer a dose of IV morphine sulfate.

c. Begin cardiopulmonary resuscitation.

d. Place the infant in a knee-to-chest position.

CRITICAL THINKING EXERCISES

1. A baby boy was born at 26 weeks' gestation to 15-year-old unmarried parents who abuse drugs. The infant weighed 1.5 kg at birth and was diagnosed with AV canal defect and Down syndrome. Discuss some of the major issues in planning for care. Include a care plan and a list of teaching needs for the family.

2. A 4-year-old boy has parents with little education, and the child has Medicaid coverage. Another child is 7 years old and has well-educated parents with private insurance coverage. Both of these children need a heart transplant, and a heart is available that is a very good match for both children. Discuss some of the issues involved in deciding which child should receive the heart.

3. A 13-year-old boy was diagnosed with hypertension over 2 years ago. He is noncompliant with his antihypertensive medication regimen. He is 5 feet tall and weighs 170 pounds. His favorite activity is video games. Develop a teaching plan for this teen, providing creative approaches at the appropriate developmental level.

STUDY ACTIVITIES

1. Teach a class of sixth graders about healthy activities to prevent high cholesterol levels, hypertension, and heart disease. Use visual materials.

2. Spend the day with a nurse practitioner in the pediatric cardiology clinic. Report to the clinical group your observations about the children's quality of life, growth, and development.

3. Observe in the pediatric cardiothoracic intensive care unit or telemetry unit. Note the different cardiac rhythms displayed by children with a variety of cardiovascular disorders.

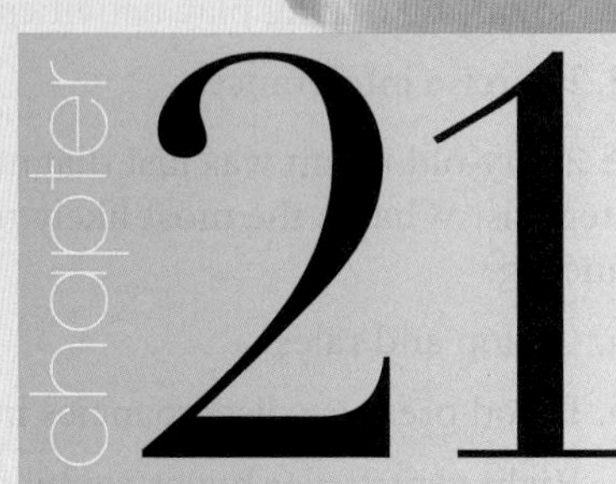

Nursing Care of the Child With a Gastrointestinal Disorder

Key TERMS

ALTE
anal fissure
anastomosis
atresia
cholestasis
cirrhosis
cleft
dysphagia
encopresis
enteral
fecal impaction
fibrosis
guarding
icteric
lethargy
protuberant
pylorus
rebound tenderness
regurgitation
steatorrhea

Learning OBJECTIVES

Upon completion of the chapter, the learner will be able to:

1. Compare the differences in the anatomy and physiology of the gastrointestinal system between children and adults.
2. Discuss common medical treatments for infants and children with gastrointestinal disorders.
3. Discuss common laboratory and diagnostic tests used to identify disorders of the gastrointestinal tract.
4. Discuss medication therapy used in infants and children with gastrointestinal disorders.
5. Recognize risk factors associated with various gastrointestinal illnesses.
6. Differentiate between acute and chronic gastrointestinal disorders.
7. Distinguish common gastrointestinal illnesses of childhood.
8. Discuss nursing interventions commonly used for gastrointestinal illnesses.
9. Devise an individualized nursing care plan for infants/children with a gastrointestinal disorder.
10. Develop teaching plans for family/patient education for children with gastrointestinal illnesses.
11. Describe the psychosocial impact that chronic gastrointestinal illnesses have on children.

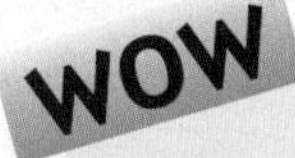

Children instinctively eat to live, and the nurse can help them devour the joys that life brings.

Ethan Richardson, 2 months old, is brought to the clinic by his mother. He has been vomiting for the past 3 days. His mother states she switched formula to see if that would help, but the vomiting worsened. Since last night she has attempted to feed him only Pedialyte. Mrs. Roberts says, "He can't keep anything down and he's very irritable." His weight at birth was 8 lbs 9 ounces, length 21 inches, and head circumference 37 cm. At his 2-month check-up last week he weighed 13 lbs.

Gastrointestinal (GI) disorders affect children of all ages. The most common result of a GI illness is dehydration, requiring fluid therapy at home or, in more extreme cases, in a hospital setting. GI illnesses range from acute to chronic problems. However, even acute, non-life-threatening illnesses (e.g., diarrhea or vomiting) can become life-threatening without proper nursing assessment and interventions. Therefore, all GI disorders should be taken seriously until symptoms are well controlled.

Patient and family education related to the treatment of GI disorders is key to preventing the illness from progressing to an emergency situation. Therefore, the nurse's knowledge of the disorders that affect the GI system is crucial. Most often, the parents or patient will contact the primary care provider in an outpatient setting to seek help. The nurse is usually the person to triage the phone call to determine the next step in the situation, which may be determining whether the patient should be managed at home, brought to the office for assessment, or sent directly to an emergency room for evaluation. The majority of GI disorders can be handled in an outpatient setting to avoid unnecessary hospitalizations, but some life-threatening problems (e.g., bowel obstruction) require emergency care in the hospital. Again, the knowledge base of the nurse is instrumental in obtaining the proper information by taking a thorough and accurate health history from the caregiver or patient.

Variations in Pediatric Anatomy and Physiology

The GI tract includes all of the structures from the mouth to the anus. The primary functions of the GI system are the digestion and absorption of nutrients and water, elimination of waste products, and secretion of various substances required for digestion. Babies are born with GI tracts that are not fully mature until age 2. Due to this immaturity, there are many differences between the digestive tract of the young child and that of the older child or adult.

Mouth

The mouth is highly vascular, making it a common entry point for infectious invaders. In addition, the infant and young child repeatedly bring objects to their mouths and explore them in that fashion. This behavior increases the infant's and young child's risk for contracting infectious agents via the mouth.

Esophagus

The esophagus provides a passageway from the mouth to the stomach for food. The lower esophageal sphincter (LES) prevents **regurgitation** of stomach contents up into the esophagus and/or oral cavity. The muscle tone of the LES is not fully developed until age 1 month, so infants less than 1 month of age frequently regurgitate after feedings. Many children less than 1 year of age continue to regurgitate for several months, but this usually disappears with age. If edema or narrowing of the esophagus occurs in a child with undeveloped esophageal muscle tone, **dysphagia** may occur.

Stomach

Newborns have a stomach capacity of only 10 to 20 mL. At age 2 months an infant has the capacity to hold up to 200 mL, though most young infants cannot tolerate 200-mL feedings. By age 16, the stomach capacity is 1,500 ml; by adulthood it is 2,000 to 3,000 mL. Levels of hydrochloric acid, which is found in gastric contents to aid in digestion, reach adult levels by age 6 months.

Intestines

A full-term infant has approximately 250 cm of small intestine; an adult has up to 600 cm. The function of the small intestine is not at a full level at birth. Fat losses may be up to 20% of intake for a newborn, as opposed to 7% for an adult. Intestinal growth occurs in rapid spurts, usually between the age of 1 and 3 years and again at 15 to 16 years. Infants who have small bowel loss during early infancy have more problems with absorption and diarrhea than adults who have the same amount of small bowel loss.

Biliary System

The liver is relatively large at birth, accounting for 5% of the infant's body weight, compared with 2% in an adult. This allows the smooth edge of the liver to be easily palpated in infancy, as much as 2 cm below the costal margin. The pancreatic enzymes all develop at certain postnatal times, not reaching adult levels until 2 years of age (Hamilton, 2000).

Fluid Balance and Losses

Children exhibit differences compared with adults that affect the ways that fluid volume is maintained. These differences are evident in body fluid balance and insensible fluid losses.

Body Fluid Balance

Infants and children have a proportionately greater amount of body water than do adults. Infants and young children require a greater relative fluid intake than adults and excrete a greater relatively larger amount of fluid. This places them at greater risk for fluid loss with illness compared to adults. Until age 2 years, the extracellular fluid makes up about half of the child's total body water. Since extracellular fluid has a larger proportion of sodium and chloride, when potential fluid-loss states occur, water loss occurs more rapidly and in larger amounts than in adults.

Insensible Fluid Losses

Fever increases fluid loss at a rate of about 7 mL/kg/24-hour period for every sustained 1-degree Celsius rise in temperature. Since children become febrile with illness more readily and their fevers are higher than those of adults, infants and young children are more apt than adults to experience insensible fluid loss with fever when ill.

Fluid loss via the skin accounts for about two thirds of insensible fluid loss. Infants have a relatively larger body surface area (BSA) than older children and adults. The newborn's BSA is about two or three times greater than the adult's, and the preterm infant's is about five times greater than the adults. This places infants, especially young infants, at increased risk of insensible fluid loss as compared to older children and adults.

The basal metabolic rate in infants and children is higher than that of adults in order to support growth. This higher metabolic rate, even in states of wellness, accounts for increased insensible fluid losses and increased need for water for excretory functions. The young infant's renal immaturity does not allow the kidneys to concentrate urine as well as in older children and adults. This puts infants at particular risk for dehydration or overhydration, depending upon the circumstances.

Common Medical Treatments

There are many different forms of medical treatment for GI disorders. In the hospital setting, most medical treatments will require a physician's order. The most common treatments and medications used for GI disorders are listed in Common Medical Treatments 21.1 and Drug Guide 21.1. Both tables provide essential information about medical treatments and medications used in pediatric GI disorders. These tables should be referred to as needed while completing the remainder of the chapter.

Nursing Process Overview for the Child With a GI Disorder

Nursing care of the child with a GI disorder includes nursing assessment, nursing diagnosis, planning, interventions, and evaluation. Each step of this process must be individualized for each patient. A general understanding of the GI tract and the most common disorders can help to individualize these nursing care plans.

> Remember Ethan, the 2-month-old with vomiting and irritability? What additional health history and physical examination assessment information should you obtain?

ASSESSMENT

The assessment of the child with a GI disorder includes a health history, physical examination, and laboratory and diagnostic testing.

Health History

A thorough health history is very important in the assessment of a child with a GI disorder. The health history includes past history (previous illnesses/surgeries), past family history, present illness (when the symptoms began and how this differs from the patient's normal status), and how the patient's symptoms have been managed up to this point (relevant medical records/home treatments). Detailed knowledge of the past medical and surgical history of the patient may reveal bowel resection, previous intestinal infections, and dietary issues and problems. The patient's growth patterns can also be an instrumental part of the health history and may help to generate a timeline for when the current problems appeared. The family history is also extremely important in identifying common genetic/familial GI symptoms or disorders such as irritable bowel syndrome, inflammatory bowel disease, or food allergies. The history of the present illness and symptoms can often distinguish chronic problems from acute disorders. All of these pieces of the health history require descriptive questions and answers from both nurses and patients. The person providing the history must be able to provide accurate details of the health history.

Physical Examination

The physical examination of the child should be done from the least invasive part of the examination to the most invasive. It is important for the child to remain as relaxed as possible during this part of the assessment.

Inspection and Observation

Inspect and observe the child's color, hydration status, abdominal size and shape, and mental status.

Color. First observe the patient's skin, eye, and lip color. Pale skin or lips in a patient with a GI disorder may be a sign of anemia or dehydration. During liver dysfunction, the bilirubin levels can rise, causing the skin to look jaundiced (yellow). The eyes can also become **icteric**, further indicating that the liver is not functioning correctly.

(text continues on page 665)

Common Medical Treatments 21.1 Gastrointestinal Disorders

Treatment	Explanation	Indication	Nursing Implications
Cleansing enema	Insertion of fluid into the rectum to soften the stool and stimulate bowel activity	Fecal impaction, severe constipation	Explain procedure to child prior to enema. With multiple enemas, observe for electrolyte imbalances.
Bowel preparation	Use of highly osmotic fluids to induce severe diarrhea to cleanse the entire bowel	Preparation for colonoscopy or bowel surgery	Some children may need to have a nasogastric tube placed so they can consume the needed amounts of fluids. Observe for signs and symptoms of dehydration/electrolyte imbalances.
Feeding tubes	Flexible tubes used for enteral feeding when the infant or child is incapable of swallowing safely or for augmenting nutrition. May be orogastric, nasogastric, gastrostomy, or jejunostomy.	Feeding difficulties, failure to thrive, gastroesophageal reflux disease, chronic illness	Orogastric and nasogastric tubes must be checked for placement prior to each use. If required long term, use a softer, flexible tube intended for long-term use. Stomahesive or Duoderm applied to the cheek may decrease risk of skin breakdown from tape. Gastrostomy tubes vary in type. Keep insertion site clean and dry.
Intravenous therapy	Administration of fluids via a catheter that delivers electrolytes and fluids into the venous system	Dehydration, bowel rest, NPO status	Monitor intravenous site for redness, swelling, and pain. Assess urine output to evaluate hydration status.
Ostomy	A portion of the intestine is brought to the level of the skin to allow passage of stool.	Imperforate anus, gastroschisis, omphalocele, Hirschsprung's disease, necrotizing enterocolitis, Crohn's disease, ulcerative colitis	Ostomy contents may be acidic and irritate the skin. Use Stomahesive or Duoderm under the pouch to avoid tape irritation to the skin. Pouch should fit the stoma correctly. Assess stoma for pinkness and moist appearance.
Oral rehydration therapy	Administration by mouth of fluids that contain certain amounts of electrolytes and glucose to prevent dehydration and/or promote rehydration	Diarrhea, acute gastroenteritis, vomiting	Fluid administration should begin prior to the onset of dehydration. Urine output should be monitored to evaluate hydration status.
Probiotics (lactobacillus, acidophilus)	Food supplement containing dormant bacteria that when activated may alter the intestinal microflora	Treatment/prevention of diarrhea	Particularly helpful in prevention of or decreasing incidence of antibiotic-induced diarrhea
Total parenteral nutrition (TPN)	Intravenous complete nutrition. Provides glucose, protein, lipids, vitamins, and minerals.	Long-term NPO status, swallowing difficulties, difficulties tolerating enteral feeding (short bowel syndrome, necrotizing enterocolitis)	Higher glucose and protein concentrations and solutions containing calcium require central venous access. Monitor blood glucose levels with initiation, rate changes, and discontinuation. Blood chemistries should be monitored on a regular basis.

Drug Guide 21.1 Common Drugs for GI Disorders

Classification	Action	Indication	Nursing Implications
Histamine-2 blockers (ranitidine, famotidine, cimetidine, nizatidine)	Decreases histamine production, thereby reducing gastric acid secretion	Heartburn, esophagitis, GERD, benign duodenal or gastric ulcers	May cause drowsiness or dizziness
Proton pump inhibitors (omeprazole, lansoprazole, esomeprazole, pantoprazole, rabeprazole)	Blocks the pump that produces gastric acids	Erosive esophagitis, symptomatic GERD, *H. pylori* eradication	Adverse effects include headache, nausea, abdominal pain, or diarrhea.
Prokinetics (metoclopramide, cisapride)	Stimulates GI motility to help empty the stomach faster and promote intestinal motility	Delayed gastric emptying, intestinal dysmotility	Metoclopramide may have central nervous system adverse effects. Cisapride available only in limited-access protocol studies.
Antibacterials/ antibiotics (metronidazole, vancomycin)	Treatment of bacterial infections of the GI tract	Suspected or proven bacterial infections of the GI tract, such as *C. difficile* or parasitic infections	May cause GI upset, diarrhea. Very important to finish entire course of treatment.
Immunosuppressants (6-mercaptopurine, azathioprine)	Suppresses the immune system to keep autoimmune disorders in remission	Crohn's disease, ulcerative colitis, autoimmune hepatitis	Drug levels should be checked to determine drug metabolite levels and potential for hepatotoxicity or bone marrow suppression.
Stimulants (senna, docusate sodium)	Stimulates peristalsis in the large intestine to produce a bowel movement	Constipation associated with slow transit through the colon	May cause cramping or diarrhea. Stool patterns should be constantly assessed.
Laxatives (polyethylene glycol, milk of magnesia, lactulose)	Softens the stool to allow for easier passage through the colon	Constipation	Stool patterns should be monitored. Doses may need to be readjusted frequently to find the correct dose for the patient.
Antidiarrheals (loperamide, diphenoxylate/ atropine)	Decreases peristalsis, thus prolonging transit time of stool through the intestines	Diarrhea related to short bowel syndrome, chronic nonspecific diarrhea, irritable bowel syndrome	May cause drowsiness or constipation
Corticosteroids (prednisone)	Acts systemically to reduce inflammation and suppress the normal immune response	Inflammatory bowel disease, autoimmune disorders	Systemic adverse effects include hirsutism, osteoporosis, GI upset, cushingoid appearance, increased intraocular pressure, irritability, and personality changes. Should be taken as directed. Stopping the medication suddenly may cause adrenal insufficiency.

(continued)

Drug Guide 21.1 Common Drugs for GI Disorders (continued)

Classification	Action	Indication	Nursing Implications
Antiemetics (promethazine, metoclopramide)	Acts on the central nervous system transmitters to prevent vomiting	Severe nausea and/or vomiting	May have central nervous system adverse effects, such as drowsiness or irritability
Anticholinergic/antispasmodics (hyoscyamine, dicyclomine, glycopyrrolate)	Used to control abdominal spasms and cramping	Irritable bowel syndrome, functional bowel disorders	May cause excessive thirst or dizziness. Encourage plenty of fluids while taking these medications.
Anti-inflammatory (mesalamine, balsalazide, hydrocortisone enemas/suppositories, olsalazine, sulfasalazine)	Reduces inflammation in the colon	Ulcerative colitis, proctitis	Stool output should be monitored to assess for presence of oral medications (indicating poor absorption).

GERD, gastroesophageal reflux disease.

Inspect the abdomen for signs of distended veins, which can indicate abdominal or vascular obstruction or distention. As in any part of a physical assessment, watch for areas of ecchymosis, which may be a sign of abuse.

Hydration Status. The child's hydration status often indicates how severe the current GI illness is. Dehydration can occur rapidly in children, especially in infants and young children. The oral mucosa should be pink and moist. Skin turgor should be elastic. Decreased turgor and tenting indicate dehydration. During crying, especially in infants, the absence of tears may indicate dehydration. Assess the amount of urine output the patient has had in the past 24 hours.

Abdominal Size and Shape. Inspect the size and shape of the abdomen while the child is standing and while lying supine. The abdomen should be flat when the child is supine. An especially **protuberant** abdomen suggests the presence of ascites, fluid retention, gaseous distention, or even a tumor, but many children (toddlers in particular) have a prominent "pot-bellied" abdomen as a normal variation of their anatomy. A depressed or concave abdomen could indicate a high abdominal obstruction or dehydration. Inspect the umbilicus for color, odor, discharge, inflammation, and herniation.

Mental Status. Perform a brief mental status examination of all GI patients. Mental status changes can occur in many instances, such as when ammonia levels are elevated with severe liver disease, severe dehydration, anaphylactic reactions to foods/medicines, tumors, and other metabolic disorders. Irritability and restlessness are usually the early signs of mental status changes. **Lethargy** and listlessness can occur much more rapidly in children than in adults and should be identified promptly and emergently treated.

Auscultation

As with all patients, both pediatric and adult, auscultate bowel sounds in all four quadrants. Hyperactive bowel sounds may be noted in children with diarrhea or gastroenteritis. Hypoactive or absent bowel sounds may signify an obstructive process and should be reported to the physician immediately. Absence of bowel sounds can be determined after a 5-minute period of auscultation. This can be extremely difficult to perform with children and infants, who may be uncooperative during the examination.

Percussion

Dullness or flatness is normally found along the right costal margin and 1 to 3 cm below the costal margin of the liver. The area above the symphysis pubis may be dull in young children with full bladders, which is a normal finding. Percussion of the remainder of the abdomen should reveal tympany. Note abnormal findings.

Palpation

Palpation should be reserved for last in the sequence of abdominal examination. First, lightly palpate the abdomen to assess for areas of tenderness, lesions, muscle tone, turgor, and cutaneous hyperesthesia (a finding in acute peritonitis). Then perform deep palpation from the lower quadrants upward to best feel the liver edge, which should be firm and smooth. In infants and children, palpate the liver during inspiration below the right costal margin. The tip of the spleen may be palpated also during inspiration; it should be 1 to 2 cm below the left costal margin. Palpable kidneys, except in neonates, may indicate tumor or hydronephrosis. The sigmoid colon can be palpated in the left lower quadrant. The cecum may be felt in the right lower quadrant as a soft mass. Areas of firmness or masses may indicate tumor or stool in the abdomen.

Tenderness in the abdomen is not a normal physical finding. Right upper quadrant tenderness could indicate liver enlargement. Right lower quadrant pain, including **rebound tenderness**, can be a warning sign of appendicitis and should be reported to a physician immediately. Palpate the external inguinal canals for presence of inguinal hernias, often elicited by having the child turn the head and cough, or blow up a balloon (Katz, 2001).

Laboratory and Diagnostic Testing

Common Laboratory and Diagnostic Tests 21.1 gives information about the tests most often ordered by physicians for children with GI illnesses. Some of these tests are ordered in the hospital setting; others are done on an outpatient basis. Typically, the nurse is involved directly in the laboratory tests while a specifically trained person performs the diagnostic tests. Regardless of who performs the test, nurses must be familiar with preparation guidelines for the patient, how each test is performed, and normal and abnormal findings and their significance so that they can provide patient and family education. Teaching Guideline 21.1 gives tips on collecting stool specimens.

(text continues on page 669)

Common Laboratory and Diagnostic Tests 21.1

Test	Explanation	Indication	Nursing Implications
Abdominal ultrasonography	Visualizes abdominal organs and related vessels	Abdominal pain, vomiting, pregnancy, abnormal liver tests, abdominal mass, enlarged organs on palpation	Barium decreases visualization of organs on ultrasound.
Abdominal x-ray (KUB)	Plain x-ray of the abdomen without contrast media	Constipation, abdominal pain, abdominal distention, ascites, foreign body, palpable mass	Usually ordered as flat and upright to allow for free air and fluid levels in the bowel to be detected
Amylase (serum)	An enzyme that changes starch to sugar, which enters the blood with inflammation of the pancreas	Acute pancreatitis, pancreatic trauma, acute cholecystitis	Increased levels are seen after 3 to 6 hours of the onset of abdominal pain.
Barium enema	After instillation of barium, fluoroscopically allows visualization of the colon	Constipation, rectal prolapse, bleeding, suspected intussusception	Bowel preparation prior to examination may be ordered. Stool will be light-colored due to barium for a few days.
Electrolytes (serum)	Sodium, potassium, CO_2, chloride, blood urea nitrogen (BUN), creatinine	To determine extent of dehydration	BUN and creatinine may be elevated with dehydration. Sodium, potassium, chloride, and CO_2 levels can be greatly affected with dehydration.
Barium swallow/ upper GI series	Visualizes the form, position, mucosal folds, peristaltic activity, and motility of the esophagus, stomach, and upper GI tract	Foreign body ingestion, abdominal pain, vomiting, dysphagia, malrotation	Females of reproductive age must be screened for pregnancy. Infants may need to be given barium via bulb syringe.

(continued)

Common Laboratory and Diagnostic Tests 21.1 (continued)

Test	Explanation	Indication	Nursing Implications
Small bowel series	Done in conjunction with upper GI series to visualize the small intestine contour, position, and motility	Suspected inflammatory bowel disease (bowel wall thickening), intussusception	Very important to encourage large amounts of water/fluids after test to avoid barium-induced constipation
Endoscopic retrograde cholangiopancreatography (ERCP)	A fiberoptic endoscope is used to view the hepatobiliary system by instilling contrast to outline the pancreatic and common bile ducts.	Pancreatitis, jaundice, pancreatic tumors, common duct stones, biliary tract disease	Monitor for infection, urinary retention, cholangitis, or pancreatitis after the procedure. Done only occasionally in children.
Esophageal manometry	Tests the esophagus for normal contractile activity and effectiveness of swallowing by measurement of intraluminal pressures and acid sensors	Abnormal esophageal muscle function, dysphagia, chest pain of unknown cause, esophagitis, vomiting	Often done in conjunction with pH probe. The manometric catheter is placed through the nose into the esophagus. May cause nasal irritation/sore throat.
Esophageal pH probe	A single- or double-channeled probe placed into the esophagus to monitor the pH of the contents that are regurgitated into the esophagus from the stomach	Vomiting, gastroesophageal reflux, correlation of symptoms to gastroesophageal reflux events and high risk for problems, as in asthma, apparent life-threatening event, sinusitis, or choking/gagging episodes	24-hour study is most accurate. Special diet during study is often used. Accurate diary of symptoms and feedings during the study is essential. May cause nasal irritation/sore throat.
Gastric emptying scan	Assesses the rate at which the stomach empties food into the small intestine by adding isotopes to food and visualizing with scans	Unexplained nausea, vomiting, diarrhea, abdominal cramping	Medications may alter gastric emptying times. Crying or stress during the examination may cause delay in emptying and should be documented.
Hemoccult	Checks for occult blood in the stool	Crohn's disease, ulcerative colitis, malabsorption syndromes, diarrhea, abdominal pain	
Hepatobiliary scan (HIDA scan)	Visualizes the gallbladder and determines patency of the biliary system by use of a radionuclide. The amount of radionuclide ejected from the gallbladder (ejection fraction) is calculated.	Differentiate between biliary atresia and neonatal hepatitis; assess liver trauma, right upper quadrant pain, and congenital malformations	Intravenous line will be established to give radionuclide. Pain during injection should be assessed and documented.
Lactose tolerance test	After ingesting lactose, this tests the hydrogen levels in the breath, which will increase with lactose build-up in the intestines.	Postprandial diarrhea, gassiness, bloating, abdominal pain	May produce similar symptoms during the test itself. A positive test will require diet modification and education regarding lactose intolerance.
Lipase (serum)	An enzyme that changes fat to fatty acids and glycerol appearing in the blood with pancreatic change	Pancreatitis, pancreatic carcinoma, cholecystitis, peritonitis	Lipase levels stay elevated longer with acute pancreatitis.

Common Laboratory and Diagnostic Tests 21.1 (continued)

Test	Explanation	Indication	Nursing Implications
Liver biopsy	A test done to evaluate the microscopic hepatic structures	Hyperbilirubinemia, jaundice, chronic liver disease, hepatitis	Monitor after procedure for bleeding complications; must maintain strict bed rest for up to 8 hours.
Liver function tests (LFTs) (AST/ALT/GGT)	Enzymes that have high concentrations in the liver	Elevations may indicate the severity of liver disease.	May be affected by drugs or viral illnesses
Lower endoscopy (colonoscopy)	Allows visualization and biopsies of the lower GI tract from the anus to the terminal ileum with a fiberoptic instrument	Rectal bleeding, lower abdominal pain, suspected tumors or strictures, foreign body removal	The child must undergo a bowel cleansing prior to the examination. Encourage fluids to prevent dehydration. Conscious sedation or anesthesia care; monitor for possible complications of perforation, bleeding, increased abdominal pain.
Meckel's scan	A gamma camera is used to identify gastric mucosa seen in the distal portion of the ileum after injection of radiopharmaceuticals.	Rectal bleeding, anemia, used only to identify a Meckel's diverticulum	Gloves are worn by nurse during and after scan when radiopharmaceuticals are given.
Oropharyngeal motility study (OPMS)	A study done with different textures to evaluate the dynamics of swallowing and reveal transient abnormalities	Dysphagia, recurrent aspiration	Usually done in combination with therapists and nutritionist
Rectal suction biopsy	Biopsy is taken of the rectum at different levels to assess for the presence of ganglion cells.	Absence of ganglion cells indicates Hirschsprung's disease.	Infants/children should be assessed for rectal bleeding after examination.
Stool culture	Stool is smeared on culture medium and assessed for growth of bacteria over a period of days.	To determine bacterial cause of diarrhea	Requires minimum of 48 hours for growth, several days to weeks in some cases. Can be done with a small amount of stool.
Stool for ova and parasites (O&P)	Checks for the presence of parasites or their eggs in the stool	To determine cause of diarrhea or abdominal pain	Requires about 2 tablespoons of stool
Upper endoscopy (EGD)	Allows visualization and biopsies of the upper GI tract (mouth to upper jejunum) with a fiberoptic instrument	Dysphagia, foreign body removal, epigastric/abdominal pain, suspected celiac disease	Conscious sedation or anesthesia care; monitor for complications of perforation/bleeding
Urea breath test	Used to detect the presence of *Helicobacter pylori* in the exhaled breath	*Helicobacter pylori* infection	Patient must not take proton pump inhibitors for 5 days, all antibiotic therapy and Pepto-Bismol for 14 days.

From Fischbach, 2003.

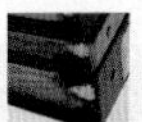

TEACHING GUIDELINE 21.1

Stool Specimen Collection Variations

- If the child is in diapers, use a tongue blade to scrape a specimen into the collection container.
- If the child has runny stool, a piece of plastic wrap in the diaper may catch the stool specimen. Very liquid stool may require application of a urine bag to the anal area to collect the stool.
- The older ambulatory child may first urinate in the toilet, and then the stool specimen may be retrieved from the new or clean collection container that fits under the seat at the back of the toilet.
- For the bedridden child, collect the stool specimen from a clean bedpan (do not allow urine to contaminate the stool specimen).
- Send the specimen to the laboratory immediately for accuracy of results.

Adapted from Berman, 2003.

NURSING DIAGNOSES, GOALS, INTERVENTIONS, AND EVALUATION

Upon completion of a thorough assessment, the nurse might identify several nursing diagnoses, including:

- Risk for deficient fluid volume
- Diarrhea
- Constipation
- Risk for impaired skin integrity
- Imbalanced nutrition: less than body requirements
- Pain
- Ineffective breathing pattern
- Risk for caregiver role strain
- Disturbed body image

After completing an assessment on Ethan, you note the following: weight 10 lbs, length 23.5 inches, head circumference 40.75 cm. Head is round with sunken anterior fontanel, eyes appear sunken, mucous membranes are dry, heart rate 158, breath sounds clear with respiratory rate of 42, positive bowel sounds in all four quadrants, difficulty palpating abdomen due to crying. Based on these assessment findings, what would your top three nursing diagnoses be for Ethan?

Nursing goals, interventions, and evaluation for the child with a GI disorder are based on the nursing diagnoses. Nursing Care Plan 21.1 can be used as a guide in planning nursing care for the child with a GI disorder. The nursing care plan should be individualized based on the patient's symptoms and needs. Refer to Chapter 15 for detailed information about pain management. Additional information will be included later in the chapter as it relates to specific disorders.

Based on your top three nursing diagnoses for Ethan, describe appropriate nursing interventions.

Stool Diversions

Children may undergo stool diversions for a variety of GI disorders. Surgical procedures involve the creation of an ostomy, primarily an *ileostomy* or *colostomy*, by bringing a portion of the small or large intestine to the surface of the abdomen (Fig. 21.1).

Ostomy pouches are worn over the ostomy site to collect stool. The pouch must be of an appropriate size and it should fit around the stoma properly (Fig. 21.2). The pouch may be tucked inside the diaper or underwear or angled to fit outside of the diaper/underwear. Contemporary pouches cannot be seen under most clothing because they are designed to lie flat against the body. Avoid tight or constricting clothing around the stoma site. Teach families to store ostomy supplies in a cool, dry place. Educate parents to inform school staff that the child should be allowed to use the water fountain and the bathroom without restriction, and the school nurse should have extra ostomy supplies available.

Ostomy care for a child can be challenging due to the child's normal growth and development as well as activity. Empty the ostomy pouch and measure for stool output several times per day. The stool may be semisolid to very liquid in consistency depending on the location of the stoma. Liquid stool output can be acidic, causing irritation and severe burn-like areas on the surrounding skin, so special attention to skin care around the ostomy site is essential. Products such as powders and pastes are available to help protect the skin.

The stoma should be moist and pink or red, demonstrating proper circulation to the intestine (Fig. 21.3). Immediately notify the physician if the stoma is not moist and pink or red. Also notify the provider if the volume of stool output is greatly increased, or if the stoma is prolapsed or retracted.

Perform ostomy care as needed; pouches usually need to be changed every 1 to 4 days (Nursing Procedure 21.1). The word "stoma" can be used as a mnemonic for the steps for changing an ostomy pouch.

Structural Anomalies of the GI Tract

Structural anomalies of the GI tract include cleft lip and palate, omphalocele and gastroschisis, hernias (inguinal and umbilical), and anorectal malformations.

(text continues on page 673)

Nursing Care Plan 21.1

Overview for the Child with a GI Disorder

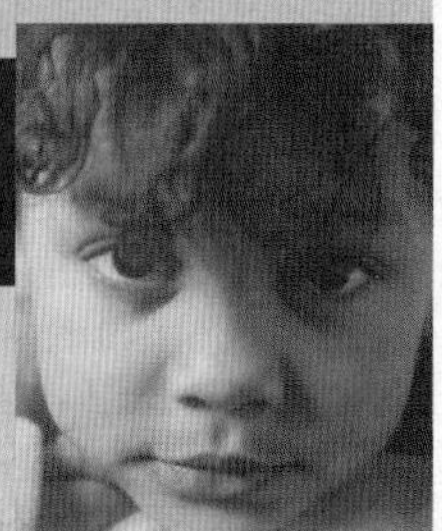

Nursing Diagnosis: Fluid volume, risk for deficit: risk factors may include excessive losses through vomiting or diarrhea, inadequate oral intake, possible NPO status (particularly in the surgical client)

Outcome identification and evaluation

Child will maintain adequate fluid volume as evidenced by *elastic skin turgor; moist, pink oral mucosa; presence of tears;* urine output 1 mL/kg/hr or more.

Intervention: maintaining fluid balance

- Maintain IV line and administer IV fluid as ordered *to maintain fluid volume.*
- Offer small amounts of oral rehydration solution frequently *to maintain fluid volume. Small amounts are usually well tolerated by children with diarrhea and vomiting.*
- When symptoms have lessened or resolved, reintroduce regular diet *to reduce number of stools, provide adequate nutrition, and shorten duration of effects of illness.*
- Avoid high-carbohydrate fluids such as Kool-aid and fruit juice, *as they are low in electrolytes, and increased simple carbohydrate consumption can decrease stool transit time.*
- Assess hydration status (skin turgor, oral mucosa, presence of tears) every 4 to 8 hours *to evaluate maintenance of adequate fluid volume.*
- Assess adequacy of urine output *to assess end-organ perfusion.*
- Maintain strict intake and output record and weigh child daily *to evaluate effectiveness of rehydration.*
- Weigh child daily: *accurate weight is one of the best indicators of fluid volume status in children.*
- Discourage fluids and milk products that contain high levels of sugar during the acute phase of illness, *as these products may worsen diarrhea.*

Nursing Diagnosis: Diarrhea; may be related to inflammation of small intestines, presence of infectious agents or toxins, possibly evidenced by loose liquid stools, hyperactive bowel sounds, or abdominal cramping

Outcome identification and evaluation

Child will experience decrease in diarrhea: *will have bulkier stool as per normal routine.*

Intervention: relieving diarrhea

- Maintain clear liquid diet no longer than 24 hours, *as prolonged clear liquids will result in continued liquid ("starvation") stools.*
- Avoid milk products until diarrhea improves: *temporary poor absorption from villus injury follows viral diarrhea.*
- Encourage complex carbohydrate foods *to bulk up the stools.*
- Add fat to carbohydrates *to increase intestinal transit time to encourage water absorption (bulks up stool).*

Nursing Diagnosis: Constipation, related to GI obstructive lesions, pain on defecation, diagnostic procedures, inadequate toileting, or behavioral stool holding, possibly evidenced by change in character or frequency of stools, feeling of abdominal or rectal fullness or pressure, changes in bowel sounds, and abdominal distention

Outcome identification and evaluation

Child will experience improvement in constipation *by passing daily soft bowel movement without pain or straining.*

Intervention: relieving constipation

- Palpate for abdominal distention, percuss for dullness, and auscultate for bowel sounds *to assess for signs of constipation.*

Overview for the Child with a GI Disorder (continued)

- Encourage adequate fluid intake *to soften the stool.*
- Administer medications as ordered *to keep stool moving on daily basis.*
- Encourage activity as tolerated: *immobility contributes to constipation.*
- The child with stool withholding should sit on the toilet twice daily, preferably after breakfast and dinner, *to maximize chances for successful stool passage by taking advantage of the gastrocolic reflex.*
- For behavioral stool holding, use rewards or stickers *to encourage appropriate toileting.*

Nursing Diagnosis: Skin integrity, risk for impaired: risk factors include frequent loose stools, poor nutritional status, presence of stoma, acidic gastric contents contact with skin if gastrostomy present

Outcome identification and evaluation

Infant's skin will remain intact: *buttocks skin will be free from rash, excoriation.*

In the child with an ostomy: skin surrounding stoma will remain intact: *free from redness, rash, excoriation.*

Intervention: maintaining skin integrity

- Change diapers frequently *to limit acidic stool content contact with skin.*
- Use barrier diaper cream *to protect skin.*
- Assess skin integrity at every diaper change *to recognize skin changes early so that corrective measures can begin.*
- Leave diaper area open to air several times a day if redness is present *so that air can circulate and skin healing can be facilitated.*
- Use plain water or only mild soap to cleanse the skin with diaper changes *to avoid pH changes that contribute to diaper area skin breakdown.*
- Avoid diaper wipes that contain fragrance or alcohol if the skin is red or has a rash, *as both alcohol and perfume cause stinging if used on non-intact skin and can worsen skin breakdown.*

For the child with an ostomy:

- Ensure proper fit of the ostomy appliance/pouch *to avoid acidic stool contact with skin.*
- Use a barrier wafer (e.g., Stomahesive or Duoderm) to attach appliance: *avoids repeated pulling of adhesive tape from skin.*
- If redness occurs, use barrier/healing cream or paste on skin around stoma *to promote healing and prevent further skin breakdown.*
- Consult enterostomal therapy nurse as needed *to provide additional support.*

Nursing Diagnosis: Nutrition: imbalanced, less than body requirements; may be related to inability to ingest, digest, or absorb nutrients; intestinal pain after eating; decreased transit time through bowel; or psychosocial factors, possibly evidenced by lack of appropriate weight gain or growth, weight loss, aversion to eating, poor muscle tone, or observed lack of intake

Outcome identification and evaluation

Nutritional status will be maximized: *child will maintain or gain weight appropriately.*

Intervention: maintaining appropriate nutrition

- Encourage favorite foods (within prescribed diet restrictions if present) *to maximize oral intake.*
- Administer enteral tube feedings as ordered *to maximize caloric intake.*
- Add butter, gravy, cheese as appropriate to foods (if allowed within diet restrictions) *to increase caloric intake.*
- Encourage high-quality, high-calorie snacks between meals, *so as not to interfere with meal intake.*
- Document response to feeding *to determine feeding tolerance.*
- Limit intake of calorie-free beverages: *beverages should contain nutrients and calories.*
- Consult nutritionist *for appropriate diet supplementation recommendations.*

(continued)

Overview for the Child with a GI Disorder (continued)

Nursing Diagnosis: Breathing pattern, ineffective, risk for: risk factors include postoperative immobility, abdominal pain interfering with breathing, use of narcotic analgesics

Outcome identification and evaluation

Child will demonstrate effective breathing pattern: *respiratory rate normal for age, absence of accessory muscle use, adequate aeration with clear breath sounds throughout all lung fields.*

Intervention: promoting effective breathing patterns

- Turn, cough, deep breathe every 2 hours *to encourage adequate aeration and discourage fluid pooling in lungs.* In the infant or toddler, turn every 2 hours and use percusser or chest physiotherapy *to prevent pooling of secretions.*
- Play games to encourage deep breathing (blow out penlight, blow cotton ball across bedside table with straw, etc.): *children are more likely to cooperate with interventions if play is involved.*
- In the developmentally able child, encourage incentive spirometer use every 2 hours *to improve lung aeration.*
- Demonstrate/encourage use of pillow splinting with coughing *to decrease abdominal pain and stress on incision.*

Nursing Diagnosis: Caregiver role strain, risk for: risk factors may include infant with congenital defect, child with chronic illness, marginal caregiver coping patterns, long-term stress, complexity and quantity of care child requires

Outcome identification and evaluation

Caregiver will exhibit emotional health: *verbalizes concerns calmly, participates in child's care, and demonstrates knowledge of resources.*

Intervention: easing caregiver role strain

- Assess parental behavior *to identify role strain.*
- Provide emotional support and encourage talking about feelings, fears, and concerns: *to promote trust in nurse as a source of emotional support.*
- Arrange for and/or encourage respite care for child: *provides parent with time away from continual care.*
- Consult social services *to identify community resources available for caregiver support (home health, support group, etc.).*
- Encourage parent to meet own needs and find personal time *to increase energy level and self-esteem, ultimately enhancing the quality of care given.*

Nursing Diagnosis: Body image disturbance; may be related to presence of stoma, loss of control of bowel elimination, scars from multiple surgical procedures, or effects of treatment regimen, possibly evidenced by verbalization of negative feelings about body, refusal to look at stoma or participate in care

Outcome identification and evaluation

Child or teen will demonstrate acceptance of change in body image *by verbalization of adjustment; looking at, touching, caring for body; returning to previous social involvement.*

Intervention: promoting proper body image

- Observe child's coping mechanisms *to reinforce their use in times of stress.*
- Acknowledge denial, anger, and other feelings as normal *to support child/teen through difficult transition.*
- Allow child gradual introduction to stoma *to ease transition.*
- Encourage child/teen to participate in care, *as this sense of control will contribute to positive self-esteem.*

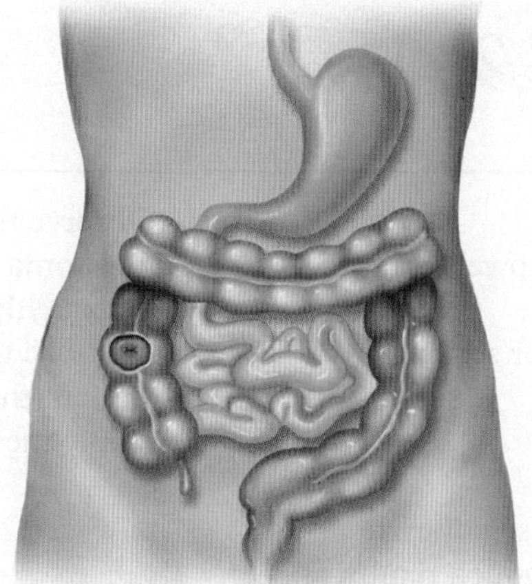
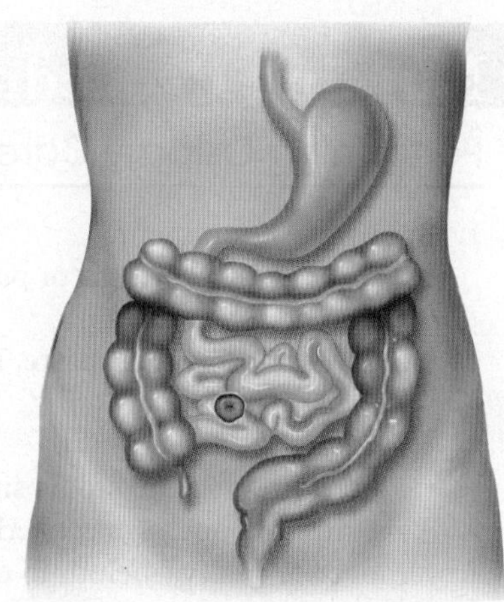

● Figure 21.1 A colostomy is a stoma from the colon; an ileostomy is a stoma from the ileum.

● CLEFT LIP AND PALATE

Cleft lip and palate (Fig. 21.4) is the most common congenital craniofacial anomaly, occurring once in every 700 births (Mitchell & Wood, 2000). It occurs frequently in association with other anomalies and has been identified in more than 300 syndromes. The most common anomalies associated with cleft lip and palate include heart defects, ear malformations, skeletal deformities, and genitourinary abnormality.

Complications of cleft lip and palate include feeding difficulties, altered dentition, delayed or altered speech development, and otitis media. The infant with cleft lip may have difficulty forming an adequate seal around a nipple in order to create the necessary suction for feeding and may also experience excessive air intake. Gagging, choking, and nasal regurgitation of milk may occur in babies with cleft palate. Excessive feeding time, inadequate intake, and fatigue contribute to insufficient growth (Cahill & Wagner, 2002). Primary or permanent teeth may be missing, malformed, or unusually positioned. Children with cleft palate may have slight delays in speech development, a nasal quality to the speech, and difficulty saying certain consonants correctly (Sharp et al., 2003). The opening in the cleft palate contributes to build-up of fluid in the middle ear (otitis media with effusion), which can lead to an acute infection (acute otitis media). Long-lasting otitis media with effusion leads to temporary and sometimes permanent hearing loss.

Pathophysiology

Development of the **cleft** occurs early in pregnancy. The tissue that forms the lip ordinarily fuses by 5 to 6 weeks of gestation, and the palate closes between 7 and 9 weeks of gestation. Therefore, if either the lip or palate does not fuse, then the infant is born with a cleft. Cleft lip or cleft palate may occur in isolation from one another, but 70% of infants born with cleft lip also have cleft palate (March of Dimes, 2004). The cleft may be unilateral (the left side is affected more often) or bilateral.

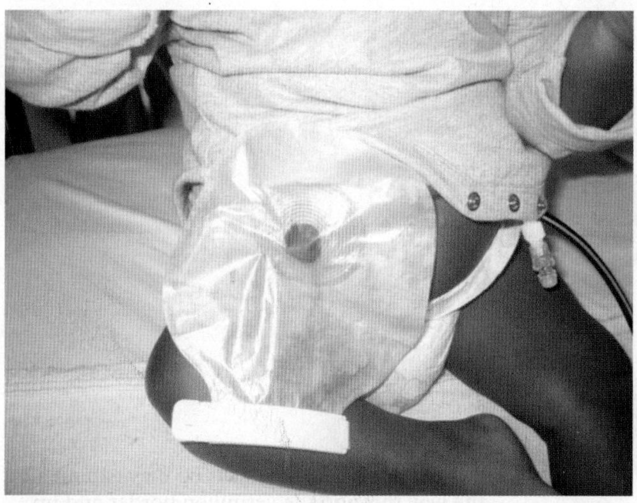

● Figure 21.2 Ensure that the ostomy pouch fits closely around the stoma to prevent irritation of the surrounding skin.

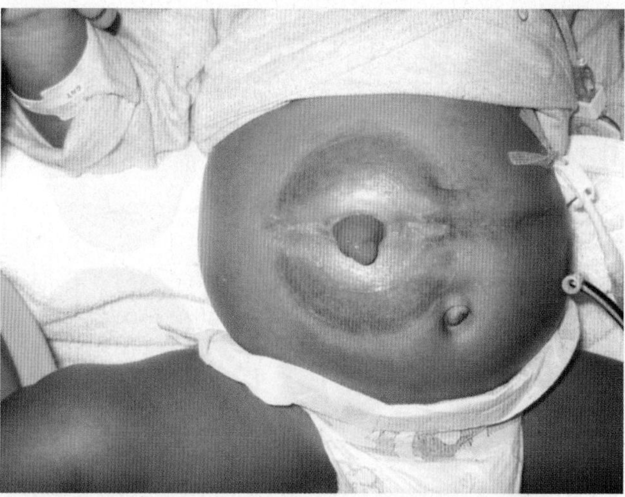

● Figure 21.3 The healthy stoma is pink and moist.

Nursing Procedure 21.1

Performing Ostomy Care

1. Set up the equipment:
   - Warm, wet washcloths or paper towels
   - Clean pouch and clamp
   - Skin barrier powder, paste, and/or sealant
   - Pencil or pen
   - Scissors
   - Pattern to measure stoma size
2. Take off the pouch (may need to use adhesive remover or wet washcloth to ease pouch removal).
3. Observe the stoma and surrounding skin. Clean the stoma and skin as needed, allowing it to dry thoroughly.
4. Measure the stoma, mark the new pouch backing, and cut the new backing to size.
5. Apply the new pouch.

Adapted from Children's Healthcare of Atlanta. (2004). *Ostomy care homecare manual.*

Therapeutic Management

Babies with cleft lip and palate are usually managed by a specialized team that may include a plastic surgeon or craniofacial specialist, oral surgeon, dentist or orthodontist, prosthodontist, psychologist, otolaryngologist, nurse, social worker, audiologist, and speech-language pathologist. Many children's hospitals offer these services in one location, such as a craniofacial specialty center. Historically, cleft lip has been repaired surgically around the age of 2 to 3 months and cleft palate at 9 to 18 months, but in recent years institutions with an experienced craniofacial team have successfully repaired clefts in the neonatal period (Sandberg et al., 2002). Early repair of the cleft lip restores a normal appearance to the child's face and may improve parent–infant bonding. Regardless of the timing of the surgical repair, however, surgical revision of the palate may be required as the child grows.

Nursing Assessment

For a full description of the assessment phase of the nursing process refer to page 662. Assessment findings pertinent to cleft lip and palate are discussed below.

Health History

For the newborn, explore pregnancy history for risk factors for development of cleft lip and palate, which include:

- Maternal smoking
- Prenatal infection
- Advanced maternal age
- Use of anticonvulsants, steroids, and other medications during early pregnancy

When an infant or child with cleft lip or palate returns for a clinic visit or hospitalization, inquire about feeding difficulties, respiratory difficulties, speech development, and otitis media.

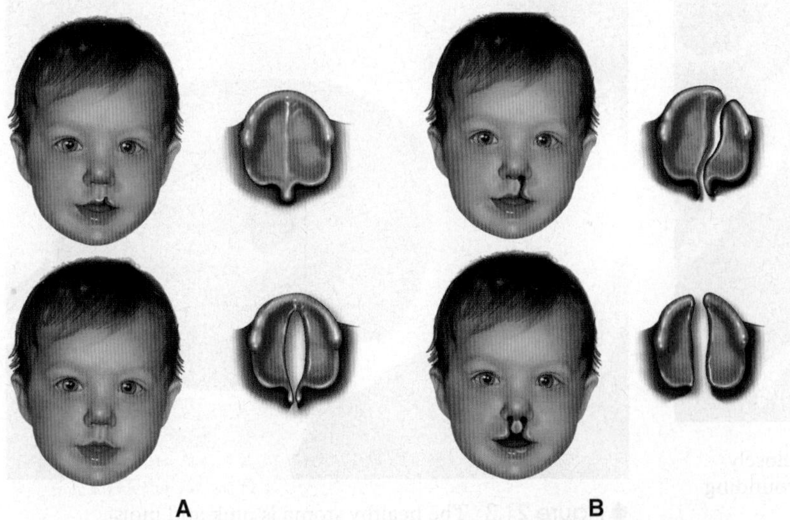

● Figure 21.4 (A) The cleft lip may extend all the way through the vermilion border and up into the nostril, or it may be significantly smaller. (B) The cleft palate may be a small opening or may involve the entire palate.

Physical Examination

Observe the infant for the presence of the characteristic physical appearance of cleft lip. The cleft may involve the lip only or extend up into the nostril (Fig. 21.5). Cleft palate may be visualized on examination of the mouth. Palpate with a gloved finger to discover mild clefts.

Laboratory and Diagnostic Tests

Cleft lip may be diagnosed by prenatal ultrasound, but it is diagnosed most commonly at birth by the classic physical appearance.

Nursing Management

Refer to the Nursing Care Plan 21.1 for nursing diagnoses and interventions related to airway maintenance, pain alleviation, fluid balance promotion, and restoration of family processes. These should be individualized for the particular situation. In addition to the nursing diagnoses and related interventions discussed in the Nursing Care Plan, interventions common to cleft lip and palate follow.

Preventing Injury to the Suture Line

It is critical to prevent injury to the facial suture line or to the palatal operative sites. Do not allow the infant to rub the facial suture line. To prevent this, position the infant in a supine or side-lying position. It may be necessary to use arm restraints to stop the hands from touching the face or entering the mouth. Clean the suture line as ordered by the surgeon. Possible care options include using petroleum jelly on the facial suture line or a lip-protective device such as a Logan bow (curved thin metal apparatus) or a butterfly adhesive, both of which protect and maintain the suture line. Protect the palate operative site. Avoid putting items in the mouth that might disrupt the sutures (e.g., suction catheter, spoon, straw, pacifier, or plastic syringe).

Prevent vigorous or sustained crying in the infant, because this may cause tension on either suture line. Ways to prevent crying include administering medications as needed for pain and providing other comfort or distraction measures, such as cuddling, rocking, and anticipation of needs.

Promoting Adequate Nutrition

Preoperatively, the baby with a cleft lip may demonstrate enhanced growth patterns if breastfed. The contour of the breast against the lip may allow for a better seal to be maintained for adequate sucking. Some infants will be fed with a special cleft lip nipple (Fig. 21.6). Parent and surgeon preference will determine the method of feeding. Burp the infant well to expel excess air taken in during difficulty with sucking.

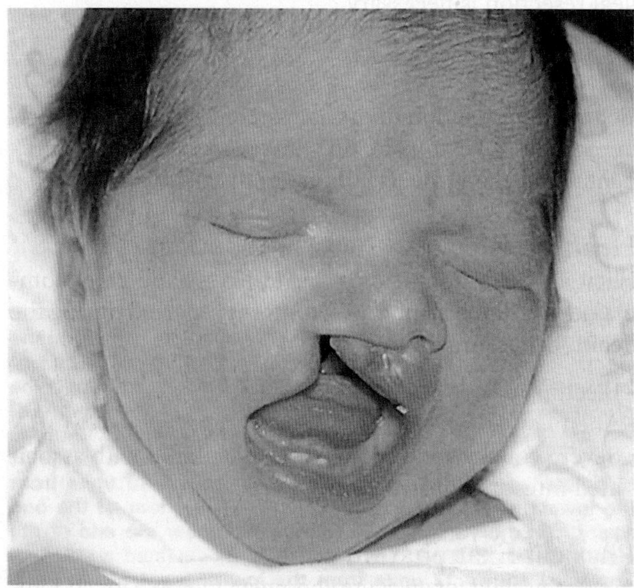

● Figure 21.5 Cleft lip.

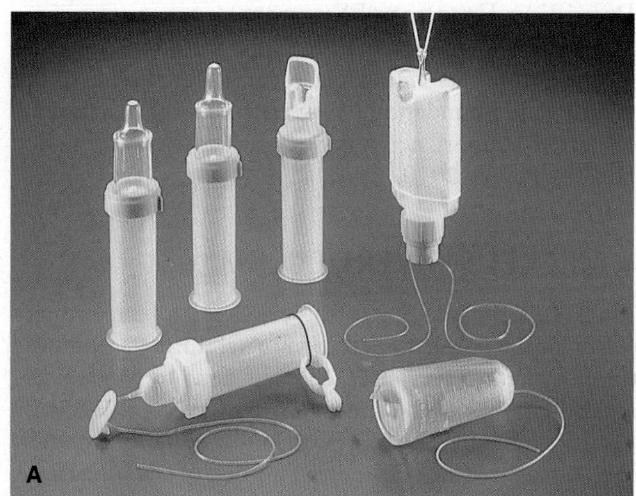

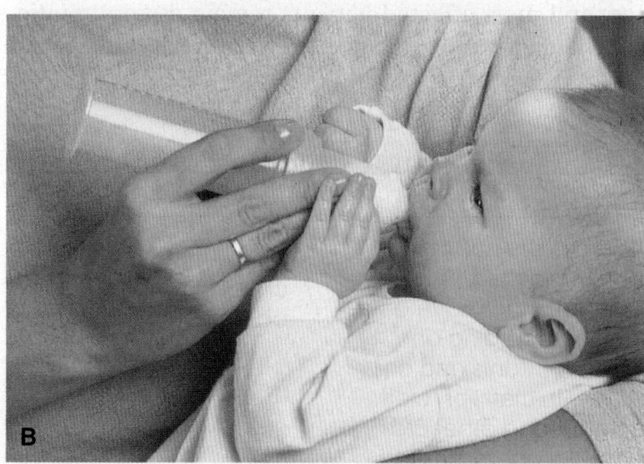

● Figure 21.6 (**A**) Specialty feeding devices used for infants with cleft lip and cleft palate. (**B**) An infant uses a Haberman Feeder.

The infant with cleft palate is at risk for aspiration with oral feeding. In some instances a prosthodontic device may be created to form a false palate covering. This device may prevent breast milk or formula from being aspirated. Breastfeeding may be effective in the infant with cleft palate due to the pliability of the breast and the fact that breast tissue may cover the opening in the palate. Postoperatively, some surgeons allow breastfeeding to be resumed almost immediately. In the bottle-fed infant special nipples or feeders may have to be used. When the suture line is healed, ordinary feeding may resume.

Encouraging Infant–Parent Bonding

For some parents, the appearance of a cleft lip is appalling. Encourage parents to hold the medically stable infant immediately after delivery to encourage bonding. Acknowledge normal feelings of guilt, anger, and sadness. Support the parents in providing care for the infant, particularly feeding, which is a viewed as a significant nurturing function. Provide education about the anticipated surgical procedure and eventual normal appearance of the child's lip.

Providing Emotional Support

Many families will benefit from support in addition to that received from the craniofacial team. Refer parents to the Cleft Palate Foundation (www.cleftline.org) or a parent-to-parent support network such as www.cleft.org. See Healthy People 2010.

• MECKEL'S DIVERTICULUM

Meckel's diverticulum is the result of an incomplete fusion of the omphalomesenteric duct during embryonic development. This causes a fibrous band to connect the small intestine to the umbilicus, known as a Meckel's diverticulum (Fig. 21.7). It is the most common congenital anomaly of the GI tract. The risk of complications from Meckel's diverticulum decreases with advancing age, and most affected patients remain asymptomatic. Thus, infants under the age of 1 year are at the greatest risk for complications (21%). The disorder is more common in males than females (Wyllie, 2004d).

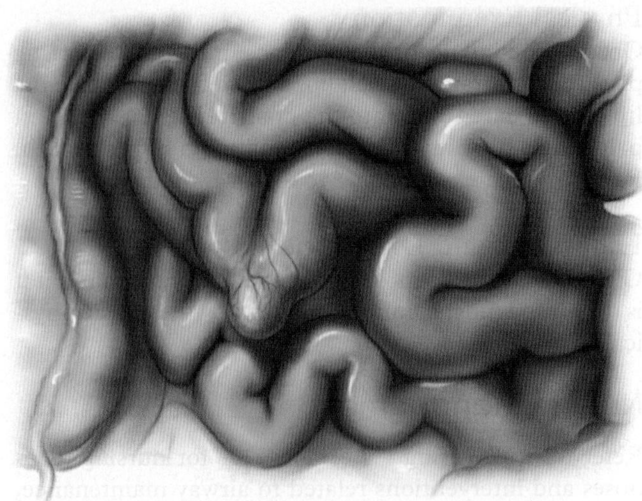

• Figure 21.7 A Meckel's diverticulum is usually found within 100 cm of the ileocecal valve.

The location of a Meckel's diverticulum is on the anterior mesenteric border of the ileum, 40 to 90 cm from the ileocecal valve. The length of the diverticulum can be up to 5 cm and the diameter up to 2 cm (Wyllie, 2004d). The diverticulum contains all of the layers of the intestinal wall, and peptic ulceration of the ileal mucosa adjacent to the ectopic gastric tissue of the diverticulum causes bleeding. Complications associated with Meckel's diverticulum include bleeding, anemia, and intestinal obstruction (most commonly seen as volvulus and intussusception in children) (Shukla, 2002).

Surgical correction of the Meckel's diverticulum is necessary in patients who have complications. The surgery is usually done to remove the diverticulum itself. At times, ileal resection is necessary.

Nursing Assessment

For a full description of the assessment phase of the nursing process refer to page 662. Assessment findings pertinent to Meckel's diverticulum are discussed below.

Health History

Elicit a description of the present illness and chief complaint. Common signs and symptoms reported during the health history might include:

- Bleeding
- Anemia
- Severe colicky abdominal pain (in children with associated intestinal obstruction)

Physical Examination

Assess the child for an acute abdomen. Observe for abdominal distention, palpate for an abdominal mass, assess for

HEALTHY PEOPLE 2010

Objective	Significance
Increase the number of states and the District of Columbia that have a system for recording and referring infants and children with cleft lips, cleft palates, and other craniofacial anomalies to craniofacial anomaly rehabilitative teams.	• Ensure that your office, clinic, or hospital participates in such a system. • If it does not, advocate for such participation.

abdominal **guarding** and rebound tenderness, and auscultate for hypoactive bowel sounds.

Laboratory and Diagnostic Tests

Common laboratory and diagnostic tests ordered for assessment of Meckel's diverticulum include:

- Abdominal x-rays to rule out an acute obstructive process
- Meckel's scan (conclusive)
- Stool tests for color, consistency, and occult blood (usually positive in Meckel's diverticulum)
- Complete blood count (CBC) to assess for anemia

Nursing Management

If anemia is significant, administer ordered blood products (packed red blood cells) to stabilize the patient before surgery. Administer intravenous fluids and maintain NPO status for symptomatic patients while further evaluation is being performed. Immediately report an acute abdomen to a physician. Postoperative care will vary depending on the surgery that was performed. Provide patient and family education as necessary to relieve anxiety related to the diagnosis and surgical intervention. Refer to the Nursing Care Plan 21.1 for additional information.

OMPHALOCELE AND GASTROSCHISIS

Anterior abdominal wall defects, such as omphalocele and gastroschisis, occur in some infants (Fig. 21.8). The diagnosis of omphalocele and gastroschisis is usually made during a prenatal ultrasound examination. Omphalocele usually is associated closely with other congenital anomalies, such as chromosomal abnormalities, diaphragmatic hernia, and heart defects. Gastroschisis tends to be associated with other anomalies less frequently. An omphalocele occurs when the intestine and other viscera, covered by a sac, herniate into the umbilical cord. In gastroschisis, the intestine and stomach herniate through the abdominal wall laterally and to the right of the normal umbilical cord (Lockridge et al., 2002).

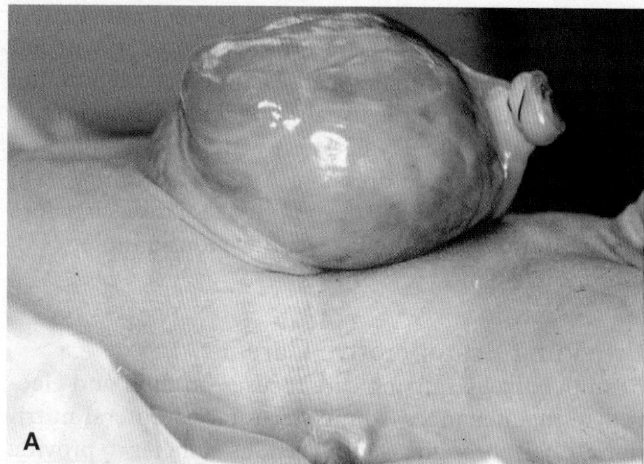

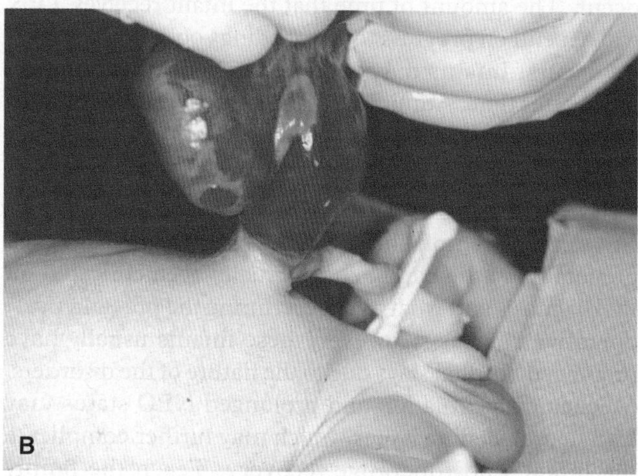

Figure 21.8 (**A**) Omphalocele: a membranous sac covers the exposed organs. (**B**) In gastroschisis, the organs are not covered by a membrane.

Therapeutic Management

A pediatric surgeon should see the baby at delivery to determine the extent of the defect and possible complications. Surgical repair of gastroschisis is done emergently due to the high risk of intestinal **atresia**, resulting in obstruction. Primary repair of gastroschisis is usually performed without incident, unless the contents cannot fit into the abdominal cavity. This occurs more often with a large omphalocele. In this situation a staged closure is performed: this entails covering the defect with a synthetic material that is sequentially "squeezed like toothpaste" to reduce the defect into the abdominal cavity. After enough of the defect is in the abdominal cavity, a surgical repair is performed (Lockridge et al., 2002). If damage to the exposed organs occurs, such as necrosis, then the necrotic sections are removed during the repair. If a significant amount of small intestine is lost, then the complication of short gut syndrome may occur.

Nursing Assessment

Assess infants born with either omphalocele or gastroschisis repeatedly for proper hydration status. Since infants with omphalocele are at much higher risk for associated congenital problems, perform a complete nursing assessment routinely to look for possible complications from undiagnosed conditions.

Nursing Management

Nursing management of the child with omphalocele and gastroschisis consists primarily of providing preoperative and postoperative care and family education.

Providing Preoperative Care

Nursing management in the postnatal/preoperative period should be focused on fluid promotion and management.

Once the infant is placed on NPO status, immediately start intravenous fluids. Before surgery, or if a staged reduction occurs, nursing care is aimed at keeping the infant warmed properly, usually under a radiant warmer. Cover the abdominal wall defect with a plastic film and wrap it with a sterile dressing. A nasogastric tube will most likely be inserted to decompress the stomach before repair. If ordered, administer intravenous antibiotics to prevent infection.

Providing Postoperative Care

Postoperatively, nursing care focuses on fluid and electrolyte maintenance. Administer total parenteral nutrition (TPN) through a central venous catheter to provide nutrition while bowel rest and healing of the surgical site occur. The amount of time that the infant receives TPN will depend on progress to oral feedings once bowel motility occurs. Infants may require mechanical ventilation during this time. Administer antibiotics to prevent or treat infection (Lockridge et al., 2002).

Providing Family Education

Most cases of omphalocele or gastroschisis are diagnosed prenatally, so the parents have usually been educated on the diagnosis and what to expect during the pre- and postoperative courses. However, these infants usually have prolonged hospital stays due to the nature of the disorders. Mechanical ventilation and prolonged NPO status may lead to oral feeding issues, which may further complicate the infant's postoperative recovery. Teach the family regarding all aspects of care to help decrease their anxiety. Refer families to a support network such as the online group at www.omphalocele.com.

INGUINAL AND UMBILICAL HERNIAS

Inguinal and umbilical hernias are defects that occur during fetal development. They are one of the most common reasons why infants and children are referred to pediatric surgeons.

Inguinal Hernia

Inguinal hernias occur in 0.8% to 4.4% of children, most commonly in premature infants. Boys are 3 to 10 times more likely to have an inguinal hernia than girls (Katz, 2001). In most cases of inguinal hernia, the processus vaginalis fails to completely close, which then allows the abdominal or pelvic viscera to enter the patent processus and travel through the internal inguinal ring into the inguinal canal. The hernia sacs that develop most often contain bowel in males and fallopian tubes or ovaries in females. Surgical correction of the inguinal hernia is usually performed when the infant is several weeks old and has been thriving.

Nursing Assessment

Assess infants and children with an inguinal hernia for the presence of a bulging mass in the lower abdomen or groin area (Fig. 21.9). It may be possible to visualize the mass, but often the mass is seen only during crying or straining, making it difficult to actually identify in the clinic setting.

Nursing Management

If a mass is felt upon palpation, the physician may attempt to reduce the hernia by pushing it back through the external inguinal ring. The nurse may be asked to help assist in a reduction, most likely helping to hold the child in a position that will allow the physician to reduce the hernia. If reduction is not possible even with patient sedation, the hernia could be incarcerated. An incarcerated hernia could eventually lead to bowel strangulation.

Reduction is only a temporary method of managing inguinal hernias; they must be corrected surgically. The hernia should be manually reduced as needed until the time of the surgery, so teach the family how to reduce the hernia. Instruct the family to contact the surgeon immediately if the hernia becomes irreducible. Routine pre- and postoperative care is expected during inguinal hernia surgical repair. Provide patient and family education to relieve anxiety.

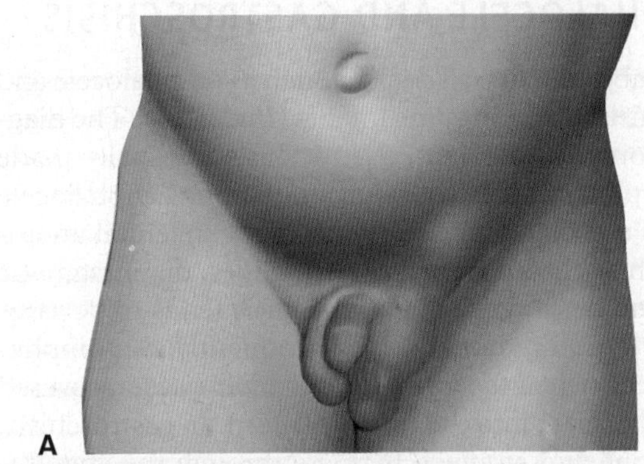

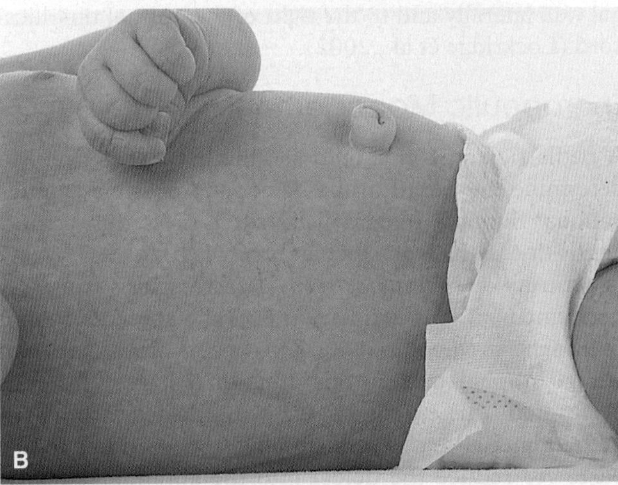

● Figure 21.9 (**A**) Inguinal hernia: note the bulge in the inguinal (groin) area. (**B**) Umbilical hernia: note the protrusion in the umbilical area.

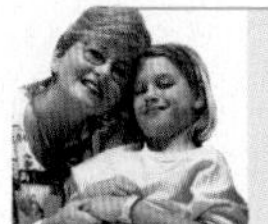

Tell the parents that if the child's inguinal hernia becomes hard, discolored, or painful (inconsolable crying), they should immediately call the physician to determine the next course of action (office visit or emergency room visit).

Umbilical Hernia

Umbilical hernia occurs in 10% to 30% of term infants but up to 75% of preterm infants (Katz, 2001). An umbilical hernia is caused by an incomplete closure of the umbilical ring, allowing intestinal contents to herniate through the opening. Unlike inguinal hernias, most umbilical hernias are not corrected surgically. Most children will have spontaneous closure of the umbilical hernia by age 5 (Katz, 2001). Surgical correction is necessary only for the largest umbilical hernias that have failed to close by age 5 years.

Nursing Assessment

Assess whether the hernia can be reduced. Notify the surgeon if the hernia will not reduce. Incarceration is extremely rare, but when it does occur, the child will report abdominal pain, tenderness, or redness at the umbilicus (see Fig. 21.9).

Nursing Management

Since operative repair is not as likely with umbilical hernias as with inguinal hernias, the aim of nursing management is education. Teach the patient and family how to reduce the hernia. The child may have some self-esteem issues related to the large protrusion of the unrepaired umbilical hernia. Teach the child coping skills to help relieve anxiety.

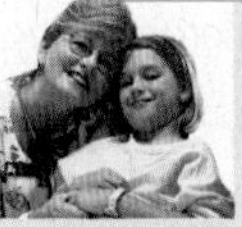

The use of home remedies to reduce an umbilical hernia should be discouraged because of the risk of bowel strangulation. This includes taping a quarter over a reduced umbilical hernia and the use of "belly bands."

ANORECTAL MALFORMATIONS

Malformations of the anal opening (imperforate anus) occur as often as 1 in 5,000 births. The obvious lack of an anal opening in the newborn is simple to recognize, but imperforate anus also occurs as a blind rectal opening. Frequently, a fistula accompanies the malformation from the distal part of the rectum into the perineum or genitourinary system. Anorectal malformations may be associated with other anomalies (Box 21.1) (Peña, 2004).

Imperforate anus can be characterized as either high or low, depending on where the lesion ends as related to the levator ani muscle complex (Fig. 21.10). High lesions may end with a fistula from the bowel to the bladder, urethra, or vagina. This type of imperforate anus necessitates a colostomy to divert the colon to a stoma for a period of time after anorectoplasty is performed in order to allow healing to occur. Low lesions have a perineal fistula, and dilation of the fistula can be performed to correct the lesion. Some infants require a staged repair in which the bowel is connected to the anal opening or an anal opening is created. Often several corrective surgeries must be performed to correct the genitourinary problems associated with imperforate anus (Peña, 2004; Wesson & Haddock, 2000).

BOX 21.1

ANOMALIES ASSOCIATED WITH ANORECTAL MALFORMATIONS

- VACTERL syndrome: **v**ertebral, **a**norectal, **c**ardiovascular, **t**racheo**e**sophageal, **r**enal, and **l**imb
- Esophageal atresia
- Intestinal atresia
- Malrotation
- Renal agenesis
- Hypospadias
- Vesicoureteral reflux
- Bladder exstrophy
- Cardiac anomalies
- Skeletal anomalies

Nursing Assessment

In the infant suspected of having an imperforate anus, assess for common signs and symptoms of intestinal obstruction, which may occur as a result of the malformation. These include abdominal distention and bilious vomiting. In the newborn, observe for an appropriate anal opening. If the anal opening exists, observe for a meconium stool to be passed within the first 24 hours of life. Assess urine output to identify genitourinary problems. Radiographic studies may be ordered to further assess for complications associated with imperforate anus.

Nursing Management

Preoperatively, provide intravenous fluids. Infants are not fed during this time in order to decrease intestinal motility. Postoperatively, teach colostomy care to the family whose child required a permanent or temporary colostomy for passage of stool. Assess for and teach the parents about postoperative complications, including strictures, prolapse, constipation, or incontinence. Review long-term care regarding bowel continence with the family; the child with a high lesion may have problems with fecal incontinence up to school age.

After the intestinal pull-through procedure is done when the infant is several months old, it will be the first time that stool has passed through the anal sphincter. The stool may be quite loose depending on the severity of the imperforate anus. The perianal skin is at significant

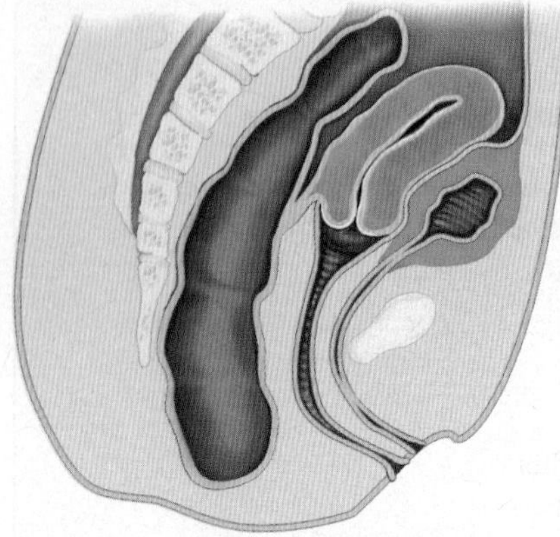

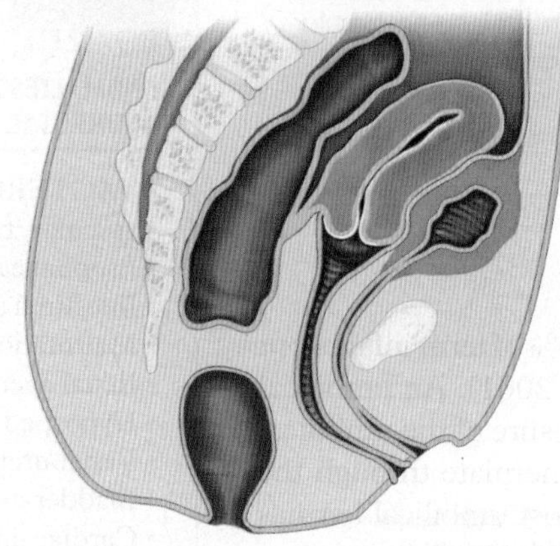

● Figure 21.10 In imperforate anus, there is not an obvious anal opening from the rectum.

risk for breakdown, so a barrier cream should be used on that area and it should be cleaned once daily with soap and water. Otherwise, wipe liquid stool off the barrier cream with mineral oil and cotton balls. Most of the barrier cream will remain intact, protecting the infant's perianal area.

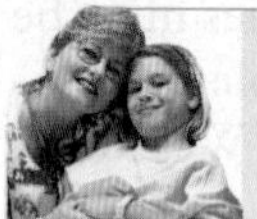

To decrease the drying associated with frequent cleaning, avoid baby wipes and frequent use of soap and water.

Acute GI Disorders

Acute GI disorders include dehydration, vomiting, diarrhea, oral candidiasis, oral lesions, hypertrophic pyloric stenosis, necrotizing enterocolitis, intussusception, malrotation and volvulus, appendicitis, and Meckel's diverticulum.

● DEHYDRATION

Dehydration occurs more readily in infants and young children than it does in adults. The risk is increased in infants and young children because they have an increased extracellular fluid percentage and a relative increase in body water compared to adults. Increased basal metabolic rate, increased body surface area, immature renal function, and increased insensible fluid loss through temperature elevation also contribute to the increased risk for dehydration in infants and young children as compared to adults. Dehydration left unchecked leads to shock, so early recognition and treatment of dehydration is critical to prevent progression to hypovolemic shock. The goals of therapeutic management of dehydration are to restore appropriate fluid balance and to prevent complications.

Nursing Assessment

For a full description of the assessment phase of the nursing process refer to page 662. Assessment findings pertinent to dehydration are discussed below.

Health History

Elicit a description of the present illness and chief complaint. Common signs and symptoms reported during the health history are included in Comparison Chart 21.1, which compares the clinical manifestations of mild, moderate, and severe dehydration.

Explore the client's current and past medical history for risk factors for dehydration such as:

- Diarrhea
- Vomiting
- Decreased oral intake
- Sustained high fever
- Diabetic ketoacidosis
- Extensive burns

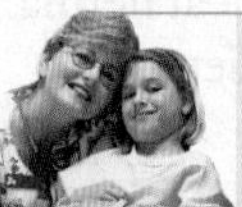

Nurses must be able to assess a child's hydration status accurately and intervene quickly. Children are at higher risk than adults for hypovolemic shock. Dehydrated children may deteriorate very quickly and experience shock.

Physical Examination and Laboratory and Diagnostic Tests

Assess the child's hydration status: heart rate, blood pressure, skin turgor, fontanels, oral mucosa, eyes, temperature and color of extremities, mental status, and urine output. Children usually compensate well initially; their heart rate increases in moderate dehydration, but blood pressure remains normal until it decreases in severe dehydration.

Nursing Management

Nursing goals for the infant or child with dehydration are aimed at restoring fluid volume and preventing progression to hypovolemia. Provide oral rehydration to children for mild to moderate states of dehydration (CDC, 2003; Dale, 2004) (Teaching Guideline 21.2). Children with severe dehydration should receive intravenous fluids. Initially, administer 20 mL/kg of normal saline or lactated Ringer's, and then reassess the hydration status (refer to Chapter 32 for further specifics regarding hypovolemic shock).

COMPARISON CHART 21.1 Dehydration

	Mild	Moderate	Severe
Mental status	Alert	Alert to listless	Alert to comatose
Fontanels	Soft and flat	Sunken	Sunken
Eyes	Normal	Mildly sunken orbits	Deeply sunken orbits
Oral mucosa	Pink and moist	Pale and slightly dry	Dry
Skin turgor	Elastic	Decreased	Tenting
Heart rate	Normal	May be increased	Increased, progressing to bradycardia
Blood pressure	Normal	Normal	Normal, progressing to hypotension
Extremities	Warm, pink, brisk capillary refill	Delayed capillary refill	Cool, mottled or dusky, significantly delayed capillary refill
Urine output	May be slightly decreased	<1 mL/kg/hour	Significantly <1 mL/kg/hour

Once initial fluid balance is restored, the physician may order intravenous fluids at the maintenance rate or as much as 1.5 times maintenance. Maintenance fluid requirements refer to the amount needed under conditions of normal hydration. Maintenance fluid requirements may be determined with the use of the formula found in Box 21.2. In the example provided in Box 21.2, a 23-kg child will need maintenance fluid equivalent to 65 mL/hr.

The same anatomic and physiologic differences that make infants and young children susceptible to dehydration also make them susceptible to overhydration. Thus, continuously evaluate hydration status and be aware of the appropriateness of intravenous fluid orders.

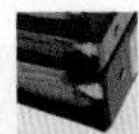

TEACHING GUIDELINE 21.2

Oral Rehydration Therapy

- Oral rehydration solution (ORS) should contain 50 mmol/L sodium and 20 g/L glucose (standard ORS solutions include Pedialyte, Infalyte, and Ricelyte).
- Tap water, milk, undiluted fruit juice, soup, and broth are NOT appropriate for oral rehydration.
- Children with mild to moderate dehydration require 50 to 100 mL/kg of ORS over 4 hours.
- After re-evaluation, oral rehydration may need to be continued if the child is still dehydrated.
- When rehydrated, the child can resume a regular diet.

From Berman, 2003.

VOMITING

Vomiting is the forceful expulsion of gastric contents through the mouth (Ulshen, 2004c). It occurs as a reflex with three different phases:

- Prodromal period: nausea and signs of autonomic nervous system stimulation
- Retching
- Vomiting

Vomiting in infants and children has many different causes and is considered to be a symptom of some other condition. Table 21.1 lists common causes of vomiting.

Therapeutic management of vomiting most often involves slow oral rehydration and at times may require administration of antiemetics.

BOX 21.2

FORMULA FOR FLUID MAINTENANCE

- 100 mL/kg for first 10 kg
- 50 mL/kg for next 10 kg
- 20 mL/kg for remaining kg
- Add together for total mL needed per 24-hour period.
- Divide by 24 for mL/hr fluid requirement.

Thus, for a 23-kg child:

- 100 × 10 = 1,000
- 50 × 10 = 500
- 20 × 3 = 60
- 1,000 + 500 + 60 = 1,560

1,560/24 = 65 mL/hr

Table 21.1 Causes of Vomiting by Temporal Pattern

Category	Acute	Chronic	Cyclic
Infectious	Gastroenteritis, otitis media, pharyngitis, sinusitis (acute), hepatitis, pyelonephritis, meningitis	*H. pylori*, *Giardia*, sinusitis (chronic)	Chronic sinusitis
GI	Intussusception, malrotation with volvulus, appendicitis, cholecystitis, pancreatitis	GERD, gastritis, peptic ulcer disease	GERD, malrotation with volvulus
Genitourinary	Ureteropelvic junction obstruction, pyelonephritis	Pregnancy, pyelonephritis	Hydronephrosis
Endocrine/Metabolic	Diabetic ketoacidosis	Adrenal hyperplasia	Diabetic ketoacidosis, Addison's disease, acute intermittent porphyria
Neurologic	Concussion, subdural hematoma, brain tumor	Brain tumor, Arnold-Chiari malformation	Migraines, Arnold-Chiari malformation, brain tumor
Other	Food poisoning, toxic ingestion	Bulimia, rumination	Cyclic vomiting syndrome

GERD, gastroesophageal reflux disease.

Nursing Assessment

For a full description of the assessment phase of the nursing process refer to page 662. Assessment findings pertinent to vomiting are discussed below.

Health History

Elicit a description of the present illness and chief complaint. Note onset and progression of symptoms. The assessment of an infant or child with vomiting should include a history of the vomiting events, including:

- Contents/character of the emesis
- Effort and force of vomiting episodes
- Timing

Contents and character of the vomitus may give clues to the cause of vomiting. Bilious vomiting is never considered normal and suggests an obstruction distal to the ampulla of Vater. Bloody emesis can signify esophageal or GI bleeding. Assess the effort and force of vomiting to identify whether the episodes are effortful and projectile, as with pyloric stenosis, or effortless, as is often seen in gastroesophageal reflux. The timing of the vomiting also is helpful in determining the cause. Vomiting that occurs several hours past meals could signify delayed gastric emptying. When vomiting occurs upon waking or in the middle of the night, particularly if it is associated with headaches, an intracranial lesion or tumor may be suspected. Note any associated events, such as diarrhea or pain.

Diarrhea may occur with viral gastroenteritis or food poisoning. Pain in the epigastric area could signify peptic ulcer disease, pancreatitis, or cholecystitis. Assess the client's past medical history to identify preexisting illnesses, drug abuse, trauma, prescribed medications, and previous abdominal surgery (Ulshen, 2004c). Risk factors for vomiting include exposure to viruses, certain medication use, and overfeeding in an infant.

Physical Examination

Perform a physical examination, noting the child's general appearance. Note hydration status, as well as mental status changes. Note the quality of bowel sounds upon auscultation. Palpate the abdomen for the presence of abdominal masses, tenderness, or signs of trauma.

Laboratory and Diagnostic Tests

Laboratory studies may be ordered to assess the child's hydration status or to rule out certain causes of vomiting, such as urinary tract infection, pancreatitis, or an acute infectious process. Common laboratory and diagnostic tests ordered for assessment of the cause of vomiting include:

- Abdominal ultrasound
- Upper GI series
- Plain abdominal radiographs

Nursing Management

Nursing management focuses on promoting fluid and electrolyte balance. Oral rehydration is accomplished successfully in most outpatient cases of simple vomiting. Teach the primary caregiver about oral rehydration (refer to Teaching Guideline 21.2). In the child with mild to moderate dehydration resulting from vomiting, oral feeding should be withheld for 1 to 2 hours after emesis, after which time oral rehydration can begin. Give the infant or child 0.5 to 2 ounces of oral rehydration solution every 15 minutes, depending on the child's age and size. Most infants and children can retain this small amount of fluid if fed the restricted amount every 15 minutes. As the child improves, larger amounts will be tolerated (CDC, 2003; Dale, 2004).

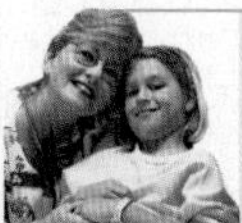

Homemade oral rehydration solution can be made by combining 1 quart of water (can be water poured from cooking rice if desired), 8 teaspoons sugar, and 1 teaspoon salt.

If oral rehydration is not possible due to continued nausea and vomiting, intravenous fluids will likely be ordered. In some cases, antiemetics may be used to help control the vomiting. Some antiemetics can cause drowsiness or other side effects and should not be used until a definitive diagnosis is made or severe pathologic processes can be excluded. Educate the family regarding the prevention of vomiting and use of antiemetic therapy.

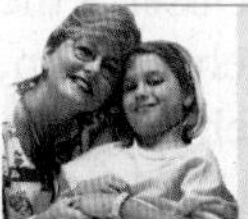

Ginger capsules, ginger tea, and candied ginger are generally useful in reducing nausea, are safe for use in children, and usually produce no side effects. Most commercially produced "ginger ale" no longer contains real ginger and so is of limited usefulness (Gardiner & Kemper, 2005).

DIARRHEA

Diarrhea is either an increase in the frequency or a decrease in the consistency of stool (Ulshen, 2004c). Diarrhea in children can either be acute or chronic. Acute infectious diarrhea (gastroenteritis) remains the leading cause of death for children worldwide. In the United States, the incidence of diarrhea varies between 1 and 2.5 episodes per child per year, leading to approximately 38 million cases, 2 to 3.7 million physician visits, 220,000 hospitalizations, and 325 to 425 deaths annually (Berman, 2003).

Pathophysiology

Acute diarrhea in children is most commonly caused by viruses, but it may also be related to bacterial or parasitic enteropathogens. Viruses injure the absorptive surface of mature villous cells, resulting in decreased fluid absorption and disaccharidase deficiency. Bacteria produce intestinal injury by directly invading the mucosa, damaging the villous surface, or releasing toxins (Berman, 2003). Acute diarrhea may be bloody or nonbloody. The viral, bacterial, and parasitic causes of acute infectious diarrhea are discussed in Box 21.3. Diarrhea may also occur in relation to antibiotic use. Risk factors for acute diarrhea include recent ingestion of undercooked meats, foreign travel, daycare attendance, and well water use.

Though most cases of diarrhea in children are of acute origin, it may also occur chronically. Chronic diarrhea is diarrhea that lasts for more than 2 weeks. This type of diarrhea is not usually caused by serious illnesses. The causes of chronic diarrhea are listed in Box 21.4 according to age groups.

Since most cases of diarrhea are acute and viral in nature, therapeutic management of diarrhea is usually supportive (maintaining fluid balance and nutrition). Probiotic supplementation may decrease the length and extent of diarrhea (Young & Huffman, 2003). Bacterial and parasitic causes of diarrhea may be treated with antibiotics or antiparasitic medications, respectively.

Nursing Assessment

For a full description of the assessment phase of the nursing process refer to page 662. Assessment findings pertinent to diarrhea are discussed below.

Health History

Elicit a description of the present illness and chief complaint. Important information related to the course of the diarrhea includes:

- Number and frequency of stools
- Duration of symptoms
- Stool volume
- Associated symptoms (abdominal pain, cramping, nausea, vomiting, fever)
- Presence of blood or mucus in the stool

Explore the client's current and past medical history for risk factors such as:

- Likelihood of exposure to infectious agents (well water, farm animals, daycare attendance)
- Dietary history
- Family history of similar symptoms
- Recent travel
- Patient age (to identify common etiology for that age group)

BOX 21.3

CAUSES OF ACUTE INFECTIOUS DIARRHEA

Viral	Bacterial	Parasitic
Rotavirus: characterized by acute onset of fever and vomiting, followed by loose, watery stools; most common cause of viral diarrhea	Salmonella: usually from ingestion of poultry, meats, or dairy products. Infants are at highest risk. Bacteria are excreted for up to 1 year. Severe cases are treated with antibiotics.	*Giardia lamblia:* the most common intestinal parasite in the United States; oral–fecal transmission; sudden onset of watery, foul-smelling stool; often causes gassiness and belching; treated with antiparasitic medications
Adenovirus 40 and 41: second most common cause of viral diarrhea illnesses, similar characteristics to rotavirus	*Escherichia coli* 0157:H7: most often associated with gross bloody stools and abdominal cramping; may lead to hemolytic-uremic syndrome	*Entamoeba histolytica:* oral–fecal transmission; more common outside of United States; colitis symptoms common
Norwalk virus: more common in older children and adults; characterized by vomiting, nausea, and cramping abdominal pain	Campylobacter: symptoms vary from mild diarrhea to dysentery; severe cases may be treated with antibiotics	*Cryptosporidium:* spread via farm animals and people; fecal–oral transmission; watery diarrhea, nausea, vomiting, and flu-like symptoms. No definitive treatment.
Caliciviruses: affected age usually 3 months to 6 years, seen in daycare settings	Shigella: high fevers and bloody stools are common; may cause seizures with fever. Treatment with antibiotics is recommended.	
Astrovirus: affected age usually 1 to 3 years, causing vomiting, diarrhea, fever, and abdominal pain	*Clostridium difficile:* usually related to antibiotic use; may cause pseudomembranous colitis in severe cases. Infants may be carriers of the bacteria and asymptomatic. Treatment with anti-infective medications may be helpful. Probiotic therapy is usually recommended.	
Cytomegalovirus (CMV): causes other medical problems, but may cause diarrhea with colitis	*Yersinia enterocolitica:* usually affects children less than 5 years of age; watery or mucoid diarrhea common, occasionally with gross blood	

BOX 21.4

CAUSES OF CHRONIC DIARRHEA BY AGE

Infants	Toddlers	School-Age Children
Intractable diarrhea of infancy	Chronic nonspecific diarrhea	Inflammatory bowel disease
Milk and soy protein intolerance	Viral enteritis	Appendiceal abscess
Infectious enteritis	*Giardia*	Lactase deficiency
Hirschsprung's disease	Tumors (secretory diarrhea)	Constipation with encopresis
Nutrient malabsorption	Ulcerative colitis	
	Celiac disease	

Physical Examination

Inspection

Assess the child with diarrhea for dehydration. Observe the child's general appearance and color. In mild dehydration, the child may appear normal. In moderate dehydration, the eyes may have decreased tear production or sunken orbits. Mucous membranes may also be dry. Mental status may be compromised with moderate to severe dehydration, as evidenced by listlessness or lethargy. Skin may be nonelastic or exhibit tenting, signifying lack of proper hydration. Abdominal distention or concavity may be present. Urine output may also be decreased if the child is dehydrated. Stool output may be available to assess for color and consistency. Inspect the anal area for presence of redness or rash related to increased stool volumes and increased frequency.

Auscultation

Auscultate bowel sounds to assess for presence of hypoactive or hyperactive bowel sounds. Hypoactive bowel sounds may indicate obstruction or peritonitis. Hyperactive bowel sounds may indicate diarrhea/gastroenteritis.

Percussion

Percuss the abdomen. Note any abnormalities; the presence of abnormalities on examination for a diagnosis of acute or chronic diarrhea would indicate a pathologic process.

Palpation

Tenderness in the lower quadrants may be related to gastroenteritis. Rebound tenderness or pain should not be found on palpation; if found, it could indicate appendicitis or peritonitis.

Laboratory and Diagnostic Tests

Common laboratory and diagnostic studies ordered for the assessment of diarrhea include:

- Stool culture: may indicate presence of bacteria
- Stool for ova and parasites (O&P): may indicate the presence of parasites
- Stool viral panel or culture: to determine presence of rotavirus or other viruses
- Stool for occult blood: may be positive if inflammation or ulceration is present in the GI tract
- Stool for leukocytes: may be positive in cases of inflammation or infection
- Stool pH/reducing substances: to see if the diarrhea is caused by carbohydrate intolerance
- Electrolyte panel: may indicate dehydration
- Abdominal x-rays (KUB): presence of stool in colon may indicate constipation or **fecal impaction**; air–fluid levels may indicate intestinal obstruction

Nursing Management

Nursing management of the child with diarrhea focuses on restoring fluid and electrolyte balance and providing family education.

Restoring Fluid and Electrolyte Balance

Continue the child's regular diet if the child is not dehydrated. Initial nursing management of the dehydrated child with diarrhea is focused on fluid and electrolyte balance restoration. Refer to the Nursing Care Plan Overview on page 670. Probiotic supplementation while a child is taking antibiotics for other disorders may reduce the incidence of antibiotic-related diarrhea (Young & Huffman, 2003). After rehydration is achieved, it is important to encourage the child to consume a regular diet to maintain energy and growth (Brunell, 2006) (see Common Medical Treatments 21.1).

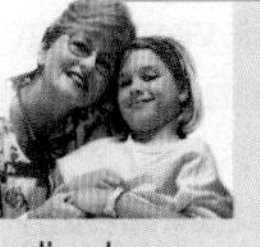

Avoid prolonged use of clear liquids in the child with diarrhea because "starvation stools" may result. Also avoid fluids high in glucose, such as fruit juice, gelatin, and soda, which may worsen diarrhea.

Providing Family Education

Teach the parents the importance of oral rehydration therapy (see Teaching Guideline 21.2). The physician may order medication therapy. In such instances, teach the importance of finishing all prescribed antibiotic therapy. After the cause of the diarrhea is known, teach the child and family how to prevent further occurrences. As most cases of acute diarrhea are infectious, provide education about proper hand washing techniques and transmission route. Chronic diarrhea is often a result of excessive intake of formula, water, or fruit juice, so teach the parents about appropriate fluid intake.

ORAL CANDIDIASIS (THRUSH)

Oral candidiasis (thrush) is a fungal infection of the oral mucosa. It is most common in newborns and infants. Children at risk for thrush include those with immune disorders and those receiving therapy that suppresses the immune system (e.g., chemotherapy for cancer). Children who use corticosteroid inhalers are also at increased risk for the development of thrush. Antibiotic use may also contribute to thrush. Fungal infection may be transmitted between the infant and breastfeeding mother.

Therapeutic management includes treatment with oral antifungal agents such as Mycostatin (nystatin) or fluconazole.

Nursing Assessment

Assess for risk factors for oral candidiasis such as young age, immune suppression, antibiotic use, use of corticosteroid inhalers, or presence of fungal infection in the mother. Inspect the oral mucosa. Thrush appears as thick white patches on the tongue, mucosa, or palate, resembling curdled milk (Fig. 21.11). Unlike milk retained in the mouth, the patches do not easily wipe off with a swab or washcloth. Also assess for presence of candidal diaper

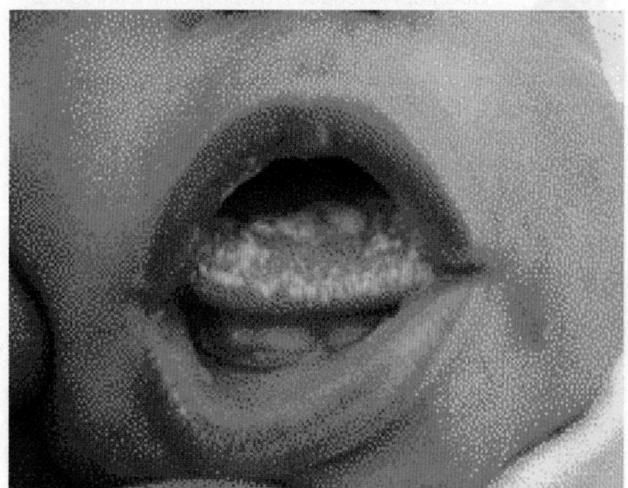

Figure 21.11 Thick white patches in the infant with oral candidiasis (thrush).

rash (beefy-red rash with satellite lesions). Determine the extent to which the presence of the lesions is interfering with the infant's ability to feed. The lesions may cause significant discomfort.

Diagnosis is usually based on clinical presentation, though a careful scraping of the lesions can be sent out for fungal culture.

Nursing Management

Nursing management of the patient with thrush includes administering medications and providing family education.

Administering Medications

Ensure appropriate administration of oral antifungal agents. Mycostatin suspension should be given four times per day following feeding to allow the medication to remain in contact with the lesions. In the younger infant, Mycostatin can be applied to the lesions with a cotton-tipped applicator. The older infant or child can easily swallow the pleasantly flavored suspension. An advantage of fluconazole is its once-daily dosing, but infants and children receiving it should be monitored for hepatotoxicity. Unlike Mycostatin, fluconazole should be administered with food to decrease the side effects of nausea and vomiting.

Educating the Family

If the mother is also infected, she must receive antifungal treatment as well. Fungal infection of the breast can cause the mother a great deal of pain with nursing, but if appropriately treated breastfeeding can continue without interruption. Appropriate hand washing should be stressed. Bottle nipples and pacifiers need to be kept clean. Infants and young children often mouth their toys, so they should also be cleaned appropriately. Parents of infants with thrush should report diaper rash because fungal infections in the diaper area often occur concomitantly with thrush and also need to be treated.

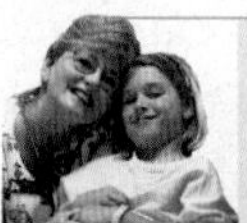

Geographic tongue is a benign, noncontagious condition. A reduction in the filiform papillae (bumps on the tongue) occurs in patches that migrate periodically, thus giving a map-like appearance to the tongue, with darker and lighter, higher and lower patches. Do not confuse the lighter patches of geographic tongue with the thick white plaques that form on the tongue with thrush.

● ORAL LESIONS

A number of oral lesions may affect infants and children. A few of the most common are aphthous ulcers, gingivostomatitis (from herpes simplex virus), and herpangina (Blevins, 2003; Leung & Kao, 2003). Table 21.2 lists the causes of common oral lesions. Regardless of type, oral lesions are often painful and can interfere with the child's ability to eat. Therapeutic management of oral lesions varies depending on the cause.

Nursing Assessment

Explore the health history for the presence of risk factors such as immune deficiency, cancer chemotherapy treatment, exposure to infectious agents, trauma, stress, or celiac or Crohn's disease. Note the onset of the lesion(s) and progression over time. Question the parent or child about presence of sore throat or dysphagia (occurs with herpangina). Inspect the oral cavity, including the tongue, buccal mucosa, palate, and hypoglossal area. Note presence of lesions and their distribution. Refer to Table 21.2 for descriptions and illustrations of various oral lesions. Inspect the pharynx, which may be red with herpangina. Generally the diagnosis is based on the history and clinical presentation, but occasionally oral lesions are cultured for herpes simplex virus (HSV).

Nursing Management

The primary concerns with oral lesions are pain management and maintenance of hydration. A corticosteroid-containing dental paste used for aphthous ulcers is formulated to "stick" to mucous membranes, so the lesion area should be as dry as possible prior to application of the paste. Children do not care for having the paste applied and will often resist. Older children with herpangina or stomatitis can "swish and spit" various formulations of "magic mouthwash" (typically a combination of liquid diphenhydramine, liquid acetaminophen, and milk of magnesia); they may offer some pain relief. Common over-the-counter medications such as Ambesol, Oragel, and Kanka may be helpful for topical pain relief, though oral analgesics are often necessary.

The child with herpangina is typically a toddler or preschooler. It may be very difficult to coach a young child to drink fluids when his or her mouth is hurting. Playing games and offering favorite fluids and Popsicles may encourage adequate oral intake. Carbonated beverages and citrus juices should be avoided when oral lesions are present as they can cause further stinging and burning.

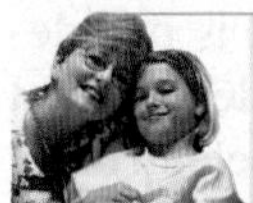

Viscous lidocaine should be used with caution as a topical treatment for numbing the lesions or as a swish-and-spit treatment, as younger children may swallow the lidocaine.

● HYPERTROPHIC PYLORIC STENOSIS

Hypertrophic pyloric stenosis is one of the most common conditions requiring surgery in the first 2 months of life. In pyloric stenosis, the circular muscle of the **pylorus** becomes hypertrophied, causing thickness in the luminal side of the pyloric canal (Fig. 21.12). This thickness creates a gastric outlet obstruction, causing nonbilious vomiting. The vomiting becomes more frequent and forceful as time goes on and is often projectile. The incidence is higher in males than females, and it occurs in whites more commonly than any other ethnic background.

Table 21.2 Oral Lesions

	Aphthous Ulcers	Gingivostomatitis	Herpangina
Cause	Trauma, vitamin deficiency, celiac disease, Crohn's disease	Herpes simplex virus	Enterovirus (Coxsackie)
Appearance	Erythematous border, often yellow appearance to the ulcer, anywhere on oral mucosa or lips	Vesicular lesions on erythematous base, anywhere in oral cavity, including lips	Bright-red ulcers, generally in posterior oral cavity
Fever	Generally absent	May have high fever with initial outbreak	Abrupt onset of high fever (up to 39.4 to 40.6 degrees C), lasting 1 to 4 days
Length of illness	Generally heal within 7 to 14 days; may recur	10 to 12 days initially; may recur with stress, febrile illness, or intense sunlight exposure (as virus lies dormant in system)	Generally resolves within 5 to 7 days
Therapeutic management	Topical corticosteroid in dental paste may help.	Acyclovir	Supportive treatment only

The cause of pyloric stenosis is unknown, though there are theories that the cause could be diet-related or even related to pyloric enervation. Infants with pyloric stenosis typically present with symptoms of nonbilious vomiting between weeks 2 and 4 of life, but infants up to 3 months of age should be considered at risk for developing pyloric stenosis (Letton, 2001).

Pyloric stenosis requires surgical intervention. A pyloromyotomy is performed to cut the muscle of the pylorus and relieve the gastric outlet obstruction (see Fig. 21.12). Postoperative complications are rare.

Nursing Assessment

For a full description of the assessment phase of the nursing process refer to page 662. Assessment findings pertinent to hypertrophic pyloric stenosis are discussed below.

Health History

Elicit a description of the present illness and chief complaint. Common signs and symptoms reported during the health history might include:

- Forceful, nonbilious vomiting, unrelated to feeding position
- Hunger soon after vomiting episode
- Weight loss due to vomiting
- Progressive dehydration with subsequent lethargy

Risk factors include a positive family history. The disorder occurs most frequently in first-born males.

Physical Examination and Laboratory and Diagnostic Tests

Palpate for a hard, moveable "olive" in the right upper quadrant (hypertrophied pylorus). If an easily palpable mass is felt, no further testing is necessary and a surgical

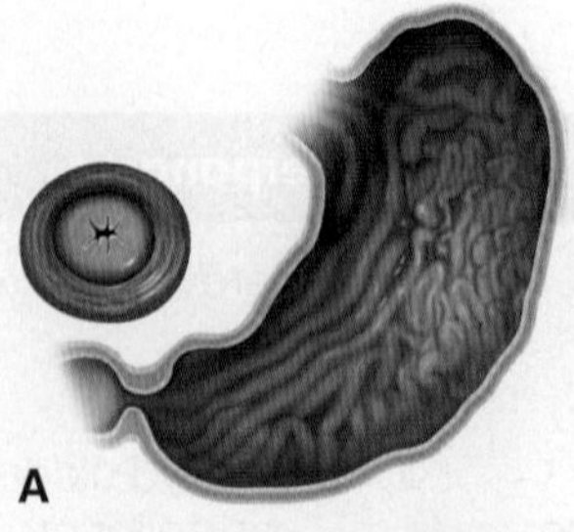

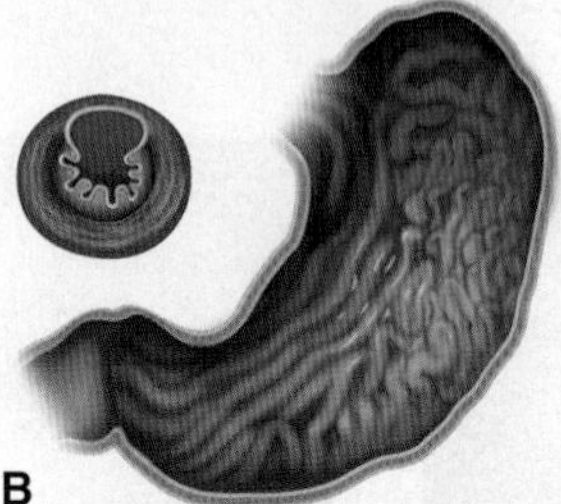

● Figure 21.12 (A) Hypertrophied pylorus muscle and narrowed stomach outlet. (B) In pyloromyotomy, the pylorus is incised, thus increasing the diameter of the pyloric outlet.

consult is called. If no mass is identified, a pyloric ultrasound may be ordered to identify a thickened hypoechoic ring in the region of the pylorus. An upper GI series may identify pyloric stenosis as well, but an ultrasound is less invasive and is considered more diagnostic of pyloric stenosis. Assess laboratory values to determine if the infant has metabolic alkalosis resulting from dehydration.

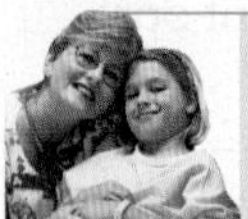

It may be difficult to examine the infant's abdomen when pyloric stenosis is suspected because of the infant's extreme irritability. A pacifier or nipple dipped in glucose water may soothe the infant long enough to obtain the abdominal examination.

Nursing Management

Preoperative management of infants with pyloric stenosis is aimed at fluid management and correcting abnormal electrolyte values. Family anxiety is high during this time because of the impending surgery for an otherwise healthy infant. Provide emotional support to the family. Teach them about the surgical procedure and what to expect postoperatively. After surgery, infants usually resume oral feedings after 1 to 2 days.

● NECROTIZING ENTEROCOLITIS

Necrotizing enterocolitis (NEC) is characterized by ulcerations and necrosis of the distal ileum and proximal colon. It is the most common and most serious acquired GI disorder among hospitalized preterm neonates and is associated with significant acute and chronic morbidity and mortality (Stoll & Kliegman, 2004). The incidence of NEC is 1 to 3 per 1,000 live births; it affects 1% to 5% of all infants in intensive care units (Stoll & Kliegman, 2004).

The pathophysiology of NEC is unknown, but it is thought that the immaturity of GI function is a predisposing factor. The lower the birthweight of the neonate, the more likely it is that he or she will develop NEC. Three factors that play a role in the development of NEC are intestinal ischemia, **enteral** feedings, and bacterial infections.

Therapeutic management of NEC initially consists of bowel rest and antibiotic therapy. Serial KUB x-rays determine resolution or progression of NEC. If medical treatment fails to stabilize the patient or if free air is present on a left lateral decubitus film, surgical intervention will be necessary to resect the portion of necrotic bowel. Surgery for NEC usually requires the placement of a proximal enterostomy until the **anastomosis** site is ready for reconnection.

Nursing Assessment

For a full description of the assessment phase of the nursing process refer to page 662. Assessment findings pertinent to NEC are discussed below.

Health History

Elicit a description of the present illness and chief complaint. Common signs and symptoms reported during the health history might include:

- Abdominal distention and tenderness
- Bloody stools
- Feeding intolerance characterized by bilious vomiting
- Signs of sepsis
- Lethargy
- Apnea
- Shock

Risk factors include prematurity, advancing enteral feedings too quickly, and a history of anoxia/hypoxia or shock.

Physical Examination

Always keep in mind the possibility of NEC when dealing with premature infants, especially when enteral feedings are being administered. Perform a GI assessment on the infant. Consider infants with noticeable abdominal distention and/or high residual gastric volumes suspicious for NEC. Assess perfusion to all vital organs and monitor closely for circulatory collapse.

Laboratory and Diagnostic Tests

Common laboratory and diagnostic tests ordered for assessment of NEC include:

- KUB of the abdomen to confirm the presence of pneumatosis intestinalis (air in the bowel wall)
- Blood laboratory values to assess for increases in the white blood cell count, thrombocytopenia, or neutropenia

Nursing Management

Nursing management of the child with NEC focuses on maintaining fluid and nutritional status, caring for the patient having surgery, and teaching the family about the prognosis.

Maintaining Fluid and Nutritional Status

If NEC is suspected, immediately stop enteral feedings until a diagnosis is made. Administer intravenous fluids initially to restore proper fluid status. If ordered, administer TPN to keep the infant supported nutritionally. Administer prescribed intravenous antibiotics to prevent sepsis from the necrotic bowel. If surgery is required, antibiotics may be needed for an extended time. Restart enteral feedings once the disease has resolved (normal abdominal examination and KUB negative for pneumatosis) or as determined postoperatively by the surgeon.

Teaching the Family About the Prognosis

The diagnosis of NEC may cause significant family anxiety. Teach the family that medically treated NEC is usually limited to a short time and resolves within 48 hours of stopping oral feedings. Surgically treated NEC, however, can involve a much lengthier process. If an extensive amount of bowel has necrosed, the infant is more likely to have long-term medical problems. Short bowel syndrome may result from a large resection (short bowel syndrome is discussed later in this chapter). Reassure the family that though some infants have more involved cases of NEC, the improved parenteral nutrition formulations have given more hope for these infants. Provide education about ostomy care if surgery is required (refer to page 699 for a discussion of ostomy care).

• INTUSSUSCEPTION

Intussusception is a process that occurs when a proximal segment of bowel "telescopes" into a more distal segment, causing edema, vascular compromise, and ultimately partial or total bowel obstruction (Fig. 21.13). Intussusception usually occurs in otherwise healthy infants under age 2. It is three times more likely in males than females. Seventy-five percent to 90% of cases of intussusception occur with no specified "lead point" (i.e., pathologic point) that causes the telescoping. When a lead point is identified, it usually occurs in children over age 5. The most common type of lead point is a Meckel's diverticulum, but other lead points may include duplication cysts, polyps, hemangiomas, tumors, the appendix, or even lymphomas (Wyllie, 2004b). Children with cystic fibrosis, celiac disease, and Crohn's disease may be at higher risk for developing intussusception.

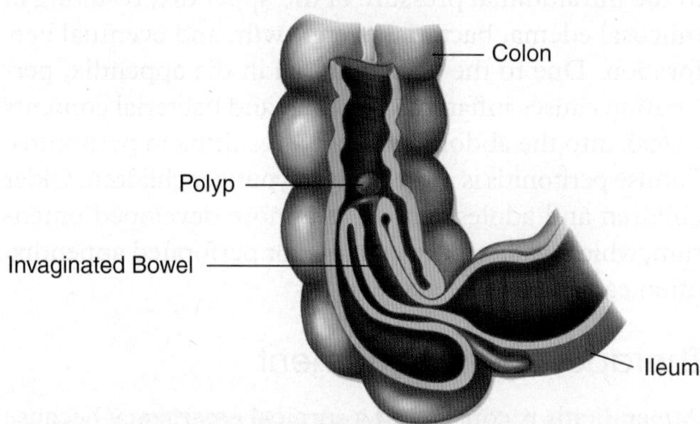

• Figure 21.13 In intussusception, the intestine telescopes upon itself.

A barium enema is successful at reducing a large percentage of intussusception cases; other cases are reduced surgically. If surgical reduction is unsuccessful or bowel necrosis has occurred, a portion of the bowel must be resected.

Nursing Assessment

For a full description of the assessment phase of the nursing process refer to page 662. Assessment findings pertinent to intussusception are discussed below.

Health History

Elicit a description of the present illness and chief complaint. Common signs and symptoms reported during the health history might include:

- Sudden onset of intermittent, crampy abdominal pain
- Severe pain (children usually draw up their knees and scream)
- Vomiting
- Diarrhea
- Currant-jelly stools, gross blood, or Hemoccult-positive stools
- Lethargy

Typically, symptoms flare and then regress. Between episodes, children may have no symptoms of intussusception. This return to a normal state is due to the intussusception reducing on its own. The child may be asymptomatic and may appear well when presenting to the pediatrician or emergency room. Again, this may be a sign that the bowel has reduced spontaneously. Assess the severity of pain, length of time the symptoms have been present, presence of vomiting, and stool patterns and color. Immediately report the presence of bilious vomiting, which occurs only in an obstructive situation. Also assess for signs and symptoms of acute peritonitis. Explore the client's current and past medical history for risk factors, such as cystic fibrosis or celiac disease.

Physical Examination

Palpate the abdomen for the presence of a sausage-shaped mass in the upper mid-abdomen: this is a hallmark sign of intussusception. Note any mental status changes.

Laboratory and Diagnostic Tests

Intussusception is usually diagnosed with an air or barium enema. Use of an enema may show the intussusception and also may reduce it, making the enema therapeutic (Wyllie, 2004b). A pediatric surgeon should be available at the time of the enema in case the enema is unsuccessful or perforation (rare) occurs. White blood cell elevation may occur and electrolytes may show signs of dehydration.

Nursing Management

Administer intravenous fluids and antibiotics before the diagnostic laboratory and radiograph studies are performed. Refer to the Nursing Care Plan 21.1 for nursing management of the postoperative child.

The parents may be very fatigued after dealing with a crying infant. They are often quite anxious about surgery in an otherwise healthy child. Offer emotional support and provide appropriate preoperative and postoperative education to the family.

MALROTATION AND VOLVULUS

Intestinal malrotation occurs during the 10th week of embryonic development. At week 10, the intestine is anchored to the abdominal wall by the base of the mesentery in a specific pattern to avoid kinking or twisting (Wyllie, 2004c). When malrotation occurs, the intestine is abnormally attached and the mesentery narrows, twisting on itself (volvulus). If the volvulus involves the entire small bowel, it is termed a mid-gut volvulus.

The main symptom of malrotation is bilious vomiting. Many children also have abdominal pain, shock symptoms, abdominal distention, tachycardia, and bloody stools. Most cases of malrotation will present in the first few weeks of life, but symptoms may not occur until the patient is well into adulthood.

Therapeutic management of malrotation and volvulus is accomplished surgically. A Ladd procedure is performed, during which the intestine is straightened out and bands contributing to the misalignment are divided. If bowel necrosis has occurred (rare), then an ostomy may be necessary.

Nursing Assessment

For a full description of the assessment phase of the nursing process refer to page 662. Assessment findings pertinent to malrotation and volvulus are discussed below.

Health History

Elicit a description of the present illness and chief complaint. Common signs and symptoms reported during the health history might include vomiting and abdominal pain. Since obstruction can occur with resulting necrosis of the bowel, immediately inform the physician if obstruction is suspected.

Physical Examination and Diagnostic and Laboratory Tests

Observe for severity of pain, palpate for abdominal guarding and rebound tenderness, and auscultate for hypoactive bowel sounds. Common laboratory and diagnostic studies ordered for the assessment of malrotation and volvulus include:

- KUB to reveal obstruction
- Upper GI series to identify the location of the duodenojejunal junction and corkscrew appearance of the twisted bowel

Nursing Management

When diagnostic testing reveals malrotation/volvulus, administer ordered intravenous fluids and intravenous antibiotics. Often a nasogastric tube is placed to decompress the stomach. Surgery is performed as soon as possible. After surgery, provide postoperative care of the child (see Nursing Care Plan 21.1). Provide continuous emotional support and family education.

APPENDICITIS

Appendicitis, an acute inflammation of the appendix, is the most common cause of emergent abdominal surgery in children. It occurs in all age groups; the median age in the pediatric population is 6 to 10 years. The incidence in the United States is 4 per 1,000 children. It occurs twice as often in males than in females.

Pathophysiology

Appendicitis is due to a closed-loop obstruction of the appendix (Fig. 21.14). It is thought that the obstruction is due to fecal material impacted into the relatively narrow appendix, though other causes such as ingested foreign bodies may exist. This causes a subsequent increase in the intraluminal pressure of the appendix, resulting in mucosal edema, bacterial overgrowth, and eventual perforation. Due to the fecal material in the appendix, perforation causes inflammatory fluid and bacterial contents to leak into the abdominal cavity, resulting in peritonitis. Diffuse peritonitis is more likely in younger children. Older children and adolescents have a more developed omentum, which walls off the inflamed or perforated appendix, often causing a focal abscess.

Therapeutic Management

Appendicitis is considered a surgical emergency because if left uncorrected, the appendix may perforate. Surgical removal of the appendix is necessary and is often accom-

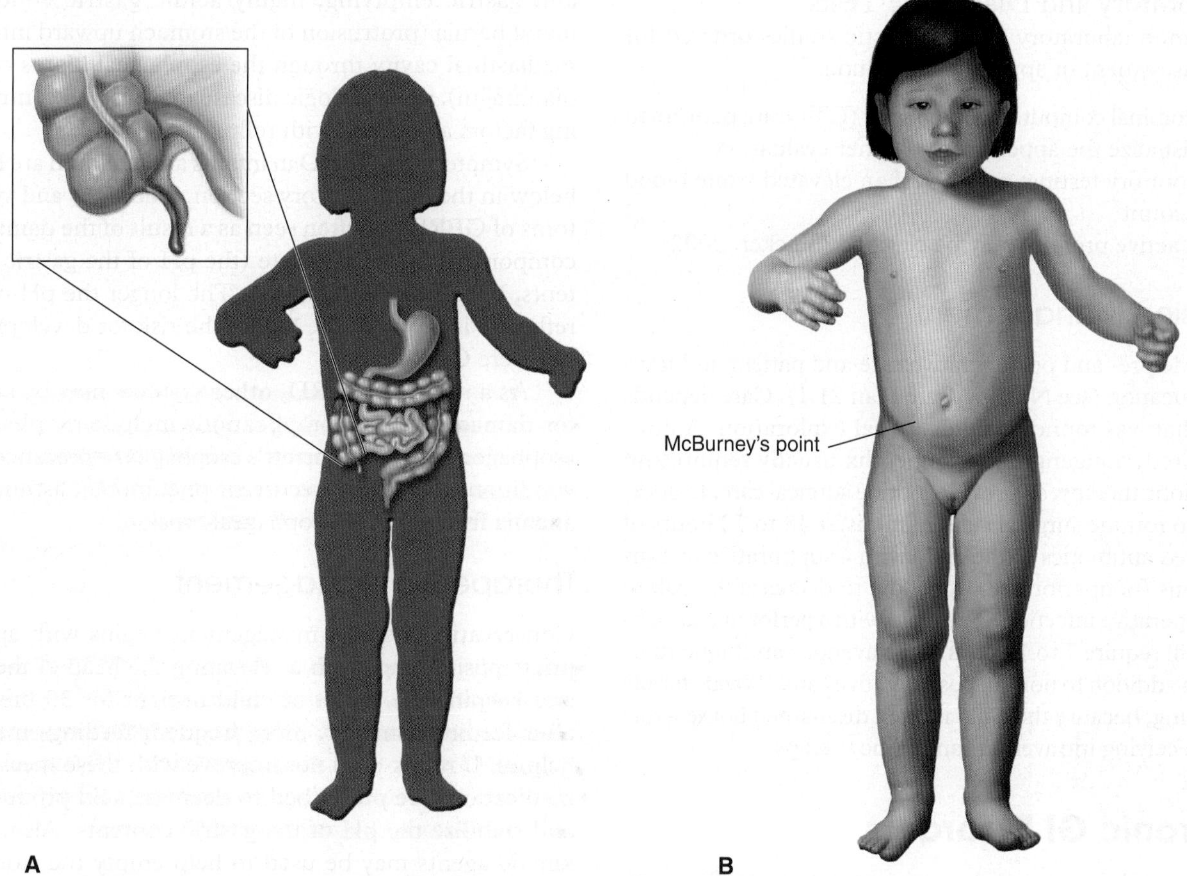

● Figure 21.14 (**A**) In appendicitis, the lumen of the appendix is obstructed, resulting in edema and compressed blood vessels. (**B**) As appendicitis progresses, pain may become localized at McBurney's point (a point midway between the anterior superior iliac crest and the umbilicus).

plished via minimally invasive laparoscopic technique. In the case of perforation, an open surgical procedure is usually required, and lavage of the abdominal cavity may be performed to cleanse it of the infected fluid released from the appendix.

Nursing Assessment

Early diagnosis and intervention are the key elements to avoid perforation. For a full description of the assessment phase of the nursing process refer to page 662. Assessment findings pertinent to appendicitis are discussed below.

Health History

Elicit a description of the present illness and chief complaint. Appendicitis may be gradual, and symptoms usually do not come and go; they remain persistent and intensify. Common signs and symptoms reported during the health history might include:

- Vague abdominal pain in the initial stages, localizing to the right lower quadrant over a few hours
- Nausea and vomiting (which usually develop after the onset of pain)
- Small-volume, frequent, soft stools, often confused with diarrhea
- Fever (usually low grade unless perforation occurs, which results in high fever)

Physical Examination

Children with appendicitis often appear anorexic and ill. They often cannot walk or climb up onto the examination table without assistance. Upon palpation, maximal tenderness occurs over McBurney's point in the right lower quadrant (Tucker, 2002) (see Fig. 21.14). Assess the abdomen for acute peritonitis, as indicated by diffuse abdominal tenderness or distention. Immediately report positive findings to a physician.

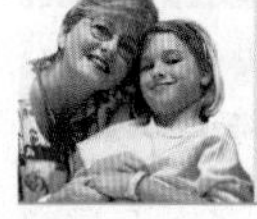

If the child's abdominal pain is suddenly relieved without intervention, suspect perforation and notify the physician immediately.

Laboratory and Diagnostic Tests

Common laboratory and diagnostic studies ordered for the assessment of appendicitis include:

- Abdominal computed tomography (CT) scan: performed to visualize the appendix for further evaluation
- Laboratory testing: may reveal an elevated white blood cell count
- C-reactive protein: may be elevated (Tucker, 2002)

Nursing Management

Provide pre- and postoperative care and patient and family education (see Nursing Care Plan 21.1). Care depends on what was found during surgical exploration. A nonruptured, nongangrenous appendix usually requires no antibiotic therapy, so provide routine surgical care. In addition to routine surgical care, administer 48 to 72 hours of ordered antibiotics to the child with a suppurative or gangrenous (nonperforated) appendix to decrease the risk of postoperative infection. The child with a perforated appendix will require 7 to 14 days of intravenous antibiotic therapy in addition to normal postoperative care. Provide family teaching, because the child is often discharged home while still receiving intravenous antibiotic therapy.

Chronic GI Disorders

Chronic GI disorders include gastroesophageal reflux, peptic ulcer disease, constipation/encopresis, Hirschsprung's disease, short bowel syndrome, inflammatory bowel disease, celiac disease, recurrent abdominal pain, failure to thrive, and chronic feeding problems.

● GASTROESOPHAGEAL REFLUX

Gastroesophageal reflux is passage of gastric contents into the esophagus. It is considered a normal physiologic process that occurs in healthy infants and children. However, when complications develop from the reflux of gastric contents back into the esophagus or oropharynx, it becomes more of a pathologic process known as gastroesophageal reflux disease (GERD). GER occurs frequently during the first year of life; most infants outgrow the reflux by age 6 months. GER is particularly common in premature infants. Other possible diagnoses that can be mistaken for GER include food allergies, formula enteropathies, gastric outlet obstruction, malrotation, cyclic vomiting, or central nervous system lesions.

Pathophysiology

The process of GER occurs during episodes of transient relaxation of the LES, which can occur during swallowing, crying, or other Valsalva maneuvers that increase intra-abdominal pressure. Delayed esophageal clearance and gastric emptying, highly acidic gastric contents, hiatal hernia (protrusion of the stomach upward into the mediastinal cavity through the esophageal hiatus of the diaphragm), or neurologic disease may also be contributing factors associated with reflux.

Symptoms of GERD in infants and children are listed below in the health history section. The signs and symptoms of GERD are often seen as a result of the damaging components of the refluxate (the pH of the gastric contents, bile acids, and pepsin). The longer the pH of the refluxate is below 4, the higher the risk for development of severe GERD.

As a result of GERD, other systems may be at risk for damage. These complications include esophagitis, esophageal stricture, Barrett's esophagus (a precancerous condition), laryngitis, recurrent pneumonia, asthma, or anemia from chronic esophageal erosion.

Therapeutic Management

Conservative medical management begins with appropriate positioning, such as elevating the head of the bed and keeping the infant or child upright for 30 minutes after feeding. Smaller, more frequent feedings may be helpful. If reflux does not improve with these measures, medications are prescribed to decrease acid production and stabilize the pH of the gastric contents. Also, prokinetic agents may be used to help empty the stomach more quickly, minimizing the amount of gastric contents in the stomach that the child can reflux.

If the GERD cannot be medically managed effectively or requires long-term medication therapy, surgical intervention may be necessary. A Nissen fundoplication is the most common surgical procedure performed for antireflux therapy. The gastric fundus is wrapped around the lower 2 to 3 cm of the esophagus (Fig. 21.15). Laparoscopic fundoplications are being performed as a way to minimize the recovery period and reduce potential complications.

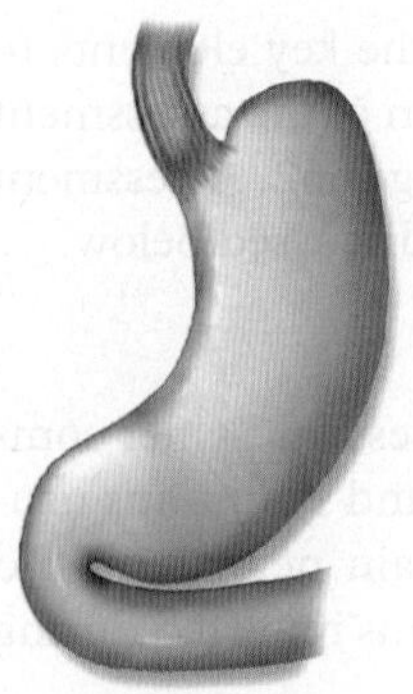

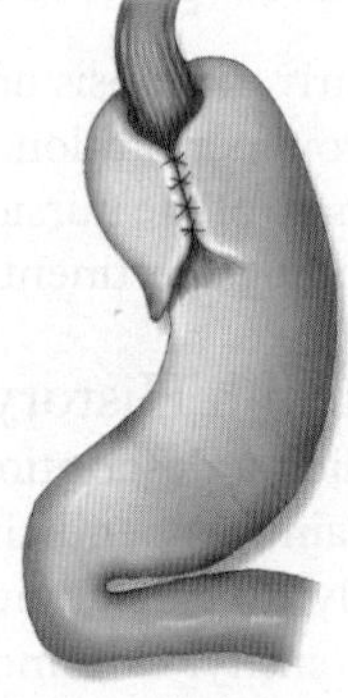

● Figure 21.15 In the Nissen fundoplication, the fundus (upper portion of the stomach) is wrapped around the lower segment of the esophagus.

Nursing Assessment

For a full description of the assessment phase of the nursing process refer to page 662. Assessment findings pertinent to gastroesophageal reflux are discussed below.

Health History

Elicit a description of the present illness and chief complaint. Note onset and progression of symptoms. Common signs and symptoms reported during the health history include:

- Recurrent vomiting or regurgitation
- Weight loss or poor weight gain
- Irritability in infants
- Respiratory symptoms (chronic cough, wheezing, stridor, asthma, apnea)
- Hoarseness/sore throat
- Halitosis (mostly in older children)
- Heartburn or chest pains
- Abdominal pain
- Abnormal neck posturing (Sandifer syndrome)
- Hematemesis
- Dysphagia or feeding refusal
- Chronic sinusitis, otitis media
- Poor dentition (caused by acid erosion)

Explore the patient's current and past medical history for risk factors such as:

- Prematurity, noting prolonged ventilator use or chronic lung disease
- Dietary habits (e.g., chocolate, coffee, spicy or fatty foods, caffeine, formula-fed or breastfed, overeating or overfeeding)
- Current medications
- Smoking/alcohol use (older children)
- Food allergies
- Other GI disorders (gastric outlet dysfunction/hiatal hernia) or congenital abnormalities
- Feeding positions and patterns (especially important in infants)
- Sleeping positions/patterns
- Other medical history, such as asthma, recurrent infections/pneumonia

Physical Examination

The physical examination consists of inspection, auscultation, percussion, and palpation.

Inspection

Observe the child's general appearance and color. Infants and children with uncontrolled GER for a period of time may appear underweight or malnourished. Infants may be irritable due to painful regurgitation/reflux events. Note breathing patterns, because reflux-induced asthma may have developed. **Acute life-threatening events** (ALTE) and apnea have been associated with severe GERD. Observe the child for cyanosis, altered mental status, and alterations in tone. Inspect emesis for blood or bile.

Auscultation

Evaluate the lung fields for the presence of complications related to GERD, such as wheezing or pneumonia. No further pathologic findings related to GERD should be auscultated on examination.

Percussion

Perform routine abdominal percussion, noting any abnormalities. No specific findings should be noted.

Palpation

Use caution when palpating the abdomen, especially with infants with GER, because it may induce vomiting. No abnormalities should be palpated.

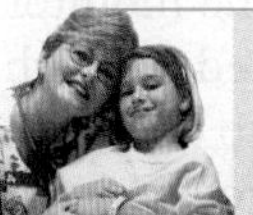

Not all infants with GERD actually vomit. Those with "silent" GERD may only demonstrate irritability associated with feeding or posturing (arching back during or after feeding) and grimacing. Episodes of GERD often cause bradycardia, so if the above signs occur, they should be reported to the physician, even if the baby is not vomiting.

Laboratory and Diagnostic Tests

Common laboratory and diagnostic studies ordered for the assessment of gastroesophageal reflux include:

- Upper GI series: though not sensitive or specific to GER, may show some reflux; used to narrow down the differential diagnosis
- Esophageal pH probe study: quantifies GER episodes as they correlate to symptoms
- Esophagogastroduodenoscopy (EGD): shows esophageal and gastric tissue damage from GERD
- Complete blood count: may demonstrate anemia if chronic esophagitis or hematemesis is present
- Hemoccult: may be positive if chronic esophagitis is present

Nursing Management

As with most GI disorders, initial nursing management is aimed at restoring proper fluid balance and nutrition. Refer to the Nursing Care Plan on page 670. Additional considerations are reviewed below.

Promoting Safe Feeding Techniques and Positioning

Feeding adjustments are an essential part of reflux management. Give infants smaller, more frequent feedings using a nipple that controls flow well. Frequently burp the infant during feeds to control reflux. Thickening of the formula with products such as rice or oatmeal cereal can significantly help keep the formula and gastric contents down. Positioning after feedings is important. Keep infants upright for 30 to 45 minutes after feeding. For infants, elevate the head of the crib 30 degrees. For older children, elevate the head of the bed as much as possible and restrict meals for several hours before bedtime. While the proper positioning of an infant with GERD for sleep is controversial, infants can be positioned safely on their sides or upright in a car seat to minimize the risk of aspiration while on their backs. However, individual physicians may have specific preferences about sleeping positions for infants with GERD.

Maintaining a Patent Airway

GERD symptoms often involve the airway. Maximize reflux precautions to keep the risk of airway involvement to a minimum. In rare instances, GERD causes apnea or an ALTE. In these cases, use an apnea or bradycardia monitor to monitor for such episodes. The monitor requires a physician's order and can be ordered through a home health company. Teach parents how to deal with these episodes, as their anxiety is very high. Provide CPR instruction to all parents whose children have had an ALTE previously.

Educating the Family and Child

The goals for the infant and child with gastroesophageal reflux are a decrease in symptoms, a decrease in the frequency and duration of reflux episodes, healing of the injured mucosa, and prevention of further complications of GERD. Teach the parents the signs and symptoms of complications. Explain that reflux is usually limited to the first year of life, though in some cases it persists. If medications are prescribed, thoroughly explain their use and their side effects (see Drug Guide 21.1).

Providing Postoperative Care

If the child requires fundoplication, a gastrostomy tube is often placed for use in the immediate postoperative period or for long-term feeding. In the immediate postoperative period, assess for pain, abdominal distention, and return of bowel sounds. If a gastrostomy tube is placed, it is often open to straight drain for a period of time postoperatively to keep the stomach empty and allow for the internal incision to heal. When bowel sounds have returned and the infant or child is stable, introduce feedings slowly (typically via the gastrostomy tube). Assess for tolerance of feedings (absence of abdominal distention or pain, minimal residual, and passage of stool). If the abdomen does become distended or the child has discomfort, open the gastrostomy tube to air to decompress the stomach. Assess the insertion site of the gastrostomy tube for redness, edema, or drainage. Keep the site clean and dry per surgeon or hospital protocol. Teach the parents how to care for the gastrostomy tube and insertion site and how to use the tube for feeding.

Promoting Family and Patient Coping

Parents can feel a great deal of anxiety. Teach the family about all aspects of GERD to help promote coping. School-age children often have reflux episodes exhibited by postprandial vomiting, which can be very embarrassing for the children. Notify the school about the medical issues related to GER to minimize the situations for the child.

● PEPTIC ULCER DISEASE

Peptic ulcer disease (PUD) is a term used to describe a variety of disorders of the upper GI tract that result from the action of gastric secretions (Fig. 21.16). Mucosal inflammation and subsequent ulceration occur as a result of either a primary or a secondary factor. In children, duodenal ulcers are more common than gastric ulcers. Primary peptic ulcers are usually associated with *Helicobacter pylori,* a gram-negative organism that causes mucosal inflammation and in some cases more severe disease. *H. pylori* is found mostly in the duodenum.

Secondary peptic ulcers may occur as a result of an identifiable factor, such as excess acid production, stress, medications, or the presence of other underlying conditions. Secondary ulcers tend to be gastric in location as opposed to duodenal.

Primary PUD is more common in children over age 10. There is a higher incidence of secondary PUD in patients under age 6, though it can be found in children of all ages (Herbst, 2004).

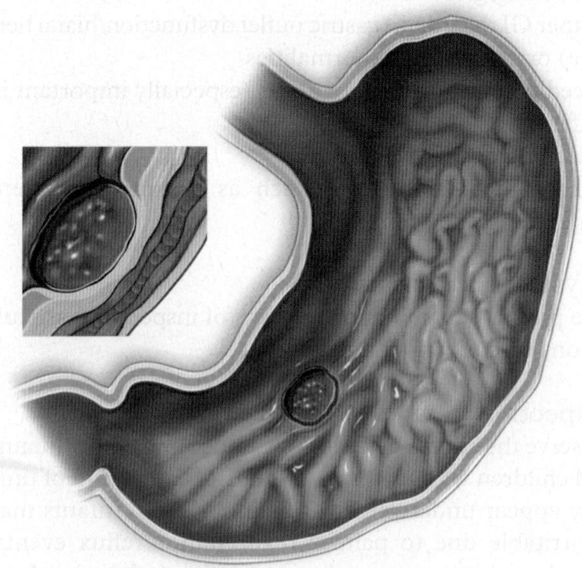

● Figure 21.16 Peptic ulcer disease.

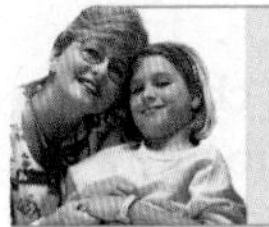

Severe stress, such as burns or another illness necessitating critical care, can contribute to the development of a peptic ulcer in children.

Therapeutic Management

PUD may be treated with antibiotics (if *H. pylori* is verified), histamine agonists, and/or proton pump inhibitors. If the child presents with a severe esophageal or gastric hemorrhage, a nasogastric tube may be placed to decompress the stomach. The patient may require intravenous infusion of a histamine H2-receptor antagonist or a proton pump inhibitor initially until the bleeding has stopped and the disease is stabilized.

Nursing Assessment

For a full description of the assessment phase of the nursing process refer to page 662. Assessment findings pertinent to PUD are discussed below.

Health History

Elicit a description of the present illness and chief complaint. Common signs and symptoms reported during the health history might include:

- Abdominal pain
- GI bleeding
- Vomiting

Abdominal pain is the most common complaint of children with PUD. It is important to characterize the abdominal pain, as many other digestive disorders may mimic PUD. The pain tends to be dull and vague, mostly epigastric or periumbilical. Most often, patients with PUD have pain that worsens after meals, and the pain may wake them at night. Vomiting may be noted in preschool and school-age children.

Explore the client's current and past medical history for risk factors such as a family history of PUD or other GI diseases, or chronic salicylate or prednisone use.

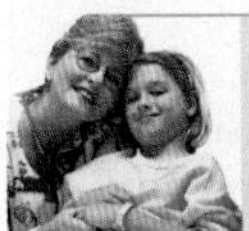

Adolescents at increased risk for the development of PUD include those who use tobacco, alcohol, and caffeine.

Physical Examination and Laboratory and Diagnostic Tests

Palpate the abdomen for the location of the pain, which is usually epigastric or periumbilical. Note the presence of blood in emesis or stools, as GI bleeding may occur (Carroll, 2002). Common laboratory and diagnostic studies ordered for the assessment of PUD include the following:

- Laboratory studies: to identify anemia or *H. pylori* antibodies
- Urea breath test: to identify *H. pylori* gastritis
- Upper GI series: to detect presence of ulcerations
- Upper endoscopy: the definitive diagnostic test to look for ulceration and nodularity in the upper GI tract
- Biopsies: to assess for *H. pylori,* granulomas, eosinophils, or corrosive agents to identify the primary cause of the PUD

Nursing Management

Hemodynamic stabilization should be the focus of nursing management if significant GI bleeding occurs. Once patients are stabilized and tolerating oral feeds, they may be discharged to home. Provide discharge instructions on the following topics:

- Medications
- Dietary management (especially when allergic gastroenteropathy is found)
- Safety precautions (in cases of ingested substances)
- Stressors
- Prevention of disease recurrence

● CONSTIPATION AND ENCOPRESIS

Constipation is a very common problem seen in a pediatric practice, reportedly representing 3% to 5% of all pediatric outpatient visits. It accounts for 25% of the referrals made to a pediatric gastroenterologist for further management of the condition (Castiglia, 2001).

Constipation is usually defined as failure to achieve complete evacuation of the lower colon. It is usually associated with difficulty in passing hard, dry stools but can sometimes be seen as small stools the size of marbles. Term newborns should pass a meconium stool within the first 24 hours of life. If this does not occur, the newborn is at risk for developing an underlying GI disorder. The bowel habits of both infants and children vary widely, so assess and treat each child on an individual basis. Breastfed infants may produce a stool with each feeding, though some will skip a few days between stools. Most bottle-fed babies will produce a stool one or two times per day, but they may go 2 to 3 days without producing a stool.

Encopresis is a term used to describe soiling of fecal contents into the underwear beyond the age of expected toilet training (4 to 5 years of age). Encopresis is often seen as a result of chronic constipation and withholding of stool. As stool is withheld in the rectum, the rectal muscle can stretch over time, and this stretching of the rectum causes fecal impactions. Patients who have a stretched rectal vault may experience diarrhea, where leakage occurs around a fecal mass. This is often an embarrassing issue that occurs with school-age children, and the child may hide his or her underwear to avoid punishment. Many psychological issues arise from chronic constipation and encopresis.

Pathophysiology

As stool passes through the colon, water is reabsorbed into the colon, resulting in a formed stool by the time it reaches the rectum. At this point, the anal sphincter relaxes to allow the passage of stool from the anus. In constipation, however, this relaxation does not occur.

Most causes of constipation are functional in nature (inorganic). Children with functional constipation usually present with this problem during the toilet-training years. Children have a painful experience during defecation, which in turn creates a fear of defecation, resulting in further withholding of stool. Organic causes of constipation rarely occur in children; however, this may be a sign of a disease such as spina bifida or sacral agenesis. The causes of pediatric constipation are discussed in Box 21.5.

Therapeutic Management

Once any organic process is ruled out as a cause for constipation, it may initially be managed with dietary manipulation such as increasing fiber and fluids. Behavior modification is necessary for most children. Children need to relearn to allow bowel evacuation when stool is present. Children with severe constipation and withholding behaviors may not benefit from dietary management and may require laxative therapy. Sometimes mechanical disimpaction is required initially, followed by the above measures.

Nursing Assessment

For a full description of the assessment phase of the nursing process refer to page 662. Assessment findings pertinent to constipation/encopresis are discussed below.

Health History

Elicit a description of the present illness and chief complaint. Note the onset of symptoms as described by the parent/child. Common signs and symptoms reported during the health history may include:

- Altered stooling patterns (size, frequency, amount, color)
- Pain with defecation
- Withholding behaviors (postures to try to withhold the stool, such as crossing the legs, squatting or hiding in a corner, or "dancing")
- Complaints of abdominal pain and cramping and poor appetite
- Diarrhea leakage
- Soiling of undergarments

It is important to note the duration of the symptoms to determine an acute onset versus a chronic disorder.

Explore the client's past and current medical history for risk factors such as:

- Family history of GI disorders
- History of rectal bleeding or **anal fissures**
- Report of first meconium stool after 24 hours of age
- History of sexual abuse

An accurate dietary history as well as a history of fluid intake should be taken. Current medication or laxative use should also be explored.

Physical Examination

Physical examination of the child with constipation consists of inspection, auscultation, percussion, and palpation.

Inspection

Observe the child's general appearance. Note whether the abdomen appears distended or rounded. Observe the

BOX 21.5

CAUSES OF PEDIATRIC CONSTIPATION BY AGE

Newborn/Infant	Toddler and Ages 2–4 Years	School Age	Adolescent	Any Age
• Meconium plug • Hirschsprung's disease • Cystic fibrosis • Congenital anorectal malformations • Pseudo-obstruction • Endocrine: hypothyroidism • Metabolic: diabetes insipidus, renal tubular acidosis • Withholding • Dietary changes	• Anal fissures • Withholding • Toilet refusal • Short-segment Hirschsprung's disease • Neurologic disorders • Spinal cord: meningomyelocele, tumors, tethered cord	• Toilet or bathroom access limited or unavailable • Limited ability to recognize physiologic cues, preoccupation with other activities • Tethered cord • Withholding	• Spinal cord injury (accidents, trauma) • Dieting • Anorexia • Pregnancy • Idiopathic slow transit constipation, particularly in females • Laxative abuse • Irritable bowel syndrome, constipation variant	• Medication side effect, dietary, post-operative state • Previous anorectal surgery • Withholding and overflow from chronic rectal distention • Relatively rapid change to sedentary state, dehydration • Hypothyroidism

lower back for a deep pilonidal dimple with hair tuft, which is suggestive of spina bifida occulta. Flat buttocks may be suggestive of sacral agenesis. Inspect the anus for signs of fissures or soiling. Inspect the child's underwear for stains or smears, which are indicative of soiling (Ulshen, 2004c).

Auscultation

Auscultate bowel sounds to determine the possibility of an obstruction (hypoactive or absent bowel sounds) in the child with an acute case of constipation.

Percussion

Percuss the abdomen to reveal dullness, which would indicate a fecal mass.

Palpation

Palpate the abdomen for any tenderness or masses. The nurse may assist the physician or practitioner with the performance of a rectal examination to assess for rectal tone and rectal vault size.

Laboratory and Diagnostic Tests

Laboratory and diagnostic tests are not routine with the diagnosis of functional constipation, but if an organic cause is suspected, the following laboratory and diagnostic tests would be ordered:

- Stool for occult blood: the presence of blood could indicate some other disease process
- Abdominal x-ray: large quantities of stool may be seen in the colon
- Sitz marker study: to detect colonic dysmotility
- Barium enema: to rule out a stricture or Hirschsprung's disease
- Rectal manometry: to evaluate rectal musculature dysfunction
- Rectal suction biopsy: to rule out Hirschsprung's disease

Nursing Management

Nursing management for the infant or child with constipation is aimed at educating the patient and family and promoting patient and family coping. Refer to the Nursing Care Plan on page 670. Additional considerations are reviewed below.

Educating the Family and Patient

Teach parents how to assess for signs of constipation and withholding behaviors. Also provide guidelines on scheduling and supervising bowel habits in reconditioning the child to use the toilet regularly. Teach parents to use positive reinforcement techniques: for example, when the child produces an adequate-volume bowel movement, reward him or her with stickers, extra playtime or television time, and so on (Schmitt, 2004).

Dietary changes may help some children. High-fiber diets help to regulate bowel activity. Increasing fluid intake may also aid in bringing extra water into the bowel, thereby softening the stool. Infants and toddlers with constipation may experience constipation from formula or milk changes. Manipulating the formula or milk may result in better bowel habits.

Educate families about the importance of compliance with medication use, if medication is ordered. Parents often are very anxious about the use of these medications, but stress to them that compliance is essential. Assess for improper laxative use based on the history of stool patterns.

Many children present to their doctor with fecal impaction or partial impaction. Teach parents how to disimpact their children at home; this often requires an enema or stimulation therapy. Nursing Procedure 21.2 gives instructions on enema administration in children. Explain the procedure to the child in developmentally appropriate terms. Enema administration can be uncomfortable, but calming measures, such as distraction and

Nursing Procedure 21.2

Administering an Enema

1. Gather supplies (enema bag, lubricant, enema solution).
2. Wash hands and apply gloves.
3. Position the child:
   - Infant or toddler on abdomen with knees bent
   - Child or adolescent on left side with right leg flexed toward chest
4. Clamp the enema tubing, remove the cap, and apply lubricant to the tip.
5. Insert the tube into the rectum:
   - 2.5 to 4 cm (1 to 1.5 inches) in the infant
   - 5 to 7.5 cm (2 to 3 inches) in the child
6. Unclamp the tubing and administer the prescribed volume of enema solution at a rate of about 100 mL per minute. Recommended volumes:
   - 250 mL or less for the infant
   - 250 to 500 mL for the toddler or preschooler
   - 500 to 1,000 mL for the school-age child
7. Hold the child's buttocks together if needed to encourage retention of the enema for 5 to 10 minutes.

praise, provide a comforting environment. After the impaction is removed, promote regular bowel habits to keep the impaction from recurring.

Promoting Patient and Family Coping

Childhood constipation can be a very stressful process for both the child and family. Behavior modification is necessary for many children. To facilitate daily bowel evacuation, the child should sit on the toilet twice a day (after breakfast and dinner) for 5 to 15 minutes. Instruct the family to keep a "star" or reward chart to encourage compliance. The star should be awarded for compliance with time sitting on the toilet and should not be reserved for successful bowel movements only. Weeks to months may be required to change the stooling pattern.

Many parents seek counselors to help the entire family deal with the issues. Counseling is geared toward allaying the fears of a child who is afraid to defecate due to pain. Also, children who are older may have behavioral issues that need to be addressed. Psychological evaluation and possible behavioral therapy may need to be implemented if constipation becomes a power struggle.

Consider THIS!

Jung Kim, 3 years old, is brought to the clinic by his parents with abdominal pain and a poor appetite. His mother states, "He cries when I put him on the toilet."

What other assessment information would you obtain?

What education and interventions may be necessary for this child and family?

HIRSCHSPRUNG'S DISEASE (CONGENITAL AGANGLIONIC MEGACOLON)

Hirschsprung's disease is the most common cause of neonatal intestinal obstruction (Fig. 21.17). The disease is most commonly characterized by constipation in newborns. This is due to a lack of ganglion cells in the bowel, which causes inadequate motility in part of the intestine. These ganglion cells can be absent from the rectosigmoid colon all the way into the small intestine. Approximately 75% of cases affect only the rectosigmoid colon (short-segment Hirschsprung's), but in 8% of the cases, total colonic involvement is seen (long-segment Hirschsprung's). The incidence is 1 in 5,000, and males are affected three times more than females. Hirschsprung's usually occurs in the absence of other associated anomalies, but there is an association with Down syndrome (Wylie, 2004a).

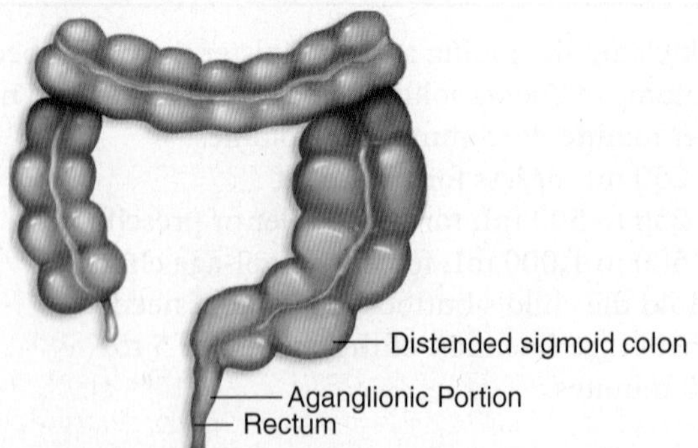

● Figure 21.17 Enlarged megacolon of Hirschsprung's disease.

Therapeutic Management

Surgical resection of the aganglionic bowel and reanastomosis of the remaining intestine is necessary to promote proper bowel function. There are several types of surgical procedures to correct this, usually performed in stages. The surgical resection requires the child to have an ostomy to divert the stool through a stoma on the abdomen. This allows the area of the resected bowel and anastomosis to heal before it is used. The ostomy is closed at a later date.

Nursing Assessment

For a full description of the assessment phase of the nursing process refer to page 662. Assessment findings pertinent to Hirschsprung's are discussed below.

Health History

Elicit a description of the present illness and chief complaint. Newborn stool patterns are a key element in recognizing this diagnosis. Assess whether the newborn passed a meconium stool: most children with Hirschsprung's do not pass a meconium stool within the first 24 to 48 hours of life. Also, newborns who required rectal stimulation to pass their first meconium stool or who passed a meconium plug should be evaluated for Hirschsprung's.

Explore the child's current and past medical history for risk factors such as a family history of Hirschsprung's or Down syndrome. Hirschsprung's may also be associated with congenital deafness, malrotation, gastric diverticulum, and intestinal atresia.

Physical Examination

Inspect and palpate the abdomen. The abdomen is typically distended, and often stool masses can be palpated in the abdomen. Perform a rectal examination to assess for rectal tone and the presence of stool in the rectum. Often with Hirschsprung's, no stool is present in the rectum, but at the end of the rectal examination, when the finger is being withdrawn, a child with Hirschsprung's may have a forceful expulsion of fecal material.

Laboratory and Diagnostic Tests

Common laboratory and diagnostic studies ordered for the assessment of Hirschsprung's include:

- Barium enema: to look for a narrowing of the intestine
- Rectal suction biopsy: to demonstrate an absence of ganglion cells (definitive diagnosis)

Nursing Management

Nursing management includes providing postoperative care, performing ostomy care, and providing patient and family education.

Providing Postoperative and Ostomy Care

Provide routine postoperative care and observe for the complication of enterocolitis (see Nursing Care Plan 21.1). Observe for the following signs and symptoms of enterocolitis:

- Fever
- Abdominal distention
- Chronic diarrhea
- Explosive stools
- Rectal bleeding
- Straining

If any of the above symptoms are noted, immediately notify the physician, maintain bowel rest, and administer intravenous fluids and antibiotics to prevent the development of shock and possibly death.

The patient with Hirschsprung's may have either a colostomy or ileostomy, depending on the extent of disease in the intestine. In either case, perform proper ostomy care to avoid skin breakdown. Accurately measure stool output to assess the child's fluid volume status.

Providing Patient and Family Education

The family may be anxious and fearful about upcoming surgeries and possible complications. Help to relieve their anxiety by providing information about the diagnosis and the stages of surgical procedures the patient will undergo. Provide postoperative teaching to educate parents on proper stoma care as well as medication management (to avoid dehydration, most Hirschsprung's patients will be prescribed medications to slow stool output). Arrange for the family to consult with a wound care nurse to help them deal with the anxieties and care of newly placed stomas. Provide education about possible postsurgical problems, emphasizing the importance of prompt medical treatment for signs of enterocolitis.

• SHORT BOWEL SYNDROME

Short bowel syndrome is a clinical syndrome of nutrient malabsorption and excessive intestinal fluid and electrolyte losses that occurs following massive small intestinal loss or surgical resection. The degree of malabsorption is usually related to the extent of resection of small bowel. The most common causes of short bowel syndrome are necrotizing enterocolitis, small intestinal atresia, gastroschisis, malrotation with volvulus, and trauma to the small intestine. A child can lose as much as 75% of the small intestine without serious long-term problems, as long as the duodenum, terminal ileum, and ileocecal valve are still functioning. However, even a 25% intestinal loss can result in significant problems if the terminal ileum and ileocecal valve are not spared (Jakubik et al., 2000). If the terminal ileum is lost, vitamin B12 deficiency and bile salt malabsorption may occur. If the ileocecal valve is lost, small bowel bacterial overgrowth is likely to occur, as well as poor intestinal motility.

Therapeutic Management

The child with short bowel syndrome is at risk for chronic complications. The goals of therapeutic management are to minimize bacterial overgrowth and to maximize the child's nutritional status. Antibiotics may be used to control bacterial overgrowth. Vitamin and mineral supplementation is necessary because the small intestine is usually where fat-soluble vitamins, calcium, magnesium, and zinc are absorbed. Antidiarrheal agents such as loperamide and gastric acid-suppressive medications may be used to decrease stool output. Many children with short bowel syndrome require TPN for extended periods to achieve adequate growth. Progression to enteral feeding may occur extremely slowly, depending upon the intestine's response. Despite a markedly improved prognosis for these patients, some will not do as well and may ultimately require intestinal and liver transplantation due to irreversible liver damage from long-term use of TPN (Jakubik et al., 2000).

Nursing Assessment

Elicit the health history, noting diarrhea, which is the primary symptom of short bowel syndrome. Note past history of bowel loss or resection as noted above. Assess the child's hydration state. Inspect the stool for consistency, color, odor, and volume. Review laboratory results, particularly chemistries, to evaluate hydration status, and liver function tests, which may reveal evolving **cholestasis** secondary to long-term TPN use.

Nursing Management

Nursing management focuses on encouraging adequate nutrition and promoting effective family coping.

Encouraging Adequate Nutrition

Treatment for short bowel syndrome can be a slow and tedious process. Most patients will require TPN until they can tolerate enteral feeds without significant malabsorption. TPN is usually required for a lengthy time, so most children will require long-term intravenous access. Long-term intravenous access places the child at high risk for infection and resulting sepsis, so closely monitor for signs and symptoms of infection. Immediately report to the physician any fevers or redness or drainage at the intravenous site.

When started, enteral feeding must be administered very slowly to avoid further malabsorption. Usually the feeding is started continuously, 24 hours per day, via a feeding pump. Most patients have long-term feeding tubes, usually gastrostomy tubes. Most of these children will require special formulas to promote absorption. Assess for feeding tube residuals and abdominal distention or discomfort. Strictly monitor intake and output to avoid dehydration. Assess the stool for signs of carbohydrate malabsorption. Administer vitamin and mineral supplementation, antidiarrheals, and antibiotics as ordered. Teach the family about use of enteral feeding tubes, feeding pumps, and medication administration. (Jakubik et al., 2000).

Promoting Effective Family Coping

Children with short bowel syndrome are considered to be medically fragile for a lengthy period. There is much anxiety related to the initial bowel resection that resulted in short bowel. Long-term hospitalization is almost always required, causing parents to miss work and cutting down on the time they have to spend with other children. This can lead to even more anxiety about finances and relationships. Encourage families to become the experts on their child's needs and condition via education and participation in care. Provide teaching so that the family is better able to care for the child in an outpatient setting. Education focuses on information about TPN and central line care, enteral feedings, assessing for hydration status, and managing medications.

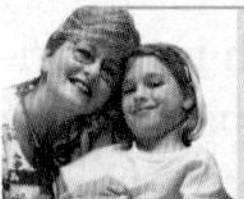

Maintaining long-term central venous access for TPN in infants can present a challenge. One-piece clothing with the central venous line (CVL) tubing exiting and secured on the back of the outfit can help discourage the infant from pulling on (and subsequently dislodging) the line.

• INFLAMMATORY BOWEL DISEASE

Crohn's disease and ulcerative colitis are the two major idiopathic inflammatory bowel diseases of children. The causes are unknown, but they may be due to an abnormal or uncontrolled genetically determined immunologic or inflammatory response to an environmental antigenic trigger, possibly a virus or bacterium. The features of Crohn's disease and ulcerative colitis are listed in Comparison Chart 21.2.

Therapeutic Management

Medication is used to control inflammation and symptoms. Medications commonly used include 5-aminosalicylates, antibiotics, immunomodulators, immunosuppressives, and anti-tumor necrosis antibody therapy. Dietary manipulation is also very important.

Failure to respond to medical therapy may result in surgical intervention. Many patients with ulcerative colitis eventually undergo a total proctocolectomy, with resulting ostomy, as a curative measure. Approximately 70% of Crohn's disease patients will require surgery to relieve obstruction, drain an abscess, or relieve intractable symptoms (Sondheimer, 2005).

Nursing Assessment

For a full description of the assessment phase of the nursing process refer to page 662. Assessment findings pertinent to Crohn's disease and ulcerative colitis are discussed below.

Health History

Elicit a description of the present illness and chief complaint. Common signs and symptoms reported during the health history include:

- Abdominal cramping
- Nighttime symptoms, including waking due to abdominal pain or urge to defecate
- Fever
- Weight loss
- Poor growth
- Delayed sexual development

Children may be reluctant or unwilling to talk about their bowel movements, so explain the importance of doing so. Assess stool pattern history, including frequency, presence of blood or mucus, and duration of symptoms.

Explore the patient's current and past medical history for risk factors, such as:

- Family history of inflammatory bowel disease
- Family history of colon cancer
- Family history of immunologic disorders

Physical Examination

Assess the child's growth using growth charts to identify any poor growth patterns. Perform a full abdominal examination, noting tenderness, masses, or fullness. Inspect the perianal area to look for skin tags or fissures, which would be highly suspicious for Crohn's disease. Assist the physician in performing a rectal examination to further assess the rectal area for blood or other lesions.

Laboratory and Diagnostic Tests

Laboratory test results may be normal. Results for children with Crohn's disease and ulcerative colitis are found in Comparison Chart 21.2. Common laboratory and diagnostic studies ordered for the assessment of inflammatory bowel disease include:

- Radiologic studies such as upper GI series with small bowel series: may identify evidence of intestinal inflammation, estimate distribution and extent of disease, and help distinguish between Crohn's disease and ulcerative colitis
- CT scan: to rule out suspected abscess

COMPARISON CHART 21.2 Features of Crohn's Disease and Ulcerative Colitis

Feature	Crohn's Disease	Ulcerative Colitis
Age at onset	10 to 20 years	10 to 20 years
Incidence	4 to 6 per 100,000	3 to 15 per 100,000
Area of bowel affected	Oropharynx, esophagus, and stomach, rare: small bowel only, 25% to 30%; colon and anus only, 25%; ileocolitis, 40%; diffuse disease, 5%	Total colon, 90%; proctitis, 10%
Distribution	Segmental; disease-free skip areas common	Continuous; distal to proximal
Pathology	Full-thickness, acute, and chronic inflammation; noncaseating granulomas (50%), extraintestinal fistulas, abscesses, stricture, and fibrosis may be present	Superficial, acute inflammation of mucosa with microscopic crypt abscess
X-ray findings	Segmental lesions; thickened, circular folds, cobblestone appearance of bowel wall secondary to longitudinal ulcers and transverse fissures; fixation and separation of loops; narrowed lumen; "sting sign"; fistulas	Superficial colitis; loss of haustra; shortened colon and pseudopolyps (islands of normal tissue surrounded by denuded mucosa) are late findings
Intestinal symptoms	Abdominal pain, diarrhea (usually loose with blood if colon involved), perianal disease, enteroenteric or enterocutaneous fistula, abscess, anorexia	Abdominal pain, bloody diarrhea, urgency, tenesmus
Extraintestinal symptoms:		
Arthritis/arthralgia	15%	9%
Fever	40% to 50%	40% to 50%
Stomatitis	9%	2%
Weight loss	90% (mean 5.7 kg)	68% (mean 4.1 kg)
Delayed growth and sexual development	30%	5% to 10%
Uveitis, conjunctivitis	15% (in Crohn's colitis)	4%
Sclerosing cholangitis	—	4%
Renal stones	6% (oxalate)	6% (urate)
Pyoderma gangrenosum	1% to 3%	5%
Erythema nodosum	8% to 15%	4%
Laboratory findings	High erythrocyte sedimentation rate; microcytic anemia; low serum iron and total iron-binding capacity; increased fecal protein loss; low serum albumin; antineutrophil cytoplasmic antibodies present in 10% to 20%; *Saccharomyces cervisiae* antibodies positive in 60%	High erythrocyte sedimentation rate; microcytic anemia; high white blood cell count with left shift; antineutrophil cytoplasmic antibodies present in 80%

From Sondheimer, 2005.

- Colonoscopy: to diagnose inflammatory bowel disease
- Upper endoscopy: to rule out affected mucosal tissue between the mouth and anus in children with upper abdominal complaints

Nursing Management

Nursing management focuses on teaching about disease management, teaching about nutritional management, teaching about medication therapy, and promoting family and child coping.

Teaching About Disease Management

The diagnosis of Crohn's disease or ulcerative colitis can be very difficult for the patient and family to comprehend. Provide teaching about the disease process and medication therapy to help the child and family understand the seriousness of the disease. The physician may discuss surgical options during uncontrolled flare-ups, but the nurse may be the person to whom the family members or patient address their questions regarding surgery. Provide the family with information to help answer some of their questions and allay fears.

Teaching About Nutritional Management

Teach the child and family about nutritional management of the disease. For example, adequate nutrition with a high-protein and high-carbohydrate diet may be recommended; when the disease is active, lactose may be tolerated poorly; and vitamin and iron supplements will most likely be recommended. Explain that in severe cases enteral feeding tubes or TPN may be needed; this is rare but often induces remission.

Teaching About Medication Therapy

Medications are extremely important in controlling inflammatory bowel disease. Provide information about the following common medications used to control the disease:

- 5-aminosalicylates (5-ASA): used to prevent relapse (usually used in ulcerative colitis)
- Antibiotics (usually metronidazole and ciprofloxacin): typically used in patients who have perianal Crohn's disease
- Immunomodulators (usually 6-mercaptopurine [6-MP] or azathioprine): used to help maintain remission. Monitor patients for neutropenia and hepatotoxicity.
- Cyclosporine or tacrolimus: used occasionally in conjunction with 6-MP or azathioprine to maintain remission in fulminant ulcerative colitis
- Methotrexate: sometimes used to manage severe Crohn's disease
- Anti-tumor necrosis antibody therapy: widely used for children with Crohn's disease; occasionally used for children with ulcerative colitis

Promoting Family and Child Coping

Inflammatory bowel disease is a chronic and often debilitating illness. Many children with this diagnosis can lead normal lives, but frequent illnesses can cause school absences, which in turn add stress to the situation. Because schools have become much less tolerant of absences and tardiness, it may be necessary to write letters to the school explaining the frequent absences or in-school needs. Bathroom privileges should be very flexible for children during flare-ups. Children tend to be of small stature due to the illness itself and steroid use, which stunts growth; this may cause psychological issues, especially for older boys. Children with ostomies as a result of surgical resection may have self-esteem issues related to the presence and care of the ostomy. Arrange for counseling for both the child and family to discuss fears and anxiety related to a chronic disease.

● CELIAC DISEASE

Celiac disease, also known as celiac sprue, is an immunologic disorder in which gluten, a product most commonly found in grains, causes damage to the small intestine. The villi of the small intestine are damaged due to the body's immunologic response to the digestion of gluten. The function of the villi is to absorb nutrients into the bloodstream. When the villi are blunted or damaged, malnutrition occurs.

Celiac disease was once considered a rare disease found only in Europe, but it is now thought to be the most prevalent genetic disorder in the world, affecting approximately 1 in 150 people. The incidence of celiac disease is much higher in people who have a relative with the disease, as high as 1 in 20 (Korn, 2002). Relatives of those diagnosed with celiac disease are often screened for the disorder, especially in the presence of GI symptoms.

The only current treatment for celiac disease is a strict gluten-free diet. Eliminating gluten will cause the villi of the intestines to heal and function normally, with subsequent improvement of symptoms. Even very small amounts of gluten introduced back into the diet can cause damage to the villi, so the patient must adhere to the diet throughout life.

Nursing Assessment

For a full description of the assessment phase of the nursing process refer to page 662. Assessment findings pertinent to celiac disease are discussed below. The child with symptoms of celiac disease often presents for evaluation by age 2.

Health History

Elicit a description of the present illness and chief complaint. The symptoms of celiac disease are very broad and are easily confused with other GI disorders. The classic symptoms of children with celiac disease are:

- Diarrhea
- **Steatorrhea**
- Constipation
- Failure to thrive or weight loss

- Abdominal distention or bloating
- Poor muscle tone
- Irritability and listlessness
- Dental disorders
- Anemia
- Delayed onset of puberty or amenorrhea
- Nutritional deficiencies

Explore the child's current and past medical history for risk factors such as Caucasian European descent and a family history of celiac disease (Allen, 2004).

Physical Examination

Assess for the typical appearance of children with celiac disease: distended abdomen, wasted buttocks, and very thin extremities (Allen, 2004) (Fig. 21.18).

Laboratory and Diagnostic Tests

Common laboratory and diagnostic studies ordered for the assessment of celiac disease include serological antibody screening and intestinal biopsy for confirmation and genetic testing. The serum antibody markers look for antibodies in the bloodstream that are specific to a patient's response to gluten. The intestinal biopsy is taken from the duodenum during an upper endoscopic procedure performed by a gastroenterologist. Pathology from the biopsy reveals partial or subtotal villous atrophy or blunting of the villi of the small intestine. A child undergoing an intestinal biopsy to confirm or rule out celiac disease must not be restricted from consuming gluten for approximately 2 months before the biopsy. However, children may become symptomatic and extremely ill with a gluten challenge; in these cases, biopsies should be obtained sooner. Genetic testing is also available for celiac disease, looking for certain human leukocyte antigen (HLA) types. This may rule out celiac disease with 99% accuracy in people who are genetically predisposed to celiac disease, obviating the need for an intestinal biopsy (Allen, 2004).

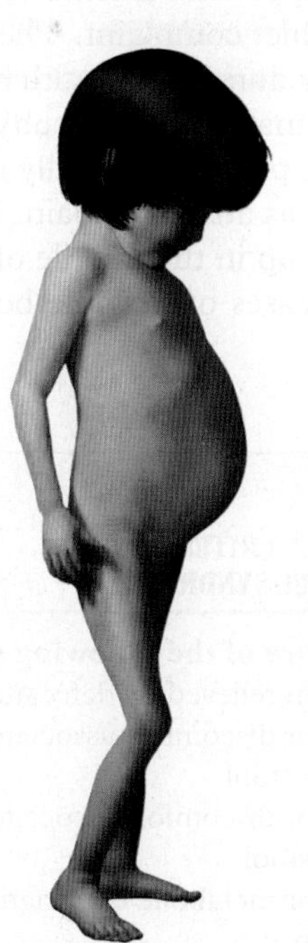

● **Figure 21.18** The child with celiac disease typically displays a distended abdomen and wasted extremities.

Nursing Management

Providing patient and family education is the key nursing role in managing children with celiac disease. The patient must adhere to a strict gluten-free diet for his or her entire life. This is often very challenging, because gluten is found in most wheat products, rye, barley, and possibly oats. Encourage the parents and child to maintain this gluten-free diet. Often, families consult a dietitian to learn about the gluten-free diet (Teaching Guideline 21.3).

Provide educational materials and resources to the parents. Many resources are available today about celiac disease because it is becoming more commonly diagnosed (Box 21.6).

● RECURRENT ABDOMINAL PAIN

Recurrent abdominal pain is a common GI complaint of children and adolescents. It affects children of all ages. The etiology remains unclear. A community-based study of middle- and high-school students showed that 13% to 17% have weekly abdominal pain (Jarrett et al., 2003). The Rome Committee is a group of specialists who are focusing on the identification, management, and treatment of both adults and children with these functional GI disorders. The three categories of recurrent abdominal pain in children are functional abdominal pain, nonulcer dyspepsia, and irritable bowel syndrome. Box 21.7 outlines the Rome Committee's criteria for distinguishing different features of irritable bowel syndrome (Longstreth, 2002).

Pathophysiology

The etiology of recurrent abdominal pain is controversial but most likely multifactorial. It is thought that the autonomic nervous system, which controls the body's response to emotions and stress, and intestinal motility are the two mechanisms. Symptoms may result from an alteration in the transmission of messages between the enteric nervous system and the central nervous system, leading to visceral hypersensitivity. Information from the GI tract is transmitted through bidirectional nerve pathways to the brain. Most neurotransmitters are found in both the brain and the gut, suggesting the potential for integrated effects of pain modulation (Jarrett et al., 2003). As different possibilities exist for the pathophysiology of recurrent abdominal pain, it is clear that there are no structural or biochemical abnormalities that are identifiable.

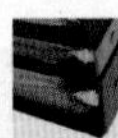

TEACHING GUIDELINE 21.3

Dietary Considerations in a Gluten-Free Diet

Foods Allowed	Foods To Avoid
Potato, soy, rice, or bean flour, rice bran, cornmeal, arrowroot, corn or potato starch, sago, tapioca, buckwheat, millet, flax, teff, sorghum, amaranth, quinoa	Wheat flour, rye, triticale, barley, oats, wheat germ or bran, graham, gluten, or durum flour, wheat starch, oat bran, bulgur, farina, spelt, kamut, malt extract, hydrolyzed vegetable protein
Plain, fresh, frozen, or canned vegetables made with allowed ingredients	Any creamed or breaded vegetables, canned baked beans, some French fries
All fruits and fruit juices	Some commercial fruit pie fillings and dried fruit
All milk and milk products except those made with gluten additives, aged cheese	Malted milk, flavored or frozen yogurt
All meat, poultry, fish, and shellfish, dried peas and beans, nuts, peanut butter, soybean, cold cuts, frankfurters or sausage without fillers	Any meats or poultry prepared with wheat, rye, oats, barley, gluten stabilizers, or fillers for meats, canned meats, self-basting turkey, some egg substitutes
Butter, margarine, salad dressings, sauces, soups, and desserts with allowable ingredients, sugar, honey, jelly, jam, hard candy, plain chocolate, coconut, molasses, marshmallows, meringues, pure instant or ground coffee, tea, carbonated drinks, wine (from the United States)	Commercial salad dressings, prepared soups, condiments, sauces, and seasonings made with avoided products, nondairy cream substitutes, flavored instant coffee, alcohol distilled from cereals, licorice

From NDDIC, 2003.

Therapeutic management most often focuses on increasing the child's coping skills. Some children may need dietary manipulation or medications to control diarrhea (irritable bowel syndrome).

Nursing Assessment

For a full description of the assessment phase of the nursing process refer to page 662. Assessment findings pertinent to recurrent abdominal pain are discussed below.

Health History

The diagnosis of recurrent abdominal pain is made on a symptom-based approach. Elicit a description of the present illness and chief complaint. The symptom reported mostly commonly during the health history is abdominal pain. The child may have difficulty providing a good description of the pain. It is usually periumbilical and is usually described as attacks of pain. It is uncommon for the child to wake up in the middle of the night with this type of pain. In cases of irritable bowel syndrome, the

BOX 21.6

RESOURCES FOR PARENTS OF CHILDREN WITH CELIAC DISEASE

- American Celiac Society: 973-325-8837
- Celiac Disease Foundation: www.celiac.org, 818-990-2354
- Celiac Sprue Association: www.csaceliacs.org, 402-558-0600
- Gluten Intolerance Group (GIG): www.gluten.net, 206-246-6652
- R.O.C.K. (Raising Our Celiac Kids) support group: www.celiackids.com, 858-395-5421

These resources can offer information on all aspects of celiac disease, including dietary guidelines and resources for food shopping and eating in restaurants.

From Korn, 2002.

BOX 21.7

ROME COMMITTEE CRITERIA FOR IRRITABLE BOWEL SYNDROME

12 weeks or more of the following symptoms:

- Abdominal pain relieved by defecation
- Onset of pain or discomfort associated with a change in frequency of stool
- Onset of pain or discomfort associated with a change in form of the stool
- No structural or metabolic explanation for this abdominal pain

From Longstreth, 2002.

pain may be relieved by defecation. Because diet may play a large role in the symptoms, obtain a dietary history. Take a detailed medication history, because abdominal pain may be an adverse effect of some medications. Identifying social and school stressors is essential (Jarrett et al., 2003).

Physical Examination

Note the child's body positioning and facial expressions. Interactions with family members during the interview may provide more details regarding social stressors. Palpate the abdomen for tenderness.

Laboratory and Diagnostic Tests

Common laboratory and diagnostic studies ordered for the assessment of recurrent abdominal pain include:

- Complete blood count: to rule out organic causes of abdominal pain
- Erythrocyte sedimentation rate: to rule out organic causes of abdominal pain
- Urinalysis: to rule out organic causes of abdominal pain
- Complete metabolic panel (CMP): to rule out organic causes of abdominal pain
- Stool studies: to assess for routine pathogens

Nursing Management

Once the diagnosis of recurrent abdominal pain with no organic cause is made, the majority of the nursing management is focused on promoting coping skills. Often the physician performs a battery of tests to rule out organic causes, especially when patient and family anxiety is high. After these tests are complete, teach the family about the factors that exacerbate the pain and how to deal with these factors.

Diet changes may need to be implemented. High-fiber diets help with bowel regulation by keeping motility regular.

Often medications are used to relieve abdominal cramps. Antidiarrheals may be used for patients with irritable bowel syndrome that is manifested by diarrhea. Occasionally pain modulators and antidepressants are used to help block the neurotransmitters in the brain–gut connection that cause pain. Encourage compliance with the medication regimen: compliance is needed to achieve beneficial results with many of these medications.

Arrange for counseling, if necessary, for children with social stressors. Children with recurrent abdominal pain may become so debilitated that they cannot function in school, possibly requiring homebound instruction. Provide education to the school, with parental permission, regarding the child's illness and how to best deal with it. Explain that this recurrent abdominal pain is a true pain that children feel and is not "in their minds" (Jarrett et al., 2003).

Hepatobiliary Disorders

Hepatobiliary disorders include pancreatitis, gallbladder disease, jaundice, biliary atresia, hepatitis, cirrhosis and portal hypertension, and liver transplantation.

• PANCREATITIS

Pancreatitis is increasingly being recognized as a childhood problem. It is classified into two categories: acute and chronic. Acute pancreatitis is an acute inflammatory process that occurs within the pancreas, with variable involvement of localized tissues and remote organ systems. Most common causes of acute pancreatitis include abdominal trauma, drugs and alcohol (though probably rare in children), multisystem disease (such as inflammatory bowel disease or systemic lupus erythematosus), infections (usually viruses such as cytomegalovirus or hepatitis), congenital anomalies (ductal or pancreatic malformations), obstruction (most likely gallstones or tumors in children), or metabolic disorders. Chronic pancreatitis is defined based on the structural and/or functional permanent changes that occur in the pancreas (Werlin, 2004).

When pancreatitis is suspected, the child is placed on immediate bowel rest (NPO). Often, a nasogastric tube placed for suction will be needed to keep the stomach decompressed. Serial monitoring of serum amylase levels will determine when oral feeding may be restarted (Werlin, 2004).

Nursing Assessment

For a full description of the assessment phase of the nursing process refer to page 662. Assessment findings pertinent to pancreatitis are discussed below.

Health History

Elicit a description of the present illness and chief complaint. Common signs and symptoms reported during the health history include:

- Acute onset of persistent midepigastric and periumbilical abdominal pain, often with radiation to the back or chest
- Vomiting, especially after meals
- Fever

Explore the child's current and past medical history for risk factors such as:

- Cystic fibrosis
- History of gallstones
- Traumatic injury
- Family history of hereditary pancreatitis

Physical Examination

On abdominal assessment, the bowel sounds may be diminished, suggesting peritonitis. The abdomen may be tender, and distention may occur in younger children and infants. In severe cases, jaundice, ascites, or pleural effusions may occur. Bluish discoloration around the umbilicus or flanks is seen in the most severe cases of pancreatitis when hemorrhage is present.

Laboratory and Diagnostic Tests

Common laboratory and diagnostic studies ordered for the assessment and monitoring of pancreatitis include:

- Serum amylase and/or lipase: levels three times the normal values are extremely indicative of pancreatitis (Werlin, 2004)
- Liver profile: often done to check for increased liver functions and/or bilirubin levels
- Blood work: leukocytosis is common with acute pancreatitis. Hyperglycemia and hypocalcemia may also be noted.
- C-reactive protein: levels may be elevated

Diagnostic imaging studies performed to identify malformations or cysts on the pancreas include:

- Plain abdominal x-ray: may show a localized ileus
- Ultrasound: allows direct visualization of the pancreas and the surrounding structures. This is used most frequently with children, as it is less invasive than a CT scan. A CT scan is usually used when there is difficulty in determining the cause of the pancreatitis during ultrasonography.
- Endoscopic retrograde cholangiopancreatography (ERCP): used in some children who may have ductal anomalies, usually with chronic pancreatitis, though complications from this procedure may occur.

Nursing Management

Maintain NPO status and nasogastric tube suction and patency. Administer intravenous fluids to keep the patient hydrated and correct any alterations in fluid and electrolyte balance. Pain management is crucial in children with pancreatitis. If hemorrhagic pancreatitis has occurred, blood products and/or intravenous antibiotics may be needed. Oral feedings are restarted only after the serum amylase level has returned to normal (usually in 2 to 4 days) (Werlin, 2004). Often, pancreatic enzymes are given with oral feedings if pain occurs after oral feeds are restarted.

Surgery is rarely needed in patients with pancreatitis, except in those with severe abdominal trauma or major ductal abnormalities.

Though chronic pancreatitis is rare in children, provide patient and family education regarding the signs and symptoms of recurrence and complications.

● GALLBLADDER DISEASE

Cholelithiasis is the presence of stones in the gallbladder. Cholesterol stones are usually associated with hyperlipidemia, obesity, pregnancy, birth control pill use, or cystic fibrosis. They are seen more often in females than males, and increased risk occurs with age and onset of puberty. These stones occur in the gallbladder and may be found in the common bile duct. Pigment stones are found in prepubertal children and occur about equally in males and females. They are usually found in the common bile duct (associated with bacterial or parasitic infections) or the gallbladder itself (associated with hemolytic anemia or liver cirrhosis). Cholecystitis is an inflammation of the gallbladder that is caused by the chemical irritation due to the obstruction of bile flow from the gallbladder into the cystic ducts (Fig. 21.19). This inflammation is typically associated with gallstones in children. The most common complication in children with gallstone disease is pancreatitis (Suchy, 2004).

If cholelithiasis results in symptomatic cholecystitis, then surgical removal of the gallbladder (cholecystectomy) will be necessary. This is often accomplished laparoscopically.

Nursing Assessment

For a full description of the assessment phase of the nursing process refer to page 662. Assessment findings pertinent to gallbladder disease are discussed below.

Health History

Elicit a description of the present illness and chief complaint. Common signs and symptoms reported during the health history include:

- Right upper quadrant pain, often radiating substernally or to the right shoulder
- Nausea and vomiting
- Jaundice and fever (with cholecystitis)

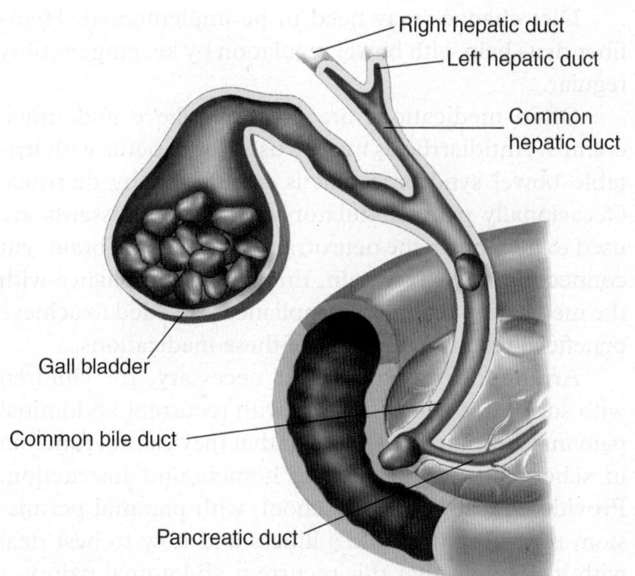

● **Figure 21.19** When gallstones block the flow of bile through the ducts, cholecystitis results.

Document a detailed diet history as it relates to the presenting symptoms. Pain episodes usually occur after meals (postprandially), especially after the ingestion of fatty or greasy foods. Younger children may present with more nonspecific symptoms, most often due to their lack of ability to communicate their symptoms to others. Explore the patient's current and past medical history for risk factors such as chronic TPN use or sickle cell disease.

Physical Examination

Palpate the abdomen for tenderness. If cholecystitis is present, the gallbladder becomes inflamed, often to the point of causing localized tenderness upon palpation. Assess skin and sclerae color for jaundice. Note presence of fever.

Laboratory and Diagnostic Tests

Common laboratory and diagnostic studies ordered for the assessment of cholecystitis include:

- Liver function tests, bilirubin, and C-reactive protein: values may be elevated if ductal stones are present
- CBC: may reveal leukocytosis
- Amylase and lipase: may be elevated if pancreatitis is also present
- Plain abdominal x-rays: may reveal radiopaque stones
- Ultrasound of the gallbladder and surrounding structures: to assess the intraluminal contents of the gallbladder as well as any anatomic alterations
- ERCP: to rule out ductal stones
- HIDA scan: to evaluate the function of the gallbladder

Nursing Management

The child with symptomatic cholecystitis will usually be hospitalized. Administer intravenous fluids, maintain NPO status and gastric decompression, and administer pain medications. If ordered, administer intravenous antibiotics to treat clinically worsening symptoms of cholecystitis, such as persistent fever. Provide routine postoperative care after cholecystectomy is performed. Provide pre- and postoperative teaching for families of children undergoing gallbladder removal.

• JAUNDICE

Jaundice is the most common clinical problem in newborns and is the most common reason for infant readmission to the hospital in the first week of life (AAP, 2004; Maisels, 2005a, b, c, d). It may also occur in older infants and children as a symptom of another disease process. Jaundice is a condition in which the skin, sclerae, body fluids, and other tissues have a yellow discoloration caused by the deposition of bile pigment resulting from excess bilirubin in the blood. It may be caused by obstruction of bile passageways, excess destruction of red blood cells (hemolysis), or disturbances in functioning of liver cells (Maisels, 2005a, b, c, d).

Newborn jaundice can be divided into two categories: physiologic and pathologic. Physiologic jaundice is the more common type, occurring usually after the first 24 hours of life. It usually lasts no longer than 1 week, and the infant shows no signs of illness. Physiologic jaundice occurs because the newborn cannot excrete bilirubin due to immaturity. Normally, the level of indirect or unconjugated bilirubin peaks at day 3 to 4 of life at 5 to 6 mg/dL. These levels may be higher in breastfed infants.

Pathologic jaundice may appear at less than 24 hours of age and lasts for longer than 1 week. In some cases, the jaundice may disappear and reappear after a period of time, as in biliary atresia. In pathologic jaundice, the conjugated or direct bilirubin value is greater than 20% of the total bilirubin value (Maisels, 2005a, b, c, d). There may be several causes for pathologic jaundice (Table 21.3).

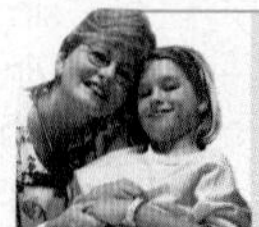

Significant jaundice in a newborn less than 24 hours of age should be immediately reported to the physician, as it may indicate a pathologic process.

Therapeutic Management

Physiologic jaundice is initially managed by increasing oral feedings to enhance bilirubin excretion. Phototherapy is indicated when jaundice fails to resolve within an acceptable time frame. In babies with hemolytic disorders, exchange therapy may be necessary to remove the sensitized red blood cells and bilirubin and exchange them with bilirubin-free blood. This is usually accomplished in the intensive care unit. Pathologic jaundice requires further investigation to determine the cause; treatment is based on the cause.

Nursing Assessment

For a full description of the assessment phase of the nursing process refer to page 662. Assessment findings pertinent to jaundice are discussed below.

Health History

Elicit a description of the present illness and chief complaint. Typically, the parents report that the infant is sleepier than usual or feeding poorly. Explore the patient's current and past medical history for risk factors such as family history of metabolic or hepatic disease; exposure to drugs, toxins, or infectious agents; Rh or ABO incompatibility; presence of large cephalhematoma or significant bruising; and polycythemia. Assess the infant's feeding history.

Physical Examination

Assess the skin, mucous membranes, sclerae, and bodily fluids (tears, urine) for a yellow color. Observe stool

Table 21.3 Causes of Pathologic Jaundice

Cause	Laboratory Values	Possible Explanations	Notable Facts
Hemolysis	Indirect bilirubin levels are elevated in the first 24 hours of life.	Rh incompatibility, sickle cell anemia, drug-induced, hemolytic-uremic syndrome, Wilson's disease, deficiencies of red blood cell enzymes (G6PD deficiency), hereditary spherocytosis	Elevated unconjugated hyperbilirubinemia
Obstructive disorders	Direct hyperbilirubinemia, usually elevations in alkaline phosphatase, serum GGT, liver enzymes, occasionally pancreatic enzymes	Biliary atresia, cholelithiasis, choledochal cysts, tumors, bile duct stenosis	Surgical correction is necessary in all obstructive disorders to avoid long-term damage to vital organs.
Infectious causes	Specific to different causes of infection	Hepatitis A, B, C, D, E, and G, cytomegalovirus, herpes simplex virus 1, 2, 6, Epstein-Barr virus, measles, varicella, human parvovirus, toxoplasmosis, syphilis, bacterial sepsis/urinary tract infection, cholecystitis	Treatment options differ with causes; bacterial causes should be identified and treated immediately.
Metabolic disorders	Specific to different disorders; elevations in conjugated bilirubin seen	Wilson's disease, alpha-1 antitrypsin deficiency, tyrosinemia, galactosemia, fructosemia, Zellweger syndrome, neonatal iron storage disease, cystic fibrosis, bile acid synthesis defects	Considered rare but should not be excluded from differential diagnosis of infant with hyperbilirubinemia
Toxic disorders	Elevations in conjugated bilirubin as well as drug levels and liver enzymes	Total parenteral nutrition (TPN), drug overdose (such as acetaminophen and ethanol), toxic drug levels (phenytoin, valproic acid)	Patients receiving hepatotoxic drugs should be monitored for toxic blood levels periodically and with dosage changes.
Idiopathic	Elevations in serum conjugated bilirubin levels	Idiopathic neonatal hepatitis, Alagille syndrome, familial intrahepatic cholestasis, cholestasis with lymphedema (Aagenaes syndrome), cholestasis with hypopituitarism	Can be infectious or hereditary

color; stools may appear acholic (white and chalky). Use digital skin blanching to determine the presence of jaundice. Infants with jaundice will appear icteric initially in the face, and then the yellowish discoloration will spread caudally to the trunk and then the extremities. Inspect the abdomen for distention (liver enlargement or ascites).

Laboratory and Diagnostic Studies

Assess laboratory values for bilirubin (both unconjugated and conjugated), alkaline phosphatase, liver enzymes, GGT, and prothrombin time (PT) and partial thromboplastin time (PTT). Many infants and children will need radiologic evaluation to determine abnormalities that may be causing the jaundice.

Nursing Management

Nursing management of the infant or child with jaundice is specific to the underlying cause. However, in all cases, proper nutrition is essential to increase bilirubin clearance. For newborns with physiologic jaundice, encourage mothers of breastfeeding infants to nurse up to 12 times in a 24-hour period (Maisels, 2005a, b, c, d). If this does not reduce jaundice, the infant's diet may need to be supplemented with formula for a specific period of time. Administer phototherapy as ordered, ensuring that appropriate precautions are taken to shield the eyes from the ultraviolet light (Fig. 21.20). Explain to parents that this therapy is used to expose the infants to light (sun or artificial) to help alter the bilirubin to a readily excreted form. Reassess the stools and feeding history of infants receiving phototherapy to ensure proper hydration. Help to relieve family anxiety regarding jaundice in the newborn or child by explaining when to notify the physician (increasing jaundice, lethargy, poor feeding, vomiting, or acute changes in the child's condition).

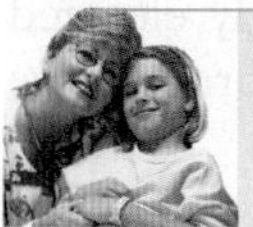

The AAP does not recommend the use of sunlight as a treatment for physiologic jaundice because of the risk for sunburn and the difficulty with regulating light exposure.

● BILIARY ATRESIA

Biliary atresia is an absence of some or all of the major biliary ducts, resulting in obstruction of bile flow. The resultant obstruction to bile flow causes cholestasis and progressive fibrosis with end-stage cirrhosis of the liver (Balistreri, 2004). In approximately 80% of the cases, biliary atresia presents around 4 weeks of age in term, healthy infants who have resolved physiologic jaundice. In approximately 20% of cases, biliary atresia presents with persistent jaundice that never disappeared from the physiologic period. This second type of biliary atresia often is associated with other congenital anomalies, such as situs inversus, malrotation, polysplenia, and cardiovascular defects (Balistreri, 2004). The etiology of biliary atresia is unknown, but there are several theories, including infectious, autoimmune, or ischemic causes.

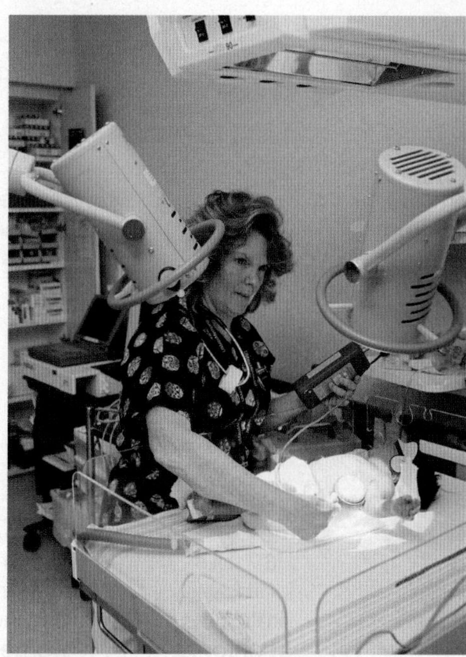

● Figure 21.20 The infant's eyes must be covered to protect them from the ultraviolet light when receiving phototherapy.

Therapeutic Management

If there is a high suspicion of biliary atresia, the infant will undergo exploratory laparotomy. If biliary atresia is found, a Kasai procedure (hepatoportoenterostomy) is performed to connect the bowel lumen to the bile duct remnants found at the porta hepatis. This procedure is usually successful only for infants up to 8 weeks of age, as bile flow restoration after this age is minimal. Infants who are not identified early enough or those who have failed to respond to the Kasai procedure will need to undergo liver transplantation, usually by age 2.

Nursing Assessment

For a full description of the assessment phase of the nursing process refer to page 662. Assessment findings pertinent to biliary atresia are discussed below.

Health History

Elicit a description of the present illness and chief complaint. Persistent or recurring jaundice is the most common symptom reported during the health history.

Physical Examination

In the initial assessment of an infant with cholestasis of unknown origin, assess the stool character. In biliary atresia, stools will be acholic (chalky and white due to the lack of bile pigment). During the physical assessment, the liver will feel enlarged and hardened. Splenomegaly may occur. In the absence of other congenital malformations, the infant will otherwise appear healthy.

Laboratory and Diagnostic Studies

Common laboratory and diagnostic studies ordered for the assessment of biliary atresia include:

- Serum bilirubin, alkaline phosphatase, liver enzymes, GGT: elevated
- Ultrasound: to identify anomalies
- Biliary scan: to distinguish whether the cholestasis is intrahepatic or extrahepatic
- Liver biopsy: to confirm the diagnosis (Balistreri, 2004)

Nursing Management

Nursing management of infants who have biliary atresia will focus on vitamin and caloric support. Administer fat-soluble vitamins A, D, E, and K. Special formulas containing medium-chain triglycerides are used because significant fat malabsorption occurs when cholestasis is present. Administer feedings via nasogastric tube as needed to ensure increased caloric intake. Identify infections as quickly as possible and administer intravenous antibiotics as ordered. Manage ascites with diuretics and dietary restrictions. Preoperative management before a Kasai procedure is focused on preparation for surgery; infants who have suspected biliary atresia require immediate surgery to optimize outcomes.

Parents and family members of these infants will have extreme anxiety due to the implications of the diagnosis and outcomes. Focus education on the diagnosis and postoperative care. Nursing Care Plan 21.1 gives information about routine postoperative care.

HEPATITIS

Hepatitis is an inflammation of the liver that is caused by a variety of agents, including viral infections, bacterial invasion, metabolic disorders, chemical toxicity, and trauma. The most common viral causes of hepatitis are listed in Table 21.4. Other viruses that may cause hepatitis are cytomegalovirus (CMV), Epstein-Barr virus (EBV), and adenovirus. Fulminant hepatitis is thought to be caused by a non-A, non-B, non-C virus. Children who present with fulminant hepatitis have acute massive hepatic necrosis, resulting in death without liver transplantation. The disease progresses rapidly to severe jaundice, coagulopathy, elevated ammonia levels, significantly elevated liver enzyme levels (AST and ALT), and progressive

Table 21.4 Hepatitis Viruses A–E

	Hepatitis A (HAV)	Hepatitis B (HBV)	Hepatitis C (HCV)	Hepatitis D (HDV)	Hepatitis E (HEV)
Transmission route	Oral–fecal route, poor sanitation, waterborne	Sexual, intravenous drug use, blood transfusion, perinatally transmitted from mother to infant	Blood product transfusion, intravenous drug use	Same as HBV; HBV markers in serum must be present	Oral–fecal, possible contact
Incubation period	15 to 30 days	50 to 150 days	30 to 160 days	50 to 150 days	15 to 65 days
Signs and symptoms	Flu-like symptoms Preicteric phase: headache, fatigue, fever, anorexia Icteric phase: jaundice, dark urine, tender liver (right upper quadrant pain)	Some cases are asymptomatic; others present with anorexia, abdominal pain, fatigue, rash, slight fever, visible jaundice, enlarged liver.	Chronic cases usually present asymptomatically; others with flu-like symptoms, jaundice, hepatosplenomegaly	Same as HBV	Same as HAV, more severe in pregnant women
Prognosis	Rarely develops into fulminant liver failure; 95% of children recover without sequelae	Chronic disease state likely; increased risk of hepatic cancer	Many will develop chronic hepatitis and cirrhosis.	Same as HBV, but increased likelihood of chronic active hepatitis and cirrhosis	Same as HAV; high mortality in pregnant women

coma. Autoimmune hepatitis is a chronic disorder, affecting mostly adolescent females. The clinical presentation of a child with autoimmune hepatitis includes hepatosplenomegaly, jaundice, fever, fatigue, and right upper quadrant pain.

Therapeutic Management

Acute hepatitis is treated with rest, hydration, and nutrition. Control of bleeding may also be necessary. Chronic hepatitis often eventually requires liver transplantation. Corticosteroids and immunosuppressants may be used for autoimmune hepatitis. The child with fulminant hepatitis usually requires intensive care with cardiorespiratory support. See Healthy People 2010.

Nursing Assessment

For a full description of the assessment phase of the nursing process refer to page 662. Assessment findings pertinent to hepatitis are discussed below. The nursing assessment for any child who presents with suspected hepatitis should be the same.

Health History

Elicit a description of the present illness and the chief complaint. Common signs and symptoms reported during the health history include:

- Jaundice
- Fever
- Fatigue
- Abdominal pain

Explore the patient's current and past medical history for risk factors such as:

- Recent foreign travel
- Sick contacts
- Medication use
- Abdominal trauma
- Sexual activity
- Intravenous drug use
- Blood product transfusion

Document onset of symptoms as well as all signs and symptoms the patient has been experiencing.

Physical Examination

Observe the skin for jaundice and the sclerae for icterus. Palpate the abdomen to reveal abnormal liver and spleen size or tenderness.

Laboratory and Diagnostic Studies

Common laboratory and diagnostic studies ordered for the assessment of hepatitis include:

- Liver enzymes, GGT: elevated
- PT/PTT: prolonged
- Ammonia: elevated in the presence of encephalopathy
- Autoimmune studies, such as antinuclear antibodies, anti–smooth muscle antibodies, and liver–kidney microsomal antibodies: may be used to diagnose autoimmune hepatitis
- Viral studies: to identify viral causes of hepatitis, such as hepatitis A–E antigens and antibodies, CMV and EBV
- Ultrasound: to assess liver or spleen abnormalities
- Liver biopsy: to determine the type of hepatitis and to assess for damage that has already been done to the liver

Nursing Management

Acute hepatitis requires rest, hydration, and nutrition. If the child develops vomiting, dehydration, elevated bleeding times (PT/PTT), or mental status changes (encephalopathy), hospitalization may be required. When caring for patients with infectious hepatitis, provide education about transmission and prevention, including proper hygiene, safe sexual activity, careful hand washing techniques, and blood/bodily fluid precautions.

Fulminant hepatitis treatment is aggressive and will require NPO status, nasogastric tube administration of lactulose to decrease ammonia levels that lead to encephalopathic conditions, TPN administration, vitamin K injections to help with coagulopathies, and, ultimately, liver transplantation. Fear and anxiety of the patient and parents will likely be very high. Teach the child and family about the diagnosis and what to expect during treatment. Provide immunoglobulin therapy and vaccinations to close contacts of infectious hepatitis patients.

HEALTHY PEOPLE 2010

Objective	Significance
Reduce or eliminate indigenous cases of vaccine-preventable diseases, hepatitis B (persons aged 2 to 18 years). Reduce hepatitis A.	• Educate families about hepatitis B and its transmission. • Encourage routine infant and childhood vaccination against hepatitis A and B as recommended. • For hepatitis A prevention, educate families about appropriate hygiene and hand washing.

● CIRRHOSIS AND PORTAL HYPERTENSION

Cirrhosis of the liver occurs as a result of the destructive processes that occur during liver damage, leading to the formation of nodules. These nodules can be small (micronodular [less than 3 mm]) or large (macronodular [greater than 3 mm]) and distort the vasculature of the liver, leading to further complications. Causes of cirrhosis in children include biliary malformations, alpha-1 antitrypsin deficiency, Wilson's disease, galactosemia, tyrosinemia, chronic active hepatitis, and prolonged TPN use (Sokol & Narkewicz, 2005). Major complications may exist due to cirrhosis of the liver, including portal hypertension. In portal hypertension, the blood flow to, through, or from the liver meets resistance, causing portal blood flow pressures to rise. As these pressures rise, collateral veins form between the portal and systemic venous circulations. The most significant complication of portal hypertension is GI bleeding, from shunting to submucosal veins (varices) in the stomach and esophagus. Esophageal varices may be treated with sclerotherapy during endoscopy to stop acute bleeding. Often blood product administration and vasopressive drugs are needed. In the long term, the only cure for cirrhosis is liver transplantation.

Nursing Assessment

For a full description of the assessment phase of the nursing process refer to page 662. Assessment findings pertinent to cirrhosis and portal hypertension are discussed below.

Health History

Elicit a description of the present illness and chief complaint. Common signs and symptoms reported during the health history include:

- Nausea and vomiting
- Jaundice
- Weakness
- Swelling
- Weight loss

Explore the patient's current and past medical history for risk factors such as hepatitis, cystic fibrosis, Wilson's disease, hematochromatosis, and biliary atresia. Assess the past medical history to identify possible causes for liver disease.

Physical Examination

Inspect for jaundice, ascites, spider angiomas, and palmar erythema. Gynecomastia is often seen in males. Palpate the liver; typically it is enlarged and hard, but occasionally it is small and shrunken. Evaluate mental status to determine the presence of hepatic encephalopathy.

Laboratory and Diagnostic Studies

Laboratory and diagnostic testing will be similar to that of a child with hepatitis. Common laboratory and diagnostic studies ordered for the assessment of cirrhosis or portal hypertension include:

- Liver biopsy: reveals regenerating nodules and surrounding **fibrosis**
- Upper endoscopy: reveals varices and bleeding (Fig. 21.21)

Nursing Management

Nursing management is very similar to the care of the patient with hepatitis. In cases of cirrhosis causing portal hypertension and bleeding varices, GI bleeding must be controlled. This is usually done by replacing blood loss and providing vasopressive therapy to constrict the shunted blood flow. As with all liver disorders and GI bleeding, address and manage family and patient anxiety. Be honest about the child's treatment plan and prognosis. Involve the family in the care of the child and educate them as needed.

LIVER TRANSPLANTATION

Hepatobiliary disorders that result in failure of the liver to function result in the need for liver transplantation. Liver transplantation in children has become increasingly successful in the past several years due to advances in immunosuppression, better selection of transplant candidates, and improvements in surgical techniques and postoperative care. Transplant centers now offer both cadaveric and living-related liver transplants for children. Rejection of the transplanted liver is the most significant complication. Most children will require immunosuppressive therapy for a lifetime, putting them at risk for infections.

Nursing Assessment

Many children will be admitted to a transplant center for a preoperative work-up to determine the best possible tissue and blood match for the patient. There is much

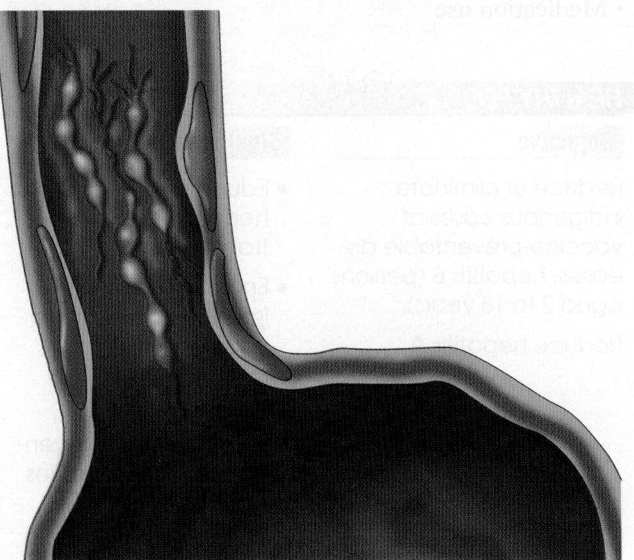

● Figure 21.21 Esophageal varices.

anxiety among family members when a cadaveric transplant is the only possibility for survival. This puts a child on a waiting list that is prioritized based on several criteria. Because there are a limited number of pediatric liver transplant centers throughout the country, there may be many issues regarding transportation, finances, job loss, and lodging. Assess the need for social work intervention; a social worker is almost always involved with these patients. A liver transplant coordinator will assist with coordinating the care for pre- and post-transplant patients.

Nursing Management

Preoperatively, assist with the transplant work-up and teach the child and family what to expect during and after the liver transplantation. Postoperatively, the child will be in the intensive care unit for several days until he or she is stabilized from the actual surgery (see Nursing Care Plan 21.1). After the child is sent to a regular unit in the hospital, monitor the child for several days to weeks for signs and symptoms of rejection and infection, including fever, increasing liver function test results and GGT, and increasing pain, redness, and swelling at the incision site.

Patient and family education is an important element of nursing management in the post-transplant patient. Assess and reassess medication knowledge throughout the entire hospitalization, as these children usually require medications for a lifetime.

References

Books and Journals

Allen, P. L. J. (2004). Guidelines for the diagnosis and treatment of celiac disease in children. *Pediatric Nursing, 30*(6), 473–476.

American Academy of Pediatrics, Subcommittee on Hyperbilirubinemia. (2004). Clinical practice guideline: Management of hyperbilirubinemia in the newborn infant 35 or more weeks of gestation. *Pediatrics, 114*(1), 297–316.

Arguin, A. L., & Swartz, M. K. (2004). Gastroesophageal reflux in infants: A primary care perspective. *Pediatric Nursing, 30*(1), 45–51, 71.

Balistreri, W. F. (2004). Cholestasis. In R. E. Behrman, R. M. Kliegman, & H. B. Jenson (Eds.), *Nelson textbook of pediatrics* (17th ed.). Philadelphia: W. B. Saunders.

Bender, B. J., Skae, C. C., & Ozuah, P. O. (2005). Oral rehydration therapy: The clear solution to fluid loss. *Contemporary Pediatrics, 22*(4), 72–76.

Berman, J. (2003). Heading off the dangers of acute gastroenteritis. *Contemporary Pediatrics, 20*(7), 57–74.

Bhutani, V. K., Johnson, L. H., & Keren, R. (2005). Treating acute bilirubin encephalopathy before it's too late. *Contemporary Pediatrics, 22*(5), 57–74.

Blevins, J. Y. (2003). Primary herpetic gingivostomatitis in young children. *Pediatric Nursing, 29*(3), 199–201.

Brent, N. B. (2001). Thrush in the breastfeeding dyad: Results of a survey on diagnosis and treatment. *Clinical Pediatrics, 40*, 503–506.

Brunnell, P. A. (2006). Winter vomiting disease, 1929–2006. *Infectious Diseases in Children, 19*(1), 6–7.

Cahill, J., & Wagner, C. (2002). Challenges in breastfeeding: Neonatal concerns. *Contemporary Pediatrics.* Accessed 5/24/04 at www.contpeds.com

Carroll, M. (2002). Peptic ulcer disease. Available at: www.emedicine.com/ped/topic2341.htm

Castiglia, P. (2001). Constipation in children. *Journal of Pediatric Health Care, 15*, 200–202.

Centers for Disease Control and Prevention. (2003). Managing acute gastroenteritis among children: Oral rehydration, maintenance, and nutritional therapy. *MMWR, 52*(No. RR-16), 1–16.

Children's Healthcare of Atlanta. (2004). *Ostomy care home care manual.* Atlanta: Children's Healthcare of Atlanta.

Cincinnati Children's Hospital Medical Center (2003). Intestinal malrotation and volvulus. www.cincinattichildrens.org/health/info/abdomen/diagnose/intestinal-malrotation.htm

Cincinnati Children's Hospital Medical Center. (2005). *Enema administration.* Retrieved May 13, 2006, from www.cincinnati childrens.org/health/info/abdomen/home/enema.htm

ConvaTec (2000). *A parent's guide to ostomy care for infants and children.* Princeton: ConvaTec, A Bristol-Myers Squibb Company.

Coughlin, E. C. (2003). Assessment and management of pediatric constipation in primary care. *Pediatric Nursing, 29*(4), 296–301.

Curtin, G. (2004). Cleft lip and cleft palate. In P. L. Jackson & J. A. Vessey (Eds.), *Primary care of the child with a chronic condition* (4th ed.). St. Louis: Mosby.

Dale, J. (2004). Oral rehydration solutions in the management of acute gastroenteritis among children. *Journal of Pediatric Health Care, 18*, 211–212.

DiPalma, J., & Gremse, D. (2003). Chronic constipation in children: Rational management. *Consultant for Pediatricians, 2*(4), 151–155.

Engel, J. (2002). *Pocket guide to pediatric assessment* (4th ed). St. Louis: Mosby.

Fischbach, F. (2003). *A manual of laboratory & diagnostic tests* (7th ed.). Philadelphia: Lippincott Williams & Wilkins.

Gallagher, C. (2003). A guidelines-based approach for managing acute gastroenteritis in children. *Journal for Specialists in Pediatric Nursing, 8*(3), 107–110.

Gardiner, P., & Kemper, K. J. (2005). For GI complaints, which herbs and supplements spell relief? *Contemporary Pediatrics, 22*(8), 51–55.

Hamilton, J. (2000). The pediatric patient: Early development and the digestive system. In W. Walker, P. Durie, J. Hamilton, J. Walker-Smith, & J. Watkins (Eds.), *Pediatric GI disease.* Hamilton, Ontario: B. C. Decker, Inc.

Herbst, J. J. (2004). Primary (peptic) ulcers. In R. E. Behrman, R. M. Kliegman, & H. B. Jenson (Eds.), *Nelson textbook of pediatrics* (17th ed.). Philadelphia: W. B. Saunders.

Holcomb, S. S. (2005). Managing jaundice in full-term infants. *Nurse Practitioner, 30*(1), 6–12.

Hollister, Inc. (2003). *Pediatric care: what's right for my baby?* Libertyville, IL: Hollister, Inc.

Howell, L. J. (2004). *Information about specific surgical procedures: ileostomy.* Retrieved May 13, 2006, from www.chop.edu/consumer/jsp/division/generic.jsp?id=72368

Jakubik, L. D., Colfer, A., & Grossman, M. B. (2000). Pediatric short bowel syndrome: Pathophysiology, nursing care, and management issues. *Journal of the Society of Pediatric Nurses, 5*(3), 111–121.

Jarrett, M., Heitkemper, M., Czyzewski, D. I., & Shulman, R. (2003). Recurrent abdominal pain in children: Forerunner to adult irritable bowel syndrome? *Journal for Specialists in Pediatric Nursing, 8*(3), 81–89.

Katz, D. A. (2001). Evaluation and management of inguinal and umbilical hernias. *Pediatric Annals, 30*(12), 729–735.

Korn, D. (2002). *Wheat-free, worry-free: The art of happy, healthy gluten-free living.* Carlsbad, CA: Hay House, Inc.

Kronemyer, B. (2003). Establish duration of mouth ulcer to successfully treat in children. *Infectious Diseases in Children, 16*, 43–44.

Letton, R. (2001). Pyloric stenosis. *Pediatric Annals, 30*(12), 745–749.

Leung, A. K., & Kao, C. P. (2003). Oral lesions in children. *Consultant for Pediatricians, 2*(2), 81–84.

Lockridge, T., Caldwell, A. D., & Jason, P. (2002). Congenital neonatal surgical emergencies: Stabilization and management. *Journal of Obstetric, Gynecologic and Neonatal Nursing, 31*, 328–339.

Longstreth, G. F. (2002). Current approach to the diagnosis of irritable bowel syndrome. [electronic version] available at www.aboutibs.org/Publications/diagnosis.html

Maisels, J. (2005a). A primer on phototherapy for the jaundiced newborn. *Contemporary Pediatrics, 22*(6), 38–57.

Maisels, J. (2005b). Jaundice. In M. G. MacDonald, M. M. K. Seshia, & M. D. Mullett (Eds.), *Avery's neonatology: Pathophysiology and management of the newborn.* Philadelphia: Lippincott Williams & Wilkins.

Maisels, J. (2005c). Jaundice in a newborn: Answers to questions about a common clinical problem. *Contemporary Pediatrics, 22*(5), 34–40.

Maisels, J. (2005d). Jaundice in a newborn: How to head off an urgent situation. *Contemporary Pediatrics, 22*(5), 41–54.

March of Dimes (2004). Cleft lip and cleft palate. Accessed May 24, 2004, at www.marchofdimes.com/professionals/681_1210.asp

Mitchell, J., & Wood, R. (2000). Management of cleft lip and palate in primary care. *Journal of Pediatric Health Care, 14*(1), 13–19.

National Digestive Diseases Information Clearinghouse (NDDIC) (2003). *Celiac disease.* http://digestive.niddk.nih.gov/ddiseases/pubs/celiac/index/htm

Peña, A. (2004). Anorectal malformations. In R. E. Behrman, R. M. Kliegman, & H. B. Jenson (Eds.), *Nelson textbook of pediatrics* (17th ed.). Philadelphia: W. B. Saunders.

Pollack, V. P., & Ravenscroft, A. D. (2004). Inflammatory bowel disease. In P. L. Jackson & J. A. Vessey (Eds.), *Primary care of the child with a chronic condition* (4th ed.). St. Louis: Mosby.

Rolstad, B. S., & Erwin-Toth, P. (2004). Peristomal skin complications: Prevention and management. *Ostomy/Wound Management, 50*(9), 68–77.

Sandberg, D., Magee, W., & Denk, M. (2002). Neonatal cleft lip and cleft palate repair. *AORN Journal, 72*(3), 490–508.

Schmitt, B. (2002). *Enema: How to give.* Broomfield, CO: McKesson Health Solutions LLC.

Schmitt, B. D. (2004). Toilet training problems: Underachievers, refusers, and stool holders. *Contemporary Pediatrics, 21*(4), 71–80.

Sehgal, S., & Allen, P. L. J. (2004). Hepatitis C in children. *Pediatric Nursing, 30*(5), 409–413.

Sharp, H. M., Dailey, S., & Moon, J. B. (2003). Speech and language development disorders in infants and children with cleft lip and palate. *Pediatric Annals, 32*(7), 476–480.

Shollenberger, D. A., & Small, C. C. (2004). GI care. In E. J. Mills (Ed.), *Nursing procedures.* Philadelphia: Lippincott Williams & Wilkins.

Shukla, P. (2002). *Meckel diverticulum.* http://www.emedicine.com/ped/topic1389.htm

Sokol, R., & Narkewicz, M. (2005). Liver & pancreas. In W. W. Hay, M. J. Levin, J. M. Sondheimer, & R. R. Deterding (Eds.), *Current pediatric diagnosis & treatment* (17th ed.). NewYork: McGraw-Hill.

Sondheimer, J. (2005). GI tract. W. W. Hay, M. J. Levin, J. M. Sondheimer, & R. R. Deterding (Eds.), *Current pediatric diagnosis & treatment* (17th ed.). New York: McGraw-Hill.

Steiner, M. J., DeWalt, D. A., & Byerley, J. S. (2004). Is this child dehydrated? *Journal of the American Medical Association, 291*(22), 2746–2754.

Stoll, B. J. & Kliegman, P. M. (2004). Neonatal necrotizing enterocolitis (NEC). In R. E. Behrman, R. M. Kliegman, & H. B. Jenson (Eds.), *Nelson textbook of pediatrics* (17th ed.). Philadelphia: W. B. Saunders.

Suchy, F. J. (2004). Diseases of the gallbladder. In R. E. Behrman, R. M. Kliegman, & H. B. Jenson (Eds.), *Nelson textbook of pediatrics* (17th ed.). Philadelphia: W. B. Saunders.

Taketokmo, C. K., Hodding, J. H., & Kraus, D. M. (2004). *Lexi-comp's pediatric dosage handbook* (11th ed.). Hudson, Ohio: Lexi-comp.

Texas Children's Hospital (2000). *What is an ostomy?* Retrieved May 13, 2006, from www2.texaschildrenshospital.org/internetarticles/uploadedfiles/174.pdf

Tucker, J. (2002). *Appendicitis.* www.emedicine.com/ped/topic127.htm

Ulshen, M. (2004a). Chronic ulcerative colitis. In R. E. Behrman, R. M. Kliegman, & H. B. Jenson (Eds.), *Nelson textbook of pediatrics* (17th ed.). Philadelphia: W. B. Saunders.

Ulshen, M. (2004b). Crohn disease (regional enteritis, regional ileitis, granulomatous colitis). In R. E. Behrman, R. M. Kliegman, & H. B. Jenson (Eds.), *Nelson textbook of pediatrics* (17th ed.). Philadelphia: W. B. Saunders.

Ulshen, M. (2004c). Major symptoms and signs of digestive tract disorders. In R. E. Behrman, R. M. Kliegman, & H. B. Jenson (Eds.), *Nelson textbook of pediatrics* (17th ed.). Philadelphia: W. B. Saunders.

Werlin, S. L. (2004). Pancreatitis. In R. E. Behrman, R. M. Kliegman, & H. B. Jenson (Eds.), *Nelson textbook of pediatrics* (17th ed.). Philadelphia: W. B. Saunders.

Wesson, D., & Hadock, G. (2000). Congenital anomalies. In W. Walker, P. Durie, J. Hamilton, J. Walker-Smith, & J. Watkins (Eds.), *Pediatric GI disease.* Hamilton, Ontario: B. C. Decker, Inc.

Wyllie, R. (2004a). Congenital aganglionic megacolon (Hirschsprung disease). In R. E. Behrman, R. M. Kliegman, & H. B. Jenson (Eds.), *Nelson textbook of pediatrics* (17th ed.). Philadelphia: W. B. Saunders.

Wyllie, R. (2004b). Intussusception. In R. E. Behrman, R. M. Kliegman, & H. B. Jenson (Eds.), *Nelson textbook of pediatrics* (17th ed.). Philadelphia: W. B. Saunders.

Wyllie, R. (2004c). Malrotation. In R. E. Behrman, R. M. Kliegman, & H. B. Jenson (Eds.), *Nelson textbook of pediatrics* (17th ed.). Philadelphia: W. B. Saunders.

Wyllie, R. (2004d). Meckel diverticulum and other remnants of the omphalomesenteric duct. In R. E. Behrman, R. M. Kliegman, & H. B. Jenson (Eds.), *Nelson textbook of pediatrics* (17th ed.). Philadelphia: W. B. Saunders.

Young, R., & Huffman, S. (2003). Probiotic use in children. *Journal of Pediatric Health Care, 17*(6), 277–283.

Websites

www.aboutkidsgi.org/ International Foundation for Functional Gastrointestinal Disorders
www.acpa.-cpf.org American Cleft Palate/Craniofacial Association
www.celiac.org Celiac Disease Foundation
www.celiackids.com R.O.C.K. (Raising Our Celiac Kids) support group
www.childliverdisease.org/ Children's Liver Disease Foundation
www.cleft.org support for families with cleft lip or palate
www.cleftline.org Cleft Palate Foundation
www.convatec.com ConvaTec
www.csaceliacs.org Celiac Sprue Association
www.gluten.net Gluten Intolerance Group
www.liverfoundation.org American Liver Foundation
www.marchofdimes.com March of Dimes
www.naspgn.org/ North American Society for Pediatric Gastroenterology, Hepatology and Nutrition
www.oley.org/ Oley Foundation, a national organization for persons dependent upon intravenous or tube-fed nutrition
www.omphalocele.com a support network for parents of infants with omphalocele
www.pullthrough.org/ Pull-Through Network
www.uoaa.org United Ostomy Associations of America
www.widesmiles.org/ Wide Smiles, a cleft lip and palate resource
www.wocn.org Wound, Ostomy and Continence Nurse Society

Chapter WORKSHEET

MULTIPLE CHOICE QUESTIONS

1. A mother brings her 6-month-old infant to the clinic. The child has been vomiting since early morning and has had diarrhea since the day before. His temperature is 38° C, pulse 140, and respiratory rate 38. He has lost 6 ounces since his well-child visit 4 days ago. He cries before passing a bowel movement. He will not breastfeed today. What is the priority nursing diagnosis?
   a. Thermoregulation alteration
   b. Pain (abdominal) related to diarrhea
   c. Fluid volume deficit related to excessive losses and inadequate intake
   d. Alteration in nutrition, less than body requirements, related to decreased oral intake
2. A child presents with a 2-day history of fever, abdominal pain, occasional vomiting, and decreased oral intake. Which finding would the nurse prioritize for immediate reporting to the physician?
   a. Temperature 101.9° F
   b. Rebound tenderness and abdominal guarding
   c. Parents will be leaving the child alone in the hospital
   d. Child can tolerate only sips of fluid without nausea
3. A 3-day-old infant presenting with physiologic jaundice is hospitalized and placed under phototherapy. Which response indicates to the nurse that the parent needs more teaching?
   a. "My infant is at risk for dehydration."
   b. "My infant needs to stay under the lights, except during feeding time."
   c. "My infant can continue to breastfeed during this time."
   d. "My infant has a serious liver disease."
4. A 3-month-old infant presents with a history of vomiting after feeding. The plan for the infant is to rule out GERD. What information from the history would lead the nurse to believe that this infant may need further intervention?
   a. Poor weight gain
   b. Has small "spits" after feeding
   c. Sleeps through the night
   d. Is difficult to burp
5. The nurse is caring for a child who has had diarrhea and vomiting for the past several days. What is the priority nursing assessment?
   a. Determine the child's weight.
   b. Ask if the family has traveled outside of the country.
   c. Assess circulation and perfusion.
   d. Send a stool specimen to the lab.

CRITICAL THINKING EXERCISES

1. A 6-month-old baby is brought to the pediatrician's office with a history of diarrhea. She has had six watery stools in the past 18 hours. She is vomiting her formula. Her mother states that she has had no fever.
   a. Upon completion of the history and physical examination, what signs and symptoms would you expect to find that would indicate that the baby is experiencing mild dehydration?
   b. What is the priority nursing diagnosis for this infant?
   c. Identify a plan for this nursing diagnosis; include a teaching plan for the mother.
2. A 14-kg child with moderate dehydration has received two boluses of normal saline in the emergency room prior to being admitted to the pediatric nursing unit. The physician orders D5 ½ NS @ 1½ maintenance.
   a. What would the intravenous fluid rate be?
   b. What will the nurse assess for to determine whether the child is becoming overhydrated?
3. An infant requires a temporary colostomy. What discharge instructions would you provide to the parents about how to take care of the colostomy and when to call their health care provider?

STUDY ACTIVITIES

1. In the clinical setting, compare the growth records of a child with celiac disease to those of a similar-aged child without disease.
2. While caring for children in the clinical setting, compare and contrast the medical history, signs and symptoms of illness, and prescribed treatment for a child with Crohn's disease and one with ulcerative colitis.
3. In the clinical setting, observe the behavioral responses of an infant or young child with inorganic failure to thrive.

chapter 22

Nursing Care of the Child With a Genitourinary Disorder

Key TERMS

amenorrhea
anasarca
anuria
azotemia
bacteriuria
dysmenorrhea
enuresis
hematuria
hyperlipidemia
menorrhagia
oliguria
proteinuria
sepsis
urgency
urinary frequency

Learning OBJECTIVES

Upon completion of the chapter, the learner will be able to:

1. Compare anatomic and physiologic differences of the genitourinary system in infants and children versus adults.
2. Describe nursing care related to common laboratory and diagnostic testing used in the medical diagnosis of pediatric genitourinary conditions.
3. Distinguish genitourinary disorders common in infants, children, and adolescents.
4. Identify appropriate nursing assessments and interventions related to medications and treatments for pediatric genitourinary disorders.
5. Develop an individualized nursing care plan for the child with a genitourinary disorder.
6. Describe the psychosocial impact of chronic genitourinary disorders on children.
7. Devise a nutrition plan for the child with renal insufficiency.
8. Develop patient/family teaching plans for the child with a genitourinary disorder.

WOW *A child's essential bodily processes of elimination can be a major event of wonder and creative accomplishment.*

Corey Bond, 5 years old, is brought to the clinic by her mother. She presents with fever and lethargy for the past 24 hours. Her mother states, "Corey has had a few accidents in her pants over the past few days, which is unusual for her. She also has been getting up at night more often to use the bathroom."

Genitourinary (GU) disorders in children and adolescents may occur as a result of abnormalities in fetal development, infectious processes, trauma, neurologic deficit, genetic influences, or other causes. Congenital disorders account for a large proportion of GU disorders in infants, while enuresis and urinary tract infection (UTI) also occur in a significant number of children. Some of the disorders directly involve the kidney from the outset, while others involve other parts of the urinary tract and may have a long-term effect on the kidneys and renal function, particularly if left untreated or treated inadequately. Disorders affecting the reproductive organs often require early diagnosis and management to preserve future reproductive capabilities.

Nurses must be knowledgeable about pediatric GU conditions to provide prompt recognition, nursing care, education, and support to children and their families. Though some disorders are acute and resolve quickly, many have a long-term effect on quality of life and will require more intense, extended support.

Management of acute or common pediatric GU disorders may be provided in the pediatric or family practice outpatient setting, while specialists such as pediatric nephrologists or urologists usually manage chronic involved GU disorders.

Variations in Pediatric Anatomy and Physiology

Though all of the urinary tract and reproductive organs are present at birth, their functioning is immature initially. Many pediatric GU disorders are congenital (present at birth). External GU malformations are easily identified at birth, but internal structural defects may not be identified until later in infancy or childhood when symptoms or complications arise. In children, chronic kidney disease is most often the result of congenital structural defects or infectious, inflammatory, or immune processes that damage the kidney, whereas in adults it usually results from hypertension or diabetes. The infant or child is at increased risk for the development of certain GU disorders because of the anatomical and physiological differences between children and adults.

Urinary Concentration

Blood flow through the kidneys (glomerular filtration rate [GFR]) is slower in the infant and young toddler compared with the adult. The kidney is less able to concentrate urine and reabsorb amino acids, placing the infant and young toddler at increased risk for dehydration during times when fluid loss or decreased fluid intake occurs. The normal range for serum blood urea nitrogen (BUN) and creatinine of the healthy infant or young toddler is usually less than the older child's or adult's. The renal system usually reaches functional maturity at around 2 years of age.

Structural Differences

The kidney is large in relation to the size of the abdomen until the child reaches adolescence. Due to this increased size, the kidneys of the child are less well protected from injury by the ribs and fat padding than they are in the adult. The urethra is naturally shorter in all ages of females than in males, placing them at increased risk for the entrance of bacteria into the bladder via the urethra. In the female infant or young child, this risk is compounded by the physical proximity of the urethral opening to the rectum. The young male's urethra is much shorter than the adult male's, placing the male infant or young child at increased risk of urinary tract infection compared with the adult male.

Urine Output

Bladder capacity is about 30 mL in the newborn; it increases to the usual adult capacity of about 270 mL by 1 year of age. The expected urine output in the infant and child is 0.5 to 2 mL/kg/hour, with the average 1-year-old voiding about 400 to 500 mL per day. The average urine output for a teenager is about 800 to 1,400 mL per day. The infant and toddler may void as often as 9 or 10 times per day. By age 3 the average number of voids per day is the same as the adult's (three to eight).

Reproductive Organ Maturity

The reproductive organs are also immature at birth. The gonads are not mature until adolescence in most children. The hormonal changes that occur with puberty account for some of the reproductive concerns, particularly for female adolescents.

Common Medical Treatments

A variety of medications as well as other medical treatments and surgical procedures are used to treat GU problems in children. Most of these treatments will require a physician's order when the child is in the hospital. The most common treatments and medications are listed in Common Medical Treatments 22.1 and Drug Guide 22.1. The nurse caring for the child with a GU disorder should

(text continues on page 721)

Common Medical Treatments 22.1 Genitourinary Disorders

Treatment	Explanation	Indication	Nursing Implications
Urinary diversion	Surgical diversion of ureters to the abdominal wall. Continent diversion uses a piece of intestine to create a bladder that can be catheterized. Noncontinent diversion involves a stoma on the abdominal wall that requires use of an ostomy pouch.	Any situation in which the bladder needs to be removed or does not function correctly (bladder exstrophy or prune belly)	Meticulous skin care is necessary to prevent breakdown around stoma. Teach families how to care for ostomy pouch or how to catheterize continent stoma. Expect mucus in urine if intestine is used for urinary reservoir. Monitor for signs of urinary tract infection.
Foley catheter	An indwelling urinary catheter stays in place by means of an inflated balloon.	Usually used only during the postoperative period	Monitor for urethral drainage or irritation. Keep area clean and dry. Monitor color, consistency, clarity, and amount of urine in drainage bag. Monitor for infection, checking results of urinalysis and urine cultures.
Ureteral stent	A thin catheter temporarily placed in the ureter to drain urine. Removed via cystoscopy when it is time for discontinuation.	Urinary tract anomalies	Monitor urine output carefully. Check for bleeding postoperatively.
Nephrostomy tube	Tube placed directly into the kidney to drain urine externally to a bag	Urinary tract anomalies	Monitor urine output carefully.
Suprapubic tube	Catheter placed in the bladder via the abdominal wall above the symphysis pubis	Postoperative urine drainage with reconstructive surgeries	Monitor for blood in urine, adequate urine output. Minimize manipulation of suprapubic tube to avoid triggering bladder spasms.
Vesicostomy	Stoma in the abdominal wall to the bladder	Urinary tract anomalies, neurogenic bladder	Constant urine drainage requires diaper use. Monitor urine output. Assess skin around stoma for breakdown.
Appendicovesicostomy (Mitrofanoff procedure)	Uses appendix to create a stoma on the abdominal wall that allows for catheterization of the bladder	Urinary tract anomalies, neurogenic bladder	Allows for urinary continence, which improves the child's self-esteem. Teach family and child how to catheterize stoma.
Bladder augmentation	Uses a piece of stomach or intestine to enlarge bladder capacity	Decreased bladder capacity	Since a portion of the GI tract is used, urine is often mucus-like.

Drug Guide 22.1 Common Drugs for GU Disorders

Medication	Action	Indication	Nursing Implications
Anticholinergic agents (oxybutynin, propantheline bromide, belladonna & opium suppository)	Cause smooth muscle relaxation of the bladder	Urinary tract spasms or contractions related to surgical procedure or use of catheters. Control of nocturnal enuresis.	Increase fluid intake (limit to during the day in the child with nocturnal enuresis). Avoid use in febrile patient.
Antibiotics (oral, parenteral)	Kill bacteria or arrest their growth	Urinary tract infection, pelvic inflammatory disease, toxic shock syndrome	Check for antibiotic allergies. Should be given as prescribed for the length of time indicated.
Desmopressin (DDAVP)	Antidiuretic hormone effects by causing renal tubule to absorb more water, decreasing volume of urine	Nocturnal enuresis	Nasal spray may cause nasal irritation, nausea, flushing, or headache. Administer at bedtime; alternate nares. Associated with a high relapse rate.
Human chorionic gonadotropin (hCG)	Stimulates production of gonadal steroids	To precipitate testicular descent	Monitor for signs of precocious puberty if used long term.
Corticosteroids	Anti-inflammatory and immunosuppressive action	Induce remission and promote diuresis in nephrotic syndrome. High-dose intravenous therapy used when nephrotic syndrome is resistant to conventional doses.	Administer with food to decrease GI upset. May mask signs of infection. Do not stop treatment abruptly, or acute adrenal insufficiency may occur. Monitor for Cushing syndrome. Doses may be tapered over time. Monitor for hypertension during infusion.
Cytotoxic drugs (cyclophosphamide (Cytoxan) and chlorambucil (Leukeran))	Interfere with normal function of DNA by alkylation	Induction of prolonged remission in nephrotic syndrome	Causes bone marrow suppression. Monitor for signs of infection. Cyclophosphamide: administer in the morning; provide adequate hydration; have child void frequently during and after infusion to decrease risk of hemorrhagic cystitis. Chlorambucil: administer with nonspicy, non-acidic foods; rarely seizures occur.

(continued)

Drug Guide 22.1 Common Drugs for GU Disorders (continued)

Medication	Action	Indication	Nursing Implications
Immunosuppressant drugs (cyclosporine A (CyA), azathioprine, tacrolimus, mycophenolate)	Inhibit production and release of interleukin II. Inhibition of T-cell activation by inhibiting calcineurin phosphatase activity. Inhibition of T- and B-cell proliferation (mycophenolate).	Prevention of rejection of renal transplants. CyA and tacrolimus may be used for steroid-dependent nephrotic syndrome.	Monitor complete blood count, serum creatinine, potassium, and magnesium. Monitor blood pressure and observe for signs of infection. Blood levels should be drawn prior to morning dose. CyA: do not give with grapefruit juice. Azathioprine and mycophenolate: give on empty stomach; do not open capsule or crush tablet. Tacrolimus: give on empty stomach, assess for development of hyperglycemia. Relapse of nephrotic syndrome may occur after withdrawal of CyA or tacrolimus therapy.
Muromonab-CD3 (Orthoclone OKT3)	Removal of all CD3 molecules from T-lymphocyte surface so it has inability to act	Treatment of acute renal transplant rejection	Monitor for development of pulmonary edema. First-dose effect may cause fever, chills, chest tightness, wheezing, nausea, and vomiting.
Angiotensin-converting enzyme (ACE) inhibitors (captopril, enalapril)	Potent vasoconstrictor, prevents conversion of angiotensin I to angiotensin II	Renal causes of hypertension	Monitor blood pressure frequently. May cause cough, hyperkalemia. Captopril: administer on empty stomach. Enalapril: administer without regard to food.
Imipramine (Tofranil) (tricyclic antidepressant)	Increases the synaptic concentration of serotonin and/or norepinephrine	Enuresis	Monitor for urinary retention. May cause decreased appetite.
Diuretics: furosemide (Lasix), hydrochlorothiazide (HCTZ)	Inhibits resorption of sodium and chloride in ascending loop of Henle (furosemide) or inhibits reabsorption of sodium in distal tubules (hydrochlorothiazide), leading to increased excretion of water and electrolytes	Nephrotic syndrome, acute glomerulonephritis, hemolytic-uremic syndrome or other instances of fluid overload with renal sufficiency	Administer with food or milk to decrease GI upset. Monitor blood pressure, renal function, and electrolytes (particularly potassium). May cause photosensitivity.

(continued)

Drug Guide 22.1 Common Drugs for GU Disorders (continued)

Medication	Action	Indication	Nursing Implications
Vasodilators: hydralazine (Apresoline), minoxidil	Direct vasodilation of arterioles, resulting in decreased systemic resistance	Renal causes of hypertension	May cause fluid retention. Hydralazine: administer with food. Monitor heart rate and blood pressure (closely with intravenous use). Minoxidil: may be administered without regard to food. May cause dizziness.
Calcium channel blocker: nifedipine (Procardia)	Prevents calcium from entering voltage-sensitive channels, resulting in coronary vasodilation	Renal causes of hypertension	Administer with food; avoid grapefruit juice. Insoluble shell of extended-release tablet may pass in stool. Use caution when administering liquid-filled capsule sublingually or by bite and swallow method, as significant hypotension may occur.
Albumin (intravenous)	Increases intravascular oncotic pressure, resulting in movement of fluid from interstitial to intravascular space	Nephrotic syndrome	May require a filter depending upon brand used. Rapid infusion can result in vascular overload. Monitor vital signs; observe for pulmonary edema and cardiac failure.

be familiar with what the procedures are, how the treatments and medications work, and common nursing implications related to use of these modalities.

Nursing Process Overview for the Child With a GU Disorder

Care of the child with a GU disorder includes assessment, nursing diagnosis, planning, interventions, and evaluation. There are a number of general concepts related to the nursing process that may be applied to GU disorders. From a general understanding of the care involved for a child with urinary, renal, or reproductive dysfunction, the nurse can then individualize the care based on client specifics.

ASSESSMENT

Assessment of urinary tract, renal, or reproductive dysfunction includes health history, physical examination, and laboratory and diagnostic testing.

> Remember Corey, the 5-year-old with fever and lethargy? What additional health history and physical examination assessment information should you obtain?

Health History

The health history comprises past medical history, including the mother's pregnancy history, family history, and history of present illness (when the symptoms started and how they have progressed), as well as medications and treatments used at home. The past medical history may be significant for maternal polyhydramnios, oligohydramnios, diabetes, hypertension, or alcohol or cocaine ingestion. Neonatal history may include the presence of a single umbilical artery or an abdominal mass, chromosome abnormality, or congenital malformation. Document past medical history of UTI or other problems with the GU tract. Family history may be significant for renal disease or uropathology, chronic UTIs, renal calculi, or a history of parental enuresis. Determine age of successful toilet training, pattern of incontinent episodes (having "accidents"), and toileting hygiene self-care routines. Note myelomeningocele or other spinal disturbance that may affect the child's ability to urinate. Note previous urologic surgeries or ongoing renal interventions (e.g., dialysis). For the adolescent girl, obtain a thorough menstrual history, including sexual behavior and pregnancy history.

When determining the history of the present illness, inquire about the following:

- Burning on urination
- Changes in voiding patterns
- Foul-smelling urine
- Vaginal or urethral discharge
- Genital pain, irritation, or discomfort
- Blood in the urine
- Edema
- Masses in the groin, scrotum, or abdomen
- Flank or abdominal pain
- Cramps
- Nausea and/or vomiting
- Poor growth
- Weight gain
- Fever
- Infectious exposure (particularly streptococcus A or *Escherichia coli*)
- Trauma

Record medications used for acute or chronic conditions, or for contraception.

Physical Examination

Physical examination of the GU system includes inspection and observation, auscultation, percussion, and palpation.

Inspection and Observation

Observe the child's general appearance, noting growth retardation or unusual weight gain. Inspect the skin for presence of pruritus, edema (generalized or periorbital), or bruising. Note pallor of the skin or dysmorphic features (associated with genetic conditions). Document presence of lethargy, fatigue, rapid respirations, confusion, or developmental delay. Observe the external genitalia area for infant diaper rash, constant urine dribble, displaced urethral opening, reddened urethral opening, or discharge. In females note vaginal irritation or labial fusion. In males observe the scrotal sac for enlargement or discoloration. Note the condition of a urinary stoma or diversion if present. With the child lying flat, observe the abdomen for distention, ascites, or slack abdominal musculature.

Auscultation

Listen carefully to heart sounds, as a flow murmur may be present in the anemic child with a renal disorder. Noted elevated heart rate. Auscultate blood pressure with the appropriate-size cuff, noting elevation or depression. In the edematous child, carefully auscultate the lungs, noting presence of adventitious sounds. Note absence of bowel sounds, as this may indicate peritonitis. In the child who receives chronic hemodialysis, auscultate the fistula for presence of a bruit (desired normal finding).

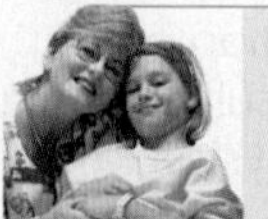

Use the bell of the stethoscope when auscultating the infant's or child's blood pressure so that you can hear the softer Korotkoff sounds more accurately.

Percussion

Percuss the abdomen. Note unusual dullness or flatness (dullness is usually heard over the spleen at the right costal margin, over the kidneys, and 1 to 3 cm below the left costal margin). A full bladder may yield dullness above the symphysis pubis.

Palpation

Palpate the abdomen. Note presence of palpable kidneys (indicating enlargement or mass, as they are usually difficult to palpate in the older infant or child). Note presence of abdominal masses or a distended bladder. Document tenderness to palpation or along the costovertebral angle. Palpate the scrotum for presence of descended testicles, masses, or other abnormalities. Note whether the foreskin, if present, can be retracted. In the child who receives chronic hemodialysis, palpate the fistula or graft for presence of a thrill (desired normal finding).

Laboratory and Diagnostic Testing

Common Laboratory and Diagnostic Tests 22.1 offers an explanation of the most commonly used laboratory and diagnostic tests used for a child suspected of having a GU disorder. The test results can help the physician to diagnose the disorder or to determine treatment. Laboratory or non-nursing personnel obtain some of the tests, while the nurse might obtain others. In either instance the nurse should be familiar with how the tests are obtained, what they are used for, and normal versus abnormal results. This knowledge will also be necessary when providing patient and family education related to the tests and results.

Urine specimens may be collected using a variety of different methods in infants and children. Suprapubic aspiration is a useful method for obtaining a sterile urine specimen from the neonate or young infant. A sterile needle is inserted into the bladder through the anterior wall of the abdomen and the urine is then aspirated. This method is generally performed by the physician or advanced practitioner. Infants and toddlers who are not toilet trained may require a urine bag for urine collection. A sterile urine bag is required for a urine culture, a clean bag for routine urinalysis. A 24-hour urine-collection bag is also available. Nursing Procedure 22.1 gives details on the use of the urine bag.

(text continues on page 725)

Common Laboratory and Diagnostic Tests 22.1 Genitourinary Disorders

Test	Explanation	Indication	Nursing Implications
Complete blood count	Evaluate hemoglobin and hematocrit, white blood cell count, and platelet count	Any condition in which anemia, infection, or thrombocytopenia is suspected	Normal values vary according to age and gender. White blood cell count differential is helpful in evaluating source of infection.
Blood urea nitrogen (BUN) (serum)	Indirect measurement of renal function and glomerular filtration in the presence of adequate liver function	Nephrotic syndrome, hemolytic-uremic syndrome, renal failure, acute glomerulonephritis or other renal diseases	BUN may be elevated with high-protein diet or dehydration, may be decreased with overhydration or malnutrition.
Creatinine (serum)	A more direct measurement of renal function, only minimally affected by liver function. Generally, doubling of the creatinine level is suggestive of a 50% reduction in glomerular filtration rate.	Used to diagnose impaired renal function	A diet high in meat may cause a transient though not pronounced increase in creatinine. There are also slight diurnal variations in levels. Draw at same time each day if serial evaluations are ordered.
Creatinine clearance (urine and serum)	A 24-hour urine collection is evaluated for the presence of creatinine, then compared with the serum creatinine level to determine creatinine clearance.	Used to diagnose impaired renal function	Discard the first void and then begin the 24-hour urine collection. Keep the specimen on ice during the collection period. Collect ALL urine passed in the 24-hour period. Ensure that a venous blood sample is drawn during the 24-hour period. The urine specimen should be sent promptly to the laboratory at the end of the 24-hour period.
Potassium (serum)	Measures the concentration of potassium in the blood	Any suspected renal disease; followed routinely in renal failure	Avoid hemolysis and allowing child to open and close the hand with a tourniquet in place, as these can cause elevation in potassium levels. Evaluate the child with increased or decreased potassium levels for cardiac arrhythmias. Immediately notify physician of critically high potassium levels.
Total protein, globulin, albumin (serum)	Protein electrophoresis separates the various components into zones according to their electrical charge.	Used to diagnose, evaluate, and monitor chronic renal disease	Significantly low levels of albumin contribute to extent of edema, as albumin is necessary in the blood to maintain colloidal osmotic pressure.

Common Laboratory and Diagnostic Tests 22.1 Genitourinary Disorders (continued)

Test	Explanation	Indication	Nursing Implications
Calcium (serum)	Measurement of calcium level in the blood; half of all calcium is protein-bound, so the level will decrease with hypoalbuminemia.	Renal diseases associated with hypoalbuminemia and edema	Avoid prolonged tourniquet use during blood draw, as this may falsely increase the calcium level.
Phosphorus (serum)	Measurement of phosphate level in the blood. Phosphorus levels are inversely related to calcium levels (they increase when calcium levels decrease).	Renal disease, ongoing monitoring, particularly in the patient with hypocalcemia	Child should be NPO past midnight prior to the morning of the blood draw. Avoid hemolysis, as it can falsely elevate the phosphate level.
Urinalysis (urine)	Evaluates color, pH, specific gravity, and odor of urine. Also assesses for presence of protein, glucose, ketones, blood, leukocyte esterase, red and white blood cells, bacteria, crystals, and casts.	Reveals preliminary information about the urinary tract. Useful in children with fever, dysuria, flank pain, urgency, or hematuria. Proteinuria may be noted in renal disorders.	Be aware of the many drugs affecting urine color and notify laboratory if child is taking one. Notify laboratory if female is menstruating. Refrigerate specimen if not processed promptly. While proteinuria may occur with various renal disorders, it may also occur as either transient or orthostatic proteinuria, both of which are benign events.
Cystoscopy	Endoscopic visualization of the urethra and bladder	Evaluate hematuria, recurrent urinary tract infection; determine ureteral reflux; measure bladder capacity	Encourage fluids. Monitor vital signs. Child may feel burning with voiding after procedure. Pink tinge to urine is common after procedure.
Urine culture and sensitivity	Urine is plated in the laboratory and evaluated every day for the presence of bacteria. A final report is usually issued after 48 to 72 hours. Sensitivity testing is performed to determine the best choice of antibiotic.	Used to diagnose urinary tract infection	Obtain culture specimen prior to starting antibiotics if at all possible. Avoid contamination of the specimen with stool. May be obtained by catheterization, clean-catch specimen, or sterile U-bag. In some institutions, suprapubic tap is performed in neonates and young infants by the physician or nurse practitioner.
Urodynamic studies	Measure the urine flow during micturition via a urine flow meter	Dysfunctional voiding	The child must have a full bladder. The child then urinates into the urine flow meter. There is no discomfort associated with the test.

(continued)

Common Laboratory and Diagnostic Tests 22.1 Genitourinary Disorders (continued)

Test	Explanation	Indication	Nursing Implications
Voiding cystourethrogram (VCUG)	The bladder is filled with contrast material via catheterization. Fluoroscopy is performed to demonstrate filling of the bladder and collapsing after emptying.	Hematuria, urinary tract infections, vesicoureteral reflux, suspected structural anomalies	Just prior to the test, insert the Foley catheter. Ensure that the adolescent female patient is not pregnant. After the test, encourage the child to drink fluids to prevent bacterial accumulation and aid in dye elimination.
Intravenous pyelogram (IVP)	Radiopaque contrast material is injected intravenously and filtered by the kidneys. X-ray films are obtained at set intervals to show passage of the dye through the kidneys, ureters, and bladder.	Urinary outlet obstruction, hematuria, trauma to the renal system, suspected kidney tumor	Contraindicated in children allergic to shellfish or iodine. If the dye infiltrates at the intravenous site, hyaluronidase (Wydase) may be used to speed absorption of the iodine. Ensure adequate hydration before and after the test. Some institutions require enema or laxative evacuation of the bowel prior to the study to ensure adequate visualization of the urinary tract.
Renal biopsy	Usually a percutaneous specimen is obtained by inserting a needle through the skin and into the kidney. The sample of kidney tissue obtained is then microscopically examined.	Diagnosis of renal disease or assessment of renal transplant rejection	After the biopsy, carefully assess for signs or symptoms of bleeding: increased heart rate, pale color, flank pain or backache, shoulder pain, lightheadedness. Inspect urine for gross hematuria. Child will be on bed rest, preferably supine for 24 hours.
Renal ultrasound	Reflected sound waves allow visualization of the kidneys, ureters, and bladder.	Useful in determining kidney size (as with hydronephrosis and polycystic kidney), presence of cysts or tumors, or rejection of kidney transplant	No fasting is required prior to the procedure. Does not require contrast material. The child should feel no discomfort during the ultrasound.

Sterile urinary catheterization is performed like that in adults. The size of the catheter varies depending on the size of the child. If a small urinary catheter is not available, a sterile 5 French or 8 French feeding tube works well.

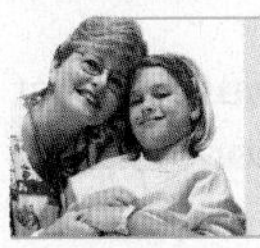

Use familiar terms such as "pee-pee," "tinkle," or "potty" to explain to the child what is needed and to gain his or her cooperation.

NURSING DIAGNOSES AND RELATED INTERVENTIONS

Upon completion of a thorough assessment, the nurse might identify several nursing diagnoses, such as:

- Impaired urinary elimination
- Fluid volume excess
- Imbalanced nutrition, less (or more) than body requirements
- Risk for infection
- Deficient knowledge of the child or family
- Urinary retention

Nursing Procedure 22.1

Applying the Urine Bag

1. Cleanse the perineal area well and pat dry. If a culture is to be obtained, cleanse the genital area with povidone–iodine (Betadine) or per institutional protocol.
2. Apply benzoin around the scrotum or the vulvar area to aid with urine bag adhesion.
3. Allow the benzoin to dry.
4. Apply the urine bag.
   - For boys: Ensure that the penis is fully inside the bag; a portion of the scrotum may or may not be inside the bag, depending upon scrotal size.
   - For girls: Apply the narrow portion of the bag on the perineal space between the anal and vulvar areas first for best adhesion, then spread the remaining adhesive section.
5. Tuck the bag downward inside the diaper to discourage leaking.
6. Check the bag frequently for urine.

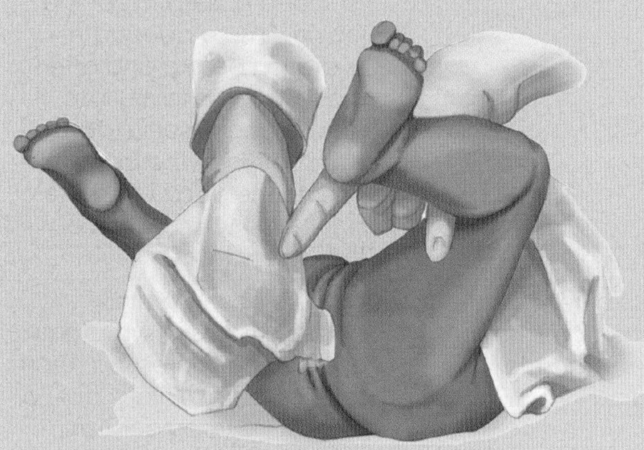

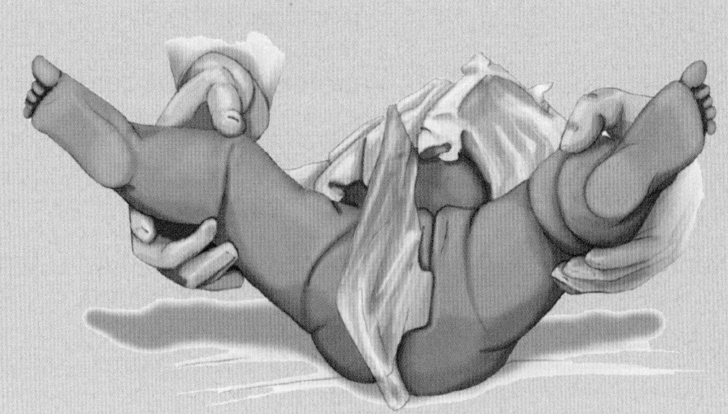

- Activity intolerance
- Interrupted family process
- Disturbed body image

> After completing an assessment of Corey, you note the following: foul-smelling urine, abdominal tenderness, redness in her perineal area, and slightly blood-tinged, cloudy urine. Based on these assessment findings, what would your top three nursing diagnoses be for Corey?

Nursing goals, interventions, and evaluation for the child with a GU disorder are based on the nursing diagnoses. Nursing Care Plan 22.1 can be used as a guide in planning nursing care for the child with a GU disorder. The care plan overview includes nursing diagnoses and interventions for urinary tract disorders as well as genital (or reproductive system) disorders. It should be individualized based on the patient's symptoms and needs. Refer to Chapter 15 for detailed information about pain management. Additional information will be included later in the chapter as it relates to specific disorders.

> Based on your top three nursing diagnoses for Corey, describe appropriate nursing interventions.

Urinary Tract and Renal Disorders

The urinary tract and renal disorders discussed below include structural disorders, UTI, enuresis, and acquired disorders that result in altered renal function.

● STRUCTURAL DISORDERS

Numerous urologic conditions occur as a result of altered fetal development. Many of these defects are apparent at birth, yet some are not recognized until later in infancy or childhood.

Bladder Exstrophy

In classic bladder exstrophy, a midline closure defect occurs during the embryonic period of gestation, leaving

(text continues on page 730)

Nursing Care Plan 22.1

Overview for the Child with a Genitourinary Disorder

Nursing Diagnosis: Activity intolerance related to generalized edema, anemia, or generalized weakness as evidenced by verbalization of weakness or fatigue, elevated heart rate, respiratory rate, or blood pressure with activity, complaint of shortness of breath with play or activity

Outcome identification and evaluation

Child will display increased activity tolerance, *desire to play without developing symptoms of exertion.*

Intervention: promoting activity

- Encourage activity or ambulation per physician's orders: *early mobilization results in better outcomes.*
- Observe child for symptoms of activity intolerance such as pallor, nausea, lightheadedness, or dizziness or changes in vital signs *to determine level of tolerance.*
- If child is on bed rest, perform range-of-motion exercises and frequent position changes, as *negative changes to the musculoskeletal system occur quickly with inactivity and immobility.*
- Cluster nursing care activities and plan for periods of rest before and after exertional activities *to decrease oxygen need and consumption.*
- Refer the child to physical therapy *for exercise prescription to increase skeletal muscle strength.*

Nursing Diagnosis: Excess fluid volume related to decreased protein in the bloodstream, decreased urine output, sodium retention, possible inappropriate fluid intake, or altered hormone levels inducing fluid retention as evidenced by edema, bloating, weight gain, oliguria, azotemia, or changes in heart and lung sounds

Outcome identification and evaluation

Child will attain appropriate fluid balance, *will lose weight (fluid), edema or bloating will decrease, lung sounds will be clear and heart sounds normal.*

Intervention: encouraging fluid loss

- Weigh child daily on same scale in similar amount of clothing; *in children, weight is the best indicator of changes in fluid status.*
- Monitor location and extent of edema (measure abdominal girth daily if ascites present): *decrease in edema indicates positive increase in oncotic pressure.*
- Auscultate lungs carefully to determine presence of crackles *(indicating pulmonary edema).*
- Assess work of breathing and respiratory rate *(increased work of breathing is associated with pulmonary edema).*
- Assess heart sounds for presence or absence of gallop *(presence of S3 may indicate fluid overload).*
- Maintain fluid restriction as ordered *to decrease intravascular volume and workload on the heart.*
- Strictly monitor intake and output *to quickly note discrepancies and provide intervention.*
- Provide sodium-restricted diet as ordered *(restricting sodium in the diet allows for better renal excretion of extra fluid).*
- Administer diuretics as ordered and monitor for side effects of those medications. *Diuretics encourage excretion of fluid and elimination of edema, reduce cardiac filling pressures, and increase renal blood flow. Side effects include electrolyte imbalance as well as orthostatic hypotension.*

(continued)

Overview for the Child with a Genitourinary Disorder (continued)

Nursing Diagnosis: Imbalanced nutrition: less than body requirements related to anorexia and protein loss as evidenced by weight, length/height, and/or BMI below average for age

Outcome identification and evaluation

Child will improve nutritional intake, resulting in *steady increase in weight and length/height.*

Intervention: promoting adequate nutrition

- Determine body weight and length/height norm for age, *to determine goal to work toward.*
- Assess child for food preferences that fall within dietary restrictions, *as the child will be more likely to consume adequate amounts of foods that he or she likes.*
- Weigh daily or weekly (according to physician order or institutional standard) and measure length/height weekly: *to monitor for increased growth.*
- Offer highest calorie meals at the time of day when the child's appetite is the greatest *(to increase likelihood of increased caloric intake).*
- Provide increased calorie shakes or puddings within diet restriction *(high calorie foods increase weight gain).*
- Administer vitamin and mineral supplements as prescribed *to attain/maintain vitamin and mineral balance in the body.*

Nursing Diagnosis: Imbalanced nutrition: more than body requirements related to increased appetite secondary to steroid therapy as evidenced by weight greater than 95th percentile for age or recent increase in weight

Outcome identification and evaluation

Child will demonstrate balanced nutritional intake, *will maintain current weight or steadily lose excess weight.*

Intervention: encouraging appropriate nutritional intake

- Determine ideal body weight and body mass index for age *to determine goal to work toward.*
- Consult dietitian *for guidance in planning nutrient-rich diet in context of restrictions.*
- Evaluate for emotional/psychological reasons for overeating *to address these concerns.*
- Formulate a contract with the child *to involve him/her in the planning process and encourage compliance with the plan.*
- With the child, plan for daily exercise/activity *to expend excess calories.*
- Instruct the child/parent about appropriate nutrient-rich foods to choose within the constraints of diet and fluid restrictions *to provide basis for ongoing diet management at home.*
- Weigh child twice weekly on same scale *to determine progress toward goal.*

Overview for the Child with a Genitourinary Disorder (continued)

Nursing Diagnosis: Impaired urinary elimination related to urinary tract infection or other urologic condition, or other factors such as ignoring urge to void at appropriate time as evidenced by urinary retention or incontinence, dribbling, urgency, or dysuria

Outcome identification and evaluation

Child will maintain continence; *will void in the toilet.*

Intervention: promoting adequate urinary elimination

- Assess the child's usual voiding pattern and success within that pattern *to determine baseline.*
- Develop a schedule for bladder emptying *to encourage voiding in the toilet.*
- Maintain adequate hydration, *as dehydration irritates the bladder.*
- Avoid constipation, *as constipation is associated with inability to adequately empty bladder.*
- Teach parents to restrict child's fluid intake after dinner *to avoid bedwetting.*
- Ensure child voids prior to going to bed *to avoid bedwetting.*
- Teach bladder-stretching exercises as prescribed per physician *to increase bladder capacity.*

Nursing Diagnosis: Urinary retention related to anatomic obstruction, sensory motor impairment or dysfunctional voiding as evidenced by dribbling, inadequate bladder emptying

Outcome identification and evaluation

Child's bladder will empty adequately, *according to pre-established quantities and frequencies individualized for the child (usual urine output is 0.5 to 2 mL/kg/hour).*

Intervention: promoting successful bladder emptying

- Assess child's ability to adequately empty bladder via history focused on character and duration of lower urinary symptoms *to establish baseline.*
- Assess for history of fecal impaction or encopresis, *as alterations in bowel elimination may have a negative impact on urinary elimination.*
- Assess for bladder distention by palpation or urinary retention by post-void residual obtained via catheterization or bladder ultrasound *to determine extent of retention.*
- Maintain adequate hydration *to avoid irritating effects of dehydration on the bladder.*
- Schedule voiding *to decrease bladder overdistention.*
- In the child with significant urinary retention, teach parents/child the technique of clean intermittent catheterization, *which allows for regular complete bladder emptying.*

Nursing Diagnosis: Disturbed body image related to anatomic differences, short stature, or effects of long-term corticosteroid use as evidenced by verbalization of dissatisfaction with the child's or adolescent's looks

Outcome identification and evaluation

Child or adolescent will display appropriate body image, *will look at self in mirror and participate in social activities.*

Intervention: promoting body image

- Acknowledge feelings of anger over body changes and illness: *venting feelings is associated with less body image disturbance.*
- Support the child's or teen's choices of comfortable, fashionable clothing *that may disguise anatomic abnormalities and dialysis tubing.*
- Involve the child and especially the teen in the decision-making process, *as a sense of control of their own body will improve body image.*
- Encourage children or teens to spend time with others their own age who have short stature or other effects of renal disorders: *a peer's opinions are often better accepted than those of persons in authority, such as parents or health care professionals.*

Overview for the Child with a Genitourinary Disorder (continued)

Nursing Diagnosis: Knowledge deficit related to lack of information regarding complex medical condition, prognosis, and medical needs as evidenced by verbalization, questions, or actions demonstrating lack of understanding regarding child's condition or care

Outcome identification and evaluation

Child and parents will verbalize accurate information and understanding about condition, prognosis, and medical needs: *Child and parents demonstrate knowledge of condition and medications and will demonstrate therapeutic procedures the child requires.*

Intervention: educating the child and parents

- Assess child's and parents' willingness to learn: *Child and parents must be open to learning for teaching to be effective.*
- Provide parents with time to adjust to diagnosis: *will facilitate adjustment and ability to learn and participate in child's care.*
- Teach in short sessions: *many short sessions are found to be more helpful than one long session.*
- Repeat information: *allows parents and child time to learn and understand.*
- Individualize teaching to the parents' and child's level of understanding (depends on age of child, physical condition, memory) *to ensure understanding.*
- Provide reinforcement and rewards *to facilitate the teaching/learning process.*
- Use multiple modes of learning involving many senses (written, verbal, demonstration, and videos) when possible: *child and parents are more likely to retain information when presented in different ways using many senses.*

the bladder open and exposed outside of the abdomen. The bony pelvis may also be malformed, resulting in an opening in the pelvic arch. Bladder exstrophy may be diagnosed by prenatal ultrasound. Complications include UTI from ascending organisms. Treatment of bladder exstrophy involves surgical repair.

Nursing Assessment

On physical examination of the infant or child, note the red appearance to the bladder seen on the abdominal wall (Fig. 22.1). Draining urine will be visible. Note excoriation of abdominal skin around the bladder resulting from contact with urine. A malformed urethra may be present in females, while males may have an unformed or malformed penis or a normal penis with an epispadias.

Nursing Management

Nursing management consists of preventing infection and skin breakdown, providing postoperative care, and catheterizing the stoma.

Preventing Infection and Skin Breakdown

Bladder exstrophy requires surgical repair. In the preoperative period, care is focused on protecting the exstrophied bladder and preventing infection. Keep the infant in a supine position; keep the bladder moist and cover it with a sterile plastic bag. Change soiled diapers immediately to prevent contamination of the bladder with feces. Sponge-bathe the infant rather than immersing him or her in water to prevent pathogens in the bath water from entering the bladder. Prevent breakdown of the surrounding abdominal skin by applying protective barrier creams. In some instances it may be necessary to consult the ostomy nurse for advice on dealing with the abdominal skin excoriation. If an orthopedic surgeon is involved due to the malformed pubic arch, follow through with recommended positioning or bracing to prevent further separation of the pubic arch.

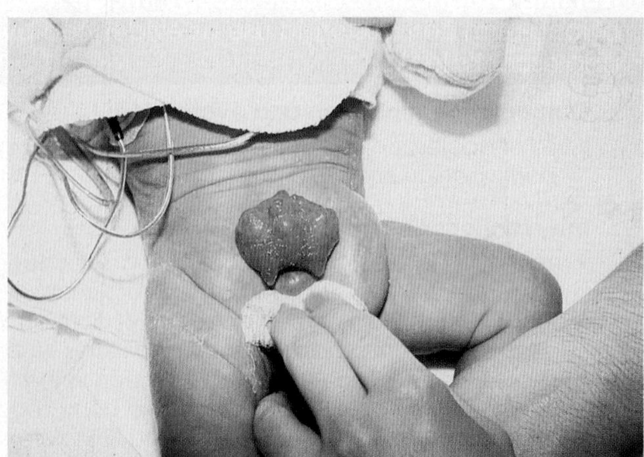

● Figure 22.1 Note the bright-red color of the bladder exstrophy.

Providing Postoperative Care

Nursing management in the postoperative period again focuses on preventing infection. Keep the infant supine and quickly change soiled diapers to prevent contamination of the incision with stool. Surgical reconstruction of the bladder within the pelvic cavity and reconstruction of a urethra are done if enough bladder tissue is present. An indwelling urethral catheter or suprapubic tube will allow urinary drainage, allowing the bladder to rest in the initial postoperative period. Ensure that catheters drain freely and do not become kinked. Sometimes tubes or catheters used in the postoperative period require irrigation. Refer to the institution's policy and the surgeon's orders for specifics related to urinary catheter irrigation.

Manage bladder spasms with oxybutynin (Ditropan) or belladonna and opioid (B & O) suppositories as ordered. Note blood-tinged urine upon return from surgery, with clearing of urine within hours to days.

Catheterizing the Stoma

If bladder tissue is insufficient for repair, then the bladder is removed and a continent urinary reservoir created. The ureters are connected to a portion of the small intestine that is separated from the gastrointestinal (GI) tract, thus creating a urinary reservoir. The intestines are reanastomosed to leave the GI tract intact and separate from the GU tract. A stoma is created on the abdominal wall; it provides access to the urinary reservoir (Fig. 22.2). The stoma is catheterized about four times per day to empty the reservoir of urine. Urine from an intestine-based urinary reservoir tends to be mucus-like and is often cloudier than urine from a urinary bladder. Teach parents the procedure for catheterizing the urinary reservoir and instruct them to call the child's urologist or pediatrician if signs or symptoms of UTI occur.

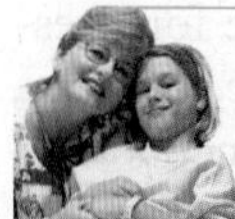

About one third of all children with urologic malformations are at high risk for the development of latex allergy. Latex allergy can result in anaphylaxis. Primary prevention of latex allergy is warranted in all children with urologic malformations, so use latex-free gloves, tubes, and catheters in these children.

Hypospadias/Epispadias

Hypospadias is a urethral defect in which the opening is on the ventral surface of the penis rather than at the end of the penis (Fig. 22.3). Epispadias is a urethral defect in which the opening is on the dorsal surface of the penis. In either case, the opening may be near the glans of the penis, midway along the penis, or near the base. If left uncorrected, the boy may not be capable of appropriately aiming a urinary stream from a standing position. The abnormal placement of the urethral opening may interfere with the deposition of sperm during intercourse, leaving the man infertile. Also, if left uncorrected, the boy's self-esteem and body image may be damaged by the abnormal appearance of his genitalia. For these reasons, the defect is usually repaired sometime after about 1 year of age. The goal of surgical correction for either condition is to provide for an appropriately placed meatus that allows for normal voiding and ejaculation. The meatus is moved to the glans penis and the urethra is reconstructed as needed. Most repairs are accomplished in one surgery. More extensive reconstructions may require two stages.

Nursing Assessment

Note history of an unusual urine stream. Inspect the penis for placement of the urethral meatus: it may be slightly off center of the glans or may be present somewhere along the shaft of the penis. Inspect for chordee, a fibrous band

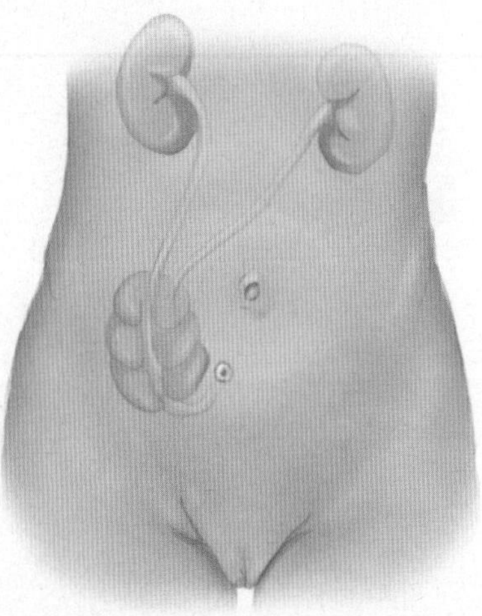

● Figure 22.2 The abdominal stoma allows for urinary continence and requires catheterization.

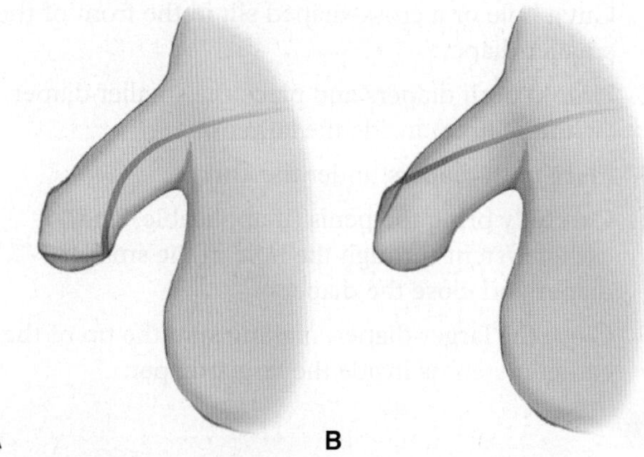

● Figure 22.3 (**A**) Hypospadias: the urethral opening is located on the ventral side of the penis. (**B**) Epispadias: the urethral opening is located on the dorsal side of the penis.

causing the penis to curve downward. Palpate for presence or absence of testicles in the scrotal sac, because cryptorchidism (undescended testicles) often occurs with hypospadias, as do hydrocele and inguinal hernia.

Nursing Management

The newborn with hypospadias or epispadias should not undergo circumcision until after surgical repair of the urethral meatus. In more extreme cases, the surgeon may need to use some of the excess foreskin while reconstructing the meatus. Nursing management of the infant who has undergone a hypospadias or epispadias repair focuses on providing routine postoperative care and parent education.

Providing Postoperative Care

Postoperatively, assess urinary drainage from the urethral stent or drainage tube, which allows for discharge of urine without stress along the surgical site. Ensure that the urinary drainage tube remains carefully taped with the penis in an upright position to prevent stress on the urethral incision. The penile dressing is usually a compression type, used to decrease edema and bruising. Administer antibiotics if prescribed. Assess for pain, which is usually not extensive, and administer analgesics or antispasmodics (oral oxybutynin or B & O suppository) as needed for bladder spasms.

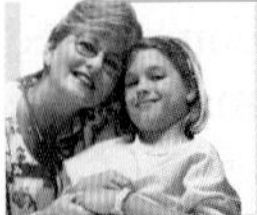

Bladder spasms may also be managed effectively through the use of epidural analgesia, which is being used more frequently in the postoperative period in the pediatric population.

Double diapering is a method used to protect the urethra and stent or catheter after surgery; it also helps keep the area clean and free from infection. The inner diaper contains stool and the outer diaper contains urine, allowing separation between the bowel and bladder output. Nursing Procedure 22.2 details the double-diapering technique. Change the outside (larger) diaper when the child is wet; change both diapers when the child has a bowel movement.

Educating the Family

If the child is to be discharged with the urinary catheter in place (which is common), teach the parents how to care for the catheter and drainage system. Have parents demonstrate their ability to irrigate the catheter should a mucus plug occur. Tub baths are generally prohibited until it is time to remove the penile dressing. Roughhousing, ride-on toys, or any activity involving straddling is not allowed for 2 to 3 weeks.

Obstructive Uropathy

Obstructive uropathy is an obstruction at any level along the upper or lower urinary tract. This discussion will focus on congenital structural defects, though obstruction can also occur as a result of other disease processes (acquired obstructive uropathy). The most common sites of obstruction are listed in Table 22.1. The defect may be unilateral or bilateral and can cause partial or complete obstruction of urine flow, resulting in dilation of the affected kidney (hydronephrosis). Complications include recurrent UTI, renal insufficiency, and progressive damage to the kidney resulting in renal failure.

Nursing Procedure 22.2

Double Diapering

1. Cut a hole or a cross-shaped slit in the front of the smaller diaper.
2. Unfold both diapers and place the smaller diaper (with the hole) inside the larger one.
3. Place both diapers under the child.
4. Carefully bring the penis (if applicable) and catheter/stent through the hole in the smaller diaper and close the diaper.
5. Close the larger diaper, making sure the tip of the catheter/stent is inside the larger diaper.

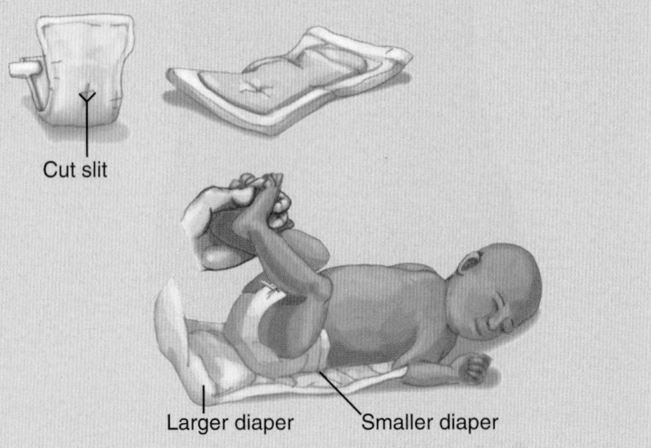

Pictures and text adapted from Children's Healthcare of Atlanta (2004). *Double diapering.*

Table 22.1 Common Sites of Obstructive Uropathy

Disorder	Site	Illustration
Ureteropelvic junction (UPJ) obstruction	Junction of the upper ureter with the pelvis of the kidney	Urinary tract with unilateral hydronephrosis and narrowing of the UPJ on that side
Ureterovesical junction (UVJ) obstruction	Junction of the lower ureter and the bladder	Urinary tract with unilateral hydronephrosis and dilated ureters with narrowing of the UVJ on that side
Ureterocele	Ureter swells into the bladder	Bladder with cystic pouch where ureters insert (unilateral)
Posterior urethral valves (males only)	Flaps of tissue in the proximal urethra	Distended proximal urethra, bladder, ureters, and hydronephrosis

Nursing Assessment

For a full description of the assessment phase of the nursing process refer to page 721. Assessment findings pertinent to obstructive uropathy are discussed below.

Health History

Elicit a description of the present illness and chief complaint. Common signs and symptoms reported during the health history might include:

- Recurrent UTI
- Incontinence
- Fever
- Foul-smelling urine
- Flank pain
- Abdominal pain
- **Urinary frequency**
- Urinary **urgency**
- Dysuria
- **Hematuria**

Explore the child's current and past medical history for risk factors such as:

- "Prune belly" syndrome
- Chromosome abnormalities
- Anorectal malformations
- Ear defects

Physical Examination and Laboratory and Diagnostic Tests

Palpate the abdomen for presence of an abdominal mass (hydronephrotic kidney). Assess the blood pressure; elevation may occur if renal insufficiency is present. Many cases of obstructive uropathy may be diagnosed with prenatal ultrasound if the obstruction has been significant enough to cause hydronephrosis or dilatation elsewhere along the urinary tract.

Nursing Management

Surgical correction is specific to the type of obstruction and generally consists of removal of the obstruction, reimplantation of the ureters as necessary, and occasionally creation of a urinary diversion. Postoperatively, assess urine output via vesicostomy, nephrostomy, suprapubic tube, or urethral catheter for color, clots, clarity, and amount. Encourage fluids once the child can tolerate them orally. Administer analgesics and/or antispasmodics as needed for bladder spasms. Teach parents care of vesicostomy or drainage tubes, with which the child may be discharged.

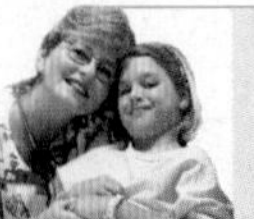

Upon return from surgery, most children have intravenous fluids without added potassium infusion. Potassium is withheld from the intravenous fluid until adequate urine output is established post-operatively to avoid the development of hyperkalemia should the kidneys fail to function properly.

Hydronephrosis

Hydronephrosis is a condition in which the pelvis and calyces of the kidney are dilated (Fig. 22.4). Hydronephrosis may occur as a congenital defect, as a result of obstructive uropathy, or secondary to vesicoureteral reflux. Congenital hydronephrosis may be revealed on prenatal ultrasound. Complications of hydronephrosis include renal insufficiency, hypertension, and eventually renal failure.

Nursing Assessment

For a full description of the assessment phase of the nursing process refer to page 721. Assessment findings pertinent to hydronephrosis are discussed below.

Health History

Elicit a description of the present illness and chief complaint. The infant may be asymptomatic, but signs and symptoms reported during the health history might include:

- Failure to thrive
- Intermittent hematuria
- Presence of an abdominal mass
- Signs and symptoms associated with a UTI such as fever, vomiting, poor feeding, and irritability

Explore the child's current and past medical history for risk factors such as:

- Maternal oligohydramnios or polyhydramnios (congenital hydronephrosis)
- Elevated levels of serum alpha-fetoprotein (congenital hydronephrosis)

Physical Examination and Diagnostic and Laboratory Tests

Monitor the blood pressure of infants and children suspected of having hydronephrosis. Palpation of the abdomen may reveal enlarged kidney(s) or a distended

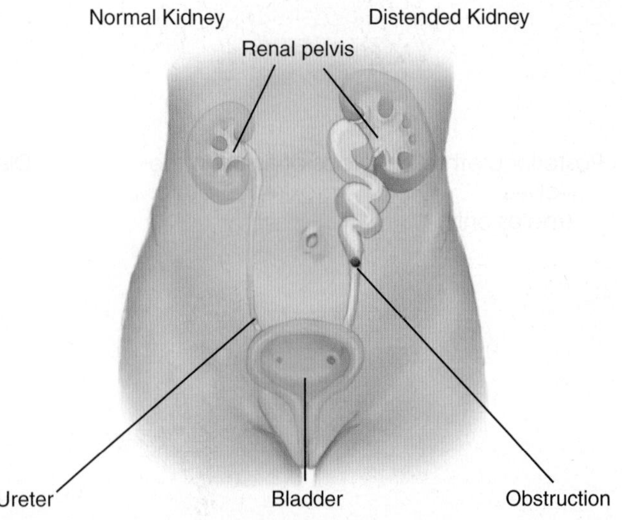

● Figure 22.4 Hydronephrosis.

bladder. A voiding cystourethrogram (VCUG) will be performed to determine the presence of a structural defect that may be causing the hydronephrosis. Other diagnostic tests, such as a renal ultrasound or an intravenous pyelogram, may also be performed to clarify the diagnosis.

Nursing Management

Teach the parents signs and symptoms of UTI and **sepsis**, as these complications may occur. The parents should observe the child for adequacy of urine output and hydration status. Teach the parents to perform appropriate perineal hygiene and to avoid using irritants in the genital area. The infant or child with hydronephrosis will need follow-up with a pediatric nephrologist or urologist.

Vesicoureteral Reflux

Vesicoureteral reflux (VUR) is a condition in which urine from the bladder flows back up the ureters. This reflux of urine occurs during bladder contraction with voiding (Fig. 22.5). Reflux may occur in one or both ureters. If reflux occurs when the urine is infected, the kidney is exposed to bacteria and pyelonephritis may result. The increased pressure placed upon the kidney with reflux can cause renal scarring and lead to hypertension later in life and, if severe, renal insufficiency or failure.

Primary VUR results from a congenital abnormality at the vesicoureteral junction that results in incompetence of the valve (Ellsworth et al., 2000). Secondary VUR is related to other structural or functional problems such as neurogenic bladder, bladder dysfunction, or bladder outlet obstruction (Roth et al., 2002). As many as 30% to 40% of all children diagnosed with UTI have primary VUR (Thompson et al., 2005).

VUR is graded according to its severity: grade 1 results in minor dilatation of the proximal ureter and grade V is severe dilatation of the ureter and pelvis of the kidney (Wald, 2006). Grade I and II VUR cases usually resolve spontaneously, but grade III to V cases are generally associated with recurrent UTIs, hydronephrosis, and progressive renal damage.

Figure 22.5 Note retrograde flow of urine up the ureter upon bladder contraction.

The goal of therapeutic management of VUR is prevention of pyelonephritis and subsequent renal scarring, which may contribute to the development of hypertension later in life (Ellsworth et al., 2000). Management includes antibiotic prophylaxis and hygiene/voiding practices to prevent UTI. Serial urine cultures are used to determine recurrence of UTI. Biannual, annual, or biennial radionuclide VCUGs are performed to determine the status of VUR.

Grade III, IV, and V cases usually warrant surgical intervention. The ureters are resected from the bladder and reimplanted elsewhere in the bladder wall to regain functionality.

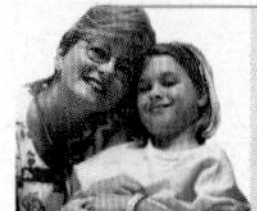

The keys to prevention of long-term sequelae such as hypertension in children with urologic conditions are early diagnosis and intervention, prevention of infection, and close clinical follow-up. Nurses play a key role in monitoring and education.

Nursing Assessment

For a full description of the assessment phase of the nursing process refer to page 721. Assessment findings pertinent to VUR are discussed below.

Health History

Elicit a description of the present illness and chief complaint. Common signs and symptoms reported during the health history might include:

- Fever
- Dysuria
- Frequency or urgency
- Nocturia
- Hematuria
- Pain in the back, abdomen, or flank

Explore the child's current and past medical history for risk factors such as:

- Recurrent UTI in the female
- Single episode of UTI in the male
- Congenital defect
- Family history of VUR

For the child who is receiving ongoing follow-up for VUR, determine whether UTIs have occurred since the last visit, as well as the name and dose of prophylactic antibiotic.

Physical Examination

Monitor the blood pressure for elevation. Palpate the abdomen for presence of a mass (if hydronephrosis is present). VCUG may be used to diagnose VUR.

Nursing Management

Nursing management for the child with VUR includes preventing infection and providing postoperative care.

Preventing Infection

When VUR is present, the goal is to avoid urine infection so that infected urine cannot gain access to the kidneys. Initially, most cases of VUR are managed medically. Teach the child to empty the bladder completely. Teach child and parents appropriate perineal hygiene as well as toileting hygiene to prevent recurrence of UTI. Teach parents about the antibiotic therapy prescribed: the child will be maintained on a low daily dose to prevent UTI. The drug is most effective when given at bedtime because of urinary stasis overnight. Inform parents of the schedule for serial urine cultures and follow-up VCUG.

Providing Postoperative Care

If VUR is severe or if UTI is recurrent, surgical correction will be necessary. In the first 24 to 48 hours after surgery, maintain the intravenous fluid rate at 1.5 times maintenance to encourage a high urinary output. Monitor urine output via the Foley catheter; urine should be bloody initially, clearing within 2 to 3 days. If ureteral stents are present, monitor urine output from those as well. Administer analgesics for incisional pain relief and antispasmodics or B & O suppositories as needed for bladder spasms. Encourage ambulation and advancement of diet as ordered to promote return of appropriate bowel function. Teach parents that prophylactic antibiotics will be given until 1 to 2 months after surgery, when the VCUG demonstrates absence of reflux (Ellsworth et al., 2000).

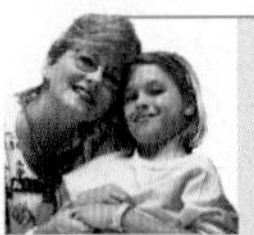

When caring for the child who has undergone urologic surgery, avoid manipulating the Foley or suprapubic catheter: catheter manipulation contributes to bladder spasms.

● URINARY TRACT INFECTION

UTI occurs most often as a result of bacteria ascending to the bladder via the urethra. UTI is the most common serious bacterial infection in children (Dulczak & Kirk, 2005), with lower tract infection (cystitis) being less serious than upper tract infection (pyelonephritis). As many as 7% of females and 2% of males will experience a UTI by age 6 years (Alper & Curry, 2005). UTI is most common in infants and young children. It occurs more frequently in males than females during infancy, but after 1 year of age is more common in females. One explanation for the more common occurrence in females is that the female's shorter urethra allows bacteria to have easier access to the bladder. The urethra is also located quite close to the vagina and anus in females, allowing spread of bacteria from those areas. The sexually active female adolescent is at risk for the development of cystitis, as bacteria may be forced in to the urethra by pressure from intercourse. The male may be somewhat protected from UTI by the antibacterial properties of prostate secretions.

UTI presents differently in infants than it does in children. Infants may exhibit fever, irritability, vomiting, failure to thrive, or jaundice. Children may also experience fever and vomiting and may have dysuria, frequency, hesitancy, urgency, or pain (Alper & Curry, 2005).

Pathophysiology

E. coli accounts for about 85% to 90% of all UTIs, as it is usually found in the perineal and anal region, close to the urethral opening (Jantuten et al., 2001). Other organisms include *Klebsiella, Staphylococcus aureus, Proteus, Pseudomonas,* and *Haemophilus.* Numerous factors may contribute to bacterial proliferation. Urinary stasis contributes to the development of a UTI once the bacteria have gained entry. Urine that remains in the bladder after voiding allows bacteria to grow rapidly. A decreased fluid intake also contributes to bacterial growth, as the bacteria become more concentrated. If the urine is alkaline, bacteria are better able to flourish. Untreated bladder infection may allow reflux of infected urine up the ureters to the kidneys and result in pyelonephritis, a more serious infection.

Therapeutic Management

UTIs are treated with either oral or intravenous antibiotics, depending on the severity of the infection. Urine culture and sensitivity determines the appropriate antibiotic. Current treatment recommendations call for a 7- to 14-day course of antibiotics; this is in contrast to adult treatment, which may involve only 1 to 3 days of treatment in certain cases (Daniels & DiCenso, 2003). Adequate fluid intake is necessary to flush the bacteria from the bladder. Fever management may also be needed.

Nursing Assessment

For a full description of the assessment phase of the nursing process refer to page 721. Assessment findings pertinent to UTI are discussed below.

Health History

Elicit a description of the present illness and chief complaint. Common signs and symptoms reported during the health history might include:

- Fever
- Nausea or vomiting
- Chills
- Abdomen, back, or flank pain
- Lethargy

- Jaundice (in the neonate)
- Poor feeding or "just not acting right" (in the infant)
- Urinary urgency or frequency
- Burning or stinging with urination (the infant may cry with urination, the toddler may grab the diaper)
- Foul-smelling urine
- Poor appetite (child)
- Enuresis or incontinence in a previously toilet-trained child
- Blood in the urine

Explore the child's current and past medical history for risk factors such as:

- Previous UTI
- Obstructive uropathy
- Inadequate toileting hygiene (often occurs with preschool girls)
- VUR
- Constipation
- Urine holding or dysfunctional voiding
- Neurogenic bladder
- Uncircumcised male
- Sexual intercourse
- Pregnancy
- Chronic illness

Physical Examination

In the neonate or young infant, observe for jaundice or increased respiratory rate. In infants and children, inspect the perineal area for redness or irritation. Observe the urine for visible blood, cloudiness, dark color, sediment, mucus, or foul odor. Note pallor, edema, or elevated blood pressure. Palpate the abdomen. Note distended bladder, abdominal mass, or tenderness, particularly in the flank area.

Laboratory and Diagnostic Tests

Common laboratory and diagnostic studies ordered for the assessment of UTI include:

- Urinalysis (clean-catch, suprapubic, or catheterized): may be positive for blood, nitrites, leukocyte esterase, white blood cells, or bacteria (bacteriuria)
- Urine culture: will be positive for infecting organism
- Renal ultrasound: may show hydronephrosis if child also has a structural defect
- VCUG: not usually performed until the child has been treated with antibiotics for at least 48 hours, as infected urine tends to reflux up the ureters anyway. VCUG performed once the urine has regained sterility may be positive for VUR.

Renal ultrasound, VCUG, and other nuclear medicine scans such as the DMSA scan may be indicated in certain populations. The physician or nurse practitioner will determine the need for radiologic testing.

Nursing Management

Goals for nursing management include eradicating infection, promoting comfort, preventing complications, and preventing recurrence of infection.

Eradicating Infection

The child who can tolerate oral intake will be prescribed an oral antibiotic. The child who has protracted vomiting related to the UTI or who has suspected pyelonephritis will require hospitalization and intravenous antibiotics. Any infant less than 3 months of age with fever and suspected UTI should also be hospitalized for administration of intravenous antibiotics. Administer oral or intravenous antibiotics as prescribed. Urge the parent to complete the entire course of oral antibiotic at home, even though the child is feeling better. Administer intravenous fluids as ordered or encourage generous oral fluid intake to help flush the bacteria from the bladder.

Promoting Comfort

Administer antipyretics such as acetaminophen or ibuprofen to reduce fever. A heating pad or warm compress may help relieve abdomen or flank pain. If the child is afraid to urinate due to burning or stinging, encourage voiding in a warm sitz or tub bath.

Preventing Recurrence of Infection

Encourage the parents to return as ordered for a repeat urine culture after completion of the antibiotic course to ensure eradication of bacteria. Teaching Guideline 22.1 gives further information on preventing UTI.

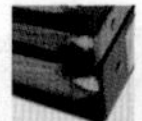

TEACHING GUIDELINE 22.1

Preventing Urinary Tract Infection in Females

- Drink enough fluid (to keep urine flushed through bladder).
- Drink cranberry juice to acidify the urine. Avoid colas and caffeine, which irritate the bladder.
- Urinate frequently and do not "hold" urine (to discourage urinary stasis).
- Avoid bubble baths (they contribute to vulvar and perineal irritation).
- Wipe from front to back after voiding (to avoid contaminating the urethra with rectal material).
- Wear cotton underwear (to decrease the incidence of perineal irritation).
- Avoid wearing tight jeans or pants.
- Wash the perineal area daily with soap and water.
- While menstruating, change sanitary pads frequently to discourage bacterial growth.
- Void immediately after sexual intercourse.

ENURESIS

Enuresis is continued incontinence of urine past the age of toilet training. Box 22.1 gives further definitions related to enuresis. Nocturnal enuresis generally subsides by 6 years of age; if it does not, further investigation and treatment may be warranted. Occasional daytime wetting or dribbling of urine is usually not a cause for concern, but frequent daytime wetting concerns both the child and the parents. Nocturnal enuresis may persist in some children into late childhood and adolescence, causing significant distress for the affected child and family.

In some children, enuresis may occur secondary to a physical disorder such as diabetes mellitus or insipidus, sickle cell anemia, ectopic ureter, or urethral obstruction. Other causes common to both diurnal and nocturnal enuresis include a urine-concentrating defect, UTI, constipation, and emotional distress (sometimes serious). The most frequent cause of daytime enuresis is dysfunctional voiding or holding of urine, though giggle incontinence and stress incontinence also occur. Nocturnal enuresis may be related to a high fluid intake in the evening, obstructive sleep apnea, sexual abuse, a family history of enuresis, or inappropriate family expectations. Physical causes of enuresis must be treated; further management of the disorder focuses on behavioral training, which may be augmented with the use of enuresis alarms or medications.

Nursing Assessment

Elicit a description of the present illness and chief complaint. Determine the age of toilet training and when or if the child achieved successful daytime and nighttime dryness. Inquire about urine-holding behaviors such as squatting, dancing, or staring as well as rushing to the bathroom (diurnal enuresis). Inquire about the amount and types of fluid the child typically consumes before bedtime (nocturnal enuresis). Assess for risk factors such as:

- Family disruption or other stressors
- Chronic constipation (carefully assess bowel movement patterns)
- Excessive family demands related to toileting patterns
- History of being difficult to arouse from sleep
- Family history of enuresis

> BOX 22.1
>
> **DEFINITIONS RELATED TO ENURESIS**
>
> - **Primary enuresis:** enuresis in the child who has never achieved voluntary bladder control
> - **Secondary enuresis:** urinary incontinence in the child who previously demonstrated bladder control over a period of at least 3 to 6 consecutive months
> - **Diurnal enuresis:** daytime loss of urinary control
> - **Nocturnal enuresis:** nighttime bedwetting

Assess the child's cognitive status: developmentally delayed children may take significantly longer to achieve urine continence than their typical same-age peers. Assess for short stature or elevated blood pressure, as these may occur when renal abnormalities are present.

Nursing Management

For the child with diurnal enuresis, encourage him or her to increase the amount of fluid consumed during the day in order to increase the frequency of the urge to void. Set a fixed schedule for the child to attempt to void throughout the day. These practices will usually be sufficient to retrain the child's voiding patterns. The child with nocturnal enuresis without a physiologic cause for bedwetting may present a management challenge.

Educating the Child and Family About Nocturnal Enuresis

Teach the family that the child is not lazy, nor does he or she wet the bed intentionally. Encourage the child and family to read books such as *Dry All Night: The Picture Book Technique That Stops Bedwetting* by Alison Mack or *Waking Up Dry: A Guide to Help Children Overcome Bedwetting* by Dr. Howard Bennett. Encourage the parents to limit intake of bladder irritants such as chocolate and caffeine. Teach parents to limit fluid intake after dinner and ensure that the child voids just before going to bed. Waking the child to void at 11 p.m. may also be helpful. Teach the parents to use bed pads and to make the bed with two sets of sheets and pads to decrease the workload in the middle of the night. When sleeping at home, the child should wear his or her usual underwear or pajamas. If away on a family vacation, pull-ups may decrease the stress on both the child and the parents.

Providing Support and Encouragement

It is important for the child to understand that he or she is not alone. Depending on the child's developmental level, explain that as many as 5 million people have enuresis (this can be done in terms the child can relate to, such as a proportion within a school or 100 times the number of children in one school, etc.). It is not only "little kids" who wet the bed, and all kids who wet the bed need help overcoming this problem. Parents should include the child in plans for nighttime urinary control; this helps to increase the child's motivation to become dry. Parents should set up a reward system for dry nights. Parents should include the child in bed linen changes when he or she does wet the bed, but should do so in a matter-of-fact manner rather than in a punitive way; in fact, punishment for bedwetting should always be avoided.

With patience, consistency, and time, dryness will be achieved. Provide ongoing emotional support and positive reinforcement to the child and family.

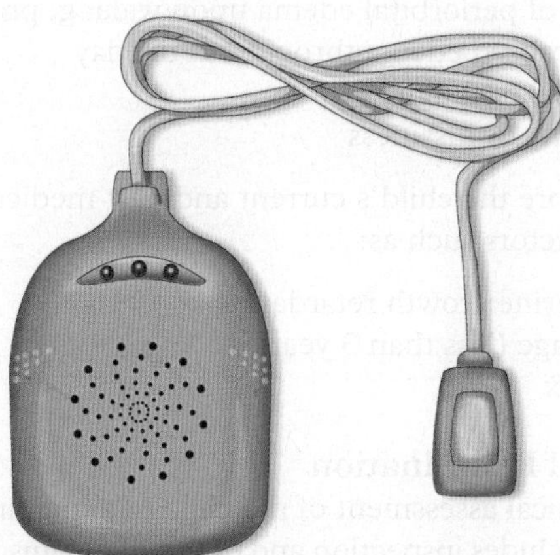

● Figure 22.6 Some children and families find great success with the use of an enuresis alarm. The alarm wakes the child at the first sign of wetness. Over time, the child learns to awaken at night in response to the sensation of a full bladder.

Decreasing Nighttime Voiding

Teach the family using an enuresis alarm system how to use the alarm as well as the previously mentioned techniques (Fig. 22.6 and Box 22.2). Most of these devices work by sounding an alarm when the first few drops of urine appear; the child then awakens and stops the urine flow. Over time the child becomes conditioned to either awaken when the bladder is full or stop the urine flow when sleeping.

When behavioral and motivational therapies are unsuccessful, particularly in the older child, medications may be prescribed. Teach the child and parents about the use of medications such as oxybutynin, imipramine, and desmopressin (DDAVP) if these are prescribed (refer to Drug Guide 22.1).

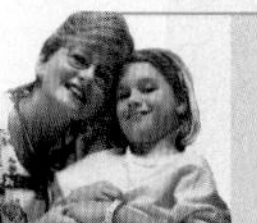

Enuresis is a source of shame and embarrassment for children and adolescents. It affects the child's life emotionally, behaviorally, and socially. The family's life is also significantly affected. Treatment failures for enuresis have been correlated with adolescent low self-esteem.

BOX 22.2

SOURCES FOR ENURESIS ALARMS

- www.bedwettingstore.com (800) 214-9605
- www.dri-sleeper.com (877) 331-2768
- www.nytone.com (801) 973-4090
- www.pediatricwarehouse.com (248) 318-6117
- www.pottypager.com (800) 497-6573

Consider THIS!

Antonio Cruise, a 7-year-old boy, is brought to the clinic by his mother for his annual examination. During your assessment the mother brings up concerns that Antonio continues to wet the bed at night. She states, "I was hoping this would end on its own, but now I'm concerned that there is a problem."

What further assessment information would you obtain?

What education and interventions may be necessary for this child and family?

What can you do to provide support and encouragement for Antonio and his family?

● ACQUIRED DISORDERS RESULTING IN ALTERED RENAL FUNCTION

A number of acquired disorders are responsible for alterations in renal function. They may occur as an autoimmune response or in relation to a bacterial infection. Renal dysfunction may also occur as a result of obstructive disorders or repeated VUR, as discussed earlier. Left untreated, these disorders may lead to renal failure; even when treated appropriately, sometimes the appropriate response is not achieved and acute or chronic renal failure develops. Renal disorders are the most frequent cause of hypertension in children.

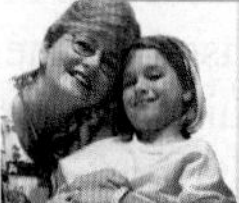

Severe hypertension (blood pressure higher than the 99th percentile for age and sex) may lead to damage of the eye or vital organs (kidney, brain, or heart), or even death. Pediatric nurses must be adept at accurately measuring blood pressure in children.

Nephrotic Syndrome

Nephrotic syndrome occurs as a result of increased glomerular basement membrane permeability, which allows abnormal loss of protein in the urine. Nephrotic syndrome generally occurs in three forms: congenital, idiopathic, and secondary. Congenital nephrotic syndrome is an inherited disorder; it is rare and occurs primarily in families of Finnish descent. The prognosis is poor, though some success has occurred with early, aggressive treatment and with the advances in kidney transplantation in infants. Nephrotic syndrome may occur secondary to another condition such as systemic lupus erythematosus, Henoch-Schonlein purpura, or diabetes. Idiopathic nephrotic syndrome is the most commonly occurring type in children and is often termed minimal change nephrotic syndrome (MCNS). MCNS occurs more frequently in males than females and is most common in children less than 3 years of age. This discussion will focus primarily on MCNS. Complications of nephrotic syndrome include anemia, infection, poor growth, peritonitis, thrombosis, and renal failure.

Pathophysiology

Increased glomerular permeability results in the passage of larger plasma proteins through the glomerular basement membrane. This results in excess loss of protein (albumin) in the urine (**proteinuria**) and decreased protein and albumin (hypoalbuminemia) in the bloodstream. Protein loss in nephrotic syndrome tends to be almost exclusively albumin. Hypoalbuminemia results in a change in osmotic pressure, and fluid shifts from the bloodstream into the interstitial tissue (causing edema). This decrease in blood volume triggers the kidneys to respond by conserving sodium and water, leading to further edema. The liver senses the protein loss and increases production of lipoproteins. **Hyperlipidemia** then develops as the excess lipids cannot be excreted in the urine. Hyperlipidemia associated with nephrotic syndrome may be quite severe, yet cholesterol levels may decrease when the nephrotic syndrome is in remission, only to rise significantly again with a relapse.

Children with nephrotic syndrome are at increased risk for clotting (thromboembolism) because of the decreased intravascular volume. They are also at increased risk for the development of serious infection, most commonly pneumococcal pneumonia, sepsis, or spontaneous peritonitis. Steroid-resistant nephrotic syndrome may result in acute renal failure.

Therapeutic Management

Medical management of MCNS usually involves the use of corticosteroids. Intravenous albumin may be used in the severely edematous child. Diuretics are also required in the edematous phase. Long-term therapy is usually required to induce remission. The nephrologist will determine the length of therapy based on the child's response. Children who have steroid-responsive MCNS generally have a favorable prognosis. Some children with MCNS exhibit a minimal response to steroid therapy or experience remissions and the MCNS is steroid-resistant. Immunosuppressive therapy such as cyclophosphamide, cyclosporine A, or mycophenolate mofetil may be necessary.

Nursing Assessment

For a full description of the assessment phase of the nursing process refer to page 721. Assessment findings pertinent to MCNS are discussed below.

Health History

Elicit a description of the present illness and chief complaint. Common signs and symptoms reported during the health history might include:

- Nausea or vomiting (may be related to ascites)
- Recent weight gain
- History of periorbital edema upon waking, progressing to generalized edema throughout the day
- Weakness or fatigue
- Irritability or fussiness

Explore the child's current and past medical history for risk factors such as:

- Intrauterine growth retardation
- Young age (less than 3 years)
- Male sex

Physical Examination

The physical assessment of the child with nephrotic syndrome includes inspection and observation, auscultation, and palpation.

Observe the child for edema (periorbital, generalized [**anasarca**], or abdominal ascites). As the disease progresses, the edema also progresses to become more generalized, eventually becoming severe. Inspect the skin for a stretched, tight appearance, pallor, or skin breakdown related to significant edema (Fig. 22.7). Document height (or length) and weight. Note increased respiratory rate or increased work of breathing related to ascites and edema.

Note the blood pressure; it may be elevated in the child with nephrotic syndrome, though it is most often either normal or decreased unless the child is progressing to renal failure. Auscultate heart and lung sounds, noting abnormalities related to fluid overload. Palpate the skin, noting tautness. Palpate the abdomen and document presence of ascites.

Laboratory and Diagnostic Tests

Urine dipstick will reveal marked proteinuria. Infrequently, mild hematuria is also present. Serum protein and albumin levels will be low (often markedly so). Serum cholesterol

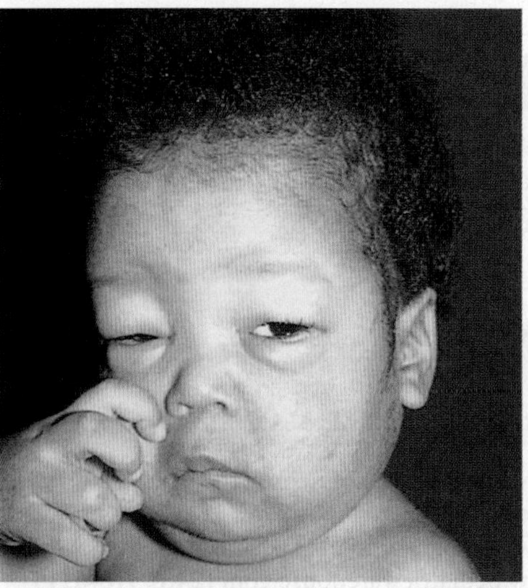

● **Figure 22.7** Note marked edema associated with nephrotic syndrome.

and triglyceride levels are elevated. With continued nephrotic syndrome, creatinine and blood urea nitrogen (BUN) may become elevated.

Nursing Management

Goals for nursing management include promoting diuresis, preventing infection, promoting adequate nutrition, and educating the parents about ongoing care at home. As with other chronic disorders, provide ongoing emotional support to the child and family.

Promoting Diuresis

Administer corticosteroids as ordered. Tapering or weaning doses are required when the time comes to stop corticosteroid therapy. Administer diuretics if ordered, usually furosemide (Lasix). Children may develop hypokalemia because of potassium loss as an adverse effect of furosemide. Those children may require potassium supplementation or a diet higher in potassium-containing foods. Monitor urine output and the amount of protein in the urine (by dipstick). Weigh the child daily on the same scale either naked or wearing the same amount of clothing. Assess for resolution of edema. Measure pulse rate and blood pressure every 4 hours to detect hypovolemia resulting from excessive fluid shifts. Enforce oral fluid restrictions if ordered.

In cases of severe hypoalbuminemia, intravenous albumin may be administered. Increases in the serum albumin level cause fluid to shift from the subcutaneous spaces back into the bloodstream. A diuretic such as furosemide administered immediately after the albumin infusion allows for optimal diuresis and prevents fluid overload. Refer to Drug Guide 22.1 for the nursing implications related to use of these medications.

Preventing Infection

Monitor the child's temperature. Viral illness may trigger a relapse in children with nephrotic syndrome who have achieved remission. Administer pneumococcal vaccine as prescribed (see Chapter 9 for information on immunizations). Administer prophylactic antibiotics, if prescribed. Live vaccines should be delayed until at least 2 weeks after corticosteroid or other immunosuppressive medication therapy ceases. Teach parents that if the child is unimmunized and is exposed to chickenpox, the pediatrician or nephrologist should be notified immediately so that the child may receive varicella zoster immunoglobulin.

Encouraging Adequate Nutrition and Growth

Encourage a nutrient-rich diet within prescribed restrictions. Fluid restriction is reserved for children with massive edema. Sodium intake may be restricted in the edematous child in an effort to prevent further fluid retention. Consultation with the dietitian is often helpful in meal planning because many of the foods that children like are high in sodium. Encourage protein-rich snacks. Consult with the child and family in planning meals and snacks that the child likes and will be likely to consume. Use of nutritional supplement shakes may be helpful in some children.

Educating the Family

Teach parents how to give medications and monitor for adverse effects. Demonstrate the urine dipstick technique for detecting protein, and encourage the family to keep a chart of dipstick results. The child may return to school but should avoid contact with sick playmates. If the child is exposed to another child with an infectious illness, the parents should monitor temperature and urine dipstick results more frequently to identify a relapse in nephrotic syndrome early so that treatment can begin.

Providing Emotional Support

Nephrotic syndrome is often a chronic condition, and children who are responsive to steroid treatment may enter remission only to experience relapse. This cycle of relapse and remission takes an emotional toll on the child and family. Frequent hospitalizations require the child to miss school and the parents to miss work; this creates further stress for the family. The child may experience social isolation because he or she must avoid exposure to infections or because of self-esteem problems. The child may be dissatisfied with his or her appearance because of edema and weight gain, short stature, and the classic "moon face" associated with chronic steroid use.

Provide emotional support to the child and family. Encourage them in their efforts to maintain the treatment plan. Introduce the child to other youngsters with chronic renal conditions. Refer families to the National Kidney Foundation (www.kidney.org) for information about local support groups and resources.

Acute Glomerulonephritis

Acute glomerulonephritis is a condition is which immune processes injure the glomeruli. Immune mechanisms cause inflammation, which results in altered glomerular structure and function in both kidneys. It often occurs following an infection, usually an upper respiratory or skin infection. The most common form is acute poststreptococcal glomerulonephritis (APSGN), and the following discussion will focus on this type. APSGN is caused by an antibody–antigen reaction secondary to an infection with a nephritogenic strain of group A beta-hemolytic streptococcus. APSGN occurs more frequently in males than females and is most common in children older than 2 years of age. The most serious complication is progression to uremia and renal failure (either acute or chronic).

There is no specific medical treatment for APSGN. Treatment is aimed at maintaining fluid volume and managing hypertension. If there is evidence of a current streptococcal infection, antibiotic therapy will be necessary.

Nursing Assessment

For a full description of the assessment phase of the nursing process refer to page 721. Assessment findings pertinent to acute glomerulonephritis are discussed below.

Health History

Elicit a description of the present illness and chief complaint. Common signs and symptoms reported during the health history might include:

- Fever
- Lethargy
- Headache
- Decreased urine output
- Abdominal pain
- Vomiting
- Anorexia

Assess the child's current and past medical history for risk factors such as a recent episode of pharyngitis or other streptococcal infection, age over 2 years, or male sex.

Physical Examination and Laboratory and Diagnostic Tests

Assess the child's blood pressure for elevation, which is common. Note the presence of mild edema. Observe for signs of cardiopulmonary congestion such as increased work of breathing or cough. Auscultate the lungs for crackles and the heart for gallop. The urine dipstick test will reveal proteinuria as well as hematuria. Inspect the urine for gross hematuria, which will cause the urine to appear tea-colored, cola-colored, or even a dirty green color. Serum creatinine and BUN may be normal or elevated, the serum complement level is depressed, and the erythrocyte sedimentation rate is elevated. Laboratory findings specific to streptococcus include an elevated anti-streptolysin (ASO) titer and an elevated DNAase B antigen titer.

Nursing Management

Administer antihypertensives such as labetalol or nifedipine and diuretics as ordered. Monitor blood pressure frequently. Maintain sodium and fluid restrictions as prescribed during the initial edematous phase. Weigh the child daily on the same scale wearing the same amount of clothing. Monitor increasing urine output and note improvement in the urine color. Document resolution of edema. Provide careful neurological evaluation, as hypertension may cause encephalopathy and seizures. Children with APSGN generally are fatigued and choose bed rest during the acute phase. Provide the child with age-appropriate activities and cluster care to allow rest periods.

Some children may be managed at home if edema is mild and they are not hypertensive. Teach the family to monitor urine output and color, take blood measurements, and restrict the diet as prescribed. The child cared for at home should not participate in strenuous activity until proteinuria and hematuria are resolved.

If renal involvement progresses, dialysis may become necessary.

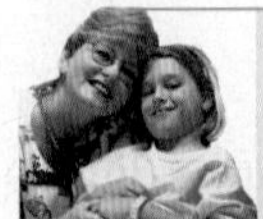

Avoid use of nonsteroidal anti-inflammatory drugs (NSAIDs) in children with questionable renal function, as the antiprostaglandin action of NSAIDs may cause a further decrease in the glomerular filtration rate.

Hemolytic-Uremic Syndrome

Hemolytic-uremic syndrome (HUS) is defined by three features: hemolytic anemia, thrombocytopenia, and acute renal failure. In 90% of cases of HUS, an illness featuring diarrhea precedes the onset of the syndrome. Other causes include idiopathic, inherited, drug-related, association with malignancies, transplantation, and malignant hypertension. This discussion will focus on typical HUS, the type preceded by a diarrheal illness. Watery diarrhea progresses to hemorrhagic colitis, then to the triad of HUS. The features of HUS, as well as effects on other organs, are caused primarily by microthrombi and ischemic changes within the organs. The thrombotic events in the small blood vessels of the glomerulus lead to occlusion of the glomerular capillary loops and glomerulosclerosis, resulting in renal failure.

A verotoxin-producing strain of *E. coli,* O157:H7, causes the majority of cases, though *Streptococcus pneumoniae, Shigella dysenteriae,* and other bacteria may also be the cause. It is thought that antibiotic treatment for the aforementioned bacteria may contribute to release of the verotoxin. Undercooked ground beef accounts for most cases of *E. coli* O157:H7 infection, but it is also transmitted via the feces of numerous animals as well as unpasteurized dairy and fruit products. Transmission also occurs via human feces, and cases have been linked to public swimming pools. HUS occurs most often in children age 6 months to 4 years. Complications include chronic renal failure, seizures and coma, pancreatitis, intussusception, rectal prolapse, cardiomyopathy, congestive heart failure, and acute respiratory distress syndrome (Varade, 2000).

Therapeutic management of HUS is directed toward maintaining fluid balance; correcting hypertension, acidosis, and electrolyte abnormalities; replenishing circulating red blood cells; and providing dialysis if needed.

Nursing Assessment

For a full description of the assessment phase of the nursing process refer to page 721. Assessment findings pertinent to HUS are discussed below.

Health History

Elicit a description of the present illness and chief complaint. Common signs and symptoms reported during the health history might include watery diarrhea accompanied by cramping and sometimes vomiting. After several days, the diarrhea becomes bloody and eventually improves.

Explore the child's current and past medical history for risk factors such as ingestion of ground beef, visits to a water park or to a petting zoo before the onset of the diarrheal illness, or use of antidiarrheal medications or antibiotics.

Physical Examination

Observe the child for pallor, toxic appearance, edema, **oliguria**, or **anuria**. Assess for elevated blood pressure and tenderness in the abdomen. Assess the child for neurologic involvement, which may include irritability, altered level of consciousness, seizures, posturing, or coma.

Laboratory and Diagnostic Tests

Urinalysis may reveal the presence of blood, protein, pus, and/or casts. Serum laboratory abnormalities are numerous and may include:

- Elevated BUN and creatinine
- Moderate to severe anemia (with the presence of Burr cells, schistocytes, spherocytes, or helmet cells), mild to severe thrombocytopenia
- Increased reticulocyte count
- Increased bilirubin and lactic dehydrogenase (LDH) levels
- Negative Coombs' test (except in cases of *S. pneumoniae* infection)
- Leukocytosis with left shift
- Hyponatremia
- Hyperkalemia
- Hyperphosphatemia
- Metabolic acidosis

Nursing Management

Nursing management of the child with HUS focuses on close observation and monitoring of the child's status. Institute and maintain contact precautions to prevent spread of *E. coli* O157:H7 to other children (bacteria are shed for up to 17 days after resolution of the diarrhea). Close attention must be paid to fluid volume status. Prevention of HUS is also an important nursing function.

Maintaining Appropriate Fluid Volume Balance

Maintain strict intake and output monitoring and recording to evaluate the progression toward renal failure. Carefully monitor intravenous infusions and blood chemistries. Administer diuretics as ordered. Assess blood pressure frequently and report elevations to the physician. Administer antihypertensives as ordered and monitor their effectiveness. Encourage adequate nutritional intake within the constraints of prescribed dietary restrictions. Monitor for bleeding as well as for fatigue and pallor. Follow the institutional protocol for transfusion of packed red blood cells and/or platelets (platelets are usually transfused only if active bleeding or severe thrombocytopenia occurs). Report progressive deterioration in laboratory findings to the physician. About 50% of children with HUS will require dialysis for at least several days.

Preventing HUS

Proper hand washing is necessary. Teach children to wash their hands after using the bathroom, before eating, and after petting farm animals. Encourage the use of "swim diapers," which contain feces, for children who are not toilet trained. Teach parents to thoroughly cook all meats to a core temperature of 155° F, or until the meat is gray or brown throughout and the juices from the meat are clear rather than pink. Wash all fruits and vegetables thoroughly. Ensure that drinking water and water used for recreation is appropriately treated. Avoid unpasteurized dairy products and fruit juices (including cider).

● RENAL FAILURE

Renal failure is a condition in which the kidneys cannot concentrate urine, conserve electrolytes, or excrete waste products. As in adults, renal failure in children may occur as an acute or chronic condition. Some cases of acute renal failure resolve without further complications, while dialysis is necessary in other children. When acute renal failure continues to progress, it becomes chronic (also known as end-stage renal disease [ESRD]). Dialysis and kidney transplantation are treatment modalities used for ESRD.

Acute Renal Failure

Acute renal failure is defined as a sudden, often reversible, decline in renal function that results in the accumulation of metabolic toxins (particularly nitrogenous wastes) as well as fluid and electrolyte imbalance. Fluid overload may lead to hypertension, pulmonary edema, and congestive heart failure. Additional complications include hyperkalemia, metabolic acidosis, hyperphosphatemia, and uremia. In children, acute renal failure most commonly occurs as a result of decreased renal perfusion, as occurs in hypovolemic or septic shock. It may also occur in children with hemolytic anemia or as a result of nephrotoxicity from medications. Complications include anemia, hyperkalemia, hypertension, pulmonary edema, cardiac failure, and altered level of consciousness or seizures, and acute renal failure may also progress to a chronic state.

Therapeutic management is aimed at treating the underlying cause and managing the fluid and electrolyte disturbances, as well as decreasing blood pressure.

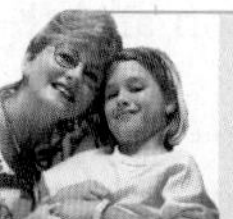

Medications commonly used in children can reduce renal function. Cephalosporins may cause a transient increase in BUN and creatinine. Truly nephrotoxic drugs often used in children include aminoglycosides, sulfonamides, vancomycin, and nonsteroidal anti-inflammatories (NSAIDs). Make sure that potentially nephrotoxic drugs are administered according to published safe guidelines (dosage, frequency, rate of administration).

Nursing Assessment

For a full description of the assessment phase of the nursing process refer to page 721. Assessment finding pertinent to acute renal failure are discussed below.

Health History

Elicit a description of the present illness and chief complaint. Common signs and symptoms reported during the health history might include:

- Nausea
- Vomiting
- Diarrhea
- Lethargy
- Fever
- Decreased urine output

Assess the child's current and past medical history for risk factors such as history of shock, trauma, burns, urologic abnormalities, renal disease, use of nephrotoxic medications, or severe blood transfusion reaction.

Physical Examination and Laboratory and Diagnostic Tests

Note decreased skin elasticity, dry mucous membranes, or edema. Auscultate lungs for crackles, which may occur with pulmonary edema. Document tachypnea. Note cardiac rhythm disturbances. Evaluate the child's level of consciousness. Laboratory tests will reveal increased serum creatinine levels and possible electrolyte disturbances, such as hyperkalemia or hypocalcemia. Urinalysis may reveal proteinuria or hematuria.

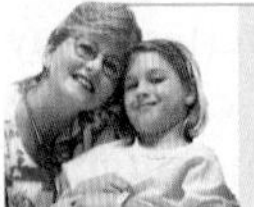

Monitor the infant or child with renal failure carefully for signs of congestive heart failure, such as edema accompanied by bounding pulse, presence of an S3 heart sound, adventitious lung sounds, and shortness of breath.

Nursing Management

Nursing care focuses on managing hypertension, restoring fluid and electrolyte balance, and educating the family.

Managing Hypertension

Carefully monitor the child's blood pressure. Administer antihypertensives as prescribed. When a fast-acting drug such as nifedipine (Procardia) sublingually or labetalol intravenously is used, stay with the child and frequently monitor blood pressure. Immediately notify the physician if high blood pressure is resistant to medication and the blood pressure remains elevated.

Restoring Fluid and Electrolyte Balance

Monitor vital signs frequently and assess urine specific gravity. Maintain strict records of intake and output. Administer diuretics as ordered. When urine output is restored, diuresis may be significant. Monitor for signs of hyperkalemia (weak, irregular pulse; muscle weakness; abdominal cramping) and hypocalcemia (muscle twitching or tetany). Administer polystyrene sulfonate (Kayexalate) as ordered orally, rectally, or through a nasogastric tube to decrease potassium levels. Kayexalate removes potassium primarily by exchanging sodium for it, which is then eliminated in the feces. Administer packed red blood cell transfusions as ordered (may need to be followed by a dose of diuretic). Dialysis may become necessary if oliguria is sustained and leads to significant fluid overload, the electrolyte imbalance reaches dangerous levels, or uremia results in depression of the central nervous system.

Providing Family Education

Educate the family about the plan of care and the need for fluid restriction if ordered. Instruct the family to save all voids for observation and measurement by the nurse. Provide education about the use of dialysis if relevant.

End-Stage Renal Disease

End-stage renal disease (ESRD) is chronic renal failure requiring long-term dialysis or renal transplantation. Chronic renal failure in children most often results from congenital structural defects such as obstructive uropathy. It may also be caused by an inherited condition such as familial nephritis or may result from an acquired problem such as glomerulonephritis; it may also follow an infectious process such as pyelonephritis or HUS. This is in contrast to chronic renal failure in adults, which primarily results from diabetes or hypertension. Uremia, hypocalcemia, hyperkalemia, and metabolic acidosis occur. Complications of ESRD are many. Uremic toxins deplete erythrocytes and the failing kidneys cannot produce erythropoietin, so severe anemia results. Hypertension is common and heart failure may occur. Hypocalcemia results in renal rickets (brittle bones). Growth is retarded and sexual maturation may be delayed or absent. Many children with ESRD experience depression, anxiety, impaired social interaction, and poor self-esteem. See Healthy People 2010.

Nursing Assessment

For a full description of the assessment phase of the nursing process refer to page 721. Assessment finding pertinent to ESRD are discussed below.

HEALTHY PEOPLE 2010

Objective	Significance
Reduce the rate of new cases of end-stage renal disease (ESRD).	• Encourage compliance with medical regimens related to urinary tract disorders in order to prevent progression to chronic renal failure

Health History

Explore the health history for low birthweight (associated with kidney dysfunction and anatomic alterations), poor growth (weight, length/height, and head circumference), and regimen of dialysis. Note decreased appetite or energy level, dry or itchy skin, or bone or joint pain.

Physical Examination and Laboratory and Diagnostic Tests

Perform a thorough physical assessment, noting any abnormalities (may vary from child to child). If present, assess the peritoneal catheter site for absence of drainage, bleeding, or redness. If the child undergoes hemodialysis, assess the fistula or graft site for the presence of a bruit and a thrill. Laboratory tests may reveal low hemoglobin and hematocrit, increased serum phosphorus and potassium levels, and decreased sodium, calcium, and bicarbonate levels. BUN, uric acid, and creatinine levels will be elevated. A 24-hour urine creatinine clearance test will show increased amounts of creatinine in the urine, reflecting decreasing kidney function.

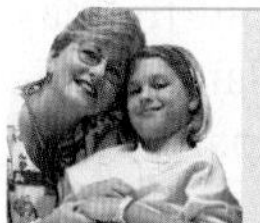

Carefully assess children with ESRD for worsening uremia or metabolic acidosis. Uremia may result in central nervous system symptoms such as headache or coma, or gastrointestinal or neuromuscular disturbances. Metabolic acidosis causes lethargy, dull headache, and confusion.

Nursing Management

Nursing goals for the child with ESRD include promoting growth and development, removing waste products and maintaining fluid balance via dialysis, encouraging psychosocial well-being, and supporting and educating the family.

Promoting Growth and Development

Encourage the child to choose foods he or she likes that are within the imposed dietary restrictions. Daily protein requirements for adequate growth range from 0.9 to 1.5 grams of protein per kilogram of weight. Sodium and/or potassium restrictions may also be necessary. Enforce fluid restrictions if prescribed. Administer medications such as erythropoietin, growth hormone, and vitamin and mineral supplements to augment nutritional status and promote growth. Table 22.2 lists medications and supplements used to support growth.

Encouraging Psychosocial Well-Being

The child with chronic renal failure and particularly ESRD often suffers from depression and anxiety. Refer children and their families to the hospital social worker or counselor as needed for depression or anxiety issues. The chronic need for dialysis (daily with peritoneal dialysis or three or four times per week with hemodialysis) confers long-term stress on the child and family. The child usually demonstrates poor growth and often suffers from body image disturbance. Frequent medical appointments and hospitalizations interfere with the child's scholastic achievements. Introduce the child to other children with ESRD (this often happens anyway at the hemodialysis center).

Ensure that the family is aware of financial and support resources within the community (refer them to the National Kidney Foundation at www.kidney.org). The American Kidney Fund (www.kidneyfund.org) provides financial aid for kidney patients and summer camps for children with renal problems. Camp is an excellent way for children to demonstrate that they have mastered some of the loss-of-control issues related to their disease.

Several websites provide forums for children and teens with kidney failure or transplantation so they can learn about their disease, access resources, and/or communicate with other children. Two of them are:

- www.kidskare.org/: created by children, for children; contains information about organ donation and transplantation
- www.transweb.org: contains information about transplantation and donation

Dialysis and Transplantation

Peritoneal dialysis or hemodialysis is required on a long-term basis for children with chronic renal failure or ESRD.

Table 22.2 Medications and Supplements Commonly Used to Treat ESRD Complications

Medication or Supplement	Purpose
Vitamin D and calcium	Correction of hypocalcemia and hyperphosphatemia
Ferrous sulfate	Treatment of anemia
Bicitra or sodium bicarbonate tablets	Correction of acidosis
Multivitamin	Augment nutritional status
Erythropoietin injections	Stimulate red blood cell growth
Growth hormone injections	Stimulate growth in stature

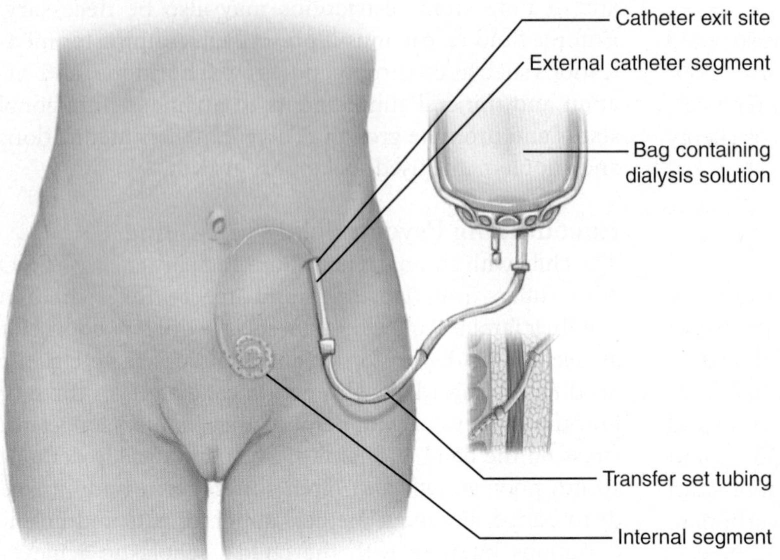

● Figure 22.8 The peritoneal dialysis catheter is tunneled under the skin into the peritoneal cavity.

Once the child has progressed to ESRD, kidney transplantation is needed for the child to progress with growth and development.

Peritoneal Dialysis

Peritoneal dialysis uses the child's abdominal cavity as a semipermeable membrane to help remove excess fluid and waste products (Figs. 22.8 and 22.9). The parent or caregiver performs peritoneal dialysis at home after completing a training course. The process is either completed overnight with the use of a machine (continuous cyclic peritoneal dialysis) or in increments throughout the day for a total of 4 to 8 hours (continuous ambulatory peritoneal dialysis). Comparison Chart 22.1 compares these two methods of peritoneal dialysis.

The advantages of peritoneal dialysis over hemodialysis include improved growth as a result of more dietary freedom, increased independence in daily activities, and a

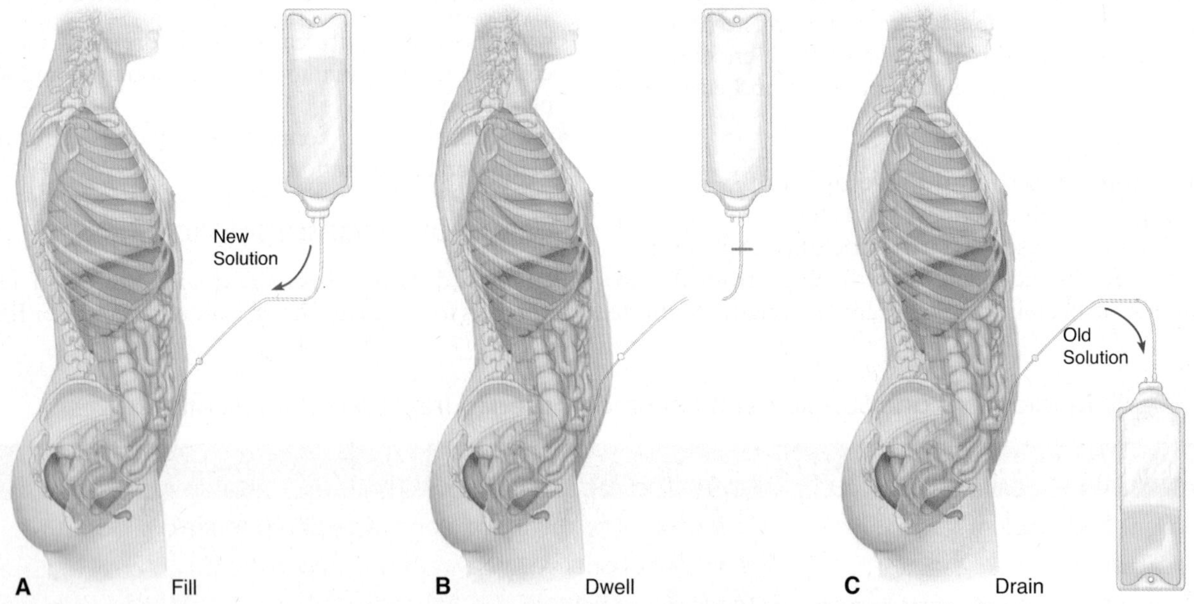

● Figure 22.9 (**A**) During the "fill" phase of peritoneal dialysis, dialysate fluid is instilled into the peritoneal cavity. (**B**) During the "dwell" phase, the child may be up out of bed with the empty dialysate bag folded up with the tubing under his clothing. (**C**) During the "drain" phase, the old dialysate is drained from the peritoneum by gravity, bringing with it waste products and excess fluid. The dialysate bags are weighed prior to filling and after draining to determine the amount of fluid removed from the child.

● COMPARISON CHART 22.1 Methods of Peritoneal Dialysis

	Continuous Ambulatory Peritoneal Dialysis (CAPD)	Continuous Cyclic Peritoneal Dialysis (CCPD)
When performed	Throughout the day, with exchanges every 3 to 6 hours. Fluid is usually allowed to dwell overnight to allow child to sleep.	Usually overnight while child is sleeping
Method	Manual instillation and draining and changing of dialysate bags with each exchange	Automated via CCPD machine; bags and tubing are attached when started, then disconnected in the morning
Dwell time	3 to 6 hours	Usually 30 minutes to 1 hour
Mobility	Allows for mobility and permits child to participate in activities between exchanges	Child is confined to bed during the night while CCPD is ongoing but completely mobile while off CCPD during the day.

steadier state of electrolyte balance. However, the risk for infection (peritonitis and sepsis) is a continual concern with peritoneal dialysis. Dialysate exchange protocols, care of the catheter in the abdomen, and dressing changes must all be performed using sterile technique to avoid introducing microorganisms into the peritoneal cavity. Box 22.3 lists additional risks associated with peritoneal dialysis.

Hemodialysis

Hemodialysis removes toxins and excess fluid from the blood by pumping the child's blood through a hemodialysis machine and then reinfusing the blood into the child. Needles to remove and reinfuse the blood are inserted into an arteriovenous fistula or graft, usually located in the child's arm (Figs. 21.10 and 21.11).

Hemodialysis frees the parent from the need to perform daily dialysis, but the procedure, which takes 3 to 6 hours, must be done two to four times per week (usually three) at a pediatric hemodialysis center. This requires time away from school and other activities for the child and from work and other family responsibilities for the parent. Since hemodialysis is usually performed only every other day, larger amounts of waste products build up in the child's blood (uremia), placing the child at higher risk for seizures. The access site may become infected, and occlusion is also possible. The child must follow a stricter diet between hemodialysis treatments, though dietary restrictions are usually lifted while the child is actually undergoing the treatment.

BOX 22.3

RISKS ASSOCIATED WITH PERITONEAL DIALYSIS

- Hypertension and other cardiac complications
- Seizures
- Obstructed catheter
- Dialysate leakage
- Hyperglycemia
- Increased triglyceride levels
- Increased protein loss
- Parental stress and burnout related to repetitive nature of daily intervention

Nursing Assessment

Refer to the section on nursing assessment of the child with chronic renal failure/ESRD, as it is similar to assessment of the child undergoing dialysis. Assess for alterations in blood pressure and laboratory values following dialysis. Monitor for signs and symptoms of infection.

Assess the child receiving peritoneal dialysis for toleration of the fluid volume instilled within the peritoneum. The abdomen will remain distended while the fluid is indwelling and will be significantly flatter when the fluid is

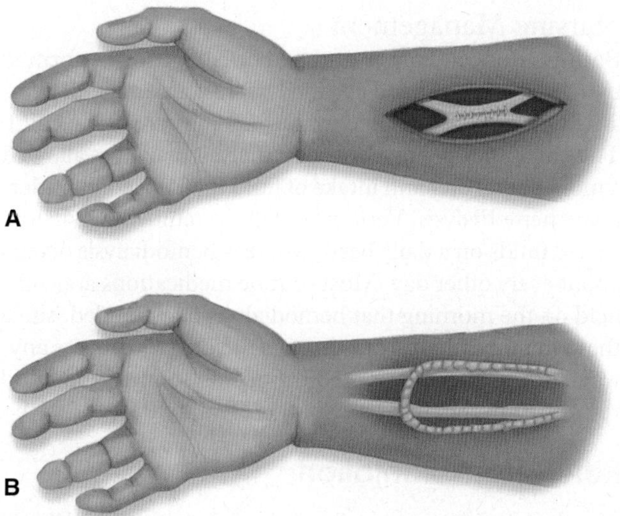

● Figure 22.10 (**A**) Arteriovenous fistula. (**B**) Arteriovenous graft.

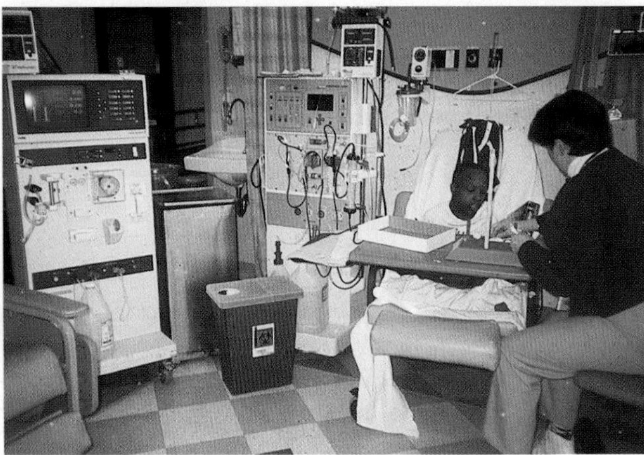

● Figure 22.11 Pediatric hemodialysis via arteriovenous fistula or graft in left arm.

HEALTHY PEOPLE 2010

Objective	Significance
Increase the proportion of new hemodialysis patients who use arteriovenous fistulas as the primary mode of vascular access. Increase the proportion of dialysis patients registered on the waiting list for transplantation.	• Educate families about the benefits of an arteriovenous fistula over other methods of hemodialysis access. • Advocate for the patient to obtain an arteriovenous fistula. • Educate families about transplantation, and if no living-related match is available, encourage the family to seek placement on the organ transplant waiting list.

drained. Assess the Tenckhoff catheter site for signs of infection. Monitor the child's temperature. Inspect the dialysate effluent for fibrin or cloudiness, which may indicate infection. Weigh the child daily (in the drain phase if on peritoneal dialysis).

For the child who receives hemodialysis, assess the arteriovenous fistula or graft site with each set of vital signs. Auscultate the site for the presence of a bruit and palpate for the presence of a thrill. Notify the physician immediately if either is absent.

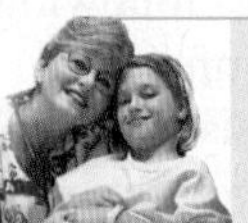

Avoid taking blood pressure, performing venipuncture, or using a tourniquet in the extremity with the arteriovenous fistula or graft: these procedures may cause occlusion and subsequent malfunction of the fistula or graft. Teach parents and children to inform all health care providers they come in contact with about the presence of the fistula or graft.

Nursing Management

Both peritoneal dialysis and hemodialysis are performed by specially trained and certified nurses. The general pediatric nurse's role is related to the ongoing care of the child. The child undergoing peritoneal dialysis usually is allowed a more liberal diet and intake of fluid than the child undergoing hemodialysis. Peritoneal dialysis removes waste and excess fluids on a daily basis, whereas hemodialysis occurs about every other day. Most routine medications are withheld on the morning that hemodialysis is scheduled, since they would be filtered out through the dialysis process anyway. Administer these medications as soon as the child returns from the dialysis unit. See Healthy People 2010.

Renal Transplantation

Renal transplantation is the optimal treatment for ESRD and offers the best opportunity for the child to live a normal life. Vigilant medication administration is necessary after the transplant to prevent organ rejection. The child may achieve 40% to 80% renal function with the transplant and demonstrate improved growth, enhanced cognitive development, and improved psychosocial development and quality of life (Milliner, 2004).

Kidneys are obtained from a cadaver (a patient declared brain-dead who had previously given consent to organ donation) or from a blood relative (living-related). The transplanted kidney must match the child's blood type and the child's human leukocyte antigens (HLA). The cadaver kidney or living-related kidney is implanted surgically in the abdomen and the blood vessels are anastomosed to the aorta and superior vena cava.

Generally, living-related transplants have a decreased rejection rate compared to cadaver transplants. Living-related kidney donation and subsequent transplantation can be planned ahead and scheduled in advance. In contrast, cadaver kidneys become available suddenly, leaving less time for preoperative preparation. For either type, last-minute blood tissue typing is required before the final decision is made to move forward with transplantation. Often the child's native kidneys are removed before or at the time of the renal transplant because of their association with hypertension in the child.

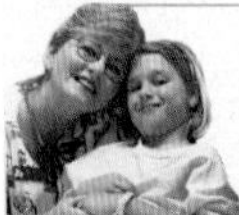

Cadaver kidneys are allocated to potential recipients based on the age of the renal failure patient, the time that he or she has been awaiting a transplant, blood type, HLA antibody matching, panel reactive antibodies, and region of the country (so that the donated kidney can be received expeditiously).

Nursing Assessment

A thorough physical assessment is warranted for any renal transplant patient, whether in the initial postoperative period, at a clinic visit, or when admitted to the hospital to rule out transplant rejection. Note recent health history, medications and their doses, and any symptoms the child has been having. In the initial postoperative period, assess the incision for redness, edema, or drainage; if any of these signs of infection or rejection occur, notify the transplant surgeon and nephrologist immediately. Monitor blood pressure and other vital signs closely. Document resolution of edema. Record intake and output accurately. Assess for signs and symptoms of transplant rejection such as malaise, fever, unexplained weight gain, or pain over the transplant area.

Nursing Management

Postoperative care focuses on preventing rejection, monitoring renal function, maintaining fluid and electrolyte balance, and educating the child and family.

Preventing Rejection and Promoting Renal Function

Administer immunosuppressants accurately and in a timely fashion. Obtain and monitor serum levels of these medications per protocol. Immediately report significant alterations in vital signs or edema at the surgical site, as they may indicate transplant rejection. Maintain strict documentation of intake and output. Once adequate urine output is established, intake is usually liberalized.

Educating the Child and Family

Develop a schedule to cluster care so that the child may receive the rest needed for recovery despite the many and frequent assessments and interventions. With the family, develop a medication schedule that will be compatible with the family's life at home as well as the restrictions related to some medications. Begin teaching with the family as soon as the child's condition is stable. Accurate medication administration and home monitoring are necessary to prevent rejection. The child may return to school when discharged from the hospital, but the family will need to communicate closely with the school nurse about the child's immunosuppressed status. The American Nephrology Nurses Association has developed a renal transplant fact sheet that can be shared with the school nurse (available at www.anna.org).

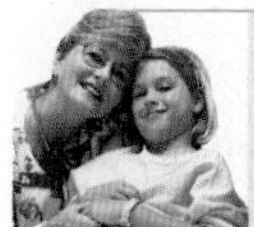

Encourage the child with a renal transplant to wear a medical alert necklace or bracelet, and urge the parents to inform community emergency services of the child's transplant status.

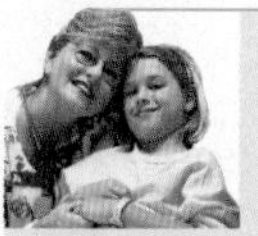

Tell the parents to inform their primary care provider about the child's long-term corticosteroid use and/or immunosuppressed status, as the child should not receive any live vaccines.

Reproductive Organ Disorders

A number of disorders may occur within the female or male genitalia and internal reproductive organs in children. These problems may be structural, infectious, or related to menstruation (in females).

● FEMALE DISORDERS

Disorders of the female reproductive organs that occur in children and adolescents include structural disorders, infectious disorders, and menstrual disorders.

Labial Adhesions

Labial adhesion or labial fusion is partial or complete adherence of the labia minora (Fig. 21.12). UTI may result from urinary stasis behind the labia; if the adhesions are left untreated, the vaginal orifice may become inaccessible, presenting difficulty with sexual intercourse in the future.

Nursing Assessment

Younger girls have a higher risk of adhesions (3 months to 4 years). Assess the history for dysuria or urinary frequency. Inspect the genitalia for fusion or adherence of the labia minora.

Nursing Management

Administer topical estrogen cream as prescribed, usually once or twice daily. Teach the parents to continue cream application until the labia separate. Encourage use of petroleum jelly daily for 1 month following labial separation to prevent recurrence of adhesion.

Vulvovaginitis

Vulvovaginitis is inflammation of the vulva and vagina. Inflammation may occur as a result of bacterial or yeast

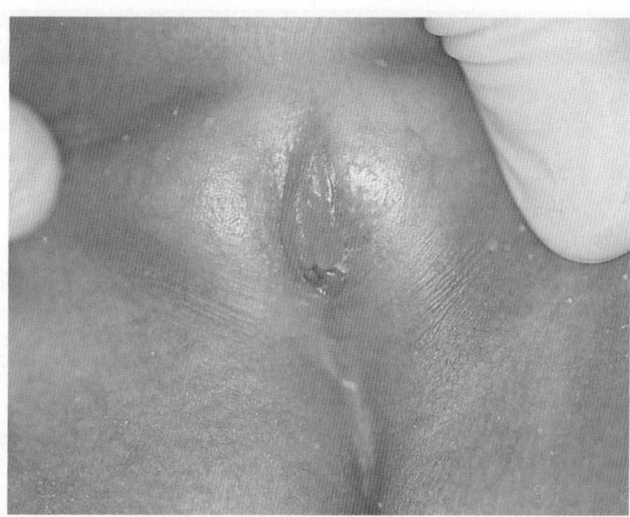

● Figure 22.12 Labial adhesions. Note fusion of the upper portion of the labia minora.

overgrowth or from chemical factors such as bubble bath, soaps, or perfumes found in personal care products. Poor hygiene may also cause vulvovaginitis. Tight clothing may cause a heat rash in the perineal area. Persistent scratching of the irritated area may result in the complication of superficial skin infection.

Nursing Assessment

Elicit a description of the present illness and chief complaint. Common signs and symptoms reported during the health history may include itching or burning in the perineal area. Explore the client's current and past medical history for risk factors, which may include:

- Young age (toilet-trained preschooler)
- Poor hygiene
- Sexual activity
- Immune disorders
- Diabetes mellitus

Inspect the perineum for redness, edema, irritation, rash, or vaginal discharge (note color, consistency, and odor).

Nursing Management

Teach appropriate hygiene (daily and toileting). Girls (or their parents) should wash the genital area thoroughly on a daily basis with mild soap and water. Rinse the area well. Encourage girls to wipe after urinating and after bowel movements to wipe in a front-to-back motion. The girl should wear cotton underwear and should change it at least once a day. Administer topical or oral medications as ordered. Table 22.3 lists treatments related to specific types of vulvovaginitis.

Pelvic Inflammatory Disease

Pelvic inflammatory disease (PID) is an inflammation of the upper female genital tract and nearby structures. The fallopian tubes, ovaries, or peritoneum may be involved, and endometriosis may also be present. PID results from bacterial invasion through the cervix and vagina, ascending into the uterus and fallopian tubes. The most common causes of PID are *Chlamydia trachomatis* and *Neisseria gonorrhoeae,* although other bacteria and normal vaginal flora may be implicated. PID may result in fever, abdominal pain, pain with intercourse, **dysmenorrhea**, and abnormal uterine bleeding. Long-term complications include chronic pelvic pain, ectopic pregnancy, and infertility related to scarring.

Nursing Assessment

For a full description of the assessment phase of the nursing process refer to page 721.

When discussing any problem related to the reproductive organs or menstruation with the pre-teen or teen, it is necessary to discuss sexuality. The girl may be reluctant to share this information with the nurse. Approaches to discussing sexuality with the adolescent that may increase the likelihood of obtaining a truthful history include:

- Discuss the girl's general health, menarche, and menstrual cycle first, and then work toward discussing sexual behavior.
- Start with questions about the girl's friends and social life, moving the conversation toward sexual behavior.
- Always discuss sexual behavior one-on-one with the adolescent (without the parent present), and then ask the adolescent's permission to discuss concerns with the

Table 22.3 Vulvovaginitis: Types and Treatments

Cause	Assessment Findings	Treatment
Unhygienic practices	Irritation of labia and vaginal opening May have foul brownish-green discharge if infected with bacteria from rectum	Good hygiene Sometimes a mild anti-inflammatory cream is prescribed. Assess for signs and symptoms of UTI, which may occur as a complication.
Candida albicans	Red bumpy perineal rash in infants White cottage-cheese–like discharge Intense itching	Antifungal cream or vaginal suppository Prevent by ingesting probiotics (found in yogurt and kefir) daily and supplementing with a probiotic such as Lactinex when taking antibiotics.
Bordetella, Gardnerella	Thin gray vaginal discharge with fishy odor	Flagyl (metronidazole) orally
Trichomonas vaginalis	Foul yellow-gray or green vaginal discharge	Flagyl (metronidazole) orally. Sexually transmitted, so can be prevented with the use of condoms.

parent. If the adolescent does not consent to parental involvement, then confidentiality must be maintained.

Assessment findings pertinent to PID are discussed below.

Health History

Elicit a description of the present illness and chief complaint. Common signs and symptoms reported during the health history might include:

- Abdominal pain (ranging from mild to severe)
- Prolonged or increased menstrual bleeding
- Dysmenorrhea
- Dysuria
- Painful sexual intercourse
- Nausea
- Vomiting

Explore the girl's current and past medical health history for risk factors such as:

- Multiple sexual partners
- Lack of consistent condom use
- Lack of contraceptive use
- History of prior sexually transmitted infection
- Douching
- Prostitution
- Alcohol or drug use (particularly if associated with sexual activity)

Physical Examination

Inspect for fever (usually over 101°F) or vaginal discharge. Palpate the abdomen, noting tenderness over the uterus or ovaries. An elevated C-reactive protein level and an elevated erythrocyte sedimentation rate indicate an inflammatory process. Cervical culture reveals the causative bacterial organism.

HEALTHY PEOPLE 2010

Objective	Significance
Reduce the proportion of females who have ever required treatment for pelvic inflammatory disease (PID).	• Educate teens that abstinence is the only way to completely avoid contracting a sexually transmitted infection. • Encourage teens to always use condoms if participating in any sexual act. • Provide an open and confidential environment so teen girls will report symptoms and seek treatment earlier.

Nursing Management

PID is often treated in the outpatient setting with intramuscular or oral antibiotic regimens. If the adolescent is severely ill or has a very high fever or protracted vomiting, then she may be hospitalized. Antibiotics are needed to eradicate the infection. Maintain hydration via intravenous fluids if necessary and administer analgesics as needed for pain. Semi-Fowler's positioning promotes pelvic drainage. A key element to treatment of PID is education to prevent recurrence (see Healthy People 2010 and Teaching Guideline 22.2).

Menstrual Disorders

Menstruation begins in most girls about 2 years after breast development starts, around the time of Tanner stage 4 breast and pubic hair development and on average at around 12 to 13 years of age. Menstruation has many effects on girls and women, including emotional and self-image issues. Adolescents may suffer from a variety of menstrual disorders, including premenstrual syndrome and several different disorders related to menstrual bleeding and cramping (Table 22.4).

In healthy girls, the menstrual period varies in the heaviness of flow. Periods may occur irregularly for up to 2 years after menarche (the onset of menstruation), but after that the regular menstrual cycle should be established. The normal cycle can vary from 21 to 45 days in length, with the period usually lasting 2 to 7 days. Girls who take oral contraceptives usually have very regular 28-day cycles, with lighter bleeding than those who do not take contraceptives.

Pathophysiology

Premenstrual syndrome is a collection of physical and/or affective symptoms that occur predictably during the luteal phase of the menstrual cycle. Symptoms begin 5 to 10 days before each period and usually resolve by the time the period begins or shortly thereafter (the timing may vary by adolescent but is consistent with each cycle). Disorders of bleeding and cramping are summarized in Table 22.4.

Nursing Assessment

For a full description of the assessment phase of the nursing process, refer to page 721. When girls present for eval-

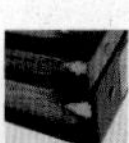

TEACHING GUIDELINE 22.2

Preventing Pelvic Inflammatory Disease

- Insist that sexual partners use condoms.
- Do not use a vaginal douche routinely, as this may lead to bacterial overgrowth.
- Get screened regularly for sexually transmitted infections.
- Make sure that each sexual partner also receives antibiotic treatment.

Table 22.4 Common Menstrual Disorders

Disorder	Definition	Cause
Primary amenorrhea	Lack of menarche within 2 years of reaching Tanner stage 4 breast development, or by 16 years of age	• Imperforate hymen • Agenesis of vulva or vagina • Turner syndrome • Chronic illness associated with delayed pubertal development (e.g., cystic fibrosis, Crohn's disease, sickle cell disease) • Suppressed levels of follicle-stimulating hormone (FSH) or luteinizing hormone (LH), as occurs with eating disorders, intense athletics, severe psychological stress, or extreme weight loss
Secondary amenorrhea	Absence of menses for 6 months in the girl who has been menstruating regularly	• Pregnancy (most common cause) • Anovulation (resulting from lack of hypothalamic-pituitary axis maturity) • Polycystic ovary syndrome (PCOS) • Suppressed levels of follicle-stimulating hormone (FSH) or luteinizing hormone (LH), as occurs with eating disorders, intense athletics, severe psychological stress, or extreme weight loss
Mittelschmerz	Abdominal pain, usually unilateral, that varies from a few sharp cramps to several hours of crampy pain	Usually occurs midway through the menstrual cycle, around the time of ovulation; is thought to be a result of egg release from the ovary
Dysmenorrhea	Pain associated with menstruation, usually abdominal cramps ranging from mild to severe	• Prostaglandin release is responsible for the smooth muscle contraction of the uterus during menstruation (primary) • Fibroids, adenomyosis, endometriosis, scar tissue (secondary)
Menorrhagia	Excessive menstrual bleeding	• Anovulatory cycles • Endometriosis • Blood dyscrasias, bleeding disorders, or use of anticoagulants • Reproductive system neoplasms
Metrorrhagia	Bleeding between menstrual periods	• Improper use of oral contraceptives • Intrauterine device • Endometriosis • Reproductive system neoplasms • Miscarriage or ectopic pregnancy

uation of menstrual concerns, a focused yet thorough nursing assessment is necessary.

Health History

Obtain a thorough and accurate menstrual history; determine age at menarche, usual length of menstrual period, usual menstrual flow, number of pads or tampons used per day, date of last normal menstrual period, premenstrual symptoms, and any pain related to the menstrual cycle. Obtain a description of the pain, what relief measures have been tried, and what the success of those measures has been. If pain occurs with menstrual periods, assess for associated symptoms such as nausea, vomiting, dizziness, or loose stools. Explore the history for symptoms of bloating, water retention, weight gain, headache, muscle aches, abdominal pain, food cravings, or breast tenderness. Determine the extent of emotional symptoms related to the menstrual cycle, such as anxiety, insomnia, mood swings, tension, crying spells, or irritability. Note the timing of these symptoms within the menstrual cycle.

Note past medical history, including any chronic illnesses and family history of gynecologic concerns. Elicit a sexual behavior history, including the type of sexual activity (oral, anal, or vaginal), number and gender of sexual partners, frequency and most recent sexual contact, history of molestation or sexual abuse, and use of contraceptives (noting type) and/or condoms.

Take a medication history, including prescription medications and contraceptives, and determine whether the girl uses anabolic steroids, tobacco, or marijuana, cocaine, or other illegal drugs.

Physical Examination

The physical assessment related to menstrual disorders includes inspection and observation, auscultation, and palpation. The bimanual pelvic examination and Pap smear are usually indicated only for more severe menstrual disorders and are usually performed by the physician or advanced practice nurse.

Inspect the breasts and pubic hair distribution to determine Tanner stage. Observe the external genitalia for vaginal discharge, redness, or irritation. Note pallor or weight gain. Document presence and extent of clots in menstrual flow. Measure orthostatic blood pressure and orthostatic pulse; decreases with position change may occur in girls with anemia. Palpate the abdomen, noting distention or tenderness.

Laboratory and Diagnostic Tests

Common laboratory and diagnostic studies ordered for the assessment of menstrual disorders include:

- Complete blood count: to determine presence of anemia with **menorrhagia** or metrorrhagia
- Human chorionic gonadotropin: to assess for pregnancy with **amenorrhea**

Nursing Management

Nursing goals for the girl with a menstrual disorder focus on normalizing menstrual flow and restoring blood volume, providing comfort, and encouraging independence in self-care.

Normalizing Menstrual Flow and Restoring Blood Volume

For the girl with mild anemia related to menorrhagia, administer iron supplements as ordered. For moderate menorrhagia, oral contraceptives may also be prescribed, since altering hormone levels decreases menstrual flow. If the contraceptive contains a high dose of estrogen, the girl may experience nausea. Administer antiemetics as ordered and encourage the girl to eat small, frequent meals to alleviate nausea. Adolescents with severe anemia may require hospitalization and blood transfusion.

Providing Comfort

Provide a heating pad or warm compress to help alleviate menstrual cramps. Administer NSAIDs such as ibuprofen or naproxen to inhibit prostaglandin synthesis, which contributes to menstrual cramps. Advise girls that beginning NSAID therapy at the first sign of menstrual discomfort is the best way to minimize discomfort. If NSAIDs are unsuccessful, oral contraceptives may be ordered; teach the girl appropriate use of oral contraceptives.

The adolescent experiencing premenstrual syndrome should keep a diary of her symptoms, their severity, and when they occur in the menstrual cycle. Like all adolescents, girls with premenstrual syndrome should eat a balanced diet that includes nutrient-rich foods so they can avoid hypoglycemia and associated mood swings. Encourage adolescent girls to participate in aerobic exercise three times a week to promote a sense of well-being, decrease fatigue, and reduce stress. Administer calcium (1,200 to 1,600 mg/day), magnesium (400 to 800 mg/day), and vitamin B6 (50 to 100 mg/day) as prescribed. In some studies, these nutrients have been shown to decrease the intensity of premenstrual symptoms. NSAIDs may be useful for painful physical symptoms, and spironolactone (Aldactone) may help reduce bloating and water retention. Herbs such as chasteberry or ginkgo may be recommended; though not found to be harmful, studies are inconclusive about their effectiveness (Dell, 2004). A recent research review proposes calcium (1,600 mg/day) and vitamin D (400 IU/day) supplementation in adolescents and women in an effort to prevent the development of premenstrual syndrome (Bertone-Johnson et al., 2005).

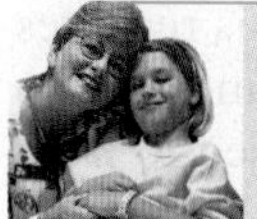

Adolescents who experience more extensive emotional symptoms with premenstrual syndrome should be evaluated for premenstrual dysphoric disorder, as they may require antidepressant therapy.

Encouraging Independence in Self-Care

Establishing a trusting relationship with the adolescent may make education about self-care more successful. Some girls have open relationships with their mothers and can discuss issues related to menses and sexuality with them, but many others cannot discuss such "embarrassing" issues with their mothers, and the nurse or other health care provider may be the only source of reliable information. Provide the adolescent with accurate information about menstruation and sexuality. Educate her about normal menstruation, the menstrual cycle, and the risk for pregnancy if sexual intercourse occurs (refer to Chapter 8 for information related to contraception). Refer girls to reliable websites (Box 22.4) if they are not comfortable with receiving information from the nurse. Encourage the girl to call or visit the office if she has additional questions.

• MALE DISORDERS

Male reproductive disorders include structural disorders and disorders caused by infection or inflammation. Circumcision will also be discussed below.

Phimosis and Paraphimosis

In phimosis, the foreskin of the penis cannot be retracted. Although this is normal in the newborn, it can be patho-

BOX 22.4

HELPFUL WEBSITES RELATED TO TEEN GIRLS' HEALTH

- www.girlpower.gov (9- to 13-year-olds)
- www.awarefoundation.org
- www.goaskalice.columbia.edu
- www.itsyoursexlife.com
- www.plannedparenthood.org/teens
- www.kidshealth.org/teen
- www.teenadviceonline.org
- www.teengrowth.com
- www.youngwomenshealth.org

logic later. Over time, the prepuce (foreskin) naturally becomes retractable. Local irritation, balanitis, or UTI may occur if urine is retained within the foreskin after voiding. Paraphimosis (fig. 22.13) is a more serious disorder characterized by retraction of the phimotic prepuce, which causes a constricting band behind the glans of the penis and results in incarceration if left untreated.

Topical steroid cream applied twice a day for 1 month may be prescribed for phimosis. Paraphimosis requires reduction of the prepuce or a small dorsal incision to release the foreskin. Circumcision may be used to treat either condition.

Nursing Assessment

Elicit a description of the present illness and chief complaint. Common signs and symptoms reported during the health history might include:

- Irritation or bleeding from the opening of the prepuce (phimosis)
- Dysuria (phimosis)
- Pain (paraphimosis)
- Swollen penis (paraphimosis)

Determine the onset of symptoms and inspect the penis for irritation, erythema, edema, or discharge.

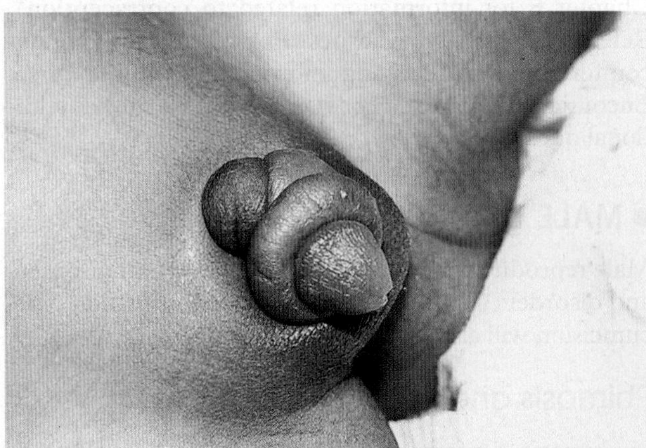

● Figure 22.13 Paraphimosis: note the swollen prepuce.

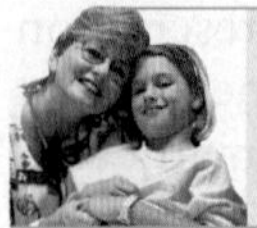

A swollen, reddened penis (paraphimosis) is a medical emergency and can quickly result in necrosis of the tip of the penis if left untreated.

Nursing Management

Apply topical steroid medication as prescribed for phimosis, following gentle retraction to stretch the foreskin back. Topical vitamin E cream may also help to soften the phimotic ring. When surgical intervention is necessary, provide routine postprocedural care and pain management (refer to the section on circumcision below). Teach the parents and uncircumcised boy proper hygiene, which will help to prevent phimosis and paraphimosis (Teaching Guideline 22.3).

Circumcision

Circumcision is the removal of the excess foreskin of the penis. Some newborn boys are circumcised shortly after birth before going home from the hospital. Some parents elect not to have their newborn boy circumcised at that time but may desire it later. Neonatal circumcision may be performed in the newborn nursery, hospital unit treatment room, or outpatient office. Circumcision is indicated later for the conditions of phimosis and paraphimosis. Circumcision done after the newborn period usually requires general anesthesia.

The benefits of circumcision include a decreased incidence of UTI, sexually transmitted diseases, acquired immune deficiency syndrome, and penile cancer, and in female partners a decreased occurrence of cervical cancer. Complications of circumcision include alterations in the urinary meatus, unintentional removal of excessive amounts of foreskin, or damage to the glans penis.

Whether to circumcise or not is a personal decision and often based on religious beliefs or social or cultural

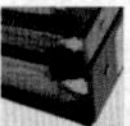

TEACHING GUIDELINE 22.3

Hygiene in the Uncircumcised Male

- The foreskin does not normally retract in the newborn boy, so do not force it to do so.
- Change the diaper frequently and wash the penis daily with water and mild soap.
- When the infant is older and the foreskin easily retracts, gently retract the foreskin and clean around the glans with water and mild soap once a week.
- Dry the area prior to replacing the foreskin.
- Always replace the foreskin after retraction.
- Teach the preschool-age boy to retract the foreskin and clean the penis during each bath or shower.

customs. Nurses should support and educate the parents in either case.

Nursing Assessment

Prior to the procedure, assess for normal placement of the urinary meatus on the glans penis (in boys with hypospadias, circumcision should be delayed until evaluation by the pediatric urologist). After the circumcision, assess for redness, edema, or active bleeding. Note signs of infection, such as purulent drainage. Assess pain level.

Nursing Management

Nursing care of the boy undergoing circumcision focuses on managing pain, providing postprocedural care, and educating the parents.

Managing Pain

Whether circumcision is performed in the obstetric area of the hospital before newborn discharge or in the outpatient setting at a few days of age, pain management during the procedure must not be neglected. Advocate for appropriate pain management for the infant undergoing circumcision. The American Academy of Pediatrics (AAP) recommends using a subcutaneous ring block with lidocaine or a dorsal nerve block to the penis. The AAP also recommends the use of EMLA (eutectic mixture of local anesthetic) cream topically to decrease pain during the circumcision. Playing calming music during the procedure may also help to soothe the infant, providing distraction. A sucrose-dipped pacifier may also be used as adjuvant therapy for pain management. To increase a sense of comfort during the procedure, restrain the infant in a padded circumcision chair with blankets covering the legs and upper body. This allows the infant to be in a semi-upright position during the procedure while still allowing for a sterile procedural field. If a padded restraint chair is not available, provide atraumatic care by padding the circumcision board and covering the infant as previously described.

Providing Postprocedural Care

Usual care after circumcision depends on the type of appliance used (Gomco or Mogan clamp or Plastibell apparatus). Cleanse the penis with clear water for the first few days and avoid using alcohol-containing wipes. To avoid irritation to the penis, fasten diapers loosely. Notify the physician if excessive redness, active bleeding, or purulent discharge occurs. Assess for the first void following the procedure, or if performed in the outpatient setting instruct parents to call the physician if the infant has not voided by 6 to 8 hours after the circumcision. Apply antibiotic ointment or petroleum jelly to the penile head with each diaper change as prescribed, based on the circumcision method used and the preference of the health care provider.

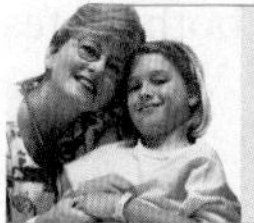

If excess bleeding occurs after the circumcision, apply direct pressure and notify the health care provider immediately.

Educating the Parents

Instruct parents to give sponge baths until the circumcision is healed. Describe the normal granulation tissue that will be present during the healing process. Teach parents to apply ointment or petroleum jelly if indicated. Instruct the parents to call the health care provider if any of the following occur:

- The infant does not urinate within 6 to 8 hours after the procedure.
- Heavy bleeding occurs (more than small spots on the diaper or bleeding that requires direct pressure to stop it).
- There is purulent or serous drainage from the circumcised area.
- There is redness or swelling of the penile shaft.

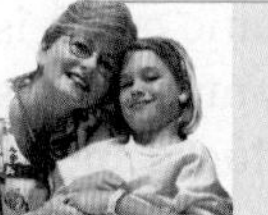

If the Plastibell is used, teach parents NOT to use petroleum jelly, as it may cause the ring to be dislodged. A yellowish crust may form that should be allowed to fall off on its own after several days.

Cryptorchidism

Cryptorchidism (also known as undescended testicles) occurs when one or both testicles do not descend into the scrotal sac. Ordinarily the testes, which in the fetus develop in the abdomen, make their descent into the scrotal sac during the seventh month of gestation. The cause for this failure to descend may be mechanical, hormonal, chromosomal, or enzymatic. The disorder may occur unilaterally or bilaterally. Up to 4% of term male infants and as many as 30% of all preterm male infants exhibit cryptorchidism (Burn et al., 2004).

Complications associated with cryptorchidism that is allowed to progress into the school-age years include sterility and an increased risk for testicular cancer in adolescence or the young adult years. Therapeutic management is surgical. An orchiopexy is performed to release the spermatic cord, and the testes are then pulled into the scrotum and tacked into place.

Nursing Assessment

Explore the health history for risk factors such as:

- Prematurity
- First-born child
- Cesarean birth
- Low birthweight
- Hypospadias

Palpate for the presence (or absence) of both testes in the scrotal sac.

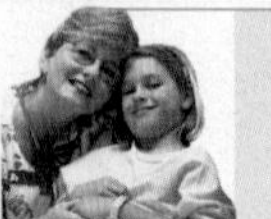

A retractile testis is one that may be brought into the scrotum, remains for a time, and then retracts back up the inguinal canal. This should not be confused with true cryptorchidism.

Nursing Management

If the testes are not descended by 6 months of age, the infant should be referred for surgical repair. The AAP recommends that orchiopexy be performed by 1 year of age. Postoperatively, observe the incision for signs of bleeding or infection.

Hydrocele and Varicocele

Hydrocele (fluid in the scrotal sac) is usually a benign and self-limiting disorder. It is usually noted early in infancy and often resolves spontaneously by 1 year of age. Varicocele (a venous varicosity along the spermatic cord) is often noted as a swelling of the scrotal sac. Complications of varicocele include low sperm count or reduced sperm motility, which can result in infertility.

Nursing Assessment

Elicit a description of the present illness and chief complaint. The boy with hydrocele will have an enlarged scrotum that may decrease in size when he is lying down. Inspect the scrotum for a fluid-filled appearance.

The boy with varicocele will have a mass on one or both sides of the scrotum and bluish discoloration. Inspect the scrotum for masses; the spermatic vein feels worm-like on palpation. The boy with varicocele may have pain.

Nursing Management

Both hydrocele and painless varicocele require watchful waiting, as these conditions will usually resolve spontaneously. If they do not resolve, or if the difference in testicular volume is marked in the boy with varicocele, refer the child to a urologist, as surgery may be indicated. Reassure parents that hydrocele is not associated with the development of infertility. Varicocele may lead to infertility if left untreated, so instruct parents to seek care if pain occurs or if there is a large difference in testicular size. Either condition may be surgically corrected on an outpatient basis. Provide routine postoperative care following either surgery.

Testicular Torsion

In testicular torsion, a testicle is abnormally attached to the scrotum and twisted. It requires immediate attention because ischemia can result if the torsion is left untreated, leading to infertility. Testicular torsion may occur at any age but most commonly occurs in boys aged 12 to 18 years (Burns et al., 2004).

Nursing Assessment

Elicit a description of the present illness and chief complaint. Signs and symptoms of testicular torsion include sudden, severe scrotal pain. Inspect the affected side for significant swelling, which may appear hemorrhagic or blue-black.

Nursing Management

Surgical correction is necessary immediately. Administer pain medication prior to surgery. Reassure the child and family that surgery will alleviate the problem and is performed to restore adequate blood flow to the testicle. After surgical repair, provide routine postoperative care.

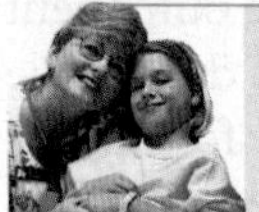

Testicular torsion is considered a surgical emergency, as necrosis of the testis may occur and gangrene may set in.

Epididymitis

Epididymitis (inflammation of the epididymis) is caused by infection with bacteria. It is the most common cause of pain in the scrotum. It rarely occurs before puberty, but if it does it may occur as a result of a urethral or bladder infection related to a urogenital anomaly (Burns et al., 2004). Therapeutic management is directed toward eradicating the bacteria. If left untreated, a scrotal abscess, testicular infarction, or infertility may occur.

Nursing Assessment

Note history of painful swelling of the scrotum, which may be gradual or acute. If the boy is sexually active, explore history of sexual encounters prior to the onset of symptoms. Document history of dysuria or urethral discharge. Note fever, which may last from days to weeks. On inspection, note edema and erythema of the scrotum. Gently palpate the scrotum for a hardened and tender epididymis. Note urethral discharge if present. Palpate the inguinal lymph nodes for enlargement. Urinalysis may be positive for bacteria and white blood cells. The culture of urethral discharge may be positive for a sexually transmitted infection such as gonorrhea or *Chlamydia.* The complete blood count may reveal an elevated white blood cell count.

Nursing Management

Encourage the boy to rest in bed with the scrotum elevated. Ice packs to the scrotum may help with pain relief. Administer pain medications such as NSAIDs or other analgesics as needed.

Administer antibiotics as prescribed. Educate the boy and his family to complete the entire course of antibiotics as prescribed to eradicate the infection. Advise the child and family to notify the physician if the condition is not improving or if the pain and swelling worsen.

References

Books and Journals

Ackley, B. J., & Ladwig, G. B. (2006). *Nursing diagnosis handbook: A guide to planning care* (7th ed.). St. Louis: Mosby.

Adelman, W. P., & Joffe, A. (2003). The adolescent with a painful scrotum. *Contemporary Pediatrics, 3,* 111.

Alper, B. S., & Curry, S. H. (2005). Urinary tract infection in children. *American Family Physician, 72*(12), 2483–2488.

American Academy of Pediatrics and American College of Obstetricians and Gynecologists. (2002). *Guidelines for perinatal care* (5th ed.). Elk Grove, IL: American Academy of Pediatrics.

American Academy of Pediatrics, Committee on Quality Improvement, Subcommittee on Urinary Tract Infection. (1999). Practice parameter: The diagnosis, treatment, and evaluation of the initial urinary tract infection in febrile infants and young children. *Pediatrics, 103*(4), 843–693.

American Academy of Pediatrics, Task Force on Circumcision. (1999). Circumcision policy statement. *Pediatrics, 103*(3), 686–693.

American Nephrology Nurses Association. (2003). Pediatric renal transplant fact sheet. *Nephrology Nursing Journal, 30*(1), 83–86.

Anderson, H. (2005). Children on the frontline against *E. coli:* Typical hemolytic uremic syndrome. *Clinical Laboratory Science, 18*(2), 90–99.

Anonymous. (2004). Information from your family doctor: Urinary tract infections in children. *American Family Physician, 69*(1), 155–156.

Balinski, W. (2000). Pediatric end-stage renal disease: Incidence, management and prevention. *Journal of Pediatric Health Care, 14*(6), 304–308.

Baylon, M. J., Butler, W., Patel, C., Kingley, J., Torres, M., Castro, E. E., & Jasovsky, D. A. (2003). Pediatric nephrotic syndrome. *Advance for Nurses, 18*(3), 31.

Bennett, H. J. (2005). Clinical tips for helping patients overcome bedwetting. *Contemporary Pediatrics, 22*(9); available at www.contemporarypediatrics.com/contpeds/article/articleDetail.jsp?id=179973&&pageID=4

Berry, A. (2005). A child with daytime wetting: Three case studies. *Urologic Nursing, 25*(3), 202–205.

Bertone-Johnson, E. R., Hankinson, S. E., Bendich, A., Johnson, S. R., Willett, W. C., & Manson, J. E. (2005). Calcium and vitamin D intake and risk of incident premenstrual syndrome. *Archives of Internal Medicine, 165,* 1246–1252.

Bortot, A. T., Risser, W. L., & Cromwell, P. F. (2004). Coping with pelvic inflammatory disease in the adolescent. *Contemporary Pediatrics, 21*(4), 33–48.

Bosarge, P. M. (November 2003). Understanding and treating PMS/PMDD. *Nursing Management,* 13–17.

Brewer, D. E., & Berry, P. L. (2006). Glomerulonephritis and nephrotic syndrome. In J. A. McMillan (Ed.), *Oski's pediatrics: Principles and practice.* Philadelphia: Lippincott Williams & Wilkins.

Broome, L. (2003). Treating pediatric nephrotic syndrome: A clinical challenge. *Nephrology Nursing Journal, 30*(6), 662–667.

Buie, M. E. (2005). Circumcision: The good, the bad and American values. *American Journal of Health Education, 36*(2), 102–108.

Burns, C. E., Dunn, A. M., Brady, M. A., Starr, N. B., & Blosser, C. (2004). *Pediatric primary care: A handbook for nurse practitioners* (3rd ed.). Philadelphia: Saunders.

Camille, C. J., Kuo, R. L., & Wiener, J. S. (2002). Caring for the uncircumcised penis: What parents (and you) need to know. *Contemporary Pediatrics, 19* [Electronic version].

Centers for Disease Control & Prevention. (2005). Guide to contraindications to vaccinations. Available at www.cdc.gov/nip/recs/contraindications.htm#immuno

Chiang, D., Ben-Meir, D., Pout, K., & Dewan, P. A. (2005). Management of post-operative bladder spasm. *Journal of Paediatrics and Child Health, 41,* 56–58.

Children's Healthcare of Atlanta. (2004). *Double diapering.* Atlanta: Children's Healthcare of Atlanta.

Cromwell, P. F., Munn, N., & Zolkowski-Wynne, J. (2005). Evaluation and management of hypertension in children and adolescents (Part 1: Diagnosis). *Journal of Pediatric Health Care, 19*(3), 172–175.

Daniels, J., & DiCenso, A. (2003). Review: Antibiotic treatment for 2–14 days reduces treatment failure in children with urinary tract infection. *Evidence-Based Nursing, 6,* accessed at http://ebn.bmjjournals.com/cgi/reprint/6/1/15

Dell, D. (2004). Premenstrual syndrome, premenstrual dysphoric disorder, and premenstrual exacerbation of another disorder. *Clinical Obstetrics and Gynecology, 47*(3), 568–575.

Dufour, J. L. (2001). Assessing and treating epididymitis. *Nurse Practitioner, 26*(3), 23–24.

Dulczak, S., & Kirk, J. (2005). Overview of the evaluation, diagnosis, and management of urinary tract infections in infants and children. *Urologic Nursing, 25*(3), 185–192.

Dunlop, A. (2005). Meeting the needs of parents and pediatric patients: Results of a survey on primary nocturnal enuresis. *Clinical Pediatrics, 44,* 297–303.

Eissa, M. A., & Cromwell, P. F. (2003). Diagnosis and management of pelvic inflammatory disease in adolescents. *Journal of Pediatric Health Care, 17*(3), 145–147.

Ellsworth, P., Cendron, M., & McCullough, M. (2000). Surgical management of vesicoureteral reflux. *AORN Journal, 71*(3), 498–513.

Farnham, S. B., Adams, M. C., Brock, J. W., & Pope, J. C. (2005). Pediatric urological causes of hypertension. *Journal of Urology, 173,* 697–704.

Flynn, J. (2003). Recognizing and managing the hypertensive child. *Contemporary Pediatrics, 20,* 38.

Frazier, J. P., Parks, D. K., & Yetman, F. J. (2001). Congenital hydronephrosis. *Journal of Pediatric Health Care, 15*(5), 260–262.

Gaines, K. K. (2004). Desmopressin (DDAVP) for enuresis, diabetes insipidus, and . . . *Urologic Nursing, 24*(6), 520–523.

Garin, E. H., Olavarrie, F., Nieto, V. G., Valenciano, B., Campos, A., & Young, L. (2006). Clinical significance of primary vesicoureteral reflux and urinary antibiotic prophylaxis after acute pyelonephritis: A multicenter, randomized controlled study. *Pediatrics, 117*(3), 626–632.

Hawkins, E. P. (2006). Renal malformations. In J. A. McMillan (Ed.), *Oski's pediatrics: Principles and practice (4th ed.).* Philadelphia: Lippincott Williams & Wilkins.

Hellerstein, S. (2002). Urinary tract infections in children: Pathophysiology, risk factors, and management. *Infections in Medicine, 19*(12), 554–560.

Herrinton, L. J., Zhao, W., & Husson, G. (2003). Management of cryptorchidism and risk of testicular cancer. *American Journal of Epidemiology, 157*(7), 602–605.

Hinds, A. C. (2004). Obstructive uropathy: Considerations for the nephrology nurse. *Nephrology Nursing Journal, 31*(2), 166–180.

Hogg, R. J., Portman, R. J., Milliner, D., Lemley, K. V., Eddy, A., & Ingelfinger, J. (2002). Evaluation and management of proteinuria and nephrotic syndrome in children: Recommendations from a pediatric nephrology panel established at the National Kidney Foundation conference on proteinuria, albuminuria, risk, assessment, detection, and elimination (PARADE). *Pediatrics, 105*(6), 1242–1249.

Lau, K. K., & Wyatt, R. J. (2005). Glomerulonephritis. *Adolescent Medicine Clinics, 16*(1), 67–85.

Kelley, K. (2004). How peritoneal dialysis works. *Nephrology Nursing Journal, 31*(5), 481–490.

Klein, N. J. (2001). Management of primary nocturnal enuresis. *Urologic Nursing, 21*(2), 71–76.

Koester, M. C. (2005). Initial evaluation and management of acute scrotal pain. *Journal of Athletic Training, 35*(1), 76–79.

Landgraf, J. M., Abidari, J., Cilento, B. G., Cooper, C. S., Schulman, S. L., & Ortenberg, J. (2004). Coping, commitment, and attitude: Quantifying the everyday burden of enuresis on children and their families. *Pediatrics, 113,* 334–344.

Lang, M. M., & Towers, C. (2001). Identifying poststreptococcal glomerulonephritis. *Nurse Practitioner, 26*(8), 34–47.

Leung, A. K., & Wong, A. L. (2003). Pediatric genital disorders. *Consultant for Pediatricians, 2*(3), 122–130.

Leung, A. K., & Wong, A. L. (2003). Pediatric scrotal swellings. *Consultant for Pediatricians, 2*(4), 172–176.

Lum, G. M. (2005). Kidney and urinary tract. In W. W. Hay, M. J. Levin, J. M. Sondheimer, & R. R. Deterding (Eds.), *Current pediatric diagnosis and treatment* (17th ed.) New York: McGraw-Hill.

Malnory, M., Johnson, T. S., & Kirby, R. S. (2003). Newborn behavioral and physiological response to circumcision. *MCN: American Journal of Maternal/Child Nursing, 28*(5), 313–319.

McEvoy, M., Chang, J., & Coupey, S. M. (2004). Common menstrual disorders in adolescence: Nursing interventions. *MCN: American Journal of Maternal-Child Nursing, 29*(1), 41–49.

Miller, D., Macdonald, D., Kolnacki, K., & Simek, T. (2004). Challenges for nephrology nurses in the management of children with chronic kidney disease. *Nephrology Nursing Journal, 31*(3), 287–295.

Milliner, D. S. (2004). Pediatric renal-replacement therapy: Coming of age. *New England Journal of Medicine, 350*(26), 2637. Retrieved May 12, 2005, from ProQuest database.

Mills, M., White, S. C., Kershaw, D., Flynn, J. T., Brophy, P. D., Thomas, S. E., & Smoyer, W. (2005). Developing clinical protocols for nursing practice: Improving nephrology care for children and their families. *Nephrology Nursing Journal, 32*(6), 599–607.

Nettina, S. M. (2005). *Lippincott manual of nursing practice.* Philadelphia: Lippincott Williams & Wilkins.

Neuhaus, T. J. (2004). Immunization in children with chronic renal failure: A practical approach. *Pediatric Nephrology, 19,* 1334–1339.

Nield, L. S., & Kamat, D. (2004). Enuresis: How to evaluate and treat. *Clinical Pediatrics, 43,* 409–415.

Pagana, K. D., & Pagana, T. J. (2006). *Mosby's manual of diagnostic and laboratory tests* (3rd ed.). St. Louis: Mosby.

Peacock, E., Jacob, V. W., & Fallone, S. M. (2001). *Escherichia coli* O157:H7: etiology, clinical features, complications, and treatment. *Nephrology Nursing Journal, 28*(5), 547–557.

Pulsifer, A. (2005). Pediatric GU examination: A clinician's reference. *Urologic Nursing, 25*(3), 163–168.

Raj, G. V., & Wiener, J. S. (2003). Varicoceles in adolescents: When to observe, when to intervene. *Contemporary Pediatrics, 21,* 39

Razmus, I. S., Dalton, M. E., & Wilson, D. (2004). Pain management for newborn circumcision. *Pediatric Nursing, 30*(5), 414–427.

Robson, W. L. M., Leung, A. K. C., & Van Howe, R. (2005). Primary and secondary enuresis: Similarities in presentation. *Pediatrics, 115*(4), 956–959.

Rogers, J. (2002). Managing daytime and night-time enuresis in children. *Nursing Standard, 16*(32), 45–52, 54, 56.

Roth, D. R., & Gonzales, E. T. (2006). Disorders of renal development and anomalies of the collecting system, bladder, penis, and scrotum. In J. A. McMillan (Ed.), *Oski's pediatrics: Principles and practice* (4th ed.). Philadelphia: Lippincott Williams & Wilkins.

Roth, K. S., Koo, H. P., Spottswood, S. E., & Chan, J. C. M. (2002). Obstructive uropathy: An important cause of chronic renal failure in children. *Clinical Pediatrics, 41,* 309–314.

Rusk, J. (2006). Proper diagnosis and treatment of UTIs in infants and young children outlined. *Infectious Diseases in Children, 19*(3), 79.

Silverstein, D. M. (2004). Enuresis in children: Diagnosis and management. *Clinical Pediatrics, 43*(3), 217–221.

Sparta, G., Kemper, M. J., Gerber, A. C., Goetschel, P., & Neuhaus, T. J. (2004). Latex allergy in children with urological malformation and chronic renal failure. *Journal of Urology, 171,* 1647–1659.

Stuart, M. (2002). Literature reviews: Minimal change nephrotic syndrome in children with intrauterine growth retardation. *Clinical Pediatrics, 41*(5), 362.

Super, E. A., Kemper, K. J., Woods, C., & Nagaraj, S. (2005). Cranberry use among pediatric nephrology patients. *Ambulatory Pediatrics, 5*(4), 249–252.

Taketokmo, C. K., Hodding, J. H., & Kraus, D. M. (2004). *Lexi-comp's pediatric dosage handbook* (11th ed.). Hudson, OH: Lexi-comp.

Thiedke, C. C. (2003). Nocturnal enuresis. *American Family Physician, 67*(7), 1499–1506.

Thompson, M., Simon, S. D., Sharma, V., & Alon, U. S. (2005). Timing of follow-up voiding cystourethrogram in children with primary vesicoureteral reflux: Development and application of a clinical algorithm. *Pediatrics, 115*(2), 426–434.

Varade, W. (2000). Hemolytic uremic syndrome: Reducing the risks. *Contemporary Pediatrics, 9,* 54.

Vogt, B. A. (2002). A newborn with a urinary tract anomaly: What role for the general pediatrician? *Contemporary Pediatrics, 19.*

Wald, E. R. (2006). Vesicoureteral reflux: The role of antibiotic prophylaxis. *Pediatrics, 117*(3), 919–922.

Wan, J., & Bloom, D. A. (2003). GU problems in adolescent males. *Adolescent Medicine, 14*(3), 717–731.

Zorzanello, M. M. (2004). Peritoneal dialysis and hemodialysis: Similarities and differences. *Nephrology Nursing Journal, 31*(5), 588–589.

Websites

aota.schipul.net American Organ Transplant Association—helps patients obtain and sustain organ transplantation

kidney.niddk.nih.gov National Kidney and Urologic Diseases Information Clearinghouse

www.aakp.org American Association of Kidney Patients—information for kidney patients, resources for dialysis and transplant patients

www.aan.com American Academy of Nephrology

www.annanurse.org American Nephrology Nurses Association—resources for nurses specializing in nephrology nursing

www.aspneph.com American Society of Pediatric Nephrology

www.auanet.org American Urologic Association

www.awarefoundation.org Adolescent Wellness and Reproductive Education Foundation

www.choa.org/default.aspx?id=516 Wellness and safety information for teens sponsored by Children's Healthcare of Atlanta

www.cota.org Children's Organ Transplant Association—fundraising for children's transplants, promotion of organ and tissue donation

www.girlpower.gov U.S. Department of Health and Human Services—a national public education campaign for adolescent girls

www.goaskalice.columbia.edu Health questions and answers sponsored by Columbia University

www.healthypeople.gov/default.htm *Healthy People 2010*

www.itns.org International Transplant Nurses Society

www.itsyoursexlife.com Guide to safe and responsible sex from the Kaiser Family Foundation

www.kidney.org National Kidney Foundation—resources for kidney patients

www.kidneyfund.org American Kidney Fund—provides financial aid for kidney patients, summer camps for children

www.kidshealth.org Nemours Foundation for Kids' Health (for kids and teens)

www.kidskare.org/ a website made by children, for children about organ donation and transplantation

www.natco1.org Organization for Transplant Professionals

www.plannedparenthood.org/teens Planned Parenthood (excellent resource on teen sexuality and reproductive health)

www.prunebelly.org Prune Belly Syndrome Network

www.suna.org Society of Urologic Nurses and Associates

www.teenadvice.org Teen Advice Online—peer counseling from other teens

www.teengrowth.com from the Pediatric Health Alliance

www.unos.org United Network for Organ Sharing—registry for donors and patients needing transplants

www.transweb.org transplantation and donation

www.youngwomenshealth.org Center for Young Women's Health, The Children's Hospital, Boston, MA

Chapter WORKSHEET

● MULTIPLE CHOICE QUESTIONS

1. The nurse is performing patient education for the parents of an infant with bladder exstrophy. Which statement by the parents would indicate an understanding of the child's future care?
   a. "Care will be no different than that of any other infant."
   b. "My infant will only need this one surgery."
   c. "My child will wear diapers all his life."
   d. "We will need to care for the urinary diversion."

2. A 4-year-old girl presents with recurrent urinary tract infection. A prior workup did not reveal any urinary tract abnormalities. What is the priority nursing action?
   a. Obtain a sterile urine sample after completion of antibiotics.
   b. Teach appropriate toileting hygiene.
   c. Prepare the child for surgery to reimplant the ureters.
   d. Administer antibiotics intramuscularly.

3. A 5-year-old who had a renal transplant 9 months ago and has no history of chickenpox presents to the pediatric clinic for his vaccinations. Which is the most appropriate set to give?
   a. DTaP, IPV
   b. DTaP, IPV, MMR, Varicella
   c. DTaP, IPV, Varicella
   d. IPV only

4. When the nurse is caring for a child with hemolytic-uremic syndrome or acute glomerulonephritis and the child is not yet toilet trained, which action by the nurse would best determine fluid retention?
   a. Test urine for specific gravity.
   b. Weigh child daily.
   c. Weigh the wet diapers.
   d. Measure abdominal girth daily.

● CRITICAL THINKING EXERCISES

1. Develop a teaching plan for an adolescent with premenstrual syndrome and dysmenorrhea.
2. Devise a meal plan for a 5-year-old child with a renal disorder that requires a 2-g sodium restriction per day. Keep in mind the child's developmental level and feeding idiosyncrasies at this age.
3. Develop a discharge teaching plan for a 3-year-old with nephrotic syndrome who will be taking corticosteroids long term.
4. Devise a developmental stimulation plan for an 11-month-old who has had significant urinary tract reconstruction surgery and is facing a prolonged period of confinement to the crib.

● STUDY ACTIVITIES

1. In the clinical setting, compare the growth and development of two children the same age, one with chronic renal failure and one who has been healthy.
2. While caring for children in the clinical setting, compare and contrast the medical history, signs and symptoms of illness, and prescribed treatments for a child with nephrotic syndrome and one with acute glomerulonephritis.
3. Observe peritoneal dialysis in the hospital or hemodialysis in a hospital or outpatient center. Record observations about the children's psychosocial and developmental status.

chapter 23

Nursing Care of the Child With a Neuromuscular Disorder

Key TERMS

atrophy
clonus
contracture
dystrophy
hypertonicity
hypotonia
neurogenic
spasticity

Learning OBJECTIVES

Upon completion of the chapter, the learner will be able to:

1. Compare differences between the anatomy and physiology of the neuromuscular system in children versus adults.
2. Identify nursing interventions related to common laboratory and diagnostic tests used in the diagnosis and management of neuromuscular conditions.
3. Identify appropriate nursing assessments and interventions related to medications and treatments used for childhood neuromuscular conditions.
4. Distinguish various neuromuscular illnesses occurring in childhood.
5. Devise an individualized nursing care plan for the child with a neuromuscular disorder.
6. Develop patient/family teaching plans for the child with a neuromuscular disorder.
7. Describe the psychosocial impact of chronic neuromuscular disorders on the growth and development of children.

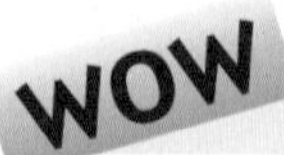

Enhancing a child's abilities may enhance his or her strength to overcome anything.

Frederick Stevens, 4 years old, seems to be falling often and has started to have difficulty climbing the stairs on his own. His mother states, "Recently he hasn't been able to keep up with his 6-year-old sister when we're playing at the park. He usually ends up sitting on the bench with me." She is concerned about the changes she has seen in her son.

A variety of neuromuscular disorders may affect children, but the result of each is muscular dysfunction. Some of the disorders result from a neurologic insult such as trauma or hypoxia to the brain or spinal cord. Others occur as a result of genetic dysfunction or structural abnormality. Still others may be autoimmune in nature, often following a simple viral infection. Many of the neuromuscular disorders are chronic, lasting the child's entire life and resulting in handicaps.

The nurse caring for a child with a neuromuscular dysfunction plays an important role in the management of these disorders. Not only must the nurse provide direct intervention in response to health alterations that result, but the nurse is often part of the larger multidisciplinary team and may serve as the coordinator of many specialists or interventions. Understanding the most common responses to these disorders gives the nurse the foundation required to plan care for any child with any neuromuscular disorder.

Variations in Pediatric Anatomy and Physiology

Neuromuscular disorders in children may occur as a congenital malformation or a genetic disorder that is present from birth but may not be identified until later in childhood or adolescence. They may also result from trauma or hypoxia or develop following a viral illness. The neurologic and musculoskeletal systems in infants and children are immature compared with adults, placing them at increased risk for the development of a neuromuscular disorder.

Brain and Spinal Cord Development

Early in gestation, around 3 to 4 weeks, the neural tube of the embryo begins to differentiate into the brain and spinal cord. If the fetus suffers infection, trauma, malnutrition, or teratogen exposure during this critical period of growth and differentiation, brain or spinal cord development may be altered. Compared with the adult, the child's spine is very mobile, especially the cervical spine region, resulting in a higher risk for cervical spine injury. The premature infant's central nervous system is less mature than the term newborn's. Such immaturity in the preterm infant places him or her at a higher risk of central nervous insult within the neonatal period, which may result in delayed motor skill attainment or cerebral palsy.

Myelinization

Though development of the structures of the nervous system is complete at birth, myelinization is incomplete. Myelinization continues to progress and is complete by about 2 years of age. Myelinization proceeds in a cephalocaudal and proximodistal fashion, allowing the infant to gain head and neck control before becoming able to control the trunk and the extremities. As the myelinization proceeds, the speed and accuracy of nerve impulses increase.

Muscular Development

The muscular system, including tendons, ligaments, and cartilage, arises from the mesoderm in early embryonic development. At birth (term or preterm), the muscles, tendons, ligaments, and cartilage are all present and functional. The newborn infant is capable of spontaneous movement but lacks purposeful control. Full range of motion is present at birth. Healthy infants and children demonstrate normal muscle tone; hypertonia or **hypotonia** is an abnormal finding. Deep tendon reflexes are present at birth and are initially brisk in the newborn and progress to average over the first few months. Sluggish deep tendon reflexes indicate an abnormality. As the infant matures and becomes mobile, the muscles develop further and become stronger. The adolescent boy, in response to testosterone release, experiences a growth spurt, particularly in the trunk and legs, and develops bulkier muscles at that time.

Common Medical Treatments

A variety of medications as well as other medical treatments are used to treat neuromuscular disorders in children. Most of these treatments will require a physician's order when the child is in the hospital. The most common treatments and medications are listed in Common Medical Treatments 23.1 and Drug Guide 23.1. The nurse caring for the child with a neuromuscular disorder should become familiar with what these procedures are and how they work as well as common nursing implications related to use of these modalities.

Nursing Process Overview for the Child With a Neuromuscular Disorder

Care of the child with a neuromuscular disorder includes assessment, nursing diagnosis, planning, interventions, and evaluation. There are a number of general concepts related to the nursing process that may be applied to neuromuscular dysfunction in children. From a general understanding of the care involved for a child with a neuro-

Common Medical Treatments 23.1

Treatment	Explanation	Indication	Nursing Implications
Skeletal or cervical traction	Traction is used to immobilize the cervical spine. Halo traction will be applied in stable injuries and allows the patient greater mobility. Cervical traction is applied by a jacket-like apparatus, and the patient can get out of bed, use a wheelchair, and even ambulate.	To minimize or prevent trauma to the spinal cord	Monitor neurologic status closely. Assess for signs and symptoms of infection or impaired skin integrity. Provide appropriate pin site care.
Physical therapy, occupational therapy, or speech therapy	Physical therapy focuses on attainment or improvement of gross motor skills. Occupational therapy focuses on refinement of fine motor skills, feeding, and activities of daily living. Speech therapy is warranted for the child with a speech impairment or feeding difficulty related to oral muscular issues.	Cerebral palsy, spina bifida, spinal cord injury, muscular dystrophy, spinal muscular atrophy	Provide follow-through with prescribed exercises or supportive equipment. Success of therapy is dependent upon continued compliance with the prescribed regimen. Ensure that adequate communication exists within the interdisciplinary team.
Orthotics, braces	Adaptive positioning devices specially fitted for each child by the physical or occupational therapist or orthotist. Used to maintain proper body or extremity alignment, improve mobility, and prevent contractures.	Cerebral palsy, spinal cord injury, spina bifida, muscular dystrophy, spinal muscular atrophy	Provide frequent assessments of skin covered by the device to avoid skin breakdown. Follow the therapist's schedule of recommended "on" and "off" times. Encourage families to comply with use.

muscular disorder, the nurse can then individualize the care based on patient specifics.

ASSESSMENT

Assessment of neuromuscular dysfunction in children includes health history, physical examination, and laboratory and diagnostic testing.

> Remember Frederick, the 4-year-old who has been falling, having difficulty climbing stairs, and seems to tire easily when playing with his sister? What additional health history and physical examination assessment information should the nurse obtain?

Health History

The health history comprises past medical history, including the mother's pregnancy history, family history, and history of present illness (when the symptoms started and how they have progressed) as well as treatments used at home. The past medical history might be significant for prematurity, difficult birth, infection during pregnancy, changes in gait, falls, delayed development, or poor growth. Family history might be significant for neuromuscular disorders that are genetic. When eliciting the history of the present illness, inquire about the following:

- Changes in gait
- Recent trauma
- Poor feeding
- Lethargy
- Fever
- Weakness
- Alteration in muscle tone

Determine the child's history of attainment of developmental milestones. Note the age that milestones such as sitting, crawling, and walking were attained, and determine whether the pace of attainment of milestones has decreased. Some children may progress normally at first and then demonstrate decreased velocity of development of achievements or even loss of abilities. Obtain a clear description of weakness; is it fatigue, or is the child truly not as strong as he or she was in the past?

Physical Examination

Physical examination of the nervous and musculoskeletal systems consists of inspection and observation and palpa-

Drug Guide 23.1 Common Drugs for Neuromuscular Disorders

Medication	Action	Indication	Nursing Implications
Benzodiazepines (diazepam, lorazepam)	Anticonvulsant; enhance the inhibition of GABA	Used adjunctively for relief of skeletal muscle spasm associated with cerebral palsy and paralysis resulting from spinal cord injury	Monitor sedation level. Assess for improvements in spasticity.
Baclofen (oral or intrathecal)	Central-acting skeletal muscle relaxant; precise mechanism unknown	Used to treat painful spasms and decrease spasticity in children with motor neuron lesions, such as cerebral palsy and spinal cord injury	Assess motor function. Monitor for a decrease in spasticity. Observe for mental confusion, depression, or hallucinations. Dosage must be tapered before discontinuing because withdrawal symptoms may occur.
Corticosteroids	Anti-inflammatory and immunosuppressive action	Duchenne muscular dystrophy, myasthenia gravis, dermatomyositis	Administer with food to decrease GI upset. May mask signs of infection. Do not stop treatment abruptly or acute adrenal insufficiency may occur. Monitor for Cushing syndrome. Dosage may be tapered over time.
Botulin toxin	Neurotoxin produced by *Clostridium botulinum* that blocks neuromuscular conduction	Relief of spasticity in cerebral palsy, occasionally for torticollis	Injected into the muscle by an advanced provider. May cause dry mouth.

tion and should also include auscultation of the heart and lungs, as the function of these organs may be affected by certain neuromuscular conditions.

Inspection and Observation

Observe the infant or child playing with toys, crawling, or walking to obtain significant information about cranial nerve, cerebellar, and motor function. Observe the child's general appearance, noting any asymmetry in muscle development. Lack of use of extremities leads to muscular **atrophy**, so a shortened limb may indicate chronic hemiparesis. Note symmetry of spontaneous movement of extremities as well as facial muscles. Determine cranial nerve function. Inspect the spine for cutaneous abnormalities such as dimples or hair tufts, which may be associated with spinal cord abnormalities. Observe the child's level of consciousness (LOC), noting decrease or significant changes. Note presence of lethargy. Refer to Chapter 17 for a complete description of evaluation of LOC.

Motor Function. Observe spontaneous activity, posture, and balance, and assess for asymmetrical movements. In the infant, observe resting posture, which will normally be a slightly flexed posture. The infant should be able to extend extremities to a normal stretch. Note position of comfort of the infant's or child's neck.

Reflexes. Note sluggish or brisk deep tendon reflexes. Note persistence of primitive reflexes in the older infant or child, such as Moro or tonic neck. Assess for development of protective reflexes, which is often delayed in infants with motor disorders.

Sensory Function. Alterations in sensory function accompany many neuromuscular disorders. Assess sensory function in a similar fashion to that used in the adult. The sensory functions of light touch, pain, vibration, heat, and cold are distinguishable by a child. In the infant, assess for response to light touch or pain. The usual response to pain will be withdrawal from the stimulus. Always prepare the child for the sensory examination in order to gain cooperation. The pinprick test may be particularly frightening, but most children will cooperate if educated appropriately.

Palpation

Assess muscle strength and tone in the infant or child. Compare strength and tone bilaterally. Evaluate neck tone by pulling the infant from a supine position to a sitting position (Fig. 23.1). By 4 to 5 months the infant should be able to maintain the head in a neutral position. Perform passive range of motion of the neck. Alterations in range of motion may indicate a neuromuscular disorder or torticollis. Note trunk tone in the infant by holding the infant under the axillae and palpating for trunk tone. The hypotonic infant will feel as though he or she is slipping through the examiner's hands. The hypertonic infant will feel rigid, extending the trunk and legs. Assess leg tone in the infant by placing the infant in the vertical position with the feet on a flat surface; the 4-month-old infant should be able to momentarily support his or her weight (Fig. 23.2). Assess the strength of the infant or child by noting ability to move the muscles against gravity. Note any hypertonia or **spasticity**, which may be an early indication of cerebral palsy or other neuromuscular disorder.

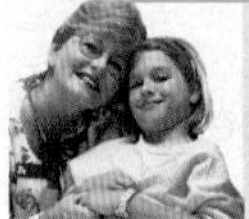

In cases of trauma or suspected trauma, do not perform any assessment that involves movement of the head and neck until cervical injury is ruled out. Maintain complete immobilization of the cervical spine until that time.

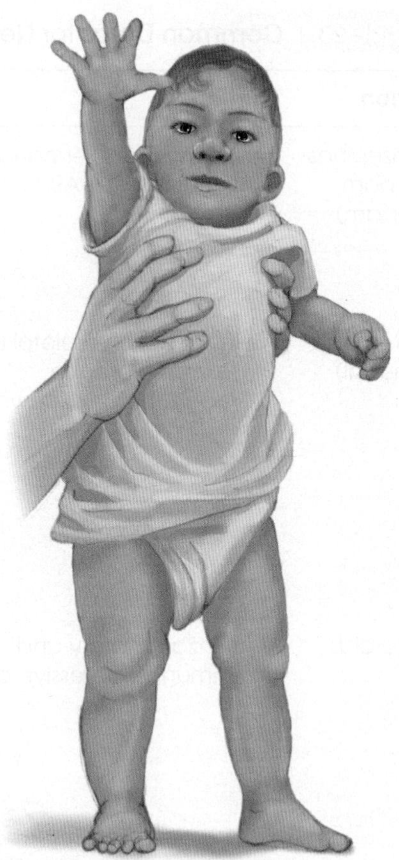

● **FIGURE 23.2** Assessing leg tone in an infant.

Auscultation

Auscultate the child's lungs; adventitious sounds are often present when respiratory muscle function is impaired.

Laboratory and Diagnostic Testing

Common Laboratory and Diagnostic Tests 23.1 offers an explanation of the laboratory and diagnostic tests most commonly used in neuromuscular disorders. The tests can assist the physician in diagnosing the disorder and/or be used as guidelines in determining ongoing treatment. Laboratory or non-nursing personnel perform some of the tests, while the nurse might perform others. In either instance the nurse should be familiar with how the tests are performed, what they are used for, and normal versus abnormal results. This knowledge will also be necessary when providing patient and family education related to the testing.

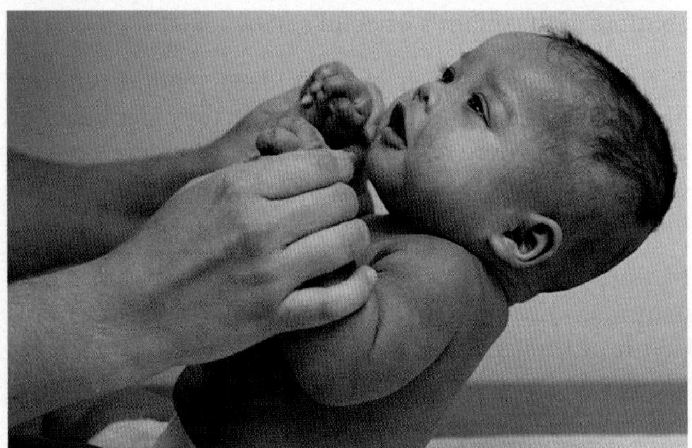

● **FIGURE 23.1** Assessing neck tone in an infant.

NURSING DIAGNOSES, GOALS, INTERVENTIONS, AND EVALUATIONS

Upon completion of a thorough assessment, the nurse might identify several nursing diagnoses, including:

- Impaired physical mobility related to spasticity, neuromuscular impairment, or weakness
- Imbalanced nutrition, less than body requirements, related to spasticity, feeding, or swallowing difficulties
- Urinary retention related to anatomic obstruction, sensory motor impairment, or dysfunctional voiding as evidenced by dribbling, inadequate bladder emptying
- Constipation related to immobility, loss of sensation

Common Laboratory and Diagnostic Tests 23.1

Test	Explanation	Indication	Nursing Implications
Cervical spine x-rays	Radiographic image of the cervical spine	Detection of spinal fractures	In the trauma victim, the cervical spine should remain immobilized until cleared after cervical spine x-rays.
Fluoroscopy	Radiographic examination that uses continuous x-rays to show live, real-time images	Assessment of cervical spine instability during movement	Children may be afraid of the x-ray machine but will need to cooperate with flexion and extension of the neck. Allow a parent or family member to accompany the child.
Myelography	X-ray study of the spinal cord allowing visualization of the cord, nerve roots, and surrounding meninges	Detection of space-occupying lesions of the spinal cord; visualization of neural tube defects; evaluation of traumatic injury	Involves injection of contrast medium into the CSF via lumbar puncture. After procedure, keep head of bed elevated for several hours. Encourage hydration. Observe for signs of meningeal irritation.
Ultrasound	Use of sound waves to locate the depth and structure within soft tissues and fluid	Assessment of spinal abnormalities	Better tolerated by nonsedated children than CT or MRI. Can be performed with a portable unit at bedside.
Computed tomography (CT)	Noninvasive x-ray study that looks at tissue density and structures. Images a "slice" of tissue.	Evaluation of congenital abnormalities such as neural tube defects, fractures, demyelinization, or inflammation	Machine is large and can be frightening to children. Procedure can be lengthy and child must remain still. If unable to do so, sedation may be necessary. If performed with contrast medium, assess for allergy. Encourage fluids after procedure if not contraindicated.
Magnetic resonance imaging (MRI)	Based on how hydrogen atoms behave in a magnetic field when disturbed by radiofrequency signals. Does not require ionizing radiation. Provides a 3D view of the body part being scanned.	Assessment of inflammation, congenital abnormalities such as neural tube defects	Remove all metal objects from the child. Child must remain motionless for entire scan; parent can stay in room with child. Younger children will require sedation in order to be still. A loud thumping sound occurs inside the machine during the procedure, which can be frightening to children.
Creatine kinase	Reflects muscle damage: it leaks from muscle into plasma as muscles deteriorate	Diagnosis of muscular dystrophy, spinal muscular atrophy	Draw sample before electromyogram or muscle biopsy, as those tests may lead to release of creatine kinase.
Electromyography	A recording electrode is placed in the skeletal muscle and electrical activity is recorded.	Differentiates muscular disorders from those that are neurologic in origin	Requires insertion of short needles into the muscles.

Common Laboratory and Diagnostic Tests 23.1 (continued)

Test	Explanation	Indication	Nursing Implications
Nerve conduction velocity	Measures the speed of nerve conduction	Differentiation of muscular disorders	Feels like mild electric shocks
Muscle biopsy	Removal of a piece of muscular tissue either by needle or by open biopsy	Determination of type of muscular dystrophy or spinal muscular atrophy	Post-biopsy care is similar to that for other types of biopsy. Involves a small incision with one or two sutures.
Dystrophin	A normal intracellular plasma membrane protein in the muscle	Determination of specific type of muscular dystrophy	Absent in Duchenne muscular dystrophy, decreased in Becker muscular dystrophy
Genetic testing	Tests for presence of the gene for the disease or for carrier status	Determination of disease or carrier status of inherited muscular disorder	Entire family should be tested, even those unaffected, because carrier status should be determined and genetic counseling related to reproduction provided.

- Self-care deficit related to neuromuscular impairment, sensory deficits
- Risk for impaired skin integrity related to immobility, braces, or adaptive devices
- Chronic sorrow related to presence of chronic disability
- Risk for injury related to muscle weakness
- Deficient knowledge related to lack of information regarding complex medical condition, prognosis, and medical needs
- Family processes, interrupted, related to child's illness, hospitalization, diagnosis of chronic illness in child, and potential long-term effects of illness

> **After completing an assessment of Fredrick,** the nurse noted the following: he started walking at 2 years of age, he has difficulty jumping, his gait has a waddling appearance, and he does not rise from the floor in the usual fashion. Based on these assessment findings, what would your top three nursing diagnoses be for Fredrick?

Nursing goals, interventions, and evaluation for the child with neuromuscular dysfunction are based on the nursing diagnoses (see Nursing Care Plan Overview 23.1). The nursing care plan may be used as a guide in planning nursing care for the child with a neuromuscular disorder. The care plan includes many nursing diagnoses that are applicable to the child or adolescent. Children's responses to neuromuscular dysfunction and its treatment will vary, and nursing care should be individualized based on the child's and family's responses to illness; see Healthy People 2010. Additional information about nursing management will be included later in the chapter as it relates to specific disorders.

Internet resources for families of children with disabilities include:

- www.acf.dhhs.gov/programs/add: Administration on Developmental Disabilities, Department of Health and Human Services
- www.childrenwithdisabilities.ncjrcs.org: Children with Disabilities
- www.childrensdefense.org: Children's Defense Fund
- www.familiesusa.org: Families USA
- www.irsc.org: Internet Resources for Special Children
- www.nicchy.org: National Information Center for Children and Youth with Disabilities

> **Based on your top three nursing diagnoses for Fredrick,** describe appropriate nursing interventions.

Congenital Neuromuscular Disorders

Several disorders with neuromuscular effects are congenital in nature. These include the neural tube defects and genetic neuromuscular disorders. The structural disorders are spina bifida occulta, meningocele, and myelomeningocele (neural tube defects). The genetic neuromuscular disorders include the various types of muscular dystrophy and spinal muscular atrophy. These disorders are not always recognized at birth, as signs and symptoms are not evident until months or even years after birth, but they are still considered to be congenital as they have a genetic basis.

(text continues on page 770)

Nursing Care Plan 23.1

Overview for the Child with a Neuromuscular Disorder

Nursing Diagnosis: Impaired physical mobility related to muscle weakness, hypertonicity, impaired coordination, loss of muscle function or control as evidenced by an inability to move extremities, to ambulate without assistance, to move without limitations

Outcome identification and evaluation

Child will be able to engage in activities within age parameters and limits of disease: *child is able to move extremities, move about environment, and participate in exercise programs within limits of age and disease.*

Intervention: maximizing physical mobility

- Encourage gross and fine motor activities *to facilitate motor development.*
- Collaborate with physical therapy, occupational therapy, and speech therapy to strengthen muscles and promote optimal mobility *to facilitate motor development.*
- Use passive and active range-of-motion exercises and teach child and family how to perform them *to prevent contractures, facilitate joint mobility and muscle development (active ROM), and help increase mobility.*
- Praise accomplishments and emphasize child's abilities *to improve self-esteem and encourage feeling of confidence and competence.*

Nursing Diagnosis: Nutrition, imbalanced, less than body requirements, related to difficulty feeding secondary to deficient sucking, swallowing, or chewing; difficulty assuming normal feeding position; inability to feed self as evidenced by decreased oral intake, impaired swallowing, weight loss or plateau.

Outcome identification and evaluation

Child will exhibit signs of adequate nutrition *as evidenced by appropriate weight gain, intake & output within normal limits, and adequate ingestion of calories.*

Intervention: promoting adequate nutrition

- Monitor height and weight: *insufficient intake will lead to impaired growth and weight gain.*
- Monitor hydration status (moist mucous membranes, elastic skin turgor, adequate urine output): *insufficient intake can lead to dehydration.*
- Use techniques to promote caloric and nutritional intake and teach family about these techniques (e.g., positioning, modified utensils, soft or blended foods, allowing extra time) *to facilitate intake.*
- Assess respiratory system frequently *to assess for aspiration.*
- Assist family to help child assume as normal a feeding position as possible *to help increase oral intake.*

Nursing Diagnosis: Urinary retention related to sensory motor impairment as evidenced by dribbling, inadequate bladder emptying

Outcome identification and evaluation

Child's bladder will empty adequately, *according to pre-established quantities and frequencies individualized for the child (usual urine output is 0.5 to 2 mL/kg/hour).*

Intervention: promoting successful bladder emptying

- Assess child's ability to empty bladder via history focused on character and duration of lower urinary symptoms *to establish baseline.*
- Assess for history of fecal impaction or constipation, *as alterations in bowel elimination may hinder urinary elimination.*

(continued)

Overview for the Child with a Neuromuscular Disorder (continued)

Intervention: promoting successful bladder emptying

- Assess for bladder distention by palpation or urinary retention by post-void residual obtained via catheterization or bladder ultrasound *to determine extent of retention.*
- Maintain adequate hydration *to avoid irritating effects that dehydration has on the bladder.*
- Schedule voiding *to decrease bladder overdistention.*
- Teach the family (and the child if old enough) with significant urinary retention the technique of clean intermittent catheterization *to allow regular, complete bladder emptying.*

Nursing Diagnosis: Risk for constipation related to immobility, loss of sensation

Outcome identification and evaluation

Child will demonstrate adequate stool passage, *will pass soft, formed stool every 1 to 3 days without straining or other adverse effects.*

Intervention: promoting appropriate bowel elimination

- Assess usual pattern of stooling *to determine baseline and identify potential problems with elimination.*
- Palpate for abdominal fullness and auscultate for bowel sounds *to assess for bowel function and presence of constipation.*
- Encourage fiber intake *to increase frequency of stools.*
- Ensure adequate fluid intake *to prevent formation of hard, dry stools.*
- Encourage activity within child's limits or restrictions: *even minimal activity increases peristalsis.*
- Administer medications or enemas as ordered *to promote bowel training/evacuation (especially in child with myelomeningocele or spinal cord injury).*

Nursing Diagnosis: Self-care deficit related to neuromuscular impairments, cognitive deficits as evidenced by an inability to perform hygiene care and transfer self independently

Outcome identification and evaluation

Child will demonstrate ability to care for self within age parameters and limits of disease: *Child is able to feed, dress, manage elimination within limits of disease and age.*

Intervention: maximizing self-care

- Introduce child and family to self-help methods as soon as possible *to promote independence from the beginning.*
- Encourage family and staff to allow child to do as much as possible *to allow child to gain confidence and independence.*
- Teach specific measures for bowel and urinary elimination as needed *to promote independence and increase self-care abilities and self-esteem.*
- Collaborate with physical therapy, occupational therapy, and speech therapy to provide child and family with appropriate tools to modify environment and methods to promote transferring and self-care *to allow for maximum functioning.*
- Praise accomplishments and emphasize child's abilities *to improve self-esteem and encourage feelings of confidence and competence.*
- Balance activity with periods to rest *to reduce fatigue and increase energy for self-care.*

Nursing Diagnosis: Risk for impaired skin integrity related to immobility, use of braces or adaptive devices

Outcome identification and evaluation

Child's skin will remain intact, *without evidence of redness or breakdown.*

Overview for the Child with a Neuromuscular Disorder (continued)

Intervention: promoting skin integrity

- Monitor condition of entire skin surface at least daily *to provide baseline and allow for early identification of areas at risk.*
- Avoid excessive friction or harsh cleaning products *that may increase risk of breakdown in child with susceptible skin.*
- Keep child's skin free from stool and urine *to decrease risk of breakdown.*
- Change child's position frequently *to decrease pressure to susceptible areas.*
- Monitor skin condition affected by braces or adaptive equipment frequently *to prevent skin breakdown related to poor fit.*

Nursing Diagnosis: Chronic sorrow related to presence of chronic disability as evidenced by child's or family's expression of sadness, anger, disappointment, or feeling overwhelmed

Outcome identification and evaluation

Child and/or family will accept situation; *child/family will appropriately identify feelings, function at a normal developmental level, and plan for the future.*

Intervention: easing sorrow

- Assess degree of sorrow *to provide baseline for intervention.*
- Identify problems with eating or sleeping, *often affected when grief or sorrow is present.*
- Spend time with the child and family; *an empathetic presence is valued by suffering families.*
- Encourage the use of positive coping techniques; *taking action, expressing feelings, intentional attempts at coping are helpful techniques.*
- Refer for spiritual counseling as desired; *many families experience grief resolution in a more timely fashion if spiritual needs are addressed.*

Nursing Diagnosis: Risk for injury related to muscle weakness

Outcome identification and evaluation

Child will remain free from injury; *child will not fall or experience other injury.*

Intervention: preventing injury

- Ensure that side rails of bed are elevated when caregiver is not directly at bedside *to prevent fall from bed.*
- Use appropriate safety restraints with adaptive equipment and wheelchairs *to prevent fall or slipping from equipment.*
- Do not leave child unattended in tub *as weakness may cause the child to slip under the water.*
- Avoid restraint use if at all possible; *close observation is more appropriate.*

Nursing Diagnosis: Deficient knowledge related to lack of information regarding complex medical condition, prognosis, and medical needs as evidenced by verbalization, questions, or actions demonstrating lack of understanding regarding child's condition or care

Outcome identification and evaluation

Child and family will verbalize accurate information and understanding about condition, prognosis, and medical needs: *Child and family demonstrate knowledge of condition and prognosis and medical needs, including possible causes, contributing factors, and treatment measures.*

Intervention: providing patient and family teaching

- Assess child's and family's willingness to learn: *Child and family must be willing to learn for teaching to be effective.*

(continued)

Overview for the Child with a Neuromuscular Disorder (continued)

Intervention: providing patient and family teaching

- Provide family with time to adjust to diagnosis *to facilitate adjustment and ability to learn and participate in child's care.*
- Repeat information *to allow family and child time to learn and understand.*
- Teach in short sessions: *many short sessions are more helpful than one long session.*
- Gear teaching to the level of understanding of the child and family (depends on age of child, physical condition, memory) *to ensure understanding.*
- Provide reinforcement and rewards *to facilitate the teaching/learning process.*
- Use multiple modes of learning involving many senses (provide written, verbal, demonstration and videos) when possible: *child and family are more likely to retain information when it is presented in different ways using many senses.*

Nursing Diagnosis: Family processes, interrupted, related to child's illness, hospitalization, diagnosis of chronic illness in child, and potential long-term effects of illness as evidenced by family's presence in hospital, missed work, demonstration of inadequate coping

Outcome identification and evaluation

Family will maintain functional system of support, demonstrate adequate coping, adaptation of roles: *Parents are involved in child's care, ask appropriate questions, express fears and concerns, and are able to discuss child's care and condition calmly.*

Intervention: promoting appropriate family functioning

- Encourage parents and family to verbalize concerns related to child's illness, diagnosis, and prognosis: *allows the nurse to identify concerns and areas where further education may be needed; demonstrates family-centered care.*
- Explain therapies, procedures, child's behaviors, and plan of care to parents: *understanding of the child's current status and plan of care helps decrease anxiety.*
- Encourage parental involvement in care *to allow parents to feel needed and valued and to have a sense of control over their child's health.*
- Identify support system for family and child: *support system is often needed by stressed families to assist with coping.*
- Educate family and child on additional resources available *to help them develop a wide base of support.*

HEALTHY PEOPLE 2010

Objective	Significance
Increase the proportion of children with special health needs who have access to a medical home.	• Educate the family that specialist care (though often consisting of frequent and multiple visits) does not replace primary care through the medical home. • Encourage families to find a primary care pediatrician with whom they feel comfortable for well-child check-ups and routine childhood illnesses.

NEURAL TUBE DEFECTS

Neural tube defects account for the majority of congenital anomalies of the central nervous system. The neural tube closes between the third and fourth week of gestation. The cause of neural tube defects is not known, but many factors, such as drugs, malnutrition, chemicals, and genetics, can hinder normal central nervous system development. Strong evidence exists that supplementation of folic acid by the mother before conception decreases the incidence of neural tube defects in pregnancies at risk by 50% (Behrman et al., 2004). In 1992 the U.S. Public Health Service recommended that all women of childbearing age who are capable of becoming pregnant take 0.4 mg of folic acid daily (Merereau et al., 2004). According to the Centers for Disease Control and Prevention (CDC), the number of pregnancies affected by neural tube defects decreased from 4,000 in 1995–1996 to 3,000 in

1999–2000 (Merereau et al, 2004). Prenatal screening of maternal serum for alpha-fetoprotein (AFP) and ultrasound at 16 to 18 weeks of gestation can help identify fetuses at risk. Neural tube defects primarily affecting spinal cord development include spina bifida occulta, meningocele, and myelomeningocele (Fig. 23.3). Neural tube defects primarily affecting brain development are discussed in Chapter 17.

Spina Bifida Occulta

Spina bifida is a term that is often used to refer to all neural tube disorders that affect the spinal cord. This can be confusing and a cause of concern for parents. There are well-defined degrees of spinal cord involvement, and use of the correct terminology is important for health care professionals.

Spina bifida occulta is a defect of the vertebral bodies without protrusion of the spinal cord or meninges. This defect is not visible externally and in most cases has no adverse affects (see Fig. 23.3). Spina bifida occulta is a common anomaly: it is estimated that it affects one fifth of the population (Pate, 2002). Children with spina bifida occulta need no immediate medical intervention. Complications may include tethered cord, syringomyelia, or diastematomyelia.

Nursing Assessment

In most cases, spina bifida occulta is benign and asymptomatic and produces no neurologic signs; it may be considered a normal variant. The defect, which is usually present in the lumbosacral area, often goes undetected. However, there may be noticeable dimpling, abnormal patches of hair, or discoloration of skin at the defect site. If so, further investigation, including magnetic resonance imaging (MRI), may be warranted.

Nursing Management

Nursing care will focus on educating the family. Inform parents of its presence and what the diagnosis means. Many times parents will confuse this diagnosis with spina bifida cystica, a much more serious defect. Occasionally, children with spina bifida occulta eventually need surgical intervention due to degenerative changes or involvement of the spine and nerve roots resulting in complications such as tethered cord, syringomyelia, or diastematomyelia. When these associated problems occur, the condition is often termed "occult spinal dysraphism" to avoid confusion.

Meningocele

Meningocele, the less serious form of spina bifida cystica, occurs when the meninges herniate through a defect in the vertebrae. The spinal cord is usually normal and there are typically no associated neurologic deficits. Treatment for meningocele involves surgical correction of the lesion (see Fig. 23.3).

Nursing Assessment

Initial assessment after delivery will reveal a visible external sac protruding from the spinal area. It is most often seen in the lumbar region but can be anywhere along the spinal canal. Most are covered with skin and pose no threat to the patient. However, assessment to ensure that the sac covering is intact remains important. Assess neurologic status carefully: most children will be asymptomatic, with no neurologic deficits. Before surgical correction the infant will be thoroughly examined to determine whether there is any neural involvement or associated anomalies. Diagnostic procedures such as computed tomography (CT), MRI, and ultrasound may be performed.

Nursing Management

If the skin covering the sac is intact, surgical correction may be delayed. However, as in a child with myelomeningocele, immediately report any evidence of leaking cerebrospinal fluid (CSF) to ensure prompt intervention to prevent infection. Nursing management will be supportive. Provide preoperative and postoperative care similar to the child with

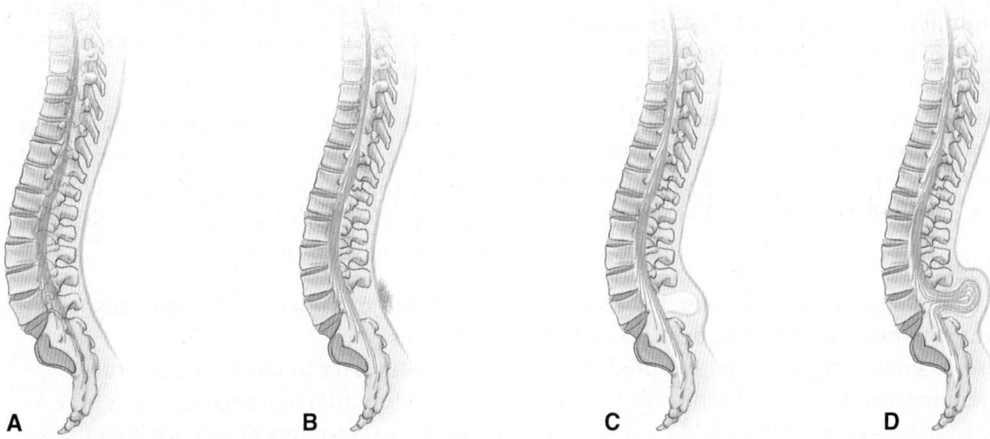

● FIGURE 23.3 (**A**) Normal spine. (**B**) Spina bifida occulta. (**C**) Meningocele. (**D**) Myelomeningocele.

myelomeningocele to prevent rupture of the sac and to prevent infection, and provide adequate nutrition and hydration. Monitor for symptoms of constipation or bladder dysfunction that may result due to increasing size of the lesion. Resulting hydrocephalus has been associated with some cases of meningocele; therefore, monitor head circumference and watch for signs and symptoms of increased intracranial pressure (ICP).

Myelomeningocele

Myelomeningocele, the most severe form of neural tube defect, occurs in approximately 1 in 4,000 live births (Behrman et al., 2004). Myelomeningocele is a type of spina bifida cystica, and clinically the term "spina bifida" is often used to refer to myelomeningocele. It may be diagnosed *in utero* via ultrasound; otherwise it is visually obvious at birth. The newborn with myelomeningocele is at increased risk for meningitis, hypoxia, and hemorrhage.

In myelomeningocele, the spinal cord often ends at the point of the defect, resulting in absent motor and sensory function beyond that point (see Fig. 23.3). Therefore, the long-term complications of paralysis, orthopedic deformities, and bladder and bowel incontinence are often seen in children with myelomeningocele. The presence of **neurogenic** bladder and frequent catheterization puts the child at an increased risk for urinary tract infections, pyelonephritis, and hydronephrosis, which may result in long-term renal damage if managed inappropriately. Accompanying hydrocephalus associated with type II Chiari defect is seen in 80% of patients with myelomeningocele (Behrman et al., 2004). Due to the improper development and the downward displacement of the brain into the cervical spine, CSF flow is blocked, resulting in hydrocephalus. The lower the deformity is on the spine, the lower the risk of developing hydrocephalus.

These children usually require multiple surgical procedures and due to frequent catheterizations are at an increased risk of developing a latex allergy. Learning problems and seizures are more common in these children than in the general population, but 70% of those with myelomeningocele have normal intelligence (Behrman et al., 2004). Ambulation is possible for some children, depending on the level of the lesion. Due to advances in medical treatment the life expectancy of children with this disorder has increased. For children born with a myelomeningocele who receive aggressive treatment, the mortality rate is 10% to 15%; most deaths occur before the age of 4 years old (Behrman et al., 2004).

Pathophysiology

The cause of myelomeningocele is unknown, but risk factors are consistent with other neural tube defects, such as maternal drug use, malnutrition, and a genetic predisposition. In myelomeningocele, the neural tube fails to close at the end of the fourth week of gestation. As a result, an external sac-like protrusion that encases the meninges, spinal fluid, and in some cases nerves is present on the spine (see Fig. 23.3). A myelomeningocele can be located anywhere along the spinal cord, but 75% are located in the lumbosacral region (Behrman et al., 2004). The degree of neurologic deficit will depend on the location. An increase in neurologic deficit is seen as the myelomeningocele extends into the thoracic region.

Therapeutic Management

Surgical closure will be performed as soon as possible after birth, especially if a CSF leak is present or if there is a danger of the sac rupturing. The goal of early surgical intervention is to prevent infection and to minimize further loss of function, which can result from the stretching of nerve roots as the meningeal sac expands after birth. A new option is becoming available but remains experimental. *In utero* fetal surgery to repair the myelomeningocele has been performed in the United States (Jobe, 2002). The benefits and risks remain uncertain at this time. Ongoing management of this disorder remains complex; a multidisciplinary approach is needed, involving specialists in neurology, neurosurgery, urology, orthopedics, therapy, and rehabilitation along with intense nursing care. The chronic nature of this disorder necessitates life-long follow-up.

Nursing Assessment

For a full description of the assessment phase of the nursing process, refer to page 762. Assessment findings pertinent to myelomeningocele are discussed below.

Health History

High-risk deliveries should be identified. Explore the pregnancy history and past medical history for risk factors such as:

- Lack of prenatal care
- Lack of preconception and/or prenatal folic acid supplementation
- Previous child born with neural tube defect or family history of neural tube defects
- Maternal consumption of certain drugs that antagonize folic acid, such as anticonvulsants (carbamazepine and phenobarbital)

The older infant or child with a history of myelomeningocele requires numerous surgical procedures and lifelong follow-up. In an infant or child returning for a clinic visit or hospitalization, the health history should include questions related to:

- Current mobility status and any changes in motor abilities
- Genitourinary function and regimen
- Bowel function and regimen
- Signs or symptoms of urinary infections
- History of hydrocephalus with presence of shunt

- Signs or symptoms of shunt infection or malfunction (refer to section on hydrocephalus)
- Latex sensitivity
- Nutritional status, including changes in weight
- Any other changes in physical or cognitive state
- Resources available and used by the family

Physical Examination

Initial assessment after delivery will reveal a visible external sac protruding from the spinal area (Fig. 23.4). Observe the baby's general appearance and assess whether the sac covering is intact. Assess neurologic status and look for associated anomalies. Assess for movement of extremities and anal reflex, which will help determine the level of neurologic involvement. Flaccid paralysis, absence of deep tendon reflexes, lack of response to touch and pain stimuli, skeletal abnormalities such as club feet, constant dribbling of urine, and a relaxed anal sphincter may be found.

In the older infant or child, perform a thorough physical examination and focus on the functional assessment. Note level of paralysis or paresthesia. Inspect skin for breakdown. Determine the child's motor capabilities.

Laboratory and Diagnostic Tests

A myelomeningocele may be detected prenatally around 16 to 18 of weeks' gestation by ultrasound, by a blood test that detects AFP increases, or by analysis of amniotic fluid for AFP increases. Common laboratory and diagnostic studies ordered for the assessment of myelomeningocele include:

- MRI
- CT
- Ultrasound
- Myelography

These diagnostic tests are used to evaluate brain and spinal cord involvement (refer to Common Laboratory and Diagnostic Tests 23.1).

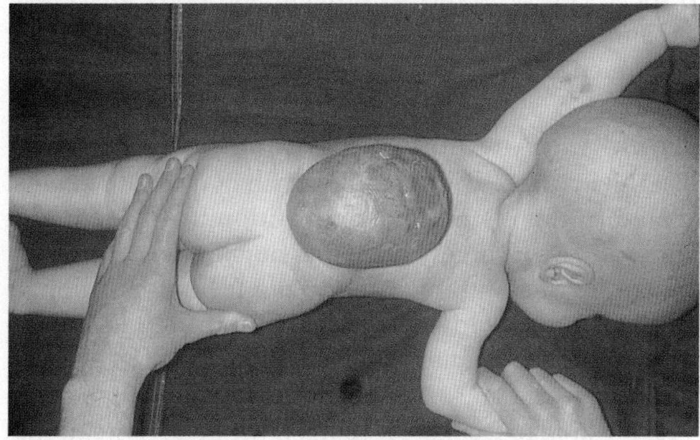

● FIGURE 23.4 Usually a sac covers the deformity of myelomeningocele and is visible at birth.

Nursing Management

Initial nursing management of the child with myelomeningocele involves preventing trauma to the meningeal sac and preventing infection before surgical repair of the defect. Refer to the Nursing Care Plan Overview in this chapter. Additional considerations are reviewed below.

Preventing Infection

Risk for infection related to the presence of the meningeal sac and potential for rupture is a central nursing concern in the newborn with myelomeningocele. Until surgical intervention occurs, the goal is to prevent rupture or leakage of CSF from the sac. Keeping the sac from drying out is important, as well as preventing trauma or pressure on the sac. Use sterile saline-soaked non-adhesive gauze or antibiotic-soaked gauze to keep the sac moist. Immediately report any seepage of clear fluid from the lesion, as this could indicate an opening in the sac and provide a portal of entry for microorganisms. Position the infant in the prone position or supported on the side to avoid pressure on the sac. To keep the infant warm, place the infant in a warmer or Isolette to avoid the use of blankets, which could exert too much pressure on the sac. Pay special attention while the infant is in a warmer or Isolette because the radiant heat can cause drying and cracking of the sac.

Keep the lesion free of feces and urine to help avoid infection. Position the infant so that urine and feces flow away from the sac (e.g., prone position, or place a folded towel under the abdomen) to help prevent infection. Placing a piece of plastic wrap below the meningocele is another way of preventing feces from coming into contact with the lesion. After surgery, position the infant in the prone or side-lying position to allow the incision to heal. Continue with precautions to prevent urine or feces from coming into contact with the incision.

Promoting Urinary Elimination

Children with myelomeningocele often have bladder incontinence, though some children may achieve normal urinary continence. The level of the lesion will influence the amount of dysfunction. Myelomeningocele remains one of the most common causes of neurogenic bladder in children. Therefore, evaluation of renal function by a pediatric urologist should be performed on each child with myelomeningocele.

Neurogenic bladder refers to the failure of the bladder to either store urine or empty itself of urine. Children with neurogenic bladder have loss of control over voiding. The spastic type of neurogenic bladder is hyperreflexive and yields frequent release of urine, but with incomplete emptying. The hypotonic neurogenic bladder is flaccid and weak and becomes stretched out; it can hold very large amounts of urine, resulting in continuous dribbling of urine from the urethra. Urinary stasis and retention occur in both types, placing the child at risk for urinary tract infection as well as reflux of bladder contents back up into the ureters and kidneys, resulting in renal scarring and insufficiency.

The goals of neurogenic bladder management are to promote optimal urinary continence and prevent renal complications. Interventions for neurogenic bladder include clean intermittent catheterization to promote bladder emptying; medications such as oxybutynin chloride (Ditropan) to improve bladder capacity; prompt recognition and treatment of infections; and in some children surgical interventions such as a continent urinary reservoir or vesicostomy to facilitate urinary elimination. Clean intermittent catheterization is addressed below. In the child with a spastic or rigid bladder, teach parents how to administer antispasmodic medications such as oxybutynin. Teach the parents that the medication is used to increase the bladder capacity and reduce the potential for reflux. Refer to Chapter 22 for additional information on nursing care related to the surgical procedures.

Assessing Urinary Function

Determine the child's pattern and success of toilet training, both for bladder and bowel. Assess the child's cognitive/developmental level. Observe the genital area for dribbling of urine from the urethra, noting odor of urine if present. Note redness of the urethra or excoriation in the diaper area. Inspect the abdomen for scars from prior surgeries and the presence of urinary diversion or continent stoma. Palpate the abdomen for presence of distended bladder, fecal mass, or enlarged kidneys. Determine the child's level of paralysis or paresthesia.

Clean Intermittent Catheterization

Depending on the level of paralysis at birth in the child with myelomeningocele, clean intermittent catheterization may be started at that time. In other children with spina bifida and in children who suffer spinal cord injury, catheterization may be started at a later age. Teach parents the technique of clean intermittent catheterization via the urethra, unless a urinary diversion or continent stoma has been created (Teaching Guideline 23.1).

Teaching the parents the techniques of clean intermittent catheterization is an important step in preserving renal functioning and preventing infection and helping the family gain some control over the child's physical condition. Until the child is able to self-catheterize, the parents will be responsible for this procedure. Children with normal intelligence and upper extremity motor skills usually learn to self-catheterize at the age of 6 years. Urinary incontinence is associated with poor self-esteem, particularly as the child gets older. Educating the child to self-catheterize the urethra or stoma as appropriate empowers the child, gives him or her a sense of control, and allows for appropriate urinary elimination when the child is away from the parents (e.g., at school).

Offer support and appropriate referrals to the child and family. Refer families to vendors in the local area for catheterization supplies.

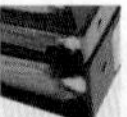

TEACHING GUIDELINE 23.1

Clean Intermittent Catheterization

- Wash hands with soap and water.
- Apply water-based lubricant to catheter.
- Perform catheterization. Insert catheter only as far as needed to obtain urine flow.
- Wash reusable catheter after use with soapy water; rinse and allow to dry.
- When dry, store in zip-top plastic bag or other clean storage container.
- Weekly, soak the catheter in a 1:1 vinegar and water solution, rinsing well before next use.
- When developmentally ready, teach the child to self-catheterize.

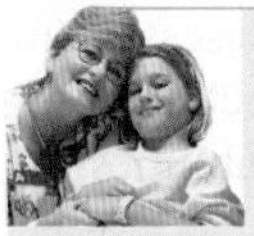

Over time, bacterial colonization of the bladder may occur; however, antibiotic prophylaxis is not recommended for these children because of the increased risk for development of antibiotic resistance.

Use only latex-free catheters and gloves for catheterization of children with myelomeningocele and/or neurogenic bladder, as these children exhibit a high incidence of latex allergy.

Promoting Bowel Elimination

Children with myelomeningocele often have bowel incontinence as well; the level of the lesion affects the amount of dysfunction. Many children with myelomeningocele can achieve some degree of bowel continence. Bowel training with the use of timed enemas or suppositories along with diet modifications can allow for defecation at predetermined times once or twice a day. Although bowel incontinence can be difficult for children as they grow older due to social concerns and self-esteem and body image disturbances, it does not pose the same health risks as urinary incontinence.

Promoting Adequate Nutrition

The risk for altered nutrition, less than body requirements, related to the restrictions on positioning of the infant before and after surgery is another nursing concern. Assist the family in assuming as normal a feeding position as possible. Preoperatively, the risk of rupture may be too high to warrant holding. Therefore, the infant's head can be turned to the side or the infant can be placed in the side-lying position to facilitate feeding. If the infant is held, special care needs to be taken to avoid pressure on the sac or postoperative incision. Encourage the parents to interact as much as possible with the infant by talking and touching the infant during feeding to help promote intake. If the mother was planning on breastfeeding the infant, assist her in meeting this goal, if possible. If the infant can be held, encourage her to do this, or assist her in pumping and saving breast milk to be given to the infant via bottle until the infant is able to be held. Feeding an infant in an unusual position can be difficult, and it is the nurse's role to provide support, education, and modeling for the parents and family when needed.

Preventing Latex Allergic Reaction

Sensitivity to latex or natural rubber is very common among children with myelomeningocele. They are at an increased risk of developing an allergy to latex related to the multiple exposures to latex products during surgical procedures and bladder catheterizations. Research has shown that up to 70% of children who require repeat surgeries due to spina bifida or bladder exstrophy are sensitive to latex (Kaplan, 2003). A latex-free environment should be created for all procedures performed on children with myelomeningocele to prevent latex allergy. Therefore, children at high risk for or with a known latex allergy must be identified and managed in a latex-free environment. Ensure that these children do not come into direct contact with latex or equipment and supplies that contain latex. Be familiar with those products and equipment at your facility that contain latex and those that are latex-free. The Food and Drug Administration now requires that all medical supplies be labeled if they contain latex, but this is not the case for consumer products. Many resources exist that list products that are latex-free, and each hospital should have such a list readily available to health care professionals. For an updated list of latex-containing products and other helpful information for parents regarding consumer products, contact the Spina Bifida Association of America (www.sbaa.org; 4590 MacArthur Blvd. NW, Suite 250, Washington D.C. 20007-4226; 1-800-621-3141 or 202-944-3285).

Children who are at a high risk for latex sensitivity should wear medical alert identification. Education programs regarding latex sensitivity and ways to prevent it need to be directed at those who care for high-risk children, including teachers, school nurses, relatives, babysitters, and all health care professionals.

Maintaining Skin Integrity

Address the risk for altered skin integrity related to the infant's prone position and impaired mobility. The prone position puts constant pressure on the knees and elbows, and it may be difficult to keep the infant clean of urine and feces. Diapering may be contraindicated preoperatively to avoid pressure on the sac. Therefore, ensure that the infant is kept as clean and dry as possible. This is made more difficult by the constant dribbling of stool and urine that may be present. Placing a pad beneath the diaper area and changing it frequently is important. Perform meticulous skin care. Place the infant on a special care mattress and place synthetic sheepskin under the infant to help reduce friction. Special attention to the infant's legs needs to occur when positioning them, since paralysis may be present. Using a folded diaper between the legs can help reduce pressure and friction from the legs rubbing together.

Educating and Supporting the Child and Family

Myelomeningocele is a serious disorder that affects multiple body systems and produces varying degrees of deficits. It is a disorder that has lifelong effects. Thanks to medical advances and technology most children born with myelomeningocele can expect to live a normal life, but challenges remain for the family and child as they learn to cope and live with this physical condition. Adjusting to the demands this condition places on the child and family is difficult. Parents may need time to accept their infant's condition, but as soon as possible they should be involved in the infant's care.

Teaching should begin immediately in the hospital. Teaching should include positioning, preventing infection, feeding, promoting urinary elimination through clean intermittent catheterization, preventing latex allergy, and the signs and symptoms of complications like increased ICP. Due to the chronic nature of this condition, long-term planning needs to begin in the hospital. These children usually require multiple surgical procedures and hospitalizations, and this can place stress on the family and their finances. The nurse has an important role in providing ongoing education about the illness and its treatments and the plan of care. As the family becomes more comfortable with the condition, they will become the experts in the child's care. Respect and recognize the family's changing needs. Providing intense daily care can take its toll on a family, and continual support and encouragement are needed. Referral to the Spina Bifida Association and a local support group for families of children with myelomeningocele is appropriate. See Healthy People 2010.

HEALTHY PEOPLE 2010

Objective	Significance
Increase the proportion of children and youth with disabilities who spend at least 80% of their time in regular education programs.	• Become familiar with local schools' offerings and capabilities so that you can refer families to an educational site appropriate for their child.

ConsiderTHIS!

A newborn has an obvious defect on his spine. Upon assessment, the nurse notes flaccid extremities and a distended bladder. The parents are devastated.

Identify additional assessments the nurse should make.

Describe nursing care for this neonate.

What teaching will the nurse do with this infant's family?

MUSCULAR DYSTROPHY

Muscular **dystrophy** refers to a group of inherited conditions that result in progressive muscle weakness and wasting. The muscles affected are primarily the skeletal (voluntary) muscles. Nine types of muscular dystrophy exist. All include muscle weakness over the lifetime; it is progressive in all cases but more severe in others. The various muscular dystrophies are most often diagnosed in childhood and affect a variety of muscle groups. The inheritance pattern for muscular dystrophy differs for each type but may be X-linked, autosomal dominant, or recessive. The genetic mutation in muscular dystrophy results in absence or decrease of a specific muscle protein that prevents normal function of the muscle. The skeletal muscle fibers are affected, yet there are no structural abnormalities in the spinal cord or the peripheral nerves. Table 23.1 gives specifics related to the various types of muscular dystrophy.

Duchenne muscular dystrophy, the most common neuromuscular disorder of childhood, is universally fatal (usually by the teens or twenties). The incidence is about 1 in 3,500 live male births (Balaban et al., 2005). For these reasons, this discussion will focus on Duchenne muscular dystrophy.

Pathophysiology

The gene mutation in Duchenne muscular dystrophy results in the absence of dystrophin, a protein that is critical for maintenance of muscle cells. The gene is X-linked recessive, meaning that mainly boys are affected and they receive the gene from their mothers (women are carriers but have no symptoms). Absence of dystrophin leads to generalized weakness of voluntary muscles, and the weakness progresses over time. The hips, thighs, pelvis, and shoulders are affected initially; as the disease progresses, all voluntary muscles as well as cardiac and respiratory muscles are affected. Rarely, males with Duchenne muscular dystrophy may survive beyond the early 30s (Muscular Dystrophy Association, 2006b).

Table 23.1 Types of Muscular Dystrophy

Type	Onset	Inheritance	Muscle Involvement
Duchenne (pseudohypertrophic)	Early childhood	X-linked recessive	Generalized weakness, muscle wasting (limb and trunk first)
Becker	Adolescence or adulthood	X-linked recessive	Similar but less severe than Duchenne
Congenital	At birth	Autosomal dominant or recessive	Generalized muscular weakness, possible joint deformities
Emery-Dreifuss	Childhood to early teens	X-linked recessive	Weakness, wasting of shoulder, upper arm, and shin muscles
Limb-girdle	Childhood to middle age	Autosomal or X-linked recessive	Weakness, wasting of shoulder and pelvic girdles first
Facioscapulohumeral	Childhood to early adulthood	Autosomal dominant	Facial muscles weaken first, then shoulders and upper arms
Myotonic	Childhood to middle age	Autosomal dominant	Generalized weakness, wasting of face, feet, hands, and neck first Delayed relaxation of muscles after contraction
Oculopharyngeal	Early adulthood to middle age	Autosomal dominant	Affects muscles of eyelid and throat first
Distal	40 to 60 years of age	Autosomal dominant	Weakness, wasting of hand, forearm, lower leg muscles

Data from www.mda.org

Boys with Duchenne muscular dystrophy are often late in learning to walk. As toddlers, they may display pseudohypertrophy (enlarged appearance) of the calves. During the preschool years they fall often and are quite clumsy. The affected child has difficulty climbing stairs and running and cannot get up from the floor in the usual fashion. The school-age child walks on the toes or balls of the feet with a rolling or waddling gait. Balance is disturbed significantly, and the child's belly may stick out when the shoulders are pulled back to stay upright and keep from falling over. During the school-age years it also becomes difficult for the child to raise his or her arms. Sometime between the ages of 7 and 12 years nearly all boys with Duchenne muscular dystrophy lose the ability to ambulate, and by the teen years any activity of the arms, legs, or trunk requires assistance or support. The most predictive factor for losing the ability to ambulate is loss of strength in hip extension and ankle dorsiflexion (Bakker et al., 2002). Most boys with Duchenne muscular dystrophy have normal intelligence, but many may exhibit a specific learning disability (Cotton et al., 2005).

Therapeutic Management

Though there is no cure for Duchenne muscular dystrophy, the use of corticosteroids may slow the progression of the disease. It is thought that prednisone helps by protecting muscle fibers from damage to the sarcolemma (defective in the absence of dystrophin). Numerous studies have shown that boys treated with prednisone demonstrate improved strength and function. The side effects of corticosteroids are many, including weight gain, osteoporosis, and mood changes (Carter & MacDonald, 2000). Calcium supplements are prescribed to prevent osteoporosis, and antidepressants may be helpful when depression occurs related to the chronicity of the disease and/or as an effect of corticosteroid use; see Healthy People 2010. Braces or orthoses and mobility and positioning aids are necessary.

As the muscles deteriorate, joints may become fixated, resulting in **contractures**. Contractures restrict flexibility and mobility and cause discomfort. Sometimes contractures require surgical tendon release. Spinal curvatures result over time. The boy with Duchenne muscular dystrophy who can still walk may develop lordosis. More frequently, scoliosis or kyphosis develops with this disorder. Surgical spinal fixation with rod implantation is often required by the age of 11 to 13 years. Additional complications include pulmonary, urinary, or systemic infections, depression, learning or behavioral disorders, aspiration pneumonia (as oropharyngeal muscles become affected), cardiac dysrhythmias, and eventually respiratory insufficiency and failure (as weakness of the chest muscles and diaphragm progresses).

HEALTHY PEOPLE 2010

Objective	Significance
Reduce the proportion of children and adolescents with disabilities who are reported to be sad, unhappy, or depressed.	• Use every encounter with the child or adolescent with a disability as an opportunity to screen for mental health concerns. • Refer these children and teens as appropriate for mental health assessment and intervention.

Nursing Assessment

For a full description of the assessment phase of the nursing process, refer to page 762. Assessment findings pertinent to Duchenne muscular dystrophy are discussed below.

Health History

Examine the health history for a family history of neuromuscular disorders. Note pregnancy and delivery history, as this information may be useful in ruling out a pregnancy problem or birth trauma as a cause for the motor dysfunction. Determine status of developmental milestone achievement. Boys with Duchenne muscular dystrophy learn to walk but over time become unable to do so. If the child was previously diagnosed with muscular dystrophy, determine progression of disease. Inquire about functional status and need for assistive or adaptive equipment such as braces or wheelchairs. Determine skills related to activities of daily living. Note history of cough or frequent respiratory infections, which occur as the respiratory muscles weaken. While talking with the child and family, determine whether psychosocial issues such as decreased self-esteem, depression, alterations in socialization, or altered family processes might be present.

Physical Examination

Perform a thorough physical examination on the child with suspected muscular dystrophy or the child with known history of the disorder. Particular findings related to inspection, observation, auscultation, and palpation are presented below.

Inspection and Observation

Observe the child's ability to rise from the floor. A hallmark finding of Duchenne muscular dystrophy is the presence of Gowers' sign: the child cannot rise from the floor in standard fashion because of increasing weakness (Fig. 23.5). Observe the child's gait. Determine effectiveness of cough.

Auscultation and Palpation

Auscultate the heart and lungs. Note tachycardia, which develops as the heart muscle weakens. Note adequacy of

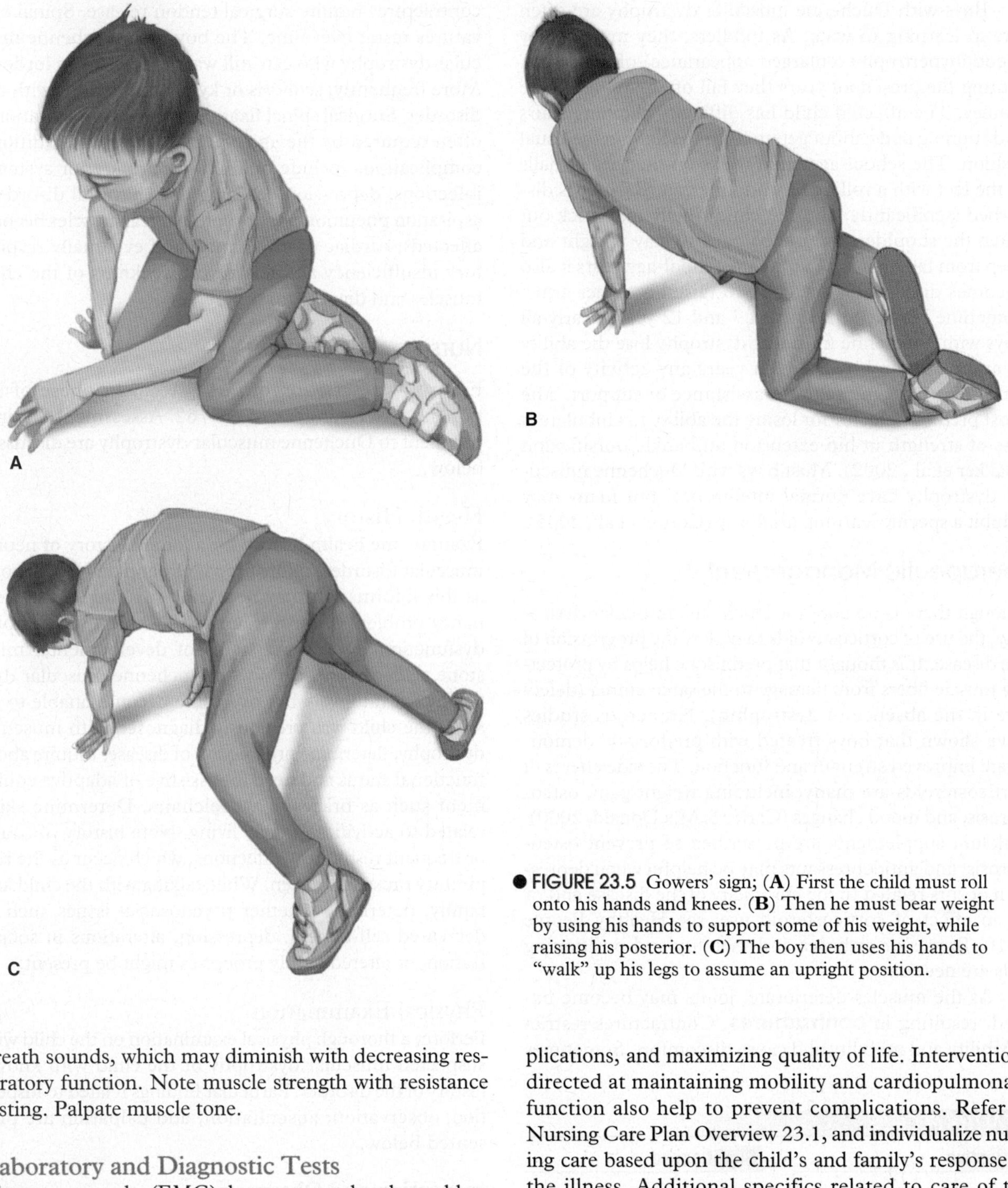

● FIGURE 23.5 Gowers' sign; (**A**) First the child must roll onto his hands and knees. (**B**) Then he must bear weight by using his hands to support some of his weight, while raising his posterior. (**C**) The boy then uses his hands to "walk" up his legs to assume an upright position.

breath sounds, which may diminish with decreasing respiratory function. Note muscle strength with resistance testing. Palpate muscle tone.

Laboratory and Diagnostic Tests

Electromyography (EMG) demonstrates that the problem lies in the muscles, not in the nerves. Serum creatine kinase levels are elevated early in the disorder, when significant muscle wasting is actively occurring. Muscle biopsy provides definitive diagnosis, demonstrating the absence of dystrophin. DNA testing reveals the presence of the gene.

Nursing Management

Nursing management is aimed at promoting mobility, maintaining cardiopulmonary function, preventing complications, and maximizing quality of life. Interventions directed at maintaining mobility and cardiopulmonary function also help to prevent complications. Refer to Nursing Care Plan Overview 23.1, and individualize nursing care based upon the child's and family's response to the illness. Additional specifics related to care of the child with muscular dystrophy are discussed below.

Promoting Mobility

Administer corticosteroids and calcium supplements as ordered. Encourage at least minimal weight-bearing in a standing position to promote improved circulation, healthier bones, and a straight spine. Boys with Duchenne muscular dystrophy may use a standing walker or standing frame to maintain an upright position. Perform passive stretching or strengthening exercises as recommended by the physical therapist. These exercises preserve mobility and may help to prevent muscle atrophy. Use orthotic supports such as hand braces or ankle–foot orthoses (AFOs) to prevent contractures of joints. Schedule activities during the part of the day when the child has the most energy. Teach parents the use of positioning, exercises, orthoses, and adaptive equipment.

Maintaining Cardiopulmonary Function

Assess respiratory rate, depth of respirations, and work of breathing. Auscultate the lungs to determine whether aeration is sufficient and to assess clarity of breath sounds. Position the child for maximum chest expansion, usually in the upright position. Teach the child and family deep-breathing exercises to strengthen or maintain respiratory muscles and encourage coughing to clear the airways. Perform chest physical therapy or assist with chest percussion. Monitor the results of pulmonary function testing. Use of intermittent positive-pressure ventilation and mechanically assisted coughing will become necessary in the teen years for some boys, possibly later for others (Gomez-Merino & Bach, 2002). Teach parents monitoring and use of these modalities in conjunction with the respiratory therapist. Monitor cardiac status closely to identify heart failure early. Assess for edema, weight gain, or crackles. Strictly monitor fluid intake and output.

Maximizing Quality of Life

Long periods of bed rest may contribute to further weakness. Work with the family and child to develop a schedule for diversional activities that provide appropriate developmental stimulation but avoid overexertion or frustration (related to inability to perform the activity). Periods of adequate rest must be balanced with activities. Walking or riding a stationary bike is appropriate for the child who has upper extremity involvement. For the child with lower extremity involvement, a wheelchair may become necessary for mobility, and the child may participate in crafts, drawing, and computer activities. Participating in the Special Olympics may be appropriate for some children (www.specialolympics.org).

Provide emotional support to the child and family. Long-term direct care is stressful for families and becomes more complex as the child gets older (Chen et al., 2002). Families often need respite from continual caregiving duties. When a child is hospitalized, the caregiver may feel comfortable allowing nurses and other health care professionals to assume more of the child's daily care; this can be an opportunity for the caregiver to obtain respite from daily care. Respite care may also be offered in the home by various community services, so explore these resources with families.

Assess the child's educational status. Some children attend school; others may opt for home-schooling.

Administer antidepressants as ordered: managing depression may increase the child's desire to participate in activities and self-care.

Refer the child and family to the Muscular Dystrophy Association (www.mda.org), which provides multidisciplinary care via clinics located throughout the United States. The association is also a clearinghouse for resources for individuals with muscular dystrophy.

Ensure that families receive genetic counseling for family planning purposes as well as determining which family members may be carriers for muscular dystrophy.

• SPINAL MUSCULAR ATROPHY

Spinal muscular atrophy (SMA) is a genetic motor neuron disease that affects the spinal nerves' ability to communicate with the muscles. It is inherited via an autosomal recessive mechanism. The motor neuron protein SMN (survival of motor neurons) is deficient as a result of a faulty gene on chromosome 5. The motor neurons are located mostly in the spinal cord. Without adequate SMN, the signals from the neurons to the muscles instructing them to contract are ineffective, so the muscles lose function and over time atrophy. The proximal muscles, those closer to the body's center, are usually more affected than the distal muscles. Emotional and mental development as well as sensation are unaffected by the disease (Muscular Dystrophy Association, 2006c).

There are several types of SMA: type 1 (Werdnig-Hoffmann disease, infantile SMA), type 2 (intermediate), and type 3 (Kugelberg-Welander disease or juvenile SMA). Table 23.2 compares these three types, their usual progression, and their prognosis.

Respiratory muscle weakness may occur with all types of SMA and is usually the cause of death in type 1 and type 2 SMA. Upper respiratory tract infections and aspiration related to dysphagia or gastroesophageal reflux often develop into pneumonia and eventual respiratory failure, as the affected child cannot effectively cough independently in order to clear the airway. Many children with severe type 1 SMA are ventilator dependent. Pectus excavatum develops in children with type 1 and 2 SMA who exhibit paradoxical breathing (use of the diaphragm without intercostal muscle support). The chest becomes funnel-shaped and the xiphoid process is retracted (pectus excavatum), further restricting respiratory development (Bach & Bianchi, 2003). Inability to appropriately suck and swallow leads to difficulty feeding in the child with type 1 SMA. Weak back muscles affect the developing spine, resulting in the complication of scoliosis, kyphosis, or both.

Therapeutic management of SMA is supportive, aimed at promoting mobility, maintaining adequate nutrition and pulmonary function, and preventing complications. Spinal fusion may be performed in older children with significant scoliosis. Supplementation with creatine and/or coenzyme Q10 is under investigation (Muscular Dystrophy Association, 2006c).

Table 23.2 Features of Spinal Muscular Atrophy

Features	Type 1 SMA (Werdnig-Hoffman disease, infantile SMA)	Type 2 SMA (Intermediate SMA)	Type 3 SMA (Kugelberg-Welander disease, juvenile SMA)
Onset	Before birth to 6 months of age	6 to 18 months of age	After 18 months of age; child has started walking or has taken at least five independent steps
Symptoms	• Generalized weakness; cannot sit without support • Weak cry • Difficulty sucking, swallowing, and breathing	• Weakness that is most severe in the shoulders, hips, thighs, and upper back • Respiratory muscles may be involved. • Scoliosis may occur.	• Weakness that is most severe in the shoulders, hips, thighs, and upper back • Respiratory muscles may be involved. • Scoliosis may occur.
Progression	Rapidly progresses to early childhood death. Use of ventilators and gastrostomy feeding tubes may prolong life expectancy.	Slower progression. Survival into adulthood common if respiratory status maintained appropriately.	Slow progression. Life span usually unaffected. Walking ability maintained until at least adolescence; may need wheelchair later in life.

Data from Muscular Dystrophy Association, 2006.

Nursing Assessment

Note history of attainment of developmental milestones, as well as loss of milestones. In the infant or child with known SMA, assess for recent hospitalizations or respiratory illness. Determine the respiratory support regimen used at home (if any). Note level of motor ability, and identify the orthoses or adaptive equipment used. Elicit history related to feeding patterns at home. Assess for floppy appearance in the infant with SMA (Fig. 23.6). Note decreased ability to initiate spontaneous muscle movement. In the infant or young child with SMA, note narrow chest with decreased excursion, relatively protuberant abdomen, and paradoxical breathing pattern (Fig. 23.7). Observe chest for formation of pectus excavatum. Auscultate lungs for diminished or adventitious breath sounds. Monitor laboratory testing, which may include:

- Creatine kinase (CK): elevated when muscular damage is occurring
- Genetic testing: identifies presence of gene for SMA
- Muscle biopsy: shows the muscle abnormality
- Nerve conduction velocity test and electromyelogram: to determine extent of involvement

Nursing Management

Nursing management of type 2 and type 3 SMA focuses on promoting mobility, maintaining pulmonary function, and preventing complications. Children with type 1 SMA need additional interventions related to prevention of complications from immobility and assistance with nutrition. Refer to Nursing Care Plan Overview 23.1 for interventions related to these areas. Individualize the nursing plan of care based on the individual child's responses to the disorder.

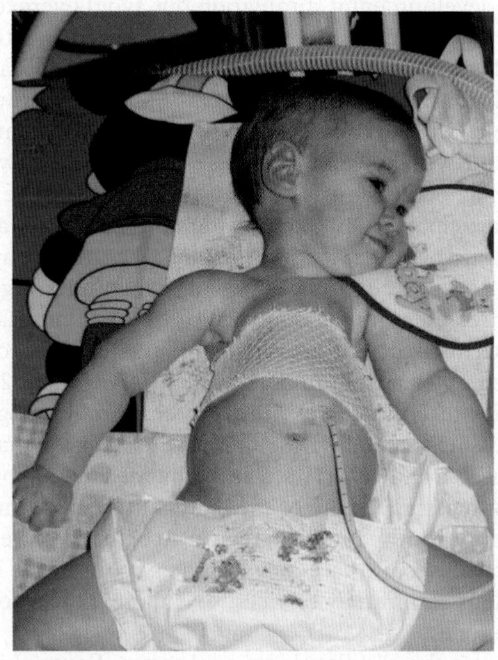

● FIGURE 23.6 Note the hypotonic (floppy) posture of this infant with type 1 SMA (rotated arms, frog-legged lower extremities). (Graphic courtesy of the Muscular Dystrophy Association, www.mda.org.)

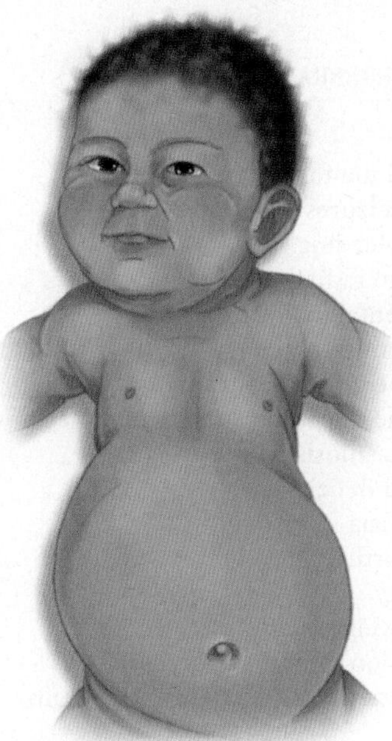

● FIGURE 23.7 Note the very narrow chest, beginning xiphoid depression, and relatively enlarged appearance of the abdomen in this infant with type 1 SMA.

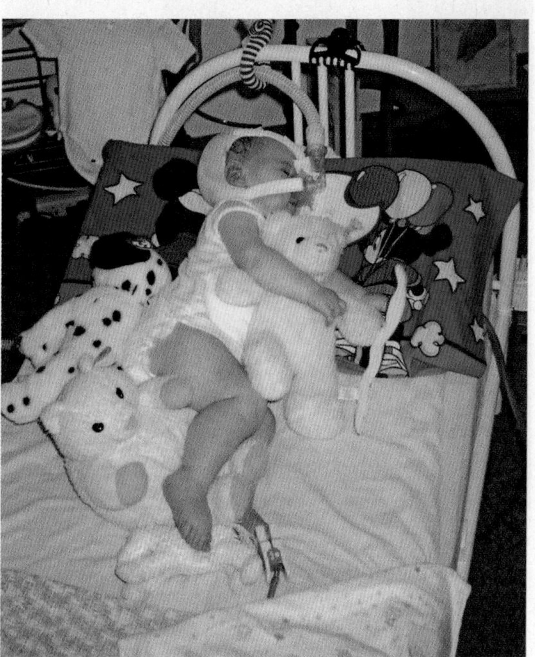

● FIGURE 23.8 Position the infant with SMA to maintain appropriate body alignment, propping extremities as needed. (Graphic courtesy of the Muscular Dystrophy Association, www.mda.org.)

Promote mobility through the use of range-of-motion exercises, lightweight orthotics, standing frames, and wheelchair use as appropriate. Support parents in their efforts to comply with physical and occupational therapy regimens. Older children may exercise with assistance in a warm pool. Position the child in a fashion that maintains appropriate body alignment (Fig. 23.8).

Provide chest percussion to assist with coughing and clearance of secretions. In collaboration with respiratory therapy, teach families the use of noninvasive ventilation support, in which positive pressure is delivered to the lungs through a mask or mouthpiece (Fig. 23.9). Provide routine tracheostomy care if the child has a tracheostomy (refer to tracheostomy sections of Chapter 14 and to Chapter 19).

Administer gastrostomy tube feedings if ordered, and teach families gastrostomy tube care. Use bracing as prescribed to prevent spinal curvature (Fig. 23.10). Make frequent inspections for skin breakdown in areas affected by bracing.

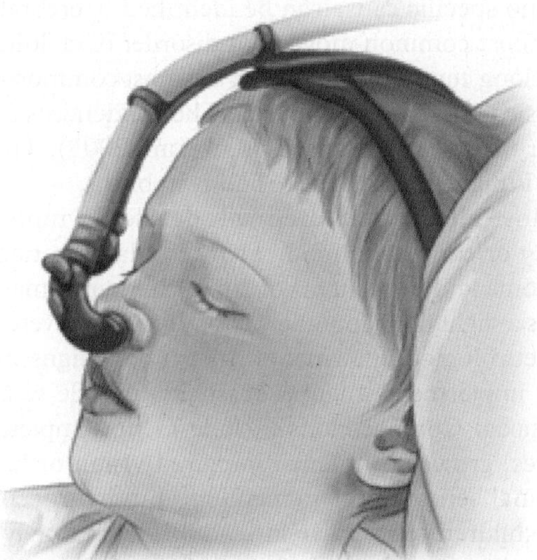

● FIGURE 23.9 Use of noninvasive positive-pressure monitoring via a mask can maximize respiration and may help prevent pulmonary complications.

Cerebral Palsy

Cerebral palsy is a term used to describe a range of nonspecific clinical symptoms characterized by abnormal motor pattern and postures caused by nonprogressive abnormal brain function. The majority of causes occur

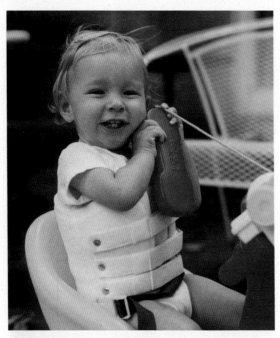

● FIGURE 23.10 Bracing may be necessary in the young child with SMA to either prevent scoliosis from developing or prevent its progression. (Graphic courtesy of the Muscular Dystrophy Association, www.mda.org.)

BOX 23.1

CAUSES OF CEREBRAL PALSY

Prenatal

- Congenital malformation
- Maternal seizures
- Maternal bleeding
- Exposure to radiation
- Environmental toxins
- Genetic abnormalities
- Intrauterine growth restriction
- Intrauterine infection, such as cytomegalovirus and toxoplasmosis
- Nutritional deficits
- Pre-eclampsia
- Multiple births
- Prematurity
- Low birthweight
- Malformation of brain structure
- Abnormalities of blood flow to the brain

Perinatal

- Prematurity (<32 weeks)
- Asphyxia
- Hypoxia
- Breech position
- Sepsis or central nervous system infection
- Placental complications
- Electrolyte disturbance
- Cerebral hemorrhage
- Kernicterus (a type of brain damage that may result from neonatal hyperbilirubinemia)
- Chorioamnionitis (infection of the placental tissues and amniotic fluid)

Postnatal

- Head trauma (e.g., motor vehicle accidents, abuse)
- Seizures
- Toxins
- Viral or bacterial infection of the central nervous system (e.g., meningitis)

before or during delivery and are often associated with brain anoxia (Box 23.1); see Healthy People 2010. Many times no specific cause can be identified. Cerebral palsy is the most common movement disorder of childhood; it is a lifelong condition and one of the most common causes of physical disability in children. The incidence is 2 to 2.5 in every 1,000 live births (Rosenbaum, 2003). The incidence is higher in premature and twin births.

Most affected children will develop symptoms in infancy or early childhood. There is a large variation in symptoms and disability. For some children it may be as mild as a slight limp; for others it may result in severe motor and neurologic impairments. Its primary signs include motor impairments such as spasticity, muscle weakness, and ataxia. Complications include mental impairments, seizures, growth problems, impaired vision or hearing, abnormal sensation or perception, and hydrocephalus. Most children can survive into adulthood but may suffer substantial impairments in function and quality of life.

Pathophysiology

Cerebral palsy is a disorder caused by abnormal development of, or damage to, the motor areas of the brain. It results in a disruption in the brain's ability to control movement and posture. It is difficult to establish an exact location of the neurologic lesion, and the lesion itself does not change; thus, the disorder is considered nonprogressive since the brain injury does not progress. However, the clinical manifestations of the lesion change as the child grows. Some children may improve, but many either plateau in their attainment of motor skills or demonstrate worsening of motor abilities, as it is difficult to maintain the ability to move over time.

Cerebral palsy is classified in several ways. One common way is by the type of movement disturbance (Table 23.3).

Therapeutic Management

Management involves multiple disciplines, including a primary physician, specialty physicians such as neurolo-

HEALTHY PEOPLE 2010

Objective	Significance
Reduce preterm births.	• Encourage appropriate birth control use among adolescents to decrease the incidence of teen pregnancy (teens have an increased incidence of preterm delivery). • If an adolescent does become pregnant, encourage early appropriate prenatal care. • Discourage substance use among pregnant teens. • Teach pregnant teens about an appropriate diet.

gist and orthopedic surgeon, nurses, physical therapists, occupational therapists, speech therapists, dietitian, psychologist, counselors, teachers, and parents. Spasticity management will be a primary concern and will be determined by clinical findings. There is no standard treatment for all children. The overall focus of therapeutic management will be to assist the child to gain optimal development and function within the limits of the disease. Treatment is mainly symptomatic, preventive, and supportive.

Medical management is focused on promoting mobility through the use of therapeutic modalities and medications. Many children will require surgical procedures to correct deformities related to spasticity. Multiple corrective surgeries may be required; they usually are orthopedic or neurosurgical. Surgery may be used to correct contractures that are severe enough to cause movement limitations. Common orthopedic procedures include tendon lengthening procedures, correction of hip and adductor muscle spasticity, and fusion of unstable joints to help improve locomotion, correct bony deformities, decrease painful spasticity, and maintain, restore, or stabilize a spinal deformity. Neurosurgical interventions may include placement of a shunt in children who have developed hydrocephalus, or surgical interventions to decrease spasticity. Selective dorsal root rhizotomy is used to decrease spasticity in the lower extremities by reducing the amount of stimulation that reaches the muscles via nerves. The effectiveness of this surgery is controversial, and research is ongoing.

Physical, Occupational, and Speech Therapy

The use of therapies such as physical therapy, occupational therapy, and speech therapy will be essential in

Table 23.3 Classification of Cerebral Palsy

Types	Description	Characteristics
Spastic	Hypertonicity and permanent contractures; different types based on which limbs are affected: • Hemiplegia: both extremities on one side • Quadriplegia: all four extremities • Diplegia or paraplegia: lower extremities	• Most common form • Poor control of posture, balance, and movement • Exaggeration of deep tendon reflexes • Hypertonicity of affected extremities • Continuation of primitive reflexes • In some children, failure to progress to protective reflexes
Athetoid or dyskinetic	Abnormal involuntary movements	• Infant is limp and flaccid. • Uncontrolled slow worm-like, writhing, or twisting movements • Affects all four extremities and possible involvement of face, neck, and tongue • Movements increase during periods of stress. • Dysarthria and drooling may be present.
Ataxic	Affects balance and depth perception	• Rare form • Poor coordination • Unsteady gait • Wide-based gait
Mixed	Combination of the above	Most common is spastic and athetoid.

promoting mobility and development in the child with CP. The earlier the treatment begins, the better chance the child has of overcoming developmental disabilities.

Physical therapists work with children to assist in the development of gross motor movements such as walking and positioning, and they help the child develop independent movement. They also assist in preventing contractures, and they instruct children and caregivers in the use of assistive devices such as walkers and wheelchairs. Occupational therapists may be responsible for fashioning orthotics and splints. AFOs are the most common orthotic used by children with cerebral palsy (Fig. 23.11). AFOs help prevent deformity from conditions such as contractures and help reduce the effects of existing deformities. They can help improve a child's mobility by assisting in control of alignment and helping to increase the efficiency of the child's gait. Spinal orthotics such as braces are used in young children with cerebral palsy to combat scoliosis that develops due to spasticity. These braces are used to delay surgical management of the scoliosis until the child reaches skeletal maturity. Splinting is used to maintain muscle length. Serial casting may also be used to increase muscle and tendon length.

Occupational therapy also assists in the development of fine motor skills and will help the child to perform optimal self-care by working on skills such as activities of daily living. Speech therapy assists in the development of receptive and expressive language and addresses the use of appropriate feeding techniques in the child who has swallowing problems. Speech therapists may teach augmented communication strategies to children who are nonverbal or who have articulation problems. Many children may not communicate verbally but can use alternative means such as communication books or boards to make their desires known or to participate in conversation.

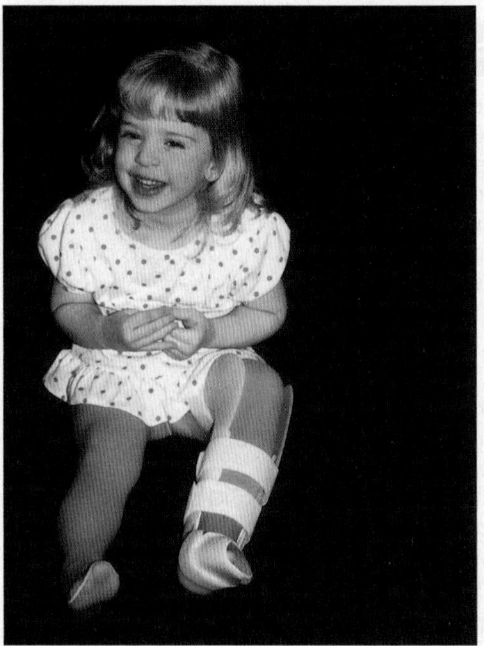

● FIGURE 23.11 The child with cerebral palsy may benefit from wearing ankle–foot orthotics to provide the support needed for independent or assisted walking.

Pharmacologic Management

Various pharmacologic options are available to manage spasticity. Medications are also used to treat seizure disorders in children with cerebral palsy (refer to Chapter 17 for information related to seizure management). Oral medications used to treat spasticity include baclofen and diazepam (see Drug Guide 23.1). Patients with athetoid cerebral palsy may be given anticholinergics to help decrease abnormal movements.

Parenterally administered medications such as botulin toxins and baclofen are also used to manage spasticity. Botulinum toxin is injected into the spastic muscle to balance the muscle forces across joints and to decrease spasticity. It is useful in managing focal spasticity in which the spasticity is interfering with function, producing pain, or contributing to a progressive deformity. Botulin toxin injection is performed by the physician or advanced practitioner and can be done in the clinic or outpatient setting.

Intrathecal administration of baclofen has been shown to decrease tone, but it must be infused continuously due to its short half-life. Surgical placement of a baclofen pump will be considered in children with general spasticity that is limiting function, comfort, activities of daily living, and endurance. To test whether it is a suitable option, an intrathecal test dose of baclofen will be administered. If the trial is successful, a baclofen pump will be implanted. Once inserted, delivery of the drug can be individualized to meet the patient's unique needs. The pump needs to be replaced every 5 to 7 years and must be refilled with medication approximately every 3 months, depending on the type of pump. Complications with baclofen pump placement include infection, rupture, dislodgement, or blockage of the catheter.

Nursing Assessment

For a full description of the assessment phase of the nursing process, refer to page 762. Assessment findings pertinent to cerebral palsy are discussed below.

Health History

Elicit a description of the present illness and chief complaint. Obtain a detailed account of gestation and perinatal events (refer to Box 23.1). Common signs and symptoms reported during the health history of the undiagnosed child might include:

- Intrauterine infections
- Prematurity with intracranial hemorrhage
- Difficult, complicated, or prolonged labor and delivery

- Multiple births
- History of possible anoxia during prenatal life or birth
- History of head trauma
- Delayed attainment of developmental milestones
- Muscle weakness or rigidity
- Poor feeding
- Hips and knees feel rigid and unbending when pulled to a sitting position
- Seizure activity
- Subnormal learning
- Abnormal motor performance, scoots on back instead of crawling on abdomen, walks or stands on toes

Children known to have cerebral palsy are often admitted to the hospital for corrective surgeries or other complications of the disease, such as aspiration pneumonia and urinary tract infections. The health history should include questions related to:

- Respiratory status: Has a cough, sputum production, or increased work of breathing developed?
- Motor function: Has there been a change in muscle tone, increase in spasticity?
- Presence of fever
- Feeding and weight loss
- Any other changes in physical state or medication regimen

Physical Examination

Observe general appearance. Pay close attention to the neurologic assessment and motor assessment. Assess for delayed development, size for age, and sensory alterations like strabismus, vision problems, and speech disorders. Abnormal postures may be present. While lying supine, the infant may demonstrate scissor crossing of the legs with plantarflexion. In the prone position the infant may raise his or her head higher than normal due to arching of the back, or the opisthotonic position may be noted. The infant may also abnormally flex the arms and legs under the trunk. Primitive reflexes may persist beyond the point at which they disappear in a healthy infant. Evolution of protective reflexes may be delayed. Watch the infant or child play, crawl, walk, or climb to determine motor function and capability. Note any movement disorder. Infants with cerebral palsy may demonstrate abnormal use of muscle groups such as scooting on their back instead of crawling or walking.

Assess active and passive range of motion. Pay particular attention to muscle tone. Though an increased or decreased resistance may be noted with passive movements, **hypertonicity** is most often seen. Increased resistance to dorsiflexion and passive hip abduction are the most common early signs. Sustained **clonus** may be present after forced dorsiflexion. Lift the child by placing your hands in the infant's or child's axillary area to assess shoulder girdle function and tone. Infants with cerebral palsy often demonstrate prolonged standing on their toes when supported in an upright standing position in this fashion. Lift the young child off the ground while the child holds your thumbs to test hand strength. Observe for presence of limb deformity, as decreased use of an extremity (as in the case of hemiparesis) may result in shortening of the extremity compared to the other one.

Laboratory and Diagnostic Tests

A complete history, physical examination, and ancillary investigations are the primary modality for establishing a diagnosis of cerebral palsy. Common supplementary laboratory and diagnostic studies ordered for the diagnosis and assessment of cerebral palsy include:

- Electroencephalogram: usually abnormal but the pattern is highly variable
- Cranial x-rays or ultrasound: may show cerebral asymmetry
- MRI or CT: may show area of damage or abnormal development but may be normal
- Screening for metabolic defects and genetic testing may be performed to help determine the cause of cerebral palsy.

These tests will help determine whether cerebral palsy is the likely cause or whether another condition may be the cause of the child's symptoms. These tests also will be important in evaluating the severity of the child's physical disabilities.

Nursing Management

Nursing management focuses on promoting growth and development by promoting mobility and maintaining optimal nutritional intake. Providing support and education to the child and family is also an important nursing function. In addition to the nursing diagnoses and related interventions discussed in the Nursing Care Plan Overview, interventions common to caring for a child with cerebral palsy follow.

Promoting Mobility

Mobility is critical to childhood development. Treatment modalities to promote mobility include physiotherapy, pharmacologic management, and surgery. Surgical procedures are discussed above. Physical or occupational therapy as well as medications may be used to address musculoskeletal abnormalities, to facilitate range of motion, to delay or prevent deformities such as contractures, to provide joint stability, to maximize activity, and to encourage the use of adaptive devices. The nurse's role in relation to the various therapies is to provide ongoing follow-through with prescribed exercises, positioning, or bracing.

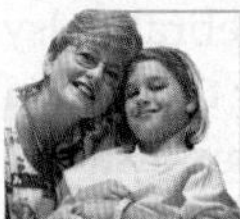

Therapeutic horseback riding has been demonstrated to improve gross motor function in children with cerebral palsy. If available in the local area, refer the child and family to the North American Riding for the Handicapped Association (NARHA) (Sterba, 2004; Sterba et al., 2002).

When casting, splinting, or orthotics are used, assess skin integrity frequently. Pain management may also be necessary. Nursing management of children receiving botulin toxin focuses on assisting with the procedure and providing education and support to the child and family. Nursing interventions related to baclofen include assisting with the test dose and providing preoperative and postoperative care if a pump is placed, as well as providing support and education to the child and family. Teaching Guideline 23.2 gives information related to baclofen pump insertion.

Promoting Nutrition

Children with cerebral palsy may have difficulty eating and swallowing due to poor motor control of the throat, mouth, and tongue. This may lead to poor nutrition and problems with growth. The child may require a longer time to eat because of poor motor control. Special diets, such as soft or puréed, may make swallowing easier. Proper positioning during feeding is essential to facilitate swallowing and reduce the risk of aspiration. Speech or occupational therapists can assist in working on strengthening swallowing muscles as well as assisting in developing accommodations to facilitate nutritional intake. Consult a dietitian to ensure adequate nutrition for children with cerebral palsy. In children with severe swallowing problems or malnutrition, a feeding tube such as a gastrostomy tube may be placed.

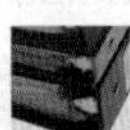

TEACHING GUIDELINE 23.2

Baclofen Pump: Patient/Family Education

- Check the incisions daily for redness, drainage, or swelling.
- Notify the physician if the child has a temperature greater than 101.5° F, or if the child has persistent incision pain.
- Avoid tub baths for 2 weeks.
- Do not allow the child to sleep on the stomach for 4 weeks after pump insertion.
- Discourage twisting at the waist, reaching high overhead, stretching, or bending forward or backward for 4 weeks.
- When the incisions have healed, normal activity may be resumed.
- Wear loose clothing to prevent irritation at the incision site.
- Carry implanted device identification and emergency information cards at all times.

Providing Support and Education

Cerebral palsy is a lifelong disorder that can result in severe physical and cognitive disability. In some cases disability may require complete intensive daily care of the child. Adjusting to the demands of this multifaceted illness is difficult. Children are frequently hospitalized and need numerous corrective surgeries, which places strain on the family and its finances. From the time of diagnosis, the family should be involved in the child's care. It is important to include parents in the planning of interventions and care of this child. In most cases they are the primary caregivers and will assist the child in development of functioning and skills as well as providing daily care. They will provide essential information to the health care team and will be advocates for their child throughout his or her life. It is important that nurses provide ongoing education for the child and family.

As the child grows, the needs of the family and child will change. Recognize and respect these needs. Providing daily intense care can be demanding and tiring. When a child with cerebral palsy is admitted to the hospital, this may serve as a time of respite for family and primary caregivers. Encourage respite care and provide support and encouragement. Because cerebral palsy is a lifelong condition, children will need meaningful education programs that emphasize independence in the least restrictive educational environment. Refer caregivers to local resources, including education services and support groups. United Cerebral Palsy, a national organization, can be accessed at www.ucp.org/ (1660 L Street, NW, Suite 700, Washington, D.C. 20036; 800-872-5827/202-776-0406). Easter Seals is an organization that helps children with disabilities and special needs and provides support to families (www.easterseals.com).

Refer children under age 3 years to the local early intervention service. Early intervention provides case management of developmental services for children with special needs. Each state has a coordinator for early intervention. The office of the early intervention coordinator can then direct the health care professional to the local or district early intervention office.

Additional resources for families of young children with special needs are available at www.zerotothree.org. For additional reading, recommend the book *Children with Cerebral Palsy: A Parent's Guide* by E. Geralis (published by Woodbine House).

Acquired Neuromuscular Disorders

A number of neuromuscular disorders may be acquired during childhood or adolescence. These include disorders resulting from trauma as well as those that are autoimmune and infectious in nature. Trauma or unintentional injury is a leading cause of childhood morbidity and mortality in the United States. Injuries are the leading cause of death in children younger than 1 year of age and account for a significant percentage of childhood morbidity. The child is at increased risk for trauma based on the developmental factors of physical and emotional immaturity. The adolescent is at increased risk because of the normal adolescent belief of invincibility. The developing neuromuscular system, if injured, may be irreparable, so the injury may result in life-threatening or lifelong effects. Neuromuscular trauma includes spinal cord injury and birth trauma. Autoimmune neuromuscular disorders include Guillain-Barré syndrome, myasthenia gravis, and dermatomyositis. Botulism, though uncommon in developed countries, is an important neuromuscular disorder resulting from infection.

SPINAL CORD INJURY

Spinal cord injury is damage to the spinal cord that results in loss of function. Frequent causes are trauma, such as car accidents, falls, diving into shallow water, gunshot or stab wounds, sports injuries, child abuse, or birth injuries. Spinal cord injuries are relatively uncommon in children, but when they do occur they have a devastating impact on the child's physical and functional status, social and emotional development, and family functioning. More spinal cord injuries are seen in adolescents due to their increased incidence of accidents, particularly motor vehicle accidents.

Spinal cord injury is a medical emergency and immediate medical attention is required. Cervical traction is often used initially and surgical intervention is sometimes necessary. Ongoing medical treatment will be based on the child's age and overall health and the extent and location of the injury. Therapeutic management focuses on rehabilitation and prevention of complications. Spinal cord injury in children is managed similarly to that in adults.

Nursing Assessment

Symptoms vary based on the location and severity of the injury. Common signs and symptoms associated with spinal cord injury include:

- Inability to move or feel extremities
- Numbness
- Tingling
- Weakness

The higher the injury in the spinal cord, the more extensive the damage and the greater the loss of function. High cervical injury will result in damage to the phrenic nerve, which innervates the diaphragm. Damage to this nerve will leave the child unable to breathe without assistance. Paralysis depends on the location of the injury to the spinal cord.

The diagnosis of spinal cord injury is made by clinical signs and diagnostic tests, which may include x-rays, CT, and MRI.

Nursing Management

Any child who requires hospitalization due to trauma should be considered at risk for a spinal cord injury, and immobilization of the spine is essential until full evaluation of the injury is complete and spinal cord damage is ruled out. Nursing management will be similar to management of the adult with a spinal cord injury and will focus on optimizing mobility, promoting bladder and bowel management, promoting adequate nutritional status, preventing complications associated with extreme immobility such as contractures and muscle atrophy, managing pain, and providing support and education to the child and family. Refer to the myelomeningocele section of this chapter for information related to urinary and bowel elimination.

The nurse plays an important role not only in the acute care of children with spinal cord injury but also during rehabilitation. Recovery from a spinal cord injury requires long-term hospitalization and rehabilitation. An interdisciplinary team of physicians, nurses, therapists, social workers, and case managers will work to manage the child's complex and long-term needs. Promoting communication among the interdisciplinary team is essential and will be a key nursing function. Rehabilitation will need to focus on the ever-changing developmental needs of the child as he or she grows.

Prevention of spinal cord injuries is an important nursing consideration. Educate the public on vehicular safety, including seat belt use and the proper use of age-appropriate safety seats. Additional education topics include bicycle, sports, and recreation safety, prevention of falls, violence prevention including gun safety, and water safety, including the risk of diving. This education can help decrease the incidence of spinal cord injury in children.

BIRTH TRAUMA

Birth traumas are injuries sustained by the newborn during the birthing process. They may result from the pressure of birth, especially in a prolonged or abrupt labor, abnormal or difficult presentation, cephalopelvic disproportion, or mechanical forces, such as forceps or vacuum used during delivery. Newborns at risk include multiple fetus deliveries, large-for-dates infants, extreme prematurity, large fetal head, or newborns with congenital anomalies. Most injuries are minor and resolve without treatment (Table 23.4).

Nursing Assessment

Assess the eyes and face for facial paralysis, observing for asymmetry of the face with crying or appearance of the

Table 23.4 Common Types of Neuromuscular Birth Trauma

Types	Description
Brachial plexus injury	• Primarily in large babies, babies with shoulder dystocia, or breech delivery • Results from stretching, hemorrhage within a nerve, or tearing of the nerve or the roots associated with cervical cord injury • Associated traumatic injuries include fracture of the clavicle or humerus or subluxations of the shoulder or cervical spine. • Erb's palsy is an upper brachial plexus injury, and the involved extremity usually presents adducted, prone, and internally rotated. • Moro, bicep, and radial reflexes are absent, but the grasp reflex is usually present. • Treatment consists of prevention of contractures, which involves immobilization of the limb gently across the abdomen for the first week and then the use of passive range-of-motion exercises. • There is usually no associated sensory loss, and this condition usually improves rapidly. • In some cases deficits persist, so observation is warranted.
Cranial nerve injury	• Most common is facial nerve palsy. • Frequently attributed to pressure resulting from forceps • May also result from pressure on the nerve *in utero*, related to fetal positioning such as the head lying against the shoulder • Physical findings include asymmetry of the face when crying; mouth may be drawn toward the normal side. • The paralyzed side may be smooth, with a swollen appearance. • Most infants begin to recover in the first week, but full resolution may take up to several months. • In most cases, treatment is not necessary, only observation. • In cases in which the eye is affected and unable to close, protection with the use of patches and synthetic tears may be necessary.

mouth being drawn to the unaffected side. Ensure that the infant spontaneously moves all extremities. Note any absence of or decrease in deep tendon reflexes or abnormal positioning of extremities.

Nursing Management

Nursing management will be mainly supportive and will focus on assessing for resolution of the trauma or any associated complications, along with providing support and education to the parents. Provide parents with explanation and reassurance that these injuries are harmless. Parents are alarmed when their newborn cannot move an extremity or demonstrates asymmetric facial movement. Reassure parents and offer support. Provide parents with education regarding the length of time until resolution and when and if they need to seek further medical attention for the condition.

● GUILLAIN-BARRÉ SYNDROME

Guillain-Barré syndrome (also called acute inflammatory demyelinating polyradiculoneuropathy or polyneuropathy) is an uncommon disorder in which an immune response within the body attacks the peripheral nervous system but does not usually affect the brain or spinal cord. Guillain-Barré syndrome results in inflammation and demyelinization of the peripheral nerves. It is not fully understood why this occurs, but it is believed to be an autoimmune condition that most commonly is triggered by a previous viral or bacterial infection, usually described as an influenza-like upper respiratory tract infection or an acute gastroenteritis with fever. In rare cases it has occurred after the patient has had an immunization. Box 23.2 lists antecedent infections and events. In most cases the causative agent remains unidentified.

Therapeutic Management

Treatment of Guillain-Barré syndrome is symptomatic and focuses on lessening the severity and speeding recovery. Plasma exchange and administration of intravenous immunoglobulins may occur, especially in severe cases. The goal of treatment is to keep the body functioning until the nervous system recovers. Guillain-Barré syndrome is a life-threatening condition, and some children will die during the acute phase due to respiratory failure. Most children will make a full recovery, but a few may have residual damage.

BOX 23.2

ANTECEDENT INFECTIONS AND EVENTS RELATED TO GUILLAIN-BARRÉ SYNDROME

Viral infections

- Cytomegalovirus
- Epstein-Barr virus
- Herpes virus
- Human immunodeficiency virus

Bacterial infections

- *Mycoplasma pneumoniae*
- Typhoid
- Paratyphoid
- Tuberculosis

Events

- Post–rabies vaccine and swine influenza vaccine
- Post–combined diphtheria, pertussis, and tetanus vaccine (DPT)
- Post–rubella, tetanus, cholera and typhoid vaccines

Data from Joseph, S. A., & Tsao, C. (2002). Guillain-Barré syndrome [electronic version]. *Adolescent Medicine, 13*(3), 487. Retrieved 6/28/04 from Proquest database.

Nursing Assessment

Early diagnosis and prompt treatment are essential since the disorder can quickly lead to respiratory failure and death from muscle paralysis. For a full description of the assessment phase of the nursing process, refer to page 762. Assessment findings pertinent to Guillain-Barré syndrome are discussed below.

Health History

Elicit a description of the present illness and chief complaint. The clinical presentation is fairly similar in children and adults. It can occur a few days or weeks after the causative infection or event. Guillain-Barré syndrome has a quick onset and begins with muscle weakness and paresthesias such as numbness and tingling. Classically it initially affects the legs and progresses in an ascending manner. Occasionally it affects the arms or face first and proceeds in a descending manner. Progression is usually complete in 2 to 4 weeks, followed by a stable period leading to the recovery phase, which lasts for a few weeks to months in most cases but can take years. Severity of the disorder ranges from mild weakness to total paralysis.

In children, pain, especially of the lower extremities, as the initial presentation preceding motor involvement has been reported. Other symptoms seen during the course of the illness include:

- Fairly symmetrical flaccid weakness or paralysis
- Ataxia
- Sensory disturbances

Physical Examination and Laboratory and Diagnostic Tests

Physical examination findings may include decreased or absent tendon reflexes. Facial weakness or difficulty swallowing may also be present. Diagnosis is usually based on clinical findings of paralysis. CSF analysis may reveal an increased level of protein, but this may not be evident until after the first week of the illness.

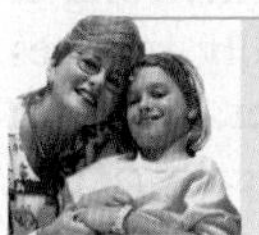

Tickling may be a successful technique for assessing the level of paralysis in the child with Guillain-Barré syndrome, either initially or in the recovery phase.

Nursing Management

Nursing management is supportive. In severe cases the child may require intensive nursing care along with mechanical ventilation. Observe the child closely for the extent of paralysis and monitor for respiratory involvement. Nursing care focuses on the same concerns as in any patient with extreme immobility or paralysis.

Prevention of complications associated with immobility is a central concern and involves maintaining skin integrity, preventing respiratory complications and contractures, maintaining adequate nutrition, and managing pain. Interventions include turning and repositioning every 2 hours, assessing the skin for redness or breakdown, performing range-of-motion exercises, keeping the skin clean and dry, encouraging intake of fluids to maintain hydration status, and encouraging coughing and deep breathing every 2 hours and as needed. Enteral feeding or parenteral nutrition may be indicated if swallowing becomes impaired. Physical therapy may be helpful in preventing complications and promoting motor skill recovery. Provide support and education to the parent and child. The rapid onset and long recovery can be difficult and can cause strain on the family and its finances. If residual disability occurs, the family will need help adjusting and caring for their child.

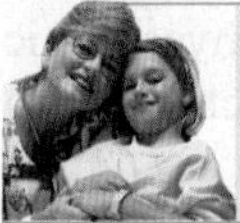

Serial measurement of tidal volumes may reveal respiratory deterioration in the child with Guillain-Barré syndrome.

● MYASTHENIA GRAVIS

Myasthenia gravis is an autoimmune disease that may be triggered by a viral or bacterial infection or by the thymus gland. The acetylcholine receptor at the neuromuscular junction is affected, inhibiting normal neuromuscular transmission. The result is progressive weakness and fatigue of the skeletal muscles. Though no gene has been discovered as responsible for myasthenia gravis, autoimmune diseases do demonstrate a genetic predisposition. Myasthenia gravis occurs in three forms: neonatal, congenital, and acquired.

Therapeutic management generally involves the use of anticholinesterase medications such as pyridostigmine, which blocks the breakdown of acetylcholine at the neuromuscular junction. Additional medications may include corticosteroids and other immunosuppressants, plasmapheresis, intravenous immunoglobulin, and, in children who have reached puberty, thymectomy (Armstrong & Schumann, 2003). Myasthenia gravis usually reaches maximum severity within 1 to 3 years of onset, and with proper treatment children can remain physically active (Muscular Dystrophy Association, 2006d). It may be aggravated by stress, exposure to extreme temperatures, and infections, resulting in a myasthenic crisis.

Nursing Assessment

Note history of fatigue and weakness; difficulty chewing, swallowing, or holding up the head; or pain with muscle fatigue. In the verbal child, note complaints of double vision. Observe the child for ptosis (droopy eyelids) or altered eye movements from partial paralysis. The neonate may display inadequate suck, weak cry, floppy extremities, and, possibly, respiratory insufficiency. Note increased work of breathing. Laboratory testing may involve the edrophonium (Tensilon) test, in which a short-acting cholinesterase inhibitor is used. Acetylcholine receptor (AchR) antibodies may be present in elevated quantities in the serum.

Nursing Management

Administer anticholinergic or other medications as ordered, teaching children and families about the use of these drugs. Anticholinergic drugs should be given 30 to 45 minutes before meals, on time and exactly as ordered. Encourage families to seek prompt medical treatment for suspected infections. Encourage appropriate stress management and avoidance of extreme temperatures. Teach families that physical activities should be performed during times of peak energy; rest periods are needed for energy conservation. Teach families to call their neurologist immediately if signs and symptoms of myasthenic crisis or cholinergic crisis appear. Encourage children to wear a medical alert bracelet.

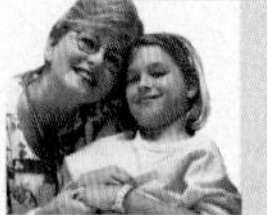

Signs and symptoms of myasthenic crisis include severe muscle weakness, respiratory difficulty, tachycardia, and dysphagia. Signs and symptoms of cholinergic crisis include severe muscle weakness, sweating, increased salivation, bradycardia, and hypotension.

• DERMATOMYOSITIS

Dermatomyositis is an autoimmune disease that results in inflammation of the muscles or associated tissues. It occurs more often in girls and is generally diagnosed between the ages of 5 and 14 years. The autoimmune response may be triggered by exposure to a virus or to certain medications. As with other autoimmune diseases, a genetic predisposition is present. The inflammatory cells of the immune system cause a vasculitis that affects the skin, muscles, kidneys, retinas, and gastrointestinal tract.

Therapeutic management involving the use of corticosteroids or other immunosuppressants is necessary to prevent the complications of painful calcium deposits under the skin, as well as joint contractures. With appropriate treatment, children may recover completely, though some children experience relapses (Muscular Dystrophy Association, 2006a).

Nursing Assessment

Elicit a health history, which commonly involves history of fever, fatigue, and rash, usually followed by muscle pain and weakness. Determine onset and progression of muscle weakness. Inspect the skin for presence of rash involving the upper eyelids and extensor surfaces of the knuckles, elbows, and knees. The rash is initially a reddish-purplish color, and then progresses to scaling with resulting roughness of the skin. Test muscle strength, noting particularly weakness in the pelvic and shoulder girdles. Laboratory and diagnostic testing may include muscle enzyme levels, a positive ANA test, and an electromyelogram to distinguish muscular weakness from other causes.

Nursing Management

Administer medications as ordered and teach families about their use; instruct them to monitor for side effects. Educate the family about the importance of maintaining the medication regimen in order to prevent calcinosis (calcium deposits) and joint deformity in the future. Encourage compliance with physical therapy regimens. Ensure that children are excused from physical education classes while the disease is active.

• BOTULISM

Botulism is a disease that is caused by a toxin produced in the immature intestines of young children resulting from infection with the bacterium *Clostridium botulinum.* It is rare but can cause serious paralytic illness. Botulism is mainly a food-borne infection but can also be contracted through wound infections or intestinal infections in infants. *C. botulinum* is common in soil and can also be found in a variety of foods, such as improperly preserved home-canned foods. It generally occurs in infants less than 6 months of age. It has been associated with feeding honey and corn syrup to infants; thus, these should be avoided in children less than 1 year of age. The disease is not infectious; to become infected, the child must ingest the bacterial spores. These spores then multiply in the intestinal tract and produce the toxin, which is absorbed in the immature intestines of the infant. It is generally not a problem for older children because the bacteria do not grow well in mature intestines due to the presence of the normal intestinal flora. Prognosis is good, but if treatment is not initiated, paralysis of the arms, legs, trunk, and respiratory system can develop. Therapeutic management is usually supportive but may involve administration of botulinum toxin.

Nursing Assessment

For a full description of the assessment phase of the nursing process, refer to page 762. Assessment findings pertinent to botulism are discussed below.

Health History

Elicit a description of the present illness and chief complaint. Signs and symptoms usually occur soon after ingestion of the bacteria. Common signs and symptoms in infants reported during the health history might include:

- Constipation
- Poor feeding
- Listlessness
- Generalized weakness
- Weak cry

Common signs and symptoms in older children reported during the health history might include:

- Double vision
- Blurred vision
- Drooping eyelids
- Difficulty swallowing
- Slurred speech
- Muscle weakness

Physical Examination and Laboratory and Diagnostic Tests

Assess for a diminished gag reflex, which is indicative of botulism. Diagnostic tests include cultures of stool and serum. Botulism is a rare disease and is difficult to diagnose since its symptoms are similar to those of other neuromuscular diseases. Therefore, assessment may include diagnostic tests to help rule out other diseases, such as Guillain-Barré syndrome, stroke, and myasthenia gravis.

Nursing Management

Treatment is mainly supportive and focuses on maintaining respiratory status and nutritional status. If ordered, administer botulinum toxin early in the disease to reduce its severity and progression.

References

Books and Journals

Anonymous (2003). Botulism—information from the World Health Organization [Electronic Version]. *Journal of Environmental Health, 65*(9), 51–53. Retrieved 6/18/04 from Proquest database.

Armstrong, S. M., & Schumann, L. (2003). Myasthenia gravis: Diagnosis and treatment. *Journal of the American Academy of Nurse Practitioners, 15*(2), 72–78.

Bach, J. R., & Bianchi, C. (2003). Prevention of pectus excavatum for children with spinal muscular atrophy type I. *Orthopedics, 82*(10), 815–819.

Bach, J. R., Vega, J., Majors, J., & Friedman, A. (2003). Spinal muscular atrophy type 1 quality of life. *American Journal of Physical Medicine and Rehabilitation, 82(*2), 137–142.

Bakker, J. P. J., de Groot, I. J. M., Beelen, A., & Lankhorst, G. J. (2002). Predictive factors of cessation of ambulation in patients with Duchenne muscular dystrophy. *American Journal of Physical Medicine & Rehabilitation, 81*(12), 906–912.

Balaban, B., Matthews, D. J., Clayton, G. H., & Carry, T. (2005). Corticosteroid treatment and functional improvement in Duchenne muscular dystrophy: Long-term effect. *American Journal of Physical Medicine and Rehabilitation, 84,* 843–850.

Bankhead, R. W., Kropp, B. P., & Cheng, E. Y. (2000). Evaluation and treatment of children with neurogenic bladders. *Journal of Child Neurology, 15*(3), 141–149.

Behrman, R. E., Kliegman, R. M., & Jenson, H. B. (2004). *Nelson's textbook of pediatrics* (17th ed.). Philadelphia: Saunders.

Blann, L. E. (2005). Early intervention for children and their families with special needs. *Maternal Child Nursing, 30*(4), 263–267.

Carter, G. T., & McDonald, C. M. (2000). Preserving function in Duchenne dystrophy with long-term pulse prednisone therapy. *American Journal of Physical Medicine & Rehabilitation, 79*(5), 455–458.

Chen, J., Chen, S., Jong, Y., Yang, Y., & Chang, Y. (2002). A comparison of the stress and coping strategies between the parents of children with Duchenne muscular dystrophy and children with fever. *Journal of Pediatric Nursing, 17*(5), 369–379.

Cooley, W. C. (2004). Providing a primary care medical home for children and youth with cerebral palsy. *Pediatrics, 114*(4), 1106–1113.

Cotton, S. M., Voudouris, N. J., & Greenwood, K. M. (2005). Association between intellectual functioning and age in children and young adults with Duchenne muscular dystrophy: Further results from a meta-analysis. *Developmental Medicine and Child Neurology, 47*(4), 257–265.

Emory University School of Medicine, Department of Pediatrics. (2005). Baclofen pump implants (intrathecal): Home care. Available online at www.pediatrics.emory.edu/NEURO/bacinfo1.htm.

Griffin, H. C., Fitch, C. L., & Griffin, L. W. (2002). Causes and interventions in the area of cerebral palsy [electronic version]. *Infants and Young Children, 14*(3), 18–24. Retrieved 6/25/04 from Proquest database.

Gomez-Merino, E., & Bach, J. R. (2002). Duchenne muscular dystrophy: Prolongation of life by noninvasive ventilation and mechanically assisted coughing. *American Journal of Physical Medicine & Rehabilitation, 81*(6), 411–415.

Halsted, M. J., & Jones, B. V. (2002). Pediatric neuroimaging for the pediatrician. *Pediatric Annals, 31*(10), 661–670.

Hernandez-Diaz, S., Werler, M. M., Walker, A. M., & Mitchell, A. A. (2001) Neural tube defects in relation to use of folic acid antagonists during pregnancy [electronic version]. *American Journal of Epidemiology, 153*(10), 961. Retrieved 6/22/04 from Proquest database.

Hobdell, E. (2001). Infant neurologic assessment [electronic version]. *Journal of Neuroscience Nursing, 33*(4), 190–194. Retrieved 5/17/04 from Proquest database.

Hollister, J. R. (2005). Rheumatic diseases. In W. W. Hay, M. J. Levin, J. M. Sondheimer, & R. R. Deterding (Eds.), *Current pediatric diagnosis & treatment* (17th ed.). New York: McGraw-Hill.

Ioos, C., Leclair-Richard, D., Mrad, S., Barois, A., & Estournet-Mathiaud, B. (2004). Respiratory capacity course in patients with infantile spinal muscular atrophy. *Chest, 126*(3), 831–837.

Jobe, A. H. (2002). Fetal surgery for myelomeningocele [electronic version]. *New England Journal of Medicine, 347*(4), 230–231. Retrieved 6/20/04 from Proquest database.

Joseph, S. A., & Tsao, C. (2002). Guillain-Barré syndrome [electronic version]. *Adolescent Medicine, 13*(3), 487. Retrieved 6/28/04 from Proquest database.

Kaplan, M. S. (2003). Impact of repeated surgical procedures on the incidence and prevalence of latex allergy: A prospective study of 1263 children [electronic version]. *Pediatrics, 112*(2), 463. Retrieved 6/20/04 from Proquest database.

Koman, L. A., Smith, B. P., & Shilt, J. S. (2004). Cerebral palsy [electronic version]. *Lancet, 363*(9421), 1619–1632. Retrieved 6/23/04 from Proquest database.

Komelasky, A. (2005). Pediatric neurologic disorders. In S. M. Nettina (Ed.), *Lippincott manual of nursing practice.* Philadelphia: Lippincott Williams & Wilkins.

Lee, L., Chuang, Y., Yang, B., Hsus, M., & Liu, Y. (2004). Botulinum toxin for lower limb spasticity in children with cerebral palsy. *American Journal of Physical Medicine & Rehabilitation, 83*(10), 766–773.

Merereau, P., Kilker, K., Carter, H., Fassett, E., et al. (2004). Spina bifida and anencephaly before and after folic acid mandate—United States, 1995–1996 and 1999–2000 [electronic version]. *Morbidity and Mortality Weekly Report, 53*(17), 362–365. Retrieved 6/19/04 from Proquest database.

Moe, P. G., & Benke, T. A. (2005) Neurologic and muscular disorders. In W. W. Hay, M. J. Levin, J. M. Sondheimer, & R. R. Deterding (Eds.), *Current pediatric diagnosis & treatment* (17th ed.). New York: McGraw-Hill.

Morantz, C., & Torrey, B. (2004). Immunotherapy in patients with Guillain-Barré syndrome [electronic version]. *American Family Physician, 69*(4), 997–999.

Muscular Dystrophy Association. (2006a). *Dermatomyositis.* Retrieved April 8, 2007 from http://www.mda.org/disease/pmdm-d.html.

Muscular Dystrophy Association. (2006b). *Duchenne muscular dystrophy (DMD).* Retrieved April 8, 2007 from http://www.mda.org/disease/dmd.html.

Muscular Dystrophy Association. (2006c). *Facts about spinal muscular atrophy (SMA).* Retrieved April 8, 2007 from http://www.mda.org/publications/fa-sma-qa.html.

Muscular Dystrophy Association. (2006d). *Myasthenia gravis.* Retrieved April 8, 2007 from http://www.mda.org/disease/mg.html.

Pate, D. (2002). Spina bifida occulta [electronic version]. *Dynamic Chiropractic, 20*(14), 44. Retrieved 6/19/04 from Proquest database.

Rosenbaum, P. (2003). Cerebral palsy: What parents and doctors want to know. *British Medical Journal, 326,* 970–974.

Schlager, T. A., Clark, M., & Anderson, S. (2001). Effect of a single-use sterile catheter for each void on the frequency of bacteriuria in children with neurogenic bladder on intermittent catheterization for bladder emptying. *Pediatrics, 108,* 71–74.

Skelly, C. L., Jackson, C. A., Wu, Y., Hill, C. B., Chwals, W. J., & Liu, D. C. (2003). Thorascopic thymectomy in children with myasthenia gravis. *American Surgeon, 69*(12), 1087–1089.

Sterba, J. A. (2004). Effect of horseback riding therapy on Gross Motor Function Measure for each level of disability for children with cerebral palsy. *Developmental Medicine and Child Neurology, 46,* 47.

Sterba, J. A., Rogers, B. T., France, A. P., & Vokes, D. A. (2002). Horseback riding in children with cerebral palsy: Effect on gross motor function. *Developmental Medicine and Child Neurology, 44*(5), 301–308.

Tang, T., & Noble-Jamieson, C. N. (2001). A painful hip as a presentation of Guillain-Barré syndrome in children [electronic version]. *British Medical Journal, 322*(7279), 149. Retrieved 6/28/04 from Proquest database.

Zickler, C. F., & Richardson, V. (2004). Achieving continence in children with neurogenic bowel and bladder. *Journal of Pediatric Health Care, 18*(6), 276–283.

Websites

www.aacpdm.org/index American Academy for Cerebral Palsy and Developmental Medicine—multidisciplinary scientific society devoted to the study of cerebral palsy, focusing on improving quality of life

www.aascin.org/ American Association of Spinal Cord Injury Nurses

www.acf.dhhs.gov/programs/add Administration on Developmental Disabilities, Department of Health and Human Services

www.childrensdefense.org Children's Defense Fund

www.childrenwithdisabilities.ncjrs.org Children with Disabilities

www.cms-kids.com Children's Medical Services program—provides family-centered, multidisciplinary, case-managed care to children with special health care needs through age 21, coordinated through offices throughout the United States

www.cpconnection.com Cerebral Palsy Connection—network for parents of children with cerebral palsy

www.familiesusa.org Families USA

www.fscip.org Foundation for Spinal Cord Injury Prevention, Care & Cure

www.irsc.org Internet Resources for Special Children

www.marchofdimes.com March of Dimes—research to prevent birth defects.

www.mdac.ca Muscular Dystrophy Canada

www.mda.org/ Muscular Dystrophy Association—research, support, resources, education, regional multidisciplinary clinics throughout the United States

www.mdff.org/ Muscular Dystrophy Family Foundation—resources and assistance for families

www.nectas.org National Early Childhood Technical Assistance System

www.nicchy.org National Information Center for Children and Youth with Disabilities

www.parentprojectmd.org/ Parent Project Muscular Dystrophy—an organization for parents of boys with Duchenne and Becker muscular dystrophy, providing education, resources, research, and advocacy

www.sbaa.org/site/PageServer?pagename=index Spina Bifida Association—dedicated to improving the lives of children with spina bifida

www.sbhac.ca/index.php?page=main Spina Bifida and Hydrocephalus Association of Canada—resources and education

www.spinalcord.org/ National Spinal Cord Injury Association

www.spinalcord.uab.edu/ Spinal Cord Injury Information Network

www.spinalcordinjury.org Spinal Cord Injury Network International

www.spinalinjury.net/ Spinal Cord Injury Resource Center

www.ucp.org United Cerebral Palsy—research, resources, education

www.zerotothree.org Zero to Three

Chapter WORKSHEET

● MULTIPLE CHOICE QUESTIONS

1. A boy with Duchenne muscular dystrophy is admitted to the pediatric unit. He has an ineffective cough. Lung auscultation reveals diminished breath sounds. What is the priority nursing intervention?
   a. Apply supplemental oxygen.
   b. Notify the respiratory therapist.
   c. Monitor pulse oximetry.
   d. Position for adequate airway clearance.
2. A 7-year-old child with cerebral palsy has been admitted to the hospital. Which information is most important for the nurse to obtain in the history?
   a. Age that the child learned to walk
   b. Parents' expectations of the child's development
   c. Functional status related to eating and mobility
   d. Birth history to identify cause of cerebral palsy
3. The nurse is caring for a 2-year-old with myelomeningocele. When teaching about care related to neurogenic bladder, what response by the parent would indicate that additional teaching is required?
   a. "Routine catheterization will decrease the risk of infection from urine staying in the bladder."
   b. "I know it will be important for me to catheterize my child for the rest of her life."
   c. "I will make sure that I always use latex-free catheters."
   d. "I will wash the catheter with warm soapy water after each use."
4. The nurse is caring for a child with cerebral palsy who requires a wheelchair to attain mobility. Which intervention would help the child achieve a sense of normality?
   a. Encourage follow-through with physical therapy exercises.
   b. Restrict the child to a special needs classroom.
   c. Encourage after-school activities within the limits of the child's abilities.
   d. Ensure the school is aware of the child's capabilities.
5. What is the priority nursing intervention for the child recently admitted with Guillain-Barré syndrome?
   a. Perform range-of-motion exercises.
   b. Take temperature every 4 hours.
   c. Monitor respiratory status closely.
   d. Assess skin frequently.

● CRITICAL THINKING EXERCISES

1. A 5-year-old girl, diagnosed with myelomeningocele, is admitted to the hospital for a corrective surgical procedure. Choose four questions from below that the nurse should ask when obtaining the health history that would assist in planning the child's care.
   a. What is the child's current mobility status?
   b. Is there a family history of myelomeningocele?
   c. What is the child's genitourinary and bowel function and regimen?
   d. Does this child have a history of hydrocephalus with presence of shunt?
   e. Does she have known latex sensitivity?
   f. Were there any complications during the pregnancy or birth of this child?
   g. Did the mother take prenatal folic acid supplementation?
2. Based on the case in the above question, develop a nursing care plan for the child with myelomeningocele.
3. A 5-year-old child is admitted to the pediatric unit with a history of cerebral palsy sustained at birth. The child is admitted for a scheduled tendon lengthening procedure. Based on your knowledge about the effects of cerebral palsy, list three priorities to focus on when planning her care. Compare this to a child admitted for surgical correction of a broken femur with no significant past medical history.

● STUDY ACTIVITIES

1. In the clinical setting, compare the growth of a child with muscular dystrophy, spinal muscular atrophy, or cerebral palsy to the growth of a similar-age child who has been healthy. What differences or similarities do you find? What are the explanations for your findings?
2. Identify the role of the registered nurse in the multidisciplinary care of the child with a debilitating neuromuscular disorder.
3. In the clinical setting, interview the parent of a child with Duchenne muscular dystrophy, myelomeningocele, spinal muscular atrophy, or severe cerebral palsy. Determine the parent's feelings about the ongoing care that he or she is responsible for. Reflect upon this interview in your clinical journal.
4. In the clinical setting, compare the cognitive abilities of two children with a severe neuromuscular disorder. What are the reasons for the similarities or differences that you find?

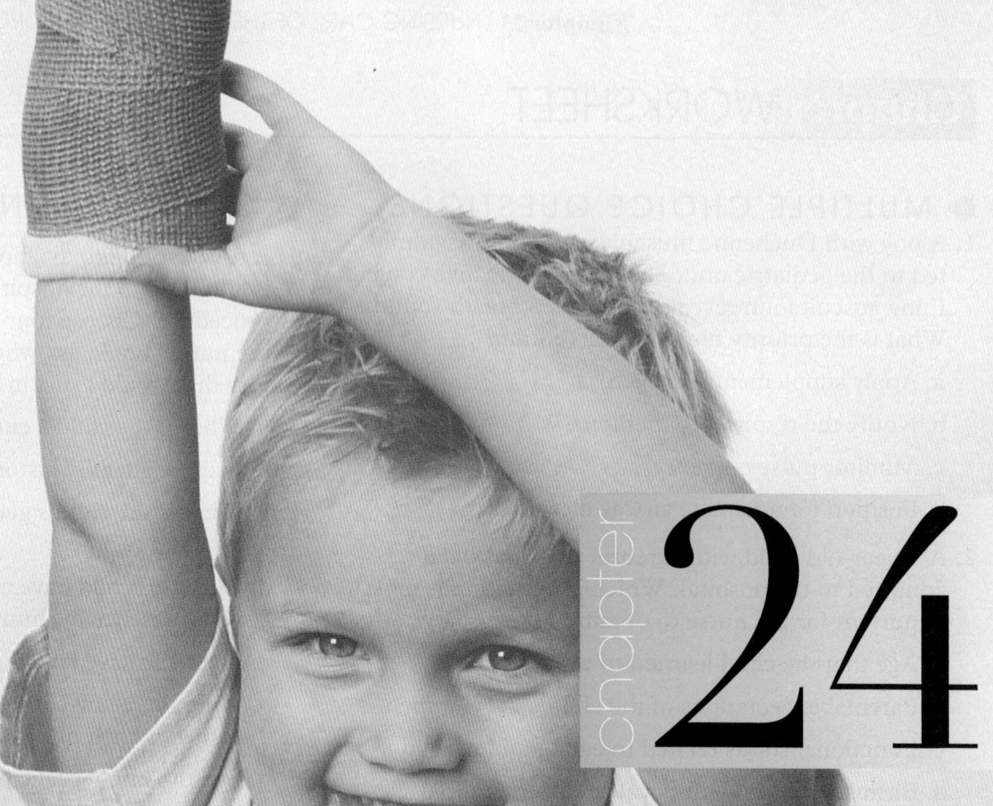

chapter 24

Nursing Care of the Child With a Musculoskeletal Disorder

Key TERMS

compartment syndrome
distraction
epiphysis
external fixation
immobilize
kyphosis
lordosis
ossification
splint
traction
Trendelenburg gait

Learning OBJECTIVES

Upon completion of the chapter, the learner will be able to:

1. Compare the anatomy and physiology of the musculoskeletal system in children versus adults.
2. Identify nursing interventions related to common laboratory and diagnostic tests used in the diagnosis and management of musculoskeletal disorders.
3. Identify appropriate nursing assessments and interventions related to medications and treatments for common childhood musculoskeletal disorders.
4. Distinguish various musculoskeletal disorders occurring in childhood.
5. Devise an individualized nursing care plan for the child with a musculoskeletal disorder.
6. Develop patient/family teaching plans for the child with a musculoskeletal disorder.
7. Describe the psychosocial impact of chronic musculoskeletal disorders on the growth and development of children.

WOW *Nursing care that heals children to take wobbly steps, run, jump, fall, and get up again provides life itself in a child's world.*

Dakota Dawes, 2 years old, is brought to the clinic by his mother. She states, "Last night Dakota said his arm hurt, but he didn't have any complaints during the day. Today when he was playing I noticed he wasn't using his right arm."

A variety of musculoskeletal disorders may affect children, but the result of each is motor dysfunction. Understanding the most common responses to these disorders gives the nurse the foundation required to plan care for any child with any musculoskeletal disorder.

Variations in Pediatric Anatomy and Physiology

Musculoskeletal disorders in children may occur as a congenital malformation or a genetic disorder that is present from birth but may not be identified until later in childhood or adolescence. Some disorders are developmental; others result from trauma. The infant and young child has resilient soft tissue, so sprains and strains are less common in this age group. Older school-age children and adolescents often participate in sports, resulting in an increased risk of injuries such as sprains, fractures, and torn ligaments. The musculoskeletal system in infants and children is immature compared with adults; thus, when a musculoskeletal problem occurs in childhood, the child's growth may be hindered. The immobility associated with most musculoskeletal disorders may affect the child's development and acquisition of motor skills.

Myelinization

Myelinization of the central nervous system continues to progress after birth and is complete by about 2 years of age. Myelinization proceeds in a cephalocaudal and proximal–distal fashion, allowing voluntary muscle control to progress as myelinization occurs. As myelinization proceeds, the speed and accuracy of nerve impulses increase. Primitive reflexes are replaced with voluntary movement.

Muscle Development

The muscular system, including tendons, ligaments, and cartilage, arises from the mesoderm in early embryonic development. At birth (term or preterm), the muscles, tendons, ligaments, and cartilage are all present and functional. The newborn infant is capable of spontaneous movement but lacks purposeful control. Full range of motion is present at birth. Healthy infants and children demonstrate normal muscle tone. As the infant matures and becomes mobile, the muscles develop further and become stronger and their mass increases. The infant's muscles account for approximately 25% of total body weight, as compared with the adult's muscle mass, which accounts for about 40% of total body weight. Muscles grow rapidly in adolescence; this contributes to clumsiness, which places the teen at increased risk for injury. In response to testosterone release, the adolescent boy experiences a growth spurt, particularly in the trunk and legs, and develops bulkier muscles. Female infants tend to have laxer ligaments than male infants, possibly due to the presence of female hormones, placing them at increased risk for developmental dysplasia of the hip.

Skeletal Development

The infant's skeleton is not fully ossified at birth. The skeleton contains increased amounts of cartilage compared with adolescents and adults. The infant and young child's bones are more flexible and more porous and have a lower mineral content than the adult's. These structural differences of a young child's bones allow for greater shock absorption, so the bones will often bend rather than break when an injury occurs. The thick, strong periosteum of the child's bones allows for a greater absorption of force than is seen in adults. As a result, the cortex of the bone does not always break, sometimes buckling or bending only. **Ossification** and conversion of cartilage to bone continue throughout childhood and are complete at adolescence.

During fetal development the spine displays **kyphosis**. Cervical **lordosis** develops as the infant starts to hold the head up. When the infant or toddler assumes an upright position, the primary and secondary curves of the spine begin to develop. The balance of the curves allows the head to be centered over the pelvis. During the toddler years, the period of early walking, lumbar lordosis may be significant (also termed toddler lordosis), and the toddler appears quite swaybacked and potbellied. As the child develops, the spine takes on more adult-like curves. During adolescence thoracic kyphosis may become evident. This is most often a postural effect, and as the teen matures, the posture appears similar to that of an adult.

Growth Plate

The ends of the bones in young children are composed of the **epiphysis** and the physis, in combination termed the growth plate. In infants, the epiphyses are cartilaginous and ossify over time. In children, the epiphysis is the secondary ossification center at the end of the bone. The physis is a cartilaginous area between the epiphysis and the metaphysis. Growth of the bones occurs primarily in the epiphyseal region. This area is vulnerable and structurally weak. Traumatic force applied to the epiphysis during injury may result in fracture in that area of the bone. Epiphyseal injury may result in early, incomplete, or partial closure of the growth plate, leading to deformity or shortening of the bone. Epiphyseal growth continues until skeletal maturity is reached during adolescence. Production of androgens in adolescence gradually causes the growth plates to fuse, and thus long bone growth is complete (Fig. 24.1).

Bone Healing

The child's bones have a thick, strong periosteum with an abundant blood supply. Bone healing occurs in the same fashion as in the adult, but because of the rich nutrient supply to the periosteum, it occurs more quickly in children. Children's bones produce callus more rapidly and in larger quantities than do adults'. As new bone cells quickly form, a bulge of new bone growth occurs at the site of the fracture. The younger the child, the more quickly the bone heals. Also, the closer the fracture is to the growth plate (epiphysis), the more quickly the fracture heals. The capacity for remodeling (the process of breaking down and forming new bone) is increased in children as compared with adults. This means that straightening of the bone over time occurs more easily in children.

Positional Alterations

The lower extremities of the infant tend to have a bowed appearance, attributed to *in utero* positioning. *In utero,* the fetus' hips are usually flexed, abducted, and externally rotated, with the knees also flexed and the lower limbs inwardly rotated (Fig. 24.2). This normal developmental variation is termed internal tibial torsion. The legs straighten with passive motion, and internal tibial torsion should not be confused with "bowlegs." Internal tibial torsion usually resolves independently some time in the second or third year of life as the toddler bears weight and the lower extremity muscles and bones mature. The bowlegged appearance is sometimes also referred to as genu varum. As internal tibial torsion or genu varum resolves, physiologic genu valgum occurs. Children usually demonstrate symmetric genu valgum (knock-knees) by the age of 2 to 3 years. In genu valgum, when the knees are touching the ankles are significantly separated, with the lower portion of the legs angled outward (Fig. 24.3). By age 7 or 8 years, genu valgum gradually resolves in most children.

The newborn's feet also display in-toeing (metatarsus adductus) as a result of *in utero* positioning (see Fig. 24.2). The feet remain flexible and may be passively moved to midline and in a straight position. This also resolves as the infant's musculoskeletal system matures. Pes planus (flat feet) is noted in infants when they begin to walk. The long arch of the foot is not yet developed and makes contact with the floor, resulting in a medial bulge. As the child

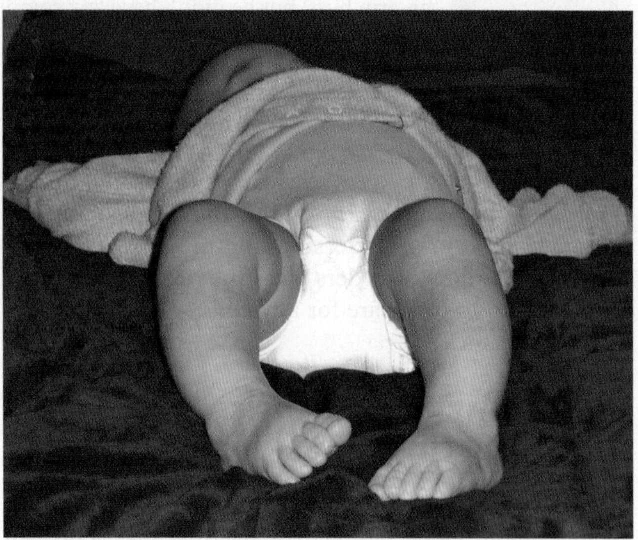

● Figure 24.2 Internal tibial torsion with metatarsus adductus—normal findings in the infant.

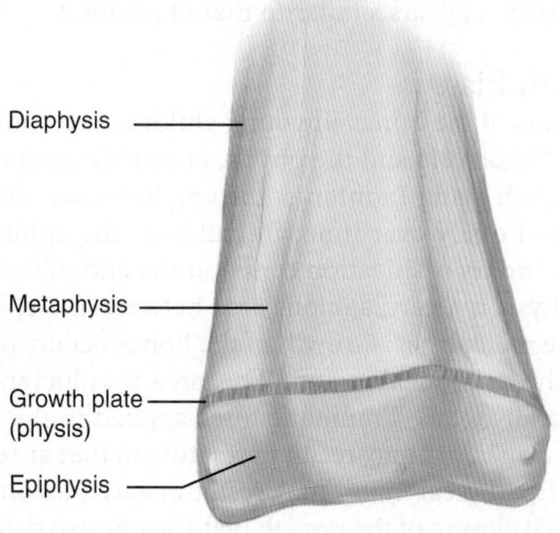

● Figure 24.1 Anatomic areas of growing bone.

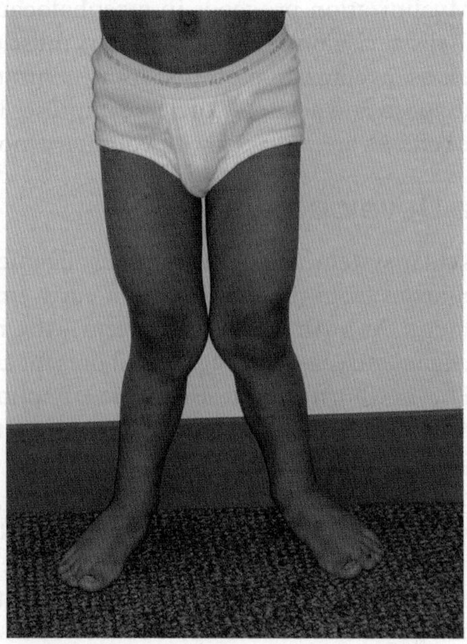

● Figure 24.3 Genu valgum (knock-knees): note knees touching at midline and outward angle of the lower half of the legs.

grows and the muscles become less lax, the arch generally develops. Some children may continue with flexible flat feet, and this is considered a normal variation.

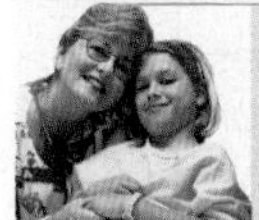

Fractures are rare in children less than 1 year of age. The infant who presents with a fracture should be carefully evaluated for child abuse or an underlying musculoskeletal disorder.

Common Medical Treatments

A variety of medications as well as other medical treatments are used to treat musculoskeletal disorders in children. Most of these treatments will require a physician's order when the child is in the hospital. The most common treatments and medications are listed in Common Medical Treatments 24.1 and Drug Guide 24.1. The nurse caring for the child with a musculoskeletal disorder should become familiar with what the procedures are, how they work, as well as common nursing implications related to use of these modalities. The treatment of musculoskeletal disorders often involves immobilization via casting, bracing, splinting, or traction to allow healing with the bones in appropriate alignment. The length of treatment with these immobilization methods varies from weeks to months depending on the type of disorder being treated and its severity. Complications related to casting and traction include neurovascular compromise, skin integrity impairment, soft tissue injury, **compartment syndrome**, and, with skeletal traction, pin site infection or osteomyelitis. The nursing care of immobilized children is similar to that of adults, yet develop-

Common Medical Treatments 24.1

Treatment	Explanation	Indication	Nursing Implications
Traction	Application of a pulling force on an extremity or body part	Fracture reduction, dislocations, correction of deformities	To maintain even, constant traction: • Ensure weights hang free at all times and ropes remain in the pulley grooves. • Keep weights out of child's reach. • Maintain prescribed weight. • Elevate head or foot of bed only with physician order. Monitor for complications: • Perform neurovascular checks at least every 4 hours. • Assess for skin impairment.
Casting	Application of plaster or fiberglass material to form a rigid apparatus to immobilize a body part	Fracture reduction, dislocations, correction of deformities	Assess frequently for neurovascular compromise, skin impairment at cast edges. Protect cast from moisture. Teach family how to care for cast at home.
Splinting	Temporary stiff support of injured area	Temporary fracture reduction, immobilization and support of sprains	Similar to cast care. Some splints are removable and are replaced when the child is up out of bed. Teach family appropriate use of splints.
Fixation	Surgical reduction of a fracture or skeletal deformity with an internal or external pin or fixation device	Fractures, skeletal deformities	No additional care for internal fixation. External fixation: perform pin care as prescribed by the surgeon. Assess for excess drainage or pin slippage, notifying physician if this occurs. Velcro or snaps on sleeves and pant legs help with dressing.

(continued)

Common Medical Treatments 24.1 (continued)

Treatment	Explanation	Indication	Nursing Implications
Cold therapy	Application of ice bags, commercial cold packs, or cold compresses	Most often used in acute injuries to cause vasoconstriction, thereby decreasing pain and swelling	Apply for 20 to 30 minutes, then remove for 1 hour, then reapply for 20 to 30 minutes. Discontinue when numbness occurs. Place a towel between the cold pack and the skin to prevent thermal injury.
Crutches	Ambulatory devices that transfer body weight from lower to upper extremities	Used whenever weight bearing is contraindicated	Top of crutch should reach 2 to 3 fingerbreadths below the axillae to prevent nerve palsy. Teach child appropriate ambulation with crutches or reinforce teaching if performed by physical therapist.
Physical therapy, occupational therapy	Physical therapy focuses on attainment or improvement of gross motor skills. Occupational therapy focuses on refinement of fine motor skills, feeding, and activities of daily living.	Restore function after injury or surgery; promote developmental activities when limb use is compromised, as in limb deficiency	Provide follow-through with prescribed exercises or supportive equipment. Success of therapy is dependent upon continued compliance with the prescribed regimen. Ensure adequate communication exists within the interdisciplinary team.
Orthotics, braces	Adaptive positioning devices specially fitted for each child by the physical or occupational therapist or orthotist. Used to maintain proper body or extremity alignment, improve mobility, and prevent contractures.	Used to immobilize a body part or prevent deformity through positioning. Used to treat developmental dysplasia of the hip and scoliosis; also may be used for a period of time after cast removal.	Provide frequent assessments of skin covered by the device to avoid skin breakdown. Cotton undergarment worn under the brace helps to maintain skin integrity. Follow the therapist's schedule of recommended "on" and "off" times. Encourage families to comply with use.

mental and age-appropriate effects must be taken into account. Prevention of complications is a key nursing function. Nursing Care Plan Overview 24.1 gives interventions related to prevention of complications. Particular care related to casts and traction is discussed below.

Casts

Casts are used to **immobilize** a bone that has been injured or a diseased joint. When a fracture has occurred, a cast serves to hold the bone in reduction, thus preventing deformity as the fracture heals. Casts are constructed of a hard material, traditionally plaster but now more commonly fiberglass. The hard nature of the cast keeps the bone aligned so that healing may occur more quickly. In a fracture that would heal on its own without specific immobilization, a cast may be used to reduce pain and to allow the child increased mobility. The choice of cast material and type of cast will be determined by the pediatrician or orthopedic surgeon. Table 24.1 shows selected casts used in children.

Cast Application

Before cast or splint application, perform baseline neurovascular assessment for comparison after immobilization. Include:

- Color (note cyanosis or other discoloration)
- Movement (note inability to move fingers or toes)
- Sensation (note whether loss of sensation is present)
- Edema
- Quality of pulses

Drug Guide 24.1 Common Drugs for Musculoskeletal Disorders

Medication	Action	Indication	Nursing Implications
Benzodiazepines (diazepam, lorazepam)	Antianxiety drugs that also have the effect of skeletal muscle relaxation	Treatment of muscle spasms associated with traction or casting	Monitor sedation level. May cause dizziness. Paradoxical excitement may occur. Assess for improvements in spasms.
Acetaminophen	Blocks pain impulses in response to inhibition of prostaglandin synthesis	Relief of mild pain if used alone, moderate or severe pain if used with a narcotic analgesic	Often combined with a narcotic such as codeine or oxycodone for increased analgesic effect. Monitor pain levels and response to medication.
Narcotic analgesics	Act on receptors in the brain to alter perception of pain	Relief of moderate to severe pain associated with injuries, orthopedic procedures	Assess pain location, quality, intensity, and duration. Assess respiratory rate prior to and periodically after administration. Monitor sedation level. May cause nausea, vomiting, constipation, pupil constriction.
Nonsteroidal anti-inflammatory drugs (NSAIDs: ibuprofen, ketorolac)	Inhibit prostaglandin synthesis, having a direct inhibitory effect on pain perception	Relief of mild to moderate pain. Treatment of Legg-Calvé-Perthes disease.	Monitor for nausea, vomiting, diarrhea, constipation. Administer with water or food to decrease GI upset.
Bisphosphonate: IV—pamidronate, zoledronic acid; oral—alendronate, risedronate	Increase bone mineral density	Decrease incidence of fractures in moderate to severe osteogenesis imperfecta	IV: given at 4-month intervals, causes a decrease in serum calcium level, influenza-like reaction with first IV dose. Oral: side effects include heartburn, regurgitation, upper abdominal discomfort.

Enlist the cooperation of the child and reduce his or her fear by showing the child the cast materials and using an age-appropriate approach to describe cast application. Premedicate as ordered to reduce pain when manual traction is applied to align the bone. Use **distraction** throughout cast application and assist with application of the cast or splint (Fig. 24.4).

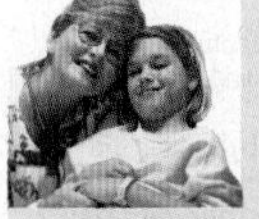

Modern fiberglass cast materials are available in a variety of colors, as well as a few patterns. Allowing the child to choose the color will increase the child's cooperation with the procedure.

After the cast or splint is applied, drying time will vary based on the type of material used. Splints and fiberglass casts usually take only a few minutes to dry and will cause a very warm feeling inside the cast, so warn the child that it will begin to feel very warm. Plaster requires 24 to 48 hours to dry. Take care not to cause depressions in the plaster cast while drying, as those may cause skin pressure and breakdown. Instruct the child and family to keep the cast still, positioning it with pillows as needed. Fiberglass casts usually have a soft fabric edge, so they usually do not cause skin rubbing at the edges of the cast. On the other hand, plaster casts require special treatment of the cast edge to prevent skin rubbing. This may be accomplished through a technique called petaling: cut rounded-edge strips of moleskin or another soft material with an adhesive backing and apply them to the edge of cast, as shown in Figure 24.5.

Table 24.1 Selected Casts Used in Children

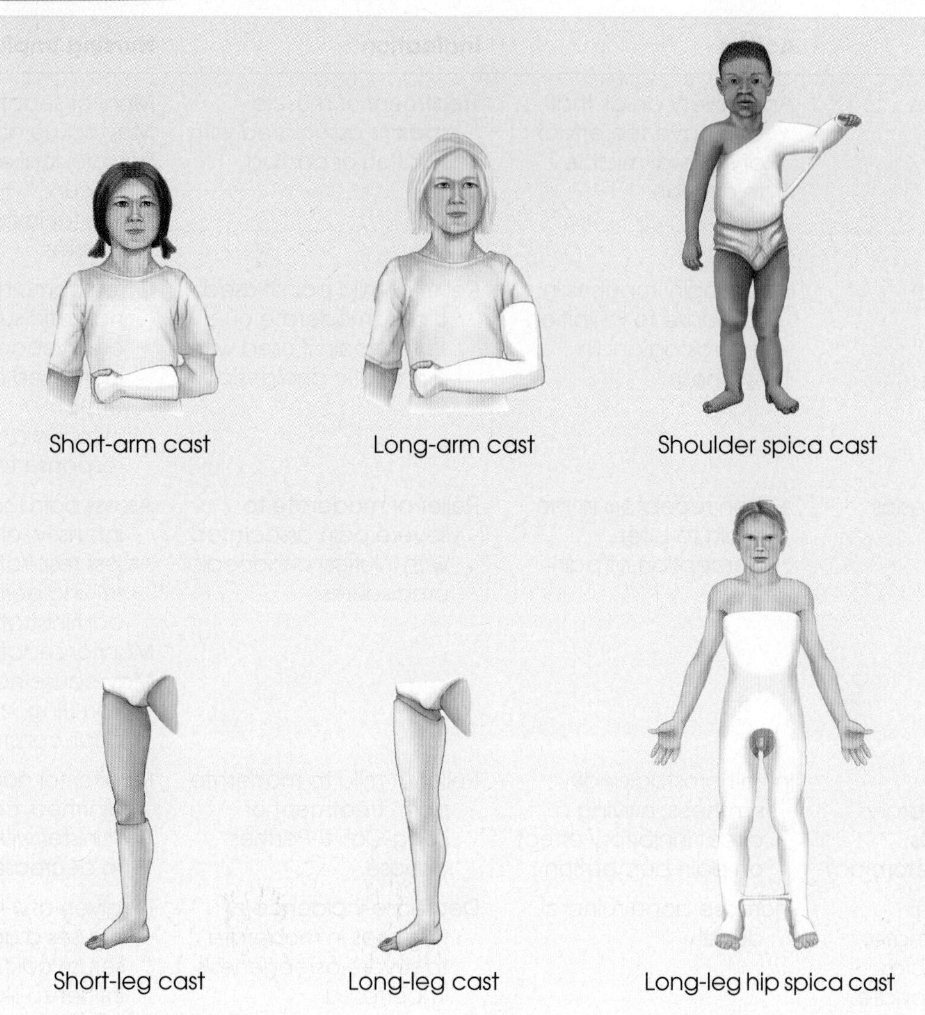

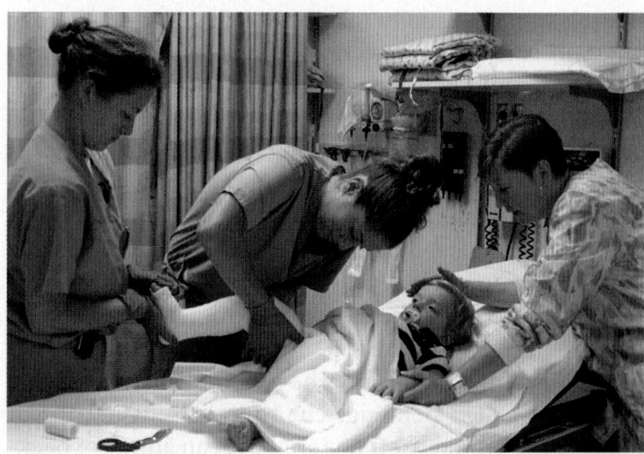

● Figure 24.4 Assist with cast application by distracting or comforting the child.

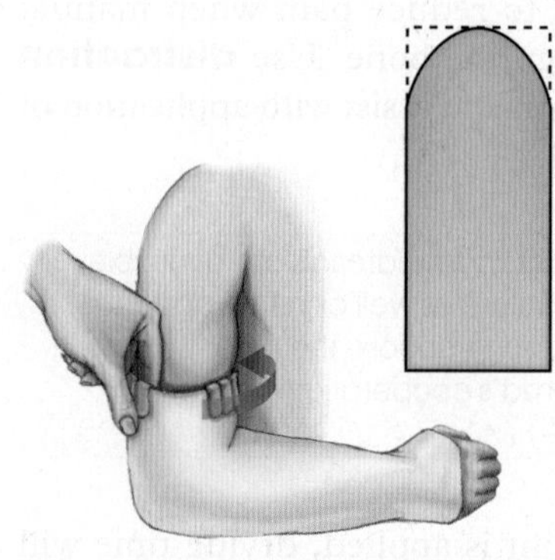

To petal a cast:
1. Cut several strips of adhesive tape or moleskin three to four inches in length. Use one inch tape for smaller areas (e.g., infant's foot) and two inch tape for larger areas (e.g., adolescent's waist).
2. Round one end of each strip to keep the corners from rolling.
3. Apply the first strip by tucking the straight end inside the cast and by bringing the rounded end over the cast edge to the outside.
4. Repeat the procedure, overlapping each additional strip, until all rough edges are completely covered.

● Figure 24.5 Petaling the cast.

Caring for the Child With a Cast

Perform frequent neurovascular checks of the casted extremity to identify signs of compromise early. These signs include:

- Increased pain
- Increased edema
- Pale or blue color
- Skin coolness
- Numbness or tingling
- Prolonged capillary refill
- Decreased pulse strength (or absence of pulse)

Notify the physician of changes in neurovascular status or odor or drainage from the cast.

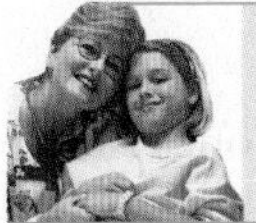

Persistent complaints of pain may indicate compromised skin integrity under the cast.

Position the child with the casted extremity elevated on pillows. Ice may be applied during the first 24 to 48 hours after casting if needed. Teaching the child to use crutches is an important nursing intervention for any child with lower extremity immobilization so that the child can maintain mobility (Fig. 24.6). Provide home care instructions to the family about cast care (Teaching Guideline 24.1).

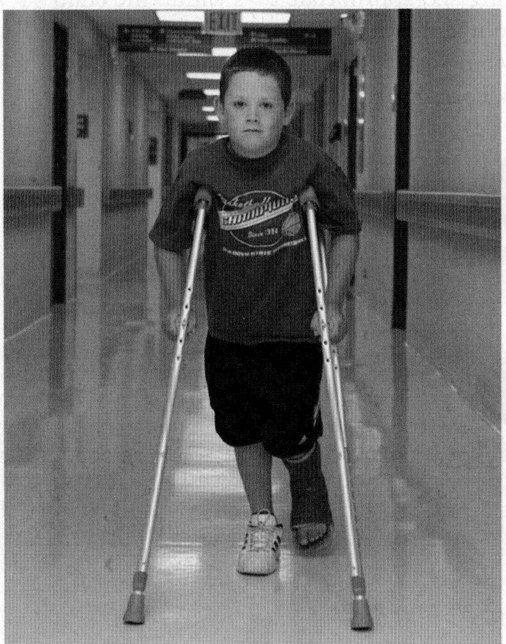

● **Figure 24.6** Reinforce appropriate crutch walking for children with lower extremity immobilization.

Assisting With Cast Removal

Children may be frightened by cast removal. Prepare the child using age-appropriate terminology:

- The cast cutter will make a loud noise (Fig. 24.7).
- The skin or extremity will not be injured (demonstrate by touching the cast cutter lightly to your palm).
- The child will feel warmth or vibration during cast removal.

Teaching Guideline 24.2 gives instructions related to skin care after cast removal.

Traction

Traction, another common method of immobilization, may be used to reduce and/or immobilize a fracture, to align an injured extremity, and to allow the extremity to be restored to its normal length. Traction may also reduce pain by decreasing the incidence of muscle spasm.

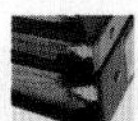

TEACHING GUIDELINE 24.1

Home Cast Care

- For the first 48 hours, elevate the extremity above the level of the heart and apply cold therapy for 20 to 30 minutes, then off 1 hour, and repeat.
- Assess for swelling, and have the child wiggle the fingers or toes hourly.
- For itching inside the cast:
  - Never insert anything into the cast for the purposes of scratching.
  - Blow cool air in from a hair dryer set on the lowest setting.
  - Do not use lotions or powders.
- Check the skin at the cast edges daily for irritation.
- Protect the cast from wetness.
- Apply a plastic bag around cast and tape securely for bathing or showering.
- Call the physician if:
  - The casted extremity is cool to the touch.
  - The child cannot move the fingers or toes.
  - Severe pain occurs when the child attempts to move the fingers or toes.
  - Persistent numbness or tingling occurs.
  - Drainage or a foul smell comes from under the cast.
  - Severe itching occurs inside the cast.
  - The child runs a fever greater than 101.5° F for longer than 24 hours.
  - Skin edges are red and swollen or exhibit breakdown.
  - The cast gets wet or is cracked, split, or softened.

Modified from DiFazio, R., & Atkinson, R. (2005). Extremity fractures in children: When is it an emergency? *Journal of Pediatric Nursing, 20*(4), 298–304.

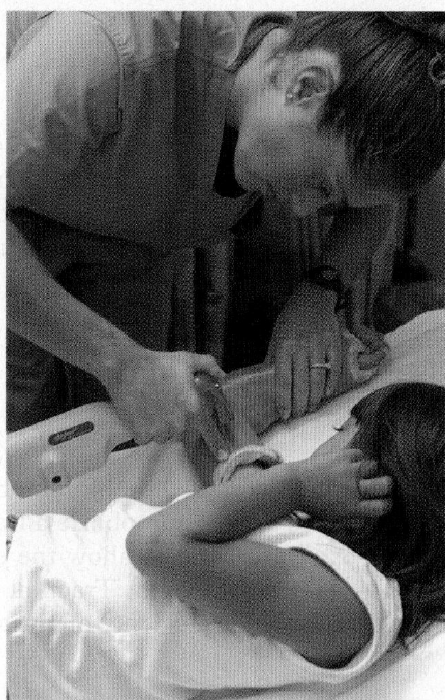

● Figure 24.7 The loud noise of the cast saw may frighten the child.

In running traction, the weight pulls directly on the extremity in only one plane. This may be achieved with either skin or skeletal traction. In balanced suspension traction, additional weights are used to provide a counterbalance to the force of traction. This allows for constant pull on the extremity even if the child changes position somewhat. Table 24.2 describes the various types of traction and nursing implications specific to each type. Comparison Chart 24.1 discusses skin versus skeletal traction.

Caring for the Child in Traction

Nursing care of the child in any type of traction focuses not only on appropriate application and maintenance of traction but also on promoting normal growth and development and preventing complications. Apply skin traction over intact skin only so that the pull of the traction is effective. Prepare the skin with an appropriate adhesive before applying the traction tapes to ensure that the tapes adhere well, preventing skin friction. After application of the traction tapes, apply the elastic bandage or use the foam boot. Attach the traction spreader block and then apply the prescribed amount of weight via a rope attached to the spreader block. Ensure that the rope moves without obstruction and that the weights hang freely without touching the floor.

In skeletal traction, apply weight via ropes attached to the skeletal pins. The pin sites should be treated as surgical wounds (see section on pin site care). Protect the exposed ends of the pins to avoid injury. Whether skin or skeletal traction is used, be sure that constant and even traction is maintained.

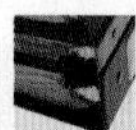

TEACHING GUIDELINE 24.2

Skin Care After Cast Removal

- Brown, flaky skin is normal and occurs as dead skin and secretions accumulate under the cast.
- Soak with warm water daily.
- Wash with warm soapy water, avoiding excessive rubbing, which may traumatize the skin.
- Discourage the child from scratching the dry skin.
- Apply moisturizing lotion to relieve dry skin.
- Encourage activity to regain strength and motion of extremity.

Preventing Complications

Refer to Nursing Care Plan 24.1 for interventions related to pain management and prevention of complications of immobility such as skin integrity impairment. To prevent contractures and atrophy that may result from disuse of muscles, ensure that unaffected extremities are exercised. Assist the child to exercise the unaffected joints and to use the unaffected extremity if this does not disrupt traction alignment. Promote use of a trapeze if not contraindicated to involve the child in repositioning and assist with movement. Encourage deep-breathing exercises to prevent the pulmonary complications of long-term immobilization.

Promote normal growth and development by:

- Placing age-appropriate toys within the child's reach
- Encouraging visits from friends
- Providing diversional activities such as drawing, coloring, or video games (Fig. 24.8)

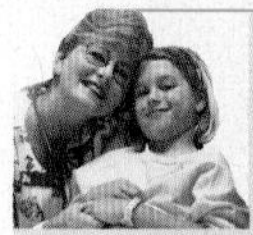

Avoid sudden bumping or movement of the bed: this can disturb traction alignment and cause additional pain to the child as the weights are jostled.

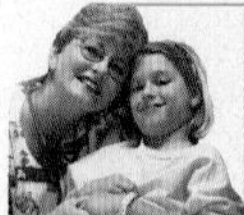

Ongoing, careful neurovascular assessments are critical in the child with a cast or in skeletal traction. Notify the physician immediately if these signs of compartment syndrome occur: extreme pain (out of proportion to the situation), pain with passive range of motion of digits, distal extremity pallor, inability to move digits, loss of pulses.

External Fixation

External fixation may be used for complicated fractures, especially open fractures with soft tissue damage. A series of pins or wires are inserted into bone and then

Table 24.2 Types of Traction and Nursing Implications

Type of Traction	Description	Nursing Implications
Bryant's traction 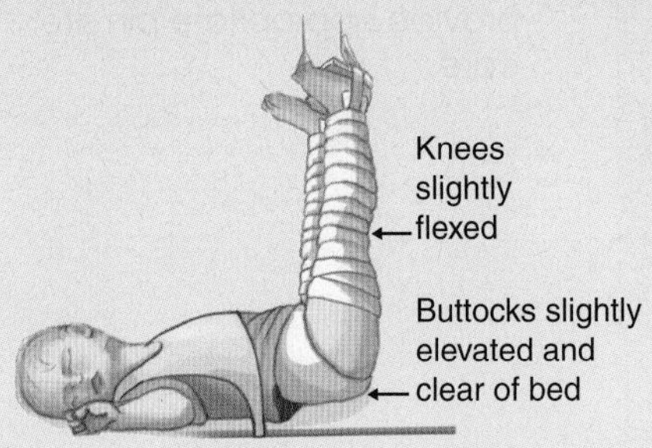 Knees slightly flexed Buttocks slightly elevated and clear of bed	Both legs are extended vertically, with child's weight serving as countertraction. Skin traction is applied to both legs. Used for infants with femur fracture or developmental dysplasia of the hip.	Maintain appropriate position. Ensure heels and ankles are free from pressure. Rewrap elastic bandages as ordered.
Russell's traction 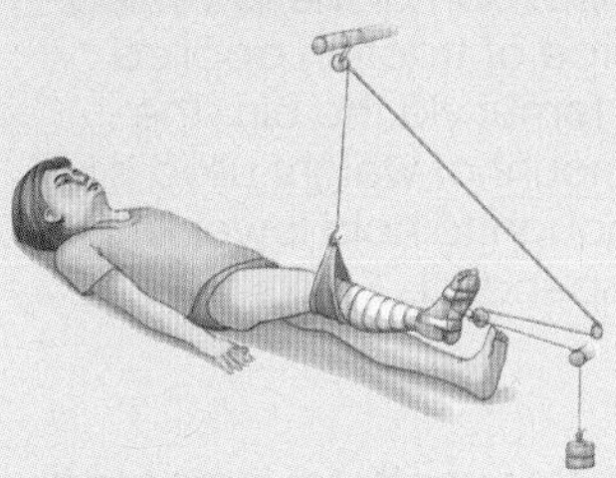	Skin traction for femur fracture, hip and knee contractures. Uses a knee sling. In split Russell's traction, a portion of the traction weight may be redistributed via a pulley from the sling to the head of the bed (used for femur fracture, Legg-Calvé-Perthes disease, slipped capital femoral epiphysis).	Wrap bandages from ankle to thigh on children less than age 2 years, from ankle to knee on children older than 2 years. Use a foot support to prevent foot drop. Ensure heel is free from bed. Assess popliteal region for skin breakdown from the sling. Mark leg to ensure proper replacement of sling.
Buck's traction 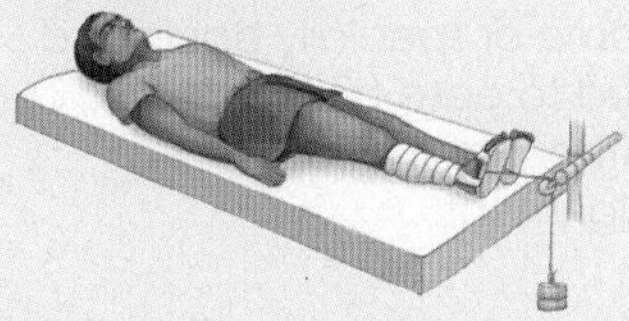	Skin traction for hip and knee contractures, Legg-Calvé-Perthes disease, slipped capital femoral epiphysis. Traction force delivered in straight line.	Remove traction boot every 8 hours to assess skin. Leg may be slightly abducted.
Cervical skin traction 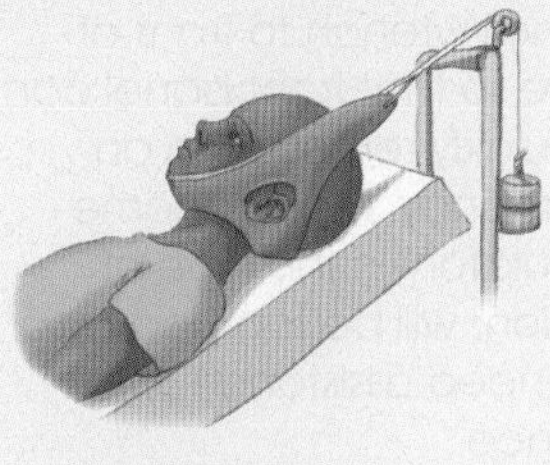	Skin traction applied with a skin strap (head halter). Used for neck sprains/strains, torticollis, or nerve trauma.	Ensure that head halter or skin strap does not place pressure on ears or throat. Limit of 5 to 7 pounds weight.
Side-arm 90-90 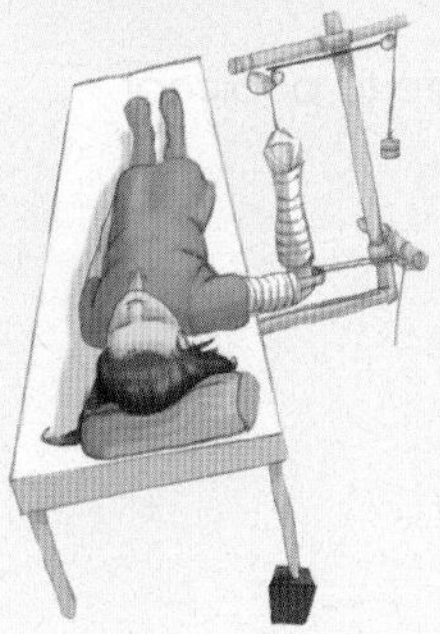	Skin traction for humerus fractures and injuries to the shoulder girdle. Used to treat fractures of the humerus and injuries in or around the shoulder girdle.	Maintain elbow flexed at 90 degrees. Fingers and hand may feel cool because of elevation. Child may turn to affected side only.

(continued)

Table 24.2 Types of Traction and Nursing Implications (continued)

Type of Traction	Description	Nursing Implications
Dunlop side-arm 00-90 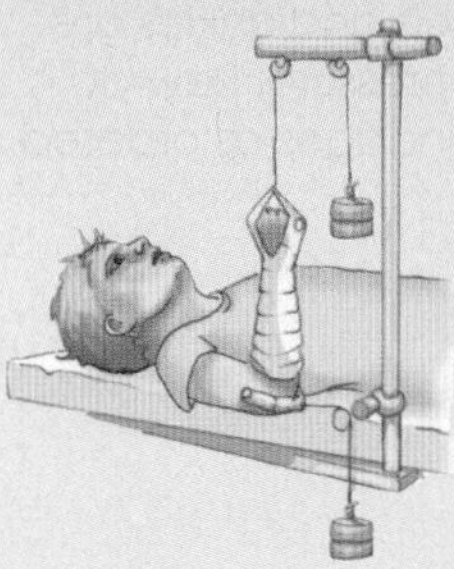	Skeletal traction through an olecranon screw or pin in distal humerus. Lower arm is held in balanced suspension.	See side-arm 90-90. In addition, provide appropriate pin site care.
90-90 traction 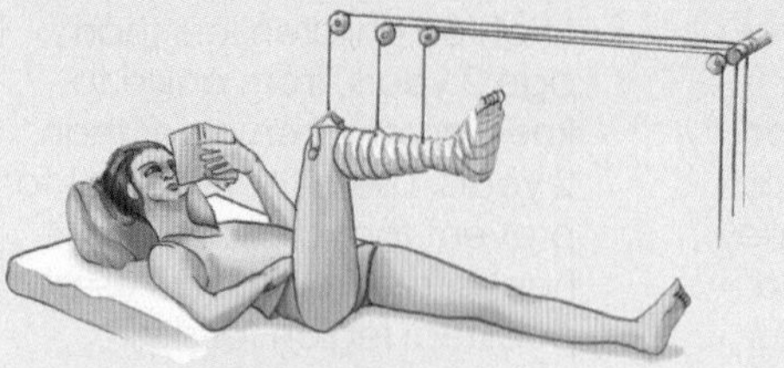	For femur fracture reduction when skin traction is inadequate. Skeletal traction with force applied through pin in distal femur.	A foam boot may be used for suspension of the lower leg. Force of traction applied to femur via the pin. The amount of weight used is just enough to hold lower limb suspended.
Cervical skeletal tongs 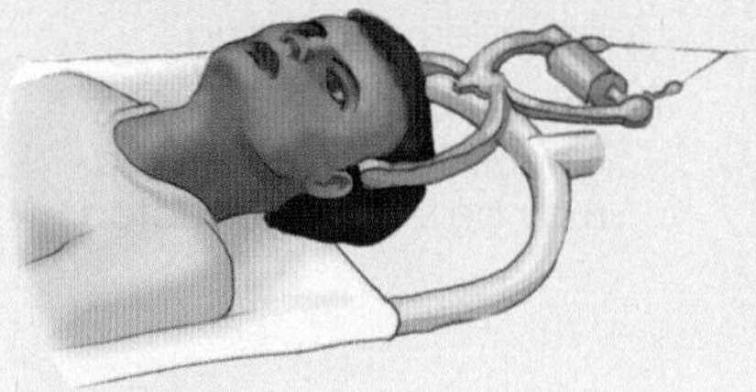	Tongs attached to skull via pins. Used with fractures or dislocations of the cervical or high thoracic vertebrae.	Assess frequently for increased pain, respiratory distress, and cranial nerve or brachial plexus injury. Place on Stryker frame or specially equipped bed to ease positioning without disruption of alignment.
Halo traction 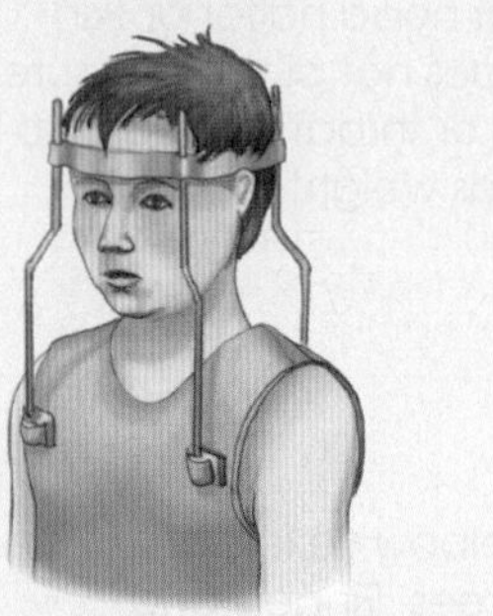	Metal halo attached to skull via pins. Used for cervical or high thoracic vertebrae fracture or dislocation and for postoperative immobilization following cervical fusion.	Refer to nursing implications for cervical tongs. Tape small wrench to front of brace so that front panel can be quickly removed in an emergency. May become ambulatory in this type of traction; will be top-heavy so may need assistance with balance.
Balanced suspension traction 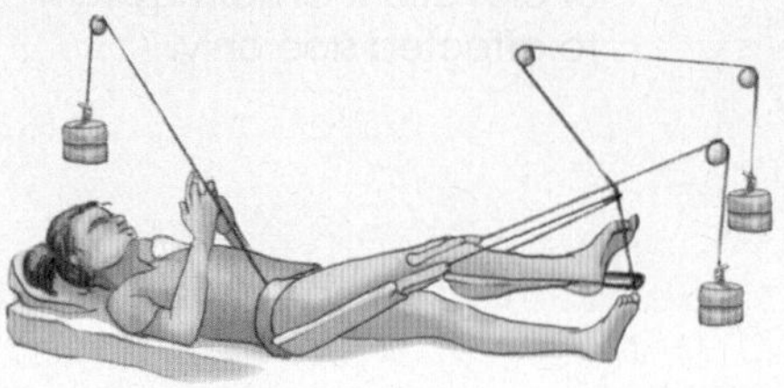	Used for femur, hip, or tibial fracture. Thomas splint suspends the thigh while the Pearson attachment allows knee flexion and supports the leg below the knee.	Avoid pressure to popliteal area.

● COMPARISON CHART 24.1 Skin Versus Skeletal Traction

	Skin Traction	Skeletal Traction
Application of force	To the skin via strips or tapes secured with Ace bandages or traction boots	To the body part directly by fixation into or through the bone
Length of treatment	Usually limited	Allows for longer periods of traction
Amount of force	Less	More

attached to an external frame. The fixator apparatus may be adjusted as needed by the health care provider. Once the desired level of correction is achieved, no further adjustment occurs and the bone is allowed to heal. Advantages of external fixation include increased patient comfort and improved function of muscles and joints when complicated fracture occurs.

Caring for the Child With an External Fixator

In addition to routine neurovascular assessment, elevate the extremity to prevent swelling. The fixator may be moved by grasping the frame, as the fixator can tolerate ordinary movement. Encourage weight bearing as prescribed. Provide appropriate education to the child and family. Encourage the child to look at the apparatus.

Providing Pin Care

Whether pins are inserted for skeletal traction or as part of an external fixator (see section on fractures), keeping the pin sites clean is important to prevent infection. Perform pin site care according to institutional policy or the physician's orders. Cleaning of the pin sites prevents infection by promoting comfort and preventing healing skin from adhering to the metal pin. Notify the orthopedic surgeon if signs of pin site infection are present or if pin slippage occurs.

Thus far, attempts to obtain evidence supporting the various types of pin site care have been unsuccessful. Certain physicians prefer the site to be cleaned with normal saline; others choose a solution with antibacterial properties. Some institutions recommend removal of all crusts formed on the skin around the pin; others do not. The rationale for crust removal is to promote free drainage and prevent the surrounding skin from adhering to the pin. A keyhole dressing may be necessary around the pin if drainage is present. No matter which procedure is ordered or preferred, perform pin care as necessary to prevent infection at the pin site. The Ilizarov fixator uses wires that are thinner than ordinary pins, so simply cleansing by showering is usually sufficient to keep the pin site clean. If drainage is present, the skin around the wires can be cleansed with a dry gauze pad.

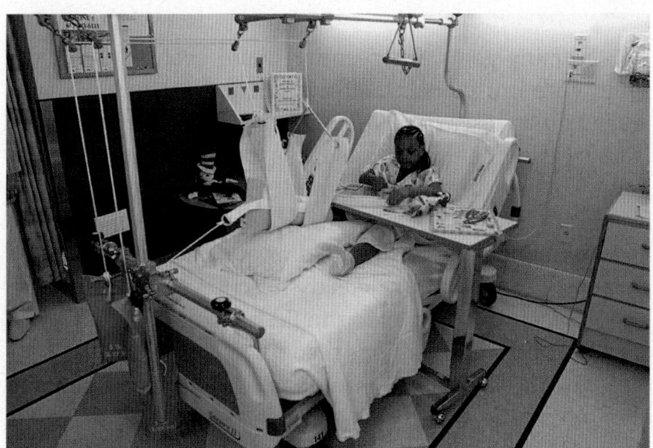

● Figure 24.8 Provide age-appropriate diversional activities and schoolwork for children confined to bed in traction.

Nursing Process Overview for the Child With a Musculoskeletal Disorder

Care of the child with a musculoskeletal disorder includes assessment, nursing diagnosis, planning, interventions, and evaluation. There are a number of general concepts related to the nursing process that may be applied to musculoskeletal dysfunction in children. From a general understanding of the care involved for a child with a musculoskeletal disorder, the nurse can then individualize the care based on patient specifics.

ASSESSMENT

Assessment of musculoskeletal dysfunction in children includes health history, physical examination, and laboratory and diagnostic testing.

> Remember Dakota, the 2-year-old with right arm pain and refusal to use his arm? What additional health history and physical examination assessment information should the nurse obtain?

Health History

The health history comprises past medical history, family history, and history of present illness (when the symptoms started and how they have progressed) as well as treatments used at home. The past medical history might be significant for musculoskeletal congenital anomaly or orthopedic injury during the birthing process. Breech delivery may be associated with developmental dysplasia of the hip. Determine history related to attainment of developmental milestones, such as walking and whether or not the child participates in sports. Inquire about the child's usual level of physical activity, participation in sports, and use of protective equipment. Family history may be positive for orthopedic problems. When eliciting the history of the present illness, inquire about the following:

- Limp or other changes in gait
- Recent trauma (determine the mechanism of injury)
- Recent strenuous exercise
- Fever
- Weakness
- Alteration in muscle tone
- Areas of redness or swelling

Physical Examination

Physical examination of the musculoskeletal system consists of inspection, observation, and palpation.

Inspection and Observation

Observe the child's posture and alignment of the trunk. Inspect extremities for symmetry and positioning and for absence, duplication, or webbing of any digits. Note any obvious extremity deformity or limb-length discrepancy. Inspect skin for redness, warmth, bruises, and puncture sites. Observe gait in the child who has achieved the developmental skill of walking. Note refusal to walk, limp, intoeing, out-toeing, or foot slap. Inspect injured joints for ecchymosis or swelling. In the injured extremity, note color of fingertips or toes. Observe spontaneous range of motion. Perform scoliosis screening to determine spinal alignment. Note symmetry of thigh folds.

Palpation

Palpate the clavicles in the newborn or young infant for tenderness or a bump that indicates callus formation with clavicle fracture. Perform active range of motion to determine if a joint position is fixed (e.g., clubfoot). Palpate the affected joint or extremity to detect warmth or tenderness. In the injured child or the child with a cast or splint, thoroughly assess the neurovascular status of the affected extremities. Palpate the fingers or toes for warmth. Determine the capillary refill time. Note presence of sensation or motion. Evaluate muscle strength. Palpate pulses distal to the injury, noting their strength and quality. Perform the Ortolani and Barlow maneuvers to assess for developmental dysplasia of the hip.

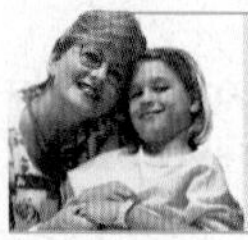

Assess the injured site last, and do so gently.

Laboratory and Diagnostic Testing

Common Laboratory and Diagnostic Tests 24.1 explains the laboratory and diagnostic tests most commonly used when considering musculoskeletal disorders. The tests can assist the physician in diagnosing a disorder and/or be used as guidelines in determining ongoing treatment. Some of the tests are obtained by laboratory or nonnursing personnel, while others might be obtained by the nurse. In either instance the nurse should be familiar with how the tests are obtained, what they are used for, and normal versus abnormal results. This knowledge will also be necessary when providing patient and family education related to the tests.

NURSING DIAGNOSES, GOALS, INTERVENTIONS, AND EVALUATION

Upon completion of a thorough assessment, the nurse might identify several nursing diagnoses, including:

- Pain related to trauma, edema, or muscle spasm (see Chapter 15)
- Impaired physical mobility related to injury, pain, or weakness
- Risk for constipation related to immobility
- Self-care deficit related to immobility
- Risk for impaired skin integrity related to immobility, braces, or adaptive devices
- Deficient knowledge related to cast care, activity restrictions, or other prescribed treatment
- Risk for developmental delay related to immobility, alterations in extremities

After completing an assessment of Dakota, the nurse noted the following: the history revealed he had been sledding with his older brother the day before. Upon examination, bruising and swelling of the right arm are noted, with point tenderness at the wrist. Based on the assessment findings, what would your top three nursing diagnoses be for Dakota?

Nursing goals, interventions, and evaluation for the child with musculoskeletal dysfunction are based on the nursing diagnoses (see Nursing Care Plan Overview 24.1). The nursing care plan may be used as a guide in planning nursing care for the child with a musculoskeletal disorder. The care plan includes many nursing diagnoses that are applicable to the child or adolescent. Children's responses to musculoskeletal dysfunction and its treatment will vary, and nursing care should be individualized based on the child's and family's responses to illness.

The nursing care of immobilized children is similar to that of adults but developmental and age-appropriate effects must be taken into account. Prevention of complications is a key nursing function. Refer to Nursing Care Plan 24.1 for interventions related to prevention of

Common Laboratory and Diagnostic Tests 24.1

Test	Explanation	Indication	Nursing Implications
X-rays	Radiographic image; usually two views are obtained of the affected extremity (lateral and anteroposterior)	To detect fractures and other anomalies	Child must cooperate and hold still. Enlist the family's help in calming the child.
Ultrasound	Use of sound waves to locate the depth and structure within soft tissues and fluid	To diagnose toxic synovitis, Legg-Calvé-Perthes disease, slipped capital femoral epiphysis, osteomyelitis, fractures, ligament or soft tissue injuries. Monitoring and follow-up of fractures and remodeling.	Better tolerated by nonsedated children than CT or MRI. Can be performed with a portable unit at bedside.
Computed tomography (CT)	Noninvasive x-ray study that looks at tissue density and structures. Images a "slice" of tissue.	To evaluate the extent of osteomyelitis, Legg-Calvé-Perthes disease, or slipped capital femoral epiphysis or to rule out other problems	Machine is large and can be frightening to children. Procedure can be lengthy and child must remain still. If unable to do so, sedation may be necessary. If performed with contrast medium, assess for allergy. Encourage fluids after the procedure if not contraindicated.
Magnetic resonance imaging (MRI)	Based on how hydrogen atoms behave in a magnetic field when disturbed by radio-frequency signals. Does not require ionizing radiation. Provides a 3D view of the body part being scanned.	To assess hard and soft tissue, as well as bone marrow, to evaluate extent of osteomyelitis, Legg-Calvé-Perthes disease, or slipped capital femoral epiphysis, or to rule out other problems	Remove all metal objects from the child. Child must remain motionless for entire scan; parent can stay in room with child. Younger children will require sedation in order to be still. A loud thumping sound occurs inside the machine during the scan procedure, and this can be frightening to children.
Arthrography	X-ray of a joint after direct injection with a radiopaque substance	To assess ligaments, muscles, tendons, and cartilage, particularly after injury	Should not be performed if joint infection is present. Apply cold therapy afterward and assess for swelling and pain. Crepitus may be present in the joint for 1 to 2 days after procedure.
Complete blood count	Evaluates hemoglobin and hematocrit, white blood cell count, platelet count	To evaluate hemoglobin and hematocrit with fracture with potential bleeding. To determine infection in osteomyelitis, septic arthritis, and toxic synovitis.	Normal values vary according to age and gender. White blood cell count differential is helpful in evaluating source of infection. May be affected by myelosuppressive drugs.

(continued)

Common Laboratory and Diagnostic Tests 24.1 (continued)

Test	Explanation	Indication	Nursing Implications
Erythrocyte sedimentation rate	Nonspecific test used to determine presence of infection or inflammation	To evaluate for osteomyelitis or septic arthritis	Send sample to laboratory immediately; if allowed to stand for longer than 3 hours, may produce falsely low result.
C-reactive protein	Measures acute-phase reactant protein indicative of inflammatory process	To evaluate for osteomyelitis or septic arthritis	Anti-inflammatory drugs may cause decreased levels. More sensitive and rapidly responsive than erythrocyte sedimentation rate.
Blood culture	To determine presence of bacteria in blood	May be positive with septic arthritis or osteomyelitis	Transport specimen to laboratory within 30 minutes. Avoid skin contamination of specimen while obtaining it. Cultures should usually be drawn before starting antibiotics, as partial antibiotic treatment may result in negative culture.
Joint fluid aspiration	Aspirated joint fluid is examined for presence of pus and white blood cells; culture is performed.	To evaluate for septic arthritis	Use cold therapy to decrease swelling after aspiration. Apply pressure dressing to prevent hematoma formation or fluid re-collection. Assess for fever and joint pain or edema, which may indicate infection. Positive fluid culture indicates a bacterial infection in the joint. May also be used to relieve pressure in the joint space.

complications. Additional information about nursing care related to certain disorders will be included later in the chapter as it relates to specific disorders. Refer to Chapter 15 for nursing interventions related to pain management. Particular care related to casts, traction, and external fixation is discussed below.

> Based on your top three nursing diagnoses for Dakota, describe appropriate nursing interventions.

Congenital and Developmental Disorders

Congenital anomalies of the musculoskeletal system are usually readily identified at birth. Congenital structural anomalies involving the skeleton include pectus excavatum, pectus carinatum, limb deficiencies, polydactyly or syndactyly, metatarsus adductus, congenital clubfoot, and osteogenesis imperfecta. A developmental anomaly that may be diagnosed at birth or later in life is developmental dysplasia of the hip. A muscular condition, torticollis, most often presents as a congenital condition but may also develop after birth. Tibia vara is a developmental disorder affecting young children. Rarely, a developmental positional alteration such as genu varum, genu valgum, or pes planus will persist past the usual age of resolution or cause the child pain. If those situations occur, bracing, orthotics, or surgical correction may become necessary.

• PECTUS EXCAVATUM

Pectus excavatum and pectus carinatum are anterior chest wall deformities. Pectus excavatum, a funnel-shaped chest, accounts for 87% of anterior chest wall deformities (Goretsky et al., 2004). A depression that sinks inward is apparent at the xiphoid process (Fig. 24.9). Pectus carinatum, a protuberance of the chest wall, accounts for only 5% of anterior chest wall deformities. The remainder are mixed deformities.

Pectus excavatum does not resolve as the child grows; rather, it progresses with growth. The chest depression may be minimal or marked. When the pectus is more pronounced, cardiac and pulmonary compression occurs.

Nursing Care Plan 24.1

Overview for the Child With a Musculoskeletal Disorder

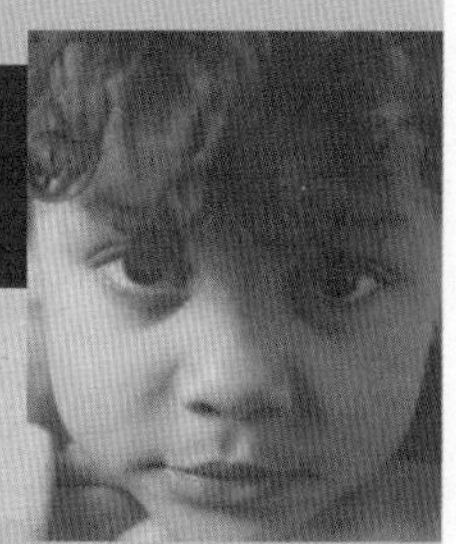

Nursing Diagnosis: Impaired physical mobility related to injury, pain, or weakness as evidenced by inability to move an extremity, to ambulate, or to move without limitations

Outcome identification and evaluation

Child will engage in physical activities within limits of injury or disease: *child will assist with transfers and positioning in bed and/or participate in prescribed bed exercises.*

Intervention: maximizing physical mobility

- Assess child's ability to move based upon injury or disease and within limits of prescribed treatment *to determine baseline.*
- Prior to prescribed exercise or major position changes, ensure that pain medication is given: *relief of pain increases child's ability to tolerate and participate in activity.*
- Use passive and active range-of-motion exercises and teach child and family how to perform them *to facilitate joint mobility and muscle development (active ROM) and to help increase mobility (within limits of restrictions related to injury or prescribed treatment).*
- Praise accomplishments and emphasize child's abilities *to improve self-esteem and encourage feelings of confidence and competence.*
- Teach child and family necessary care related to mobility issues *so the family can continue with these measures at home.*

Nursing Diagnosis: Risk for constipation related to immobility and/or use of narcotic analgesics

Outcome identification and evaluation

Child will demonstrate adequate stool passage, *will pass soft, formed stool every 1 to 3 days without straining or other adverse effects.*

Intervention: promoting appropriate bowel elimination

- Assess usual pattern of stooling *to determine baseline and identify potential problems with elimination.*
- Palpate for abdominal fullness and auscultate for bowel sounds *to assess for bowel function and presence of constipation.*
- Encourage fiber intake *to increase frequency of stools.*
- Ensure adequate fluid intake *to prevent formation of hard, dry stools.*
- Encourage activity within child's limits or restrictions *as even minimal activity increases peristalsis.*

Nursing Diagnosis: Self-care deficit related to immobility as evidenced by inability to perform hygiene care and transfer self independently

Outcome identification and evaluation

Child will demonstrate ability to care for self within age parameters and limits of disease: *child is able to feed, dress, and manage elimination within limits of injury or disease and age.*

Intervention: maximizing self-care

- Introduce child and family to self-help methods as soon as possible *to promote independence from the beginning.*
- Encourage family and staff to allow child to do as much as possible *to allow child to gain confidence and independence.*
- Collaborate with physical therapy and occupational therapy as needed to provide child and family with appropriate tools to modify environment and methods to promote transferring and self-care *to allow for maximum functioning.*
- Praise accomplishments and emphasize child's abilities *to improve self-esteem and encourage feelings of confidence and competence.*
- Balance activity with periods to rest *to reduce fatigue and increase energy available for self-care.*

(continued)

Overview for the Child With a Musculoskeletal Disorder (continued)

Nursing Diagnosis: Risk for impaired skin integrity related to immobility, casting, traction, use of braces or adaptive devices

Outcome identification and evaluation

Child's skin will remain intact, *without evidence of redness or breakdown.*

Intervention: promoting skin integrity

- Monitor condition of entire skin surface at least daily *to provide baseline and allow for early identification of areas at risk.*
- Avoid excessive friction or harsh cleaning products *that may increase risk of breakdown in child with susceptible skin.*
- Keep child's skin free from stool and urine *to decrease risk of breakdown.*
- Keep linen free from food crumbs and wrinkles *to prevent pressure areas from forming.*
- Change child's position frequently *to decrease pressure on susceptible areas.*
- Monitor condition of skin affected by braces or adaptive equipment frequently *to prevent skin breakdown related to poor fit.*

For the child in traction:

- Pad bony prominences with cotton padding before applying traction *to protect skin from injury.*
- Gently massage child's back and sacrum with lotion *to stimulate circulation.*

For the child in a spica cast:

- Apply plastic wrap to the perineal edges of the cast *to prevent soiling of cast edges, which can contribute to cast breakdown.*
- Use a fracture bedpan *to facilitate toileting without soiling cast.*
- For the child still in diapers, tuck a smaller diaper under the perineal edges of cast and cover with a larger diaper *to prevent cast soiling.*

Nursing Diagnosis: Deficient knowledge related to cast care, activity restrictions, or other prescribed treatment as evidenced by verbalization, questions, or actions demonstrating lack of understanding regarding child's condition or care

Outcome identification and evaluation

Child and family will demonstrate accurate understanding about condition and course of treatment *through verbalization and return demonstration.*

Intervention: providing patient and family teaching

- Assess child's and family's willingness to learn: *child and family must be willing to learn for teaching to be effective.*
- Provide teaching at an appropriate level for the child and family (depends on age of child, physical condition, memory) *to ensure understanding.*
- Teach in short sessions: *many short sessions are more helpful than one long session.*
- Repeat information *to give family and child time to learn and understand.*
- Provide reinforcement and rewards *to facilitate the teaching/learning process.*
- Use multiple modes of learning involving many senses (provide written, verbal, demonstration, and videos) when possible: *child and family are more likely to retain information when presented in different ways using many senses.*

Overview for the Child With a Musculoskeletal Disorder (continued)

Nursing Diagnosis: Risk for delayed development related to immobility, alterations in extremities

Outcome identification and evaluation

Development will be enhanced; *child will make continued progress toward developmental milestones and will not show regression in abilities.*

Intervention: promoting development

- Screen for developmental capabilities *to determine child's current level of functioning.*
- Offer age-appropriate toys, play, and activities (including gross motor) *to encourage further development.*
- Perform exercises or interventions as prescribed by physical or occupational therapist: *repeat participation in those activities helps to promote function and acquisition of developmental skills.*
- Provide support to families: *immobility and extremity deficits may lead to slow progress in achieving developmental milestones, so ongoing motivation is needed.*

Symptoms of this compression most often present during puberty, when the pectus quickly worsens. Children may complain of shortness of breath, withdraw from physical activities, and have a poor body image.

Therapeutic Management

Therapeutic management of pectus excavatum involves surgical correction, preferably before puberty, when the skeleton is more pliable. Various surgical techniques may be used and generally involve either the placement of a surgical steel bar or using a piece of bone in the rib cage to lift the depression. This discussion will focus on care of the child who undergoes surgical steel bar placement for pectus correction.

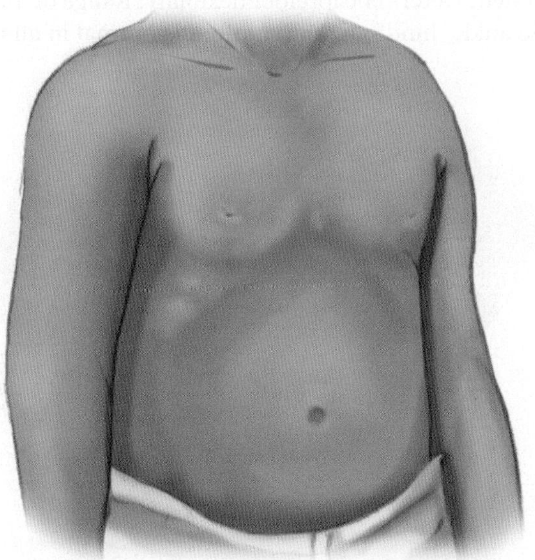

● Figure 24.9 Pectus excavatum: note the depression in the chest wall at the xiphoid process.

Nursing Assessment

Elicit the health history, noting progression of the defect and effects on the child's cardiopulmonary function. Note shortness of breath, exercise intolerance, or chest pain. Observe the child's chest for anterior wall deformity, noting depth and severity. Auscultate the lungs to determine the adequacy of aeration. X-rays, computed tomography (CT), or magnetic resonance imaging (MRI) may be used to determine the extent of the anomaly and compression of inner structures.

Nursing Management

Prepare the child preoperatively by allowing a tour of the surgical area and the pediatric intensive care unit. Introduce the child to the pain scale that will be used in the postoperative period.

Postoperatively, nursing management focuses on assessment, protection of the surgical site, and pain management. Auscultate lung sounds frequently to determine the adequacy of aeration and to monitor for development of the complication of pneumothorax. Assess for signs of wound infection that would necessitate removal of the curved bar. Do not allow the child to lie on either side and do not log-roll the child (these positions may disrupt the bar's position). Administer analgesics as needed either intravenously or via the epidural catheter. Teach families that the child will not be allowed to lie on his or her side at home for 4 weeks after the surgery to ensure that the band does not shift. Encourage aerobic activity at home after cleared by the surgeon (this will increase the child's vital capacity, previously hindered by the pectus). The bar will be removed 2 to 4 years after the initial placement.

LIMB DEFICIENCIES

Limb deficiencies, either complete absence of a limb or a portion of it or deformity, occur as the fetus is developing. These defects are attributed to an amniotic band constricting the limb, resulting in either incomplete development or amputation of the limb. Many children born with limb deformities also have developmental craniofacial abnormalities (Morrissy et al., 2001).

Therapeutic management is aimed at improving the child's functional ability. Physical therapy and occupational therapy may be helpful. Adaptive equipment such as a prosthesis may also be prescribed.

Nursing Assessment

Note the extent of limb deformity, providing an accurate description of the presence or absence of a portion of the arm or leg, or missing fingers or toes. Assess the child's ability to use the extremity as a helper (arms) or in ambulation (legs). Determine status of acquisition of developmental skills.

Nursing Management

Reinforce prescribed activities that are meant to improve the child's function. Provide activities in which the child is capable of participating. If the limb deficiency is significant, refer the infant to the local early intervention office as soon as possible after birth. Early intervention, available in all 50 states, is designed to promote development from birth to age 3 years. Absence of a limb or a significant portion of a limb will have a considerable impact on the child's ability to meet developmental milestones as expected.

POLYDACTYLY/SYNDACTYLY

Polydactyly is the presence of extra digits on the hand or foot (Fig. 24.10). It occurs equally in both genders and affects African-Americans more frequently than Caucasians. One third of the time, polydactyly occurs in both the hand and foot (Gore & Spencer, 2004). It usually involves digits at the border of the hand or foot, near the fifth finger or toe. Syndactyly is webbing of the fingers and toes.

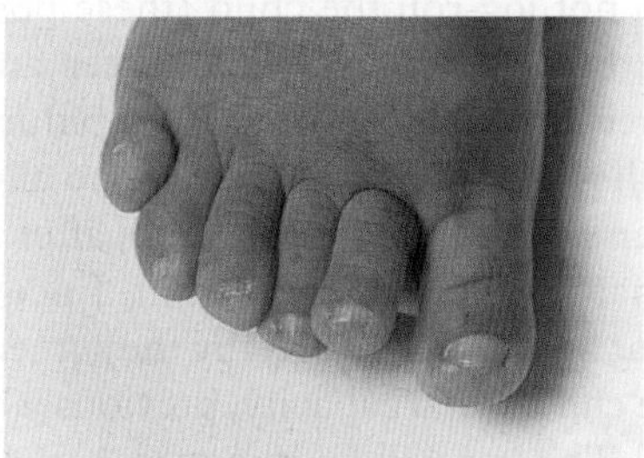

Figure 24.10 Note additional digits (toes) of polydactyly.

Treatment includes tying off the additional digit until it falls off or surgical removal of the digit. No treatment is usually required for syndactyly, though surgical repair is sometimes performed for cosmetic reasons.

Nursing Assessment

Inspect the hands and feet for the presence of extra digits. Note whether the additional digits are soft (without bone) or are full or partial digits with bone present. Note location of webbing.

Nursing Management

If the digit is tied off, observe for expected necrosis of tissue and eventually loss of the extra digit. When surgical removal is necessary, provide routine pre- and postoperative care as appropriate.

METATARSUS ADDUCTUS

Metatarsus adductus, a medial deviation of the forefoot, is one of the most common foot deformities of childhood (Fig. 24.11). It occurs as a result of *in utero* positioning. It occurs in one in 1,000 live births, affects boys and girls equally, and is bilateral in half of all cases and unilateral in the remainder (Gilmore & Thompson, 2003). Type I and Type II are usually benign deformities, resolving spontaneously by the age of 3 years. Children with type III deformity usually require manipulation and serial casting, preferably before the age of 8 months. Surgical intervention is rarely needed.

Nursing Assessment

The deformity is usually noted at birth. Note inward deviation of the forefoot. The great and second toes might be separated. Determine forefoot flexibility. Range of motion of the ankle, hindfoot, and midfoot is normal in all three

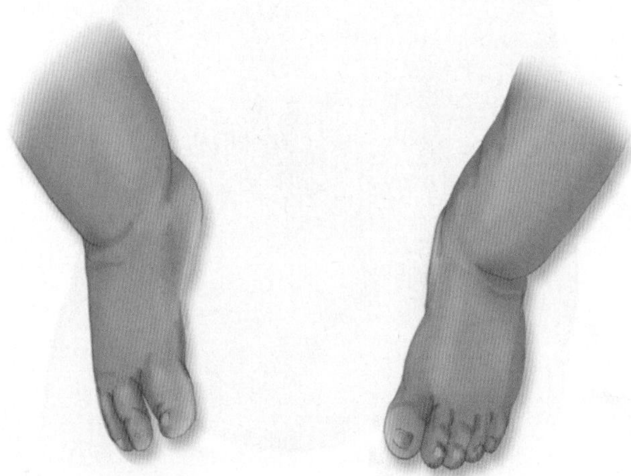

Figure 24.11 Metatarsus adductus: note medial deviation of the forefoot.

BOX 24.1

TYPES OF METATARSUS ADDUCTUS

- Type I: Forefoot is flexible past neutral actively and passively.
- Type II: Forefoot is flexible passively past neutral, but only to midline actively.
- Type III: Forefoot is rigid and does not correct to midline even with passive stretching.

types. Box 24.1 describes the three types based on flexibility of the forefoot.

Nursing Management

Nursing care for children with type I and II metatarsus adductus is aimed at education and reassurance of the parents. The nursing care for the child with type III is similar to that of the child with clubfoot (see below).

● CONGENITAL CLUBFOOT

Congenital clubfoot (also termed congenital talipes equinovarus) is a congenital anomaly that occurs in one out of 1,000 live births (Gilmore & Thompson, 2003). Clubfoot consists of:

- Talipes varus (inversion of the heel)
- Talipes equinus (plantarflexion of the foot; the heel is raised and would not strike the ground in a standing position)
- Cavus (plantarflexion of the forefoot on the hindfoot)
- Forefoot adduction with supination (the forefoot is inverted and turned slightly upward) (Mosca, 2001)

The foot resembles the head of a golf club (Fig. 24.12). Half of all cases occur bilaterally. Males are affected two and a half times more frequently than females. The exact etiology of clubfoot is unknown.

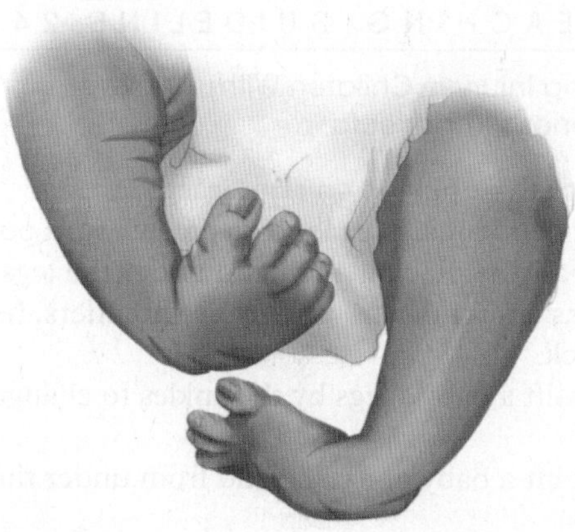

● Figure 24.12 Note inverted heel, ankle equinus, and forefoot adduction in this infant with bilateral clubfoot.

Clubfoot may be classified into four categories: postural, neurogenic, syndromic, and idiopathic. Postural clubfoot often resolves with a short series of manipulative casting. Neurogenic clubfoot occurs in infants with myelomeningocele. Clubfoot in association with other syndromes (syndromic) is often resistant to treatment. Idiopathic clubfoot occurs in otherwise normal healthy infants. The approach to treatment is similar regardless of the classification.

Therapeutic Management

The goal of therapeutic management of clubfoot is achievement of a functional foot; treatment starts as soon after birth as possible. Weekly manipulation with serial cast changes is performed; later, cast changes occur every 2 weeks. This approach is successful in about half of all cases. The other infants require corrective shoes or bracing; in some infants, surgical release of soft tissue may be necessary. Following surgery, the foot is immobilized with a cast for up to 12 weeks, and then ankle–foot orthoses or corrective shoes are used for several years.

Complications of clubfoot and its treatment include residual deformity, rocker-bottom foot, awkward gait, weight bearing on the lateral portion of the foot if uncorrected, and disturbance to the epiphysis.

Nursing Assessment

Note family history of foot deformities and obstetric history of breech position. Inspect the foot for position at rest. Perform active range of motion, noting inability to move foot into normal positioning at midline. X-rays are obtained to determine bony abnormality and note progress during treatment.

Nursing Management

Perform neurovascular assessment and cast care as for any disorder requiring casting. Provide emotional support, as treatment often begins in the newborn period and families may have a difficult time adjusting to the diagnosis and treatment required for their new baby. Teach families cast care and later the use of orthotics or braces as prescribed.

● OSTEOGENESIS IMPERFECTA

Osteogenesis imperfecta is a genetic bone disorder that results in low bone mass, increased fragility of the bones, and other connective tissue problems such as joint hypermobility, resulting in instability of the joints that may further contribute to fracture occurrence. Dentinogenesis imperfecta may also occur: the tooth enamel wears easily and the teeth become discolored.

The disorder usually occurs as a result of a defect in the collagen type 1 gene, usually through an autosomal recessive or dominant inheritance pattern. The types of osteogenesis imperfecta range from mild to severe connective tissue and bone involvement (Table 24.3). In children with moderate to severe disease, fractures are more likely to occur, and short stature is common. In addition to multiple fractures, additional complications include early hearing loss, acute and chronic pain, scoliosis, and respiratory problems.

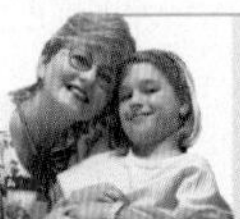

Blue sclera is not diagnostic of osteogenesis imperfecta, but it is a common finding. The sclerae of newborns tend to be bluish, progressing to white over the first few weeks of life. There are some individuals with blue sclerae who do not have osteogenesis imperfecta.

Therapeutic Management

The goal of medical and surgical management is to decrease the incidence of fractures and maintain mobility. Bisphosphonate administration is used for moderate to severe disease. Fracture care is often required. Physical therapy and occupational therapy prevent contractures and maximize mobility. Standing with bracing is encouraged. Lightweight splints or braces may allow the child to bear weight earlier. Severe cases may require surgical insertion of rods into the long bones.

Table 24.3 Classification of Osteogenesis Imperfecta

Classification	Characteristics
I	Common and mild Autosomal dominant Blue sclera Fragile bones, early fractures (by preschool age) Type A without dentinogenesis imperfecta, type B with dentinogenesis
II	Lethal in perinatal period Autosomal recessive Dark-blue sclera
III	Severe Autosomal recessive Normal sclera Fractures at birth with progressive deformity
IV	Moderately severe Autosomal dominant Normal sclera Fragile bones Type A without dentinogenesis imperfecta, type B with dentinogenesis

Zaleske, D. J. (2001). Metabolic and endocrine abnormalities. In R. T. Morrissy & S. L. Weinstein (Eds.), *Lovell & Winter's pediatric orthopaedics* (5th ed.). Philadelphia: Lippincott Williams & Wilkins.

Nursing Assessment

Elicit a health history, which may reveal a family history of osteogenesis imperfecta, a pattern of frequent fractures, or screaming associated with routine care and handling of the newborn. Inspect the eyes for sclerae that have a blue, purple, or gray tint. Note abnormalities of the primary teeth. Inspect skin for bruising and note joint hypermobility with active range of motion. Laboratory tests may include a skin biopsy (which reveals abnormalities in type 1 collagen) or DNA testing (locating the genetic mutation).

Nursing Management

Handle the child carefully and teach the family to avoid trauma (Teaching Guideline 24.3). Refer families to the Osteogenesis Imperfecta Foundation (www.oif.org), which provides access to multiple resources as well as clinical trials. An excellent book for families of children with osteogenesis imperfecta is *Children with OI: Strategies to Enhance Performance* by H. L. Cintas and L. H. Gerber.

Encourage safe mobility. Reinforce physical and occupational therapists' recommendations for promotion of fine motor skills and independence in activities of daily living, as well as use of adaptive equipment and appropriate promotion of mobility. Adapted physical education is important to promote mobility and maintain bone and muscle mass. If the child is ambulatory, even with adaptive equipment use, walking is a good form of exercise.

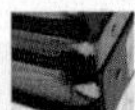

TEACHING GUIDELINE 24.3

Preventing Injury in Children With Osteogenesis Imperfecta

- Never push or pull on an arm or leg.
- Do not bend an arm or leg into an awkward position.
- Lift a baby by placing one hand under the legs and buttocks and one hand under the shoulders, head, and neck.
- Do not lift a baby's legs by the ankles to change the diaper.
- Do not lift a baby or small child from under the armpits.
- Provide supported positioning.
- If fracture is suspected, handle the limb minimally.

Swimming and water therapy are appropriate, allowing independent movement with little fracture risk.

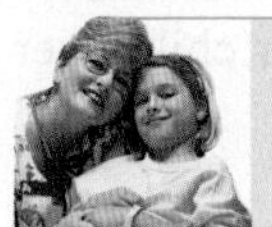

Use caution when inserting an intravenous line or taking a blood pressure measurement, as pressure on the arm or leg can lead to bruising and fractures.

DEVELOPMENTAL DYSPLASIA OF THE HIP

Developmental dysplasia of the hip (DDH) refers to abnormalities of the developing hip that include dislocation, subluxation, and dysplasia of the hip joint. In DDH, the femoral head has an abnormal relationship to the acetabulum. Frank dislocation of the hip may occur, in which there is no contact between the femoral head and acetabulum. Subluxation is a partial dislocation, meaning that the acetabulum is not fully seated within the hip joint. Dysplasia refers to an acetabulum that is shallow or sloping instead of cup-shaped. DDH may affect just one or both hips. The dysplastic hip may be provoked to subluxation or dislocated and then reduced again. DDH affects females eight times more often than males (Fig. 24.13).

Pathophysiology

While dislocation may occur during a growth period *in utero,* the laxity of the newborn's hip allows dislocation and relocation of the hip to occur. The hip can develop normally only if the femoral head is appropriately and deeply seated within the acetabulum. If subluxation and periodic or continued dislocation occur, then structural changes in the hip's anatomy occur. Continued dysplasia of the hip leads to limited abduction of the hip and contracture of muscles. DDH is more common in females, probably because female hormones contribute to laxity of the ligaments. Mechanical factors such as breech positioning or the presence of oligohydramnios also contribute to the development of DDH. Genetic factors also play a role: there is an increased incidence of DDH among persons of Native American and Lapp descent, with very low rates among people of African or southern Chinese heritage. Complications of DDH include avascular necrosis of the femoral head, loss of range of motion, recurrently unstable hip, femoral nerve palsy, leg-length discrepancy, and early osteoarthritis.

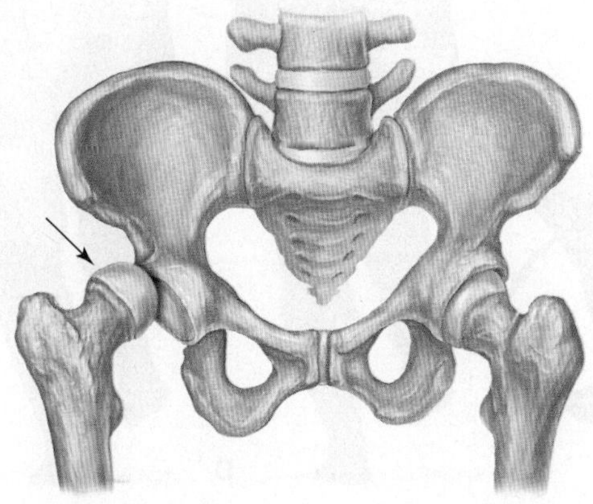

● Figure 24.13 Developmental dysplasia of the hip.

Therapeutic Management

The goal of therapeutic management is to maintain the hip joint in reduction so that the femoral head and acetabulum can develop properly.

Treatment varies based upon the child's age and the severity of DDH. Infants younger than 6 months of age may be treated with a Pavlik harness, which reduces and stabilizes the hip by preventing hip extension and adduction. The Pavlik harness is successful in the treatment of DDH in the majority of infants less than 6 months of age if it is used on a full-time basis and applied properly (Weinstein, 2001). Children from 6 months to 2 years of age often require closed reduction. Skin or skeletal traction may be used first to gradually stretch the associated soft tissue structures. Closed reduction occurs under general anesthesia, with the hip being gently maneuvered back into the acetabulum. A spica cast worn for 12 weeks maintains reduction of the hip. After the cast is removed, the child must wear an abduction brace full-time (except for baths) for 2 months. Then the brace is worn at night and during naps until development of the acetabulum is normal. Children over 2 years of age or those who have failed to respond to prior treatment require an open surgical reduction followed by a period of casting (Weinstein, 2001).

Nursing Assessment

Nursing assessment of children with DDH includes obtaining a health history and inspecting, observing, and palpating for findings common to DDH.

Health History

Assess the health history for risk factors such as:

- Family history of DDH
- Female gender
- Oligohydramnios or breech birth
- Native American or Laplander descent
- Associated lower limb deformity or other congenital musculoskeletal deformity

Previously undiagnosed older children may complain of hip pain.

Physical Assessment

The physical examination for DDH includes inspection, observation, and palpation. Since DDH is a developmental process, ongoing screening assessments are required throughout at least the first several months of the infant's life.

Inspection and Observation

Ensure that the infant is on a flat surface and is relaxed. Note asymmetry of thigh or gluteal folds with the infant in a prone position. Document shortening of affected femur observed as limb-length discrepancy. Older children may exhibit **Trendelenburg gait**. Figure 24.14 illustrates these assessments.

Palpation

Note limited hip abduction when passive range of motion is performed. Abduction should ordinarily occur to 75 degrees and adduction to within 30 degrees with the infant's pelvis stabilized. Perform Barlow and Ortolani tests, noting a "clunk" as the femoral head dislocates or reduces back into the acetabulum. Force is not necessary when performing the Barlow and Ortolani maneuvers (see Fig. 24.14).

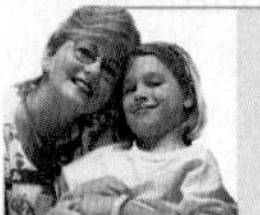

A higher-pitched "click" may occur with flexion or extension of the hip. When assessing for DDH, do not confuse this benign, adventitial sound with a true "clunk."

Diagnostic Testing

Ultrasound of the hip allows for visualization of the femoral head and the outer edge of the acetabulum. Plain hip x-rays may be used in the infant or child over 6 months of age.

Nursing Management

Earlier recognition of hip dysplasia with earlier harness use results in better correction of the anomaly. Excellent assessment skills and reporting of any abnormal findings are critical. Initially, the infant will need to wear the Pavlik harness continuously (Fig. 24.15). The physician makes all appropriate adjustments to the harness when applied so that the hips are held in the optimal position for appropriate development. Teach parents use of the harness and assessment of the baby's skin. If started early, harness use usually continues for about 3 months (Teaching Guideline 24.4). Breastfeeding can continue throughout the harness treatment period, but creative positioning of the infant may be needed.

For infants or children diagnosed later than 6 months of age or those who do not improve with harness use,

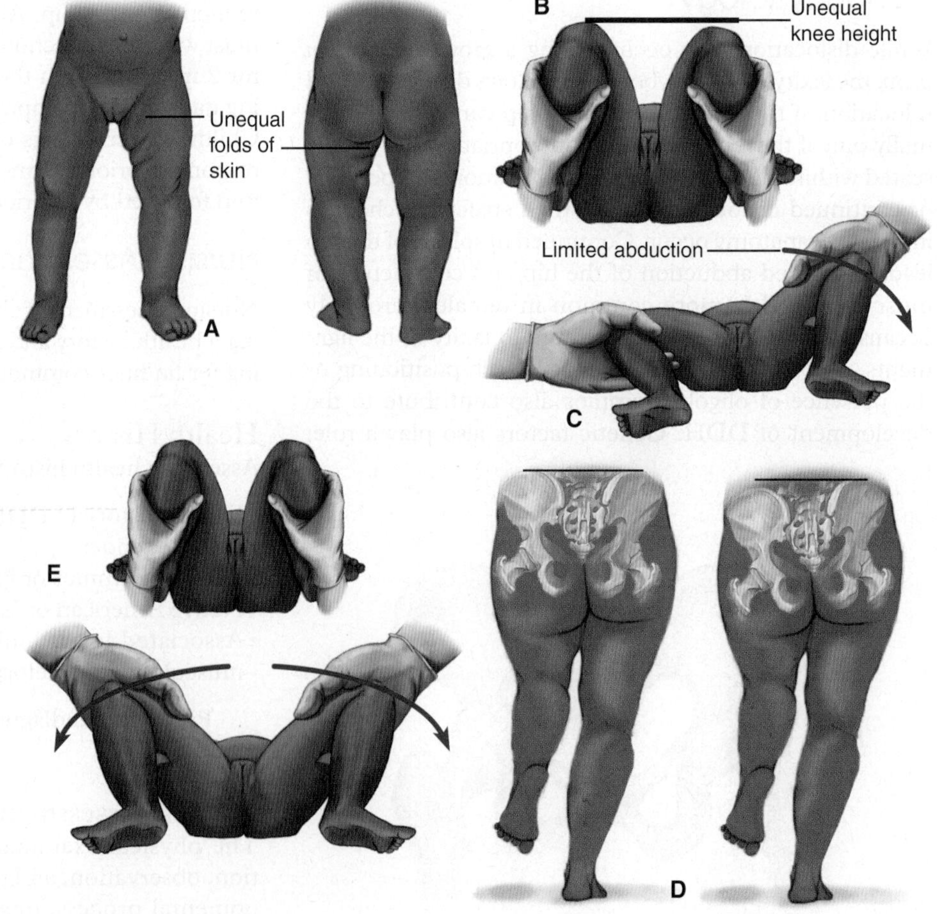

Unequal folds of skin
A
B
Unequal knee height
Limited abduction
C
E
D
Normal
Positive
A. Assess for asymmetry of thigh and gluteal folds.
B. Assess for unequal knee height related to femur shortening.
C. Note limitation in hip abduction.
D. Positive Trendelenburg sign: note pelvis/hip drops when leg is raised.
E. Assess for "clunk" with the Ortolani maneuver.

● Figure 24.14 Assessment techniques for developmental dysplasia of the hip.

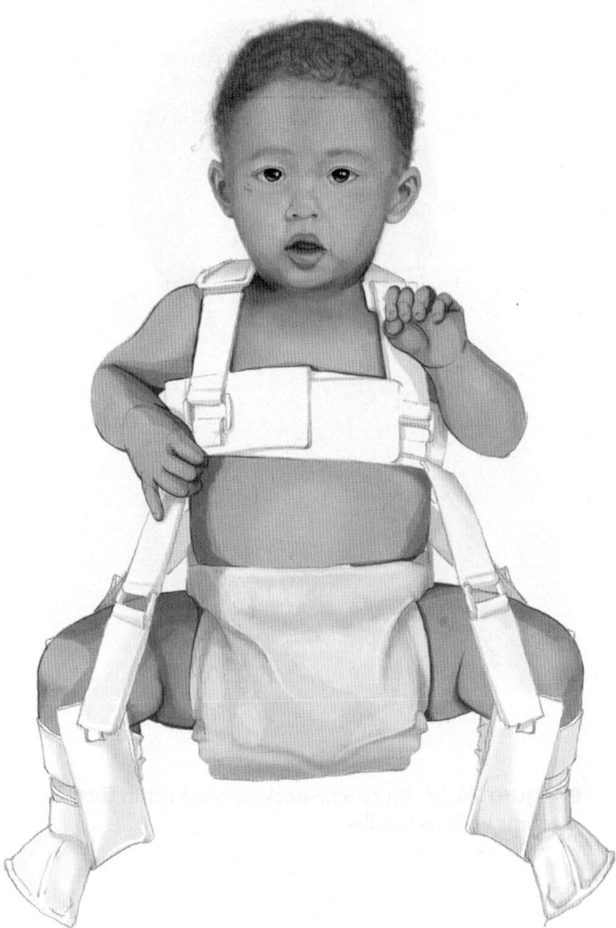

● Figure 24.15 Pavlik harness for treatment of developmental dysplasia of the hip.

surgical reduction may be performed after a period of traction. Postoperative casting followed by bracing or orthotic use is common. Caring for the child in the postoperative period is similar to care of any child in a cast. Pain management and monitoring for bleeding are priority activities. Teach families care of the cast at home.

● TIBIA VARA (BLOUNT'S DISEASE)

Tibia vara (Blount's disease) is a developmental disorder affecting young children. The normal physiologic bowing or genu varum becomes more pronounced in the child with tibia vara. The cause of tibia vara is unknown, but it is considered to be a developmental disorder as it occurs most frequently in children who are early walkers. Most cases occur in African-Americans. In addition to early walking, obesity is also a risk factor. If left untreated, the growth plate of the upper tibia ceases bone production. Asymmetric growth at the knee then occurs and the bowing progresses. Severe degenerative arthritis of the knee is an additional long-term complication.

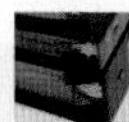

TEACHING GUIDELINE 24.4

Caring for a Child in a Pavlik Harness

- Do not adjust the straps without checking with the physician first.
- Until your physician instructs you to take the harness off for a period of time each day, it must be used continuously (for the first week or sometimes longer).
- Change your baby's diaper while in the harness.
- Place your baby to sleep on his or her back.
- Do not place clothes under the harness during the period of continuous use.
- Once the baby is permitted to be out of the harness for a short period, you may bathe your baby while the harness is off.
- Long knee socks and an undershirt are recommended to prevent rubbing of the skin against the brace.
- Note location of the markings on the straps for appropriate placement of the harness.
- Wash the harness with mild detergent by hand and air dry. If using the dryer, use *only* the air fluffing setting (no heat).

Therapeutic management is aimed at stopping the progression of the disease through bracing or surgical treatment. Medical or surgical treatment should begin early, before 4 years of age.

Nursing Assessment

Elicit a health history and determine the age at which the child started walking. Assess growth parameters to determine whether the risk factor of obesity is present. Note significant bowing of the legs in standing and while ambulating (Fig. 24.16).

Nursing Management

Bracing may include a modified knee–ankle–foot orthosis that relieves the compression forces on the growth plate, allowing bone growth resumption and correction of bowlegs. To be successful, bracing must be continued for months to years and the brace must be worn 23 hours per day. Compliance is the most significant barrier to successful treatment. Parents have a difficult time forcing their toddler to stay in a brace that inhibits mobility for the bulk of the day (particularly a bilateral brace). Support parents by encouraging and praising their compliance with bracing. Teach parents to assess for potential skin impairment from brace rubbing.

When surgical treatment is required, the leg(s) will be immobilized in a long-leg bent knee or spica cast after the osteotomy is performed. Perform routine cast care. Refer to Nursing Care Plan 24.1 for additional interventions related to care of the immobilized child.

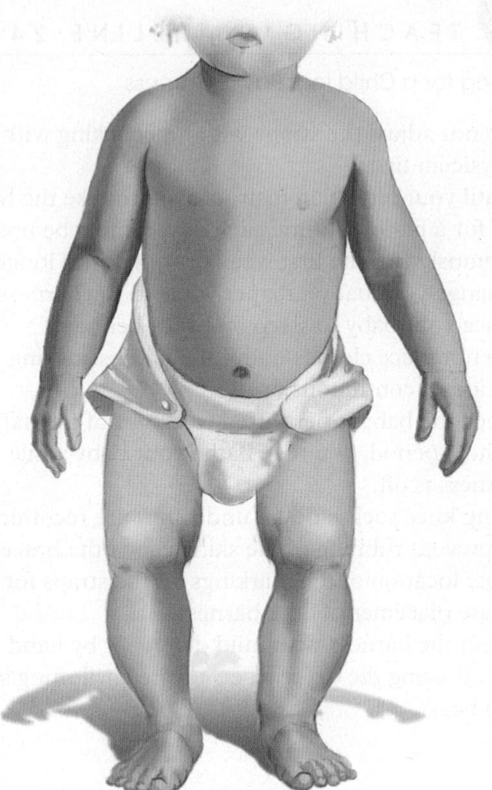

● Figure 24.16 Note extreme bowing of the legs in tibia vara.

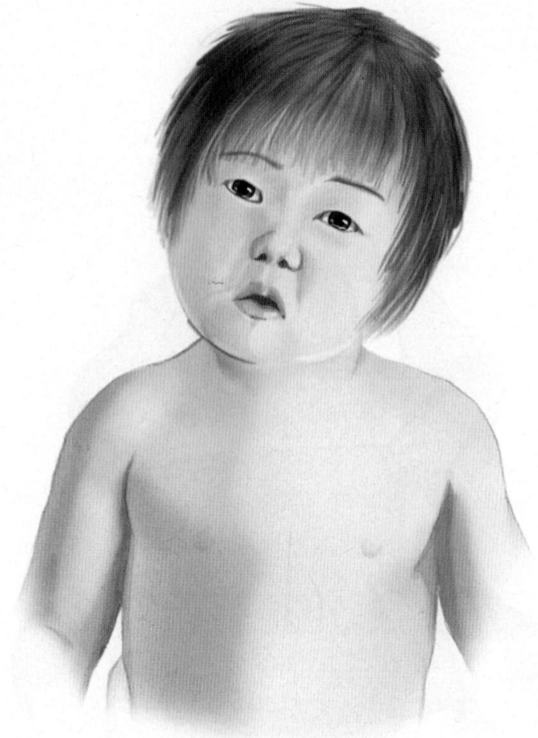

● Figure 24.17 Note wry-neck or head tilt in the infant with torticollis.

● TORTICOLLIS

Torticollis is a painless muscular condition presenting in infants or in children with certain syndromes. Congenital muscular torticollis may result from *in utero* positioning or difficult birth. Preferential turning of the head to one side while in the supine position after birth may also lead to torticollis. Torticollis results from tightness of the sternocleidomastoid muscle, resulting in the infant's head being tilted to one side.

Medical treatment involves passive stretching exercises, which are effective in 90% of affected infants (Luther, 2002). Botulinum toxin injection has been used recently with success in cases of torticollis that have not improved with stretching exercises. Plagiocephaly may result from the continued pressure on the side of the skull to which the neck is turned.

Nursing Assessment

Note history of head tilt and infant's lack of desire to turn the head in the opposite direction. Observe the infant for wry-neck (tilting of the head to one side; Fig. 24.17). Note limited movement of the neck when passive range of motion is performed. Palpate the neck, noting a mass in the sternocleidomastoid muscle on the affected side. Examine the head for evidence of plagiocephaly.

Nursing Management

Teach parents gentle neck-stretching exercises to be performed several times a day. While immobilizing the shoulder on the affected side, gently sustain a side-to-side stretch toward the unaffected side, holding the stretch for 10 to 30 seconds. Repeat 10 to 15 times per session. Perform an ear-to-shoulder stretch in a similar fashion. To prevent the development of torticollis in the unaffected infant, positional plagiocephaly must be prevented. Prevent flatness of one side of the head by varying the baby's head position, and do not always turn the head to one side while in the infant seat or swing or lying supine. Refer families to the National Infant Torticollis Foundation (www.infant-torticollis.org), a parent support network.

Acquired Disorders

Several acquired musculoskeletal disorders may affect children. Nutritional deficits or malabsorption of fats may lead to rickets. Slipped capital femoral epiphysis and Legg-Calvé-Perthes disease affect mainly school-age and adolescent boys. Osteomyelitis, septic arthritis, and toxic synovitis are common infectious musculoskeletal disorders. Spinal curvature may occur as a result of a neuromuscular disorder or idiopathically.

● RICKETS

Rickets is a condition in which there is softening or weakening of the bones. Childhood rickets may occur as a result of nutritional deficiencies such as inadequate consumption of calcium or limited exposure to sunlight (required for adequate production of vitamin D). Rickets may also occur if the body cannot regulate calcium and phosphorus in the appropriate balance, such as in chronic renal disease. Gastrointestinal disorders in which fat absorption is altered (e.g., Crohn's disease and cystic fibrosis) may lead to rickets, as vitamin D is a fat-soluble vitamin. Vitamin D regulates calcium absorption from the small intestine and levels of calcium and phosphate in the bones. Calcium is primarily laid down in the bones of the fetus during the third trimester. Premature infants miss this period of calcium accumulation and also suffer from inadequate calcium intake in the neonatal period and often demonstrate rickets of prematurity. When calcium and phosphate levels in the blood are imbalanced, then calcium is released from the bones into the blood, resulting in loss of the supportive bony matrix. Rickets is most likely to occur during periods of rapid growth.

Therapeutic Management

Treatment of rickets is aimed at correcting the calcium imbalance so that the skeleton may develop properly and without deformity. Calcium and phosphorus supplements are given, and some children also require vitamin D supplements. If rickets is not corrected while the child is still growing, permanent skeletal deformities and short stature may result.

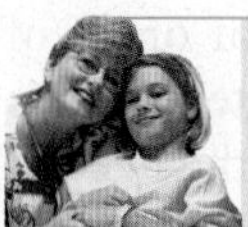

Children who do not receive adequate daily exposure to sunlight require supplementation with 5 micrograms of vitamin D per day.

Nursing Assessment

Obtain a health history, determining risk factors such as:

- Limited exposure to sunlight
- Strict vegetarian diet or lactose intolerance (either one without milk product ingestion)
- Exclusive breastfeeding by a mother who has a vitamin D deficiency
- Dark-pigmented skin
- Prematurity
- Malabsorptive gastrointestinal disorder
- Chronic renal disease

Note history of fractures or bone pain. Observe for dental deformities and bowlegs. Decreased muscle tone may also be present. Note low serum calcium and phosphate levels and high alkaline phosphatase levels. X-rays may show changes in the shape and structure of the bone.

Nursing Management

Administer calcium and phosphorus supplements at alternate times to promote proper absorption of both of these supplements. Encourage exposure to moderate amounts of sunlight and administer vitamin D supplements as prescribed. Teach families that good dietary sources of vitamin D are fish, liver, and processed milk.

● SLIPPED CAPITAL FEMORAL EPIPHYSIS

Slipped capital femoral epiphysis (SCFE) is a condition in which the femoral head dislocates from the neck and shaft of the femur at the level of the epiphyseal plate. The epiphysis slips downward and backward. SCFE occurs most frequently in obese males, 9 to 16 years of age; it is more common in African-American boys than in Caucasians (Leung & Lemay, 2004). The exact cause is unknown, but it is thought that during the teenage growth spurt the femoral growth plate weakens and becomes less resistant to stressors. Hormonal alterations during this period may also play a role.

SCFE is classified based upon its severity and whether the slip is acute or chronic. Chronic SCFE may lead to shortening of the affected leg and thigh atrophy.

Therapeutic Management

Promptly refer the child with SCFE to an orthopedic surgeon, as early surgical intervention will decrease the risk of long-term deformity. The goals of therapeutic management are to prevent further slippage, minimize deformity, and avoid the complications of cartilage necrosis (chondrolysis) and avascular necrosis of the femoral head. Surgical intervention may include in situ pinning, in which a pin or screw is inserted percutaneously into the femoral head to hold it in place. Osteotomy may be used for more severe cases. Osteoarthritis may be a long-term complication of SCFE.

Nursing Assessment

Elicit a health history, determining the onset and extent of pain. In acute SCFE, the pain is usually sudden in onset and results in inability to bear weight. Chronic SCFE may present with an insidious onset of pain and limp. Note risk factors of age 9 to 16 years, African-American race, and obesity. Observe ambulation, noting Trendelenburg gait. Assess for pain that is in the hip or that is referred to the groin, medial thigh, or knee. Note decreased range of motion in the affected hip with external rotation. X-rays will be obtained to confirm the diagnosis (anteroposterior and lateral frog-leg views of hips). Bone scan can rule out avascular necrosis, and CT scan helps define the extent of slippage.

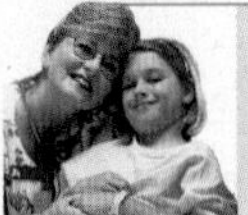

Do not attempt to perform passive range of motion to determine the extent of limitation in the child with SCFE; this may cause worsening of the condition.

Nursing Management

Enforce bed rest and activity restriction. If traction is used for a period before surgery, perform routine traction care and neurovascular assessments. Assess pain and administer analgesics as needed. After in situ pinning, assist the child with crutch walking. Teach the family that weight bearing is usually resumed about a week after the surgery and that the pin will be removed later. Prolonged immobility may isolate the adolescent from usual peer interactions, so encourage phone calls and visits with friends. Provide books, games, electronic devices, and magazines for distraction during the period of immobility. Provide family support.

● LEGG-CALVÉ-PERTHES DISEASE

Legg-Calvé-Perthes disease is a self-limiting condition that involves avascular necrosis of the femoral head. It occurs most often in small, active Caucasian boys or those of Asian descent, usually aged 4 to 10 years, with peak incidence between 6 and 9 years of age (Gunner & Scott, 2001). The disease affects girls much less frequently. The etiology is unknown, but the interruption of the blood supply to the femoral head results in bone death, and the spherical shape of the femoral head may be lost. Swelling of the soft tissues around the hip may occur. As new blood vessels develop, the area is supplied with circulation, allowing bone resorption and deposition to take place. During this period of revascularization, which takes 18 to 24 months, the bone is soft and more likely to fracture. Over time, the femoral head reforms.

Therapeutic Management

The goal of therapeutic management is to maintain normal femoral head shape and to restore appropriate motion. Treatment of Legg-Calvé-Perthes disease includes anti-inflammatory medication to decrease muscle spasms around the hip joint and to relieve pain. Activity limitation may be prescribed, and sometimes bracing is recommended to contain the femoral head. Serial x-ray follow-up determines progress of the disease. If surgery becomes warranted, then osteotomy may be performed. Complications include joint deformity, early degenerative joint disease, persistent pain, loss of hip motion or function, and gait disturbance.

Nursing Assessment

Explore the health history for short stature, delayed bone maturation, or a family history of Legg-Calvé-Perthes disease. Note painless limp, which may be intermittent over a period of months. Mild hip pain may result and may be referred to the knee or the thigh. Pain may be aggravated by exercise. Observe the child walking and note Trendelenburg gait. Perform range of motion, noting internal rotation of the hip and limited abduction. Muscle spasm may result with hip extension and rotation. Hip x-rays are obtained to evaluate the extent of epiphyseal involvement. MRI or bone scan may also be used to differentiate Legg-Calvé-Perthes disease from other disorders.

Nursing Management

Nursing care of Legg-Calvé-Perthes disease is highly variable and depends on the stage of the disease and its severity. Administer anti-inflammatory medications, noting their effect on pain. If activities are restricted, exercise the unaffected body parts. Assist families with use of the brace if prescribed. The brace may be wiped with a damp cloth if it becomes dirty. Some children will be prescribed no treatment other than avoidance of contact or high-impact sports. Swimming and bicycle riding help to maintain range of motion with little risk. If mobility equipment is needed, educate the child and family on its use. If osteotomy is performed, provide routine postoperative care, with education and support of the child and family.

● OSTEOMYELITIS

Osteomyelitis is a bacterial infection of the bone and soft tissue surrounding the bone. The long bone metaphysis is the most common location. Children usually present for evaluation within a few days to a week of onset of symptoms, though some may present later. Osteomyelitis is most often diagnosed in children between the ages of 3 and 12 years. *Staphylococcus aureus* accounts for 90% of cases in infants and children who are otherwise healthy (Carek et al., 2001). Additional causes in infants include group B streptococcus and *Escherichia coli*; in children, *Streptococcus pyogenes* and *Haemophilus influenzae* are also implicated.

Osteomyelitis is acquired hematogenously. Bacteria from the bloodstream mainly invade the most rapidly growing portion of the bone. The invading bacteria trigger an inflammatory response, formation of pus and edema, and vascular congestion. Small blood vessels thrombose and the infection extends into the metaphyseal marrow cavity. As the infection progresses, the inflammation extends throughout the bone and blood supply is disrupted, resulting in death of the bone tissues (Fig. 24.18).

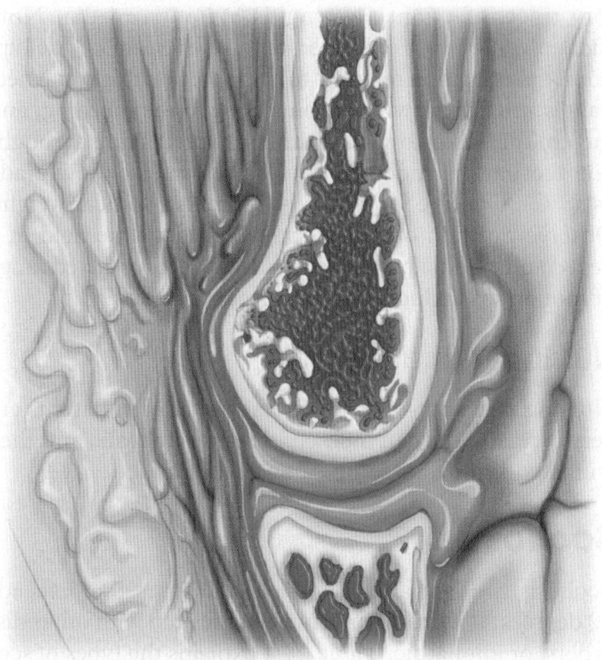

● Figure 24.18 In osteomyelitis, bacterial invasion leads to infection within the bone.

Therapeutic Management

Treatment includes a 4- to 6-week course of antibiotics. Some children may receive 1 to 2 weeks of intravenous antibiotics and then be switched to oral antibiotics for the remainder of the course. Surgical débridement is rarely necessary. Early treatment may prevent the complications of bone destruction, fracture, and growth arrest. Additional complications include recurrent infection, septic arthritis, and systemic infection.

Nursing Assessment

For a full description of the assessment phase of the nursing process, refer to page 805. Assessment findings pertinent to osteomyelitis are discussed here. Explore the health history for risk factors and symptoms. Risk factors include impetigo, infected varicella lesions, furunculosis, infected burns, and prolonged intravenous line use. Note history of irritability, lethargy, possible fever, and onset of pain or change in activity level. The child usually refuses to walk and demonstrates decreased range of motion in the affected extremity. Inspect the affected extremity for swelling. Palpate for local warmth and tenderness. Note point tenderness over affected bone.

Laboratory and diagnostic testing may reveal:

- Elevated white blood cell count, erythrocyte sedimentation rate, and C-reactive protein level
- Positive blood cultures (present in 50% of children; Carek et al., 2001)
- Deep soft tissue swelling on x-ray
- Changes on ultrasound or CT scan

Nursing Management

Nursing management of osteomyelitis focuses on assessment, pain management, and maintenance of intravenous access for administration of antibiotics. Individualize care based on the child's and family's response to the illness; see Nursing Care Plan Overview 24.1. Maintain bed rest initially to prevent injury and promote comfort. Administer antipyretics as ordered if the child is febrile in the initial stage of the illness. Encourage use of unaffected extremities by providing developmentally appropriate toys and games. Instruct child and family on safe and proper use of crutches or walker if prescribed. Some children will be discharged home on intravenous antibiotics, while others will finish an oral antibiotic course. Teach parents proper administration of medications and maintenance of a peripherally inserted central catheter or central line at home if the child is finishing the antibiotic course intravenously.

● SEPTIC ARTHRITIS

Acute septic arthritis is a condition in which bacteria invade the joint space, most often the hip. Its usually occurs in children less than 10 years old, with 3- to 7-year-olds being most frequently affected. Bacteria gain access to the joint in one of three ways:

- Directly from a puncture of the joint or via venipuncture or wound infection
- Seeding from a distal infection site (e.g., otitis media or respiratory infection)
- Compression of the joint capsule from adjacent osteomyelitis

S. aureus, H. influenzae type B, and various streptococci are the most commonly responsible organisms. Sepsis of the hip joint may cause avascular necrosis of the femoral head due to pressure on blood vessels and cartilage within the joint space. Septic arthritis is considered a medical emergency, as this destruction may occur within just a few days. Additional complications of septic arthritis include permanent deformity, leg-length discrepancy, and long-term decreased range of motion and disability.

The goals of treatment of septic arthritis are to prevent destruction of the joint cartilage and maintain function, motion, and strength. Septic arthritis is treated rapidly with joint aspiration or arthrotomy, followed by intravenous antibiotic therapy while in the hospital and oral antibiotics at home.

Nursing Assessment

Note history of predisposing factors such as respiratory infection or otitis media, skin or soft tissue infections, or, in the neonate, traumatic puncture wounds and femoral venipunctures. The history is usually significant for sudden onset of fever and moderate to severe pain.

Upon physical examination, the infant or child appears ill. Note extent of fever, refusal to bear weight or straighten the hip, and limited range of motion (the child usually maintains the joint in flexion and will not allow the leg to be straightened). Palpate the affected joint for warmth and swelling.

Laboratory findings may include:

- White blood cell count normal or elevated with elevated neutrophil counts
- Elevated erythrocyte sedimentation rate and C-reactive protein levels
- Fluid from joint aspiration demonstrates elevated white blood cell count; culture determines responsible organism.
- Joint x-ray may show subtle soft tissue changes or increase in the joint space.
- Positive blood culture for the causative organism (15% of cases)

Nursing Management

Refer to Nursing Care Plan Overview 24.1 for interventions related to musculoskeletal disorders. Assess aspiration wound for signs of infection. Monitor vital signs for resolution of fever. Pain management with ibuprofen or acetaminophen will be sufficient for some children; others may initially require codeine or morphine. Assess the affected joint for decrease in swelling, increasing range of motion, and decreasing or absent pain. The child may be discharged after 72 hours of intravenous antibiotics following joint aspiration if he or she is improving and can tolerate oral antibiotics. At discharge, if the child cannot ambulate, physical therapy may be consulted for short-term use of crutches or a wheelchair. Teach families how to assess for signs and symptoms of wound infection, how to administer oral antibiotics and pain medication, and how to assist their child with crutch walking.

TRANSIENT SYNOVITIS OF THE HIP

Transient synovitis of the hip (also termed toxic synovitis) is the most common cause of hip pain in children (Kehl, 2001). It occurs in children as young as 9 months of age through adolescence, most commonly affecting children 3 to 8 years old. Boys are affected twice as often as girls and African-Americans exhibit the lowest incidence. The exact cause is unclear, but it is thought to be associated with recent or active infection or with trauma. A self-limiting disease, most cases resolve within a week, but it may last as long as 4 weeks. Therapeutic management involves nonsteroidal anti-inflammatory medications and bed rest to relieve weight bearing on the affected hip joint.

Nursing Assessment

Explore the health history for risk factors such as antecedent trauma, concurrent or recent upper respiratory tract infection, pharyngitis, or otitis media. Note sudden acute onset of moderate to severe pain of one hip. Sometimes pain is referred to the anterior thigh or knee. Pain is usually the worst upon arising in the morning, and the child refuses to walk, with pain decreasing throughout the day. Temperature will be normal or low-grade (<38°C). Observe for a limp or for refusal to bear weight. Observe position of the affected hip: it will be held in a flexed and externally rotated position. Note restricted range of motion for abduction and internal rotation.

Nursing Management

Nursing care focuses on educating the family. Parents are very concerned when their child refuses to walk, and they will need significant support and reassurance.

Scoliosis

Scoliosis is a lateral curvature of the spine that exceeds 10 degrees. It may be congenital, associated with other disorders, or idiopathic. Table 24.4 explains the types of scoliosis. Idiopathic scoliosis accounts for 65% of all cases of scoliosis, with the majority of those occurring during adolescence (Zak, 2005). Hence, this discussion will focus on adolescent idiopathic scoliosis. The etiology of idiopathic scoliosis is not known, but genetic factors, growth abnormalities, and bone, muscle, disk, or central nervous system disorders may contribute to its development. Early screening and detection of scoliosis result in improved outcomes.

Pathophysiology

In the rapidly growing adolescent, the involved vertebrae rotate around a vertical axis, resulting in lateral curvature.

Table 24.4 Types of Scoliosis

Type	Associated Factors
Idiopathic	Unknown cause Infantile: occurs in the first 3 years of life Juvenile: diagnosed between age 4 and 10 years, or prior to adolescence Adolescent: age 11 to 17 years
Neuromuscular	Associated with neurologic or muscular disease such as cerebral palsy, myelomeningocele, spinal cord tumors, spinal muscular atrophy
Myopathic	Associated with certain types of muscular dystrophy
Congenital	Results from anomalous vertebral development

The vertebrae rotate to the convex side of curve, with the spinous processes rotating toward the concave side. Wedge-shaped vertebral bodies and disks develop because growth is suppressed on the concave side of the curve (Newton & Wenger, 2001). As the curve progresses, the shape of the thoracic cage changes and respiratory and cardiovascular compromise may occur (the main complications of severe scoliosis).

Therapeutic Management

Treatment of scoliosis is aimed at preventing progression of the curve and decreasing the impact on pulmonary and cardiac function. Treatment is based on the age of the child, expected future growth, and severity of the curve. Observation with serial examinations and spine x-rays is used to monitor curve progression. For curves of 20 to 50 degrees, bracing may be sufficient to decrease progression of the curve. Some curves will progress despite appropriate bracing and compliance. Box 24.2 describes types of scoliosis braces and Figure 24.19 shows examples. The choice of brace will depend on the location and severity of the curve.

Surgical correction is often required for curves greater than 45 degrees; it is achieved with rod placement and bone grafting. Partial spinal fusion accompanies many of the corrective surgeries. Multiple surgical approaches and techniques exist for fusion and rod placement. The surgical approach may be anterior, posterior, or both. Traditional rod placement (Harrington rod) involved a single rod fused to the vertebrae, resulting in curve correction but also a flat-backed appearance. Newer rod instrumentations allow for scoliosis curve correction with maintenance of normal back curvature. The rods are shorter, and several are wired or grafted to the appropriate vertebrae to achieve correction. Figure 24.20 shows one example of surgical rod instrumentation.

Nursing Assessment

For a full description of the assessment phase of the nursing process, refer to page 805. Assessment findings pertinent to scoliosis are discussed below.

Health History

Determine why the child is presenting for evaluation of scoliosis. Commonly the child or adolescent will not report back pain, as only mild discomfort is associated with idiopathic scoliosis until the curve becomes severe. Often the family recognizes asymmetry in the hips or shoulders or the child is screened for scoliosis at school and determined to be at risk. Explore the client's current and past medical history for risk factors such as:

- Family history of scoliosis
- Recent growth spurt
- Physical changes related to puberty

Determine the age of development of secondary sex characteristics and the age of menarche, as these signs of pubertal development indicate the expected velocity and length of remaining growth.

Physical Examination

The physical assessment of a child with possible or actual scoliosis involves mainly inspection and observation. Auscultate the heart and lungs to determine compromise related to severe curvature.

Observe the child at rest, sitting, and standing for evidence of poor posture. Inspect the child's back in a standing position. Note asymmetries such as shoulder elevation, prominence of one scapula, uneven curve at the waistline, or a rib hump on one side. Measure shoulder levels from the floor to the acromioclavicular joints. Note the difference between the height of the high and low shoulder in centimeters. Measure heights of anterior and posterior iliac spines and note the difference in centimeters. View the patient from the side, noting abnormalities in the spinal curve. With the child bending forward, arms hanging freely, note asymmetry of the back (pronounced hump on one side). Figure 24.21 shows scoliosis noted upon visual inspection. Note leg-length discrepancy if present. During the neurologic examination, balance, motor strength, sensation, and reflexes should all be normal.

Laboratory and Diagnostic Tests

Full-spine x-rays are necessary to determine the degree of curvature. The radiologist will determine the extent of the curve based on specific formulas and techniques of measurement.

Nursing Management

Nursing Care Plan 24.1 lists general interventions; nursing care should be tailored based on the adolescent's response to the disease and its treatment. Additional nursing interventions specific to scoliosis are discussed here.

Encouraging Compliance With Bracing

Bracing is intended to prevent progression of the curve but does not correct the current curve. Although mod-

BOX 24.2

TYPES OF BRACES USED TO TREAT SCOLIOSIS

- Underarm (Boston, Wilmington): less conspicuous, no visible neckpiece
- Milwaukee: traditional standard, has a visible neckpiece
- Nighttime bending (Charleston): creates a curve so severe that walking is not possible, so can be worn only at night

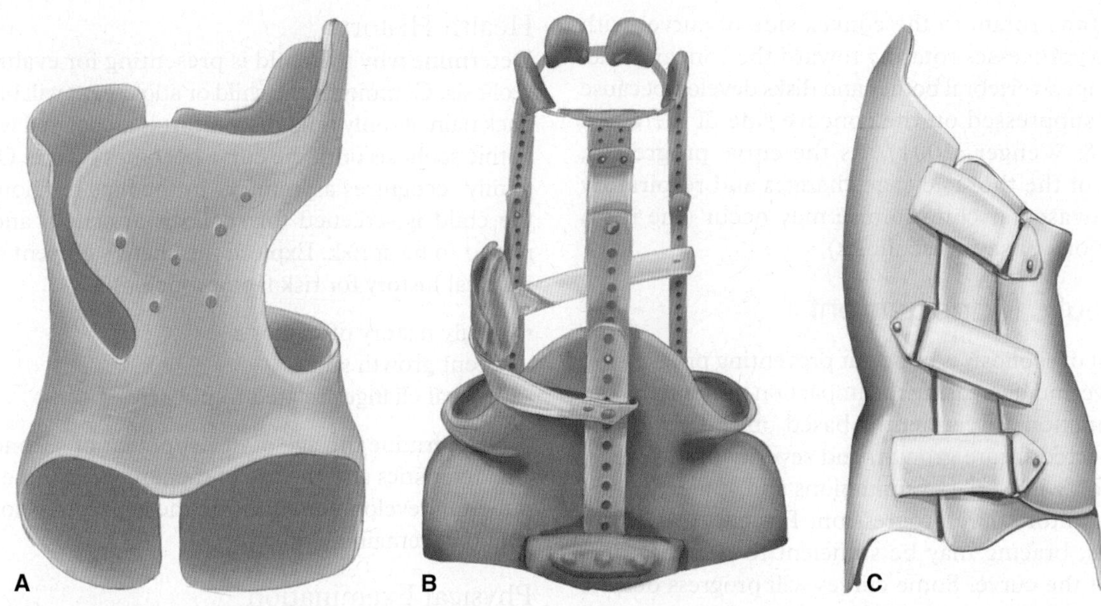

● Figure 24.19 (A) Boston brace. (B) Milwaukee brace. (C) Nighttime bending brace.

ern braces display an improved appearance, with no visible neckpiece, and can be worn under clothes, many adolescents are not compliant with brace wear. The brace must be worn 23 hours per day to prevent curve progression. Many factors may contribute to noncompliance, including the discomfort associated with brace wear such as pain, heat, and poor fit. The family environment may not be conducive to compliance with brace wear, and teenagers are very concerned about body image.

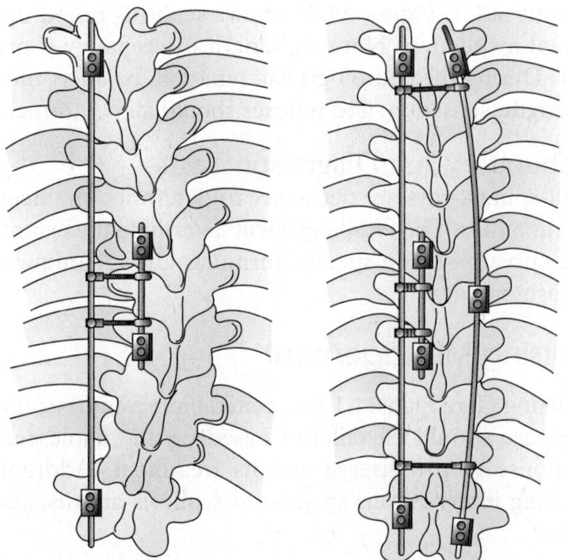
● Figure 24.20 Rods are fused to the vertebrae and connected to a distracting rod to rotate the vertebral column (Cotrel-Dubousset method is shown).

Inspect the skin for evidence of rubbing by the brace that may impair skin integrity. Teach families appropriate skin care and recommend they check the brace daily for fit and breakage. Encourage the teen to shower during the 1 hour per day that the brace is off and to ensure that the skin is clean and dry before putting the brace back on. Wearing a cotton T-shirt under the brace may decrease some of the discomfort associated with brace wear. Exercises to strengthen back muscles may prevent muscle atrophy from prolonged bracing and maintain spine flexibility.

Promoting Positive Body Image

Encourage the teen to express his or her feelings or concerns about wearing the brace. Give the teen ways to explain scoliosis and its treatment to his or her peers. Wearing stylish baggy clothes may help the teen to conceal the brace if desired. Refer teens and their families to the National Scoliosis Foundation (www.scoliosis.org) for additional support.

Providing Preoperative Care

If the curve progresses despite bracing or causes pulmonary or cardiac compromise, surgical intervention will be warranted. In the preoperative period, teach the teen the importance of turning, coughing, and deep breathing in the postoperative period. Explain the tubes and lines that will be present immediately after the surgery. Review positioning guidelines: back flexion or extension will not be allowed. Introduce the child to the patient-controlled analgesia pump and explain pain scales. There is a high risk for significant blood loss with spinal fusion and instrumentation, so if possible arrange for preoperative autologous blood donation.

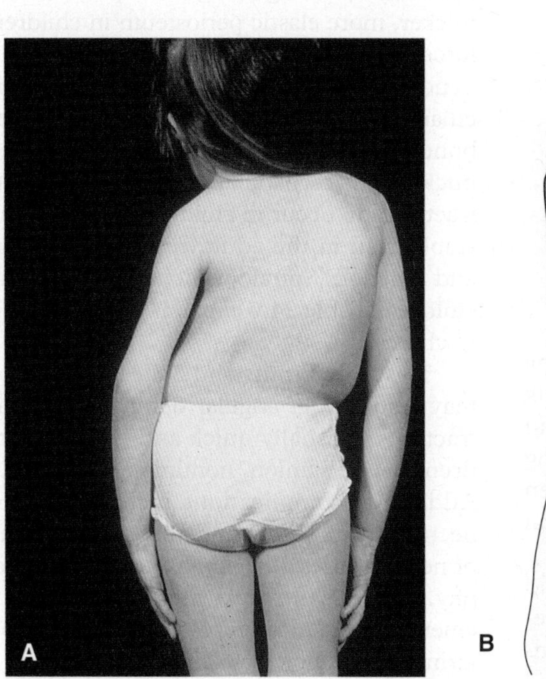

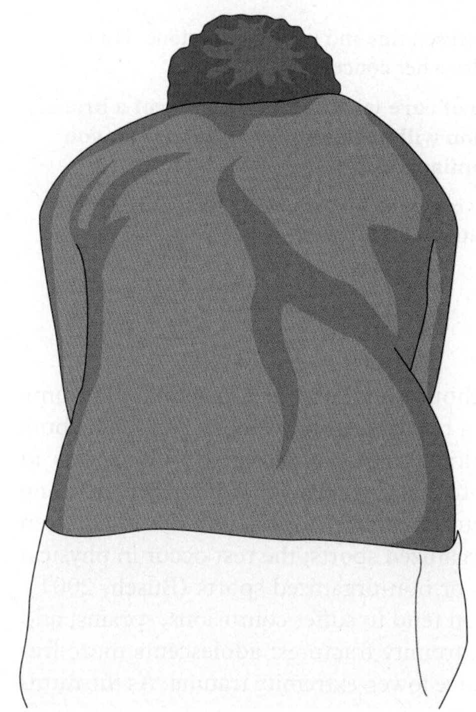

● Figure 24.21 (**A**) Note right shoulder, scapula, and hip elevation as well as discrepancy in waist curvature. (**B**) Note right upper back hump.

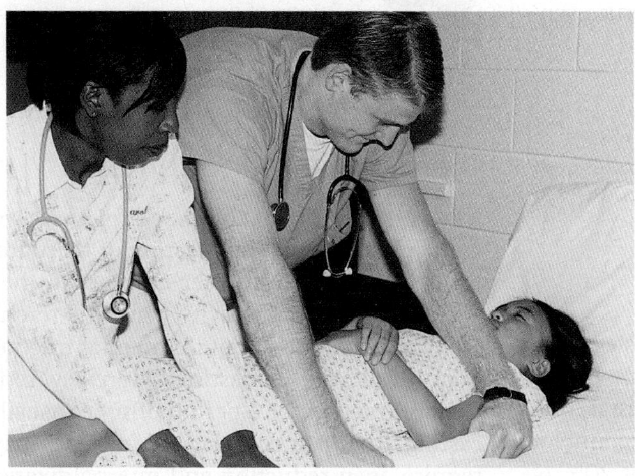

● Figure 24.22 Log-roll the postoperative spinal fusion patient to prevent spine flexion.

Providing Postoperative Care

The goal of nursing management in the postoperative period after spinal fusion with or without instrumentation is to avoid complications. Perform neurovascular checks with each set of vital signs. When turning the child, use the log-roll technique to avoid flexion of the back (Fig. 24.22). Administer prophylactic intravenous antibiotics if ordered. Assess for drainage from the operative site and for excess blood loss via the Hemovac or other drainage tube. Maintain Foley patency, as the child will be confined to bed for the first couple of days. Maintain strict recording of fluid intake and output. Administer transfusions of packed red blood cells if ordered. Ambulation, once ordered, should be done slowly to avoid orthostatic hypotension. Assist the family with arrangements to continue the teen's school work while hospitalized and/or arrange for home tutoring during the several-week recovery period.

Consider THIS!

Angela Hernandez, a 15-year-old girl, is being seen in the clinic after she was found to be at high risk for scoliosis during a school screening. Upon assessment the nurse notes asymmetry of the hips, with shoulder elevation and prominence of one scapula. She is visibly upset and wants to know what caused this and what can be done. How would you address her concerns?

Angela's plan of care will include wearing of a brace. What education will be necessary and how can you promote compliance?

Describe nursing care for Angela if surgical correction is necessary.

Injuries

Injuries throughout childhood are inevitable. Trauma often occurs as a result of motor vehicle injury. The bulk of trauma resulting from physical activity or sports in children is due to running, skateboarding, and climbing trees. Only about one third of sports injuries in children occur during organized sports; the rest occur in physical education class or non-organized sports (Busch, 2001). Younger children tend to suffer contusions, sprains, and simple upper extremity fractures; adolescents more frequently experience lower-extremity trauma. As the number of children participating in youth sports increases and the intensity of training and the level of competition also increase, the incidence of injury is also likely to increase.

Many types of musculoskeletal injuries exist. This discussion will focus on fractures, sprains, overuse syndromes, and dislocated radial head.

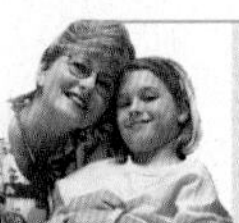

Fracture in the newborn or infant should raise a high index of suspicion for abuse, as fractures are very unusual in children who cannot yet walk.

• FRACTURE

Fractures occur frequently in children and adolescents; 40% of boys and 25% of girls will suffer a fracture by age 16 years. About 50% of fractures occur in the distal forearm and hand. Greenstick and buckle fractures account for about half of pediatric fractures, and only about 20% of childhood fractures require reduction (Price et al., 2001).

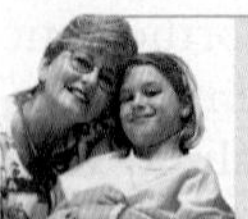

Do not attempt to straighten or manipulate an injured limb.

Pathophysiology

Fractures result most frequently from accidental trauma (DiFazio & Atkinson, 2005). Nonaccidental trauma (child abuse) and other disease processes are the other causes of fractures. The growth plate is the most vulnerable portion of the child's bone and is frequently the site of injury. The Salter-Harris classification system is used to describe fractures involving the growth plate (Table 24.5). The thicker, more elastic periosteum in children yields to the force encountered with trauma, resulting more frequently in nondisplaced fractures in children. The increased vascularity and decreased mineral content make the child's bones more flexible. Plastic or bowing deformities and buckle and greenstick fractures are the result. Complete fractures do occur in children, but they tend to be more stable than in the adult, resulting in improved healing and function. Spiral, pelvic, and hip fractures are rare in children. Table 24.6 explains common types of fractures in children.

Plastic deformity and Salter-Harris type IV fractures may result in an angular deformity. Though healing of fractures is usually quick and without incident in children, delayed union, nonunion, or malunion can occur. Additional complications include infection, avascular necrosis, bone shortening from epiphyseal arrest, vascular or nerve injuries, fat embolism, reflex sympathetic dystrophy, and compartment syndrome, which is an orthopedic emergency. Later in life, osteoarthritis may occur as a long-term complication from childhood fracture.

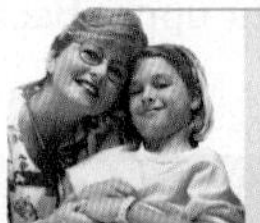

Spiral femur fractures and humerus fractures, particularly in the child less than 2 years of age, should always be thoroughly investigated to rule out the possibility of child abuse.

Therapeutic Management

The vast majority of childhood fractures would heal well with splinting only, but casting of these fractures is performed to provide further comfort to the child and to allow for increased activity while the fracture is healing. Displaced fractures require manual traction to align the bones, followed by casting. More severe fractures may require traction for a period of time, usually followed by casting. Severe or complicated fractures may alternatively require open reduction and internal fixation for healing to occur. Complex fractures are often treated with external fixation (Fig. 24.23).

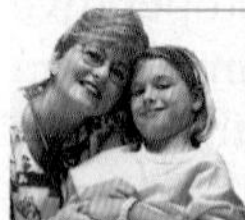

Significant swelling may occur initially after immobilization with a splint. Splinting and then delaying casting for a few days provides time for some of the swelling to subside, allowing for successful casting a few days after the injury.

Nursing Assessment

For a full description of the assessment phase of the nursing process, refer to page 805. Assessment findings pertinent to fractures are discussed below.

Table 24.5 The Salter-Harris Classification System

Type	Description	Illustration
I	Fracture is through the physis, widening it.	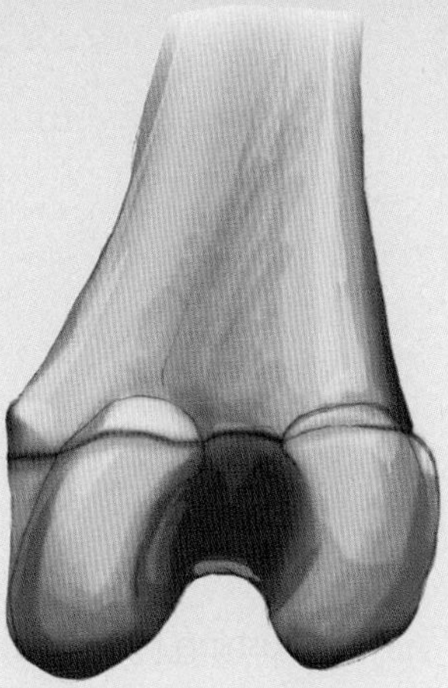
II	Fracture is partially through the physis, extending into the metaphysis.	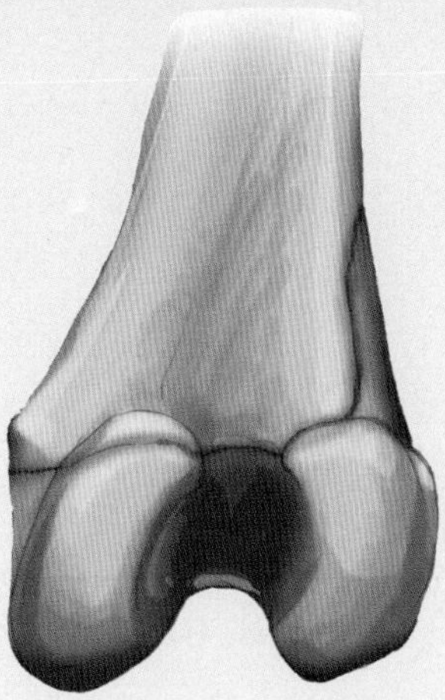
III	Fracture is partially through the epiphysis, extending into the epiphysis.	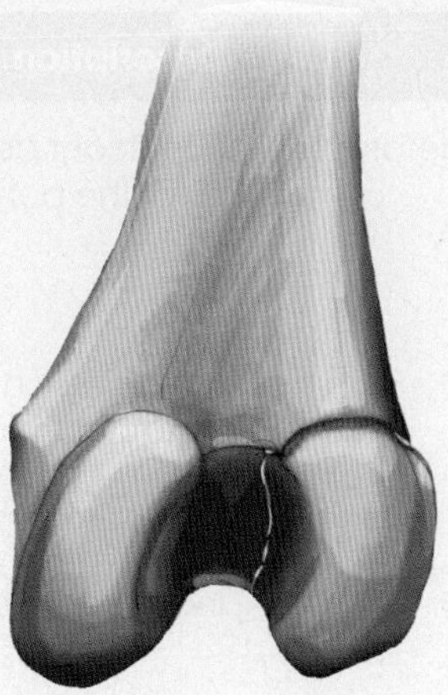

(continued)

Table 24.5 The Salter-Harris Classification System (continued)

Type	Description	Illustration
IV	Fracture is through the metaphysis, physis, epiphysis.	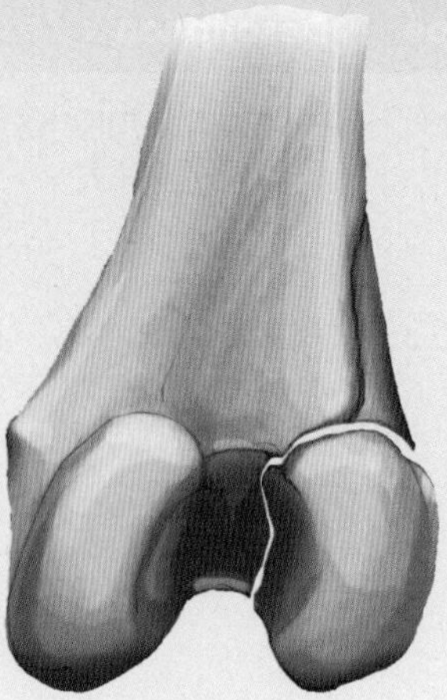
V	Crushing injury to the physis	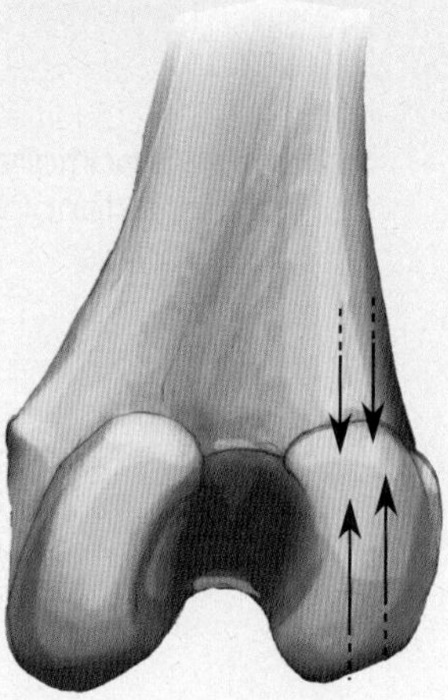

Table 24.6 Types of Fractures in Children

Fracture Type	Description	Illustration
Plastic or bowing deformity	Significant bending without breaking of the bone	A 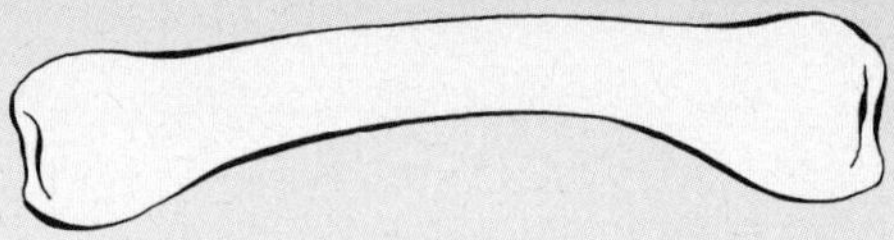
Buckle fracture	Compression injury; the bone buckles rather than breaks	B 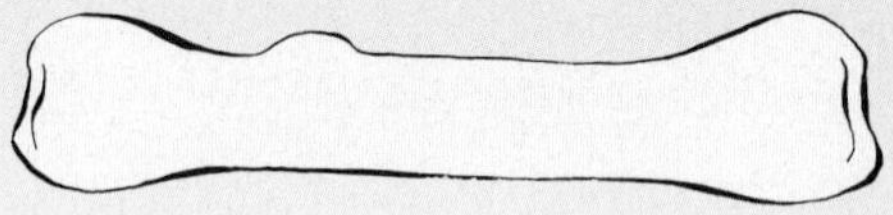
Greenstick fracture	Incomplete fracture of the bone	C 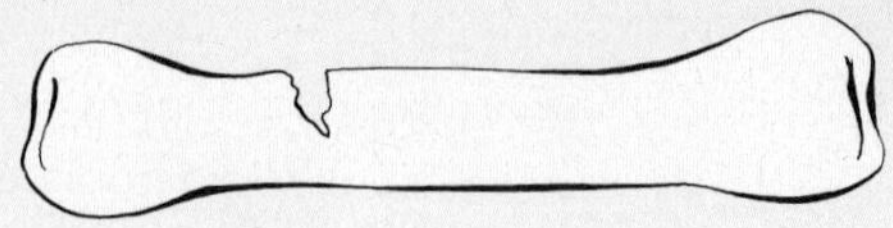
Complete fracture	Bone breaks into two pieces	D 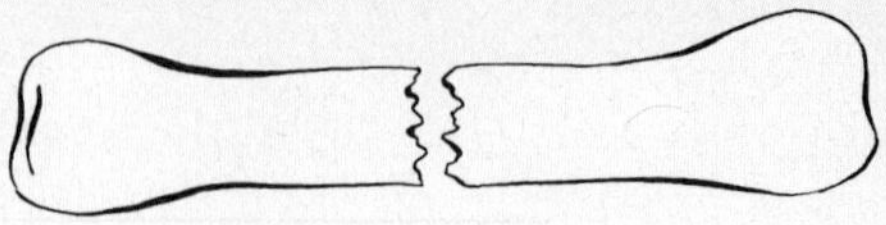

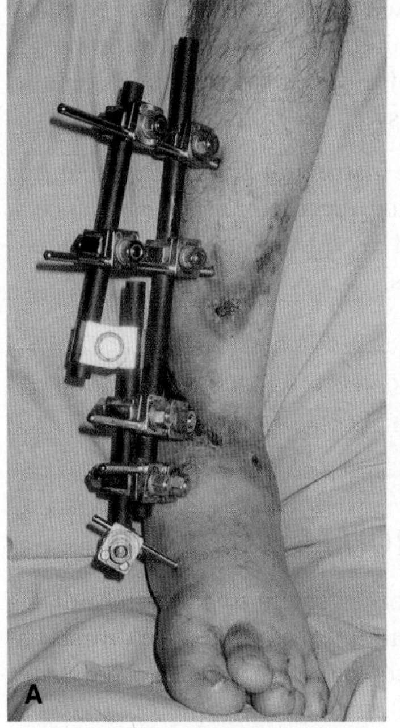

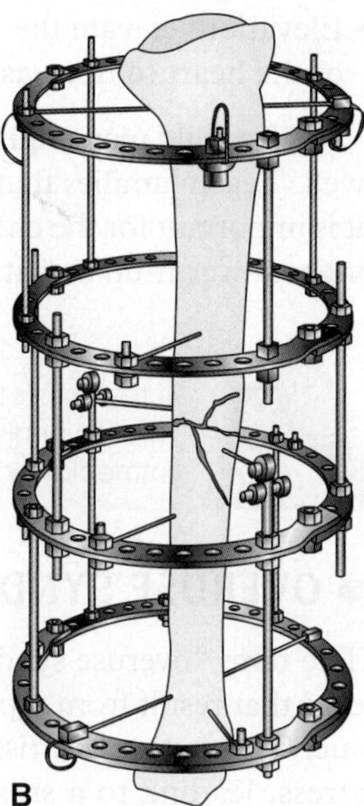

● Figure 24.23 (A) External fixation is required for complicated fractures. (B) The Ilizarov fixator is a circular apparatus usually used for complicated lower extremity fractures. The pins are smaller in diameter, more like wires, than those used in other fixators.

Health History

Elicit a description of the present illness and chief complaint. Common signs and symptoms reported during the health history might include recent trauma or fall, complaint of pain, difficulty bearing weight, limp, or refusal to use an extremity. Young children often demonstrate sudden onset of irritability and refusal to bear weight. Ask about the mechanism of injury and obtain a description of the traumatic event. Be alert to inconsistencies between the history and the clinical picture or mechanism of injury, as such inconsistency may be an indicator of child abuse. Explore the patient's current and past medical history for risk factors such as:

- Rickets
- Renal osteodystrophy
- Osteogenesis imperfecta
- Participation in sports, particularly contact sports
- Failure to use protective equipment as recommended for various physical activities and sports (e.g., wrist guards while rollerblading)

Physical Examination

Perform the physical examination of the child with a potential fracture carefully, so as not to cause further pain or trauma. The physical examination particular to fractures includes inspection, observation, and palpation.

Inspection and Observation

Inspect the skin for bruising, erythema, or swelling. Observe the extremities for deformity. Note neglect of an extremity or inability to bear weight. If ambulating, note any limp.

Palpation

Carefully palpate the joint or injured part. Distract the young child with a toy or activity while palpating. Note point tenderness, which is a reliable indicator of fracture in children. Assess neurovascular status, noting distal extremity temperature, spontaneous movement, sensation, numbness, capillary refill time, and quality of pulses. The neurovascular assessment is critical to providing a baseline so that any changes associated with compartment syndrome can be quickly identified.

Laboratory and Diagnostic Tests

Usually plain x-ray films are all that is required to identify a simple fracture. Complicated fractures that require surgical intervention may require further evaluation with CT or MRI.

Nursing Management

Immediately after the injury, immobilize the limb above and below the site of injury in the most comfortable position with a splint. Use cold therapy to reduce swelling in the first 48 hours after injury. Elevate the injured extremity above the level of the heart. Perform frequent neurovascular checks. Assess pain level and administer pain medications as needed. Administer tetanus vaccine in the child with an open fracture if he or she has not received a tetanus booster within the past 5 years.

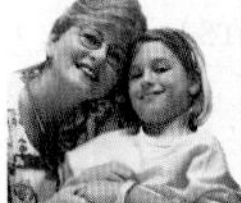

Assess the injured, splinted, or casted extremity frequently for the "5 P's," which may indicate compartment syndrome: pain (increased out of proportion), pulselessness, pallor, paresthesia, paralysis. Report these findings immediately.

Providing Family Education

Unless bed rest is prescribed, children with upper extremity casts and "walking" leg casts can resume increased levels of activity as the pain subsides. Children who require crutches while in a cast may return to school, but those in spica casts will be at home for several weeks. Providing distraction and finding ways to keep up with school work are important. Families must also learn to care for the cast (see Teaching Guideline 24.1).

Preventing Fractures

Discourage risky behavior such as climbing trees and performing tricks on bicycles. Provide appropriate supervision, particularly with outdoor activity. Encourage appropriate use of protective equipment, such as wrist guards with rollerblading and shin guards with soccer. Ensure that playground equipment is in good working order and intact; there should not be protruding screws or unbalanced portions of equipment, which may increase the risk for falling.

● SPRAINS

Sprains result from a twisting or turning motion of the affected body part. The tendons and ligaments stretch excessively and may tear slightly. They may occur at any joint, but the most common are ankle and knee sprains. Therapeutic management of sprains includes rest, ice, compression, and elevation (RICE). On initial evaluation, sprains need to be differentiated from torn ligaments and meniscal tears, as those conditions are more serious and may require surgical intervention.

Nursing Assessment

Elicit a health history, determining the mechanism of injury (whether it occurred during sports or simply a misstep or fall). Determine what treatment the family has used so far. Inspect the affected body part for edema, which is frequently present, and bruising, which sometimes occurs. Note limp or inability to bear weight. Do not attempt to perform passive range of motion on the affected body part. Assess neurovascular status distal to the injury (usually normal).

Nursing Management

Instruct the child and family in appropriate treatment of sprains, which includes:

- Rest: limit activity.
- Ice: apply cold packs for 20 to 30 minutes, remove for 1 hour, and repeat (for the first 24 to 48 hours).
- Compression: apply an Ace wrap or other elastic bandage or brace; check skin for alterations when rewrapping.
- Elevation: elevate the injured extremity above the level of the heart to decrease swelling (Fig. 24.24).

The child may require instruction in crutch walking as well. Teach families that to prevent sprains during sports, it is important for the child to perform appropriate stretching and warm-up activities.

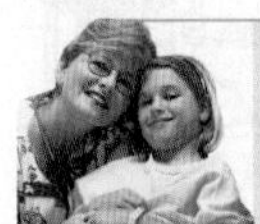

If the child's fingers or toes become increasingly swollen or discolored, remove the Ace wrap immediately.

● OVERUSE SYNDROMES

The term "overuse syndrome" refers to a group of disorders that result from repeated force applied to normal tissue. The connective tissues fail in response to repetitive stress, leading to a small amount of tissue breakdown. They develop over the course of weeks to months. There is usually no identifiable injury associated with overuse syndromes. Pain is usually associated with the activity and worsens with continued participation in the activity. Table 24.7 gives details on several common overuse syndromes. Therapeutic management is aimed at reassurance, pain management, and limiting rather than eliminating activity.

Nursing Assessment

Elicit a health history to determine the extent of involvement in sports. Note onset of pain, duration, intensity,

RICE

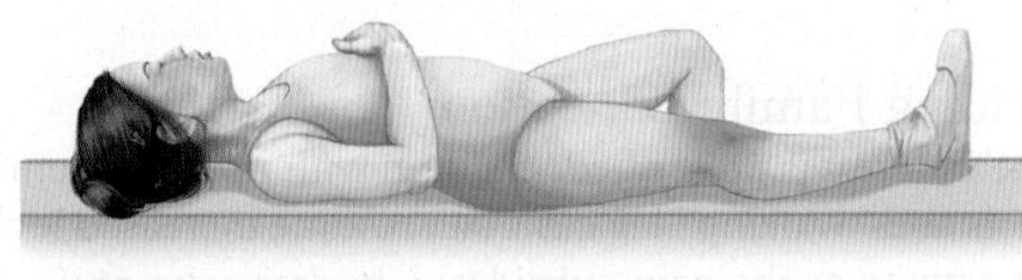

Rest

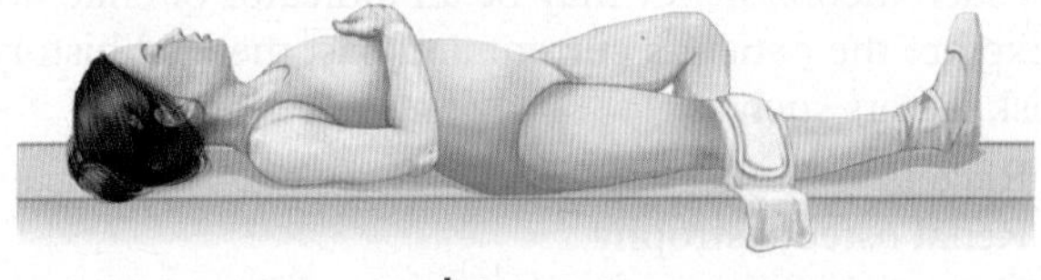

Ice

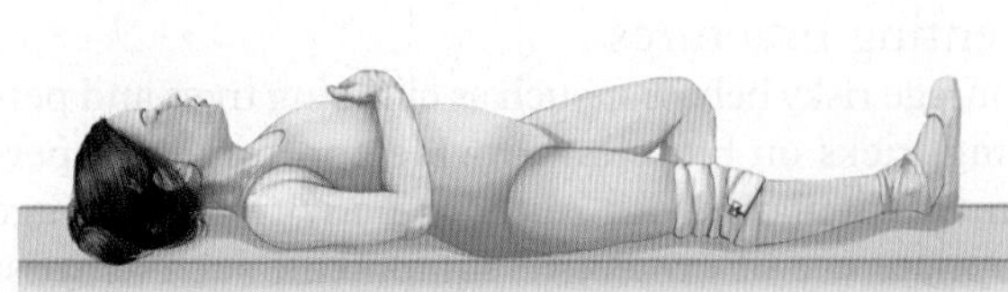

Compression

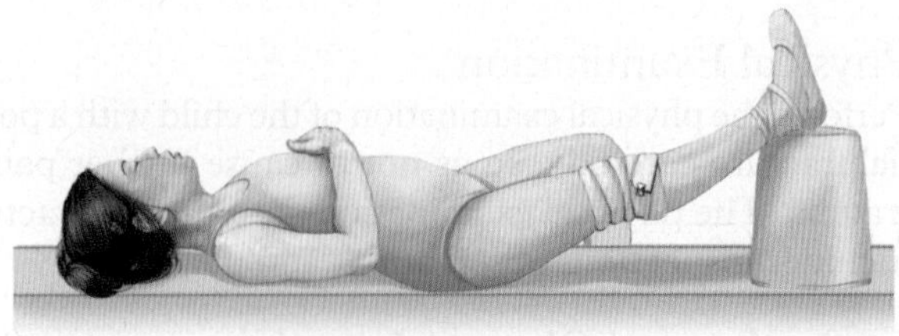

Elevation

● Figure 24.24 RICE (rest, ice, compression, elevation) is the appropriate treatment for sprains.

Table 24.7 Overuse Disorders

Disorder	Anatomic Area Affected	Most Commonly Occurs in	Symptoms
Osgood-Schlatter disease	Partial avulsion of the ossification center of the tibial tubercle	Active adolescents, most often boys. Most frequently during periods of rapid growth.	• Mild to moderate pain, activity-related • Tibial tubercle is tender when palpated. • Painful swelling or prominence of the anterior portion of the tibial tubercle
Epiphysiolysis of proximal humerus	Proximal humerus (widening of growth plate)	Occurs with rigorous upper extremity activity, such as baseball pitching	• Tenderness in the shoulder or proximal humerus • Pain with active internal rotation • Full shoulder range of motion continues.
Epiphysiolysis of distal radius	Distal radius (widening of growth plate)	Occurs with overuse of the distal radius, such as in gymnasts	• Wrist pain that worsens with activity
Sever's disease (calcaneal apophysitis)	Calcaneus (heel)	Usually in 9- to 14-year-olds	• Pain over the posterior aspect of the calcaneus • Limited active and passive dorsiflexion of foot
Shin splints	Refers to a variety of overuse syndromes associated with the shin (stress fracture, tibial stress, muscular issues)	Occurs with activities that place repeated exertion on the lower leg, as in runners, ballerinas, elite soccer players	• Exercise-induced pain of the anterior aspect of the middle part of the lower leg • May be sharp pain • Worsens with exercise • With stress fracture, may have a limp that worsens with activity

aggravating factors, and treatments used at home. Examine the painful part, noting findings similar to those noted for each syndrome in Table 24.7.

Nursing Management

Initially, apply ice when pain is severe. Anti-inflammatory medications such as ibuprofen may be helpful. The child should limit exercise and participate in a different activity. After a few weeks, most overuse syndromes resolve; at that point, the athlete may resume the prior activity. Osgood-Schlatter disease is the exception and may require 12 to 18 months to resolve. Using pads or braces that are appropriate to the painful body part is also helpful. Supporting the arm with a sling may relieve stress on the proximal humerus when epiphysiolysis occurs. Heel cups used in athletic shoes help relieve stress on the heels associated with Sever's disease. To prevent overuse syndromes, encourage athletes to perform appropriate stretching exercises during a 20- to 30-minute warm-up period before each practice or game. Also encourage several weeks of conditioning training before the season begins.

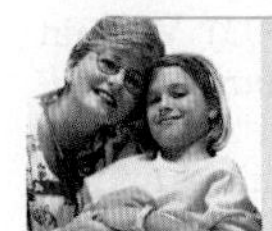

"Energy healing" such as therapeutic touch and Reiki may provide a nonpharmacologic adjunct to pain management for musculoskeletal injuries.

● DISLOCATED RADIAL HEAD

Dislocation of the radial head ("nursemaid's elbow") occurs when a pulling motion on the arm causes the ligament surrounding the radial head to become entrapped within the joint. It usually occurs in children less than 7 years of age and is a common injury in children aged 1 to 4. To reduce the injury, the elbow is flexed to 90 degrees and then the forearm is fully and firmly supinated, causing the ligament to snap back into place. With appropriate reduction of the radial head, no complications result.

Nursing Assessment

The child will hold the arm slightly flexed at the side and refuse to move it. When the arm is still, the child apparently has no discomfort. Assess neurovascular status (intact).

Nursing Management

After treatment, usually hyperpronation to reduce the dislocation, assess the child's ability to use the arm without pain. Teach parents to avoid pulling up on the child's arm, particularly in an abrupt jerking fashion, to prevent recurrence.

References

Books and Journals

Ackley, B. J., & Ladwig, G. B. (2004). *Nursing diagnosis handbook: A guide to planning care* (6th ed.). St. Louis: Mosby.

Allard, P., Chavet, P., Barbier, F., Gatto, L., Labelle, H., & Sadeghi, H. (2004). Effect of body morphology on standing balance in adolescent idiopathic scoliosis. *American Journal of Physical Medicine and Rehabilitation, 83,* 689–697.

American Academy of Pediatrics, Committee on Quality Improvement, Subcommittee on Developmental Dysplasia of the Hip. (2000). Clinical practice guideline: Early detection of developmental dysplasia of the hip. *Pediatrics, 105*(4), 896–905.

Bernardo, L. M. (2001). Evidence-based practice for pin site care in injured children. *Orthopedic Nursing, 20*(5), 29–34.

Bernardo, L. M., Gardner, M. J., & Seibel, K. (2001). Playground injuries in children: A review and Pennsylvania trauma center experience. *Journal of the Society of Pediatric Nurses, 6*(1), 11–20.

Brown, D., & Fisher, E. (2004). Femur fractures in infants and young children. *American Journal of Public Health, 94*(4), 558–560.

Bulloch, B., Neto, G., Plint, A., Lim, R., Lidman, P., Reed, M., Nijssen-Jordan, C., Tenebein, M., Klassen, T. P., & Bhargava, R. (2003). The Ottawa knee rules accurately identified fractures in children with knee injuries. *Annals of Emergency Medicine, 42,* 48–55.

Busch, M. T. (2001). Sports medicine in children and adolescents. In R. T. Morrissy & S. L. Weinstein (Eds.), *Lovell & Winter's pediatric orthopaedics* (5th ed.). Philadelphia: Lippincott Williams & Wilkins.

Carakushansky, M., O'Brien, K. O., & Levine, M. A. (2003). Vitamin D and calcium: Strong bones for life through better nutrition. *Contemporary Pediatrics, 20*(3), 37–50.

Carek, P. J., Dickerson, L. M., & Sack, J. I. (2001). Diagnosis and management of osteomyelitis. *American Family Physician, 63*(12), 2413–2420.

Cartwright, C. C. (2002). Assessing asymmetrical infant head shapes. *Nurse Practitioner, 27*(8), 33–39.

Chin, K. R., Price, J. S., & Zimbler, S. (2001). A guide to early detection of scoliosis. *Contemporary Pediatrics, 18*(9), 77 [electronic version] available at www.contemporarypediatrics.com.

Clark, C. (2001). Osteogenesis imperfecta: An overview. *Nursing Standard,* 16(5), 47–52.

DiFazio, R., & Atkinson, R. (2005). Extremity fractures in children: When is it an emergency? *Journal of Pediatric Nursing, 20*(4), 298–304.

DiNucci, E. M. (2005). Energy healing: A complementary treatment for orthopaedic and other conditions. *Orthopaedic Nursing, 24*(4), 259–269.

Eiff, M. P., & Hatch, R. L. (2003). Boning up on common pediatric fractures. *Contemporary Pediatrics, 20*(11), 30–59.

Eilert, R. E. (2007). Orthopedics. In Hay, W. W., Levin, M. J., Sondheimer, J. M., & Deterding, R. R. (Eds.), *Current pediatric diagnosis and treatment* (18th ed.). New York: McGraw-Hill.

Falk, M. J., Heeger, S., Lynch, K. A., DeCaro, K. R., Bohach, D., Gibson, K. S., & Warman, M. L. (2003). Intravenous bisphosphonate therapy in children with osteogenesis imperfecta. *Pediatrics, 111*(3), 573–578.

Frasier, L. D. (2003). Child abuse or mimic? *Consultant for Pediatricians, 2,* 212–215.

Ganel, A., Dudkiewicz, I., & Grogan, D. P. (2003). Pediatric orthopedic physical examination of the infant: A 5-minute assessment. *Journal of Pediatric Health Care, 17*(1), 39–41.

Gilmore, A., & Thompson, G. H. (2003). Common childhood foot deformities. *Consultant for Pediatricians, 2*(2), 63–71.

Godley, D. R. (2002). A practical approach to the child that limps. *Contemporary Pediatrics, 19*(2), 56 [electronic version] available at www.contemporarypediatrics.com.

Gore, A. I., & Spencer, J. P. (2004). The newborn foot. *American Family Physician, 69*(4), 865–872.

Goretsky, M. J., Kelly, R. E., Croitoru, D., & Nuss, D. (2004). Chest wall anomalies: Pectus excavatum and pectus carinatum. *Adolescent Medicine Clinics, 15*(3), 455–471 [electronic version]. Accessed 10/1/05.

Greene, J. (2001). Fractures at an early age: "It's just bad luck." *Journal of Pediatric Health Care, 15,* 318–328.

Gris, M., Van Nieuwenhove, O., Gehanne, C., Quintin, J., & Burny, F. (2004). Treatment of supracondylar humeral fractures in children using external fixation. *Orthopedics, 27*(11), 1146–1150.

Gunner, K. B., & Scott, A. C. (2001). Evaluation of the child with a limp. *Journal of Pediatric Health Care, 15,* 38–40.

Hennrikus, W. L. (1999). Developmental dysplasia of the hip: Diagnosis and treatment in children younger than 6 months. *Pediatric Annals, 28*(12), 740–746.

Howard, A. W., MacArthur, C., Willan, A., Rothman, L., Moses-McKeag, A., & MacPherson, K. (2005). The effect of safer play equipment on playground injury rates among school children. *Canadian Medical Association Journal, 172*(11), 1443–1446 [electronic version]. Accessed via Proquest database 10/1/05.

Kehl, D. K. (2001). Developmental coax vara, transient synovitis and idiopathic chondrolysis of the hip. In R. T. Morrissy & S. L. Weinstein (Eds.), *Lovell & Winter's pediatric orthopaedics* (5th ed.). Philadelphia: Lippincott Williams & Wilkins.

Killian, J. T., Mayberry, S., & Wilkinson, L. (1999). Current concepts in adolescent idiopathic scoliosis. *Pediatric Annals, 28*(12), 755–761.

Kocher, M. S., Mandiga, R., Murphy, J. M., Goldman, D., Harper, M., Sundel, R., Ecklund, K., & Kasser, J. R. (2003). A clinical practice guideline for treatment of septic arthritis in children: Efficacy in improving process of care and effect on outcome of septic arthritis of the hip. *Journal of Bone and Joint Surgery, 85*(6), 994–999.

Kocher, M. S., Mandiga, R., Zurakowski, B. C., & Kasser, J. R. (2004). Validation of a clinical prediction rule for the differentiation between septic arthritis and transient synovitis of the hip in children. *Journal of Bone and Joint Surgery, 86*(8), 1629–1638.

Koester, M. C. (2003). Making the preparticipation athletic evaluation more than just a "sports physical." *Contemporary Pediatrics, 20*(9), 85–121.

Koester, M., & Mangus, B. C. (2005). Heads up for soccer injuries! What you need to know. *Contemporary Pediatrics, 22*(5), 75–88.

Labbe, A. C., Demers, A. M., Rodrigues, R., Arlet, V., Tanguay, K., & Moore, D. (2003). Surgical-site infection following spinal fusion: A case-control study in a children's hospital. *Infection Control & Hospital Epidemiology, 24*(8), 591–595.

Lazzarini, L., Mader, J. T., & Calhoun, J. H. (2004). Current concepts review: Osteomyelitis in long bones. *Journal of Bone and Joint Surgery, 86*(10), 2305–2318.

Lee, L. H., & Hall, C. B. (2000). Recognizing infection-related arthritis. *Contemporary Pediatrics, 17*(5), 119–130.

Leung, A. K. C., & Lemay, J. F. (2004). The limping child. *Journal of Pediatric Health Care, 18,* 219–223.

Luther, B. L. (2002). Congenital muscular torticollis. *Orthopedic Nursing, 21*(3), 21–28.

Mayrl, J. M., Grechenig, W., & Hollwarth, M. E. (2004). Musculoskeletal ultrasound in pediatric trauma. *European Journal of Trauma, 3,* 150–160 [electronic version]. Accessed 10/1/05 via Proquest database.

Metzl, J. D., & Metzl, J. A. (2004). Shin pain in an adolescent soccer player: A case-based look at "shin splints." *Contemporary Pediatrics, 21*(9), 36–48.

Molczan, K. A. (2001). Triaging pediatric orthopedic injuries. *Journal of Emergency Nursing, 27,* 297–300.

Moreland, M. S. (2001). Special concerns of the pediatric athlete. In F. H. Fu & D. A. Stone (Eds.), *Sports injuries: Mechanisms, prevention, treatment* (2nd ed.). Philadelphia: Lippincott Williams & Wilkins.

Morrissy, R. T., Giavedoni, B. J., & Coulter-O'Berry, C. (2001). The limb-deficient child. In R. T. Morrissy & S. L. Weinstein (Eds.), *Lovell & Winter's pediatric orthopaedics* (5th ed.). Philadelphia: Lippincott Williams & Wilkins.

Mosca, V. S. (2001). The foot. In R. T. Morrissy & S. L. Weinstein (Eds.), *Lovell & Winter's pediatric orthopaedics* (5th ed.). Philadelphia: Lippincott Williams & Wilkins.

Newton, P. O., & Wenger, D. R. (2001). Idiopathic and congenital scoliosis. In R. T. Morrissy & S. L. Weinstein (Eds.), *Lovell & Winter's pediatric orthopaedics* (5th ed.). Philadelphia: Lippincott Williams & Wilkins.

Pagana, K. D., & Pagana, T. J. (2002). *Mosby's manual of diagnostic and laboratory tests* (2nd ed.). St. Louis: Mosby.

Parikh, S. N., Crawford, A. H., & Choudhury. (2004). Magnetic resonance imaging in the evaluation of infantile torticollis. *Orthopedics, 27*(5), 509–515.

Patel, D. R., Greydanus, D. E., & Pratt, H. D. (2001). Youth sports: More than sprains and strains. *Contemporary Pediatrics, 18*(3), 45–74.

Pierce, M. C., Bertocci, G. E., Janosky, J. E., Aguel, F., Deemer, E., Moreland, M., Boal, D., Garcia, S., Herr, S., Zuckerbraun, N., & Vogeley, E. Femur fractures resulting from stair falls among young children: An injury plausibility study. *Pediatrics,* 115(6), 1712–1722.

Price, C. T., Phillips, J. H., & Devito, D. P. (2001). Management of fractures. In R. T. Morrissy & S. L. Weinstein (Eds.), *Lovell & Winter's pediatric orthopaedics* (5th ed.). Philadelphia: Lippincott Williams & Wilkins.

Rauch, F., & Glorieux, F. H. (2004). Osteogenesis imperfecta. *Lancet, 363,* 1377–1385.

Ryan, L. M., DePiero, A. D., Sadow, K. B., Warmink, C. A., Chamberlin, J. M., Teach, S. J., & Johns, C. M. S. (2004). Recognition and management of pediatric fractures by pediatric residents. *Pediatrics, 114*(6), 1530–1533.

Sadovsky, R. (2000). Oral antibiotic therapy for septic arthritis in children. *American Family Physician, 61*(11), 3434 [electronic version]. Accessed 10/1/05.

Sakkers, R., Kok, D., Engelbert, R., van Dongen, A., Jansen, M., Pruijs, H. Verbout, A., Schweitzer, D., & Uiterwaal, C. (2004). Skeletal effects and functional outcome with olpadronate in children with osteogenesis imperfecta: A 2-year randomized placebo-controlled study. *Lancet, 363,* 1427–1431.

Salzbach, R. (1999). Pediatric septic arthritis. *AORN Journal, 70*(6), 986–1010 [electronic version]. Accessed via Proquest database 10/1/05.

Santy, J. (2000). Nursing the patient with an external fixator. *Nursing Standard, 14*(31), 47–52, 54.

Sapountzi-Krepia, D. S., Valavanis, J., Panteleakis, G. P., Zangana, D. T., Vlachojiannis, P. C., & Sapkas, G. S. (2001). Perceptions of body image, happiness and satisfaction in adolescents wearing a Boston brace for scoliosis treatment. *Journal of Advanced Nursing, 35*(5), 683–690.

Stellwagen, L. M., Hubbard, E., & Vaux, K. (2004). Look for the 'stuck baby' to identify congenital torticollis. *Contemporary Pediatrics, 21*(5), 55 [electronic version]. Available at www.contemporarypediatrics.com.

Swoveland, B., Medvick, C., Kirsh, M., Thompson, K., & Nuss, D. (2001). The Nuss procedure for pectus excavatum correction. *AORN Journal, 74*(6), 827–850 [electronic version]. Accessed via Proquest database 10/1/05.

Taft, E., & Francis, R. (2003). Evaluation and management of scoliosis. *Journal of Pediatric Health Care, 17*(1), 42–44.

Taketokmo, C. K., Hodding, J. H., & Kraus, D. M. (2004). *Lexi-comp's pediatric dosage handbook* (11th ed.). Hudson, Ohio: Lexi-comp.

Tice, A., Rehm, S. J., Dalovisio, J. R., Bradley, J. S., Martinelli, L. P., Graham, D. R., Gainer, R. B., Kunkel, M. J., Yancey, R. W., & Williams, D. N. (2004). Practice guidelines for outpatient parenteral antimicrobial therapy. *Journal of Infusion Nursing, 27*(5), 339–359.

Weinstein, S. L. (2001). Developmental hip dysplasia and dislocation. In R. T. Morrissy & S. L. Weinstein (Eds.), *Lovell & Winter's pediatric orthopaedics* (5th ed.). Philadelphia: Lippincott Williams & Wilkins.

Zak, M. (2005). Pediatric orthopedic problems. In S. M. Nettina (Ed.), *Lippincott manual of nursing practice.* Philadelphia: Lippincott Williams & Wilkins.

Zaleske, D. J. (2001). Metabolic and endocrine abnormalities. In R. T. Morrissy & S. L. Weinstein (Eds.), *Lovell & Winter's pediatric orthopaedics* (5th ed.). Philadelphia: Lippincott Williams & Wilkins.

Websites

www.cincinnatichildrens.org/health/yh/archives/2002/summer/sports-injury.htm How to prevent sports injuries in children

www.infant-torticollis.org/ National Infant Torticollis Association

www.marchofdimes.com March of Dimes (birth defects foundation)

www.mliles.com/pedortho/index.shtml an index to a variety of pediatric orthopedic websites

www.momsteam.com/index.shtml youth sports information for parents

www.niams.nih.gov/hi/topics/childsports/child_sports.htm National Institute of Arthritis and Musculoskeletal and Skin Diseases/National Institutes of Health, section on child sports

www.oif.org Osteogenesis Imperfecta Foundation

www.orthoseek.com/ pediatric orthopedics and pediatric sports medicine for parents

www.pectus.org/ United Kingdom pectus excavatum and pectus carinatum information site

www.peds-ortho.com/ pediatric orthopedic surgery resource site

www.scoi.com/peds.htm pediatric orthopedic information from the Southern California Orthopedic Institute

www.scoliosis.com information on nonsurgical correction of scoliosis

www.scoliosis.org/ National Scoliosis Foundation

www.sportssafety.org/ National Center for Sports Safety

www.usa.safekids.org/index.cfm USA Safe Kids

Chapter WORKSHEET

● MULTIPLE CHOICE QUESTIONS

1. The nurse is evaluating a parent's understanding of treatment for torticollis. Which response best indicates that the parent understands the appropriate treatment?
   a. Encourages the infant to turn the head to the unaffected side
   b. States that prone positioning for sleep will be needed
   c. Places the infant on the affected side
   d. Stretches the infant's neck to the opposite side and holds it for 5 seconds
2. The nurse is providing patient education related to use of a brace that the orthopedic surgeon has ordered as treatment for idiopathic scoliosis in an adolescent girl. Which statement by the teen best indicates an understanding of appropriate use of the brace?
   a. "I can take my brace off only for special occasions."
   b. "I will take my brace off for only 1 hour per day, for showering."
   c. "I do not need to wear my brace at night while I am sleeping."
   d. "It is most important for me to wear my brace during the day, while I am upright."
3. The nurse is caring for orthopedic patients who are in the postoperative period following spinal fusion. What is the most appropriate activity to delegate to unlicensed assistive personnel?
   a. Ambulate the children twice daily to promote mobility.
   b. Encourage commode use to promote bowel function.
   c. Provide diversionary activities, as the children must stay flat on their backs.
   d. Assist with log-rolling the children every 2 hours.
4. The nurse is caring for a child with a fractured left femur who has been in skeletal traction for several days. Upon assessment, she notes that the left foot is pale, with a nonpalpable pedal pulse. What is the priority nursing intervention?
   a. Release the traction, as there may be too much weight on it.
   b. Nothing; alterations in circulation are expected with skeletal traction.
   c. Immediately notify the physician of this abnormal finding.
   d. Massage the foot immediately to increase circulation.

● CRITICAL THINKING EXERCISES

1. Develop a teaching plan for the family of an infant with developmental dysplasia of the hip or clubfoot.
2. Develop a discharge teaching plan for a 2-year-old who will be in a hip spica cast for 10 more weeks at home.
3. Devise a developmental/education plan for a child who will be confined to traction for 6 weeks. Choose a child in the clinical area whom you have cared for or choose a particular age group and develop the plan.

● STUDY ACTIVITIES

1. In the clinical setting, compare the growth and development of a child with osteogenesis imperfecta or rickets with that of typical healthy child. What differences or similarities do you find? What are the explanations for your findings?
2. Attend a pediatric orthopedic clinic or the local clinic of Children's Medical Services. Identify the role of the registered nurse in this setting.

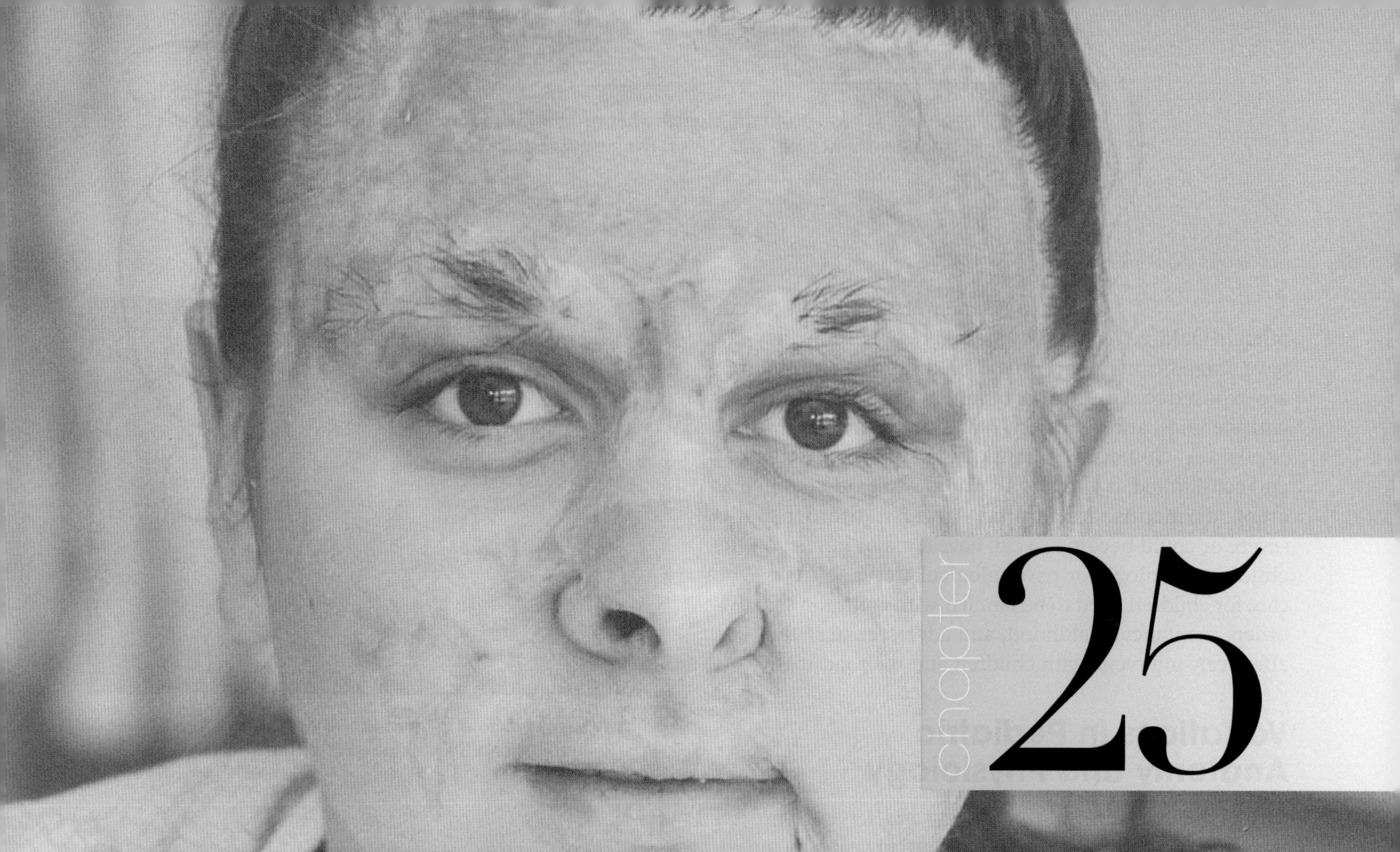

chapter 25

Nursing Care of the Child With an Integumentary Disorder

Key TERMS

annular
dermatitis
erythema
macule
papule
pruritus
scaling
vesicle

Learning OBJECTIVES

Upon completion of the chapter, the learner will be able to:

1. Compare anatomic and physiologic differences of the integumentary system in infants and children versus adults.
2. Describe nursing care related to common laboratory and diagnostic tests used in the medical diagnosis of integumentary disorders in infants, children, and adolescents.
3. Distinguish integumentary disorders common in infants, children, and adolescents.
4. Identify appropriate nursing assessments and interventions related to pediatric integumentary disorders.
5. Develop an individualized nursing care plan for the child with an integumentary disorder.
6. Describe the psychosocial impact of a chronic integumentary disorder on children or adolescents.
7. Develop patient/family teaching plans for the child with an integumentary disorder.

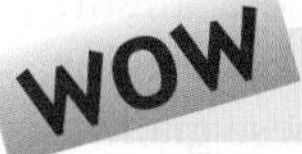

To a nurse the child's skin is life's gift wrapping, but to the child the skin is the space suit for life.

Eva Lopez, 1 year old, is brought to the clinic by her mother, who states, "Eva has dry patches of skin, her wrists bleed from her scratching, and she's having trouble sleeping at night."

Integumentary disorders occur often in children, and if they are severe or chronic they can have a significant impact on the child. Infants and children are exposed to a multitude of infectious microorganisms and allergens, and their skin is sometimes affected by these exposures. Some integumentary disorders are as mild and self-limited as a minor abrasion, while others, such as atopic dermatitis, are chronic. Any skin disorder that is severe or could become so can have a major impact on the child's physiologic or psychological status. Nurses who care for children need to be familiar with common skin disorders of infancy, childhood, and adolescence so they can effectively intervene with children and their families.

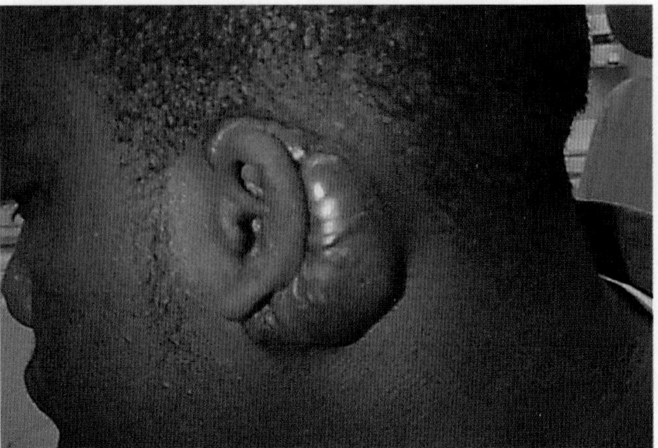

● Figure 25.1 Keloid formation is more common in dark-skinned than light-skinned children.

Variations in Pediatric Anatomy and Physiology

Skin is the largest organ of the body and serves to protect the underlying tissues from trauma and invasion by microorganisms. The skin's health also reflects the internal well-being of the body (Cole & Gray-Miceli, 2002). The skin is also important for the perception of pain, heat, and cold and for the regulation of body temperature.

Differences in the Skin Between Children and Adults

The infant's epidermis is thinner than the adult's, and the blood vessels lie closer to the surface because there is a decreased amount of subcutaneous fat. Thus, the infant loses heat more readily through the skin's surface than the older child or adult does. The thinness of the infant's skin also allows substances to be absorbed through the skin more readily than they would be in an adult. Bacteria can gain access via the infant's and younger child's skin more readily than they can through the adult's skin. The infant's skin contains more water than in adults, and the epidermis is loosely bound to the dermis. This means that friction may easily cause separation of the layers, resulting in blistering or skin breakdown. The infant's skin is also less pigmented than that of the adult (in all races), placing the infant at increased risk of skin damage from ultraviolet radiation. Over time, the infant's skin toughens and becomes less hydrated and thus is less susceptible to microorganism invasion. The skin thickness and characteristics reach adult levels in the late teenage years (Starr, 2004).

Differences in Dark-Skinned Children

Children with dark skin tend to have more pronounced cutaneous reactions compared to children with lighter skin (Starr, 2004). Hypopigmentation or hyperpigmentation in the affected area following healing of a dermatologic condition is common in dark-skinned children. This change in pigmentation may be temporary (a few months following a superficial skin disorder) or permanent (following a more involved skin condition). Dark-skinned children tend to have more prominent papules, follicular responses, lichenification, and vesicular or bullous reactions than lighter-skinned children with the same disorder. Hypertrophic scarring and keloid formation (Fig. 25.1) occurs more often in dark-skinned children.

Sebaceous and Sweat Glands

Sebaceous glands function immaturely at birth. The sebum secreted serves to lubricate the skin and hair. Sebum production increases in the preadolescent and adolescent years, which is why acne develops at that time. The infant's eccrine sweat glands are somewhat functional and will produce sweat as a response to emotional stimuli and heat. They become fully functional in the middle childhood years. Until that time, temperature regulation is less effective compared to older children and adults. The apocrine sweat glands are small and nonfunctional in the infant. They mature during puberty, at which time body odor develops in response to the fluid secreted by these glands.

Common Medical Treatments

A variety of medications as well as other medical treatments are used to treat integumentary disorders in children. Most of these treatments will require a physician's order when the child is in the hospital. The most common treatments and medications are listed in Common Medical Treatments 25.1 and Drug Guide 25.1. The nurse caring for the child with an integumentary disorder should be familiar with the procedures and medications, how they work, as well as common nursing implications related to their use.

Nursing Process Overview for the Child With a Integumentary Disorder

Nursing management of the child with an integumentary disorder requires astute assessment skills, development of accurate nursing diagnoses and expected outcomes, implementation of appropriate interventions, and evaluation of the entire process. Many skin rashes may be associated with other, often serious, illnesses, so the nurse must use comprehensive and excellent assessment skills when evaluating rashes in children. Certain integumentary conditions are chronic and require ongoing care related to health maintenance, education, and psychosocial needs.

ASSESSMENT

Nursing assessment of the child with an integumentary disorder includes obtaining the health history and performing a physical examination. Assisting with or obtaining laboratory tests may also be necessary.

> **Remember Eva,** the 1-year-old with the dry patches, itching, and trouble sleeping? What additional health history and physical examination assessment information should the nurse obtain?

Health History

Determine the child's or parent's chief complaint, which is most often related to pruritus, **scaling**, or a cosmetic disruption. Document the history of the present illness, noting onset, location, duration, characteristics, other symptoms and relieving factors, particularly as related to a rash or lesion. Also ask about the quantity and quality of any discharge from the rash or lesions. Document accompanying symptoms. Note the child's general state of health, history of chronic medical conditions, recent

Common Medical Treatments 25.1

Treatment	Explanation	Indication	Nursing Implications
Wet dressing	Dressing moistened with lukewarm water (sterile water may be required in certain cases)	In the presence of itching, crusting, or oozing—helps to remove crusts	May use Burow's, Domeboro, or saline solutions in certain cases Provide atraumatic care by giving premedication before dressing change.
Sunscreen	Lotion, gel, or cream with a sun-protective factor (SPF)	All children over 6 months of age	Use a fragrance-free, para-aminobenzoic acid (PABA)–free preparation with an SPF of 15 or higher. Apply at least 30 minutes prior to sun exposure. Reapply at least every 2 hours while exposed (every 60 to 80 minutes while in the water). Sweat- and water-resistant preparations are available yet still require reapplication as noted above. Use daily in summer and in warm climates, even on overcast and cloudy days.
Bathing	Use of lukewarm water (with or without soap) to bathe	Itchy and irritating skin conditions	Recommend fragrance-free, dye-free soaps such as Dove, Aveeno, Basis, Lubriderm. Colloid (oatmeal baths) are especially helpful. Pat the child dry; do not rub the skin. Leave the child moist before applying medication, dressing, or moisturizer.

Drug Guide 25.1 Common Drugs for Integumentary Disorders

Medication	Action	Indication	Nursing Implications
Antibiotics (topical)	Decrease skin colonization with bacteria	Mild acne vulgaris, impetigo, folliculitis	Apply as prescribed to clean skin or a cleansed wound. Be alert for neomycin allergy.
Antibiotics (systemic)	Bactericidal and bacteriostatic against a variety of organisms, depending on the preparation	Moderate to severe acne vulgaris, extensive impetigo, cellulitis, scalded skin syndrome	Check for medication allergies prior to administration. Teach families to finish entire course of antibiotics.
Corticosteroids (topical)	Anti-inflammatory effect	Atopic dermatitis, certain kinds of contact dermatitis	Do not use moderate- or high-potency cortico-steroid preparations on the face or genitals. Do not cover with an occlusive dressing. Absorption is increased in the young infant.
Antifungals (topical)	Fungicidal	Tinea, candidal diaper rash	Apply a thin layer as pre-scribed. Comply with length of treatment as prescribed to prevent re-emergence of the rash.
Antifungals (systemic): griseofulvin, ketoconazole	Kills fungus; binds to human keratin, making it resistant to fungus	Tinea capitis, severe or widespread fungal skin infections	Griseofulvin: give with fatty food to increase absorption. Requires minimum 4-week course. Monitor liver function tests and CBC. May cause photosensitivity. Ketoconazole: administer with food to decrease GI upset.
Benzoyl peroxide	Decreases colonization of *P. acnes*	Mild acne vulgaris	Available in combination with topical antibiotics. Apply sparingly. Shake before application. Avoid contact with eyes and mucous membranes.
Retinoids (topical): tretinoin, adapalene, tazarotene	Anticomedogenic activity	Moderate to severe acne vulgaris	Adverse effects: dryness, burning, photosensitivity. Instruct child to use SPF 15 or higher sunscreen.
Topical immune modulators (tacrolimus, pimecrolimus)	Inhibits T-lymphocyte action at the skin level	Moderate to severe atopic dermatitis, or in conditions resistant to topical steroids	Use only in children over 2 years old. Avoid sunlight exposure. May cause burning, pruritus, flu-like symp-toms, or headache.

Drug Guide 25.1 Common Drugs for Integumentary Disorders (continued)

Medication	Action	Indication	Nursing Implications
Antihistamines (diphenhydramine, chlorpheniramine, hydroxyzine)	Antihistaminic effect, results in sedation	Hypersensitivity reactions, atopic dermatitis or contact dermatitis that is severely pruritic	May give three or four times a day unless sedation effect interferes with activities of daily living or school
Systemic corticosteroids (prednisone, dexamethasone, methylprednisolone)	Anti-inflammatory and immunosuppressive action	Severe contact dermatitis	Administer with food to decrease GI upset. May mask signs of infection. Monitor blood pressure, urine for glucose. Do not stop treatment abruptly or acute adrenal insufficiency may occur. Monitor for Cushing syndrome. Doses may be tapered over time.
Isotretinoin (Accutane)	Reduces sebaceous gland size, decreases sebum production, and regulates cell proliferation and differentiation	Cystic acne or severe acne that is resistant to 3 months of treatment with oral antibiotics	Ensure that the adolescent girl is not pregnant and does not become pregnant. Monitor CBC, lipid profiles, liver function tests, and beta-human chorionic gonadotropin monthly. Monitor for suicide risk.
Coal tar preparations	Antipruritic and anti-inflammatory effect	Psoriasis, atopic dermatitis	May stain fabrics; strong and unpleasant odor. Apply at bedtime and rinse off in the morning to improve compliance.
Silver sulfadiazine 1% (Silvadene)	Bactericidal against gram-positive and gram-negative bacteria and yeasts	Burns	Cover with occlusive dressing. Apply BID. Do not use in patients with sulfa allergy. Forms a gel on the burn that is painful to remove. May cause transient neutropenia. Do not use on the child's face or on an infant less than 2 months of age.

surgeries, hospitalizations, medications, or immunizations. Has there been a recent change in the child's food intake or environment? Is there a family history of chronic or acute skin conditions? Does anyone in the home have a similar concern at this time? Does the family have pets that go outdoors? Does the child play in the woods or garden? Note usual skin care routines, as well as types of soaps, cosmetics, or other skin care products used. Determine the amount of daily sun exposure and whether the child consistently uses sunscreen.

Physical Examination

Perform a complete physical examination, noting any abnormalities. Perform a focused and thorough examination of the skin. The best lighting for examination of the skin is natural daylight. Look at the skin in general, noting distribution of any obvious lesions. Inspect the mucous membranes, noting and describing lesions if present. Examine all surfaces of the skin and scalp carefully. Note temperature, moisture, texture, and fragility of the skin. If a rash or lesions are present, note their location and provide a detailed description of them. Describe whether a rash is macular, papular, pustular, or vesicular. Provide a description of vascular lesions if present (refer to Chapter 10 for additional information on vascular lesions). Describe lesions according to the following criteria:

- Linear: in a line
- Shape: Are the lesions round, oval, **annular** (ring around central clearing)?
- Morbilliform: a rosy, maculopapular rash
- Target lesions: like a bull's-eye

If lesions are present on the scalp, has hair loss in that region occurred? If drainage is present, describe it as clear, purulent, honey-colored, or otherwise. Note scaling or lichenification of the skin. Palpate for regional lymphadenopathy.

Laboratory and Diagnostic Testing

Common Laboratory and Diagnostic Tests 25.1 details the laboratory and diagnostic tests most commonly used when considering integumentary disorders. The tests can assist the physician or nurse practitioner in diagnosing the disorder or can be used as guidelines in determining ongoing treatment. Some of the tests are obtained by laboratory or non-nursing personnel, while others might be obtained by the nurse. In either instance the nurse should be familiar with how the tests are obtained, what they are used for, and normal versus abnormal results. This knowledge will also be necessary when providing patient and family education related to the testing.

NURSING DIAGNOSES AND RELATED INTERVENTIONS

Upon completion of a thorough assessment, the nurse might identify several nursing diagnoses, such as:

- Impaired skin integrity
- Pain
- Risk for infection

Common Laboratory and Diagnostic Tests 25.1

Test	Explanation	Indication	Nursing Implications
Complete blood count (CBC) with differential	Evaluate hemoglobin and hematocrit, WBC count (particularly the percentage of individual WBCs), and platelet count	Infection or inflammatory process	Normal values vary according to age and gender. WBC differential is helpful in evaluating source of infection. May be affected by myelosuppressive drugs. Eosinophils may be elevated in the child with atopic dermatitis.
Erythrocyte sedimentation rate (ESR)	Nonspecific test used to detect presence of infection or inflammation	Infection or inflammatory process	Send sample to laboratory immediately; if allowed to stand for longer than 3 hours, may result in falsely low result.
Potassium hydroxide (KOH) prep	Reveals branching hyphae (fungus) when viewed under microscope	To identify fungal infection	Place skin scrapings on a microscope slide and add KOH 20% drop.
Culture of wound or skin drainage	Allows for microbial growth and organism identification	Identification of specific organism	Note sensitivities.
Immunoglobulin E (IgE)	Measurement of serum IgE	Atopic dermatitis	Often elevated in allergic or atopic disease, though this is a nonspecific finding. May be increased if the child takes systemic corticosteroids.
Patch or skin testing	Needle prick testing with allergens	Atopic or contact dermatitis	Have emergency equipment available in the event of anaphylaxis (rare).

- Disturbed body image
- Risk for fluid volume deficit
- Altered nutrition

> **After completing an assessment of Eva,** the nurse noted the following: hypopigmentation of the skin behind her knees, dry patches on her wrists and face, and slight wheezing heard bilaterally on auscultation. Based on these assessment findings, what would your top three nursing diagnoses be for Eva?

Desired outcomes and interventions are based on the nursing diagnoses. Nursing Care Plan 25.1 can be used as a guide in planning nursing care for the child with an integumentary disorder. Individualize the plan of care based on the child's and family's responses to the health alteration; see Chapter 15 for information about pain management. Additional information will be included later in the chapter as it relates to specific disorders.

> **Based on your top three nursing diagnoses for Eva,** describe appropriate nursing interventions.

Infectious Disorders

Infectious disorders of the skin include those caused by viral, bacterial, or fungal infection. The viral exanthems are discussed in Chapter 16. Bacterial and fungal infections of the skin are discussed below.

• BACTERIAL INFECTIONS

Bacterial infections of the skin include bullous and nonbullous impetigo, folliculitis, cellulitis, and staphylococcal scalded skin syndrome. These bacterial skin infections are often caused by *Staphylococcus aureus* and group A beta-hemolytic streptococcus, which are ordinarily normal flora on the skin. Impetigo, folliculitis, and cellulitis are usually self-limited disorders that rarely become severe.

Impetigo is a readily recognizable skin rash (Fig. 25.2). Nonbullous impetigo generally follows some type of skin trauma or may arise as a secondary bacterial infection of another skin disorder, such as atopic dermatitis. Bullous impetigo demonstrates a sporadic occurrence pattern and develops on intact skin, resulting from toxin production by *S. aureus.*

Folliculitis, infection of the hair follicle, most often results from occlusion of the hair follicle. It may occur as a result of poor hygiene, prolonged contact with contaminated water, maceration, or a moist environment or from use of occlusive emollient products.

Cellulitis is a localized infection and inflammation of the skin and subcutaneous tissues and is usually preceded by skin trauma of some sort (Fig. 25.3).

Staphylococcal scalded skin syndrome results from infection with *S. aureus* that produces a toxin, which then causes exfoliation. It has an abrupt onset and results in diffuse erythema and skin tenderness. Scalded skin syndrome is most common in infancy and rare beyond 5 years of age (Marino & Fine, 2007).

Of particular concern are bacterial skin infections caused by methicillin-resistant *S. aureus* (MRSA). In children these infections most commonly occur after an insect or spider bite or other cause of cellulitis (Siberry, 2005). Additional risk factors for community-acquired MRSA are turf burns, towel-sharing, shaving, improper disinfection of sports protective equipment and locker rooms, and poor hygiene (Romero et al., 2006). Community outbreaks of MRSA became widespread throughout the United States by 2004 (Siberry, 2005). If the child presents with a moderate to severe skin infection or with an infection that is not responding as expected to therapy, it is important to culture the infected area for MRSA.

Therapeutic management of bacterial skin infections includes topical or systemic antibiotics and appropriate hygiene (Table 25.1).

Nursing Assessment

Obtain the history as noted in the nursing process overview section. Note history of skin disruption such as a cut, scrape, or insect or spider bite (nonbullous impetigo and cellulitis). Note body piercing in the adolescent, which can lead to impetigo or cellulitis. Measure the child's temperature: fever may occur with bullous impetigo or cellulitis and is common with scalded skin syndrome. Inspect the skin, noting abnormalities, documenting their location and distribution, and describing drainage if present. Table 25.1 gives specific clinical manifestations of the various bacterial skin infections. Palpate for regional lymphadenopathy, which may be present with impetigo or cellulitis. Blood cultures are indicated in the child with cellulitis with lymphangitic streaking and in all cases of periorbital or orbital cellulitis.

Nursing Management

Administer antibiotics topically or systemically as prescribed. Teach the family about antibiotic administration and care of the lesions or rash. Soak impetiginous lesions with cool compresses or Burow's solution to remove crusts before applying topical antibiotics. Though impetigo is considered a contagious disorder among vulnerable populations, removal from school or day care is not necessary unless the condition is widespread or actively weeping (Watkins, 2005). Prevent transmission of nosocomial MRSA by appropriately isolating children according to the institution's policy when the child is hospitalized. In children with scalded skin syndrome, the risk of scarring may be reduced by minimal handling, avoidance of

(text continues on page 845)

Nursing Care Plan 25.1

Overview for the Child With an Integumentary Disorder

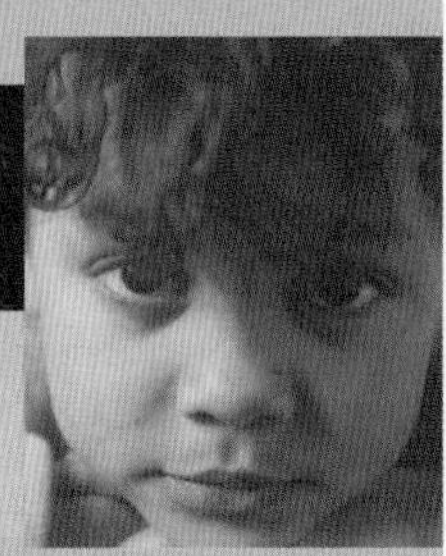

Nursing Diagnosis: Impaired skin integrity related to infectious process, hypersensitivity reaction, injury, or mechanical factors as evidenced by rash, inflammation, abrasion, laceration, or disrupted epidermis

Outcome identification and evaluation

Integrity of skin surface will be restored; *rash, abrasion, laceration, or other skin disruption will heal.*

Interventions: restoring skin integrity

- Assess site of skin impairment *to determine extent of involvement and plan care.*
- Monitor skin impairment every shift for changes in color, warmth, redness, or other signs of infection *to identify problems early.*
- Determine the child's and family's skin care practices *to determine need for education related to skin care.*
- Individualize the child's skin care regimen depending on the child's particular skin condition *to most appropriately care for skin in light of the child's disorder.*
- In the immobile child, use a risk assessment tool (such as a modified Norton or Braden scale) *to identify risk for skin breakdown.*
- Position the child on the opposite side of the skin impairment *to avoid further skin breakdown.*
- Encourage appropriate nutritional intake *as adequate nutrients are necessary for appropriate immune function and skin healing.*
- Consult the wound and ostomy care nurse specialist *to determine best approach for individualized wound care.*
- Provide dressing change and wound care as prescribed *to promote wound or burn healing.*

Nursing Diagnosis: Risk for infection related to disruption in protective skin barrier

Outcome identification and evaluation

Child will remain free of local or systemic infection, *will remain afebrile, without additional redness or warmth at skin disruption site.*

Interventions: preventing infection

- Use appropriate hand hygiene *to decrease transmission of infectious organisms.*
- Assess the skin impairment site for increased warmth, redness, discharge, or new purulence *to identify infection early.*
- Assess temperature every 4 hours or more frequently if needed, *as children develop fever quickly in response to infection.*
- Note WBC and culture results, *reporting unexpected values to the primary care provider so that appropriate treatment may be started.*
- Follow prescribed therapies for skin alteration *to maintain skin moisture and prevent further breakdown, which may lead to infection.*
- Encourage appropriate nutritional intake *as adequate nutrients are necessary for appropriate immune function and skin healing.*

Overview for the Child With an Integumentary Disorder (continued)

Nursing Diagnosis: Disturbed body image related to chronic skin changes caused by disease process, burns, or other skin alteration as evidenced by child's verbalization, reluctance to participate in activities, or social withdrawal

Outcome identification and evaluation

Child will verbalize or demonstrate acceptance of alteration in body, *will return to previous level of social involvement.*

Interventions: promoting appropriate body image

- Assess child or teen for feelings about alteration in skin *to determine baseline.*
- Acknowledge feelings of anger or depression related to skin changes *to provide an outlet for feelings.*
- Encourage the child or teen to participate in skin care *to give some sense of control over what is occurring.*
- Help the child or teen to accept self *as the perception of self is tied to knowing oneself and identifying what the self values.*

Nursing Diagnosis: Risk for deficient fluid volume related to burns

Outcome identification and evaluation

Fluid volume status will be balanced, *child will maintain urine output of 1 to 2 mL/kg/hour, oral mucosa will be moist and pink, heart rate will remain within age- and situation-specific parameters.*

Interventions: promoting fluid balance

- Assess fluid volume status at least every shift, more frequently if disrupted, *to obtain baseline for comparison.*
- Strictly monitor intake and output *to detect imbalance or need for additional fluid intake.*
- Weigh the child daily on the same scale, at the same time, in the same amount of clothing *as changes in weight are an accurate indicator of fluid volume status in children.*
- Provide intravenous fluid resuscitation in initial period, followed by encouragement of oral fluid intake in the burned patient, *to compensate for fluid loss through burned areas.*

Nursing Diagnosis: Imbalanced nutrition, less than body requirements, related to increased metabolic state (burns) as evidenced by poor wound healing, difficulty gaining or maintaining body weight

Outcome identification and evaluation

Child will demonstrate balanced nutritional state, *will maintain or gain weight as appropriate for situation, will demonstrate improvement in wound healing.*

Interventions: promoting nutrition

- Assess the child's food preferences and ability to eat *to provide a baseline for planning nursing care.*
- Consult the nutritionist *because nutritional needs are increased related to altered metabolic state as a result of burns.*
- Collaborate with the nutritionist, child, and parents to plan meals that appeal to the child *to increase the child's intake.*
- Administer vitamin and mineral preparations as prescribed *to supplement nutrients.*
- Provide smaller, more frequent meals and snacks *to promote increased intake.*
- Weigh the child daily *to determine progress.*

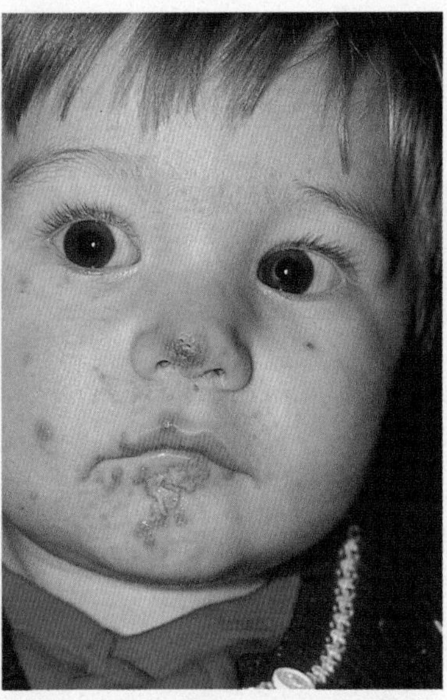

● Figure 25.2 Note honey-colored crusting with impetigo.

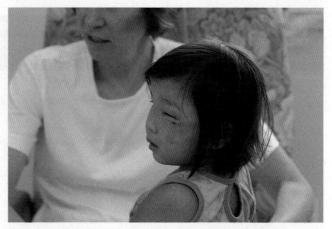

● Figure 25.3 Note erythema and edema associated with cellulitis.

Table 25.1 Bacterial Skin Infections

Disorder	Skin Findings	Usual Treatment
Nonbullous impetigo	• **Papules** progressing to **vesicles**, then painless pustules with a narrow erythematous border • Honey-colored exudate when the vesicles or pustules rupture, which forms a crust on the ulcer-like base (see Fig. 25.2)	• Limited amount: treat topically with mupirocin ointment. • If numerous lesions, oral first-generation cephalosporin is indicated (Marino & Fine, 2007). • Clindamycin may be needed for MRSA. • Remove honey-colored crust with cool compresses BID.
Bullous impetigo	• Red macules and bullous eruptions on an erythematous base • Size may be from a few millimeters to several centimeters.	• Oral first-generation cephalosporin • Good hygiene
Folliculitis	• Red, raised hair follicles	• Treat with aggressive hygiene: warm compresses after washing with soap and water several times a day. • Topical mupirocin is indicated; occasionally oral antibiotics are required.
Cellulitis	• Localized reaction: **erythema**, pain, edema, warmth at site of skin disruption (see Fig. 25.3)	• Mild cases are usually treated with cephalexin or amoxicillin/clavulanic acid. • More severe cases and periorbital or orbital cellulitis require IV cephalosporins.
Staphylococcal scalded skin syndrome	• Flattish bullae that rupture within hours • Red, weeping surface is left, most commonly on face, groin, neck, and axillary region	• Mild to moderate cases are treated with oral cephalexin, dicloxacillin, or amoxicillin/clavulanic acid. • Severe cases are managed similar to burns with aggressive fluid management and IV oxacillin or clindamycin.

corticosteroids, and application of soothing ointments as the skin heals (Starr, 2004).

Educate the family about prevention of bacterial skin infections. Stress the importance of cleanliness and hygiene. Teach the family to keep the child's fingernails cut short and to clean the nails with a nail brush at bath time. When a skin disruption such as a cut, scrape, or insect bite occurs, teach the family to clean the area well to prevent the development of cellulitis. Folliculitis may be prevented with diligent hygiene and avoidance of occlusive emollients. Table 25.1 gives additional information about specific treatments for bacterial skin infections.

● FUNGAL INFECTIONS

Fungi also cause infections on children's skin. *Tinea* is a fungal disease of the skin occurring on any part of the body. The part of the body affected determines the second word in the name; for instance, tinea pedis refers to a fungal infection on the feet. The three organisms most often responsible for tinea are *Epidermophyton, Microsporum,* and *Trichophyton,* though *Malassezia furfur* causes tinea versicolor. *Candida albicans* may cause an infection of the skin, particularly in a warm, moist area such as the diaper area; in fact, 80% of diaper rashes lasting longer than 4 days are colonized with *C. albicans* (Marino & Fine, 2007). All fungal skin infections may occur year-round, but tinea versicolor is more common in warm weather.

Therapeutic management of fungal infections involves appropriate hygiene and administration of an antifungal agent. Table 25.2 gives further information about treatment.

Nursing Assessment

Elicit the health history, noting exposure to another person with a fungal infection or exposure to a pet (fungi are often carried by pets). Note onset of the rash and whether it is itchy. Determine if the child has recently visited the barber (tinea capitis). Note contact with damp areas such as locker rooms and swimming pools, use of nylon socks or nonbreathable shoes, or minor trauma to the feet (tinea pedis). Document a history of wearing tight clothing or participating in a contact sport such as wrestling (tinea cruris). Inspect the skin and scalp, noting the location, description, and distribution of the rash or lesions (Figs. 25.4, 25.5, and 25.6). Table 25.2 describes the clinical findings associated with various types of tinea.

Scraping and KOH preparation show branching hyphae. For tinea capitis, Wood's lamp will fluoresce yellow-green if it is caused by *Microsporum,* but not with

Table 25.2 Manifestations and Management of Fungal Infections

Disorder	Skin Findings	Usual Treatment
Tinea corporis (ringworm)	• Annular lesion with raised peripheral scaling and central clearing (looks like a ring) (see Fig. 25.4)	• Topical antifungal cream is required for at least 4 weeks.
Tinea capitis	• Patches of scaling in the scalp with central hair loss • Risk of kerion development (inflamed, boggy mass that is filled with pustules) (see Fig. 25.5)	• Oral griseofulvin for 4 to 6 weeks • Selenium sulfide shampoo may be used to decrease contagiousness (adjunct only). • No school or daycare for 1 week after treatment initiated
Tinea versicolor	• Superficial tan or hypopigmented oval scaly lesions, especially on upper back and chest and proximal arms • More noticeable in the summer with tanning of unaffected areas	• Apply selenium sulfide shampoo all over body (from face to knees) and allow to stay on skin overnight, rinsing in the morning, once a week for 4 weeks (this may cause skin irritation). • Topical antifungals in the imidazole family may be used instead.
Tinea pedis (athlete's foot)	• Red, scaling rash on soles and between the toes	• Topical antifungal cream, powder, or spray • Appropriate foot hygiene
Tinea cruris	• Erythema, scaling, maceration in the inguinal creases and inner thighs (penis/scrotum spared)	• Topical antifungal preparation for 4 to 6 weeks
Diaper candidiasis (also called monilial diaper rash)	• Fiery red lesions, scaling in the skin folds, and satellite lesions (located further out from the main rash) (see Fig. 25.6)	• Topical nystatin with diaper changes for several days • See section on diaper dermatitis for additional information.

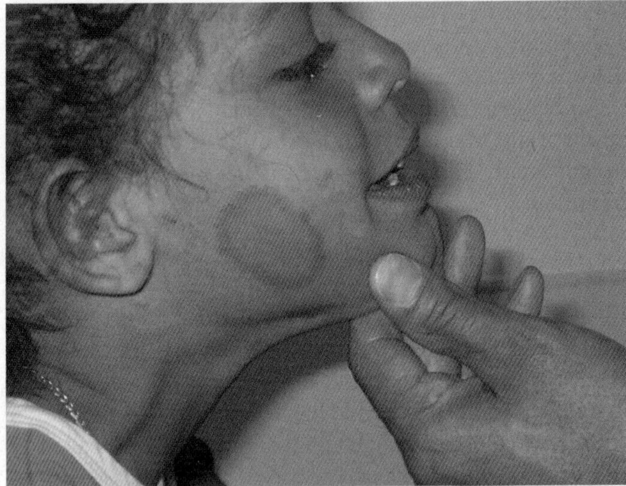

● Figure 25.4 Tinea corporis: note raised scaly border with clearing in center.

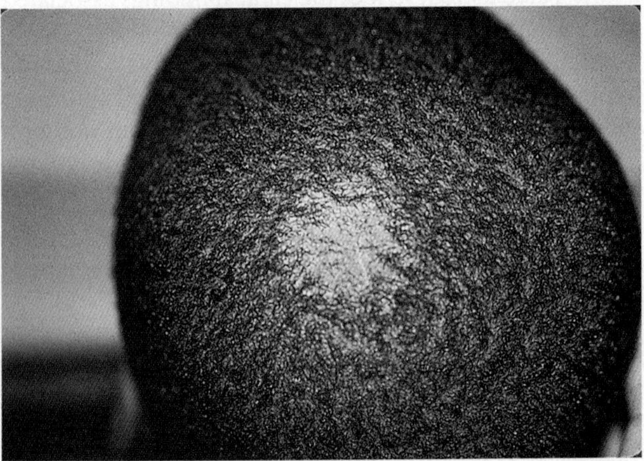

● Figure 25.5 Note hair breakage and loss with tinea capitis.

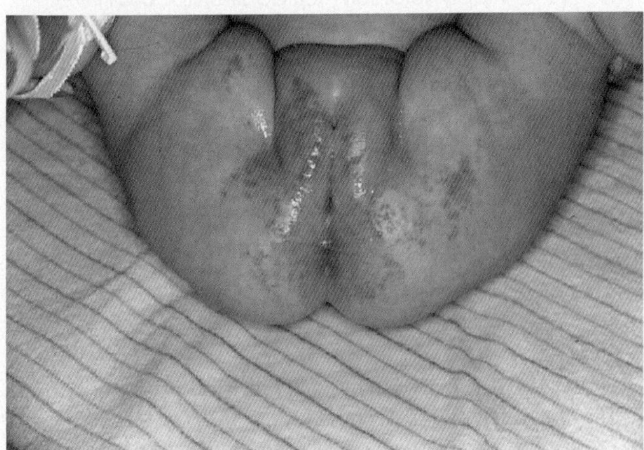

● Figure 25.6 A bright red rash with satellite lesions occurs with diaper candidiasis.

Trichophyton. A fungal culture of a plucked hair is more reliable for diagnosis of tinea capitis.

Nursing Management

Maintain appropriate hygiene and administer antifungal agents as prescribed (see Table 25.2). Additional specifics related to the individual fungal disorders are as follows:

- Tinea corporis is contagious, but the child may return to daycare or school once treatment has begun. Identify and treat family members or other contacts.
- Counsel the child with tinea capitis and parents that hair will usually regrow in 3 to 12 months. Wash sheets and clothes in hot water to decrease the risk of the infection spreading to other family members.
- Instruct the child with tinea pedis to keep the feet clean and dry. Feet should be rinsed with water or a water/vinegar mixture and dried well, especially between the toes. The child should wear cotton socks and shoes that allow the feet to breathe. Going barefoot at home is allowed, but flip-flops should be worn around swimming pools and in locker rooms.
- Inform the child with tinea versicolor that return to normal skin pigmentation may take several months.
- Counsel the boy with tinea cruris to wear cotton underwear and loose clothing. It is important to maintain good hygiene, particularly after sports practice or a sporting event.
- For management of diaper candidiasis, follow the suggestions listed below in the section on diaper dermatitis.

Hypersensitivity Reactions

Skin disorders caused by hypersensitivity reactions include diaper dermatitis, atopic dermatitis, contact dermatitis, erythema multiforme, and urticaria. Drug reactions may result in skin rashes, or as erythema multiforme or urticaria.

● DIAPER DERMATITIS

Diaper dermatitis is an inflammatory reaction of the skin in the area covered by a diaper (Nield & Kamat, 2006). It is a nonimmunologic response to a skin irritant that results in skin cell hydration disturbance (Allen, 2004). Prolonged exposure to urine and feces may lead to skin breakdown (Fig. 25.7). Diaper wearing increases the skin's pH, activating fecal enzymes that further contribute to skin maceration.

Nursing Assessment

Determine from the history whether the infant or child wears diapers. Ask about the onset and progression of the rash, as well as any treatments and response. Inspect the skin in the diaper area for erythema and maceration (see Fig. 25.7). Ordinary diaper dermatitis does not usu-

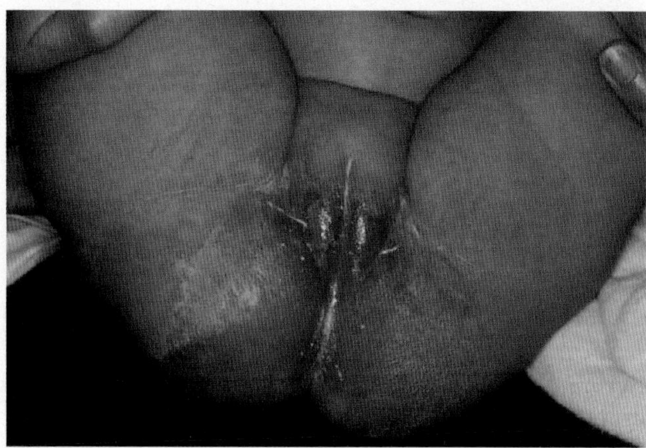

● Figure 25.7 Diaper dermatitis.

ally result in a bumpy rash, but starts as a flat red rash in the convex skin creases. It may appear red and shiny and may or may not also have papules. Untreated, it may become more widespread or severe. Some cases of diaper dermatitis are caused by overgrowth of *C. albicans* (see Fig. 25.6 and the section on fungal infections).

Nursing Management

Prevention is the best management. Topical products such as ointments or creams containing vitamins A, D, and E, zinc oxide, or petrolatum are helpful to provide a barrier to the skin. Teaching Guideline 25.1 gives further information on diaper dermatitis. See above for treatment of diaper rash caused by *C. albicans* infection.

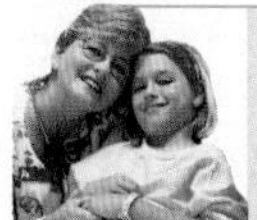

Discourage parents from using any type of baby powder to avoid the risk of aspiration, which may result in pneumonitis.

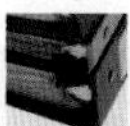

TEACHING GUIDELINE 25.1

Diaper Dermatitis

- Change diapers frequently. Stool-soiled diapers should be changed as soon as possible.
- Gently wash the diaper area with a soft cloth, avoiding harsh soaps.
- Baby wipes may be used in most children, but avoid wipes that contain fragrance or preservatives.
- Once the rash has occurred, allow the infant or child to go diaperless for a period of time each day to allow the rash to heal.
- Blow-dry the diaper area with the dryer set on the warm (not hot) setting for 3 to 5 minutes.
- Avoid rubber pants.

● ATOPIC DERMATITIS

Atopic dermatitis (eczema) is one of the disorders in the atopy family (along with asthma and allergic rhinitis). Atopic dermatitis affects 10% of the population as a whole (Marino & Fine, 2007). About half of the children who have atopic dermatitis also have asthma (Marino & Fine, 2007). Seventy-five percent of persons with atopic dermatitis have a family history of the disorder, and as many as 60% to 65% of children with the disorder show signs of it in the first year of life (Garfunkel et al., 2002; Yetman & Parks, 2002). The average age of onset is 3 months (Shwayder, 2003), and 90% of children with atopic dermatitis develop symptoms before 5 years of age (Yetman & Parks, 2002).

The chronic itching associated with atopic dermatitis causes a great deal of psychological distress. The child's self-image may be affected, particularly if the rash is extensive. Difficulty sleeping may occur because of the itching. The child is irritable and has difficulty concentrating, and family life is disrupted (Hansen, 2003). Parents' stress related to the child's condition may increase the child's anxiety and lead to an increase in itching and scratching. The child may outgrow atopic dermatitis, its severity may decrease as the child approaches adulthood, or the child may continue to have difficulties into the adult years (Cheigh, 2003). Bacterial superinfection may occur as a complication.

Therapeutic management includes good skin hydration, application of topical corticosteroids or immune modulators, oral antihistamines for sedative effects, and antibiotics if secondary infection occurs.

Pathophysiology

Atopic dermatitis is a chronic disorder characterized by extreme itching and inflamed, reddened, and swollen skin (Yetman & Parks, 2002). It has a relapsing and remitting nature. The skin reaction occurs in response to specific allergens, usually food (especially eggs, wheat, milk, and peanuts) or environmental triggers (e.g., molds, dust mites, and cat dander). Other factors, such as high or low ambient temperatures, perspiring, scratching, skin irritants, or stress, may contribute to flare-ups. When the child encounters a triggering antigen, antigen-presenting cells stimulate interleukins to begin the inflammatory process. The skin begins to feel pruritic and the child starts to scratch. The sensation of itchiness comes first, and then the rash becomes apparent. The itching causes the rash to appear. Sweating causes atopic dermatitis to worsen, as does excessively humid or dry environments.

Nursing Assessment

For a full description of the assessment phase of the nursing process, refer to page 837. Assessment findings pertinent to atopic dermatitis are discussed below.

Health History

Elicit a description of the present illness and chief complaint. Common signs and symptoms reported during the health history might include:

- Wiggling or scratching
- Dry skin
- Scratch marks noticed by the parents
- Disrupted sleep
- Irritability

Explore the child's current and past medical history for risk factors such as:

- Family history of atopic dermatitis, allergic rhinitis, or asthma
- Child's history of asthma or allergic rhinitis
- Food or environmental allergies

Determine the onset of the rash, its location, progression, severity, and response to treatments used so far. Note medications used to treat the rash, as well as other medications the child may be taking.

Physical Examination

Physical examination consists of inspection and observation and auscultation.

Inspection and Observation

Observe whether the infant is wiggling or the child is actively scratching. Carefully inspect the skin. Document dry, scaly, or flaky skin, as well as hypertrophy and lichenification (Fig. 25.8). If lesions are present they may be dry lesions or weepy papules or vesicles. In children under 2 years old, the rash is most likely to occur on the face, scalp, wrists, and extensor surfaces of the arms or legs. In older children it may occur anywhere on the skin, but is found more commonly on the flexor areas. Note erythema or warmth, which may indicate associated secondary bacterial infection. Document areas of hyperpigmentation or hypopigmentation, which may have resulted from a prior exacerbation of atopic dermatitis or its treatment. Inspect the eyes, nose, and throat for symptoms of allergic rhinitis.

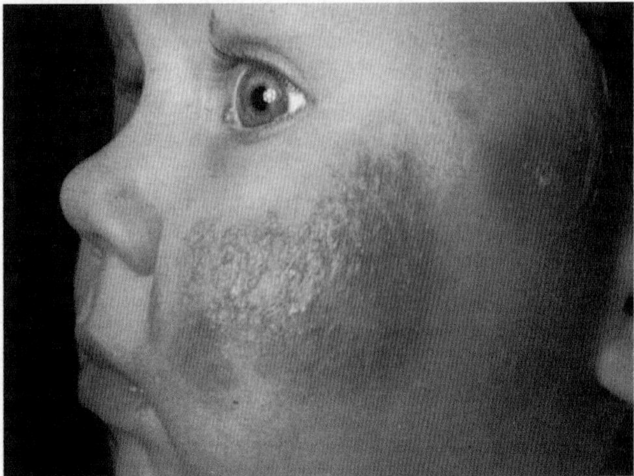

● Figure 25.8 Atopic dermatitis rash is red, dry, and scaly.

Auscultation

Auscultate the lungs for wheezing (commonly found in the associated condition of asthma).

Laboratory and Diagnostic Tests

Serum IgE levels may be elevated in the child with atopic dermatitis. Skin prick allergy testing may determine the food or environmental allergen to which the child is sensitive.

Nursing Management

Nursing management of the child with atopic dermatitis focuses on promoting skin hydration, maintaining skin integrity, and preventing infection.

Promoting Skin Hydration

First and foremost, avoid hot water and any skin or hair product containing perfumes, dyes, or fragrance. Bathe the child twice daily in warm (not hot) water. Use a mild soap to clean only the dirty areas. Recommended mild soaps or cleansing agents include:

- Unscented Dove or Dove for sensitive skin
- Tone
- Caress
- Oil of Olay
- Cetaphil
- Aquanil

Slightly pat the child dry after the bath, but do not rub with the towel. Leave the child moist. Apply topical ointments or creams as prescribed to the affected area. Apply fragrance-free moisturizer over the prescribed topical medication and all over the child's body. Recommended moisturizers include:

- Eucerin, Moisturel, Curel (cream or lotion)
- Aquaphor
- Vaseline
- Crisco

Apply moisture multiple times throughout the day. Avoid clothing made of synthetic fabrics or wool. Avoid triggers known to exacerbate atopic dermatitis.

Evening primrose oil and other essential fatty acid supplements over a period of at least 6 weeks may produce an improvement in the atopic dermatitis. Headache and nausea are rare adverse effects of these supplements and if they occur are usually mild (Gardiner et al., 2001). Chamomile preparations for topical use may also be effective and are generally considered safe.

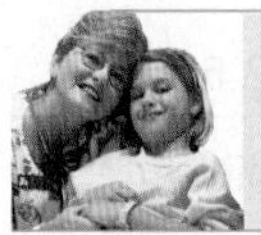

Vaseline or generic petrolatum is an inexpensive, readily available moisturizer.

Maintaining Skin Integrity and Preventing Infection

Cut the child's fingernails short and keep them clean. Avoid tight clothing and heat. Use 100% cotton bed sheets and pajamas. In addition to keeping the child's skin well moisturized, it is extremely important to prevent the child from scratching. Scratching causes the rash to appear and further scratching may lead to secondary infection. Antihistamines given at bedtime may sedate the child enough to allow him or her to sleep without awakening because of itching.

During the waking hours, behavior modification may help to keep the child from scratching. Have the parent keep a diary for 1 week to determine the pattern of scratching. Help the parent to determine specific strategies that may raise the child's awareness of scratching. A hand-held clicker or counter may help to identify the scratching episode for the child, thus raising awareness. The use of diversion, imagination, and play may help to distract the child from scratching. The parent and child may create a game together that results in the child participating in a behavior rather than scratching. Pressing the skin or clenching the fist may replace scratching. It is important for the child to stay active to distract his or her mind from the itching. The parent should positively reinforce and reward the desired behaviors (Buchanan, 2001).

• CONTACT DERMATITIS

Contact dermatitis is a cell-mediated response to an antigenic substance exposure. The first exposure is the sensitization phase. The antigen attaches to cells that migrate to regional lymph nodes and have contact with T lymphocytes, where recognition of antigen is developed. During the second phase, elicitation, contact with the antigen results in T-lymphocyte proliferation and release of inflammatory mediators. An allergic response occurs within 24 to 48 hours after contact with the substance (Allen, 2004).

One of the more common causes of contact dermatitis in children results from exposure to highly allergenic plants and thus will be the focus of this discussion. *Toxicodendron radican* (poison ivy), *Toxicodendron quercifolium* (Eastern poison oak), *Toxicodendron diversilobum* (Western poison oak), and *Toxicodendron vernix* (poison sumac) are the typical offenders. Contact with the plant's oil (urushiol), which is found in the leaves, stems, and roots, results in an allergic reaction in 50% to 70% of people (Allen, 2004). Even contact with dormant plants or plants perceived to be dead may cause an allergic response. The rash is extremely pruritic and may last for 2 to 4 weeks, and lesions continue to appear during the illness.

Contact dermatitis is not contagious and does not spread either to other parts of the affected child's skin or to other people. Scratching does not spread the rash, but it may cause skin damage or secondary infection. Complications of contact dermatitis include secondary bacterial skin infections and lichenification or hyperpigmentation, particularly in dark-skinned people.

Therapeutic management is directed toward management of itching and the use of topical corticosteroids. Moderate-potency topical glucocorticoid cream or ointment is used for mild to moderate contact dermatitis, and high-potency preparations are used for more severe cases. Some severe cases of contact dermatitis, may require the use of systemic steroids.

Nursing Assessment

Elicit the health history, noting time spent in the woods or noncultivated areas within 1 to 2 days before the onset of the rash. Note contact with a family pet that spends time outdoors. Note onset, description, location, and progression of the rash, which will be intensely pruritic in most children (Fig. 25.9). Document treatment used thus far, and the child's response to it. Examine the skin, noting an erythematous papulovescicular rash at the site of contact. Some lesions may be weeping; others erupt and form a crust. The lesions are often distributed in an asymmetric linear pattern on exposed body parts. If the child's shirt came in contact with the plant and then the shirt was removed by pulling it over the head, there may be widespread lesions over both sides of the face. Lesions near the eyes often cause significant eyelid edema.

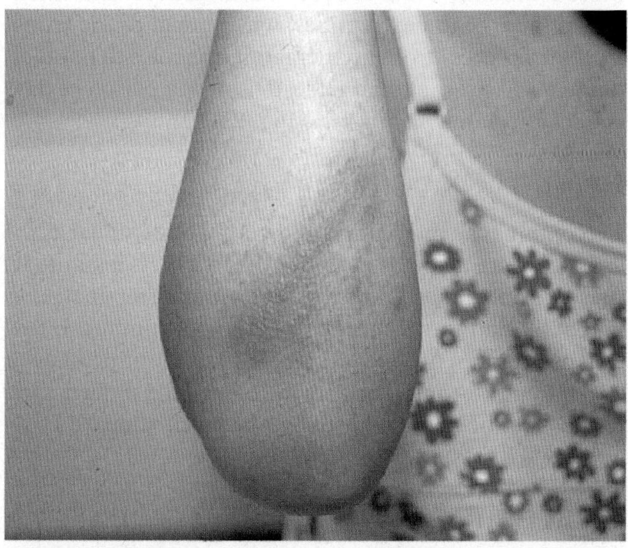

● Figure 25.9 Note vesicular rash in linear formation characteristic of poison ivy.

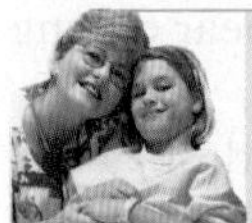

Nickel dermatitis may occur from contact with jewelry, eyeglasses, belts, or clothing snaps. Infants may display a small red circle with scaling at the site of contact with sleeper snaps.

Nursing Management

Contact dermatitis may be prevented by avoiding contact with the allergen. When the condition does occur, nursing management focuses on relieving the discomfort associated with the rash. Administer topical or systemic corticosteroids as prescribed and teach the family about use of the medications. Teaching Guideline 25.2 gives more information about the treatment and prevention of contact dermatitis.

• ERYTHEMA MULTIFORME

Erythema multiforme, though uncommon in children, is an acute, self-limiting hypersensitivity reaction. It may occur in response to viral infections, such as adenovirus or Epstein-Barr virus, *Mycoplasma pneumoniae* infection, or a drug (especially sulfa drugs, penicillins, or immunizations) or food reaction. Stevens-Johnson syndrome is the most severe form of erythema multiforme and most often occurs in response to certain medications or to *Mycoplasma* infection (Box 25.1). Therapeutic management of erythema multiforme is generally supportive, as it resolves on its own.

Nursing Assessment

Note history of fever, malaise, and achiness (myalgia). Determine onset and progression of rash, and presence of **pruritus** and burning. Document the child's temperature upon assessment. Inspect the skin for lesions, which most commonly occur over the hands and feet and extensor surfaces of the extremities, with spread to the trunk. Lesions progress from erythematous macules to papules, plaques, vesicles, and target lesions over a period of days (hence the name *multiforme*) (Fig. 25.10).

Nursing Management

Discontinue the medication or food if it is identified as the cause. Ensure that treatment for *Mycoplasma* is instituted if present. Encourage oral hydration. Administer analgesics and antihistamines as needed to promote comfort. If oral lesions are present, encourage soothing mouthwashes or use of topic oral anesthetics in the older child or teen. Oral lesions may be débrided with hydrogen peroxide.

• URTICARIA

Urticaria, commonly called hives, is a type I hypersensitivity reaction caused by an immunologically mediated antigen–antibody response of histamine release from mast cells. Vasodilation and increased vascular permeability result, and erythema and wheals then occur. Urticaria usually begins rapidly and may disappear in a few days or may take up to 6 or 8 weeks to resolve. The most common causes of this reaction are foods, drugs, animal stings, infections, environmental stimuli (e.g., heat, cold, sun, tight clothes), and stress. Therapeutic management focuses on identifying and removing the cause as well as providing antihistamines or steroids.

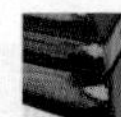

TEACHING GUIDELINE 25.2

Prevention and Treatment of Contact Dermatitis

Prevention

- Wear long sleeves and long pants on outings in the woods.
- Identify and remove offending plants in the yard by using a commercial weed or underbrush killer.
- Vinyl gloves (not rubber or latex) are an effective barrier.
- The plant's oil residue may be on clothes, pets, garden and sports equipment, and toys; wash those well with soap and water.
- If contact occurs, wash vigorously with soap and water within 10 minutes of contact.
- Zanfel and Tecnu Oak-N-Ivy Outdoor Skin Cleanser (both soap mixtures) may prevent rash if used to wash the skin soon after exposure.
- Ivy Block (an organoclay) is the only FDA-approved preventive treatment for contact dermatitis related to poison ivy, oak, or sumac (www.enviroderm.com). It is applied to the skin before possible exposure.

Treatment

- Wash lesions daily with mild soap and water.
- Mildly débride crusted lesions.
- Tepid baths (colloidal oatmeal such as Aveeno) are helpful to decrease itching.
- Avoid hot baths or showers, as they aggravate itching.
- Apply corticosteroid preparations topically as directed (if using high-potency preparations, do not cover with an occlusive dressing).
- Weeping lesions may be wrapped lightly; avoid occlusion.
- Burow's or Domeboro solutions with a dressing applied twice daily for 20 minutes may help to dry weepy lesions.
- Over-the-counter preparations such as calamine lotion or Ivy Rest may reduce itching and help the lesions to dry.
- Do not use topical antihistamines, benzocaine, or neomycin because of the potential for sensitization.

Data from Allen, P. L. J. (2004). Leaves of three, let them be: If it were only that easy! *Pediatric Nursing, 30*(2), 129–135; and Guin, J. D., & Bruckner, A. L. (2005). Compendium on poison ivy dermatitis: The insidious plants, the resulting lesions, the treatment options. *Contemporary Pediatrics, 22*(1 suppl.), 4–15.

BOX 25.1
STEVENS-JOHNSON SYNDROME

- 1- to 14-day history of fever, malaise, headache, generalized aching, emesis, and diarrhea
- Sudden onset of high fever with rash appearing
- Rash is characteristic of erythema multiforme with the addition of inflammatory bullae on at least two types of mucosa (lips, oral mucosa, bulbar conjunctivae, or anogenital region).
- Mortality rate of 10% (Marino & Fine, 2007), particularly when the genitourinary, gastrointestinal, and respiratory tracts are involved
- Treatment: hospitalization, isolation, fluid and electrolyte support, treatment of secondary infection of the lesions
- Ophthalmologic consult to determine if corneal ulceration, keratitis, uveitis, or panophthalmitis is present

Nursing Assessment

Obtain a detailed history of new foods, medications, symptoms of a recent infection, changes in environment, or unusual stress. Inspect the skin, noting raised, edematous hives anywhere on the body or mucous membranes. The hives are pruritic, blanch when pressed, and may migrate. Angioedema may also be present and is identifiable as subcutaneous edema and warmth, occurring most frequently on the extremities, face, or genitalia. Carefully assess airway and breathing, as hypersensitivity reactions may affect respiratory status.

Nursing Management

Identify and remove the offending trigger. Discontinue antibiotics. Administer antihistamines, corticosteroids, and topical antipruritics as prescribed. Inform the child and family that the episode should resolve within a few days. If it lasts up to 6 weeks, the child should be re-evaluated.

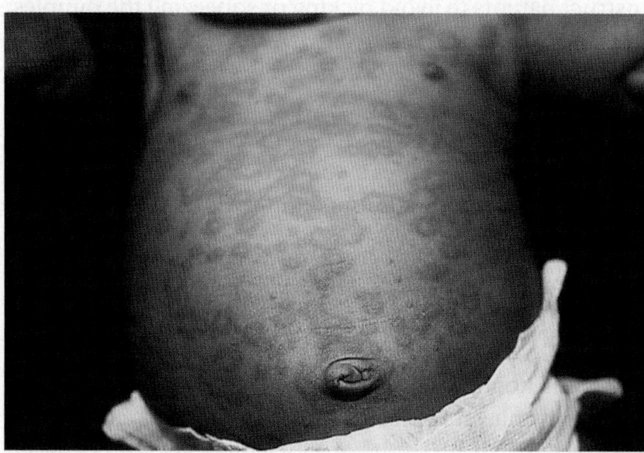

● Figure 25.10 Erythema multiforme.

Advise the family to obtain a medical alert bracelet for the child if the reaction is severe.

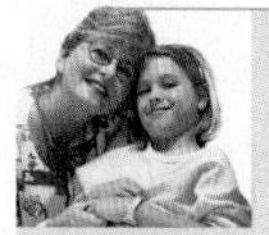

In an emergency situation when airway and breathing are compromised, subcutaneous epinephrine followed by IV diphenhydramine and steroids is necessary.

Seborrhea

Seborrhea is a chronic inflammatory dermatitis that may occur on the skin or scalp. In infants it occurs most often on the scalp and is commonly referred to as cradle cap. Infants may also manifest seborrhea on the nose or eyebrows, behind the ears, or in the diaper area. It usually resolves completely by 8 to 12 months of age (Krowchuk & Tunnessen, 2006). Adolescents manifest seborrhea on the scalp (dandruff) and on the eyebrows and eyelashes, behind the ears, and between the shoulder blades. Skin lesions are treated with corticosteroid creams or lotions. Anti-dandruff shampoos containing selenium sulfide, ketoconazole, or tar are used to treat the scalp. It is thought that seborrhea is an inflammatory reaction to the fungus *Pityrosporum ovale* and is worsened by sebaceous involvement related to maternal hormones in the infant and androgens in the adolescent (Krowchuk & Tunnessen, 2006).

Nursing Assessment

Elicit the health history, determining onset and progression of skin and scalp changes. Note response to treatment used so far. In the infant, inspect the scalp and forehead, behind the ears, and the neck, trunk, and diaper area for thick or flaky greasy yellow scales (Fig. 25.11). In the adolescent,

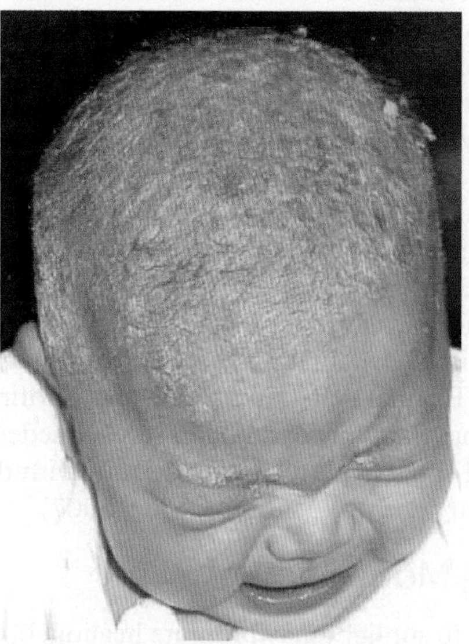

● Figure 25.11 Severe cradle cap (yellow, greasy-appearing plaques).

note mild flakes in the hair with yellow greasy scales on the scalp, forehead, and eyebrows, behind the ears, or between the scapulae.

Nursing Management

Wash or shampoo the affected areas with a mild soap. Apply anti-inflammatory cream to skin lesions if prescribed. In the infant, apply mineral oil to the scalp, massage it in well with a washcloth, and then shampoo 10 to 15 minutes later, using a brush to gently lift the crusts; do not forcibly remove the crusts. If needed, selenium sulfide shampoo may safely be used on the infant, following the aforementioned procedure. The adolescent may require daily shampooing with an anti-dandruff shampoo.

Psoriasis

Psoriasis is a chronic skin disease with periods of remission and exacerbation (Marino & Fine, 2007). Control is possible with conscientious therapy. Psoriasis does occur in children, but the peak onset is between 15 and 25 years of age (Wong & Rogers, 2006). Psoriasis demonstrates a multifactorial inheritance pattern (Marino & Fine, 2007), with up to 50% of patients having a family history of psoriasis (Wong & Rogers, 2006).

Hyperproliferation of the epidermis occurs, with a rash developing at sites of mechanical, thermal, or physical trauma. Therapeutic management includes skin hydration, use of tar preparations, ultraviolet light, or tazarotene (a topical retinoid). Narrow-band ultraviolet light has been used with some success in children with severe psoriasis (Wong & Rogers, 2006).

Nursing Assessment

Note family history of psoriasis. Determine onset and progression of rash, as well as treatments used and the response to treatment. Question the child about pruritus, which is usually absent with psoriasis. Inspect the skin for erythematous papules that coalesce to form plaques, most frequently found on the scalp, elbows, genital area, and knees. Facial plaques may also occur and are more common in children than adults (Wong & Rogers, 2006). The plaques have a silvery or yellow-white scale and sharply demarcated borders. Layers of scale may be present, which, when removed, result in pinpoint bleeding (referred to as the Auspitz sign). Plaques on the scalp may result in alopecia. Examine the palms and soles, noting fissures and scaling. Skin biopsy, though rarely needed for diagnosis, will show hyperplastic epidermis, with thinning of the papillary dermis (Marion & Fine, 2007).

Nursing Management

Exposure to sunlight may promote healing, but take care not to allow the child to become sunburned. Apply skin moisturizers or emollients daily to prevent dry skin and flare-ups. Apply topical anti-inflammatory creams as prescribed during flare-ups. Apply tar shampoos or skin preparations. Use mineral oil and warm towels to soak and remove thick plaques.

Acne

Acne, the most common skin condition occurring in childhood, is a disorder that affects the pilosebaceous unit. It affects males and females, as well as all ethnic groups. Overall, males tend to have more severe disease than females, probably because of the androgen influence. Acne that persists past the usual course of time for infantile or adolescent acne may be caused by endocrine abnormalities. It may also occur in response to the use of certain types of drugs such as corticosteroids, androgens, phenytoin, and others. The usual presentation and nursing management of acne neonatorum and acne vulgaris is presented below.

● ACNE NEONATORUM

Acne neonatorum occurs as a response to the presence of maternal androgens and affects about 20% of newborns (Holmes & Krusinski, 2006). It generally appears between 2 and 4 weeks of age and lasts up to 4 to 6 months, sometimes lasting until 2 to 3 years of age. Neonatal acne affects boys more often than girls and tends to be more severe in boys. Usually no treatment is necessary, but in severe cases there is a risk of scarring, so a topical preparation may be prescribed. If acne persists in the infant or young child, an endocrine disorder resulting in hyperandrogenism may be present (Rudy, 2003).

Nursing Assessment

Note oily face or scalp. Examine the face (especially the cheeks), upper chest, and back for inflammatory papules and pustules. Document absence of fever.

Nursing Management

Instruct parents to avoid picking or squeezing the pimples; to do so places the infant at risk for secondary bacterial infection and cellulitis. Teach parents to wash the affected areas daily with clear water. Avoid using fragranced soaps or lotions on the area with acne. Inform the parents that as the newborn's hormones stabilize over time, the acne usually resolves without additional intervention.

● ACNE VULGARIS

Acne vulgaris occurs in 50% to 80% of adolescents between the ages of 12 and 16 years, and endogenous androgens play a role (Rudy, 2003). It may start as early as between 7 and 10 years of age, with peak onset between 15 and 18 years of age (Silverberg et al., 2005). Acne vulgaris may also continue into the 20s and 30s. It occurs most frequently on the face, chest, and back. Risk factors for the development of acne vulgaris include preadolescent or adolescent age, male gender (due to the presence of androgens), an oily complexion, Cushing syndrome, or another disease process resulting in increased androgen production (Marino & Fine, 2007).

Pathophysiology

The sebaceous gland produces sebum and is connected by a duct to the follicular canal that opens on the skin's surface. Androgenous hormones stimulate sebaceous gland proliferation and production of sebum. These hormones exhibit increased activity during the pubertal years. Abnormal shedding of the outermost layer of the skin (the stratum corneum) occurs at the level of the follicular opening, resulting in a keratin plug that fills the follicle. The sebaceous glands increase sebum production. Bacterial overgrowth of *Proprionibacterium acnes* occurs because the presence of sebum and keratin in the follicular canal creates an excellent environment for growth. Inflammation occurs as the follicular wall perforates, allowing the contents to leak into nearby tissue (Rudy, 2003).

Therapeutic Management

Therapeutic management focuses on reducing *P. acnes*, decreasing sebum production, normalizing skin shedding, and eliminating inflammation (AAD, 2005). The skin should be cleansed gently twice a day. Medication therapy may include a combination of benzoyl peroxide, salicylic acid, retinoids, and topical or oral antibiotics. Isotretinoin (Accutane) may be used in severe cases. Drug Guide 25.1 gives further information on these medications. In girls, oral contraceptives may help lessen acne by decreasing the effects of androgens on the sebaceous glands (Keri, 2006). Diode laser or blue ultraviolet light therapy may also be used. CO_2 lasers and dermabrasion may be used to treat pitted scarring (Silverberg et al., 2005).

Nursing Assessment

Note history of onset of acne lesions, as well as family history of acne. Determine medication use; certain medications may hasten the onset of acne or worsen it when already present. In particular, note use of corticosteroids, androgens, lithium, phenytoin, and isoniazid. Document history of an endocrine disorder, particularly one that results in hyperandrogenism. In girls, note worsening of acne 2 to 7 days before the start of the menstrual period. Inspect the skin for lesions (particularly on the face and upper chest and back, which are the areas of highest sebaceous activity). Note presence, distribution, and extent of noninflammatory lesions, such as open and closed comedones, as well as inflammatory lesions such as papules, pustules, nodules, or cysts (open comedones are commonly referred

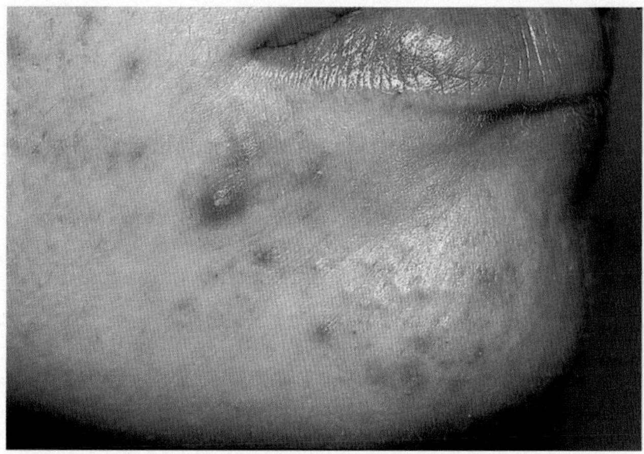

● Figure 25.12 Acne vulgaris.

to as blackheads and closed comedones as whiteheads; see Fig. 25.12). Examine the skin for hypertrophic scarring resulting from inflammatory lesions. Table 25.3 explains the acne classification. Note oily skin and oily hair, which result from increased sebum production. Determine remedies that have been used and the extent of success of those treatments. Assess the child's or teen's feelings about the disorder.

Nursing Management

Avoid oil-based cosmetics and hair products, as their use may block pores, contributing to noninflammatory lesions. Look for cosmetic products labeled as noncomedogenic. Headbands, helmets, and hats may exacerbate the lesions by causing friction. Dryness and peeling may occur with acne treatment, so encourage the child to use a humectant moisturizer. Mild cleansing with soap and water twice daily is appropriate. Avoid excessive scrubbing and harsh chemical or alcohol-based cleansers (Berson, 2005). Avoid

Table 25.3 Classification of Acne

Classification	Manifestations
Mild acne	Primarily noninflammatory lesions (comedones)
Moderate acne	Comedones plus inflammatory lesions such as papules or pustules (localized to face or back)
Severe acne	Lesions similar to moderate acne, but more widespread, and/or presence of cysts or nodules. Associated more frequently with scarring.

picking or squeezing the lesions. Using a noncomedogenic sunscreen with an SPF of 30 or higher may reduce the risk of postinflammatory discoloration from acne lesions (Silverberg et al., 2005). Teach adolescents that the prescribed topical medications must be used daily and that it may take 4 to 6 weeks to see results. Avoid the use of over-the-counter preparations because they are irritating and aggravate the drying effect of prescription acne treatments (Rudy, 2003). Boys should shave gently and avoid using dull razors, so as not to further irritate the condition. Adolescent girls taking isotretinoin (Accutane) who are sexually active must be on a pregnancy prevention program because the drug causes defects in fetal development (Box 25.2).

Patients interested in complementary medicine approaches may try topical use of a tea tree oil preparation. Fewer adverse effects may occur with tea tree oil preparations than with benzoyl peroxide preparations, but local reactions may still occur (Gardiner et al., 2001).

If the acne is severe, depression may occur as a result of body image disturbances. Provide emotional support to adolescents undergoing acne therapy. Refer teens for counseling if necessary.

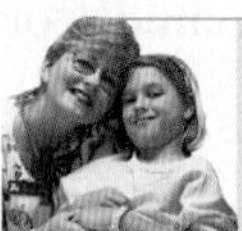

Chocolate, skim milk, and French fries have not been proven to contribute to the incidence or severity of acne. However, advise teens to wash their hands after eating greasy finger foods to avoid spreading additional oil to the surface of the face.

BOX 25.2

DECREASING RISK OF FETAL EXPOSURE TO ISOTRETINOIN: IPLEDGE

- As of 2006, physicians, pharmacists, and patients are required to register in the iPLEDGE program before they prescribe, dispense, or receive isotretinoin (Accutane).
- The iPLEDGE program is a central registry requiring monthly input as noted below in order to continue isotretinoin treatment.
- Monthly input includes the following:
  - Females of childbearing age are using two forms of contraception.
  - Pregnancy test results are negative.
  - Isotretinoin users do not donate blood during or for 1 month after completion of treatment.
  - Additional information is available at http://www.fda.gov/cder/drug/infopage/accutane/default.htm

Data from Cuzzell, J. Z. (2005). FDA approves mandatory risk management program for isotretinoin. *Dermatology Nursing, 17*(5), 383; and U.S. Food and Drug Administration, Center for Drug Evaluation and Research. (2006). *Isotretinoin (marketed as Accutane) capsule information.* Retrieved 7/25/06 from http://www.fda.gov/cder/drug/infopage/accutane/default.htm.

Consider THIS!

Paxton Herman, age 16, comes to the clinic with complaints of acne on his face and back. What assessment information should the nurse obtain? What education will be important for Paxton?

Injuries

Children, by their inquisitive natures, developmental immaturity, and skin's properties, are prone to experience a variety of skin injuries. Pressure ulcers are most likely to occur in hospitalized or otherwise immobile children. Typical healthy, active children are likely to suffer cuts, abrasions, and foreign body penetration, burns and other thermal injuries, bites, and stings.

PRESSURE ULCERS

Skin breakdown involves changes in intact skin, which may range from blanchable erythema to deep pressure ulcers. The term "pressure ulcer" refers to damage to the skin resulting in skin loss and development of a crater that may be mild or deep (Suddaby et al., 2006). The incidence of pressure ulcers in children remains unknown. Pressure ulcers develop from a combination of factors, including immobility or decreased activity, decreased sensory perception, increased moisture, impaired nutritional status, inadequate tissue perfusion, and the forces of friction and shear. Common sites of pressure ulcers in hospitalized children include the occiput and toes, while children who require wheelchairs for mobility have pressure ulcers in the sacral or hip area more frequently.

Nursing Assessment

Note history of immobility (chronic, related to a condition such as paralysis) or lengthy hospitalization, particularly in intensive care. Inspect the skin for areas of erythema or warmth. Note ulceration of the skin. Use the facility's wound assessment scale to document the extent of the ulcer. Take a photo of the ulcer if possible.

Nursing Management

Position the child to alleviate pressure on the area of the ulcer. Use specialized beds or mattresses to prevent further pressure areas from developing. Perform prescribed wound care meticulously, noting the formation of granulation tissue as the ulcer begins to heal. Prevent pressure ulcers in the child who is hospitalized for long periods of time by turning the child frequently, assessing the entire surface of the child's skin at least every shift, using pressure-alleviating beds and mattresses, and maintaining the child's nutritional status.

MINOR INJURIES

Children suffer minor injuries very frequently. These include minor cuts and abrasions, as well as skin penetration of foreign bodies such as splinters or glass fragments. Because of their developmental immaturity and inquisitive nature, children often attempt tasks they are not yet capable of or take risks that an adult would not, often resulting in a fall or other accident. The break in the skin allows an entry point for bacteria, and the complication of cellulitis may occur. Treatment is directed at cleaning the wound and preventing infection.

Nursing Assessment

Obtain the history from the child or caregiver to determine whether dirt or a foreign object may be present in the wound. Inspect the wound, noting depth of injury, a foreign body, and bleeding.

Nursing Management

Cleanse the wound with mild soap and water or with an antibacterial cleanser. Wet gauze helps to scrub away fine and large sand particles. Remove pieces of loose skin with sterile scissors, foreign particles with sterile forceps, and road tar with petrolatum. Small abrasions and minor, well-approximated cuts may be left open to the air. Apply a small amount of antibacterial ointment and cover large abrasions with a loose dressing. Change the dressing 12 hours later and redress after cleaning the wound. Leave it open to air after 24 hours have passed from the time of injury.

Calendula preparations are presumed to be safe for topical use and may speed wound healing. Chamomile may help to dry a weeping wound, and allergic reactions to the herb are rare (Gardiner et al., 2001).

Assess the wound daily for signs of infection, which include purulence, warmth, edema, increasing pain, and erythema that extends past the margin of the cut or abrasion.

BURNS

Over 1 million people experience a burn injury each year in the United States, and 35% of those burn injuries are to children (Shriners Hospital for Children, 2005). Burns are the second-leading cause of death from unintentional injury in children between 1 and 4 years of age and the third-leading cause in all persons under 19 years old. Children less than 6 years of age are at highest risk for burns (Schweich, 2006), and the mortality rate from burns in young children is twice that of older children (National Safe Kids Campaign, 2004).

Most pediatric burn-related injuries do not result in death, but injuries from burns often cause extreme pain and extensive burns can result in serious disfigurement. While most pediatric burns are tragic unintentional injuries, about 75% of them could have been prevented, and child abuse is the cause of about 15% to 30% of serious pediatric burns (American Medical Student Association, 2006). See Healthy People 2010.

Carbon monoxide poisoning often occurs in conjunction with burns as a result of smoke inhalation, and infants and children are at greater risk for carbon monoxide poisoning than adults.

Great advances have been made in the care of children with serious burns. As a result of improved burn care, children who in the past would have died as a result of burns over large body surface areas have a much greater chance of survival. These improved outcomes for seriously burned children are thought to be the result of refinements in:

- Resuscitation
- Operative techniques
- Critical care (mechanical ventilation, monitoring, and vascular access)
- Pain control
- Nutritional support
- Skin and blood banking
- Antibiotic therapy (Sheridan et al., 2000)

Conventional wisdom is that children with severe burns should be transferred to a specialized burn unit. The Committee on Trauma of the American College of Surgeons (1999) has developed the following criteria for referral of burned persons to a burn unit:

- Partial thickness burns greater than 10% of total body surface area
- Burns that involve the face
- Burns that involve the hands and feet, genitalia, perineum, or major joints
- Electrical burns, including lightning injury
- Chemical burns
- Inhalation injury
- Burn injury in patients who have pre-existing conditions that might affect their care
- Persons with burns and traumatic injuries
- Persons who will require special social, emotional, or long-term rehabilitative care
- Burned children in a hospital without qualified personnel or equipment for the care of children

HEALTHY PEOPLE 2010

Objective	Significance
Reduce residential fire deaths. Increase functioning residential smoke alarms.	• Question all families about smoke detectors and if they are working. • Provide families with resources related to fire prevention.

Burns are classified according to the extent of injury. Superficial burns involve only epidermal injury and usually heal without scarring or other sequelae within 4 to 5 days. In partial-thickness burns, injury occurs not only to the epidermis but also to portions of the dermis. These burns usually heal within about 2 weeks and carry a minimal risk of scar formation. Deep partial-thickness burns take longer to heal, may scar, and result in changes in nail and hair appearance as well as sebaceous gland function in the affected area. They may require surgical intervention. Full-thickness burns result in significant tissue damage as they extend through the epidermis, dermis, and hypodermis. Extensive scarring results, as hair follicles and sweat glands are destroyed. Full-thickness burns require a significant time to heal. If underlying tendons and/or bone are involved, the burn may be termed fourth degree. Contractures and limited function may occur as a complication of full-thickness burns. Skin grafting is usually necessary. Full or partially circumferential burns may result in ischemia from loss of blood flow related to progressive swelling of the area.

Pathophysiology

Burned tissue begins to coagulate after the injury, and direct coagulation and microvascular reactions in the adjacent dermis may extend the burn. The blood vessels demonstrate increased capillary permeability, resulting in vasodilatation. This leads to increased hydrostatic pressure in the capillaries, causing water, electrolytes, and protein to leak out of the vasculature and result in significant edema. Edema forms very rapidly in the first 18 hours after the burn, peaking at around 48 hours. Capillary permeability then returns to normal between 48 and 72 hours after the burn and the lymphatics can reabsorb the edema fluid. Diuresis occurs, ridding the body of the excess fluid. Fluid loss from burned skin occurs at an amount that is 5 to 10 times greater than that from undamaged skin, and this fluid loss continues until the damaged surface is healed or grafted (Merz et al., 2003).

Initially, the severely burned child experiences a decrease in cardiac output, with a subsequent hypermetabolic response during which cardiac output increases dramatically. During this heightened metabolic state, the child is at risk for insulin resistance and increased protein catabolism. Children who are burned during an indoor or chemical fire are at an increased risk of respiratory injury. Children who have aspirated hot liquids are particularly at risk for airway-altering edema.

Therapeutic Management

Therapeutic management of burns focuses on fluid resuscitation, wound care, prevention of infection, and restoration of function. Burn infections are treated with antibiotics specific to the causative organism. If invasive burn damage occurs, surgery may be necessary.

Nursing Assessment

For a full description of the assessment phase of the nursing process, refer to page 837. Upon arrival, the pediatric burn client should be evaluated to determine if he or she will require intensive management. Remove any smoldering clothing. Obtain a brief history of the burn circumstances while you are assessing the child and providing care.

Health History

If the burn is severe or there is a potential for respiratory compromise, obtain a brief history while simultaneously evaluating the child and providing emergency care. If the burn does not appear to pose an immediate life-threatening risk, obtain an in-depth history. Elicit a description of how the burn occurred, noting date, time, and cause. Determine if smoke inhalation or an associated fall may have occurred. Document treatment that the parent or caregiver has provided to the child's burn so far. Note the child's recent health status, current medications, recent or chronic illness, and immunization status, in particular noting the date of the most recent tetanus vaccination. Determine whether the history being given sounds consistent with the type of burn injury that has occurred. Inquire about what caused the burn and if the event was witnessed by anyone. Spatter-type burns resulting from the child pulling a source of hot fluid onto himself or herself usually yield a non-uniform, asymmetric distribution of injury. In contrast, intentional scald injuries usually yield a uniform "sock" or "glove" distribution when the child's extremity is held under very hot water as punishment. It is important for the nurse to pick up on clues in the health history that may indicate that the burn is a result of child abuse, rather than an accident (Box 25.3). Children are also burned by curling irons, gasoline, fireworks, room heaters, ovens, and ranges. Obtain a detailed history about the circumstances surrounding these types of burns. Ask the parent what the home hot water heater temperature is.

Physical Examination

Emergency examination of the burned child consists of a primary survey followed by a secondary survey. The primary survey includes evaluation of the child's airway, breathing, and circulation; the secondary survey focuses on evaluation of the burns and other injuries. Box 25.4 gives information about emergency assessment of the burned child. Inspect the child's skin, noting erythema, blistering, weeping, or eschar (charred skin).

The old terms used to describe the depth of burns as first, second, and third degree have been replaced by the contemporary terminology. Classify the burn according to its severity. Superficial burns are painful, red, dry and possibly edematous (Fig. 25.13). Partial-thickness and deep partial-thickness burns are very painful

BOX 25.3
SIGNS OF CHILD ABUSE–INDUCED BURNS

- Inconsistent history given when caregivers are interviewed separately
- Delay in seeking treatment by caregiver
- Uniform appearance of the burn, with clear delineation of burned and nonburned area (as with a hot object applied to the skin)
- In the case of a scald-induced burn, lack of spattering of water but evidence of so-called "porcelain-contact sparing," where the portion of the child's skin that was in contact with the tub or sink is not burned (commonly seen with a forced immersion in extremely hot water used as punishment).
- Flexor-sparing burns or burns that involve the dorsum of the hand
- A stocking/glove pattern on the hands or feet (circumferential ring appearing around the extremity, resulting from a caregiver forcefully holding the child under extremely hot water)

and edematous and have a wet appearance or blisters (Fig. 25.14). Full-thickness burns may be very painful or numb or pain-free in some areas. They appear red, edematous, leathery, dry, or waxy and may display peeling or charred skin (Fig. 25.15). Note whether the burn is circumferential (encircling a body part) or partially circumferential.

BOX 25.4
EMERGENCY ASSESSMENT OF THE BURNED CHILD

Primary Survey
- Assess the child's airway, noting whether it is patent, maintainable, or unmaintainable.
    - Suspect airway injury from burn or smoke inhalation if any of the following are present: burns around the mouth, nose, or eyes; carbonaceous (black-colored) sputum; hoarseness or stridor.
- Evaluate the child's skin color, respiratory effort, symmetry of breathing, and breath sounds.
- Determine the pulse strength, perfusion status, and heart rate. Note extent and location of edema.

Secondary Survey
- Determine burn depth.
- Estimate burn extent by determining the percentage of body surface area affected. Use a chart for estimation (see Fig. 25.16) or rapidly estimate by using the child's palm size, which is equivalent to about 1% of the child's body surface area.
- Inspect the child for other traumatic injuries (children who have jumped or fallen from a house fire may suffer cervical spine or internal injuries).

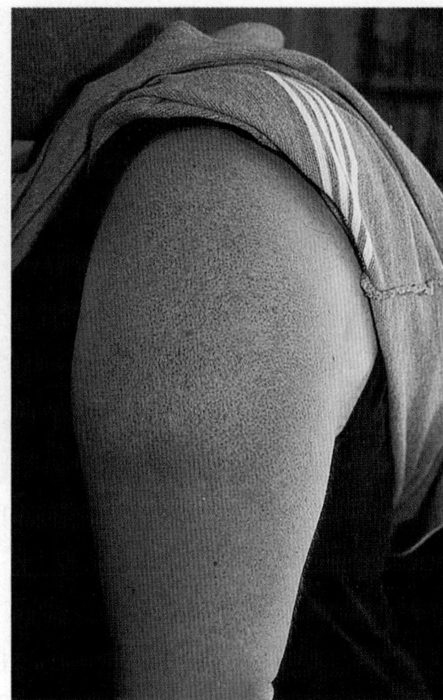

● Figure 25.13 Superficial burn—painful but without blisters.

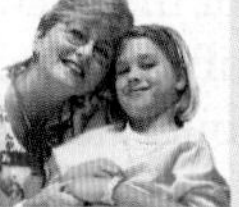

Due to overlying blistering, it is difficult to accurately distinguish between partial- and full-thickness burns. In addition, in the case of third-degree burns, it is difficult to estimate burn depth during the initial evaluation.

Laboratory and Diagnostic Tests

In the child with more extensive burns, electrolytes and complete blood count are used to measure fluid and electrolyte balance and to determine the possibility of infection, respectively. If wound infection is suspected, culture of the drainage will determine the particular bacteria. Nutritional indices such as albumin, transferrin, carotene, retinol, copper, cholesterol, calcium, thiamine, riboflavin, pyridoxine, and iron may be evaluated when the child has severe or

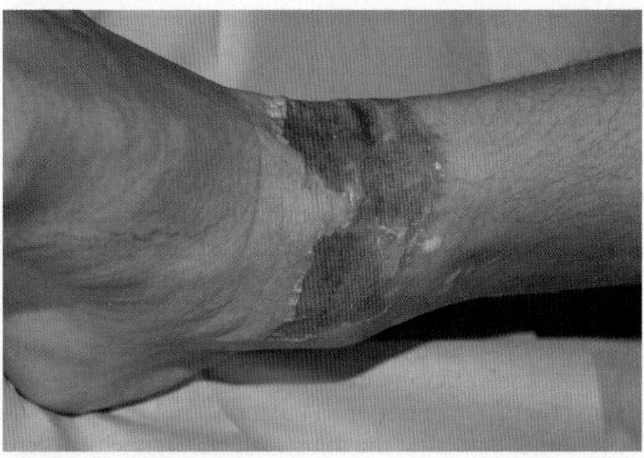

● Figure 25.14 Partial-thickness burn—very painful, with blistering.

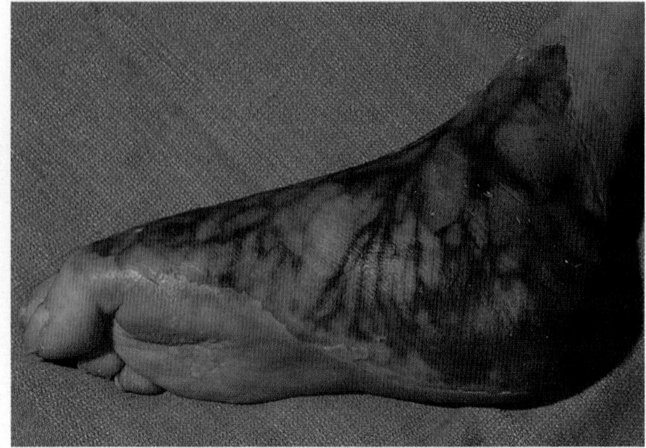

● Figure 25.15 Full-thickness burn—color ranges from red to charred, or white, minimal pain, marked edema.

extensive burns. Pulmonary status may be evaluated via pulse oximetry and end-tidal CO_2 monitoring, arterial blood gases, carboxyhemoglobin levels, and chest x-ray. Fiberoptic bronchoscopy and xenon ventilation–perfusion scanning may be used to evaluate inhalation injury. Electrocardiographic monitoring is important for the child who has suffered an electrical burn to identify cardiac arrhythmias, which can be noted for up to 72 hours after a burn injury.

Nursing Management

Nursing management of the child who has been burned focuses first on stabilizing the child. Place the child on a cardiac/apnea monitor, measure the child with the Broselow tape, monitor pulse oximetry, and apply an end-tidal CO_2 monitor if the child is ventilated. Further management focuses on cleansing the burn, pain management, and prevention and treatment of infection. Fluid status and nutrition are important components of burn care, particularly in the early stages. Rehabilitation of the child with severe burns is also an important nursing function. Providing patient and family education about the prevention of burns as well as care of burns at home is critical. Nursing Care Plan 25.1 gives additional interventions related to fluid and nutritional management.

Promoting Oxygenation and Ventilation

Institute emergency airway management as needed. If the child requires intubation, make sure that the tracheal tube is taped in a very secure manner, as reintubations in these patients will become increasingly difficult as the edema spreads. The burned child's respiratory status warrants vigilant evaluation and re-evaluation, as airway edema that is secondary to a burn may not become evident until 2 days after the injury. All children with severe burns should receive 100% oxygen via nonbreather mask or bag-valve-mask ventilation. Continue to reassess the child's pulmonary status, adjusting the interventions as necessary (refer to Chapter 32 for further information about respiratory emergency care).

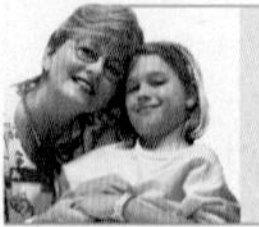

High levels of carboxyhemoglobin as a result of smoke inhalation may contribute to falsely high pulse oximetry readings.

Restoring and Maintaining Fluid Volume

Several formulas are available for the calculation of resuscitative fluids in children. Most experts recommend that pediatric burn therapy include:

- Fluid calculation based on the body surface area burned (Fig. 25.16)
- Use of a crystalloid (Ringer's lactate) during the first 24 hours; in smaller children, a small amount of dextrose may be added
- Administration of most of the volume during the first 8 hours (amounts and timing of fluid volume resuscitation will vary from child to child)
- Reassessment of the child and adjustment of the fluid rate accordingly; fluid requirements greatly decrease after 24 hours and should be adjusted to reflect this
- Administration of a colloid fluid later in therapy once capillary permeability is less of a concern
- Monitoring of the child's urine output as part of ongoing assessment of response to therapy, expecting at least 1 mL/kg per hour
- Daily weights obtained at the same time each day (the best indicator of fluid volume status)
- Monitoring of electrolyte levels (particularly sodium and potassium) for their return to normal levels

Preventing Hypothermia

Due to the loss of the protective dermis, children who are burned are at high risk for hypothermia and secondary infection. Therefore, care should be taken to keep the child warm. Warm intravenous fluids prior to their administration. Maintain a neutral thermal environment and monitor the child's temperature frequently.

Cleansing the Burn

Initially, burning must be stopped, so remove charred clothing. Wash and rinse the burn thoroughly with mild soap and water from the tap. Cool water may be used, but ice should never be applied. Children who are burned with tar require special care. Tar can be removed with cool water and mineral oil. Blisters that are intact should not routinely be removed as they provide a protective barrier; however, débridement is recommended in certain cases where large blisters impede wound care. Wounds that are open require débridement. Débridement involves the removal of loose skin and eschar (dead, charred skin). This procedure is usually performed with sterile scissors

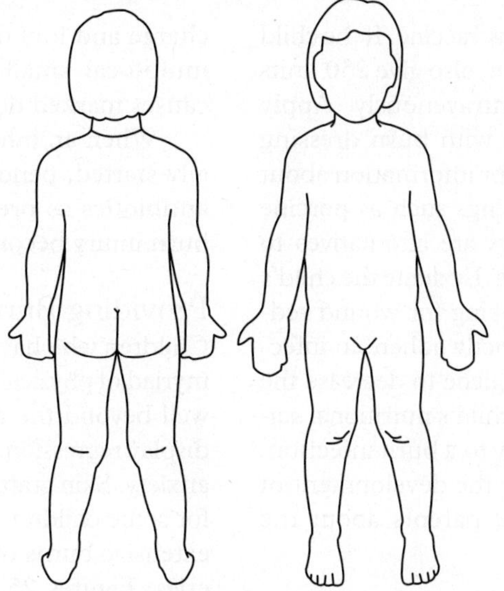

EXAMPLE

Calculating TBSA By Age (Total Body Surface Area)

Color Code
Red - 3°
Blue - 2°

Area	Birth 1 yr	1-4 yrs	5-9 yrs	10-14 yrs	15 yrs	Adult	2	3	Total
Head	19	17	13	11	9	7	—	8	8.0
Neck	2	2	2	2	2	2	—	1	1.0
Ant.Trunk	13	13	13	13	13	13	1	12	13.0
Post. Trunk	13	13	13	13	13	13	—	—	—
R. Buttock	2 1/2	2 1/2	2 1/2	2 1/2	2 1/2	2 1/2	—	—	—
L. Buttock	2 1/2	2 1/2	2 1/2	2 1/2	2 1/2	2 1/2	—	—	—
Genitalia	1	1	1	1	1	1	—	—	—
R.U. Arm	4	4	4	4	4	4	—	3.5	3.5
L.U. Arm	4	4	4	4	4	4	1	2.5	3.5
R.L. Arm	3	3	3	3	3	3	—	3	3
L.L. Arm	3	3	3	3	3	3	—	3	3
R. Hand	2 1/2	2 1/2	2 1/2	2 1/2	2 1/2	2 1/2	—	2.5	2.5
L. Hand	2 1/2	2 1/2	2 1/2	2 1/2	2 1/2	2 1/2	—	2.5	2.5
R. Thigh	5 1/2	6 1/2	8	8 1/2	9	9 1/2	1	2	3
L. Thigh	5 1/2	6 1/2	8	8 1/2	9	9 1/2	—	2	2
R. Leg	5	5	5 1/2	6	6 1/2	7	—	—	—
L. Leg	5	5	5 1/2	6	6 1/2	7	—	—	—
R. Foot	3 1/2	3 1/2	3 1/2	3 1/2	3 1/2	3 1/2	—	—	—
L. Foot	3 1/2	3 1/2	3 1/2	3 1/2	3 1/2	3 1/2	—	—	—
						Total	3%	42%	45%

● **Figure 25.16** Calculate total body surface area (TBSA) affected by using the child's age and the area affected, as well as whether the burned area is second degree (partial thickness) or third degree (full thickness).

and a pair of forceps or with a gauze sponge. The burned area should be gently cleansed; there is no advantage to aggressive scrubbing, and this technique only makes the pain more intense for the child. The nurse should wear a gown, mask, head covering, and gloves during dressing changes. Débridement is a necessary but often excruciatingly painful procedure, so the pain management needs of the child are of utmost importance (refer to the pain management section below).

When children return for evaluation of a wound that was previously seen in your facility, the dressing must be removed. Soak the dressing in lukewarm tap water to ease the removal of gauze, which may be stuck to the wound. The nurse plays an important role in ensuring that the dressing change goes smoothly. Be sure to:

- Have all dressing supplies ready.
- Provide pain medication as ordered.
- Promote good infection control technique among your colleagues.
- Assist with restraining young children, using the positions of comfort previously discussed in relation to atraumatic care.
- Encourage participation by the child's parents.
- Talk soothingly to the child, explain what you are going to do, and provide distraction during the procedure.

Preventing Infection

Prevention of infection is critical to successful outcomes for burned children. If the child's immunization status is unknown or if it has been 5 years or longer since the last tetanus vaccine, administer the tetanus vaccine. If the child has never received tetanus vaccination, also give 250 units tetanus human immunoglobulin intravenously. Apply antibiotic ointment in conjunction with burn dressing changes. Refer to Drug Guide 25.1 for information about topical antibiotics. Membrane dressings such as porcine xenograft and hydrocolloid dressings are alternatives to topical antibiotics and sterile dressings. Evaluate the child's wound during dressing changes, looking for wound redness, swelling, odor, or drainage. Strictly adhere to infection control procedures and hand hygiene to decrease the risk of burn infection. Maximize the child's nutritional status to decrease his or her susceptibility to a burn infection. Monitor the child's temperature for the development of fever. Upon discharge, instruct the parents about the signs of a wound infection.

Managing Pain

Pain management is of the utmost importance, and several options are available for the treatment of burn-related pain. Local anesthesia, sedatives, and systemic analgesics are commonly used. Children who have less severe burns that are managed at home can be given oral medications such as acetaminophen with codeine 30 to 45 minutes before dressing changes. In burns that result in more severe pain, the child should be hospitalized and given intravenous pain control with medications such as morphine sulfate. Recent research has shown that intranasal midazolam (a sedative) in conjunction with an oral pain medication was effective in reducing pain during dressing changes in burned children (Hansen et al., 2001).

Pain may also occur at any time of the day or night, not just in relation to dressing changes. Assess the child's pain status frequently using an age-appropriate pain assessment scale. Administer pain medications as prescribed and/or use nonpharmacologic techniques to alleviate or decrease the child's perception of pain. Nontraditional therapies such as virtual-reality therapy have been shown to alleviate pain during dressing changes. Virtual-reality therapy programs allow the child to immerse himself or herself in a three-dimensional computer-generated world, an extremely effective method of distraction from the pain (Hoffman, 2004).

Treating Infected Burns

The potential for burn infection increases if the child has a large, open burn wound and if there are other sources of infection, such as multiple intravenous lines. In addition, children who are immunocompromised have an increased risk of burn infection. *S. aureus* is the usual bacterium implicated in burn cellulitis and burn impetigo, though *Pseudomonas aeruginosa* may also cause cellulitis. In burn wound cellulitis, the area around the burn becomes increasingly red, swollen, and painful early in the course of burn management. With invasive burn cellulitis, the burn develops a dark brown, black, or purplish color, with a discharge and foul odor. Burn impetigo is characterized by multifocal small superficial abscesses. Burn impetigo causes marked destruction of skin-grafted areas.

When an infection is suspected, antibiotics are usually started, pending wound culture results. Administer antibiotics as prescribed (or antifungals if an extensive burn injury becomes infected with a fungus).

Providing Burn Rehabilitation

Children who have suffered a significant burn injury face a myriad of physical and psychological challenges that extend well beyond the acute injury phase. These children may display regression behaviors because of injury, pain, fear, or anxiety. Skin grafting or special burn dressings are required for some children (Box 25.5). Children who have suffered extensive burns often require multiple skin-grafting surgeries. Figures 25.17 and 25.18 show healed skin grafts. Extensive burns may also result in the need for pressure garments to decrease the risk of extensive scarring. Pressure garments are not comfortable and they must be worn continuously for at least 1 year, sometimes 2, but they have been shown to be very effective in reducing hypertrophic scarring resulting from significant burn injury.

Physical therapy will usually be initiated in the critical care setting and will continue long after hospital discharge, sometimes throughout life. Positioning, exercise, and range of motion are necessary to maintain joint flexibility (Merz et al., 2003).

Nurses play a key role in smoothing the transition from the acute care phase of life-saving interventions and frequent dressing changes to normal activities such as school and play. Body image considerations may have a significant impact on the child when he or she returns to school and should be addressed. Children with altered body image as a result of a burn might benefit from reg-

BOX 25.5

SKIN GRAFTING AND SPECIAL BURN CARE

- Biologic skin coverings are used for extensive burns or in cases of no donor.
- Autograft allows for permanent coverage of a deep partial-thickness or full-thickness burn.
  - Consists of patient's own skin
  - Split-thickness consists of epidermis and superficial layers of dermis. The donor site heals completely.
  - Full-thickness consists of full dermal thickness. Cover the donor site with fine-mesh gauze or synthetic wound coverings to allow the site to heal.
- Kaltostat (calcium alginate dressing) is a brown seaweed extract that is spun into a fiber that is highly absorbent. It reacts with exudate on the wound to form a protective gel.

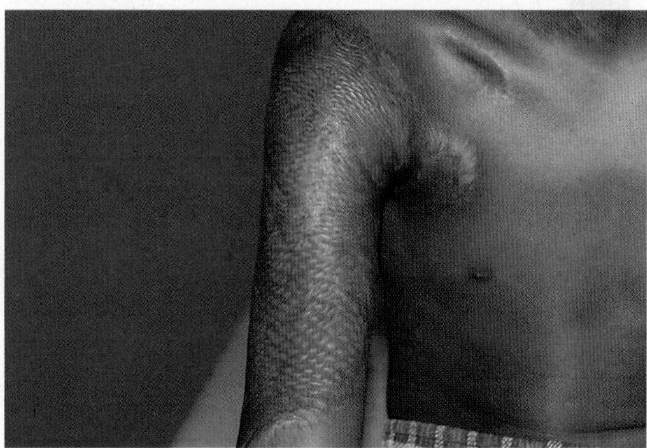

● **Figure 25.17** Healed mesh graft.

ular counseling and group therapy. Parents often need assistance with the behavioral challenges of caring for a child who is recovering from a burn injury. Various websites are available for support of persons who are burned:

- www.burnsupportgroupsdatabase.com: Burn Support Group Database
- www.burnsurvivor.com: Burn Resource Center
- www.survivingburns.org: mentor services for burn survivors

Navigating through life after suffering a serious burn injury can be difficult for the child and family, and a skilled nurse can provide valuable assistance to families during the equally important but less acute phase of the journey.

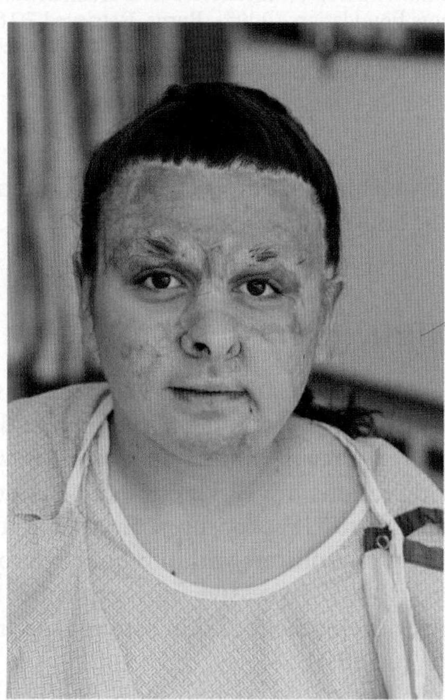

● **Figure 25.18** Extensive grafting to the face.

Preventing Burns and Carbon Monoxide Poisoning

Instruct parents about prevention of burns. All homes should have working smoke detectors, and batteries should be changed yearly. All homes should be equipped with fire extinguishers, and adults and older teenagers should be taught how to operate them. Children should sleep in fire-retardant sleepwear. Parents should not smoke in the house or the car, and they should keep lighters and matches out of children's reach. Young children are particularly susceptible to burns that occur in the kitchen, such as scalds from hot liquids and foods and burns from contact with hot burners or oven doors. Caution parents about the extreme danger that fireworks present to children. Teaching Guideline 25.3 gives additional information for parents related to burn prevention. The booklet "Burn Prevention Tips," which includes a coloring book, is available from the Shriners Hospitals for Children (www.shrinershq.org).

Children are at significant risk for burns related to hot water. Scald burns can occur when hot water comes into contact with the child's skin, even for a relatively short time. Since hot water presents such a serious risk to children, the temperature on all hot water heaters should be 120° F or lower. Figure 25.19 is a graph that shows how long a child can be exposed to water of various temperatures before a burn occurs. For example:

- If the water is 150°, a child can receive a third-degree burn within 2 seconds.

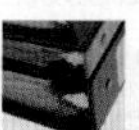

TEACHING GUIDELINE 25.3

Burn Prevention

- Keep hot water heater temperature lower than 120° F.
- Test bath water temperature before bathing children.
- Keep children away from open flames, stoves, and candles.
- Cook with pots on the inside of the stove with the handles turned in.
- Keep children away from the stove while cooking.
- Place hot liquids out of reach of children.
- Avoid drinking hot beverages while holding a child.
- Keep curling irons out of reach of children.
- Teach older children how to safely get out of the house in case of fire.
- Practice fire drills.
- Teach children to "stop, drop, and roll" if their clothes catch on fire.

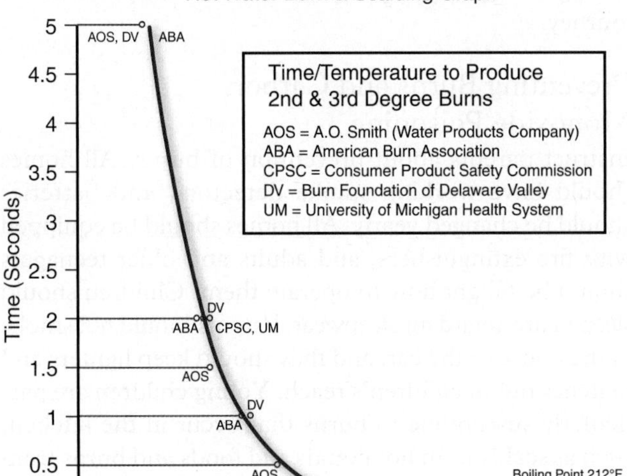

● Figure 25.19 Length of hot water exposure that results in significant burns based on water temperature.

- If the water is 140°, it takes 6 seconds of exposure to cause a significant burn.
- If the water is 130°, a child can be burned significantly in only 30 seconds.
- At 120°, the recommended maximal home hot water heater temperature, it takes as long as 5 minutes of exposure to burn a person (plenty of time to get out of the tub!).

Instruct parents about prevention of carbon monoxide poisoning. All homes should have working carbon monoxide detectors, and batteries should be changed yearly. Teach parents the signs of carbon monoxide poisoning: headaches, dizziness, disorientation, and nausea. If the carbon monoxide detector sounds, turn off any potential sources of combustion, if possible, and evacuate all occupants immediately. Do not attempt to re-enter the home until a qualified professional repairs the source of the carbon monoxide leak.

Providing Burn Care at Home

Teach parents about proper burn care in the home. Seek medical attention for burns when:

- The child has a second- or third-degree burn.
- Burns result from a fire, an electrical wire or socket, or chemicals.
- The child has a burn on the face, scalp, hands, feet, or genitals or over the joints.
- The burn appears to be infected.
- The burn is causing prolonged and significant pain.
- Concern exists that the burn was a result of abuse.

If the burn is very extensive, even if it appears to be a first-degree burn, seek medical attention immediately.

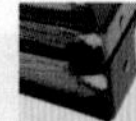

TEACHING GUIDELINE 25.4

Providing Burn Care

For first-degree (superficial) burns

- Run cool water over the burned area until the pain lessens.
- Do not apply ice to the skin.
- Do not apply butter, ointment, or cream.
- Cover the burn lightly with a clean, non-adhesive bandage.
- Administer acetaminophen or ibuprofen for pain.
- Have the child seen by the primary care provider within 24 hours.
- Ongoing care: clean in tub or shower with fragrance-free mild soap; pat or air dry.
  - Apply a thin layer of antibiotic ointment.
  - Cover with a nonadherent dressing such as Adaptic, and then cover with dry gauze.

For more extensive burns

- Remove clothing only if it comes off easily or if it is still smoldering.
- Check the child's ABCs and perform CPR if necessary.
- Do not apply butter, ointment, or any other type of cream.
- Cover the burn with a clean, lint-free bandage or sheet.
- Avoid applying large, wet sheets, as this can cause the child to become too cold.
- Do not attempt to break any blisters.
- If the child appears to be in shock, elevate the legs while protecting the burn and call 911.

Data from Frank, K. (2005). *Preventing and treating burns.* Retrieved 7/16/06 from www.kidsgrowth.com/resources/articledetail.cfm?id=2029; and Nemours Foundation. (2005). Burns. Retrieved 7/16/06 from http://www.kidshealth.org/teen/safety/first_aid/burns_sheet.html.

Teaching Guideline 25.4 gives specific information about burn care at home.

● SUNBURN

Sunburn occurs as a result of overexposure to the ultraviolet (UV) rays of the sun. The erythema and eventual blisters occur as a result of the skin's blood flow changes as well as alterations in cell kinetics and pigment products in response to UV exposures. Erythema may occur within 4 hours and blisters within 6 hours (Krowchuk & Tunnessen, 2006). Excessive sun exposure has been linked to the development of skin cancer later in life. See Healthy People 2010.

Sunburn is usually treated with cool compresses, cooling lotions, and oral nonsteroidal anti-inflammatory agents.

HEALTHY PEOPLE 2010

Objective	Significance
(Developmental) Increase the proportion of adolescents in grades 9 through 12 who follow protective measures that may reduce the risk of skin cancer.	• Encourage use of sunscreen in all children over 6 months of age, to form a life-long habit. • Discourage sun exposure between 10 a.m. and 2 p.m. • Inform teens of the hazards of ultraviolet light (even artificial) and discourage the use of tanning beds.

Nursing Assessment

Obtain the health history, noting recent sun exposure. Determine length of exposure and whether any type of sunscreen or sun block product was used. Note redness of the skin on the exposed areas. More severe areas will have a darker red, slightly purple hue. Blisters may be noted with more severe sunburn.

Nursing Management

Cool compresses may help to cool the burn. Aloe vera gel applied topically may provide significant soothing. Rarely are adverse effects reported with the use of aloe vera gel (Gardiner et al., 2001). Administer a nonsteroidal anti-inflammatory such as ibuprofen. Discourage hot showers or baths. Instruct the child to wear loose clothing and to ensure that burned areas are covered when going outside (until they are healed). If skin flaking occurs, discourage the child from "peeling" the flaked skin in order to prevent further injury. Refer to Chapter 9 for further information about safe sun exposure.

● COLD INJURY

The term "frostbite" implies freezing of the tissues. It is described on a continuum from first to fourth degree. When a child is exposed to an extremely cold environment, changes in cutaneous circulation help to maintain the core body temperature. As circulation is shunted to the core, the most peripheral body parts are those at highest risk for frostbite. Local damage occurs when the tissue temperature drops to 32° F (0° C). Initially skin sensation is lost, the vasculature constricts, and plasma leakage occurs. Ice crystals develop in the extracellular fluid, and eventually vascular stasis leads to endothelial cell damage, necrosis, and sloughing of dead tissue (Nield & Nanda, 2005).

Nursing Assessment

Note history of cold exposure. Inquire about pain or numbness. Examine the skin for indications of frostbite. First-degree frostbite results in superficial white plaques with surrounding erythema. Second-degree frostbite demonstrates blistering with erythema and edema. In third-degree frostbite, hemorrhagic blisters occur, progressing to tissue necrosis and sloughing in fourth-degree frostbite (Nield & Nanda, 2005).

Nursing Management

Remove wet or tight clothing. Avoid vigorous massage to decrease the chance of damaging the skin further. Immerse the affected part in 104° F water for 15 to 30 minutes. Thawing may cause significant pain, so administer analgesics. Keep the thawed part loosely covered, warm, and dry. Splinting may be used to help decrease associated edema. Consult the wound care specialist or plastic surgeon for further management.

Preventing frostbite may be achieved by:

- Dressing warmly in layers, and keeping warm and dry
- Avoiding exertion
- Not playing outside when wind chill advisories are in effect, and locking doors with high locks to prevent toddlers from going outside (Nield, & Nanda, 2005)

● HUMAN AND ANIMAL BITES

About 1% of emergency department visits yearly are due to bites from mammals (Starr, 2006). Children may be bitten by other children, or animals that are pets or strays such as dogs, cats, or ferrets. The hand and face are common locations for animal bites. About 50% of dog bites occur in children 5 years of age or younger (Bernardo et al., 2000). A dog is most often provoked to bite a child when the child is playing with the dog or when the child hits, kicks, hugs, grabs, or chases the dog (Melnick, 2005).

Therapeutic management involves cleansing and irrigation of the wound, wound suturing or stapling if necessary, and topical and/or systemic antibiotic therapy. Rabies prophylaxis is indicated if the rabies status of the dog is unknown. Secondary bacterial infection of the bite wound with streptococci, staphylococci, or *Pasteurella multocida* may occur. Cat and human bites are the most likely to become infected.

Nursing Assessment

Determine the history of the attack and whether it was provoked. Determine the child's tetanus vaccination status. Inspect the bite to determine the extent of laceration, avulsion, or crushing injury.

Nursing Management

Provide rabies immunoprophylaxis and a tetanus booster vaccination if indicated. Thoroughly cleanse the wound with soap and water or a povidone–iodine solution. Irrigate the wound well with normal saline after cleansing (Villani, 2006). If the animal may be rabid, cleanse the wound for at least 10 minutes with a virucidal agent such as povidone–iodine solution (Behrman, 2004). Administer antibiotics as prescribed.

Prevention of animal bites is important. Teach children the following:

- Never provoke a dog with teasing or roughhousing.
- Get adult permission before interacting with a dog, cat, or other animal that is not your pet.
- Do not bother an eating, sleeping, or nursing dog.
- Avoid high-pitched talking or screaming around dogs.
- Display a closed fist first for the dog to sniff.
- Keep ferrets away from the face.
- If a cat hisses or lashes out with the paw, leave it alone (American Veterinary Medical Association, 2006; Melnick, 2005).

Never leave a child under 5 years of age alone with a dog. Contact the local humane society for a dog bite prevention program that is appropriate for school-age children.

Children may suffer significant emotional distress after being bitten. Nightmares and increased anxiety are common (Villani, 2006). Help children through this period by talking about the incident or reading books about this type of event.

● INSECT STINGS AND SPIDER BITES

Members of the Hymenoptera class of insects sting. This class includes bees, wasps, ants, yellow jackets, and hornets. Spiders inject their venom when they bite. Stings and bites usually result in a local reaction. A systemic or anaphylactic reaction to a Hymenoptera sting may also occur, possibly resulting in airway compromise (refer to Chapter 27 for additional information on anaphylaxis). Serious reactions may occur with brown recluse or black widow spider bites. This discussion will focus on local reactions.

Local reactions to insect stings and spider bites include pruritus, pain, and edema. A hypersensitivity reaction thought to be mediated by immunoglobulin E occurs in response to the venom. This may be a physiological response to the antigens present in the insect's or spider's saliva and other fluids that are transmitted during stinging or biting. Bacterial superinfection may occur as a complication and as a result of scratching (Bircher, 2005).

Therapeutic management includes antihistamines to decrease itching and in some cases corticosteroids to decrease inflammation and swelling (Golden, 2003).

Nursing Assessment

Obtain the history of the bite or sting. Children are usually acutely aware when they have been stung by an insect, but spiders are generally not observed before the bite. Inspect the bite or sting, noting an urticarial wheal or papular reaction. A large local reaction may be mistaken for cellulitis. Note whether a stinger remains present. Assess the child's work of breathing to determine if a systemic reaction or anaphylaxis is occurring (refer to Chapter 27).

Nursing Management

Remove jewelry or constrictive clothing if the sting is on an extremity. Cleanse the wound with mild soap and water. If the stinger is present, scrape it away with your fingernail or a credit card. Apply ice intermittently to decrease pain and edema (Brinker et al., 2003). Administer diphenhydramine as soon as possible after the sting in an attempt to minimize the reaction.

Prevent insect stings and spider bites by wearing protective clothing and shoes when outdoors. Use insect repellants (with a maximum concentration of 30% DEET in infants and children older than 2 months). Teach children never to disturb a bee or wasp nest or an ant hill.

References

Books and Journals

Accurate Building Inspectors. (2006). *Water temperature thermometry.* Retrieved 7/23/06 from www.accuratebuilding.com/services/legal/charts/hot_water_burn_scalcing_graph.html.

Allen, P. L. J. (2004). Leaves of three, let them be: If it were only that easy! *Pediatric Nursing, 30*(2), 129–135.

American Medical Student Association. (2007). *Child abuse and neglect.* Retrieved May 19, 2007 from http://www.amsa.org/programs/gpit/child.cfm.

American Veterinary Medical Association. (2006). *Don't worry, they won't bite.* Retrieved 7/23/06 from http://www.avma.org/pubhlth/dogbite/dogbitebroc.asp.

Aninda, D., & Kim, K. (2000). Infections in burn injury. *Pediatric Infectious Disease Journal, 19*(8), 737–738.

Balkrishnan, R., Manuel, J., Clarke, J., Carroll, C. L., Housman, T., & Fleischer, A. B. (2003). Effects of an episode of specialist care on the impact of childhood atopic dermatitis on the child's family. *Journal of Pediatric Health Care, 17,* 184–189.

Behram, R. E., Kliegman, R. M. & Jenson, H. B. (2004). *Nelson's textbook of pediatrics* (17th ed.). Philadelphia: Saunders.

Bernardo, L. M., Gardner, M. J., O'Connor, J., & Amon, N. (2000). Dog bites in children treated in a pediatric emergency department. *Journal of the Society of Pediatric Nurses, 5*(2), 87–95.

Berson, D. S. (2005). Cosmetic management of patients with acne vulgaris and acne rosacea. *Pediatric News (supplement), 7–8,* 12.

Bircher, A. (2005). Systemic immediate allergic reactions to arthropod stings and bites. *Dermatology, 210,* 119–127.

Borkowski, S. (2004). Diaper rash care and management. *Pediatric Nursing, 30*(6), 467–470.

Brinker, D., Hancox, J. D., & Bernardon, S. O. (2003). Assessment and initial treatment of lacerations, mammalian bites and insect stings. *AACN Clinical Issues, 14*(4), 401–410.

Buchanan, P. I. (2001). Behavior modification: A nursing approach for young children with atopic eczema. *Dermatology Nursing, 13*(1), 15–16, 18, 21–25.

Casale, T. B., & Stokes, J. R. (2006). Urticaria and angioedema. In J. A. McMillan (Ed.), *Oski's pediatrics: Principles and practice* (pp. 2410–2416). Philadelphia: Lippincott Williams & Wilkins.

Cheigh, N. H. (2003). Managing a common disorder in children: Atopic dermatitis. *Journal of Pediatric Health Care, 17,* 84–88.

Chen, N., & Cunningham, B. B. (2001). Psoriasis: Finding the right approach for your patients. *Contemporary Pediatrics, 18*(8), 86–93.

Cohen, B. (2004). A baby, a cutaneous lesion—and an efficient approach to recognition and management. *Contemporary Pediatrics, 21*(7), 28–48.

Cole, J. M., & Gray-Micely, D. (2002). The necessary elements of a dermatologic history and physical examination. *Dermatology Nursing, 14*(6), 377–384.

Committee on Trauma, American College of Surgeons. (1999). Guidelines for the operation of burn units. In *Resources for optimal care of the injured patient* (pp. 55–62). Chicago: Author.

Corrarino, J. E., Walsh, P. J., & Nadel, E. (2001). Does teaching scald burn prevention to families of young children make a difference? A pilot study. *Journal of Pediatric Nursing 16*(4), 256–262.

Cuzzell, J. Z. (2005). FDA approves mandatory risk management program for isotretinoin. *Dermatology Nursing, 17*(5), 383.

Drago, D. A. (2005). Kitchen scalds and thermal burns in children five years and younger. *Pediatrics, 115*(1), 10–16.

Epstein, W. L., Guin, J. D., & Maibach, H. (2000). Poison ivy update. *Contemporary Pediatrics, 17*(4), 54–74.

Esselman, P. C., Thombs, B. D., Magyar-Russell, G., & Fauerbach, J. (2006). Burn rehabilitation: State of the science. *American Journal of Physical Medicine & Rehabilitation, 85*(4), 383–413.

Frank, K. (2005). *Preventing and treating burns.* Retrieved 7/16/06 from www.kidsgrowth.com/resources/articledetail.cfm?id=2029.

Gardiner, P., Coles, D., & Kemper, K. J. (2001). The skinny on herbal remedies for dermatologic disorders. *Contemporary Pediatrics, 18*(7), 103–114.

Garfunkel, L. C., Kaczorowski J., & Christy, C. (Eds). (2002). *Mosby's pediatric clinical advisor: instant diagnosis and treatment.* St. Louis: Mosby.

General Practice Notebook (2005). *Thermal injury.* Retrieved 10/24/05 from www.gpnotebook.co.uk/simplepage.cfm?ID=93991733&linkI.

Golden, D. B. K. (2003). Stinging insect allergy. *American Family Physician, 67*(12), 2541–2546.

Guin, J. D., & Bruckner, A. L. (2005). Compendium on poison ivy dermatitis: The insidious plants, the resulting lesions, the treatment options. *Contemporary Pediatrics, 22*(1 suppl.), 4–15.

Hansen, R. C. (2003). Atopic dermatitis: Taming "the itch that rashes." *Contemporary Pediatrics, 20*(7), 79–97.

Hansen, S. L., Voigt, D. W., & Chester, N. (2001). A retrospective study on the effectiveness of intranasal midazolam in pediatric burn patients. *Journal of Burn Care & Rehabilitation, 22*(1), 6–8.

Hoffman, H. G. (2004). Virtual reality therapy. *Scientific American, 291*(2), 58–65.

Holmes, T. E., & Krusinski, P. A. (2006). Dermatologic diseases. In J. A. McMillan (Ed.), *Oski's pediatrics: Principles and practice* (p. 462). Philadelphia: Lippincott Williams & Wilkins.

Kaplan, D. L. (2004). A photo quiz to hone dermatologic skills. *Consultant for Pediatricians, 3*(4), 169–176.

Keri, J. E. (2006). Acne: Improving skin and self-esteem. *Pediatric Annals, 35*(3), 174–179.

Krowchuk, D. P., & Tunnessen, W. W. (2006). Pediatric dermatology. In J. A. McMillan (Ed.), *Oski's pediatrics: Principles and practice* (pp. 827–878). Philadelphia: Lippincott Williams & Wilkins.

Lee, P. J. (2004). Preschooler with slowly progressing rash on one arm. *Consultant for Pediatricians, 3*(3), 114–116.

Leung, A. K. C., & Kao, C. P. (2004). What's your diagnosis? *Consultant for Pediatricians, 3*(4), 188–191.

Lyder, C. H. (2006). Effective management of pressure ulcers: A review of proven strategies. *Advances for Nurse Practitioners, 14*(7), 32–38.

Mannenbach, M., & Bechtel, K. (2005). Patterns of injury that should raise suspicion for child abuse. *Pediatric Emergency Medicine Reports.* Retrieved 4/10/06 from Health and Wellness Resource Center.

Marino, B. S., & Fine, K. S. (2007). *Blueprints: Pediatrics.* Philadelphia: Lippincott Williams & Wilkins.

McGuinness, T. M. (2006). Teens and body art. *Journal of Psychosocial Nursing & Mental Health Services, 44*(4), 13–16.

Melnick, A. (2005). "Dog bites man" is news: How pediatricians can spread the word to parents and patients. *Contemporary Pediatrics.* Retrieved 7/23/06 from http://www.contemporarypediatrics.com/contpeds/article/articleDetail.jsp?id=257429&pageID=1&sk=&date.

Merz, J., Mertens, D., & Porter, K. (2003). Wound care of the pediatric burn patient. *AACN Clinical Issues, 14*(4), 429–441.

Mondozzi, M. (2006). *Burns.* Retrieved 7/16/06 from http://www.kidshealth.org/parent/firstaid_safe/emergencies/burns.html.

Morgan, E., Bledsoe, C., & Barker, J. (2000). Ambulatory management of burns. *American Family Physician, 11,* 2015–2032.

National Institute of Arthritis and Musculoskeletal and Skin Diseases. (2006). *Questions and answers about acne.* Retrieved 7/8/06 from http://www.niams.nih.gov/hi/topics/acne/acne.htm.

National SAFE KIDS Campaign (2004). *Burn injury fact sheet.* Retrieved 11/5/06 from http://www.preventinjury.org/PDFs/BURN_INJURY.pdf.

Nemours Foundation. (2005). Burns. Retrieved 7/16/06 from http://www.kidshealth.org/teen/safety/first_aid/burns_sheet.html.

Nield, L. S., & Kamat, D. M. (2006). Diaper dermatitis: From 'A' to 'Pee.' *Consultant for Pediatricians, 5*(6), 373–380.

Nield, L. S., & Nanda, S. (2005). Cold injuries: A guide to preventing and treating hypothermia and frostbite. *Consultant for Pediatricians, 4*(9), 427–434.

Romero, D. V., Treston, J., & O'Sullivan, A. L. (2006). Hand-to-hand combat: Preventing MRSA. *Nurse Practitioner, 31*(3), 16–23.

Rudy, S. J. (2003). Overview of the evaluation and management of acne vulgaris. *Pediatric Nursing, 29*(4), 287–293.

Safe Kids. (2006a). *Facts about childhood burns.* Retrieved 11/5/06 from http://www.usa.safekids.org/content_documents/Burn_facts.pdf.

Safe Kids. (2006b). *Fire and burns safety.* Retrieved 12/26/06 from http://www.safekids.org/tips/tips_fire.htm.

Schweich, P. J. (2006). Selected topics in emergency medicine. In J. A. McMillan (Ed.), *Oski's pediatrics: Principles and practice.* Philadelphia: Lippincott Williams & Wilkins.

Sheridan, R. L. (2002). Burns. *Critical Care Medicine, 30*(11 suppl.), S500-S514.

Sheridan, R. L., Hinson, M. I., Liang, M. H., et al. (2000). Long-term outcome of children surviving massive burns. *JAMA, 283*(1), 69–73.

Shriners Hospital for Children. (2005). *Emergency treatment of burns and burn prevention.* Retrieved 10/25/05 from http://www.shrinershq.org/prevention/burntips/treatment.html.

Shwayder, T. (2003). Five common skin problems and a string of pearls for managing them. *Contemporary Pediatrics, 20*(7), 34–54.

Siberry, G. K. (2005). Fighting a rising tide of MRSA infection in the young. *Contemporary Pediatrics, 22*(7), 44–53.

Silverberg, N. B., Silverberg, J. I., & Silverberg, A. I. (2005). Eradicating acne vulgaris of puberty: What makes for optimal therapy? *Contemporary Pediatrics, 22*(10, suppl.), 12–22.

Sockrider, M. M. (2006). Respiratory complications of burns and smoke inhalation (respiratory burns). In J. A. McMillan (Ed.), *Oski's pediatrics: Principles and practice.* Philadelphia: Lippincott Williams & Wilkins.

Starr, N. B. (2004). Dermatologic diseases. In C. E. Burns, A. M. Dunn, M. A. Brady, et al. (Eds.), *Pediatric primary care: a handbook for nurse practitioners* (3rd ed.). Philadelphia: Saunders.

Suddaby, E. C., Barnett, S., & Facteau, L. (2006). Skin breakdown in acute care pediatrics. *Dermatology Nursing, 18*(2), 155–161.

Tanghetti, E. A. (2005). The importance of vehicle in acne therapy. *Pediatric News (supplement),* 1–3.

Titus, M. O., Baxter, A. L, & Starling, S. P. (2003). Accidental scald burns in sinks. *Pediatrics, 111*(2), e191-e194. Retrieved 7/16/06 from http://pediatrics.aappublications.org/cgi/content/full/111/2/e191.

U.S. Fire Administration. (2006). Exposing an invisible killer: The dangers of carbon monoxide. Retrieved 6/24/06 from http://www.usfa.dhs.gov/safety/co/fswy17.shtm.

U.S. Food and Drug Administration, Center for Drug Evaluation and Research. (2006). *Isotretinoin (marketed as Accutane) capsule information.* Retrieved 7/25/06 from http://www.fda.gov/cder/drug/infopage/accutane/default.htm.

Villani, N. M. (2006). Treating dog and cat bites. *Advance for Nurse Practitioners, 14*(7), 44–45.

Watkins, P. (2005). Impetigo: Aetiology, complications and treatment options. *Nursing Standard, 19*(36), 50–54.

Weed, R. O., & Berens, D. E. (2005). Basics of burn injury: Implications for case management and life care planning. *Lippincott's Case Management, 10*(1), 22–29.

Williams, J. V., Godfrey, J. C., & Friedlander, S. F. (2003) Superficial fungal infections: Confronting the fungus among us. *Contemporary Pediatrics, 20*(1), 58–80.

Willock, J., & Maylor, M. (2004). Pressure ulcers in infants and children. *Nursing Standard, 24*(18), 56–62.

Wong, L., & Rogers, M. (2006). Psoriasis: Varied presentations, individualized treatment. *Contemporary Pediatrics, 23*(1), 33–39.

Yen, K., Bank, D., O'Neill, A., & Yurt, R. (2001). Household oven doors: A burn hazard in children. *Archives in Pediatrics and Adolescent Medicine, 155*(1), 84–86.

Yetman, R. J., & Parks, D. (2002). Diagnosis and management of atopic dermatitis. *Journal of Pediatric Health Care, 16*, 143–145.

Websites

www.aad.org American Academy of Dermatology
www.burnsupportgroupsdatabase.com Burn Support Group Database
www.burnsurvivor.com Burn Resource Center
www.eczema.org National Eczema Society
www.herbalgram.org American Botanical Council and Herb Research Foundation (a peer-reviewed journal of herbal medical research)
www.herbmed.org HerbMed, an interactive electronic database of information on herbs
www.nationaleczema.org National Eczema Association
www.psoriasis.org National Psoriasis Foundation
www.safekids.org SafeKids
www.skincarephysicians.com/acnenet/FAQ.html Acne Net (comprehensive online acne information resource)
www.survivingburns.org mentor services for burn survivors

Chapter WORKSHEET

MULTIPLE CHOICE QUESTIONS

1. The nurse is teaching about skin care for atopic dermatitis. Which statement by the parent indicates that further teaching may be necessary?
   a. "I will use Vaseline or Crisco to moisturize my child's skin."
   b. "A hot bath will soothe my child's itching when it is severe."
   c. "I will buy cotton rather than wool or synthetic clothing for my child."
   d. "I will apply a small amount of the prescribed cream after the bath."
2. The nurse is caring for a child who has received significant partial-thickness burns to the lower body. What is the priority assessment in the first 24 hours after injury?
   a. Fluid balance
   b. Wound infection
   c. Respiratory arrest
   d. Separation anxiety
3. The nurse is caring for a child in the emergency department who was bitten by the family dog, who is fully immunized. What is the priority nursing action?
   a. Administer rabies immunoglobulin.
   b. Refer the child to a counselor.
   c. Assess the depth and extent of the wound.
   d. Administer a tetanus booster.
4. The nurse is caring for an infant on the pediatric unit who has a very red rash in the diaper area, with red lesions scattered on the abdomen and thighs. What is the priority nursing intervention?
   a. Administer griseofulvin with a fatty meal.
   b. Institute contact isolation precautions.
   c. Apply topical antibiotic cream.
   d. Apply topical antifungal cream.
5. A varsity high-school wrestler presents with a "rug burn" type of rash on his shoulder that is not healing as expected, despite use of triple antibiotic cream. Two other wrestlers on his team have a similar abrasion. What infection should the nurse be most concerned about, based on the history?
   a. Tinea cruris
   b. MRSA
   c. Impetigo
   d. Tinea versicolor

CRITICAL THINKING EXERCISES

1. A 4-year-old presents with his mother for evaluation of a yellowish, runny sore on his head. What questions would be most appropriate to ask the mother when taking the history? Should this child be placed in isolation? If so, why?
2. An 11-month-old comes to the primary care office with his mother for evaluation of a significant flaking red rash on both cheeks. The child is diagnosed with atopic dermatitis. What additional information should be obtained in the health history? What information should be included in the teaching plan for this family?

STUDY ACTIVITIES

1. Plan an educational activity:
   a. For parents of babies about the treatment and prevention of diaper dermatitis
   b. For parents of school-age children about prevention of contact dermatitis (related to poison ivy)
2. During your clinical rotation, spend a day with the wound and ostomy care nurse in a children's hospital. Report to the clinical group about what you learned that day.
3. Talk to teenagers with severe acne, atopic dermatitis, or psoriasis about their feelings about their skin's appearance. Reflect on this information in your clinical journal.

chapter 26

Nursing Care of the Child With a Hematologic Disorder

Key TERMS

anemia
chelation therapy
erythropoietin
hematocrit
hemoglobin
hemosiderosis
hypochromic
macrocytic
microcytic
platelet
platelet count
poikilocytosis
polycythemia
purpura
red blood cell
splenomegaly
thrombocytopenia
white blood cell (WBC)

Learning OBJECTIVES

Upon completion of the chapter, the learner will be able to:

1. Identify major hematologic disorders that affect children.
2. Determine priority assessment information for children with hematologic disorders.
3. Identify priority interventions for children with hematologic disorders.
4. Analyze laboratory data in relation to normal findings and report abnormal findings.
5. Provide nursing diagnoses appropriate for the child and family with hematologic disorders.
6. Develop a teaching plan for the family of children with hematologic disorders.
7. Identify resources for children and families with hematologic disorders or nutrition deficits.

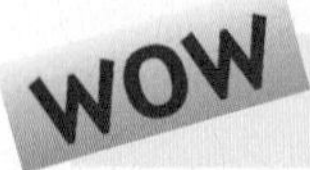

Blood is just red to the child, but to the nurse, blood is life.

Shaun O'Malley, 10 months old, is being admitted to the pediatric unit after being brought to the clinic by his father for a small laceration that he thought needed stitches. His father states, "I didn't think the cut was very deep. I was surprised how long it bled."

The hematologic system consists of the blood and blood-forming tissues of the body. These typically function together in a balance that affects the metabolism of the body. The three categories of cells are erythrocytes, or **red blood cells** (RBCs); thrombocytes, or **platelets**; and leukocytes, or **white blood cells** (WBCs). RBCs are responsible for transporting nutrients and oxygen to the body tissues and waste products from the tissues. The thrombocytes (platelets) are responsible for clotting. WBCs are responsible for fighting infection. WBCs are further divided into granulocytes (neutrophils, eosinophils, and basophils) and agranulocytes (lymphocytes and monocytes) (Kimball, 2005).

All blood cells originate from a single type of cell called a multipotent stem cell, which goes on to differentiate into the various types of blood cells. Thrombopoietin (TPO) and interleukin-7 (IL-7) act on the cell and differentiate the cell into either myeloid or lymphoid progenitor cells. The lymphoid cells either, under the influence of IL-6, become B lymphocytes, or change directly into T lymphocytes. The myeloid cells are differentiated in one of two ways, either by the action of **erythropoietin** (EPO) or granulocyte–monocyte colony-stimulating factor (GM-CSF). When the cell is acted upon by EPO, which is produced by the kidneys, the cell becomes the megakaryocyte, also known as the erythroid progenitor cell. The megakaryocyte is acted on by either EPO, to become the red blood cell, or TPO and IL-11, to become a megakaryocyte that goes on to form platelets. GM-CSF influences the cell to become the granulocyte, also known as the macrophage progenitor cell. These cells further differentiate under various influences to become the WBCs (Kimball, 2005) (Fig. 26.1).

Certain conditions may allow problems to develop within this system. These problems are related to either the production of the blood cells (too much or too little) or loss and destruction of these cells.

Nursing care for the child with a hematologic disorder is often multifaceted. A child who has iron deficiency anemia requires adequate oxygenation and may require packed red blood cells; a child with hemophilia requires factor replacement and monitoring for safety.

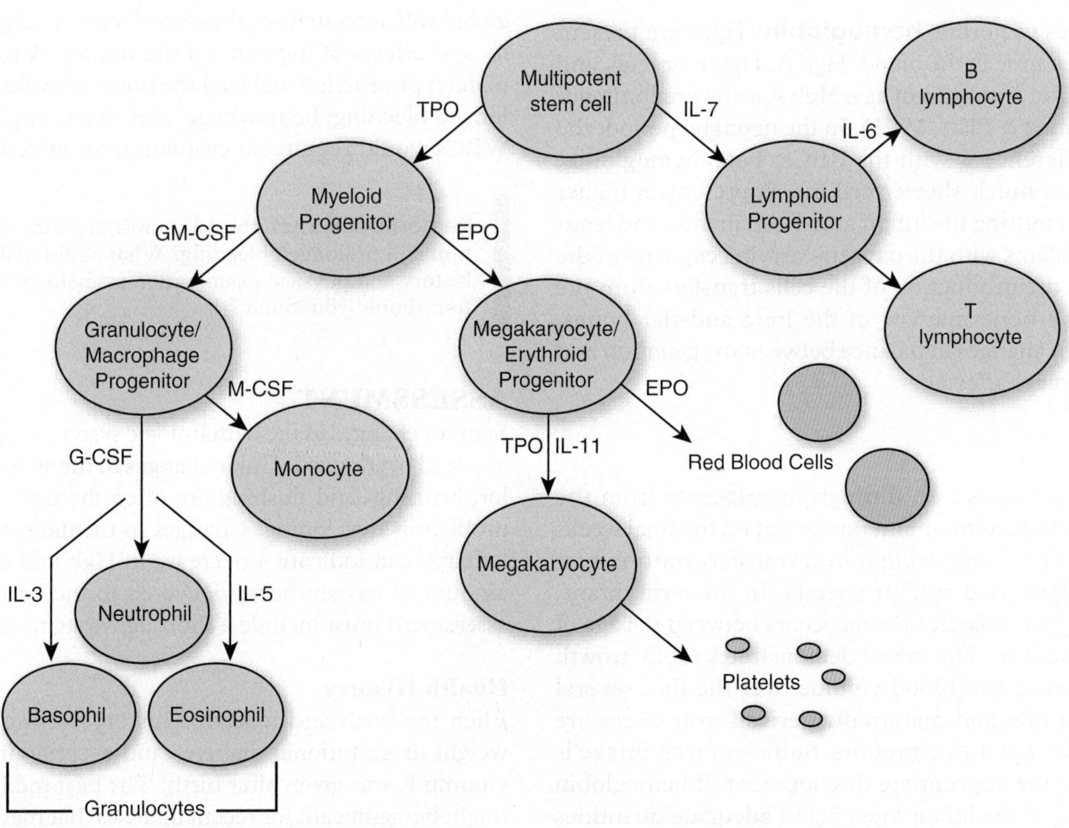

● **Figure 26.1** Process of blood cell formation.

Each condition may be life-threatening but requires different interventions.

Variations in Pediatric Anatomy and Physiology

Many factors are involved in the development of hematologic disorders, ranging from genetic causes to disorders resulting from injury, infection, or nutritional deficit. In the absence of a congenital defect, the hematologic system is intact and functional at birth. RBC and hemoglobin production as well as iron stores undergo changes in the first few months of life, after which time hematologic function is stable.

RBC Production

The production of blood cells in the embryo begins by 8 weeks' gestation. In the embryo, blood cells primarily form in the liver; this continues until a few weeks before delivery. Some cell production, lymphoid cells in particular, takes place in the spleen of the embryo, and the thymus is a site for some transient lymphocyte production. EPO, the hormone that regulates RBC production, is derived primarily from the liver in the fetus, and after birth the kidneys take over this production (Irwin & Kirchner, 2001).

Hemoglobin

Three types of normal **hemoglobin** (Hgb) are present at any given time in the blood: Hgb A, Hgb F or fetal, and Hgb A_2. After 6 months of age, Hgb A is the predominant type (Eckman & Platt, 1991). In the neonatal period, the largest difference is with the RBCs. Fetal hemoglobin, which has a much shorter cell life, is present in higher quantities, putting the infant at risk for anemia and leading to problems with the oxygen-carrying capacity of the blood. As the production of the cells transfers from the liver to the bone marrow of the long and flat bones, response to changes in balance between oxygenation and production are affected.

Iron

The fetus receives iron through the placenta from the mother. The preterm infant misses out on the final weeks or months of transplacental iron transfer, putting him or her at increased risk for anemia. In the term infant, a period of physiologic anemia occurs between the age of 2 and 6 months. The infant demonstrates rapid growth and an increase in blood volume over the first several months of life, and maternally derived iron stores are depleted by age 4 to 6 months. Sufficient iron intake is critical for the appropriate development of hemoglobin and RBCs, so the infant must ingest adequate quantities of iron either from breast milk or from iron-fortified formula in early infancy and other food sources in later infancy. Adolescence is also a time of rapid growth, and intake of iron must increase.

Common Medical Treatments

Various medications as well as other medical treatments are used to treat hematologic disorders in children. Most of these treatments will require a physician's order when the child is in the hospital. The most common treatments and medications are listed in Common Medical Treatments 26.1 and Drug Guide 26.1. The nurse caring for the child with a hematologic disorder should be familiar with what procedures are used, how the medications work, and common nursing implications related to their use.

Nursing Process Overview for the Child With a Hematologic Disorder

Care of the child with a hematologic disorder includes assessment, nursing diagnosis, planning, interventions, and evaluation. There are a number of general concepts related to the nursing process that may be applied to hematologic dysfunction in children.

Development of a plan of care will depend upon which component of the blood is changed. A decrease in hemoglobin will necessitate evaluation of oxygen-carrying capacity and effects of hypoxia on the tissues. A reduction in platelet production will lead the nurse to evaluate for prolonged bleeding, hemorrhage, and shock. An elevation in WBCs would require an evaluation for infection.

> **Remember Shaun,** the 10-month-old with the laceration and prolonged bleeding? What additional health history and physical examination assessment information should you obtain?

ASSESSMENT

Signs of changes in the hematologic system are often insidious and overlooked. Color changes to the skin such as pallor, bruising, and flushing are often the first signs that a problem is developing. Changes in mental status such as lethargy can indicate a decrease in Hgb and a decreased amount of oxygen being delivered to the brain. Nursing assessment must include a thorough systems approach.

Health History

Elicit the birth and maternal history, noting low birthweight or gestational diabetes and ascertaining whether vitamin K was given after birth. The past medical history might be significant for recent illnesses that may contribute

(*text continues on page 873*)

Common Medical Treatments 26.1

Treatment	Explanation	Indication	Nursing Implications
Blood product transfusion	Intravenous administration of whole blood, packed red blood cells (PRBCs), platelets, or plasma	PRBCs: severe anemia, thalassemia, sickle cell disease. Whole blood: acute hemorrhage or trauma. Fresh-frozen plasma: hemophilia.	Follow institution's transfusion protocol. Double-check blood type and product label with a second nurse. Use only leukodepleted, CMV-negative blood products in the child with a hemoglobinopathy. Monitor vital signs and assess child frequently to detect adverse reaction to blood transfusion. If adverse reaction suspected, immediately discontinue transfusion, run normal saline IV, reassess the child, and notify the physician. Some children require premedication with diphenhydramine and/or acetaminophen before receiving blood products.
Supplemental oxygen	Administration of oxygen via mask, cannula, or blow-by	Hypoxia associated with sickle cell crisis or severe anemia	Frequently monitor work of breathing, oxygen saturation via pulse oximetry, cardiopulmonary status, and level of consciousness.
Splenectomy	Surgical removal of the spleen	Life-threatening or recurrent splenic sequestration of sickle cell disease; thalassemia	Provide immunization against the following organisms, because they place the patient at risk for overwhelming infection: *S. pneumoniae*, *N. meningitidis*, and *H. influenzae* type B. Monitor carefully for signs of infection. Administer prophylactic antibiotics. Instruct child or teen to wear medical alert bracelet. Teach families to seek medical treatment at first sign of infection or fever.
Hematopoietic stem cell transplantation	Bone marrow transplant: transfer of healthy bone marrow into a child with disease; the transplanted cells can then develop into functional cells. Stem cell transplant: peripheral stem cells are removed from the donor via apheresis, or stem cells are retrieved from the umbilical cord and placenta. The stem cells are then transplanted into the recipient.	Sickle cell disease, aplastic anemias, thalassemia	Maintain medical asepsis and protective isolation to prevent infection. Monitor closely for graft-versus-host disease. Provide meticulous oral care. Avoid taking rectal temperatures and inserting suppositories. Encourage appropriate nutrition. Administer immunosuppressive medications as ordered.

Drug Guide 26.1 Common Drugs for Hematologic Disorders

Medication	Action	Indication	Nursing Implications
Iron supplements (ferrous sulfate, ferrous fumarate)	Supplemental iron in deficient child	Iron deficiency anemia	Dosage is based on mg of elemental iron. Do not administer with milk or milk products. May color stools and urine black Liquid can stain the teeth; mix with a small amount of juice; drinking with straw decreases tooth staining. May cause constipation; increase fiber and fluid intake
Deferoxamine (Desferal)	Binds with iron, which is removed via the kidneys	Iron toxicity	Rotate subcutaneous injection sites to decrease local reactions. Apply corticosteroid cream to irritation.
Factor (VIII or IX) replacement	Replaces deficient clotting factors	Hemophilia	Use filter needle to draw up medication. Administer IV when bleeding occurs.
Penicillin VK	Kills susceptible bacteria	Prophylaxis of infection in asplenia	Determine whether penicillin allergy is present. Monitor renal and hematologic function during prolonged use.
Folic acid	Replaces the vitamin	Folic acid deficiency; questionable use with sickle cell anemia	Administer without regard to meals. Monitor hematologic function.
Intravenous immune globulin (IVIG) (multiple manufacturers)	Provides exogenous IgG antibodies	Idiopathic thrombocytopenic purpura	Do not mix with IV medications or with other IV fluids. Do not give IM or SQ. Monitor vital signs and watch for adverse reactions frequently during infusion. Child may require antipyretic or antihistamine to prevent chills and fever during infusion. Have epinephrine available during infusion.
Chelating agents: dimercaprol (BAL), edentate calcium disodium (CaEDTA), succimer (Chemet)	Remove lead from soft tissues and bone, allowing for its excretion via the renal system	Used for blood lead levels >45 mcg/dL	Monitor intake and output closely to ensure adequacy of renal system. Encourage adequate oral hydration or provide IV hydration if required. Follow lead levels as prescribed. Ensure that lead is being removed from the child's home.

to a change in blood cell distribution. Determine the child's sleep/wake patterns and bowel elimination patterns, which may be affected by alterations in circulating blood volume or changes in oxygenation. Explore the family history for inherited disorders such as hemophilia, sickle cell disease, and thalassemia. Evaluate the child's typical diet for possible nutritional deficits. Determine risk for lead exposure based on the use of a standard questionnaire. When eliciting the history of the present illness, inquire about the following:

- Fatigue or malaise
- Paleness of the skin
- Unusual bruising
- Excessive bleeding or difficulty stopping bleeding
- Pain: location, onset, duration, quality, relieving factors

Physical Examination

A child's general appearance gives great insight into his or her health and can indicate potential problems such as malnutrition or lead poisoning. Physical examination of the child with a hematologic disorder includes inspection and observation, palpation, and auscultation.

Inspection and Observation

Note the child's general appearance, including thin or emaciated appearance or obesity, as well as color. Measure weight and height (or length) and plot on standardized growth charts. Observe the nail beds, palms, and soles for pallor. Evaluate the fingertips for clubbing, which occurs with chronic decreases in oxygen. Document the location and extent of bruises, petechiae, or purpura. Count respiratory rate and observe for work of breathing. Obtain a pulse oximeter reading to determine oxygen saturation of tissues. Note conjunctival color as well as color and moisture of oral mucosa. Determine urinary output, which may be altered with decreases in circulatory blood volume or inadequate oxygenation. Note the child's responsiveness to stimuli, movement of extremities, and quality of gait.

Auscultation

Auscultate breath sounds, noting adequacy of air movement and depth of respiration. Note adventitious sounds or absence of breath sounds (which would occur in an area of the lung filled with blood). Auscultate heart sounds, listening closely for murmurs (which can develop with changes in blood viscosity and volume). Note the rate and rhythm of the heart tones. Auscultate bowel sounds, noting presence and normalcy.

Palpation

Measure blood pressure (may change with alterations in blood volume). Palpate peripheral pulses for strength and equality. Determine capillary refill time (may be prolonged when circulating blood volume is decreased). Carefully palpate the abdomen for tenderness, hepatomegaly, or splenomegaly (increased spleen size). Note temperature of the skin. Determine elasticity of skin, noting decreased turgor. Palpate the joints for tenderness. Determine extent of limitation of range of motion.

Laboratory and Diagnostic Testing

The nurse must understand the main elements of the complete blood count (CBC; hemogram) to recognize critical values and intervene as appropriate. In evaluating the CBC, the nurse must take into account the presenting clinical picture of the child. For instance, the RBC count may be truly elevated (erythrocytosis or **polycythemia**) in certain diseases or in the case of dehydration from diarrhea or burns. When anemia is present, the RBC count is low. When the mean corpuscular volume (MCV) is elevated, the RBCs are larger than normal (**macrocytic**). When the MCV is decreased, the RBCs are smaller than normal (**microcytic**). A decrease in the mean corpuscular hemoglobin concentration (MCHC) means that the Hgb is diluted in the cell and less of the red color is present (**hypochromic**). When the Hgb concentration is increased in the RBC, then the pigmentation (red color) is increased (hyperchromic). The components of the CBC are further defined below:

- RBC count: the actual number of counted RBCs in a certain volume of blood
- Hgb: measure of the protein made up of heme (iron surrounded by protoporphyrin) and globin, alpha and beta-polypeptide chains, primarily responsible for the transport of nutrients and oxygen to the tissues
- **Hematocrit** (Hct): an indirect measure of red blood cells (number and volume)
- RBC indices
    - MCV: average size of the RBC
    - Mean corpuscular hemoglobin (MCH): a calculated value of the oxygen-carrying capacity of the Hgb in the RBCs
    - MCHC: a calculated value that reflects the concentration of Hgb inside the RBC
    - Red cell distribution width (RDW): a calculated value that is a measure of the width of RBCs
- WBC count: actual count of the number of WBCs in a volume of blood
- **Platelet count**: number of platelets per blood volume
    - Mean platelet volume (MPV): a measurement of the size of the platelets

Tables 26.1 and 26.2 give age-related values for the CBC and leukocyte count (Carey et al., 2005).

WBCs are the body's defense against infection or injury. The specific types of WBCs are discussed in Chapter 27. Platelets are necessary for clot formation, and if changes occur, problems may develop: elevations can indicate an increase in clotting, while decreases can indi-

Table 26.1 Normal Hemogram Values

Age	WBC ($\times 10^3/mm^3$)	RBC ($\times 10^6/mm^3$)	Hgb (g/dL)	Hct (%)	MCV (fL)	MCH (pg/cell)	MCHC (g/dL)	Platelets ($\times 10^3/mm^3$)	RDW (%)	MPV (fL)
Birth–2 weeks	9.0–30.0	4.1–6.1	14.5–24.5	44–54	98–112	34–40	33–37	150–450	—	—
2–8 weeks	5.0–21.0	4.0–6.0	12.5–20.5	39–59	98–112	30–36	32–36	—	—	—
2–6 months	5.0–19.0	3.8–5.6	10.7–17.3	35–49	83–97	27–33	31–35	—	—	—
6 months–1 year	5.0–19.0	3.8–5.2	9.9–14.5	29–43	73–87	24–30	32–36	—	—	—
1–6 years	5.0–19.0	3.9–5.3	9.5–14.1	30–40	70–84	23–29	31–35	—	—	—
6–16 years	4.8–10.8	4.0–5.2	10.3–14.9	32–42	73–87	24–30	32–36	—	—	—
16–18 years	4.8–10.8	4.2–5.4	11.1–15.7	34–44	75–89	25–31	32–36	—	—	—
>18 years (males)	5.0–10.0	4.5–5.5	14.0–17.4	42–52	84–96	28–34	32–36	140–400	11.5–14.5	7.4–10.4
>18 years (females)	5.0–10.0	4.0–5.0	12.0–16.0	36–48	84–96	28–34	32–36	140–400	11.5–14.5	7.4–10.4

Data from Fischbach, F. T. (2004). *A manual of laboratory and diagnostic tests* (7th ed., p. 47). Philadelphia: Lippincott Williams & Wilkins.

Table 26.2 Normal Differential for Leukocytes (White Blood Cell Differential)

Age	Bands/Stab (%)	Segs/Polys (%)	Eos (%)	Basos (%)	Lymphs (%)	Monos (%)
Birth–1 week	10–18	32–62	0–2	0–1	26–36	0–6
1–2 weeks	8–16	19–49	0–4	0	38–46	0–9
2–4 weeks	7–15	14–34	0–3	0	43–53	0–9
4–8 weeks	7–13	15–35	0–3	0–1	41–71	0–7
2–6 months	5–11	15–35	0–3	0–1	42–72	0–6
6 months–1 year	6–12	13–33	0–3	0	46–76	0–5
1–6 years	5–11	13–33	0–3	0	46–76	0–5
6–16 years	5–11	32–54	0–3	0–1	27–57	0–5
16–18 years	5–11	34–64	0–3	0–1	25–45	0–5
>18 years	3–6	50–62	0–3	0–1	25–40	3–7

Data from Fischbach, F. T. (2004). *A manual of laboratory and diagnostic tests* (7th ed., p. 51). Philadelphia: Lippincott Williams & Wilkins.

cate the risk for increased bleeding. Decreases can result if the platelets are being used up when bleeding is present, if an inherited disorder is present, or if the spleen holds them, as in hypersplenism. Platelets are larger when they are new; thus, an elevation in the mean platelet volume indicates that an increased number of platelets are being produced in the bone marrow (Carey et al., 2005).

Common Laboratory and Diagnostic Tests 26.1 explains the most commonly used laboratory and diagnostic tests used when considering hematologic disorders. The tests can assist the physician in diagnosing the disorder and/or be used as guidelines in determining ongoing treatment. Laboratory or non-nursing personnel obtain some of the tests, while the nurse might obtain others. In either instance the nurse should be familiar with how the tests are obtained, what they are used for, and normal versus abnormal results. This knowledge will also be necessary when providing patient and family education related to the testing.

NURSING DIAGNOSES, GOALS, INTERVENTIONS, AND EVALUATION

Upon completion of a thorough assessment, the nurse might identify several nursing diagnoses, including:

- Fatigue related to decreased oxygen supply in the body
- Pain related to vaso-occlusive event or bleeding into tissues
- Impaired physical mobility related to pain from sickle cell crisis or acute bleeds, or imposed activity restrictions
- Ineffective health maintenance related to knowledge and skill acquisition regarding nutritional and medical treatment of anemia, prevention of infection, home administration of intravenous clotting factors, or protection from injury
- Anxiety related to diagnostic testing
- Ineffective family coping related to hospitalization of child, or chronic, possibly life-threatening genetic disorder

After completing an assessment of Shaun, you note the following: the history revealed he bled with all four of the teeth he has cut. Upon examination numerous bruises are noted. Based on the assessment findings, what would your top three nursing diagnoses be for Shaun?

Nursing goals, interventions, and evaluation for the child with hematologic dysfunction are based on the nursing diagnoses. Nursing Care Plan Overview 26.1 may be used as a guide in planning nursing care for the child with a hematologic disorder. Children's responses to hematologic disorders and their treatments will vary, and nursing care should be individualized based on the child's and family's responses to illness. Other conditions may contribute to these nursing diagnoses and must also be considered when prioritizing care. Additional information about nursing management will be included later in the chapter as it relates to specific disorders.

Based on your top three nursing diagnoses for Shaun, describe appropriate nursing interventions.

Anemia

Anemia is a condition in which levels of RBCs and Hgb are lower than normal. Hgb levels vary throughout child-

(text continues on page 879)

Common Laboratory and Diagnostic Tests 26.1

Test	Explanation	Indication	Nursing Implications
Blood type and cross-match	Determines ABO blood type as well as presence of antigens. Cross-match is performed on RBC-containing products to avoid transfusion reaction.	Trauma victim or any person in whom blood loss is suspected, in preparation for transfusion	Avoid hemolysis of specimen. Appropriately sign and date specimen. Apply "type and cross" or "blood band" to child the time of blood draw if indicated by the institution. Most type and cross-match specimens expire after 48 to 72 hours.
Clotting studies	Prothrombin time (PT), partial thromboplastin time (PTT), activated partial thromboplastin time (aPTT), International Normalized Ratio (INR)	Evaluation of common pathway in clotting mechanism. PT, INR: evaluation of extrinsic system. PTT, aPTT: evaluation of intrinsic system.	Apply pressure to venipuncture site. Assess for bleeding (gums, bruising, blood in urine or stool).
Coagulating factor concentration	Measures concentration of specific coagulating factors in the blood	Hemophilia, DIC	Apply pressure to venipuncture site. Assess for bleeding (gums, bruising, blood in urine or stool). Deliver specimen to laboratory as soon as possible (unstable at room temperature).
Complete blood count (CBC) with differential	Evaluates hemoglobin and hematocrit, WBC count (particularly the percentage of individual WBCs), and platelet count	Anemia, infection, bleeding disorder, clotting disorder	Normal values vary according to age and gender. WBC differential is helpful in evaluating source of infection. May be affected by certain medications.
Hemoglobin electrophoresis	Measures percentage of normal and abnormal hemoglobin in the blood	Sickle cell anemia, thalassemia	Blood transfusions within the previous 12 weeks may alter test results.
Iron	Evaluates iron metabolism	Iron deficiency anemia, hemosiderosis with chronic transfusion or hemoglobinopathies	Recent blood transfusions increase level. Child should fast for 12 hours before the test. Avoid hemolysis (will falsely elevate result).
Lead	Measures level of lead in blood	Lead poisoning	Normal amount in blood is zero.
Reticulocyte count	Measures the amount of reticulocytes (immature RBCs) in the blood	Indicates bone marrow's ability to respond to anemia with production of RBCs	Rises quickly in response to iron supplementation in the iron-deficient child
Serum ferritin	Measures the level of ferritin (the major iron storage protein) in the blood	Most sensitive test for determining iron deficiency anemia	Elevated in hemolytic disease and if transfused recently. Iron supplementation increases ferritin levels.

Nursing Care Plan 26.1

Overview for the Child With a Hematologic Disorder

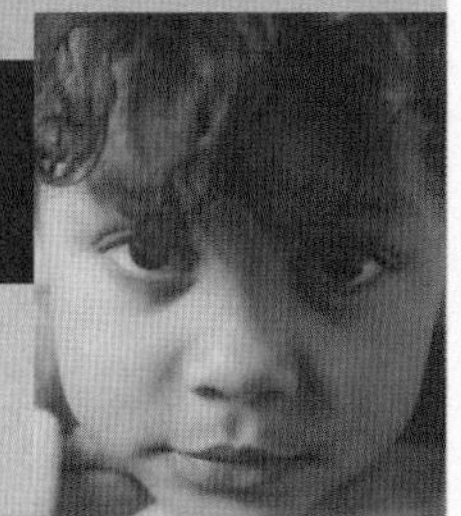

Nursing Diagnosis: Fatigue related to decreased oxygen supply in the body as evidenced by lack of energy, increased sleep requirements, or decreased interest in play activities

Outcome identification and evaluation

Child will display increased endurance, *desire to play without developing symptoms of exertion.*

Intervention: decreasing fatigue

- Cluster nursing care activities and plan for periods of rest before and after exertional activities *to decrease oxygen need and consumption.*
- Encourage activity or ambulation per physician's orders; *early mobilization results in better outcomes.*
- Observe child for symptoms of activity intolerance such as pallor, nausea, lightheadedness, or dizziness, or changes in vital signs *to determine level of tolerance.*
- If child is on bed rest, perform range-of-motion exercises and frequent position changes, *as negative changes to the musculoskeletal system occur quickly with inactivity and immobility.*
- Refer the child to physical therapy *for exercise prescription to increase skeletal muscle strength.*

Nursing Diagnosis: Impaired physical mobility related to pain from sickle cell crisis or acute bleeds or imposed activity restrictions as evidenced by guarding of painful extremity, resistance to activity

Outcome identification and evaluation

Child will be able to engage in activities within age parameters and limits of disease: *child is able to move extremities, move about environment, and participate in exercise programs within limits of age and disease.*

Intervention: promoting physical mobility

- Encourage gross and fine motor activities as able within constraints of pain/bleed *to facilitate motor development.*
- Collaborate with physical therapy to strengthen muscles and promote optimal mobility *to facilitate motor development.*
- Use passive and active range-of-motion exercises and teach child and family how to perform them: *these exercises prevent contractures and facilitate joint mobility and muscle development (active ROM) to help increase mobility.*
- Praise accomplishments and emphasize child's abilities *to improve self-esteem and encourage feelings of confidence and competence.*

Nursing Diagnosis: Ineffective health maintenance related to knowledge and skill acquisition regarding nutritional and medical treatment of anemia, prevention of infection, home administration of intravenous clotting factors, or protection from injury as evidenced by new diagnosis and inability to verbalize appropriate treatment regimen or demonstrate medication administration skills

Outcome identification and evaluation

Child's health will be maintained; *child will receive supplements, medications as prescribed and will take in an appropriate diet.*

(continued)

Overview for the Child With a Hematologic Disorder (continued)

Intervention: educating parents about effective health maintenance

- Educate the family about iron-rich foods *to be promoted in the child with iron deficiency anemia and limited in the child with thalassemia.*
- Limit cow's milk intake in the child with iron deficiency anemia *to decrease risk of microscopic GI bleeding and increase appetite for other foods.*
- Provide ongoing evaluation of nutritional intake *to ensure that appropriate dietary restrictions are followed.*
- Ensure that parents can verbalize understanding of home medication regimen: iron or folic acid supplementation for anemia, prophylactic antibiotics for sickle cell anemia, chelation for thalassemia and factor replacement for hemophilia.
- Have parents provide return demonstration of subcutaneous infusion of deferoxamine or intravenous factor as appropriate *to ensure accuracy and independence in the home environment.*
- Educate families about when to call or visit medical provider *to ensure timely intervention when signs and symptoms develop.*

Nursing Diagnosis: Anxiety related to diagnostic testing as evidenced by parent verbalization, child resistance or crying with procedures

Outcome identification and evaluation

Child's anxiety will be minimized; *child will verbalize less fear, experience less pain with procedures.*

Intervention: relieving anxiety

- Use topical anesthetic creams or agents for non-emergency lab draws *to decrease stress related to needlesticks or venipunctures.*
- Maintain a quiet and calm environment *to reduce the child's stress.*
- Educate the child, as appropriate, and the family regarding the need for obtaining any laboratory specimens: *knowledge helps to alleviate anxiety related to the unknown.*
- Identify the need for the specific test and explain the procedure before obtaining the specimen *to decrease the anxiety and time required for the procedure.*
- Provide developmentally appropriate activities for the child. *(Activities can reduce stress and also provide stimulus for children; the use of safe and developmentally appropriate activity acts as a role model for the family).*

Nursing Diagnosis: Ineffective family coping related to hospitalization of child or chronic, possibly life-threatening genetic disorder as evidenced by excessive tearfulness or denial statements, withdrawal, or verbalization of inadequate coping skills

Outcome identification and evaluation

Child and/or family will demonstrate adequate coping skills, *will verbalize feeling supported and demonstrate healthy family interactions.*

Intervention: promoting effective family coping

- Provide emotional support to the child and family *to improve coping abilities.*
- Actively listen to the child's and family's concerns *to validate the child's and family's feelings and establish trust.*
- Encourage parents to talk about their child and the illness; *verbalization brings feelings out in the open.*
- Validate feelings of guilt, shock, frustration, resentment, or depression *to promote trusting communication and begin avenue for appropriate coping.*
- Provide open communication with the child and siblings: *children appreciate honesty about their illness, and coping is improved.*

Overview for the Child With a Hematologic Disorder (continued)

- Refer families to community resources such as parent support groups, grief counseling (*involvement with emotional and instrumental support improves coping abilities*).
- Encourage role-playing and play activities *to identify the child's fears and provide a method for working through feelings.*

Nursing Diagnosis: Risk for injury related to alteration in peripheral sensory perception, decreased platelet count, deficient coagulation factor, or excessive iron load

Outcome identification and evaluation

Child will not experience hemorrhage; *will experience decreased bruising or episodes of prolonged bleeding.*

Intervention: preventing injury

- Assess for petechiae, purpura, bruising, or bleeding (*provides baseline data for comparison; if present, may warrant intervention*).
- Encourage quiet activities or play *to avoid trauma with active play.*
- Avoid rectal temperatures and examinations. Post sign at head of bed "no rectal temperatures or medications" *to avoid rectal mucosa damage resulting in bleeding.*
- Avoid intramuscular injections and lumbar puncture if possible *to decrease risk of bleeding from a puncture site.*
- If bone marrow aspiration must be performed, apply pressure dressing to site *to prevent bleeding.*
- Teach families about preferred physical activities for the child with ITP or hemophilia *to provide safe physical activity and decrease risk for injury.*

hood and should be monitored to ensure that adequate growth and development will be achieved. Anemia may develop as a result of decreased production of RBCs or loss and destruction of RBCs. The loss of production can be related to lack of dietary intake of the nutrients needed to produce the cells, alterations in the cell structure, or malfunctioning tissues, such as the bone marrow. Anemia related to nutritional deficiency includes iron deficiency, folic acid deficiency, and pernicious anemia. Anemia may also result from toxin exposure (lead poisoning) or as an adverse reaction to a medication (aplastic anemia). Blood loss may result from surgery or trauma, and destruction of cells occurs in certain genetic and cellular development disorders.

Anemia caused by the alteration or destruction of the RBC is termed hemolytic anemia. There are several types of hemolytic anemia, such as sickle cell disease and thalassemia (these two disorders are discussed under Hemoglobinopathies).

Anemia related to insufficient intake of specific nutrients is the most common type of anemia in children. Nutrient intake may be reduced in children due to food dislikes or conditions that produce malabsorption.

IRON DEFICIENCY ANEMIA

Iron deficiency anemia occurs when the body does not have enough iron to produce Hgb. In the United States 7% of children between the ages of 1 and 2 years, 5% of children between 3 and 5 years old, and 4% of children between 6 and 11 years of age developed iron deficiency anemia from 1999 to 2000. Five percent of boys and 9% of girls between the ages of 12 and 15 years have iron deficiency anemia (CDC, 2002). One of the factors that contributes to iron deficiency anemia in older infants is the consumption of cow's milk. Infants between the ages of 9 and 12 months who drank more than 500 g of cow's milk per day had reduced Hgb levels (Zetterstrom, 2004).

The heme portion of Hgb consists of iron surrounded by protoporphyrin. When not enough iron is available to the bone marrow, Hgb production is reduced. Adequate dietary intake of iron is required for the body to make enough Hgb. As Hgb levels decrease, the oxygen-carrying capacity of the blood is decreased, resulting in weakness and fatigue. Iron deficiency anemia has been associated with diminished cognitive function, changes in behavior, delayed growth and development in infants, increased fatigability, and less engagement in children (Lozoff et al., 2003). See Healthy People 2010.

Therapeutic Management

Iron supplements are usually provided in the form of ferrous sulfate or ferrous fumarate and are available over the

HEALTHY PEOPLE 2010

Objective	Significance
Reduce iron deficiency among young children and females of child-bearing age.	• Encourage use of iron-fortified formulas and infant cereal. • Encourage iron supplementation in the second half of infancy for the breast-fed infant. • Educate parents about iron-containing foods. • Encourage adolescent females to consume a diet high in iron-rich foods.

counter. Dosage is based on the amount of elemental iron. The recommended amounts of elemental iron are:

- For prophylaxis: 1 to 2 mg/kg/day, up to a maximum of 15 mg elemental iron per day
- Mild to moderate iron deficiency: 3 mg/kg/day of elemental iron in one or two divided doses
- Severe iron deficiency anemia: 4 to 6 mg/kg/day of elemental iron in three divided doses

In more severe cases, blood transfusions may be indicated. Transfusion of packed red blood cells (PRBCs) is reserved for the most severe cases. When PRBC administration is warranted, follow specific blood bank guidelines for administration. Monitor subsequent laboratory results for improvement.

Nursing Assessment

For a full description of the assessment phase of the nursing process, refer to page 870. Assessment findings pertinent to iron deficiency anemia are discussed below.

Health History

Elicit a description of the current illness and chief complaint. Common signs and symptoms reported during the health history may include irritability, headache, dizziness, weakness, shortness of breath, pallor, and fatigue. Other symptoms may be subtle and difficult for the clinician to identify; these include difficulty feeding, pica, muscle weakness, or unsteady gait.

Explore the health history for risk factors such as:

- Maternal anemia during pregnancy
- Poorly controlled diabetes during pregnancy
- Prematurity, low birthweight, or multiple birth
- Cow's milk consumption before 12 months of age
- Excessive cow's milk consumption (greater than 24 ounces a day)
- Infant consumption of low-iron formula
- Lack of iron supplementation after age 6 months in breastfed infants
- Excessive weight gain
- Chronic infection or inflammation
- Chronic or acute blood loss
- Restricted diets
- Use of medication interfering with iron absorption, such as antacids
- Low socioeconomic status
- Recent immigration from a developing country (Carley, 2003)

Evaluate the child's diet to identify adequate intake of iron-rich foods. Recommended dietary daily intake for iron in children is:

- 0 to 6 months: 6 mg
- 6 to 12 months: 10 mg
- 1 to 10 years: 10 mg
- Boys 11 to 18 years: 12 mg
- Girls 11 to 18 years: 15 mg (Abrams, 2004).

Physical Examination

Observe the child for fatigue and lethargy. Inspect the skin, conjunctivae, oral mucosa, palms, and soles for pallor. Note spooning of the nails (concave shape) (Fig. 26.2). Obtain a pulse oximeter reading. Evaluate the heart rate for tachycardia. Auscultate the heart for the presence of a flow murmur. Palpate the abdomen for splenomegaly.

Laboratory and Diagnostic Tests

Laboratory evaluation will reveal decreased Hgb and Hct, decreased reticulocyte count, microcytosis and hypochromia, decreased serum iron and ferritin levels, and an increased free erythrocyte protoporphyrin (FEP) level.

Nursing Management

Nursing management of the child with iron deficiency focuses on promoting safety, ensuring adequate iron intake, and educating the family.

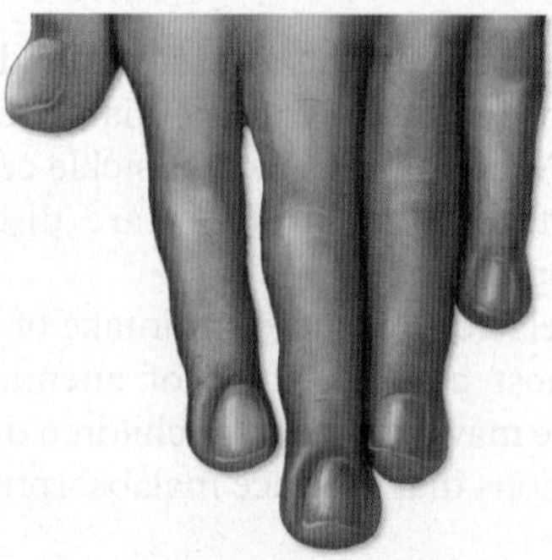

● **Figure 26.2** Note the concave shape of nails ("spooning") that occurs with iron deficiency anemia.

Promoting Safety

The child with anemia is at risk for changes in neurologic functioning related to the decreased oxygen supply to the brain. This can lead to fatigue and inability to eat enough. Neurologic effects may be manifested when the child's ability to sit, stand, or walk is impaired. Provide close observation of the anemic child. Assist the older child with ambulation. Educate the parents on how to protect the child from injury due to an unsteady gait or dizziness.

Providing Dietary Interventions

Ensure that iron-deficient infants are fed only formulas fortified with iron. Interventions for breastfed infants include beginning iron supplementation around the age of 4 or 5 months. Iron supplementation may range from adding iron-fortified cereals to the child's diet to giving iron-containing drops. Encourage breastfeeding mothers to increase their dietary intake of iron or take iron supplements when breastfeeding so that the iron may be passed on to the infant. For children over 1 year of age, limit cow's milk intake to 24 ounces per day. Limit fast-food consumption and encourage intake of iron-rich foods such as red meats, tuna, salmon, eggs, tofu, enriched grains, dried beans and peas, dried fruits, leafy green vegetables, and iron-fortified breakfast cereals (iron from red meat is the easiest for the body to absorb).

Teach the parents about dietary intake, and encourage them to provide a variety of foods for iron support and vitamins and other minerals necessary for growth. A big problem for toddlers is their "picky" eating. This often becomes a means of control for the child, and parents should guard against getting involved in a power struggle with their child. Referring parents to a developmental specialist who can assist them in their approach to diet may prove beneficial.

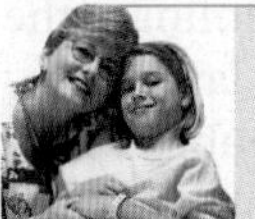

Dietary intake of more than 500 g/day of cow's milk in children has been shown to produce decreased Hgb levels. This study also found that children with lower iron levels had increased weight gain from birth to 2 years of age (Gunnarsson et al., 2004).

Refer families who meet the financial limits and who have children age 5 and under to the Women, Infants and Children (WIC) program, which provides for supplementation of infant's and children's diets.

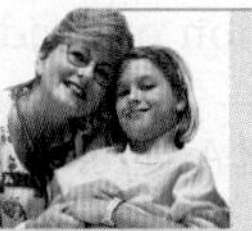

Parents are often concerned that a diagnosis of iron deficiency anemia or referral to the WIC program may lead to interventions from children's services. Assure the family that as long as appropriate measures are taken to address the anemia, referrals of this nature are not generally made.

Teaching About Iron Supplement Administration

The use of iron supplements in infants begins with the use of formula fortified with iron in the formula-fed infant. Oral supplements may be necessary as well if the baby's iron levels are extremely low. Oral supplements or multivitamin formulas that contain iron are often dark in color, as the iron is pigmented. Teaching the parents to measure precisely the amount of iron to be administered is an important nursing role. Parents should place the liquid behind the teeth, as iron in liquid form can stain the teeth. Iron supplementation can also cause constipation. In some cases reducing the amount of iron can resolve this problem, but stool softeners may be necessary to control painful or difficult-to-pass stools. Encourage parents to increase their child's fluid intake and include adequate dietary fiber to avoid constipation.

● OTHER NUTRITIONAL CAUSES OF ANEMIA

Other forms of anemia related to nutritional deficit include folic acid deficiency and pernicious anemia. Comparison Chart 26.1 discusses the causes, assessment, and management of these disorders.

● LEAD POISONING

Lead poisoning, though not as common as it once was, affected between 890,000 children (Morrissey-Ross, 2000) and 1 million children (Velsor-Friedrich, 2002) in the year 2000. Lead exerts toxic effects on the bone marrow, erythroid cells, nervous system, and kidneys. The presence of lead in the bloodstream interferes with the enzymatic processes of the biosynthesis of heme. The process results in hypochromic, microcytic anemia, and children may exhibit classic signs of anemia. Risk factors for lead poisoning are related to lead exposure in the home, school, or local environment. Sources of lead include:

- Paint in homes built before 1978, at which time lead was banned as an additive to paint used in houses
- Dust from windowsills, walls, and plaster in older homes
- Soil where cars that used leaded gas have been in the past (lead was removed from all gasoline in the United States as of 1996)
- Glazed pottery
- Stained glass products
- Lead pipes supplying water to the home
- On the clothing of parents who work in certain manufacturing jobs (battery makers, cable makers)
- Certain folk remedies, such as *greta* or *arzacon*
- Old painted toys or furniture (Environmental Protection Agency, 2005)

Complications of lead poisoning include behavioral problems and learning difficulties and, with higher lead levels, encephalopathy, seizures, and brain damage.

COMPARISON CHART 26.1 Folic Acid Deficiency Versus Pernicious Anemia

	Folic Acid Deficiency	Pernicious Anemia
Cause	Low dietary intake of green leafy vegetables, liver, and citrus. Malabsorption from medication such as phenytoin (Dilantin) or parasitic infection.	Deficiency in vitamin B12
Assessment	Determine risk factors such as prematurity, low socioeconomic status, and history of malabsorption disease. Determine dietary history, noting dislike of fresh vegetables or fruit, ingestion of overcooked foods, or lack of family purchase of fruits and vegetables. Note history of fatigue, headache, poor growth, anorexia, or diarrhea. Inspect the skin for pallor or jaundice, and note presence of a sore on the mouth or tongue.	Note history of anorexia, irritability, or chronic diarrhea. Observe the skin or conjunctivae for pallor and the tongue for smooth texture and bright-red color.
Laboratory analysis	RBC Hgb Hct	RBC Hgb Hct Low vitamin B12 level
Management	Encourage parents to include green leafy vegetables, liver, and citrus in diet. Ensure that parents comply with dietary changes.	Administer monthly injections of vitamin B12. Inform parents injections will be required throughout the child's life. Provide emotional support related to the chronic nature of this disorder.

Treatment for high blood levels of lead is **chelation therapy**, either orally or intramuscularly. Drug Guide 26.1 gives further information on chelating agents.

Nursing Assessment

Explore the health history for subtle signs such as anorexia, fatigue, or abdominal pain. Determine whether behavioral problems, irritability, hyperactivity, or lack of ability to meet developmental milestones have occurred in recent months. Screen children for risk of exposure to lead in the home. Refer to Chapter 9 for a simple screening questionnaire that can be used to determine the need for lead screening in young children. Blood levels of lead greater than 10 mcg/dL require conscientious follow-up. Note pallor of the skin. See Healthy People 2010.

HEALTHY PEOPLE 2010

Objective	Significance
Eliminate elevated blood lead levels in children.	• Appropriately screen infants and young children for lead exposure at each health care visit.

Nursing Management

Prevention of elevated lead levels is key. Screen children for lead exposure risk. The American Academy of Pediatrics recommends screening in high-risk children at ages 12 and 24 months. Table 26.3 gives recommendations for appropriate follow-up depending on lead levels.

Removing old paint is the best way to eliminate the most significant source of lead exposure for a large number of children. If the family rents or lives in public housing, the landlord or owner is responsible for following the guidelines set forth by local and state governmental agencies to correct the problem. The Enterprise Foundation has made recommendations for healthy and affordable housing; visit www.enterprisefoundation.org (Proscio, 2004).

Educate families about how to prevent exposure to lead, particularly in young children. Additional resources for families include:

- www.leadsafe.org/: Coalition to End Childhood Lead Poisoning
- www.thearc.org/faqs/leadqa.html: information on lead poisoning from the Arc
- www.epa.gov/lead/index.html: National Lead Awareness Program
- 1 (800) 424-5323 (LEAD): National Lead Information Program

Table 26.3 Interventions Based on Blood Lead Level

Blood Lead Level (in mcg/dL)	Recommended Action
<10	None required
10–14	Confirm with repeat test in 1 month and educate parents to decrease lead exposure. Repeat test within 3 months.
15–19	Confirm with repeat test in 1 month and educate parents to decrease lead exposure. Repeat test within 2 months.
20–44	Confirm with repeat test within 1 week and educate parents to decrease lead exposure. Refer to local health department for investigation of home for lead reduction, with referrals for support services.
45–69	Confirm with repeat test within 2 days and educate parents to decrease lead levels. Begin chelation therapy and refer to health department as above.
>70	Hospitalize child and begin chelation therapy. Ensure lead is removed from the home.

Adapted from American Academy of Pediatrics, Committee on Environmental Health. (1998). Screening for elevated blood lead levels. *Pediatrics, 101*(6), 1172–1178.

- www.aeclp.org: Alliance for Healthy Homes (originally the Alliance to End Childhood Lead Poisoning), 1-202-543-1147
- www.cdc.gov/nceh/lead/lead.htm: Childhood Lead Poisoning Prevention Program
- www.cehrc.org: Community Environmental Health Resource Center
- www.hud.gov: U.S. Department of Housing and Urban Development, 1-800-HUDS-FHA

If the child is undergoing chelation therapy, ensure adequate fluid intake and monitor intake and output closely. Refer children with elevated lead levels and developmental or cognitive deficits to developmental centers. These children may need an early intervention program for further evaluation and treatment of developmental delays.

APLASTIC ANEMIA

Aplastic anemia (failure of the bone marrow to produce cells) is characterized by bone marrow aplasia and pancytopenia (decreased numbers of all blood cells). Most cases are acquired, but there are a few rare types of inherited aplastic anemias. The inherited types present as congenital bone marrow failure; the best known is Fanconi's anemia, an autosomal recessive disorder. Acquired aplastic anemia is thought to be an immune-mediated response. Most cases are idiopathic, meaning the trigger remains unidentified. Other causes include exposure to environmental toxins, viruses, myelosuppressive drugs, or radiation.

Aplastic anemia may be classified as severe or nonsevere. In the severe form, the granulocyte count is less than 500, the platelet count is less than 20,000, and the reticulocyte count is less than 1%. In nonsevere aplastic anemia, the granulocyte count is about 500, the platelet count is over 20,000, and the reticulocyte count is over 1%. Complications of aplastic anemia include severe overwhelming infection, hemorrhage, and death. Therapeutic management of aplastic anemia in children involves hematopoietic stem cell transplantation from an HLA-matched sibling donor; if one is not available, immunosuppressive therapy or high-dose cyclophosphamide can be given.

Nursing Assessment

Determine history of exposure to myelosuppressive medications or radiation therapy. Obtain a detailed family, environmental, and infectious disease history. Note history of epistaxis, gingival oozing, or increased bleeding with menstruation. Anemia may lead to headache and fatigue. On physical examination, note ecchymoses, petechiae or purpura, oral ulcerations, tachycardia, or tachypnea. In addition to suppression of all blood cells, laboratory and diagnostic testing may reveal:

- Guaiac-positive stool
- Blood in the urine
- Severe decrease in or absence of hematopoietic cells on bone marrow aspiration

Nursing Management

Safety is of the utmost concern in children with aplastic anemia. Injury must be prevented to avoid hemorrhage. Stool softeners may be used to prevent anal fissures associated with constipation. Administer only irradiated and leukocyte-depleted packed red blood cells or platelet transfusions as necessary. This limits exposure to HLA antigens should the child require bone marrow transplantation in the future. For the child who does require hematopoietic stem cell transplantation, refer to Chapter 29 for additional nursing management information.

Refer families whose child has only mild or moderate disease to agencies for resources and support. These include the Aplastic Anemia and Myelodysplastic Syndrome International Foundation (www.aamds.org) and the Aplastic Anemia Foundation of America (www.aplastic.org).

Hemoglobinopathies

Hemoglobinopathy is a condition in which abnormal hemoglobin is present. A large percentage of the newborn's hemoglobin is fetal hemoglobin (Hgb F). Hgb F can exchange oxygen molecules at lower oxygen tensions compared to adult hemoglobin. Over the first several months of life, Hgb F diminishes and is replaced with Hgb A (adult hemoglobin). The healthy older infant then displays the presence of Hgb AA. In hemoglobinopathies, this normal hemoglobin configuration is disturbed. Causes of hemoglobinopathies are genetic and include sickle cell anemia, hemoglobin SC disease, alpha-thalassemia, and beta-thalassemia. This discussion will focus on sickle cell disease and beta-thalassemia (Cooley anemia).

● SICKLE CELL DISEASE

Sickle cell disease is a group of inherited hemoglobinopathies in which the RBCs do not carry the normal adult hemoglobin, but rather a less effective type. In the United States, the most common types of sickle cell disease are hemoglobin SS disease (sickle cell anemia), hemoglobin SC disease, and hemoglobin sickle–beta thalassemia. Among the sickle cell diseases, sickle cell anemia is the most common and will be the focus of this discussion.

Sickle cell anemia is a severe chronic blood disorder that affects 2,000 infants born in the United States each year; approximately 80,000 Americans have the disease. It is most common in individuals of African, Mediterranean, Middle Eastern, and Indian decent (American Academy of Pediatrics, 2002). One in 500 African-Americans has sickle cell anemia (Human Genome Management Information System, 2004). Instead of Hgb AA, individuals with sickle cell anemia have Hgb SS: rather than mostly hemoglobin A (adult hemoglobin) being present in the blood, mainly hemoglobin S (sickle hemoglobin) is present. In hemoglobin S, glutamic acid is replaced with valine in the hemoglobin molecule. This results in an elongated RBC with a shortened life span. The elongated cell is more rigid than a normal cell and becomes sickled in shape (Fig. 26.3). Persons with heterozygous representation (Hgb AS) are said to have sickle cell trait and are carriers for the disorder. One in 12 African-Americans has sickle cell trait (Human Genome Management Information System, 2004). Generally, persons with sickle cell trait have only minimal health problems.

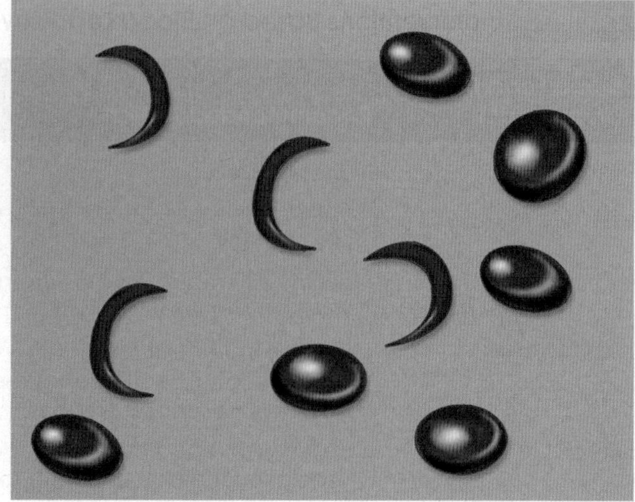

● **Figure 26.3** This peripheral blood smear demonstrates the elongated sickle-shaped red blood cell seen in sickle cell disease.

The recessive genes for sickle cell are passed on from both parents who have the gene or trait. Each parent has the gene Hgb AS. Hgb A refers to normal adult hemoglobin and Hgb S refers to sickle hemoglobin. These recessive genes for sickle cell may be passed on to the child. The risk for developing Hgb SS is one in four, or 25%, in each child from this union. With each pregnancy the risk is 25% that the child will have disease, 25% that the child will have normal hemoglobin, and 50% that the child will have the trait (Hgb AS) and will be a carrier. Figure 26.4 illustrates the inheritance probability. Infants with sickle cell anemia are usually asymptomatic until 3 to 4 months of age because Hgb F protects against sickling.

Complications of sickle cell anemia include recurrent vaso-occlusive pain crises, stroke, sepsis, acute chest syndrome, splenic sequestration, reduced visual acuity related to decreased retinal blood flow, chronic leg ulcers,

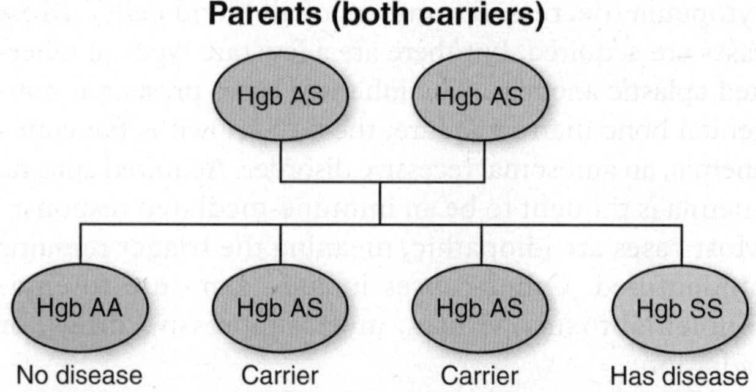

● **Figure 26.4** Simplified genetic scheme for sickle cell disease. A denotes adult hemoglobin; S denotes sickle hemoglobin. Hemoglobin AA = normal hemoglobin, hemoglobin AS = sickle cell trait, hemoglobin SS = sickle cell disease.

cholestasis and gallstones, delayed growth and development, delayed puberty, and priapism (the sickled cells prevent blood from flowing out of an erect penis) (National Heart, Lung and Blood Institute, 2005). Children with sickle cell anemia have an increased incidence of enuresis because the kidneys cannot concentrate urine effectively. As children reach adulthood, multiple organ dysfunction is common.

Pathophysiology

Significant anemia may occur when the RBCs sickle. Sickling may be triggered by any stress or traumatic event, such as infection, fever, acidosis, dehydration, physical exertion, excessive cold exposure, or hypoxia. As the cells sickle, the blood becomes more viscous because the sickled cells clump together and prevent normal blood flow to the tissues of that area. The sickle-shaped RBCs cannot pass through the smaller capillaries and venules of the circulatory system (Fig. 26.5). This vaso-occlusive process leads to local tissue hypoxia followed by ischemia and may result in infarction. Pain crisis results as circulation is decreased to the area. Pain can occur in any part of the body but is most common in the joints. Pain causes increased metabolic need by resulting in tachycardia and sometimes tachypnea, which leads to further sickling. Clumping of cells in the lungs (acute chest syndrome) results in decreased gas exchange, producing hypoxia, which leads to further sickling. Sequestration of blood in the spleen leads to splenomegaly and abdominal pain. Hemolysis follows sickling and leads to further anemia. The increased activity of the spleen related to RBC hemolysis leads to splenomegaly, then fibrosis and atrophy. Functional asplenia may develop as early as 3 months of age (American Academy of Pediatrics, 2002).

Therapeutic Management

The therapeutic management of children with sickle cell anemia focuses on preventing sickling crisis and preventing infection and other complications. Prevention of infection is critical because the child with sickle cell anemia is at increased risk for serious infection related to alterations in splenic function. Functional asplenia (decrease in the ability of the spleen to function appropriately) places the child at significant risk for serious infection related to *Streptococcus pneumoniae* or other encapsulated organisms. Prophylactic antibiotics in the young child and appropriate immunization in all children with sickle cell anemia can reduce the risk of serious infection.

Treatment of sickle cell crisis is directed toward control of pain. Oxygen administration is necessary during episodes of crisis to prevent additional cell sickling. Adequate hydration with intravenous fluids is critical. Close monitoring of Hgb, Hct, and reticulocytes determines the point at which transfusion of packed red blood cells becomes necessary. Electrolyte analysis is also necessary to ensure that appropriate amounts of electrolytes are present in the serum. When RBCs are administered, there is the potential for hemolysis of the cells, thus increasing the potassium level in the serum. Antibiotic therapy is necessary when infection is present. Box 26.1 describes additional medical treatments that are necessary in some children.

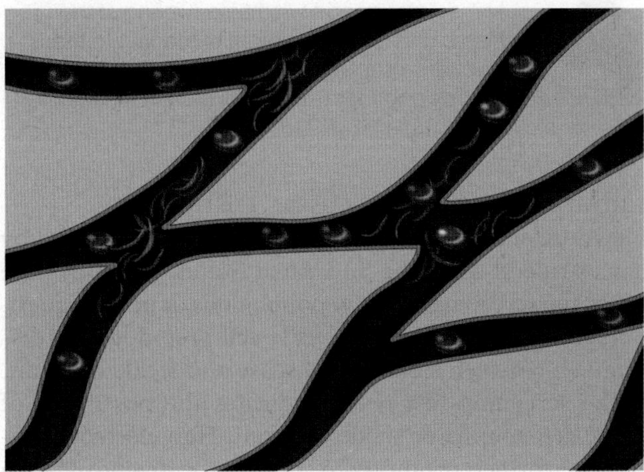

● Figure 26.5 Clumping of sickle-shaped cells.

Nursing Assessment

Children with sickle cell anemia experience a significant number of acute and chronic manifestations of the condition (Comparison Chart 26.2). For a full description of the assessment phase of the nursing process, refer to page 870. Assessment findings pertinent to sickle cell anemia are discussed below.

BOX 26.1

ADDITIONAL MEDICAL TREATMENTS FOR SOME CHILDREN WITH SICKLE CELL ANEMIA

- Cholecystectomy may become necessary if gallstones develop.
- Splenectomy may be performed to prevent recurrence of splenic sequestration if it is life-threatening.
- Administration of hydroxyurea may increase the percentage of fetal hemoglobin, but this is considered an investigational treatment.
- Blood transfusions, though not routinely given to children with sickle cell disease, are indicated in children with prolonged or widespread pain, aplastic crisis, or splenic sequestration.
- Partial exchange transfusion may be used to rapidly lower the circulating amount of Hgb SS in the event of stroke or acute chest syndrome.
- Hematopoietic stem cell transplantation is usually reserved for children with an identical HLA-matched sibling (risk of death and incidence of graft-versus-host disease is high).

● COMPARISON CHART 26.2 Acute Versus Chronic Manifestations of Sickle Cell Anemia

Acute	Chronic
*Acute chest syndrome	Anemia
*Aplastic crisis	Avascular necrosis of the hip
*Bacterial sepsis or meningitis	Cardiomegaly, functional murmur
Bone infarction	Cholelithiasis
Dactylitis	Delayed growth and development
Hematuria	Delayed puberty
Recurrent pain episodes	Functional asplenia
Pain crisis	Hyposthenuria (low urine specific gravity) and enuresis
*Splenic sequestration	Jaundice
*Stroke	Leg ulcers
Priapism	Proteinuria
	*Pulmonary hypertension
	*Restrictive lung disease
	Retinopathy

*Often life-threatening.

Health History

Elicit the health history, noting growth and development, frequency and extent of vaso-occlusive crises, past hospitalizations, and treatment for pain crises. Note history of immunizations, including pneumococcal, flu, and meningococcal vaccinations. Determine history of blood transfusions. Document current medication regimen. Note history of recurrent infections. Determine history of present illness that results in a precipitating event, such as hypoxia, infection, or dehydration. Note onset, character, and quality of pain, as well as factors that relieve it.

Physical Examination

Perform a thorough physical examination, because sickling, hypoxia, and tissue ischemia affect most areas of the body (Fig. 26.6). Note the physical findings discussed below that can be detected using inspection, observation, auscultation, and palpation.

Inspection and Observation

Inspect the conjunctivae, palms, and soles for pallor and skin for pallor or lesions or ulcers. Note jaundice of the skin or scleral icterus. Document color and moisture of oral mucosa. Measure temperature to evaluate for infection (which can precipitate a sickling crisis). Note blood pressure (may be decreased with severe anemia or increased with sickle cell nephropathy). Measure temperature, noting elevation. Determine baseline mental status. Perform a neurologic assessment frequently, as about 8% to 17% of children with sickle cell anemia experience a stroke.

Auscultation

Auscultate heart sounds for a murmur. The heart rate is often elevated with pain, hyperthermia, or dehydration. Listen to breath sounds, noting the rate and depth of respiration as well as the adequacy of aeration. Adventitious breath sounds may be present if a respiratory infection has triggered the sickle cell crisis or in the case of acute chest syndrome.

Palpation

Palpate the joints for warmth, tenderness, and range of motion. Note swelling of the hands or feet in the infant. Palpate the abdomen for areas of tenderness. Note hepatomegaly or splenomegaly.

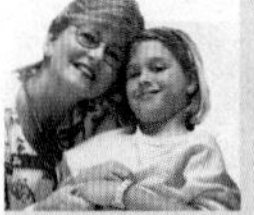

Immediately report symmetric swelling of the hands and feet in the infant or toddler. Termed dactylitis, aseptic infarction occurs in the metacarpals and metatarsals. This is often the first vaso-occlusive event seen (Fig. 26.7).

Laboratory and Diagnostic Testing

Newborn screening for sickle cell anemia is required by law or rule in 49 of the 50 United States; the 50th state offers the screening to select populations or upon request. Screening by Sickledex or sickle cell prep does not distinguish between sickle cell disease and sickle cell trait. If the screening test result indicates the possibility of sickle cell anemia or sickle cell trait, Hgb electrophoresis is performed promptly to confirm the diagnosis. Hgb electrophoresis is the only accurate test for sickle cell

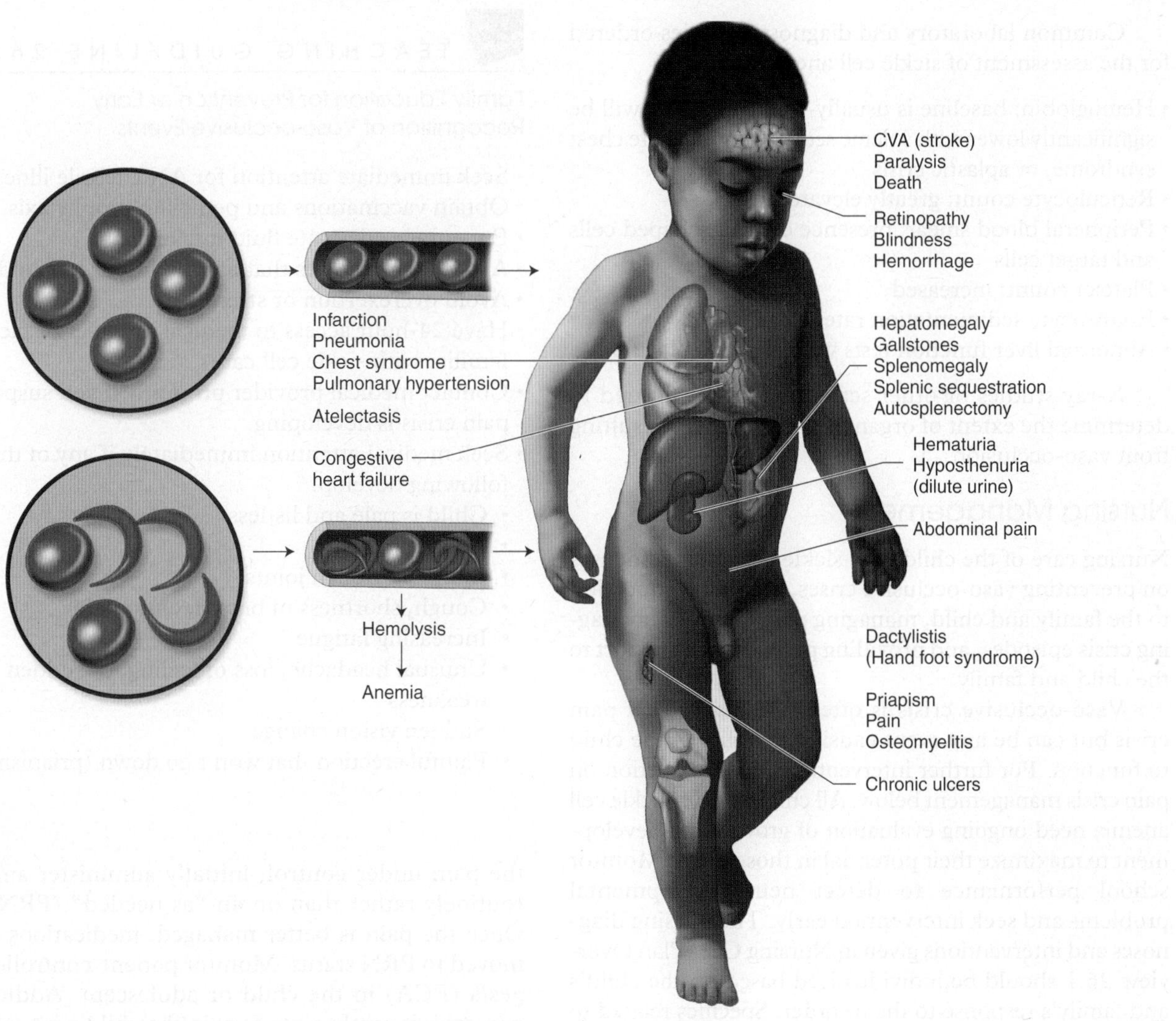

● **Figure 26.6** Effects of sickle cell anemia on various parts of the body.

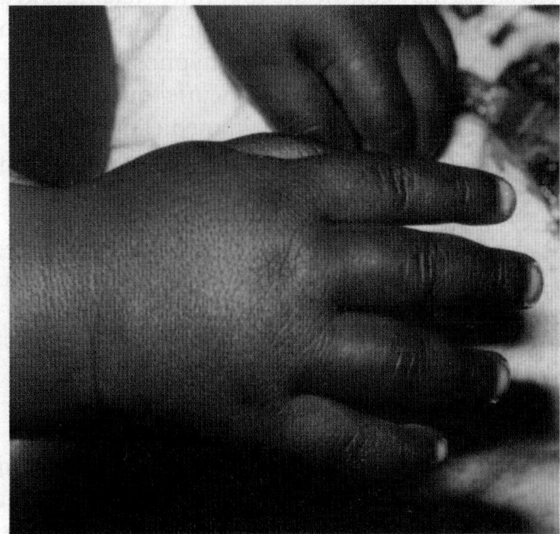

● **Figure 26.7** Swelling of the hands and feet (dactylitis) in a toddler.

disease. Hgb electrophoresis will demonstrate the presence of Hgb S and Hgb F only in the young infant; in the older infant or child, the result will be Hgb SS. See Healthy People 2010.

HEALTHY PEOPLE 2010

Objective	Significance
(Developmental) Ensure appropriate newborn bloodspot screening, follow-up testing, and referral to services.	• Follow up with state agencies at first contact with infant to ascertain results of newborn screening. • If screening not done at birth, ensure Hgb electrophoresis obtained.

Common laboratory and diagnostic studies ordered for the assessment of sickle cell anemia include:

- Hemoglobin: baseline is usually 7 to 10 mg/dL; will be significantly lower with splenic sequestration, acute chest syndrome, or aplastic crisis
- Reticulocyte count: greatly elevated
- Peripheral blood smear: presence of sickle-shaped cells and target cells
- Platelet count: increased
- Erythrocyte sedimentation rate: elevated
- Abnormal liver function tests with elevated bilirubin

X-ray studies or other scans may be performed to determine the extent of organ or tissue damage resulting from vaso-occlusion.

Nursing Management

Nursing care of the child with sickle cell anemia focuses on preventing vaso-occlusive crises, providing education to the family and child, managing pain episodes, managing crisis episodes, and providing psychosocial support to the child and family.

Vaso-occlusive crisis is often referred to as a pain crisis but can be any event causing inability of the child to function. For further interventions, see the section on pain crisis management below. All children with sickle cell anemia need ongoing evaluation of growth and development to maximize their potential in those areas. Monitor school performance to detect neurodevelopmental problems and seek intervention early. The nursing diagnoses and interventions given in Nursing Care Plan Overview 26.1 should be individualized based on the child's and family's response to the disorder. Specifics related to sickle cell disease are discussed below.

Educating the Family and Child

Education should begin immediately after the diagnosis of sickle cell anemia is confirmed. Initially, teach the family about the genetics of the disease and encourage family members to be tested for carrier status. Educate families about the disease process. Emphasize the importance of regularly scheduled health maintenance visits and immunizations. Teach families how to administer prophylactic penicillin. Encourage families to seek medical evaluation urgently for any febrile illness. Educate families about how to prevent and recognize vaso-occlusive events (Teaching Guideline 26.1). Discuss complications such as delayed growth and development, delayed puberty, stroke, cholelithiasis, retinopathy, avascular necrosis, priapism, and leg ulcers.

Managing Pain Crisis

Initiate pain assessment with a standardized pain scale upon admission. Provide frequent evaluations of pain. Always believe the child's report of pain: only the person suffering the pain knows what it feels like. Moderate to severe pain usually requires opioid medication. To bring the pain under control, initially administer analgesics routinely rather than on an "as needed" (PRN) basis. Once the pain is better managed, medications may be moved to PRN status. Monitor patient-controlled analgesia (PCA) in the child or adolescent. Addiction to narcotics is rarely a concern in the child with sickle cell anemia if the narcotic is used to alleviate severe pain. Nonsteroidal anti-inflammatory medications and acetaminophen are often used for less severe pain. Adequate pain management helps to decrease the child's stress level; elevated stress may contribute to further sickling and additional pain. Use nonpharmacologic pain management techniques such as relaxation or hypnosis, music, massage, play, guided imagery, therapeutic touch, or behavior modification to augment the pain medication regimen.

Box 26.2 gives a summary of sickle cell pain management.

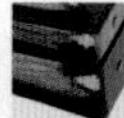

TEACHING GUIDELINE 26.1

Family Education for Prevention or Early Recognition of Vaso-occlusive Events

- Seek immediate attention for ANY febrile illness.
- Obtain vaccinations and penicillin prophylaxis.
- Encourage adequate fluid intake daily.
- Avoid temperatures that are too hot or too cold.
- Avoid overexertion or stress.
- Have 24-hour access to medical provider or facility familiar with sickle cell care.
- Contact medical provider promptly if you suspect a pain crisis is developing.
- Seek medical attention immediately if any of the following develop:
  - Child is pale and listless
  - Abdominal pain
  - Limp or swollen joints
  - Cough, shortness of breath, chest pain
  - Increasing fatigue
  - Unusual headache, loss of feeling, or sudden weakness
  - Sudden vision change
  - Painful erection that won't go down (priapism)

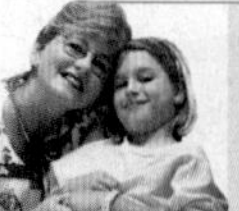

Avoid repeated use of meperidine (Demerol) for pain management during sickle cell crisis because it has been associated with an increased risk of seizures when used in children with sickle cell anemia (Sickle Cell Disease Care Consortium, 2002).

Managing Sickle Cell Crisis

Treat any underlying conditions such as infection or injury. Deficient fluid volume occurs as a result of decreased intake, increased fluid requirements during sickle cell crisis, and the kidney's inability to concentrate urine. Increasing fluid intake will dilute the blood and decrease its

BOX 26.2

ABCs OF MANAGING SICKLE CELL PAIN

A: Assess the pain (use a pain assessment tool)
B: Believe the patient's report of pain
C: Complications or cause of pain (look for complications)
D: Drugs and distraction: pain medication (opiates and NSAIDs, if no contraindications); use fixed dosing; give on a timed schedule; no prn dosing for pain medications; distraction with music, TV, relaxation techniques
E: Environment (rest in quiet area with privacy)
F: Fluids (hypotonic—D5W or D5 with 0.25 normal saline solution)

Adapted from Platt, A., Eckman, J. R., Beasley, J., & Miller, G. (2002). Treating sickle cell pain: An update from the Georgia Comprehensive Sickle Cell Center. *Journal of Emergency Nursing, 28*(4), 297–303, with permission.

viscosity. To promote hemodilution, provide 150 mL/kg of fluids per day or as much as double maintenance, either orally or intravenously. Maintain appropriate electrolyte and pH balance.

Risk for ineffective tissue perfusion related to the effects of RBC sickling and infarction of tissues is another concern. Frequently evaluate respiratory and circulatory status. Administer supplemental oxygen for a pulse oximetry reading of 90% or less to promote adequate oxygenation. Supplementation with oxygen in the absence of hypoxia is unnecessary and may inhibit erythropoiesis. Monitor level of consciousness and immediately report changes.

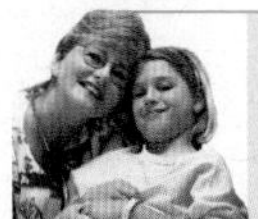

The child's temperature should be maintained as close to normal as possible without the use of cooling mattresses; a cooling mattress can cause localized circulation reduction or shivering, which may lead to increased metabolic needs and sickling of the red blood cells.

Preventing Infection

To prevent severe infection in the child with sickle cell anemia, a variety of interventions are necessary. By 2 months of age, begin administration of oral penicillin V potassium (also used to prevent pneumococcal infection). In the penicillin-allergic child, erythromycin may be used. Continue penicillin or erythromycin prophylaxis until at least age 5 years (American Academy of Pediatrics, 2002). Administer childhood immunizations according to the currently recommended schedule. To prevent overwhelming sepsis or meningitis as a result of infection with *S. pneumoniae,* the child should receive not only the 7-valent pneumococcal vaccine series in infancy but also the 23-valent pneumococcal conjugate vaccine annually after age 2 years. Meningococcal vaccination is also warranted (refer to Chapter 9 for additional information on these vaccines). Before the onset of flu season, provide influenza immunization annually (after 6 months of age).

Supporting the Family and Child

As with any chronic illness, families of children with sickle cell anemia need significant support. They often feel guilty or responsible for the disease. Reassure the family and provide education (see Healthy People 2010). Refer families to a regional sickle cell disease center for multidisciplinary care. Additional resources for families include:

- Sickle Cell Information Center, P.O. Box 109, Grady Memorial Hospital, 80 Jesse Hill Jr. Drive, SE, Atlanta, GA 30303 (www.scinfo.org)
- Sickle Cell Disease Association of America, 16 S. Calvert Street, Suite 600, Baltimore, MD 21202; 410-528-1555 or 1-800-421-8453 (www.sicklecelldisease.org)
- SickleCellKids.org, 740 Drewry Street, Atlanta, GA, 30306 (www.sicklecellkids.org/)
- American Sickle Cell Anemia Association, 10300 Carnegie Avenue, Cleveland Clinic, Cleveland, OH 44106; 1-216-229-8600 (www.ascaa.org)

Consider THIS!

A 3-year-old boy with sickle cell disease is being admitted to the pediatric unit. He has had a runny nose, slight fever, and vomiting over the past 2 to 3 days. He has not been eating well and is complaining of pain in the right leg and refusing to walk. On assessment you find his vital signs to be temperature 101.7° F, pulse 132, respirations 32, blood pressure 88/52. He is coughing, he has slightly dusky mucous membranes, and his capillary refill is 4 seconds.

1. **List nursing assessment findings in order of priority.**
2. **Identify at least three nursing interventions, prioritize them, and list the rationale for the prioritization and the intervention itself.**
3. **List teaching you will perform with this family.**

THALASSEMIA

Thalassemia is a genetic disorder that most often affects those of African descent, but it also affects individuals of Caribbean, Middle Eastern, South Asian, and Mediter-

HEALTHY PEOPLE 2010

Objective	Significance
Reduce stroke deaths.	• Educate families appropriately to decrease incidence of vaso-occlusive episodes in children with sickle cell anemia.

ranean descent (Catlin, 2003). The genetics of thalassemia are similar to those of sickle cell disease in that it is inherited via an autosomal recessive process. Children with thalassemia have reduced production of normal hemoglobin.

There are two basic types of thalassemia, alpha and beta. In alpha-thalassemia, synthesis of the alpha chain of the hemoglobin protein is affected. Problems with the beta chain occur more often, and the condition beta-thalassemia can be divided into three subcategories based on severity:

- Thalassemia minor (also called beta-thalassemia trait): leads to mild microcytic anemia; often no treatment is required
- Thalassemia intermedia: child requires blood transfusions to maintain adequate quality of life
- Thalassemia major: to survive the child requires ongoing medical attention, blood transfusions, and iron removal (chelation therapy) (Catlin, 2003)

The focus of this discussion will be on beta-thalassemia major (Cooley's anemia).

In beta-thalassemia major, the beta-globulin chain in hemoglobin synthesis is reduced or entirely absent. A large number of unstable globulin chains accumulate, causing the RBCs to be rigid and hemolyzed easily. The result is severe hemolytic anemia and chronic hypoxia. In response to the increased rate of RBC destruction, erythroid activity is increased. The increased activity causes massive bone marrow expansion and thinning of the bony cortex. Growth retardation, pathologic fractures, and skeletal deformities (frontal and maxillary bossing) result.

Hemosiderosis (excessive supply of iron) is an additional complication of significant concern. It occurs as a result of rapid hemolysis of RBCs, the decrease in hemoglobin production, and the increased absorption of dietary iron in response to the severely anemic state. The excess iron is deposited in the body's tissues, causing bronze pigmentation of the skin, bony changes, and altered organ function, particularly in the cardiac system. Additional complications include splenomegaly, endocrine abnormalities, osteoporosis, liver and gallbladder disease, and leg ulcers.

Left untreated, beta-thalassemia major is fatal, but the use of chelation therapy has increased the life expectancy of these children to beyond their teen years (Catlin, 2003).

Therapeutic Management

The therapeutic management for children with beta-thalassemia includes monitoring hemoglobin and hematocrit and transfusing packed red blood cells at regular intervals. Blood iron levels are monitored and iron chelation therapy is provided.

Nursing Assessment

Infants are usually diagnosed by 1 year of age and have a history of pallor, jaundice, failure to thrive, and hepatosplenomegaly. Determine the history of the present illness or whether the child is presenting for a routine blood transfusion. Note medications taken at home and any concerns that have arisen since the last visit. Inspect the skin, oral mucosa, conjunctivae, soles, and/or palms for pallor. Note icteral sclerae or jaundice of the skin. Measure weight and height or length and plot on an appropriate growth chart. Observe the child for bony deformities and frontal bossing (prominent forehead) (Fig. 26.8). Measure oxygen saturation via pulse oximetry. Evaluate neurologic status, determining level of consciousness and developmental abilities.

Laboratory testing may reveal:

- Significantly decreased hemoglobin and hematocrit
- Peripheral blood smear shows prominence of target cells, hypochromia, microcytosis and extensive anisocytosis and **poikilocytosis** (variation in the size and shape of the RBCs, respectively).
- Elevated bilirubin
- Hgb electrophoresis shows presence of Hgb F and Hgb A_2 only (Catlin, 2003).
- Elevated iron level

Nursing Management

The nursing care of the child with thalassemia is primarily aimed at supporting the family and minimizing the effects of the illness. This includes administering blood transfusions and making sure that the family can obtain appointments for laboratory studies.

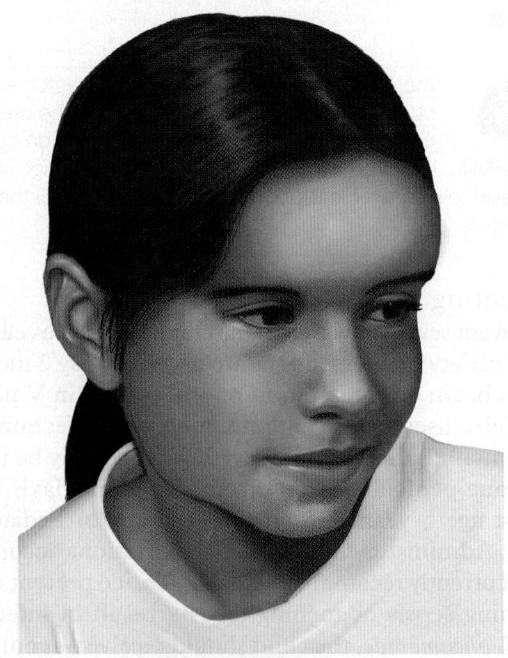

● **Figure 26.8** Iron overload related to thalassemia leads to bony changes such as frontal bossing and maxillary prominence.

Administering Packed Red Blood Cell Transfusions

Administer packed red blood cell transfusions as prescribed to maintain an adequate level of hemoglobin for oxygen delivery to the tissues and to suppress erythrocytosis in the bone marrow. Monitor for reactions to the transfusions.

Providing Chelation

Excess iron (hemosiderosis) is removed by chelation therapy. Administer the chelating agent Desferal (deferoxamine) with the transfusion. Deferoxamine binds to the iron and allows it to be removed through the stool or urine.

Educating the Family

Educate the child and family about the recommended regimen. Ensure that families understand that adhering to the prescribed blood transfusion and chelation therapy schedule is essential to the child's survival. Chelation therapy must be maintained at home to continuously decrease the iron levels in the body. Teach family members to administer deferoxamine subcutaneously with a small battery-powered infusion pump over a several-hour period each night (usually while the child is sleeping).

Refer the family for genetic counseling and family support as needed. Resources for families of children with thalassemia include:

- Cooley's Anemia Foundation: 1-800-522-7222 (www.thalassemia.org)
- Thalassemia Action Group, 129-09 26th Avenue, #203, Flushing, NY 11354; 1-800-522-7222

Glucose-6-Phosphate Dehydrogenase (G6PD) Deficiency

G6PD is an enzyme that is responsible for maintaining the integrity of RBCs by protecting them from oxidative substances. G6PD deficiency is an X-linked recessive disorder that occurs when the RBCs have insufficient G6PD, or the enzyme is abnormal and does not function properly. The RBCs are then affected by oxidative stress more easily. Triggers that may result in oxidative stress and hemolysis include bacterial or viral illness or exposure to certain substances (Miller, 2002), such as medications (e.g., sulfonamides, sulfones, malaria-fighting drugs [such as quinine], or methylene blue for treating urinary tract infections), naphthalene (an agent in mothballs), or fava beans (Pradell, 2003).

G6PD deficiency is most common in males of African decent. Other groups with G6PD deficiency are from the Mediterranean basin, including Italians, Greeks, Arabs, and Sephardic Jews. The condition tends to be less severe in those of African decent and more severe in those of Mediterranean decent. Complications include prolonged neonatal jaundice and life-threatening acute episodes of hemolysis. Therapeutic management is primarily aimed at avoiding triggers that cause oxidative stress.

Nursing Assessment

Note health history, including fatigue. Determine the parents' understanding of the disorder and the medications and foods to avoid. Inspect the skin for pallor or jaundice. Evaluate neurologic status, as it may also be affected. Measure heart rate and respiratory rate, noting elevations. Determine oxygen saturation via pulse oximeter or blood gas analysis. Note tea-colored urine. Palpate the abdomen for splenomegaly. Laboratory studies will reveal anemia (Pradell, 2003).

Nursing Management

Administer oxygen and treat the symptoms. Once the trigger agent is removed or the child recovers from an illness, the child will improve. Provide further education to the child and family about triggers and advise them that the child should avoid contact with these agents.

Clotting Disorders

Clotting is a process that occurs after injury. The blood clotting system requires certain factors in the blood and platelets to perform adequately. Individuals with deficiencies of these factors or platelets tend to bleed; they do not bleed more easily than people without these conditions, but it is just more difficult for the clot to form, and bleeding cannot be stopped easily. Factors that are most often involved in problems with clotting include factor VIII, factor IX, and factor XI. Each plays a role in clot formation. Platelets also play a role in the clotting cascade and are necessary for clot formation. Some processes can lead to destruction of the platelets and may lead to a reduction in clotting. Bleeding times are prolonged when a clotting disorder is present. Table 26.4 gives usual values for clotting studies.

Conditions affecting clotting include idiopathic thrombocytopenia purpura, Henoch-Schonlein purpura, disseminated intravascular coagulation, and factor deficiencies such as hemophilia A (factor VIII deficiency), von Willebrand disease, hemophilia B (Christmas disease, factor IX deficiency), and hemophilia C (factor XI deficiency). Table 26.5 reviews the proteins involved in coagulation.

• IDIOPATHIC THROMBOCYTOPENIA PURPURA

Idiopathic thrombocytopenia purpura (ITP) is thought to be an immune response following a viral infection that produces antiplatelet antibodies. These antibodies destroy platelets, which then leads to the development of petechiae, purpura, and excessive bruising. Petechiae are pinpoint

Table 26.4 Clotting Studies

Test	Measure
Prothrombin time (PT)	11.0–13.0 seconds (may vary by laboratory)
Partial thromboplastin time (PTT) Activated partial thromboplastin time (aPTT)	21–35 seconds
International Normalized Ratio (INR) (used to evaluate coagulation)	2.0–3.0 usual target in thromboembolic conditions

Data from Fischbach, F. T. (2004). *A manual of laboratory and diagnostic tests* (7th ed.). Philadelphia: Lippincott Williams & Wilkins.

hemorrhages that occur anywhere on the body and do not blanch to pressure (Fig. 26.9). **Purpura** are larger areas of hemorrhage in which blood collects under the tissues. They are purplish (see Fig. 26.9). ITP usually develops about 1 to 4 weeks after a viral infection. Remission is seen in 80% to 90% of the children in 6 to 9 months (Yetman, 2003). Complications include severe hemorrhage and bleeding into vital organs and intracranial hemorrhage, although these rarely occur.

For children with platelet counts below 20,000/mm^3, corticosteroids or intravenous immunoglobulin may be used. Prednisone or prednisolone is administered for 2 to 3 weeks, or until platelet counts increase above 30,000/mm^3. Intravenous immunoglobulin (IVIG) will be infused for 1 to 3 days. Platelet transfusions are not indicated unless a life-threatening condition such as intracranial hemorrhage is present. Refer the child for follow-up care with a pediatric hematologist. ITP is

Table 26.5 Select Proteins Involved in Coagulation (Factors)

Protein	Synonym	Concentration in Plasma (mg/dL)	Function
Fibrinogen	Factor I	200–400	Converted fibrin along with platelets to form clot
Factor II	Prothrombin	10–15	Is converted to thrombin (IIa), splits fibrinogen into fibrin
Factor V	Proaccelerin; labile factor	0.5–1.0	Supports Xa activation of II to IIa
Factor VII	Stable factor; proconvertin	0.2	Activates X
Factor VIII:C	Antihemophilic factor (AHF); platelet cofactor I	1.0–2.0	Supports IXa activation of X
Factor IX	Christmas factor; plasma thromboplastin component (PTC)	0.3–0.4	Activates X
Factor X	Stewart-Prower factor (AVTD prothrombin III)	0.6–0.8	Activates II
Factor XI	Plasma thromboplastin antecedent (anti-hemophilic factor C)	0.4	Activates XII and prekallikrein
Factor XII	Hageman factor	2.9	Activates XI and prekallikrein
Factor XIII	Fibrin-stabilizing factor; Laki-Lorand factor	2.5	Cross-links fibrin and other proteins
von Willebrand factor	Factor VIII–related antigen (VIII:VWD)	1.0	Stabilizes VIII, mediates platelet adhesion

Data from Fischbach, F. T. (2004). *A manual of laboratory and diagnostic tests* (7th ed.). Philadelphia: Lippincott Williams & Wilkins.

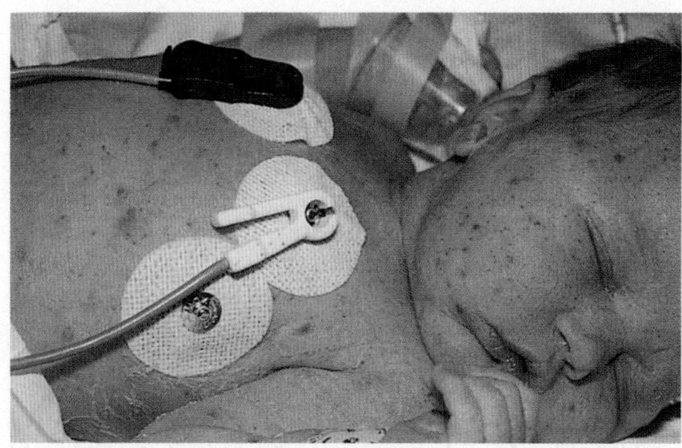

● Figure 26.9 Pinpoint hemorrhages (petechiae) and large purplish areas of discoloration (purpura) in an infant with ITP.

usually self-limiting, but if it persists for a year or longer, splenectomy may be indicated (Yetman, 2003).

Nursing Assessment

Elicit the child's health history (usually a previously healthy child who recently has developed increased bruising, epistaxis, or bleeding of the gums). Note history of blood in the stool. Note risk factors such as recent viral illness, recent MMR immunization, or ingestion of medications that can cause thrombocytopenia. Inspect for petechiae, purpura, and bruising, which may progress rapidly within the first 24 to 48 hours of the illness. Document the size and location of each lesion. Inspect the lips and buccal mucosa for petechiae. The remainder of the physical examination is usually within normal limits.

Usual laboratory findings include extremely low platelet count (<50,000), normal WBC count and differential, and normal hemoglobin and hematocrit unless hemorrhage has occurred (rare). Bone marrow aspiration may be performed to rule out leukemia.

Nursing Management

Many children require no medical treatment except observation and re-evaluation of laboratory values. Educate the family about avoiding aspirin, non-steroidal anti-inflammatory drugs (NSAIDs), and antihistamines because these medications may precipitate the development of anemia in these children. The use of acetaminophen for pain control is more appropriate when necessary. Teach the family to prevent trauma by avoiding activities that may cause injury; participating in contact sports is not recommended, specifically activities where direct contact can lead to injury or trauma. Activities such as swimming provide physical activity with less risk of trauma. Parents also need to know the signs and symptoms of serious bleeding and whom to call if it is suspected.

● HENOCH-SCHONLEIN PURPURA

Henoch-Schonlein purpura is a condition that in children develops in association with a viral or bacterial infection; in adults, drugs or toxins usually cause it. The classic presentation is vasculitis with IgA-dominant immune deposits affecting small vessels. These small vessels are generally in the skin, gut, and kidney (Fervenza, 2003). In most children the course of the disease is benign and the prognosis is good. In a few, however, ongoing nephrotic syndrome may occur as a result of renal injury, and those children may have hypertension. Pulmonary, cardiac, and neurologic complications can also occur.

No specific treatment exists for Henoch-Schonlein purpura, since most of the cases resolve without treatment. Treatment with corticosteroids, such as prednisone, is reserved for children with persistent symptoms. If renal injury occurs, children may require renal function testing, and evaluation for hypertension and treatment when present.

Nursing Assessment

Note history of viral or bacterial infection. Determine the onset of the complaint and how it has progressed or changed. Note history of joint or abdominal pain. Measure blood pressure. Inspect the skin for a purpuric palpable rash, and document the size and location of lesions. Palpate the rash to determine its extent (Fig. 26.10). Gently palpate the joints for tenderness. Palpate the abdomen for location of tenderness. Note visible or occult blood in the stool. Note cherry- or tea-colored urine, indicating the presence of blood in the urine. Urinalysis can verify the amount of blood present in the urine. Serum IgA levels may be elevated (Fervenza, 2003).

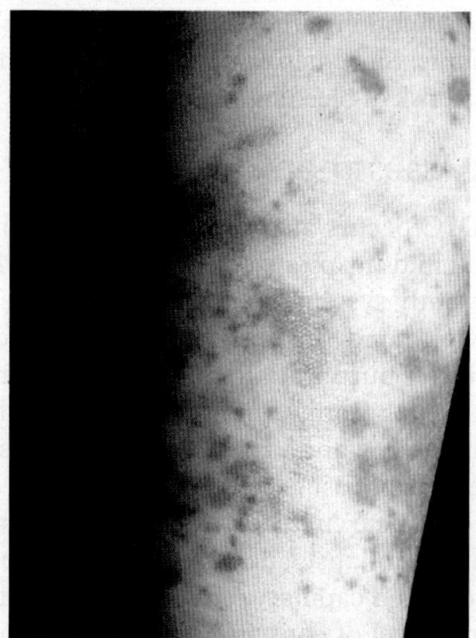

● Figure 26.10 Palpable purpura on an adolescent's arm.

Nursing Management

Treatment of the symptoms is the focus. In patients with severe joint or abdominal pain, administer analgesics as prescribed and note the response to pain medications. If the child has normal renal function, maintaining hydration is the most important intervention. Monitor intake and output. Note the color of urine. Administer corticosteroids and anticoagulants, alone or together, if ordered to reduce renal impairment (Fervenza, 2003). Teach the child and family about the therapy, such as management of hypertension with medications, and sodium restriction. Teach them about signs of renal injury such as blood in the urine and changes in weight, as well as frequency and volume of urine output.

DISSEMINATED INTRAVASCULAR COAGULATION

Disseminated intravascular coagulation (DIC) is a complex condition that leads to activation of coagulation; it usually occurs in critically ill children. Common triggers of DIC include septic shock, presence of endotoxins and viruses, tissue necrosis or injury, and cancer treatment. In DIC, thrombin is generated, fibrin is deposited in the circulation, and platelets are consumed. Deficiencies of coagulation and anticoagulation pathways occur. Hemorrhage and organ tissue damage result and can be irreversible if not recognized and treated immediately (Franchini & Manzato, 2004).

Therapeutic management of children with DIC requires careful consideration of the etiology. Initial treatment focuses on treating the underlying cause. For example, if DIC occurs secondary to an infection, appropriate antibiotics would be used to treat the infection. Heparin is also used at lower doses to counteract the deficiency in the coagulation/anticoagulation pathway. Heparin reduces consumption of the platelets, resulting in improved platelet counts. Since heparin is an anticoagulant, there is an increased risk of bleeding.

Nursing Assessment

Because DIC occurs as a secondary condition, it may occur in a child hospitalized for any reason. DIC may affect any body system, so a thorough physical examination is warranted. Inspect for signs of bleeding such as petechiae or purpura, blood in the urine or stool, or persistent oozing from venipuncture or from the umbilical cord in the newborn. Evaluate respiratory status and determine level of tissue oxygenation via pulse oximetry. Perform a complete circulatory assessment and note signs of circulatory collapse such as poor perfusion, tachycardia, prolonged capillary refill, and weak distal pulses. Note altered level of consciousness and decreased urine output. Careful abdominal palpation may reveal hepatomegaly or splenomegaly.

Laboratory testing may reveal prolonged prothrombin time (PT), partial thromboplastin time (PTT) or activated partial thromboplastin time (aPTT), bleeding time, and thrombin time and decreased levels of fibrinogen, platelets, clotting factors II, V, VIII, and X, and antithrombin III. Increases will be noted in levels of fibrinolysin, fibrinopeptide A, positive fibrin split products, and D-dimers (Fischbach, 2004).

Nursing Management

Continue to provide nursing care related to the triggering event. Assess the patient's status frequently. If bleeding is observed, apply pressure to the area along with cold compresses. Elevate the affected body part if this does not affect the patient's overall stability. If neurologic deficits are assessed, report the findings immediately so that treatment to prevent permanent damage can be started. Administer anticoagulation therapy (even though hemorrhage is a concern) to interrupt the coagulation process present in this condition. Provide ventilatory support as needed and provide continuous cardiac monitoring. Administer clotting factors, platelets, and cryoprecipitate as prescribed to prevent severe hemorrhage (Franchini & Manzato, 2004). Report changes in laboratory values to the physician. Changes can occur rapidly, and vigilance is necessary to prevent further tissue damage to the affected system.

HEMOPHILIA

Hemophilia is a group of X-linked recessive disorders that result in deficiency in one of the coagulation factors in the blood. X-linked recessive disorders are transmitted by carrier mothers to their sons, so usually only males are affected by hemophilia. The coagulation factors in the blood are essential for clot formation either spontaneously or from an injury, and when factors are absent bleeding will be difficult to stop. There are several types of hemophilia, including factor VIII deficiency (hemophilia A), factor IX deficiency or Christmas disease (hemophilia B), and factor XI deficiency (hemophilia C) (Curry, 2004; Miller, 2004). The most common is hemophilia A, and it will be the focus of this discussion. Hemophilia A occurs when there is a deficiency of factor VIII in an individual. Factor VIII is essential in the activation of factor X, which is required for the conversion of prothrombin into thrombin, resulting in an inability of the platelets to be used in clot formation.

Hemophilia is classified according to the severity of the disease, ranging from mild to severe. The more severe the disease, the more likely there will be bleeding episodes. When bleeding occurs the vessels constrict and a platelet plug forms, but because of the deficient factor the fibrin will not solidify, and thus bleeding continues (Miller, 2004).

Therapeutic Management

The primary goal is to prevent bleeding. This is best accomplished by avoiding activities with a high potential for injury (e.g., football, riding motorcycles, skateboarding) and instead participating in those with the least amount of contact (e.g., swimming, running, tennis). Limiting activities does not mean the child should do nothing; activities that promote health without increased exposure to injury are best.

If bleeding or injury occurs, factor administration is prescribed; this practice has been common in outpatient facilities or the patient's home for many years. Once the deficient factor is replaced, clotting factors return to fairly normal levels for a period of time. Factor replacement should be given prior to any surgeries or other traumas that can lead to bleeding, such as intramuscular injections and dental care.

Nursing Assessment

For a full description of the assessment phase of the nursing process, refer to page 870. Assessment findings pertinent to hemophilia in children are discussed below.

Health History

Elicit the health history, determining the nature of the bleeding episode or bruise. Include in the history any hemorrhagic episodes in other systems, such as the gastrointestinal tract (e.g., black tarry stools, hematemesis) or as a result from injury resulting in joint hemorrhage, or hematuria (Fig. 26.11). Inquire about length of bleeding and amount of blood loss. Because hemophilia A results in difficulty with clotting, the child may bleed for a longer period when injury occurs.

Physical Examination

Focus the physical examination on identification of any bleeding. This is of particular concern after injury, but a nosebleed or other spontaneous bleed can occur if factor levels are extremely low. Assess circulation by evaluating pulses and heart sounds if severe or prolonged bleeding is identified; without intervention, hypovolemia could follow, leading to shock. Note chest pain or abdominal pain, which may indicate internal bleeding. Report these findings immediately so that the underlying condition can be diagnosed and treated rapidly.

Laboratory and Diagnostic Testing

Laboratory findings may include decreased hemoglobin and hematocrit if bleeding is prolonged or severe. Factor levels may be quantified with blood testing.

Nursing Management

Nursing management includes preventing bleeding episodes, managing bleeding episodes, and providing education and support.

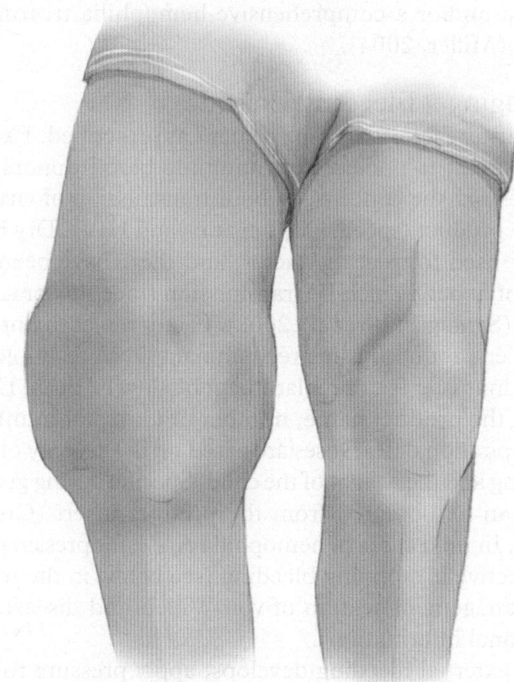

● Figure 26.11 Significant swelling and discoloration associated with a bleeding episode in a hemophiliac's knee.

Preventing Bleeding Episodes

All patients with hemophilia should attempt to prevent bleeding episodes. Major bleeds into the joints may limit range of motion and function, eventually decreasing physical abilities and crippling some boys. Teach children and families that regular physical activity or exercise helps to keep the muscles and joints stronger, and children with stronger joints and muscles experience fewer bleeding episodes (see Teaching Guideline 26.2). Refer the child with moderate to severe hemophilia to a pediatric hema-

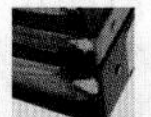

TEACHING GUIDELINE 26.2

Preventing Bleeding in the Child With Hemophilia

- Protect toddlers with soft helmets, padding on the knees, carpets in the home, and softened or covered corners.
- Children should stay active: swimming, baseball, basketball, and bicycling (wearing a helmet) are good physical activities.
- Avoid intense contact sports such as football, wrestling, soccer, and high diving.
- Avoid trampoline use and riding all-terrain vehicles (ATVs).
- Arrange premedication with Amicar if oral surgery is indicated.

tologist and/or a comprehensive hemophilia treatment center (Miller, 2004).

Managing a Bleeding Episode

Administer factor VIII replacement as prescribed. Factor replacement is pooled from multiple blood donors, so families may be concerned about transmission of viruses via the product (specifically hepatitis and HIV). Dry heat is now used to treat the factor, and there have been no cases of hepatitis or HIV transmission since this practice began (Santagostino et al., 2002). Factor replacement has also been produced using recombinant DNA technology.

Administer factor replacement by slow IV push. Document the product name, number of units, lot number, and expiration date. Doses are based on the severity of the bleeding and the weight of the child. Specific dosing guidelines can be obtained from the product insert (Curry, 2004). In mild cases of hemophilia A, desmopressin may be effective in stopping bleeding (see below in the nursing management section of von Willebrand disease for additional information).

If external bleeding develops, apply pressure to the area until bleeding stops. If it is inside a joint, apply ice or cold compresses to the area and elevate any injured extremities, except when contraindicated by further injury. Make sure that all cases of bleeding are followed up to identify whether factor replacement is necessary.

Providing Education

Inform the family that the child should wear a health alert bracelet. Families should notify the school nurse and teachers of the child's diagnosis and share precautions with them; they should be instructed to call the parent immediately if the child sustains a head, abdominal, or orbit injury at school. Teach parents and caregivers how to administer the intravenous infusion of factor VIII. Administration in the home is the preferred method for factor infusion, as the child will be able to receive treatment in the most timely and efficient manner when a bleeding episode occurs. Alternatives to the parent giving the infusion is to arrange for a home care nursing visit or for the family to keep their own supply of factor VIII that they take to the local emergency room for infusion if bleeding occurs. Involve children as developmentally appropriate in the infusion process. Young children may hold and apply the Band-Aid; older children may assist with dilution and mixing of the factor; and teens should be taught to administer their own factor infusions.

Children with severe hemophilia may need factor infusions so often that implantation of a central venous access port is warranted. Teach the family access, care, and flushing of the implanted port.

Providing Support

Children with hemophilia may be able to lead a fairly normal life, with the exception of avoiding a few activities. However, accepting the diagnosis of a bleeding disorder in their child is very difficult for parents. They fear the worst (bleeding that won't stop) as well as complications such as infection with blood-borne viruses. Reassure parents that since 1986, when factor replacement began to be treated with heat, there have been no reports of virus transmission from factor infusion. Educate and support the parents. Factor replacement is expensive and bleeding episodes often cause parents to miss work, both of which create financial strains. Refer families to the National Hemophilia Foundation (116 West 32nd Street, 11th Floor, New York, NY 10001; 1-800-42-HANDI or 1-212-328-3700; www.hemophilia.org/). Children may benefit from the services provided by NHF Youthworld (www.nhfyouthworld.org/), which offers support, education, youth leadership, scholarships, and a directory of camps for children with hemophilia and other bleeding disorders.

VON WILLEBRAND DISEASE

von Willebrand disease (vWD) is a genetically transmitted bleeding disorder that may affect both genders and all races. The disorder is a deficiency in von Willebrand factor (vWF). Under ordinary circumstances vWF serves two functions: to bind with factor VIII, protecting it from breakdown, and to serve as the "glue" that attaches platelets to the site of injury. Deficiency in this factor results in a mild bleeding disorder. Children with vWD bruise easily, have frequent nosebleeds (epistaxis), and tend to bleed after oral surgery. Pubescent girls often have menorrhagia.

Therapeutic management of vWD is similar to that of hemophilia. Prevention of injury is important. When bleeding or injury does occur, vWF is administered. Desmopressin may also be used to release the factors necessary for clotting. Desmopressin (DDAVP) raises the plasma level from stores in the endothelium of blood vessels (Curry, 2004; Santagostino et al., 2002). This releases factor VIII and vWF from these stores into the bloodstream. These may also be administered prior to dental work or surgery.

Nursing Assessment

Nursing assessment of the child with vWD is similar to the assessment of the child with hemophilia, though severe bleeding occurs much less frequently.

Nursing Management

Nursing management is also similar to the management of the child with hemophilia. The major difference is the administration of desmopressin. Administer desmopressin nasal spray as prescribed when a bleeding episode occurs. Desmopressin may also be given via an intravenous infusion or subcutaneously (less common). Stimate is the only brand of desmopressin nasal spray that is used for controlling bleeding; the other brands are used for homeostasis and enuresis (Curry, 2004). Desmopressin is an antidiuretic hormone, so closely monitor fluid balance. It should be used for 3 days in a row only, as lessening of the response (tachyphylaxis) occurs with frequent use. vWD may also be treated with intravenous infusion of vWF, similar to factor VIII infusion for hemophilia A. Teach children and their families how to avoid or minimize bleeding episodes (see Teaching Guidelines 26.2).

References

Books and Journals

Abrams, A. C. (2004). *Clinical drug therapy: Rationales for nursing practice* (7th ed.). Philadelphia: Lippincott Williams & Wilkins.

Ackley, B. J., & Ladwig, G. B. (2004). *Nursing diagnosis handbook: A guide to planning care* (6th ed.). St. Louis: Mosby.

Adams, W. G., Geva, J., Coffman, J., Palfry, S., & Bauchner, H. (1998). Anemia and elevated lead levels in underimmunized inner-city children. *Pediatrics, 101.*

Ambruso, D. R., Hays, T., Lane, P. A., & Nuss, R. (2005). Hematologic disorders. In W. W. Hay, M. J. Levin, J. M. Sondheimer, & R. R. Deterding (Eds.), *Current pediatric diagnosis & treatment* (17th ed.). New York: McGraw-Hill.

American Academy of Pediatrics, Committee on Drugs. (1995). Treatment guidelines for lead exposure in children. *Pediatrics, 96*(1), 155–160.

American Academy of Pediatrics, Committee on Environmental Health. (1998). Screening for elevated blood lead levels. *Pediatrics, 101*(6), 1172–1178.

American Academy of Pediatrics, Committee on Environmental Health. (1999). Iron fortification of infant formulas. *Pediatrics, 104*(1), 119–123.

American Academy of Pediatrics, Committee on Practice and Ambulatory Medicine. (2005). *Recommendations for preventive pediatric health care.* Available online at www.aap.org.

American Academy of Pediatrics, Section on Hematology/Oncology and Committee on Genetics. (2002). Health supervision for children with sickle cell disease. *Pediatrics 109*(3), 526–535.

Anonymous. (1999). Anaemia. Retrieved 8/31/05 from www.fortunecity.com/greenfield/rattler/46/Anaemia.html.

Anonymous. (1999). Formation of blood cells (haemopoiesis). Retrieved 8/31/05 from http://greenfield.fortunecity.com/rattler/46/haemopoiesis.htm.

Carey, R. G., Dufour, R., Farkas, D. H., Jamieson, B., Kurec, A., Kafka, M. T., et al. (2005). Complete blood count. Retrieved 8/26/05 from http://www.labtestsonline.org/understanding/analytes/cbc/glance.html.

Carley, A. (2003). Anemia: When is it iron deficiency? *Pediatric Nursing, 29*(2), 127–133.

Catlin, A. J. (2003). Thalassemia: The facts and the controversies. *Pediatric Nursing, 29*(6), 447–451.

Centers for Disease Control and Prevention. (2002). Iron deficiency—United States, 1999–2000. *Morbidity and Mortality Weekly Report, 51*(40), 897–899.

Curry, H. (2004). Bleeding disorder basics. *Pediatric Nursing, 30*(5), 402–429.

Eckman, J. R., & Platt, A. F. (1991). *Problem-oriented management of sickle syndromes.* Atlanta: Grady Memorial Hospital.

Environmental Protection Agency. (2005). Where lead is found [electronic version]. Available at http://www.epa.gov/lead/leadinfo.htm#where.

Fervenza, F. C. (2003). Henoch-Schonlein purpura nephritis. *International Journal of Dermatology, 42,* 170–177.

Fischbach, F. T. (2004). *A manual of laboratory and diagnostic tests* (7th ed.). Philadelphia: Lippincott Williams & Wilkins.

Franchini, M., & Manzato, F. (2004). Update on the treatment of disseminated intravascular coagulation. *Hematology, 9*(2), 81–85.

Gunnarsson, B. S., Thorsdottir, I., & Palsson, G. (2004). Iron status in 2-year-old Icelandic children and associations with dietary intake and growth. *European Journal of Clinical Nutrition, 58,* 901–906.

Gustafson, M. P. (2001). An adolescent with a polymorphous rash. *Nurse Practitioner, 26*(7), 48, 50–52.

Human Genome Management Information System. (2004). Genetic disease profile: Sickle cell anemia. Retrieved 12/15/05 from http://www.ornl.gov/sci/techresources/Human_Genome/posters/chromosome/sca.shtml.

Irwin, J. J., & Kirchner, J. T. (2001). Anemia in children. *American Family Physician, 64*(8), 1379–1386.

Jones, R. J., & Brodsky, R. A. (2005). Aplastic anemia. *Lancet, 365,* 1647–1656.

Kimball, J. W. (2005). Blood. Retrieved August 26, 2005, from http://users.rcn.com/jkimball.ma.ultranet/BiologyPages/B/Blood.html.

Lozoff, B., DeAndraca, I., Castillo, M., Smith, J. B., Walter, T., & Pino, P. (2003). Behavioral and developmental effects of preventing iron-deficiency anemia in healthy full-term infants. *Pediatrics, 112*(4), 846–854.

Martin, P. L., & Pearson, H. A. (1999). Hemoglobinopathies and thalassemias. In J. A. McMillan (Ed.), *Oski's pediatrics: Principles and practice.* Philadelphia: Lippincott Williams & Wilkins.

Miller, K. L. (2004). Factor products in the treatment of hemophilia. *Journal of Pediatric Health Care, 18,* 156–157.

Miller, R. (2002). Anemia. Retrieved 8/26/05 from http://www.kidshealth.org/parent/medical/heart/anemia.html.

Morrissey-Ross, M. (2000). Lead poisoning and its elimination: An opportunity for success. *Public Health Nursing, 17*(4), 229–230.

Myer, S. A., & Oliva, J. (2002). Severe aplastic anemia and allogeneic hematopoietic stem cell transplantation. *AACN Clinical Issues, 13*(2), 169–191.

National Heart, Lung and Blood Institute (NHLBI) of the National Institutes of Health, Diseases and Conditions Index. (2005). Sickle cell anemia. Retrieved 8/26/05 from http://www.nhlbi.nih.gov/health/dci/Diseases/Sca/SCA_All.html.

National Newborn Screening and Genetics Resource Center. (2005). National newborn screening and status report [electronic version] available at http://genes-r-us.uthscsa.edu/nbsdisorders.pdf.

Nead, K. G., Halterman, J. S., Kaczorowski, J. M., Auinger, P., & Weitzman, M. (2004). Overweight children and adolescents: A risk group for iron deficiency. *Pediatrics, 114*(1), 104–108.

Pagana, K. D., & Pagana, T. J. (2002). *Mosby's manual of diagnostic and laboratory tests* (2nd ed.). St. Louis: Mosby, Inc.

Pradell, L. (2003). G6PD deficiency. Retrieved 9/4/05 from www.kidshealth.org/parent/general/aches/g6pd.html.

Platt, A., Eckman, J. R., Beasley, J., & Miller, G. (2002). Treating sickle cell pain: An update from the Georgia Comprehensive Sickle Cell Center. *Journal of Emergency Nursing, 28*(4), 297–303.

Proscio, T. (2004). Healthy housing, healthy families: Toward a national agenda for affordable healthy homes. Retrieved 8/29/05 from http://www.enterprisefoundation.org.

Ruble, K. (2005). Pediatric hematologic disorders. In S. M. Nettina (Ed.), *Lippincott manual of nursing practice.* Philadelphia: Lippincott Williams & Wilkins.

Santagostino, E., Gringeri, A., & Mannucci, P. M. (2002). State of care for hemophilia in pediatric patients. *Pediatric Drugs, 4*(3), 149–157.

Sickle Cell Disease Care Consortium. (2002). *Outpatient evaluation and management of pain in child with sickle cell disease.* Retrieved March 28, 2007 from http://www.scinfo.org/protpainOP.htm.

Taketokmo, C. K., Hodding, J. H., & Kraus, D. M. (2004). *Lexi-comp's pediatric dosage handbook* (11th ed.). Hudson, OH: Lexi-comp.

Tomlinson, D., & Kline, N. E. (eds.) (2005). *Pediatric oncology nursing.* New York: Springer.

Trigg, M. E. (2004). Hematopoietic stem cells. *Pediatrics, 113*(4), 1051–1057.

Velsor-Friedrich, B. (2002). The silent epidemic: Lead poisoning. *Journal of Pediatric Nursing, 17*(1), 59–61.

Yetman, R. J. (2003). Evaluation and management of childhood idiopathic (immune) thrombocytopenia. *Journal of Pediatric Health Care, 17*(5), 261–263.

Zetterstrom, R. (2004). Iron deficiency and iron deficiency anaemia during infancy and childhood. *Acta Paediatrica, 93,* 436–439.

Websites

www.aeclp.org Alliance for Healthy Homes (originally the Alliance to End Childhood Lead Poisoning)—resources for the prevention of lead poisoning

www.aplastic.org Aplastic Anemia and Myelodysplasia International Foundation—resources for patient assistance and emotional support

www.ascaa.org American Sickle Cell Anemia Association—resources, education, and support

www.cdc.gov Centers for Disease Control and Prevention (CDC)—multiple health resources available

www.cehrc.org Community Environmental Health Resource Center—resources for prevention of lead poisoning

www.enterprisefoundation.org resources for lead removal from homes

www.epa.gov/lead/index.html National Lead Awareness Program

www.fns.usda.gov/wic/ Women, Infants and Children program of the Food and Nutrition Service of the U.S. Department of Agriculture—provides supplemental foods to low-income children up to 5 years of age

www.healthypeople.gov *Healthy People 2010*

www.hematology.org American Society of Hematology—provides information related to blood, blood-forming tissues, and blood diseases

www.hemophilia.org/ National Hemophilia Foundation—resources, education, research, and support

www.hud.gov U.S. Department of Housing and Urban Development—resources for lead removal from homes

www.irondisorders.org Iron Disorders Institute—mission is to reduce pain, suffering, and death related to disorders involving iron

www.leadsafe.org/ Coalition to End Childhood Lead Poisoning

www.nhfyouthworld.org/ National Hemophilia Foundation Youthworld—website for children with bleeding disorders

www.nhlbi.nih.gov National Heart, Lung, and Blood Institute—education and research related to heart, blood vessel, lung, and blood diseases

www.scinfo.org Sickle Cell Information Center—patient and professional education, news, research updates, and sickle cell resources.

www.sicklecelldisease.org Sickle Cell Disease Association of America—resources, support, and education

www.sicklecellkids.org website for children with sickle cell disease

www.thalassemia.org Cooley's Anemia Foundation—education, resources, and support

www.thearc.org/faqs/leadqa.html information on lead poisoning from the Arc

Chapter WORKSHEET

MULTIPLE CHOICE QUESTIONS

1. A child on the hematology unit has the following a.m. laboratory results: Hgb 10.0, Hct 30.2, WBC 24,000, platelets 20,000. What is the priority nursing assessment?
   a. Assess for pallor, fatigue, and tachycardia.
   b. Monitor for fever.
   c. Assess for bruising or bleeding.
   d. Determine intake and output.
2. A child with hemophilia fell while riding his bicycle. He was wearing a helmet and did not lose consciousness. He has a mild abrasion on his knee that is not oozing. He is complaining of abdominal pain. What is the priority nursing assessment?
   a. Perform neurologic checks.
   b. Assess ability to void frequently.
   c. Carefully assess abdomen.
   d. Examine his knee frequently.
3. A 14-year-old with thalassemia asks for your assistance in choosing her afternoon snack. Which choice is the most appropriate?
   a. Peanut butter with rice cake
   b. Small spinach salad
   c. Apple slices with cheddar cheese
   d. Small burger on wheat bun
4. The nurse is caring for a child who has just been admitted to the pediatric unit with sickle cell crisis. He is complaining that his right arm and leg hurt. What is the priority nursing intervention?
   a. Administer pain medication every 3 hours intravenously until pain is controlled.
   b. Perform passive range of motion of the arm and leg to maintain function.
   c. Try acetaminophen for pain first, moving up to opioids only if needed.
   d. Use narcotic analgesics and warm compresses as needed to control the pain.

CRITICAL THINKING EXERCISES

1. Develop a discharge teaching plan for the parent of a toddler who has just been diagnosed with hemophilia and received factor infusion treatment for a bleeding episode.
2. An 8-year-old girl has been diagnosed with iron deficiency anemia. Formulate a nutrition plan for this child.
3. A 5-year-old with beta-thalassemia is resistant to nightly chelation therapy at home. Devise a developmentally appropriate teaching plan for this child.
4. Develop a nursing care plan for a child with sickle cell disease who experiences frequent vaso-occlusive crises.

STUDY ACTIVITIES

1. Visit your local WIC office. Meet with the staff and learn about the services offered for prevention of and nutritional support for anemia. Provide a written report of your learning experience or provide a presentation to your classmates.
2. In the clinical setting, compare the growth and development of a child with sickle cell disease to that of a similarly aged child who has been healthy.
3. Talk to a teenager with hemophilia about his life experiences and feelings about his disease and his health. Reflect upon this conversation in your clinical journal.
4. Visit a public health clinic that provides primary care to children. Spend time with the registered nurse, the advanced practice nurse, and the unlicensed assistive personnel. Write a summary of the roles of the registered nurse in screening for and managing hematologic disorders in children, noting roles that are reserved for the advanced practice nurse and activities that the RN would delegate to unlicensed assistive personnel.

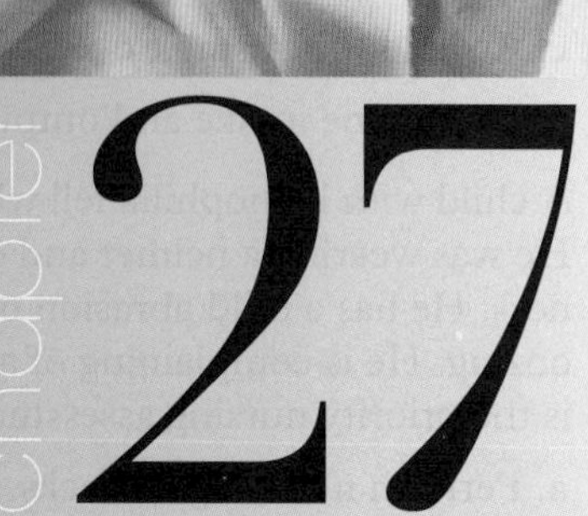

Nursing Care of the Child With an Immunologic Disorder

Key TERMS

antibodies
antigen
autoantibodies
B cells
cellular immunity
chemotaxis
complement
graft-versus host disease
humoral immunity
immunity
immunodeficiency
immunoglobulins
immunosuppressive
lymphocyte
neutrophil
opsonization
phagocytosis
stem cells
T cells

Learning OBJECTIVES

Upon completion of the chapter, the learner will be able to:

1. Explain anatomic and physiologic differences of the immune system in infants and children versus adults.
2. Describe nursing care related to common laboratory and diagnostic testing used in the medical diagnosis of pediatric immune and autoimmune disorders.
3. Distinguish immune and autoimmune disorders common in infants, children, and adolescents.
4. Identify appropriate nursing assessments and interventions related to medications and treatments for pediatric immune, autoimmune, and allergic disorders.
5. Develop an individualized nursing care plan for the child with an immune or autoimmune disorder.
6. Describe the psychosocial impact of chronic immune disorders on children.
7. Devise a nutrition plan for the child with immunodeficiency.
8. Develop patient/family teaching plans for the child with an immune or autoimmune disorder.

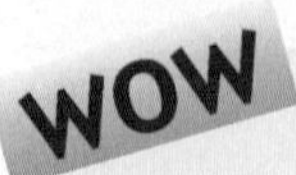

Resistance to disease can be a child's battle for life.

Lakeisha Harris, 15 years old, is brought to the clinic by her mother. She presents with complaints of pain and swelling in her joints, weight gain, and fatigue. Lakeisha states, "I'm just very tired all the time, and my knees and ankles ache."

Immunodeficiency, autoimmune, and allergic disorders have a significant impact on the lives of affected children. Infants and children are exposed to many infectious microorganisms and allergens and thus need a functional immune system to protect themselves. Temporary immune deficiencies may follow a common viral infection, surgery, or a blood transfusion. They may also be caused by malnutrition or smoking. Temporary immune depression returns to normal over a period of time. Primary or secondary immune deficiencies are the focus of this discussion, along with allergy and anaphylaxis. These immune disorders are chronic, and affected children have more infections than healthy children do. Recurrent viral or bacterial infections may cause the child to miss significant amounts of school or playtime with other children. Many immunodeficiencies require chronic and frequent clinic visits as well as daily medications. This can be a stress on the family as well. Autoimmune disorders are also chronic, causing significant disruption to the child's and family's life. Allergic disorders in some children may cause significant stress for the child and family. Nurses who care for children need to be familiar with common immunodeficiencies, autoimmune disorders, and allergies to intervene effectively with children and their families.

Variations in Pediatric Anatomy and Physiology

Normal immune function is a complex process involving **phagocytosis**, **humoral immunity**, **cellular immunity**, and activation of the **complement** system. The lymphatic system and the white blood cells (WBCs) are the primary "players" in the immune response. Though these structures and cells are present at birth, the healthy full-term infant's immune system is still immature. The newborn exhibits a decreased inflammatory response to invading organisms, and this increases his or her susceptibility to infection. Cellular immunity is generally functional at birth, and as the infant is exposed to various substances over time, humoral immunity develops. Comparison Chart 27.1 provides more information on humoral and cellular immunity.

Lymph System

Lymph nodes in the newborn are relatively small, soft, and difficult to palpate. As the infant is exposed to various germs or illnesses, the lymph system passively filters plasma for bacteria or other foreign material before returning it to the bloodstream and back to the heart. As WBCs infiltrate the lymph nodes to attack the foreign substance, the nodes enlarge. Young children have frequent episodes of localized enlarged lymph nodes because of their frequent exposure to viral illnesses. The spleen is functional at birth and also filters the blood for foreign cells. The thymus, responsible for the production of **lymphocyte T cells** as well as for the development and maturation of peripheral lymphoid tissue, is quite enlarged at birth and remains so until about 10 years of age. It then involutes slowly throughout adulthood. The tonsils are also often enlarged throughout early childhood. The bone marrow is functional at birth, producing **stem cells** capable of differentiating into various blood cells.

Phagocytosis

The newborn and infant under conditions of stress may have decreased phagocytic activity. The complement system, which is responsible for **opsonization** and **chemotaxis**, is immature in the newborn but reaches adult levels of activity by 3 to 6 months of age. The infant's phagocytic cells (**neutrophils** and monocytes) demonstrate decreased

COMPARISON CHART 27.1 Humoral Versus Cellular Immunity

Humoral Immunity (antibody protection)	Cellular Immunity (cell-mediated immune response)
• Lymphocytes: B cells	• Lymphocytes: T cells
• Secrete antibodies to viruses and bacteria	
• Recognize antigens	• Do not recognize antigens
• Antibodies mark the antigen cell for destruction.	• Direct and regulate immune response (helper T cells)
• Do not destroy the foreign cell	• Attack infected or foreign cells (killer T cells and natural killer cells)
• Crosses the placenta in the form of IgG	• Does not cross the placenta

chemotaxis, reaching adult levels when the child is several years old. With complement levels being only 50% to 75% of adult levels in the full-term infant, decreased opsonization may be responsible for decreased phagocytic activity compared with adults.

Cellular Immunity

Maternal T cells do not cross the placenta, so the fetal thymus begins production of T cells early in gestation, and the newborn demonstrates a relative lymphocytosis compared with the adult, probably due to increased amounts of T-cell lymphocytes. Though cellular immunity does not cross the placenta, the fetal T cells may become sensitized to antigens that do cross the placenta. Viral infection, hyperbilirubinemia, and drugs taken by the mother late in pregnancy may contribute to depressed T-cell function in the newborn. Since delayed hypersensitivity reactions are mediated by T cells rather than antibodies, skin test responses (such as PPD for tuberculosis detection) are diminished until about 1 year of age, probably due to the infant's decreased ability to mount an inflammatory response.

Humoral Immunity

The newborn's **B cells** do not respond as well to infection as do adults'. B cells are responsible for the formation of **antibodies** (specific immunity). The antibodies bind to the **antigen**, thus disabling the specific toxin. The fetus is normally in an antigen-free environment and so produces only trace amounts of IgM. Most of the newborn's IgG is acquired transplacentally from the mother. Hence, the newborn exhibits passive **immunity** to antigens to which the mother had developed antibodies. These antibodies wane over the first months of life as the transplacental IgG is catabolized, having a half-life of only about 25 days. The newborn begins to make IgG but ordinarily experiences a physiologic hypogammaglobulinemia between 2 and 6 months of age until self-production of IgG reaches higher levels. The breastfed infant will acquire passive transfer of maternal immunity via the breast milk and will be better protected during the physiologic hypogammaglobulinemia phase. By 1 year of age IgG is 70% of the adult level, and by 8 years of age it should reach the adult level.

IgA, IgD, IgE, and IgM do not cross the placenta; they require an antigenic challenge for production. IgD and IgE constitute a very small percentage of the **immunoglobulins** in all ages. IgA increases slowly to about 30% of the adult level at 1 year of age, reaching the adult level by age 11 years. IgM is close to the adult level by 1 year of age.

Common Medical Treatments

A variety of medications and other medical treatments are used to treat immune deficiencies and autoimmune problems in children. Most of these treatments will require a physician's order when the child is in the hospital. The most common treatments and medications are listed in Common Medical Treatments 27.1 and Drug Guide 27.1. The nurse caring for the child with an immune deficiency or autoimmune disorder should be familiar with what the procedures and medications are, how they work, and common nursing implications related to use of these modalities.

Nursing Process Overview for the Child With an Immunologic Disorder

Care of the child with an immunologic or allergic disorder includes assessment, nursing diagnosis, planning, interventions, and evaluation. There are a number of general concepts related to the nursing process that may be applied to immunodeficiencies and autoimmune disorders. From a general understanding of the care involved for a child with immune dysfunction, the nurse can then individualize the care based on patient specifics.

ASSESSMENT

Assessment of children with immunodeficiency, autoimmune disorders, or allergy includes health history, physical examination, and laboratory and diagnostic testing.

> Remember Lakeisha, the 15-year-old with joint pain and swelling, fatigue, and weight gain? What additional health history and physical examination assessment information should you obtain?

Health History

The health history comprises past medical history, including the mother's pregnancy history, family history, and history of present illness (when the symptoms started and how they have progressed), as well as medications and treatments used at home. The past medical history may be significant for maternal HIV infection; frequent, recurrent infections such as otitis media, sinusitis, or pneumonia; chronic cough; recurrent low-grade fever; two or more serious infections in early childhood; recurrent deep skin or organ abscesses; persistent thrush in the mouth; extensive eczema; or growth failure. Family history may be positive for primary immune deficiency or autoimmune disorder. Document history of known allergy. Note the response that occurs when the child encounters the allergen.

Physical Examination

Physical examination of the child with immunodeficiency or autoimmune disorder includes inspection and observation, auscultation, percussion, and palpation.

Inspection and Observation

Plot weight and length or height on appropriate growth charts. Inspect the oropharynx for tonsillar size. Note

Common Medical Treatments 27.1

Treatment	Explanation	Indication	Nursing Implications
Immunizations	Killed or modified microorganisms, or components of them, cause the immune system to develop antibodies to the microorganism without developing disease.	Prevention of certain viral and bacterial infections	Do not administer live vaccines to immunosuppressed persons. Refer to the individual vaccine for method of administration and contraindications. Report adverse reactions via the Vaccine Adverse Reaction (VAR) reporting system.
Bone marrow or stem cell transplantation	Bone marrow transplant: Transfer of healthy bone marrow into the bones of a person with immune malfunction; the transplanted cells can then develop into functional B and T cells. Stem cell transplant: Peripheral stem cells are removed from the donor via apheresis or stem cells are retrieved from the umbilical cord and placenta. The stem cells are then transplanted into the recipient.	Wiskott-Aldrich syndrome, SCID	Administer immunosuppressive medications as ordered. Maintain medical asepsis and protective isolation to prevent infection. Monitor closely for graft-versus-host disease. Provide meticulous oral care. Avoid rectal temperatures and suppositories. Encourage appropriate nutrition.

eczematous or other skin lesions, which may occur with allergic diseases or Wiskott-Aldrich syndrome. Document presence of thrush, which occurs frequently in children with immunodeficiency. Observe gait for unexplained ataxia (neurologic alterations occur with HIV infection).

Auscultation, Percussion, and Palpation

Auscultate the lungs for adventitious sounds, which may be present with a concurrent respiratory infection or as wheezing with an allergic reaction. Percuss the abdomen and determine liver span. Palpate for unusually enlarged lymph nodes, particularly in nonadjacent locations. Palpate the abdomen for enlarged spleen or liver.

Laboratory and Diagnostic Testing

Common Laboratory Diagnostic Tests 27.1 explains the laboratory and diagnostic tests most commonly used when considering immune disorders. Results of these tests may assist the physician in diagnosing the disorder and/or be used as guidelines in determining ongoing treatment. Laboratory or non-nursing personnel obtain some of the tests, while the nurse might obtain others. In either instance the nurse should be familiar with how the tests are obtained, what they are used for, and normal versus abnormal results. This knowledge will also be necessary when providing patient and family education related to the testing.

NURSING DIAGNOSES AND RELATED INTERVENTIONS

Upon completion of a thorough assessment, the nurse might identify several nursing diagnoses. These may include:

- Ineffective protection
- Imbalanced nutrition, less than body requirements
- Pain
- Impaired skin integrity
- Activity intolerance
- Delayed growth and development

> After completing an assessment of Lakeisha, you note the following: alopecia, abdominal tenderness, and oral ulcers. Based on these assessment findings, what would your top three nursing diagnoses be for Lakeisha?

Nursing goals, interventions, and evaluation for the child with an immunologic disorder are based on the nursing diagnoses. Nursing Care Plan Overview 27.1 can be used as a guide in planning nursing care for the child with an immunologic disorder, autoimmune disorder, or allergic response. It should be individualized based on the patient's symptoms and needs. Additional information will

Drug Guide 27.1 Common Drugs for Immunologic Disorders

Medication	Action	Indication	Nursing Implications
Intravenous immune globulin (IVIG); multiple manufacturers	Provides exogenous IgG antibodies	Primary immune deficiencies, HIV infection	Do not mix with IV medications or with other IV fluids. Do not give IM or SQ. Monitor vital signs and watch for adverse reactions frequently during infusion. May require antipyretic or antihistamine to prevent chills and fever during infusion. Have epinephrine available during infusion.
Nucleoside analogue reverse transcriptase inhibitors (NRTIs): abacavir, lamivudine, zidovudine	Inhibits reverse transcription of the viral DNA chain	Treatment of HIV-1 infection as part of a 3-drug regimen. Zidovudine is also used to prevent perinatal transmission of HIV.	Notify physician of muscle weakness, shortness of breath, headache, insomnia, rash, or unusual bleeding. Give IV zidovudine over 1 hour. Fatal hypersensitivity reaction may occur with abacavir.
Non-nucleoside analogue reverse transcriptase inhibitors (NNRTIs): efavirenz, nevirapine	Binds to HIV-1 reverse transcriptase, blocking DNA polymerase activity and disrupting the virus life cycle	Treatment of HIV-1 infection as part of a 3-drug regimen	*Nevirapine:* Avoid St. John's wort. Shake suspension gently before administration. Observe for symptoms of Stevens-Johnson syndrome. *Efavirenz:* May cause drowsiness
Protease inhibitors: amprenavir, atazanavir, indinavir, lopinavir, nelfinavir, ritonavir, saqinavir	Inhibits protease activity in the HIV-1 cell, resulting in immature, noninfectious viral particles	Treatment of HIV-1 infection as part of a 3-drug regimen	Multiple drug interactions. Review specific medication for adverse effects and administration implications.
Nonsteroidal anti-inflammatory drugs (NSAIDs): aspirin, trisalicylate, ibuprofen, naproxen, others	Inhibits prostaglandin synthesis, anti-inflammatory action	Juvenile idiopathic arthritis	Administer with food to decrease GI upset. May cause gastric bleeding, increased liver enzymes, decreased renal function. Monitor liver enzymes. Do not crush or chew extended-release or timed-release preparations. *Aspirin and trisalicylate:* Follow serum salicylate levels. Observe for signs of toxicity, including hyperventilation with heavy breathing, drowsiness, nausea, vomiting, bruising, tinnitus, hearing loss.
Corticosteroids (usual dosage)	Anti-inflammatory and immunosuppressive action	Juvenile idiopathic arthritis, SLE. Also used for immunosuppression in bone marrow or stem cell transplant patients.	Administer with food to decrease GI upset. May mask signs of infection. Monitor blood pressure, urine for glucose. Do not stop treatment abruptly or acute adrenal insufficiency may occur.

Drug Guide 27.1 Common Drugs for Immunologic Disorders (continued)

Medication	Action	Indication	Nursing Implications
			Monitor for Cushing syndrome. Doses may be tapered over time.
Intravenous pulse corticosteroids	Anti-inflammatory and immunosuppressive effects	Severe SLE or juvenile arthritis	As noted above. Monitor for hypertension during infusion.
Cytotoxic drugs (cyclophosphamide [Cytoxan])	Interferes with normal function of DNA by alkylation	Severe SLE	Causes bone marrow suppression. Monitor for signs of infection. *Cyclophosphamide:* Administer in the morning. Provide adequate hydration and have child void frequently during and after infusion to decrease risk of hemorrhagic cystitis.
Immunosuppressant drugs (cyclosporine A [CyA], azathioprine)	Inhibition of production and release of interleukin II (CyA). Antagonizes purine metabolism (azathioprine)	Severe steroid-resistant autoimmune disease	Monitor CBC, serum creatinine, potassium, and magnesium. Monitor blood pressure and watch for signs of infection. Draw blood levels before morning dose. *CyA:* Do not give with grapefruit juice.
Antimalarial drugs: hydroxychloroquine sulfate (Plaquenil)	Impairs complement-dependent antigen–antibody reactions	Control of arthritis and arthralgia in juvenile arthritis, SLE; control of skin disease in SLE; prevention of serious flares of juvenile arthritis and SLE	Funduscopic eye exam and visual field testing every year
Disease-modifying antirheumatic drugs (DMARDs): methotrexate, etanercept	Methotrexate: antimetabolite that depletes DNA precursors, inhibits DNA and urine synthesis. Etanercept: binds to tumor necrosis factor (TNF), rendering it ineffective.	Severe polyarticular juvenile arthritis	*Methotrexate:* Do not give oral form with dairy products. Approximate time to benefit in treatment of arthritis is 3 to 6 weeks. Salicylates may delay clearance. Protect IV preparation from light. Monitor CBC, renal and liver function, and symptoms of infection. *Etanercept:* Monitor closely for infection. Do not give live vaccines. Give SQ, twice weekly; effect in 1 week to 3 months.

Refer to Chap. 15 for a thorough explanation of assessment and management of pain.

be included later in the chapter as it relates to specific disorders.

> Based on your top three nursing diagnoses for Lakeisha, describe appropriate nursing interventions.

Primary Immunodeficiencies

More than 100 primary immunodeficiencies have been identified. They are mostly hereditary or congenital. About half of primary immunodeficiencies are humoral deficiencies. The remainder are combined (B- and T-cell

(text continues on page 909)

Common Laboratory and Diagnostic Tests 27.1

Test	Explanation	Indication	Nursing Implications
Complete blood count (CBC) with differential	Evaluate hemoglobin and hematocrit, WBC count (particularly the percentage of individual WBCs), and platelet count.	Infection, inflammatory process, immunosuppression	Normal values vary according to age and gender. WBC count differential is helpful in evaluating source of infection. May be affected by myelosuppressive drugs.
Immunoglobulin electrophoresis	Determines level of individual immunoglobulins (IgA, IgD, IgE, IgG, IgM) in the blood	Immune deficiency, autoimmune disorders	Normal levels vary with age. IVIG administration and steroids alter levels.
IgG subclasses	Measures the levels of the 4 subclasses of IgG (1, 2, 3, and 4)	Determine immune deficiency	Normal levels vary with age. IVIG administration and steroids alter levels.
Lymphocyte immunophenotyping T-cell quantification	Measures level of T cells (T-helper (CD4), T-suppressor (CD8)), B cells, and natural killer cells in the blood	Ongoing monitoring of progressive depletion of CD4 T lymphocytes in HIV disease	Do not refrigerate specimen. Steroids may elevate and immunosuppressive drugs may depress lymphocyte levels.
Delayed hypersensitivity skin test	Measures the presence of activated T cells that recognize certain substances	Immune disorders	Administered intradermally. Read and document size of reaction at 48 to 72 hours (tuberculosis, mumps, candida, tetanus).
Human immunodeficiency virus (HIV) antibodies	Used to detect antibodies to HIV	Determining HIV infection when suspected	ELISA method detects only antibodies, so may remain negative for several weeks up to 6 months (false-negative). False-positive may result with autoimmune disease. Requires serial testing. HIV test results are confidential.
Polymerase chain reaction (PCR)	Used to detect HIV DNA and RNA	Diagnosis of HIV infection in children over 1 month old	Sensitive and specific for presence of HIV in blood. Poor accuracy on samples obtained at birth. Sequential testing needed to determine perinatal transmission.
Complement assay (C3 and C4)	Measures the level of total complement in the blood, as well as levels of C3 and C4	Monitor SLE. Determine complement deficiency.	Send to laboratory immediately (unstable at room temperature). Usually sent out to a reference laboratory.
Erythrocyte sedimentation rate (ESR)	Nonspecific test used to determine presence of infection or inflammation	Immune disorder initial workup, ongoing monitoring of autoimmune disease	Send to laboratory immediately; if allowed to stand >3 hours, falsely low result may occur.
Rheumatoid factor (RF)	Determines the presence of RF in the blood	Juvenile idiopathic arthritis, SLE	Positive RF is also sometimes seen in chronic infectious disorders.
Antinuclear antibody (ANA)	Tests for presence of autoantibodies that react against cellular nuclear material	SLE	Check for signs of infection at venipuncture site. Steroid use can cause false-negative result. May be weakly positive in about 20% of healthy individuals.

Nursing Care Plan 27.1

Overview for the Child With an Immunologic Disorder

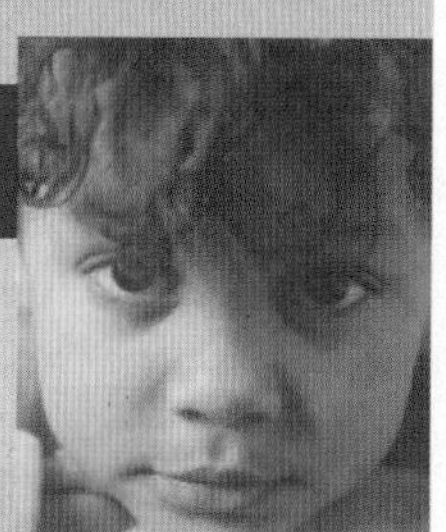

Nursing Diagnosis: Ineffective protection related to inadequate body defenses, inability to fight infection as evidenced by deficient immunity

Outcome identification and evaluation

Child will not experience overwhelming infection, *will be infection-free or able to recover if he or she becomes infected.*

Intervention: preventing infection

- Maintain meticulous hand washing procedures (include family, visitors, staff) *to minimize spread of infectious organisms.*
- Maintain isolation as prescribed *to minimize exposure to infectious organisms.*
- Clean frequently touched surfaces with an appropriate cleanser *to minimize spread of infectious organisms.*
- Educate family and visitors that child should be restricted from contact with known infectious exposures (in hospital and at home) *to encourage cooperation with infection control.*
- Strictly observe medical asepsis *to avoid unintentional introduction of microorganisms.*
- Promote nutrition and appropriate rest *to maximize body's potential to heal.*
- Educate family to contact health care provider if child has known exposure to chickenpox or measles *so that preventive measures (e.g., VZIG) can be taken.*
- Administer vaccines (not live) as prescribed *to prevent common childhood communicable diseases.*
- Administer prophylactic antibiotics as prescribed *to prevent infection with opportunistic organisms.*

Nursing Diagnosis: Imbalanced nutrition, less than body requirements, related to poor appetite, chronic illness, debilitated state, concurrent illness as evidenced by poor growth, weight gain and stature increases less than expected, poor head growth

Outcome identification and evaluation

Child will consume adequate intake, *will demonstrate appropriate weight gain and growth of length/height and/or head circumference.*

Intervention: promoting adequate nutritional intake

- Monitor growth (weight and height/length weekly) *to determine progress toward goal.*
- Determine realistic goal for weight gain for age (consulting dietitian if necessary) *to have a specific outcome to work toward.*
- Observe child's physical ability to eat *(if pain from candidiasis or motor impairment is present, will need additional interventions).*
- Provide nutrient-rich meals and snacks *to maximize caloric intake.*
- Supplement milkshakes with protein powder or other additives *to maximize caloric intake.*
- Provide child's favorite foods *to encourage increased intake.*
- Provide smaller, more frequent meals *to reduce sensation of fullness and increase overall intake.*
- If vomiting is an issue, administer antiemetics as ordered prior to meals *to provide optimal state for success at mealtime.*

(continued)

Overview for the Child With an Immunologic Disorder (continued)

Nursing Diagnosis: Impaired skin integrity related to disease process or photosensitivity as evidenced by skin rash or alopecia

Outcome identification and evaluation

Skin integrity will be maintained; *secondary infection will not occur, rash will not increase.*

Intervention: preventing skin impairment

- Assess and monitor extent and location of rash *to provide baseline information and evaluate success of interventions.*
- Keep skin clean and dry *to prevent secondary infection.*
- For the child with eczema, apply topical medications as ordered *to decrease inflammatory response.*
- For the child with limited mobility, turn frequently and use specialty mattress or bed *to prevent pressure ulcers.*
- Implement a written plan of care directed toward topical treatment of skin integrity impairment *to provide consistency of care and documentation.*
- Educate child and family to limit direct sun exposure and use sunscreen *to prevent sun damage.*

Nursing Diagnosis: Activity intolerance related to joint pain, fatigue or weakness, concurrent illness as evidenced by dyspnea, lack of desire to participate in play, inability to maintain usual routine

Outcome identification and evaluation

Child will participate in activities; *will demonstrate easy work of breathing and participate in daily routine and play.*

Intervention: promoting activity

- Cluster care *to decrease disturbances and allow for longer uninterrupted rest periods.*
- Pace activities and encourage regular rest periods *to conserve energy.*
- Administer early morning warm bath *to ease AM stiffness (juvenile arthritis).*
- Use assistive devices such as splints and orthotics *to improve physical function.*
- Plan developmentally appropriate activities that the child can participate in while in bed *to encourage play and continued development.*
- Schedule activities for time of day child usually has the most energy *to encourage successful participation.*

Nursing Diagnosis: Delayed growth and development related to physical effects of chronic illness, or physical disability (juvenile arthritis) as evidenced by delay in meeting expected milestones

Outcome identification and evaluation

Development will be enhanced: *child will make continued progress toward expected developmental milestones.*

Intervention: enhancing growth and development

- Screen for developmental capabilities *to determine child's current level of functioning.*
- Offer age-appropriate toys, play, and activities (including gross motor) *to encourage further development.*
- Encourage peer contact through telephone, e-mail, or letters *to promote/continue socialization.*
- Perform interventions as prescribed by physical or occupational therapist: *repeat participation in those activities helps child improve function and acquire developmental skills.*
- Provide support to families of children with developmental delay *(progress in achieving developmental milestones can be slow, and ongoing motivation is needed).*
- Encourage child to continue schoolwork *so that child will not fall behind.*
- Reinforce positive attributes in the child *to maintain motivation.*

deficiencies), phagocytic system defects, and T-cell defects (cellular immunity deficiencies), with only 2% related to complement deficiencies (Petry et al., 2004). This discussion will focus on a few of the more common and/or severe primary immunodeficiencies in children. Box 27.1 lists 10 warning signs that a child may need further evaluation for the possibility of primary **immunodeficiency**.

HYPOGAMMAGLOBULINEMIA

Hypogammaglobulinemia refers to a variety of conditions in which the child does not form antibodies appropriately. It results in low or absent levels of one or more of the immunoglobulin classes or subclasses. Table 27.1 provides an overview of several types of hypogammaglobulinemia. Therapeutic management of most types of hypogammaglobulinemia is periodic administration of intravenous immunoglobulin (IVIG).

Nursing Assessment

Note history of recurrent respiratory, gastrointestinal, or genitourinary infections. Palpate for enlarged lymph nodes and spleen in the child with X-linked hyper-IgM syndrome. In children presenting for routine administration of IVIG, determine whether any infections have occurred since the previous infusion.

Nursing Management

Nursing management of hypogammaglobulinemia involves IVIG administration and the provision of education and support to the child and family.

Administering IVIG

Determine the amount of IVIG to be given and reconstitute the product according to the manufacturer's directions (available on the package insert). Many IVIG products are packaged as two vials, one of IVIG powder and one of sterile diluent (Fig. 27.1). After the diluent is added to the powder, gently roll the vial between your hands to mix. Reconstituted IVIG may be refrigerated overnight but should be brought to room temperature prior to infusion. Assess baseline serum blood urea nitrogen (BUN) and creatinine, as acute renal insufficiency may occur as a serious adverse reaction. Though less common in children than adults, assess for risk factors associated with a thromboembolic event, such as history of stroke, hypertension, diabetes, hypercholesterolemia, impaired cardiac output, monoclonal gammopathy, clotting disorder, obesity, or immobility.

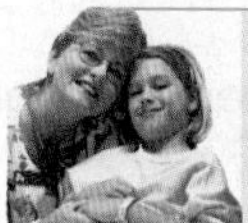

Do not shake the IVIG, as this may lead to foaming and may cause the immunoglobulin protein to degrade.

Ensure that the child is well hydrated prior to the infusion to decrease the risk for rate-related reactions and aseptic meningitis after the infusion. Premedication with diphenhydramine or acetaminophen may be indicated in children who have never received IVIG, have not had an infusion in more than 8 weeks, have had a recent bacterial infection, have a history of serious infusion-related adverse reactions, or are diagnosed with agammaglobulinemia or hypogammaglobulinemia.

The rate for infusion of IVIG is generally prescribed as milligrams of IVIG per kilogram of body weight per minute. Carefully calculate the infusion rate. Obtain a baseline physical assessment and set of vital signs. Begin the infusion slowly, increasing to the prescribed rate as tolerated (see Fig. 27.1). Assess vital signs and check for adverse reactions every 15 minutes for the first hour, then every 30 minutes throughout the remainder of the infusion (the frequency of assessments may vary according to institutional protocol). IVIG is a plasma product, so observe closely for signs of anaphylaxis such as headache, facial flushing, urticaria, dyspnea, shortness of breath, wheezing, chest pain, fever, chills, nausea, vomiting, increased anxiety, or hypotension. If these symptoms occur, discontinue the infusion and notify the physician or nurse practitioner. The infusion may be restarted after the symptoms have subsided. Have oxygen and emergency medications such as epinephrine, diphenhydramine, and intravenous corticosteroids available in case of anaphylactic reaction. If the child complains of discomfort at the intravenous site, a cold compress may be helpful (Murphy et al., 2005).

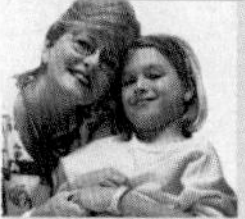

Many children who have had previous reactions to IVIG can tolerate the infusion without reaction if they are premedicated and if the infusion is given at a slower rate.

Providing Education and Support

Provide education and support to the child and family. An excellent book for children with an immune deficiency is

---

BOX 27.1

TEN WARNING SIGNS OF PRIMARY IMMUNODEFICIENCY

- 8 or more episodes of acute otitis media in 1 year
- 2 or more episodes of severe sinusitis in 1 year
- Treatment with antibiotics for 2 months or longer with little effect
- 2 or more episodes of pneumonia in 1 year
- Failure to thrive
- Recurrent deep skin or organ abscesses
- Persistent oral thrush or skin candidiasis after 1 year of age
- History of infections that do not clear with IV antibiotics
- 2 or more serious infections
- Family history of primary immunodeficiency

From the Jeffrey Modell Foundation, 2005.

Table 27.1 Types of Hypogammaglobulinemia

Type	Definition	Characteristics	Treatment
Selective IgA deficiency	Serum IgA <7 mg/dL, normal IgG and IgM	May be asymptomatic. Child is more prone to allergies due to lack of the mucosal protection that IgA offers. Recurrent infections of respiratory, gastrointestinal, and genitourinary tracts, development of autoimmune disorders.	No specific gammaglobulin treatment available. Treat infections or autoimmune disorders. Severe anaphylactic reaction can occur if child receives transfusion of blood containing IgA and IgA antibodies.
X-linked agammaglobulinemia	Markedly reduced or absent IgG, IgM, and IgA. Absence of B cells.	Males only. Recurrent respiratory and gastrointestinal infections.	Routine IVIG. Treat infections.
X-linked hyper-IgM syndrome	Defect in protein found on T-cell surface, resulting in decreased IgG and IgA levels with significant increase in IgM levels	Males only. Recurrent respiratory infections, diarrhea, malabsorption. Neutropenia, autoimmune disorders.	Routine administration of IVIG. Subcutaneous granulocyte colony-stimulating factor (G-CSF) when neutropenic. Bone marrow transplantation. Treatment of autoimmune disorders.
IgG subclass deficiency	Low levels of one or more of the subclasses of IgG	Recurrent respiratory infections. Some children outgrow this condition.	Treatment of respiratory infections. Administration of IVIG is helpful in some children.

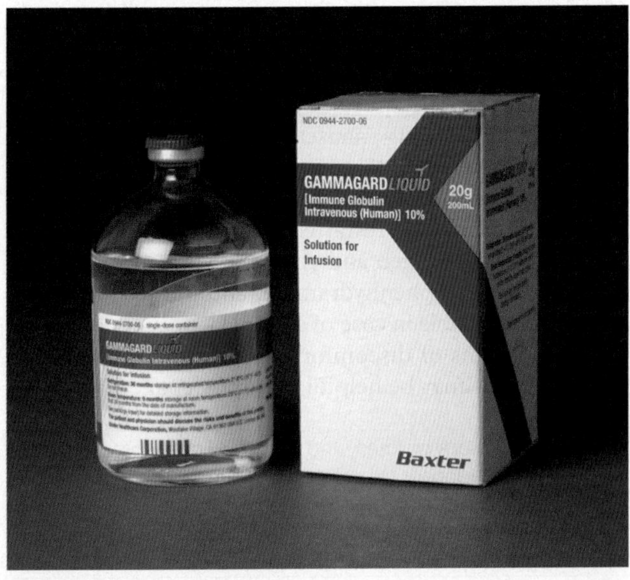

A

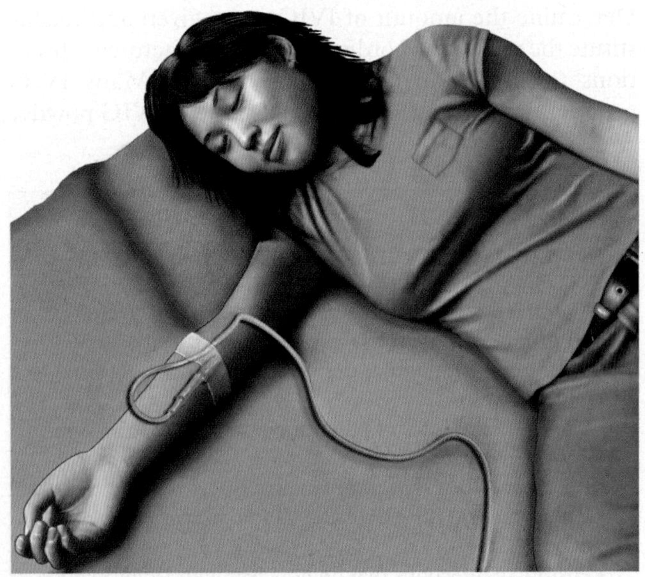

B

● **Figure 27.1** (**A**) Intravenous IVIG. (**B**) Intravenous administration of exogenous immunoglobulin every several weeks can decrease the frequency and severity of infections in children with various forms of hypogammaglobulinemia.

Our Immune System (1993) by Sara le Bien (available from the Immune Deficiency Foundation at www.primaryimmune.org).

WISKOTT-ALDRICH SYNDROME

Wiskott-Aldrich syndrome is an X-linked genetic disorder that results in immunodeficiency, eczema, and thrombocytopenia. It affects males only. The defective gene responsible for this disorder has been identified recently and is called the Wiskott-Aldrich syndrome protein (WASp). Complications include autoimmune hemolytic anemia, neutropenia, skin or cerebral vasculitis, arthritis, inflammatory bowel disease, and renal disease.

Autoimmune disease may require high-dose steroids, azathioprine, or cyclophosphamide. Splenectomy may be performed to correct thrombocytopenia. The only cure is bone marrow or cord blood stem cell transplantation.

Nursing Assessment

Note history of petechiae, bloody diarrhea, or bleeding episode in the first 6 months of life. Note any history of hematemesis or intracranial or conjunctival hemorrhages. Observe the skin for eczema, which usually worsens with time and tends to become secondarily infected (Fig. 27.2). Laboratory findings include low IgM concentration, elevated IgA and IgE concentrations, and normal IgG concentrations.

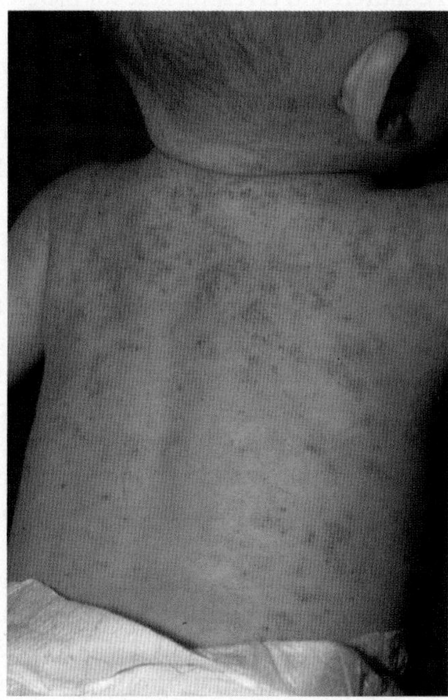

Figure 27.2 Boys with Wiskott-Aldrich syndrome often have worsening of eczema over time.

An episode of prolonged bleeding such as after circumcision may be the first sign of Wiskott-Aldrich syndrome in the male infant.

Nursing Management

Administer IVIG as ordered to help decrease the frequency of bacterial infections. Perform good skin care and frequently assess eczematous areas to detect secondary infection (refer to Chapter 25 for care of eczema). If the patient undergoes splenectomy, in addition to providing routine postoperative care, be aware of the additional risk for development of infection in the asplenic patient. Explain to the patient that severe cutaneous papillomavirus infection may occur after stem cell transplantation (even years later).

SEVERE COMBINED IMMUNE DEFICIENCY

Severe combined immune deficiency (SCID) is a rare X-linked or autosomal recessive disorder; it can occur in girls or boys. SCID is characterized by absent T-cell and B-cell function. There are at least five types of SCID, classified according to the exact genetic defect. Infants with SCID normally present in the first 2 to 7 months of life, when maternally acquired immunity wanes. SCID is a potentially fatal disorder requiring emergency intervention at the time of diagnosis. Gene therapy provides some promise for the future treatment of SCID, but until then bone marrow or stem cell transplantation is necessary. IVIG infusions may help decrease the number of infections until bone marrow or stem cell transplantation can be done. Certain children with SCID (adenosine deaminase enzyme deficiency) may benefit from ongoing subcutaneous adenosine deaminase enzyme replacement. These injections will be required throughout life. Long-term antibiotic therapy helps to contain chronic infections.

Nursing Assessment

Note history of chronic diarrhea and failure to thrive. Note history of severe infections beginning early in infancy. Inspect the mouth for persistent thrush. Auscultate the lungs, noting adventitious sounds related to pneumonia. Laboratory findings include very low levels of all of the immunoglobulins.

Nursing Management

Prevention of infection is critical. Teach the family to practice good hand washing. The child must not be exposed to persons outside the family, particularly young children. Instruct families to administer prophylactic antibiotics if prescribed. Encourage adequate nutrition; supplemental enteral feedings may be necessary in the child with poor appetite. Administer IVIG infusions as prescribed and monitor for adverse reactions (refer to the nursing management section for hypogammaglobulinemia for further information related to IVIG administration). If the child receives a bone marrow transplant (HLA-matched sibling is preferred), provide post-transplant care as outlined in Chapter 29. Refer the family for genetic counseling. Provide ongoing support; this is a difficult situation for families to cope with and the therapy required is life-long.

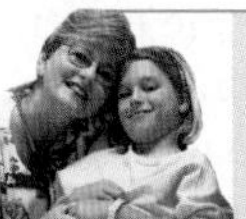

Monitor the bone marrow or stem cell transplant patient closely for a maculopapular rash that usually starts on the palms and soles; this is an indication that **graft-versus-host disease** (GVHD) is developing. Use only cytomegalovirus (CMV)-negative, irradiated blood or platelets if transfusion is necessary in the infant with SCID. CMV-positive blood could cause an infection in the infant, and T lymphocytes in blood products may cause fatal GVHD to occur.

Secondary Immunodeficiencies

Secondary immunodeficiency may occur as a result of chronic illness, malignancy, use of **immunosuppressive** medication, malnutrition or protein-losing state, prematurity, or HIV infection. This discussion will focus on HIV infection.

• HIV INFECTION

Worldwide, 3.2 million children less than 15 years old are living with HIV infection and an additional 1,800 to 2,000 become infected with HIV each day (UNICEF, 2005). In the United States, 15% of all newly diagnosed HIV patients are 13 to 24 years old, and HIV is the sixth leading cause of death among 15- to 24-year-olds (National Association of Pediatric Nurse Practitioners, 2001). More than 10,000 children in the United States have HIV infection or AIDS, and at least 100 of those children die each year (Moylett & Shearer, 2006). Infants primarily become infected through their mothers, whereas adolescents primarily contract HIV infection through sexual activity.

Pathophysiology

HIV affects immune function via alterations mainly in T-cell function, but it also affects B-cells, natural killer cells, and monocyte/macrophage function. HIV infects the CD4 (T-helper) cells. The virus replicates itself via the CD4 cell and renders the cell dysfunctional. Immune deficiency results as the number of normal, functioning CD4 cells drops. Initially, as CD4 counts decrease, the T-suppressor (CD8) counts increase, but as the disease progresses, CD8 counts also fall. The helper T-cell function declines even in asymptomatic infants and children who have not experienced significant decreases in the CD4 cell count. The T cells lose response to recall antigens, and this loss is associated with an increased risk of serious bacterial infection.

B-cell defects also occur in HIV-infected children, contributing to high rates of serious bacterial infections. The B-cells demonstrate impaired response to mitogens and antigens. They also exhibit defective antibody production in response to antigen exposure or vaccination. Also, infants lack a pool of memory B cells for recall antigens (simply from lack of exposure). Natural killer cells also are affected by HIV infection, as they are dependent upon cytokines secreted by the CD4 cells for development of functionality. Functional killer cells play a role in fighting viruses and are critical to immunity in the newborn while the T-cell line develops. Decreased function of the natural killer cells then contributes to increased severity of viral infection in the HIV-infected child or infant. Though the virus does not destroy monocytes and macrophages, their function is affected. Macrophages in the HIV-infected child exhibit decreased chemotaxis and the antigen-presenting capability of the monocytes is defective.

Without appropriate T-cell, B-cell, natural killer cell, monocyte, and macrophage function, the infant's or child's immune system cannot fight infections it ordinarily could. Recurrent infection with ordinary organisms occurs more frequently in children with HIV infection, and the infections are more severe than in noninfected children. Opportunistic infections also occur in HIV-infected children, similar to those in adults with HIV.

HIV rapidly invades the central nervous system in infants and children and is responsible for progressive HIV encephalopathy. As a result of encephalopathy, acquired microcephaly, motor deficits, or loss of previously achieved developmental milestones may occur. In children with progressive HIV encephalopathy, neurologic symptoms may present before immune suppression. Currently, there is no cure for HIV infection.

Children acquire HIV either vertically or horizontally. Vertical transmission refers to perinatal (*in utero* or during birth) transmission or via breast milk. Vertical transmission accounts for about 90% of all cases of pediatric HIV infection (Khoury & Kovacs, 2001). Horizontal transmission refers to transmission via nonsterile needles (as in intravenous drug use or tattooing) or via intimate sexual contact. With nationwide screening of blood products, HIV transmission via transfused blood products has become rare.

The Centers for Disease Control and Prevention (CDC) has developed a classification system for HIV infection in children entitled "The 1994 Revised Classification System for Human Immunodeficiency Virus Infection in Children Less Than 13 years of Age." The classification ranges from the HIV-exposed newborn to the infant or child with AIDS and is based on the severity of the child's clinical symptoms as well as extent of immunologic suppression. The system is useful for determining the severity of illness and for choosing the medication regimen. The classification system may be viewed online at www.cdc.gov/mmwr/preview/mmwrhtml/00032890.htm.

Therapeutic Management

Current recommendations for treatment of HIV infection in children include the use of a combination of antiretroviral drugs. Medication therapy ranges from single-drug therapy in the asymptomatic HIV-exposed newborn to highly active antiretroviral therapy (HAART), consisting of a combination of antiretroviral drugs. Medications are prescribed based on the severity of the child's illness using the CDC classification system (see below). One of the goals of HAART is to prevent or arrest progressive HIV encephalopathy.

Nursing Assessment

For a full description of the assessment phase of the nursing process, refer to page 902. Assessment findings pertinent to HIV infection and AIDS in children are discussed below.

Health History

Elicit a description of the present illness and chief complaint. Common signs and symptoms reported during the health history might include:

- Failure to thrive
- Recurrent bacterial infections
- Opportunistic infections
- Chronic or recurrent diarrhea
- Recurrent or persistent fever
- Developmental delay
- Prolonged candidiasis

These signs and symptoms may be present in either the child who is undergoing initial diagnosis or the child with known HIV infection. Explore the child's current and past medical history for risk factors such as maternal HIV infection or AIDS, receipt of blood transfusions before current nationwide screening policies, adolescent or childhood sexual abuse, substance use or abuse (including intravenous drug use), or participation in vaginal or anal sex without the use of a condom. Document who the primary caregiver is, as many children with HIV have lost their parents to the disease. In addition, for the child with known HIV infection, determine the child's medications and dosages as well as the outcome of any recent health care visits or hospitalizations.

Physical Examination

A thorough and complete physical examination should be performed on the child with AIDS or suspected HIV infection.

Inspection and Observation

Note presence of fever. Measure weight, height or length, and head circumference (in children less than 3 years old) and plot this information on standard growth charts, noting whether the measurements fall within the average or below the lower percentiles. Perform a developmental screening test to detect developmental delay. Inspect the oral cavity for candidiasis. Observe work of breathing (may be increased if pneumonitis or pneumonia is present). Determine level of consciousness (may be depressed if HIV encephalopathy is present).

Auscultation and Palpation

Auscultate the lungs, noting adventitious breath sounds associated with pneumonia or pneumonitis. Palpate for the presence of enlarged lymph nodes (lymphadenopathy) or swollen parotid glands. Palpate the abdomen, noting hepatosplenomegaly.

Laboratory and Diagnostic Tests

Common laboratory and diagnostic studies ordered for the assessment of HIV infection include:

- Polymerase chain reaction test (PCR): positive in infected infants over 1 month of age. PCR is the preferred test to determine HIV infection in infants and to exclude HIV infection as early as possible. Box 27.2 gives recommendations for testing.
- Enzyme-linked immunosorbent assay (ELISA) test: positive in infants of HIV-infected mothers because of transplacentally received antibodies. These antibodies may persist and remain detectable up to 24 months of age, making the ELISA test less accurate at detecting HIV infection in infants and toddlers than the PCR.
- Platelet count: above 500,000 (in severe HIV infection)
- CD4 counts (low in HIV infection)

Nursing Management

Nursing care of the child with HIV infection or AIDS is directed at avoiding infection, promoting compliance with the medication regimen, promoting nutrition, providing pain management and comfort measures, educating the child and caregivers, and providing ongoing psychosocial support. Children with HIV infection may access health

BOX 27.2

VIROLOGIC TESTING FOR HIV-EXPOSED INFANTS (WITH PCR)

- At birth
- 4 to 7 weeks of age
- 8 to 16 weeks of age
- Serologic testing at 12 months of age or older to document disappearance of the HIV-1 antibody

services through funding provided by the Ryan White Comprehensive AIDS Resources Emergency Act. This federal funding provides for primary health care and other services to persons with HIV infection. The Nursing Care Plan Overview lists appropriate nursing diagnoses and interventions. In addition, nursing management specific to HIV infection is covered below.

Preventing HIV Infection in Children

All pregnant women should be offered routine HIV counseling and voluntary testing. Depending upon the stage of pregnancy, the mother should be treated with an antiretroviral drug if she is HIV positive. Children born to HIV-positive mothers should receive a 6-week course of zidovudine (ZDV) therapy. Discourage breastfeeding in the HIV-infected mother and instruct her about safe alternatives to breastfeeding. Early recognition of infection is crucial so that treatment can begin and progression to AIDS can be prevented. Educate sexually active adolescents about HIV transmission and urge them to use condoms. Counsel teens about the increased risk of HIV transmission with all forms of sexual activity, with vaginal and anal sex being even riskier than oral sex. Urge teens to limit the number of sexual partners. Discourage substance use, as the effects of drugs and alcohol often impair the teen's ability to make wise choices about sexual conduct (Morrison-Beedy et al., 2005). Warn teens of the risk of contracting HIV infection via shared needles (as with intravenous drug use). See Healthy People 2010.

Promoting Compliance With Antiretroviral Therapy

Before HAART was available as a treatment option, progressive HIV encephalopathy was inevitably fatal, usually within 2 years of diagnosis. To prevent progression of HIV disease and prevent encephalopathy, compliance with the HAART regimen is required. Educate the family about the importance of complying with the medication regimen. Help the caregivers develop a schedule for medication administration that is compatible with the family's home routine. See Healthy People 2010.

HEALTHY PEOPLE 2010

Objective	Significance
(Developmental) Reduce new cases of perinatally acquired HIV infection. (Developmental) Increase the proportion of pregnant females screened for sexually transmitted diseases (including HIV infection and bacterial vaginosis) during prenatal health care visits, according to recognized standards.	• Encourage sexually active adolescents to seek appropriate reproductive health care and screening. • For the pregnant adolescent, encourage HIV testing to determine status. • Encourage the HIV-positive pregnant adolescent to comply with HIV treatment as prescribed.

HEALTHY PEOPLE 2010

Objective	Significance
(Developmental) Reduce the number of cases of HIV infection among adolescents and adults. (Developmental) Reduce HIV infections in adolescent and young adult females aged 13 to 24 years that are associated with heterosexual contact.	• Encourage abstinence in adolescents. • If adolescents are sexually active, educate about the risks of HIV transmission; encourage condom use with all sexual activity.

Reducing Risk for Infection

In the newborn whose mother is infected with tuberculosis, syphilis, toxoplasmosis, cytomegalovirus, hepatitis B or C, or herpes simplex virus, testing and treatment should be provided. To prevent infection with *Pneumocystis jiroveci*, administer prophylactic antibiotics as prescribed in any HIV-exposed infant in whom HIV infection has not yet been excluded. Provide tuberculosis screening and childhood immunization in accordance with national guidelines.

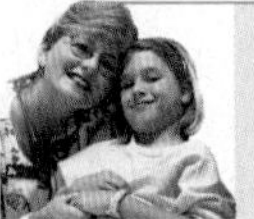

Do not administer live vaccines to the immunocompromised child without the express consent of the infectious disease or immunology specialist. Immunosuppression is a contraindication to vaccination with live vaccines.

Promoting Nutrition

For the infant, provide increased-calorie formula as tolerated. For the child, provide high-calorie, high-protein meals and snacks. Supplements may be added to milkshakes to increase the protein intake. Ensure that the child is able to choose foods that he or she prefers from the hospital menu.

HEALTHY PEOPLE 2010

Objective	Significance
Reduce deaths from HIV infection. (Developmental) Extend the interval of time between an initial diagnosis of HIV infection and AIDS diagnosis in order to increase years of life of an individual infected with HIV.	• Educate families about the importance of complying with medication therapy (HAART) and receiving regularly scheduled medical evaluations.

Document growth through weekly measurements of weight and height.

Promoting Comfort

Children with HIV infection experience pain from infections, encephalopathy, adverse effects of medications, and the numerous procedures and treatments that are required, such as venipuncture, biopsy, or lumbar puncture. Refer to Chapter 15 for detailed information about pain assessment and management.

Providing Family Education and Support

Educate caregivers about the medication regimen, the ongoing follow-up that is needed, and when to call the infectious disease provider. Families of HIV-infected children experience a significant amount of stress from many sources: the diagnosis of an incurable disease, financial difficulties, multiple family members with HIV, HIV-associated stigmas, desire to keep HIV infection confidential, and multiple medical appointments and hospitalizations. Parents of HIV-infected children often die of AIDS themselves, leaving care of the child to another relative or foster parent. The daycare center or school that the child attends will need education about HIV, which can be provided only if the parent or caretaker consents to divulging the child's diagnosis to that agency. Provide education to the school or daycare center about how the infection is transmitted (i.e., not through casual contact).

Disclosure of the diagnosis of HIV to the child is another source of stress for the family. The timing of this disclosure will vary considerably depending on the child's and family's situation. Generally, children over 6 years of age will eventually need to have their diagnosis disclosed to them in an age-appropriate manner. They begin to ask questions and often seem to sense that something is going on other than what they've been told so far. When made aware of the diagnosis and educated about the disease, the child may exhibit a variety of reactions. Anger, depression, or school problems may occur. The child may experience a spiritual dilemma. The nurse should continue to provide emotional support to the child and family. If the disclosure results in significant emotional turmoil, refer the child and caregivers to a counselor, social worker, or psychologist.

Anticipatory grieving also may occur. Parents or caregivers may express guilt or anger over the diagnosis of HIV infection. At the other end of the spectrum, families may use denial as their method for coping. Use therapeutic communication with open-ended questions to discover the family's thoughts and fears. Provide emotional support and allow for crying and verbalization. If needed, refer the caregivers to the appropriate professional for additional psychological and emotional intervention.

Many children with HIV have psychosocial, emotional, and cognitive problems. These contribute to a lower quality of life. They are affected by the stigma of their diagnosis and often by the social isolation associated with it. They may suffer multiple losses within the family related to deaths caused by HIV infection. Children with HIV infection need significant psychosocial support and intervention. Resources for families of HIV-infected children are listed in Box 27.3.

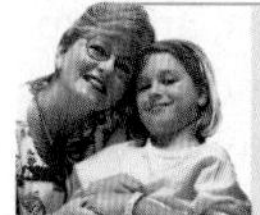

Family-centered care of the HIV-exposed child and HIV-infected mother may involve a multidisciplinary approach and can result in improved outcomes for both the mother and the child.

Consider THIS!

Jake Reddington, a 2-year-old diagnosed with HIV infection, is brought to the clinic by his aunt for his regular check-up. His aunt has recently taken over the care of Jake since his mother is too ill with HIV infection to care for him.

What education will be important for Jake's aunt and her family?

Discuss some of the psychosocial issues and concerns that face a child with HIV and his or her family.

Autoimmune Disorders

Autoimmune disorders result from the immune system's malfunction. The body manufactures T cells and antibodies against its own cells and organs (**autoantibodies**). The development of an autoimmune disorder is thought to be multifactorial. Potential influencing factors include heredity, hormones, self-marker molecules, and environmental influences such as viruses and certain drugs.

• SYSTEMIC LUPUS ERYTHEMATOSUS

Systemic lupus erythematosus (SLE) is a multisystem autoimmune disorder that affects both humoral and cellular immunity. SLE can affect any organ system, so the

BOX 27.3

RESOURCES FOR HIV-INFECTED CHILDREN AND THEIR FAMILIES

- www.hivpositive.com/f-Nutrition/f-3-PediatricNeut/n-Zafonte.html: Nutrition in Pediatric HIV Infection
- www.pedsaids.org: Elizabeth Glaser Pediatric AIDS Foundation—resources for HIV-infected children and their families
- www.vachss.com/help_text/hiv_aids_ped.html—Pediatric HIV infection and AIDS resources
- www.womenchildrenhiv.org/: Women, Children and HIV—resources for prevention and treatment

onset and course of the disease are quite variable. SLE is usually diagnosed after age 5 years (usually between 15 and 45 years of age), but onset can occur at any age. Before puberty, girls with SLE outnumber boys with SLE by a 3-to-1 margin. After puberty the incidence is nine times greater in females than it is in males (Gottlieb & Ilowite, 2000). SLE is more common in non-Caucasians, and typically black and Hispanic patients experience more severe effects from SLE than other racial or ethnic groups.

Pathophysiology

In SLE, autoantibodies react with the child's self-antigens to form immune complexes. The immune complexes accumulate in the tissues and organs, causing an inflammatory response resulting in vasculitis. Injury to the tissues and pain occur. Since SLE may affect any organ system, the potential for alterations or damage to tissues anywhere in the body is significant. In some cases, the autoimmune response may be preceded by a drug reaction, an infection, or excessive sun exposure. In children, the most common initial symptoms are hematologic, cutaneous, and musculoskeletal in origin. The disease is chronic, with periods of remission and exacerbation (flares). Common complications of SLE include ocular or visual changes, cerebrovascular accident (CVA), transverse myelitis, immune complex–mediated glomerulonephritis, pericarditis, valvular heart disease, coronary artery disease, seizures, and psychosis.

Therapeutic Management

Therapeutic management focuses on treating the inflammatory response. NSAIDs, corticosteroids, and antimalarial agents are often prescribed for the child with mild to moderate SLE. The child with severe SLE or frequent flare-ups of symptoms may require high-dose (pulse) corticosteroid therapy or immunosuppressive drugs. When end-stage renal failure develops as a result of glomerulonephritis, dialysis becomes necessary.

Nursing Assessment

For a full description of the assessment phase of the nursing process, refer to page 902. Assessment findings pertinent to SLE in children are discussed below.

Health History

Elicit a description of the present illness and chief complaint. Common signs and symptoms reported during the health history are history of fatigue, fever, weight changes, pain or swelling in the joints, numbness, tingling or coolness of extremities, or prolonged bleeding. Assess for risk factors, which include female sex; family history (only 10% of cases); African, Native American, or Asian descent; recent infection; drug reaction; or excessive sun exposure.

Physical Examination

Measure temperature and document the presence of fever. Observe the skin for malar rash (a butterfly-shaped rash over the cheeks); discoid lesions on the face, scalp, or neck; changes in skin pigmentation; or scarring (Fig. 27.3). Document alopecia. Inspect the oral cavity for painless ulcerations and the joints for edema. Measure blood pressure, as hypertension may occur with renal involvement. Auscultate the lungs; adventitious breath sounds may be present if the pulmonary system is involved. Palpate the joints, noting tenderness. Palpate the abdomen and note areas of tenderness (abdominal involvement is more common in children with SLE than in adults). Box 27.4 lists common clinical findings in SLE.

Laboratory and Diagnostic Findings

Laboratory findings may include decreased hemoglobin and hematocrit, decreased platelet count, and low WBC count. Complement levels, C3 and C4, will also be decreased. Though not specific to SLE, the ANA is usually positive in patients with SLE.

Nursing Management

Nursing management of the child or adolescent with SLE is long term and supportive. Management focuses on preventing and monitoring for complications. Educate the child and family about the importance of a healthy diet, regular exercise, and adequate sleep and rest. Administer NSAIDs, corticosteroids, and antimalarial agents as ordered for the child with mild to moderate SLE and pulse corticosteroid therapy or immunomodulators to the child with severe SLE or frequent flare-ups. Refer families to support services such as the Lupus Alliance of America (www.lupusalliance.org) and the Lupus Foundation of America (www.lupus.org).

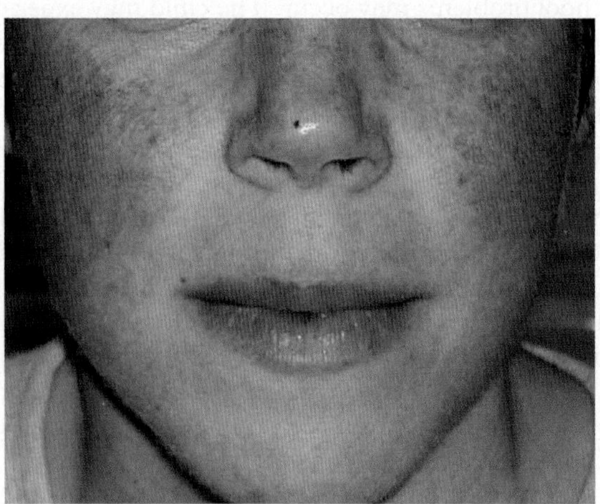

● **Figure 27.3** The malar or butterfly rash (erythema over the cheeks in the shape of a butterfly) is typical in SLE.

BOX 27.4

MOST COMMON CLINICAL MANIFESTATIONS OF SLE

- Alopecia
- Anemia
- Arthralgia
- Arthritis
- Fatigue
- Lupus nephritis
- Photosensitivity
- Pleurisy
- Raynaud's phenomenon
- Seizures
- Skin rashes, including malar rash
- Stomatitis
- Thrombocytopenia

Preventing and Monitoring for Complications

Teach families to apply sunscreen (minimum SPF 15) to their child's skin daily to prevent rashes resulting from photosensitivity. Instruct the child and family to protect against cold weather by layering warm socks and wearing gloves when outdoors in the winter. If the child is outside for extended periods during the winter months, the fingers and toes should be inspected for discoloration. Watch for the development of nephritis by evaluating blood pressure, serum BUN and creatinine levels, and urine output and monitoring for hematuria or proteinuria. Ensure that yearly vision screening and ophthalmic examinations are performed to preserve visual function should changes occur.

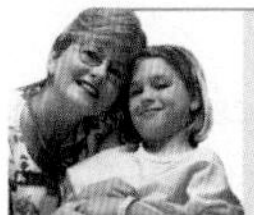

Avascular necrosis (lack of blood supply to a joint, resulting in tissue damage) may occur as an adverse effect of long-term or high-dose corticosteroid use. Teach families to report new onset of joint pain, particularly with weight bearing, or limited range of motion to their physician or nurse practitioner.

JUVENILE IDIOPATHIC ARTHRITIS

Juvenile idiopathic arthritis is an autoimmune disorder in which the autoantibodies mainly target the joints. Inflammatory changes in the joints cause pain, redness, warmth, stiffness, and swelling. Stiffness usually occurs after inactivity (as in the morning, after sleep). Some forms also affect the eyes or other organs. Table 27.2 explains the three most common types. Juvenile idiopathic arthritis is a chronic disease: the child may experience healthy periods alternating with flare-ups. In some children the disease resolves as they approach adolescence or adulthood, while others will have more severe disease that continues throughout the adult years. Juvenile idiopathic arthritis was formerly termed "juvenile rheumatoid arthritis," but unlike adult rheumatoid arthritis, few types of juvenile arthritis actually demonstrate a positive rheumatoid factor.

Therapeutic management focuses on inflammation control, pain relief, promotion of remission, and maintenance of mobility. NSAIDs, corticosteroids, and antirheumatic drugs such as methotrexate and etanercept are prescribed, depending on the type and severity of the disease. NSAIDs are helpful with pain relief, but disease-modifying (antirheumatic) drugs are necessary to prevent disease progression.

Nursing Assessment

Note history of irritability or fussiness, which may be the first sign of this disease in the infant or very young child. Note complaints of pain, though children do not always communicate this. Document history of withdrawal from play or difficulty getting the child out of bed in the morning (joint stiffness after inactivity). Inquire about history of fever (above 39.5° C for 2 weeks or more in systemic disease).

Measure temperature (fever is present with systemic disease). Inspect skin for evanescent, pale red, nonpruritic

Table 27.2 Types of Juvenile Idiopathic Arthritis

Type	Definition	Non-Joint Manifestations	Complications
Pauciarticular	Involvement of four or fewer joints; quite often the knee is involved. Most common type.	Eye inflammation, malaise, poor appetite, poor weight gain	Iritis, uveitis, uneven leg bone growth
Polyarticular	Involvement of five or more joints; frequently involves small joints and often affects the body symmetrically	Malaise, lymphadenopathy, organomegaly, poor growth	Often a severe form of arthritis; rapidly progressing joint damage, rheumatoid nodules
Systemic	In addition to joint involvement, fever and rash may be present at diagnosis.	Enlarged spleen, liver, and lymph nodes; myalgia; severe anemia	Pericarditis, pericardial effusion, pleuritis, pulmonary fibrosis

macular rash, which may be present at diagnosis of systemic disease. Observe the gait, noting limping or guarding of a joint or extremity. Document growth, which may be delayed. Inspect and palpate each joint for edema, redness, warmth, and tenderness (Fig. 27.4). Note positioning of joints (usually flexed in position of comfort). Mild to moderate anemia and an elevated erythrocyte sedimentation rate are common. Young children with the pauciarticular form may demonstrate a positive antinuclear antibody, and adolescents with polyarticular disease may have a positive rheumatoid factor.

Nursing Management

Nursing management focuses on managing pain, maintaining mobility, and promoting a normal life. Refer the child to a pediatric rheumatologist to ensure that he or she receives the most up-to-date treatment. Disease-modifying medications approved for use in children may produce better long-term outcomes than were possible in the past. Clinical research trial information is available through the Childhood Arthritis & Rheumatology Research Alliance. Encourage regular eye examinations and vision screening to allow for early treatment of visual changes and to prevent blindness.

Managing Pain and Maintaining Mobility

Administer medications as prescribed to control inflammation and prevent disease progression. Refer to Drug Guide 27.1 for information related to NSAIDs, corticosteroids, and disease-modifying antirheumatic drugs. Maintain joint range of motion and muscle strength via exercise (physical or occupational therapy). Swimming is a particularly useful exercise to maintain joint mobility without placing pressure on the joints. Teach families appropriate use of splints prescribed to prevent joint contractures. Monitor for pressure areas or skin breakdown with splint or orthotic use.

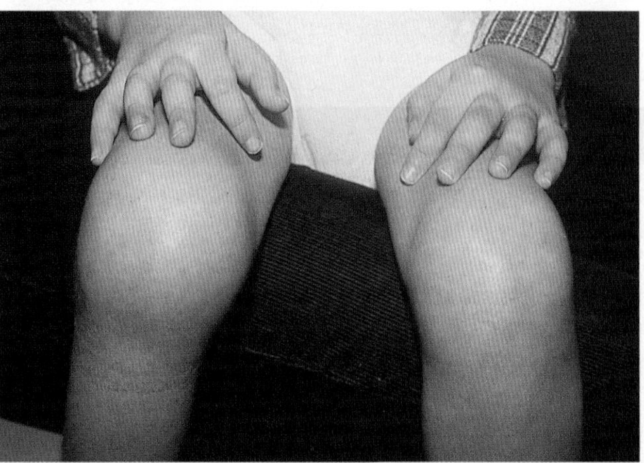

● Figure 27.4 Note the swollen, reddened joints of this child with juvenile arthritis.

Promoting Normal Life

Chronic pain and decreased mobility may reduce the child's psychological and emotional status significantly, both during childhood and adulthood. Providing adequate pain relief and promoting compliance with the disease-modifying medication regimen may allow the child to have a more normal life in the present as well as in the future. In addition to measures described in the previous section, encourage adequate sleep to allow the child to cope better with symptoms and to function better in school. Sleep may be promoted by a warm bath at bedtime and warm compresses to affected joints or massage. To prevent social isolation, encourage the child to attend school and ensure that teachers, the school nurse, and classmates are educated about the child's disease and any limitations on activity. Having two sets of books (one at school and one at home) allows the child to do homework without having to carry heavy books home. Modifications such as allowing the child to leave the classroom early in order to get to the next class on time may seem small but can have a significant impact on the child's life.

Encourage children and families to become involved with local support groups so they can see that they are not alone. Assist children to set and achieve goals to increase their sense of hopefulness. Special summer camps for children with juvenile arthritis allow the child to socialize and belong to a group and have been shown to promote self-esteem in the child with chronic illness. Encourage appropriate family functioning and refer the family to support groups such as those sponsored by the American Juvenile Arthritis Organization. See Healthy People 2010.

Allergy and Anaphylaxis

Allergy is an immune-mediated response resulting in an adverse physiologic event or reaction (Sampson & Eggleston, 2006). Allergy affects about 20% to 25% of the U.S. population; the extent of the allergic response is determined by the duration, rate, and amount of exposure to the allergen as well as environmental and host factors (American College of Allergy, Asthma and Immunology, 2006; Fletcher-Janzen & Reynolds, 2003). IgE-mediated

HEALTHY PEOPLE 2010

Objective	Significance
(Developmental) Increase the proportion of persons with arthritis who have had effective, evidence-based arthritis education as an integral part of the management of their condition.	• Educate children and families about juvenile arthritis, its treatments, and interventions for improving mobility. Begin at diagnosis and provide continual reinforcement.

allergy will be the focus of this discussion. This type of allergic response is mediated by antigen-specific IgE antibodies. When the antibody is exposed to the antigen (allergen), rapid cell activation occurs and potent mediators and cytokines are released, resulting in changes in the blood vessels, bronchi, and mucus-secreting glands. In addition to the atopic diseases (asthma, allergic rhinitis, atopic dermatitis), urticaria, digestive allergy, and systemic anaphylaxis are also IgE-mediated (Fletcher-Janzen & Reynolds, 2003; Sampson & Eggleston, 2006). Though any allergen has the potential to trigger an anaphylactic response, food and insect sting allergies are most common.

• FOOD ALLERGIES

A true food hypersensitivity or allergy is defined as an immunologic reaction resulting from the ingestion of a food or food additive (Burks, 2001). This type of reaction is an IgE-mediated response to a particular food. Food allergy affects approximately 6% to 8% of children under the age of 3 and can lead to significant medical complications (Sicherer et al., 2003). During the first few years of life, the most common food allergens are milk, eggs, peanuts, tree nuts, fish and shellfish, wheat, and soy. Typically, allergies to these foods are acquired in childhood, and for most children only allergies to peanuts, tree nuts, and fish and shellfish persist into adulthood (Vadas, 2003). Most reactions occur within minutes of exposure, but they may occur up to 2 hours after ingestion. Signs and symptoms of a food allergy reaction include hives, flushing, facial swelling, mouth and throat itching, and runny nose. Many children also have a gastrointestinal reaction, including vomiting, abdominal pain, and diarrhea. In extreme cases, swelling of the tongue, uvula, pharynx, or upper airway may occur. Wheezing can be an ominous sign that the airway is edematous. Rarely, cardiovascular collapse occurs. Though the risk for anaphylaxis is small, parents, caregivers, and health care providers should be vigilant when caring for children with food allergies (Macdougall et al., 2002).

Therapeutic Management

Therapeutic management involves verifying the food allergy, avoiding the allergen, and treating the reaction with epinephrine or antihistamines. Preventing the development of food allergies is also a key intervention.

It is important to discern a true food allergy from intolerance to certain foods. "Food intolerance" is a general term that describes an abnormal physiologic response to an ingested food or food additive that has not been proven to be immunologic (Burks, 2001). Often a milk allergy is confused with lactose intolerance. Therefore, a detailed dietary history is important when distinguishing a true allergy versus intolerance.

To prevent the development of food allergies, infants should be breastfed for at least the first 6 months of life and the following common food allergens should be avoided in children under 1 year of age (Chamberlain, 2006; Muraro et al., 2004):

- Cow's milk
- Eggs
- Peanuts
- Tree nuts
- Sesame seeds
- Kiwi fruit
- Fish and shellfish

Nursing Assessment

Patients with food allergy reactions must be assessed accurately. In the initial nursing assessment, the child should be immediately assessed for airway, breathing, or circulation problems (see Chapter 32). If the child's condition is stable, the nurse should finish the assessment. The history should include a detailed food history and documentation of the reaction, including the food suspected of causing the reaction, the quantity of food ingested, the length of time between ingestion and development of symptoms, the symptoms, what treatment has been administered, and the subsequent response. Note gastrointestinal symptoms such as:

- Burning in the mouth or throat
- Bloating
- Nausea
- Diarrhea

Assess for risk factors such as previous exposure to the food, history of poorly controlled asthma, or an increase in atopic dermatitis flare-ups in relation to food intake (Roberts et al., 2003).

Inspect the skin for color, rash, hives, or edema. Auscultate the heart and lungs to determine heart rate and to assess for wheezing.

The American College of Allergy, Asthma & Immunology's new practice parameter recommends food-specific IgE testing if the child has a history of food allergy. Food avoidance is recommended for those who have a highly predictive reaction to testing or a history of anaphylactic response. If the child has episodic symptoms, an oral challenge may be appropriate. If symptoms are chronic, a trial elimination diet may be indicated. If symptoms resolve without the food, true allergy may be present (American College of Allergy, Asthma & Immunology, 2006). On an elimination diet, the child should stop eating all suspicious foods for 1 to 2 weeks and then retry the foods one at a time, over a period of several days, to see whether a similar reaction occurs. Often this is done in the pediatrician's office or hospital setting if severe reactions have occurred in the past. If a similar reaction occurs, it is very suggestive of a food allergy. Allergy skin prick tests and RAST blood tests are widely used by pediatricians to look for reactions. However, these tests may have false-positive results, and children may need to avoid many foods unnecessarily.

Nursing Management

Initial nursing management is aimed at stabilizing the child's condition if an acute reaction to a food allergen is present (see Chapter 32). Medications used in the treatment of a food allergy reaction include histamine blockers and, in anaphylactic reactions, epinephrine. Teach the child (if appropriate) and the parents how and when to use these medications during an allergic reaction. Since these reactions can be so sudden (unknown ingestion of allergen) and severe, it is helpful for the family to have an emergency written plan in case of a reaction.

Managing the Child's Diet

Dietary teaching is aimed at educating the family on how to avoid the offending foods. Families should be extremely careful when reading food labels. A dietitian may be helpful in this teaching process. Teaching Guideline 27.1 gives information about hidden allergens in food. Teach the parents what "safe" foods can be substituted for offensive ones (Box 27.5). Children with peanut allergy should not eat tree nuts, as up to 50% of children who are allergic to peanuts are also allergic to tree nuts (Jackson, 2002).

Having a child with a food allergy can be very anxiety-producing for parents: they often live in fear that the child may accidentally ingest an allergen (Sicherer et al., 2001). Educating the child and family about allergic reactions may help to decrease their anxiety. Teach the child and family how to recognize the signs and symptoms of an allergic reaction. The nurse may need to provide information to daycare providers as well as schoolteachers, staff, and camp counselors (Munoz-Furlong, 2003). Refer families to the Food Allergy & Anaphylaxis Network (www.foodallergy.org).

BOX 27.5
FOOD SUBSTITUTIONS

- Replace milk with water, fruit juice, rice milk, or soy milk.
- Replace each egg with 1.5 tablespoons each of water and oil and 1 teaspoon baking powder; OR 1 packet plain gelatin with 2 tablespoons warm water added at time of use; OR 1 teaspoon yeast and a quarter-cup warm water.
- Replace peanuts or tree nuts with raisins, dates, or crispy cereal.

Munoz-Furlong, A. (2003). Daily coping strategies for patients and their families. *Pediatrics, 111*(6), 1654–1661.

● ANAPHYLAXIS

Anaphylaxis is an acute IgE-mediated response to an allergen that involves many organ systems and may be life-threatening (Sampson, 2006). As many as 1% to 2% of the population is at risk for anaphylaxis due to food allergies or insect stings (McIntyre et al., 2005). In addition to nuts, shellfish, eggs, and bee or wasp stings, drugs such as penicillin and NSAIDs, radiopaque dyes, and latex are the leading causes of anaphylaxis (Sampson, 2003; Tang, 2003). The reaction is severe and usually starts within 5 to 10 minutes of exposure, though delayed reactions are possible. Histamines and secondary mediators are released from the mast cells and eosinophils in response to contact with an allergen. Cutaneous, cardiopulmonary, gastrointestinal, and neurologic symptoms occur. Vasodilation results in a rapid decrease in plasma volume, leading to the risk of circulatory collapse (Dreskin, 2005). Prolonged resuscitation may be needed, and death may occur.

Therapeutic management focuses on assessment and support of the airway, breathing, and circulation. Epinephrine is usually required, and intramuscular or

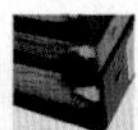

TEACHING GUIDELINE 27.1

Allergens Hidden in Food

If Child is Allergic to:	Teach Families to Avoid:	Unexpected Locations of Common Ingredients
Milk	Artificial butter flavor, casein, lactalbumin, nougat, pudding, whey, yogurt, ghee	Some deli meats and hot dogs, nondairy products, coffee whiteners
Wheat	Cereal extract, couscous, durum, semolina, spelt	
Eggs	Albumin, globulin, ovalbumin	
Peanuts	Fast food cooked in peanut oil, many Asian foods, baked goods with nuts or processed on equipment that also processes peanuts	Brown gravy, barbeque sauce, meat sauce, egg rolls, enchilada sauce, hot chocolate

Data from Munoz-Furlong, A. (2003). Daily coping strategies for patients and their families. *Pediatrics, 111*(6), 1654–1661; and Vadas, P. (2003). Food allergens and anaphylaxis. *Canadian Journal of Dietetic Practice and Research, 64*(2), insert.

intravenous diphenhydramine is used secondarily. Late-onset reactions can be prevented with corticosteroids.

Nursing Assessment

Assess patency of the airway and adequacy of breathing. Determine if circulation is sufficient. Note level of consciousness. Obtain a brief history, inquiring specifically about allergen exposure. Determine whether the child has received any medication (e.g., epinephrine or diphenhydramine) since the onset of the reaction and what effect the medication had on the symptoms. Table 27.3 gives additional signs and symptoms of anaphylaxis.

Nursing Management

Nursing management initially focuses on supporting airway, breathing, and circulation. Provide supplemental oxygen by mask or bag-valve-mask ventilation. Ensure that bronchodilator inhalation treatment (albuterol) is given if bronchospasm is present. Administer intravenous fluids to provide volume expansion. Administer epinephrine, diphenhydramine, and/or corticosteroids as ordered to reverse the allergic process (Sampson, 2003).

Preventing and Managing Future Episodes

Education of the family about preventing and managing future episodes is critical. Teach the family how to use injectable epinephrine in case of subsequent allergen exposure. Intramuscular epinephrine may be given via the Epipen or Epipen Jr. Dosage is based on the child's weight. The gray safety release on the Epipen should never be removed until just before use. The thumb, fingers, or hand should not be placed over the black tip. Nursing Procedure 27.1 gives further instructions related to Epipen use. Instruct the child and family to call 911 and seek immediate medical attention after using the Epipen. Warn the child that the epinephrine may make him or her feel as if the heart is racing (Clark & Ewan, 2003).

Daycare providers, school nurses, teachers, and staff who interact with the child must know how to recognize an anaphylactic event. In 2004, Public Law No. 108-377, Asthmatic Schoolchildren's Treatment and Health Management Act, was passed by the U.S. Congress. This law is intended to ensure that students with severe allergies can carry prescribed medications (i.e., Epipen) with them. All children with allergies should have an action plan in place at the school or daycare center (Clark & Ewan, 2003; Frost & Chalin, 2005; Watura, 2002). Advise the child to wear a medical alert bracelet or necklace at all times (Tang, 2003).

Teach children and families to avoid known food allergens. Avoid stings from bees and wasps (Hymenoptera) by being alert when eating outdoors, wearing long sleeves and pants when in fields, and removing hives or nests. Desensitization is available for children with severe penicillin allergy. Avoid use of cephalosporins in children with severe penicillin allergy (Ellis & Day, 2003).

• LATEX ALLERGY

Latex allergy is an IgE-mediated response to exposure to latex, a natural rubber product used in many common items (especially gloves in the health care setting). The pathophysiology of latex allergy is similar to that of food allergy. Avoidance of latex products is recommended for those who are allergic to it. An immediate allergic reaction may occur if a latex-allergic child comes in to contact with latex. Latex allergy can also result in anaphylaxis (refer to section above on anaphylaxis).

Table 27.3 Clinical Manifestations of Anaphylaxis

Body Area or System	Manifestation
Oral	• Lip, tongue, or palate pruritus • Lip or tongue edema
Cutaneous	• Urticaria (hives), flushing, pruritus, angioedema
Respiratory	• Nasal pruritus, congestion, sneezing, rhinorrhea • Stridor, tightness in the throat, dysphagia, dysphonia, hoarseness • Shortness of breath, dyspnea, tight chest, wheeze
Cardiovascular	• Tachycardia, chest pain, arrhythmia, hypotension
Neurologic	• Syncope, feeling faint, aura of doom, lethargy, disorientation
Gastrointestinal	• Bloating, abdominal pain, diarrhea, vomiting

Data from Clark, A. T., & Ewan, P. W. (2003). Food allergy in childhood. *Archives of Disease in Childhood, 88* (1), 79–81; Sampson, H. A. (2003). Anaphylaxis and emergency treatment. *Pediatrics, 111*(6), 1601–1908; Dreskin, S.C. (2005). Anaphylaxis. Available at http:www.emedicine.com/med/topic/28.htm.

Nursing Procedure 27.1

Use of the Epipen or Epipen Jr.

1. Grasp the Epipen or Epipen Jr. with the black tip pointing downward, forming a fist.
2. With the other hand, pull off the gray safety release.

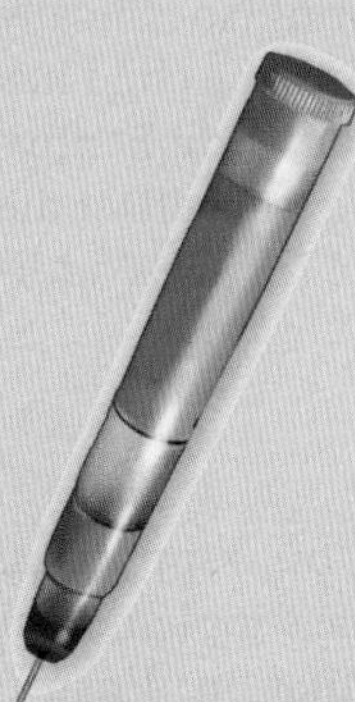

3. Swing and jab the epipen firmly into the outer thigh at a 90-degree angle and hold firmly there for 10 seconds

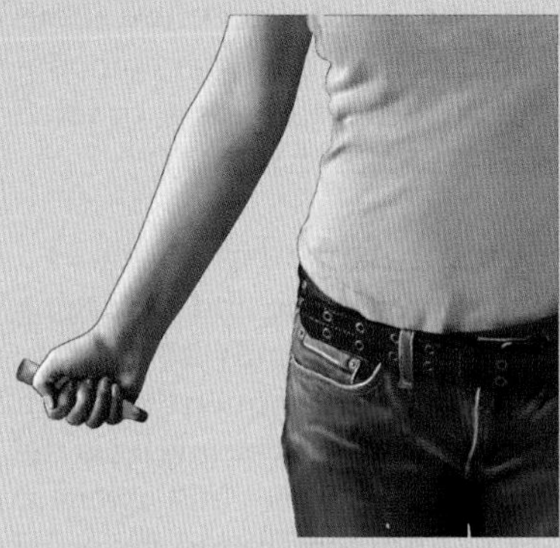

4. Remove the Epipen and massage the thigh for 10 seconds.

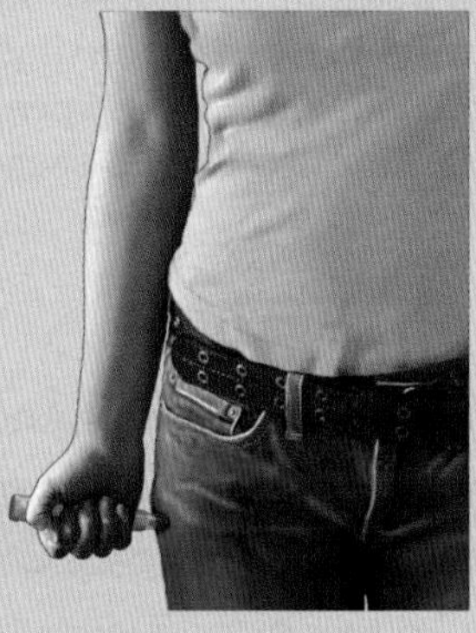

Adapted from the Epipen website (www.epipen.com/howtouse/aspx).

Nursing Assessment

Screen all children who visit a health care facility of any kind for latex allergy. Ask if the child is allergic to rubber gloves or has ever developed hives after exposure to them. Ask the parent if the child has symptoms such as coughing, wheezing, or shortness of breath after glove exposure. Has the child ever had swelling in the mouth or complained that the mouth itched after a dental examination? Determine whether the child has ever had allergic symptoms after eating foods with a known cross-reactivity to latex, such as pear, peach, passion fruit, plum, pineapple, kiwi, fig, grape, cherry, melon, nectarine, papaya, apple, apricot, banana, chestnut, carrot, celery, avocado, tomato, or potato. For the child who has come into contact with latex, assess for symptoms of a reaction such as hives;

wheeze; cough; shortness of breath; nasal congestion and rhinorrhea; sneezing; nose, palate, or eye pruritus; or hypotension.

Nursing Management

Nursing management of latex allergy focuses on preventing exposure to latex products. Instruct children and their families to avoid foods with a known cross-reactivity to latex such as those listed above (Binkley et al., 2003; Ellis & Day, 2003; Tang, 2003). If the child is exposed to latex, remove the irritating substance and cleanse the area with soap and water. Assess for the need for resuscitation and perform it if needed (Binkley et al., 2003). Become familiar with your institution's latex allergy policy. Know which products contain latex and which do not. Document latex allergy on the chart, patient identification band, the medication administration record, and the physician's order sheet. Refer families to resources for persons with latex allergy, such as:

- www.latexallergyresources.org: American Latex Allergy Association
- latexallergylinks.tripod.com/: comprehensive listing of latex allergy websites and documents

References

Books and Journals

Ackley, B. J., & Ladwig, G. B. (2004). *Nursing diagnosis handbook: A guide to planning care* (6th ed.). St. Louis: Mosby.

American Academy of Pediatrics, Committee on Pediatric AIDS. (2000). Education of children with human immunodeficiency virus infection. *Pediatrics, 105*(6), 1358–1360.

American Academy of Pediatrics, Committee on Pediatric AIDS and Committee on Adolescence. (2001). Adolescents and human immunodeficiency virus infection: The role of the pediatrician in prevention and intervention. *Pediatrics, 107*(1), 188–190.

American College of Allergy, Asthma, & Immunology (ACAAI). (2006). Food allergy: A practice parameter. *Annals of Allergy, Asthma, & Immunology, 96*(3 Suppl. 2), S1–68.

Anderson, V. L. (2006). Uncovering a pediatric immunodeficiency, part 1. *Journal for Nurse Practitioners, 2*(3), 186–193.

Bader-Meunier, B., Armengaud, J. B., Haddad, E., Salomon, R., Desche'nes, G., Kone-Paut, I., et al. (2005). Initial presentation of childhood-onset systemic lupus erythematosus: A French multicenter study. *Journal of Pediatrics, 146*, 648–653.

Baxter Healthcare Corporation. (2006). *Primary immunodeficiency (e-textbook)*. Accessed 4/29/06 at www.immunedisease.com/US/hcp/etextbook/index.html.

Berrien, V. M., Salazar, J. C., Reynolds, E., & McKay, K. (2004). Adherence to antiretroviral therapy in HIV-infected pediatric patients improves with home-based intensive nursing intervention. *AIDS Patient Care and STDs, 18*(6), 355–363.

Binkley, H. M., Schroyer, T., & Catalfano, J. (2003). Latex allergies: a review of recognition, evaluation, management, prevention, education, and alternative product use. *Journal of Athletic Training, 38*(2), 133–140.

Bonilla, F. A., & Geha, R. S. (2003). Primary immunodeficiency disease. *Journal of Allergy and Clinical Immunology, 111*(2), S571–S581.

Buckley, R. H. (2006). Combined immunodeficiency diseases. In J. A. McMillan (Ed.), *Oski's pediatrics: Principles and practice* (4th ed.). Philadelphia: Lippincott Williams & Wilkins.

Burks, W. (2001). Diagnosing pediatric food allergies. *Pediatric Basics, 95*, 2–13.

Camm, J. (2005). Allergic reaction. *Community Practitioner, 78*(7), 234–235.

Casale, T. B., & Stokes, J. R. (2006). Urticaria and angioedema. In J. A. McMillan (Ed.), *Oski's pediatrics: Principles and practice* (4th ed.). Philadelphia: Lippincott Williams & Wilkins.

Cassidy, J. T. (2006). Rheumatic diseases of childhood. In J. A. McMillan (Ed.), *Oski's pediatrics: Principles and practice* (4th ed.). Philadelphia: Lippincott Williams & Wilkins.

Centers for Disease Control & Prevention (1994). *1994 Revised classification system for human immunodeficiency virus infection in children less than 13 years of age* [electronic version]. Available at www.cdc.gov/mmwr/preview/mmwrhtml/00032890.htm.

Chamberlain, J. (2006). Preventing food allergies in children: Some effective measures, but many unknown. *Infectious Diseases in Children, 19*(2), 72.

Champi, C. (2002). Primary immunodeficiency disorders in children: Prompt diagnosis can lead to lifesaving treatment. *Journal of Pediatric Health Care, 16*(1), 16–21.

Chiappini, E., Galli, L., Gabiano, C., Tovo, P., & de Martino, M. (2006). Early triple therapy vs. mono or dual therapy for children with perinatal HIV infection. *Journal of the American Medical Association, 295*(6), 626–628.

Chiriboga, C. A., Fleishman, J. S., Champion, S., Gaye-Robinson, L., & Abrams, E. J. (2005). Incidence and prevalence of HIV encephalopathy in children with HIV infection receiving highly active anti-retroviral therapy (HAART). *Journal of Pediatrics*, 402–407.

Clark, A. T., & Ewan, P. W. (2003). Food allergy in childhood. *Archives of Disease in Childhood, 88*(1), 79–81.

Coleman, M., Toledo, C., & Wallinga, C. (2000). Stress responses of child care providers to classroom activities and childhood behaviors involving HIV/AIDS. *Journal of Pediatric Nursing, 15*(6), 356–363.

Collura, J. M., & Kraus, D. M. (2000). New pediatric antiretroviral agents. *Journal of Pediatric Health Care, 14*(4), 183–192.

Connelly, T. W. (2005). Family functioning and hope in children with juvenile rheumatoid arthritis. *Maternal Child Nursing, 30*(4), 245–250.

Crow, M. E. (1995). Intravenous immune globulin for prevention of bacterial infections in pediatric AIDS patients. *American Journal of Health-System Pharmacy, 52*(8), 803–811.

Dall'Era, M., & Davis, J. (2003). Systemic lupus erythematosus. *Postgraduate Medicine, 114*(5), 31–40.

Domek, G. J. (2006). Social consequences of antiretroviral therapy: Preparing for the unexpected futures of HIV-positive children. *Lancet, 367*, 1367–1369.

Dominguez, K. L. (2006). Prophylaxis for exposure to human immunodeficiency virus. In J. A. McMillan (Ed.), *Oski's pediatrics: Principles and practice* (4th ed.). Philadelphia: Lippincott Williams & Wilkins.

Dreskin, S. C. (2005). *Anaphylaxis.* Retrieved April 22, 2007 from http://www.emedicine.com/med/topic128.htm.

Dupuis-Girod, S., Medioni, J., Haddad, E., Quartier, P., Cavazzana-Calvo, M., Le Deist, F., et al. (2003). Autoimmunity in Wiskott-Aldrich syndrome: Risk factors, clinical features, and outcome in a single-center cohort of 55 patients. *Pediatrics, 111*(5), e622–e626.

Ellaurie, M. (2004). Thrombocytosis in pediatric HIV infection. *Clinical Pediatrics, 43*(7), 627–629.

Ellis, A. K., & Day, J. H. (2003). Diagnosis and management of anaphylaxis. *Journal of the Canadian Medical Association, 169*(4), 307–312.

Farland, E. J. (2005). Human immunodeficiency virus infection. In W. W. Hay, M. J. Levin, J. M. Sondheimer, & R. R. Deterding (Eds.), *Current pediatric diagnosis & treatment* (17th ed.). New York: McGraw-Hill.

Fletcher-Jantzen, E., & Reynolds, C. R. (2003). *Childhood disorders: Diagnostic desk reference.* Hoboken, NJ: John Wiley and Sons.

Frost, D. W., & Chalin, C. G. (2005). The effect of income on anaphylaxis preparation and management plans in Toronto primary schools. *Canadian Journal of Public Health, 96*(4), 250–253.

Gelfand, E. W. (2005). Critical decisions in selecting an intravenous immunoglobulin product. *Journal of Infusion Nursing, 28*(6), 366–374.

Gerson, A. C., Joyner, M., Fosarelli, P., Butz, A., Wissow, L., Lee, S., et al. (2001). Disclosure of HIV diagnosis to children: When, where, why, and how. *Journal of Pediatric Health Care, 15*(4), 161–167.

Gottlieb, B. S., & Ilowite, N. T. (2000). Meeting the challenge of rheumatologic diseases in teens. *Contemporary Pediatrics* [electronic version]. Available at www.contemporarypediatrics.com.

Guay, L. A., & Ruff, A. J. (2001). HIV and infant feeding: An ongoing challenge. *Journal of the American Medical Association, 286*(19), 2462–2464.

Hashkes, P. J., & Laxer, R. M. (2005). Medical treatment of juvenile idiopathic arthritis. *Journal of the American Medical Association, 294,* 1671–1684.

Hayward, A. R. (2005). Immunodeficiency. In W. W. Hay, M. J. Levin, J. M. Sondheimer, & R. R. Deterding (Eds.), *Current pediatric diagnosis & treatment* (17th ed.). New York: McGraw-Hill.

Health Resources and Services Administration, The HIV/AIDS Bureau. (2006). *Ryan White CARE Act.* Washington, DC: United States Department of Health and Human Services. Accessed 4/29/06.

Hollister, J. R. (2005). Rheumatic diseases. In W. W. Hay, M. J. Levin, J. M. Sondheimer, & R. R. Deterding (Eds.), *Current pediatric diagnosis & treatment* (17th ed.) New York: McGraw-Hill.

Houck, J. (2005). HIV disease and AIDS. In S. M. Nettina (Ed.), *Lippincott manual of nursing practice.* Philadelphia: Lippincott Williams & Wilkins.

Hughes, W. T., Dankner, W. M., Yogev, R., Huange, S., Paul, M. E., Flores, M. S., et al. (2005). Comparison of atovaquone and azithromycin with trimethoprim-sulfamethoxazole for the prevention of serious bacterial infections in children with HIV infection. *Clinical Infectious Diseases, 40,* 136–145.

Ilowite, N. (2002). Current treatment of juvenile rheumatoid arthritis. *Pediatrics, 109*(1), 109–115.

Immune Deficiency Foundation. (2003). *The clinical presentation of the primary immunodeficiency diseases (physician's primer).* Retrieved 3/12/06 from http://www.primaryimmune.org/pubs/book_phys/phys_p01.htm.

Immune Deficiency Foundation. (2005). *IDF patient and family handbook for the primary immune deficiency diseases* (3rd ed.). Retrieved 3/12/06 from http://www.primaryimmune.org/pubs/book_pats/book_pats.htm.

Ivey, J., & Corley, B. (2003). Pediatric management problems. *Pediatric Nursing, 29*(5), 370–371.

Jackson, P. L. (2002). Peanut allergy: An increasing health risk for children. *Pediatric Nursing, 28*(5), 496–498, 504.

Jones, K., & Walsek, C. (2005). Pediatric immunologic disorders. In S. M. Nettina (Ed.), *Lippincott manual of nursing practice.* Philadelphia: Lippincott Williams & Wilkins.

Khoury, M., & Kovacs, A. (2001). Pediatric HIV infection. *Clinical Obstetrics and Gynecology, 44*(2), 243–275.

King, S. M. (2004). Evaluation and treatment of the human immunodeficiency virus-1-exposed infant. *Pediatrics, 114*(2), 497–505.

Klunklin, P., & Harrigan, R. C. (2002). Child-rearing practices of primary caregivers of HIV-infected children: An integrative review of the literature. *Journal of Pediatric Nursing, 17*(4), 289–296.

Kuska, B. (2000). Wiskott-Aldrich syndrome: Molecular pieces slide into place. *Journal of the National Cancer Institute, 92*(1), 9–11.

Labyak, S. E., Bourguignon, C., & Docherty, S. (July/August 2003). Sleep quality in children with juvenile rheumatoid arthritis. *Holistic Nursing Journal,* 193–200.

Laffort, C., Le Deist, F., Favre, M., Caillat-Zucman, S., Radfore-Weiss, I., Debre, M., et al. (2004). Severe cutaneous papillomavirus disease after haemopoietic stem-cell transplantation. *Lancet, 363,* 2051–2054.

Lederman, H. M. (2006). Primary immunodeficiency diseases. In J. A. McMillan (Ed.), *Oski's pediatrics: Principles and practice* (4th ed.). Philadelphia: Lippincott Williams & Wilkins.

Lederman, H. M. (2006). Disorders of humoral immunity. In J. A. McMillan (Ed.), *Oski's pediatrics: Principles and practice* (4th ed.). Philadelphia: Lippincott Williams & Wilkins.

Lederman, H. M. (2006). The immune system. In J. A. McMillan (Ed.), *Oski's pediatrics: Principles and practice* (4th ed.). Philadelphia: Lippincott Williams & Wilkins.

Lee, G. M., Gortmaker, S. L., McIntosh, K., Hughes, M. D., Oleske, J. M., & Pediatric AIDS Clinical Trials Group Protocol 219C Team. (2006). Quality of life for children and adolescents: Impact of HIV infection and antiretroviral treatment. *Pediatrics, 117*(2), 273–283.

Levin, M. J., Gershon, A. A., Weinberg, A., Blanchard, S., Nowak, B., Palumbo, P., Chan, C. Y., & the AIDS Clinical Trials Group 265 Team. (2001). Immunization of HIV-infected children with varicella vaccine. *Journal of Pediatrics, 139*(2), 305–310.

Lynch, D. A., Krantz, S., Russell, J. M., Hornberger, L. L., & Van Ness, C. J. (2000). HIV infection: A retrospective analysis of adolescent high-risk behaviors. *Journal of Pediatric Health Care, 14*(1), 20–25.

Macdougall, C., Cant, A., & Colver, A. (2002). How dangerous is food allergy in childhood? The incidence of severe and fatal allergic reactions across the United Kingdom and Ireland. *Archives of Diseases of Childhood, 86,* 236–239.

McIntyre, C. L., Sheetz, A. H., Carroll, C. R., & Young, M. C. (2005). Administration of epinephrine for life-threatening allergic reactions in school settings. *Pediatrics, 116*(5), 1134–1140.

McKinney, R. E. (2006). Antiretroviral therapy in pediatric acquired immunodeficiency syndrome. In J. A. McMillan (Ed.), *Oski's pediatrics: Principles and practice* (4th ed.). Philadelphia: Lippincott Williams & Wilkins.

Meier, E. (2003). The growth of AIDS orphans and policy solutions. *Pediatric Nursing, 29*(1), 75–76.

Miller-Hoover, S. (2005). Juvenile idiopathic arthritis: Why do I have to hurt so much? *Journal of Infusion Nursing, 28*(6), 385–391.

Mofensen, L. M. (2002). U.S. public health service task force recommendations for use of antiretroviral drugs in pregnant HIV-1 infected women for maternal health and interventions to reduce perinatal HIV-1 transmission in the United States. *Morbidity and Mortality Weekly Report, 51,* RR-18, 1–43.

Morantz, C., & Torrey, B. (2004). Treatment of infants with HIV-1 infection. *American Family Physician, 70*(6), 1171–1172.

Morrison-Beedy, D., Nelson, L. E., & Volpe, E. (2005). HIV risk behaviors and testing rates in adolescent girls: Evidence to guide clinical practice. *Pediatric Nursing, 31*(6), 508–512.

Moylett, E. H., & Shearer, W. T. (2002). Diagnosis of human immunodeficiency virus infection in children. *Pediatric Asthma, Allergy & Immunology, 15*(3), 125–131.

Moylett, E. H., & Shearer, W. T. (2006). Pediatric human immunodeficiency virus infection. In J. A. McMillan (Ed.), *Oski's pediatrics: Principles and practice* (4th ed.). Philadelphia: Lippincott Williams & Wilkins.

Munoz-Furlong, A. (2003). Daily coping strategies for patients and their families. *Pediatrics, 111*(6), 1654–1661.

Muraro, A., Dreborg, S., Halken, S., Host, A., Niggemann, B., Aalberse, R., et al. (2004). Dietary prevention of allergic diseases in infants and small children, part III: Critical review of published peer-reviewed observational and interventional studies and final recommendations. *Pediatric Allergy and Immunology, 15,* 291–307.

Murphy, E., Martin, S., & Patterson, J. V. (2005). Developing practice guidelines for the administration of intravenous immunoglobulin. *Journal of Infusion Nursing, 28*(4), 265–272.

National Association of Pediatric Nurse Practitioners. (2001). Position Statement: Pediatric HIV disease. *Journal of Pediatric Health Care, 15*(1), 24a.

National Institute of Child Health and Human Development, National Institute of Health, Department of Health and Human Services. (1999). *Primary immunodeficiency (99-4149).* Washington, DC: U.S. Government Printing Office.

Nehring, W. M., Lashley, F. R., & Malm, K. (2000). Disclosing the diagnosis of pediatric HIV infection: Mothers' views. *Journal of the Society of Pediatric Nurses, 5*(1), 5–14.

Otto, S. E. (2003). Understanding the immune system: Overview for infusion assessment. *Journal of Infusion Nursing, 26*(2), 79–85.

Pagana, K. D., & Pagana, T. J. (2002). *Mosby's manual of diagnostic and laboratory tests* (2nd ed.). St. Louis: Mosby.

Patel, S. J., & Lundy, D. C. (2002). Ocular manifestations of autoimmune disease. *American Family Physician, 66,* 991–998.

Patrick, C. C. (2006). Opportunistic infections in the compromised host. In J. A. McMillan (Ed.), *Oski's pediatrics: Principles and practice* (4th ed.). Philadelphia: Lippincott Williams & Wilkins.

Petry, L., Mathur, A., & Kamat, D. M. (2004). Immunodeficiency disorders: What should primary care providers know? *Consultant for Pediatricians, 3*(5), 228–232.

Roberts, G., Patel, N., Levi-Schaffer, F., Habibi, P., & Lack, G. (2003). Food allergy as a risk factor for life-threatening asthma in childhood: A case-controlled study. *Journal of Allergy and Clinical Immunology, 112*(1), 168–174.

Sampson, H. A. (2002). Peanut allergy. *New England Journal of Medicine, 346*(17), 1294–1299.

Sampson, H. A. (2003). Anaphylaxis and emergency treatment. *Pediatrics, 111*(6), 1601–1908.

Sampson, H. A. (2006). Food allergies. In J. A. McMillan (Ed.), *Oski's pediatrics: Principles and practice* (4th ed.). Philadelphia: Lippincott Williams & Wilkins.

Sampson, H. A., & Eggleston, P. A. (2006). General considerations of allergies in childhood. In J. A. McMillan (Ed.), *Oski's pediatrics: Principles and practice* (4th ed.). Philadelphia: Lippincott Williams & Wilkins.

Shah, I. (2005). Age-related clinical manifestations of HIV infection in Indian children. *Journal of Tropical Pediatrics, 51*(5), 300–303.

Sicherer, S. H., Munoz-Furlong, A., Murphy, R., Wood, R. A., & Sampson, H. A. (2003). Symposium: Pediatric food allergy. *Pediatrics, 111*(6), 1591–1594.

Sicherer, S., Noone, S., & Munoz-Furlong, A. (2001). The impact of childhood food allergy on quality of life. *Annals of Allergy and Immunology, 87,* 461–464.

Simmons, F. E. R., Gu, S., Silver, N. A., & Simons, K. J. (2002) Epipen Jr versus Epipen in young children weighing 15 to 30 kg at risk for anaphylaxis. *Journal of Allergy and Clinical Immunology, 109,* 171–175.

Skoda-Smith, S., & Barrett, D. B. (2000). When earaches and sore throats are more than a pain in the neck. *Contemporary Pediatrics* [electronic version]. Available at www.contemporarypediatrics.com.

Stringer, J. R., Beard, C. B., Miller, R. F., & Wakefield, A. E. (2002). A new name (*Pneumocystis jiroveci*) for Pneumocystis from humans. *Emerging Infectious Diseases, 8*(9), 891–896.

Sullivan, J. L., & Luzuriaga, K. (2001). Editorial: The changing face of pediatric HIV-1 infection. *New England Journal of Medicine, 345*(21), 1568–1569.

Symmons, D. (2005). Juvenile idiopathic arthritis: Issues of definition and causation. *International Journal of Epidemiology, 34,* 671–672.

Taketokmo, C. K., Hodding, J. H., & Kraus, D. M. (2004). *Lexi-comp's pediatric dosage handbook* (11th ed.). Hudson, OH: Lexi-comp.

Tang, A. W. (2003). A practical guide to anaphylaxis. *American Family Physician, 68*(7), 1325–1332.

Tani, M., Nagase, M., & Nishiyama, T. (2002). The effects of long-term herbal treatment for pediatric AIDS. *American Journal of Chinese Medicine, 30*(1), 51–64.

Tretheway, P. (2004). Systemic lupus erythematosus. *Dimensions in Critical Care Nursing, 23*(3), 111–115.

UNICEF. (2004). *The state of the world's children 2005: Childhood under threat.* New York: The United Nations Children's Fund.

UNICEF. (2005). *The state of the world's children 2006: Excluded and invisible.* New York: The United Nations Children's Fund.

United States House of Representatives. (2004). *Public Law No. 108-377 Asthmatic Schoolchildren's Treatment and Health Management Act of 2004.* Washington, DC: Library of Congress. Accessed 5/3/06 at http://frwebgate.access.gpo.gov/cgi-bin/getdoc.cgi?dbname=108_cong_public_laws&docid=f:publ377.108.pdf.

Vadas, P. (2003). Food allergens and anaphylaxis. *Canadian Journal of Dietetic Practice and Research, 64*(2), insert.

Watson, D. C., & Counts, D. R. (October, 2004). Growth hormone deficiency in HIV-infected children following successful treatment with highly active antiretroviral therapy. *Journal of Pediatrics,* 549–551.

Watura, J. C. (2002). Nut allergy in schoolchildren: A survey of schools in the Severn NHS trust. *Archives of Diseases of Childhood, 86,* 240–244.

Weglarz, M., & Boland, M. (2005). Family-centered nursing care of the perinatally infected mother and child living with HIV infection. *Journal for Specialists in Pediatric Nursing, 10*(4), 161–170.

Working Group on Antitetroviral Therapy and Medical Management of HIV-Infected Children. (2005). *Guidelines for the use of antiretroviral agents in pediatric HIV infection* [electronic version]. Available at http://aidsinfo.nih.gov/.

Zingernagel, R. M. (2001). Maternal antibodies, childhood infections, and autoimmune diseases. *New England Journal of Medicine, 345*(18), 1331–1335.

Websites

http://aidsinfo.nih.gov/ U.S. Department of Health and Human Services offers information on HIV/AIDS treatment, prevention, and research

www.aaaai.org American Academy of Allergy, Asthma, & Immunology

www.aafa.org Asthma & Allergy Foundation of America

www.aanma.org Allergy & Asthma Network Mothers of Asthmatics

www.anaphylaxis.org Anaphylaxis Canada

www.arthritis.org Arthritis Foundation—education, research, resources for patients, local chapters, and a juvenile arthritis division: American Juvenile Arthritis Organization

www.carragroup.info/ Childhood Arthritis & Rheumatology Research Alliance

www.cdcnpin.org/ Centers for Disease Control's National Prevention and Information Network

www.cincinnatichildrens.org/Research/Divisions/Rheumatology/default.htm coordinating center for the Pediatric Rheumatology Collaborative Research Group (PRCRG)—research and clinical trials

www.csaci.medical.org Canadian Society of Allergy and Clinical Immunology

www.eatright.org American Dietetic Association

www.foodallergy.org Food Allergy & Anaphylaxis Network—focuses on education, advocacy, research, and awareness

www.hivpositive.com/f-Nutrition/f-3-PediatricNeut/n-Zafonte.html nutrition in pediatric HIV infection

www.info4pi.org National Primary Immunodeficiency Research Center—increasing public awareness

www.jmfworld.org Jeffery Modell Foundation—dedicated to research, physician and patient education, patient support, and public awareness

www.lupusalliance.org Lupus Alliance of America—support, education, and resources for lupus patients

www.lupus.org Lupus Foundation of America—support, education, resources for lupus patients, local support chapters

www.medicalert.org MedicAlert Foundation

www.niams.nih.gov/index.htm National Institute of Arthritis and Musculoskeletal and Skin Diseases through the National Institutes of Health—health information, research, and training

www.pedsaids.org Elizabeth Glaser Pediatric AIDS Foundation—resources for HIV-infected children and their families

www.primaryimmune.org Immune Deficiency Foundation—a national organization dedicated to research, education, and advocacy for the primary immune deficiency diseases; has patient and family resources

www.rheumatology.org American College of Rheumatology—educational materials, guidelines, and referrals

www.scid.net education, support, resources on severe combined immunodeficiency

www.thebody.com/ complete HIV/AIDS resource

www.vachss.com/help_text/hiv_aids_ped.html pediatric HIV infection and AIDS resources

www.womenchildrenhiv.org/ resources for prevention and treatment of HIV infection

Chapter WORKSHEET

● MULTIPLE CHOICE QUESTIONS

1. The nurse is caring for a 6-year-old with juvenile idiopathic arthritis. The mother states that she has trouble getting her daughter out of bed in the morning and believes the girl's behavior is due to a desire to avoid going to school. What is the best advice by the nurse?
   a. Refer the girl to a psychologist for evaluation of school phobia related to chronic illness.
   b. Administer a warm bath every morning before school.
   c. Give the child her prescribed NSAIDs 30 minutes before getting out of bed.
   d. Allow her to stay in bed some mornings if she wants.
2. A 14-year-old with systemic lupus erythematosus wants to know how to care for her skin. What should the nurse teach this adolescent?
   a. Careful sun tanning will give your skin an attractive color.
   b. No special skin care is needed.
   c. Use sunscreen daily to avoid rashes.
   d. Use makeup to camouflage the butterfly rash on her face.
3. The mother of a child with hypogammaglobulinemia reports that her child had a fever and slight chills with an intravenous gammaglobulin infusion last month. She wants to know what other course of treatment might be available. What is the best response by the nurse?
   a. Administration of acetaminophen or diphenhydramine prior to the next infusion may decrease the incidence of fever or chills.
   b. Giving the gammaglobulin intramuscularly is recommended to prevent a reaction.
   c. Talk to her physician about alternative medications that may be used to boost the gammaglobulin level in the blood.
   d. If the child is no longer experiencing frequent infections, then the IV infusions may not be necessary.
4. A 4-month-old infant born to an HIV-infected mother is going into foster care because the mother is too ill to care for the child. The foster mother wants to know if the infant is also infected. What is the best response by the nurse?
   a. "It's too early to know; we have to wait until the infant has symptoms."
   b. "Since the mother is so ill, it's likely the child is also infected with HIV."
   c. "The ELISA test is positive, so the child is definitely infected."
   d. "The PCR test is positive; this indicates HIV infection, which may or may not progress to AIDS."
5. A mother has received instructions about avoiding wheat and soy allergens. Which response by the mother would indicate that further education is needed?
   a. "I will not feed my child any breads made with wheat flour."
   b. "I will allow my child to eat semolina pasta, the kind he loves."
   c. "I will not feed my child shakes made with soy protein."
   d. "I will read labels to be sure I am avoiding wheat and soy."

● CRITICAL THINKING EXERCISES

1. Develop a discharge teaching plan for a 14-year-old with systemic lupus erythematosus who will be taking corticosteroids long term.
2. Devise a developmental stimulation plan for a 22-month-old with HIV infection and encephalopathy with developmental delay (to the level of a 9-month-old).
3. Determine an appropriate nursing plan of care for an infant who has undergone bone marrow transplantation for severe combined immune deficiency.
4. Develop a prioritized list of nursing diagnoses for a child with HIV infection, candidiasis, poor growth, and pneumonia requiring oxygen.
5. A child with recurrent infections is being evaluated. Other than information about onset of symptoms and events leading up to this present episode, what other types of information would the nurse ask while obtaining the history?

● STUDY ACTIVITIES

1. In the clinical setting, compare the growth and development of two children the same age, one with HIV infection and one who has been healthy.
2. Attend an outpatient clinic that provides care to children with HIV infection. Observe the physician or nurse practitioner during office visits and attend a multidisciplinary planning meeting. Identify the role

of the registered nurse in providing family education, coordination of care, and referrals.

3. Conduct an Internet search to determine the educational material available to children and their families related to immune deficiencies, autoimmune disorders, or allergies.

4. Research your clinical institution's policies related to latex allergy, alternative products available at the institution, and how to obtain them for a latex-allergic patient. Provide a presentation to your clinical group about your findings.

chapter 28

Nursing Care of the Child With an Endocrine Disorder

Key TERMS

adrenarche
beta cells
constitutional delay
diabetic ketoacidosis (DKA)
exophthalmos
gland
glucose
glycosylated hemoglobin
goiter
gonad
hirsutism
hormone
hyperfunction/hypersecretion
hypofunction/hyposecretion
ketoacidosis
ketone
Kussmaul respiration
menarche
polydipsia
polyphagia
polyuria
tetany

Learning OBJECTIVES

Upon completion of the chapter, the learner will be able to:

1. Describe the major components and functions of a child's endocrine system.
2. Differentiate between the anatomic and physiologic differences of the endocrine system in children versus adults.
3. Identify the essential assessment elements, common diagnostic procedures, and laboratory tests associated with the diagnosis of endocrine disorders in children.
4. Identify the common medications and treatment modalities used for palliation of endocrine disorders in children.
5. Distinguish specific disorders of the endocrine system affecting children.
6. Link the clinical manifestations of specific disorders in the endocrine system of a child with the appropriate nursing diagnoses.
7. Establish the nursing outcomes, evaluative criteria, and interventions for a child with specific disorders in the endocrine system.
8. Develop child/family teaching plans for the child with an endocrine disorder.

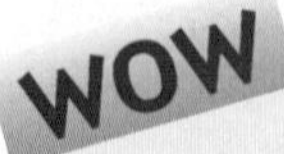

Endocrine disorders in children often elude the medical radar screen.

Carlos Rodriguez, 12 years old, is seen in the clinic today with complaints of weakness, fatigue, blurred vision, and headaches. His mother states, "Carlos' teacher has noticed mood changes and is concerned about his behavior at school. He's always been a good boy. I'm not sure what's going on."

The endocrine system consists of various **glands**, tissues, or clusters of cells that produce and release hormones. **Hormones** are chemical messengers that stimulate and/or regulate the actions of other tissues, organs, or other endocrine glands that have specific receptors to a hormone. Along with the nervous system, the endocrine milieu influences all physiologic effects such as growth and development, metabolic processes related to fluid and electrolyte balance and energy production, sexual maturation and reproduction, and the body's response to stress. The release patterns of the hormones vary, but the level in the body is maintained within specified limits to preserve health.

Problems develop in the endocrine system when there is a deficiency (**hypofunction**) or excess (**hyperfunction**) of a specific hormone. In children, endocrine conditions often develop insidiously and result from an insufficient production of hormones. If the problem is not diagnosed and treated early, delayed growth and development, cognitive impairments, or death may result. Generally, the treatment plan involves correction of the underlying reason for the dysfunction, such as surgical removal of a tumor, and supplementation of missing hormones or adjustment of specific hormone levels. This allows most children to live normal lives.

Variations in Anatomy and Physiology

The organs or tissues of the endocrine system include the hypothalamus, pituitary gland, thyroid gland, parathyroid glands, adrenal glands, gonads, and the islets of Langerhans located in the pancreas. Figure 28.1 shows the location of the organs or tissues involved in the endocrine system. Typically, most endocrine glands begin to develop during the first trimester of gestation, but their development is incomplete at birth. Thus, complete hormonal control is lacking during the early years of life, and the infant cannot appropriately balance fluid concentration, electrolytes, amino acids, **glucose**, and trace substances.

Hormone Production and Secretion

The hypothalamic-pituitary axis produces a number of releasing and inhibiting hormones that regulate the function of many of the other endocrine glands, including the thyroid gland, the adrenal glands, and the male and female gonads. Some glands regulate their function in connection with the nervous system, such as the islets of Langerhans in the pancreas and the parathyroid glands. Many other cells in the body secrete hormones such as the pineal gland, the scattered epithelial cells in the gastrointestinal tract, and the thymus. Disorders related to these other cells as well as gonad dysfunction are discussed in other chapters in this textbook.

Figure 28.1 shows the major glands, the hormones produced by the glands, and the effect each hormone has on the target cell, tissue, or organ. The process of hormone production and secretion involves the principle of feedback control. One gland produces a hormone that affects another endocrine gland. Once the physiologic effect is achieved, this gland, known as the target organ, inhibits the further release of the original hormone. The reverse occurs when the first gland detects low levels of the target gland hormone. If the original gland does not release enough of the hormone, the inhibition process stops so that the gland increases the production of the hormone. The endocrine system and the nervous system work closely together to maintain an optimal internal environment for the body, known as homeostasis.

Common Medical Treatments

Primarily, the treatment of endocrine disorders involves decreasing hormone production (in cases of hypersecretion) or replacing the hormones (in cases of hypofunction). The first step in treating many of these disorders is to screen for potential problems, especially when familial patterns are present. Since the proper functioning of the endocrine system is critical to growth and development, the child's growth is affected by endocrine dysfunction and lack of treatment may lead to mental retardation. Early treatment is often associated with better prognosis and prevention of long-term problems. The next step in treatment involves identifying underlying causes for the dysfunction (e.g., a tumor or growth that requires surgical removal or irradiation). The use of supplemental hormone in cases of hypofunction is generally successful in children, as is the use of inhibiting substances in cases of hyperfunction.

Common Medical Treatments 28.1 describes the common treatments used in children with endocrine disorders. The table explains and gives indications for each treatment as well as relevant nursing implications. Advances in technology and our understanding of molecular biology continue to increase our knowledge of these disorders and the modalities needed to prevent them or improve quality of life for affected children. These advances are vital, since the whole body is influenced by the endocrine milieu.

Drug Guide 28.1 lists the medications most commonly used to treat endocrine disorders. The table gives the actions and indications of each drugs, as well as pertinent nursing implications. Many of the medications are synthetic preparations of the actual hormones. It is impor-

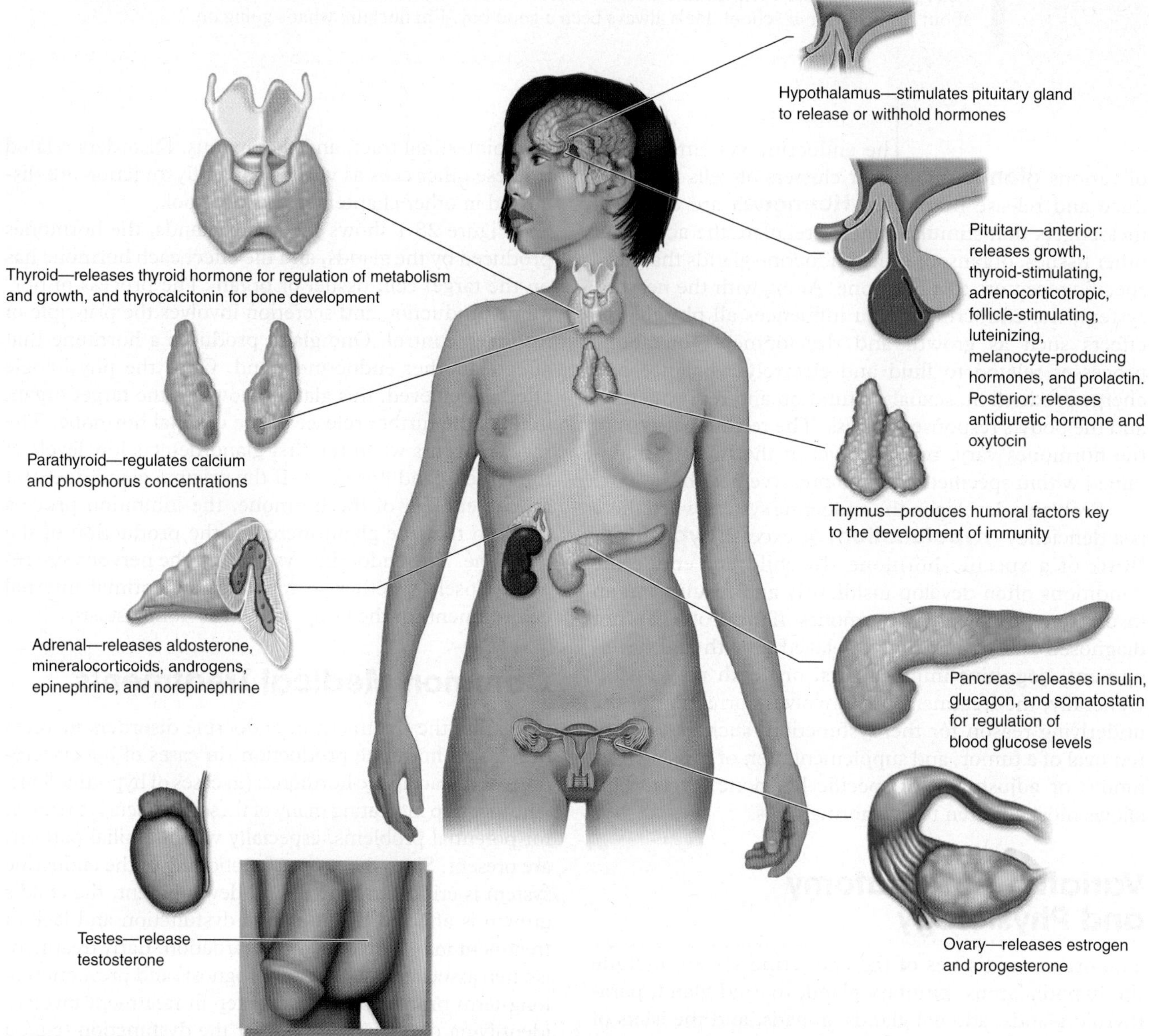
Hypothalamus—stimulates pituitary gland to release or withhold hormones
Pituitary—anterior: releases growth, thyroid-stimulating, adrenocorticotropic, follicle-stimulating, luteinizing, melanocyte-producing hormones, and prolactin. Posterior: releases antidiuretic hormone and oxytocin
Thyroid—releases thyroid hormone for regulation of metabolism and growth, and thyrocalcitonin for bone development
Parathyroid—regulates calcium and phosphorus concentrations
Thymus—produces humoral factors key to the development of immunity
Adrenal—releases aldosterone, mineralocorticoids, androgens, epinephrine, and norepinephrine
Pancreas—releases insulin, glucagon, and somatostatin for regulation of blood glucose levels
Testes—release testosterone
Ovary—releases estrogen and progesterone

● **Figure 28.1** Location of the endocrine glands in the body, with the major effects of the glands listed.

tant to maintain specific blood levels of the drugs to mimic the actual hormone in the body. Nurses must monitor for side effects of too little or too much of the hormone in the child's system. Most endocrine disorders in children require treatment and follow-up with a pediatric endocrinologist as well as a multidisciplinary team that includes a registered nurse who specializes in this area.

Nursing Process Overview for the Child With an Endocrine Disorder

The nursing care of the child with an endocrine disorder requires astute assessment skills, accurate nursing diagnoses and expected outcomes, skilled interventions, and evaluation of the entire process. Children, especially very young ones, easily develop imbalances such as fluid and electrolyte disturbances that can cause further problems. Most of the endocrine disorders are chronic conditions that require ongoing care related to health maintenance, education, developmental issues, and psychosocial needs. These conditions are sometimes complex and range from mild to profound. Early diagnosis and treatment can improve the long-term outcomes for these children.

> Remember Carlos, the 12-year-old with weakness, fatigue, blurred vision, headaches, and mood changes? What additional health history and physical examination assessment information should the nurse obtain?

(text continues on page 934)

Common Medical Treatments 28.1

Treatment	Explanation	Indication	Nursing Implications
Newborn metabolic screening programs	Newborn blood testing to identify certain disorders	Identification of newborns so that treatment can begin early to prevent impact of disorder, such as severe cognitive impairment or death	• Refer to each state's protocol for fetal/newborn screening for endocrine disorders. • Explain to family the rationale and procedure. • Infant should be feeding for 24 hours prior to collection. • Collect blood sample accurately. • IV antibiotic use in newborn may affect results. • Ensure screening is done for early discharges.
Administration of hormone	Give hormone if hypofunction exists or give blocking agent if hyperfunction exists to establish normal growth and development and specific function disrupted by disorder.	Most endocrine disorders, such as diabetes mellitus or growth hormone deficiency	• Follow specific administration requirements for each hormone/drug. • Monitor serum levels carefully to detect appropriate levels. • Observe for adverse effects of too little or too much hormone. • Carefully monitor growth and development patterns.
Surgery	Surgical removal of tumors or cysts	Any endocrine malfunction caused by the presence of a mass	• Provide routine preoperative and postoperative care, depending on location and extent of surgery. • Keep family informed of choices.
Irradiation/radioactive iodine	Radiation is used to influence the hormone secretion of a gland; it is less invasive than surgery.	Hyperfunction of an endocrine gland; may be used when surgery is not possible	• Prepare child for specific procedures following protocols. • Explain the procedure. • Check to ensure child has no sensitivity to iodine preparations.
Glucose monitoring	Fingerstick blood sample several times per day	Monitoring of glucose control	• Teach family appropriate procedure. • Refer family to sources for equipment and supplies. • Assist family to develop a system of record-keeping that works for them.
Dietary interventions	Restriction or manipulation of dietary intake	Diabetes mellitus	• Refer family to a dietitian specializing in pediatric diabetes mellitus. • Reinforce teaching related to special diets.

Drug Guide 28.1 Common Drugs for Endocrine Disorders

Medication	Action	Indication	Nursing Implications
Insulin	Used to replace body's natural insulin, which is necessary for proper glucose use	Diabetes mellitus	• Monitor vital signs and blood glucose levels. • Educate child and family on proper techniques, actions, and adverse effects. • Rotate site of injections to prevent adipose hypertrophy.
Oral hypoglycemic drugs (glipizide, glyburide, metformin)	Assists body's production of insulin by stimulating beta cells to secrete more insulin	Diabetes mellitus type 2	• Monitor vital signs and glucose levels. • Administer with food to minimize gastric upset. • Instruct child and family on use of drug and adverse effects. • Warn family that some over-the-counter or other drugs may increase hypoglycemic effect.
Growth hormone (GH)/somatropin (Humatrope)	Elicits same responses produced by natural GH: stimulates linear bone, skeletal muscle, and organ growth	GH deficiency, growth failure related to inadequate pituitary hormone	• Monitor blood sugar and electrolyte levels. • Administer before epiphyses are fused. • Monitor growth with accurate measurements. • Instruct child and family on appropriate route and method of administration. • Periodic thyroid function tests will be needed. • May interact with glucocorticoid therapy • Monitor for limping or complaints in knee or hip related to slipped epiphysis.
Octreotide acetate (Sandostatin)	Suppresses GH release	Acromegaly	• Monitor for biliary tract abnormalities, glucose tolerance, and hypothyroidism. • Give subcutaneous injections between meals to decrease gastric effects. • Refer family to www.pap.novartis.com for assistance with covering cost of drug.
Corticosteroids (dexamethasone or hydrocortisone)	Elicits same response as natural cortisol: helps control blood sugar, increase protein and fat metabolism, responds to stressors	Cortisol replacement in congenital adrenal hyperplasia, absence of adrenal glands. Also used to close epiphyseal plates in hyperpituitarism.	• Give with milk or food. • May need to increase dose if child is ill or runs fever • Monitor for edema, weight gain, glycosuria, signs of infection, and symptoms of peptic ulcer development. • Do not decrease dose or abruptly stop drug to avoid adrenal crisis.

(continued)

Drug Guide 28.1 Common Drugs for Endocrine Disorders (continued)

Medication	Action	Indication	Nursing Implications
Desmopressin acetate (DDAVP)	Synthetic antidiuretic hormone that promotes reabsorption of water by action on renal tubules	Diabetes insipidus	• Contraindicated in nephrogenic diabetes insipidus • Monitor for water intoxication and adverse effects such as nasal irritation, headache, nausea, increased blood pressure. • Record input and output and weigh child daily. • Titrate dose until appropriate output is obtained. • Instruct child and family in proper intranasal administration. • Avoid over-the-counter cough/hay fever preparations, as they may decrease the drug response. • Store in refrigerator.
Levothyroxine (Synthroid)	Thyroid hormone replacement; increases metabolic rate, controls protein synthesis, and increases cardiac output	Hypothyroidism	• Check blood pressure and pulse before each dose. • Monitor input and output and daily weights. • Watch for thyroid storm. • Report irritability or anxiety. • Instruct child and family to avoid over-the-counter preparations with iodine or foods such as soybeans, iodized salt, tofu, turnips. • Administer at same time each day.
Methimazole, propylthiouracil	Antithyroid drug; blocks synthesis of T3 and T4	Hyperthyroidism	• Check pulse and blood pressure before each dose. • Monitor input and output, daily weights, serum T3 and T4 levels; watch for edema, leukopenia, thrombocytopenia, or agranulocytosis. • Administer with meals to decrease gastric upset. • Give at the same time each day. • Store in light-resistant container. • Instruct child and family to report sore throat, mouth lesions, unusual bleeding or bruising. • Signs of overdose: periorbital edema, cold intolerance, mental depression • Signs of inadequate dose: tachycardia, diarrhea, fever, or irritability
Mineralocorticoid (Florinef)	Promotes reabsorption of Na and K, water from distal renal tubules	Adrenal insufficiency	• Monitor daily weights, blood pressure, intake and output. • Observe for potassium depletion. • Titrate dose to lowest effective dose. • Adverse effects include flushing, sweating, headache, increased blood pressure.

ASSESSMENT

Nursing assessment of a child with endocrine dysfunction includes obtaining a thorough health history, performing a physical assessment, and assisting with or obtaining laboratory and diagnostic tests. The clinical manifestations of endocrine disorders occur as a result of the altered control of the bodily processes normally regulated by the gland or hormone. These manifestations present in many areas of the body because of the diverse functions associated with the endocrine system.

Health History

Focus the health history on the possibility of a family history of an endocrine disorder, prenatal history, history of chronic childhood disease, and growth and development patterns. Use a genogram or family tree to detail the information about the family history in a clear and concise manner.

Endocrine disorders often cause problems in normal growth and development as well as behavioral changes. Question the parent or caregiver about prior growth patterns, achievement of developmental milestones, and the child's behavior. Have the child and family describe the child's activities on a typical day, including school performance, to identify subtle variations in the child's behavior or moods. For example, a child who is typically quiet might ordinarily be less active than average children of that age, and the child with decreased endocrine function also often displays inactivity and fatigue. By having the family and child describe a typical day, the nurse can distinguish between what is appropriate for that child and what may be a change related to endocrine dysfunction.

In addition, obtain a history of dietary and elimination habits. Note extreme thirst, excessive appetite, vomiting, or frequent voiding. Children with endocrine disorders may have some of these symptoms. Table 28.1 lists the types of questions to ask or areas to review when obtaining a health history on a child with possible endocrine dysfunction.

Physical Examination

Table 28.2 lists key physical examination findings that may be present in the child with endocrine dysfunction.

Inspection and Observation

Note a fatigued appearance, cool or dry skin, poor muscle tone, sweatiness, faintness, nervousness, or confusion. Inspect the head and face, noting coarse or brittle hair, excessive hair growth, a rounded face, a protuberant

Table 28.1 Health History Questions Related to Endocrine Disorders

General demographics	Gender, age
Present illness	Gradual or sudden onset of symptoms Changes in child's lifestyle, physical appearance, sleep patterns, appetite, thirst, vision, bowel and urinary habits, or nausea and vomiting Recent increases or decreases in weight and height, muscle weakness, cramps, twitching, or headaches
Past medical history	Birth: any neonatal screening done and results, trauma during birth, birth size, feeding difficulties Prenatal history: maternal factors that may affect growth and development such as substance abuse, use of tobacco or alcohol, Graves' disease Past health: treated for any endocrine problem in the past, recent gastroenteritis or viral syndrome Current immunization status
Allergies	History of allergies to medications, foods, milk or formula
Current medications	Prescribed, over-the-counter, or home remedies
Family history	Any endocrine disorders or growth and development difficulties
Environmental exposure	Exposure to exogenous steroids or gonadotropins
Social history	Normal daily activities; activity level; family resources such as insurance and support systems to maintain long-term treatment regimen
Growth and development milestones	History of growth patterns Presence of learning disabilities, cognitive delays, early or late development of secondary sexual characteristics

Table 28.2 Key Physical Examination Findings Related to Endocrine Problems

Height and weight	Below third percentile or above 90th percentile (pituitary, thyroid, adrenal, or diabetes mellitus)
Hair	Coarse, brittle, excessive (hypothyroidism) Abnormal distribution (adrenal disorders)
Face	Round with hair growth (Cushing's syndrome) Deformities or abnormal features (hypoparathyroidism)
Eyes	Blurred or changes in vision (diabetes mellitus, pituitary tumors, precocious puberty)
Mouth	Delayed dentition (hypocalcemia, hypopituitarism) Fruity breath (ketoacidosis)
Neck	Goiter (hyperthyroidism)
Skin	Cool to touch, dry (hypothyroidism) Changes in color or texture (pituitary disorders) Easy bruising, striae (Cushing's syndrome)
Chest	Tachycardia (hyperthyroidism) Palpitations, sweating (thyroid disorders) Deep, labored breathing (ketoacidosis) Hypertension (Cushing's syndrome)
Abdomen	Extreme weight loss (diabetes mellitus) Extreme fat (Cushing's syndrome) Changes in bowel habits (SIADH, diabetes insipidus, diabetes mellitus)
Fingers	Trembling (hyperthyroidism, parathyroid disorders)
Genitals	Excessive growth (adrenogenital syndrome) Early growth (precocious puberty) Delayed growth (hypopituitarism)

tongue, drooping eyelids, or **exophthalmos** (protrusion of the eyeballs). On inspection of the mouth, note delayed dentition or a fruity breath odor. Note early, excessive, or delayed growth of the genitals. Plot the child's height and weight on growth charts to determine abnormal growth velocity, which occurs in many of these disorders.

Auscultation

Auscultate the heart and lungs. Note tachycardia or irregular heart rhythm. During auscultation of the lungs, note labored respiratory effort, such as Kussmaul breathing, which occurs in diabetic ketoacidosis. Document the blood pressure.

Percussion and Palpation

Percuss and then palpate the abdomen. Dull (nontympanic) sounds or the presence of masses may indicate constipation or a tumor of the ovaries.

Laboratory and Diagnostic Testing

Common Laboratory and Diagnostic Tests 28.1 describes the diagnostic tests and procedures frequently used in identifying and monitoring endocrine disorders in children. Serum and urine hormone and other levels are used to determine whether amounts are adequate, deficient, or excessive. Radiographic studies are used to evaluate bone maturation and growth potential as well as density or tissue calcification. Genetic studies may be used to determine enzyme deficiencies or chromosome defects. Stimulation studies provide a more accurate or definitive test for identifying the disorder after preliminary serum levels are abnormal. Serial blood sampling identifies peak or trough levels of hormones. Computed tomography (CT) scans, magnetic resonance imaging (MRI), nuclear medicine studies, and ultrasonography are used to look for tumors, cysts, or structural defects.

NURSING DIAGNOSES, GOALS, INTERVENTIONS, AND EVALUATION

After completing the assessment, the nurse identifies nursing diagnoses with related goals/outcomes, interventions, and evaluations. The nursing diagnoses for a child with endocrine dysfunction may include:

- Delayed growth and development
- Disturbed body image
- Deficient knowledge
- Interrupted family processes
- Imbalanced nutrition: less than or more than body requirements
- Deficient or excess fluid volume
- Noncompliance

Common Laboratory and Diagnostic Tests 28.1

Diagnostic Test or Procedure	Explanation	Indication	Nursing Implications
Random serum hormone levels	Serum levels of various hormones; immuno-assay measures levels with very small amounts of blood	High or low levels are used to evaluate the function of the specific gland.	• May need to draw specimens at specific times. • Keep child NPO after midnight before test if ordered. • Diurnal variations and episodic secretion of many hormones may require special directions or further testing.
Genetic testing	Identify DNA sequencing	Determines genetic involvement of any disorder	• Explain procedure and the expense involved. • Refer for genetic counseling if needed.
Serum chemistry levels	Serum blood urea nitrogen (BUN), creatinine, sodium, potassium, glucose, calcium, phosphorus, alkaline phosphatase, etc.	To rule out chronic renal failure or other chronic illnesses; to monitor effects of treatment	• BUN levels may be elevated with high-protein diet or dehydration, may be decreased with overhydration or malnutrition. • A diet high in meat may cause a transient but not pronounced increase in creatinine. There are also slight diurnal variations in levels. • Avoid hemolysis of specimen, as this may cause elevation in potassium levels. • Calcium and phosphorus: avoid prolonged tourniquet use during blood draw, as this may falsely increase levels. Child should be NPO past midnight prior to the morning of the blood draw.
Growth hormone stimulation	Stimulate release of GH in response to administration of insulin, arginine, or clonidine	Evaluate and diagnose GH deficiency	• Keep child NPO for specified time. • Obtain serial blood samples at specific times. • Monitor blood glucose levels during study. • Observe for signs of hypoglycemia, diaphoresis, somnolence. • Provide cookies and punch at end of test.
Water deprivation study	Child is deprived of fluids for several hours, and serum sodium and urine osmolality are monitored.	Diabetes insipidus	• Stop test if child exhibits extreme weight loss or changes in vital signs or neurologic status. • Weigh child before, during, and after test. • Rehydrate child after test. • Monitor for orthostatic hypotension.

Common Laboratory and Diagnostic Tests 28.1 (continued)

Diagnostic Test or Procedure	Explanation	Indication	Nursing Implications
Bone age radiograph	Radiographic study of wrist or hand to determine bone maturation compared to national standards	Determine if bone age is consistent with chronologic age to rule out GH deficiency or excess or hypothyroidism	• Explain procedure to child because child must hold still for the x-ray. • Allow family to accompany child. Enlist the family's help if needed to calm child during x-ray.
Other nuclear medicine studies	Contrast media uptake is assessed with serial radiographs.	To visualize an ectopic, enlarged, absent, or nodular gland	• Assess child for allergy to iodine or shellfish. • Explain procedure to child.
Computed tomography or magnetic resonance imaging of brain	Noninvasive imaging methods to identify abnormalities of brain or other areas as necessary	Evaluate presence of tumors, cysts, or structural abnormalities that may affect specific gland or structure	• Machine is large and can be frightening to children. • Scan may be lengthy and the child must remain still, so sedation may be necessary. • If contrast medium is to be used, assess for allergy. • Encourage fluids after procedure if not contraindicated.
Ultrasonography	Noninvasive sound waves are used to visualize structures such as thyroid or pelvic region.	Evaluate presence of tumors or cysts in specific gland, such as the adrenal glands or ovaries, to rule out disorders	• Requires full bladder if in pelvic region

After completing an assessment of Carlos, the nurse noted the following: history reveals Carlos has had episodes of bedwetting over the past month and has had polydipsia and polyphagia. His weight continues to be greater than the 95th percentile on the growth chart. Based on these assessment findings, what would your top three nursing diagnoses be for Carlos?

Because of the gradual, insidious onset of many of these disorders, the child may first be seen in an acute situation. It may be easier for the child and family to work with short-term goals until they accept the chronic situation. A major goal will be to achieve compliance with medical management. The goals for the child with a disorder of the endocrine system generally include re-establishing homeostasis, promoting adequate growth and development, establishing appropriate body image, promoting health-seeking behaviors, and providing education so the family can manage the condition.

Nursing Care Plan 28.1 can be used as a guide in planning care for the child with a disorder of the endocrine system. Of course, this plan will need to be individualized based on the child's symptoms, needs, and disorder as well as the family's requirements. A key element to include in any care plan for the child with an endocrine disorder involves preparing the child, based on his or her developmental needs, for invasive procedures and tests. Provide an opportunity for the family and child to express their concerns and fears during diagnosis and treatment. Reinforce realistic expectations for treatment and prospects for improvement with the family and child. The care plan also needs to address developmental, acute, chronic, and home care issues as well as patient and family education. Families will need assistance with managing the condition from a multidisciplinary team.

Based on your top three nursing diagnoses for Carlos, describe appropriate nursing interventions.

Pituitary Disorders

Because of the close anatomic and functional relationships between the hypothalamus and pituitary gland, we will discuss them together. The hypothalamus affects the

(text continues on page 941)

Nursing Care Plan 28.1

Overview for the Child with an Endocrine Disorder

Nursing Diagnosis: Delayed growth and development related to hypo- or hyperfunction of gland/hormone as evidenced by weight and/or height less than expected for age, failure to meet expected age-appropriate developmental milestones

Outcome identification and evaluation

Nutritional status will be maximized and development will be enhanced: *child will maintain or gain weight appropriately and will make continued progress toward expected developmental milestones.*

Interventions: enhancing growth and development

- Monitor growth parameters using standard growth charts.
- Encourage favorite foods (within prescribed diet restrictions if present) *to maximize oral intake.*
- Consult dietitian *for appropriate diet supplementation recommendations.*
- Encourage compliance with hormone supplementation *to enhance ability to achieve appropriate growth.*
- Provide care related to any complications of dysfunction *such as correcting fluid and electrolyte imbalances or diarrhea.*
- Screen for developmental capabilities *to determine child's current level of functioning.*
- Offer age-appropriate toys, play, and activities (including gross motor) *to encourage further development.*
- Provide support to families of children with developmental delay (*progress in achieving developmental milestones can be slow and ongoing motivation is needed*).
- Reinforce positive attributes in the child *to maintain motivation.*

For the child with diabetes mellitus:

- Provide a calorie-appropriate, nonrestricted, well-balanced diet *to maintain appropriate growth.*
- Encourage three meals with two or three snacks with consistent carbohydrates *to maintain appropriate blood glucose levels and promote growth.*

Nursing Diagnosis: Disturbed body image related to abnormal growth and development/changes in physical appearance due to hormone dysfunction as evidenced by verbalization of dissatisfaction with the child's or adolescent's looks

Outcome identification and evaluation

Child demonstrates appropriate self-esteem in relation to body image; *expresses positive feelings about self and participates in social activities.*

Interventions: promoting healthy body image

- Provide opportunities for child to explore feelings related to appearance: *venting feelings is associated with less body image disturbance.*
- Relate to child on age level, not appearance level: *"babying" a child who looks younger due to his or her small size reduces self-image.*
- Involve the child and especially the teen in the decision-making process: *a sense of control will improve body image.*
- Encourage the child to spend time with peers who have similar endocrine disorders: *peers' opinions are often better accepted than those of persons in authority, such as parents or health care professionals.*
- Refer to counseling or support groups *to further support the child.*

Overview for the Child with an Endocrine Disorder (continued)

Nursing Diagnosis: Deficient knowledge related to therapeutic regimen as evidenced by questions about endocrine disorder and self-management

Outcome identification and evaluation

Child and family will demonstrate sufficient understanding and skills for self-management; *verbalize information about disorder, complications/adverse effects, home care regimen, and long-term needs, and provide return demonstrations of medication administration or other procedures.*

Interventions: promoting knowledge required for self-management

- Assess child's developmental level and family's ability to absorb instruction *to determine how to approach teaching sessions.*
- Establish teaching plan with child and family *to gain cooperation and involvement.*
- Teach and give printed instructions on disorder, complications, home care, and follow-up requirements *so family has source to refer to at home.*
- Evaluate teaching with return demonstrations *to determine whether child/family is skilled enough for home management of the disorder.*

For the child with diabetes mellitus:

- First teach "survival skills" (e.g., glucose and urine testing, administering insulin, record-keeping, food guidelines, when to call physician) *to provide initial base of knowledge for self-management.*
- Implement second-phase home management program with more extensive instruction; *providing additional teaching over time is necessary for management of a significant chronic illness.*
- Monitor outcomes of teaching with every contact *to ensure progress with patient/family education.*

Nursing Diagnosis: Interrupted family processes or adjustment issues related to lifestyle changes required to manage chronic illness and possible lifestyle changes as evidenced by family's presence in the hospital, missed work, demonstration of inadequate coping

Outcome identification and evaluation

Family will maintain functional system of support; demonstrate adequate coping, adaptation of roles and functions, and decreased anxiety: *Parents are involved in child's care, ask appropriate questions, express fears and concerns, identify needs, seek appropriate resources and support, can discuss child's care and condition calmly.*

Interventions: encouraging healthy family processes

- Encourage parents and family members to verbalize concerns related to child's illness, diagnosis, and prognosis: *allows the nurse to identify concerns and areas where further education may be needed.*
- Explain treatments, medications, procedures, child's behaviors, and plan of care to parents: *Understanding of the child's current status and plan of care helps decrease anxiety.*
- Identify support system for family and child: *helps nurse identify needs and resources available for coping.*
- Provide family with information about support groups, financial resources, and special clinics in the area for the particular type of disorder *to provide family with a wide base of support.*
- Encourage parents to become involved in care: *allows parents to feel needed and valued and gives them a sense of control over their child's health.*
- Evaluate coping processes on follow-up visits *to determine restoration of family processes.*

(continued)

Overview for the Child with an Endocrine Disorder (continued)

Nursing Diagnosis: Imbalanced nutrition: less than or more than body requirements related to pathophysiology of dysfunction as evidenced by growth parameters significantly less or more than expected for age

Outcome identification and evaluation

Child's nutritional status is balanced; *child adheres to nutritional guidelines, demonstrates adequate growth (weight and height) pattern within normal range for age and gender or, in the child who has difficulty growing, a progressive increase over time.*

Interventions: maintaining adequate nutrition

- Determine body weight and length/height norm for age or what the child's pretreatment measurements were *to determine goal to work toward.*
- Weigh daily or weekly (according to physician order or institutional standard) and measure length/height weekly *to monitor for appropriate growth.*
- Determine child's food preferences and provide favorite foods as able *to increase the likelihood that the child will consume appropriate amounts of foods.*
- Instruct child and family about nutritional requirements *so that they are involved and are prepared for home care.*
- Refer to dietitian *for more detailed information and assistance.*

For the child who needs to gain weight:

- Offer highest-calorie meals at the time of day when the child's appetite is the greatest *to increase likelihood of increased caloric intake.*
- Provide increased-calorie shakes or puddings within dietary restrictions *(high-calorie foods increase weight gain).*
- Administer vitamin and mineral supplements as prescribed *to attain/maintain vitamin and mineral balance in the body.*

Nursing Diagnosis: Deficient or excess fluid volume related to pathophysiology of endocrine dysfunction as evidenced by signs and symptoms of dehydration (deficient fluid volume) or edema and excessive urine output (excess fluid volume)

Outcome identification and evaluation

Child will maintain adequate fluid volume *as evidenced by elastic skin turgor; absence of edema; moist, pink oral mucosa; presence of tears; urine output 1 mL/kg/hr or more; vital signs within normal range for age; and normal electrolyte/hormone serum levels.*

Interventions: maintaining adequate fluid volume

- Assess hydration status (skin turgor, oral mucosa, presence of tears) every 4 to 8 hours *to evaluate maintenance of adequate fluid volume.*
- Assess adequacy of urine output *to evaluate end-organ perfusion.*
- Maintain strict intake and output record *to evaluate effectiveness of rehydration.*
- Weigh child daily: *accurate weight is one of the best indicators of fluid volume status in children.*
- Administer specific hormone, fluid, and electrolyte requirements as ordered *to aid in fluid balance.*

Fluid volume deficit:

- Maintain IV line and administer IV fluid as ordered *to maintain fluid volume.*

Fluid volume excess:

- Maintain fluid restriction as ordered *to restore homeostasis.*

Overview for the Child with an Endocrine Disorder (continued)

Nursing Diagnosis: Noncompliance related to long-term/complex management of some disorders as evidenced by failure to keep appointments, development of complications or exacerbation of symptoms, or child/family verbalization of inability to maintain treatment plan

Outcome identification and evaluation

Child and family will comply with treatment regimen; *child and family will list treatment expectations and agree to follow through.*

Interventions: encouraging compliance

- Listen nonjudgementally while child/family describe reasons for noncompliance; *assessment of problem should begin with nonthreatening discussion.*
- Help child/family develop a schedule for medication administration and other home regimens that works best for them; *involving child and family in planning care will increase compliance by making them feel respected and valued.*
- Work with the child and family to develop a written treatment plan or schedule that best suits their needs *to provide support for maintenance of treatment plan.*
- Establish follow-up visits to fit family's situation *to promote compliance.*
- Encourage monitoring with pediatric endocrinologist and specialists: *multidisciplinary involvement has been shown to increase compliance.*
- Recognize that behavioral change comes slowly; *allows time for child and family to adjust to chronic nature of illness.*

pituitary by releasing and inhibiting hormones and may be the cause of pituitary disorders. In general, disorders of the pituitary fall into two major groups: the anterior pituitary hormones and the posterior pituitary hormones. Anterior pituitary primary disorders in children include growth hormone deficiency, hyperpituitarism, and precocious puberty. Posterior pituitary disorders include diabetes insipidus and syndrome of inappropriate antidiuretic hormone secretion.

● GROWTH HORMONE DEFICIENCY

Growth hormone deficiency, also known as hypopituitarism or dwarfism, is characterized by poor growth and short stature. It is generally a result of the failure of the anterior pituitary to produce sufficient growth hormone (GH). GH is vital for postnatal growth. It is released throughout the day, with most secreted during sleep. GH stimulates linear growth, bone mineral density, and growth in all body tissues.

GH deficiency occurs in approximately 0.25 per 1,000 live births (Radovick & MacGillivray, 2003). Although it occurs with the same frequency in both genders, society often expects boys to be a certain height, and as a result families may more often request an evaluation in boys. Often this condition is first identified when the health care provider assesses growth patterns. Children may start with a normal birthweight and length, but within a few years the child is less than the third percentile on the growth chart (Radovick & MacGillivray, 2003).

Possible complications related to GH deficiency and its treatment include slipped capital femoral epiphysis, pseudotumor cerebri, increased glucose levels, infection at the injection site, edema, and sodium retention (Behrman et al., 2004; Burg et al., 2002). Recent reports have found no evidence linking GH therapy to higher rates of neoplastic diseases (Behrman et al., 2004; Burg et al., 2002).

Pathophysiology

Primary causes of GH deficiency include an injury or destruction of the anterior pituitary gland because of a tumor such as craniopharyngioma, infection, infarction, or irradiation. Secondary causes of GH deficiency include primary hypothalamic dysfunction related to a deficiency of the hypothalamic releasing or inhibitory factors or insulin-like growth factor (IGF-1) deficiency. A genetic factor such as a dominant or recessive inheritance or genetic mutation may also play a role. For example, mutations in growth hormone–releasing hormone (GHRN) occur in larger numbers in individuals from Pakistan, India, and Brazil (Behrman et al., 2004).

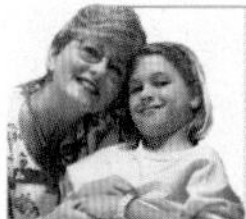

Psychosocial dwarfism results from emotional deprivation that causes suppression of production of the pituitary hormones, resulting in decreased growth hormone. The child is withdrawn, has bizarre eating and drinking habits such as drinking from toilets, and has primitive speech. The treatment involves removing the child from the dysfunctional environment and providing normal dietary intake. With normalized eating and behavioral habits, pituitary secretion is restored and the child dramatically catches up in growth parameters.

Therapeutic Management

Treatment of primary GH deficiency involves the use of supplemental GH. Secondary GH deficiency requires removal of any tumors that might be the underlying problem, followed by GH therapy. Biosynthetic GH, derived from recombinant DNA, is given by subcutaneous injection. The weekly dosage is 0.18 to 0.3 mg/kg, divided into equal doses. The first year of treatment results in 8 to 10 cm of growth, followed by normal growth (Behrman et al., 2004, Sperling, 2002). Daily administration of GH appears to be more effective than schedules such as three times a week (Sperling, 2002).

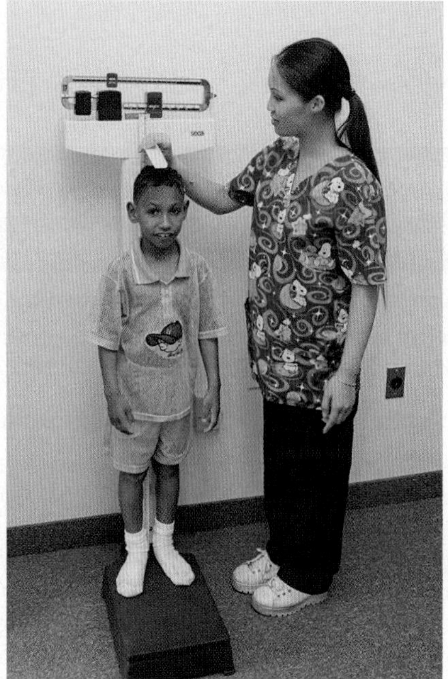

● Figure 28.2 The child with growth hormone deficiency displays short stature.

Nursing Assessment

The focus of the evaluation for GH deficiency is to rule out chronic illnesses such as renal failure, liver disorders, and thyroid dysfunction. For a full description of the assessment phase of the nursing process, refer to page 934. Assessment findings pertinent to GH deficiency are discussed below.

Health History

The health history may reveal a familial pattern of short stature or a prenatal history of maternal disorders such as malnutrition. The past history may be significant for birth history of intrauterine growth retardation or past history of severe head trauma or a brain tumor such as craniopharyngioma. Evaluate previous and current growth patterns. Note history of chronic illness such as cardiac, kidney, or intestinal disorders that may contribute to a decreased growth pattern. Assess the child's feelings about being short.

Physical Examination

In addition to the linear height being at or below the third percentile on standard growth charts, the physical assessment findings may show that the child has a higher weight-to-height ratio (Fig. 28.2). Other physical findings may include prominent subcutaneous deposits of abdominal fat, a childlike face with a large, prominent forehead, a high-pitched voice, delayed sexual maturation (e.g., micropenis and undescended testes in boys), delayed dentition, and decreased muscle mass.

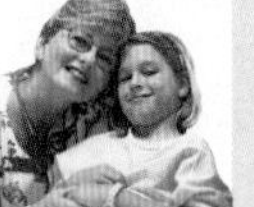

Infants with congenital defects of the pituitary gland or hypothalamus may present as a neonatal emergency. The symptoms include apnea, cyanosis, severe hypoglycemia with possible seizures, and prolonged jaundice.

Laboratory and Diagnostic Testing

The child will undergo laboratory tests to rule out chronic illnesses such as renal failure or liver and thyroid dysfunction. Laboratory and diagnostic tests used in children with suspected GH deficiency include:

- Bone age (as shown by radiographs) will be two or more deviations below normal.
- CT or MRI rules out tumors or structural abnormalities.
- Pituitary function testing confirms the diagnosis. This test consists of providing a GH stimulant such as glucagon, clonidine, insulin, arginine, or L-dopa to stimulate the pituitary to release a burst of GH. Peak GH levels below 7 to 10 ng/mL in at least two tests confirm the diagnosis. A new trend in diagnosing this condition also involves determining whether serum concentrations of insulin-like growth factor are low (Behrman et al., 2004; Sperling, 2002).

Nursing Management

Nursing management for the child with GH deficiency focuses on promoting growth, enhancing the child's self-esteem related to short stature, and providing appropriate education about the disorder.

Promoting Growth

The goal of growth promotion is for the child to demonstrate an improved growth rate, as evidenced by at least 3 to 5 inches in linear growth in the first year of treatment without complications. With early diagnosis and treatment, the child has a better prognosis for reaching a normal adult height. Growth is usually excellent in the first year of therapy compared to later years. Treatment stops when the epiphyseal growth plates fuse.

At the beginning of treatment, monitor for height increase and possible side effects related to the medications. Measure the child's height at least every 6 months and plot growth over time on standardized growth charts. Provide information to the child and family about normal development and growth rates, bone age, and growth potential. Explore with the family and child the expectations and their understanding of what is normal so they will have realistic expectations of treatment. Consult a dietitian if the child and family need assistance in providing adequate nutrition for growth and development.

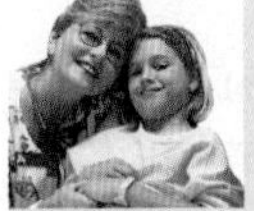

Many children are measured inaccurately in primary care centers. Improved accuracy, especially in performing linear measurements, could yield earlier detection and diagnosis of growth disorders (Lipman et al., 2004).

Enhancing the Child's Self-Esteem

The child with GH deficiency often has younger-looking features and is shorter than his or her peers. Encourage the child to express positive feelings about his or her self-image, as shown by comments during health care visits as well as involvement with peers. Encourage the child to voice concerns. Emphasize the child's strengths and assets. Provide information about community support groups or websites related to GH deficiency. Evaluate for long-term learning problems that may develop if the child had a tumor and surgery or irradiation to remove it. Unidentified learning problems can have a negative impact on the child's self-esteem. Treat and communicate with the child in an age-appropriate manner even though he or she may appear younger.

Educating the Family

GH is a powder that is mixed with packaged diluents. Explain how to prepare it and give the correct dosage. Have the family provide a return demonstration to make sure they understand correct dilution and administration of GH. Instruct the family to report headaches, rapid weight gain, or painful hip joints as possible adverse reactions. The child should visit the pediatric endocrinologist every 3 to 6 months to monitor for potential adverse effects and for compliance with therapy; the family should know that these frequent visits will be needed. Stress the importance of complying with the GH replacement therapy and frequent supervision by a pediatric endocrinologist. Educate the family about the financial costs of therapy, which may be around $15,000 to treat a child weighing 20 kg (Behrman et al., 2004; Sperling, 2002); the family may need help in obtaining assistance and require referral to social services.

Guide the family and child in setting realistic goals and expectations based on age, personal abilities and strengths, and the effectiveness of the GH replacement therapy. For example, the family may want to encourage the child to choose sports that are not dependent on height. Encourage the family to dress the child according to age, not size. Refer the child and family to counseling if indicated. Inform families about support groups such as the Short Stature Foundation (1-800-243-9273) or the Human Growth Foundation (www.hgfound.org/, 1-800-451-6434).

HYPERPITUITARISM (PITUITARY GIGANTISM)

Hyperpituitarism, an extremely rare disorder in children, results from an excessive secretion of GH that leads to an increased growth rate greater than the 95th percentile (Sperling, 2002). The cause of this overproduction of GH is most often a tumor of the anterior pituitary, a pituitary adenoma, or, if combined with precocious puberty, a tumor of the hypothalamus (Sperling, 2002). If this overproduction occurs before the epiphyseal plates close, the child may grow to 7 to 8 feet in height. If the overproduction occurs after they close, acromegaly occurs. Acromegaly is an enlargement of the bones of the head and soft parts of the feet and hands. Being tall is valued in today's society, so assessment for accelerated growth is often delayed, especially in boys.

Therapeutic management includes removing the tumor, restoring the GH patterns to normal, and preventing recurrence. Treatment depends on the cause and may involve surgery, radiation therapy, radioactive implants, or pituitary hormone replacement after surgery. Alternatively, treatment may involve administration of somatostatin analogs to suppress GH production.

Complications of hyperpituitarism include hypogonadism, visual loss, and heart failure.

Nursing Assessment

In addition to excessive height, physical findings include coarse facial features and enlarged hands and feet. Some patients display behavioral and visual problems. Typically, the condition presents at puberty, but it has been found as early as the newborn period (Sperling, 2002). Increased levels of IGF-1 establish the diagnosis of hyperpituitarism. The gold standard for making the diagnosis of GH excess is failure to suppress serum GH levels after an oral glucose challenge test (Spelling, 2002). A bone scan determines whether the epiphyseal plates are closed. Radiologic studies, including MRI, are used to detect any tumors.

Nursing Management

Nursing management depends on which treatment the child undergoes. If surgical removal of a tumor is required, provide routine pre- and postoperative care. Administer somatostatin analog (e.g., octreotide acetate) if ordered. It is usually given as a subcutaneous injection every 12 hours; refer to Drug Guide 28.1 for further information. Treat the child according to chronologic age rather than according to height. Assess the child's self-image, teach the child and family about the disorder and the treatment plan, and provide emotional support. Monitor for and report signs of potential complications such as hypogonadism, visual loss, or heart failure.

● PRECOCIOUS PUBERTY

In precocious puberty, the child develops sexual characteristics before the usual age of pubertal onset. Puberty, also known as sexual maturation, occurs when the gonads produce increased amounts of sex hormones. Typically, this occurs around 10 to 12 years of age for girls and 11 to 14 years of age for boys. In precocious puberty, breasts develop before age 7 years in white girls or before age 6 years in African-American girls, or secondary sex characteristics develop in boys younger than 9 years (Burg et al., 2002). The incidence appears to be 0.1 to 0.5 per 1,000 children; the disorder is five times more common in girls, and 95% of the cases have idiopathic etiologies (Burg et al., 2002). Other causes include benign hypothalamic tumor, brain injury or radiation, a history of infectious encephalitis, meningitis, congenital adrenal hyperplasia, and tumors of the ovary, adrenal gland, or testes.

Pathophysiology

True precocious puberty develops as a result of premature activation of the hypothalamic-pituitary-gonadal axis that results in the production of gonadotropin-releasing hormone (GnRH), which stimulates the pituitary to produce luteinizing hormone (LH) and follicle-stimulating hormone (FSH). These hormones in turn stimulate the gonads to secrete the sex hormones (estrogen or testosterone). The child develops sexual characteristics, shows increased growth and skeletal maturation, and has reproductive capability. Pseudoprecocious puberty presents with no early secretion of gonadotropin or maturation of gonads but rather early overproduction of sex hormones. The condition results in increased end-organ sensitivity to low levels of circulating sex hormones and leads to premature pubic hair and breast development. If left untreated, the child may become fertile. In addition, the hormones stimulate the closure of the epiphyseal plates, which results in overall short stature.

Therapeutic Management

The clinical treatment for precocious puberty first involves determining the cause. For example, if the etiology is a tumor of the central nervous system, the child undergoes surgery, radiation, or chemotherapy. The treatment for central precocious puberty involves administering a GnRH analog. This is available as a depot injection given every 3 to 4 weeks, a subcutaneous injection given daily, or an intranasal compound given two or three times each day. This analog stimulates gonadotropin release initially but when given on a long-term basis will suppress gonadotropin release. With this treatment, the growth rate slows and secondary sexual development stabilizes or regresses. When treatment is discontinued, puberty resumes according to appropriate developmental stages. Medroxyprogesterone (Depo-Provera) reduces secretion of gonadotropins and prevents menstruation. The overall aim of treatment is to halt or even reverse sexual development and rapid growth as well as promote psychosocial well-being.

Nursing Assessment

For a full description of the assessment phase of the nursing process, refer to page 934. Pertinent assessment findings related to precocious puberty are discussed below.

Health History

The health history may reveal complaints of headaches, nausea, vomiting, and visual difficulties due to the circulating hormones. The psychosocial development is typical for the child's age, but the child may show emotional lability, aggressive behavior, and mood swings. Information from the child and family may also reveal risk factors such as exposure to exogenous hormones, history of central nervous system trauma or infection, or a family history of early puberty.

Physical Examination

Physical examination may reveal acne and an adult-like body odor. The child will present with an accelerated rate of growth. The Tanner staging of breasts, pubic hair, and genitalia reveals advanced maturation for the child's age, but the child does not typically display sexual behavior.

Laboratory and Diagnostic Testing

Radiologic examinations and pelvic ultrasound identify advanced bone age, increased uterus size, and development of ovaries consistent with the diagnosis of precocious puberty. Laboratory studies include screening radioimmunoassays for LH, FSH, estradiol, or testosterone. The child's response to GnRH stimulation confirms the diagnosis of central precocious puberty versus gonadotropin-independent puberty. This test involves administering synthetic GnRH intravenously and drawing serial blood levels, about every 2 hours, of LH, FSH, and estrogen or testosterone. A positive result is defined as pubertal or adult levels of these hormones in response to the GnRH administration. CT, MRI, or skull radiography reveals any lesions in the central nervous system.

Nursing Management

In general, nursing management of the child with precocious puberty focuses on administering medications, helping the child to deal with self-esteem issues related to the accelerated growth and development of secondary sexual characteristics, and educating the child and family. Goals of nursing management include appropriate physical development and pubertal progression appropriate for age. Refer to Nursing Care Plan 28.1, and individualize care based on the child's and family's response to this disorder.

Nursing care involves assessing and documenting the physical changes the child is experiencing and administering medications. Demonstrate correct administration of medication and observe for potential adverse effects (teach this information to the family as well). Encourage the family to comply with follow-up appointments, which typically occur every 6 months and include scheduled stimulation tests. Inform families that pharmacologic intervention stops when the child reaches the age appropriate for pubertal development. Provide appropriate sex education, but reassure parents that precocious puberty does not usually involve precocious sexual behavior.

Dealing With Self-Esteem Issues

Often these children develop self-esteem issues and anxiety related to body image disturbances and impaired social interactions. The goal is for the child to exhibit normal psychosocial development and understand the physical and emotional changes that occur with early onset of puberty. Communicate with the child on an age-appropriate level, even when physical characteristics make the child appear older. Maintain a calm, supportive atmosphere and provide for privacy during examinations. Refer the child and family for counseling if behavioral or psychological disturbances develop. Since the child may have issues with self-image and may be self-conscious, encourage him or her to express his or her feelings about the changes, and use role-playing to show the child how to handle teasing from other children. Let the child know that everyone develops sexual characteristics in time.

• DELAYED PUBERTY

Delayed puberty is a condition of delayed secondary sexual development. In girls, it exists if the breasts have not developed by age 13, pubic hair has not appeared by age 14, or **menarche** has not occurred by age 16. In boys, it exists when no testicular enlargement or scrotal changes have occurred by age 14 or pubic hair has not appeared by age 15 followed by testicular enlargement. The most common cause for delayed puberty is a hereditary condition known as **constitutional delay** (Radovick & MacGillivray, 2003). Hypogonadism also may result when there is decreased stimulation of the gonads due to dysfunction in the hypothalamus or pituitary gland as well as from tumors, irradiation, or genetic syndromes such as Turner or Klinefelter syndrome. Another common cause is a chronic condition such as anorexia or cystic fibrosis.

Management involves administering testosterone or estradiol in low dosages if there is no underlying situation to address. This is usually necessary for only a short time to get puberty started.

Nursing Assessment

Assessment involves obtaining a health history to identify the indications for this condition. Assessment of the growth pattern using correct techniques and standards for comparison is essential. On physical assessment, note absence of secondary sex characteristics as noted above. Laboratory and diagnostic testing rules out other causes for delayed puberty. Blood levels of reproductive hormones may also be evaluated.

Nursing Management

In addition to the general interventions presented in Nursing Care Plan 28.1, instruct the child and family about the medication therapy. Educate the child and family about the different stages of puberty. Help the family develop a home management schedule for the administration of medication. Answer the family's questions about the condition or potential complications (e.g., infertility), depending on the cause of the condition.

• DIABETES INSIPIDUS

Diabetes insipidus is a disorder of the posterior pituitary gland resulting from a deficiency in the secretion of antidiuretic hormone (ADH). This hormone, also known as vasopressin, is produced in the hypothalamus and stored in the pituitary gland. ADH is involved in concentrating the urine from the kidneys by stimulating reabsorption of water in the renal collecting tubules through increased membrane permeability. This conserves water and maintains normal osmolality. With a deficiency in ADH, the kidney loses massive amounts of water and retains sodium in the serum.

Typically, this disorder occurs in children as a result of complications from head trauma or cranial surgery to remove hypothalamic-pituitary tumors such as craniopharyngioma (Behrman et al., 2004) Other causes include granulomatous disease, infections such as meningitis or encephalitis, vascular anomalies, congenital malformations, infiltrative disease such as leukemia, or drug administration; 10% of the cases in children are idiopathic (Behrman et al., 2004). A rare variant, nephrogenic diabetes insipidus, tends to be transmitted genetically (e.g., sex-linked, autosomal dominant, or autosomal recessive forms); it is not associated with the pituitary gland and displays vasopressin insensitivity at the level of the kidneys (Behrman et al., 2004).

Diabetes insipidus is usually permanent and requires treatment throughout life.

Therapeutic Management

Unless a tumor is present (in which case it is removed by surgery), the usual treatment involves daily replacement of ADH in older children. In neonates and young infants, the treatment is fluid therapy at 3 L/m^2 per 24 hours (Behrman et al., 2004). The drug of choice for home treatment is desmopressin acetate (DDAVP), 25 to 300 mcg, a long-acting vasopressin analog. It is given intranasally, subcutaneously, or orally every 8 to 12 hours. The dose depends on the child's age, urine output, and urine specific gravity. The use of DDAVP in infants is controversial. In the hospital, the child receives aqueous vasopressin, 8-arginine vasopressin (Pitressin), intravenously. This is a short-acting drug, so the dosage can be quickly adjusted. Both types of the medication decrease urinary output and thirst but need to be titrated.

For nephrogenic diabetes insipidus, the treatment involves diuretics, high fluid intake, and restricted sodium intake as well as a high-protein diet.

Nursing Assessment

For a full description of the assessment phase of the nursing process, refer to page 934. Assessment findings pertinent to diabetes insipidus are discussed below.

Health History

Nursing assessment involves obtaining a history of any conditions that led to the development of the disorder. This review includes information about the neonatal period as well as a current history of infections such as meningitis, diseases such as leukemia, or familial patterns. Most symptoms of endocrine disorders develop slowly, but the onset of this disorder is abrupt. The health history usually elicits the cardinal symptoms as well as complaints representing the early signs of dehydration.

The most common initial symptoms reported are polyuria and polydipsia. Except for unconscious patients, the child typically maintains adequate perfusion by drinking water (Perkin et al., 2003). The parent or child may report frequent trips to the bathroom, nocturia, or enuresis. When the child cannot compensate for the excessive loss of water by increasing fluid intake, other symptoms will be reported, such as weight loss or signs of dehydration. For example, irritability may be due to the early signs of dehydration or the frustration the child feels at being unable to quench his or her thirst. Other signs may be intermittent fever, vomiting, and constipation.

Physical Examination

Observation and inspection may reveal weight loss or failure to thrive in the young infant. Inspection may also reveal signs of dehydration, such as dry mucous membranes or decreased tears. The child may excrete greater than 3 L/m^2 of urine per day. On auscultation, tachycardia or increased respiratory rate may be signs of compensation for the decrease in fluid volume. Palpation reveals slightly depressed fontanels or decreased skin turgor.

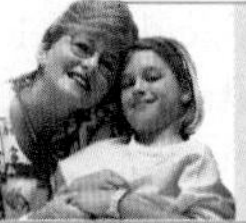

The cardinal signs of diabetes insipidus are **polyuria** (excessive urination) and **polydipsia** (excessive thirst).

Laboratory and Diagnostic Testing

Diagnostic tests used to evaluate diabetes insipidus include:

- Radiographic studies such as CT scan or ultrasound of the skull and kidneys to determine whether a lesion or tumor is present
- Urinalysis: urine is dilute, osmolarity is less than 3000 mOsm/L, specific gravity is less than 1.005
- Serum osmolarity is greater than 300 mOsm/L.
- Serum sodium is elevated.
- Fluid deprivation test measures vasopressin release from the pituitary in response to water deprivation. Normal results will show decreased urine output, increased urine specific gravity, and no change in serum sodium.

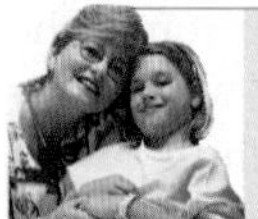

During a fluid deprivation test, the child may be irritable and frustrated because fluid is being withheld. Don't drink in front of the child.

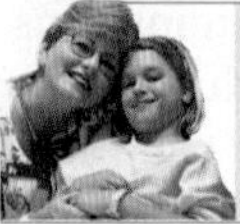

Stop the fluid deprivation test if 3% to 5% of body weight is lost, because complications may occur (Dveirin & Tunnessen, 2000).

Nursing Management

Refer to Nursing Care Plan 28.1, and individualize the plan of care based on the child's and family's response to the illness. Specific interventions related to nursing care of the child with diabetes insipidus are discussed below.

Promoting Hydration

The goal of treatment is to achieve hourly urine output of 1 to 2 mL/kg and urine specific gravity of at least 1.010.

Maintain fluid intake regimens as ordered. Monitor fluid status by measuring vital signs, fluid intake and output, and daily weights (using the same scale at the same time of day). If fluids are stopped too soon, the child may become hypernatremic, which can lead to seizures. Feed infants more frequently, since they excrete more dilute urine, consume larger volumes of free water, and secrete lower amounts of vasopressin than older children. Monitor for signs and symptoms of dehydration during the fluid deprivation test as well as when starting the treatment regimen. If the child is unconscious or has brain injury, maintain hydration and nutrition with nasogastric or gastrostomy feedings.

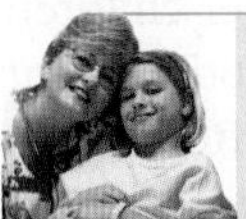

Monitor blood pressure closely when initiating vasopressin.

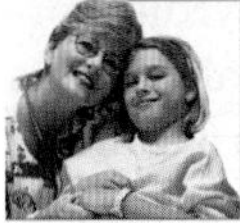

Notify the physician if the urine output is greater than 1,000 mL per hour for two consecutive voids.

Promoting Activity

Establish appropriate activity for the child, and allow time for him or her to regain strength and the desire to increase level of activity. Assess the child's abilities daily, schedule frequent bathroom breaks, keep fluids the child likes available at all times, and fit the treatment plan to the child's activity.

Educating the Family

Involve the family in development of the fluid intake regimens. A journal or daily log is essential in maintaining the regimen and identifying problems. Children with intact thirst centers can self-regulate their need for fluids, but if this is not the situation, help the family develop a plan for 24-hour fluid replacement. This may require instruction on nasogastric or gastrostomy feedings. Infants will need fluid intake at night. Educate the family about the symptoms of water intoxication and dehydration. Help the family develop a plan to inform the school and other individuals in the child's life about the need for liberal bathroom privileges and extra fluids to prevent accidents or dehydration. Teaching Guideline 28.1 gives tips on educating the family about the medication regimen. Recommend that the family obtain a medical alert bracelet or necklace for the child. Encourage compliance with follow-up appointments, which will probably be every 6 months.

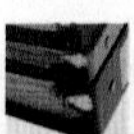

TEACHING GUIDELINE 28.1

DDAVP Administration

- Keep DDAVP in the refrigerator at all times.
- Clear the nostrils (the medication may be poorly absorbed if the child has nasal congestion).
- Insert the measuring tube into the bottle.
- Fill to proper dosage and hold the top of the tube closed while inserting the medication-filled end into the nostril.
- Blow the liquid out of the tubing into the nostril.
- If the child sneezes, repeat the dosage.
- Measure urine specific gravity to monitor effectiveness of the drug.

SYNDROME OF INAPPROPRIATE ANTIDIURETIC HORMONE (SIADH)

SIADH occurs when ADH (vasopressin) is secreted in the presence of low serum osmolality because the feedback mechanism that regulates ADH does not function properly. ADH continues to be released, and this leads to water retention, decreased serum sodium due to hemodilution, and extracellular fluid volume expansion. SIADH is often caused by central nervous system infections such as meningitis, head trauma, brain tumors, intracranial surgery, and certain medication such as analgesics, barbiturates, or chemotherapy. SIADH may also result from excessive administration of vasopressin during the treatment of diabetes insipidus (Nelson, 2004).

Management of SIADH includes correcting the underlying disorder in addition to fluid restriction and intravenous sodium chloride administration to correct hyponatremia and increase serum osmolality.

Nursing Assessment

Obtain a health history, noting history of a central nervous system infection or tumor, intracranial surgery, head trauma, or use of the above-mentioned medications. Note symptoms such as decreased urine output and weight gain, or gastrointestinal symptoms such as anorexia, nausea, and vomiting. Assess neurologic status, noting lethargy, behavioral changes, headache, altered level of consciousness, seizure, or coma. Neurologic signs develop as the sodium level decreases. Diagnostic tests reveal low serum sodium and osmolality, as well as decreased urea, creatinine, uric acid, and albumin levels. Urine samples demonstrate elevated osmolality, high sodium concentrations, and specific gravity greater than 1.030. Adrenal, thyroid, and renal function studies may be used to rule out other causes of hyponatremia.

Nursing Management

Nursing goals focus on restoring fluid balance and preventing injury. Institute safety precautions if altered level of consciousness, confusion, or seizures are present. Notify the physician if headache or irritability is present. Monitor intake and output and weigh the child daily. An indwelling urinary catheter may be needed to allow for hourly monitoring of urine volume and specific gravity. Help the child cope with fluid restriction by offering sugarless candy, a wet washcloth, or maybe ice chips. Administer electrolyte replacement as necessary to correct imbalances.

Comparison Chart 28.1 compares diabetes insipidus with SIADH.

Disorders of Thyroid Function

Disorders of the thyroid gland are relatively common in infancy and childhood (Burg et al., 2002). These disorders can be serious because thyroid hormones are important for growth and development: they regulate metabolism of nutrients and energy production.

CONGENITAL HYPOTHYROIDISM

Congenital hypothyroidism, also known as cretinism, usually results from failure of the thyroid gland to migrate during fetal development. This results in malformation or malfunction of the thyroid gland, which leads to insufficient production of the thyroid hormones that are required to meet the body's metabolic and growth and development needs. Congenital hypothyroidism leads to low concentrations of circulating thyroid hormones (T3 and T4). Before newborn screening for the disorder in North America began in the 1970s, the diagnosis was often not made until 8 to 12 weeks; the delay produced irreversible brain damage and loss of intellectual function (Burg et al., 2002).

Congenital hypothyroidism occurs in 0.25 per 1,000 live births (Burg et al., 2002). It occurs more often in girls, infants of Hispanic or Far Eastern origin, and children with Down syndrome and is less common in African-American infants (Burg et al., 2002).

Pathophysiology

Congenital hypothyroidism is due to a defect in the development of the thyroid gland in the fetus due to a spontaneous gene mutation, an inborn error of thyroid hormone synthesis resulting from an autosomal recessive trait, pituitary dysfunction, or failure of the central nervous system–thyroid feedback mechanism to develop (Burg et al., 2002). Transient primary hypothyroidism may also occur; it results from transplacental transfer of maternal antithyroid drugs, topical iodine exposure, or maternal thyroid-blocking antibodies (Eugster et al., 2004).

Therapeutic Management

To prevent mental retardation and restore normal growth and motor development, thyroid hormone replacement with sodium L-thyroxine (Synthroid, synthetic thyroxine or Levothroid) begins. The recommended starting dosage is 10 to 15 mcg/kg per day; infants and younger children typically require a higher dosage per unit of body weight (Burg et al., 2002). There are no adverse effects with physiologic doses, but thyroid function tests are performed initially every 2 weeks to closely monitor for effects and to ensure proper dosing. Since thyroid hormone is vital to the infant's developing central nervous system, the goal is to normalize thyroid function as quickly as possible. This treatment will be needed lifelong to maintain normal metabolism and normal physical and mental growth and development.

Nursing Assessment

Nursing assessment of the child with congenital hypothyroidism includes health history, physical examination, and laboratory testing.

Health History

Determine whether the neonatal metabolic screening test was performed early or whether it was not performed shortly after birth. Inquire about maternal history that may indicate a connection to hypothyroidism, such as maternal exposure to iodine. Additional history findings may include sensitivity to cold, constipation, feeding problems, or lethargy. Since parents like babies to sleep well, the parents may not complain that the baby is sleeping too much; rather, they may remark that it is difficult to keep the baby awake.

COMPARISON CHART 28.1 Diabetes Insipidus Versus SIADH

Diabetes Insipidus	Syndrome of Inappropriate Antidiuretic Hormone
• "High and dry" • Increased urination • Hypernatremia • Serum osmolality > 300 mOsm/kg • Urine specific gravity 1.005 • Decreased urine osmolality • Dehydration, thirst	• "Low and wet" • Decreased urination • Hyponatremia • Serum osmolality < 280 mOsm/kg • Urine specific gravity > 1.030 • Increased urine osmolality • Fluid retention, weight gain, and hypertension

Physical Examination

Most infants are asymptomatic until the first month, when they begin to develop clinical signs. Inspection and observation reveal a lethargic baby or a child with hypotonia, hypoactivity, and a dull expression. A combination of lethargy and irritability may exist, with an overall delayed mental responsiveness. Measurements of weight and height may reveal delayed growth. Other findings may include a persistent open posterior fontanel, coarse facies with short neck and limbs, periorbital puffiness, enlarged tongue, and poor sucking response (Fig. 28.3). The skin may appear pale with mottling or yellow from prolonged jaundice, or it may be cool, dry, and scaly to the touch, with sparse hair development on the older child. Auscultation of the chest might reveal bradycardia. Signs of respiratory distress and decreased pulse pressure may also be present. On palpation of the abdomen, there may be evidence of an umbilical hernia or a mass due to constipation.

Laboratory and Diagnostic Testing

States mandate newborn screening for thyroid hormone levels before discharge from the hospital or 2 to 6 days after birth. When the test is performed within the first 24 to 48 hours along with other metabolic screenings, the result may be inaccurate because of the immediate increase in thyroid-stimulating hormone (TSH) shortly after birth. Radioimmunoassay is used to measure levels of thyroxine (T4), which accurately reflects the child's thyroid status. If the T4 level is less than 6.5 μU/mL (normal is 6.5 to 13 μU/mL), then a second confirming laboratory test is performed, as well as determining whether the TSH is greater than 5 μU/mL through a non-isotopic, time-released fluoroimmunoassay (TR-FIA). A thyroid scan may also be used to check for the absence or ectopic placement of the gland. In addition to serum measurement of T4, other diagnostic tests include serum T3, radioiodine uptake, thyroid-bound globulin, and ultrasonography.

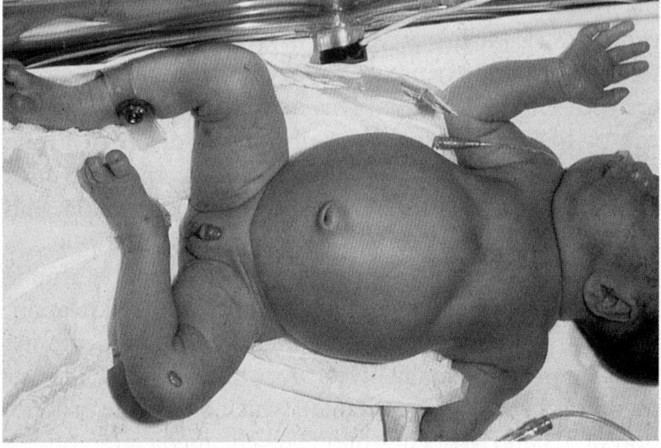

● Figure 28.3 Newborn with congenital hypothyroidism.

Nursing Management

The overall goal of nursing management of the infant or child with congenital hypothyroidism is to establish a normal growth pattern without complications such as mental retardation or failure to thrive. Individualize the nursing care plan based on the infant's responses to the illness.

Promoting Appropriate Growth

Measure and record growth at regular intervals. Thyroid levels are measured every 2 to 4 weeks until the target range is reached on a stabilized dose of medication. Tests are then obtained every 3 to 4 months for the first several years of life, changing to every 6 to 12 months during adolescence. Monitor for signs of hypo- or hyperfunction, including changes in vital signs, thermoregulation, and activity level. Provide adequate rest periods and meet thermoregulation needs. If the infant's tongue is unusually large, observe feeding ability, prevent airway obstruction, and position the infant on the side. Fluid restrictions or a low-salt diet may be ordered.

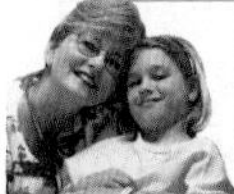

Observe for signs of thyroid hormone overdose (irritability, rapid pulse, dyspnea, sweating, fever) or ineffective treatment (fatigue, constipation, decreased appetite).

Educating the Family

Since many infants are asymptomatic, the diagnosis may be unexpected, so reassure and convey realistic expectations to the family. Developmental screening may be required if the child showed any symptoms initially or as the child gets older to ensure that drug therapy is appropriate. Educate the family about the disorder, the medication and method of administration, and adverse effects such as increased pulse rate (which may indicate an overdose of thyroid hormone). Instruct the family to check the pulse before giving the medication.

L-Thyroxine is an oral medication that is available as a pill. It must be crushed for infants and young children. It can be mixed with a small amount of formula and placed in the nipple, but it should not be placed in a full bottle of formula because the infant will not ingest all the medication if he or she does not finish the bottle. The medication can also be mixed with a small amount of liquid and given with a dropper. Medication absorption is affected by soy-based formulas and iron preparations (Burg et al., 2002), so carefully evaluate before starting the infant on formulas such as Alsoy, Isomil, Nursoy, ProSobee, and Soyalac. If the child vomits within 1 hour of administration, instruct the family to repeat the dose, since many missed doses may lead to developmental delays and poor growth.

Inform the family that this medication will be needed throughout the child's life. Tell them that frequent blood tests will be needed to evaluate thyroid function and the child's growth rate; genetic counseling may be needed. Current recommendations include monitoring by a pediatric endocrinologist every 1 to 2 months for the first year of life, every 2 to 3 months between 1 and 3 years of age, and every 2 to 12 months until growth is completed (Kemper & Foster, 2003). The nurse may need to help the family to find a laboratory nearby or to handle financial issues related to the therapy. Educate the family about infant stimulation programs if the child shows cognitive problems, retarded physical growth, or slow intellectual development. Some information may need to be reinforced during school-age or adolescent stages of development. Finally, encourage the family to obtain a medical identification bracelet or necklace for the child.

ConsiderTHIS!

Asha Virani, 1 week old, is brought to the clinic. Her newborn screening test was positive for hypothyroidism. Her parents are shocked and upset by the news. Her mother states, "My daughter's been doing so well since she came home from the hospital. She seems to be doing everything she should be. She's a great sleeper. I just can't believe anything's wrong with her."

1. **How would you address the parents' concerns?**
2. **What teaching will be appropriate for this family?**

● ACQUIRED HYPOTHYROIDISM

Hypothyroidism also occurs as an acquired condition. This disorder most commonly results from an autoimmune chronic lymphocytic thyroiditis known as Hashimoto's thyroiditis (Sperling, 2002). As a genetic condition, antibodies develop against the thyroid gland, causing the gland to become inflamed, infiltrated, and progressively destroyed. It occurs more often in girls during childhood and adolescence (Sperling, 2002). Less common etiologies include hypothyroidism associated with pituitary or hypothalamic dysfunction or exposure to drugs or substances such as lithium that interfere with thyroid hormone synthesis.

Management involves oral sodium L-thyroxine, which is given at 2 to 5 mcg/kg per day to maintain T4 in the upper half of the normal range and to suppress TSH.

Nursing Assessment

Interview the family and child to determine activity tolerance and behavior changes. The symptoms may develop over a period of time and may be subtle. Note vague complaints of fatigue, weakness, weight gain, cold intolerance, constipation, and dry skin. The severity of symptoms depends on the length of time that the hormone deficiency has existed and its extent. Reviewing the growth pattern may reveal a slowed or arrested growth rate (height) and increased weight.

Physical examination may reveal a **goiter** (enlargement of the thyroid gland). Deep tendon reflexes may be sluggish and the face, eyes, and hands may be edematous. Note thinning or coarse hair, muscle hypertrophy with muscle weakness. and signs of delayed or precocious puberty. The diagnostic evaluation involves serum thyroid function studies (TSH, T3, and T4) as well as serum thyroid antibodies to confirm autoimmune thyroiditis. MRI and a thyroid uptake test and scan may also be necessary.

Nursing Management

Work with the family to establish a daily schedule for administering L-thyroxine, which should be taken 30 to 60 minutes before a meal for optimal absorption. Explain to the family that growth is related to the child's response to the treatment, and there are no specific strategies to aid in this growth. The family should understand the diagnosis, should be able to recognize signs and symptoms of hypo- and hyperfunction, and should know when to notify the physician. The family and child may need assistance in accepting the therapy as well as the experience of catch-up growth that may occur at the beginning of therapy. The child with chronic or severe hypothyroidism may be at risk for adverse effects such as restlessness, insomnia, or irritability. The child's thyroid levels should be evaluated every 3 to 6 months by a pediatric endocrinologist.

● HYPERTHYROIDISM

Hyperthyroidism is the result of hyperfunction of the thyroid gland. This leads to excessive levels of circulating thyroid hormones. This condition is uncommon in children; the peak incidence in children occurs in adolescence as a result of Graves' disease (Radovick & MacGillivray, 2003). Graves' disease is an autoimmune disorder that causes excessive amounts of thyroid hormone to be released in response to human thyroid stimulator immunoglobulin (TSI). It occurs five times more often in girls than in boys. A goiter usually develops in this condition. There is a genetic marker in the individuals, with 60% of affected persons having a family history of autoimmune thyroid problems (Radovick & MacGillivray, 2003). A congenital form, neonatal thyrotoxicosis, occurs in infants of mothers with Graves' disease. This neonatal condition, which can be life-threatening, is a self-limiting disorder lasting 2 to 4 months (Burg et al., 2002). Less common causes are thyroiditis, thyroid hormone–producing tumors, and pituitary adenomas.

Management is aimed at decreasing thyroid hormone levels. Current treatment involves antithyroid medication, radioactive iodine therapy, and subtotal thyroidectomy. First-line treatment involves propylthiouracil (PTU) or methimazole (MTZ, Tapazole), which blocks the production of T3 and T4. The child takes the medication once a day, generally in a dosage of 0.5 to 1 mg/kg per day (Burg et al., 2002). Adjunct therapy with beta-adrenergic blockers (Inderal) may also be used if the child has marked symptoms. Radioactive iodine therapy is becoming acceptable for children as a long-term therapy (Burg et al., 2002). This therapy is administered orally and results in tissue damage and destruction of the thyroid gland within 6 to 18 weeks, but it can result in hypothyroidism. Subtotal thyroidectomy is used when drug therapy is not possible or other treatments have failed. Risks include hypothyroidism, hypoparathyroidism, or laryngeal nerve damage.

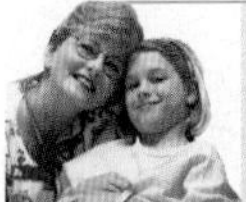

The sudden release of high levels of thyroid hormones results in thyroid storm, which progresses to heart failure and shock. Immediately report the signs of thyroid storm: sudden onset of severe restlessness and irritability, fever, diaphoresis, and tachycardia (Burg et al., 2002).

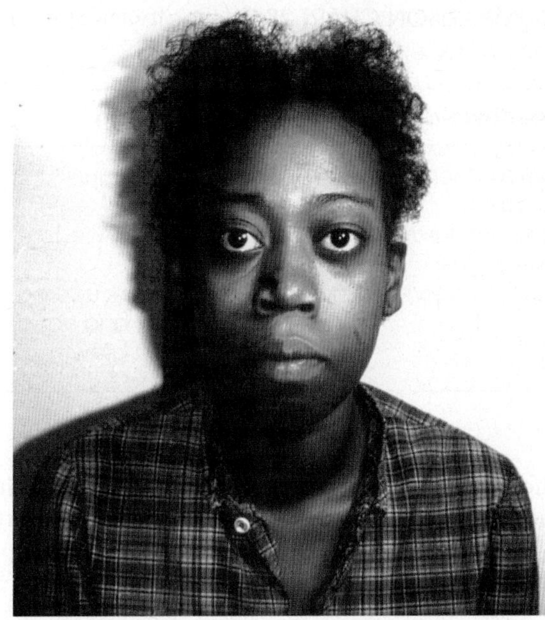

● Figure 28.4 Adolescent with Graves' disease.

Nursing Assessment

Most of these children are seen in the outpatient setting with a history of a problem with sleep, school performance, and distractibility. They become easily frustrated and overheated and fatigued during physical education class. The child may complain of diarrhea, excessive perspiration, and muscle weakness. The history may also reveal hyperactivity, heat intolerance, emotional lability, and insomnia. Initially, the symptoms are mild and often overlooked. Physical examination of the older child may reveal an increased rate of growth; weight loss despite an excellent appetite; hyperactivity; warm, moist skin; tachycardia; fine tremors; an enlarged thyroid gland or goiter; and ophthalmic changes (exophthalmos, which is less pronounced in children; proptosis; lid lag and retraction; staring expression; periorbital edema; and diplopia) (Fig. 28.4). Elevated pulse and blood pressure may also be noted. Serum T4 and T3 levels are markedly elevated. TSH levels are suppressed.

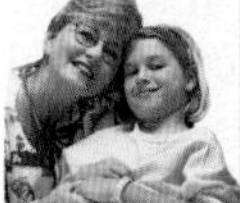

Infants with neonatal thyrotoxicosis present with low birthweight, failure to gain weight, hyperphagia, microcephaly, irritability, tachycardia, tachypnea, ophthalmopathy, enlarged thyroid, vomiting, diarrhea, jaundice, hepatosplenomegaly, and thrombocytopenia. Cardiac failure and dangerous central nervous system sequelae result if treatment is delayed.

Nursing Management

Once the treatment plan is initiated, educate the family and child about the medication and potential adverse effects, the goals of treatment, and possible complications. Monitor for adverse effects such as rash, mild leukopenia, loss of taste, sore throat, gastrointestinal disturbances, and arthralgia. If surgical intervention is chosen, provide appropriate preoperative teaching and postoperative care. Provide supportive measures such as fluid maintenance, nutritional support, and electrolyte correction. Monitor red blood cell count and liver function tests. Provide family education related to the medication. If the medication is given two or three times a day, teach the family to use a pill dispenser and alarm clock. Inform the family of the need for routine blood tests and follow-up visits with the pediatric endocrinologist every 2 to 4 months until normal levels are reached; then visits may be decreased to once or twice a year. Instruct the parents to contact the health care provider if the child has tachycardia or extreme fatigue.

Help the child and family to cope with symptoms such as heat intolerance, emotional lability, or eye problems. Ensure that this information is passed on to school or daycare personnel. The child should take more frequent rest breaks, in a cool environment, and should avoid physical education classes until normal hormone levels are attained. Encourage the family to have the child consume a healthy diet with an appropriate level of calories; the child may need to eat five or six meals a day. Provide community referrals such as to the National Graves' Disease Foundation (www.ngdf.org/ or 1-904-278-9488). Encourage the family to obtain a medical identification bracelet or necklace.

Comparison Chart 28.2 compares hypothyroidism and hyperthyroidism.

Disorders Related to Parathyroid Gland Function

The parathyroid glands secrete parathyroid hormone (PTH), which, along with vitamin D and calcitonin, regulates calcium/phosphate homeostasis by increasing osteoclastic activity, absorption of calcium and excretion

COMPARISON CHART 28.2 Hypothyroidism Versus Hyperthyroidism

Hyperthyroidism	Hypothyroidism
• Nervousness/anxiety • Diarrhea • Heat intolerance • Weight loss • Smooth, velvety skin	• Tiredness/fatigue • Constipation • Cold intolerance • Weight gain • Dry, thick skin; edema of face, eyes, and hands • Decreased growth

of phosphate by the kidneys, and absorption of calcium in the gastrointestinal tract. The two disorders associated with this gland are hypoparathyroidism and hyperparathyroidism.

HYPOPARATHYROIDISM

Hypoparathyroidism is the result of a deficiency in PTH secretion, which usually functions to maintain serum calcium. The impaired secretion affects calcium and phosphorus metabolism, leading to hypocalcemia and hyperphosphatemia. It is a very uncommon disorder in children and can be congenital (the result of aplasia or hypoplasia of the parathyroid gland) or acquired (due to inadvertent removal of the glands during thyroidectomy) (Perkin et al., 2003). It may occur in the newborn as a result of maternal hyperparathyroidism, maternal diabetes mellitus, or a diet of formula with a high phosphate-to-calcium ratio (Behrman et al., 2004; Perkin et al., 2003).

Emergency treatment involves giving intravenous calcium gluconate 10% solution at a dose of 0.5 mL/kg (up to 10 mL) over 15 minutes, followed by a continuous intravenous infusion of 500 mg/kg per 24 hours for neonates and 200 mg/kg per 24 hours for infants and children (Perkin et al., 2003). The goal is to maintain normal serum calcium and phosphate levels without complications. The treatment for less acute situations involves oral calcium gluconate and vitamin D with supplemental magnesium to help normalize PTH secretion (Perkin et al., 2003).

Nursing Assessment

Determine health history, noting poor eating, lethargy, muscle cramps progressing to numbness, and tingling in the hands and feet or around the mouth. The child may be irritable, have a history of unexplained convulsions, or complain of constipation, nausea, vomiting, or diarrhea. Physical examination may reveal **tetany**, stridor, Chvostek's sign (facial muscle spasm elicited by tapping the facial nerve), Trousseau's sign (carpopedal spasm that results from oxygen deficiency), papilledema, and dental enamel hypoplasia. The skeleton is affected over time, which may lead to permanent bone deformities and limited growth.

On palpation the child may complain of vague bone pain or abdominal discomfort. Skin may be dry, scaly, and coarse with eruptions. Laboratory testing reveals decreased serum calcium and PTH levels and increased serum phosphorus levels, which confirms the diagnosis. Bone age radiographs are usually normal, but if the condition has existed long term there may be evidence of increased bone density and suppressed growth.

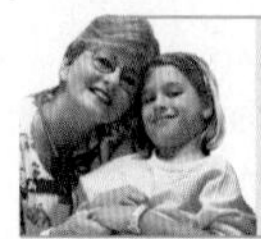

The neonate with hypoparathyroidism presents with jittery movements, convulsions, and apnea.

Nursing Management

Administer intravenous calcium gluconate for acute or severe tetany. Monitor the child for the development of cardiac arrhythmias. Ensure that the intravenous site is patent; if extravasation occurs, tissue damage or cardiac arrhythmias may result. Monitor fluid and electrolyte status, weigh the child daily, and measure urinary calcium excretion to prevent nephrocalcinosis. Institute seizure precautions and reduce environmental stimuli (e.g., loud or sudden noises, bright lights, or stimulating activities). Observe for signs and symptoms of laryngospasm (e.g., stridor, hoarseness, or a feeling of tightness in the throat). Teach the child and family about the need for continuous daily administration of calcium salts and vitamin D. Have the family observe for vitamin D toxicity by observing for signs such as weakness, fatigue, lassitude, headache, nausea and vomiting, and diarrhea.

HYPERPARATHYROIDISM

Hyperparathyroidism is an extremely rare disorder in children; the most common cause is an adenomatous disorder of the parathyroid gland (Behrman et al., 2004; Perkin et al., 2003). Chronic renal disease or congenital anomalies of the urinary tract are the causes of secondary hyperparathyroidism.

Management depends on the cause of the disorder. Surgery may be done to remove a tumor, and an attempt is made to place half of the parathyroid gland in the forearm to maintain normal calcium homeostasis (Burg et al., 2002). Phosphorus-mobilizing aluminum hydroxide may be given to reduce phosphate absorption, and intravenous fluids and furosemide at a dosage of 1 mg/kg every 6 hours may be given in an attempt to decrease calcium (Burg et al., 2002).

Nursing Assessment

The health history includes determining whether the child has a history of renal failure or congenital anomalies of the urinary tract. Note history of failure to thrive, headaches, poor school performance, and irritability. Inspection and observation may identify somnolence, stupor, or difficulty concentrating. Auscultation may reveal irregular heart rate, possibly related to cardiac dysrhythmias. Palpation of the abdomen may elicit pain, a mass due to constipation, or flank pain related to renal stones. Testing range of motion and strength may reveal muscle weakness. Blood studies are used to identify elevated calcium and decreased phosphorus levels. Serum measurements of PTH and radiographic studies are used to identify specific causes.

Nursing Management

Increase the child's fluid intake to minimize renal calculi formation. Provide fruit juices to maintain low urinary pH, acidity of body fluids, and calcium absorption. Strain the urine for renal casts. Monitor for safety by placing the child on seizure precautions, checking for fractures, and assessing the child's level of muscular weakness. If the child develops renal rickets (osteodystrophy), long-term braces may be required, so provide family education and encourage compliance. Keep the diet low in phosphorus and watch for hypocalcemia after surgery.

Disorders Related to Adrenal Gland Function

Disorders of the adrenal gland include acute and chronic adrenal insufficiency and disorders of hyperfunction such as Cushing syndrome. The adrenal cortex is the site of production of glucocorticoids, mineralocorticoids, and androgenic and estrogenic steroid compounds. The adrenal medulla is the site of production of the catecholamines and is under neuroendocrine control. When production of these compounds is altered, disease results.

• CONGENITAL ADRENAL HYPERPLASIA

Congenital adrenal hyperplasia (CAH) is a group of autosomal recessive inherited disorders in which there is an insufficient supply of the enzymes required for the synthesis of cortisol and aldosterone. The incidence is 0.06 to 0.08 per 1,000 live births (Burg et al., 2002; Sperling, 2002). Many children with CAH do not synthesize aldosterone; this results in adrenal crisis with hyponatremia and shock fairly soon after birth (Sperling, 2002). Other complications of CAH include hypertension, hypoglycemia, short adult stature, and adult testicular tumor in males.

Pathophysiology

Ninety percent to 95% of the cases of CAH are caused by a deficiency of 21-hydroxylase (21-OH) enzyme (Burg et al., 2002; Sperling, 2002). This defect results in the reduction of cortisol, which leads to increased ACTH production by the anterior pituitary. Prolonged oversecretion of ACTH causes enlargement or hyperplasia of the adrenal glands and excess production of androgens.

In males, the enzyme deficiency of 21-OH with excessive androgen secretion leads to a slightly enlarged penis, which may become adult-sized by school age, and a hyperpigmented scrotum. The female fetus develops male secondary sexual characteristics; thus, CAH causes pseudohermaphroditism, or ambiguous genitalia, in girls. The clitoris is enlarged and may resemble the penis, the labia have a rugated appearance, and the labial folds are fused, but the ovaries, fallopian tubes, and uterus are normal. The atypical form of 21-OH deficiency becomes evident later, in the toddler or preschool years, with premature **adrenarche**, pubic hair development, accelerated growth velocity, advanced bone age, early closure of the epiphyseal plates, acne, and hirsutism (Burg et al., 2002).

Therapeutic Management

The goal of treatment is to stop excessive adrenal secretion of androgens while maintaining normal growth and development. Most children with 21-OH deficiency will take a glucocorticoid such as hydrocortisone and the mineralocorticoid fludrocortisone (Florinef) for life. Infants may also require sodium supplementation. When the medications are taken at physiologic doses there are no adverse effects, but if the levels become elevated, hypertension, growth impairment, and acne become a problem. Regular follow-up care and appropriate titration maintain the dose at appropriate levels to allow normal growth and development.

In the past when girls were born with ambiguous genitalia, standard medical treatment was to correct the external genitalia and establish adequate sexual functioning. Typically, a reduction of the clitoris and opening of the labial folds were done within the first few months of life, with further surgeries at puberty. There is a trend today, however, to wait until the child can make the decision, since the surgery often results in a loss of nerve endings in the clitoris, which impairs sexuality and sexual experiences (Burg et al., 2002). The decision to intervene immediately or to delay treatment is a complex one that raises many concerns for the family. The exciting news is that with technological advances, the fetus can now be treated to prevent ambiguous genitalia (Radovick & MacGillivray, 2003).

Nursing Assessment

Nursing assessment of the child with CAH includes health history, physical examination, and laboratory and diagnostic testing. Specific findings related to CAH are presented below.

Health History and Physical Examination

Obtain the health history, noting history of abnormal genitalia at birth in the infant.

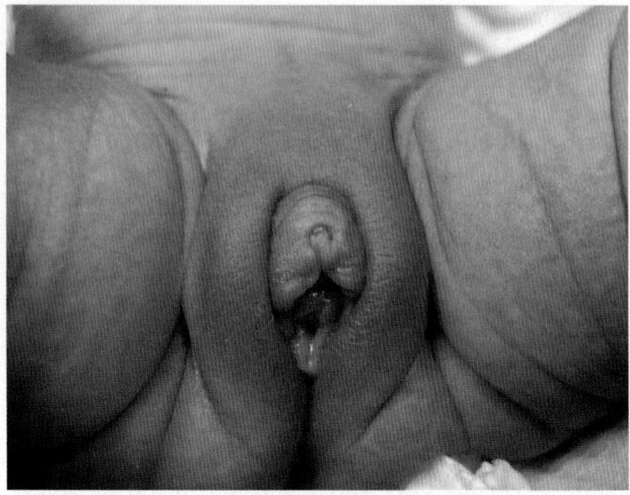

● Figure 28.5 Newborn with ambiguous genitalia.

In the toddler or preschooler, note history of accelerated growth velocity and signs of premature adrenarche. Upon inspection of the infant's genitalia, note a large penis in the boy and ambiguous genitalia in the girl (Fig. 28.5). When observing the toddler or preschooler, note pubic hair development, acne, and hirsutism.

Laboratory and Diagnostic Testing

The most common type of CAH, 21-OH enzyme deficiency, is detected by newborn metabolic screening. If this test has not been done or the results are unavailable, random hormone levels or levels associated with ACTH stimulation may be obtained. Bone age is advanced and premature closure of epiphyseal plates is noted on radiographs of the long bones. See Healthy People 2010.

Nursing Management

In addition to the common interventions associated with endocrine disorders in childhood (see Nursing Care Plan 28.1), nursing management of the infant or child with CAH focuses on helping the family to understand the child's response to disease and the importance of maintaining hormone supplementation. Supporting the family is also a key nursing focus. Provide ongoing assessment of the ill or hospitalized child with a history of CAH to recognize the development of life-threatening acute adrenal crisis. If signs and symptoms of adrenal crisis develop, the child will receive fluid resuscitation with an intravenous bolus of 0.9% normal saline (20 mL/kg). Further rehydration will occur with D5NS at twice the recommended maintenance rate. Intravenous hydrocortisone will also be given.

HEALTHY PEOPLE 2010

Objective	Significance
(Developmental) Ensure appropriate newborn bloodspot screening, follow-up testing, and referral to services.	• Follow up with state agencies at first contact with infant to ascertain results of newborn screening.

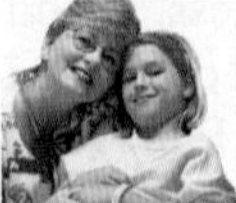

Signs and symptoms of acute adrenal crisis include persistent vomiting, dehydration, hyponatremia, hyperkalemia, hypotension, tachycardia, and shock. Monitor children with CAH and notify the physician if adrenal crisis is suspected.

Educating the Family

Medication will be required throughout the child's life, as cortisone is necessary to sustain life. Teach the family the appropriate oral dosages of hydrocortisone and fludrocortisone. It is critical to maintain tight control over the levels of these medications in the bloodstream, as either underdosing or overdosing may lead to short adult stature. Low levels of the hormones may also result in adrenal crisis. These drugs are usually given orally but in some instances will need to be given via intramuscular injections. Teach families how to give hydrocortisone intramuscularly if the child is vomiting and cannot keep down oral medication. If the child becomes ill, is under stress, or needs surgery, additional doses of medications may be required. Encourage the family to obtain an identification bracelet or necklace for the child.

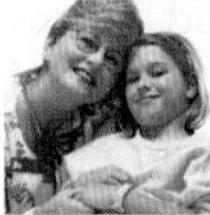

Families must keep extra Solu-Cortef (injectable form) at home to give during an emergency. The dosage is 25 mg for infants, 50 mg for children 1 to 4 years of age, and 100 mg for older children (Sperling, 2002).

Providing Family Support

Make sure the family of a newborn with ambiguous genitalia feels comfortable asking questions and exploring their feelings. There are many issues to consider, such as whether the family will reassign the child's sex or raise the child with the original assignment at birth. The birth certificate may pose a problem if the state requires identification of sex. Cultural attitudes, the parents' expectations, and the extent of family support influence the family's response to the child and the decision-making process related to sex assignment and surgical correction. If corrective surgery is immediately decided upon, then typical surgical concerns for newborns will need to be addressed.

In general, laypeople do not understand adrenal function and what this diagnosis may mean to the family. Provide families with privacy to discuss these issues, and offer emotional support. When referring to the infant, use terms such as "your baby" instead of the pronouns "he," "she," or "it" and describe the genitals as "sex organs" instead of "penis" or "clitoris." Refer families to the CARES (Congenital Adrenal Hyperplasia Research, Education, and Support) Foundation (www.caresfoundation.org, 1-866-227-3737) and the Magic Foundation (www.magicfoundation.org, 1-800-362-4423) for additional support and resources. Local parent-to-parent support groups are also helpful.

ADDISON'S DISEASE

Addison's disease (primary adrenal insufficiency) is rare in children. It results from damage or destruction of the adrenal glands caused by infections such as tuberculosis, fungal infections, or HIV-related infections; hemorrhage or surgical removal of both glands; or dysfunction of the hypothalamus or pituitary gland. Generally, the etiology in children is an autoimmune process that is familial or sporadic (Sperling, 2002). Destruction of the adrenal glands by the circulating antibodies leads to deficiency in the adrenal steroids, glucocorticoids (cortisol), and mineralocorticoids (aldosterone).

Management involves replacing deficient or absent hormones. In the acute situation this is accomplished with intravenous hydrocortisone, as well as restoring and maintaining fluid, electrolyte, and glucose balance (Behrman et al., 2004). Treatment for the chronic form of Addison's disease is oral hydrocortisone at a dosage of 10 to 15 mg/m^2 in three divided doses and Florinef at 0.05 to 0.30 mg as necessary to maintain renin levels (Behrman et al., 2004). This is a lifelong condition, and illness, stress, or surgery will require adjustment in the medication dosage to meet the body's physiologic needs. Potential complications include diabetes, thyrotoxicosis, reproductive malfunction, hypoparathyroidism, and pernicious anemia.

Nursing Assessment

Note history of gradual onset of weight loss, fatigue, anorexia, syncope, nausea, vomiting, and diarrhea. Observe the skin for hyperpigmentation and note decreased blood pressure. Addisonian crisis is an acute onset that presents during a febrile illness, infection, extreme stress, or any condition that results in increase adrenal steroid release. It is potentially life-threatening; the symptoms include sudden penetrating pain in the lower back, abdomen, or legs with severe weakness, vomiting and diarrhea, dehydration, hypotension, electrolyte imbalances, decreased cardiac output, fever, mental status changes, and hypoglycemia.

Laboratory testing reveals low serum sodium, elevated serum potassium, and low fasting glucose levels. Blood urea nitrogen and creatinine levels are increased. The blood test that confirms the diagnosis is a low fasting morning cortisol level 30 to 60 minutes after stimulation with intravenous synthetic ACTH (Sperling, 2002). In addition, the adrenal antibodies are positive in Addison's disease but negative with other causes for the condition.

Nursing Management

Nursing management of Addison's disease is similar to that of congenital adrenal insufficiency. A critical aspect of the education plan for this disorder, however, is to teach the parents to increase the dosage of cortisol during periods of illness and to use the injectable form of hydrocortisone during periods of extreme nausea or vomiting. Information about the child's condition should always be available to emergency personnel.

CUSHING'S SYNDROME

Cushing's syndrome is characterized by a cluster of signs and symptoms resulting from excess levels of glucocorticoids (excessive circulating free cortisol). Usually this condition is due to a small ACTH-producing pituitary adenoma. There are two to five new cases of Cushing's syndrome for every 1 million people each year, with about 10% of these new cases occurring in children or teenagers (National Institute of Child Health and Human Development, 2004). The most common cause in older children is prolonged or excessive use of corticosteroid therapy (Burg et al., 2003). Excessive cortisol suppresses the release of GH, so linear growth is decreased in these patients.

Management varies depending on the cause. The goal is to restore hormone balance and reverse Cushing's syndrome. If the cause is an adrenal or pituitary tumor, then surgical removal of the tumor alone or the entire adrenal gland is performed. If the cause is long-term steroid therapy, then the corticosteroid dose is reduced to the lowest dose that is effective in treating the underlying disorder. Ketoconazole may also be given to suppress adrenocortical function.

Nursing Assessment

Note history of rapid weight gain, decreased velocity of linear growth, fatigue, irritability, and sleep disturbance. The child may also have a history of long-term corticosteroid use, water retention, poor wound healing, frequent infections, and in teenage girls, missed menstrual periods. Upon observation of the child's general status, note weight gain around the abdomen, round face (moon face), and a cervical fat pad (buffalo hump) developing over time (Fig. 28.6). The skin may be thin and fragile, with a tendency to bruise. Acne and hirsutism may be present. Note reddish-purple striae on the abdomen. Test muscle strength, noting weakness. Measure the blood pressure, noting hypertension.

Laboratory testing reveals reduced serum levels of potassium and phosphorus, elevated serum calcium and sodium levels, increased 24-hour urinary levels of free cortisol and 17-hydroxycorticosteroid (17-OHCs), loss of diurnal rhythm in serum cortisol levels, chronic hyperglycemia, and elevated glycosylated hemoglobin levels.

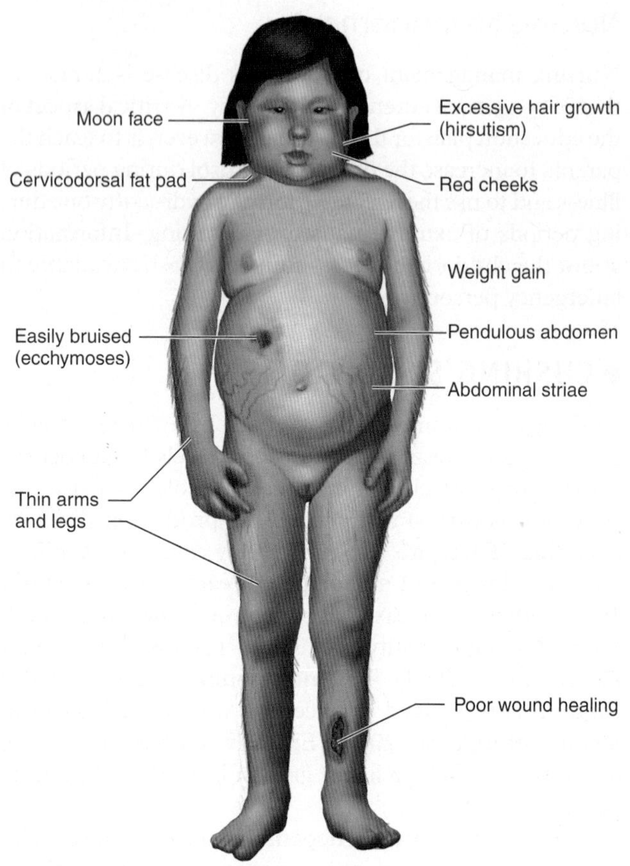

● Figure 28.6 Cushing's syndrome.

The adrenal suppression test using low-dose dexamethasone is used initially to screen for adrenocortical hyperfunction. CT and MRI are used to detect tumors in the adrenal and pituitary glands that may cause Cushing's syndrome.

Nursing Management

Provide routine yet individualized nursing interventions as outlined in Nursing Care Plan 28.1. In addition, counsel the family that the cushingoid appearance is reversible with appropriate treatment. Be alert for signs of adrenal insufficiency if the child has surgery or if corticosteroid withdrawal occurs quickly.

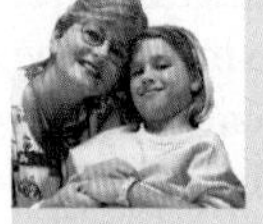

Watch for signs of shock if the adrenal gland is removed, since without epinephrine from the adrenal gland, the body's ability to maintain blood pressure is severely compromised.

Polycystic Ovary Syndrome

Polycystic ovary syndrome (PCOS), also referred to as functional ovarian hyperandrogenism or ovarian androgen excess, is an endocrine order that produces a variety of symptoms in adolescent girls and women. Testosterone production by the ovaries and adrenal cells is excessive, causing hirsutism, balding, acne, increased muscle mass, and decreased breast size. Polycystic ovaries may or may not be present. There is a genetic predisposition for PCOS, and most women with PCOS are obese. Complications of excess androgen production in women include infertility, and insulin resistance and hyperinsulinemia, leading to diabetes mellitus. Management involves the administration of oral contraceptives for their hormonal effects, as well as insulin-sensitizing medications such as metformin (Glucophage).

Nursing Assessment

Explore the health history for oligomenorrhea (irregular, infrequent periods) or amenorrhea. Note weight in relation to standardized growth charts and calculate body mass index (BMI) to determine whether the girl is overweight or obese. Inspect the skin for acne, acanthosis nigricans (darkened, thickened pigmentation, particularly around the neck or in the axillary region), and **hirsutism** (excess body hair growth). Assist with collection of timed blood specimens for glucose and insulin levels (which will often show unexpectedly elevated insulin levels in relation to the glucose level). Laboratory tests may show elevated levels of free testosterone and other androgenic hormones.

Nursing Management

One of the most important functions of the nurse in relation to PCOS is to assist with early recognition and treatment. Educate the adolescent girl about the use of oral contraceptives to normalize hormone levels, which will decrease androgenic effects. Support the teen in her efforts to diet and exercise to lose weight. Oral insulin-sensitizing drugs such as metformin (Glucophage) may be prescribed, and the teen should be encouraged to comply with the medication regimen. Routinely measure weight to determine progress with weight loss. Measure blood pressure to screen for hypertension, which may develop as a complication of PCOS. Online support groups and education are available at:

- www.kidshealth.org/teen/sexual_health/girls/pcos.html (Nemours Foundation)
- www.youngwomenshealth.org/pcos_resources.html (Children's Hospital Boston)
- www.pcosupport.org (Polycystic Ovarian Syndrome Foundation)

Diabetes Mellitus

In the most common disorder of the pancreas, the islets of Langerhans, specifically the **beta cells**, fail to produce adequate insulin. This results in diabetes mellitus (DM). DM is a chronic disorder in which carbohydrate, protein, and lipid metabolism is impaired. It is one of the leading health problems in the United States and now the most common childhood endocrine disorder (Behrman et al., 2004; Burg et al., 2002). "Primarily, DM represents a spectrum of insulin dysfunction, ranging from an autoimmune destruction of insulin-secreting beta cells (Type 1) at one end to a lack of tissue responsiveness to circulating insulin (Type 2) at the other" (Perkin et al., 2003, p. 529). If the condition goes unrecognized, **diabetic ketoacidosis (DKA)** or fat catabolism develops, resulting in anorexia, nausea and vomiting, presence of **ketones** in urine, sweet-smelling breath, Kussmaul respirations, air hunger, and, if left untreated, coma and death. Approximately 30% to 40% of children with type 1 DM present with DKA on initial evaluation (Burg et al., 2002). Eventually, the lack of insulin and resulting problems produce structural abnormalities in various tissues and organs. Long-term complications of DM include failure to grow, poor wound healing, recurrent infections, retinopathy, neuropathy, vascular complications, nephropathy, microaneurysms, and cardiovascular disease.

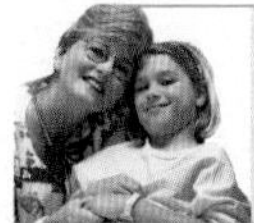

Signs and symptoms of DKA include lethargy, stupor, decreased skin turgor, abdominal pain, Kussmaul respirations and air hunger, and tachycardia.

DIABETES MELLITUS TYPE 1

DM type 1 is an autoimmune disorder that occurs in genetically susceptible individuals who may also be exposed to one of several environmental factors, such as chemicals, viruses, or other toxic agents implicated in the development process. The long arm of chromosome 14 at the 14q24 locus is the type 1 diabetes-11 marker. Approximately 5% of children have a first- or second-degree relative with DM type 1 (ADA, 2000). The incidence is 0.14 to 0.17 per 1,000 children under 20 years old in North America, with a higher incidence in African-American and Hispanic children (Perkin et al., 2003). There is equal distribution between the genders, with the peak incidence occurring in school-age children.

As the genetically susceptible individual is exposed to environmental factors, the immune system begins a T-lymphocyte–mediated process that damages and destroys the beta cells of the pancreas, resulting in inadequate insulin secretion. Insulin cannot alter peripheral cells to transport glucose across the cell membrane. The end result is hyperglycemia, glucose accumulation in the blood, and the body's inability to use its main source of fuel efficiently. By the time symptoms are present and the diagnosis is made, 90% of the beta cells have been destroyed. Immunologic markers, islet cells antibodies (ICA), insulin autoantibodies (IAA), and other antibodies may be present for years before the child develops signs and symptoms (Perkin et al., 2003).

DIABETES MELLITUS TYPE 2

In DM type 2 the pancreas usually produces insulin but the body is resistant to the insulin or there is an inadequate compensatory insulin secretion response. Eventually, insulin production decreases, with a result similar to DM type 1. Historically, DM type 2 occurred mostly in adults, with only 2% to 3% of cases occurring in children. Since the early 1990s, however, the incidence has increased: today, 8% to 45% of children with newly diagnosed diabetes have type 2 (Behrman et al., 2004). Many of these children have a relative with DM type 2 or they are overweight or from an African-American, Hispanic-American, Asian-American, or Native American background (Behrman et al., 2004). See Healthy People 2010.

SECONDARY DIABETES MELLITUS

Secondary DM, or exacerbation of insulin deficiency and resistance forms, develops as a result of conditions such as diseases of the exocrine gland (e.g., cystic fibrosis), endocrine pathologies (e.g., Cushing's syndrome), drug-induced problems (e.g., corticosteroid overuse), genetic defects of insulin action (e.g., congenital lipodystrophy), infection (e.g., congenital rubella), and gestational diabetes (Perkin et al., 2003).

Therapeutic Management

Treatment involves a multidisciplinary health care team, with the family and child as a central part of that team. In the past the children would be admitted to the hospital for 3 to 5 days for stabilization and education, but today the trend is toward treating children on an outpatient basis. The general goals for therapeutic management include:

- Achieving normal growth and development
- Promoting optimal serum glucose regulation, including fluid and electrolyte levels and near-normal **glycosylated hemoglobin** levels

HEALTHY PEOPLE 2010

Objective	Significance
Prevent diabetes. Reduce the overall rate of diabetes that is clinically diagnosed.	• Screen all children periodically for the development of overweight and obesity using body mass index on the CDC growth charts. • Educate families about appropriate diet and exercise beginning in toddlerhood in order to prevent the development of obesity.

- Preventing complications
- Promoting positive adjustment to the disease, with ability to self-manage in the home

The key to success is to educate the child and family so they can self-manage this chronic condition. Treatment involves blood glucose monitoring; daily injections of insulin for DM type 1 or oral hypoglycemic medications for DM type 2; a realistic diet; an exercise program; and self-management and decision-making skills.

Glucose Monitoring

With the advent of home blood glucose monitoring in the late 1970s, daily glucose monitoring replaced urine testing for glucose levels. Urine testing does not supply enough quantitative data to make adequate decisions about insulin doses. Glucose monitoring allows for tighter glucose control because supplemental insulin can be used to correct or prevent hyperglycemia; it also enables patients and health care providers to provide better management. The frequency of blood glucose monitoring is based on the patient's goals. Children who are in the hospital for management of their DM require blood glucose monitoring before meals, at bedtime, and at 2 a.m., if not more frequently. Additional glucose checks, such as mid-morning or mid-afternoon, should be made if glycemic control has not occurred (Perkin et al., 2003).

Insulin Replacement Therapy

Insulin replacement therapy is the cornerstone of management of DM type 1. Insulin is administered daily by subcutaneous injections into adipose tissue over large muscle masses using a traditional insulin syringe or a subcutaneous injector (Fig. 28.7). U-100 insulin may also be administered using a portable insulin pump. The frequency, dose, and type of insulin are based on how much the child needs to achieve a normal, average blood glucose concentration and to prevent hypoglycemia. Typically, two or four daily injections are commonly used, with newly diagnosed children receiving 1 unit of insulin per kilogram of body weight per day, but the dosage depends on the needs of the child (Perkin et al., 2003). The dose may need to be increased during the pubertal growth spurt.

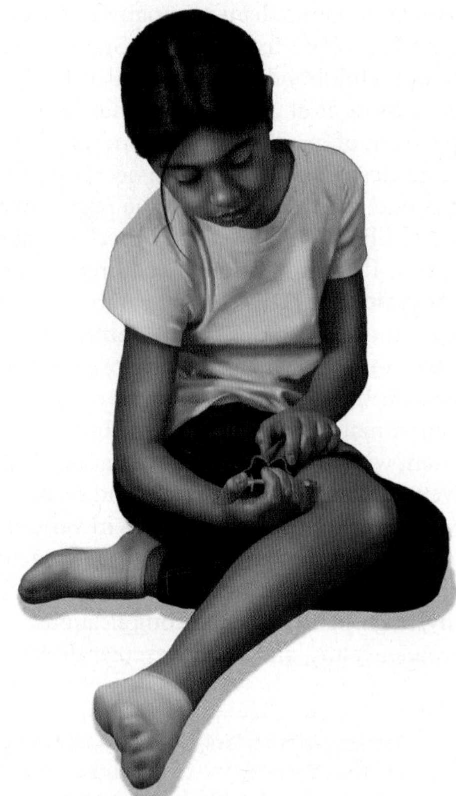

● Figure 28.7 The subcutaneous injector uses pressure jets to deliver insulin safely and accurately.

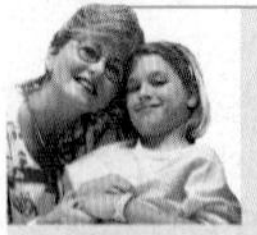

An insulin pump is a device that administers a continuous infusion of rapid-acting insulin. It comprises a computer, a reservoir of rapid-acting insulin, thin tubing through which the insulin is delivered, and a small needle inserted into the abdomen. A continuous basal rate of insulin is maintained, and a bolus of insulin can be delivered if glucose testing results show it is needed.

Types of insulin include rapid-acting, short-acting, intermediate-acting, long-acting, and fixed combinations (Table 28.3). They can be kept at room temperature but should be discarded 1 month after opening even if refrigerated. The child may receive only one type or a mixture of short-acting and intermediate-acting. Again, this depends on the child's needs. Insulin is either animal (pork) or synthetic human, produced through recombinant DNA technology, which is better for children.

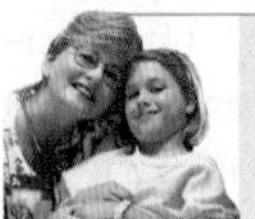

Lantus is usually given in a single dose at bedtime. Lantus may not be mixed with other insulins.

Oral Hypoglycemic Medications

In DM type 2, oral hypoglycemic medications such as sulfonylureas and meglitinides are used to increase insulin response to glucose. Another group, the biguanides, reduces glucose production from the liver, but because this group causes hypoglycemia it is not used as often in children. Insulin sensitizers improve the body's ability to use insulin in the liver and skeletal tissues. Common adverse effects of these oral agents include headache, dizziness, edema, and liver enzyme elevation. If the oral hypoglycemics fail to maintain a normal glucose level, then insulin injections will be required. These children may also be prescribed antilipidemic medication since hyperglycemia results in transient hyperlipidemia (Perkin et al., 2003).

Table 28.3 Insulin Type, Action, and Duration

Type	Onset	Peak	Duration
Lispro: ultra-short-acting	15–30 minutes	60–90 minutes	3–4 hours
Regular: short-acting	30 minutes	2–3 hours	3–6 hours
NPH or Lente: intermediate-acting	Lente: 1–2.5 hours NPH: 1–1.5 hours	7–15 hours 6–10 hours	12–24 hours 10–18 hours
Ultralente: long-acting	4–8 hours	Variable; 10–16 hours	24–36 hours
Lantus	1–2 hours	Does not truly peak; offers continual steady coverage	20–24 hours

Other Therapies

Other therapies involve diet and exercise protocols and management of complications. The American Dietetic Association in conjunction with the American Diabetes Association recommends goals that do not exclude any foods and reflect the growth needs of the child. The recommendations suggest that approximately 50% to 60% of calories come from carbohydrates, such as grains, breads, fruit, milk, and vegetables; 10% to 20% from protein, such as meat, beans, eggs, cheese, and legumes; and 20% to 30% from fats, such as butter, oil, or mayonnaise (ADA, 2001).

Exercise has an important influence on the hypoglycemic effects of insulin, so the child should maintain or increase his or her activity levels. If the child is taking insulin, the family should know how to change the dosage or add food to maintain blood glucose control. Children with DM type 2 are often overweight, so the exercise plan is very important in helping the child to lose weight as well as assisting with the hypoglycemic effects of the medications.

Nursing Assessment

Assessment involves understanding the ever-changing needs of children as they grow and develop. The first phase of assessment involves identifying the child who may have DM. The second phase involves identifying problems that might develop in the child with DM. The nurse should always be aware of this when observing for complications or management problems and should always be alert for opportunities to provide education that will expand the understanding and skills of the child and family.

Health History and Physical Examination

During the initial diagnosis of DM, obtain a detailed history of family patterns and problems in school related to some of the mental and behavior changes that may occur in a hyperglycemic state (e.g., weakness, fatigue, mood changes). The child may also complain of blurred vision, headaches, or bedwetting. The child with DM type 1 may have a history of poor growth. Comparison Chart 28.3 gives information about common history and physical examination findings in children with type 1 versus type 2 DM.

In the child who is known to have DM, the health history includes any problems with hyperglycemia or hypoglycemia, diet, activity and exercise patterns, and ability to administer insulin and monitor blood glucose levels. Perform a thorough physical examination, noting any abnormal findings.

Laboratory and Diagnostic Testing

A random glucose level above 200 mg/dL, a fasting glucose level above 126 mg/dL, and a 2-hour postprandial blood glucose level above 200 mg/dL are laboratory criteria for the diagnosis of DM. Other laboratory and diagnostic tests include glycosylated hemoglobin; hemoglobin A_{1c}, which reflects the percentage of hemoglobin to which glucose is attached; and serum measurements of islet cell antibodies. Serum levels of urea nitrogen, creatinine, calcium, magnesium, phosphate, and electrolytes such as potassium and sodium may be drawn. Additional tests include a complete blood count, urinalysis, and immunoassay to measure levels of C-peptides after a glucose challenge to verify endogenous insulin secretion.

Nursing Management

Nursing management is focused on regulating glucose control, monitoring for complications, and educating and supporting the child and family. Individualize the general nursing care discussed in Nursing Care Plan 28.1 based on the child's and family's response to illness. Additional nursing care topics related to DM are discussed below.

Regulating Glucose Control

If the child presents with DKA, monitor the glucose level hourly to prevent it from falling more than 100 mg/dL per hour. A too-rapid decline in blood glucose predisposes the child to cerebral edema. Administration of regular insulin, given intravenously, is preferred during DKA; a bolus dose of 0.1 unit/kg is given, followed by a continuous infu-

COMPARISON CHART 28.3 Type 1 Versus Type 2 Diabetes Mellitus

History and Physical Findings Usually Present at Diagnosis	Type 1	Type 2
Polydipsia, polyuria, **polyphagia**	Yes	Yes
Weight	Possibly weight loss	Obese
Age of onset	Usually younger children	Usually pubertal children
Incidental finding on screening urinalysis	Rare	Common
Antecedent flu-like illness	Common	Possible
Autoimmune antibodies	Yes	No
Diabetic ketoacidosis	Common	Possible
Hypertension	No	Common
Acanthosis nigricans	No	Common
Vaginal infection	No	Common
Dyslipidemia	No	Common

Pinhas-Hamiel, O., & Zeitler, P. (2001). Type 2 diabetes: Not just for grownups anymore. *Contemporary Pediatrics, 1,* 102 (electronic version). Available at www.contemporarypediatrics.com.

sion of 0.1 unit/kg per hour. Usually the child with DKA is treated in the pediatric intensive care unit.

The subcutaneous route of insulin administration is used once the serum glucose level reaches 250 mg/dL, serum pH is 7.35, dehydration is corrected, and the child is no longer NPO. Many times the regimen consists of three injections of intermediate-acting insulin, with the addition of rapid-acting insulin before breakfast and dinner. Insulin doses are typically ordered on a sliding scale related to the serum glucose level and how the insulin works. Two thirds of the dose is usually given before breakfast and one third before dinner (Perkin et al., 2003).

Teach the child and family to use proper subcutaneous injection techniques to avoid injecting into muscle or vascular spaces. Figure 28.8 shows appropriate sites for subcutaneous injection of insulin. Sites should be rotated to avoid adipose hypertrophy (fatty lumps that absorb insulin poorly).

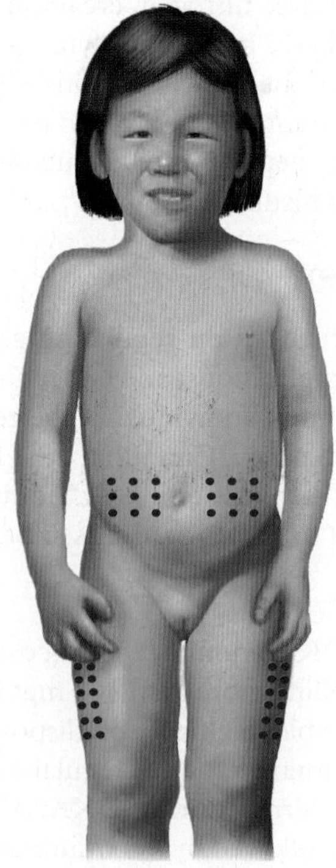
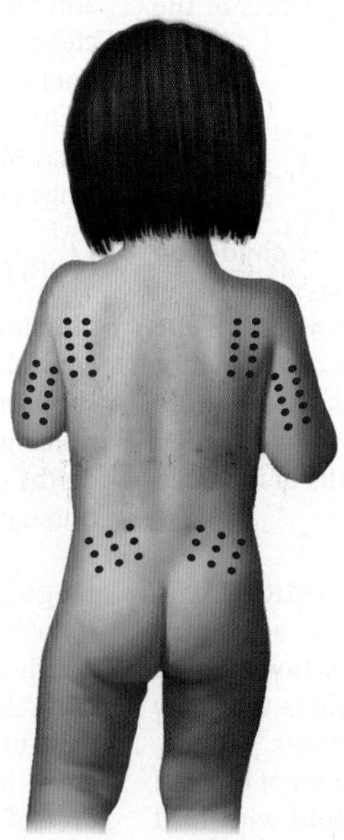

● Figure 28.8 Insulin injection sites.

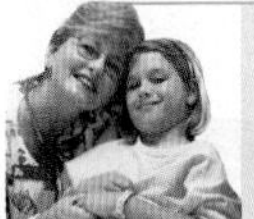
When giving a combination of short- and long-acting insulin, draw up the clear (short-acting) insulin first to prevent contamination with the long-acting insulin. Rotate the vial instead of shaking it to prevent air bubbles.

Monitoring for Complications

While the child is in the hospital, monitor for signs of complications such as acidosis, coma, hyperkalemia or hypokalemia, hypocalcemia, cerebral edema, or hyponatremia and assess for the development of hypoglycemia or hyperglycemia every 2 hours (Comparison Chart 28.4). Monitor the child's status closely during peak times of insulin action. Perform blood glucose testing as ordered or as needed if the child develops symptoms.

When the child is having a hypoglycemic reaction, administer glucagon (a hormone produced by the pancreas and stored in the liver) either subcutaneously or intramuscularly. Children under 7 years of age receive 0.5 mg; children over 7 years of age receive 1 mg. Dextrose (50%) may be given intravenously if needed. If the child is coherent, glucose paste or tablets may be used. Offer 10 to 15 g of a simple carbohydrate such as orange juice if the child feels some symptoms and glucose monitoring indicates a drop. Follow this with a more complex carbohydrate such as peanut butter and crackers to maintain the glucose level.

The hyperglycemic child requires insulin; the dosage is usually based on a sliding scale or determined after consultation with the physician.

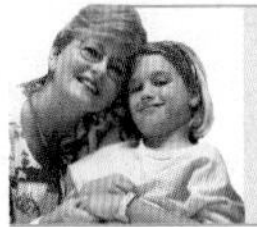
Double-check all insulin doses against the order sheet and with another nurse to ensure accuracy.

Educating the Family

Education is the priority intervention because it will enable the child and family to self-manage this chronic condition. The child and family first need time to adjust to the diagnosis of a chronic illness that will require self-management. DM is a life-long condition that requires regular follow-up visits (three or four times a year) to a diabetes specialty clinic. Because approximately 150,000 school-age children and adolescents have diabetes, this becomes a health issue for the community, especially the schools (National Institutes of Health, National Diabetes Education Program, 2004). With appropriate management, involvement of the community, and confidence and compliance by the family, the child can maintain a happy, productive life. See Healthy People 2010.

Challenges related to educating children with diabetes include:

- Children lack the maturity to understand the long-term consequences of this serious chronic illness.
- Children do not want to be different from their peers, and having to make lifestyle changes may result in anger or depression.
- Poor families may not be able to afford appropriate food, medication, transportation, and telephone service.
- Families may demonstrate unhealthy behaviors, making it difficult for the child to initiate change because of the lack of supervision or role modeling.
- Family dynamics are affected because management of diabetes must occur all day, every day.

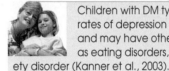

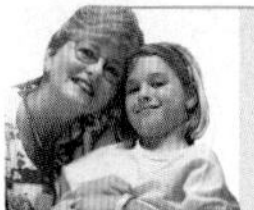
Children with DM type 1 have significantly higher rates of depression than the general population and may have other comorbid conditions, such as eating disorders, adjustment disorders, or anxiety disorder (Kanner et al., 2003).

The initial goal of education is for the family to develop basic management and decision-making skills. Assess the family's ability to learn the basic concepts, and offer psychological support. Teach about specific topics in sessions lasting 15 to 20 minutes for the children and 45 to 60 minutes for the caregivers. Teaching must be geared

COMPARISON CHART 28.4 Hypoglycemia Versus Hyperglycemia

Hypoglycemia	Hyperglycemia
Behavioral changes, confusion, slurred speech, belligerence	Mental status changes, fatigue, weakness
Diaphoresis	Dry, flushed skin
Tremors	Blurred vision
Palpitations, tachycardia	Abdominal cramping, nausea, vomiting, fruity breath odor

HEALTHY PEOPLE 2010

Objective	Significance
Increase the proportion of persons with diabetes who receive formal diabetes education.	• Begin diabetes education with child and family upon knowledge of diagnosis. • Use developmentally appropriate education with children. • Increase the self-management skills taught as the child progresses in age and cognitive development.

Table 28.4 Developmental Issues Related to Diabetes Mellitus

Age Group	Child and Family Implications	Nursing Implications
Infants and toddlers	Management falls on parents/caretakers; signs and symptoms are sometimes difficult to assess in infants and young toddlers.	Attempt to achieve consistent dietary intake. Let toddler choose foods. Get toddler to find a word or phrase to use to describe feelings when hypoglycemic. Establish rituals/routines with home management.
Preschoolers	Increased motor maturity; widening social circle, so the child will notice that he or she is "different." Magical thinking presents some issues. Some children can began to perform blood glucose testing with the newer devices.	Use simple explanations and play therapy when instructing or preparing for a procedure.
School-age children	Can perform finger/blood glucose testing, choose injection sites and give injections, perform ketone testing, recognize need to eat and treat for hypoglycemia. Must incorporate management into school day, and plan for field trips.	Use concise and concrete terms when instructing. Allow child to proceed at his or her own rate. Assist family to incorporate the testing and injections into school day and plan for field trips. Involve the school nurse in helping with the school plan.
Adolescents	Conflicts develop with self-management, body image, and peer group acceptance; must assume more of the care with supervision. Teens do not always foresee the consequences of their activity.	Slowly care is turned over to the adolescent with minor supervision from the family. Watch for depression.

toward the child's level of development and understanding (Table 28.4).

Among the topics to include when teaching children and their families about diabetes management are:

- Fingerstick method and blood glucose measurement (Fig. 28.9)
- Urine ketone testing
- Medication use (Fig. 28.10)
  - Oral hypoglycemic agents
  - Subcutaneous insulin injection or insulin pump use
  - Subcutaneous site selection and rotation
  - When to alter insulin dosages
  - Use of glucagon

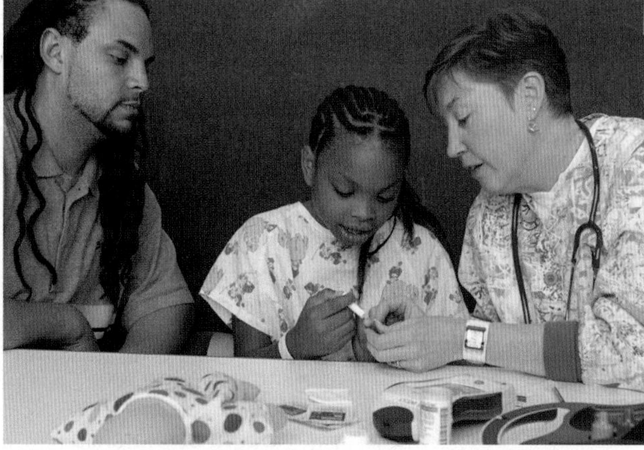

● Figure 28.9 The school-age child has developed the psychomotor skills needed for blood glucose monitoring and insulin injection.

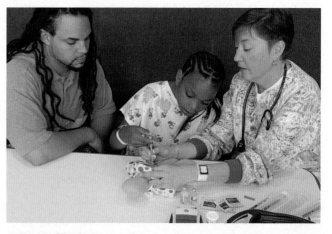

● Figure 28.10 The school-age child may first practice insulin injections on a doll.

- Signs and symptoms of hypoglycemia and hyperglycemia
- Complications
- Sick-day instructions
- Laboratory testing and follow-up care

Teaching Guideline 28.2 presents information to cover when teaching the family about blood glucose monitoring. Teach families how to give insulin, how to use the insulin pump, and how to rotate injection sites (see above). Sick-day instructions may include the following:

- Contact the physician.
- Perform blood glucose monitoring more often.
- Use a sliding scale to calculate the insulin dosage.

A dietitian can help the family with detailed meal planning and dietary guidelines. Review basic nutritional information with the child and family and provide sample meals. Incorporate the family's cultural preferences when planning meals. Encourage the child and family to keep a food diary. For the child who needs to lose weight, suggest low-carbohydrate snacks and encourage appropriate daily physical activity (Teaching Guideline 28.3).

Supporting the Child and Family

Children with diabetes and their families may have difficulty coping if they lack confidence in their self-management skills. Assess the ability of the child and family to handle situations. Role-play specific situations related to symptoms or complications to help them see different ways to solve problems. Work with the child and family to enhance their conflict resolution skills. Provide opportunities for them to express their feelings. Observe for signs of depression, especially in adolescents.

To enhance the child's confidence and promote feelings of mastery and inclusion, refer him or her to a special camp for children with diabetes (see www.diabetescamps.org/ or www.childrenwithdiabetes.com/camps/). Also refer families to local support groups, parent-to-parent networks, or one of many national support resources and foundations, such as:

- www.diabetes.org: American Diabetes Association
- www.childrenwithdiabetes.com/index_cwd.htm: Children with Diabetes (online community)
- www.mychildhasdiabetes.com/ (parenting and diabetes resources)
- www.jdf.org/: Juvenile Diabetes Research Foundation International

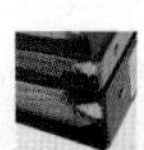

TEACHING GUIDELINE 28.2

Blood Glucose Monitoring

- Obtain glucose levels before meals and bedtime snacks.
- Perform monitoring more often during prolonged exercise, if you are ill, if you have eaten more food than usual, or if you suspect nighttime hypoglycemia.
- Use the manufacturer's recommendations and perform quality control measures as directed.
- Look for patterns. For example, 3 to 4 days of a consistent pattern of glucose values above 200 mg/dL before dinner indicates a need to adjust the insulin dose.
- Blood glucose measurements are the best way to determine daily insulin dosages.
- Normal levels are as follows: nondiabetics, 70 to 110 mg/dL; children with type 1 DM, 80 to 150 mg/dL; infants and toddlers, 100 to 200 mg/dL.

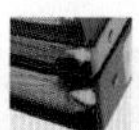

TEACHING GUIDELINE 28.3

Diet and Exercise for Children With Diabetes Mellitus

- Provide sufficient calories and good nutrition for normal growth and development. The diet should be low in saturated fats and concentrated carbohydrates (1,000 kcal/day + 100 kcal for each year, up to 2,500 kcal).
- Learn to identify carbohydrate, protein, and fat foods.
- Make adjustments during periods of rapid growth and issues such as travel, school parties, and holidays.
- Consult a dietitian with expertise in diabetes education as needed.
- Provide three meals per day and mid-afternoon and bedtime snacks. Consistency of intake can help prevent complications and maintain near-normal blood glucose levels.
- Encourage the child to exercise routinely to help the body use insulin efficiently, thus reducing the insulin requirement.
- Encourage the child to participate in age-appropriate sports.
- When exercising, monitor insulin dose and nutritional and fluid intake, and observe for hypoglycemic reactions. Add an extra snack containing 15 to 30 g carbohydrate for each 45 to 60 minutes of exercise. Avoid exercising excessively when insulin is peaking.

References

Books and Journals

Amer, K. S. (2005). Advances in assessment, diagnosis, and treatment of hyperthyroidism in children. *Journal of Pediatric Nursing, 20*(2), 119–126.

American Diabetes Association. (2005). All about diabetes. Accessed 12/20/05 at www.diabetes.org/about-diabetes.jsp.

Behrman, R., Kliegman, R. M., & Jenson, H. B. (2004). *Nelson textbook of pediatrics* (17th ed., pp. 1845–1968). Philadelphia: W. B. Saunders.

Burg, F. D., Polin, R. A., Ingelfinger, J. R., & Gershon, A. A. (2002). *Gellis & Kagan's current pediatric therapy* (pp. 677–727). Philadelphia: W. B. Saunders.

Caravalho, J. Y., & Saylor, C. R. (2000). An evaluation of a nurse case-managed program for children with diabetes. *Pediatric Nursing, 26*(3), 296. Retrieved 5/21/2004 from the ProQuest database.

Collett-Solberg, P. F. (2001). Congenital adrenal hyperplasia: From genetics and biochemistry to clinical practice, part 1. *Clinical Pediatrics, 40*(1), 1–16.

Collett-Solberg, P. F. (2001). Congenital adrenal hyperplasia: From genetics and biochemistry to clinical practice, part 2. *Clinical Pediatrics, 40*(3), 125–132.

Devendra, D., & Eisenbarth, G. S. (2003). Immunologic endocrine disorders. *Journal of Allergy & Clinical Immunology, 111*(2), part 3.

Dveirin, K., & Tunnessen, W. W. (2000). A 14-month old with polyuria and polydipsia: Searching for buried treasure. *Contemporary Pediatrics, 17*(10), 23–30.

Edwards, E. (2004). Addison's disease, case study. Retrieved 5/21/04 from www.pens.org/articles/edwards-3.htm.

Eugster, E. A., LeMay, D., Zern, M., & Pescovitz, O. H. (2004). Definitive diagnosis in children with congenital hypothyroidism. *Journal of Pediatrics, 144*(5), 643–646.

Everly, D., Kaplan, B. S., & Meyers, K. (2003) Treating NDI: Emphasizing the first year of life. Retrieved 5/24/04 from www.diabetesinsipidus.org/4di_treating_ndi_firstyear.htm.

Farthing, N., & Sadler, J. (2004). Working together with diabetes. *Pediatric Nursing, 16*(4), 20. Retrieved 5/17/04 from ProQuest database.

Floyd, J. (2002). Hypoparathyroidism, case study. Retrieved 5/21/04 from www.pens.org/articles/floyd-j.htm.

Gaines, K. K. (2004). Desmopressin (DDAVP®) for enuresis diabetes insipidus. *Urologic Nursing, 24*(6), 520–523.

Hanberg, A. (2005). Common disorders of the pituitary gland: Hyposecretion versus hypersecretion. *Journal of Infusion Nursing, 28*(1), 36–44.

Kanner, S., Hamrin, V., & Grey, M. (2003). Depression in adolescents with diabetes. *Journal of Child & Adolescent Psychiatric Nursing, 16*(1), 15–24.

Kemper, A. R., & Foster, C. M. (2003). Congenital hypothyroidism: A guide for the general pediatrician. *Contemporary Pediatrics, 20,* 32 [electronic version]. Available at www.contemporarypediatrics.com.

Keresztes, P. A., & Brick, K. (2003). Lantus: A new insulin. *MedSurg Nursing, 12*(6), 408–410.

Klingensmith, G., Kaufman, F., Schatz, D., & Clarke, W. (2004). Diabetes care in the school and day care setting. *Diabetes Care, 27,* S122. Retrieved 5/17/2004 from ProQuest database.

Leonard, B. J., Garwick, A., & Adwan, J. Z. (2005). Adolescents' perceptions of parental role involvement in diabetes management. *Journal of Pediatric Nursing, 20*(6), 405–414.

Lipman, T. H., Hench, K. D., Benyi, T., et al. (2004). A multicentre randomized controlled trial of an intervention to improve the accuracy of linear growth measurement. *Archives of Diseases of Childhood, 89*(4), 342–346.

Lloyd-Puryear, M. A., & Forsman, I. (2002). Newborn screening and genetic testing. *Journal of Obstetric, Gynecologic, and Neonatal Nursing, 31,* 200–207.

Maghnie, M., Cosi, G., Genovese, E., et al. (2000) Central diabetes insipidus in children and young adults. *New England Journal of Medicine, 343*(14), 988. Retrieved 5/4/04 from Proquest database.

Markham, L. A., & Stevens, D. L. (2003). A case report of neonatal thyrotoxicosis due to maternal autoimmune hyperthyroidism. *Advances in Neonatal Care, 3*(6), 272–282.

McDougal, J. (2002). Promoting normalization in families with preschool children with type 1 diabetes. *Journal for Specialists in Pediatric Nursing, 7*(3), 113–120.

Miller, S. M. (2003). Diabetes: Get a clearer picture. *Medical Laboratory Observer, 35*(7), 10. Retrieved 5/17/04 from ProQuest database.

National Institutes of Health, National Diabetes Education Program (n.d.). Retrieved 6/8/04 from http://ndep.nih.gov/diabetes/youth/youth_FS.htm.

National Institute of Child Health & Human Development, Cushing's Syndrome (last modified, 5/5/2004). Retrieved 6/6/04 from http://www.nichd.nih.gov/publications/pubs/cushings.htm.

O'Neal, K. J., Jonnalagadda, S. S., Hopkins, B. L., & Kicklighter, J. R. (2005). Quality of life and diabetes knowledge of young persons with type 1 diabetes: Influence of treatment modalities and demographics. *Journal of the American Dietetic Association, 105*(1), 85–91.

Pagana, K. D., & Pagana, T. J. (2006). *Mosby's manual of diagnostic and laboratory tests* (3rd ed.). St. Louis: Mosby.

Perkin, R. M., Swift, J. D., & Newton, D. A. (2003). *Pediatric hospital medicine: Textbook of inpatient management* (pp. 527–556). Philadelphia: Lippincott Williams & Wilkins.

Pinhas-Hamiel, O., & Zeitler, P. (2001). Type 2 diabetes: Not just for grownups anymore. *Contemporary Pediatrics, 1,* 102 [electronic version]. Available at www.contemporarypediatrics.com.

Plotnick, L. P., Clark, L. M., Brancati, F. L., & Earlinger, T. (2003). Safety and effectiveness of insulin pump therapy in children and adolescents with type 1 diabetes. *Diabetes Care, 26*(4), 1142–1147.

Preston, A., Storch, E. A., Lewin, A., Geffken, G. R., Baumeister, A. L., Strawser, M. S., et al. (2005). Parental stress and maladjustment in children with short stature. *Clinical Pediatrics, 44,* 327–331.

Radovick, S., & MacGillivray, M. H. (2003). *Pediatric endocrinology: A clinical guide.* Totowa, NJ: Humana Press.

Ramchandani, N. (2004). Type 2 diabetes in children. *American Journal of Nursing, 104*(3), 65–68.

Sechrist, B. (2005). Who's helping the children? Successful practices in pediatric practices in pediatric diabetes. *Lippincott's Case Management, 10*(1), 53–56.

Sperling, M. A. (2002). *Pediatric endocrinology* (2nd ed.). Philadelphia: W. B. Saunders.

Standards of Medical Care in Diabetes (Jan. 21, 2004). *Diabetes Care,* S15. Retrieved 5/17/04 from the ProQuest database.

Sullivan-Bolyai, S., Deatrick, J., Gruppuso, P., Tamborlane, W., & Grey, M. (2000). Raising young children with type 1 diabetes. *Journal for Specialists in Pediatric Nursing, 7*(3), 93–104.

Taketomo, C. K., Hodding, J. H., & Kraus, D. M. (2004). *Lexi-comp's pediatric dosage handbook* (11th ed.). Hudson, OH: Lexi-comp.

Umpaichitra, V., Bastian, W., & Castells, S. (2003). Hypocalcemia in children: Pathogenesis and management. *Clinical Pediatrics, 40*(6), 305–312.

Wilson, J. D. (2001). Prospects for research for disorders of the endocrine system. *Journal of the American Medical Association, 285*(5), 624. Retrieved 5/21/2004 from the ProQuest database.

Wise-Faberowski, L., Soriano, S. G., Ferrari, L., et al. (2004) Perioperative management of diabetes insipidus in children. *Journal of Neurosurgical Anesthesiology, 16*(2), 14–19.

Websites

www.caresfoundation.org CARES (Congenital Adrenal Hyperplasia Research, Education, and Support) Foundation, Inc.

www.childrenwithdiabetes.com/index_cwd.htm Children with Diabetes (online community for kids, families, and adults with diabetes; multiple resources)

www.diabetes.org American Diabetes Association (resources for diabetes information)

www.genetests.org (maintains current catalog of commercially available and research-based tests for genetic disorders)

www.healthypeople.gov *Healthy People 2010*

www.hgfound.org/ Human Growth Foundation (research, education, support, and advocacy for children with disorders of growth)

www.hormone.org Hormone Foundation (the education affiliate of the Endocrine Society)

www.jdk.org Juvenile Diabetes Research Foundation International

www.magicfoundation.org (resources for families with long-term conditions)

www.mychildhasdiabetes.com/ (parenting and diabetes resources)

www.ndep.nih.gov/ National Diabetes Education Program (information and resources on diabetes in children)

www.newchf.org/ Maria I. New Children's Hormone Foundation

www.ngdf.org/ National Graves' Disease Foundation

www.pedinfo.org (general information about many endocrine issues)

www.pens.org Pediatric Endocrinology Nursing Society

www.us.sandostatin.com/index.jsp (resource for octreotide acetate)

Chapter WORKSHEET

MULTIPLE CHOICE QUESTIONS

1. A young mother brings her new baby, diagnosed with congenital hypothyroidism, to the clinic so she can learn how to administer levothyroxine. The nurse should include which of the following instructions?
   a. Crush the medication and place it in a full bottle of formula to disguise the taste.
   b. Administer the medication every other day.
   c. Use an oral dispenser syringe or nipple to give the crushed medication mixed with a small amount of formula.
   d. Tell the mother that the medication will not be needed after the age of 7.
2. The nurse is instructing a 14-year-old boy about the different types of insulin. Since he takes NPH insulin every morning at 7:30 a.m., at what time could he possibly have an insulin reaction?
   a. When he goes to school at 9 a.m.
   b. When he takes a test at 11 a.m.
   c. When he eats lunch at noon
   d. When he works out after school at 3 p.m.
3. A child diagnosed with Graves' disease begins to take propylthiouracil (PTU). What symptoms should the parents and child observe for to determine if the dose is too high?
   a. Weight loss
   b. Lethargy
   c. Difficulty in school
   d. Tachycardia
4. Which endocrine disorder is considered the most common one observed in early childhood?
   a. Hypothyroidism
   b. Hyperthyroidism
   c. Diabetes mellitus
   d. Cushing's disease
5. When should growth hormone be given in a child who has growth hormone deficiency?
   a. Before meals
   b. After meals
   c. At bedtime
   d. First thing in the morning

CRITICAL THINKING EXERCISES

1. A 12-year-old boy with DM type 1 has the flu. His mother calls the diabetes clinic to report that he stayed home from school and does not have an appetite, so he is not eating. The mother asks the nurse how much insulin the boy should take. He is currently taking three injections daily with Regular and NPH in the morning before breakfast, Regular and NPH in the evening after dinner, and Regular before bedtime. What questions should the nurse ask before answering the mother's question? Based on the answers to these questions, how would you instruct the mother?
2. The mother of Robin, a 5-year-old girl, reports that Robin has a body odor. She is developing breasts and some pubic hair and was teased when she had a sleepover with friends. The review of her growth charts reveals that Robin went from the 50th percentile to the 93rd percentile in the past 6 months. Based on this information, what are the three major nursing diagnoses to begin establishing a plan of care for the child and family? What are the expected outcomes and major interventions associated with the nursing diagnosis of knowledge deficit?
3. A mother brings her baby to the clinic after receiving a phone message from the clinic saying there was a problem with the baby's thyroid test. She says the trip on the bus took a long time, but the infant slept the entire way. She says that the baby is sleeping much of the time and does not want to eat very much. The baby was discharged from the hospital 2 weeks ago. The birth was without difficulty and there were no problems during labor. Why is this visit urgent? What would the test show if the disorder was due to a pituitary gland problem and not the thyroid gland?

STUDY ACTIVITIES

1. During your clinical experiences, ask to be on an inpatient unit that provides care for children with alterations in endocrine function. Compare and contrast the health histories, assessments, laboratory tests, diagnostic procedures, and plans of care for these children with those for the care of children on other units. Participate in the teaching plan for these children and their families.
2. Attend an outpatient clinic that provides care to children with endocrine disorders. Identify the role of the registered nurse in providing coordination of

care, health teaching, and referrals for these children and their families.

3. Shadow a diabetes nurse educator to observe the teaching methods and strategies he or she uses to provide an education plan for a child with diabetes mellitus. Observe how the nurse educator includes the family in the plan. Are there any differences between the teaching plans for type 1 and type 2 DM?

4. Conduct a literature review for one of the common endocrine disorders to research current management practices. Are there evidence-based practice guidelines for nursing interventions?

5. Conduct an Internet search to research the information that is available to children and their families related to diabetes mellitus.

chapter 29

Nursing Care of the Child With a Neoplastic Disorder

Key TERMS

biopsy
biotherapy
chemotherapy
clinical trial
extravasation
malignant
metastasis
neoplastic
staging

Learning OBJECTIVES

Upon completion of the chapter, the learner will be able to:

1. Compare childhood and adult cancers.
2. Describe nursing care related to common laboratory and diagnostic testing used in the medical diagnosis of pediatric cancer.
3. Identify types of cancer common in infants, children, and adolescents.
4. Identify appropriate nursing assessments and interventions related to medications and treatments for pediatric cancer.
5. Develop an individualized nursing care plan for the child with cancer.
6. Describe the psychosocial impact of cancer on children and their families.
7. Devise a nutrition plan for the child with cancer.
8. Develop patient/family teaching plans for the child with cancer.

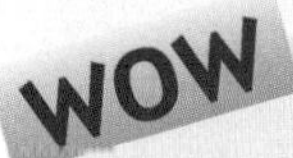

Be inspired by the courage of a child with cancer and reflect it in the care you provide.

John Shaw, 4 years old, is brought to the clinic by his parents with a fever. His father states, "John seems to get fevers and colds more often than our other children. He's also very tired these days. He hardly ever wants to go out and play with his friends. He complains of headaches frequently and just doesn't really seem like himself."

Cancer accounts for the most deaths from disease in children over age 1 year. Cure has been achieved in some children with childhood leukemia and other cancers, but there is no universal long-term cure available for any of the childhood cancers. The 5-year survival rate for all cancers in children younger than 15 years is 72% (Ritchie, 2001).

Cancer is a life-threatening illness that involves emotional distress, fear of the unknown, and changes in life priorities for the child and family. Children with cancer are at a significant risk for depression because they have a life-threatening illness and must undergo frequent and stressful tests and treatments (Cavusoglu, 2001). Initial and ongoing diagnostic testing and the adverse effects of chemotherapy, radiation, or other treatments are often painful as well.

Treatment for cancer has a significant psychosocial impact on the child or adolescent. The child often feels isolated from his or her peers, and the adolescent may have difficulty achieving independence, which is the core developmental task of the teenage years. Children and teens with cancer often demonstrate poorer school performance than healthy peers (Hokkanen et al., 2004). Nurses caring for children with cancer need to be knowledgeable about the medical treatment of the disease and must also be particularly aware of the psychosocial and emotional impact of cancer on the child and family.

Childhood Cancer Versus Adult Cancer

Cancers in children differ greatly from cancers in adults. Pediatric cancers most often arise from primitive embryonal (mesodermal) and neuroectodermal tissues, resulting in leukemias, lymphomas, sarcomas, or central nervous system (CNS) tumors. This is in direct contrast to adult cancers, which mostly arise from epithelial cells, resulting in carcinomas. The most common childhood cancers, in order of frequency, are leukemia, CNS tumors, lymphoma, neuroblastoma, rhabdomyosarcoma, Wilms' tumor, bone tumors, and retinoblastoma. Comparison Chart 29.1 explains how cancer is different in children versus adults.

In children, warning signs of cancer are most often related to changes in blood cell production or as a result of compression, infiltration, or obstruction caused by the tumor. Changes in blood cell production may result in fatigue, pallor, frequent or severe infection, or easy bruising. Infiltration, obstruction, or compression by a tumor may result in bone or abdominal pain, pain elsewhere, swelling, or unusual discharge.

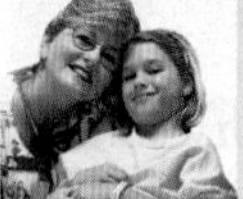

Research is underway to determine whether a statistically significant link exists between the use of supplemental oxygen in the neonatal period and the development of childhood cancer. Studies thus far have proven to be equivocal.

COMPARISON CHART 29.1 Childhood Cancer Versus Adult Cancer

	Childhood Cancer	**Adult Cancer**
Cancer usually affects	Tissues	Organs
Histologic type	Embryonal, leukemia, lymphoma	Epithelial in origin
Most common sites	Blood, lymph, brain, bone, kidney, muscle	Breast, lung, prostate, bowel, bladder
Environmental and lifestyle factors	Only a small amount of environmental influence proven	Strong influence on cancer development
Cancer prevention	Little known	80% preventable
Detection	Usually incidental or accidental	Very early detection possible if screening recommendations followed
Latent period	Relatively short	Can be very long (20 years or greater)
Extent of disease	Metastasis often present at diagnosis	Metastasis less often present at diagnosis
Response to treatment	Very responsive	Less responsive

HEALTHY PEOPLE 2010

Objective	Significance
Increase the proportion of persons who use at least one of the following protective measures that may reduce the risk of skin cancer: avoid the sun between 10 a.m. and 4 p.m., wear sun-protective clothing when exposed to sunlight, use sunscreen with a sun-protective factor (SPF) of 15 or higher, and avoid artificial sources of ultraviolet light.	• Educate families to start skin protection from the sun in childhood to reduce the risk of skin cancer as an adult. • Teach parents to use PABA-free sunscreen (formulated specifically for children) after age 6 months with an SPF of 15 or greater and to reapply sunscreen frequently while the child is out of doors. • Advocate for schools to encourage a sun-safe environment.

Common Medical Treatments

Deciding on a course of medical treatment for cancer in a developing child is complicated. Some of the treatments can impair the child's growth and development. Many pediatric oncologists and cancer treatment centers are active members of the Children's Oncology Group (COG), a National Cancer Institute–supported group that approves and administers clinical trials devoted exclusively to childhood and adolescent cancer research. A **clinical trial** is a carefully designed research study that assesses the effectiveness of a treatment as well as its acute and long-term effects on the patient. Current cancer care in children is a result of the knowledge gained through clinical trials. A clinical trial may include existing medications or treatments in combination with new drugs or may involve a different approach to sequencing or dosing of medications and treatment.

To provide optimal outcomes, the child with cancer should be treated at an institution with multidisciplinary cancer care specialists that can provide the most advanced care available. Each case of pediatric cancer should be considered individually, with the oncology health care team and the family reaching treatment decisions together, whether the treatment plan is standard or involves enrollment in a clinical trial.

In the child with cancer, particularly advanced disease, the decision to provide treatment ("let's do everything we can") or to withhold treatment in the event of an extremely poor prognosis is extraordinarily challenging in an ethical sense. A mature older child or adolescent may have a strong desire to continue or discontinue treatment, and sometimes this desire conflicts with the parents' desires or choices. The American Academy of Pediatrics, Committee on Bioethics (1995), recommends that decision making for older children and adolescents should include the assent of the patient (Box 29.1).

BOX 29.1

AMERICAN ACADEMY OF PEDIATRICS, COMMITTEE ON BIOETHICS, RECOMMENDATIONS REGARDING PEDIATRIC ASSENT

- Give consideration to each child's developmental capacity, rationality, and autonomy.
- Help each child to achieve a developmentally appropriate understanding of the illness.
- Tell the child what s/he can expect regarding testing procedures and treatments.
- Assess the child's understanding of the situation and how s/he is responding.
- Note if there is inappropriate pressure to assent to testing or treatment.
- Seriously solicit the child's expression of willingness to accept the proposed plan of care.

Hospice or palliative care may be needed for the child with cancer. Children facing the end of life experience the same effects that adults do, such as pain, fatigue, nausea, and dyspnea. Standards for end-of-life care are still in development, but all dying children have the right to die comfortably and with palliation of symptoms, as has been well established in adult hospice programs. Children's Hospice International (CHI) has demonstration models in several U.S. states that focus on enhancing the quality of life of children with life-threatening conditions. Formerly, only children with a life expectancy of less than 6 months had access to hospice care, and they were required to forego curative care to enroll in hospice. CHI's goal is to provide a comprehensive, interdisciplinary continuum of care to the child and family from the time of diagnosis with a life-threatening condition through the time of death, if cure is not achieved. For further information related to nursing care of the dying child, refer to Chapter 15.

A variety of medications and treatments are used to treat **neoplastic** disorders in children. Most of these treatments will require a physician's order when the child

HEALTHY PEOPLE 2010

Objective	Significance
Reduce the overall cancer death rate. Increase the proportion of cancer survivors who are living 5 years or longer after diagnosis.	• Teach adolescent boys testicular self-examination. • Reinforce the importance of this self-screening measure at subsequent visits.

is in the hospital. The most common treatments and medications are listed in Common Medical Treatments 29.1 and Drug Guide 29.1. Commonly, chemotherapy and radiation therapy are used to treat childhood cancers. In some instances, hematopoietic stem cell transplantation is used. The nurse caring for the child with cancer should be familiar with the procedures, how the treatments and medications work, and common nursing implications related to use of these modalities.

(text continues on page 976)

Common Medical Treatments 29.1

Treatment	Explanation	Indication	Nursing Implications
Biopsy	A small piece of the tumor is removed with a needle or via an open incision.	Solid tumors	Monitor for bleeding at the needle biopsy site. Provide routine incision care for open biopsy site.
Surgical removal of tumor	The tumor is completely or partially resected surgically.	Solid tumors	Provide routine postoperative nursing care based on the location of the tumor excision.
Leukapheresis	Whole blood is removed from the body, the WBCs are extracted, and then the blood is retransfused into the child.	Hyperviscosity with leukemia (WBC > 100,000)	Performed by specially trained personnel. Monitor blood pressure and other vital signs.
Blood product transfusion	Administration of whole blood, packed red blood cells, platelets, or plasma intravenously	Anemia, thrombocytopenia, bleeding	Follow institution's transfusion protocol. Double-check blood type and product label with a second nurse. Use only irradiated, leukodepleted, CMV-negative blood products in the pediatric cancer patient. Monitor vital signs and assess child frequently to detect adverse reaction to blood transfusion. If adverse reaction is suspected, immediately discontinue transfusion, run normal saline IV, reassess child, and notify physician. Some children require premedication with diphenhydramine and/or acetaminophen before receiving blood products.
Radiation therapy	Ionizing radiation (high-energy x-ray) is delivered to the cancerous area. The radiation damages all cells in the locally treated area (normal and cancerous), but the normal cells are able to repair themselves. Usually administered several times a week for several weeks (a short rest between treatments allows the normal cells time to regenerate). The lowest possible dose of radiation is used and it is directed to a specific area.	Solid tumors, before or after surgical resection, leukemia, lymphoma	Do not wash off radiation marking. Keep skin clean and dry. Fatigue is a common side effect. Skin at the site of radiation may become red, dry, or pruritic or may peel; eventually may become moist and red. Mucositis, dry mouth, and loss of taste may occur if head or neck radiated. Radiation may also have adverse affects on the organ irradiated, such as the brain; monitor for changes.

Common Medical Treatments 29.1 (continued)

Treatment	Explanation	Indication	Nursing Implications
Hematopoietic stem cell transplantation	*Bone marrow transplant:* transfer of healthy bone marrow into a child with cancer. The transplanted cells can then develop into functional cells. *Stem cell transplant:* peripheral stem cells are removed from the donor via apheresis, or stem cells are retrieved from the umbilical cord and placenta. The stem cells are then transplanted into the recipient.	Leukemia, lymphoma, other cancers	Maintain medical asepsis and protective isolation to prevent infection. Monitor closely for GVHD. Provide meticulous oral care. Avoid rectal temperatures and suppositories. Encourage appropriate nutrition. Administer immunosuppressive medications as ordered.
Central venous catheter (Fig. 29.1)	IV catheters inserted into the central circulation for the purpose of administering medications, total parenteral medication, or blood products	Any child with cancer who will require long-term IV medications or parenteral nutrition	Complaints of shortness of breath or chest pain may indicate air entry into the central venous catheter. Have child lie on left side, and notify physician immediately. Keep dressing clean and dry. Perform sterile dressing change per institution policy or physician order. Monitor for fever. Monitor insertion site for erythema or drainage. Maintain sterile technique when accessing line, performing dressing change, or administering any fluid through catheter.
Implanted port (Fig. 29.2)	A needle-accessible port is implanted under the skin, usually on the chest. The port has a thin catheter exiting it that is tunneled under the skin into the superior vena cava or subclavian vein.	Any child with cancer who will require long-term IV medications or parenteral nutrition	Flush non-accessed port with prescribed heparin dose per institution policy. Use sterile technique to access port with Huber needle. Monitor port site for erythema or warmth.

Drug Guide 29.1 Common Drugs for Neoplastic Disorders

Medication	Action	Indication	Nursing Implications
Chemotherapy			
Alkylating agents: busulfan, carboplatin, cisplatin, ifosfamide, temozolomide, thiotepa. Nitrosoureas: carmustine, lomustine. Nitrogen mustard: chlorambucil, cyclophosphamide, mechlorethamine, melphalan.	Interferes with DNA replication and RNA transcription by alkylation (replacing the hydrogen ion with an alkyl group), cross-links DNA. Cell cycle–nonspecific. The nitrosoureas are highly lipid-soluble and easily cross the blood–brain barrier.	A variety of cancers	Causes myelosuppression, nausea, vomiting, alopecia, mucositis. Monitor for signs of infection. Provide adequate hydration. Cyclophosphamide, ifosfamide: administer in the morning, provide adequate hydration, and have child void

(continued)

Drug Guide 29.1 Common Drugs for Neoplastic Disorders (continued)

Medication	Action	Indication	Nursing Implications
			frequently during and after infusion to decrease risk of hemorrhagic cystitis. Cisplatin, mechlorethamine, melphalan: avoid extravasation. Temozolomide: avoid opening capsules. Thiotepa: if contact with skin occurs, wash thoroughly with soap and water.
Antitumor antibiotics: bleomycin, dactinomycin, daunorubicin, doxorubicin, idarubicin, mitomycin, mitoxantrone	Interfere with cellular metabolism, causing disruptions in DNA and/or RNA synthesis. Cell cycle–nonspecific.	A variety of cancers	May cause alopecia, nausea, vomiting, myelosuppression. Bleomycin: fever and chills may occur 20 hours after infusion. Dactinomycin, mitomycin: avoid extravasation. Daunorubicin, doxorubicin, idarubicin: may turn urine red-orange, monitor for arrhythmias, congestive heart failure; avoid extravasation. Mitoxantrone: may color urine, sweat, tears, skin, sclera blue-green; monitor for arrhythmias, congestive heart failure.
Antimetabolites: cladribine, cytarabine, fludarabine, fluorouracil, mercaptopurine, methotrexate, thioguanine	Substitute for a natural metabolite in the molecule, altering the cell's function and ability to replicate. Cell cycle–specific (S phase), cladribine is cell cycle–nonspecific.	A variety of cancers	May cause alopecia, nausea, vomiting, mucositis, and myelosuppression. Cladribine: monitor for fever. Cytarabine: use corticosteroid eye drops to prevent conjunctivitis with high doses. Fludarabine: monitor for visual changes and neurotoxicity; maintain adequate hydration. Fluorouracil: maintain adequate hydration; may cause photosensitivity. Mercaptopurine: do not give oral doses with meals; may cause drug fever; avoid extravasation.

Drug Guide 29.1 Common Drugs for Neoplastic Disorders (continued)

Medication	Action	Indication	Nursing Implications
			Methotrexate: intensive hydration with high doses; may cause photosensitivity. Thioguanine: maintain hydration; administer on empty stomach.
Antimicrotubulars: paclitaxel	Inhibits mitotic cellular function in late G2 and M phases of cell cycle	Refractory leukemia, recurrent Wilms' tumor	May cause alopecia, nausea, vomiting, mucositis, myelosuppression. May cause drowsiness. Avoid extravasation.
Miscellaneous: asparaginase, pegaspargase	Inhibits protein synthesis by depriving tumor cells of the essential amino acid asparagine	Acute lymphocytic leukemia, lymphomas	May cause alopecia, nausea, vomiting, and myelosuppression. Monitor for vital signs during infusion and for signs of anaphylaxis. Have emergency equipment, oxygen, epinephrine, antihistamines, and steroids available at bedside.
Miscellaneous: dacarbazine, procarbazine	Inhibits DNA and RNA synthesis via cross-linking or suppression of mitosis	A variety of cancers	May cause alopecia, nausea, vomiting, myelosuppression. Monitor for flu-like symptoms. Dacarbazine: photosensitivity may occur; avoid extravasation.
Mitotic inhibitors: etoposide, vinblastine, vincristine	Inhibits mitotic activity by inhibiting DNA topoisomerase (etoposide). Causes metaphase arrest by binding to the mitotic spindle (vinblastine, vincristine).	A variety of cancers	May cause alopecia, nausea, vomiting, myelosuppression (only minimal with vincristine). Etoposide: monitor for anaphylaxis; have emergency equipment, oxygen, epinephrine, antihistamines, and steroids available at bedside. Vinblastine, vincristine: maintain hydration; administer allopurinol; avoid extravasation.
Topoisomerase inhibitors: irinotecan, topotecan	Binds to DNA complex, preventing religation of single-strand DNA breaks	Refractory solid tumors	May cause alopecia, nausea, vomiting, myelosuppression, severe diarrhea (irinotecan), hypotension (topotecan).

(continued)

Drug Guide 29.1 Common Drugs for Neoplastic Disorders (continued)

Medication	Action	Indication	Nursing Implications
			Maintain hydration. Avoid extravasation. Monitor blood pressure during topotecan infusion.
Corticosteroids: prednisone, dexamethasone	Suppresses immune system by decreasing lymphatic activity and volume. Also decreases edema caused by tumor or tumor necrosis.	Leukemia, some other cancers	Administer with food to decrease GI upset. May mask signs of infection. Monitor blood pressure; monitor urine for glucose. Do not stop treatment abruptly or acute adrenal insufficiency may occur. Monitor for Cushing syndrome. Doses may be tapered over time.
Biotherapy			
Colony-stimulating factors: darbepoetin alfa, epoetin alfa, filgrastim, sargramostim	Stimulates production of red blood cells (epoetin) or granulocytes (filgrastim, sargramostim)	Counteract myelosuppressive effects of chemotherapy	Administer SC or IV. Filgrastim, sargramostim: may cause bone pain. Sargramostim may cause hypotension and a first-dose reaction.
Interleukins: aldesleukin	Recombinant DNA interleukin-2 product that recruits T, B, and natural killer cells	Non-Hodgkin's lymphoma	Adverse effects are dose-dependent. May cause capillary leak syndrome within 2 to 12 hours of start of treatment: hypotension and decreased organ perfusion result.
Tumor necrosis factor (protein cytokine)	Increases effectiveness of immune cells, stops cancer cells from dividing, damages tumor blood vessels	A variety of cancers	May cause fever, chills, rigors, nausea, vomiting
Monoclonal antibodies: rituximab, gemtuzumab	Binds to CD20 antigen on B lymphocytes	CD20-positive non-Hodgkin's lymphoma, post-transplant lymphoproliferative disorder	Monitor blood pressure for hypotension. Monitor for anaphylaxis and infusion-related reaction. Have epinephrine, antihistamines, and steroids available at bedside for treatment of reaction.

Drug Guide 29.1 Common Drugs for Neoplastic Disorders (continued)

Medication	Action	Indication	Nursing Implications
Interferons: alpha, gamma	Alter cancer cell proliferation (alpha), stimulate macrophage production to fight bacteria and fungus (gamma)	A variety of cancers	May cause flu-like symptoms. Maintain adequate hydration.
Allopurinol	Decreases production of uric acid	Treatment of secondary hyperuricemia occurring during leukemia or tumor treatment	Give PO after meals with plenty of food. Cardiovascular adverse effects may occur with IV administration. Maintain adequate hydration.
Antibiotics (oral, parenteral)	Treatment or prophylaxis of bacterial infections	Prophylaxis of *Pneumocystis jiroveci.* Treatment of documented infection. Neutropenia.	Check for antibiotic allergies. Should be given as prescribed for the length of time prescribed. Start IV antibiotics as soon as possible in the neutropenic child admitted with fever.
Antiemetics: promethazine, metoclopramide, ondansetron	Acts on the CNS transmitters to prevent vomiting	Nausea and/or vomiting	May cause CNS side effects, such as drowsiness or irritability. Ondansetron: may cause dry mouth.
Antifungal agents: nystatin, amphotericin B (conventional and lipid complex)	Invades fungal cell wall, enabling its destruction	Mucositis, systemic fungal infection	Nystatin: administer after meals. Amphotericin B: may cause fever, chills, rigors, cardiovascular adverse effects; monitor patient closely throughout infusion; note dose differences between conventional and lipid complex.
Immunosuppressant drugs: cyclosporine A (CyA), mycophenolate, tacrolimus	Inhibition of production and release of interleukin II (CyA). Inhibition of T- and B-cell proliferation (mycophenolate). Inhibition of T-cell activation (tacrolimus).	Treatment of GVHD after HSCT	Monitor CBC, serum creatinine, potassium, and magnesium. Monitor blood pressure and for signs of infection. Draw blood levels prior to morning dose. CyA: do not give with grapefruit juice. Mycophenolate: give on empty stomach; do not open capsule or crush tablet.

(continued)

Drug Guide 29.1 Common Drugs for Neoplastic Disorders (continued)

Medication	Action	Indication	Nursing Implications
			Tacrolimus: give on empty stomach; monitor for anaphylaxis with first IV dose.
Mesna	Binds with and detoxifies cyclophosphamide and ifosfamide metabolites in the urinary bladder	Antidote to cyclophosphamide- or ifosfamide-induced hemorrhagic cystitis	Maintain adequate hydration. Administer concurrently and after cyclophosphamide or ifosfamide. May cause hypotension.
Methotrexate antidote: leucovorin	Reduces toxic effects of methotrexate	Leucovorin rescue with methotrexate treatment	May cause skin disturbances, wheezing, thrombocytosis. Dose depends on methotrexate level. Dose increased with increased creatinine levels.

Chemotherapy

To understand how **chemotherapy** works to destroy cancer cells, it is necessary to review the normal cell cycle. All cells progress through this cycle (Fig. 29.3). The cell cycle comprises five phases:

- G0 phase: the resting phase; lasts from a few hours to a few years; cells have not started to divide
- G1 phase: cell makes more protein in preparation for dividing; lasts 18 to 30 hours
- S phase: chromosomes are copied so that newly formed cells have the appropriate DNA; lasts 18 to 20 hours
- G2 phase: just before the cell splits into two cells; lasts 2 to 10 hours
- M phase: mitosis, the actual splitting of the cell into two new cells; lasts 30 minutes to 1 hour

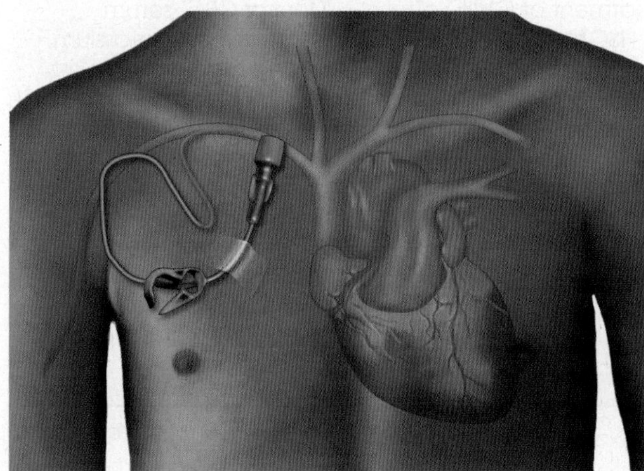

● Figure 29.1 The central venous access catheter is tunneled under the skin and secured with a cuff.

Chemotherapy drugs work in two different ways in relation to the cell cycle. Cell cycle–specific agents exert their actions during a specific phase of the cell cycle. Cell cycle–nonspecific drugs exert their effect on the cells regardless of which phase the cell is in. Chemotherapy protocols often call for a combination of drugs that act on different phases of the cell cycle, thus maximizing the destruction of cancer cells.

Chemotherapeutic medications disrupt the cell cycle of not only cancer cells but also normal rapidly dividing cells, resulting in a significant number of adverse effects. The cells most likely to be affected by chemotherapy are those in the bone marrow, the digestive tract (especially the mouth), the reproductive system, and hair follicles.

Chemotherapy drugs are divided into classes that exert slightly different actions and have an effect on different portions of the cell cycle. Drug Guide 29.1 gives further explanation about the different classes of chemotherapy drugs.

Adverse effects common to chemotherapeutic drugs include immunosuppression, infection, myelosuppression, nausea, vomiting, constipation, oral mucositis, alopecia, and pain (Bryant, 2003; Woolery et al., 2006). Long-term complications include microdontia and missing teeth as a result of damage to developing permanent teeth (Lund, 2005); hearing and vision changes; hemato-

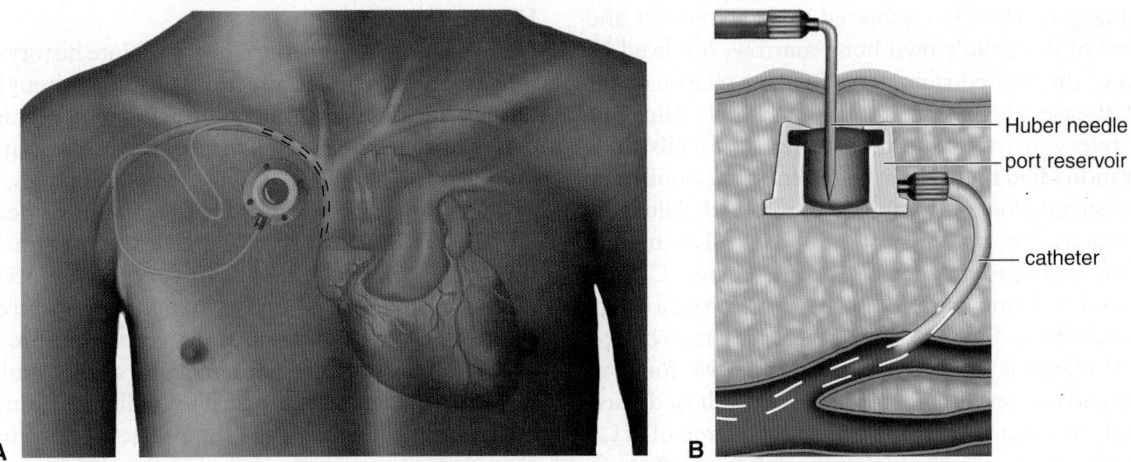

● Figure 29.2 (**A**) The implanted port consists of a reservoir under the skin for ready access. The catheter exiting the port is threaded into the subclavian vein or right atrium. (**B**) A 90-degree Huber needle is used to access the port.

poietic, immunologic, or gonadal dysfunction; endocrine dysfunction, including altered growth and precocious or delayed puberty; various alterations of the cardiorespiratory, gastrointestinal, and genitourinary systems; as well as a second cancer as an adolescent or adult (Bottomley & Kassner, 2003).

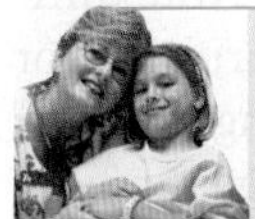

Acupuncture as an adjuvant therapy has been demonstrated to decrease nausea, vomiting, constipation, stress, aversion to chemotherapy, and psychological damage and to result in an increase in oral intake and the self-confidence needed to cope with cancer (Kurishima et al., 2002).

Radiation Therapy

Radiation therapy uses high-energy radiation to damage or kill cancer cells. Radiant energy in either a gamma or particle form is emitted during the treatment (Tomlinson & Kline, 2005). Radiation affects not only cancer cells but also any rapidly growing cells that they are in contact with. It may be used as a curative, adjuvant, or palliative treatment, either alone or in combination with chemotherapy. Radiation therapy is also used to shrink a tumor prior to surgical resection. The area to be treated is marked carefully to minimize damage to normal cells.

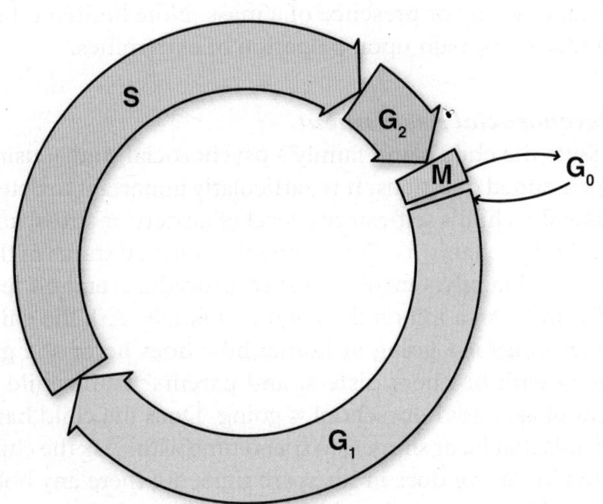

● Figure 29.3 Phases of the cell cycle.

Adverse effects of radiation therapy include fatigue, nausea, vomiting, oral mucositis, myelosuppression, and alterations in skin integrity at the site of irradiation. Long-term complications are related to the area of the body that was irradiated and include alterations in growth; hormone dysfunction; hearing and vision alterations; learning problems; cardiac dysfunction; pulmonary fibrosis; hepatic, sexual, or renal dysfunction; osteoporosis; and development of secondary cancer (particularly at the site of irradiation) (Bottomley & Kassner, 2003).

Hematopoietic Stem Cell Transplantation

Hematopoietic stem cell transplantation (HSCT), also called bone marrow transplantation, is a procedure in which hematopoietic stem cells are infused intravenously into the patient. This follows a period of purging of abnormal cells in the patient that is accomplished through high-dose chemotherapy or irradiation. The use of high-dose chemotherapy and total body irradiation kills the tumor cells but also destroys the child's bone marrow. The transplanted cells migrate to the empty spaces in the child's bone marrow and re-establish normal hematopoiesis in the child.

HSCT is used for a variety of childhood cancers, including leukemia, lymphoma, brain tumors, neuroblastoma, and other solid tumors. For most pediatric cancers, it is not the first line of treatment but is used for refractory or advanced disease.

Autologous HSCT is achieved through harvest and treatment of the child's own bone marrow, followed by infusion of the treated stem cells. Risk for relapse of the original disease is highest in autologous HSCT. Allogenic HSCT refers to transplantation using stem cells from another individual that are harvested from the bone marrow, peripheral blood, or umbilical cord blood. Allogenic HSCT requires human leukocyte antibody (HLA) matching for antigen-specific sites on the leukocytes. Closely matched HLA donors may be difficult to find from a donor listing, and sibling donors are often the closest match. The degree of match is inversely related to the risk for graft rejection and the development of graft-versus-host disease (GVHD). In other words, the lesser the degree of HLA matching in the donor, the higher the risk for graft rejection and GVHD. GVHD occurs to at least some extent in up to 70% of all allogenic HSCT recipients (Graham et al., 2005).

In addition to graft rejection and GVHD, additional initial complications of HSCT are infection, electrolyte imbalance, bleeding, and organ, skin, and mucous membrane toxicities. Long-term complications include impaired growth and fertility related to endocrine dysfunction, developmental delay, cataracts, pulmonary and cardiac disease, avascular necrosis of the bone, and the development of secondary malignancies.

Nursing Process Overview for the Child With a Neoplastic Disorder

Care of the child with a neoplastic disorder includes assessment, nursing diagnosis, planning, interventions, and evaluation. There are a number of general concepts related to the nursing process that may be applied to cancers in children. From a general understanding of the care involved for a child with cancer, the nurse can then individualize the care based on patient specifics. Children with cancer often suffer many physical effects as a result of the disease and its treatment. The nurse must be diligent when assessing for these effects and should involve the parents as a reliable source for reporting the child's physical symptoms.

ASSESSMENT

Assessment of children with neoplastic disorders includes health history, physical examination, and laboratory and diagnostic testing.

> Remember John, the 4-year-old with fever, fatigue, and headaches? What additional health history and physical examination assessment information should you obtain?

Health History

Determine current medical history. Note history of recurrent fever or frequent infections. Inquire about bleeding tendencies, such as unusual bruising or petechiae. Note early-morning headache with nausea or vomiting, gait or behavior changes, or visual disturbances. Inquire about changes in bowel or bladder habits or decrease in appetite. Note history of bone fractures unrelated to trauma. Explore the health history for the presence of risk factors such as previous malignancy and treatment; synthetic chemical exposures; parental exposure to radiation, chemicals, or chemotherapeutic agents; and a family history of malignancy (especially childhood), immune disorder, or genetic disorders such as neurofibromatosis or Down syndrome.

Physical Examination

A complete physical examination should be performed on any child with or suspected of having cancer. Note particular findings as discussed below.

Inspection and Observation

Observe the child's overall appearance and energy level. Note thin, frail appearance, fatigue, or altered level of consciousness. Document visible masses or asymmetry of the face, thorax, abdomen, or extremities. Note difficulty breathing. Inspect the skin for pallor, bruising, or petechiae. Examine the oral cavity for bleeding gums or pale mucous membranes. Observe the child's gait, noting ataxia or limp. Note rectal bleeding or vaginal discharge.

Auscultation, Percussion, and Palpation

Auscultate the heart, lungs, and abdomen, noting any abnormalities. Percuss the abdomen, noting dullness over a mass if present. Palpate for lymphadenopathy; in particular, note nontender or firm lymph nodes. Palpate any unusual area of swelling anywhere on the body, noting size and absence of tenderness. Palpate the abdomen, noting organomegaly or presence of a mass. Note limited range of motion or pain upon palpation of extremities.

Psychosocial Assessment

Assess the child's and family's psychosocial status, using open-ended questions. It is particularly important to determine the child's self-esteem, level of anxiety or stress, and coping mechanisms. Determine the spiritual status of the child and family. Ongoing medical procedures and the fear of dying take a toll on the child and family. Ask the child how things are going at home; how does he or she get along with brothers, sisters, and parents? If the child is school age, ask how school is going. Does the child have friends that he or she gets to spend time with? Ask the child what he or she does in his spare time; are there any hobbies? These types of queries will provide the nurse with information about how well the child is coping.

Assess the parents' status as well. Ask about the marital relationship and how the other children are doing. Determine whether certain stressors may need to be addressed.

Laboratory and Diagnostic Testing

Common Laboratory and Diagnostic Tests 29.1 explains the laboratory and diagnostic tests most commonly used for neoplastic disorders. The tests can assist the physician in diagnosing the disorder or can be used as guidelines in determining treatment. Laboratory or non-nursing personnel obtain some of the tests, while the nurse might obtain others. In either instance the nurse should be familiar with how the tests are obtained, what they are used for, and normal versus abnormal results. This knowledge will also be necessary when providing patient and family education about the testing.

Common Laboratory and Diagnostic Tests 29.1

Test	Explanation	Indication	Nursing Implications
Complete blood count (CBC) with differential	Evaluate hemoglobin and hematocrit, WBC count (particularly the percentage of individual WBCs), and platelet count	Infection, immunosuppression, to determine neutropenia in myelosuppression	Normal values vary according to age and gender. WBC count differential is helpful in evaluating source of infection. May be affected by myelosuppressive drugs.
Alpha-fetoprotein (AFP)	Produced by the fetal liver and yolk sac; normally decreases to very low levels by 1 year of age	May be elevated in Hodgkin's disease and other cancers. Used to determine tumor burden.	No food or fluid restriction required
Urine catecholamines (VMA, HVA)	Catabolism of catecholamines causes elevated levels in urine.	Diagnosis of neuroblastoma (produces catecholamines)	24-hour urine collection. Levels may be altered with certain foods and drugs or vigorous exercise.
Chest x-ray	Radiograph of the chest	Identify tumor or metastasis in the thorax	Chest must be held stationary for a brief time.
Computed tomography (CT scan)	Multiple films taken in successive layers to provide a 3D view of the body part being scanned	Identify tumor location or metastasis	Some CT scans are done with oral or IV contrast (notify physician if child has iodine or shellfish allergy). May require a several-hour period of NPO if contrast is used (contrast may cause nausea). Encourage fluid intake after scan to facilitate excretion of contrast dye.
Magnetic resonance imaging (MRI)	Based on how hydrogen atoms behave in a magnetic field when disturbed by radiofrequency signals. Does not require ionizing radiation. Provides a 3D view of the body part being scanned.	Identify extent of tumor or metastatic spread	Remove all metal objects from the child. Child must remain motionless for entire scan; parent can stay in room with child. Younger children will require sedation to keep still. A loud thumping sound occurs inside the machine during the scan procedure; this can be frightening to children.

(continued)

Common Laboratory and Diagnostic Tests 29.1 (continued)

Test	Explanation	Indication	Nursing Implications
Bone scan	Administration of IV radionuclide material, which is taken up by the bone and is visible on the scans	Identifies metastasis to bone	Requires patent IV for injection. Encourage fluid intake after injection to increase uptake of injected radionuclide. Scan will be performed 1 to 3 hours after injection.
Ultrasound	High-frequency sound waves are directed at internal organs and structures, and an image is made of the waves as they are reflected back through the tissues.	Identify tumor presence, especially in abdomen or on kidney	Fasting for a few hours may be required when certain organs are to be visualized.
Bone marrow aspiration and biopsy	A needle is inserted through the cortex of the bone into the bone marrow (most often the iliac spine), bone marrow is aspirated, and the cells are evaluated.	Evaluation for leukemia or metastasis of other cancers to bone marrow	Use EMLA or lidocaine to decrease pain with procedure. Often performed under conscious sedation. Apply a pressure dressing to arrest bleeding. Assess for tenderness or erythema. May require mild analgesia for post-procedure pain.
Lumbar puncture (LP)	A needle is placed in the subarachnoid space of the spinal column, below the base of the cord, and cerebrospinal fluid is withdrawn for analysis.	Evaluation of tumor or metastasis to brain or spinal cord. Also used to administer intrathecal medications.	Use EMLA before the procedure to decrease pain. May be performed under conscious sedation. Position child appropriately. Use distraction techniques in the older child or teen. Encourage child to recline for up to 12 hours after LP.

NURSING DIAGNOSIS, GOALS, INTERVENTIONS, AND EVALUATION

Upon completion of a thorough assessment, the nurse might identify several nursing diagnoses, including:

- Risk for infection
- Pain
- Impaired oral mucous membranes
- Nausea
- Imbalanced nutrition
- Constipation
- Diarrhea
- Risk for impaired skin integrity
- Activity intolerance
- Disturbed body image
- Situational low self-esteem
- Compromised family coping
- Anticipatory grieving

> After completing an assessment of John, you note the following: history of recurrent infections, unusual bruising, and enlarged lymph nodes. Based on the assessment findings, what would your top three prioritized nursing diagnoses be for John?

Nursing goals, interventions, and evaluation for the child with cancer are based on the nursing diagnoses. Nursing Care Plan 29.1 may be used as a guide in planning

(text continues on page 986)

Nursing Care Plan 29.1

Overview for the Child With a Neoplastic Disorder

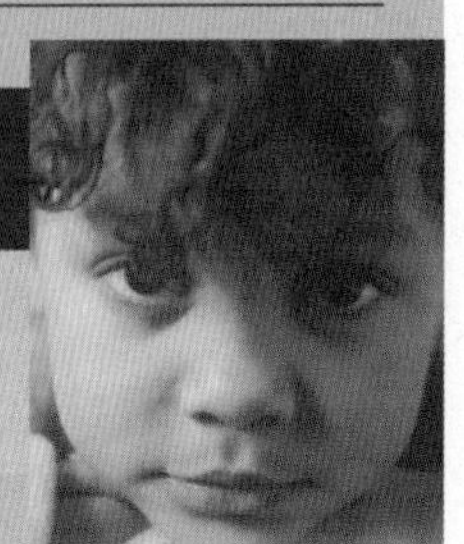

Nursing Diagnosis: Risk for infection related to neutropenia and immunosuppression

Outcome identification and evaluation

Child will not experience overwhelming infection; *will be free from infection or able to recover if becomes infected.*

Interventions: preventing infection

- Assess for fever, pain, cough, tachypnea, adventitious breath sounds, skin ulceration, stomatitis, and perirectal fissures *to identify potential infection.*
- Administer antibiotics for temperature >38.4° C *to decrease likelihood of overwhelming sepsis.*
- Maintain meticulous handwashing procedures (include family, visitors, staff) *to minimize spread of infectious organisms.*
- Maintain isolation as prescribed *to minimize exposure to infectious organisms.*
- Avoid rectal temperatures and examinations, intramuscular injections, and urinary catheterization when child is neutropenic *to decrease possibility of introducing microorganisms.*
- Educate family and visitors that child should be restricted from contact with known infectious exposures (in hospital and at home) *to encourage cooperation with infection control.*
- Strictly observe medical asepsis *to avoid unintentional introduction of microorganisms.*
- Promote nutrition and appropriate rest *to maximize body's potential to heal.*
- Inform family to contact provider if child has known exposure to chickenpox or measles *so that preventive measures (e.g., VZIG) can be taken.*
- Administer vaccines (not live) as prescribed (after clearance with oncologist) *to prevent common childhood communicable diseases.*
- Teach family to monitor for fever at home and report temperature elevations to oncologist immediately *so that antibiotic therapy may be instituted as soon as possible.*

Nursing Diagnosis: Pain related to invasive diagnostic testing, surgical procedure, neuropathy, disease progression, or adverse effects of treatment as evidenced by verbalization of pain, elevated pain scale ratings, guarding, withdrawal from play or refusal to participate in activities of daily living, or physiologic indicators such as elevated heart rate, diaphoresis, muscle tension or rigidity

Outcome identification and evaluation

Child will demonstrate pain relief, *in amount sufficient to allow participation in play, activities of daily living, or therapeutic interventions. Use the age-appropriate pain scale to set the goal and set a time frame for achievement of the goal.*

Interventions: promoting comfort

- Determine level of pain using child interview, pain scale, and assessment of physiologic variables *to determine baseline.*
- Document location, intensity, description of pain *to determine baseline.*
- Discuss with the child and parent techniques that have helped alleviate pain in the past *to incorporate successful interventions into the plan of care.*
- Administer acetaminophen for mild pain *(avoid salicylate and nonsteroidal anti-inflammatory drugs due to increased risk for bleeding).*
- Administer medications as ordered *using the least invasive method possible to avoid pain (intramuscular, subcutaneous, and rectal route should be avoided in the child with thrombocytopenia).*
- Monitor frequently for adverse effects (particularly respiratory effects) of opioid analgesics, *as opioids reduce responsiveness of carbon dioxide receptors in the brain's respiratory center.*

(continued)

Overview for the Child With a Neoplastic Disorder (continued)

- Use nonpharmacologic measures such as play therapy, games, TV, guided breathing, imagery, hypnosis, or meditation as appropriate *(distracts child's attention from the pain).*
- Use massage, positioning, or heat *to relieve pain in a particular area.*
- Use EMLA before needlesticks and conscious sedation with lumbar puncture and bone marrow aspiration *to reduce recurrent acute painful episodes associated with frequent blood draws and diagnostic/treatment procedures.*
- Have the child lie flat for 30 minutes after a lumbar puncture and increase fluid intake for 24 hours after the procedure *to decrease incidence of headache.*

Nursing Diagnosis: Impaired oral mucous membranes related to chemotherapy, radiation therapy, immunocompromise, decreased platelet count, malnutrition, or dehydration as evidenced by oral lesions, ulcers, plaques, hyperemia or bleeding, difficulty eating or swallowing, or complaint of oral discomfort

Outcome identification and evaluation

Child will maintain intact, moist mucosa, *free from redness, ulceration, or debris.*

Interventions: restoring healthy oral mucosa

- Frequently assess oral cavity for redness, lesions, ulcers, plaques, or bleeding *to provide baseline for comparison and identify alterations early.*
- Offer ice chips frequently while NPO *to maintain hydration of mucosa.*
- Use only a soft toothbrush or toothette for dental care, avoiding excessive pressure with brushing, *to decrease incidence of bleeding with mouth care.*
- Keep lips lubricated with petroleum jelly or fragrance-free lip balm *to maintain moist, hydrated lips.*
- Rinse with salt solution or mouthwash every 1 to 2 hours *to keep oral cavity clean and moist.*
- Administer glutamine and/or beta-carotene supplements, *which have been shown to decrease the incidence and severity of mucositis.*
- Have child swish and spit 1:1 Benadryl/Maalox solution *to decrease pain.*
- Administer antifungal solution *to prevent or treat oral candidiasis.*
- Avoid spicy, acidic, or very hot or very cold foods *to decrease pain.*
- Administer pain medication (usually acetaminophen or codeine) as ordered *to decrease pain.*

Nursing Diagnosis: Nausea related to adverse effects of chemotherapy or radiation therapy as evidenced by verbalization of nausea, increased salivation, swallowing movements, or vomiting

Outcome identification and evaluation

Child will experience decreased nausea, *will verbalize symptom relief and will be free from vomiting.*

Interventions: alleviating nausea and vomiting

- Administer antiemetics prior to chemotherapy and as needed thereafter *to decrease frequency of nausea.*
- Assess frequency of vomiting and level of hydration *to provide baseline data and recognize alterations early.*
- Offer frequent, smaller meals or snacks; *smaller amounts are less likely to be vomited.*
- Avoid spicy foods *to avoid stomach upset.*
- Allow bubbles to dissipate from carbonated beverages before they are ingested *(carbonation may contribute to nausea).*
- Remove cover from meal tray before entering child's room *(this will allow the food odor to dissipate outside of the room; food odors may trigger nausea and vomiting).*

Overview for the Child With a Neoplastic Disorder (continued)

Nursing Diagnosis: Imbalanced nutrition: less than body requirements related to anorexia, nausea, vomiting, or mucosal irritation associated with chemotherapy or radiation as evidenced by decreased oral intake and weight, length/height, and/or BMI below average for age or individual child's usual measures

Outcome identification and evaluation

Child will improve nutritional intake, resulting in *steady increase in weight and length/height.*

Interventions: promoting adequate nutrition

- Determine body weight and length/height norm for age or find out what the child's pretreatment measurements were *to determine goal to work toward.*
- Determine child's food preferences and provide favorite foods as able *to increase the likelihood that the child will consume adequate amounts of foods.*
- Administer antiemetics as ordered *to increase the likelihood that the child will retain the food he or she ingests.*
- Weigh child daily or weekly (according to physician order or institutional standard) and measure length/height weekly *to monitor for growth.*
- Offer highest-calorie meals at the time of day when the child's appetite is the greatest *(to increase likelihood of increased caloric intake).*
- Provide increased-calorie shakes or puddings within diet restriction *(high-calorie foods increase weight gain).*
- Administer vitamin and mineral supplements as prescribed *to attain/maintain vitamin and mineral balance in the body.*
- Administer total parenteral nutrition and intravenous lipids as ordered *to provide adequate nutrition for healing.*

Nursing Diagnosis: Constipation related to effects of vinca alkaloids, opioid use, decreased activity, and dietary changes as evidenced by hard stool or stool that is difficult to pass

Outcome identification and evaluation

Child's bowel function will return to usual pattern, *child will pass a formed, soft stool every day (or modify this criterion according to child's usual pattern).*

Interventions: preventing or managing constipation

- Ensure that child increases fluid intake *to provide enough water in the intestines for soft stool formation.*
- Increase fiber in the diet *to provide bulk for stool formation.*
- Administer stool softeners such as mineral oil, docusate sodium; *these help soften the stool, aiding in passage.*
- Provide motivator laxatives such as magnesium hydroxide, lactulose, or sorbitol *to stimulate stool passage.*
- Use stimulant laxatives such as senna or bisacodyl only intermittently rather than on a daily basis *to avoid dependency and diarrhea.*

Nursing Diagnosis: Diarrhea related to effects of radiation therapy as evidenced by loose or watery stools, possibly frequent

Outcome identification and evaluation

Child's bowel function will return to usual pattern, *child will pass a formed, soft stool daily (or modify this criterion according to child's usual pattern).*

Interventions: managing diarrhea

- Assess frequency of diarrhea and level of hydration *to provide data about severity.*
- Obtain weight daily on same scale *to determine extent of fluid loss.*
- Maintain accurate intake and output records *to determine extent of fluid loss.*

(continued)

Overview for the Child With a Neoplastic Disorder (continued)

- Administer oral rehydration solutions or intravenous fluids as ordered *to maintain or restore adequate hydration.*
- Restrict roughage and residue in diet *to decrease likelihood of diarrhea.*
- Avoid milk products during acute diarrheal phase *(lactose often worsens diarrhea).*
- Provide an elemental diet to relieve symptoms *(absorbed in the upper small bowel).*
- Provide meticulous perineal care *to avoid skin breakdown related to frequent or loose stools.*
- Administer antidiarrheal medications if ordered *to decrease frequency of stools.*
- If severe and related to radiation therapy, may require a 3- to 4-day rest period from radiation *to begin recovery of normal absorptive capabilities of bowel.*

Nursing Diagnosis: Risk for impaired skin integrity related to radiation therapy

Outcome identification and evaluation

Child's skin will remain intact, *areas of redness in radiation field will not progress to desquamation.*

Interventions: promoting skin integrity

- Assess skin frequently for erythema, erosions, ulcers, or blisters *to provide baseline data and intervene early if skin is impaired.*
- Use a mild soap for cleansing and pat dry rather than rubbing *to avoid skin irritation.*
- Use aloe vera lotion *to moisturize the skin.*
- Avoid perfumed lotions, soaps, heat, cold, or sun, *as these will further irritate the skin in the irradiated area.*
- Do not scrub ink from marked radiation field, and avoid adhesive tape in that area, *to avoid further skin irritation.*
- Administer diphenhydramine or apply hydrocortisone 1% cream *to reduce itching and urge to scratch.*
- For areas of desquamation related to radiation, apply Silvadene cream once or twice a day *to hasten skin repair.*

Nursing Diagnosis: Activity intolerance related to treatment adverse effects, anemia, or generalized weakness as evidenced by verbalization of weakness or fatigue, elevation of heart rate, respiratory rate, or blood pressure with activity, complaint of shortness of breath with play or activity

Outcome identification and evaluation

Child will display increased activity tolerance, *desire to play without developing symptoms of exertion.*

Interventions: promoting activity

- Encourage activity or ambulation per physician's orders; *early mobilization results in better outcomes.*
- Observe child for symptoms of activity intolerance such as pallor, nausea, lightheadedness or dizziness, or changes in vital signs *to determine level of tolerance.*
- If child is on bed rest, perform range-of-motion exercises and frequent position changes: *negative changes to the musculoskeletal system occur quickly with inactivity and immobility.*
- Cluster nursing care activities and plan for periods of rest before and after exertion *to decrease oxygen need and consumption.*
- Refer the child to physical therapy *for exercise prescription to increase skeletal muscle strength.*

Overview for the Child With a Neoplastic Disorder (continued)

Nursing Diagnosis: Disturbed body image related to hair loss as evidenced by verbalization of dissatisfaction with appearance

Outcome identification and evaluation

Child or adolescent will display appropriate body image, *will look at self in mirror and participate in social activities.*

Interventions: promoting body image

- Acknowledge child's feelings of anger over body changes and illness; *venting feelings is associated with less body image disturbance.*
- Encourage the child or teen to choose a wig or hats and scarves *to involve the child in making decisions about appearance.*
- Support the child's or teen's choices of comfortable, fashionable clothing *to disguise weight loss or scarring while promoting self-esteem.*
- Involve the child in the decision-making process, *as a sense of control will improve body image.*
- Encourage the child to spend time with peers who have experienced hair, limb, or weight loss, *as peers' opinions are often better accepted than those of persons in authority, such as parents or health care professionals.*

Nursing Diagnosis: Risk for situational low self-esteem related to loss of control and inability to progress with quest for independence (adolescents)

Outcome identification and evaluation

Adolescent will maintain or increase self-esteem, *will display increased coping responses and verbalize control as appropriate as well as discuss plans for future.*

Interventions: promoting self-esteem

- Identify the adolescent's positive abilities *to promote self-esteem.*
- Give genuine and honest positive feedback, *as the child or adolescent desires honesty.*
- Explore strengths and weaknesses with the adolescent: *helps the teen to see similarities and differences with healthy peers of the same age.*
- Encourage the teen to perform self-care as possible *to promote independence.*
- Offer emotional support *(reduces psychological distress and increases coping abilities).*
- Encourage participation in a support group *to allow teens to discuss body changes and the reactions they perceive in others.*
- When the adolescent is physically able, encourage attendance at camp or an adventure/wilderness event *(these programs have been shown to improve mental health and coping skills).*

Nursing Diagnosis: Compromised family coping related to potentially life-threatening illness and stressors involved with cancer treatment

Outcome identification and evaluation

Child and/or family will demonstrate adequate coping skills, *will verbalize feeling supported and demonstrate healthy family interactions.*

Interventions: promoting child and family coping

- Provide emotional support to child and family *(improves coping abilities).*
- Actively listen to the child's and family's concerns *(validates their feelings, establishes trust).*
- Provide open communication with the child and siblings; *children appreciate honesty about their illness, and coping is improved.*
- Refer families to community resources such as parent support groups and grief counseling *(such support improves coping abilities).*

(continued)

Overview for the Child With a Neoplastic Disorder (continued)

- Give terminally ill children the permission to discuss their feelings about their illness, *allowing them to conquer fears and express love for their family and friends.*
- Encourage families to be honest with siblings about the treatment and prognosis of the child with cancer *(children often sense what is going on and cope better when they are prepared and are given an honest explanation of events).*
- Prepare siblings for the death of the child with cancer, using the child life specialist and chaplain as necessary: *the bereavement period is eased when siblings are prepared.*

Nursing Diagnosis: Anticipatory grieving (family) related to diagnosis of cancer in a child and impending loss of child as evidenced by crying, disbelief of diagnosis, and expressions of grief

Outcome identification and evaluation

Family will express feelings of grief; *seek help in dealing with feelings, plan for future one day at the time.*

Intervention: supporting the grieving family

- Use therapeutic communication with open-ended questions *to encourage an open and trusting relationship for better communication.*
- Actively listen to family's expression of grief; *just being present and listening conveys support.*
- Encourage the family to cry and express feelings away from the child *to work through feelings while not upsetting the child.*
- Assess for spiritual distress *and refer the family to the hospital chaplain or clergy of choice for support.*
- Educate the family about the child's condition honestly: *knowing what is going on, what is to be expected, and what the treatment plan is gives the family a sense of control.*
- Support the family through discussions with the child about anticipated death *when the illness is deemed terminal.*

nursing care for the child with a neoplastic disorder. The care plan includes many nursing diagnoses that are applicable to the child or adolescent, but not all children will have the same effects from cancer and its treatment. Nursing care should be individualized based on the child's and family's responses to illness. Additional information about nursing management related to specific types of cancer will be included later in the chapter as it relates to specific disorders.

Provide education to families of all children with cancer as outlined in Teaching Guideline 29.1.

> Based on your top three nursing diagnoses for John, describe appropriate nursing interventions.

Administering Chemotherapy

All chemotherapy medications have the potential to cause toxicities in the child as well as the persons handling or preparing the medication. General guidelines related to the preparation and administration of chemotherapy include:

- Chemotherapy should be prepared and administered only by specially trained personnel.
- Personal protective equipment (PPE) in the form of double gloves and nonpermeable gowns should be worn when preparing or administering chemotherapy. If splashing is possible or a spill occurs, then a face shield and/or mask may also be necessary.
- Dispose of all equipment used in chemotherapy preparation and administration in a puncture-resistant container.

It is critical to calculate the chemotherapy dose correctly. Chemotherapy medication doses in children are based on body surface area (BSA). A nomogram is a commonly used device for determining BSA. To use the nomogram, draw a straight line between the child's height on the left and the child's weight on the right. The point at which the straight line crosses the center is the child's BSA expressed in meters squared (Fig. 29.4).

An alternative to using the nomogram is to use the following formula: BSA (m^2) = the square root of (height [in centimeters] × weight [in kilograms] divided by 3,600). For example, for a child 140 cm tall and weighing 30 kg: 140 × 30 = 4,200; 4,200/3,600 = 1.167; and the square root of 1.167 is 1.08. The BSA would be 1.08.

Managing Adverse Effects of Chemotherapy

Chemotherapy can result in multiple adverse effects. Myelosuppression leads to low blood counts in all cell lines, placing the child at risk for infection, hemorrhage,

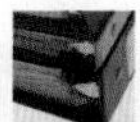

TEACHING GUIDELINE 29.1

Education for Families of Children With Cancer

- Obtain a printed or written copy of the child's treatment plan.
- Keep a calendar of all appointment times, blood count lab draw days, and phone numbers of all physicians, home care companies, laboratory, and hospital.
- Seek medical care IMMEDIATELY if the child's temperature is 38.3° C (101° F) or higher.
- Call the oncologist or seek medical care if any of the following occur:
  - Cough or rapid breathing
  - Increased bruising, bleeding or petechiae, pallor or increased levels of fatigue
  - Earache, sore throat, nuchal rigidity
  - Blisters, rashes, ulcers
  - Red, irritated skin on the child's buttocks
  - Abdominal pain, difficulty or pain with eating, drinking or swallowing
  - Constipation or diarrhea
  - For children with central venous catheters:
    - Pus, redness, or swelling at the site
    - Breakage of the catheter
- Do not give the child aspirin.

Baggott, C. R., Kelly, K. P., Fochtman, D., & Foley, G. V. (2002). *Nursing care of children and adolescents with cancer* (3rd ed.). Philadelphia: W. B. Saunders.

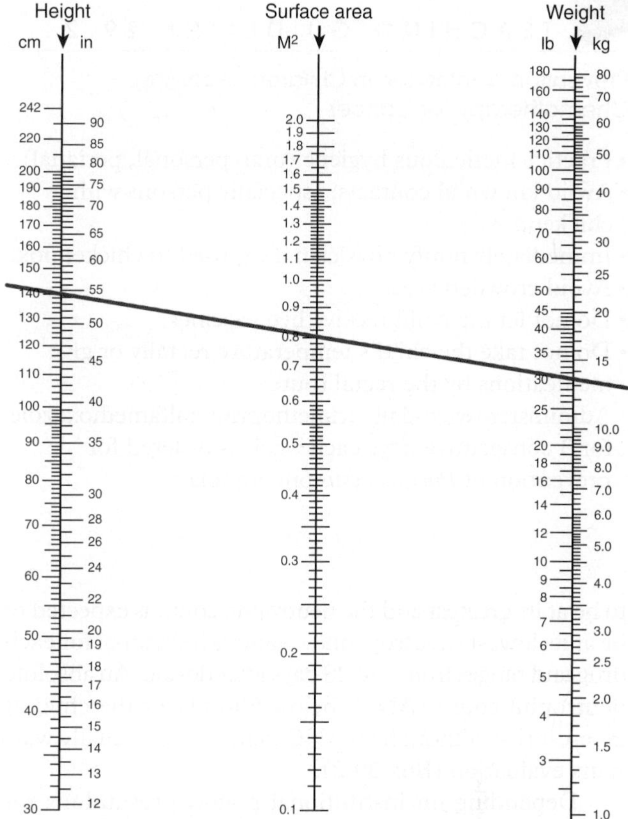

● Figure 29.4 A child who weighs 13.2 kg and is 140 cm tall has a BSA of 0.80 m².

and anemia. Nausea, vomiting, and anorexia may hinder the child's growth. Alopecia and facial changes may affect the child's self-esteem (Fig. 29.5). Nursing interventions related to the effects of myelosuppression, nausea, vomiting, and anorexia are discussed below. Refer to Nursing Care Plan 29.1 for nursing interventions related to altered body image.

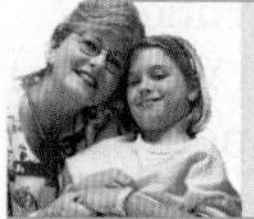

Cooling the scalp during chemotherapy administration with the use of a cooling cap may decrease hair loss. (Tomlinson & Kline, 2005).

Preventing Infection

Many chemotherapeutic drugs cause significant bone marrow suppression and decreased amounts of circulating mature neutrophils ("segs," or segmented neutrophils). Administer granulocyte colony-stimulating factor (GCSF) as ordered to promote neutrophil growth and maturation. Administer varicella zoster immunoglobulin (VZIG) within 72 hours of exposure to active chickenpox. If the child is actively infected with chickenpox, administer intravenous acyclovir as ordered. Children receiving treatment for acute lymphoblastic leukemia are at risk for opportunistic infection with *Pneumocystis jiroveci,* as most children are colonized with this fungus. Administer prophylactic antibiotics as ordered and teach the parents to administer them at home. Teaching Guideline 29.2 gives further information about infection prevention at home.

As neutrophils are the primary means of fighting bacterial infection, when the neutrophil count is low, the chance for developing an overwhelming bacterial infection is high. Each drug that causes bone marrow suppression has a point of nadir. *Nadir* is the time after administration of the drug when bone marrow suppression is expected

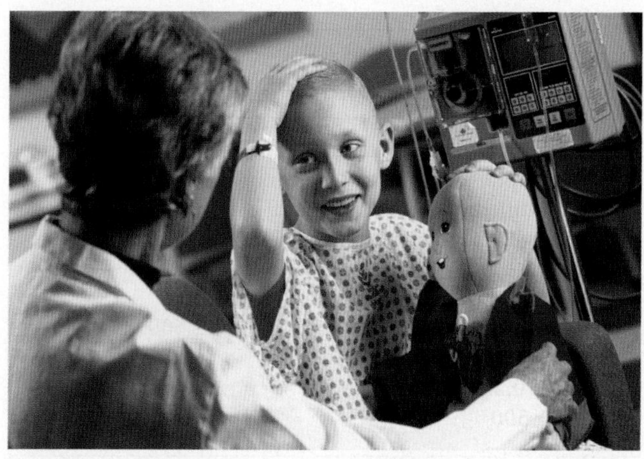

● Figure 29.5 Chemotherapy often causes alopecia.

TEACHING GUIDELINE 29.2

Prevention of Infection in Children Receiving Chemotherapy for Cancer

- Practice meticulous hygiene (oral, personal, perianal).
- Avoid known ill contacts, especially persons with chickenpox.
- Immediately notify physician if exposed to chickenpox.
- Avoid crowded areas.
- Do not let the child receive live vaccines.
- Do not take the child's temperature rectally or give medications by the rectal route.
- Administer twice-daily trimethoprim-sulfamethoxazole for 3 consecutive days each week as ordered for prevention of *Pneumocystis* pneumonia.

to be at its greatest and the neutrophil count is expected to be at its lowest (neutropenia). Nadir is individual for each drug and ranges from 7 to 28 days after dosing. An absolute neutrophil count (ANC) below 500 places the child at greatest risk, although an ANC below 1,500 usually warrants evaluation (Box 29.2).

Depending on institutional policy, precautions for neutropenia will be followed if the ANC is depressed. Precautions related to neutropenia generally include:

- Perform hand hygiene before and after each patient contact.
- Place the child in a private room.
- Monitor vital signs every 4 hours.
- Assess for signs and symptoms of infection at least every 8 hours.
- Avoid rectal suppositories, enemas, or examinations; urinary catheterization; and invasive procedures.
- Restrict visitors with fever, cough, or other signs/symptoms of infection.
- Do not permit raw fruits or vegetables or fresh flowers or live plants in the room.

BOX 29.2

CALCULATING THE ABSOLUTE NEUTROPHIL COUNT (ANC)

1. Add together the percentage of banded and segmented neutrophils reported on the complete blood count with differential (CBC with diff).
2. Multiply the total number of white blood cells reported on the CBC by the sum above. This yields the ANC (total number of neutrophils present).

Example: Bands 5%, Segs 15%, WBCs 2,500
5% + 15% = 20% (0.20)
2,500 × 0.20 = 500
ANC = 500

- Place a mask on the patient when he or she is being transported outside of the room.
- Perform dental care with a soft toothbrush if the platelet count is adequate.

Children with neutropenia and fever must be started on intravenous broad-spectrum antibiotics without delay to avoid overwhelming sepsis.

Preventing Hemorrhage

Assess for petechiae, purpura, bruising, or bleeding. Determine changes from baseline that warrant intervention. Encourage quiet activities or play to avoid trauma. Avoid rectal temperatures and examinations to avoid rectal mucosal damage that results in bleeding. Post a sign at the head of the bed stating "no rectal temperatures or medications." Avoid intramuscular injections and lumbar puncture if possible to decrease the risk of bleeding from a puncture site. If bone marrow aspiration must be performed, apply a pressure dressing to the site to prevent bleeding.

For active or uncontrolled bleeding, transfuse platelets as ordered to control bleeding.

Preventing Anemia

To maintain blood volume, limit blood draws to the minimum volume required. Encourage the child to eat an appropriate diet that includes adequate iron. Administer erythropoietin injections as ordered. Teach families to give the injections at home if prescribed.

Managing Nausea, Vomiting, and Anorexia

Many chemotherapeutic drugs produce the adverse effect of nausea and vomiting. The cycle of nausea, vomiting, and anorexia is difficult to break once it begins. Prevent nausea by administering antiemetics prior to the administration of chemotherapy and on a routine schedule around the clock for the first 1 to 2 days rather than on an as-needed (PRN) basis. Bright lights and noise may worsen nausea, so the child's environment should be dimly lit and calm. Relaxation therapy and guided imagery may also be helpful in preventing or treating nausea and vomiting. Refer to Nursing Care Plan 29.1 for additional interventions.

Taste alterations are common in children who have received chemotherapy. During or after chemotherapy, children may develop an aversion to a food that was previously their favorite (Tomlinson & Kline, 2005).

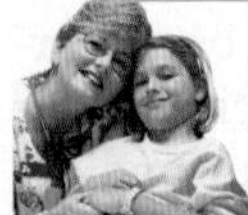

Ginger capsules, ginger tea, and candied ginger have been used as a nausea remedy for centuries. (Ginger ale is usually artificially flavored, so it would not have the same effect.) Though ginger is considered safe, instruct families to check with the oncologist before using this remedy.

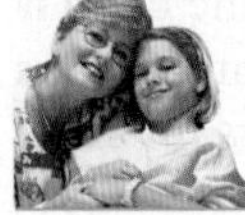

Foot massage has been demonstrated to decrease the nausea and pain associated with chemotherapy.

Monitoring the Child Receiving Radiation Therapy

Radiation causes damage to the cells in a localized area, which may include normal cells in addition to the cancerous ones. Assess the child's skin daily, particularly at the treatment site. Provide good hygiene, but gently. Encourage moisture retention in the skin by applying aqueous creams or moisturizers. Do not apply deodorants or perfumed lotions on the radiation treatment site. Avoid the use of heat or ice packs at the site. Instruct the child and family that clothing should fit loosely so as not to irritate the site. During and for 8 weeks after the radiation treatment, the skin will be more photosensitive. Protect the skin with a high-SPF sunscreen.

Providing Care to the Child Undergoing Stem Cell Transplantation

Stem cell transplantation is performed at limited specialty centers in the United States, and special training is required for all personnel caring for the transplanted child. The intent of this discussion is to provide only a brief introduction to and overview of nursing management related to HSCT.

Care may be divided into three phases: the pretransplant phase, the post-transplant phase, and the lengthy supportive care phase. Nursing management of each phase is briefly discussed below.

Pretransplant Phase

In the pretransplant phase, the child is being prepared to receive the transplant. The child's own bone marrow cells are eradicated through high-dose chemotherapy and total body irradiation. This phase usually occurs over 7 to 10 days. The child will be hospitalized because he or she is at extreme risk for serious infection. Maintain protective isolation in a positive-pressure room and limit visitors. Administer gammaglobulin, acyclovir, or antibiotics as ordered to prevent or treat infection. Lymphohematopoietic rescue occurs with infusion of the donor or autologous cells.

Post-transplant Phase

The post-transplant phase is also a time of high risk for the child. Monitor closely for symptoms of GVHD such as severe diarrhea and maculopapular rash progressing to redness or desquamation of the skin (especially palms or soles) (Fig. 29.6). If GVHD occurs, administer immunosuppressive drugs such as cyclosporine, tacrolimus, or mycophenolate (which place the child at further risk for infection).

Supportive Care

During the supportive care phase, which lasts several months after the transplant, continue to monitor for and prevent infection. Administer packed red blood cells or

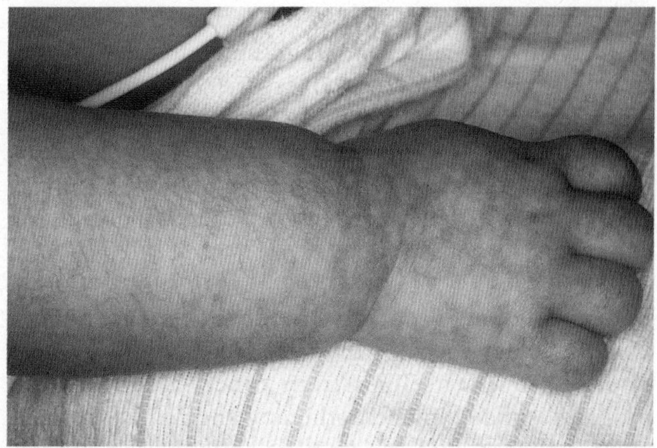

● Figure 29.6 The first sign of GVHD may be a maculopapular rash.

platelets and granulocyte colony-stimulating factor as needed.

Families and children who undergo HSCT need prolonged and extensive emotional and psychosocial support. A medical social worker and psychologist or counselor are usually members of the transplant team and are excellent resources for these families' needs.

Promoting a Normal Life

Children and teens want to be normal and to experience the things that other children their age do. The child should attend school when he or she is well enough and the white blood cell counts are not dangerously low. Children, their families, and their teachers should be aware that cancer and its treatment can affect scholastic abilities. Education-related problems include memory processing, speed, and attention (White, 2003).

Maintain other activities if the child is able and if platelet counts are within normal limits. Special camps are available for children with cancer. These camps offer an opportunity for children and adolescents to experience a variety of activities safely and to network with youngsters who are experiencing similar physical and emotional challenges. The Children's Oncology Camping Association (http://www.cocaintl.org/membercamps/location_usa.html) and the Candlelighter's Childhood Cancer Foundation (http://www.candlelighters.org/supportcamps.stm) provide lists of camps throughout the United States and Canada and internationally for children and teens with cancer.

Promoting Growth

Promote growth in children with cancer by encouraging an appropriate diet and preventing nausea and vomiting and also by addressing concerns such as diarrhea and constipation. Chronic diarrhea related to radiation therapy may prevent the child from gaining weight and growing properly (see Nursing Care Plan 29.1). The use of vinca alkaloids and opioids, as well as the decreased activity level of the child with cancer, may contribute to constipation. Constipation increases the pain experience, contributes to the child's malaise, and decreases quality of life. It directly affects the child's ability to grow by increasing anorexia, nausea, and vomiting (Tomlinson & Kline, 2005). Nursing Care Plan 29.1 details interventions related to preventing and managing constipation.

Preventing and Treating Oncologic Emergencies

Oncologic emergencies may occur as an effect of the disease process itself or from cancer treatment. As progress is made in chemotherapy and radiation treatment, children with cancer have an increased survival rate, but they still face the risk of developing an oncologic emergency. Nurses caring for children with cancer need to be familiar with signs and symptoms of oncologic emergencies as well as with their treatment. All of these problems warrant careful, frequent monitoring of respiratory, cardiovascular, neurologic, and renal status. Table 29.1 provides information about oncologic emergencies.

Caring for the Dying Child

Of the 12,000 children diagnosed with cancer annually in the United States, about 2,200 will die from the disease each year (Houlahan et al., 2006). A "do not resuscitate" (DNR) order for the child with progressive cancer is obtained in many situations. This order helps to optimize care in the terminal phase of cancer (Postovksy et al., 2004). Nurses serve as patient and family advocates, clarifying terminology and providing support as needed during the discussion of DNR orders and throughout the rest of the terminal phase.

Children with terminal cancer often experience a great deal of pain, particularly when death is imminent. Pain is often accompanied by agitation and dyspnea, which further contribute to the child's discomfort. Whether the

Table 29.1 Oncologic Emergencies

Emergency	Associated with	Signs and Symptoms	Laboratory or Diagnostic Test Findings	Management
Sepsis	Neutropenia resulting from bone marrow suppression due to chemotherapy	• Fever or low temperature • Respiratory distress • Poor perfusion • Altered level of consciousness	• ANC < 500 • Positive blood culture • Increased BUN, creatinine, potassium, clotting times • Decreased platelet count • Metabolic acidosis	• Airway and ventilation maintenance • Fluid volume resuscitation • Inotropic support • Broad-spectrum antibiotics and antifungals • Dialysis if needed
Tumor lysis syndrome	ALL, lymphoma, neuroblastoma	• Nausea, vomiting, diarrhea, anorexia • Lethargy • Increased heart rate and blood pressure • Decreased or absent urine output • Altered level of consciousness	• Hyperuricemia • Hyperkalemia • Hyperphosphatemia • Hypocalcemia • Hypoxia	• Prevent by giving allopurinol for several days prior to chemotherapy (also treat with allopurinol). • Double IV fluid maintenance • Sodium bicarbonate
Hyperleukocytosis	Leukemia with high WBC count	• Respiratory distress • Murmur, increased heart rate	• WBC count > 100,000 • Hyperkalemia, hyperphosphatemia • Hyperuricemia • Decreased pH and bicarbonate	• Leukapheresis • Respiratory support • Double IV fluid maintenance with sodium bicarbonate added • Diuretics

Table 29.1 Oncologic Emergencies (continued)

Emergency	Associated with	Signs and Symptoms	Laboratory or Diagnostic Test Findings	Management
Typhlitis (neutropenic enterocolitis)	Inflammatory process of GI tract occurring with induction phase of leukemia chemotherapy	• Acute abdominal pain • Nausea, vomiting • Bloody diarrhea and emesis • Fever • Anorexia	• KUB: scarcity of bowel gas, possibly ileus • CT (abdominal): inflammation, bowel wall thickening, peritoneal fluid	• Bowel rest (NPO status) • IV nutrition • Assess for bowel perforation/shock. • Broad-spectrum antibiotics and antifungals • Comfort measures
Superior vena cava syndrome	Compression on the SVC by NHL or other mediastinal mass, such as neuroblastoma	• Dyspnea and cyanosis • Large cervical lymph nodes • Wheezing, diminished breath sounds	• Chest x-ray or CT shows mediastinal mass. • Pleural effusion	• Intubation and ventilation • Comfort measures • Treat cause (usually surgical removal of mass).
Spinal cord compression	Tumor or metastasis compresses spinal cord	• Back, neck, or leg pain • Sensory or autonomic dysfunction • Extremity weakness or paralysis	• MRI reveals location of tumor or metastasis to epidural space.	• Dexamethasone • Careful assessment • Radiation therapy • Comfort measures
Increased intracranial pressure	Brain tumor or metastasis to brain causing compression of brain; may result in herniation	• Headache, visual disturbances • Morning vomiting • Infants: increased head circumference • Altered level of consciousness • Cushing's triad • Seizure activity	• Head CT or MRI reveals extent of mass.	• Frequent, careful neurologic assessment • Limit fluids. • Dexamethasone • Anticonvulsants • Tumor resection, radiation or chemotherapy • Comfort measures
Massive hepatomegaly	Obstruction caused by neuroblastoma filling a large portion of the abdominal cavity	• Distended, enlarged abdomen • Respiratory distress, hypoxia • Poor perfusion • Tachycardia, hypotension	• Abdominal CT reveals extent of tumor. • Coagulopathy	• Tumor resection or debulking • Mechanical ventilation, inotropic support • Nasogastric decompression • Position to minimize abdominal pressure. • Blood transfusions • Comfort measures

child has a DNR order or the status remains that of "full code," pain management is central to the nursing care of the child who is dying from cancer. The Association of Pediatric Oncology Nurses' position paper entitled "Pain Management for the Child with Cancer in End-of-Life Care" outlines the following recommendations for managing children's pain at the end of life:

- Prevention and alleviation of pain is a primary goal of care in the child dying of cancer.
- Children and parents are equal partners with members of the health care team in managing the patient's pain.
- Children dying of cancer may require aggressive dosing of analgesics. Medications that do not have a dose maximum should be escalated, sometimes rapidly, to achieve

adequate pain control or to maintain pain control when tolerance has occurred.

- The nurse's role in caring for children who are in pain at the end of life includes assessment, identifying expected outcomes, and planning, performing, and evaluating interventions (Hooke et al., 2001).

Interventions related to pain management may be found in Nursing Care Plan 29.1. Further discussion related to care of the dying child is found in Chapter 13.

Leukemia

Leukemia is a primary disorder of the bone marrow in which the normal elements are replaced with abnormal white blood cells. Normally, lymphoid cells grow and develop into lymphocytes, and myeloid cells grow and develop into red blood cells, granulocytes, monocytes, and platelets. Leukemia may develop at any time during the usual stages of normal lymphoid or myeloid development. Leukemia may be classified as acute or chronic, lymphocytic or myelogenous (Table 29.2). Acute leukemias are rapidly progressive diseases affecting the undifferentiated or immature cells; the result is cells without normal function. Chronic leukemias progress more slowly, permitting maturation and differentiation of cells so that they retain some of their normal function. Acute leukemias, including acute lymphoblastic leukemia (ALL) and acute myelogenous leukemia (AML), account for about 95% of all cases of leukemia in children and adolescents (Colby-Graham & Chordas, 2003), so they will be the focus of the discussion below.

Complications of leukemia include metastasis to the blood, bone, CNS, spleen, liver, or other organs and alterations in growth. Late effects include problems with neurocognitive function and ocular, cardiovascular, or thyroid dysfunction. With advances in treatment over the past 50 years, most cases of childhood leukemia are curable, though children who experience relapse or present with advanced disease have a poorer prognosis (Colby-Graham & Chordas, 2003).

Table 29.2 Incidence of Types of Leukemia in Children and Adolescents

Type	Incidence
Acute lymphoblastic leukemia	75% to 80%
Acute myelogenous leukemia	20% to 25%
Chronic lymphoblastic leukemia	Rare
Chronic myelogenous leukemia	<5%

From Colby-Graham, M. F., & Chordas, C. (2003). The childhood leukemias. *Journal of Pediatric Nursing, 18*(2), 87–95.

● ACUTE LYMPHOBLASTIC LEUKEMIA

ALL is the most common form of cancer in children. It most often occurs in children between 2 and 10 years of age (Albano et al., 2005). It is more common in white children than in other races. ALL is classified according to the type of cells involved: T cell, B cell, early pre-B cell, or pre-B cell. Most children will achieve initial remission if appropriate treatment is given. The overall cure rate of ALL is 65% to 75%. Relapse is rare after 7 years from diagnosis.

Prognosis is based upon the white blood cell (WBC) count at diagnosis, the type of cytogenetic factors and immunophenotype, the age at diagnosis, and the extent of extramedullary involvement. Generally, the higher the WBC at diagnosis, the worse the prognosis. Children ages 2 to 10 years at diagnosis usually have the best prognosis. Infants less than 12 months of age at diagnosis generally have a poorer prognosis. When a child experiences a relapse, the prognosis becomes poorer. Complications include infection, hemorrhage, poor growth, and CNS, bone, or testicular involvement.

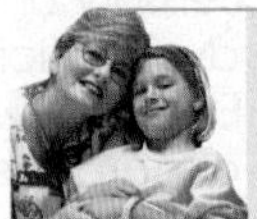

Growth hormone replacement therapy using recombinant human growth hormone may improve the long-term growth of children with leukemia.

Pathophysiology

The exact cause of ALL remains unknown. Genetic factors and chromosome abnormalities may play a role in its development. In ALL, abnormal lymphoblasts abound in the blood-forming tissues. The lymphoblasts are fragile and immature, lacking the infection-fighting capabilities of the normal WBC. In ALL, the growth of lymphoblasts is excessive and the abnormal cells replace the normal cells in the bone marrow. The proliferating leukemic cells demonstrate massive metabolic needs, depriving normal body cells of needed nutrients and resulting in fatigue, weight loss or growth arrest, and muscle wasting. The bone marrow becomes unable to maintain normal levels of red blood cells, WBCs, and platelets, so anemia, neutropenia, and thrombocytopenia result. As the bone marrow expands or the leukemic cells infiltrate the bone, joint and bone pain may occur. The leukemic cells may permeate the lymph nodes, causing diffuse lymphadenopathy, or the liver and spleen, resulting in hepatosplenomegaly. With spread to the CNS, vomiting, headache, seizures, coma, vision alterations, or cranial nerve palsies may occur.

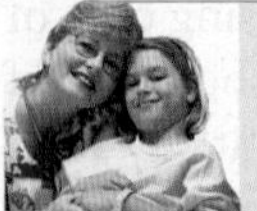

Changes in behavior or personality, headache, irritability, dizziness, persistent nausea or vomiting, seizures, gait changes, lethargy, or altered level of consciousness may indicate CNS infiltration with leukemic cells. Immediately report these findings to the pediatric oncologist.

Therapeutic Management

Therapeutic management of the child with ALL focuses on giving chemotherapy to eradicate the leukemic cells and restore normal bone marrow function. Treatment is divided into three stages. CNS prophylaxis is provided at each stage; without CNS prophylaxis, leukemia would spread to the CNS in up to 50% of children with ALL. The length of treatment and choice of medications are based on the child's age, risk category, and subtype determined by bone marrow analysis. Table 29.3 discusses the stages of leukemia treatment. For relapsed or less responsive leukemia, HSCT may be necessary.

Nursing Assessment

For a full description of the assessment phase of the nursing process, refer to page 978. Assessment findings pertinent to ALL are discussed below.

Health History

Elicit a description of the present illness and chief complaint. Common signs and symptoms reported during the health history might include:

- Fever (may be persistent or recurrent, with unknown cause)
- Recurrent infection
- Fatigue, malaise, or listlessness
- Pallor
- Unusual bleeding or bruising
- Abdominal pain
- Nausea or vomiting
- Bone pain
- Headache

Explore the child's current and past medical history for risk factors such as:

- Male gender
- Age 2 to 5 years
- Caucasian race
- Down syndrome, Shwachman syndrome, or ataxia-telangiectasia
- X-ray exposure *in utero*
- Previous radiation-treated cancer

Determine the child's history of varicella zoster immunization or disease. Chickenpox infection in the leukemic child may lead to disseminated, overwhelming infection.

Physical Examination

Take the child's temperature (fever may be present), and look for petechiae, purpura, or unusual bruising (due to decreased platelet levels). Inspect the skin for signs of infection. Auscultate the lungs, noting adventitious breath sounds, which may indicate pneumonia (present at diagnosis or due to immunosuppression during treatment). Note location and size of enlarged lymph nodes. Palpate the liver and spleen for enlargement. Document tenderness on abdominal palpation.

Laboratory and Diagnostic Tests

Common laboratory and diagnostic studies ordered for the assessment of ALL include:

- Abnormal complete blood counts: low hemoglobin and hematocrit, decreased red blood cell count, decreased platelet count, and elevated, normal, or decreased WBC count
- Peripheral blood smear may reveal blasts.
- Stained smear from bone marrow aspiration will show greater than 25% lymphoblasts. Bone marrow aspirate is also examined for immunophenotyping (lymphoid vs. myeloid, and level of cancer cell maturity) and cytogenetic

Table 29.3 Stages of Leukemia Treatment

Stage	Purpose	Length	Usual Medications
Induction	Rapid induction of complete remission	3 to 4 weeks	Oral steroids, IV vincristine, IM L-asparaginase, daunomycin (high-risk)
Consolidation (intensification)	Strengthen remission, reduce leukemic cell burden	Varies	High-dose methotrexate, 6-mercaptopurine; possibly cyclophosphamide, cytarabine, asparaginase, thioguanine, epipodophyllotoxins
Maintenance	Eliminate all residual leukemic cells	2 to 3 years	Low-dose: daily 6-mercaptopurine, weekly methotrexate, intermittent IV vincristine and oral steroids
CNS prophylaxis	Reduce risk of development of CNS disease	Given periodically in all stages	Intrathecal chemotherapy; cranial radiation is used infrequently

analysis (determines abnormalities in chromosome number and structure). Immunophenotyping and cytogenetic analysis are used in the classification of the leukemia, which helps guide treatment.

- Lumbar puncture will reveal whether leukemic cells have infiltrated the CNS.
- Liver function tests and blood urea nitrogen (BUN) and creatinine levels determine liver and renal function, which if abnormal may preclude treatment with certain chemotherapeutic agents.
- Chest x-ray may reveal pneumonia or a mediastinal mass.

Nursing Management

Nursing care of children with ALL focuses on managing disease complications such as infection, pain, anemia, bleeding, and hyperuricemia and the many adverse effects related to treatment. Many children require blood product transfusion for the treatment of severe anemia or low platelet levels with active bleeding.

Individualize nursing care based on the diagnoses, interventions, and outcomes presented in Nursing Care Plan 29.1, depending on the child's response to the disease and chemotherapy. Refer to the nursing process overview section for further information related to managing the adverse effects of chemotherapy.

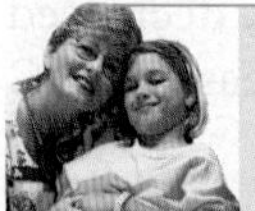

Blood products administered to children with any type of leukemia should be irradiated, cytomegalovirus (CMV) negative, and leukodepleted. This treatment of blood products before transfusion will decrease the amount of antibodies in the blood, an important factor in preventing GVHD should HSCT become necessary at a later date.

Reducing Pain

Children and teens with leukemia suffer pain related to the disease as well as the treatment. Chemotherapy drugs commonly used in leukemia may cause peripheral neuropathy and headache. Lumbar puncture and bone marrow aspiration, which are periodically performed throughout the course of treatment, also cause pain. The most common areas of pain are the head and neck, legs, and abdomen (probably from protracted vomiting with chemotherapy). Distraction techniques such as listening to music, watching TV, or playing games may take the child's mind off the pain. Administer mild analgesics such as acetaminophen for acute episodes of pain. The use of EMLA cream prior to venipuncture, port access, lumbar puncture, and bone marrow aspiration may decrease procedure-related pain events. Application of heat or cold to the painful area is usually acceptable. Narcotic analgesics may be used for episodes of acute severe pain or for palliation of chronic pain.

ACUTE MYELOGENOUS LEUKEMIA

AML is the second most common type of leukemia in children. Its incidence peaks during the adolescent years. AML affects the myeloid cell progenitors or precursors in the bone marrow, resulting in malignant cells. The French-American-British (FAB) classification system identifies eight subtypes of AML (MO to M7), depending on myeloid lineage involved and the degree of cell differentiation. These subtypes are useful for determining treatment. The overall cure rate for childhood AML is about 50%. Complications include treatment resistance, infection, hemorrhage, and metastasis.

The induction phase of AML requires intense bone marrow suppression and prolonged hospitalization because AML is less responsive to treatment than ALL. Toxicity from treatment is more common in AML and is likely to be more serious than with ALL. Empiric broad-spectrum antibiotics and prophylactic platelet transfusions may be prescribed. After remission is achieved, children require intensive chemotherapy to prolong the duration of remission. HSCT is often required in children with AML, depending on the subtype.

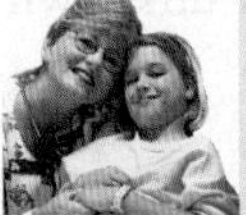

At the time of diagnosis, about 25% of children with AML present with a WBC count above 100,000 (hyperleukocytosis); this results in venous stasis and backup of blast cells in small vessels, causing hypoxia, hemorrhage, and lung or brain infarction. Hyperleukocytosis is a medical emergency. These children require leukapheresis to decrease hyperviscosity by quickly decreasing the number of circulating blasts.

Nursing Assessment

Explore the health history for common signs and symptoms, including recurrent infections, fever, or fatigue. Explore the medical history for risk factors, such as Hispanic race, previous chemotherapy, and genetic abnormalities such as Down syndrome, Fanconi anemia, neurofibromatosis type I, Shwachman syndrome, Bloom syndrome, and familial monosomy 7.

Perform a thorough physical examination. Note skin pallor and salmon-colored or blue-gray papular lesions. Palpate the skin for subcutaneous rubbery nodules. Palpate for lymphadenopathy. Note headache, visual disturbance, or signs of increased intracranial pressure, such as vomiting, that may indicate CNS involvement. Upon diagnosis of AML, the child's WBC count is typically extremely elevated. Bone marrow aspiration will reveal greater than 30% blast cells.

Nursing Management

Nursing management of the child with AML is similar to that of the child with ALL. Nursing interventions focus on managing the adverse effects of treatment and preventing infection. Refer to the nursing process overview section and to Nursing Care Plan 29.1 for appropriate interventions.

Lymphomas

Lymphomas, or tumors of the lymph tissue (lymph nodes, thymus, spleen), account for about 12% of cases of childhood cancer. Lymphomas may be divided in to two categories: Hodgkin's disease (or Hodgkin's lymphoma) and non-Hodgkin's lymphoma (NHL), which includes more than a dozen types. Hodgkin's disease tends to affect lymph nodes located closer to the body's surface, such as those in the cervical, axillary, and inguinal areas, whereas NHL tends to affect lymph nodes located more deeply inside the body.

HODGKIN'S DISEASE

In Hodgkin's disease, malignant B lymphocytes grow in the lymph tissue, usually starting in one general area of lymph nodes. The presence of Reed-Sternberg cells (giant transformed B lymphocytes with one or two nuclei) differentiates Hodgkin's disease from other lymphomas. As the cells multiply, the lymph nodes enlarge, compressing nearby structures, destroying normal cells, and invading other tissues. The cause of Hodgkin's disease is still being researched, but there appears to be a link with Epstein-Barr virus infection. Hodgkin's disease is rare in children under 5 years of age and is most common in adolescents and young adults; it is more common in boys than girls.

In addition to the traditional **staging** (I through IV, depending on the amount of spread; Table 29.4), Hodgkin's is also classified as A (asymptomatic) or B (presence of symptoms of fever, night sweats, or weight loss of 10% or more). Prognosis depends on the stage of the disease, tumor bulk, and A or B classification (disease classified as A generally carries a better prognosis). Hodgkin's stages I and II are associated with a 10-year survival rate of 95%. Stages III and IV have a poorer prognosis, as does a tumor bulk of greater than 6 cm and the presence of B symptoms.

Table 29.4 Staging of Hodgkin's Disease

Stage	Clinical Findings
I	One group of lymph nodes is affected.
II	Two or more groups on the same side of the diaphragm are affected.
III	Groups of lymph nodes above and below the diaphragm are affected.
IV	Metastasis to organs such as the liver, bone, or lungs

Complications of Hodgkin's disease include liver failure and secondary cancer such as acute non-lymphocytic leukemia and NHL.

Chemotherapy, usually with a combination of drugs, is the treatment of choice for children with Hodgkin's disease. Radiation therapy may also be necessary. In the child with disease that does not go into remission or in the child who experiences relapse, HSCT may be an option.

Nursing Assessment

Explore the health history for common signs and symptoms, which may include recent weight loss, fever, drenching night sweats, anorexia, malaise, fatigue, or pruritus. Elicit the health history, determining risk factors such as prior Epstein-Barr virus infection, family history of Hodgkin's disease, genetic immune disorder, or HIV infection.

Evaluate respiratory status, as the presence of a mediastinal mass may compromise respiration. Palpate for enlarged lymph nodes; they may feel rubbery and tend to occur in clusters (most common sites are cervical and supraclavicular). Palpate the abdomen for hepatomegaly or splenomegaly, which may be present with advanced disease. The chest x-ray may reveal a mediastinal mass. The complete blood count may be normal or reflect anemia. Tissue sampling will reveal Reed-Sternberg cells.

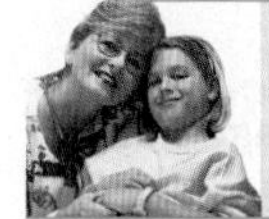

Significant pain in the affected lymph nodes has sometimes been noted after alcohol ingestion.

Nursing Management

Nursing management of the child with Hodgkin's lymphoma focuses on addressing the adverse effects of chemotherapy or radiation. Refer to the nursing process overview section and Nursing Care Plan 29.1 to develop an individualized nursing care plan based on the child's response to treatment.

NON-HODGKIN'S LYMPHOMA

NHL results from mutations in the B and T lymphocytes that lead to uncontrolled growth. NHL tends to affect lymph nodes located more deeply within the body. NHL spreads by the bloodstream and in children is a rapidly proliferating, aggressive malignancy that is very responsive to treatment. Prognosis depends on the cell type involved and the extent of the disease at diagnosis. Seventy percent to 90% of children with treated NHL have disease-free long-term survival. Complications include metastasis and the development of a secondary malignancy later in life.

Remission is induced with chemotherapy and followed with a maintenance phase of chemotherapy lasting about

2 years. NHL tends to spread easily to the CNS, so CNS prophylaxis similar to that used in leukemia is warranted. Autologous bone marrow transplantation may be used in some children.

Nursing Assessment

Children with NHL are usually symptomatic for only a few days or a few weeks before diagnosis because the disease progresses so quickly. Note onset and location of pain or lymph node swelling. Document history of abdominal pain, diarrhea, or constipation. Explore the health history for risk factors such as congenital or acquired immune deficiency.

Observe for increased work of breathing, facial edema, or venous engorgement (mediastinal mass). Palpate for the presence of lymphadenopathy and palpate the abdomen for the presence of a mass. Lymph node biopsy and bone marrow aspiration determine the diagnosis. CT scan, chest x-ray, and bone marrow results may be used to determine the extent of metastasis.

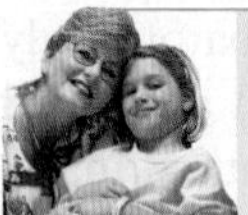

Cough, dyspnea, orthopnea, facial edema, or venous engorgement may indicate mediastinal disease in the child with NHL. This is an emergency requiring rapid treatment.

Nursing Management

As with Hodgkin's lymphoma, nursing management of NHL is directed toward managing the adverse effects of chemotherapy. Refer to the Nursing Process Overview section and Nursing Care Plan 29.1 to plan nursing care for the child and family based on the responses they exhibit.

Brain Tumors

Brain tumors are the most common form of solid tumor and the second most common type of cancer in children (Kline & Sevier, 2003). Slightly more than half of brain tumors arise in the posterior fossa (infratentorial); the rest are supratentorial in origin. The cause of brain tumors in children is unknown. Some tumors are localized, while others are of higher grade and more invasive. The prognosis depends on the location and extent of tumor. Low-grade tumors and those that are fully resectable have a better prognosis than tumors that are located deeper within the brain, making them difficult to resect. For example, low-grade astrocytomas have a 5- to 10-year survival rate of 60% to 90% (Albano et al., 2005), but the rate for the highly malignant medulloblastoma is not as positive. There are many different types of childhood brain tumors; Table 29.5 explains the most common ones.

Complications of brain tumors include hydrocephalus, increased intracranial pressure, brain stem herniation, and negative effects of radiation such as neuropsychological, intellectual, and endocrinologic sequelae.

Pathophysiology

Though the cause of brain tumors is generally not known, the effects of brain tumors are predictable. As the tumor grows within the cranium, it exerts pressure on the brain tissues surrounding it. The tumor mass may compress vital structures in the brain, block cerebrospinal fluid flow, or

Table 29.5 Childhood Brain Tumors

Tumor	Location	Characteristics
Medulloblastoma (most common)	Cerebellum	Invasive, highly malignant, grows rapidly. Less favorable outcome with disseminated disease. Progresses quickly to increased intracranial pressure, seeds on CNS pathways. Half occur in children <6 years old.
Brain stem glioma	Brain stem	Aggressive, difficult to resect, resistant to chemotherapy. Spreads widely within the brain stem but rarely extends outside of brain stem area. Affects cranial nerve function.
Ependymoma	Frequently arises from floor of fourth ventricle	Varying speed of growth. Often causes hydrocephalus. Usually diagnosed before it spreads to other parts of the brain or spinal cord.
Astrocytoma	Cerebellum, cerebral hemispheres, thalamus, hypothalamus	Slow course with insidious onset. Responsive to chemotherapy, often resectable. Causes slowly increasing intracranial pressure. Low-grade tumor may be removed completely. High-grade tumors have poor prognosis.

cause edema in the brain. The result is an increase in intracranial pressure. Presenting symptoms vary according to location and type of tumor.

Therapeutic Management

The type of tumor may be identified at the time of surgery. The location of the tumor within the brain will determine the extent to which it can safely be resected. Children with hydrocephalus may require a ventriculoperitoneal shunt (see Chapter 17 for further information on hydrocephalus). Radiation is reserved for children over age 2 years because it can have long-term neurocognitive effects. Chemotherapy is being used increasingly in the treatment of pediatric brain tumors in an attempt to avoid the use of radiation therapy.

Nursing Assessment

For a full description of the assessment phase of the nursing process, refer to page 978. Assessment findings pertinent to CNS tumors are discussed below.

Health History

Elicit a description of the present illness and chief complaint. Common signs and symptoms reported during the health history might include:

- Nausea or vomiting
- Headache
- Unsteady gait
- Blurred or double vision
- Seizures
- Motor abnormality or hemiparesis
- Weakness, atrophy
- Swallowing difficulties
- Behavior or personality changes
- Irritability, failure to thrive or developmental delay (in very young children)

Explore the patient's current and past medical history for risk factors such as history of neurofibromatosis, tuberous sclerosis, or prior treatment for CNS leukemia.

Physical Examination

Inspection and Observation

Observe for strabismus or nystagmus, "sunsetting" eyes, head tilt, alterations in coordination, gait disturbance, or alterations in sensation. Note alteration in gag reflex, cranial nerve palsy, lethargy, or irritability. Note the child's posture. Check pupillary reaction, noting size, equality, reaction to light, and accommodation.

Palpation

Measure blood pressure, which may decrease with increasing intracranial pressure. In the infant, palpate the anterior fontanel for bulging. Assess deep tendon reflexes, noting hyperreflexia.

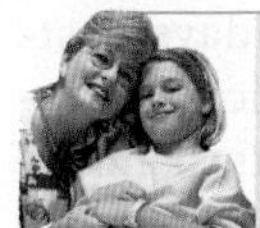

A fixed and dilated pupil is a neurosurgical emergency.

Laboratory and Diagnostic Tests

Common laboratory and diagnostic studies ordered for the assessment of CNS tumors include:

- CT, MRI, or positron-emission tomography (PET) will demonstrate evidence of the tumor and its location within the intracranial cavity.
- Lumbar puncture with cerebrospinal fluid cell evaluation may show tumor markers or the presence of alpha-fetoprotein or human chorionic gonadotropin, which may assist in the diagnosis.

Nursing Management

Nursing management of the child with a brain tumor includes preoperative and postoperative care, as well as interventions to manage adverse effects related to chemotherapy and radiation. Refer to the nursing process overview section for a discussion of nursing interventions related to chemotherapy adverse effects. Nursing Care Plan 29.1 provides additional interventions that may be individualized depending on the child's response to the brain tumor and its treatment.

Providing Preoperative Care

Preoperatively, care focuses on monitoring for additional increases in intracranial pressure and avoiding activities that cause transient increases in intracranial pressure. Administer dexamethasone as prescribed to decrease intracranial inflammation. Prevent straining with bowel movements by use of a stool softener. Assess the child's pain level as well of level of consciousness, vital signs, and pupillary reaction to determine subtle changes as soon as possible. Provide a tour of the intensive care unit, which is where the child will wake up after the surgery. Instruct the child and family about the possibility of intubation and ventilation in the postoperative period. If a ventriculoperitoneal shunt will be placed for the treatment of hydrocephalus caused by the tumor, provide education about shunts to the child and family (see Chapter 17).

Shave the portion of the head as determined by the neurosurgeon. Some children may choose to have the entire head shaved. Sometimes children with long hair may feel better about losing it if they donate it to Locks of Love (www.locksoflove.org), an organization that provides hairpieces for financially disadvantaged children.

Providing Postoperative Care

Regulate fluid administration, as excess fluid intake may cause or worsen cerebral edema. Administer mannitol or hypertonic dextrose to decrease cerebral edema. Assess vital signs frequently, along with checking pupillary reactions and determining level of consciousness. Extreme lethargy or coma may be present for several days postoperatively. Increases in temperature may indicate infection or may be caused by cerebral edema or disturbance of the hypothalamus. Treat hyperthermia with antipyretics such as acetaminophen and with sponge baths, as increases in temperature increase metabolic need. Reduce the temperature slowly.

Monitor for signs of increased intracranial pressure. Headache is common in the postoperative period. Assess pain level and provide analgesics as prescribed. Minimize environmental stimuli, providing a calm and quiet atmosphere. Check the head dressing for cerebrospinal fluid drainage or bleeding. Assess for and document the extent of head, face, or neck edema. Administer eye lubricant if edema prevents complete closure of the eyelids. Apply cool compresses to the eyes to decrease swelling.

As the child begins to regain consciousness, he or she may be confused or combative. Restrain the child if needed to keep him or her in bed and prevent dislodging of tubes and lines.

Positioning the Child in the Postoperative Period

Position the child on the unaffected side with the head of the bed flat or at the level prescribed by the neurosurgeon. Side positioning is usually preferred, as the child may have difficulty handling oral secretions if the level of consciousness is decreased. Do not elevate the foot of the bed, as this may increase intracranial pressure and contribute to bleeding. When changing the child's position, maintain the head in alignment with the remainder of the body. Children with paralyzed or spastic extremities will need additional positioning support.

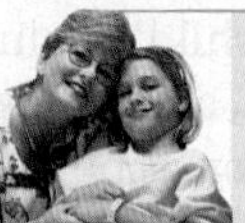

Observe preoperatively and postoperatively for signs of brain stem herniation such as opisthotonos (see Fig. 17.13), nuchal rigidity, head tilt, sluggish pupils, increased blood pressure with widening pulse pressure, change in respirations, bradycardia, irregular pulse, and changes in body temperature.

Consider THIS!

Alice Tice, 6 years old, is scheduled to receive chemotherapy for a brain tumor. As the nurse caring for her, how can you prepare Alice for this? What nursing interventions are important when caring for a child receiving chemotherapy (discuss reducing pain, reducing risk of infection, promoting adequate nutrition, and managing nausea and vomiting)?

Neuroblastoma

Neuroblastoma, a tumor that arises from embryonic neural crest cells, is the most common extracranial solid tumor in children. It most frequently occurs in the abdomen, mainly in the adrenal gland, but it may occur anywhere along the paravertebral sympathetic chain in the chest or retroperitoneum (Lofthouse et al., 2003). By the time of diagnosis, the neuroblastoma has usually already metastasized. Neuroblastoma is the most common cancer-related cause of death in children between the ages of 1 and 4 years and the most common neoplastic tumor diagnosed in infancy (Lofthouse et al., 2003).

Staging of the tumor at diagnosis determines the course of treatment and prognosis. Table 29.6 discusses the staging of neuroblastomas. Survival rates range from 40% to 90%. Prognosis depends on the tumor stage, age at diagnosis, location of tumor, and location of **metastasis**. Infants less than 12 months of age and children with stage I disease have the best survival rates. Children with tumors above the diaphragm tend to have a better prognosis than those with abdominal tumors. Metastasis to the bone is a worse prognostic factor than metastasis to the skin, liver, or bone marrow. Children who relapse after initial treatment also tend to have a dismal prognosis (Kline & Sevier, 2003). In addition to metastasis, complications may include nerve compression, resulting in neurologic deficits.

The neuroblastoma must be surgically removed. Radiation and chemotherapy are administered to all children with neuroblastoma except those with stage I disease, in whom the tumor is completely resected.

Nursing Assessment

For a full description of the assessment phase of the nursing process, refer to page 978. Assessment findings pertinent to neuroblastoma are discussed below.

Health History

Presenting signs and symptoms of neuroblastoma depend on the location of the primary tumor and the extent of

Table 29.6 Staging of Neuroblastoma

Stage	Clinical Findings
I	Tumor confined to organ or structure of origin
II	Tumor extends beyond organ or structure, not beyond midline, and regional nodes on the same side may be involved
III	Tumor invasively extends beyond the midline with bilateral lymph node involvement
IV	Metastasis to bone, bone marrow, other organs, distant lymph nodes
IV-S	Tumor would have been considered a stage I or II, but remote metastasis to one or more sites (liver, skin, or bone marrow) has occurred, but does not involve skeleton

metastasis. Often parents are the first to notice a swollen or asymmetric abdomen. Elicit the health history, documenting bowel or bladder dysfunction, especially watery diarrhea, neurologic symptoms (brain metastasis), bone pain (bone metastasis), anorexia, vomiting, or weight loss.

Physical Examination

Note neck or facial swelling, bruising above the eyes, or edema around the eyes (metastasis to skull bones). Inspect the skin for pallor or bruising (bone marrow metastasis) and document cough or difficulty breathing. Auscultate the lungs for wheezing. Palpate for lymphadenopathy, especially cervical. Palpate the abdomen, noting a firm, nontender mass. Palpate for and note hepatomegaly or splenomegaly if present.

Laboratory and Diagnostic Testing

Laboratory and diagnostic testing may reveal the following:

- CT scan or MRI to determine site of tumor and evidence of metastasis
- Chest x-ray, bone scan, and skeletal survey to identify metastasis
- Bone marrow aspiration and biopsy to determine metastasis to the bone marrow
- 24-hour urine collection for homovanillic acid (HVA) and vanillylmandelic acid (VMA); levels will be elevated, as 90% to 95% of all neuroblastomas secrete catecholamines, which are then excreted in the urine (Kline & Sevier, 2003).

Nursing Management

Postoperative nursing care depends on the site of tumor removal, which is most often the abdomen. Routine care after abdominal surgery will be needed. Refer to the nursing process overview section and Nursing Care Plan 29.1 related to the effects of chemotherapy and radiation. As the disease has often metastasized significantly by the time of diagnosis, these children and families will need emotional support and possibly referrals to help them cope with the poor prognosis.

Bone and Soft Tissue Tumors

Bone and soft tissue tumors account for about 10% to 15% of malignant tumors in children. Bone tumors are most often diagnosed in adolescence, whereas soft tissue tumors tend to occur in younger children. This discussion will focus on the most common bone and soft tissue tumors occurring in childhood. The most common bone tumors in children are osteosarcoma and Ewing sarcoma. These bone tumors often initially go undiagnosed, as adolescents frequently seek care for traumatic events and the pain suffered with a bone tumor may initially be attributed to trauma (Widhe & Widhe, 2000). Rhabdomyosarcoma is the most common soft tissue tumor in childhood.

OSTEOSARCOMA

Osteosarcoma is the most common **malignant** bone cancer in children, occurring most frequently in adolescents at the peak of the growth spurt. Osteosarcoma occurs slightly more often in females and is rare among African-Americans. It presumably arises from the embryonic mesenchymal tissue that forms the bones. The most common sites are in the long bones, particularly the proximal humerus, proximal tibia, and distal femur. Survivors of retinoblastoma who suffer a secondary malignancy are most frequently diagnosed with osteosarcoma. Complications include metastasis, particularly to the lungs and other bones, and recurrence of disease within 3 years, primarily affecting the lungs (Kline & Sevier, 2003).

Surgical removal of the tumor is necessary. Chemotherapy is often administered before surgery to decrease the size of the tumor; it is usually administered after surgery to treat or prevent metastasis. The type of surgery performed depends on the tumor size, extent of disease outside of the bone, distant metastasis, and skeletal maturity. Radical amputation may be performed, but often teens undergo a limb salvage procedure. Radical amputation may include the entire extremity or the entire affected bone. Limb-sparing surgery entails removing only the affected portion of the bone, replacing it with either an endoprosthesis or cadaver bone.

Nursing Assessment

Obtain the health history, ascertaining when pain, limp, or limitation of motion was first noticed. Dull bone pain may be present for several months, eventually progressing to limp or gait changes.

Inspect the affected limb for erythema and swelling. Palpate the affected area for warmth and tenderness and to determine the size of the soft tissue mass, if present. As with other pediatric cancers, a thorough physical examination is warranted to detect other abnormalities that may indicate metastasis.

Laboratory and diagnostic testing may include:

- CT scan or MRI to determine the extent of the lesion and to identify metastasis
- Bone scan to determine the extent of malignancy
- Elevated alkaline phosphatase levels: these may or may not be helpful, as the quickly growing adolescent often normally has elevated levels as a response to rapid bone growth

Nursing Management

The adolescent will generally be quite anxious about the possibility of amputation and even about the limb salvage procedure. Present preoperative teaching at the adolescent's developmental level and ensure that he or she is included in planning treatment. Regardless of the type of surgery performed, provide routine orthopedic postoperative care. Educate the adolescent and parents on the care of the stump, if amputation is necessary, and ensure that the teen becomes competent in crutch walking. A prosthesis may be ordered. The adolescent will need time to adjust to these significant body image changes and may benefit from talking with another teen who has undergone a similar procedure. Support the teen in choosing clothing that may camouflage the prosthesis while still allowing the teen to appear fashionable. Provide emotional support, as the teen's maturity level allows him or her to understand the severity of the disease. Peer support groups are often helpful, as teens value their peers' opinions and enjoy being part of a group. Examples of comprehensive online support groups are www.teenslivingwithcancer.org/ and www.grouploop.org/default_flash.php.

EWING SARCOMA

Ewing sarcoma is a highly malignant bone tumor. It is rarer than osteosarcoma, accounting for only about 10% of childhood bone tumors (Albano et al., 2005). It occurs most frequently in the pelvis, chest wall, vertebrae, and long bone diaphyses (midshaft). About 25% of children demonstrate metastasis; the lung, bone, and bone marrow are the most common sites (Albano et al., 2005). The prognosis depends on the extent of metastasis. Only about 30% of children with metastasis survive, despite traditional chemotherapy and surgery or augmentation with total body irradiation and HSCT (Miser et al., 2004).

Radiation, chemotherapy, and surgical excision are usually used in combination. Treatment varies depending on the site of the primary tumor and the extent of metastasis at diagnosis. Myeloablative chemotherapy (which destroys the child's marrow) may be used for metastatic disease, followed by a stem cell rescue transplant.

Nursing Assessment

Explore the history for unexplained febrile episodes, which occur in up to 33% of patients with Ewing sarcoma (Widhe & Widhe, 2000). Intermittent periods of pain may also be revealed in the history. Eventually the pain becomes constant and severe, sometimes interrupting sleep.

Note the presence of swelling or erythema at the tumor site. CT scan or MRI of the affected area will reveal the extent of the tumor. Serum LDH levels are usually elevated. CT scan of the chest, bone scan, and bilateral bone marrow aspiration with biopsy determine the extent of metastasis.

Nursing Management

Before treatment begins, discourage active play or weight bearing on the affected extremity to avoid pathologic fracture at the tumor site. Nursing management focuses on addressing the adverse effects of treatment (refer to the nursing process overview section). Teens with Ewing sarcoma need honest and direct answers to questions about their disease. These children will undergo intensive therapy and spend a great deal of time in the hospital. Depending on the age of the child, fantasy play, art or pet therapy, drama, writing, humor, and/or music may help the child to work through the psychological impact of this disease. Refer to Nursing Care Plan 29.1 for additional interventions, which should be individualized depending on the child's and family's response to the disease process and treatment.

RHABDOMYOSARCOMA

Rhabdomyosarcoma is a soft tissue tumor that usually arises from the embryonic mesenchymal cells that would ordinarily form striated muscle. The most common locations for the tumor are the head and neck, genitourinary tract, and extremities (Fig. 29.7). The tumor is highly malignant and spreads via local extension or through the venous or lymphatic system, with the lung being the most

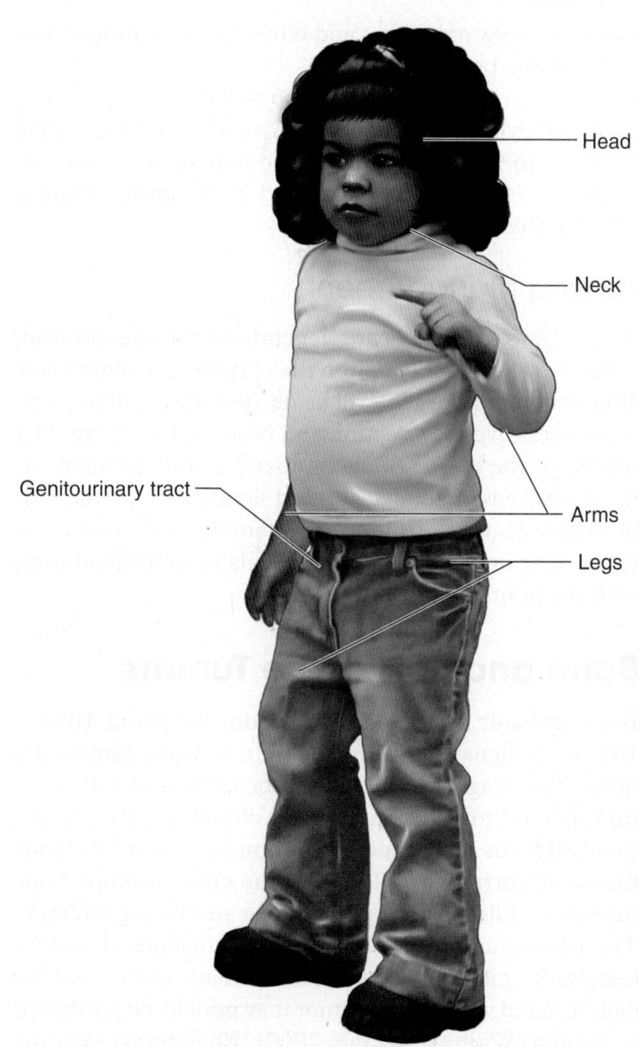

● Figure 29.7 The most common sites of rhabdomyosarcoma.

BOX 29.3

STAGING OF RHABDOMYOSARCOMA

- Stage I: completely resectable localized tumor
- Stage II: after local tumor resection, microscopic residual disease remains
- Stage III: after local tumor resection, gross residual disease remains
- Stage IV: metastasis present at diagnosis

common site for metastasis. Diagnosis is usually made between 2 and 5 years of age, with 70% of all rhabdomyosarcomas diagnosed by age 10 years (Albano et al., 2005). The prognosis is based on the stage of the disease at diagnosis. Box 29.3 explains the staging of rhabdomyosarcoma. Prognosis is generally favorable for stage I disease (Stevens et al., 2005). Children with metastatic disease have about a 40% survival rate (Breneman et al., 2003). Complications of rhabdomyosarcoma include metastasis to lung, bone, or bone marrow and direct extension into the CNS, resulting in brain stem compromise or cranial nerve palsy.

Surgical removal of the primary tumor is generally performed. At the time of the surgery, the lesion is biopsied and the stage of disease determined. Radiation and chemotherapy may be used to shrink the tumor to avoid disability, depending on the site and size of the tumor (especially head, neck, and pelvis).

Nursing Assessment

The child or parent will often discover an asymptomatic mass and seek medical attention at that time. Obtain a health history, noting recent illness, when the mass was discovered, and whether it has changed since first noted. Examine the history for risk factors such as parental smoking, exposure to environmental chemicals, family history of cancer, or neurofibromatosis. Note respiratory effort and cough, and auscultate the lungs for adventitious sounds. Palpate for lymphadenopathy. Palpate the abdomen for a mass or hepatosplenomegaly. Abnormalities found on physical examination depend on the location of the rhabdomyosarcoma (Table 29.7).

Laboratory and diagnostic testing may include:

- CT scan or MRI of primary lesion and the chest for metastasis
- Open biopsy of the primary tumor for definitive diagnosis
- Bone marrow aspiration and biopsy, bone scan, and skeletal survey to determine metastasis

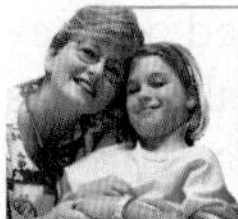

Primary tumors arising in the neck region may compress the child's airway. Assess work of breathing and lung sounds.

Nursing Management

Provide routine postoperative care, depending on the site of surgery. Assess for adverse effects of high-dose radiation, which is generally used to treat the primary tumor as well as metastatic sites. Administer chemotherapy as ordered and assess for adverse effects. Refer to the nursing process overview section and Nursing Care Plan 29.1 to determine an individualized plan of care based on the child's response to the treatment.

Wilms' Tumor

Wilms' tumor is the most common renal tumor in children. About 75% of all cases occur in children less than 5 years old. It usually affects only one kidney, but it is

Table 29.7 Presenting Signs and Symptoms Related to Location of Rhabdomyosarcoma

Location of Tumor	Presenting Signs and Symptoms
Orbit	Proptosis
Middle ear	Drainage, pain, facial nerve palsy
Sinuses	Discharge, pain, sinusitis, facial swelling
Nasopharynx	Pain, epistaxis, dysphagia, nasal quality to speech, airway obstruction
Neck	Dysphagia, hoarseness
Thorax, testicle, extremities	Enlarging mass, painless
Retroperitoneum	Gastrointestinal and urinary tract obstruction, pain, weakness, paresthesia
Bladder, prostate	Hematuria, urinary obstruction
Vagina	Mass, vaginal bleeding or chronic discharge

bilateral in 5% to 10% of cases (Fig. 29.8). The etiology is unknown, but some cases occur via genetic inheritance. Associated anomalies may occur with Wilms' tumor. Wilms' tumor demonstrates rapid growth and is usually large at diagnosis. Metastasis occurs via direct extension or through the bloodstream. Wilms' tumor most commonly metastasizes to the perirenal tissues, liver, diaphragm, lungs, abdominal muscles, and lymph nodes. The prognosis depends on staging at diagnosis and the extent of metastasis (Box 29.4). The overall survival rate is about 90%. Complications include metastasis or complications from radiation therapy such as liver or renal damage, female sterility, bowel obstruction, pneumonia, or scoliosis.

Therapeutic Management

Surgical removal of the tumor and affected kidney (nephrectomy) is the treatment of choice and also allows for accurate staging and assessment of tumor spread. Radiation or chemotherapy may be administered either before or after surgery.

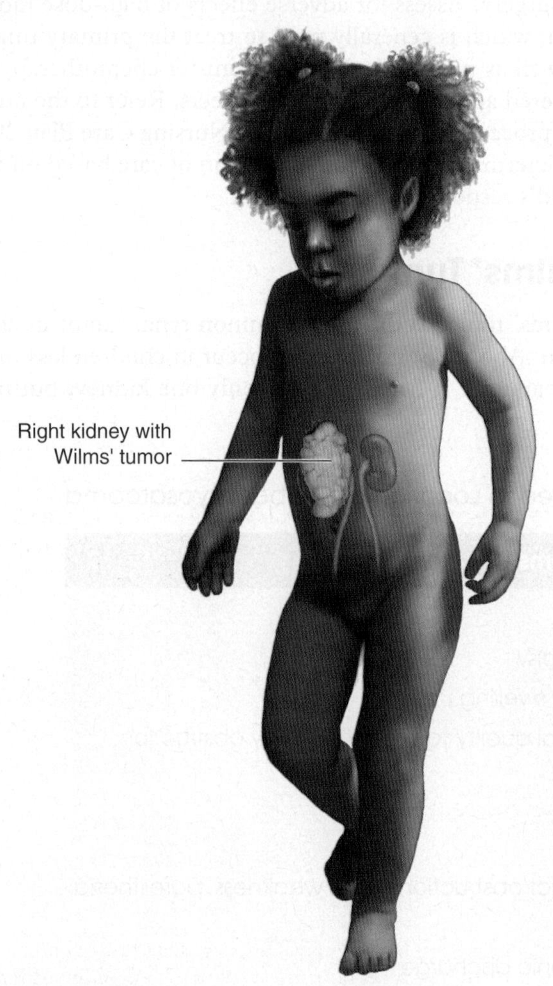

● Figure 29.8 Wilms' tumor is usually unilateral.

BOX 29.4

STAGING OF WILMS' TUMOR

- Stage I: unilateral, limited to kidney, completely resectable
- Stage II: unilateral, tumor extends beyond kidney but is completely resectable
- Stage III: unilateral, tumor has spread outside of kidney, located in abdominal cavity only, not fully removed
- Stage IV: unilateral with metastasis in liver, lung, bone, or brain
- Stage V: bilateral kidney involvement

Nursing Assessment

For a full description of the assessment phase of the nursing process, refer to page 978. Assessment findings pertinent to Wilms' tumor are discussed below.

Health History

Parents typically initially observe the abdominal mass associated with Wilm's tumor and then seek medical attention. Elicit the health history, noting when the mass was discovered. Note abdominal pain, which may be related to rapid tumor growth. Document history of constipation, vomiting, anorexia, weight loss, or difficulty breathing. Determine risk factors such as hemihypertrophy of the spine, Beckwith-Wiedemann syndrome, genitourinary anomalies, absence of the iris, or family history of cancer.

Physical Examination

Measure blood pressure: hypertension occurs in 25% of children with Wilms' tumor (Albano et al., 2005). Inspect the abdomen for asymmetry or a visible mass. Observe for associated anomalies as noted above. Auscultate the lungs for adventitious breath sounds associated with tumor metastasis. Palpate for lymphadenopathy.

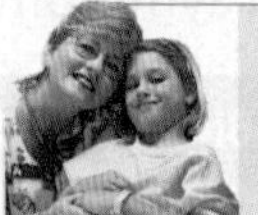

Avoid palpating the abdomen after the initial assessment preoperatively. Wilms' tumor is highly vascular and soft, so excessive handling of the tumor may result in tumor seeding and metastasis.

Laboratory and Diagnostic Testing

Laboratory and diagnostic testing may include:

- Renal or abdominal ultrasound to assess the tumor and the contralateral kidney
- CT scan or MRI of the abdomen and chest to determine local spread to lymph nodes or adjacent organs, as well as any distant metastasis
- Complete blood count, BUN, and creatinine: usually within normal limits
- Urinalysis: may reveal hematuria or leukocytes

- 24-hour urine collection for HVA and VMA to distinguish the tumor from neuroblastoma (levels will not be elevated with Wilms' tumor)

Nursing Management

Postoperative care of the child with Wilms' tumor resection is similar to that of children undergoing other abdominal surgery. Assessment of remaining kidney function is critical. The child may have adverse effects related to chemotherapy or radiation. Refer to the nursing process overview section and Nursing Care Plan 29.1 to individualize care for the child based on the child's response to therapy.

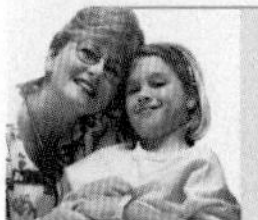

To avoid injuring the remaining kidney, children with a single kidney should not play contact sports.

Retinoblastoma

Retinoblastoma is a congenital, highly malignant tumor that arises from embryonic retinal cells. It accounts for 5% of cases of blindness in children (Albano et al., 2005). Most children are diagnosed by age 3, and the overall survival rate is 90%. When retinoblastoma extends outside of the eye, the mortality rate is very high (DiCiommoa et al., 2000). Retinoblastoma may be hereditary or nonhereditary. Nonhereditary retinoblastoma may be associated with advanced paternal age and always presents with unilateral involvement. Hereditary retinoblastoma is inherited via the autosomal dominant mode. These cases may be unilateral or bilateral. The tumor may grow forward into the vitreous cavity of the eye or extend into the subretinal space, causing retinal detachment. The tumor may extend into the choroid, the sclera, and the optic nerve.

Complications include spread to the brain and the opposite eye, as well as metastasis to lymph nodes, bone, bone marrow, and liver. Second tumors, most often sarcomas, may also occur in children who have been treated for retinoblastoma. Table 29.8 explains the staging of retinoblastoma.

The goals of treatment are to eradicate the tumor, preserve vision, and provide a good cosmetic outcome (Brady, 2003). Retinoblastoma may be treated with radiation, chemotherapy, laser surgery, cryotherapy, or a combination. Moderate vision may be preserved for most children without advanced disease (DiCiommoa et al., 2000). In advanced disease or in the case of a massive tumor with retinal detachment, enucleation (removal of the eye) is necessary (Brady, 2003).

Nursing Assessment

Parents are often the first to notice the "cat's eye reflex" or "whitewash glow" to the child's affected pupil. Obtain the health history, determining when other associated symptoms such as strabismus, orbital inflammation, vomiting, or headache began. Inquire about risk factors such as a family history of retinoblastoma or other cancer or the presence of chromosomal anomalies. Assess pupils for size and reactivity to light. Note presence of leukocoria ("cat's eye reflex," a whitish appearance of the pupil) in the affected eye (Fig. 29.9). Assess the eyes for associated signs, which may include erythema, orbital inflammation, or hyphema.

Table 29.8 Staging of Retinoblastoma

Stage	Description
A	Small tumors (<3 mm; about 0.1 inch) confined to the retina
B	Larger tumors confined to the retina
C	Localized seeding of the vitreous or under the retina <6 mm (0.2 inches) from the original tumor
D	Widespread vitreous or subretinal seeding, may have total retinal detachment
E	No visual potential, eye cannot recover

From American Cancer Society. (2005). How is retinoblastoma staged? Available online at http://www.cancer.org/docroot/CRI/content/CRI_2_4_3X_How_is_retinoblastoma_staged_37.asp?sitearea=.

Diagnostic evaluation includes an ophthalmologic examination under anesthesia. CT, MRI, or ultrasound of the head and eyes will help to visualize the tumor. The infant or toddler may also undergo lumbar puncture and bone marrow aspiration to determine the presence and extent of metastasis.

Nursing Management

Provide routine postoperative care to the infant or toddler. If the eye is enucleated, observe the large pressure dressing on the eye socket for bleeding. Dressing changes to the socket may include sterile saline rinses and/or antibiotic ointment application. If disease occurs outside of the eye or if metastasis is present, inform the parents that

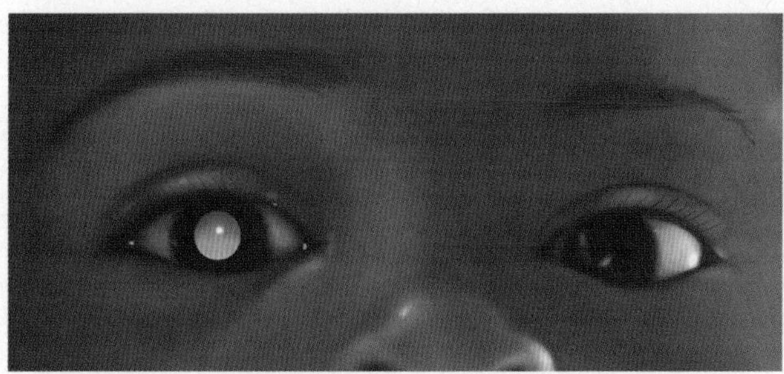

● Figure 29.9 Note the whitish appearance of this child's pupil (leukocoria). (Photo courtesy of The Childhood Eye Cancer Trust of the United Kingdom.)

chemotherapy will be necessary. Monitor for side effects of chemotherapy (see the nursing process overview section). Follow-up will include eye examinations every 3 to 6 months until age 6 and then annually to check for further tumor development (Brady, 2003). If the eye is enucleated, several weeks after removal, a prosthetic eye will be fitted. Teach families use of the prosthetic eye; it does not require daily removal.

Provide parents with support and encouragement. Refer the family for genetic counseling. Subsequent children will need ophthalmologic examination under anesthesia at 2 months of age and frequent examinations until age 3 years. Children treated for retinoblastoma will also need genetic counseling as they reach puberty, as about half of the offspring of children with retinoblastoma have bilateral disease.

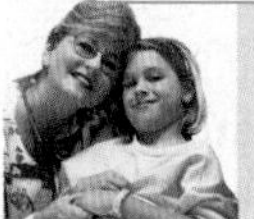

Educate parents about protecting vision in the remaining eye: routine eye checkups, protection from accidental injury, use of safety goggles during sports, and prompt treatment of eye infections. Generally, children with one eye should not participate in contact sports.

Screening for Reproductive Cancers in Adolescents

Increasingly, reproductive cancers are being diagnosed in adolescents. Cervical cancer and testicular cancer may be discovered early with appropriate screening, and earlier discovery leads to better outcomes. Starting screening in the teenage years may also instill a life-long healthy habit in the adolescent.

CERVICAL CANCER

Risk factors for cervical cancer include young age at first intercourse, infection with a sexually transmitted disease, and a history of multiple sex partners, and more and more teenagers are presenting with these risk factors. Counsel all sexually active adolescents to seek reproductive care, which is available without parental consent in most states. The screening Papanicolaou (Pap) smear is efficient and reliable at determining abnormal cervical cells and is a key part of screening for cervical cancer (if cancer is present, the parent will have to be notified). Cervical cancer has a very high response to therapy and rate of cure if treated in its early stages, so nurses should encourage teenage girls to be responsible for their sexual health by seeking appropriate examination and screening.

HEALTHY PEOPLE 2010

Objective	Significance
Increase the proportion of women who receive a Pap test.	• When an adolescent girl makes the decision to become sexually active, counsel her about the importance of getting annual Pap smears.

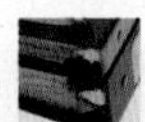

TEACHING GUIDELINE 29.3

Testicular Self-Examination

- Perform the examination once a month, after a shower.
- Be familiar with the size and weight of your testicles.
- Roll the testicle between your fingers. The small ropelike structure is the epididymis; this is normal.
- Report any lump, swelling, or heaviness of one testicle to your health care provider.

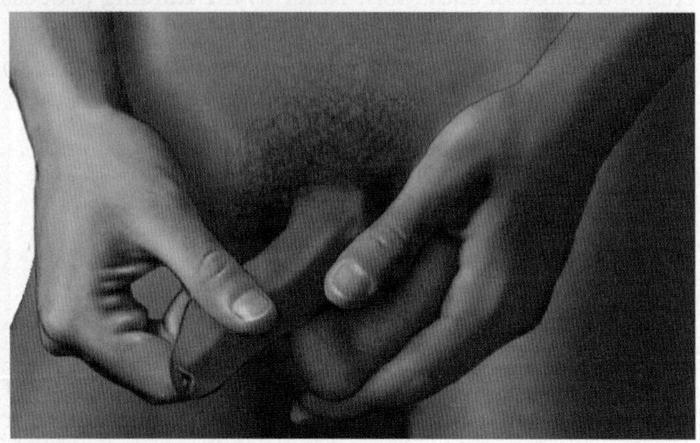

TESTICULAR CANCER

Although uncommon in teens, testicular cancer is the most frequently diagnosed cancer in males age 15 to 35. It is one of the most curable cancers if diagnosed early. To get into the habit of screening for testicular lumps, adolescent boys should begin performing testicular self-examinations monthly (Teaching Guideline 29.3).

References

Books and Journals

Ackley, B. J., & Ladwig, G. B. (2006). *Nursing diagnosis handbook: A guide to planning care* (7th ed.). St. Louis: Mosby.

Albano, E. A., Bassal, M., Porter, C. C., Greffe, B. S., Foreman, N. K., & Stork, L. C. (2005). Neoplastic disease. In W. W. Hay, M. J. Levin, J. M. Sondheimer, & R. R. Deterding (Eds.), *Current pediatric diagnosis & treatment* (17th ed.). New York: McGraw-Hill.

Alcoser, P. W., & Rodgers, C. (2003). Treatment strategies in childhood cancer. *Journal of Pediatric Nursing, 18*(2), 103–112.

American Academy of Pediatrics, Committee on Bioethics. (1995). Informed consent, parental permission, and assent in pediatric practice. *Pediatrics, 95*(2), 314–317.

American Cancer Society. (2005). How is retinoblastoma staged? Available online at http://www.cancer.org/docroot/CRI/content/CRI_2_4_3X_How_is_retinoblastoma_staged_37.asp?sitearea=.

Baggott, C. R., Kelly, K. P., Fochtman, D., & Foley, G. V. (2002). *Nursing care of children and adolescents with cancer* (3rd ed.). Philadelphia: W. B. Saunders.

Ballard, K. (2004). Meeting the needs of siblings of children with cancer. *Pediatric Nursing, 30*(5), 394–401.

Bottomley, S. J., & Kassner, E. (2003). Late effects of childhood cancer therapy. *Journal of Pediatric Nursing, 18*(2), 126–133.

Bowden, V. R., Byock, I., Conway-Orgel, M., Cormier, A. B., Dulzack, S., Frader, J., et al. (2003). Precepts of palliative care for children, adolescents, and their families. Available at www.lastacts.org.

Brady, G. (2003). Retinoblastoma: Care and support of the pediatric patient and family. *Insight, Journal of the American Society of Ophthalmic Registered Nurses, 28*(3), 67–69.

Breneman, J. C., Lyden, E., Pappo, A. S., Link, M. P., Anderson, J. R., Parham, D. M., et al. (2003). Prognostic factors and clinical outcomes in children and adolescents with metastatic rhabdomyosarcoma: A report from the Intergroup Rhabdomyosarcoma Study IV. *Journal of Clinical Oncology, 21*, 78–84.

Bryant, R. (2003). Managing side effects of childhood cancer. *Journal of Pediatric Nursing, 18*(2), 113–125.

Cantril, C. A., & Haylock, P. J. (2004). Tumor lysis syndrome. *American Journal of Nursing, 104*(4), 49–52.

Cavusoglu, H. Depression in children with cancer. (2001). *Journal of Pediatric Nursing, 16*(5), 380–385.

Cheng, K. K. F., & Chang, A. M. (2003). Palliation of oral mucositis symptoms in pediatric patients treated with cancer chemotherapy. *Cancer Nursing, 26*(6), 476–484.

Clerici, C. A., Ferrari, A., Massimino, M., Terenziani, M., Casanova, M., Luksch, R., et al. (2004). Five questions for assessing psychological problems in pediatric patients cured of neoplastic disease. *Pediatric Hematology and Oncology, 21*, 481–487.

Colby-Graham, M. F., & Chordas, C. (2003). The childhood leukemias. *Journal of Pediatric Nursing, 18*(2), 87–95.

Cordier, S., Monfort, C., Filippini, G., Preston-Martin, S., Lubin, F., Mueller, B. A., et al. (2004). Parental exposure to polycyclic aromatic hydrocarbons and the risk of childhood brain tumors. *American Journal of Epidemiology, 159*(12), 1109–1116.

DiCiommoa, D., Gallie, B. L., & Bremner, R. (2000). Retinoblastoma: the disease, gene and protein provide critical leads to understand cancer. [Electronic version] Available at http://www.retinoblastoma.ca/docs/retino.pdf.

Eiser, C. (2004). *Children with cancer: The quality of life.* Mahwah, NJ: Lawrence Erlbaum Associates.

Feudtner, C. (2004). Perspective on quality at the end of life. *Archives of Pediatric and Adolescent Medicine, 158*, 415–418.

Florin, T. A., & Hinkle, A. S. (2005). A guide to caring for cancer survivors. *Contemporary Pediatrics, 22*(8), 31–48.

Gardiner, P., & Kemper, K. J. (2005). For GI complaints, which herbs and supplements spell relief? *Contemporary Pediatrics, 22*(8), 50–55.

Graham, D. K., Giller, R. H., & Quinones, R. R. (2005). Hematopoietic stem cell transplantation. In W. W. Hay, M. J. Levin, J. M. Sondheimer, & R. R. Deterding (Eds.), *Current pediatric diagnosis & treatment* (17th ed.). New York: McGraw-Hill.

Grealish, L., Lomasney, A., & Whiteman, B. (2000). Foot massage: A nursing intervention to modify the distressing symptoms of pain and nausea in patients hospitalized with cancer. *Cancer Nursing, 23*(3), 237–243.

Haut, C. (2005). Oncological emergencies in the pediatric intensive care unit. *AACN Clinical Issues, 16*(2), 232–245.

Heiferty, C. M. (2004). Spiritual development and the dying child: The pediatric nurse practitioner's role. *Journal of Pediatric Health Care, 18*, 271–275.

Hendershot, E. (2005). Treatment approaches for metastatic Ewing's sarcoma: A review of the literature. *Journal of Pediatric Oncology Nursing, 22*(6), 339–352.

Hilden, J. M., Watterson, J., & Chrastek, J. (2003). Tell the children. *Classic Papers, supplement to Journal of Clinical Oncology, 21*, 9, 37s–39s.

Hokkanen, H., Eriksson, E., Ahonen, O., & Salantera, S. (2004). Adolescents with cancer: Experience of life and how it could be made easier. *Cancer Nursing, 27*(4), 325–335.

Hooke, C., Hellsten, M. B., Stutzer, C., & Forte, K. (2001). Pain management for the child with cancer in end of life care: APON position paper. Available at www.apon.org.

Houlahan, K. E., Branowicki, P. A., Mack, J. W., Dinning, C., & McCabe, M. (2006). Can end-of-life care for the pediatric patient suffering with escalating and intractable symptoms be improved? *Journal of Pediatric Oncology Nursing, 23*, 45–51.

Hugger, L. (2005). The psychological treatment of children recovering from leukemia. *Journal of Infant, Child, and Adolescent Psychotherapy, 4*(4), 408–423.

Hurwitz, C. A., Duncan, J., & Wolfe, J. (2004). Caring for the child with cancer at the close of life: "There are people who make it, and I'm hoping I'm one of them." *Journal of the American Medical Association, 292*(17), 2141–2149.

Jones, S. E., & Saraiya, M. (2006). Sunscreen use among U.S. high school students, 1999–2003. *Journal of School Health, 76*(4), 150–153.

Kingston, J. (2005). Thyroid cancer after neck irradiation during childhood. *Lancet, 365*, 1987–1988.

Kline, N. E., & Sevier, N. (2003). Solid tumors in children. *Journal of Pediatric Nursing, 18*(2), 96–102.

Koontz, B. F. (2006). Palliative radiation therapy for metastatic Ewing sarcoma. *Cancer, 106*(8), 1790–1793.

Kreitler, S., & Arush, M. W. B. (eds.). (2004). *Psychosocial aspects of pediatric oncology.* West Sussex, England: John Wiley and Sons.

Kurishima, A., Chang, W. T., Shimda, S., Lopes, A., & de Carmargo, B. (2002). The use of acupuncture to control side effects and pain during treatment for childhood cancer. *Journal of Pediatric Oncology Nursing, 19*(2), 49–50.

Kushner, B. H., & Cheung, N. V. (2005). Neuroblastoma: From genetic profiles to clinical challenge. *New England Journal of Medicine, 353*(21), 2215–2217.

Kutluk, M. T., Yalcin, B., Akyuz, C., Varan, A., Ruacan, S., & Buyukpamukcu, M. (2004). Treatment results and prognostic factors in Ewing sarcoma. *Pediatric Hematology and Oncology, 21*, 597–610.

Lievkovsky, Y. E., Donaldson, S. S., Torres, M. A., Wong, R. M., Amylon, M. D., Link, M. P., & Agarwal, R. (2004). High-dose therapy and autologous hematopoietic stem-cell transplantation for recurrent or refractory pediatric Hodgkin's disease: Results and prognostic indices. *Journal of Clinical Oncology, 22*(22), 4532–4540.

Lofthouse, C. M., Akobeng, A. K., Adamski, J., & Brennan, B. (2003). A 2-year-old boy with diarrhoea and failure to thrive. *Lancet, 361*, 1012.

Lund, A. E. (2005). Cancer therapies in childhood can damage developing teeth. *Journal of the American Dental Association, 10*, 1370.

Mabbott, D. J., Speigler, B. J., Greenberg, M. L., Rutka, J. T., Hyder, D. J., & Bouffet, E. (2005). Serial evaluation of academic and behavioral outcome after treatment with cranial radiation in childhood. *Journal of Clinical Oncology, 23*(10), 2256–2263.

MacDonald, D. J., & Lessick, M. (2000). Hereditary cancers in children and ethical and psychosocial implications. *Journal of Pediatric Nursing, 15*(4), 217–225.

Marcoux, K. K. (2005). Management of increased intracranial pressure in the critically ill child with acute neurological injury. *AACN Clinical Issues, 16*(2), 212–231.

Marinsek, Z. P. (2006). Ewing sarcoma/PNET: 27 years of experience in Slovenia. *Pediatric Hematology and Oncology, 23*(4), 355–367.

McCaffrey, C. N. (2006). Major stressors and their effect on the well-being of children with cancer. *Journal of Pediatric Nursing, 21*(1), 59–66.

McCubbin, M., Balling, K., Possin, P., Frierdich, S., & Bryne, B. (2002). Family resiliency in childhood cancer. *Family Relations, 51*(2), 103–111.

Melamud, A., Palekar, R., & Singh, A. (2006). Retinoblastoma. *American Family Physician, 73*(6), 1039–1044.

Metzler, L. J., & Rourke, M. T. (2005). Oncology summer camp: Benefits of social comparison. *Children's Health Care, 34*(4), 305–314.

Miser, J. S., Krailo, M. D., Tarbell, N. J., Link, M. P., Fryer, J. H., Pritchard, D. J., et al. (2004). Treatment of metastatic Ewing's sarcoma or primitive neuroectodermal tumor of bone: Evaluation of combination ifosfamide and etoposide: A Children's Cancer Group and Pediatric Oncology study. *Journal of Clinical Oncology, 22*(14), 2873–2876.

Mosher, R. B. (2006). This is the best life yet: Life at Camp Friendship. *Pediatric Nursing, 32*(1), 84–87.

Murray, J. S. (2000). A concept analysis of social support as experienced by siblings of children with cancer. *Journal of Pediatric Nursing, 15*(5), 313–322.

Nelson, M. B., & Meeske, K. (2005). Recognizing health risks in childhood cancer survivors. *Journal of the American Academy of Nurse Practitioners, 17*(3), 96–103.

Pagana, K. D., & Pagana, T. J. (2006). *Mosby's manual of diagnostic and laboratory tests* (3rd ed.). St. Louis: Mosby.

Paulino, A. C., & Fowler, B. Z. (2005). Secondary neoplasms after radiation for a childhood solid tumor. *Pediatric Hematology and Oncology, 22,* 89–101.

Postovsky, S., Levenzon, A., Ofir, R., & Arush, M. W. B. (2004). "Do not resuscitate" orders among children with solid tumors at the end of life. *Pediatric Hematology and Oncology, 21,* 661–668.

Ritchie, M. A. (2001). Self-esteem and hopefulness in adolescents with cancer. *Journal of Pediatric Nursing, 16*(1), 35–42.

Roye, C. F., Stanis, P., & Nelson, J. (2003). Evidence of the need for cervical cancer screening in adolescents. *Pediatric Nursing, 29*(3), 224–232.

Ruble, K. (2005). Pediatric oncology. In S. M. Nettina (Ed.), *Lippincott manual of nursing practice.* Philadelphia: Lippincott Williams & Wilkins.

Rushton, C. H. (2000). Pediatric palliative care: Coming of age. *Innovations in End-of-Life Care, 2*(2). Available at www2.edc.org/lastacts/archives/archivesMarch00/editorial.asp

Spector, L. G., Klebanoff, M. A., & Feusner, J. H. (2005). Childhood cancer following neonatal oxygen supplementation. *Journal of Pediatrics, 147,* 27–31.

Speigler, B. J., Bouffet, E., Greenberg, M. L., Rutka, J. T., & Mabbott, D. J. (2004). Change in neurocognitive functioning after treatment with cranial radiation in childhood. *Journal of Clinical Oncology, 22*(4), 706–713.

Susman, E. (2005). Cancer pain management guidelines issues for children; adult guidelines updated. *Journal of the National Cancer Institute, 97*(10), 711–719.

Stevens, M. C. G., Rey, A., Bouvet, N., Ellershaw, C., Flamant, F., Habrand, J. L., et al. (2005). Treatment of nonmetastatic rhabdomyosarcoma in childhood and adolescence: Third study of the International Society of Pediatric Oncology. *Journal of Clinical Oncology, 23*(12), 2618–2628.

Stringer, J. R., Beard, C. B., Miller, R. F., & Wakefield, A. E. (2002). A new name (*Pneumocystis jiroveci*) for pneumocystis from humans. *Emerging Infectious Disease, 8.* [electronic version] http://www.cdc.gov/ncidod/EID/vol8no9/02-0096.htm.

Taha, D. R., Bastian, W., & Castells, S. (2001). Growth hormone replacement therapy in children with leukemia in remission. *Clinical Pediatrics, 40,* 441–445.

Taketokmo, C. K., Hodding, J. H., & Kraus, D. M. (2004). *Lexi-comp's pediatric dosage handbook* (11th ed.). Hudson, OH: Lexi-comp.

Tomlinson, D., & Kline, N. E. (eds.) (2005). *Pediatric oncology nursing.* New York: Springer.

Trigg, M. E. (2004). Hematopoietic stem cells. *Pediatrics, 113*(4), 1051–1057.

Turkoski, B. B. (2005). When a child's treatment decisions conflict with the parents. *Home Healthcare Nurse, 23*(2), 123–126.

Ulster, A. A., & Antle, B. J. (2005). In the darkness there can be light: A family's adaptation to a child's blindness. *Journal of Visual Impairment & Blindness, 99*(4), 209–218.

U.S. Cancer Statistics Working Group. (2004). *United States cancer statistics: 2001 incidence and mortality.* Atlanta: Department of Health and Human Services, Centers for Disease Control and Prevention and National Cancer Institute [electronic version]. Available at http://www.cdc.gov/cancer/npcr/uscs/pdf/USCS.pdf.

Van Cleve, L., Bossert, W., Beecroft, P., Adlard, K., Alvarez, O., & Savedra, M. C. (2004). The pain experience of children with leukemia during the first year after diagnosis. *Nursing Research, 53*(1), 1–10.

Van Larebeke, N. A., Birnbaum, L. S., Boogaerts, M. A., Bracke, M., Davis, D. L., Demarini, D. M., et al. (2005). Unrecognized or potential risk factors for childhood cancer. *International Journal of Occupational and Environmental Health, 11*(2), 199–201.

White, N. C. (2003). Education-related problems for children with cancer. *Journal of Pediatric Oncology Nursing, 20*(2), 50–55.

Widhe, B., & Widhe, T. (2000). Initial symptoms and clinical features of osteosarcoma and Ewing sarcoma. *Journal of Bone and Joint Surgery, 82*(5), 667–674.

Wohlschlaeger, A. (2004). Prevention and treatment of mucositis: A guide for nurses. *Journal of Pediatric Oncology Nursing, 21*(5), 281–287.

Woodgate, R. L. (2005). Adolescents' experiences with cancer. *Cancer Nursing, 28*(1), 8–15.

Woolery, M., Carroll, E., Fenn, E., Weiland, H., Jarosinski, P., Corey, B., & Wallen, E. R. (2006). A constipation assessment scale for use in pediatric oncology. *Journal of Pediatric Oncology Nursing, 23*(2), 65–73.

Websites

kidshealth.org/teen/sexual_health/guys/tse.html information for teen boys on testicular self-examination

home.ccr.cancer.gov/oncology/pediatric Pediatric Oncology Branch of the National Cancer Institute; clinical protocol childhood cancer treatment on the NIH campus in Bethesda, MD

www.acor.org/ped-onc Pediatric Oncology Resource Center

www.allianceforchildhoodcancer.org Alliance for Childhood Cancer, a forum of national patient advocacy groups interested in advancing research, public education, survivorship of children and teens with cancer

www.apon.org Association of Pediatric Oncology Nursing

www.aspho.org American Society of Pediatric Hematology and Oncology

www.bearnecessities.org Bear Necessities Pediatric Cancer Foundation (patient and family services, research and support)

www.campdream.org Camp Mak-a-Dream, a cost-free camp in Montana for children with cancer

www.cancer.gov National Cancer Institute of the U.S. National Institutes of Health

www.cancer.org American Cancer Society (research, education, referrals, help finding a pediatric cancer center)

www.candlelighters.org Candlelighters Childhood Cancer Foundation (support and education for children with cancer and their families)

www.cbtf.org Children's Brain Tumor Foundation (education, research, and parent-to-parent network for family support)

www.chect.org.uk/index.php Childhood Eye Cancer Trust (United Kingdom), charity for those with retinoblastoma

www.childhoodbraintumor.org Childhood Brain Tumor Foundation (public awareness, research, improvement of quality of life)

www.childrenscause.org/about/donate.shtml Children's Cause for Cancer Advocacy (resources for research and treatment, addresses needs and concerns of survivors)

www.childrensoncologygroup.org the Children's Oncology Group (cancer treatment clinical trials)

www.chionline.org Children's Hospice International (hospice and palliative care support for children through pediatric care facilities, hospice and home care programs)

www.cureourchildren.org Ewing sarcoma and pediatric cancer support group resources page from the "Cure Our Children" Foundation (extensive resources and links)

www.curesearch.org combined effort of the National Childhood Cancer Foundation and the Children's Oncology Group for prevention and treatment of childhood cancers

www.florida-FEAR.org Florida's Enhanced Awareness of Retinoblastoma

www.grouploop.org/default_flash.php The Wellness Community (national cancer support, education and hope for teens)

www.healthypeople.gov *Healthy People 2010*

www.hopestreetkids.org education, support, and advocacy for children with cancer and their families

www.leukemia.org Leukemia and Lymphoma Society (research, education and patient services)

www.leukemia-research.org Leukemia Research Foundation

www.locksoflove.org Locks of Love (provides hairpieces to financially disadvantaged children)

www.marrow.org National Marrow Donor Program (information and resources for donors, patients, and physicians about bone marrow and stem cell transplantation)

www.msc-worldwide.com Penguin cold cap therapy
www.mskcc.org/mskcc/html/2718.cfm Memorial Sloan Kettering Cancer Center (information on diseases, treatment, and resources)
www.nationalchildrenscancersociety.com National Children's Cancer Society (financial and in-kind assistance, advocacy, support services and education)
www.oncolink.org cancer resource sponsored by Abramson Cancer Center of the University of Pennsylvania
www.ontumor.com Cancer Information Network
www.pbtc.org Pediatric Brain Tumor Consortium (multidisciplinary cooperative research organization focusing on central nervous system tumors of childhood)
www.retinoblastoma.ca Canadian resources for retinoblastoma
www.retinoblastoma.net Retinoblastoma International (education, research, resources, focusing on early diagnosis and treatment)
www.starbright.org Starlight, Starbright Children's Foundation (dedicated to brightening the lives of seriously ill children and their families)
www.stjude.org Saint Jude Children's Research Hospital
www.tbts.org Brain Tumor Society (education, research, support, family networking)
www.teenslivingwithcancer.org Melissa's Living Legacy Foundation/Helping Teens Live with Cancer
www.wish.org Make-A-Wish Foundation (granting wishes of children with life-threatening illnesses)

Chapter WORKSHEET

● MULTIPLE CHOICE QUESTIONS

1. A 5-year-old has been diagnosed with Wilms' tumor. What is the priority nursing intervention for this child?
   a. Educate the parents about dialysis, as the kidney will be removed.
   b. Measure abdominal girth every shift.
   c. Avoid palpating the child's abdomen.
   d. Monitor BUN and creatinine every 4 hours.

2. A child with leukemia has the following a.m. laboratory results: Hgb 8.0, Hct 24.2, WBC 8,000, platelets 150,000. What is the priority nursing assessment?
   a. Monitor for fever.
   b. Assess for bruising or bleeding.
   c. Determine intake and output.
   d. Assess for pallor, fatigue, tachycardia.

3. A child with leukemia received chemotherapy about 10 days ago. She presents today with a temperature of 100.4 degrees F, an absolute neutrophil count of 500, and mild bleeding of the gums. What is the priority nursing intervention?
   a. Administer IV antibiotics as ordered.
   b. Provide vigorous oral care frequently with a firm toothbrush.
   c. Monitor pulse and blood pressure for changes.
   d. Administer packed red blood cell transfusion.

4. A child with cancer is receiving chemotherapy, and his mother is concerned that the nausea and vomiting associated with chemotherapy are reducing his ability to eat and gain weight appropriately. What is the most appropriate nursing action?
   a. Administer an antiemetic at the first hint of nausea.
   b. Offer the child's favorite foods to encourage him to eat.
   c. Start antiemetic drugs prior to the chemotherapy infusion.
   d. Maintain IV fluid infusion to avoid dehydration.

● CRITICAL THINKING EXERCISES

1. Develop a discharge teaching plan for a child who has just completed the induction phase of chemotherapy for acute lymphocytic leukemia.
2. A 17-year-old girl has recently been diagnosed with osteosarcoma. She is worried about how treatment will affect her plans for college, marriage, and children. How will you respond to her concerns?
3. A 3-year-old is going to be starting chemotherapy for rhabdomyosarcoma. Develop an age-appropriate teaching plan for this child.
4. Develop a nursing care plan for an adolescent with cancer who is undergoing radiation and chemotherapy and experiencing a significant number of adverse effects from his treatment.

● STUDY ACTIVITIES

1. While in the clinical area, care for a young child who has undergone therapy for a brain tumor. Compare this child's growth and development to those of a healthy similar-age child who you know or have cared for.
2. During your clinical rotation, care for a child who has received several chemotherapy treatments. After establishing a therapeutic relationship, talk with the child about his or her understanding of the disease and the experience the child has had with diagnosis and treatment thus far. If time allows, ask the child to draw a picture describing this experience. Record your observations in your clinical journal and reflect on the emotions you feel about this experience.
3. Attend the pediatric oncology clinic. Determine the role of the advanced practice nurse (nurse practitioner or clinical nurse specialist), compared to the role of the registered nurse in the outpatient care of children with cancer. Determine which activities the nurse appropriately delegates to unlicensed assistive personnel in that setting.
4. Talk to the hospital chaplain about his or her experiences with dying children. Reflect on this conversation in your clinical journal.

chapter 30

Nursing Care of the Child With a Genetic Disorder

Key TERMS

allele
chromosome
consanguinity
gene
genetics
genome
genotype
heterozygous
homozygous
karyotype
nondisjunction
phenotype

Learning OBJECTIVES

Upon completion of the chapter, the learner will be able to:

1. Discuss various inheritance patterns, including nontraditional patterns of inheritance.
2. Discuss ethical and legal issues associated with genetic testing.
3. Discuss genetic counseling and the role of the nurse.
4. Identify nursing interventions related to common laboratory and diagnostic tests used in the diagnosis and management of genetic conditions.
5. Distinguish various genetic disorders occurring in childhood.
6. Devise an individualized nursing care plan for the child with a genetic disorder.
7. Develop patient/family teaching plans for the child with a genetic disorder.

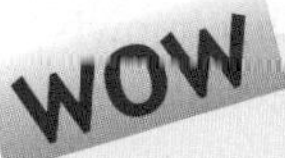

Nursing includes care for the helpless and brave child victim of heredity.

Julie Woods, a 5-year-old, is brought to the clinic for her annual examination. Her mother states, "She's so much smaller than all of the other kindergartners."

Genetics is the study of heredity and its variation (Venes, 2005). Many disorders of childhood have a genetic or inherited cause. Common disorders suspected to be caused or influenced by genetic factors include birth defects, chromosomal abnormalities, neurocutaneous disorders, mental retardation, many types of short stature, connective tissue disorders, and inborn errors of metabolism. According to the Centers for Disease Control and Prevention, birth defects and genetic disorders are a significant cause of morbidity and mortality in infancy and childhood: "Twenty-five to thirty-nine percent of admissions to children's hospitals involve children with genetically determined or partially genetically determined disorders; 11% of all deaths in childhood are related to an underlying genetic condition" (Behrman et al., 2004, p. 367).

Our ability to diagnose genetic conditions is far superior to our ability to cure or treat them. However, accurate diagnosis leads to improved treatment and outcomes. Nurses should have a basic knowledge of genetics, common genetic disorders in children, genetic testing, and genetic counseling so that they can provide support and information to families and can promote an improved quality of life.

Inheritance

A **gene** is the basic unit of heredity. Genes occupy a specific location on a **chromosome** (a long, continuous strand of DNA that carries genetic information) and determine the organism's physical and mental characteristics. In humans each somatic cell (a cell forming the body of an organism) has 46 chromosomes: 22 pairs of non-sex chromosomes (autosomes) and 1 pair of sex chromosomes. The **genotype** is the specific genetic makeup of an individual; it is the internally coded inheritable information and refers to the particular **allele** (one of two or more alternative versions of gene at a given position on a chromosome that imparts the same characteristic of that gene). For example, each human has a gene that controls height, but there are variations of these genes (alleles) that can produce a height of 5 feet or one of 6 feet, 2 inches. A gene that controls eye color may have an allele that can produce blue eyes or an allele that produces brown eyes. The genotype, together with environmental variation that influences the individual, determines the **phenotype** (the outward characteristics of the individual).

A human inherits two genes, one from each parent; therefore one allele comes from the mother and one from the father. These alleles may be the same for the characteristic (**homozygous**) or different (**heterozygous**). If the two alleles differ, the dominant one will usually be expressed in the individual's phenotype.

The Human Genome

The **genome** of an organism is its entire hereditary information encoded in the DNA. The Human Genome Project (HGP), an international effort to produce a comprehensive sequence of the human genome, was coordinated by the U.S. Department of Energy and the National Institutes of Health. It began in October 1990 and was completed in May 2003. Its goals included:

- Identify all of the approximately 20,000 to 25,000 genes in human DNA.
- Determine the sequences of the 3 billion chemical base pairs that make up human DNA.
- Store this information in databases to make it accessible for further study.
- Improve tools for data analysis.
- Transfer related technologies to the private sector.
- Address the ethical, legal, and social implications of this discovery.

The HGP has led to the discovery of the genetic basis for hundreds of disorders and has advanced our understanding of basic genetic processes at the molecular level. More information is available at http://www.ornl.gov/sci/techresources/Human_Genome/home.shtml.

One goal of the HGP was to translate the findings into new and more effective strategies for the prevention, diagnosis, and treatment of genetic disorders. Current and potential applications for the HGP to health care include rapid and more specific diagnosis of disease, with hundreds of genetic tests available in research or clinical practice; earlier detection of genetic predisposition to disease; less emphasis on treating the symptoms of a disease and more emphasis on seeking the fundamental causes of the disease; new classes of drugs; avoiding environmental conditions that may trigger disease; and repair or replacement of defective genes using gene therapy. This knowledge, along with the commercialization of the technology, will change our approach to genetic disorders.

Although these advances have many current and potential benefits to children, they also raise serious ethical, legal, and social issues. The HGP recognized this and developed a branch, called Ethical, Legal, and Social Issues, that was responsible for addressing and overseeing these issues while determining how to use this information in the safest, most beneficial manner. Some of these issues include privacy and confidentiality of genetic information; who should have access to personal genetic information;

psychological impact and stigmatization due to individual genetic differences; use of genetic information in reproductive decision making and reproductive rights; and whether testing should be performed if no cure is available. More information on these issues is available at http://www.ornl.gov/sci/techresources/Human_Genome/research/elsi.shtml.

Patterns of Inheritance

Diagnosis of a genetic disorder is usually based on clinical signs and symptoms or on laboratory confirmation of an altered gene associated with the disorder. Accurate diagnosis can be aided by identifying the pattern of inheritance within a family. Also, nurses must understand the pattern of inheritance so they can teach and counsel families about the risks of future pregnancies. Some genetic disorders occur in multiple family members; others may occur in only a single family member. A genetic disorder is caused by completely or partially altered genetic material; in contrast, a familial disorder is more common in relatives of the affected individual but may be caused by environmental influences, not genetic alterations.

Mendelian or Monogenic Disorders

A genetic disorder is a disease caused by an abnormality in an individual's genetic material or genome. Patterns of inheritance dictate how this abnormality can be passed onto offspring. Principles of inheritance of single-gene disorders are the same that govern the inheritance of other traits, such as eye and hair color. These are known as Mendel's laws of inheritance, named for Gregor Mendel, an Austrian naturalist who conducted genetic research. These patterns occur because a single gene is defective and are referred to as monogenic or sometimes mendelian disorders. They include autosomal dominant, autosomal recessive, X-linked dominant, and X-linked recessive patterns.

Autosomal Dominant Inheritance

Autosomal dominant inheritance occurs when a single gene in the heterozygous state is capable of producing the phenotype. In other words, the abnormal or mutant gene overshadows the normal gene and the individual will demonstrate signs and symptoms of the disorder. The affected person generally has an affected parent, and an affected person has a 50% chance of passing the abnormal gene to each of his or her children (Fig. 30.1). Affected individuals are present in every generation. Males and family members who are phenotypically normal (do not show signs or symptoms of the disorder) do not transmit the condition to their offspring. Females and males are equally affected and a male can pass the disorder on to his son. This male-to-male transmission is important in distinguishing autosomal dominant inheritance from X-linked inheritance. There are varying degrees of presentation among individuals in a family: a parent with a mild form could have a child with a more severe form. Common types of genetic disorders that follow the autosomal dominant pattern of inheritance include neurofibromatosis, Huntington disease, achondroplasia, and polycystic kidney disease.

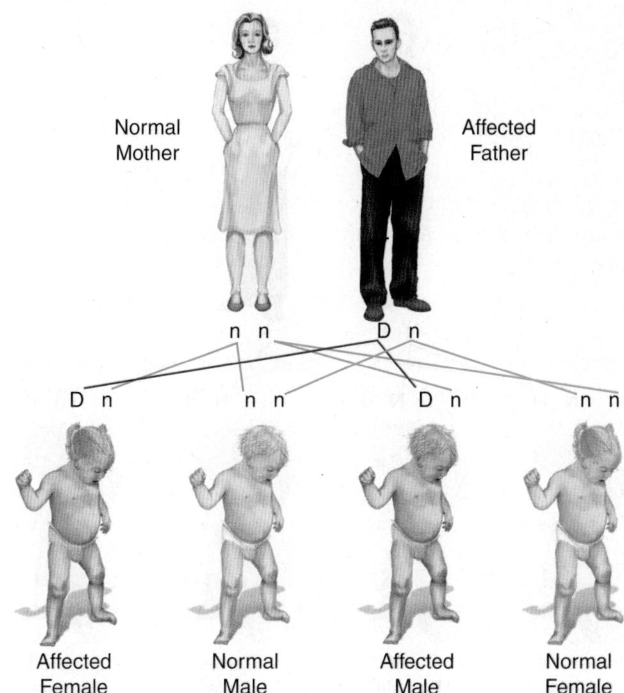

● Figure 30.1 Autosomal dominant inheritance pattern.

Autosomal Recessive Inheritance

Autosomal recessive inheritance occurs when two copies of the mutant or abnormal gene in the homozygous state are necessary to produce the phenotype. In other words, two abnormal genes are needed for the individual to demonstrate signs and symptoms of the disorder. These disorders are generally less common than autosomal dominant disorders (Behrman et al., 2004). Both parents of the affected person must be heterozygous carriers of the gene (clinically normal but carry the gene) and their offspring have a 25% chance of being homozygous (a 50% chance of getting the mutant gene from each parent and therefore a 25% chance of inheriting two mutant genes). If the child is clinically normal, there is a 50% chance the child is a carrier (Fig. 30.2). Affected individuals are usually present in only one generation of the family. Females and males are equally affected, and a male can pass the disorder on to his son. The chance that any two parents will both be carriers of the mutant gene is increased if the couple have **consanguinity** (relationship by blood or common ancestry). Common types of genetic disorders that follow the autosomal recessive inheritance pattern include cystic fibrosis, phenylketonuria, Tay-Sachs, and sickle cell disease.

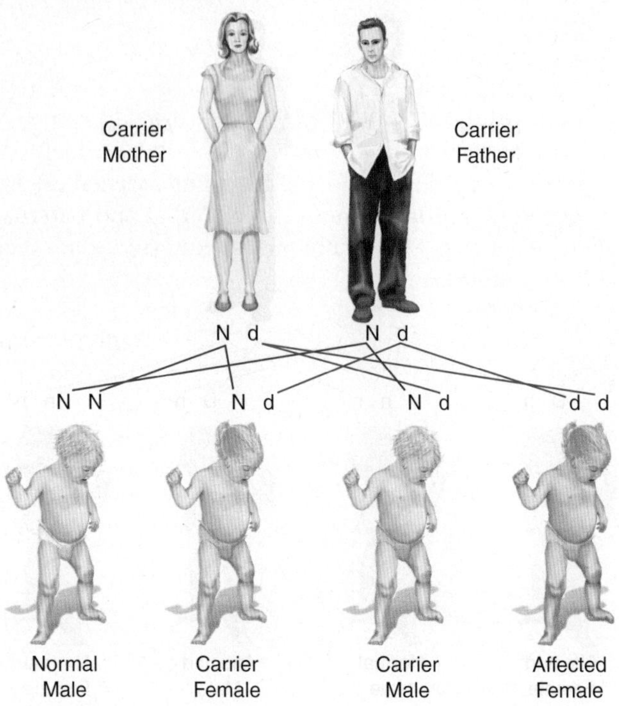

● Figure 30.2 Autosomal recessive inheritance pattern.

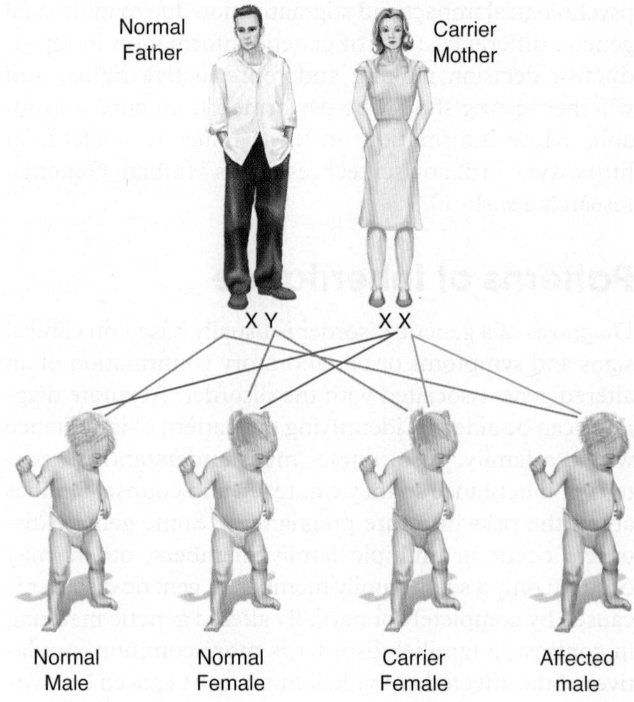

● Figure 30.3 X-linked recessive inheritance pattern.

X-Linked Inheritance

X-linked inheritance disorders are those associated with altered genes on the X chromosome. They differ from autosomal disorders. If a male inherits an X-linked altered gene, he will express the condition. Since a male has only one X chromosome, all the genes on his X chromosome will be expressed (the Y chromosome carries no normal allele to compensate for the altered gene). Because females inherit two X chromosomes, they can be either heterozygous or homozygous for any allele. Therefore, X-linked disorders in females express similarly to autosomal disorders.

X-Linked Recessive Inheritance

Most X-linked disorders demonstrate a recessive pattern of inheritance. There are more affected males than females; since a male has only one X chromosome, all the genes on his X chromosome will be expressed, whereas a female will usually need both X chromosomes to carry the disease. There is no male-to-male transmission (since no X chromosome from the male is transmitted to male offspring), but any man who is affected will have carrier daughters. If a woman is a carrier, there is a 50% chance her sons will be affected and a 50% chance that her daughters will be carriers (Fig. 30.3). Common types of genetic disorders that follow X-linked recessive inheritance patterns include hemophilia, color blindness, and Duchenne muscular dystrophy.

X-Linked Dominant Inheritance

X-linked dominant inheritance is present if heterozygous female carriers demonstrate signs and symptoms of the disorder. All of the daughters and none of the sons of an affected male have the condition, while both male and female offspring of an affected woman have a 50% chance of inheriting and presenting with the condition (Fig. 30.4). X-linked dominant disorders are rare; the most common is hypophosphatemic (vitamin D–resistant) rickets.

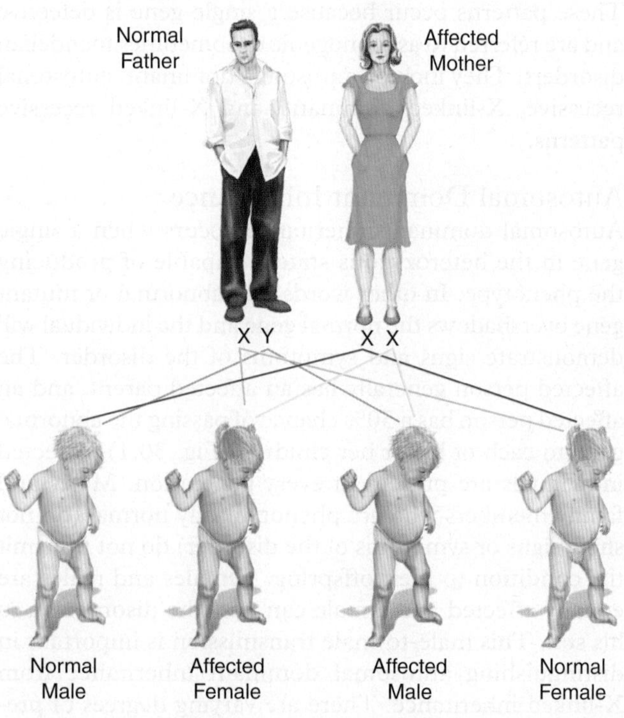

● Figure 30.4 X-linked dominant inheritance pattern.

Multifactorial Inheritance

Many of the common congenital malformations, such as cleft lip, cleft palate, spina bifida, pyloric stenosis, clubfoot, congenital hip dysplasia, and cardiac defects, are attributed to multifactorial inheritance. These conditions are thought to be caused by multiple gene and environmental factors. A combination of genes from both parents, along with unknown environmental factors, produces the trait or condition. An individual may inherit a predisposition to a particular anomaly or disease. The anomalies or diseases vary in severity and often a sex bias is present. For example, pyloric stenosis is seen more often in males, while congenital hip dysplasia is much more likely in females. Multifactorial conditions tend to run in families, but the pattern of inheritance is not as predictable as with single-gene disorders. The chance of recurrence is also less than in single-gene disorders, but the degree of risk is related to the number of genes in common with the affected individual. The closer the degree of relationship, the more genes an individual has in common with the affected family member, and thus the higher risk that the individual's offspring will have a similar defect. In multifactorial inheritance the likelihood that both identical twins will be affected is not 100%, indicating that there are nongenetic factors involved.

Nontraditional Inheritance Patterns

Molecular studies have revealed that some genetic disorders are inherited in ways that do not follow the typical patterns of dominant, recessive, X-linked, or multifactorial inheritance. Examples of nontraditional inheritance patterns include mitochondrial inheritance and genomic imprinting. As the science of molecular genetics advances and we learn more about inheritance patterns, other nontraditional patterns of inheritance may be discovered or may be found to be relatively common.

Mitochondrial Inheritance

Certain diseases result from mutations in the mitochondrial DNA. Mitochondria (the part of the cell responsible for energy production) are inherited almost exclusively from the mother. Therefore, mitochondrial inheritance is usually passed from the mother to the offspring, regardless of the offspring's sex (differentiating mitochondrial inheritance from X-linked recessive inheritance). These mutations are often deletions and abnormalities and are often seen in one or more organs, such as the brain, eye, and skeletal muscle. They are often associated with energy deficits in cells with high energy requirements, such as nerve and muscle cells. These disorders tend to be progressive and the age of onset can vary from infancy to adulthood. There is an extreme amount of variability in symptoms within a family. Examples of disorders that follow mitochondrial inheritance include Kearns-Sayre syndrome (a neuromuscular disorder) and Leber's hereditary optic neuropathy (which causes progressive visual impairment).

Genomic Imprinting

Another nontraditional inheritance pattern results from a process called genomic imprinting. Genomic imprinting plays a critical role in fetal growth and development and placental functioning. It is a phenomenon by which the expression of a gene is determined by its parental origin. In genomic imprinting both the maternal and paternal alleles are present, but only one is expressed; the other is inactive. Genomic imprinting does not alter the genetic sequence itself but affects the phenotype observed. In these cases, the altered genes in a certain region of the genome have very different expressions depending on whether they were inherited from the mother or the father. Several human syndromes are known to be associated with defects in gene imprinting. Disorders that result from a disruption of imprinting usually involve a growth phenotype and include varying degrees of developmental problems. Common examples include Prader-Willi syndrome (a condition resulting in severe hypotonia and hyperphagia, leading to obesity and mental retardation), Angelman syndrome (a neurodevelopmental disorder associated with mental retardation, jerky movements, and seizures), and Beckwith-Wiedemann syndrome (characterized by somatic overgrowth, congenital malformations, and a predisposition to embryonic neoplasia).

Chromosomal Abnormalities

In some cases of genetic disorders, the abnormality occurs due to problems with the chromosomes. Chromosomal abnormalities do not follow straightforward patterns of inheritance. Sperm and egg cells each have 23 unpaired chromosomes. When they unite during conception they form a fertilized egg with 46 chromosomes. Sometimes before pregnancy begins, an error has occurred during the process of cell division, leaving an egg or sperm with too many or too few chromosomes. If this egg or sperm cell joins with a normal egg or sperm cell, the resulting embryo has a chromosomal abnormality. Chromosomal abnormalities can also occur due to an error in the structure of the chromosome. Small pieces of the chromosome may be deleted, duplicated, inverted, misplaced, or exchanged with part of another chromosome. Most chromosomal abnormalities occur due to an error in the egg or sperm. Therefore, the abnormality is present in every cell of the body. Some abnormalities can happen after fertilization during mitotic cell division and result in mosaicism. Mosaicism or mosaic form is when the chromosomal abnormalities do not show up in every cell; only some cells or tissues carry the abnormality. In mosaic forms of the disorder the symptoms are usually less severe than if all the cells were abnormal.

Chromosomal abnormalities occur in 0.4% of live births (Behrman et al., 2004). There is a much higher frequency of chromosomal abnormalities in spontaneous abortions and stillbirths. Congenital anomalies and mental retardation are often associated with chromosomal abnormalities. These abnormalities occur on autosomal or non-sex chromosomes as well as sex chromosomes and can result from abnormalities of either chromosome structure or chromosome number.

A **karyotype** is a pictorial analysis of chromosomes. It depicts a systematic arrangement of chromosomes of a single cell by pairs (Fig. 30.5). Karyotyping is often used in prenatal testing to diagnose or predict genetic diseases.

Abnormalities of Chromosome Number

Chromosomal abnormalities of number often result due to **nondisjunction** (failure of separation of the chromosome pair) during cell division, meiosis, or mitosis. Few chromosomal numerical abnormalities are compatible with full-term development and most result in spontaneous abortion. Some numerical abnormalities, however, can support development to term because the chromosome on which the abnormality is present carries relatively few genes (e.g., chromosome 13, 18, 21, or X). Two common abnormalities of chromosome number are monosomies or trisomies. In monosomies there is only one copy of a particular chromosome instead of the usual pair; in these cases all fetuses spontaneously abort in early pregnancy. Survival occurs only in mosaic forms of these disorders. In trisomies, there are three of a particular chromosome instead of the usual two. The most common trisomies include trisomy 21 (Down syndrome), trisomy 18, and trisomy 13 (see below for further discussion). Trisomies may be present in every cell or may present in the mosaic form.

Abnormalities of Chromosome Structure

Abnormalities of chromosome structure usually occur when there is a breakage and loss of a portion of one or more chromosomes, and during the repair process the broken ends are rejoined incorrectly. Structural abnormalities usually lead to having too much or too little genetic material. Altered chromosome structure can take on several forms. Deletions occur when a portion of the chromosome is missing, resulting in a loss of that portion of the chromosome. Duplications are seen when a portion of the chromosome is duplicated and an extra chromosomal segment is present. Clinical findings vary depending on how much chromosomal material is involved. Inversions occur when a portion of the chromosome breaks off at two points and is turned upside down and reattached; therefore, the genetic material is inverted. With inversion, there is no loss or gain of chromosomal material and carriers are phenotypically normal, but they do have an increased risk for miscarriage and having chromosomally abnormal offspring. Ring chromosomes are seen when a portion of a chromosome has broken off in two places and has formed a circle or ring. The most clinically significant structural

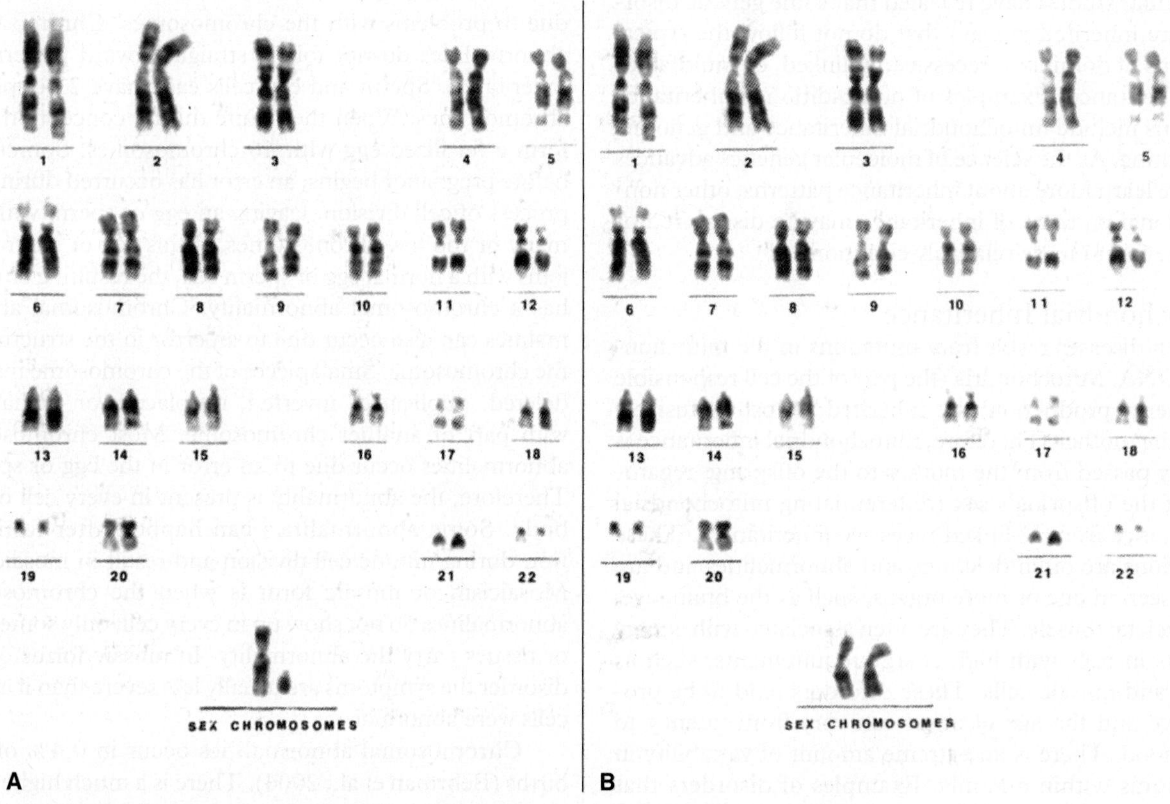

● Figure 30.5 Chromosomes in a karyotype are arranged and numbered by size, from largest to smallest. The normal human karyotype has 46 chromosomes: 22 pairs of autosomes and 2 sex chromosomes. (**A**) A normal male. (**B**) A normal female.

abnormality is a translocation. This occurs when a portion of one chromosome is transferred to another chromosome and an abnormal rearrangement is present.

Structural abnormalities can be balanced or unbalanced. Balanced abnormalities involve the rearrangement of genetic material with neither an overall gain nor loss. Individuals who inherit a balanced structural abnormality are usually phenotypically normal but are at a higher risk for miscarriages and having chromosomally abnormal offspring. Examples of structural rearrangements that can be balanced include inversions, translocations, and ring chromosomes. Unbalanced structural abnormalities are similar to numerical abnormalities because genetic material is either gained or lost. Unbalanced structural abnormalities can encompass several genes and result in severe clinical consequences.

Sex Chromosome Abnormalities

Chromosomal abnormalities can also involve sex chromosomes. These cases usually have milder clinical effects than autosomal chromosomal abnormalities. Sex chromosome abnormalities are gender-specific and involve a missing or extra sex chromosome. They affect sexual development and may cause infertility, growth abnormalities, and possibly behavioral and learning problems. Many affected individuals lead essentially normal lives. Examples are Turner syndrome in females and Klinefelter syndrome in males (see discussion later in this chapter).

Genetic Evaluation and Counseling

Genetic counseling has been defined as "an educational process that seeks to assist affected and/or at-risk individuals to understand the nature of a genetic disorder, its transmission, and the options available to them in management and family planning" (Behrman et al., 2004, p. 395). There are a variety of reasons an individual should be referred for genetic counseling (Box 30.1). In many cases, geneticists and genetic counselors provide information to families regarding genetic diseases. However, an experienced family physician, pediatrician, or nurse who has received special training in genetics may also provide the information. A genetic consultation involves evaluation of an individual or a family. Its purpose is to confirm, diagnose, or rule out genetic conditions, identify medical management issues, calculate and communicate genetic risks to a family, discuss ethical and legal issues, and assist in providing and arranging psychosocial support. Genetic counselors serve as educators and resource people for other health care providers and the general public.

The ideal time for genetic counseling is before conception. Preconception counseling allows couples to identify and reduce potential pregnancy risks, plan for known risks, and establish early prenatal care. Unfortunately, many woman delay seeking prenatal care until their second or third trimester, after the crucial time of organogenesis has occurred. Preconception counseling should be offered to all women as they seek health care throughout their childbearing years, especially if they are contemplating pregnancy. Health care providers should assume an active role. Nurses are often the first health care providers to encounter women with preconception and prenatal issues, so nurses play an important role in beginning the preconception counseling process and referring women and their partners for further genetic testing when indicated.

BOX 30.1

THOSE WHO MAY BENEFIT FROM GENETIC COUNSELING

- Maternal age 35 years or older when the baby is born
- Paternal age 50 years or older
- Previous child, parents, or close relatives with an inherited disease, congenital anomalies, metabolic disorders, developmental disorders, or chromosomal abnormalities
- Consanguinity or incest
- Pregnancy screening abnormality, including alpha-fetoprotein, triple screen, amniocentesis, or ultrasound
- Stillborn with congenital anomalies
- Two or more pregnancy losses
- Teratogen exposure or risk
- Concerns about genetic defects that occur frequently in their ethnic or racial group (e.g., those of African descent are most at risk for having a child with sickle cell anemia)
- Abnormal newborn screening
- Child born with one or more major malformations in a major organ system
- Child with abnormalities of growth
- Child with developmental delay, mental retardation, blindness, or deafness

Preconception screening and counseling can raise serious ethical and moral issues for a couple. Prenatal genetic testing can lead to the decision to terminate a pregnancy based on the results, even if the results may not be conclusive but indicate a strong possibility that the child will have an abnormality. The severity of the abnormality may not be known, and some may find the decision to terminate unethical. Another difficult situation is when a mother finds that she is a carrier for a disorder that affects only one gender. If no prenatal screening test is available, the couple may decide to terminate any pregnancy in which the fetus is the affected sex, even though there is a 50% chance of the child not inheriting the disorder. The choice is the couple's, and information and support must be provided in a nondirective manner.

An accurate and thorough family history is an essential part of preconception counseling. Information is obtained about congenital anomalies, mental retardation, genetic diseases, reproductive history, general health, and causes of death, ideally for three generations. After careful analysis of the data, the couple are referred to a genetic counselor when indicated.

Genetic counseling is particularly important if a congenital anomaly or genetic disease has been diagnosed prenatally or when a child is born with a life-threatening congenital anomaly or genetic disease. In these cases families need urgent information because they need to make immediate decisions. If a diagnosis with genetic implications is made later in life, if a couple with a family history or a previous child with a genetic disorder is planning a family, or if there is suspected teratogen exposure, urgency of information is not such an issue; in these situations the family needs to take in all the information and explore all their options. This may occur during several meetings over a longer period of time.

Genetic counseling involves extensive information gathering about birth history, past medical history, and current health status. A detailed family history is imperative and in most cases will include the development of a pedigree, which is like a family tree (Fig. 30.6). Information is ideally gathered on three generations, but if the family history is complicated, information from more distant relatives may be needed. Families receiving genetic counseling should be told that this information will be necessary so that they can discuss these sensitive issues with family members in advance. When necessary, medical records may be requested for family members, especially those who have a genetic disorder. Sometimes the process of preparing a pedigree may reveal information that is not known by all family members, such as an adopted child, a child conceived through in vitro fertilization, or a husband not being the father of a baby. Therefore, it is extremely important to take steps to maintain confidentiality.

Medical genetic knowledge has increased dramatically over the past few decades. It is possible not only to detect specific diseases with genetic mutations, but also

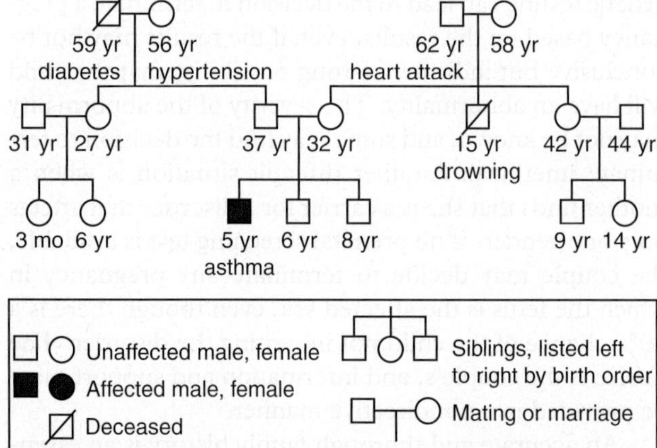

● **Figure 30.6** A pedigree is a diagram that shows the links between family members and includes medical information for each relative.

to test for a genetic predisposition to various diseases or conditions and certain physical characteristics. This leads to complex ethical, moral, and social issues. Health care providers need to maintain client privacy and confidentiality and administer care in a nondiscriminatory manner while maintaining sensitivity to cultural differences. It is essential to respect the patient's autonomy and present information in a nondirective manner.

Nurse's Role and Responsibilities

Pediatric nurses will encounter children with genetic disorders in every clinical specialty area. This includes clinics, hospitals, schools, and community-based centers. Talking with families who have recently been diagnosed with a genetic disorder or who have had a child born with congenital anomalies is very difficult. Many times the nurse is the one who has first contact with these parents and will be the one to provide follow-up care. Genetic disorders are significant, life-changing, and possibly life-threatening situations. The information is highly technical and the field is still evolving, so the family should probably be referred to a health care provider who specializes in genetics. The nurse should understand who will benefit from genetic counseling and should be able to discuss the role of the genetic counselor with families. Families at risk should be informed that genetic counseling is available before they attempt to have another baby. Nurses play an essential role in providing emotional support to the family throughout this challenging time. Nurses should also refer the family to appropriate agencies, support groups, and resources.

Common Medical Treatments

A variety of medications and other medical treatments are used to treat the symptoms of genetic disorders in children. Genetic disorders do not have specific treatments and there is no cure, so treatment focuses on the specific symptoms of each disorder. Genetic disorders often involve multiple organ systems and the patients have complex medical needs, so a multidisciplinary approach and good communication are imperative. See below for a discussion on common genetic disorders and their management.

Nursing Process Overview for the Child With a Genetic Disorder

Care of the child with a genetic disorder includes assessment, nursing diagnosis, planning, interventions, and evaluation. There are a number of general concepts related to the nursing process that may be applied to the care of children with genetic disorders. From a general understanding of the care involved for a child with a genetic disorder, the nurse can then individualize the care based on patient specifics.

ASSESSMENT

Assessment of the child with a genetic disorder includes health history, physical examination, and laboratory and diagnostic testing.

> Remember Julie, the 5-year-old brought in for her annual examination? What additional health history and physical examination information should you obtain?

Health History

The health history comprises past medical history, including the mother's pregnancy history, family history, neonatal history, history of present illness (when the symptoms started and how they have progressed), as well as treatments used at home. Explore the patient's current and past medical history for risk factors such as:

- Family history of genetic disorders
- Any complications during the prenatal, perinatal, or postnatal periods
- Changes in developmental status or delays in developmental milestones

The pregnancy history can be extremely relevant when identifying a genetic disorder. The pregnancy history may be significant for maternal age over 35 years, repeated premature births, breech delivery, congenital hip dysplasia, abnormalities found on ultrasound, abnormalities in prenatal blood screening tests (e.g., triple/quadruple screen, alpha fetoprotein), amniotic fluid abnormalities (polyhydramnios, oligohydramnios), multiple births, exposure to medications and known teratogens, and decreased fetal movement.

A focused neonatal history can also help identify a genetic problem. The neonatal history may be significant for symmetric intrauterine growth restriction, large for gestational age without a reason, hearing impaired, persistent hyperbilirubinemia, poor adaptation to the extrauterine environment (demonstrated by temperature and heart rate instability and poor feeding), hypotonia or hypertonia, seizures, and abnormal newborn screening results.

The family history plays a critical role in identifying genetic disorders. Data should be gathered for three generations. If there is a positive family history, the likelihood of a genetic disorder in the patient is increased. It is helpful to create a family pedigree (refer to the genetic counseling section above). The family history may be significant for major congenital anomalies, mental retardation, genetic diseases, metabolic disorders, multiple miscarriages or stillbirths, developmental delays, significant learning disabilities, psychiatric problems, consanguinity, and chronic serious illness (e.g., diabetes, hypertension, renal disease, hearing impairment, blindness, asthma, seizures, and unexplained death).

When eliciting the history of the present illness, inquire about:

- Developmental delay
- Seizures
- Hypotonia or hypertonia
- Feeding problems
- Lethargy
- Failure to thrive
- Septic appearance
- Vomiting

Children known to have a genetic disorder are often admitted to the hospital for other health-related issues or complications and management of the genetic disorder. The health history should include questions related to:

- Age when the disorder was diagnosed
- Developmental delay
- Complications of the disorder (e.g., thyroid problems, cardiac problems, respiratory problems, leukemia, seizures, cognitive impairment)
- Medications the child takes for complications associated with the disorder
- Dietary restrictions
- Compliance with management regimen

Once complications have been identified, further investigation into their severity, frequency, and management is essential to the care of this child while in the hospital.

Physical Examination

Physical examination of the child with a genetic disorder includes inspection and observation, palpation, and auscultation.

Inspection and Observation

Inspect and observe for congenital anomalies, either major or minor. A major anomaly is an anomaly or malformation that creates significant medical problems and requires surgical or medical management (Box 30.2). Minor anomalies are features that vary from those seen in the general population but do not cause an increase in morbidity in and of themselves (Box 30.3).

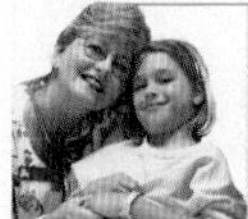

> Low-set ears are associated with numerous genetic dysmorphisms. If noted, assess thoroughly for other abnormalities.

When three or more minor anomalies are present, the risk for a major anomaly or mental retardation is approximately 20% (Siegel & Milunsky, 2004). When one major anomaly is present, the possibility of a genetic cause must be investigated. In children with three or more minor

BOX 30.2

MAJOR CONGENITAL ANOMALIES

- Cleft lip
- Cleft palate
- Congenital heart disease, structural and conduction disorders
- Neural tube defects
- Brain anomalies
- Omphalocele
- Hepatosplenomegaly
- Asymmetry of face, skeleton, or limb
- Generalized dysmorphism
- Specific skin lesions, such as café-au-lait macules, hypopigmented macules, or cutaneous hemangiomas

Adapted from Siegel, B., & Milunsky, J. (2004). When should the possibility of a genetic disorder cross your radar screen? *Contemporary Pediatrics, 21*(5), 37.

anomalies, selected major anomalies, a recognized pattern of anomalies, or a combination of major and minor anomalies, a genetic diagnostic workup is recommended (Siegel & Milunsky, 2004).

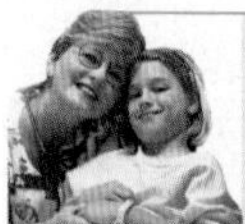

Cleft lip and cleft palate are associated with many syndromes. If noted, assess for other anomalies.

BOX 30.3

MINOR CONGENITAL ANOMALIES

- Flat occiput
- Prominent occiput
- Widow's peak
- Triple hair whorl
- Flat-bridged nose
- Nostrils anteverted
- Ear lobe crease
- Ear lobe notched
- Forward displacement or protruding ears
- Cleft uvula
- Webbed neck
- Extra nipples
- Single umbilical artery
- Umbilical hernia
- Tapered fingers
- Overlapping digits
- Broad thumb or great toe
- Increased space between toes
- Syndactyly
- Polydactyly

Adapted from Siegel, B., & Milunsky, J. (2004). When should the possibility of a genetic disorder cross your radar screen? *Contemporary Pediatrics, 21*(5), 37.

Table 30.1 Inborn Errors of Metabolism and Associated Odor

Inborn Error of Metabolism	Associated Odor
Phenylketonuria	Mousy or musty
Maple syrup urine disease	Maple syrup
Tyrosinemia	Cabbage-like, rancid butter
Trimethylaminuria	Rotting fish

Inspect and observe for an abnormal or foul odor of the child's excretions, as certain metabolic disorders or inborn errors of metabolism are associated with specific odors (Table 30.1).

Auscultation

Physical examination includes auscultation of the heart. Murmurs or dysrhythmias may have a genetic cause. In a patient with a congenital heart problem (e.g., ventricular septal defect) and a strong family history of cardiac structural problems, a genetic cause needs to be considered. Approximately 3% of all cases of congenital heart disease are caused by a single mutant gene, and 5% of congenital heart defects are caused by chromosomal abnormalities (Siegel & Milunsky, 2004).

Palpation

Palpation can be used to detect hepatosplenomegaly (an enlarged spleen and liver), but because this requires skill and experience, this assessment may be performed by advanced practitioners or physicians. Hepatosplenomegaly may indicate a metabolic disorder.

Laboratory and Diagnostic Testing

Common Laboratory and Diagnostic Tests 30.1 explains the laboratory and diagnostic tests used most commonly to detect genetic disorders. The tests can assist the physician in diagnosing the disorder or can be used as guidelines in determining treatment. Laboratory or non-nursing personnel obtain some of the tests, while the nurse might obtain others. In either instance the nurse should be familiar with how the tests are obtained, what they are used for, and normal versus abnormal results. This knowledge will also be necessary when providing patient and family education related to the testing. Due to the nature of the information, a referral to genetic counseling before testing may be appropriate. Advances in genetic technology, including information obtained from the Human Genome Project, have led to dramatic increases in the number of diagnostic and screening tests.

(text continues on page 1021)

Common Laboratory and Diagnostic Tests 30.1

Test	Explanation	Indication	Nursing Implications
Amniocentesis	Ultrasound-guided (to determine placental location) insertion of a needle through the abdomen and into the uterine cavity of a pregnant woman to obtain a sample of amniotic fluid. The fluid contains skin cells that have been shed by the fetus and can be isolated and grown in the laboratory to provide enough genetic material for testing.	Tests for chromosomal abnormality or specific genetic conditions of the fetus. Performed if considered high risk for a genetic disorder or abnormal ultrasound. Most common prenatal test used to diagnose chromosomal and congenital anomalies.	Usually not performed before 14 to 16 weeks. Some clinicians offer early amniocentesis (between 11 and 14 weeks), but this is still considered experimental and may be riskier than second-trimester amniocentesis. Complications include miscarriage, fetal injury, amniotic fluid leakage, infection, spontaneous abortion, premature labor, maternal hemorrhage, amniotic fluid embolism, abruptio placentae, and damage to the bladder or intestines. Results are usually not available for 2 weeks, but this varies by laboratory. Monitor fetus before and after procedure.
Chorionic villi sampling (CVS)	Involves the removal of a small amount of tissue directly from the chorionic villi (minute vascular projections of the fetal chorion that combine with maternal uterine tissue to form the placenta). In the laboratory, the chromosomes of the fetal cells are analyzed for number and type. Extra chromosomes, such as are present in Down syndrome, can be identified. Additional laboratory tests can be performed to look for specific disorders.	Tests for chromosomal abnormality or specific genetic conditions of the fetus. Performed if considered high risk for a genetic disorder or abnormal ultrasound.	Performed at 8 to 12 weeks of gestation, so provides early detection of genetic abnormalities. Complications include accidental abortion, infection, bleeding, amniotic fluid leakage, fetal limb deformities. Results are usually available within a week, but this varies depending on the laboratory and location of procedure (results are usually available sooner than with an amniocentesis). Monitor fetus before and after procedure.
Triple/quadruple screen	A maternal serum laboratory test that measures the level of 3 substances made by the developing baby and placenta: alpha-fetoprotein (AFP), human chorionic gonadotropin (hCG), and unconjugated estriol (uE3). Dimeric inhibin-A has been added to make the "quadruple test." The addition of dimeric inhibin-A increases the detection rate of Down syndrome in the quadruple screen.	A screening test for low-risk pregnant women to determine pregnancies at an increased risk for open neural tube defects, Down syndrome, and trisomy 18	Performed between 16 and 19 weeks of gestation. Educate mothers that a normal test does not guarantee a healthy baby. Quadruple test identifies 3 out of 4 Down syndrome pregnancies, 4 out of 5 open spina bifida pregnancies, and 1 out of 2 trisomy 18 pregnancies (MSU Division of Human Genetics, 2002). Conversely, an abnormal result does not guarantee the baby has a problem. Additional testing will be necessary to confirm or rule out a specific genetic condition.

(continued)

Common Laboratory and Diagnostic Tests 30.1 (continued)

Test	Explanation	Indication	Nursing Implications
Ultrasound	Safe, noninvasive, accurate investigation of the fetus. A transducer is placed in contact with the mother's abdomen and high-frequency sound waves are directed at the fetus. The sound waves are reflected back through the tissues and recorded and displayed in real time on a screen.	To screen for structural malformations	Usually performed at 18 to 20 weeks of gestation; routinely done. Early ultrasound can be performed at 13 to 14 weeks to evaluate for Down syndrome.
Percutaneous umbilical blood sampling	An ultrasound-guided needle is inserted through the abdominal and uterine wall to the umbilical cord and a sample of blood is retrieved and sent to the laboratory for analysis. Procedure is similar to amniocentesis but requires a higher level of expertise and experience.	To detect chromosome abnormalities. Usually done when diagnostic information cannot be obtained through amniocentesis, CVS, or ultrasound or the results of these tests were inconclusive.	Performed at or after 18 weeks. Complications include miscarriage, blood loss, infection, premature rupture of membranes. The risk to the pregnancy is greater than with other prenatal procedures such as amniocentesis and CVS. Not performed as often due to risks and since discovery of fluorescent in situ hybridization (FISH).
Fetoscopy	Endoscopic procedure that allows direct visualization of the fetus through the insertion of a tiny flexible instrument called a fetoscope. It is inserted through the abdominal wall and into the uterine cavity. Ultrasound is used to guide the placement of the scope. Direct visualization can evaluate the fetus for severe congenital anomalies such as neural tube defects. Fetal blood samples from the umbilical cord can be obtained and tested for congenital blood disorders such as hemophilia and sickle cell anemia. Fetal tissue samples (usually skin) can be collected and tested for genetic diseases.	Indicated for any woman at risk for delivering a baby with significant congenital anomalies; can be used to perform corrective surgery (e.g., shunt placement) on the fetus	Performed during or after the 18th week of pregnancy. Complications include spontaneous abortion, premature delivery, premature rupture of membranes, amniotic fluid leak, intrauterine fetal death, infection. Monitor fetus before and after procedure.
Gene testing	Gene testing is currently available for over 950 inherited diseases. It involves analysis of DNA, RNA, chromosomes, proteins, metabolites, and biochemical agents.	To detect abnormalities that may indicate actual disease or predict future disease. Indicated in the evaluation of congenital anomalies, mental retardation, growth retardation, recurrent	Provide support, information, and resources to family. Refer to genetic counseling before and after test.

Common Laboratory and Diagnostic Tests 30.1 (continued)

Test	Explanation	Indication	Nursing Implications
	Specimens for gene testing can be obtained from numerous sources; leukocytes from blood are the most common and easily obtained site, during pregnancy, amniocentesis and chorionic villus sampling, and fetal tissue or products of conception after a miscarriage Most common use is DNA or chromosomes isolated from blood Direct detection of abnormalities in genes and chromosomes is performed using DNA based test or cytogenetic tests (which look at chromosome) and other methods. Cytogenetic tests also include a relatively new technology, fluorescent in situ hybridization (FISH), to assist in detecting chromosomal abnormalities such as duplication, deletion, rearrangements and translocations	miscarriage to determine reason for the loss of a fetus, prenatal diagnosis of genetic disease.	
Newborn screening	Blood screening performed shortly after birth, used to identify many life threatening genetic illnesses that have no immediate visible effects but can lead to physical problems, mental retardation and even death.	Every U.S. state routinely screens all newborns, but each state dictates which disorders to screen for, so components of the screening vary from state to state.	Ideally performed after 24 hours of age; obtain specimen as close to time of discharge from newborn or labor and delivery unit as possible and no later than 7 days of age. The test is less accurate if done before 24 hours of age and should be repeated by 2 weeks of age if the newborn is less than 24 hours old. Ensure appropriate follow-up with newborn screening results; results are available in 2 to 3 weeks.

NURSING DIAGNOSES, GOALS, INTERVENTIONS, AND EVALUATION

Upon completion of an assessment, the nurse might identify several nursing diagnoses, including:

- Deficient knowledge
- Decisional conflict
- Risk for delayed growth and development
- Fear
- Interrupted family processes

After completing an assessment of Julie, the nurse noted the following: short stature for age and a low posterior hairline. Based on these assessment findings, what would your top three nursing diagnoses be for Julie?

Nursing goals, interventions, and evaluation for the child with a genetic disorder are based on the nursing diagnoses. Nursing Care Plan 30.1 provides a general

(text continues on page 1024)

Nursing Care Plan 30.1

Overview for the Child With a Genetic Disorder

Nursing Diagnosis: Deficient knowledge related to lack of information regarding complex, technical medical condition, prognosis, and medical needs as evidenced by verbalization, questions, or actions demonstrating lack of understanding about child's condition or care

Outcome identification and evaluation

Child and family will verbalize accurate information and understanding about condition, prognosis, and medical needs: *Child and family demonstrate knowledge of condition, prognosis, and medical needs, including possible causes, contributing factors, and treatment measures.*

Intervention: providing patient and family teaching

- Assess child's and family's willingness to learn: *Child and family must be willing to learn for teaching to be effective.*
- Provide family with time to adjust to diagnosis: *will facilitate adjustment and ability to learn and participate in child's care.*
- Repeat information: *allows family and child time to learn and understand.*
- Teach in short sessions: *many short sessions are more helpful than one long session.*
- Gear teaching to the child and family's level of understanding (depends on age of child, physical condition, memory) *to ensure understanding.*
- Provide reinforcement and rewards: *facilitates the teaching/learning process.*
- Use multiple modes of learning involving many senses (written, verbal, demonstration, and videos) when possible: *child and family are more likely to retain information when presented in different ways using many senses.*
- Refer child and family to a genetics specialist: *genetic information is highly technical; the field is advancing at a rapid pace, and information needs to be the most current and accurate. A genetic specialist can provide this along with expertise, support, and resources.*

Nursing Diagnosis: Decisional conflict related to treatment options, conflicting values, and ethical, legal, and social issues surrounding genetic testing as evidenced by verbalization of uncertainty about choices, verbalization of undesired consequences of alternative actions being considered, delayed decision making, physical signs of stress

Outcome identification and evaluation

Family will state they are able to make an informed decision: *Family will state advantages and disadvantages of choices and share fears and concerns regarding choices.*

Intervention: providing decision-making support

- Give family time and encourage them to express their feelings associated with decision making: *the decision-making process becomes more difficult if feelings are not expressed.*
- Encourage family to list advantages and disadvantages of each alternative: *aids in problem solving and helps family recognize all alternatives.*
- Initiate health teaching and referral to genetic specialist when needed: *genetic testing information is often technical and complex. Families need accurate and up-to-date information to aid in decision making.*
- Maintain a nondirective manner: *this is a difficult decision that the family must make for themselves; the nurse should provide all the necessary information while maintaining an unobtrusive role.*
- Validate the family's feelings regarding the decisional conflict: *Validation is a therapeutic communication technique that promotes the nurse–patient relationship.*

Overview for the Child With a Genetic Disorder (continued)

Nursing Diagnosis: Risk for delayed growth and development related to physical disability, cognitive deficits, activity restrictions secondary to genetic disorder

Outcome identification and evaluation

Child's growth and development will be enhanced; child will demonstrate adequate growth patterns within parameters of disease, child will make continued progress toward attainment of developmental milestones and will not suffer regression in abilities.

Child will demonstrate developmental milestones within age parameters and limits of disease.

Child will make steady gains in growth patterns (e.g., height and weight) within disease parameters. Child expresses interest in the environment and people around him or her, interacts with environment appropriately for developmental level.

Intervention: promoting growth and development

- Screen for developmental capabilities *to determine child's current level of functioning.*
- Offer age-appropriate toys, play, and activities (including gross motor) *to encourage further development.*
- Perform exercises or interventions as prescribed by physical or occupational therapist: *these activities promote function and developmental skills.*
- Provide support to families: *due to immobility and extremity deficits, the child's progress toward developmental milestones may be slow.*
- Use therapeutic play and adaptive toys *to facilitate developmental functioning.*
- Provide stimulating environment when possible *to maximize potential for growth and development.*
- Praise accomplishments and emphasize child's abilities *to improve self-esteem and encourage feeling of confidence and competence.*
- Monitor height and weight and plot on growth chart *to identify growth patterns and deviations in these patterns.*

Nursing Diagnosis: Fear related to outcome of genetic testing as evidenced by reports of apprehension and increased tension

Outcome identification and evaluation

Family will state they can cope with the results of the genetic testing or demonstrate reduced fear. *Family accurately discusses chances of offspring having genetic disease, demonstrates positive coping, asks questions about genetic testing and meaning of results.*

Intervention: managing fear

- Empathize with the family and avoid false reassurances; be truthful: *allows family to recognize that fear is a reasonable response. Giving false information or reassurance will actually increase fear.*
- Explore coping skills used previously by the family to cope with fear. Reinforce these skills and explore other outlets, such as relaxation, breathing, and physical activity: *encourages use of coping mechanisms that help control fear.*
- Encourage verbalization of feelings and concerns about genetic testing. Allow time for questions: *provides a safe outlet to express feelings and encourages open communication between the family members.*
- Explain all procedures and review results as available: *Knowledge deficit contributes to fear.*
- Refer to appropriate support groups and genetic counseling: *talking with families who have gone through similar situations can help decrease fear and provide methods of coping. Genetic counseling provides information along with support and additional resources.*

(continued)

Overview for the Child With a Genetic Disorder (continued)

Nursing Diagnosis: Family processes, interrupted, related to child's illness, hospitalization, diagnosis of genetic illness in child, and potential long-term effects of illness as evidenced by family's presence in hospital and clinic, missed work, demonstration of inadequate coping

Outcome identification and evaluation

Family will maintain functional system of support, demonstrate adequate coping, adaptation of roles and functions, and decreased anxiety. *Parents are involved in child's care, ask appropriate questions, express fears and concerns, and can discuss child's care and condition calmly.*

Intervention: promoting family coping

- Encourage family to verbalize concerns about child's illness, diagnosis, and prognosis: *allows the nurse to identify concerns and areas where further education may be needed and demonstrates family-centered care.*
- Explain therapies, procedures, child's behaviors, and plan of care to parents: *Understanding the child's current status and plan of care helps decrease anxiety.*
- Encourage parental involvement in care: *allows parents to feel needed and valued and gives them a sense of control over their child's health.*
- Identify support system for family and child: *helps nurse identify needs and resources available for coping.*
- Educate family about resources available *to help them develop a wide base of support.*

guide for planning care for a child with a genetic disorder. Additional information about nursing management will be included later in the chapter as it relates to specific disorders.

No matter what the genetic abnormality is, the news may be shattering to the family. It is difficult for nurses to even begin to understand what the family is going through. When providing support and education to families of children with serious genetic abnormalities, use these guiding principles:

- Build a trusting relationship.
- Stress the authenticity of the parents' feelings.
- Reject your own personal biases.
- Recognize that individuals cope in various ways; the family's behavior may not be what you would expect.
- Help the family to identify their own strengths and supports, building on those as able.
- Know that the family's emotions may exhaust and disorganize them.
- Assist the family members to maintain open communication among themselves.
- Provide referrals to local parent groups or other families with a child with a similar disorder.
- Allow the family to verbalize their emotions and ask questions.
- Always ask the parents how *they* are doing (Lashley, 2005).

Based on your top three nursing diagnoses for Julie, describe appropriate nursing interventions.

Common Chromosomal Abnormalities

Chromosomal abnormalities are seen in 1 in 200 babies. Many children with chromosomal abnormalities have associated mental retardation, learning disabilities, behavioral problems, and distinct features, including physical birth defects. The risk for autosomal trisomies increases with advanced maternal age. The most common chromosomal abnormalities will be discussed below. New techniques in chromosome analysis have made it possible to identify tiny abnormalities that could not be seen before. Therefore, more chromosomal abnormalities are being identified in children (Table 30.2).

TRISOMY 21 (DOWN SYNDROME)

Trisomy 21 (Down syndrome) is the most common chromosomal abnormality associated with mental retardation. One in 600 to 800 live births result in trisomy 21 (Van Riper & Cohen, 2001). More than half of trisomy 21 conceptions result in spontaneous abortion (Van Riper &

Table 30.2 Less Common Chromosomal Abnormalities

Chromosomal Abnormality	Features
Prader-Willi syndrome	Severe hypotonia, obesity, short stature, small hands and feet, hypogonadism, hyperphagia, and mental retardation (varies from mild to severe)
Angelman syndrome	Hypotonia, microbrachycephaly, fair hair, midface hypoplasia, deep-set eyes, large mouth with tongue protrusion, seizures, jerky ataxic movements (resembling a puppet gait), uncontrolled bouts of laughter/smiling, happy demeanor, easily excitable personality, developmental delay and speech impairment, and severe mental retardation www.angelman.org: Angelman Syndrome Foundation, Inc.
Cri-du-chat syndrome	Hypotonia, short stature, slow growth, low birthweight, characteristic weak, cat-like cry, microcephaly with protruding metopic suture, moon-like round face, bilateral epicanthal folds (folds of skin over the eyelids), high-arched palate, wide and flat nasal bridge, micrognathia (small receding chin), simian crease, and mental retardation www.fivepminus.org: 5p- Society
Velocardiofacial/DiGeorge syndrome	Hypoplasia or agenesis of the thymus and parathyroid glands, hypoplasia of auricle and external auditory canal, cardiac anomalies, cleft palate, short stature, distinctive facial appearance (elongated face, almond-shaped eyes, wide nose, small ears), and learning, speech, feeding, and behavioral problems www.vcfsef.org/: Velo-Cardio-Facial Syndrome Educational Foundation, Inc.

Cohen, 2001). Trisomy 21 is seen in all ages, races, and socioeconomic levels, but a higher incidence is found with a maternal age above 35 years: the likelihood of having a baby with Down syndrome is 1 in 400 at age 35, 1 in 60 at age 42, and 1 in 12 by age 49 (National Institutes of Health, 2006).

Trisomy 21 is associated with some degree of mental retardation, characteristic facial features (e.g., slanted eyes and depressed nasal bridge), and other health problems (e.g., cardiac defects, visual and hearing impairment, intestinal malformations, and an increased susceptibility to infections). The severity of these problems varies.

The prognosis has been improving over the past few decades. Fundamental changes in the care of these children have resulted in longer life expectancy (around 55 years of age) and an improved quality of life.

Pathophysiology

Trisomy 21 is a disorder caused by nondisjunction (an error in cell division) prior to or at conception. Each egg and sperm cell normally contains 23 chromosomes. When they join, this results in 23 pairs or 46 chromosomes. Sometimes, due to nondisjunction, a cell contributes an extra critical portion of chromosome number 21, resulting in an embryo with three chromosome 21s in all cells (Fig. 30.7). This results in the characteristic features and birth defects of Down syndrome. This error in cell division and the presence of three chromosome 21s in all cells is responsible for 95% of cases of Down syndrome (Behrman et al., 2004).

In approximately 1% of cases of Down syndrome, the nondisjunction occurs after fertilization and a mixture of two cell types is seen (Behrman et al., 2004). In these

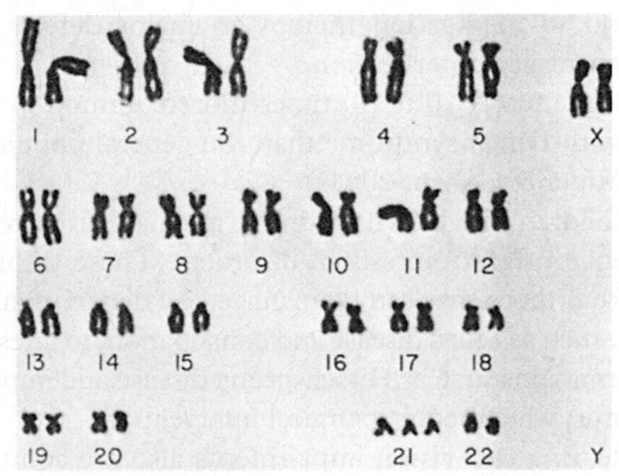

● Figure 30.7 Down syndrome karyotype. Note the third chromosome located at chromosome 21.

cases some cells have 47 chromosomes (due to three chromosome 21s), while others have the normal 46 chromosomes (with the normal two chromosome 21s present). This is referred to as the mosaic form of Down syndrome. Children with mosaic Down syndrome may have a milder form of the disorder, but this is not a general finding.

About 4% of Down syndrome cases involve a translocation, in which part of the number 21 chromosome breaks off during cell division prior to or at conception and attaches to another chromosome. The cells will remain with 46 chromosomes, but this extra portion of the number 21 chromosome results in the clinical findings of Down syndrome. Cases of translocation are not associated with older maternal age, as is the situation with nondisjunction errors, and 25% of cases are the result of a hereditary translocation (American Academy of Pediatrics, 2001).

Therapeutic Management

Management of Down syndrome will involve multiple disciplines, including a primary physician, specialty physicians such as cardiologist, ophthalmologist, and gastroenterologist, nurses, physical therapists, occupational therapists, speech therapists, dietitian, psychologist, counselors, teachers, and of course the parents. There is no standard treatment for all children, and there is no cure or prevention. The overall focus of therapeutic management will be to promote the child's optimal growth and development and function within the limits of the disease. Treatment is mainly symptomatic and supportive.

Managing Complications

Children with Down syndrome need the usual immunizations, well-child care, and screening recommended by the American Academy of Pediatrics. In addition, medical management will focus on complications associated with Down syndrome.

Congenital heart disease occurs in 40% to 60% of children with Down syndrome (Van Riper & Cohen, 2001). Cardiac problems vary from minor defects that respond to medication therapy to major defects that require surgical intervention.

Leukemia is 10 to 30 times more common in children with Down syndrome than the general population (Van Riper & Cohen, 2001).

Children with Down syndrome also have an increased incidence of gastrointestinal disorders. These disorders vary from those that can be managed by dietary manipulation, such as celiac disease and constipation, to intestinal malformations such as Hirschsprung disease and imperforate anus, which require surgical intervention.

Hearing and vision impairments also are common. More than 60% of children with Down syndrome have a hearing loss (Van Riper & Cohen, 2001), so regular evaluation of vision and hearing is essential.

Obstructive sleep apnea is present in 50% to 75% of children with Down syndrome (American Academy of Pediatrics, 2001). Often parents are unaware their child is having sleep disturbances, so baseline testing in young children may be warranted (Groch, 2006).

Children with Down syndrome have a higher incidence of thyroid disease, which can affect growth and cognitive function. Most of these children have hypothyroidism (an underactive thyroid), but sometimes hyperthyroidism (an overactive thyroid) occurs. Periodic thyroid testing may be warranted.

Atlanto-axial instability (increased mobility of the cervical spine at the first and second vertebrae) is seen in about 14% of children with Down syndrome (Van Riper & Cohen, 2001). In most cases these children are asymptomatic, but symptoms may appear if spinal cord compression occurs. Screening for atlanto-axial instability may be appropriate, especially if the child is involved in sports.

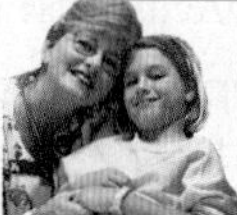

If neck pain, unusual posturing of the head and neck (torticollis), change in gait, loss of upper body strength, abnormal reflexes, or change in bowel or bladder functioning is noted in the child with Down syndrome, immediate attention is required.

Children with Down syndrome also have a higher susceptibility to infection and a higher mortality rate from infectious diseases, so precautions to prevent and monitor for infection are needed (Van Riper & Cohen, 2001).

Due to their increased risk for certain congenital anomalies and diseases, children with Down syndrome will need to be monitored closely, and regular medical care is essential.

Early Intervention Therapy

Early intervention refers to a variety of specialized programs and resources available to young children with developmental delay or other impairment. These programs may involve an array of health care professionals such as physical, occupational, and speech therapists, special educators, and social workers. The programs focus on providing stimulation and encouragement to children with Down syndrome. They help encourage and accelerate development and may help to prevent some developmental delays. The earlier the intervention can begin, the more beneficial it will be. The programs are individualized to meet the specific needs of each child.

Children with Down syndrome progress through the same developmental stages as typical children, but they do so on their own timetable. For example, children with Down syndrome will learn to walk, but the average child with Down syndrome walks at 24 months (versus 12 months for a child without Down syndrome). Conditions such as hypotonia, ligament laxity, decreased strength, enlarged tongue, and short arms and legs are common in children with Down syndrome, and early intervention can help in the development of gross and fine motor skills, language, and social and self-care skills.

Parents also benefit from early intervention programs in terms of support, encouragement, and information. Early intervention programs teach parents how to interact with their child while meeting the child's specific needs and encouraging development.

Nursing Assessment

For a full description of the assessment phase of the nursing process, refer to page 1017. Assessment findings pertinent to Down syndrome are discussed below.

Health History

Down syndrome is often diagnosed prenatally using perinatal screening and diagnostic tests. If not diagnosed prenatally, most cases are diagnosed in the first few days of life based on the physical characteristics associated with Down syndrome. High-risk deliveries should be identified. Explore the pregnancy history and past medical history for risk factors such as:

- Lack of prenatal care
- Abnormal prenatal screening or diagnostic tests for Down syndrome (e.g., triple/quadruple screen, ultrasound, amniocentesis)
- Maternal age over 35 years

The older infant or child known to have Down syndrome is often admitted to the hospital for corrective surgeries or other complications of the disease, such as infections. Elicit a description of the present illness and chief complaint. In an infant or child returning for a clinic visit or hospitalization, the health history should include questions related to:

- Cardiac defects or disease (treatment regimen, surgical repair)
- Hearing or vision impairment (last hearing and vision evaluation, any corrective measures)
- Developmental delays (speech, gross and fine motor skills)
- Sucking or feeding problems
- Cognitive abilities (degree of mental retardation)
- Gastrointestinal disorders such as vomiting or absence of stools (special dietary management, surgical interventions)
- Thyroid disease
- Leukemia
- Atlanto-axial instability
- Seizures
- Infections such as recurrent or chronic respiratory infections, otitis media
- Growth (height and weight changes, feeding problems, unexplained weight gain)
- Signs and symptoms of sleep apnea, such as snoring, restlessness during sleep, daytime sleepiness
- Any other changes in physical state or medication regimen

Physical Examination

The initial assessment after birth may reveal certain physical features characteristic of Down syndrome (Box 30.4 and Fig. 30.8).

Observe the child's general appearance. Note lack of muscle tone and loose joints; this is usually more pronounced in infancy, and the infant has a floppy appearance. Observe growth and development. Plot growth on appropriate growth charts. Because children with Down syndrome grow at a slower rate, special growth charts have been developed (see http://thepoint.lww.com for an example).

When assessing achievement of developmental milestones in children with Down syndrome, it may be more useful to look at the sequence of milestones rather than the age at which they were achieved. Each milestone represents a skill that is needed for the next stage of development.

Perform a subjective assessment of hearing and refer the child for further evaluation if indicated. Assess vision, especially for cataracts. Assess respiratory status and cardiac status. Auscultate for murmurs and pulmonary changes, which can indicate congenital heart disease.

BOX 30.4

COMMON CLINICAL MANIFESTATIONS OF DOWN SYNDROME

- Flattened occiput
- Small (brachycephalic) head
- Flat facial profile
- Depressed nasal bridge and small nose
- Oblique palpebral fissures (an upward slant to the eyes)
- Brushfield spots (white spots on the iris of the eye)
- Low-set ears
- Abnormally shaped ears
- Small mouth
- Protrusion of tongue; tongue is large compared to mouth size
- Arched palate
- Hands with broad, short fingers
- A single deep transverse crease on the palm of the hand (simian crease)
- Congenital heart defect
- Short neck, with excessive skin at the nape
- Hyperflexibility and looseness of joints (excessive ability to extend the joints)
- Dysplastic middle phalanx of fifth finger (one flexion furrow instead of two)
- Epicanthal folds (small skin folds on the inner corner of the eyes)
- Excessive space between large and second toe
- Hypotonia

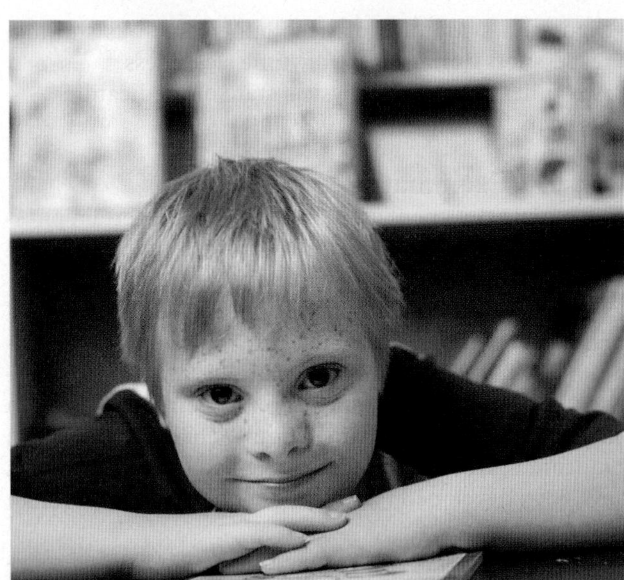

● Figure 30.8 Child with Down syndrome.

Chronic or recurrent respiratory infections, such as pneumonia and otitis media, may be found.

Laboratory and Diagnostic Tests

Down syndrome can be detected prenatally around 16 to 18 weeks of gestation using ultrasound, a blood test to detect increases in alpha fetoprotein, or analysis of amniotic fluid or tissue from chorionic villi to detect chromosomal abnormalities. Down syndrome can be confirmed after birth using chromosome analysis (see Common Laboratory and Diagnostic Tests 30.1).

Common laboratory and diagnostic studies ordered for the diagnosis and assessment of complications associated with Down syndrome include:

- Echocardiogram: to detect cardiac defects
- Vision and hearing screening: to detect vision and hearing impairments
- Thyroid hormone level: to detect thyroid disease
- Cervical x-rays: to assess for atlanto-axial instability
- Ultrasound: to assess gastrointestinal malformations

These tests will be important in evaluating the severity of the child's physical disabilities.

Nursing Management

Due to the high incidence of Down syndrome and the complex medical needs of these children, most pediatric nurses are likely to care for these children in their practice. Nursing management focuses on providing supportive measures such as promoting growth and development, preventing complications, promoting nutrition, and providing support and education to the child and family. In addition to the nursing diagnoses and related interventions discussed in Nursing Care Plan 30.1, additional considerations are reviewed below.

Promoting Growth and Development

Children with Down syndrome tend to grow more slowly, learn more slowly, have shorter attention spans, and have trouble with reasoning and judgment. Their personality tends to be one of genuine warmth and cheerfulness along with patience, gentleness, and a natural spontaneity. Growth and developmental milestones for children with Down syndrome have been developed as a guide for health care providers. Table 30.3 gives examples of the average age at which these children reach selected milestones versus typical children.

Nurses play a key role in connecting families with appropriate resources that can facilitate the child's growth and development. The sooner early intervention programs can begin, the better for the child (see the above discussion on early intervention). Speech and language therapy, occupational therapy, and physical therapy will be important in promoting the child's growth and development. Special education should fit the child's individual needs, and the child should be integrated into mainstream education whenever possible.

Preventing Complications

Children with Down syndrome are at risk for certain health problems (see above). Even though most nurses will encounter a child with Down syndrome in their practice, only a few nurses will become experts in their care. The needs of these children are complex, and guidelines have been established that can help the nurse care for these children and their families (http://www.denison.edu/collaborations/dsq/health99.html). Nurses also play a key role in educating parents and caregivers about how to prevent the complications of Down syndrome (Teaching Guideline 30.1).

Promoting Nutrition

Children with Down syndrome may have difficulty sucking and feeding due to lack of muscle tone. They tend to have small mouths; a smooth, flat, large tongue; and due to the underdeveloped nasal bone, chronically stuffy noses. This may lead to poor nutritional intake and problems with growth. These problems usually improve as the child gains tongue control. Use of a bulb syringe, humidification, and changing the infant's position can lessen the problem. Breastfeeding a baby with Down syndrome is usually possible, and the antibodies in breast milk can help the child fight infections. The caregiver's hand can be used to provide additional support of the chin and throat. Speech or occupational therapists can work on strengthening muscles and assisting in feeding accommodations. Other feeding problems and failure to thrive can be related to cardiac defects and usually improve after medical management is initiated or corrective surgery performed.

Children with Down syndrome do not need a special diet unless underlying gastrointestinal disease is present,

Table 30.3 Average Age of Skill Acquisition in Children With Down Syndrome

Developmental Milestone	Average Age of Acquisition, Children with Down Syndrome	Average Age of Acquisition, Typical Children
Smile	2 months	1 month
Roll over	6 months	4 months
Sit alone	9 months	7 months
Crawl	11 months	9 months
Walk	21 months	13 months
Speak words	14 months	10 months
Speak in sentences	24 months	21 months
Feed self with fingers	12 months	8 months
Use spoon	20 months	13 months
Bladder training	48 months	32 months
Bowel training	42 months	29 months
Undress	40 months	32 months
Put on clothes	58 months	47 months

Adapted from Pueschel, S. M. (2001). *A parent's guide to Down syndrome: Toward a brighter future.* Baltimore: Paul H. Brookes Publishing Company, Inc.

such as celiac disease. A balanced, high-fiber diet and regular exercise are important. Research has suggested that children with Down syndrome have lower basal metabolic rates, which can lead to problems with obesity, so it is important in the early years to develop appropriate eating habits and a regular exercise routine. High fiber intake is important for children with Down syndrome because their lack of muscle tone may decrease gastric motility, leading to constipation.

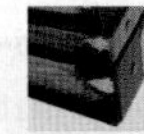

TEACHING GUIDELINE 30.1

Health Guidelines for Children With Down Syndrome

- Have your child evaluated by a pediatric cardiologist before 3 months of age, including an echocardiogram.
- Take your child for routine vision and hearing tests.
- Make sure your child gets regular medical care, including a yearly thyroid test.
- Have your child follow a regular diet and exercise routine.
- Make sure all family members perform proper hand hygiene to prevent infection.
- Monitor for signs and symptoms of respiratory infections, such as pneumonia and otitis media.
- Discuss with your pediatrician the use of pneumococcal, respiratory syncytial virus, and influenza vaccines.
- Begin early interventions, therapy, and education as soon as possible.
- Make sure your child brushes his or her teeth regularly. He or she should visit the dentist every 6 months.
- Make sure the child gets a cervical x-ray between 3 to 5 years of age to screen for atlanto-axial instability.

Providing Support and Education for the Child and Family

Down syndrome is a life-long disorder that can result in health problems and cognitive disability. The diagnosis is usually made prenatally or shortly after birth. Parents and caregivers will need support and education during this difficult time. The range of mental impairment varies from mild to moderate; severe deficits occur occasionally. Some families may see having a child with Down syndrome as a life-long tragedy; others may view it as a positive growing experience (Van Riper & Cohen, 2001). Evaluate how the family defines and manages this experience. Base the plan of care on each individual family's values, beliefs, strengths, and resources (Van Riper & Cohen, 2001).

Family members may have trouble meeting the demands of caring for a child with Down syndrome. These children have complex medical needs, which place strain on the family and its finances. From the time of diagnosis, the family should be involved in the child's care. Include parents in planning interventions and care for the child. In most cases they are the primary caregivers and will provide daily care as well as assisting the child in the development of functioning and skills. They can provide essential information to the health care team and will be advocates for their child throughout his or her life.

As the child grows, the needs of the family and child will change. Recognize and respect these needs and provide ongoing education and support for the child and family. Children with Down syndrome will need meaningful education programs. Many children with Down syndrome begin formal education in infancy and continue through high school. Full integration is recommended when possible.

The outlook is brighter than it once was for children with Down syndrome. Many go on in adulthood to obtain jobs, to receive secondary education, and to live on their own or in semi-independent housing. Be familiar with local and national resources for families of children with Down syndrome so that you can help them fulfill their potential (Box 30.5).

ConsiderTHIS!

Charles Faust, a 10-month-old with Down syndrome, is seen in the clinic for a well-child examination. The parents have questions about his growth and development. They are concerned because Charles can't pick up finger foods such as Cheerios and put them in his mouth.

How would you address their concerns?

Discuss ways the family can encourage Charles's growth and development.

In addition to usual well-child care, what other medical management will you want to discuss with the family to prevent complications associated with Down syndrome?

BOX 30.5

RESOURCES FOR FAMILIES OF CHILDREN WITH DOWN SYNDROME

- March of Dimes, 1275 Mamaroneck Avenue, White Plains, NY 10605
  1-888-MODIMES (1-888-663-4637)
  http://www.marchofdimes.com/
- National Association for Down Syndrome, P.O. Box 206, Wilmette, IL 60091
  1-630-325-9112
  http://www.nads.org/
- National Down Syndrome Congress, 1370 Center Drive, Suite 102, Atlanta, GA 30338
  1-800-232-6372
  http://www.ndsccenter.org
- National Down Syndrome Society, 666 Broadway, New York, NY 10012
  1-800-221-4602
  http://www.ndss.org/
- Canadian Down Syndrome Society, 811- 14 Street NW, Calgary, Alberta T2N 2A4
  1-800-883-5608
  http://www.cdss.ca

• TRISOMY 18 AND TRISOMY 13

Trisomy 18 (also known as Edwards syndrome) and trisomy 13 (also known as Patau syndrome) are two other common trisomies. The incidence of trisomy 18 (the presence of three number 18 chromosomes) is 1 in 6,000 births; the incidence of trisomy 13 (the presence of three number 13 chromosomes) is 1 in 10,000 births (Behrman et al., 2004). As in Down syndrome, they usually result from nondisjunction (failure of a chromosome pair to separate) during cell division. Trisomy 18 and trisomy 13 can be present in all cells or may occur in mosaic forms. Both are associated with a characteristic set of anomalies and mental retardation.

The prognosis for trisomy 18 and trisomy 13 is usually poor; these children usually do not survive beyond the first year of life. There is no cure for trisomy 18 or trisomy 13. Therapeutic management will focus on managing the various congenital anomalies and health issues associated with the disorders.

Nursing Assessment

Nursing assessment will include a general observation for characteristic anomalies (Table 30.4 and Figs. 30.9 and 30.10).

Prenatal screening and diagnostic tests for trisomy 18 and 13 exist. If not diagnosed during the prenatal period, most cases are diagnosed in the first few days of life based on the physical characteristics associated with the disorders.

Nursing Management

Nursing management will be mainly supportive. This will be a difficult time for the family, so providing support and resources for the family will be an important nursing function. SOFT is a support organization for families who have had a child with a chromosome abnormality; they can be reached at http://www.trisomy.org/; 2982 South Union Street, Rochester, NY 14624; (800) 716-SOFT (7638).

• TURNER SYNDROME

Turner syndrome is a common abnormality of the sex chromosome. The phenotype is female. It occurs in about 1 in 4,000 live female births (Behrman et al., 2004). Affected fetuses are often aborted spontaneously. The abnormality is due to a loss of all or part of one of the sex chromosomes. About half of the affected individuals have only one X chromosome; the other half have a variety of abnormalities of one of their sex chromosomes and may present with the mosaic form. In about 5% to 10% of cases of Turner syndrome the individual presents with some Y chromosome material in some or all of her cells. These females may present with some masculinization. The risk of recurrence in future pregnancies is not

Table 30.4 Clinical Manifestations of Trisomy 18 and Trisomy 13

Chromosomal Abnormality	Clinical Manifestations
Trisomy 18	Prominent occiput, low-set ears, short eyelid fissures, severe mental retardation, severe hypotonia, webbing, clenched fist with index finger over third digit and fifth digit overlapping the fourth, hypoplasia of fingernails, narrow hips with limited abduction, short sternum, congenital cardiac defects
Trisomy 13	Microcephalic head, wide sagittal suture and fontanels, malformed ears, small eyes, extra digits, severe hypotonia, severe mental retardation, congenital heart defects, cleft lip, cleft palate

increased, as Turner syndrome appears to be a sporadic event.

There is no cure for Turner syndrome. Therapeutic management will focus on managing the health issues associated with the syndrome. Children with Turner syndrome are more prone to cardiovascular problems, kidney and thyroid problems, skeletal disorders such as scoliosis and osteoporosis, hearing and eye disturbances, and obesity. They have normal intelligence, although 70% have some learning disability (Sybert & McCauley, 2004). Infertility is usually present, but some women with mosaic Turner syndrome may be fertile. Growth hormone administration is a standard of care and usually begins when the child's height falls below the fifth percentile for healthy girls. Hormone replacement therapy may also be given to initiate puberty and complete growth.

Nursing Assessment

On assessment, note patterns of growth; short stature and slow growth will be a characteristic finding and often the first indication. Other physical characteristics include a webbed neck, low posterior hairline, wide-spaced nipples, edema of the hands and feet, amenorrhea, no development of secondary sex characteristics, sterility, and perceptual and social skill difficulties (Fig. 30.11).

Turner syndrome can be suspected prenatally by ultrasound findings such as fetal edema or redundant nuchal skin or by abnormal results of the triple screen. It can be diagnosed by chromosomal analysis, either prenatally or after birth. Most children are diagnosed at birth or in early childhood when slow growth or growth failure is noted.

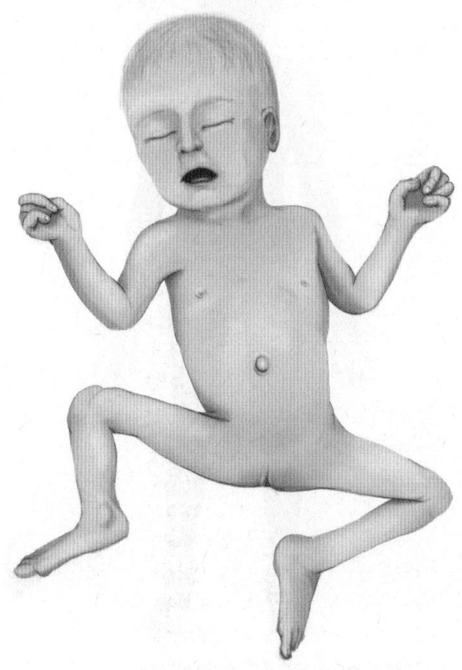

● **Figure 30.9** Trisomy 18.

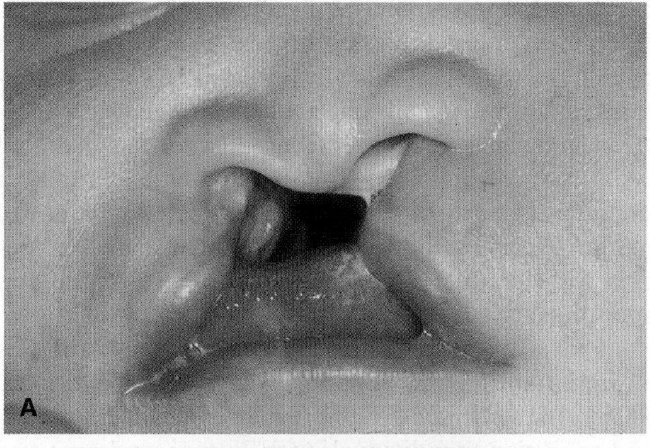

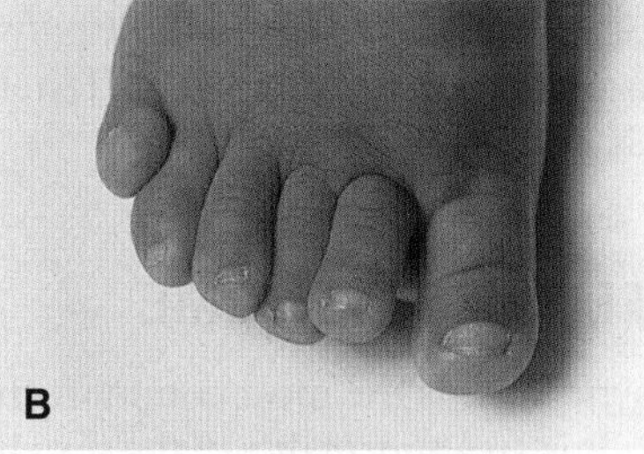

● **Figure 30.10** Trisomy 13.

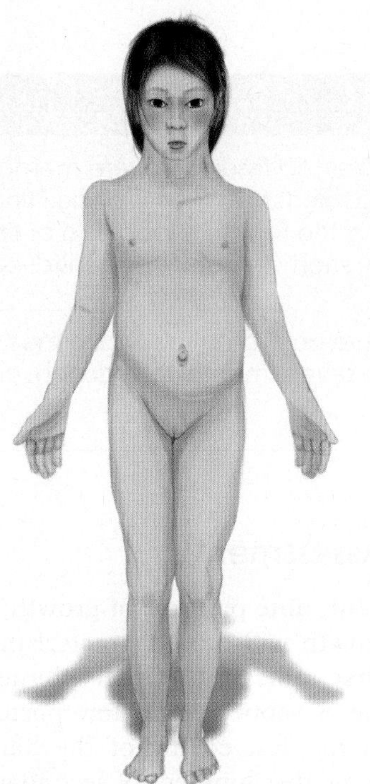

● Figure 30.11 Note the webbed neck of the child with Turner syndrome.

Some cases will not be diagnosed until the pubertal growth spurt does not occur.

Nursing Management

Nursing management is mainly supportive. Provide education and support to the family; they need to understand that short stature and infertility are likely. Explain that mental retardation is unlikely, but some learning disabilities may be present. Emphasize that with medical supervision and support, girls with Turner syndrome may lead healthy, satisfying lives. Counseling about infertility is important. Parents may be upset that their daughter will not be able to reproduce, so explain that many alternatives for reproduction, such as in vitro fertilization and adoption, are available.

Providing support and resources for the family is an important nursing function. The Turner Syndrome Society of the United States provides assistance, support, and education to individuals with Turner syndrome and their families and can be accessed at http://www.turner-syndrome-us.org/about/ or 14450 T. C. Jester, Suite 260, Houston, TX 77014, (800) 365-9944.

• KLINEFELTER SYNDROME

Klinefelter syndrome is the most common chromosomal abnormality. It is an abnormality of the sex chromosome: the karyotype and phenotype are male, but one or more extra X chromosomes is present. The abnormality is usually caused by nondisjunction during meiosis, but mosaic forms do present. The incidence of Klinefelter syndrome is 1 in 1,000 males (Wattendorf & Muenke, 2005). Males present with some female-like physical features that are caused by testosterone deficiency. The risk of recurrence in future pregnancies in not increased.

There is no cure for Klinefelter syndrome. Therapeutic management will focus on interventions to enhance masculine characteristics, such as testosterone replacement. Early recognition and hormonal treatment are important to improve quality of life and prevent serious consequences. Cosmetic surgery may be performed to minimize female characteristics such as gynecomastia (increased breast size).

Nursing Assessment

Due to nonspecific findings during childhood, the diagnosis is not usually made until adolescence or adulthood. Prenatal diagnosis is rare unless amniocentesis was performed for genetic testing. Many males with Klinefelter syndrome go through life without being diagnosed. The diagnosis is confirmed by chromosomal analysis.

On assessment, lack of development of secondary sex characteristics may be found. The individual may have decreased facial hair, gynecomastia, decreased pubic hair, and hypogonadism or underdeveloped testes, which leads to infertility. The individual may be taller than average by 5 years of age, with long legs and a short torso (Fig. 30.12).

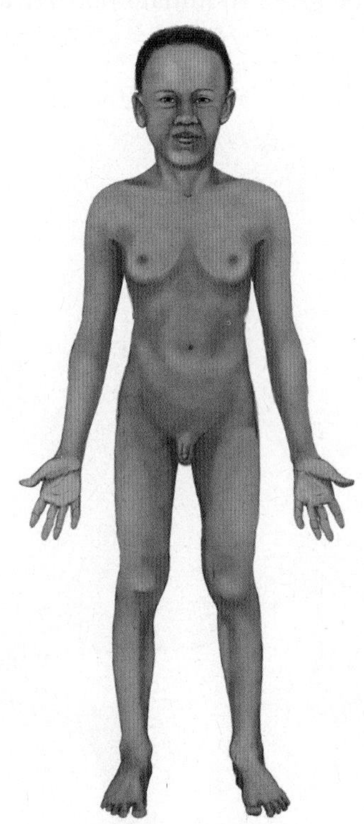

● Figure 30.12 Klinefelter syndrome.

Mental retardation is not present, but cognitive impairments of varying degree, such as motor delay, speech or language difficulties, attention deficits, and learning disabilities, may be found.

Nursing Management

Nursing management will be mainly supportive. Provide education and support to the family. The American Association for Klinefelter Syndrome Information & Support can be accessed at http://www.aaksis.org or at 1-888-466-KSIS, the Klinefelter Syndrome Support Group at http://klinefeltersyndrome.org/, or Klinefelter Syndrome and Associates at http://genetic.org/ks/.

Counseling about infertility is important. Educate patients and families that marriage and sexual relations are possible. Parents may be upset that their son will not be able to reproduce, so explain that many alternatives for reproduction are available and technology is advancing in the field of infertility.

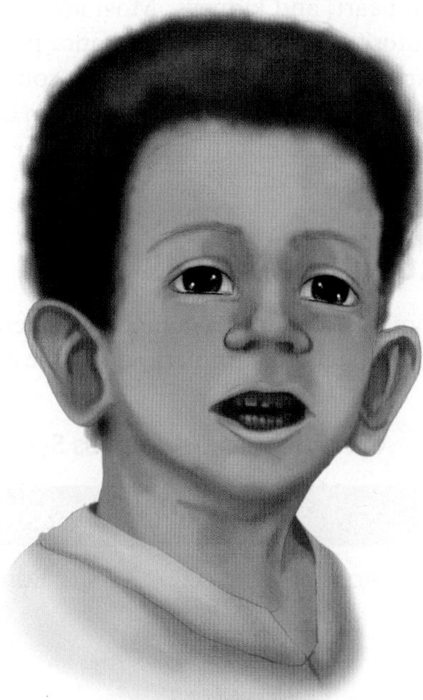

● Figure 30.13 Fragile X syndrome.

● FRAGILE X SYNDROME

Fragile X syndrome is the most common inherited cause of mental retardation. It is the outcome of a mutation of a gene (FMR1 [fragile X mental retardation]) on the X chromosome. This mutation essentially "turns off" the gene, triggering fragile X syndrome. The exact number of children affected by the mutation or premutation is not known. Males and females are both affected, but females usually have milder symptoms. The inheritance of fragile X is complex and is less straightforward than single-gene or Mendelian inheritance. Some carrier females are affected, and not all males with the gene abnormality show symptoms. Males and females are both fertile and can transmit the disorder to their offspring, so genetic counseling is appropriate. The prognosis for individuals with fragile X is good, and they tend to live a normal life span.

There is no cure for fragile X syndrome. Therapeutic management will be multidisciplinary and aimed at interventions to improve cognitive, emotional, and behavioral impairments.

Nursing Assessment

During childhood, clinical manifestations are subtle, with minor dysmorphic features and developmental delay. Problems with sensation, emotion, and behavior often are the first signs. A delay in attaining developmental milestones will most likely be the first clue found on assessment. Intellectual impairment can range from subtle learning disabilities to severe mental retardation and autistic-like behaviors. In adolescence, boys tend to present with characteristic features such as an elongated face, prominent jaw, large, protruding ears, large size, macroorchidism (large testes), and a range of behavioral abnormalities and cognitive deficits (Fig. 30.13). There is a characteristic pattern to the cognitive deficits, with problems in abstract reasoning, sequential processing, and mathematics. Typical behavior problems include attention deficits, hand flapping and biting, hyperactivity, shyness, social isolation, low self-esteem, and gaze aversion. In females the clinical manifestations are similar but are more varied and often present in a milder form.

The average age at diagnosis is 8 years. Diagnosis is confirmed by molecular genetic testing. Fragile X can be diagnosed prenatally if inheritance is suspected.

Nursing Management

Nursing management will be mainly supportive. Early diagnosis and intervention with developmental therapies and an individualized education plan are ideal. Care of these children will be the same as care of other children with mental retardation (see Chapter 31 for further information on mental retardation).

Provide education and support to the family. The National Fragile X Foundation provides education and emotional support and works to increase awareness and advance research for fragile X (http://www.fragilex.org/).

Neurocutaneous Disorders

Neurocutaneous disorders, also referred to as hamartoses, are a group of disorders characterized by abnormalities of both the skin and the central nervous system. Many neurologic conditions are associated with cutaneous manifestations, since the skin and the nervous system share a common embryologic origin. They are complex conditions and most also affect other organ systems such as eyes, bones, heart, and kidneys. Most are hereditary and follow an autosomal dominant inheritance pattern or sporadic occurrence. Neurofibromatosis is a common neurocutaneous syndrome and will be discussed in detail below. Table 30.5 provides information on other neurocutaneous syndromes.

NEUROFIBROMATOSIS

Neurofibromatoses are neurocutaneous genetic disorders of the nervous system that primarily affect the development and growth of neural cell tissues. There are two distinct types: neurofibromatosis 1 and neurofibromatosis 2. Neurofibromatosis 1 (von Recklinghausen disease) is the more common type. This disorder causes tumors to grow on nerves and produce other abnormalities such as skin changes and bone deformities. Complications associated with neurofibromatosis include scoliosis, cardiac defects, hypertension, seizures, vision and hearing loss, learning disabilities, attention deficit disorder, abnormalities of speech, and a higher risk for neoplasms. In lay circles this is often referred to as "Elephant Man"

Table 30.5 Other Neurocutaneous Syndromes

Disorder	Incidence	Clinical Manifestations	Nursing Considerations
Tuberous sclerosis	1 in 6,000 (Behrman et al., 2004)	Benign tumors present in the brain and skin. Presents most often as a generalized seizure disorder. Tumors can also involve heart, kidney, eyes, lung, and bones. Developmental delay and behavioral problems may be noted. Usually evident in early childhood. Wide clinical spectrum from severe mental retardation with incapacitating seizures to normal intelligence and no seizures.	Treatment will be mainly symptomatic. Seizure control will be a primary concern. Provide support and education to the family. Referral for genetic counseling (it follows an autosomal dominant inheritance pattern and half the cases are due to a new mutation) and appropriate resources. www.tsalliance.org: Tuberous Sclerosis Alliance
Sturge-Weber syndrome	1 in 50,000 (Behrman et al., 2004)	Facial nevus (port wine stain) most often seen on the forehead and on one side of the face, seizures, hemiparesis, intracranial calcifications. In many cases mental retardation, behavioral and emotional problems, and learning disabilities are present. Seizures usually begin in infancy and may worsen with age. Convulsions are usually noted on the side of the body opposite the facial nevus. Muscle weakness may be present on the same side. Most affected individuals have glaucoma at birth or will develop it later in life.	Treatment will be mainly symptomatic. Seizure control will be a primary concern (use of anticonvulsants or surgery). Seizures due to Sturge-Weber are often difficult to control. Laser treatment may be used to lighten or remove the facial nevus. Surgery may be performed on more serious cases of glaucoma. Physical therapy should be considered for infants and children with muscle weakness. Educational therapy is often prescribed for those with mental retardation or developmental delays. Provide support and education to the family. Refer to appropriate resources. Genetic counseling may be appropriate (inheritance is unclear and sporadic). www.sturge-weber.com: Sturge-Weber Foundation

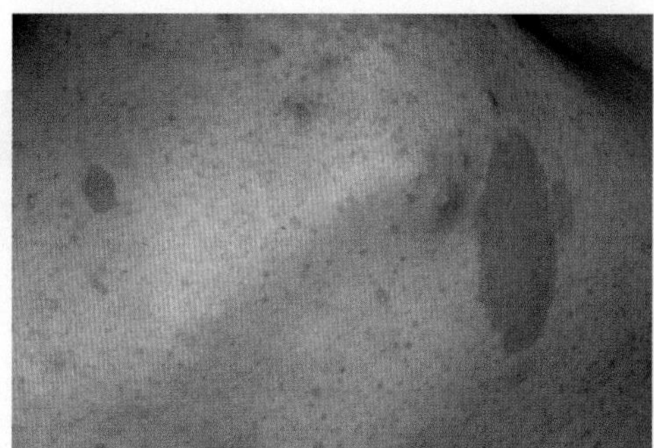

● Figure 30.14 Café-au-lait spots associated with neurofibromatosis.

disease, but health care providers should avoid this term. Many assume that the disease will result in horrible disfigurement, but in reality most patients present with fairly mild disease.

Although many affected persons inherit the disorder, nearly half of the cases are due to a new mutation. The inheritance pattern is autosomal dominant; therefore, offspring of affected individuals have a 50% chance of inheriting the altered gene and presenting with symptoms. Neurofibromatoses are due to a mutation of the neurofibromin gene on chromosome 17. The estimated prevalence is 1 in 3,000 live births (Behrman et al., 2004; Jones, 2006).

There is no cure for neurofibromatosis. Therapeutic management is aimed at controlling symptoms. Surgical intervention can help reduce some of the bone malformations and remove painful or disfiguring tumors. The American Academy of Pediatrics recommends that these children have a yearly physical, including blood pressure, scoliosis screening, and an ophthalmology examination, developmental screening, and a neurologic examination (Behrman et al., 2004).

The disease is progressive and symptoms usually worsen over time, but it is difficult to predict the course. Most affected individuals develop mild to moderate symptoms, with non-life-threatening complications, and live a normal, productive life.

Nursing Assessment

On assessment the nurse may find café-au-lait spots (light-brown macules), which are the hallmark of neurofibromatosis (Fig. 30.14). These are usually present at birth but can appear during the first year of life and usually increase in size, number, and pigmentation. They are present all over the body, particularly the trunk and extremities, while usually sparing the face. Pigmented nevi, axillary freckling, slow-growing cutaneous, subcutaneous, or dermal neurofibromas, which are benign tumors, are other signs of neurofibromatosis. Many children with neurofibromatosis have larger-than-normal head circumference and are shorter than average. Enough features are usually present by 6 years of age to make a diagnosis. The severity of symptoms varies greatly, but the diagnosis is made if two or more of the clinical signs in Box 30.6 are present.

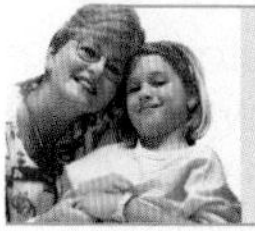

If more than six café-au-lait spots are present, neurofibromatosis should be suspected.

Nursing Management

Nursing management will be mainly supportive. Early detection of treatable conditions and complications is a priority. Provide support and education to the child and family. Discuss genetic counseling with the family. Referral to appropriate resources is essential. The Children's Tumor Foundation can be accessed at http:// www.ctf.org/ or 95 Pine Street, 16th Floor, New York, NY 10005, (800) 323-7938. Neurofibromatosis, Inc. can be accessed at http://www.nfinc.org/ or P.O. Box 18246, Minneapolis, MN 55418, (800) 942-6825.

Other Genetic Disorders

Thousands of genetic disorders are known, and new ones are being discovered, but most of them are rare. Table 30.6 lists other genetic disorders that the pediatric nurse may encounter. Nursing management of these disorders will be mainly supportive and will focus on providing support and

(text continues on page 1038)

BOX 30.6

CLINICAL SIGNS OF NEUROFIBROMATOSIS

Diagnosis is made if two or more of the following are present:

- Six or more café-au-lait macules (light brown spots) >5 mm in diameter in children and >15 mm in diameter in adolescents and adults
- Two or more neurofibromas (benign tumors) or one plexiform neurofibroma (tumor that involves many nerves)
- Freckling in the armpit or groin
- Presence of an optic glioma (a tumor on the optic nerve)
- Two or more growths on the iris of the eye (Lisch nodules or iris hamartomas)
- Abnormal development of the spine (scoliosis), the temple bone of the skull, or the tibia
- A first-degree relative (parent, sibling, or child) with neurofibromatosis 1

Table 30.6 Other Genetic Disorders, Syndromes, and Associations

Disorder	Inheritance/Cause	Signs and Symptoms	Management
CHARGE syndrome (a recognizable pattern of congenital anomalies seen) **C: C**oloboma **H: H**eart disease **A: A**tresia (choanal) **R: R**etarded growth and development and/or CNS anomalies **G: G**enital anomalies, hypogonadism **E: E**ar anomalies and deafness Incidence is 1 in 10,000 to 12,000 (Griffin et al., 2004).	Autosomal dominant inheritance; most cases are due to new mutation of the gene. Mutations in the gene CDH7 have been indicated in some cases.	Coloboma is a lesion or defect of the eye, usually a fissure or cleft in the iris, ciliary, or choroid; can also see microphthalmos (small eyes) and cryptophthalmos (absent eye). Can lead to vision impairments. Heart anomaly can include any type but most common are aortic arch anomalies and tetralogy of Fallot. Atresia (choanal) is blocked or narrowed passages from the nose to the throat, which can lead to aspiration. Retarded growth or cognitive development can range from mild to severe. Genital anomaly may include micropenis, undescended testes, and hypoplastic labia. Ear anomalies include short, wide ears with little or no lobe, prominent inner fold, floppy appearance, asymmetry; can have hearing impairment. Each feature occurs in a spectrum from absent to severe; no single feature is present in all individuals.	Focus is on identifying and treating all defects; early diagnosis is important. www.chargesyndrome.org: CHARGE Syndrome Foundation
Marfan syndrome: disorder of connective tissue Incidence is 1 in 5,000 to 10,000 (Behrman et al., 2004).	Autosomal dominant inheritance; caused by a mutation in the gene fibrillin-1, which results in changes in connective tissue	Tall stature with long slim limbs, minimal subcutaneous fat, muscle hypotonia, loose joints, long and narrow face, abnormalities of skeletal system (e.g., pectus excavatum (funnel chest) or pectus carinatum (pigeon breast)), ocular system (e.g., enlarged cornea or lens subluxation), and cardiovascular system (e.g., dilation of the aorta or mitral valve prolapse). Delayed achievement of gross and fine motor milestones may occur.	Focus is on preventing complications. www.marfan.org: National Marfan Foundation www.marfan.ca: Canadian Marfan Association

Table 30.6 Other Genetic Disorders, Syndromes, and Associations (continued)

Disorder	Inheritance/Cause	Signs and Symptoms	Management
VATER association (not a diagnosis, but refers to a non-random association of defects found to occur together) **V: V**ertebral defects **A: A**nal atresia **TE:** Tracheoesophageal fistula with esophageal atresia **R**adial and **R**enal dysplasia May also occur as VACTERL association, with **C: C**ardiac anomalies **L: L**imb abnormalities added	Sporadic inheritance. Cause is unknown. Can occur with other chromosomal abnormalities such as trisomy 18. Frequently seen in the offspring of diabetic mothers.	3 or more anomalies are present. Anomalies seen include hypoplastic (small) vertebrae or hemivertebra (only half the bones are formed). These anomalies lead to an increased risk of scoliosis. With imperforate anus or anal atresia, the anus does not open to the outside of the body. Incomplete formation of one or more kidneys, obstruction of urine flow out of kidneys, or severe reflux back into kidneys can all lead to kidney failure later in life. Cardiac anomalies: most common are ventricular septal defects, atrial septal defects, and tetralogy of Fallot. Absent or displaced thumb, polydactyly (extra digits), syndactyly (fusion of digits). A single umbilical artery at birth is often present. Failure to thrive and slow development in early infancy due to anomalies. Usually normal intelligence.	Focus is on identifying and treating all defects. www.tefvater.org: TEF VATER National Support Network
Apert syndrome (named for the French physician who described the syndrome) Incidence is 1 in 65,000 live births (Jones, 2006).	Autosomal dominant inheritance. Cases are sporadic and have been associated with older paternal age.	Craniosynostosis, bilateral symmetrical syndactyly, and craniofacial anomalies such as prominent forehead, midface hypoplasia resulting in sunken appearance, short anteroposterior diameter, down-slanting eyelids. Small nasopharynx can lead to upper airway obstruction and sleep apnea. Learning disabilities and mental deficiency.	Early surgery for craniosynostosis when increased intracranial pressure is noted. Vigorous early management should occur with a multidisciplinary approach to address multiple anomalies. www.aboutfaceusa.org: About Face USA www.ccakids.com: Children's Craniofacial Association www.faceit.org: Let's Face It, Inc. www.faces-cranio.org: National Craniofacial Association www.nffr.org: National Foundation for Facial Reconstruction

(continued)

Table 30.6 Other Genetic Disorders, Syndromes, and Associations (continued)

Disorder	Inheritance/Cause	Signs and Symptoms	Management
Achondroplasia (most common chondrodysplasia (diseases resulting in disordered growth)) Incidence is 1 in 15,000 (Jones, 2006).	Autosomal dominant inheritance pattern. Caused by mutations in fibroblast growth factor receptor 3 (FGFR3). 90% new gene mutation. Older paternal age may be a contributing factor.	Characterized by abnormal body proportion. Small stature (average adult height is 4 feet for both men and women), short limbs with normal-size torso, low nasal bridge with prominent forehead. Midface hypoplasia, caudal narrowing of spinal canal, megalocephaly, small foramen magnum; hands are short and stubby with separation between middle and ring finger ("trident hand"). Delayed motor skills, problems with persistent middle ear dysfunction and infections, and bowing of lower legs. Less common complications include hydrocephalus, craniocervical junction compression, upper airway obstruction, and thoracolumbar kyphosis. Usually present with normal intelligence and lead independent, productive lives.	Medical management of symptoms. Monitor height, weight, and head circumference. Manage and prevent complications (careful and thorough neurologic exam, assessment for sleep apnea). Growth hormone therapy is controversial and still experimental. Limb-lengthening surgeries may be performed. www.lpaonline.org: Little People of America, Inc. www.shortsupport.org: Short Persons Support

education to the family and child, with an emphasis on developmental and educational needs. Referral to genetic counseling and appropriate resources is an important nursing function.

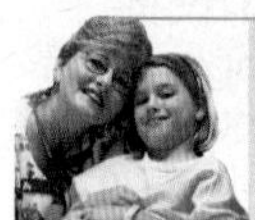

Children with VATER syndrome who have only one kidney should not play contact sports.

Inborn Errors of Metabolism

Inborn errors of metabolism are a group of hereditary disorders. They are collectively common but individually rare. Most follow an autosomal recessive inheritance pattern. They are caused by gene mutations that result in abnormalities in the synthesis or catabolism of proteins, carbohydrates, or fats. The body cannot convert food into energy as it normally would. Most inborn errors are due to a defect in an enzyme or transport protein that results in a block in the metabolic pathway. The blocked metabolic pathway allows for accumulation of the damaging byproduct of the impaired metabolic process or may be responsible for a deficiency or absence of a necessary product. Presentation can occur at any time, even in adulthood, but many affected individuals exhibit signs in the newborn period or shortly after. Most inborn errors of metabolism presenting in the neonatal period are lethal if specific treatment is not initiated immediately.

Newborn screening is used to detect these disorders before symptoms develop. Recent developments in screening techniques (tandem mass spectrometry) allow dozens of metabolic disorders to be detected from a single drop of blood. A child who tests positive will require additional testing to confirm the diagnosis (see Chapter 9 for more information on newborn screening).

Therapeutic management of these disorders varies depending on the cause of the error of metabolism, but dietary management is often a key component.

Nursing Assessment

Clinical signs and symptoms vary with each disorder. Table 30.7 gives information on some common inborn errors of metabolism seen in children.

Table 30.7 Inborn Errors of Metabolism

Disorder/Explanation	Incidence*	Clinical Manifestations	Management
Phenylketonuria (PKU): deficiency in a liver enzyme leading to inability to process the essential amino acid phenylalanine properly. Phenylalanine accumulation can lead to brain damage unless PKU is detected soon after birth and treated.	>1 in 25,000	No symptoms at birth. Most cases are identified before symptoms are present due to newborn screening (PKU is screened for in all states). If undiagnosed, newborn may present with vomiting, irritability, eczema-like rash, and mousy odor to urine.	Low-phenylalanine diet. Phenylalanine is found mostly in protein-containing foods such as meat and milk (including breast milk and formula). www.pkunetwork.org: Children's PKU Network www.pku-allieddisorders.org: National Coalition for PKU & Allied Disorders www.pkunews.org: National PKU News
Galactosemia: deficiency in the liver enzyme needed to convert galactose, the breakdown product of lactose, which is commonly found in dairy products, into glucose. Galactose accumulation leads to damage to vital organs.	>1 in 50,000	No symptoms at birth. If undiagnosed, newborn will have jaundice, diarrhea, and vomiting and will not gain weight. If untreated, can lead to liver disease, blindness, severe mental retardation, and death.	Ingestion of galactose can produce sepsis in an affected child; therefore, septic workup and antibiotics may be necessary in a child if galactose ingestion has occurred. Elimination of galactose and lactose from the diet is the only treatment. Therefore, milk and dairy products will be eliminated for life. www.galactosemia.org: Parents of Galactosemic Children
Maple sugar urine disease: affects the metabolism of amino acids. A deficiency in the enzyme that metabolizes leucine, isoleucine, and valine, which are components of protein often referred to as the branch chain amino acids. These amino acids then accumulate in the blood and cause damage to the brain.	<1 in 100,000	No symptoms at birth, but if untreated newborns soon begin to show neurologic signs, vomiting, poor feeding, increased reflex action, and seizures. If untreated, can lead to life-threatening neurologic damage.	Special low-protein diet, will vary based on severity of symptoms. Thiamine supplements may be given. Diet must be continued throughout life. www.msud-support.org: Maple Syrup Urine Disease Family Support Group

(continued)

Table 30.7 Inborn Errors of Metabolism (continued)

Disorder/Explanation	Incidence*	Clinical Manifestations	Management
Biotinidase deficiency: lack of the enzyme biotinidase results in biotin deficiency	>1 in 75,000	No symptoms at birth; in first weeks or months of life, symptoms such as hypotonia, uncoordinated movement, seizures, developmental delay, alopecia, seborrheic dermatitis, hearing loss, optic nerve atrophy, and mental retardation develop. Metabolic acidosis can lead to death.	Daily oral free biotin www.kumc.edu/gec/support/metaboli.html: Association for Neuro-Metabolic Diseases
Medium-chain acyl-CoA dehydrogenase deficiency (MCAD): lack of an enzyme required to metabolize fatty acids	>1 in 25,000	Recurrent episodes of metabolic acidosis and hypoglycemia, lethargy, seizures, liver failure, brain damage, coma, and cardiac arrest. Can lead to serious and fatal illness in children not eating well.	Avoid fasting; have frequent meals. Special considerations during illness. If unable to tolerate food, IV dextrose is required. www.fodsupport.org: Fatty Oxidation Disorders (FOD) Family Support Group
Homocystinuria: deficiency in the enzyme needed to digest a component of food called methionine (an amino acid)	<1 in 100,000	If undetected and untreated can lead to mental retardation, psychiatric disturbances, developmental delays, displacement of the lens of the eye, abnormal thinning and weakness of bones, and formation of thrombi in veins and arteries that can lead to life-threatening complications such as stroke.	Methionine-restricted diet and cystine supplements; vitamin B6 and B12 supplements and possibly other supplements, such as betaine and folic acid. www.rarediseases.org: National Organization for Rare Disorders
Tyrosinemia: deficiency in an enzyme essential in the metabolism of tyrosine; accumulation of the byproducts results in liver and kidney damage	<1 in 100,000	Symptoms usually appear in the first months of life: poor weight gain, enlarged liver and spleen, increased bleeding tendency, distended abdomen, jaundice, cirrhosis, and liver failure.	Diet low in phenylalanine, methionine, and tyrosine. www.liverfoundation.org: American Liver Foundation

Table 30.7 Inborn Errors of Metabolism (continued)

Disorder/Explanation	Incidence*	Clinical Manifestations	Management
Tay-Sachs: caused by insufficient activity of an enzyme called hexosaminidase A, which is necessary for the breakdown of certain fatty substances in brain and nerve cells	Occurs more frequently among persons of Central and Eastern European and Ashkenazi Jewish descent. ~1 in every 27 Jews is a carrier, whereas in the general population 1 in 250 people is a carrier (National Human Genome Research Institute, 2007). Non-Jewish French Canadians from the East St. Lawrence River Valley of Quebec and members of the Cajun population in Louisiana are also at an increased risk. These groups have about a 100 times higher incidence than other ethnic groups (March of Dimes, 2006*b*).	Infants appear normal and healthy for the first few months of life. Then, as harmful quantities of the fatty substances (called gangliosides) build up in tissues and nerve cells and cause damage, mental and physical deterioration occurs. The child becomes blind, deaf, and unable to swallow; muscles begin to atrophy; and paralysis sets in. Dementia, seizures, and an increased startle reflex may be seen. There is a late-onset type of Tay-Sachs seen in persons in their 20s and early 30s, but this is much rarer.	No treatment or cure. Medical management will focus on managing symptoms and maintaining comfort. Anticonvulsants may be given to control seizures. Death usually occurs in early childhood, by age 4 or 5. Carriers can be identified by a blood test and prenatal testing is available. www.ntsad.org: National Tay-Sachs & Allied Diseases Association

*Incidence data from March of Dimes (2006*c*). *Recommended newborn screening tests: 29 disorders.* Retrieved on March 1, 2006, from http://www.marchofdimes.com/professionals/14332_15455.asp.

Saving Babies through Screening Foundation, Inc. (2005). *Disease description.* Retrieved on March 1, 2006, at http://www.savebabies.org/diseasedescriptions.php

Because of newborn screening and early identification and management, it is rare to see an untreated newborn with clinical signs and symptoms of the disease. If seen, in many cases a newborn who was healthy at birth will present with lethargy, poor feeding, apnea or tachypnea, recurrent vomiting, altered consciousness, failure to thrive, seizures, septic appearance, or developmental delay. Physical changes that may be seen include dysmorphology, cardiomegaly, rashes, cataracts, retinitis, optic atrophy, corneal opacity, deafness, skeletal dysplasia, macrocephaly, hepatomegaly, jaundice, or cirrhosis.

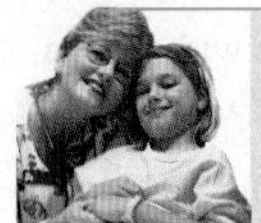

When a previously healthy newborn presents with a history of deterioration, an inborn error of metabolism should be suspected.

The diagnostic workup usually requires a variety of specific laboratory studies and may include:

- Glucose: may be elevated
- Ammonia: may be elevated
- Blood gases: may have low bicarbonate and low pH, metabolic acidosis (respiratory alkalosis may also be seen, especially when high ammonia levels are present)

Early diagnosis is the key to saving and improving the lives of these children.

When a child who has previously been diagnosed with an inborn error of metabolism is hospitalized, the nurse must determine the prescribed diet and medications so these may be continued while in the hospital setting.

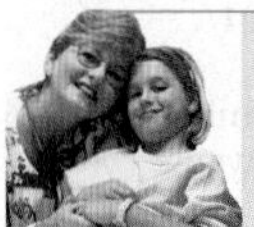

If an inborn error of metabolism is suspected, feedings will usually be stopped until the test results are received.

Nursing Management

Ensure that the diet prescribed for the infant or child is followed. For amino acid disorders (e.g., phenylketonuria [PKU]), urea cycle defects (e.g., tyrosinemia type I), and organic acidemia (e.g., maple syrup urine disease), nutritional therapy is the major intervention. Dietary intake of specific amino acids is restricted according to the disorder. Ensure that overall protein and calorie needs are still met, as children need sufficient calories for proper growth. In children with urea cycle defects and organic acidemia, anorexia is common and severe, and the child may need gastrostomy tube feeding supplementation. In fatty acid oxidation disorders (e.g., medium-chain acyl-CoA dehydrogenase deficiency), the goal is to avoid prolonged periods of fasting and to provide frequent feeds when the child is sick. Supplementation with specific vitamins may also be important in the treatment of these disorders. Strict adherence to the diet is necessary and will require close supervision by registered dietitians, physicians, and nurses and the cooperation of both the parent and child.

Nursing management will focus on education and support for the family, who will need thorough knowledge about the child's disease and management. Referral to a dietitian and appropriate resources, including support groups, will be important. The nurse should also monitor the child's developmental progress and begin therapies as soon as a concern arises.

References

Books and Journals

Ackley, B. J., & Ladwig, G. B. (2006). *Nursing diagnosis handbook: A guide to planning care.* (7th ed.). St. Louis: Mosby.

American Academy of Pediatrics, Committee on Genetics. (1996). Newborn screening fact sheet. *Pediatrics, 98*(3), 473–501.

American Academy of Pediatrics, Committee on Genetics. (2001). Health supervision for children with Down syndrome. *Pediatrics, 107*(2), 442–449.

Behrman, R. E., Kliegman, R. M., & Jenson, H. B. (2004). *Nelson's textbook of pediatrics* (17th ed.). Philadelphia: Saunders.

Blacher, J. (2003). Recent news about fragile X: What's all the fuss about? *The Exceptional Parent, 33*(4), 70–75.

CHARGE Syndrome Foundation. (2006). *About CHARGE.* Retrieved July 22, 2006, from http://www.chargesyndrome.org/about-charge.asp.

Cohen, W. (1999). Health care guidelines for individuals with Down syndrome: 1999 revision [Reprinted from *Down Syndrome Quarterly, 4*(3)]. Retrieved July 22, 2006, from http://www.denison.edu/collaborations/dsq/health99.html.

Cunniff, C., Hersh, J. H., Hoyme, H. E., et al. (2003). Health supervision for children with Turner's syndrome. *Pediatrics, 111*(3), 692–703.

Griffin, H. C., Davis, M. L., & Williams, S. C. (2004). CHARGE Syndrome: Educational and technological interventions. *RE:view: Rehabilitation and Education for Blindness and Visual Impairment, 35*(4), 149–158. Retrieved July 22, 2006, from www.findarticles.com/p/articles/mi_hb4327/is_200401/ai_n15081011.

Groch, J. (2006). Sleep apnea tests advised for Down's children. *Medpage Today.* Retrieved July 22, 2006, from http://www.medpagetoday.com/tbindex2.cfm?tbid=3111.

Human Genome Project. (2004). *Ethical, legal, and social issues research.* Retrieved July 22, 2006, from http://www.ornl.gov/sci/techresources/Human_Genome/research/elsi.shtml.

Human Genome Project. (2006). *Human Genome Project information.* Retrieved July 22, 2006, from http://www.ornl.gov/sci/techresources/Human_Genome/home.shtml.

Johnson, M., & Robin, N. H. (2000). Pediatrics and the human genome project. *Contemporary Pediatrics, 17*(5), 100–112.

Jones, K. L. (2006). *Smith's recognizable patterns of human malformation* (6th ed.). Philadelphia: Elsevier Saunders.

Kam, J. R., & Helm, T. N. (2005). Neurofibromatosis. *eMedicine.* Retrieved July 22, 2006, from http://www.emedicine.com/DERM/topic287.htm.

Keku, T. O., Rakhra-Burris, T., & Millikan, R. (2003). Gene testing: What the health professional needs to know. *Journal of Nutrition, 133,* 3754S–3757S.

Korson, M. S. (2000). Advances in newborn screening for metabolic disorders: What the pediatrician needs to know. *Pediatric Annals, 29*(5), 294–301.

Lashley, F. R. (2005). *Clinical genetics in nursing practice.* New York: Springer Publishing.

March of Dimes. (2006*a*). *Quick reference and fact sheet: Chromosomal abnormalities.* Retrieved July 22, 2006, from www.marchofdimes.com/professionals/681_1209.asp.

March of Dimes. (2006*b*). *Quick reference and fact sheet: Tay-Sachs.* Retrieved July 22, 2006, from http://www.marchofdimes.com/professionals/681_1227.asp.

March of Dimes. (2006*c*). *Recommended newborn screening tests: 29 disorders.* Retrieved July 22, 2006, from http://www.marchofdimes.com/professionals/14332_15455.asp.

MSU Division of Human Genetics (2002) *Maternal serum screening.* Retrieved July 22, 2006, from http://www.healthteam.msu.edu/clinics/Genetics/documents/PRENATAL%20GENETICS.pdf.

National Human Genome Research Institute. (2007). *Learning about Tay-Sachs disease.* Retrieved April 22, 2007 from http://www.genome.gov/10001220.

National Institutes of Health, National Institute of Child Health and Human Development. (2006). *Facts about Down syndrome.* Retrieved July 22, 2006, from http://www.nichd.nih.gov/publications/pubs/downsyndrome/down.htm#TheOccurrence.

National Institute of Neurological Disorders and Stroke (2006). *Neurofibromatosis fact sheet.* Retrieved July 22, 2006, from www.ninds.nih.gov/disorders/neurofibromatosis/detail_neurofibromatosis.htm.

National Institute of Neurological Disorders and Stroke (2006). *NINDS Tay-Sachs disease information page.* Retrieved July 22, 2006, from www.ninds.nih.gov/disorders/taysachs/taysachs.htm.

Pagana, K. D., & Pagana, T. J. (2006). *Mosby's manual of diagnostic and laboratory tests* (3rd ed.). St. Louis: Mosby.

Paoloni-Giacobino, A., & Chaillet, J. R. (2004). Genomic imprinting and assisted reproduction. *Reproductive Health, 1*(6). Retrieved July 22, 2006, from http://www.reproductive-health-journal.com/content/1/1/6.

Pueschel, S. M. (2001). *A parent's guide to Down syndrome: Toward a brighter future.* Baltimore: Paul H. Brookes Publishing Company, Inc.

Saving Babies through Screening Foundation, Inc. (2006). *Disease descriptions.* Retrieved July 22, 2006, from http://www.savebabies.org/diseasedescriptions.php.

Siegel, B., & Milunsky, J. (2004). When should the possibility of a genetic disorder cross your radar screen? *Contemporary Pediatrics, 21*(5), 30–45.

Skinner, D., & Schaffer, R. (2005). Families and genetic diagnoses in the genomic and internet age. *Infants and Young Children, 19*(1), 16–24.

Stroop, J. (2000). The family history as a screening tool. *Pediatric Annals, 29*(5), 279–282.

Sybert, V. P., & McCauley, E. (2004). Turner's syndrome. *New England Journal of Medicine, 351*(12), 1227–1241.

Trotter, T. L., Hall, J. G., American Academy of Pediatrics Committee on Genetics. (2005). Health supervision for children with achondroplasia. *Pediatrics, 116*(3), 771–784.

Van Riper, M., & Cohen, W. (2001). Caring for children with Down syndrome and their families. *Journal of Pediatric Health, 15*(3), 123–131.

Venes, D. (2005). *Taber's cyclopedic medical dictionary* (20th ed.). Philadelphia: F. A. Davis.

Vernon, P. (2000). Neurofibromatosis: An elephant by another name. *Journal of Pediatric Health Care, 14*(5), 244–247.

Wattendorf, D. J., & Muenke, M. (2005). Klinefelter syndrome. *American Family Physician, 72*(11), 2259–2263.

Wattendorf, D. J., & Muenke, M. (2005). Diagnosis and management of fragile X syndrome. *American Family Physician, 72*(1), 111–114.

Weiner, D. L. (2005). Pediatrics, inborn errors of metabolism. *eMedicine.* Retrieved July 22, 2006, from http://www.emedicine.com/emerg/topic768.htm.

Wille, M. C., Weitz, B., Kerper, P., & Frazier, S. (2004). Advances in preconception genetic counseling. *Journal of Perinatal & Neonatal Nursing, 18*(1), 28–41.

Websites

www.aboutfaceusa.org About Face USA
www.angelman.org Angelman Syndrome Foundation, Inc.
www.ccakids.com Children's Craniofacial Association
www.cdss.ca Canadian Down Syndrome Society
www.chargesyndrome.org CHARGE Syndrome Foundation
www.ctf.org/ Children's Tumor Foundation (dedicated to neurofibromatosis research)
www.faceit.org Let's Face It, Inc.
www.faces-cranio.org National Craniofacial Association
www.fivepminus.org 5p- Society (cri-du-chat syndrome)
www.fodsupport.org Fatty Oxidation Disorders (FOD) Family Support Group
www.fragilex.org/ National Fragile X Foundation
www.galactosemia.org Parents of Galactosemic Children
www.kumc.edu/gec/support/metaboli.html Association for Neuro-Metabolic Diseases
www.liverfoundation.org American Liver Foundation
www.lpaonline.org Little People of America, Inc.
www.marchofdimes.com/ March of Dimes (information on birth defects, genetic disorders and inborn errors of metabolism)
www.marfan.ca Canadian Marfan Association
www.marfan.org National Marfan Foundation
www.msud-support.org Maple Syrup Urine Disease Family Support Group
www.nads.org/ National Association for Down Syndrome
www.ndsccenter.org/ National Down Syndrome Congress
www.ndss.org/ National Down Syndrome Society
www.nffr.org National Foundation for Facial Reconstruction
www.nfinc.org/ Neurofibromatosis, Inc. (dedicated to education, advocacy, and research)
www.ntsad.org National Tay-Sachs & Allied Diseases Association
www.pkunetwork.org Children's PKU Network
www.pkunews.org National PKU News
www.rarediseases.org National Organization for Rare Disorders
www.shortsupport.org Short Persons Support
www.sturge-weber.com Sturge-Weber Foundation
www.tefvater.org TEF VATER National Support Network
www.trisomy.org/ Support Organization for Trisomy 18, 13, and Related Disorders
www.tsalliance.org Tuberous Sclerosis Alliance
www.turner-syndrome-us.org/about/ Turner Syndrome Society of the United States
www.vcfsef.org/ Velo-Cardio-Facial Syndrome Educational

Chapter WORKSHEET

MULTIPLE CHOICE QUESTIONS

1. You are counseling a couple, one of whom is affected by neurofibromatosis, an autosomal dominant disorder. They want to know the risk of transmitting the disorder. The nurse should tell them that each offspring has a:
   a. One in four (25%) chance of getting the disease
   b. One in eight (12.5%) chance of getting the disease
   c. One in one (100%) chance of getting the disease
   d. One in two (50%) chance of getting the disease
2. The nurse working in a women's health clinic determines that genetic counseling may be appropriate for a woman:
   a. Who just had her first miscarriage at 10 weeks
   b. Who is 30 years old and planning to conceive
   c. Whose history reveals a close relative with fragile X syndrome
   d. Who is 18 weeks pregnant and whose triple screen came back normal
3. A child born with a single transverse palmar crease, a short neck with excessive skin at the nape, a depressed nasal bridge, and cardiac defects is most likely to have which autosomal abnormality?
   a. Trisomy 21
   b. Trisomy 18
   c. Trisomy 14
   d. Trisomy 13
4. A mother brings her 4-day-old infant to the clinic with vomiting and poor feeding. The newborn was healthy at birth. The nurse should suspect:
   a. Sturge-Weber syndrome
   b. An inborn error of metabolism
   c. Trisomy 18
   d. Turner syndrome

CRITICAL THINKING EXERCISES

1. An 8-month-old is seen in the clinic. On assessment the nurse finds eight café-au-lait spots on the child's trunk and extremities. What other assessment findings may be pertinent?
2. A child's newborn screen came back positive for phenylketonuria. After further testing, the diagnosis is confirmed. What instructions would you give the parents regarding care of their child?
3. A 6-year-old boy with Down syndrome is admitted to the hospital with pneumonia. Choose three pieces of information that the nurse should seek when obtaining the health history:
   a. Presence of cardiac defects or disease
   b. Last hearing and vision evaluation
   c. Mother's pregnancy history
   d. Presence of thyroid disease
   e. Mother's immunization history

STUDY ACTIVITIES

1. Develop a nursing care plan for a child with Down syndrome.
2. Shadow a genetic counselor. Identify ways he or she helps families understand and cope with genetic disorders.
3. Attend a meeting of an ethics committee at a local hospital. Identify some of the ethical, legal, and social issues in health care that they discuss, particularly related to genetic testing and genetic disorders.

chapter 31

Nursing Care of the Child With a Cognitive or Mental Health Disorder

Key TERMS

abuse
affect
anxiety
bingeing
comorbidity
neglect
purging
suicide
violence

Learning OBJECTIVES

Upon completion of the chapter, the learner will be able to:

1. Discuss the impact of alterations in mental health upon the growth and development of infants, children, and adolescents.
2. Describe techniques used to evaluate the status of mental health in children.
3. Identify appropriate nursing assessments and interventions related to therapy and medications for the treatment of childhood and adolescent mental health disorders.
4. Distinguish mental health disorders common in infants, children, and adolescents.
5. Develop an individualized nursing care plan for the child with a mental health disorder.
6. Develop patient/family teaching plans for the child with a mental health disorder.

WOW *A child's sense often exceeds all human intellect.*

John Howard, age 6 years, is brought to the clinic for his annual examination. His father states, "John has frequent emotional outbursts and his mood seems to switch from happy to sad rather quickly. His teachers have said his performance at school has been poor."

Mental health issues make up the bulk of the "new morbidity" of children. Such issues include academic difficulties, psychiatric disorders, **violence**, school hostility, substance abuse, and adverse effects of the media (Reasor & Farrell, 2004). As many as 13 million children may be suffering from mental health-related problems (American Academy of Pediatrics [AAP], 2000). Up to 80% of children with social, emotional, or behavioral problems fail to receive the services they need, leading to further academic and social difficulties. Mental illness manifested in the early years increases the risk of adolescent emotional issues, use of firearms, reckless driving, substance abuse, and promiscuous sexual activity. Some cognitive or neurobehavioral disorders may have a genetic or physiologic cause, whereas others result from family or environmental stressors.

Usually children with cognitive or mental health disorders are treated in the community or on an outpatient basis, but sometimes the disorder has such a significant impact on the child and family that hospitalization is required. Many hospitalized children also suffer from cognitive or mental health disorders. When a child is diagnosed with a neurobehavioral disorder, the family may become overwhelmed by the multifaceted services that he or she requires.

The scope of mental health issues among children, adolescents, and their families has become so extensive that the U.S. Surgeon General has published a "National Agenda for Action." The Surgeon General's Conference on Children's Mental Health has set the following goals:

1. Promote public awareness of children's mental health issues and reduce the stigma associated with mental illness.
2. Continue to develop, disseminate, and implement scientifically proven prevention and treatment services in the field of children's mental health.
3. Improve the assessment of and recognition of mental health needs in children.
4. Eliminate racial/ethnic and socioeconomic disparities in access to mental health care services.
5. Improve the infrastructure for children's mental health services, including support for scientifically proven interventions across professions.
6. Increase access to and coordination of quality mental health care services.
7. Train front-line providers to recognize and manage mental health issues, and educate mental health care providers about scientifically proven prevention and treatment services.
8. Monitor the access to and coordination of quality mental health care services (U.S. Public Health Service, 2004).

Mental health problems in children are real and painful and can be severe. For affected children to have a chance at a healthy future, nurses must participate in the early identification and referral of children with potential cognitive deficits or other mental health issues.

Effects of Mental Health Issues on Health and Development

Children's behavior is influenced by biologic or genetic characteristics, nutrition, physical health, developmental ability, environmental and family interactions, the child's individual temperament, and the parents' or caregiver's responses to the child's behavior (Goldson & Reynolds, 2007). The changes that occur with normal growth and development are often a source of stress for children, and in some children they may lead to dysfunction. Children progress at very different rates, so it is often difficult to identify subtle abnormalities. When stress, fatigue, or pain occurs in children, they may quickly regress to earlier patterns of behavior. These regressive behaviors may continue if a mental health concern is present. It is possible that stress placed on developing neurons leads to decreased coping abilities later in life. Children learn through their experiences; therefore, they may develop maladaptive behaviors through life interactions.

Common Medical Treatments

A variety of medications and other medical treatments are used to treat mental health disorders in children. Most of these treatments will require a physician's order when the child is in the hospital. The most common medications are listed in Drug Guide 31.1. The nurse caring for the child with a mental health disorder should become familiar with how the treatments and medications work, as well as medication adverse effects to monitor for. Many mental health disorders are treated with some type of therapy. Table 31.1 reviews the types of therapies commonly used. These therapies are generally carried out only by specially trained personnel.

Behavior management techniques are also used to help children alter negative behavior patterns. The methods may be used outside of therapy sessions, in the hospital,

Drug Guide 31.1 Drugs Used for Pediatric Mental Health Disorders

Medication	Action	Indication	Nursing Implications
Psychostimulants: methylphenidate (Ritalin), dextro-amphetamine (Adderall), pemoline (Cylert), long-acting methylphenidate (Concerta, Metadate CD, Ritalin LA), long-acting dextroamphetamine (Dexedrine Spansules, Adderall XR)	Increases synaptic levels of dopamine and norepinephrine	ADHD	• Methylphenidate has a short half-life; give TID (a.m., mid-day at school, at home after school) • Long-acting preparations are given once daily in the a.m. • Adverse effects: decreased appetite, headache, abdominal pain, difficulty sleeping, irritability, social withdrawal, motor tics. If dose is too high, child may have flat affect. • Pemoline is only rarely used because of hepatotoxicity.
Antianxiety agent: buspirone (BuSpar)	Highly blocks reuptake of dopamine	Anxiety, rage, mania, psychosis, depression, Tourette syndrome	• Administer in consistent relation to food (either with or without). • May cause drowsiness • Monitor for disinhibition, agitation, confusion, depression.
Antimanic agent: lithium (Eskalith, Lithobid)	Influences reuptake of serotonin and/or norepinephrine	Bipolar disorder, depression, hyperaggression	• Monitor closely. • May cause polyuria, polydipsia, tremor, nausea, weight gain, diarrhea
Selective serotonin reuptake inhibitors: fluoxetine (Prozac), paroxetine (Paxil), sertraline (Zoloft)	Potentiates serotonin activity in the brain	Depression, obsessive-compulsive disorder, anxiety	• Observe for irritability, insomnia, GI distress, nausea, headache. • Monitor BP for increase.
Atypical antidepressants: trazodone (Desyrel)	Inhibits reuptake of serotonin	Depression	• Monitor BP for postural hypotension. • Observe for sedation and drowsiness; avoid alcohol use. • Administer after meals or with a snack.
Nonstimulant norepinephrine reuptake inhibitors: atomoxetine (Straterra)	Enhances norepinephrine activity	ADHD	• Administer without regard to food once or twice daily. • Monitor weight, height, BP, heart rate. • May cause dizziness, dry mouth
Alpha-agonist antihypertensive agents: clonidine (Catapres), guanfacine (Tenex)	Activates inhibitory neurons in the brain stem	ADHD, Tourette syndrome, self-abuse, aggression	• Clonidine is strongly sedating. • Monitor BP and pulse. • Observe for dry mouth, confusion, depression, urinary retention, constipation.

(continued)

Drug Guide 31.1 Drugs Used for Pediatric Mental Health Disorders (continued)

Medication	Action	Indication	Nursing Implications
Antipsychotic agents: thioridazine (Mellaril), chlorpromazine (Thorazine), haloperidol (Haldol)	Reversibly block type 2 dopamine receptors in the central nervous system	Psychosis, mania, self-harm, violent or destructive behavior	• May cause drowsiness • Monitor for anticholinergic effects, drowsiness and dystonia (extrapyramidal effects), dizziness. • Evaluate for the development of orthostatic hypotension, tachycardia. • Observe closely for the development of tardive dyskinesia, particularly early in treatment.
Atypical antipsychotics: risperidone (Risperdal), clozapine (Clozaril), olanzapine (Zyprexa)	Reversibly block type 2 dopamine receptors in the central nervous system	Psychosis, bipolar disorder, autism spectrum disorder, Tourette syndrome	• Monitor for seizures, agitation, headache, nausea, sedation. • Olanzapine may cause weight gain. • Note WBC.
Tricyclic antidepressants: amitriptyline (Elavil), desipramine (Norpramin), imipramine (Tofranil), nortriptyline (Pamelor)	Enhances synaptic concentration of serotonin and/or norepinephrine	Depression, ADHD, tics, anxiety	• Monitor for anticholinergic effects, weight loss. • Check blood levels. • Monitor ECG for arrhythmias.

Table 31.1 Types of Therapy

Treatment	Explanation
Behavioral therapy	Uses stimulus and response conditioning to manage or alter behavior. Reinforces desired behaviors, replacing the inappropriate ones. Consistency is of utmost importance.
Play therapy	Designed to change emotional status. Encourages the child to act out feelings of sadness, fear, hostility, or anger.
Cognitive therapy	Teaches children to change reactions so that automatic negative thought patterns are replaced with alternative ones
Family therapy	Exploration of the child's emotional issue and its effect on family members
Group therapy	May be conducted in a school, hospital, treatment facility, neighborhood center. Feelings are expressed and participants gain hope, feel a part of something, and benefit from role modeling. Takes advantage of peer relationships as developmental focus in preteen and teen groups.
Milieu therapy	A specially structured setting designed to promote the child's adaptive and social skills. A safe and supportive environment for those at risk of self-harm or those who are very ill or very aggressive.
Individual therapy	The child and therapist work together to resolve the conflicts, emotions, or behavior problems. Trust is central. Structured based on the child's developmental level (e.g., may use play therapy for a younger child).
Hypnosis	Deep relaxation with suggestibility remarks

clinic, or classroom. Behavior management techniques include the following:

- Set limits with the child, holding him or her responsible for his or her behavior.
- Do not argue, bargain, or negotiate about the limits once established.
- Provide consistent caregivers (unlicensed assistive personnel and nurses for the hospitalized child) and establish the child's daily routine.
- Use a low-pitched voice and remain calm.
- Redirect the child's attention when needed.
- Ignore inappropriate behaviors.
- Praise the child's self-control efforts and other accomplishments.
- Use restraints only when necessary.

Nursing Process Overview for the Child With a Mental Health Disorder

Care of the child with a mental health disorder includes assessment, nursing diagnosis, planning, interventions, and evaluation. There are a number of general concepts related to the nursing process that may be applied to mental health concerns in children. From a general understanding of the care involved for a child with a mental health disorder, the nurse can then individualize the care based on patient specifics.

ASSESSMENT

A careful and thorough health history forms the basis of the nursing assessment of a child with a mental health or cognitive disorder. The physical examination may yield clues to the type of disorder but is often completely normal.

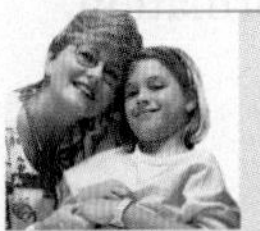

Observe a child's play or drawings; if you suspect cognitive or psychological issues from the play or artwork, refer the child for further mental health evaluation.

Health History

Elicit the health history, noting the child's prenatal and birth history, past medical history, including previously diagnosed cognitive or mental health disorders, history of neurologic injury or disease, and family history of mental health disorder. Perform a developmental history, noting age of attainment (or loss) of milestones. Question the child and/or parent about behavior changes such as:

- Altered sleep
- Difference in eating patterns, weight loss or gain, change in appetite
- Problems at school
- Participation in risk-taking behaviors
- Alterations in friendships
- Changes in extracurricular activity participation

Note results of any developmental testing performed. Ask the family about progression of the child's skills. Note any unusual deficits or capabilities. Question the family about recent stress, trauma, or change in family structure; are any family members chronically ill? Note medications the child takes routinely, and any allergies to food, drugs, medications, or environmental agents.

Interview the child at an age-appropriate level to determine his or her self-perception, future plans, and stressors and how he or she copes with them. Determine the child's perception of his relationship with his parents, siblings, friends, peers, pets, inanimate objects, and transitional or security objects. What is the child's predominant mood? Determine whether the child likes himself or herself, asking such questions as "What do you like most about yourself?" and "What would you like to change about yourself?" Determine the child's gender identity status. Does the child have a sense of pride in his or her accomplishments? Has the child developed an appropriate conscience (with understanding of right and wrong)?

Note history of complaints that may be associated with certain mental health disorders, such as sore throat, difficulty swallowing, or genital burning or itching. Document if the child displays any of the following during the health interview:

- Hallucinations
- Aggression
- Impulsivity
- Distractibility
- Intolerance to frustration
- Lack of sense of humor or fun
- Inhibition
- Poor attention span
- Potential cognitive or learning disabilities
- Unusual motor activities

Remember John, the 6-year-old brought in for his annual examination? What additional health history and physical examination assessment information should the nurse obtain?

Physical Examination

Observe the child's clothing, noting whether it is appropriate for age, developmental level, and setting. Note the child's facial expression and response to the parent or caretaker and the nurse. Does the child make appropriate eye contact? Determine the child's level of consciousness and extent of interest in and interaction with surroundings. Note the child's posture, **affect**, and mood. How appropriate to the situation are the child's emotional reactions? Does the child communicate well?

Measure the child's weight and height/length, as well as head circumference if he or she is less than 3 years old.

Perform a thorough physical examination, noting any physical abnormalities or signs of other physical health disorders. Note abnormal findings that may be associated with particular mental health disorders, such as bruising, burns, contusions, cuts, abrasions, unusual skin marks, soft/sparse body hair, split fingernails, inflamed oropharynx, eroded tooth enamel, reddened gums, or genitourinary discharge or bleeding.

Laboratory and Diagnostic Testing

Mental health disorders are generally diagnosed based upon clinical features. Brain imaging such as computed tomography or magnetic resonance imaging may be used to evaluate for a congenital abnormality or alterations in the brain tissue that may lead to developmental delay. A blood or urine toxicology panel is useful in the diagnosis of drug abuse or overdose, or instances of bizarre behavior.

Nursing Diagnoses and Related Interventions

The overall goal of nursing management of cognitive and mental health disorders in children is to help the child and family to reach an optimal level of functioning. This may be achieved through interventions designed to decrease the impact of stressors upon the child's life. Upon completion of a thorough assessment of the child and family, the nurse might identify several nursing diagnoses, including:

- Impaired social interaction
- Delayed growth and development
- Ineffective individual coping
- Hopelessness
- Imbalanced nutrition, less than body requirements
- Disturbed thought processes
- Caregiver role strain

> **After completing an assessment of John,** the nurse noted the following: difficulty sitting still for the examination, easily distracted, and frustrated, labile mood. Based on the assessment findings, what would your top three nursing diagnoses be for John?

Nursing goals, interventions, and evaluation for the child with a mental health disorder are based on the nursing diagnoses. Nursing Care Plan Overview 31.1 provides a general guide for planning care for a child with a mental health disorder. Children's responses to a mental health issue and its treatment will vary, and nursing care should be individualized based on the child's and family's responses to illness. Additional information about nursing management will be included later in the chapter as it relates to specific disorders. See Healthy People 2010.

> **Based on your top three nursing diagnoses for John,** describe appropriate nursing interventions.

Developmental and Behavioral Disorders

Developmental and behavioral disorders make up a large proportion of mental health disorders in children. They include learning disabilities, mental retardation, autism spectrum disorder, and attention-deficit/hyperactivity disorder.

● LEARNING DISABILITIES

About 5% to 10% of children and adolescents have learning disabilities; some estimates are as high as 17% (Aylward, 2002). About half of the children with a learning disability have at least one other comorbid condition (usually a mental health or behavioral disorder). The National Center for Learning Disabilities (2006) defines a learning disability as "a neurological disorder that affects the brain's ability to receive, process, store, and respond to information." Learning disabilities become evident when a child of average intelligence has difficulty mastering basic academic skills. Learning disabilities can affect the child's ability to listen, speak, read, write, and perform mathematics:

- Children with dyslexia have difficulty with reading, writing, and spelling.
- Dyscalculia leads to problems with mathematics and computation.
- Problems with manual dexterity and coordination result when a child has dyspraxia.
- Children with dysgraphia have difficulty producing the written word (composition, spelling, and writing).

Sensory integration dysfunction may be mistaken for a learning disability, but it is not and should be treated differently. Box 31.1 provides additional information.

Nursing Assessment

Elicit the health history, noting risk factors such as a family history of learning disability, problems during pregnancy or birth, prenatal alcohol or drug use, low birthweight, premature or prolonged labor, head injury, poor nutritional status or failure to thrive, or lead poisoning. Obtain detailed information about the educational difficulties the child is experiencing (e.g., he seems to do fine in math but always reverses letters when reading). A thorough physical examination may reveal clues to comorbid conditions. Ensure that the child has undergone a comprehensive education evaluation with assessment testing to diagnose the specific learning disability. Testing may be performed by a school, educational, developmental, or clinical psychologist, occupational therapist, speech and language therapist, or other developmental specialist, depending on the areas of learning with which the child is experiencing difficulty.

Nursing Care Plan 31.1

Overview for the Child With a Mental Health Disorder

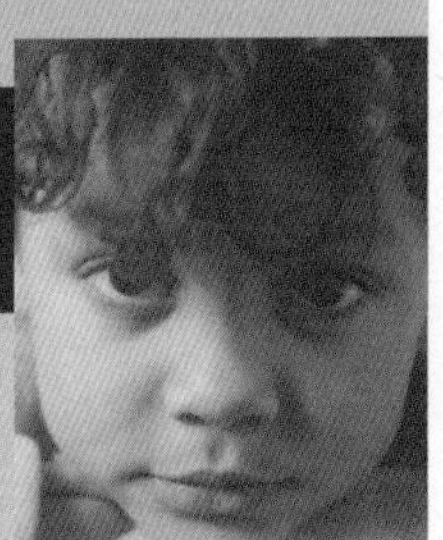

Nursing Diagnosis: Impaired social interaction related to altered social skills as evidenced by impulsivity, intrusive behavior, inability to follow through, anxiety, depressed mood, feelings of unattractiveness or unworthiness

Outcome identification and evaluation

The child will demonstrate socially acceptable skills, *interacting successfully with peers and in the educational setting, completing tasks as required.*

Interventions: promoting appropriate social interaction

- Identify factors that may aggravate the child's performance *to minimize stimuli that exacerbate the child's undesired behaviors.*
- Modify the environment to decrease distracting stimuli *as child's ability to deal with external stimuli may be impaired.*
- Ensure that the child hears his name and makes eye contact prior to conversing or instructions *so that child is engaged and has increased ability to follow through.*
- State expectations for tasks or behaviors clearly *as understanding is necessary to ensure completion.*
- Provide positive feedback for appropriate behaviors or task completion, *encouraging the child to adopt expectations into his behaviors and routine.*

Nursing Diagnosis: Ineffective individual coping related to inability to deal with life stressors as evidenced by few or no meaningful friendships, inability to empathize or give/receive affection, low self-esteem, or maladaptive coping behaviors such as substance abuse

Outcome identification and evaluation

The child will demonstrate improved coping, *verbalize feelings, socially engage, demonstrate problem-solving skills.*

Interventions: promoting coping skills

- Encourage discussion of thoughts and feelings, *as this is an initial step toward learning to deal with them appropriately.*
- Provide positive feedback for appropriate discussion, *as this increases the likelihood of continuing performance.*
- Demonstrate unconditional acceptance of the child as a person *to increase self-esteem in the child who has been feeling rejection.*
- Set clear limits on behavior as needed *so the child has a structure to adhere to.*
- Teach the child problem-solving skills *as an alternative to acting-out behaviors.*
- Role-model appropriate social and conversation skills *so the child can see what is expected in a nonthreatening manner.*

Nursing Diagnosis: Imbalanced nutrition, less than body requirements, related to intake insufficient to meet metabolic needs as evidenced by weight loss, failure to gain weight, less-than-expected increases in stature and weight, loss of appetite, or refusal to eat

Outcome identification and evaluation

The child or adolescent will demonstrate appropriate growth, *making gains in weight and stature as appropriate.*

Interventions: improving nutritional intake

- Provide favorite foods *to encourage the child with poor appetite to eat more.*
- Assist families to choose nutrient-rich foods *so that the food the child does eat is most beneficial.*

(continued)

Overview for the Child With a Mental Health Disorder (continued)

For the child with an eating disorder:

- Mutually establish a contract related to treatment *to promote the child's sense of control.*
- Provide mealtime structure, *as clear limits let the child know what the expectations are.*
- Encourage the child to choose foods and timing of meals *to develop independence in eating habits.*
- Ensure the eating environment is pleasant and relaxed, with minimal distractions, *to minimize the child's anxiety and guilt about not eating.*
- Withdraw attention if child refuses to eat *(secondary gain is minimized if refusal to eat is ignored).*
- Provide continuous supervision during the meal and for 30 minutes following it *so that the child cannot conceal or dispose of food or induce vomiting.*

Nursing Diagnosis: Delayed growth and development related to disability, behavioral disorder, or altered nutrition as evidenced by lack of attainment of age-appropriate skills, regression in skills, or altered intellectual functioning

Outcome identification and evaluation

Child will demonstrate progress toward developmental milestones: *Child expresses interest in the environment and people around him, interacts with environment in an age-appropriate way.*

Interventions: promoting development

- Use therapeutic play and adaptive toys *to facilitate developmental functioning.*
- Provide stimulating environment when possible *to maximize potential for growth and development*
- Praise accomplishments and emphasize child's abilities *to improve self-esteem and encourage feeling of confidence and competence.*
- Follow through with physical, occupational, and speech therapists' recommendations *to maximize exposure to exercises designed to increase the child's skills.*
- Determine parents' expectations of child's future achievement *to help them work toward these goals.*

Nursing Diagnosis: Disturbed thought processes related to behavioral disorder, depression, anxiety, abusive situation, or substance abuse as evidenced by distractibility, non-reality-based thinking, hypervigilance, or inaccurate interpretation of interactions of others

Outcome identification and evaluation

Child's thought processes will improve; *child will demonstrate appropriate orientation, remain free from physical harm, and perform activities of daily living as able.*

Interventions: improving thought processes

- Observe for causes of altered thought processes *to provide a baseline for assessment and intervention.*
- Perform an age-appropriate mental status examination *to determine extent of altered thinking.*
- Adjust communication style based on child's cues *to improve communication.*
- Listen carefully and seek clarification *to determine basis for child's agitation or other behaviors.*
- Provide validation of the child's thoughts and feelings *to improve trust in the relationship.*
- Establish a daily routine *to provide the child with a sense of security.*

Overview for the Child With a Mental Health Disorder (continued)

Nursing Diagnosis: Hopelessness related to child's perception of his life situation, negative life view, or alteration in mental well-being as evidenced by passivity, verbalization, alterations in sleep, or lack of initiative

Outcome identification and evaluation

Child will display a sense of hope, *will verbalize feelings, participate in care, make positive statements.*

Interventions: promoting hope

- Monitor and document potential for suicide, *as hopelessness often leads to suicidal ideation.*
- Assist the child to identify reasons for hope and for living, *so the nurse is aware of the child's values.*
- Help the child to set goals that are important to him *to allow the child to see possibilities.*
- Encourage simple decision making on a daily basis, *as hopelessness often occurs as a response to loss of control.*
- Assist the child to identify positive qualities in himself and his life *to facilitate the development of hope.*
- Involve parents or others the child loves in the child's care *as social support is critical to the development of hope.*

Nursing Diagnosis: Caregiver role strain related to long-term care of the child with a chronic mental health disorder as evidenced by fatigue, inattention to own needs, conflict, or ambivalence

Outcome identification and evaluation

The child's caregiver will participate in the child's care, *verbalizing the child's needs and treatment plan and demonstrating skills necessary for care.*

Interventions: decreasing role strain

- Teach the parent or caregiver about the child's illness, treatments, and medications *to clarify expectations for the child and parent.*
- Role-model appropriate interaction behaviors with the child *so the parent can learn these techniques by watching.*
- Encourage structure in daily routines *to allow the parent to meet own needs and allow for adequate rest.*
- Gradually increase the parent's responsibility related to care of the child *to help the parent feel less overwhelmed.*
- Allow the parent to move at his or her own pace in assuming care *to enhance the chances for success.*
- Help the parent to identify a back-up caregiver *so the parent has times of respite from constant involvement with the child.*

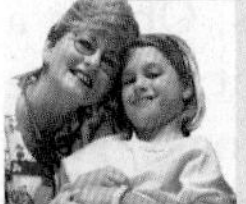

If a child cannot speak in sentences by 30 months of age, does not have understandable speech 50% of the time by age 3 years, cannot sit still for a short story by 3 to 5 years of age, or cannot tie shoes, cut, button, or hop by 5 to 6 years of age, refer the child to be evaluated for a learning disability.

Nursing Management

Ensure that families are aware of their child's rights under the Individuals with Disabilities Act (IDEA), which was reapproved in 2004. IDEA offers protection from discrimination and the right to assistance in the school or workplace. Each child will need an individualized education plan (IEP) that reflects his or her particular needs, which then must be provided for through the school system. Offer encouragement and support to families as they advocate for their child. Follow up at subsequent health care visits to determine that the child is receiving the services he or she needs to optimize his or her potential for success. Refer families for additional resources through the

HEALTHY PEOPLE 2010

Objective	Significance
(Developmental) Increase the proportion of children with mental health problems who receive treatment.	• Screen all children and adolescents for mental health problems. • Encourage children and adolescents to participate in treatment planning as is developmentally appropriate, allowing them to make choices about intervention as possible.

National Center for Learning Disabilities (www.ncld.org), Learning Disabilities Online (www.ldonline.org), or the Center for Learning Differences (www.centerforlearningdifferences.org).

MENTAL RETARDATION

Mental retardation refers to a functional state in which significant limitations in intellectual status and adaptive behavior (functioning in daily life) develop before the age of 18 years. Up to 3% of the population may be designated as mentally retarded (Accardo et al., 2006; Wickham, 2004).

As defined by the American Association on Intellectual and Developmental Disabilities (AAIDD, 2007), mental retardation includes:

- Deviations in IQ of two or more standard deviations (IQ of less than 70 to 75)
- Coexisting deficits in at least two adaptive skills: communication, community use, functional academics, health and safety, home living, leisure, self-care, self-direction, social skills, and work
- Occurring before the age of 18 years

BOX 31.1

SENSORY INTEGRATION DYSFUNCTION (ALSO CALLED SENSORY PROCESSING DISORDER)

- A neurologic disorder in which the child cannot organize sensory input used in daily living
- Hyposensitivity or hypersensitivity to sensory input
- Results in overreaction to different textures, decreasing the child's ability to participate in the world
- Preterm and low-birthweight infants are at increased risk compared with typical infants.
- Occupational and other therapies may increase the child's ability to function.

Long ago mentally retarded persons were confined to institutions and were thought to be harmful to society. In the early 21st century, most children with mental retardation are receiving their education in public schools with their peers and living at home with their families or elsewhere in the community. Only the most severely affected individuals require separate classrooms or schools.

Pathophysiology

In many instances of mental retardation the exact cause remains unknown. Prenatal errors in central nervous system development may be responsible, or an insult or damage to the brain may occur in the prenatal, perinatal, or postnatal period from a variety of causes. Motor problems such as hypotonia, tremor, ataxia, or clumsiness, visual motor problems, or other issues may occur concomitantly with mental retardation. When a learning disability or sensory processing impairment is also present, functioning at a higher intellectual level may be prevented. Mental retardation is generally categorized according to severity:

- Mild: IQ 50 to 70
- Moderate: IQ 35 to 50
- Severe: IQ 20 to 35
- Profound: IQ less than 20

Therapeutic Management

The primary goal of therapeutic management of children with mental retardation is to provide appropriate educational experiences that allow the child to achieve a level of functioning and self-sufficiency needed for existence in the home, community, work, and leisure settings. The child's conceptual, social, practical, and intellectual abilities will drive school placement and the focus of the educational experience. The student's success is also dependent upon community and family influences. The majority of mentally retarded individuals require only minimal support, and these individuals are able to achieve some level of self-sufficiency. Only a few children and adults with mental retardation require extensive support.

Nursing Assessment

Perform developmental screening at each health care visit to identify developmental delays early. Elicit the health history, determining the mental and adaptive capacities of the child's parents and other family members. Obtain a detailed pregnancy and birth history. Document sequence and age of attainment of developmental milestones. Note history of motor, visual, or language difficulties. Assess the child's health history for risk factors such as preterm or postterm birth, low birthweight, birth injury, prenatal or neonatal infection, prenatal alcohol or drug exposure, genetic syndrome, chromosomal alteration, metabolic disease, exposure to toxins (e.g., lead), head injury or other trauma, nutritional deficiency, cerebral malformation, and other brain disease or mental health disorder. Note history of or concomitant seizure disorder, orthopedic problems, speech problems, or vision or hearing deficit.

For the child with known mental retardation, assess language, sensory, and psychomotor functioning. Determine the child's ability to toilet, dress, and feed himself or herself. Ask the parents about involvement with school and community services and support.

On physical examination note dysmorphic features (possibly very mild) consistent with certain syndromes (e.g., fetal alcohol syndrome; Box 31.2). Evaluate the newborn or metabolic screening results. Computed tomography or magnetic resonance imaging of the head may be performed to evaluate the brain structure. Thyroid function tests may be ordered to rule out thyroid problems leading to developmental delay.

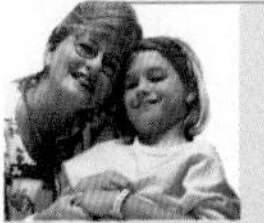

Due to the extent of cognition required to understand and produce speech, the most sensitive early indicator of intellectual disability is delayed language development.

Nursing Management

When children with mental retardation are admitted to the hospital (usually for some other physical or medical condition), it is important for the nurse to continue the child's usual home routine. Follow through with feeding and motor supports that the child uses. Ensure that the child is closely supervised and remains free from harm. Allow parents time to verbalize frustrations or fears. For some families the caretaking burden is extensive and lifelong; arrange for respite care as available. Support the child's strengths, and assist the child and family to follow through with therapy or treatment designed to enhance the child's functioning. Assist with the development of the child's IEP as appropriate.

AUTISM SPECTRUM DISORDER

Autism spectrum disorder (ASD), also termed pervasive developmental disorder, has its onset in infancy or early childhood. One child in 500 is diagnosed with autism (Choueiri & Bridgemohan, 2005; Oliver, 2003), though some sources estimate the incidence to be as frequent as 1 in 250 children (Dumont-Mathieu et al., 2005). The spectrum of autism disorder ranges from mild (e.g., Asperger syndrome) to severe. Autistic behaviors may be first noticed in infancy as developmental delays or between the age of 12 and 36 months when the child regresses or loses previously acquired skills. Parental concerns about development may be sensitive indicators of the development of autism (Beauchesne & Kelly, 2004).

BOX 31.2

FETAL ALCOHOL SYNDROME

- Results from *in utero* alcohol exposure
- Typical facial features include low nasal bridge with short upturned nose, flattened midface, long philtrum with narrow upper lip
- Poor coordination, skeletal abnormalities
- Microcephaly
- Failure to thrive
- Hearing loss

Pathophysiology

The exact etiology of autism continues to elude scientists, but it may be due to genetic makeup, brain abnormalities, altered chemistry, a virus, or toxic chemicals (Oliver, 2003). Children with ASD display impaired social interactions and communication and display perseverative or stereotypic behaviors. They may fail to develop interpersonal relationships and experience social isolation. Most children with autism are mentally retarded, requiring lifelong supervision (Choueiri & Bridgemohan, 2005), though some are gifted.

Therapeutic Management

There are no medications or treatments available to cure autism. Each child's treatment is individualized; behavioral and communication therapies are very important. Children with ASD respond very well to highly structured educational environments. Stimulants may be used to control hyperactivity, and antipsychotic medications are sometimes helpful in children with repetitive and aggressive behaviors.

Many families are drawn to the use of complementary and alternative medical therapies in attempts to treat their autistic child. They may use vitamins and nutritional supplements, herbs or restrictive diets, music therapy, art therapy, and sensory integration techniques. To date, these therapies have not been scientifically proven to improve autism.

The goal of therapeutic management is for the child to reach optimal functioning within the limitations of the disorder.

Nursing Assessment

Elicit the health history, noting delay or regression in developmental skills, particularly speech and language abilities. The child may be mute, utter only sounds (not words), or repeat words or phrases over and over. The parent may report that the infant or toddler spends hours in repetitive activity and demonstrates bizarre motor and stereotypic behaviors. The infant may resist cuddling, lack eye contact, be indifferent to touch or affection, and have little change in facial expression. Toddlers may display hyperactivity, aggression, temper tantrums, or self-injury behaviors, such as head-banging or hand-biting. The history may also reveal hypersensitivity to touch or hyposensitivity to pain. Assess the child's functional status, including behavior, nutrition, sleep, speech and language, education needs, and developmental or neurologic limitations (Giarelli et al., 2005). Assist with screening, using an approved autism screening tool such as:

- Checklist for Autism in Toddlers (CHAT)
- Modified Checklist for Autism in Toddlers (M-CHAT)
- Social Communication Questionnaire (SCQ)
- Pervasive Developmental Disorders Screening Test-II (PDDST-II)

Perform a thorough physical examination. Observe the infant or toddler for lack of eye contact, failure to look at objects pointed to by the examiner, failure to point to himself, failure to let his needs be known, perseverative play activities, and unusual behavior such as hand-flapping or spinning. Measure growth parameters, in particular noting head circumference (macrocephaly or microcephaly may be associated with ASD). Note the presence of large, prominent, or posteriorly rotated ears. Examine the skin for hypo- or hyperpigmented lesions. Note asymmetry of nerve function or palsy, hypertonia, hypotonia, alterations in deep tendon reflexes, toe-walking, loose gait, or poor coordination. Obtain hearing screening results and ascertain that lead screening has been performed.

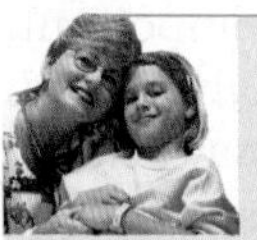

Screen all infants and toddlers for warning signs of autism:

- Not babbling by 12 months
- Not pointing or using gestures by 12 months
- No single words by 16 months
- No two-word utterances by 24 months
- Losing language or social skills at any age

Nursing Management

When children are initially diagnosed with autism, parents need an extensive amount of emotional support, professional guidance, and education about the disorder while they are attempting to adjust to the diagnosis (Giarelli et al., 2005). Assess the "fit" between the child's developmental needs and the treatment plan. Help parents overcome barriers to obtain appropriate education, developmental, and behavioral treatment programs. Ensure that the child younger than 36 months of age receives services via the local early intervention program and children 3 years and over have an IEP in place if enrolled in the public school system. Stress the importance of rigid, unchanging routines, as children with ASD often act out when their routine changes (which is likely to occur if the child must be hospitalized for another condition). Many special schools exist for children with significant developmental disorders, though some are extremely expensive. Assess the parents' need for respite care and make referrals accordingly. Provide positive feedback to parents for their perseverance in working with their child.

ATTENTION-DEFICIT/ HYPERACTIVITY DISORDER

Attention-deficit/hyperactivity disorder (ADHD) is one of the most common mental health disorders diagnosed in childhood: it affects 3% to 7% of all children, and up to 70% of children with ADHD will manifest symptoms throughout adulthood (DeNisco et al., 2005). ADHD is characterized by inattention, impulsivity, distractibility, and hyperactivity. Three subtypes of ADHD exist: hyperactive–impulsive, inattentive, and combined. The child with ADHD has a disruption in learning ability, socialization, and compliance, placing significant demands on the child, parents, teachers, and community (Hunt et al., 2001). About two thirds of children with ADHD also have a **comorbidity** such as oppositional defiant disorder, conduct disorder, an anxiety disorder, depression, a less severe developmental disorder, an auditory processing disorder, or learning or reading disabilities (DeNisco et al., 2005; Stein, 2002; Vlam, 2006). Comparison Chart 31.1 gives information about oppositional defiant disorder and conduct disorder to distinguish them from ADHD.

COMPARISON CHART 31.1

Oppositional Defiant Disorder	Conduct Disorder
• Excessive arguing with adults • Frequent temper tantrums • Active defiance • Revenge-seeking behaviors • Frequent resentment or anger • Touchiness; easily annoyed • Noncompliance with adult requests or limits • Blaming of others for misbehavior or mistakes	• Bullying and threatening of others • Initiation of physical fights • Weapon use to cause others harm • Physical cruelty to animals or people • Destruction of property or arson • Lying and stealing • Serious violation of rules: staying out past curfew, truancy, running away • Use of force in sexual activity

Pathophysiology

Though the exact cause of ADHD remains unidentified, current thought includes as its etiology an alteration in the dopamine and norepinephrine neurotransmitter system. The symptoms of impulsivity, hyperactivity, and inattention begin before 7 years of age and persist longer than 6 months. Symptoms exist in the school and home settings, impairing family and social interactions. Children and teens with ADHD experience frustration, labile moods, emotional outbursts, peer rejection, poor school performance, and low self-esteem. They may also have poor metacognitive abilities such as organization, time management, and the ability to break a project down into a series of smaller tasks (Leslie, 2002). They are not lazy or unmotivated, but simply have poor skills in these areas. Box 31.3 provides criteria for the diagnosis of ADHD.

Therapeutic Management

Medication management of ADHD includes the use of psychostimulants, nonstimulant norepinephrine reuptake inhibitors, and/or alpha-agonist antihypertensive agents. These medications are not a cure for ADHD, but help to increase the child's ability to pay attention and decrease the level of impulsive behavior. The child's activity level is not usually affected. Since ADHD manifests into young adulthood, treatment should continue throughout adolescence (Barbaresi et al., 2006). Concomitant disorders, such as anxiety, should also be treated. Behavior therapy and classroom restructuring may be useful.

BOX 31.3

DIAGNOSIS OF ADHD

Presence of six or more of the following:
- Failure to pay close attention
- Careless mistakes on schoolwork
- Difficulty paying attention to tasks or play
- Doesn't listen
- Doesn't follow through
- Doesn't complete tasks
- Doesn't understand instructions
- Poorly organized
- Avoids, dislikes, or fails to engage in activities requiring mental effort
- Loses things needed for task completion
- Easily distracted
- Forgetful

Presence of six or more of the symptoms of hyperactivity or impulsivity:
- Fidgety or squirmy
- Often out of seat
- Activity inappropriate to the situation
- Cannot engage in quiet play
- Always on the go
- Talks excessively
- Blurts out answers
- Has difficulty waiting his turn
- Often interrupts or intrudes on others (Stevens, 2005)

Nursing Assessment

For a full description of the assessment phase of the nursing process, refer to page 1049. Assessment findings pertinent to ADHD are discussed below.

Health History

Elicit a description of the behavioral issue or school performance problem. Explore the child's history for risk factors such as head trauma, lead exposure, cigarette smoke exposure, prematurity, or low birthweight. The past history may also reveal a larger-than-usual number of accidents. Determine if there is a family history of ADHD. Question the parent about school behavior. The school-age child may be unable to stay on task, talks out of turn, leaves his desk frequently, and either neglects to complete in-class and homework assignments or forgets to turn them in. The adolescent may be inattentive in school, poorly organized, and forgetful.

Several behavioral checklists are available that may assist in the diagnosis of ADHD. They may be completed by the child's teacher and/or parent and focus on behavior patterns related to conduct or learning problems, social competence, anxiety, activity level, and attention. Obtain the completed behavioral checklists (usually one from the parent and one from the teacher) as well as any school records or testing performed.

Physical Examination

Perform vision and hearing screening to rule out vision or hearing impairment as the cause of poor school performance. Observe the preschool child's behavior, noting quickness, agility, fearlessness, and the desire to touch or explore everything in the room.

Laboratory and Diagnostic Tests

No definitive laboratory or diagnostic test is available for the identification of ADHD. A complete blood count may be performed to rule out anemia, and thyroid hormone levels may be drawn to determine whether they are normal.

Nursing Management

Having a child with ADHD can be frustrating as the child's inattention, high activity level, impulsivity, and distractibility are often very difficult to deal with. Parents may doubt their ability to be effective parents or may view their child as somehow defective. Children with ADHD may also feel they are bad, faulty, stupid, or retarded (DeMarle et al., 2003). Provide emotional support, allowing enough time for the family to air their concerns. Work with the child and family to develop goals such as completion of homework, improved communication, or increasing independence in self-care.

Assist the family to advocate for their child's needs through the public school system. The child is entitled to a developmentally appropriate education via an IEP as necessary (refer to Chapter 13 for additional information about special education). The IEP should be updated as needed. Ensure coordination of health and school services. Flag the child's chart and set up a schedule for systematic communication with the family and school. Teach families and school personnel to use behavioral techniques such as time-out, positive reinforcement, reward or privilege withdrawal, or a token system. The token system rewards appropriate behavior with a token and results in a token being taken away if inappropriate behavior occurs. At the end of a specified period of time, the tokens may be exchanged for a prize or privilege (Stein, 2002). Refer families to local support groups and the national ADHD support group www.chadd.org.

Stimulant medications should be taken in the morning to decrease the adverse effect of insomnia. Some children may experience decreased appetite, so giving the medication with or after the meal may be beneficial. The child may feel "different" from his peers if he has to visit the school nurse for a lunchtime dose of ADHD medication; this may lead to noncompliance and a subsequent increase in ADHD symptoms, with deterioration in schoolwork. In this situation, encourage the family to explore with their physician the option of one of the newer extended-release or once-daily ADHD medications.

Tourette Syndrome

Tourette syndrome is estimated to affect about 1% of children (Zinner, 2004a). Its onset is before 18 years of age. The syndrome consists of multiple motor tics and one or more vocal tics occurring either simultaneously or at different times. Children are not tic-free for longer than 3 months. Tics are defined as sudden rapid recurrent stereotypical movements and/or sounds over which the child appears to have no control. Comorbid conditions such as ADHD and obsessive-compulsive disorder occur in 90% of children with Tourette syndrome (Zinner, 2004a). The exact pathophysiologic mechanism of Tourette syndrome has yet to be identified, though genetics does seem to play a part. Therapeutic management is highly individualized and involves psychopharmacology and behavioral therapies. Habit reversal training may help in some children.

Nursing Assessment

Evaluate the health history for the occurrence of tics. The child may be embarrassed or ashamed about the tics and the parents may feel fearful, angry, or guilty. Determine the presence of comorbid symptoms. Elicit the child's past health history, noting a family history of tics. Assess the child's psychosocial history to determine the extent to which the tics interfere with friendship, school performance, and self-esteem. Observe the child for simple or complex motor tics. Vocal tics such as sniffling, grunting, clicking, or word utterance may occur. Perform a thorough physical examination, which is usually normal.

Nursing Management

Inform families that the tics become more noticeable or severe during times of stress and less pronounced when the child is focused on an activity such as watching TV, reading, or playing a video game. Help the family to build on the child's functional behaviors and adaptive skills to improve the child's self-esteem. Encourage the family to pursue classroom accommodations such as allowing for "tic breaks," taking untimed tests or tests in another room, or using note-takers or tape recording. Support the family's decisions related to medication use and provide appropriate education about the particular drugs. "Teaching the Tiger" by M. P. Dornbush and S. K. Pruitt (Hope Press) is useful for teachers of the child with Tourette syndrome. For additional support refer families to www.tsa-usa.org (Tourette Syndrome Association), www.tourette.ca (Tourette Syndrome Foundation of Canada), or www.tourettesyndrome.net (Tourette Syndrome Plus).

Eating Disorders

Eating disorders affect a significant number of children, especially adolescents. Pica, which occurs most frequently in 2- to 3-year-olds, is an eating disorder in which the child ingests (over at least a 1-month period) a non-nutritive material such as paint, clay, or sand. Rumination is an eating disorder occurring in infants in which the baby regurgitates partially digested food or formula and expels or swallows it. The numbers of children affected by pica and rumination is not known.

Anorexia nervosa and bulimia are common eating disorders affecting primarily adolescents, though younger children may also be affected. In American society, being thin is highly valued, compounding the problem. Anorexia nervosa occurs in about 1 of 200 adolescent females; bulimia affects about 1% to 3% (Marino & Fine, 2007). Anorexia nervosa is characterized by dramatic weight loss as a result of decreased food intake and sharply increased physical exercise. Bulimia refers to a cycle of normal food intake, followed by binge-eating and then purging; the adolescent remains at a near-normal weight. Complications include fluid and electrolyte imbalance, decreased blood volume, cardiac arrhythmias, esophagitis, rupture of the esophagus or stomach, tooth loss, and menstrual problems. The mortality rate for anorexia is about 4% (Marino & Fine, 2007).

Nursing Assessment

Determine the health history, noting risk factors such as family history, female gender, Caucasian race, preoccupation with appearance, obsessive traits, or low self-esteem. Adolescents with anorexia may have a history of constipation, syncope, secondary amenorrhea, abdominal pain, and periodic episodes of cold hands and feet. Parents usually note the chief complaint as weight loss. Note history of depression in the child with bulimia. Evaluate the child's self-concept, noting multiple fears, high need for acceptance, disordered body image, and perfectionism. Perform a thorough physical examination. The anorexic is usually severely underweight, with a body mass index (BMI) less than 17. Note cachetic appearance, dry sallow skin, thinning scalp hair, soft sparse body hair, and nail pitting. Measure vital signs, noting low temperature, bradycardia, or hypotension. Auscultate the heart, noting murmur as a result of mitral valve prolapse (occurs in about one third of patients). The adolescent with bulimia will be of normal weight or slightly overweight. Inspect the hands for calluses on the backs of the knuckles and split fingernails. Inspect the mouth and oropharynx for eroded dental enamel, red gums, and inflamed throat from self-induced vomiting. Careful evaluation of serum electrolytes and electrocardiogram is needed in anorexics, as severe electrolyte disturbances and cardiac arrhythmias often occur.

Nursing Management

Most children with eating disorders can be treated successfully on an outpatient basis. Those with anorexia who display severe weight loss, unstable vital signs, food refusal, or arrested pubertal development or who require enteral nutrition will need to be hospitalized. Refeeding syndrome (cardiovascular, hematologic, and neurologic complications) may occur in the severely malnourished patient if rapid nutritional replacement is given, so slow refeeding is essential to avoid complications. Phosphorus supplements are given as ordered. Assess vital signs frequently for orthostatic hypotension, irregular and decreased pulse, or hypothermia.

Consult the nutritionist for assistance with calculating caloric needs and determining an appropriate diet. Aim for a weight gain goal of 0.5 to 2 pounds per week. Instruct the child and family to keep a daily journal of intake, bingeing and purging behaviors, mood, and exercise. The journal may be used as an assessment tool as well as to document progress toward recovery. Assist the child and family to plan a suitably structured routine for the child that includes meals, snacks, and appropriate physical activity.

Use the physical findings associated with anorexia to educate the child about the consequences of malnutrition and how they can be remedied with adequate nutrient intake. Behavior or group therapy may also be needed. Assess the child's need for intervention for concomitant depression or **anxiety** (some anorexics also require psychotropic medications). Provide emotional support and positive reinforcement to the child and family. Refer the family to local support groups or online resources such as the Academy for Eating Disorders (www.aedweb.org) or the National Eating Disorders Association (www.nationaleatingdisorders.org). See Healthy People 2010.

ConsiderTHIS!

Nicole Ashton, 16 years old, is seen in your clinic due to weight loss. Her mother states that she has lost noticeable weight over the past few months and has stopped menstruating. What additional assessment information would be necessary?

After further examination it is determined that Nicole has anorexia nervosa. Her treatment is to take place on an outpatient basis beginning immediately. Discuss ways the family can encourage and assist in Nicole's recovery.

Mood Disorders

Mood disorders in children include depressive disorders and bipolar disorder. During childhood the incidence of depressive disorders is approximately equal between boys and girls, but they affect more girls during adolescence. Major depressive disorder affects 1% to 3% of children and 8% of adolescents. Dysthymic disorder occurs in 1% of children and 8% of adolescents (Shoaf et al., 2001). Bipolar disorder refers to a condition of alternating manic and depressive episodes. During the manic episode, mood is significantly elevated and the patient displays excess energy.

Depression may cause significant alterations in school performance and social relationships. Anxiety disorders and disruptive behavior disorders occur together with depression at rates of 70% and 50% respectively (Shoaf et al., 2001). Substance abuse also occurs about 25% of the time with depression. Divorce and serious family issues may contribute to the development of depression because

HEALTHY PEOPLE 2010

Objective	Significance
(Developmental) Reduce the relapse rate for persons with eating disorders, including anorexia nervosa and bulimia nervosa.	• Provide appropriate follow-up for all children recovering from anorexia or bulimia. • Ensure that psychotherapy is available to children with eating disorders.

of the ongoing stress they place on the child and their strong psychological impact (Mahon et al., 2003; Pompili et al., 2005).

Depressed children are at risk for suicide, which is the third leading cause of death among teens age 15 to 19 years (McClain, 2003). The 2005 Centers for Disease Control and Prevention Youth Risk Behavior Surveillance Report revealed that nearly 17% of teens had seriously considered suicide and 8.4% had attempted it (CDC, 2006).

Pathophysiology

Both norepinephrine and dopamine play a role in mood. Norepinephrine is considered to be important in the areas of energy and alertness, dopamine in the areas of pleasure and motivation. When alterations in the neurotransmission of norepinephrine and dopamine occur, the symptoms of depression (apathy, loss of interest and pleasure) result. Decreased levels of serotonin have also been implicated in depressive symptoms. In addition, circadian rhythm disturbances may play a role in the development of depression (Castiglia, 2000).

Therapeutic Management

Children with mood disorders usually benefit from psychotherapy. This helps the child to deal with the psychosocial consequences of his or her behavior on his or her interpersonal relationships with others. Crisis management, parental counseling, and individual, group, or family therapy may be useful. Major depressive disorder warrants the use of pharmacologic antidepressants. Bipolar disorder may be treated with neuroleptic agents or mood stabilizers.

Nursing Assessment

Children with untreated depression are at high risk for suicide as well as the development of comorbid disorders such as anxiety, substance abuse, and disruptive behavioral disorders. The nurse must screen all children for the development of depression.

Health History

Obtain a health history from the child and separately from the parent. Evaluate the child for history of recent changes in behavior, changes in peer relationships, alterations in school performance, withdrawal from previously enjoyed activities, sleep disturbances, changes in eating behaviors, increase in accidents, or sexual promiscuity (Castiglia, 2000). If possible, use a standardized depression screening questionnaire; there are many available.

Ask about potential stressors such as school concerns, conflicts with parents, dating issues, and **abuse** (physical or sexual) (McClain, 2003). When bipolar disorder is suspected, the history may reveal rapid, pressured speech, increased energy, decreased sleep, flamboyant behavior, or irritability during the manic episodes.

Note history of weight loss, failure to thrive, or increased incidence of infections in the infant. For the toddler, note delay or regression in developmental skills, increase in nightmares, or parental reports of clinginess. The preschooler may have a history of loss of interest in newly acquired skills; manifest encopresis, enuresis, anorexia, or binge-eating; or make frequent negative self-statements. The parents of a school-age child may report that he or she has a depressed, irritable, or aggressive mood.

Assess for risk factors for suicide, which include:

- Previous suicide attempt (Pompili et al., 2005)
- Change in school performance, sleep, or appetite
- Loss of interest in formerly favorite school or other activities
- Feelings of hopelessness or depression
- Statements about thoughts of suicide (McClain, 2003)

Physical Examination

Observe the infant for weepiness, withdrawn behaviors, or a frozen facial expression. Note a sad or expressionless face in the toddler or preschooler. In any age child, observe for apathy. Inspect the entire body surface for self-inflicted injuries, which may or may not be present. The remainder of the physical examination is generally normal unless the depressed child also has a chronic medical condition.

Nursing Management

Nursing management of children and adolescents with mood disorders focuses on education, support, and prevention.

Educating and Supporting the Child and Family

Teach families that mood disorders are biologic conditions, not personality flaws. Teach families how to administer antidepressant medication and to monitor for adverse effects. Encourage and praise their efforts at following through with cognitive and behavioral therapies. Support the family throughout the process, as sometimes treatment may be lengthy. Refer parents to local support resources or to the Depression and Bipolar Support Alliance (http://www.ndmda.org) or the Child and Adolescent Bipolar Foundation (www.bpkids.org).

Preventing Depression and Suicide

Establish a trusting relationship with the children and adolescents with whom you interact, particularly in the primary care setting, school, or chronic illness clinic. This trusting relationship may encourage children or adolescents to confide feelings or problems earlier than they may do with their parents. Screen all healthy and chronically ill preteens and teens for the development of depression. Use standardized screening tools such as those listed in Box 31.4. When a potential problem is identified, immediately refer the child for mental health assessment and

BOX 31.4
SCREENING TOOLS FOR DEPRESSION

- Children's Depression Rating Scale-Revised (CDRS-R): available at http://portal.wpspublish.com
- Center for Epidemiological Studies Depression Scale Modified for Children (CES-DC): available at http://www.brightfutures.org/mentalhealth/pdf/tools.html
- Weinberg Depression Scale for Children and Adolescents (WDSCA): available at http://www.proedaust.com.au/psyc.cfm
- Children's Depression Inventory (CDI): available at http://www.pearsonassessments.com/tests/cdi.htm
- Beck Depression Inventory for Youth (BDI-Y): available at http://harcourtassessments.com

intervention. It is important to identify depression early so that treatment can start. When a grief-inducing event is impending (such as the death of a family member), begin preventive intervention to help the child to deal with it. Provide appropriate observation for any child exhibiting suicidal ideation. See Healthy People 2010.

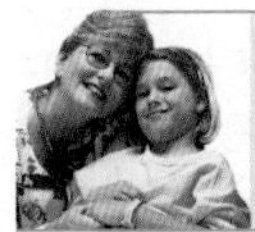

Closely observe children taking antidepressants for the development of presuicidal behavior.

Anxiety Disorders

Anxiety disorders are the most commonly diagnosed psychiatric conditions among children and adolescents (Williams & Hodgman, 2001). As many as 6% to 20% of children experience at least one anxiety disorder (American Academy of Child and Adolescent Psychiatry, 2007a). Anxiety often occurs together with other mental health disorders, especially depression. Normal children experience fear, worry, and shyness. Infants fear loud noises, being startled, and strangers. Toddlers are afraid of the dark and of separation. Preschoolers fear imaginary creatures and body mutilation. School-age children worry about injury and natural events, whereas adolescents are anxious about school and social performance. These normal fears produce a certain level of anxiety that is tolerated by most children, but it is important to distinguish normal developmentally appropriate anxiety from problematic anxiety.

Anxiety is considered to be a reaction to a perceived or actual threat. The threat may or may not be distorted by the child, and emotional distress leads to behavioral responses. The "fight-or-flight" response results in tachycardia, increased blood pressure, sweating, enhanced arousal and reactivity, tremors, and increased blood flow to the muscles.

HEALTHY PEOPLE 2010

Objective	Significance
(Developmental) Reduce the rate of suicide attempts by adolescents.	• Screen all children and adolescents for the development of depression. • When depression or excess stress is present, refer the child to the appropriate support.

Types of Anxiety Disorders

Generalized anxiety disorder (GAD) is characterized by unrealistic concerns over past behavior, future events, and personal competence. Social phobia may result, in which the child or teen demonstrates a persistent fear of speaking or eating in front of others, using public restrooms, or speaking to authorities. Selective mutism may also occur. Separation anxiety is more common in children than adolescents; the child may need to remain close to the parents, and the child's worries focus on separation themes. Obsessive-compulsive disorder (OCD) is characterized by compulsions (repetitive behaviors such as cleaning, washing, checking something), which the child performs to reduce anxiety about obsessions (unwanted and intrusive thoughts). Post-traumatic stress disorder (PTSD) is an anxiety disorder that occurs after a child experiences a traumatic event, later experiencing physiologic arousal when a stimulus triggers memories of the event.

Pathophysiology

Anxiety disorders are thought to occur as a result of disrupted modulation within the central nervous system. Underactivation of the serotonergic system and overactivation of the noradrenergic system are thought to be responsible for dysregulation of physiologic arousal and the resulting emotional experience. Disruption of the gamma-butyric acid (GABA) system may also play a role. Recently, the role of corticosteroids in behaviors related to stress and the way the brain processes fear-inducing stimuli have been explored.

Therapeutic Management

Therapeutic management of anxiety disorders generally involves the use of pharmacologic agents and psychological therapies. Anxiolytics or antidepressants are the most common pharmacologic approaches. Cognitive-behavioral therapy, individual, family, or group psychotherapy, and other behavioral interventions such as relaxation techniques may also be useful.

Nursing Assessment

Children and adolescents do not usually express anxiety directly, so it is very important for the nurse to evaluate somatic complaints and perform a careful history.

Health History

Explore the patient's current and past medical history for risk factors such as depression, anxious temperament, family history of anxiety disorders, certain environmental or life experiences (such as parental dysfunction or significant stressful event or trauma), or unstable parental attachment. Elicit the health history, noting history of social inhibition, panic, or "heart racing." Young children may display overactivity, acting out, sleep difficulties, or separation issues. Older children may describe feelings of nervousness, anger, fear, or tension and may display disruptive behavior. Ask the child to choose a number on a scale from 0 to 10 to describe how much he or she worries about things. Have the parent rank the child's worry in the same fashion, and ask the parent what the child worries about most. Determine frequency of headaches and stomachaches. Use a standardized screening tool such as:

- Multidimensional Anxiety Scale for Children (MASC), available at http://harcourtassessment.com
- Spence Children's Anxiety Scale (SACS), available at http://www2.psy.uq.edu.au/%7Esues/scas/
- Preschool Anxiety Scale, available at http://www2.psy.uq.edu.au/%7Esues/scas/preschool.html
- Beck Anxiety Inventory for Youth, available at http://harcourtassessment.com

Physical Examination

Perform a complete physical examination to rule out physiologic causes of the child's symptoms. Note patches of hair loss that occur with repetitive hair twisting or pulling associated with anxiety. Evaluate for evidence of nail biting, sucking blisters, or skin erosion from finger-rubbing. Inspect the entire body for signs of self-injury, which may or may not be present.

Nursing Management

Screen children at well-child or other health care visits, as well as upon admission to the hospital, for anxiety symptoms. If an anxiety disorder is suspected, refer the child to the appropriate mental health provider for further evaluation. When the child is diagnosed with an anxiety disorder and medication is prescribed, teach families about medication administration and adverse effects. Encourage and praise them for follow-through related to cognitive and behavioral therapy or psychotherapy. Provide emotional support to the child and family. Assess the family for the presence of parental anxiety or insecure attachment. Note parenting style and parent–child interactions. Not only the child but also the family will benefit from interventions that improve parent–child relationships, decrease parental anxiety, and foster parenting skills that promote autonomy in the child. Thus, ensure that concurrent family therapy occurs if needed.

Abuse and Violence

Abuse and violence contribute significantly to mental illness in children. Children may suffer from physical or sexual abuse, Münchausen syndrome, or substance abuse.

● PHYSICAL AND SEXUAL ABUSE

Physical abuse refers to injuries that are intentionally inflicted and that result in morbidity or mortality. Sexual abuse refers to involvement of the child in any activity meant to provide sexual gratification to an adult. **Neglect** is defined as failure to provide a child with appropriate food, clothing, shelter, medical care, and schooling. A history of childhood abuse is associated with the development of depressive disorders, suicidal ideation and attempts, and alcohol and drug use (Lesser & Koniak-Griffin, 2000). The Youth Risk Behavior Surveillance Survey reveals some startling statistics about the extent of abuse and violence in the United States:

- 6% of youths have not gone to school on at least one occasion because they thought they would be unsafe.
- Almost 14% have been involved in a physical fight at school.
- 8% have been threatened with a weapon one or more times on school property.
- 9% of youths have been slapped, hit, or intentionally physically hurt by their boyfriend or girlfriend.
- 7.5% have been physically forced to have sexual intercourse when they did not want to (CDC, 2006).

Statistics related to family violence as well as child physical and sexual abuse are difficult to determine, as the perpetrator usually forces the victim into silence. Children usually do not want to admit that their parent or relative has hurt them, partly from feelings of guilt and partly because they do not want to lose that parent. Abuse and violence occur across all socioeconomic levels but are more prevalent among the poor. Despite the lack of adequate statistics, it is well known that the problem of abuse and violence is widespread. Infants represent almost half of all children brought for medical treatment related to abuse (Marino & Fine, 2007). Parents, boyfriends of the child's mother, and stepparents are the most frequent perpetrators. Abuse places children at risk for low self-esteem, depressive disorders, and poor academic achievement. Long-term sequelae of abuse and violence include mood and anxiety disorders, post-traumatic stress disorder, reactive attachment disorder, later substance abuse, perpetuation of the violence cycle, and unknown neurobiologic effects.

Therapeutic management of victims of abuse and violence involves physical treatment of the injury, palliative care in some cases, and intervention to preserve or restore the child's mental well-being as well as family functioning. To protect children, all states require by law that health care professionals report suspected cases of abuse or neglect.

Nursing Assessment

Elicit the health history, noting the chief complaint and timing of onset. Pay particular attention to statements made by the child's parent or caretaker. Is the history given consistent with the injury? Identify abuse and violence by screening all children and families using these questions:

- Questions for children:
  Are you afraid of anyone at home?
  Who could you tell if someone hurt you or touched you in a way that made you uncomfortable?
  Has anyone hurt you or touched you in that way?
- Ask parents:
  Are you afraid of anyone at home?
  Do you ever feel like you may hit or hurt your child when frustrated? (Melnyk et al., 2003)

Note inappropriate sexual behavior for developmental age, such as seductiveness, as this may indicate sexual abuse. Determine if the child has a history of hurting self or others, running away, attempting suicide, or being involved in high-risk behaviors. Assess for risk factors such as poverty, prematurity, cerebral palsy, chronic illness, or mental retardation. Risk factors in parents or caretakers include a history of being abused themselves, alcohol or substance abuse, or extreme stress. Note history of chronic sore throat or difficulty swallowing, which may occur with forced oral sex or sexually transmitted infections. Document history of genital burning or itching (associated with sexual abuse).

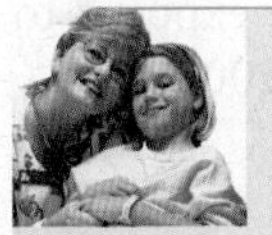

A delay in seeking medical treatment, a history that changes over time, or a history of trauma that is inconsistent with the observed injury all suggest child abuse.

Physical Examination

Perform a gentle but thorough physical examination, using a soft touch and calm voice. Observe the parent–child interaction, noting fear or an excessive desire to please. Note the infant's level of consciousness. Vigorous shaking in the infant leads to intracranial hemorrhage and shaken baby syndrome. Inspect the skin for bruises, burns, cuts, abrasions, contusions, scars, and any other unusual or suspicious marks. Current or healed scratches or cuts may be found on parts of the body ordinarily covered by clothing in the child who self-mutilates. Burns that occur in a stocking or glove pattern, or only to the soles or palms, are highly suspicious for inflicted burns. Injuries in various stages of healing are also indicative of abuse. Bruises on the chest, head, neck, or abdomen are suspicious for abuse. Nonambulatory children infrequently experience bruises or fractures. Figure 31.1 shows injury sites usually indicative of abuse; Figure 31.2 is a photograph of a child who

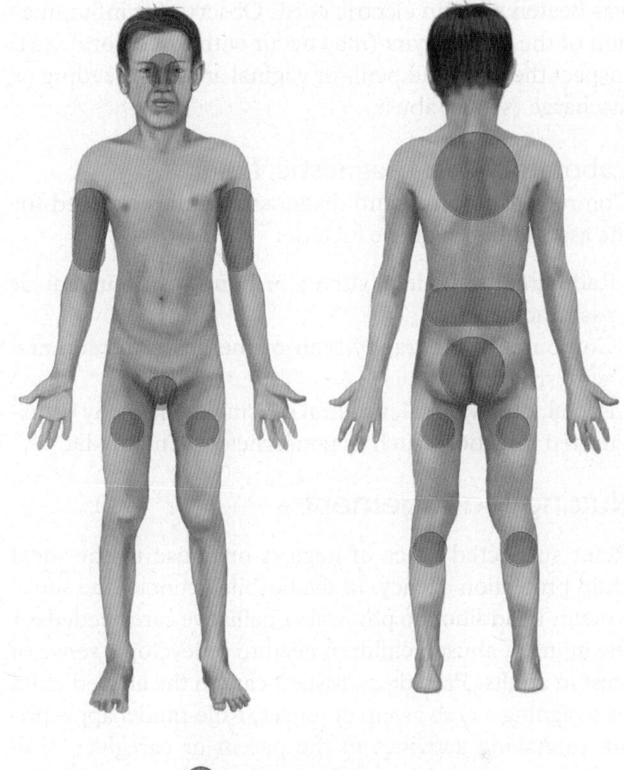

● Figure 31.1 Injury sites that are suspicious for abuse.

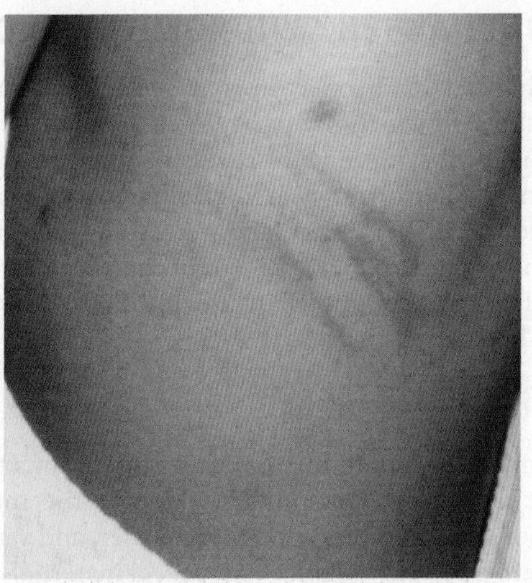

● Figure 31.2 Note the mark left from a looped electric cord.

was beaten with an electric cord. Observe for inflammation of the oropharynx (may occur with forced oral sex). Inspect the anus and penis or vaginal area for bleeding or discharge (sexual abuse).

Laboratory and Diagnostic Tests

Common laboratory and diagnostic studies ordered for the assessment of abuse include:

- Radiographic skeletal survey or bone scan: current or past fractures
- Computed tomography scan of the head: intracranial hemorrhage
- Rectal, oral, vaginal, urethral specimens: sexually transmitted infections such as gonorrhea or Chlamydia

Nursing Management

Refer suspected cases of neglect or abuse to the local child protection agency. In the hospital, contact the social worker. In addition to physical or palliative care needed for the injuries, abused children need to redevelop a sense of trust in adults. Provide consistent care to the abused child by assigning a core group of nurses. Role-model appropriate caretaking activities to the parent or caregiver. Call attention to normal growth and development activities noted in the infant or child, as sometimes parents have expectations of child behavior that may be unrealistic based on the child's age, leading to the abuse. Praise parents and caretakers for taking appropriate steps toward getting help and for providing appropriate care to the child. Refer parents to Parents Anonymous, an organization dedicated to the prevention of child abuse through strengthening of the family (www.parentsanonymous.org). If the child is removed from the family temporarily or permanently, provide the foster or adoptive family with education necessary to assume the child's care.

● MÜNCHAUSEN SYNDROME BY PROXY

Münchausen syndrome by proxy (MSBP) is a type of child abuse in which the parent creates physical and/or psychological symptoms of illness or impairment. The adult meets her own psychological needs by having an ill child. MSBP is difficult to detect and may remain hidden for years. Ninety percent of the perpetrators are biological mothers, mostly white and 20 to 30 years of age (Thomas, 2003).

Nursing Assessment

Determine the health history, using quotations to document the parent's responses. Observe the mother's behavior with the child, spouse or partner, and staff. Use of covert video surveillance may reveal maternal actions causing illness in the child. Warning signs of MSBP include:

- Child with one or more illnesses that do not respond to treatment or that follow a puzzling course; a similar history in siblings
- Symptoms that do not make sense or that disappear when the perpetrator is removed or not present; the symptoms are witnessed only by the caregiver (e.g., cyanosis, apnea, seizure)
- Physical and laboratory findings that do not fit with the reported history
- Repeated hospitalizations failing to produce a medical diagnosis, transfers to other hospitals, discharges against medical advice
- Parent who refuses to accept that the diagnosis is not medical

Nursing Management

Management of MSBP is complex. Detailed documentation of the history and physical examination is the basis for determining that MSBP is present. Observe the caregiver–child interactions closely, using covert video surveillance if available. When an actual abusive activity is identified, notify the social services and risk management departments of the hospital. Ensure that the local child protection team and the caregiver's family or support system is present when the caregiver is confronted. Inform the caregiver of the plan of care for the child and of the availability of psychiatric assistance for the caregiver.

● SUBSTANCE ABUSE

According to the Youth Risk Behavior Survey, over 40% of students drink alcohol, and 25% of them take their first alcoholic drink before age 13. Among youths, 20% use marijuana, almost 8% use some form of cocaine, and about 2% use injectable illegal drugs. In addition, youths report having used heroin, hallucinogenic drugs, methamphetamines, inhalants, and Ecstasy (CDC, 2006). Twenty-five percent of children under 18 years of age are exposed to alcohol abuse in their families (Melnyk et al., 2003).

Nursing Assessment

Note risk factors for substance abuse, such as family history, current parental substance use, dysfunctional family relationships, concurrent mental health disorder, negative life events, or peers who use substances. Determine the child's history, noting altered school performance or attendance, changes in peer group participation, frequent mood swings, changes in physical appearance, or an altered relationship with or perception of parents. Document history of insomnia, appetite loss, excessive itching, sleepiness or extreme fatigue, dry mouth, or shakiness. Note violent behavior, drunkenness, stupor, blank expression, drowsiness, lack of coordination, confusion, incoherent speech, extremes in emotions, aggressive behavior, silly behavior, or rapid speech. Observe for an odor of alcohol or marijuana smoke. Assess the eyes, noting wateriness or dilated pupils. Inspect the nares, noting rhinorrhea or absence of nasal hair. Inspect the fingers for glue smears or discoloration and the skin for needle marks or tracks. Palpate the hands and feet for coolness. Toxicology studies such as urine screening can determine the presence of stimulants, sedative-hypnotics, barbiturates, Quaaludes, opiates, cocaine, and marijuana.

Nursing Management

Help the adolescent to acknowledge that he or she has a problem. Explain the negative consequences of substance use and raise the teen's awareness of risks. Remain empathetic, yet leave responsibility with the adolescent.

Promoting Participation in Treatment Programs

Refer the adolescent to a substance abuse program. Outpatient or day treatment programs are useful in most situations. Family-based programs produce the highest level of recovery. Self-help or 12-step groups are an important element in the recovery process. Serious addiction, the presence of one or more comorbid psychiatric conditions, or suicidal ideation requires residential treatment or hospitalization. See Healthy People 2010.

Preventing Substance Abuse

Teach all children, beginning at the elementary school level, that all chemicals have the potential to be harmful to the body, including tobacco, alcohol, and illicit drugs. Help children to learn problem-solving skills that they can call upon in the future rather than relying on drugs or other substances. Teach children to "just say no." Reinforce that they are the ones who have control over their body and what they expose it to. Educate children and adolescents that no matter which administration route is used, the drug still enters the body and affects it. Encourage children to participate in the local DARE program (Drug Abuse Resistance Education) and praise them for completing it.

HEALTHY PEOPLE 2010

Objective	Significance
(Developmental) Increase the proportion of persons with co-occurring substance abuse and mental disorders who receive treatment for both disorders.	• Screen all children and adolescents with mental health disorders for the coexistence of substance abuse (and vice versa). • Refer clients to appropriate treatment programs and therapy.

References

Books and Journals

Accardo, P. J., Accardo, J. A., & Capute, A. J. (2006). Mental retardation. In J. A. McMillan (Ed.), *Oski's pediatrics: Principles and practice.* Philadelphia: Lippincott Williams & Wilkins.

American Academy of Child and Adolescent Psychiatry. (2007a). Practice parameter for the assessment and treatment of children and adolescents anxiety disorders. *Journal of the American Academy of Child and Adolescent Psychiatry, 46*(2), 267–283.

American Academy of Child and Adolescent Psychiatry. (2007b). Practice parameter for the assessment and treatment of children and adolescents with oppositional defiant disorder. *Journal of the American Academy of Child and Adolescent Psychiatry, 46*(1), 126–141.

American Academy of Pediatrics. (2000). Insurance coverage of mental health and substance abuse service of children and adolescents: a consensus statement. *Pediatrics, 106,* 860–862.

American Academy of Pediatrics, Committee on Children with Disabilities. (2001). The pediatrician's role in the diagnosis and management of autistic spectrum disorder in children. *Pediatrics, 107*(5), 1221–1226.

American Academy of Pediatrics, Committee on Psychosocial Aspects of Child and Family Health. (2001). The new morbidity revisited: A renewed commitment to the psychosocial aspects of pediatric care. *Pediatrics, 108,* 1227–1230.

American Association on Intellectual and Developmental Disability. (2007). The AAMR definition of mental retardation. Retrieved January 22, 2007, from http://www.aamr.org/Policies/faq_mental_retardation.shtml.

Aylward, G. P. (2002). Learning disabilities. In N. J. Salkind (Ed.), *Child development* (pp. 240–243). New York: Macmillan.

Barbaresi, W. J., Katusic, S. K., Colligan, R. C., et al. (2006). Long-term stimulant medication treatment of attention-deficit/hyperactivity disorder: Results from a population-based study. *Journal of Developmental and Behavioral Pediatrics, 27*(1), 1–10.

Beauchesne, M. A., & Kelly, B. R. (2004). Evidence to support parental concerns as an early indicator of autism in children. *Pediatric Nursing, 30*(1), 57–67.

Bernal, P. (2003). Hidden morbidity in pediatric primary care. *Pediatric Annals, 3*(6), 413–418.

Castiglia, P. T. (2000). Depression in adolescents. *Journal of Pediatric Health Care, 14,* 180–182.

Centers for Disease Control and Prevention. (2006). Youth risk behavior surveillance—United States, 2005. *Morbidity and Mortality Weekly Report, 55*(SS-5), 1–112.

Choueiri, R., & Bridgemohan, C. (2005). To make the biggest difference, screen early for autism spectrum disorders. *Contemporary Pediatrics, 22*(10), 54–64.

Clift, G. (2002). Anxiety disorders in children: Intervention strategies for the primary care setting. *Journal of Pediatric Health Care, 16,* 253–255.

Davis, D. W., Burns, B., Snyder, E., et al. (2004). Parent–child interaction and attention regulation in children born prematurely. *Journal for Specialists in Pediatric Nursing, 9*(3), 85–94.

DeMarle, D. J., Denk, L., & Ernsthausen, C. S. (2003). Working with the family of a child with attention deficit hyperactivity disorder. *Pediatric Nursing, 29*(4), 302–308, 330.

DeNisco, S., Tiago, C., & Kravitz, C. (2005). Evaluation and treatment of pediatric ADHD. *Nurse Practitioner, 30*(8), 14–23.

Dumont-Mathieu, T., Fein, D., & Kleinman, J. (2005). *Screening for autism in young children: The modified checklist for autism in toddlers (M-CHAT).* Retrieved December 27, 2006, from www.dbpeds.org/articles/detail.cfm?TextID=377.

Ellis, C. R., & Schnoes, C. J. (2006). *Eating disorder: Pica.* Retrieved February 18, 2007, from www.emedicine.com/ped/topic1798.htm.

Ellis, C. R., & Schnoes, C. J. (2006). *Eating disorder: Rumination.* Retrieved February 18, 2007, from http://www.emedicine.com/ped/topic2652.htm.

Ferren, P. M. (2006). Demystifying the black box warning on antidepressants: A protocol for safe prescribing in your office. *Contemporary Pediatrics, 23*(2), 28–35.

Ford-Martin, P. (2006). Stanford-Binet intelligence scales. *Gale encyclopedia of medicine, vol. 4* (3rd ed., pp. 3517–3518). Detroit: Gale.

Giarelli, E., Souders, M., Pinto-Martin, J., et al. (2005). Intervention pilot for parents of children with autistic spectrum disorder. *Pediatric Nursing, 31*(5), 389–398.

Goldson, E., & Reynolds, A. (2007). Child development and behavior. In W. W. Hay, M. J. Levin, J. M. Sondheimer, & R. R. Deterding, *Current pediatric diagnosis and treatment* (8th ed.). New York: McGraw-Hill Companies, Inc.

Gracious, B. L., & Findling, R. L. (2001). Antipsychotic medications for children and adolescents. *Pediatric Annals, 30*(3), 138–145.

Harris, J. C. (2006). Depression in childhood and adolescence. In J. A. McMillan (Ed.), *Oski's pediatrics: Principles and practice.* Philadelphia: Lippincott Williams & Wilkins.

Harris, J. C. (2006). Disruptive behavior disorders. In J. A. McMillan (Ed.), *Oski's pediatrics: Principles and practice.* Philadelphia: Lippincott Williams & Wilkins.

Harris, J. C. (2006). Emotional disorders with childhood onset. In J. A. McMillan (Ed.), *Oski's pediatrics: Principles and practice.* Philadelphia: Lippincott Williams & Wilkins.

Harris, J. C. (2006). Mental disorders and psychological stress. In J. A. McMillan (Ed.), *Oski's pediatrics: Principles and practice.* Philadelphia: Lippincott Williams & Wilkins.

Harris, J. C. (2006). Pervasive developmental disorder and autistic disorder. In J. A. McMillan (Ed.), *Oski's pediatrics: Principles and practice.* Philadelphia: Lippincott Williams & Wilkins.

Harris, J. C. (2006). Psychosocial interview. In J. A. McMillan (Ed.), *Oski's pediatrics: Principles and practice.* Philadelphia: Lippincott Williams & Wilkins.

Harris, J. C. (2006). Suicide. In J. A. McMillan (Ed.), *Oski's pediatrics: Principles and practice.* Philadelphia: Lippincott Williams & Wilkins.

Hunt, R. D., Paguin, A., & Payton, K. (2001). An update on assessment and treatment of complex attention-deficit hyperactivity disorder. *Pediatric Annals, 30*(3), 162–171.

Kelly, K. (2003). Lesson from Eric: Learning from an autistic child. *American Journal of Nursing, 103*(5), 64F–64G.

Kreipe, R. E. (2006). Eating disorders. In J. A. McMillan (Ed.), *Oski's pediatrics: Principles and practice.* Philadelphia: Lippincott Williams & Wilkins.

Lansford, A. H. (2005). The importance of recognizing a child with bipolar disorder. *Contemporary Pediatrics, 22*(2), 69–78.

Leonard, H. L., Freeman, J., Garcia, A., et al. (2001). Obsessive-compulsive disorder and related conditions. *Pediatric Annals, 30*(3), 154–160.

Leslie, L. K. (2002). The role of primary care physicians in attention-deficit/hyperactivity disorder. *Pediatric Annals, 31*(8), 475–484.

Lesser, J., & Koniak-Griffin, D. (2000). The impact of physical or sexual abuse on chronic depression in adolescent mothers. *Journal for Specialists in Pediatric Nursing, 15*(6), 378–387.

Mahon, N. E., Yarcheski, A., & Yarcheski, T. J. (2003). Anger, anxiety, and depression in early adolescents from intact and divorced families. *Journal for Specialists in Pediatric Nursing, 18*(4), 267–273.

Malatack, J. J, Consolini, D., Mann, K., & Rabb, C. (2006). Taking on the parent to save a child: Munchausen syndrome by proxy. *Contemporary Pediatrics, 23*(6), 50–63.

Marino, B. S., & Fine, K. S. (2007). *Blueprints: Pediatrics.* Philadelphia: Lippincott Williams & Wilkins.

McClain, N. (2003). Adolescent suicide attempt: Undisclosed secrets. *Pediatric Nursing, 29*(1), 52–53.

Melnyk, B. M., Brown, H. E., Jones, D. C., et al. (2003). Improving the mental/psychosocial health of U.S. children and adolescents: Outcomes and implementation strategies from the national KySS summit. *Journal of Pediatric Health Care, 17*(6), S1–S24.

National Center for Learning Disabilities. (2006). *LD at a glance.* Retrieved January 22, 2007, from www.ncld.org/content/view/448/391/.

Oliver, C. J. (2003). Triage of the autistic spectrum child utilizing the congruence of case management concepts and Orem's nursing theories. *Lippincott's Case Management, 8*(2), 66–82.

Pinto-Martin, J. A., Souders, M. C., Giarelli, E., & Levy, S. E. (2005). The role of nurses in screening for autistic spectrum disorder in pediatric primary care. *Journal of Pediatric Nursing, 20*(3), 163–169.

Pompili, M., Mancinelli, I., Girardi, P., et al. (2005). Childhood suicide: A major issue in pediatric health care. *Issues in Comprehensive Pediatric Nursing, 28,* 63–68.

Reasor, J. E., & Farrell, S. P. (2004). Early childhood mental health: Services that can save a life. *Journal of Pediatric Nursing, 19*(2), 140–144.

Reid, B., & Long, A. (2002). Suspected child abuse: Communicating with a child and her mother. *Journal of Pediatric Nursing, 17*(3), 229–235.

Scarpa, A., & Raine, A. (2004). The psychophysiology of child misconduct. *Pediatric Annals, 33*(5), 297–304.

Scheid, J. M. (2003). Recognizing and managing long-term sequelae of childhood maltreatment. *Pediatric Annals, 32*(6), 391–401.

Schultz, J. M., & Videbeck, S. L. (2005). *Lippincott's manual of psychiatric nursing care plans.* Philadelphia: Lippincott Williams & Wilkins.

Semrud-Clikeman, M., & Higgins, K. (2003). Learning disabilities. In J. J. Ponzetti, Jr. (Ed.), *International encyclopedia of marriage and families, vol. 3* (2nd ed., pp. 1034–1041). New York: Macmillan.

Shoaf, T. L., Emslie, G. J., & Mayes, T. L. (2001). Childhood depression: Diagnosis and treatment strategies in general pediatrics. *Pediatric Annals, 30*(3), 130–137.

Snell, M. E. (2002). Education of individuals with mental retardation. In J. W. Guthrie (Ed.), *Encyclopedia of education, vol. 5* (2nd ed., pp. 1616–1617). New York: Macmillan.

Stein, M. A., & Baren, M. (2003). Welcome progress in the diagnosis and treatment of ADHD in adolescence. *Contemporary Pediatrics, 20*(8), 83–84, 87–90, 93–98, 100–110.

Stein, M. T. (2002). The role of attention-deficit/hyperactivity disorder diagnostic and treatment guidelines in changing physician practices. *Pediatric Annals, 31*(8), 496–504.

Stevens, S. (2005). Attention deficit/hyperactivity disorder: Working the system for better diagnosis and treatment. *Journal of Pediatric Nursing, 20*(1), 47–51.

Thomas, K. (2003). Münchausen syndrome by proxy: Identification and diagnosis. *Journal of Pediatric Nursing, 18*(3), 174–180.

U.S. Public Health Service. (2004). Report of the Surgeon Generals' Conference on Children's Mental Health: A national action agenda. Washington, D.C.: Department of Health and Human Services. Retrieved January 2, 2007, from www.surgeongeneral.gov/topics/cmh/childreport.htm.

Vlam, S. L. (2006). Attention-deficit/hyperactivity disorder: Diagnostic assessment methods used by advanced practice registered nurses. *Pediatric Nursing, 31*(1), 18–24.

Wickham, P. (2004). Retardation. In P. S. Fass (Ed.), *Encyclopedia of children and childhood in history and society, vol. 2* (pp. 712–714). New York: Macmillan.

Williams, T., & Hodgman, C. (2001). Medication for the management of anxiety disorders in children and adolescents. *Pediatric Annals, 30*(3), 146–153.

Zinner, S. H. (2004a). Tourette syndrome—much more than tics: Management tailored to the entire patient. *Contemporary Pediatrics, 21*(8), 38–49.

Zinner, S. H. (2004b). Tourette syndrome—much more than tics: Moving beyond misconceptions to a diagnosis. *Contemporary Pediatrics, 21*(8), 22–36.

Zinner, S. H. (2006c). Tourette syndrome in infancy and early childhood. *Infants and Young Children, 19*(4), 353–370.

Websites

www.aacap.org American Academy of Child and Adolescent Psychiatry

www.aamr.org American Association of Intellectual and Developmental Disability

www.aedweb.org Academy for Eating Disorders

www.afsp.org American Foundation for Suicide Prevention

www.autism-society.org American Autism Society

www.autismonline.org Autism Online

www.bpkids.org Child and Adolescent Bipolar Foundation

www.centerforlearningdifferences.org Center for Learning Differences

www.chadd.org Children and Adults with Attention-Deficit/Hyperactivity Disorder

http://child-abuse.com Child Abuse Prevention Network

www.childwelfare.gov Child Welfare Information Gateway

www.dbpeds.org Developmental and Behavioral Pediatrics Online
www.edjj.org National Center on Education, Disability, and Juvenile Justice
www.ed.gov/about/offices/list/osdfs/index.html Office of Safe and Drug-Free Schools
http://endabuse.org Family Violence Prevention Fund
www.firstsigns.org First Signs, Inc., educating parents and professionals about early detection of autism and other developmental delays—Modified Checklist for Autism in Toddlers (M-CHAT)
www.getreadytoread.org Get Ready to Read!
www.harcourtassessment.com to order the Pervasive Developmental Disorders Screening Test-II (PDDST-II)
www.helpautismnow.com Help Autism Now Society
www.ldonline.org web site for learning disabilities and ADHD
www.ispn-psych.org/html/acapn.html Association of Child and Adolescent Psychiatric Nurses
http://mentalhealth.samhsa.gov/child/childhealth.asp Substance Abuse and Mental Health Services Administration's (SAMHSA) National Mental Health Information Center
http://ncadi.samhsa.gov alcohol and drug information from Prevention Online
www.nationaleatingdisorders.org National Eating Disorders Association
www.ncld.org National Center for Learning Disabilities
www.ncmhjj.com National Center for Mental Health and Juvenile Justice
www.nctsnet.org/nccts/nav.do?pid=hom_main National Child Traumatic Stress Network
www.niaaa.nih.gov National Institute on Alcohol Abuse and Alcoholism
www.nimh.nih.gov National Institute of Mental Health
www.parentsanonymous.org Parents Anonymous (child abuse prevention)
www.preventchildabuse.org Prevent Child Abuse U.S.A.
www.shakenbaby.com Shaken Baby Alliance
www.stopfamilyviolence.org Stop Family Violence
www.wpspublish.com Western Psychological Services (the Social Communication Questionnaire [SCQ])

Chapter WORKSHEET

MULTIPLE CHOICE QUESTIONS

1. The nurse is caring for a child with ADHD. Which behavior would the nurse **not** expect the child to display?
   a. Moody, morose behavior with pouting
   b. Interruption and inability to take turns
   c. Forgetfulness and easy distractibility
   d. Excessive motor activities and fidgeting
2. An adolescent girl who has been receiving treatment for anorexia nervosa has failed to gain weight over the past week despite eating all of her meals and snacks. What is the priority nursing intervention?
   a. Increase the teen's daily caloric intake by at least 500 calories.
   b. Ensure that the teen's entire fluid intake includes calories.
   c. Supervise the teen for 2 hours after all meals and snacks.
   d. Assess the teen's anxiety level to determine need for medication.
3. A 15-year-old patient has been making demands all day, exaggerating her every need. She is now crying, saying she has nothing to live for and threatening to kill herself. What is the priority nursing action?
   a. Ignore her continued exaggerated and melodramatic behavior.
   b. Consult with the physician to increase her antidepressant dose.
   c. Leave the girl alone for a little while until she composes herself.
   d. Take the girl's suicidal threat seriously and provide close supervision.
4. When trying to manage aggressive or impulsive behaviors in children or adolescents, what is the best nursing intervention?
   a. Train the child to be assertive.
   b. Provide consistency and limit-setting.
   c. Allow the child to negotiate the rules.
   d. Encourage the child to express feelings.

CRITICAL THINKING EXERCISES

1. A mother tells you that her son's behavior is unmanageable, and she is having difficulty coping with it. The boy is argumentative and is bullying others. He is struggling with his schoolwork because he has difficulty staying on task, gets out of his chair often, and frequently distracts others. What additional assessments should you obtain? What interventions would be helpful in managing the boy's behavior?
2. A 14-year-old moderately retarded boy is able to feed himself but is incontinent. Discuss the issues his family must deal with.

STUDY ACTIVITIES

1. Explore several of the websites related to child abuse prevention listed at the end of this chapter. Develop a list of resources for families in your local area.
2. Attend a group therapy session during your pediatric clinical rotation. Observe the children's verbal and nonverbal communication, noting inconsistencies or other interesting observations.
3. Visit a school for autistic children. Spend time with the various specialists who work with children with ASD, determining their roles and the effect the treatment they are providing has on the children. Report your findings to your classmates.
4. Attend a local CHADD meeting. Talk to parents about having a child with ADHD.

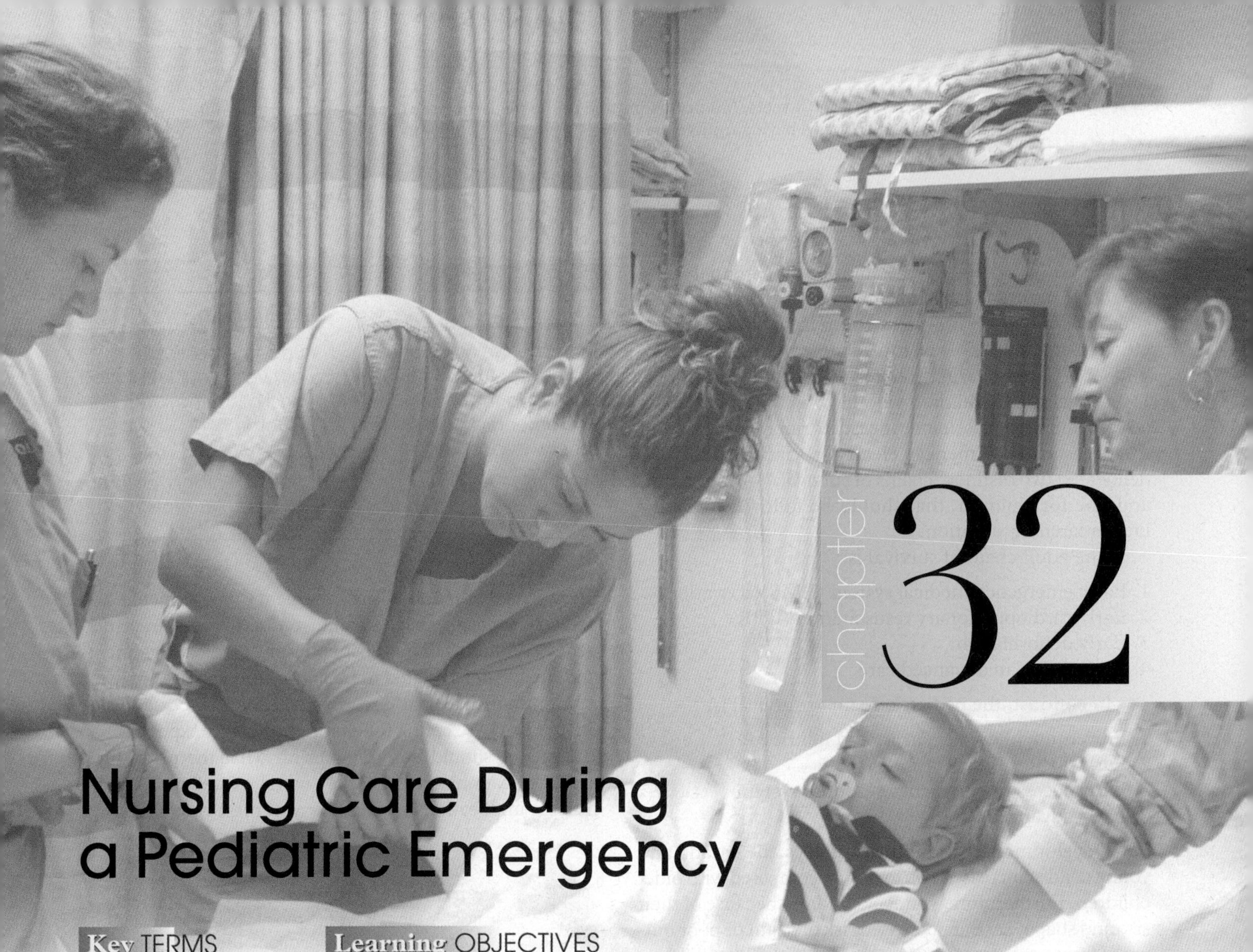

chapter 32

Nursing Care During a Pediatric Emergency

Key TERMS

asystole
barotrauma
bradycardia
cardioversion
cricoid pressure
defibrillation
hypercapnia
hyperventilation
hypocapnia
hypoventilation
intubation
periodic breathing
tachycardia
tachypnea
tracheal (endotracheal) tube

Learning OBJECTIVES

Upon completion of the chapter, the learner will be able to:

1. Identify various factors contributing to emergency situations among infants and children.
2. Discuss common treatments and medications used for a child experiencing an emergency.
3. Conduct a health history of a child experiencing an emergency situation, specific to the emergency.
4. Perform a rapid cardiopulmonary assessment.
5. Discuss common laboratory and other diagnostic tests used during pediatric emergencies.
6. Integrate the principles of the American Heart Association (AHA) and Pediatric Advanced Life Support (PALS) in the comprehensive management of a child with an emergent medical situation.

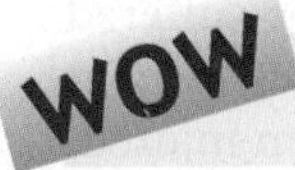

A nurse must possess knowledge and skills to aid an acutely ill child.

Alma Anderson, age 8 years, has been admitted to the pediatric unit. Her mother calls the nurse into the room, stating, "Alma's having trouble breathing!"

Children are uniquely vulnerable to a diverse range of emergency situations. These situations are often life-threatening if not treated in an efficient manner. For example, most pediatric cardiopulmonary arrests result from respiratory failure or shock. Data suggest that children who have a cardiopulmonary arrest requiring resuscitative measures rarely fare well. For these reasons, the American Heart Association (AHA) has delineated two distinct "chains of survival," one for adults and one for children, that should be followed during a life-threatening situation.

The adult chain of survival is:

1. Early emergency medical system (EMS) activation
2. Early cardiopulmonary resuscitation (CPR)
3. Early defibrillation
4. Early access to advanced care

In contrast, the pediatric chain of survival is:

1. Prevention of cardiac arrest and injuries
2. Early CPR
3. Early access to emergency response system
4. Early advanced care

Developmental immaturity places the infant and young child at increased risk for injury compared with older children. Furthermore, younger children, because of their size and shape, have an increased risk of death or poor outcome from traumatic injury compared with older children (American College of Surgeons, 2004; MacLachlan, 2003). Near-drowning and poisoning are two additional emergency situations for which children are at increased risk.

Considering the special risks that threaten children, the AHA has also developed specific guidelines for Pediatric Advanced Life Support (PALS). Courses in PALS are offered for health care professionals so that they can provide expert care for children in emergencies. This chapter emphasizes the principles of PALS in its discussion of the pediatric nurse's role in the management of pediatric emergencies.

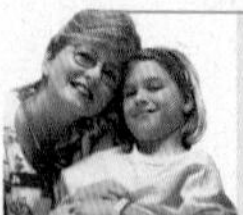

New PALS guidelines published in 2005 define the pediatric patient as any child up to about 16 to 18 years of age. Children in this age group or younger should be managed using the PALS guidelines rather than those for adults (AHA, 2005e). See Healthy People 2010.

HEALTHY PEOPLE 2010

Objective	Significance
Increase the number of states and the District of Columbia that have implemented guidelines for prehospital and hospital pediatric care.	• Become politically active in your local area and at the national level. • Advocate for optimum care for infants, children, and adolescents.

Common Medical Treatments

A variety of medications as well as other medical treatments are used to treat pediatric emergencies. Most of these treatments will require a physician's order when the child is in the hospital, though some emergency departments and pediatric units may have standing orders for pediatric emergency conditions. The most common medical treatments and medications related to pediatric emergencies are listed in Common Medical Treatments 32.1 and Drug Guide 32.1. The nurse caring for children who may experience an emergency should be familiar with what the procedures and medications are, how they work, as well as common nursing implications related to use of these modalities.

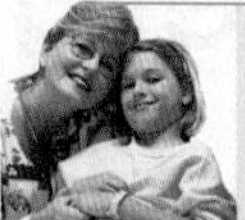

Certain code drugs for children may be given via a **tracheal tube** (a tube inserted into the trachea that serves to maintain the airway and facilitate artificial respiration). Use the mnemonic LEAN (lidocaine, epinephrine, atropine, and naloxone) to remember which drugs may be given via the tracheal route (AHA, 2001b). In certain cases, when an emergency drug is given via the tracheal tube, the dosage must be increased. In addition, drugs given via this route should usually be diluted with 2 to 5 mL of sterile saline and followed by multiple positive-pressure ventilations to ensure that the drugs are delivered.

Nursing Process Overview for the Child Experiencing an Emergency Situation

The nurse may encounter a child who is experiencing an emergency in a variety of settings. As a member of a trauma team at a pediatric hospital, the nurse may participate in the stabilization of a child who has suffered a near-drowning or trauma. The emergency department nurse may encounter a child who has just been injured, such as from a fall, accident, or sports. On the hospital unit, a child with asthma may suffer respiratory distress or stop breathing. Regardless of the setting or how the emergency developed, the principles for managing pediatric emergencies are the same.

(text continues on page 1075)

Common Medical Treatments 32.1 Pediatric Emergencies

Treatment	Explanation	Indication	Nursing Implications
Suctioning (oropharyngeal, nasopharyngeal, tracheal, or tracheostomy)	Removal of secretions via bulb syringe or suction catheter	Excessive airway secretions affecting airway patency	Use caution and suction only as far as recommended for age, tracheal tube size, or tracheostomy tube size or until coughing or gagging occurs.
Oxygen	Supplementation via mask, nasal cannula, hood, or tent or via tracheal/nasotracheal tube	Hypoxemia, respiratory distress, shock, trauma	Monitor response via color, work of breathing, respiratory rate, oxygen saturation levels via pulse oximetry, and level of consciousness.
Bag-valve-mask ventilation	Provision of ventilation via a bag-valve-mask device, manual ventilation	Apnea, ineffective ventilation and oxygenation with spontaneous breaths, extremely slow respiratory rate	Ensure adequate chest rise with ventilation. Do not overventilate or bag aggressively to avoid barotrauma. Maintain a seal on the child's face with the appropriate-sized mask. Ensure the oxygen supply tubing is connected to 100% oxygen.
Intubation	Insertion of a tube into the trachea to provide artificial ventilation	Apnea, airway that is not maintainable, need for prolonged assisted ventilation	Determine adequacy of breath sounds with bagging immediately upon insertion of the tracheal tube. Assess for symmetrical chest rise. Tape tube securely in place and note number marking on the tube. Connect to ventilator when available.
Needle thoracotomy	Insertion of a needle between the ribs into the pleural space to remove air	Tension pneumothorax	There should be a rush of air as the needle reaches the air space. Monitor breath sounds, work of breathing, pulse oximetry.
IV fluid therapy	Administration of crystalloid or colloid solutions to provide hydration or improve perfusion	Altered perfusion states such as respiratory distress, shock, trauma, cardiac disturbances	Insure patency of IV catheter. Use intraosseous route if a peripheral IV cannot be obtained quickly in the young child in shock. Reassess respiratory and circulatory status frequently after each IV fluid bolus and during continuous infusion.
Blood product transfusion	Administration of whole blood, packed red blood cells, platelets, or plasma intravenously	Trauma, hemorrhage	Follow institution's transfusion protocol. Double-check blood type and product label with a second nurse. Monitor vital signs and assess child frequently to determine adverse reaction to blood transfusion.

(continued)

Common Medical Treatments 32.1 Pediatric Emergencies (continued)

Treatment	Explanation	Indication	Nursing Implications
			If adverse reaction is suspected, immediately discontinue transfusion, infuse normal saline solution IV, reassess the child, and notify the physician.
Cervical stabilization	Maintenance of the cervical spine in an immobile position	Trauma, near-drowning	Use the jaw-thrust maneuver without head tilt to open the airway. Maintain cervical stabilization until the cervical spine x-rays are cleared by the physician or radiologist.
Defibrillation and synchronized cardioversion	Provision of electrical current to alter the heart's electrical rhythm	Defibrillation: ventricular fibrillation and pulseless ventricular tachycardia. Synchronized cardioversion: supraventricular tachycardia and ventricular tachycardia with a pulse	In the pulseless patient, always ensure CPR is ongoing while the defibrillator is being readied. Ensure adequate oxygenation. Provide lidocaine or epinephrine if indicated before defibrillation. Sedate the child if time allows.

Drug Guide 32.1 Common Medications Used in Pediatric Emergency Situations

Medication	Action	Indication	Nursing Implications
Adenosine (antiarrhythmic)	Slows conduction through AV node, restoring normal sinus rhythm	Supraventricular tachycardia (SVT)	• Administer IV at a dose ranging from 0.05 to 0.1 mg/kg. • Administer very rapidly (1 to 2 seconds) followed by a rapid, generous saline flush. • Repeat every 1 to 2 minutes, increasing by 0.05 to 0.1 mg/kg with each dose (maximum dose 0.3 mg/kg). • Monitor for shortness of breath, dyspnea, worsening of asthma.
Atropine (anticholinergic)	Increases cardiac output, dries secretions, inhibits serotonin and histamine	Sinus bradycardia, asystole, pulseless electrical activity	• Administer via IV, IO, or ET route at a dose of 0.02 mg/kg (maximum dose 0.5 mg child, 1 mg adolescent). • Repeat every 5 minutes PRN.

Drug Guide 32.1 Common Medications Used in Pediatric Emergency Situations (continued)

Medication	Action	Indication	Nursing Implications
			• Give undiluted over 30 seconds for IV or IO route. • Dilute with 3 to 5 mL normal saline for ET route; follow with five positive-pressure ventilations. • Do not mix with sodium bicarbonate (incompatible).
Dobutamine (synthetic cathecholamine)	Beta-adrenergic agent primarily affecting beta-1 receptors; increases myocardial contractility and heart rate	Ongoing short-term management of shock (hypovolemic and cardiogenic)	• Administer via IV or IO route at 2 to 20 mcg/kg/minute via a continuous infusion. Monitor for development of ventricular arrhythmias. • Expect to titrate infusion rate based on cardiac output and BP. • Administer via central line if possible due to risk of extravasation. • Monitor child closely, preferably in an ICU setting.
Dopamine (inotropic)	Increases cardiac output, BP, and renal perfusion (beta-adrenergic agonist)	Bradycardia, hypotension, and poor cardiac output	• Administer via IV or IO route at a dose of 2 to 20 mcg/kg/minute via continuous infusion. • Ensure that child has received adequate fluid resuscitation prior to administration. • Due to risk of extravasation, give via central line if possible. • Monitor child closely, preferably in an ICU setting. • Assess for ventricular arrhythmias.
Epinephrine (adrenergic)	Stimulates alpha- and beta-adrenergic receptors, increasing heart rate and systemic vascular resistance	Bradycardia, anaphylaxis	• Administer via IV or IO route at a dose of 0.01 mg/kg (0.1 mL/kg of 1:10,000 solution) or via ET route at 0.1 mg/kg (0.1 mL/kg of 1:1,000 solution). • During CPR, repeat every 3 to 5 minutes. • Monitor for ventricular arrhythmias. • High doses may cause tachycardia in newborns.

(continued)

Drug Guide 32.1 Common Medications Used in Pediatric Emergency Situations (continued)

Medication	Action	Indication	Nursing Implications
			• Due to risk of extravasation and subsequent tissue necrosis, give through a central line if possible. • May also be used as a bronchodilator IV or via inhalation (racemic epinephrine)
Glucose	Increases blood glucose level	Hypoglycemia	• Administer via IV or IO route at a dose of 1 to 2 mL/kg (D50%); maximum dose 2 to 4 mL/kg. • When administering via a peripheral IV line, dilute 1:1 with sterile water to make D25%. Monitor IV site for infiltration and tissue extravasation. • Monitor blood glucose levels closely.
Lidocaine (antidysrhythmic)	Decreases automaticity of conduction tissues of the heart	Ventricular arrhythmias	• Administer via IV or IO route at a dose of 1 mg/kg; administer via ET route at dose 2 times IV dose diluted with 3 to 5 mL normal saline, followed by positive-pressure ventilation. Maximum dose 5 mg/kg or 100 mg/dose. • Monitor ECG continuously. • Contraindicated in complete heart block • With larger-than-normal doses, monitor for hypotension or seizures.
Naloxone (Narcan)	Antagonizes action of narcotic agents	Reversal of respiratory depression related to narcotic effects	• Administer via IV, IO, SC, or ET route at a dose of 0.01 to 0.1 mg/kg in children <5 years old or <20 kg or at a dose of 2 mg in children >5 years old or >20 kg. Onset of action is within 2 to 5 minutes. • May repeat dose as necessary; narcotic effects outlast therapeutic effects of naloxone.

Care of the child who is experiencing an emergency includes all components of the nursing process: assessment, nursing diagnosis, planning, interventions, and evaluation. In an emergency situation, the nurse must act quickly, intervening immediately when an abnormality is determined upon assessment. When evaluating a child who presents emergently, always follow the AHA's guidelines for basic life support: evaluate airway, then breathing, then circulation. No matter what the cause of the emergency, the general approach to managing the child is universal, with minimal specific variations. Once the child's cardiopulmonary status is stabilized or the child is resuscitated, assessment and management will vary depending on the cause of the emergency.

ASSESSMENT

Nursing assessment of the child who presents emergently includes health history, physical examination, and laboratory and diagnostic testing. However, the initial history may be focused and very brief if the child is critically ill, necessitating that the nurse proceed immediately to rapid cardiopulmonary assessment. Once a child is stabilized, a more comprehensive history is obtained. Laboratory tests, while often important, should never take priority over the stabilization of the child from a cardiopulmonary and hemodynamic standpoint.

> Remember Alma, the 8-year-old with breathing trouble? What additional health history and physical examination assessment information should the nurse obtain?

Health History

Obtain the health history rapidly while simultaneously evaluating the child and providing life-saving interventions. A brief history is needed initially, followed by a more thorough history after the child is stabilized. The parents or caregiver will provide information about the child's "chief complaint." Record the information using the caregiver's own words. For example, the caregiver might say, "He's been having trouble breathing" if the child is presenting in respiratory distress. If the child suffered a traumatic injury from a bicycle accident, the caregiver might say, "She was riding her bike down the hill and lost control." This brief statement provides direction for obtaining more in-depth information about the nature of the emergency.

Ask about any significant past history that may affect the care of the child. For example, children who are medically fragile, who have a history of prematurity, or who have been diagnosed with a significant genetically linked disease (e.g., sickle cell anemia) may require special consideration in planning for and executing their care.

Physical Examination

In an emergency, the nurse must perform a rapid cardiopulmonary assessment and intervene immediately when alterations are noted. The remainder of the physical examination then follows.

Rapid Cardiopulmonary Assessment

As the brief history is being obtained, begin to evaluate the ABCs. The ABCs of the rapid cardiopulmonary assessment are A, airway; B, breathing; and C, circulation. Since pediatric arrests are usually related primarily to airway and breathing, and usually only secondarily to the heart, focus the assessment and interventions using the ABCs of resuscitation. Always perform the assessment and interventions in that order. In most circumstances, if the pediatric airway is properly managed and breathing is assisted, the child may not experience a full arrest requiring chest compressions.

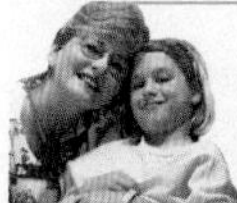

Assessment and management of the airway of a pre-arresting or arresting child is ALWAYS the first intervention in a pediatric emergency situation. Intervene if there is an airway problem before moving on to assessment of breathing. If an intervention for breathing is required, start it before progressing to assessment of circulation.

A: Airway Evaluation and Management. First evaluate the airway. Assess the patency of the airway. If no concern related to cervical spine injury exists, position the airway in a manner that promotes good air flow. If secretions are obstructing the airway, suction the airway to remove them. If the child is unconscious or has just been injured, open the airway using the head tilt–chin lift maneuver. Place the fingertips on the bony prominence of the child's chin and lift the chin to open the airway. Simultaneously, place one hand on the forehead and tilt the child's head back (Fig. 32.1). If the airway is not maintainable, reposition the airway for appropriate airflow. Place the child immediately on oxygen at 100% and apply a pulse oximeter to monitor oxygen saturation levels.

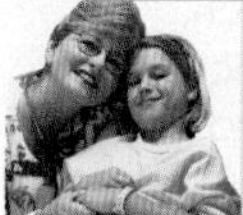

If cervical spine injury is a possibility, do not use the head tilt–chin lift maneuver; only use the jaw-thrust technique for opening the airway (see trauma section for explanation and illustration).

B: Breathing Evaluation and Management. After establishing an open airway, look for signs of respiration. Turn your head and place your ear over the child's mouth to "look, listen, and feel" for spontaneous respirations. Look to see if the child's chest is rising, listen for air escaping, and note if you feel any air coming out of the child's nose or mouth. If the child is breathing, evaluate the quality of the respirations: Is there spontaneous breathing, or is the child simply gasping ineffectively for air? Count the respiratory rate. Observe the child's color. Note adequacy of air flow in all lung fields, depth of respiration, chest rise, and presence of adventitious sounds. Evaluate for increased work of breathing and the use of accessory muscles.

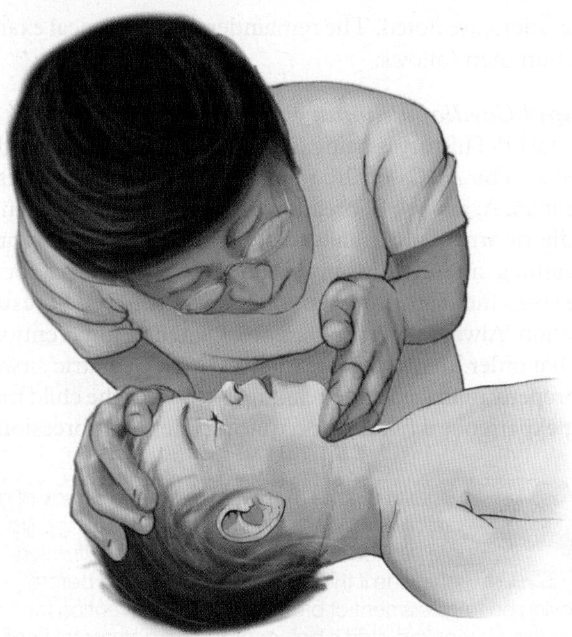

● Figure 32.1 Head tilt–chin lift maneuver in a child.

When signs of respiratory distress are noted, immediately place the child on oxygen at 100% and apply a pulse oximeter to monitor oxygen saturation levels. If the child is breathing shallowly and has poor respiratory effort, attempt to reposition the airway to promote better airflow. For the child receiving 100% oxygen who does not improve with repositioning, begin assisted ventilation with a bag-valve-mask (BVM) device. A need for ongoing BVM ventilation may require airway **intubation** (process by which a breathing tube, such as a tracheal tube, is inserted into a child's airway to assist with breathing).

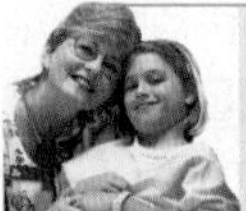

Attempts to insert a tracheal tube should last no longer that 20 to 30 seconds each. After each attempt, the child should receive multiple ventilations by the BVM method using 100% oxygen.

C: Circulation Evaluation and Management. The next step is to evaluate C, or circulation. During this phase, evaluate the heart rate, pulses, perfusion, skin color and temperature, blood pressure, cardiac rhythm, and level of consciousness. Determine the heart rate via direct auscultation or palpation of central pulses. Radial and brachial pulses are more difficult to palpate, especially in infants and young children. If perfusion is poor, such as with shock or cardiac arrest, the child may have a weak pulse or no pulse. In the young infant, check the brachial artery for a pulse. In the child and adolescent, evaluate the carotid pulse. If there is a pulse, note its quality. Is it barely palpable or weak? Is it strong or bounding? Compare strength and quality of central and peripheral pulses. Assess capillary refill time.

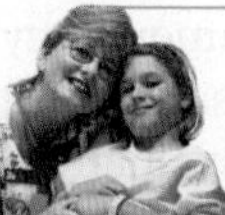

ALWAYS evaluate the presence of a heart rate by auscultation of the heart or by palpation of central pulses. NEVER use the cardiac monitor to determine if the child has a heart rate. The presence of a cardiac rhythm is not a reliable way to evaluate the ability to perfuse the body. In certain circumstances a rhythm continues but there is no pulse (pulseless electrical activity). If the child has no heart rate (pulse) despite adequate respiratory interventions, begin cardiac compressions.

Evaluate the child's perfusion by noting skin temperature and color. Is the skin pink? Is it warm to touch? The child's skin may be cool to the touch and may appear pale, mottled, or cyanotic. As the child's condition worsens with developing shock and cardiovascular compromise, note a line of demarcation of skin temperature warmth. In this situation, the distal extremities will feel cooler than the proximal regions of the body. Measure the blood pressure (BP) and place the child on a cardiac monitor to evaluate the cardiac rhythm. Note the child's sensorium or level of consciousness; if circulation is poor, the child will demonstrate an altered level of consciousness as the perfusion to the brain becomes diminished.

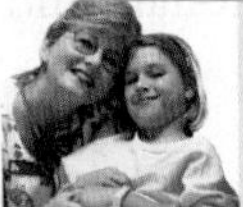

According to PALS, calculate minimum acceptable systolic BP by using this formula: 70 + (2 times the age in years). For example, a 4-year-old should have a minimal systolic BP of 78: $70 + (2 \times 4) = 78$.

If the circulation or perfusion is compromised, then fluid resuscitation is necessary. Establish large-bore intravenous (IV) access immediately and administer isotonic fluid rapidly. Provide 20 mL/kg of normal saline (NS) or lactated Ringer's (LR) as an IV bolus (if the infant is less than 1 month old, administer 10 mL/kg). If peripheral IV access cannot be obtained in the child with altered perfusion within three attempts or 90 seconds, assist with insertion of an intraosseous needle for fluid administration (refer to shock section for further information about intraosseous access). Central venous lines or cutdown access may also be used, but these measures take longer to accomplish.

Additional Physical Examination Components

In addition to assessing and stabilizing the child's airway, breathing, and circulation, perform a thorough physical examination and assess pain.

Neurologic Evaluation. Quickly evaluate the sensorium in an older child. Ask the child to state his or her name. Ask what happened to the child. Does the child know what day it is? Is the child aware of where he or she is?

If the child is an infant, evaluate his or her interest in the environment and response to parents. An infant who is not interested in the environment or seems unable to recognize his or her parents is a cause for concern. In contrast, an infant who enjoys sucking on a finger and making eye contact with the nurse during the assessment is reassuring.

Evaluate the child's head. In the infant or young toddler, palpate the anterior fontanel to determine if it is normal (soft and flat), depressed, or full. A sunken fontanel is associated with volume depletion from dehydration or blood loss. If the fontanel is full, note if it is bulging or tense, which may indicate increased intracranial pressure. Next assess the eyes. Are they open or closed? If closed, do they open spontaneously, to voice, to pain? Does the child focus on and follow your movements? Evaluate the pupils for equality and reactivity. Sluggish pupillary reaction may occur with increased intracranial pressure.

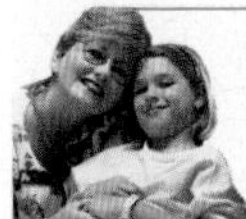

A nonreactive pupil is an ominous sign indicating a need for immediate relief of increased intracranial pressure.

Evaluate the child's face. Does the child smile or cry? Does the child react to playfulness with a laugh? Does the young infant cry vigorously? Are facial movements equal? In a child, a normal or near-normal neurologic examination can be a reassuring sign. Conversely, children who are obtunded or muted in their responses to environmental stimuli are a cause for concern.

Next evaluate for spontaneous movement of the extremities. Young infants are nonambulatory, so assess their ability to move their arms and legs and grossly evaluate the tone of their extremities. Does the infant vigorously and equally move the arms and legs? Is the muscle tone normal, or does the infant appear floppy or flaccid? When evaluating the older child, note whether he or she is ambulatory alone, ambulatory with assistance, or unable to walk. Note whether the child has use of the upper extremities. In the case of trauma, the child may arrive immobilized on a backboard. In this scenario, evaluate the child's motor responsiveness and sensation in each extremity, comparing findings bilaterally while the child is in the supine position. Ask the child if he or she feels you touching each extremity. Request that the child squeeze your fingers and then ask the child to wiggle the toes. The information obtained from these assessment techniques will provide information about cerebral integrity and perfusion, cerebellar health, and spinal cord integrity.

The Pediatric Glasgow Coma Scale may also be used to evaluate the neurologic status in children. Chapter 17 provides a more in-depth discussion of this scale.

Skin and Extremity Evaluation. Remove the child's clothing and thoroughly examine the skin for bruising, lesions, or rashes. If the child has a rash, note the size, shape, color, configuration, and location. Apply pressure to the rash with the fingertips to evaluate for the ability to blanch. Inspect the trunk, abdomen, and extremities for abrasions or deformities.

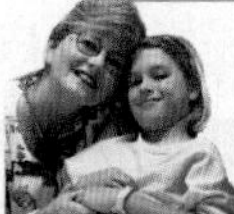

Rashes that do not blanch may be classified as petechiae or purpura. This type of rash may be associated with certain serious conditions, such as meningococcemia. Report this finding to the physician or nurse practitioner immediately.

Pain Assessment. In emergency situations, children may experience pain as a direct result of the injury or disease. Life-saving interventions such as resuscitation, insertion of IV lines, and administration of medications may cause further pain. The child's pain may also be exaggerated by light, noise, movement of the stretcher or bed, and the sensations of cold or heat (Holleran, 2002). Nurses play a key role in minimizing the child's pain, and this may help decrease the child's future distress (Johnston et al., 2005; Probst et al., 2005). If the child is awake and verbal, use an age-appropriate pain assessment scale to determine the child's pain level. If the child is sedated or unconscious, assess pain with a standardized scale that relies on physiologic measurements as well as behavioral parameters. Refer to Chapter 15 for additional information on pain assessment in children.

Laboratory and Diagnostic Testing

A number of laboratory and diagnostic tests may be ordered in a pediatric emergency. Laboratory tests can help to distinguish the cause of the emergency or additional problems that need to be treated. Standard laboratory tests obtained in most emergency departments include:

- Arterial blood gases (ABG), obtained initially and then serially to assess for status changes
- Electrolytes and glucose levels
- Complete blood count (CBC)
- Blood cultures
- Urinalysis

If ingestion is suspected, then a toxicology panel will be obtained. In suspected sepsis, erythrocyte sedimentation rate (ESR), C-reactive protein (CRP), and urine and spinal fluid cultures may also be obtained. The pediatric trauma victim may have additional laboratory tests performed, including amylase, liver enzymes, and blood type and cross-match.

Diagnostic tests may include radiologic tests, computed tomography (CT) scanning, and magnetic resonance imaging (MRI). One advantage of radiologic diagnostic testing is that the tests are relatively noninvasive. A disadvantage associated with CT and MRI testing is that before either CT or MRI can be performed, the patient must be stabilized. Common Laboratory and Diagnostic Tests 32.1 gives further information about the tests most commonly used in pediatric emergency situations.

After completing an assessment of Alma, the nurse noted the following: a patent airway, anxious but able to speak in short sentences, and skin temperature cool on the extremities. Based on these assessment findings, what would your top three nursing diagnoses be for Alma? Describe appropriate nursing interventions.

Common Laboratory and Diagnostic Tests 32.1 Pediatric Emergencies

Test	Explanation	Indications	Nursing Implications
Chest x-ray	Radiograph used to evaluate heart and lung structures	To identify: • Infections (such as pneumonia) • Foreign body • Injury • Endotracheal tube placement • Central line placement • Pneumothorax Re-evaluation of lungs after chest tube placement	• X-rays can be obtained quickly during resuscitation; usually available in emergency department. • Assist the child to lie still if necessary.
Computed tomography (CT)	Use of high radiation (equivalent to about 100 to 150 chest x-rays) with computer processing targeting specific body areas	Rapid evaluation of tissues and skeletal areas Superior test for the evaluation of internal bleeding	• Expect the child to be transported out of the area for the study. • Accompany the child to provide continued observation and management, especially if child's condition is unstable.
Magnetic resonance imaging (MRI)	Incorporation of responses of hydrogen protons to a dynamic magnetic field	Superior test for the evaluation of the spinal cord and the cerebrospinal fluid spaces; less useful in emergency situations	• Administer sedation as ordered. • Assist child in remaining still; MRI requires child to remain still for a longer period than for a CT. • Assist the conscious child to deal with fear related to loud banging noise of the machine.
Arterial blood gases (ABG)	Evaluation of blood pH and arterial blood levels of oxygen and carbon dioxide	Evaluation of quality of respiration. Evaluation of acid–base balance, such as in a child who may be acidotic due to volume loss with resultant electrolyte imbalance.	• Anticipate serial ABGs to assess for status changes. • Never delay resuscitation efforts pending blood gas results.
Serum electrolytes	Evaluation of electrolyte levels, such as sodium, potassium, and chloride, in the blood	Useful for determining baseline and if dehydration is hypertonic or isotonic	• Hemolysis of specimen may lead to falsely elevated potassium levels.
Glucose	Evaluation of glucose level in the blood	Valuable for determining need for supplementation, as in the case of hypoglycemia	• Use Accucheck or other rapid glucose test at the bedside or obtain serum blood specimen. • Elevated glucose levels can be associated with stress or with use of corticosteroids.

Common Laboratory and Diagnostic Tests 32.1 Pediatric Emergencies (continued)

Test	Explanation	Indications	Nursing Implications
Toxicology panel (blood and/or urine)	Determination of most commonly abused mood-altering medications, as well as commonly ingested drugs	Drug abuse, overdose, or poisoning	• Standard toxicology panel varies with the agency. • Follow agency protocol; may require special handling or labeling of specimen. • Use a blood specimen that is best for determining overdose or poisoning.
Complete blood count (CBC)	Evaluation of hemoglobin and hematocrit, white blood cell count, and platelet count	Any condition in which anemia, infection, or thrombocytopenia is suspected. Trauma if blood loss suspected.	• Be aware of normal values and how they vary with age and gender. • Hemoglobin and hematocrit may be elevated secondary to hemoconcentration in the case of hypovolemia.
Blood type and cross-match	Determination of ABO blood typing as well as presence of antigens. Cross-match performed on RBC-containing products to avoid transfusion reaction.	Trauma victim or any person with suspected blood loss as preparation for transfusion	• Handle specimen gently to avoid hemolysis. • Ensure that specimen request and label are appropriately signed and dated. • Apply "type and cross" or "blood band" to child at time of specimen collection if required by agency. • Most type & cross-match specimens expire after 48 to 72 hours.
Urinalysis	Evaluation of color, pH, specific gravity, and odor of urine. Assessment for evidence of protein, glucose, ketones, blood, leukocyte esterase, RBCs, WBCs, bacteria, crystals, and casts.	Patients with fever, dysuria, flank pain, urgency, hematuria or those who have experienced trauma to provide information about the urinary tract	• Many drugs can affect urine color; notify the laboratory if the child is taking one. • Notify the laboratory and document on the laboratory form if the female child is menstruating. • Refrigerate the specimen if it is not processed promptly. • Specimen may be obtained by catheterization, clean-catch voiding sample, or via a U-bag.

NURSING DIAGNOSES AND RELATED INTERVENTIONS

Upon completion of a thorough assessment and initial stabilization of the child, the nurse might identify several nursing diagnoses, including:

- Airway clearance, ineffective
- Breathing pattern, ineffective
- Gas exchange, impaired
- Fluid volume, deficient
- Cardiac output, decreased
- Tissue perfusion (cardiopulmonary, peripheral cerebral, or renal), ineffective
- Knowledge, deficient
- Fear
- Family processes, interrupted

Specific nursing goals, interventions, and evaluation for the child who is experiencing an emergency are based on the nursing diagnoses. Additional information about nursing management will be included later in the chapter as it relates to specific disorders.

Providing Cardiopulmonary Resuscitation

Always evaluate and manage the airway first, unless this is an out-of-hospital, witnessed, sudden collapse of a child. Call for help and assign someone to obtain the automatic external defibrillator (AED). Open the airway and assess for adequate breathing. If the child is not breathing, begin rescue breathing. Check for a pulse. In the child, the carotid or femoral pulses are easiest to assess. In the past, it was recommended that the brachial pulse be checked in the infant; however, this is often difficult, so an alternative is to check the femoral pulse. Carefully assess for signs of a pulse, but do not spend more than 10 seconds checking the pulse. If there is not a pulse or if the heart rate is less than 60 beats per minute, begin chest compressions.

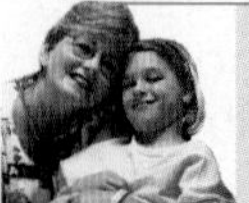

When the arrest occurs out of the hospital and is a witnessed, sudden collapse, initial management is slightly different than that for other arrests. In these sudden, witnessed events, phone first, get the AED, and return to start CPR.

Table 32.1 presents the most recent recommendations for rates of breaths to compressions. The most recent AHA recommendations stress the importance of properly performed chest compressions. Therefore, several changes have been made to the guidelines:

- Rescuers must provide compressions of adequate rate and depth.
- Chest recoil should be allowed.
- Minimal interruptions of chest compressions should be the goal.
- For infant CPR, two-person infant CPR can be performed with two thumbs encircling the chest and simultaneously using the hands to provide a thoracic squeeze.
- For two-person CPR, no pauses should occur for ventilation, with the compressing health care provider giving continuous compressions.

Providing Defibrillation or Synchronized Cardioversion

In some cases, the child experiences an abnormal life-threatening cardiac rhythm or an arrhythmia that does not respond to pharmacologic therapy or leads to hemodynamic instability. In these cases, electrical therapy, in the form of defibrillation or synchronized cardioversion, may be needed.

Defibrillation is the use of electrical energy to depolarize the cells of the myocardium to terminate an abnormal life-threatening cardiac rhythm, such as ventricular fibrillation. Defibrillation is used in conjunction with oxygen, CPR, and medications. The effects of defibrillation are enhanced in an oxygen-rich environment coupled with good artificial circulation (CPR). **Cardioversion**, another means of applying electrical current to the heart, is used when the child has supraventricular tachycardia (SVT) or ventricular tachycardia with a pulse. Cardioversion may also be enhanced with medications. Cardioversion is delivered as synchronized—that is, the electrical current is applied on the R wave of the electrocardiogram (ECG).

The basic defibrillator is equipped with adult- and pediatric-sized paddles. A switch turns the machine on and controls are used to select the amount of energy (joules). Typically, the initial energy amount is 2 joules/kg and can be increased up to 4 joules/kg for defibrillation. Energy for cardioversion is delivered at 0.5 to 1 joule/kg.

When the defibrillator is being used in an acute care setting, the leader of the code team will take charge of defibrillator use. He or she is responsible for ensuring that only the patient receives the energy from the defibrillator. The code team leader will count to 4 before delivering a shock to the patient to ensure that all personnel and other equipment are clear of the bed, so as to avoid accidental shock.

Using Automated External Defibrillation

In cases of sudden, witnessed, out-of-hospital collapse, an arrhythmia is often the cause. Therefore, the AHA has

Table 32.1 Rates of Breaths to Compressions

Age	One-Person CPR	Two-Person CPR
Infant	• 30 compressions to 2 breaths • Hand placement: two fingers, placed one fingerbreadth below the nipple line	• 15 compressions to 2 breaths • Hand placement: two thumbs encircling the chest at the nipple line
Child	• 30 compressions to 2 breaths • Hand placement: heel of hand or two hands (adult position in larger child), pressing on the sternum at the nipple line	• 15 compressions to 2 breaths • Hand placement: heel of one hand or two hands (adult position in larger child), pressing on the sternum at the nipple line

American Heart Association. (2005d). Part 11: Pediatric basic life support. *Circulation, 112,* 156–166.

revised its recommendations about the use of AED. AED is an alternative to manually defibrillating a patient. The AED device consists of electrodes that are applied to the chest. These electrodes are used to monitor the heart rhythm and deliver the electrical current. AED devices are readily available in a variety of locations, such as airports, sports facilities, and businesses. Traditionally, the AED was designed for use in adults, but newer-model AEDs with smaller paddles and the ability to alter energy delivery are now more readily available. Therefore, the AHA has recommended that an AED be used for children who are older than age 1 year who have no pulse and have suffered a sudden, witnessed collapse.

The AED is designed to be used by persons in the prehospital setting. Once the AED is turned on, the machine uses auditory commands to guide laypersons and health care professionals alike through the correct placement of the electrodes and the administration of energy. The AED periodically evaluates the arrest victim's cardiac rhythm and instructs the user about checking the pulse, continuing CPR, and delivering shocks. Nurses who care for children should be able to operate an AED and be prepared to use it in nontraditional settings.

Determining Medication Doses and Equipment Sizes

Many pediatric acute care facilities initiate code reference sheets when a pediatric patient is admitted. This sheet uses the child's actual weight to determine medication doses and equipment sizes. The reference sheet is then kept on a clipboard at the child's bedside or taped on the wall at the head of the bed. An additional copy is placed in the child's chart.

Ambulatory care providers often rely on the Broselow tape for estimating the child's weight based on the child's length as measured with the tape (Fig. 32.2). The tape is color-coded and emergency equipment for a child of that size is stored in corresponding color-coded packages or in color-coded drawers on the pediatric emergency cart (DeBoer et al., 2005). Medication doses and equipment sizes are also located on the tape. The most accurate calculation for code medications is based on the child's weight, but in numerous research studies, use of the Broselow tape for estimation in the absence of true weight has been shown to be successful (Hofer et al., 2002).

Managing Pain

Depending on the child's status and pain level, individualize pain management interventions. For the alert child, nonpharmacologic measures may be used in addition to medications. Provide atraumatic care for procedures and use aggressive pharmacologic treatments to manage pain as the child's condition allows. Refer to Chapter 15 for additional information on pain management strategies.

Ensuring Stabilization

After a child has been resuscitated, the nurse plays a key role in stabilization and transport. Thoroughly document the interventions that were performed as well as the ongoing assessment of the child in response to the interventions. Provide continued monitoring of the child while awaiting transport. Copy and assemble any pertinent documentation, such as the resuscitation record, nurses' notes, and laboratory test results, that will be given to the receiving institution. Ensure that all lines are taped securely and that vascular access sites are dressed and labeled with the date and time of insertion. As soon as possible, bring the child's family in to visit with the child. Provide explanations about the IV lines, monitoring equipment, and other medical equipment and devices. Encourage the family to talk to and touch the child.

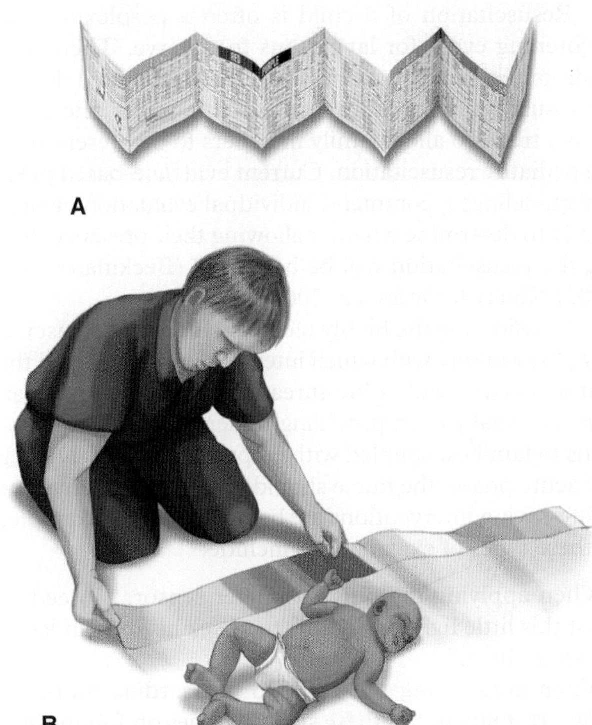

● Figure 32.2 (A) Broselow tape. (B) Measure the child's length with the Broselow tape to determine medication doses and tracheal tube size.

Providing Support and Education to the Child and Family

The experience of respiratory distress, oxygen deprivation, and an emergency situation is a frightening one for persons of all ages. The life-saving interventions involved with an emergency can be especially intimidating and frightening to children. Infants and young children cannot understand explanations about the interventions that are being provided in an emergent situation. Older children and adolescents may feel frightened and angry about the loss of control. The caregivers of the acutely ill or injured child may feel fear, anger, guilt, and sadness. They may be concerned about the very real possibility that their child might die.

Resuscitation of a child is often a perplexing and frightening event for laypersons to observe. Therefore, traditionally family members have been excluded during the resuscitation of children. Of late, however, there has been a trend to allow family members to be present during pediatric resuscitation. Current evidence-based practice guidelines recommend individual evaluation of each family to determine whether allowing their presence during the resuscitation will be beneficial (Beckman et al., 2002; Nibert & Ondrejka, 2005).

Considering the highly technical nature of resuscitation, the rapidity with which interventions occur, and the fear associated with a life-threatening event, nurses can play a crucial role in providing understandable explanations to families, coupled with empathic support. During the acute phase, the nurse should give brief explanations as life-saving interventions are being provided. Examples of these types of explanations include:

- When applying the pulse oximeter sensor: "I need to put this little light on Johnny to check his oxygen level; it won't hurt."
- When connecting the child to the cardiac monitor: "We're going to put these sticky patches on Johnny and connect them so we can monitor his heart rate on this screen."
- When preparing for intubation and ventilation: "Johnny can't breathe on his own right now, so we're going to give him some extra help with this tube. This tube will go through his breathing passage and this machine will help him to breathe."

The nurse plays a key role in providing empathy and support. Do not provide false reassurance and say, for example, "He's going to be alright." The outcome is never certain. Rather, communicate empathically. For example, say, "This must be very difficult for you. We're doing everything we can to help Johnny." Provide honest answers in a reassuring manner. Respect each family's diversity and observe their strengths and weaknesses. Be nonjudgmental in all interactions with families, even when the child's emergency situation may have resulted from family neglect.

Parents often feel very helpless when their child is in a high-tech environment. Suddenly overwhelmed with all the equipment and monitoring devices, they no longer are the persons who are the most skilled in caring for their child. Integrate the child's parents into the health care team. Suggest ways the parents can make the hospital experience more normal for their child. For example, simply allowing a father to read a story to his daughter or encouraging a mother to hold her child's hand is therapeutic both for the child and the parents. Be aware of this dramatic change and how it affects the parents. Always ensure that they feel like they are a welcome part of their child's care.

Providing the child with familiar comfort objects helps to decrease stress. Once the intubated child is alert and stabilized, assist him or her with communication. Some children can lift one finger for yes and two fingers for no. If the child is old enough to write, provide paper and pencil. Play is essential to the work of the child, and even if he or she is immobile, play is still possible. Puppets at the bedside and books help give the child a more normal experience in a scary situation that is far from the norm. Teenagers may enjoy listening to music through headphones. Even children who are comatose should be talked to and allowed to listen to familiar music.

Even if the outcomes are serious, the nurse can provide critical support to children and families. Whether hugging a crying mother or playing "peek-a-boo" with an intubated child, the nurse will be the one who can make a difference during a frightening experience.

Nursing Management of Children Experiencing Emergencies

Nurses caring for children must be adept at identifying when a child is experiencing the beginning stages of an emergency so they can quickly and appropriately intervene to prevent deterioration to cardiopulmonary arrest. Assessment and management of the most common types of emergencies in children are discussed below. The topics covered include respiratory arrest, shock, cardiac arrhythmias and arrest, near-drowning, traumatic injury, and poisoning.

RESPIRATORY ARREST

Respiratory emergencies may lead to respiratory failure and eventual cardiopulmonary arrest in children. Infants and young children are at greater risk for respiratory emergencies than adolescents and adults because they have smaller airways and underdeveloped immune systems, resulting in a diminished ability to combat serious respiratory illnesses. Young children often lack coordination, making them susceptible to choking on foods and small objects, which may also lead to cardiopulmonary arrest. In addition, sudden infant death syndrome (SIDS) is a leading cause of cardiopulmonary arrest in young infants and thus is one of the leading causes of post-neonatal mortality in the United States. For these reasons, nurses caring for children must be skilled at recognizing the signs of pediatric respiratory distress so they can prevent progression to eventual cardiopulmonary arrest. Table 32.2 lists some of the more common causes of pediatric respiratory arrest.

Nursing Assessment

If the child has severe respiratory compromise, obtain a brief history while simultaneously providing respiratory interventions. To obtain the history, use the following questions as a guide:

- When did the symptoms begin and when do they occur?

Table 32.2 Causes of Respiratory Arrest in Children

Condition	Cause
Upper airway	Burns Croup Epiglottitis Foreign body aspiration Reflux Strangulation or near-strangulation Tracheomalacia Vascular ring
Lower airway	Asthma Bronchiolitis Burns Foreign body aspiration Pertussis infection Pneumonia Pneumothorax Reflux
Nonrespiratory origins	Septic shock HIV
Neurologic	CNS infection Guillain-Barré syndrome Poliomyelitis Seizures Sleep apnea Spinal cord trauma Sudden infant death
Chronic illness	Complications of severe prematurity Cystic fibrosis Bone marrow transplant Neutropenia
Metabolic/endocrine disorders	Diabetic ketoacidosis Mitochondrial disorders
Cardiac conditions	Arrhythmia Congenital cardiac problems Acquired cardiac problems
Traumatic/unintentional injury/ intentional injury	Asphyxia Child abuse/"shaken baby syndrome" Drowning Electrocution Gunshot wound Toxic ingestion Vehicular-related trauma

Adapted from Balwin, G. (2001). *Handbook of pediatric emergencies.* Philadelphia: Lippincott Williams & Wilkins; Behrman, R. E., Kliegman, R. M., & Jenson, H. B. (2004). *Nelson's textbook of pediatrics* (17th ed.). Philadelphia: Saunders.

- Did the symptoms have a sudden onset, as with a foreign body aspiration?
- Were the symptoms initially less severe, with mild upper respiratory symptoms that progressed to paroxysmal coughing, as is commonly seen in pertussis?
- Is the cough continual, intermittent, or worse at night or with exercise?
- Has there been any stridor? (Stridor is heard upon inhalation and may be associated with swelling of the trachea [as with croup] or with a foreign body in the upper airway.)
- Is there wheezing? If so, is the wheezing on inspiration or on expiration, or both?
- What makes the symptoms better and what makes them worse?

- Does drinking from a bottle induce the symptoms, as with gastroesophageal reflux–induced aspiration?
- Is the child taking any medication for the symptoms? Does the child or do any members of the immediate family have a history of chronic respiratory disease, such as asthma?
- Are the child's immunizations up to date?
- Was the child born prematurely? If so, did the child require mechanical ventilation? If so, for how long?
- Were there any respiratory problems during the first few days of life?
- When did the child last eat? (This question is important because a recent meal will increase the child's risk of aspiration in the event of a respiratory arrest. In addition, the presence of food in the stomach will increase the risk of aspiration during tracheal intubation.)

If the child can communicate, ask how he or she is feeling. Is he short of breath? Does his chest hurt? Observe the child while speaking. Children who are in respiratory distress may speak in short sentences with gasping between words.

Physical Examination

In an emergency, physical examination is often limited to inspection, observation, and auscultation. First, quickly survey the respiratory status. Determine if the child is breathing.

Inspection and Observation

Establish if the airway is patent, maintainable, or unable to be maintained. The child with a patent airway is breathing without signs of obstruction. The maintainable airway remains patent independently by the child or with interventions such as a towel roll under an infant's neck or the insertion of a nasal trumpet. The airway that cannot be maintained does not sustain patency unless a more aggressive intervention, such as the insertion of a tracheal tube, is performed.

Look at the child's posture. Is the child sitting up, leaning forward, and drooling, as with epiglottitis? Observe the child's face: does he or she appear anxious or relaxed? Persons who are in respiratory distress often appear anxious. Look at the nose and mouth: are the nares patent? Is there noticeable nasal congestion or mucus coming from the nose? Note nasal flaring or mouth breathing. Observe for head bobbing. Listen for audible expiratory grunting or inspiratory stridor. Note the child's color. Does the child appear pale, mottled, dusky, or cyanotic? Children may appear mottled in response to poor oxygenation, hypothermia, or stress. Children with severe respiratory compromise may appear dusky. Look for cyanosis around the mouth or on the trunk. Cyanosis is a late and often ominous sign of respiratory distress. Central cyanosis is more likely to be associated with respiratory or cardiac compromise. In contrast, peripheral cyanosis is more likely to be associated with circulatory alteration.

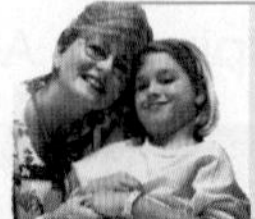

Closely inspect the color of the area around the mouth. Is there paleness (circumoral pallor)? Circumoral pallor is a sign of poor oxygenation.

Evaluate the pattern and quality of respiration, noting the respiratory rate. **Tachypnea** (increased respiratory rate) is often noted in children in respiratory distress. However, seriously ill children grunt and may have normal or subnormal respiratory rates. **Hypoventilation**, a decrease in the depth and rate of respirations, is noted in very ill children or children who have central respiratory depression secondary to narcotics. If the child is a young infant (less than 2 months) or premature, periodic breathing may occur. **Periodic breathing** is regular breathing with occasional short pauses (brief periods of apnea). After the apneic pause, the infant will breathe rapidly (up to 60 breaths per minute) for a short period and then will resume a normal respiratory rate. In general, the infant who has periodic breathing looks pink and has a normal heart rate. Observe for the use of accessory muscles in the neck or retractions in the chest, determining the extent and severity of the retractions.

Auscultation

Auscultate the lungs with the diaphragm of the stethoscope. Breath sounds over the tracheal region are higher-pitched and are described as "vesicular," while breath sounds over the peripheral lung fields tend to be lower-pitched, known as "bronchial." Instruct the child to take deep breaths with the mouth open. To encourage the young child to exhale strongly, instruct him or her to "blow out" the penlight (as with a candle) or to blow on a tissue. Encourage the child not to breathe more rapidly than normal (to prevent **hyperventilation** [increased depth and rate of respirations]) and to avoid making any noises with the mouth.

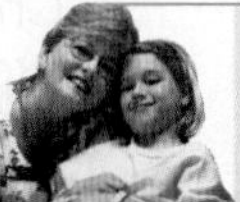

Significant upper respiratory congestion often interferes with assessment of the lower airways because the sound is easily transmitted throughout the chest. Differentiate between the upper and lower airway noises by listening with the stethoscope over the nose. You may be able to determine whether the noise is nasal or bronchial by using this technique.

Auscultate the child's chest systematically. Listen in all anterior, axillary, and posterior regions, comparing the left to the right sides. Note any decreased or absent breath sounds, which may be the result of bronchial obstruction (as with mucous infection) or air trapping (as in children with asthma). Unilateral absent breath sounds are associated with foreign body aspiration and pneumothorax.

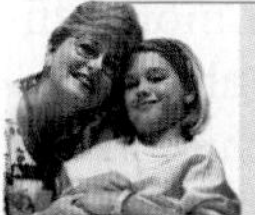

Sometimes a child's respiratory status is so severely compromised that little or no air movement is noted. This commonly occurs in a child experiencing a severe asthma exacerbation. Minimal or no air movement requires immediate intervention.

Note the presence and location of adventitious breath sounds such as crackles, wheezes, or rhonchi. Document presence of a pleural friction rub (a low-pitched, grating sound), a sound resulting from inflammation of the pleura (RNCEUS, 2006).

Palpation

Palpate the chest for any abnormalities. In the older, less severely ill and cooperative child, assess for tactile fremitus. Using the palm of the hand, palpate over the lung regions in the same manner as for auscultation and percussion while the child says, "ninety-nine." Increased vibrations elicited during this maneuver are associated with consolidating conditions, such as pneumonia.

Percussion

Percuss the interspaces of the chest between the ribs in the same systematic fashion as with auscultation. Normally, percussion over an air-filled lung reveals resonant sounds. Note the presence of hyperresonance, which may indicate an acute problem such as a pneumothorax or a chronic disease such as asthma. In contrast, percussion sounds will be dull over a lobe of the lung that is consolidated with fluid, infectious organisms, and blood cells, as in the case of pneumonia.

Laboratory and Diagnostic Testing

Use continuous pulse oximetry to monitor any child whose respiratory status is a concern. Note and report oxygen saturation levels below 95%. (See Chapter 10 for additional information about use of the pulse oximeter.)

Additional tests may reveal:

- Arterial or capillary blood gases: hypoxemia, hypercarbia, altered pH
- Chest x-ray: alterations in normal anatomy or lung expansion, or evidence of pneumonia, tumor, or foreign body
- Metal detector: evidence of metallic foreign body. Novel as it may sound, metal detectors have been found to be highly accurate (99%) in detecting the presence of ingested coins in children (Lee et al., 2005).

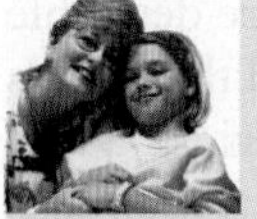

Children with cardiac conditions resulting in cyanosis often have baseline oxygen saturations that are relatively low because of the mixing of oxygenated with deoxygenated blood.

Nursing Management

The basic principle of pediatric emergency care and PALS is prevention of cardiopulmonary arrest. Therefore, the nurse must rapidly assess and appropriately manage children who are exhibiting signs of respiratory distress. PALS stresses the fact that when children in respiratory distress deteriorate and suffer a pulseless cardiac arrest, "their outcome is poor" (AHA, 2001b). In contrast, the data overwhelmingly demonstrate that children who receive prompt and proper treatment in cases of respiratory distress and respiratory arrest have a high likelihood of survival (AHA, 2001b).

Nursing management of the child in respiratory distress involves maintaining a patent airway, providing supplemental oxygen, monitoring for changes in status, and in some cases assisting ventilation. In addition to providing these life-saving measures and monitoring the child's progress, offer support and education to the child and family.

Maintaining a Patent Airway

When a child exhibits signs of respiratory distress, make a quick decision about whether it will be safe to allow the child to stay with the parent or whether the child must be placed on the examination table or bed. For example, in the case of croup, the child will often breathe more comfortably and experience less stridor while in the comfort of the parent's lap. Many children in respiratory distress often are most comfortable sitting upright, as this position helps to decrease the work of breathing by allowing appropriate diaphragmatic movement. In contrast, a child with a decreasing level of consciousness may need to be placed in the supine position to facilitate positioning of the airway.

The infant will benefit from a small sheet or towel folded under the shoulders. This will facilitate positioning the infant's airway in the "sniff" position, as is recommended by AHA's Basic Cardiac Life Support (BCLS) guidelines (Fig. 32.3). Avoid neck flexion or hyperextension, which may completely occlude the infant's airway. In children over age 1 year, the optimal method for opening the airway is to hyperextend the neck, as recommended by AHA BCLS. If a cervical spine injury is not suspected, use the head tilt–chin lift technique to open the airway. If the child has suffered head or neck trauma and cervical spine instability is a concern, use the jaw-thrust maneuver by placing three fingers under the child's lower jaw and lifting the jaw upward and outward (Fig. 32.4). In either case, never place the hand under the neck to open the airway.

Often the nurse encounters an acutely ill child who cannot maintain an airway independently but may be able to do so with some assistance. For example, sometimes simply opening the airway and moving the tongue away from the tracheal opening is all that is required to regain airway patency. In certain conditions, a nasopharyngeal or oropharyngeal airway may be necessary for airway

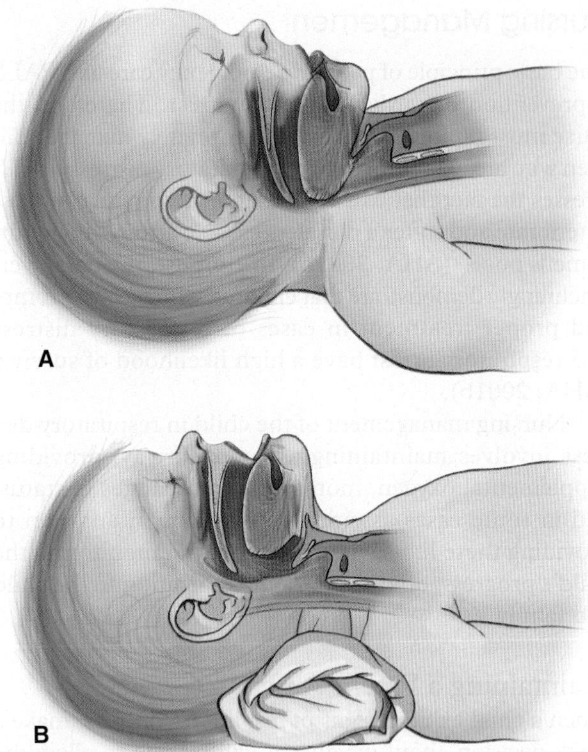

● Figure 32.3 (A) The infant and young child's prominent occiput encourages flexion of the neck and may result in airway occlusion. (B) Putting a towel roll under the shoulders helps to open the infant's or young child's airway by placing it in the neutral or "sniff" position.

maintenance. Comparison Chart 32.1 provides additional information about these types of airways.

Assisting Ventilation

The child in respiratory distress may ventilate poorly, hypoventilate, or tire and become apneic. In this case, the child may require assistance with ventilation through BVM ventilation, tracheal intubation, or a laryngeal mask airway. Table 32.3explains these methods.

Providing Bag-Valve-Mask Ventilation

The technique of BVM ventilation is used in the management of children who cannot ventilate or oxygenate effectively on their own. This technique is a more efficient way of ensuring ventilation than using only supplemental oxygen. In addition, resuscitating a child in this manner is superior to mouth-to-mouth resuscitation as it provides higher oxygen concentrations and protects the nurse from exposure to oral secretions. However, this technique requires proper training and practice. The proper procedure involves appropriate opening of the airway followed by providing breaths with the BVM.

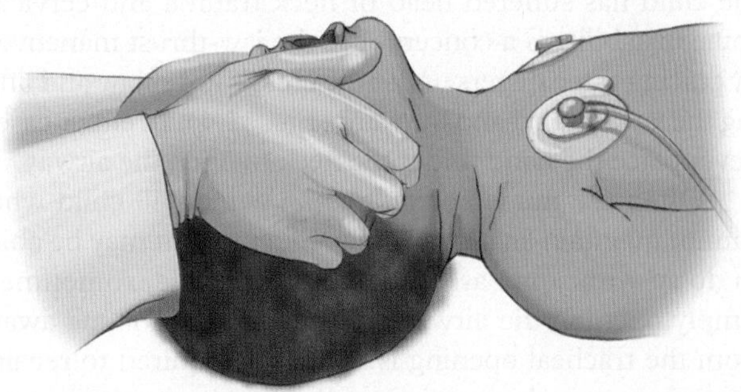

● Figure 32.4 Jaw-thrust technique for opening the airway.

Ventilation with the BVM may be performed with either one or two rescuers. First, choose an appropriate-sized bag and a corresponding face mask that fits the infant or child (Fig. 32.5). Self-inflating bags are usually available in neonatal, infant, child, and adult sizes. Corresponding masks are available. Choose a face mask that properly fits the child's face and that provides a seal over the nose and mouth and excludes the eyes, thus preventing any pressure on the eyes (Fig. 32.6).

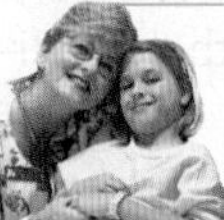

Face masks should be clear so that the nurse can see the child's lip color and identify any emesis during resuscitation. Older face masks were black and should no longer be used.

Connect the BVM via the tubing to the oxygen source and turn on the oxygen. When resuscitating infants and children, set the flow rate at approximately 10 L/minute. For an adolescent who is adult-sized, set the flow rate at 15 L/minute or higher to compensate for the larger-volume bag. Check to make sure that the oxygen is flowing through the tubing to the bag. Self-inflating bags do not provide "free-flow" oxygen out of the face mask; manual pumping of the bag is necessary. However, the bags have a corrugated plastic tail that allows oxygen to freely flow. Therefore, check over the tail for oxygen flow through the bag.

After opening the airway appropriately (see above), place the mask over the child's face. When one rescuer is providing ventilation (commonly referred to as "bagging"), the person must provide a seal with the mask over the child's face with one hand and use the other hand to manipulate the resuscitator bag. The hand used to provide the mask seal will simultaneously maintain the airway in an open position. Generally, use the left thumb and index finger to hold the mask on the child's face. While maintaining a good seal with the mask, use upward pressure on the jaw angle while pressing downward on the mask below the child's mouth to keep the mouth open (Fig. 32.7). Take care not to put pressure on the neck with the fourth and fifth fingers.

If adequate personnel are available, a more desirable situation involves one person standing behind the child's head who maintains an open airway and provides a seal of the mask over the face with a hand on each side (usually the thumbs and second fingers). A second rescuer

COMPARISON CHART 32.1 Oropharyngeal Versus Nasopharyngeal Airways

Oropharyngeal airway (used only in unconscious children)	• Consists of a simple plastic curved body that has a central air channel to allow for aeration • Is used when an unconscious child has difficulty maintaining airway patency due to upper airway obstruction, such as from the tongue • Allows for oral suction • Determine the correct size of the airway by placing it next to the child's cheek with the tip pointing down. An airway that is too large will extend past the angle of the child's mandible and can obstruct the glottic opening when inserted. • Choose the airway that best fits the child to decrease the risk of injury to the structures of the mouth.
Nasopharyngeal airway (may be used in conscious children and children who have an intact gag reflex)	• Consists of a flexible curved tube that is inserted nasally • Is used when the child has difficulty maintaining airway patency due to tongue obstruction or palate problems, when neurologic impairment causes poor pharyngeal tone, or in the child with impaired consciousness • Allows for nasopharyngeal suction • When selecting this airway, keep in mind that the diameter of the airway should not be so large that it puts too much pressure on the internal nasal tissue. There are two common methods for measuring this airway: 1) measure the distance from the end of the child's nose to the tragus of the ear; 2) look at the child's fifth digit, which is usually the approximate diameter of the nasopharyngeal airway. • Monitor for mucosal irritation, nasal septum swelling, and laceration of the adenoids. • Do not use this type of airway in children with a history of bleeding disorders and basilar skull fractures. • This airway's small diameter can easily become obstructed with secretions and blood.

stands on one side of the child and compresses the bag to ventilate the child using both hands. If the child is more difficult to ventilate, the two-rescuer method allows the ventilating nurse to provide better ventilation than with the one-rescuer method. In addition, the two-rescuer method ensures the best possible mask seal, as the rescuer holding the mask can use both hands to maintain the seal.

Regardless of the number of persons present, proper placement of the face mask is critical and a good seal must be maintained during the entire course of the resuscitation. In addition, during ventilation, use only the force and tidal volume necessary to cause a chest rise, no more. If a good chest rise is not observed, attempt to open the airway again. It may be necessary to adjust the position of the airway a few times to achieve a patency conducive to ventilation.

Compress the bag to deliver breaths at the amount recommended in infants and children. Initially, provide two rescue breaths and observe for a chest rise. Rescue breaths should not overinflate the lungs. Breaths should be delivered over 1 second. After the first two rescue ventilations, perform rescue breathing at a rate of one breath every 3 to 5 seconds, or about 12 to 20 breaths per minute. Delivering each breath should be a steady, one-inhalation-to-one-exhalation ratio. This means that the amount of time delivering the inspiratory ventilation is equal to the amount of time that expiration is allowed. While ventilating the infant or child, work with, not against, any spontaneous respiratory effort; in other words, if the child is breathing out, do not attempt to force air in at the same time.

If the child is unconscious and a third rescuer is available, that person can apply cricoid pressure. **Cricoid pressure** (also known as the Sellick maneuver) is the use of gentle pressure to occlude the esophagus, preventing air from entering the stomach (Fig. 32.8). Cricoid pressure may help to prevent vomiting secondary to gastric distention. Vomiting during resuscitative efforts can complicate the situation because the child is at risk of aspirating abdominal contents.

Monitoring Effectiveness of Ventilation

During the course of the resuscitation, continually reassess the child's response to the resuscitative efforts, noting:

- Adequacy of chest rise
- Absence or minimal presence of abdominal distention
- Improved heart rate and pulse oximetry readings

Table 32.3 Airway and Ventilation Methods

Method	Description	Comments
Anesthesia bag or flow-inflating ventilation systems	A small, collapsible bag that consists of a reservoir bag, an overflow port, and a fresh gas inflow port	• Adjustment of the oxygen flow and of the outlet control valve is necessary. • Useful in providing positive end-expiratory pressure (PEEP) or continuous positive airway pressure (CPAP) • Adequate training and significant skill are needed to properly operate this device. • Hypercapnia and barotrauma may result with improper use. • Used more commonly in the post-anesthesia care unit (PACU) and in the neonatal intensive care unit
Bag-valve-mask device or manual resuscitator	A self-inflating oxygen delivery bag that does not require an oxygen source for resuscitation and ventilation. The bag can be connected to oxygen to provide higher oxygen levels than room air. When the child exhales, the non-rebreathing valve closes allowing exhaled, deoxygenated air to escape.	• Effective in providing oxygenation to a child who is in severe respiratory distress or who has suffered a respiratory arrest • A more efficient method of respiratory resuscitation than mouth-to-mouth resuscitation; decreased rescuer exposure to communicable disease • Most medical personnel can be trained to perform resuscitation with this method. • Possibly tiring for the rescuer when used to ventilate a child for long periods of time (see discussion on bag-mask ventilation)
Laryngeal mask airway	An inflatable silicone mask and rubber connecting tube that is inserted blindly into the airway, forming a seal	• The airway is introduced into the pharynx and advanced until it meets resistance; balloon cuff is then inflated. • Easier insertion than a tracheal tube • Usually used in the unconscious child who benefits from bag-valve-mask ventilation but does not require intubation • Improvement in patient comfort
Tracheal intubation	A plastic tube inserted in the trachea to establish and maintain an airway when the airway cannot be maintained effectively using other measures (e.g., nasal trumpet or bag-valve-mask ventilation)	• Skilled medical professional (physician, nurse practitioner, respiratory specialist, EMT, or physician's assistant) necessary for insertion • The nurse acts as a valuable assistant during the intubation procedure.

- Improved color
- Capillary refill less than 3 seconds with strengthening pulses

If the child's status deteriorates and he or she becomes pulseless, then CPR must be started. In addition, periodically and briefly stop ventilating to evaluate for signs of spontaneous respirations.

Preventing Complications Related to Bag-Valve-Mask Ventilation

During a resuscitation situation, health care personnel usually exhibit high energy levels, a normal physiologic response that facilitates resuscitative efforts as the rescuers act quickly. However, this heightened state can lead to overzealousness while ventilating an infant or child.

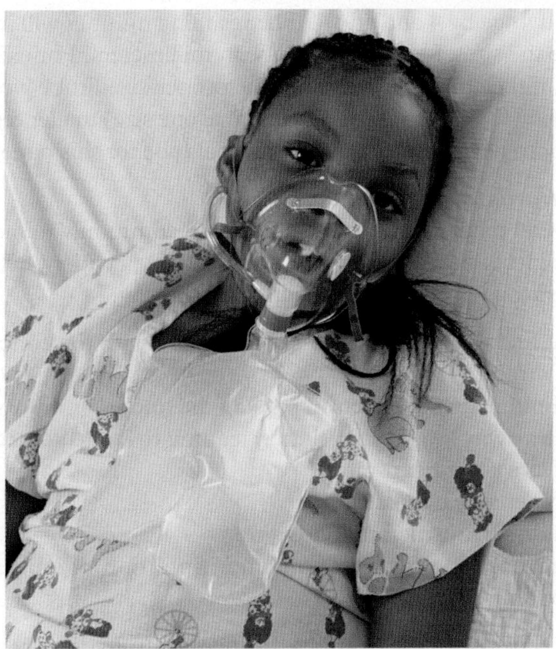

● Figure 32.5 The non-rebreather mask allows exhalation of carbon dioxide while inhibiting entrainment of room air and is capable of delivering 80% to 100% oxygen.

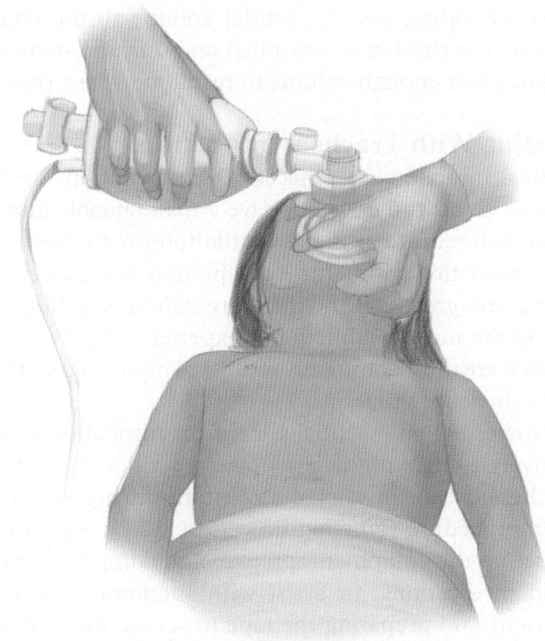

● Figure 32.7 Proper hand placement for maintaining airway and adequate mask seal using one-rescuer technique.

Health care providers may inadvertently ventilate the patient too rapidly using too much tidal volume, leading to excessive ventilation volume and increased airway pressure. This poor technique can be detrimental to the patient, causing:

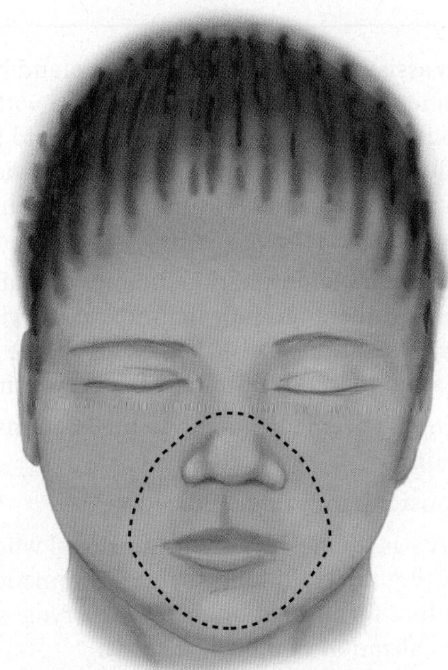

● Figure 32.6 The mask should form a seal over the nose and mouth, across the chin and nose bridge.

- Reduced cardiac output (due to increased intrathoracic pressure and increased cardiac afterload)
- Air trapping
- **Barotrauma** (trauma caused by changes in pressure)
- Air leak (thus reducing the oxygen delivered to the patient)

In addition, children with head injury who receive excessive ventilation volumes and high rates may develop:

- Decreased cerebral blood flow
- Cerebral edema
- Neurologic damage (adapted from AHA, Pediatric Advanced Life Support, 2001b)

Thus, nurses must be mindful of their technique during bagging, not exceeding the recommended respiratory

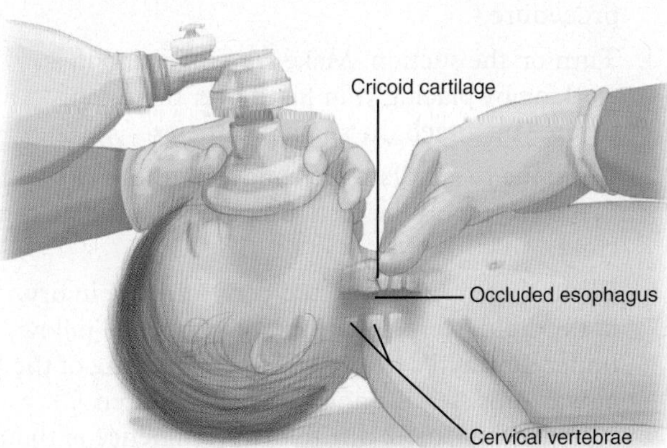

● Figure 32.8 Applying cricoid pressure.

rate or providing too much tidal volume to the child. Ventilate the child in a controlled and uniform manner, providing just enough volume to result in a chest rise.

Assisting With Tracheal Intubation

Tracheal intubation is a necessary intervention for the infant or child who does not have a maintainable airway or who will require artificial ventilation for a prolonged time. Intubation of infants and children is a procedure that requires great skill and therefore should be performed by only the most qualified and experienced personnel. Children are most commonly intubated orally, rather than nasally, in acute situations.

Nurses are an essential part of the intubation team, usually assisting a physician, nurse practitioner, respiratory therapist, or physician's assistant during the intubation procedure (Nursing Procedure 32.1). The nurse may set up the equipment, prepare and administer intubation medications, or assist with suctioning the oral secretions and preparing the tape to secure the tracheal tube. In a child in full arrest, the nurse might be responsible for performing ongoing chest compressions while other team members manage the child's airway.

Setting Up Equipment

Appropriate setup and preparation of equipment is essential (Table 32.4). The tracheal tube size used depends on the child's size. To calculate tracheal tube size, divide the child's age by 4 and add 4. The resulting number will indicate the size of the tracheal tube in millimeters. For example, if the child is 2 years old, the proper-sized tube would be 4.5 ($[2/4] + 4 = 4.5$). Always have one size smaller ready also, so have a 4.0 and a 4.5 tracheal tube for this patient.

Administering Medications

Several medications are administered commonly to facilitate intubation of children. Premedicating a patient before passing a tracheal tube aids in the following:

- Reducing pain and anxiety (consistent with the concept of atraumatic care)
- Minimizing the effects of passing the tracheal tube down the airway (vagal stimulation leading to **bradycardia** [decrease in heart rate])
- Preventing hypoxia
- Reducing intracranial pressure
- Preventing airway trauma and aspiration of stomach contents

The use of medications during the intubation process is known as rapid sequence intubation (Table 32.5). Typically, these medications are used in controlled settings such as the emergency department or the intensive care unit. Rapid sequence intubation is done only in children who are not experiencing cardiac arrest. If the intubation is expected to be particularly difficult, paralyzing medication should not be used.

Nursing Procedure 32.1

Assisting With Tracheal Intubation

1. Prepare equipment and supplies.
2. Draw up medications (for rapid sequence intubation).
3. Turn up the volume on the cardiac monitor so that members of the team can easily hear the audible QRS indication of the child's heart rate and note any bradycardia with the procedure.
4. Turn on the suction. Make sure that suction is working by placing your hand over the tubing before you attach the suction catheter.
5. Continue to ventilate the child with the BVM and 100% oxygen as the team prepares to intubate the child.
6. When there is no suspected cervical spine injury, in the child over age 2 years, place a small pillow under the child's head to facilitate opening of the airway; this step is unnecessary in children younger than age 2 due to the prominence of their occiput.
7. When assisting with the intubation, stand beside the patient's head and prepare to assist with suctioning of oral secretions, applying cricoid pressure during the insertion of the tube, providing BVM as needed, and assisting with securing the tube with tape.
8. Before the initial intubation attempt and after each subsequent attempt to intubate, provide several inhalations of 100% oxygen via the BVM ventilation method (optimally for a few minutes).
9. Administer premedication and medications for sedation.
10. Administer paralyzing medication.
11. Observe as the health care professional who is intubating the child follows the recommended procedure for intubation using the laryngoscope for visualization of the vocal cords.
12. As the tracheal tube is inserted, apply gentle cricoid pressure (too much pressure can block the trachea) if appropriate.

Table 32.4 Equipment and Supplies for Tracheal Intubation

Laryngoscope blades	Straight blades (Miller) are usually used for infants and young children. A curved-blade laryngoscope (Macintosh) may be used for older children and adolescents. The blade has a little light bulb attached to it for visualization of the trachea. The light bulb should be bright and attached securely.
Tracheal tubes	Three sizes should be readily available: the estimated size, a size smaller, and a size larger. A stylet may be used to guide the tube through the child's vocal cords (it is then removed after the intubation procedure).
Oxygen	100% oxygen is provided using a bag-valve-mask before intubation and after unsuccessful intubation attempts.
Suction	Properly working wall or portable suction with appropriate-sized suction catheters (that fit the tracheal tube) should be prepared; the package is opened, leaving the sterile-tipped end inside the package and connecting the other end to the suction tubing. A Yankauer suction catheter (large catheter) should also be available if copious secretions are present in the mouth that interfere with the ability to visualize the airway.
Monitors	Pulse oximeter and cardiac monitor with an audible tone indicating the QRS complex should be in place. Exhaled CO_2 device is needed to detect increased CO_2 levels after the intubation.
Nasogastric tube	Placing a nasogastric (NG) tube will help to mitigate abdominal distention. Patients who are manually ventilated typically have some abdominal distention as some air passes into the stomach.
Personal protective equipment	Usually just gloves, goggles, and a mask are necessary to protect health care workers. In the case of copious bleeding, health care workers should wear gowns also.
Tape, etc.	Tape should be prepared for securing the tube. Benzoin, a sticky substance, is usually applied under the tape for enhanced security of the tape. For children who have had multiple intubations, a protective barrier (as used to protect the skin around an ostomy) may be applied under the tape to protect the skin. Gauze pads should be available to clean up excess secretions that may interfere with taping the tracheal tube.

The nurse must be aware of the differences in the various medication classes, their advantages, disadvantages, and adverse effects. The nurse must also be able to distinguish between medications that produce sedation and ones that produce analgesia. Children who are paralyzed and sedated may be suffering severe pain. The pain control needs of children who are acutely ill are of paramount importance and cannot be overstated. Do not mistake a child who is immobilized as a result of sedative and paralytic medications for a child who is pain-free.

Ensuring and Maintaining Correct Tube Placement

To assess for correct placement once the tracheal tube is inserted, observe for symmetrical chest rise and auscultate over the lung fields for equal breath sounds. Inspect the tracheal tube for the presence of water vapor on the inside, indicating that the tube is in the trachea. To rule out accidental esophageal intubation, auscultate over the abdomen while the child is being ventilated: there should not be breath sounds in the abdomen. Note improvement in the oxygen saturation level via pulse oximetry.

Once tracheal tube placement is verified, mark the tube with an indelible pen at the level of the child's lip and secure it with tape. Document the number on the tracheal tube at the level of the child's mouth. Anticipate a chest x-ray to confirm correct placement of the tracheal tube.

After placement is confirmed, the tracheal tube is connected to the ventilator by respiratory personnel. The ventilator will provide continuous artificial ventilation and oxygenation. Exhaled CO_2 monitoring is recommended as it provides an indication of appropriate ventilation (Box 32.1). If an exhaled CO_2 monitor is being used, the exhaled CO_2 should be yellow.

Table 32.5 Medications for Rapid Sequence Intubation

Medications	Desired Effects	Undesirable Effects
Anticholinergic: atropine	Decreases respiratory secretions and mitigates the vagal affects of intubation, thus decreasing the risk of bradycardia	Doses that are too low (<0.1 mg) can cause a paradoxical bradycardia. Young infants are more prone to the bradycardic effects of atropine, so its use is generally contraindicated in this population.
Sedatives: barbiturates—thiopental (short-acting barbiturate)	Has very rapid onset and short duration of action; reduces intracranial pressure and oxygen demand	Hypotensive effects of this drug are more severe in the dehydrated patient. When given in combination with narcotics, respiratory depression is potentiated.
Sedatives: benzodiazepines—midazolam (Versed)	Has a slightly slower onset than thiopental but is associated with fewer adverse effects. Also causes amnesia. Can be titrated up or down (at lower doses it causes conscious sedation; at higher doses it can induce anesthesia).	When given in combination with narcotics, respiratory depression is potentiated.
Anesthetic agent: ketamine	Has a rapid onset with sedative, amnesic, and analgesic affects. Can be dissociative (child is awake but unaware). May improve BP and cause bronchodilation (helpful for children with status asthmaticus).	Ketamine can cause increased intracranial pressure and increased ocular pressure. Therefore, children who have suffered head trauma or globe injury should not receive this medication. Because of ketamine's sympathetic effects, hypertension can result from its use. Ketamine tends to cause increased secretions, often necessitating the concomitant use of atropine to counteract this adverse affect. May cause hallucinations and is therefore contraindicated in children with psychiatric problems.
Anesthetic agent: lidocaine	Can decrease intracranial pressure at higher doses. Has an advantage when used in the management of hypovolemia because it is less likely to cause hypotension.	Lidocaine can cause adverse cardiac effects (bradycardia, hypotension, dysrhythmias) in high doses. May be associated with CNS depression and seizures.
Narcotic analgesic: fentanyl citrate (Sublimaze)	A highly concentrated opioid that causes fewer adverse effects than other opioids, such as pruritus. Also exerts a less hypotensive effect.	Constipation and urinary retention (as is common with opioids) may occur. Increases risk for respiratory depression, increased intracranial pressure, and hypotension. Chest wall rigidity is common with this drug and may cause difficulty with ventilation.

Table 32.5 Medications for Rapid Sequence Intubation (continued)

Medications	Desired Effects	Undesirable Effects
Paralyzing or neuromuscular blocking agents: rocuronium (Zemuron), succinylcholine (Anectine), vercuron (Norcuron)	Used for short-term paralysis during the intubation process. May be used for extended paralysis in ICU for patient in whom movement would be detrimental. For example, a child with epiglottitis has a very precarious airway and must remain intubated until the epiglottis decreases in size. In certain respiratory conditions, spontaneous respiratory effort would interfere with the ventilation of a patient and therefore prolonged paralysis is desirable.	Succinylcholine (a depolarizing agent) has always been the gold standard for paralysis because it has a relatively rapid onset and is short-acting. However, it has a greater risk of adverse effects (bradycardia, hyperkalemia, hypertension, increased intracranial and ocular pressure) and is contraindicated in a variety of clinical conditions. The contemporary approach to paralysis involves the use of longer-acting agents, such as rocuronium and vercuron, because patients have fewer adverse effects with these medications. In addition, rocuronium and vercuron may be used for extended paralysis (not an option with succinylcholine).

The nurse plays a key role in ensuring that the tracheal tube remains taped securely in place by the following:

- Using soft wrist restraints if necessary to prevent the child from removing the tracheal tube
- Providing sedative and/or paralyzing medications
- Using caution when moving the child for x-rays, changing linens, and performing other procedures

Monitoring the Child Who Is Intubated

Provide ongoing and frequent monitoring of the intubated child to determine adequacy of oxygenation and ventilation as noted earlier. Once the child is intubated, the ventilatory support being provided should result in improvement in oxygen saturation and vital signs. If the child begins to exhibit signs of poor oxygenation, perform a quick assessment. Auscultate the lungs for equal air entry and determine the child's heart rate. Are the breath sounds equal? Is the heart rate normal for age? Perform a quick survey of the equipment and look for any disconnected tubes or kinks in the tubing. Determine oxygen saturation levels via pulse oximeter and evaluate the end-tidal CO_2 color (see Box 32.1). Use the PALS mnemonic "DOPE" for troubleshooting when the status of a child who is intubated deteriorates:

D = Displacement. The tracheal tube is displaced from the trachea.

O = Obstruction. The tracheal tube is obstructed, with a mucous plug, for example.

P = Pneumothorax. Usually a pneumothorax results in a sudden change in the child's assessment. The signs of a pneumothorax include decreased breath sounds and decreased chest expansion on the side of the pneumothorax. Subcutaneous emphysema may be noted over the chest. In the case of tension pneumothorax, the child may have a sudden drop in heart rate and blood pressure.

E = Equipment Failure. Relatively simple problems as previously discussed, such as a disconnected oxygen supply, can cause the child to deteriorate. Culprits such as a leak in the ventilator circuit or a loss of power are other types of equipment failure that may be responsible.

BOX 32.1

EXHALED CO_2 MONITORING OR END-TIDAL CO_2 MONITORING

- Device that connects to the child's ventilator circuit to detect CO_2 in the tubing. CO_2 should be noted in the tubing after six ventilations.
- Devices are usually color-coded. In the case of tracheal intubation, observe the color on the device change from purple to tan to yellow.
- The AHA's Pediatric Advanced Life Support (2002) suggests the following method to remember how the colors on the end-tidal CO_2 device correspond with tracheal tube placement:
  - Purple = Problem (little or no CO_2 detected)
  - Tan = Think about a problem.
  - Yellow = Yes, CO_2 is definitely detected and the tube is in the trachea.

Make sure all equipment is appropriately connected and functional. When obstruction with secretions is suspected, suction the tracheal tube. If the tracheal tube is displaced from the trachea, remove the tube if it remains in the child's mouth and begin BVM ventilation. In the case of pneumothorax, prepare to assist with needle thoracotomy.

Preparing the Intubated Child for Transport

Once the child is stabilized with a secure tracheal tube in place, prepare to transport the child. The child will be moved by stretcher to an intensive care unit in the acute care facility or by air or land ambulance to another facility that specializes in the care of acutely ill children. To facilitate transport, make sure that all tubes are securely taped. During transport, use portable oxygen and manually ventilate with the BVM. As the "sending" nurse, ensure that all laboratory results are obtained and provided to your "receiving" colleagues. If the child is going to another facility, complete a detailed summary of the resuscitation or provide a copy of the nurse's and/or progress notes. Complete the appropriate transfer forms as determined by the institution.

If the child is being transported by ambulance, the parents may not be able to accompany their child. In this case, find out as much as possible about the transport and assist the parents by giving directions to the receiving institution.

SHOCK

Shock is defined as a "clinical state characterized by inadequate tissue perfusion resulting in delivery of oxygen and metabolic substrates that is insufficient to meet tissue metabolic demands," according to the AHA (2001b). If shock is left untreated, cardiopulmonary arrest will result. Shock, which may be further classified as compensated or decompensated, is the result of a variety of clinical problems. Compensated shock occurs when poor perfusion exists without a decrease in BP. In decompensated shock, inadequate perfusion is accompanied by a drop in BP. Unchecked decompensated shock leads to cardiac arrest and death. The principles of PALS stress the early evaluation and management of children in compensated shock with the goal of preventing decompensated shock. Once the child in shock is hypotensive, organ perfusion is dramatically impaired and a dire clinical scenario ensues.

Pathophysiology

Shock is the result of dramatic respiratory or hemodynamic compromise. Shock is caused by impaired cardiac output or impaired systemic vascular resistance (SVR) or a combination of both. Cardiac output (CO) is equal to heart rate (HR) times ventricular stroke volume (SV) ($CO = HR \times SV$). Stroke volume is how much blood is ejected from the heart with each beat. Stroke volume is related to left ventricular filling pressure, the impedance to ventricular filling, and myocardial contractility. Left ventricular filling pressure is also known as preload, and the impedance to ventricular filling is commonly called afterload. Young children and infants have relatively small stroke volumes compared to older children and adults. Therefore, infants and young children are different from their adult counterparts in that their cardiac output depends on their heart rate, not their stroke volume. Clinically, in cases of circulatory compromise and compensated shock in infants and children, the heart rate is increased. The exception to this is a paradoxical phenomenon in neonates, who may have bradycardia rather than tachycardia.

Systemic vascular resistance or afterload is the impediment to the heart's ventricular ejection. Increased SVR will result in a decrease in blood flow unless the ventricular pressure increases. Increased vascular resistance is a common problem in shock. In children who have shock-related increased SVR, cardiac output will fall unless the ventricle can compensate by increasing pressure. In cardiac insufficiency, the child's heart will have impaired ability to compensate for the increased afterload.

Types of Shock

The most common types of shock are hypovolemic, septic, cardiogenic, and distributive. Hypovolemic shock, the most common type of shock in children, occurs when systemic perfusion decreases as a result of "inadequate intravascular volume in relation to vascular space" (AHA, 2002). Children commonly have hypovolemic shock that occurs in association with fluid losses. For example, hypovolemic shock may occur with viral or bacterial gastroenteritis that results in vomiting and diarrhea, medications such as diuretics, and heat stroke. Other causes of hypovolemia in children include blood loss, such as from a major traumatic injury, and third spacing of fluid, such as with burns.

Septic shock is related to a systemic inflammatory response in which there may be increased cardiac output with a low SVR, known as "warm shock." More commonly in children, septic shock results in a decrease in cardiac output with an increase in SVR, known as "cold shock."

Cardiogenic shock results from an ineffective pump, the heart, with a resultant decrease in stroke volume. Children who have congenital or acquired cardiac abnormalities with a poorly functioning heart are at risk for cardiogenic shock.

Distributive shock is the result of a loss in the SVR. A relative hypovolemia occurs, most often with neurogenic injury-related shock and anaphylaxis. In relative hypovolemia, the vascular compartment expands due to systemic vasodilation. This results in a relatively larger vasculature requiring more fluid to maintain cardiac output despite no actual loss of fluid.

Lastly, toxic drug ingestions may also lead to shock.

Altered microcirculatory status is common in all types of shock. Compensatory mechanisms are activated in response to decreased blood flow. Sympathetic nervous system response results in marked contraction of larger vessel sphincters and arterioles. This compression results in dramatically impaired capillary blood flow. Blood is redirected away from less important body systems, such as the skin and the kidneys, to the vital organs (the heart and brain). During compensated shock, the body can maintain some level of blood flow to the vital organs. Peripheral vasoconstriction, the body's compensatory response to diminished blood flow, often results in the child's ability to maintain a normal or near-normal BP. As shock continues, capillary beds become obstructed by cellular debris, and platelets and white blood cells aggregate. Endothelial damage occurs as a result of capillary congestion. Poor blood flow to the capillaries results in anaerobic metabolism. Lactic acid accumulates, and this can lead to acidosis. In addition, children with septic shock sustain marked endothelial damage as a result of exposure to bacterial toxins.

The cumulative affect of capillary obstruction and dramatically impaired blood flow is tissue ischemia. As tissue ischemia progresses, the child will show signs of altered perfusion to vital organs. For example, as blood flow to the brain is diminished, the child will demonstrate an altered level of consciousness. Altered blood flow to the kidneys will result in decreased urine output or absence of urine output (oliguria). Commonly, the heart rate will increase in the early stages of shock, but as the heart becomes compromised as a result of poor perfusion, the child will become bradycardic. The child will demonstrate an increased respiratory rate in the initial phase of shock. Tachypnea is seen in septic shock as well. In fact, the child may demonstrate marked hyperventilation in an effort to "blow off" carbon dioxide in response to the acidosis that is associated with septic shock.

Nursing Assessment

Nursing assessment of the child in shock includes the health history and physical examination as well as laboratory and diagnostic testing. The nursing assessment must be performed quickly and accurately so that resuscitation can be expedited.

Health History

In shock, the health history is based on the child's presentation. Children with shock are critically ill and require emergent intervention. Therefore, the history is obtained as life-saving interventions are provided. Determine when the child first became ill and treatments that have been given thus far. Inquire about sources of volume loss, such as:

- Vomiting
- Diarrhea
- Decreased oral intake
- Blood loss

Ask when the child last urinated. Investigate for other related symptoms such as behavioral changes or lethargy. Has the child had a fever or rash, complained of headache, or been exposed to anyone with similar symptoms? Inquire about daycare attendance and whether the family has recently traveled outside of the country. Determine if the child has a history of a congenital heart defect or other heart condition or if the child has severe allergies. Ask the parent about accidental ingestion of medications or other substances and, for the older child or adolescent, about the possibility of illicit substance use.

Physical Examination

The key to successful shock management is early recognition of the signs and symptoms. Obtain vital signs, noting any alterations. Measure BP, but this is not a reliable method of evaluating for shock in children. Children tend to maintain a normal or slightly less-than-normal BP in compensated shock while sacrificing tissue perfusion until the child suffers a cardiopulmonary arrest. Therefore, other components of the circulatory evaluation will be more valuable when assessing a child.

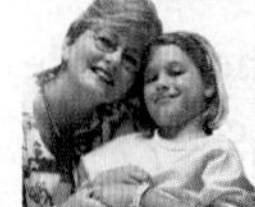

Bradycardia is a serious sign in neonates and may occur with respiratory compromise, circulatory compromise, and/or overwhelming sepsis.

As with any emergency, evaluate the airway first. Is it patent? Then determine if the child is breathing. The child in shock will often demonstrate signs of respiratory distress, such as grunting, gasping, nasal flaring, tachypnea, and increased work of breathing. Auscultate breath sounds to determine the adequacy of air entry and airflow. If the child shows signs of respiratory distress, manage the airway and breathing problem first, as discussed earlier in the chapter.

Assess the skin color. Palpate the skin temperature and determine quality of pulses. Except in special cases, such as distributive shock, the child in shock will generally have darker and cooler extremities with delayed capillary refill. Note the line of demarcation if present. This refers to the point on the distal extremity where cool temperature begins (the proximal portion of the extremity may continue to be warm). In distributive shock, the initial assessment will reveal full and bounding pulses and warm, erythemic skin. Evaluate the pulse quality. Distal pulses will likely be weaker than central pulses.

Evaluate the child's hydration state and check skin turgor. Decreased elasticity is associated with hypovolemic states, though this is usually a late sign. Observe the child's face; in compensated shock the child may be awake but obtunded and demonstrate signs of distress. The child in decompensated shock may have his or her eyes closed and may be responsive only to voice or other stimulation. Evaluate pupillary responses. Determine urinary output, which will be decreased in the child with shock.

After having evaluated and provided initial life-saving management for airway, breathing, and circulation, evaluate the child's entire body for other disabilities. Traumatic injuries warrant vigilant evaluation for ongoing blood loss, keeping in mind that traumatic injuries may also result in internal blood loss, such as in the child with a femur fracture. Look for signs of malformation, swelling, redness, or pain of the extremities, which may suggest internal blood loss. Also inspect for any open wounds and active sites of bleeding. Children with abdominal injuries also may lose copious amounts of blood internally. Inspect the abdomen for redness, skin discoloration, or distention. Auscultate for bowel sounds in all four quadrants.

Laboratory and Diagnostic Testing

As the child is being resuscitated, laboratory tests and radiographs will be ordered and obtained. However, no diagnostic test should replace the priority of respiratory support, vascular access, and fluid administration. Laboratory results will guide ongoing management. Common laboratory and diagnostic tests used for children with shock include:

- Blood glucose levels: usually performed at the bedside using a glucose meter (e.g., Chem-strip or Accucheck) to obtain a rapid result
- Electrolytes: to evaluate for electrolyte abnormalities
- Complete blood count with differential: to assess for viral or bacterial infection (septic shock) and to evaluate for anemia and platelet abnormalities
- Blood culture: to evaluate for sepsis; preliminary results will not be available for 1 to 2 days
- C-reactive protein: to evaluate for infection
- Arterial blood gases: to assess oxygen and carbon dioxide levels and to provide information about acid–base balance
- Toxicology panel (if ingestion is suspected)
- Lumbar puncture: to evaluate the cerebrospinal fluid for meningitis
- Urinalysis: to evaluate for glucose, ketones, and protein; concentration (specific gravity) is increased in dehydration states
- Urine culture: to evaluate for urinary tract or kidney infection
- Radiographs: to evaluate heart size, to evaluate the lungs for pneumonia or pulmonary edema (present with cardiogenic shock)

Nursing Management

Signs of shock in children warrant an emergent response. Always evaluate and manage the airway and breathing and check for pulses. Initiate CPR if the child is pulseless. All children who have signs and symptoms of shock should receive 100% oxygen via mask. If the child has poor respiratory effort or is apneic, administer 100% oxygen via BVM or tracheal tube (refer to the section on respiratory emergencies for more specific information about management of airway and breathing). As part of ongoing monitoring, institute cardiac and apnea monitoring and assess oxygen saturation levels via pulse oximetry.

Obtaining Vascular Access

Once the airway and breathing are addressed, nursing management of shock focuses on obtaining vascular access and restoring fluid volume. Children with signs of shock should receive generous amounts of isotonic IV fluids rapidly. However, obtaining vascular access in critically ill children can be challenging. Vascular access must be obtained using the quickest route possible in children whose condition is markedly deteriorated, such as those in decompensated shock.

Various forms of vascular access available for the management of the critically ill child include:

- Peripheral IV route: A large-bore catheter is used to give large amounts of fluid. This route may not be feasible in children with significant vascular compromise.
- Central IV route: Central lines can be inserted into the jugular vein and threaded into the superior vena cava. The femoral route is best for obtaining central venous access while CPR is in progress because the insertion procedure will not interfere with life-saving interventions involving the airway and cardiac compressions. The subclavian vein, located under the clavicle, is an alternative route for central access.
- Saphenous vein: The saphenous vein (found in the ankle) is an alternative route for venous access that is obtained using a surgical incision.
- Intraosseous access: Intraosseous access, obtained by cannulating the child's bone marrow, is recommended in cases of decompensated shock or cardiac arrest if IV access cannot be attained rapidly. The preferred site is the anterior tibia. Special intraosseous needles are used (generally a 15-gauge needle for older children, 18-gauge for younger children). The needle is inserted using a firm twisting motion slightly away from the growth plate. Any medications or fluids that can be administered using an IV site can be given using this route. Alternative sites include the femur, the iliac crest, the sternum, and the distal tibia.

Restoring Fluid Volume

Administer IV isotonic fluids, such as Ringer's lactate or normal saline (the isotonic fluids of choice) rapidly. Administer 20 mL/kg of the prescribed fluid as a bolus, infusing the fluid as rapidly as possible. In general a large-bore syringe, such as a 35- to 60-cc syringe attached to a three-way stopcock, is the preferred method for rapid fluid delivery in children. Infusing the fluid via gravity is too slow. The fluid bolus may be repeated up to two times (for a total of three times) if required.

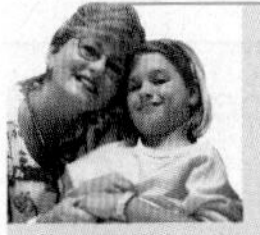

Dextrose solutions are contraindicated in shock because of the risk of complications such as osmotic diuresis, hypokalemia, hyperglycemia, and worsening of ischemic brain injury.

Children in septic shock will often require larger volumes of fluid as a result of the increased capillary permeability. Children in shock due to trauma will usually receive a colloid, such as blood, when there is an inadequate response to crystalloid isotonic fluid. After each fluid bolus, reassess the child for signs of positive response to the fluid administration.

Insert an indwelling urinary catheter to allow for accurate and frequent measurement of urine output. Indicators of improvement include:

- Improved cardiovascular status: The central and peripheral pulses are stronger. The line of demarcation of extremity coolness is diminishing and capillary refill is improved (time is decreased). BP is improved.
- Improved mental status: The child is more alert. For example, the child's eyes are open and watching personnel. If the child is younger, he or she may be pulling at the IV line.
- Improved urine output: This may not be noted initially but should be noted over the next few hours; the goal is 1 to 2 mL/kg/hour.

The process of fluid resuscitation involves giving the fluid, assessing and reassessing the child, and documenting findings in the nurses' notes. Children in shock may require as much as 100 to 200 mL/kg of resuscitative fluid during the initial hours of shock management. Most children in shock need and can tolerate this large volume of fluid. Continued reassessment will determine if the child is beginning to experience fluid overload in the form of pulmonary edema (this is rare but may occur in children with pre-existing cardiac conditions or severe chronic pulmonary disease) (AHA, 2001b; Prentiss et al., 2007).

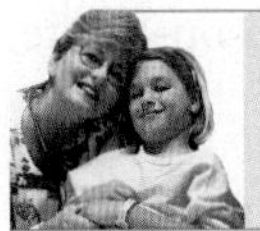

Be careful not to focus solely on the child's circulatory status; you may overlook signs and symptoms indicating respiratory deterioration.

Administering Medications

In some circumstances, such as septic shock or distributive shock, fluid alone does not adequately improve the child's status and medications may be ordered adjunctively. Vasoactive medications are used either alone or in combination to improve cardiac output, to increase SVR or to decrease SVR. The selection of medications is dictated by the child's cardiac and vascular status. For example, dobutamine is a medication with significant beta-adrenergic effects and thus can improve cardiac contractility. Epinephrine, which affects the heart muscle, is also a powerful vasoconstrictor. Dopamine affects the heart at lower doses but increasingly affects the vasculature with increased doses. These medications may be given as a loading dose, followed by a continuous infusion. When vasoactive drugs are administered, monitor for improvement in heart rate, BP, perfusion, and urine output.

CARDIAC ARRHYTHMIAS AND ARREST

Unlike adults, in whom cardiopulmonary arrest is most often caused by a primary cardiac event, children typically have healthy hearts and thus rarely experience primary cardiac arrest. More commonly they experience cardiopulmonary arrest from gradual deterioration of respiration and/or circulation (AHA, 2005e). In particular, children experiencing a respiratory emergency or shock may deteriorate and eventually demonstrate cardiopulmonary arrest. Thus, the standard of care for managing a child in this situation is vastly different from that for an adult.

Nurses who care for children should be skilled in evaluating and managing respiratory alterations and shock in children, as discussed in previous sections. Overwhelming evidence suggests that if primary respiratory compromise or shock is identified and treated in the critically ill child, a secondary cardiac arrest can be prevented. Rare exceptions do exist, however. For example, electrolyte abnormalities and toxic drug ingestions are primary insults to the cardiovascular system that may lead to a sudden cardiac arrest rather than a gradual progression. Other exceptions in which the child is at risk for a primary and sudden cardiac arrest include:

- History of a serious primary congenital or acquired cardiac defect
- Potentially lethal arrhythmias, such as prolonged QT syndrome
- Hyper- or hypotrophic cardiomyopathy
- Traumatic cardiac injury or a sharp blow to the chest, known as "commotion cordis," as can occur when a high-velocity ball impacts the chest

The overwhelming majority of children rarely experience cardiac arrhythmias, so it is beyond the scope of this chapter to discuss the myriad of possible complex rhythm disturbances. Therefore, this discussion will be limited to the management of emergent cardiac conditions that are more typically found in children.

Pathophysiology

The AHA has simplified the nomenclature used to describe pediatric cardiac compromise and has established three major categories of cardiac rhythm disturbances:

"Slow": bradyarrhythmias
"Fast": tachyarrhythmias
"Absent": pulseless, cardiovascular collapse

● COMPARISON CHART 32.2 Causes of Sinus Bradycardia Versus Heart Block

	Sinus Bradycardia	Heart Block
Causes	• Pathologic: medications such as digoxin, hypoxia, hypothermia, head injury • Nonpathologic: well-conditioned athlete	• Congenital: associated with cardiac anomalies • Acquired: endocarditis, rheumatic fever, Kawasaki disease

The pathophysiology, causes, and therapeutic management of each of the categories of rhythm disturbances are discussed below.

Bradyarrhythmias

Bradycardia is a heart rate significantly slower than the patient's normal heart rate for age. Bradycardia in children is most commonly "sinus bradycardia"—in other words, there is not a cardiac nodal abnormality associated with the slowed heart rate. In sinus bradycardia, the P waves and QRS complex remain normal on the ECG. Brief dips in heart rates can be normal, such as when the child sleeps. Children are also susceptible to brief drops in heart rate that are associated with vagal stimulation. For example, passing an orogastric tube down the esophagus of a young infant may induce a temporary bradycardic response. These normal decreases in the child's heart rate should recover with or without stimulation and are not normally associated with signs of altered perfusion.

Less commonly, children manifest bradycardia as a result of cardiac abnormalities and heart block. Infants with bradycardia related to heart block may exhibit poor feeding and tachypnea, whereas older children may demonstrate fatigue, dizziness, and syncope. Comparison Chart 32.2 compares the causes of sinus bradycardia and heart block in children.

In contrast, the child with a serious and possible life-threatening bradyarrhythmia will have a heart rate below 60 beats per minute, with signs of altered perfusion. The most common causes of profound bradycardia in children are respiratory compromise, hypoxia, and shock. Sustained bradycardia is commonly associated with arrest. It is an ominous sign and should be taken seriously.

Tachyarrhythmias

Children normally have faster heart rates than adults, and fever, fear, and pain are common explanations for significant increases in the heart rate of a child, **tachycardia**. This normal elevation in heart rate is known as sinus tachycardia. However, once the fever is reduced, the child is comforted, or the pain is managed, the heart rate should return close to the child's baseline. Hypoxia and hypovolemia are pathological reasons for tachycardia in the child. The signs, symptoms, and management of these concerns were discussed in previous sections. If the child has sinus tachycardia that results from any of these causes, the focus is on the underlying cause. It is inappropriate and dangerous to treat sinus tachycardia with medications aimed at decreasing the heart rate or with a defibrillation device.

Tachyarrhythmias in children that are associated with cardiac compromise have unique characteristics that present differently from sinus tachycardia. Examples of these include supraventricular tachycardia (SVT) and ventricular tachycardia. SVT is a cardiac conduction problem in which the heart rate is extremely rapid and the rhythm is very regular, often described as "no beat-to-beat variability." The most common cause of SVT is a re-entry problem in the cardiac conduction system. Comparison Chart 32.3 explains the differences between SVT and sinus tachycardia. Commonly, SVT is the result of a genetic cardiac conduction problem such as Wolff-Parkinson-White.

● COMPARISON CHART 32.3 Distinguishing SVT From Sinus Tachycardia

	SVT	Sinus Tachycardia
Rate (bpm)	Infants >220, children >180	Infants <220, children <180
Rhythm	Abrupt onset and termination	Beat-to-beat variability
P waves	Flattened	Present and normal
QRS	Narrow (<0.08 seconds)	Normal
History	Usually no significant history	Fever, fluid loss, hypoxia, pain, fear

SVT may also be associated with medications such as caffeine and theophylline. Children often can tolerate the characteristically higher heart rate that is associated with SVT for short periods of time. However, the increased demand that is placed on the cardiovascular system usually overtaxes the child and results in signs of congestive heart failure if the SVT continues unchecked for a prolonged time.

Ventricular tachycardia is a rhythm involving an elevation of the heart rate and a wide QRS (greater than 0.08 seconds) that is the result of an abnormal, rapid firing of one or both of the ventricles. Ventricular tachycardia is a rare arrhythmia in children and usually is associated with a congenital or acquired cardiac abnormality. In addition, prolonged QT syndrome is a conduction abnormality that can result in ventricular tachycardia and sudden death in children. Less commonly, ingestion of medications and toxins, acidosis, hypocalcemia, abnormalities of potassium, and hypoxemia have been associated with the development of ventricular tachycardia in children.

Collapsed Rhythms (Pulseless Rhythms)

A collapsed rhythm, as defined by PALS, is one that produces cardiac arrest with no palpable pulse and no signs of perfusion (cardiac arrest). Typically, the most common pulseless arrest rhythms in children are asystole or pulseless electrical activity (PEA). **Asystole** occurs when there is no cardiac electrical activity, commonly referred to as "a straight line" on the ECG. The child with PEA has some appreciable rhythm on the ECG but no palpable pulses. PEA may be caused by hypoxemia, hypovolemia, hypothermia, electrolyte imbalance, tamponade, toxic ingestion, tension pneumothorax, or thromboembolism. Ventricular tachycardia may also present as pulseless. Ventricular fibrillation, once thought to be rare in children, occurs in serious cardiac conditions in which the ventricle is not pumping effectively. It may develop from ventricular tachycardia. Ventricular fibrillation is characterized by variable, high-amplitude waveforms (coarse VF) or a finer, lower-amplitude waveform with no discernible cardiac rhythm (fine VF). In either case, cardiac output is insufficient.

Nursing Assessment

Nursing assessment of the child with a cardiac emergency includes the health history and physical examination as well as laboratory and diagnostic testing. The nursing assessment must be performed quickly and accurately so that resuscitation can be instituted if needed.

Health History

Obtain a brief health history of the child with a cardiac emergency while simultaneously assessing the child and providing life-saving interventions. Key areas to inquire about include:

- History of cardiac problems, asthma, chromosomal anomaly, delayed growth
- Symptoms such as syncope, dizziness, palpitations or racing heart, chest pain, coughing, wheezing, increased work of breathing
- Activity tolerance with play or feeding: Does the child get out of breath, turn blue, or squat during play? Can the child keep up with playmates? Does the infant tire with feedings?
- Precipitating illness, fever, unexplained joint pains, ingested medications
- Participation in a sport before the cardiac event occurred or injury to the chest
- Family history of cardiac problems, sudden death from a cardiac condition, heart attacks at a young age, chromosomal abnormalities

Determine treatment measures performed at the scene. Was CPR initiated? Was an AED used?

Physical Examination

Quickly establish the child's status. A child who is obviously in distress or is arresting must receive emergent life-saving interventions. Briefly perform the assessment while simultaneously providing life-saving interventions.

Inspection and Observation

Assess the child's airway patency and efficiency of breathing. Observe the child's color, noting circumoral pallor or duskiness or central pallor, mottling, duskiness, or cyanosis. Note any increased work of breathing, grunting, head bobbing, or apnea. Inspect the chest for barrel shape, which may be associated with chronic pulmonary or cardiac disease. Observe the pericardium for the presence of lifts or heaves. Note diaphoresis, anxious appearance, or dysmorphic features (50% of children with Down syndrome also have a congenital cardiac defect). Determine if neck vein distention is present. Inspect the fingertips for clubbing, which is indicative of chronic tissue hypoxemia.

Auscultation

Auscultate the breath sounds, noting any crackles or wheezes. Auscultate the heart rate. If the child does not have an adequate pulse, initiate CPR. If the child has a strong, perfusing pulse, complete the cardiac assessment. Auscultate with the diaphragm of the stethoscope first and then listen with the bell. Evaluate all of the auscultatory areas, listening first over the second right interspace (aortic valve) and then over the second left interspace (pulmonic valve); next move to the left lower sternal border (tricuspid area); and finally auscultate over the fifth interspace, midclavicular line (mitral area). Evaluate the rate and rhythm of the heart. Listen for any extra sounds or murmurs. Note and describe the quality, intensity, and location of any cardiac murmurs.

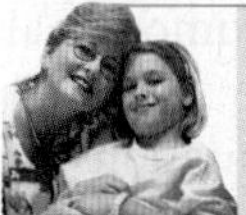

Murmurs are most often systolic and can be benign or associated with pathology. Murmurs that radiate to the back and are grade III or louder are more likely to be due to a cardiac defect. True diastolic murmurs are rare and almost always have a pathologic origin.

Percussion and Palpation

Percuss between the costal interspaces and note the heart's size. Palpate the heart to find the point of maximal impulse (PMI) and to evaluate for an associated thrill. A thrill feels like a fluttering under the fingers and is associated with cardiac pathology. Palpate and note the quality of the pulses. Evaluate each of the pulses bilaterally and note whether they are absent, faint, normal, or bounding. Compare the quality of pulses on each side of the body and also those of the upper and lower body. Note the skin temperature and evaluate the capillary refill.

Laboratory and Diagnostic Testing

The major diagnostic test used is the ECG. Identify the arrhythmia according to the ECG reading (Fig. 32.9).

Nursing Management

Provide oxygen at 100%. Institute cardiac monitoring and assess oxygen saturation levels via pulse oximeter. Obtain the child's preprinted code drug sheet or use the Broselow tape to obtain the child's height to estimate the tracheal tube sizes and medication dosages that are appropriate for the child. Always remember to intervene in this order: first airway, then breathing, then circulation. The remainder of this discussion will assume that the nurse has initiated interventions for airway and breathing as discussed earlier in the chapter.

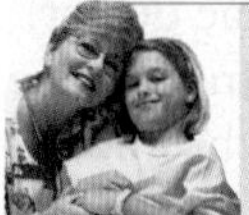

Pay attention to the rhythm on the monitor, but continually monitor the child's pulse. If the child does not have a pulse or has a pulse of less than 60 bpm, perform cardiac compressions despite the monitor reading.

Managing Bradyarrhythmias

The management of sinus bradycardia is focused on remedying the underlying cause of the slow heart rate. Since hypoxia is the most common cause of sustained bradycardia, oxygenation and ventilation are necessary. The newborn is particularly susceptible to bradycardia in relation to hypoxemia. Continue to reassess the child to determine if the bradycardia improves with adequate oxygenation and ventilation. If bradycardia persists, administer epinephrine and/or atropine as ordered. Epinephrine is the drug of choice for the treatment of persistent bradycardia.

Other causes of bradycardia such as hypothermia, head injury, and toxic ingestion are managed by addressing the underlying condition. Warming the hypothermic child may restore a normal sinus rhythm. Patients with head injury may have bradycardia without any cardiac involvement, and with successful management of the head injury, the bradycardia will resolve. Antidotes to toxins may be necessary in children whose bradycardia is the result of a toxic ingestion.

Managing Tachyarrhythmias

The tachyarrhythmias include SVT (stable or unstable) and ventricular tachycardia with a pulse. Examine the ECG to determine if the child is experiencing ventricular tachycardia or SVT. Clinically, determine whether the child in SVT is showing signs that require emergent intervention or if the child is stable. In compensated SVT, the child will appear to be alert, breathing comfortably, and well perfused. The child who is demonstrating signs of compromise, such as a change in consciousness, respiratory status, and perfusion, is considered to be in uncompensated SVT. Uncompensated SVT requires emergent intervention. The child who has ventricular tachycardia with a pulse will have poor perfusion and also requires immediate intervention. The evaluation and approaches to the tachyarrhythmias are discussed in Table 32.6.

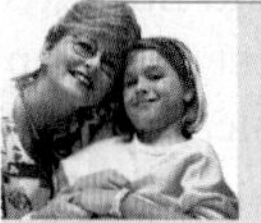

Adenosine has a rapid onset of action and an extremely short half-life. Administer it extremely rapidly with a generous amount of IV flush; otherwise, it will be ineffective.

Managing Collapsed Rhythms

As in any pediatric emergency, support the ABCs by managing the airway, providing oxygen, and giving fluids. In addition, if the child is pulseless or has a heart rate that is less than 60 bpm, initiate cardiac compressions. The pulseless rhythms include ventricular tachycardia, ventricular fibrillation, asystole, and pulseless electrical activity (PEA). ECG characteristics and management of these rhythms are summarized in Table 32.7. Also treat the underlying causes of the arrhythmia, if known.

The AHA emphasizes the importance of cardiac compressions in pulseless patients with arrhythmias. Give compressions before and immediately after defibrillation. In the past it was recommended that patients who required defibrillation be given three shocks in a row, but recent research findings have shown that the patient should be defibrillated only once, followed by five cycles of CPR. For defibrillation to be most effective, cardiac compressions must be performed effectively with minimal interruptions (AHA, 2006d).

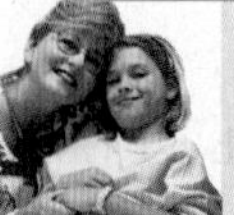

Previously, multiple doses of epinephrine were given in pediatric emergency situations. Recently, however, the AHA has recommended against this practice, as multiple doses of epinephrine have not been shown to be helpful and may actually cause harm to the child.

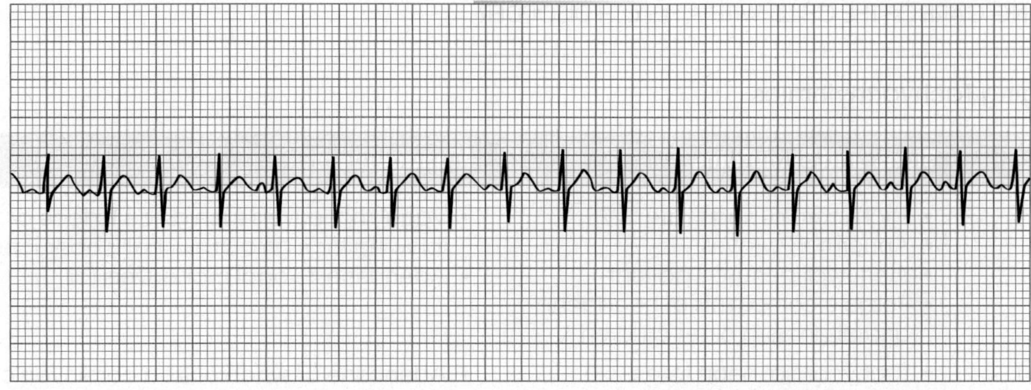

A

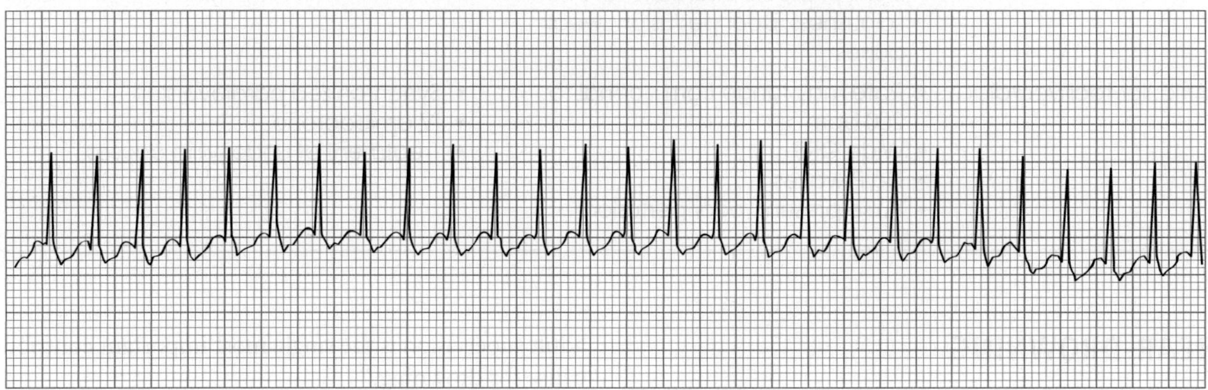

B

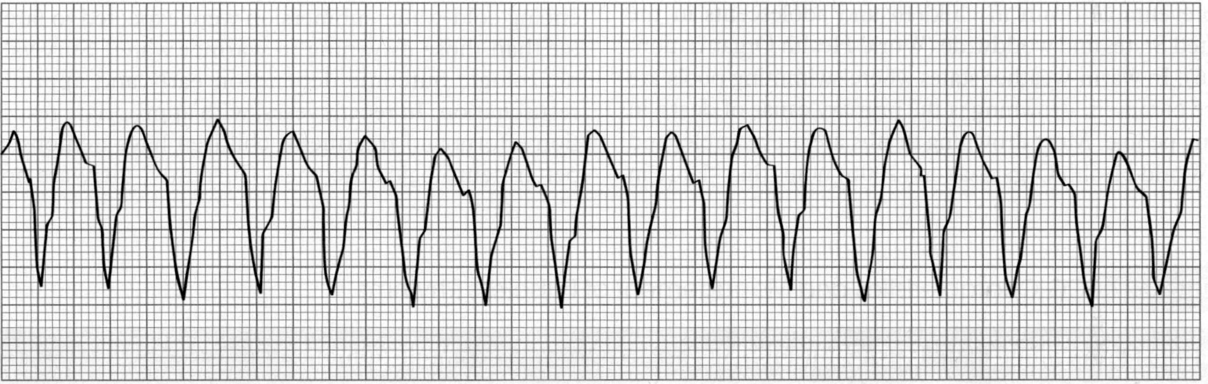

C

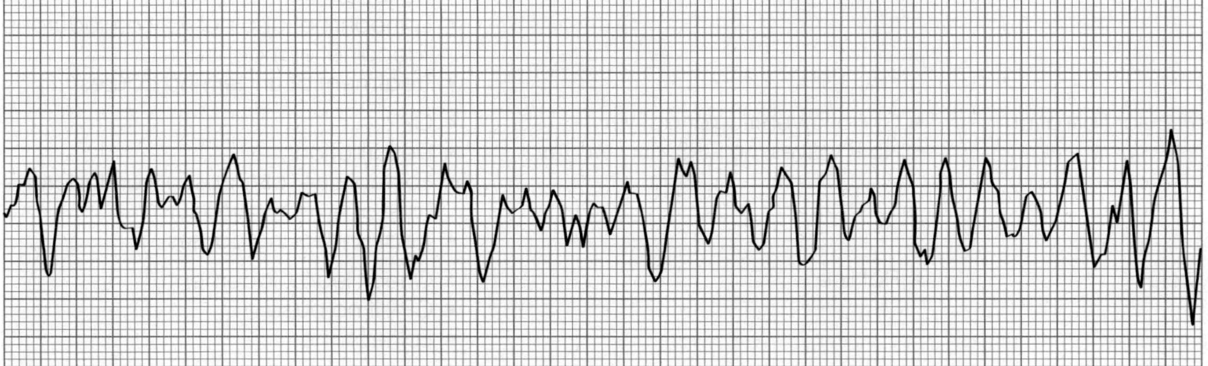

D

● Figure 32.9 Arrhythmias. (**A**) Sinus tachycardia: normal QRS and P waves, mild beat-to-beat variability. (**B**) Supraventricular tachycardia: note rate above 220, abnormal P waves, no beat-to-beat variability. (**C**) Ventricular tachycardia: rapid and regular rhythm, wide QRS without P waves. (**D**) Coarse ventricular fibrillation: chaotic electrical activity.

Table 32.6 Managing Tachyarrhythmias

Tachyarrhythmia	Signs and Symptoms	Management
Compensated SVT	• Tachycardia, heart rate >220 • Abnormal P waves • Alert, well-perfused patient • Possible complaints of headache and dizziness in older children	• Vagal maneuvers such as ice to face or blowing through a straw that is obstructed • Adenosine if vagal maneuvers fail
Uncompensated SVT	• Tachycardia, heart rate >220 • Abnormal P waves • Signs of shock: altered level of consciousness, poor perfusion, weak pulses	• Adenosine or synchronized cardioversion
Ventricular tachycardia	• Rate may range from normal to 200 bpm • Wide QRS • No P waves • Pulse present, poor perfusion	• Synchronized cardioversion • IV amiodarone • Treatment of underlying causes

NEAR-DROWNING

Water can be a great source of fun and exercise for children and adolescents, but drowning is the second-leading cause of preventable death in children and adolescents in the United States and worldwide (World Health Organization, 2006). In warm-weather states where swimming pools are more common, drowning is the primary cause of death in young people. Most drowning deaths are preventable, and the World Health Organization (2006) notes that "lapse in adult supervision is the single most important contributory cause for drowning."

Near-drowning is defined as a submersion injury in which the child survives. Traditionally, children experiencing cold-water submersion were expected to fare better than those drowning in warmer water. Survival and neurologic outcome depend on early and appropriate resuscitation. In recent years, with appropriate resuscitation efforts and treatment, children have demonstrated better neurologic outcomes. Currently, there are no fac-

Table 32.7 ECG Characteristics and Management of Pulseless Rhythms

Pulseless Arrhythmia	ECG Characteristics	Management
Ventricular tachycardia	• Wide QRS, no P waves	• CPR • Defibrillation • Epinephrine; also possibly amiodarone, lidocaine, or magnesium • Treatment of underlying causes
Ventricular fibrillation	• Chaotic ventricular activity • No P waves, no QRS, no T waves	• CPR • Defibrillation • Epinephrine; also possibly amiodarone, lidocaine, or magnesium • Treat underlying causes
Asystole	• Flat line	• Check lead placement • CPR if no pulse • Epinephrine
Pulseless electrical activity	• Electrical activity that is not consistent with ventricular tachycardia or ventricular fibrillation	• Check lead placement • CPR if no pulse • Treatment of underlying cause • Epinephrine

tors to predict whether the child's long-term neurologic status will be affected after surviving a near-drowning incident (Minto & Woodward, 2005).

Typically, a child who is drowning will struggle to breathe and eventually will aspirate water. Aspiration of relatively small amounts of water leads to poor oxygenation, with retention of carbon dioxide. Alveolar surfactant is depleted during the drowning event and pulmonary edema commonly occurs. Hypoxemia results in increased capillary permeability and resultant hypovolemia. Even small amounts of aspirated water may lead to pulmonary edema within a 24- to 48-hour period after the near-drowning episode. A near-drowning survivor is also at risk for renal complications due to altered renal perfusion during the hypoxemic state.

Nursing Assessment

Nursing assessment of the near-drowning survivor is crucial and must take place quickly and accurately.

Health History

Obtain the history rapidly while providing life-saving interventions. Ask about the circumstances of the event:

- Where did the drowning occur?
- Was the child in a lake, river, ocean, or swimming pool?
- Was the child submerged in a toilet, bucket, or bathtub?
- Did someone witness the child's entry into the water?
- Was the water fresh or salty? Cold or warm?
- Is it likely the water was contaminated?
- Were there any extenuating circumstances, such as a diving or automobile accident, associated with the near-drowning?
- What was the approximate length of time of the submersion? Was the child conscious or unconscious when rescued?
- What was done at the scene? Was CPR initiated? If so, when?
- If a cervical spine injury was suspected, was the cervical spine immobilized?
- Was an AED used?
- When did the child last eat (to prepare for possible intubation)?

Physical Examination

Evaluate airway patency and breathing. Auscultate all lung fields for signs of pulmonary edema, such as coarseness or crackles. Evaluate the heart rate, pulses, and perfusion. Note the cardiac rhythm on the monitor and report evidence of arrhythmias. Evaluate the child's neurologic status. Use a pen light to determine pupillary reaction. Use the pediatric coma score to further assess the neurologic status. Does the child open the eyes spontaneously, to stimuli, or not at all? Is there any spontaneous movement? Is the younger child crying? Can the older child speak? Measure the child's temperature, as hypothermia often occurs with near-drowning.

Laboratory and Diagnostic Testing

While awaiting laboratory and diagnostic testing results, continue resuscitative efforts as addressed below. Laboratory and diagnostic tests typically include the following:

- Arterial blood gases: hypoxemia, acidosis
- ECG: cardiac arrhythmias
- Chest x-ray: pulmonary edema, infiltrates
- Serum electrolytes: imbalance related to development of shock

Nursing Management

Because of the potentially devastating effects that drowning-related hypoxia has on the child's brain, airway interventions must be initiated immediately after retrieving a child from the water. Every second counts. Initial interventions in a near-drowning event are always focused on airway, breathing, and circulation; commonly, resuscitative efforts have begun before the child arrives at the acute care facility.

If a cervical spine injury is suspected (as in the case of a diving accident), provide stabilization either manually or with a cervical collar. As with any suspected neck injury, do not remove the cervical collar until injury to the cervical spine has been ruled out through an x-ray and clinical evaluation. Suction the airway to ensure airway patency. The child may have aspirated particles from a contaminated water source or emesis, a relatively common complication associated with near-drowning. A large-bore suction catheter such as a Yankauer suction catheter is an effective tool for clearing the upper airway. Administer supplemental oxygen at 100%. Children who have poor or absent respiratory effort most likely will require intubation. Insert a nasogastric tube to decompress the stomach and prevent aspiration of stomach contents. Initiate chest compressions if a pulse is not present.

Usually, the child exhibits some degree of hypothermia and will require warming. Generally, the core body temperature should be raised slowly, as warming a drowning victim too quickly may have deleterious effects. Remove any wet clothing, dry the child, and cover him or her with warmed blankets. Warm IV fluids and use other warming methods as prescribed.

Consider THIS!

Eva Dawson, a 2-year-old girl, is rushed into the emergency room by ambulance personnel after experiencing a near-drowning in the family swimming pool. Eva was resuscitated at the scene and is now breathing spontaneously, is lethargic, and coughs occasionally.

What health history information would you obtain from the parents or caregivers? What immediate management is necessary?

What education may be necessary for this family?

POISONING

Emergency care of the pediatric poisoning patient consists of rapid nursing assessment and prompt management.

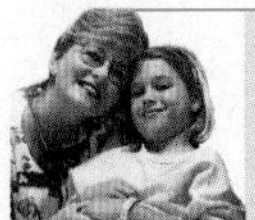

If a normally healthy child (particularly a young child) suddenly deteriorates without a known cause, suspect a toxic ingestion.

Nursing Assessment

Nursing assessment of the poisoning victim focuses on a thorough health history, followed by physical examination and laboratory and diagnostic testing.

Health History

Obtain the health history from the parents or caregiver or, in the case of an older child or teenager, from the child. Inquire about the approximate time of poisoning and the nature of the toxin. Was the toxin ingested, inhaled, or applied to the skin? In the case of pill ingestion, does the caregiver have the medication bottle with him or her? Did the child experience nausea, vomiting, anorexia, abdominal pain, or neurologic changes such as disorientation, slurred speech, or altered gait? Determine the progression of the symptoms. Did the parent or caregiver call the poison control center? Has any treatment been given? In the case of older children and teens, inquire about any history of depression or threatened suicide.

Physical Examination

Ingestion of medications or chemicals may result in a wide variety of clinical manifestations. Perform a thorough physical examination, noting alterations that may occur with particular ingestions, such as:

- Hyper- or hypotension
- Hyper- or hypothermia
- Respiratory depression or hyperventilation
- Miosis (pupillary contraction) or mydriasis (pupillary dilatation)

Pay particular attention to the child's mental status, skin moisture and color, and bowel sounds (Barry, 2005; Osterhoudt, 2000).

Laboratory and Diagnostic Testing

The suspected poison may direct the focus of laboratory and diagnostic testing. A variety of blood tests may be performed:

- Chemistry panel: to detect hypoglycemia or metabolic acidosis and assess renal function
- ECG: to identify arrhythmias or conduction delay
- Liver function tests: to assess for liver injury
- Urine and blood toxicology screens (available for a limited number of medications; may vary per institution)
- Specific drug levels if the substance ingested is known or highly suspected

Nursing Management

Management should focus on prevention of poisoning, but when poisoning does occur, give priority to airway, breathing, and circulation, treating alterations as discussed earlier in this chapter. Monitor vital signs frequently and provide supportive care. Few specific antidotes are available for medications or other toxins. Ipecac is rarely used in the health care setting to induce vomiting and it is no longer recommended for use in the home setting. Gastric lavage, administration of activated charcoal (binds with the chemical substance in the bowel), or whole bowel irrigation with polyethylene glycol electrolyte solutions may be used. Occasionally, dialysis is required to lower the level of toxin in the bloodstream. The intervention is based on the source of the ingestion. For example, activated charcoal is an effective method for preventing the absorption of many medications but is not effective in the case of an iron overdose.

If opiate or other narcotic ingestion is suspected, administer naloxone to reverse the effects of respiratory depression or alterations in level of consciousness. Treatment of seizures and alterations in thermoregulation may also be needed.

Specific treatment of the poisoning will be determined when the toxin is identified and poison control is queried. Maintain ongoing assessment of the poisoned child because many toxins exhibit very late effects.

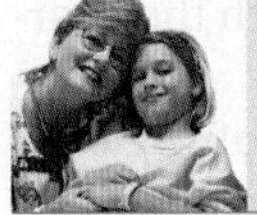

The National Poison Control number is 1-800-222-1222.

TRAUMA

The leading cause of death in persons between 3 and 33 years of age is unintentional injuries (Centers for Disease Control and Prevention [CDC], 2006e). Childhood trauma results from such events as automobile accidents, pedestrian accidents, falls, sporting injuries, and firearm use. Falls are the most common cause of pediatric injury. Children of varying ages are susceptible to various forms of injury due to their developmental level as well as their environmental exposure. Young children rely on their caregivers to promote their safety. Young children also are not developmentally equipped to be able to recognize dangerous situations.

Automobile accidents continue to cause the deaths of about five children daily, with significant numbers experiencing injury (National Highway Traffic Safety Administration, 2006). Pedestrian injuries cause 25% of traffic-related deaths in children (CDC, 2005a), and annually about 280,000 children are evaluated in emergency rooms following bicycle accidents (SafeKids,

2006e). Because pediatric injury is so common, nurses must become adept at assessment and intervention in the pediatric trauma victim.

Nursing Assessment

The trauma survey includes a brief health history as the child is being assessed and life-saving measures are being instituted.

Health History

Begin the health history by asking when the injury happened. If the child sustained a motor vehicle–related injury, ask how fast the vehicle was going. Determine if the child was appropriately restrained in the automobile. If the child was riding a bicycle, skateboarding, or using in-line skates, was he or she wearing a helmet, knee pads, and wrist guards? Determine what interventions were performed at the scene. Was the child immobilized on a backboard to protect the cervical spine? If the child is bleeding, ask the person who transported the child to estimate the amount of blood lost.

If the child experienced a fall, ask if the fall was witnessed and the height from which the child fell. Did the child fall onto a hard surface such as concrete? How did the child land: on his head or back, or did he catch himself with his hands? Younger children and boys are at higher risk for injuring their head. Did the child lose consciousness at the scene? What kind of behavior did the child exhibit after the fall? Since the fall, has the child complained of a headache or been vomiting?

While obtaining a detailed history about the fall, think about the child's developmental stage. For example, does it seem plausible that a toddler might fall down the stairs? In contrast, what is the likelihood that a 2-month-old would suffer a fractured femur from a fall? Keep in mind the possibility of child abuse. Critically evaluate the reported circumstances and try to determine if the history, developmental stage of the child, and the type of injury sustained match. In addition, evaluate the type of injury that the child sustained and the history given by the caregiver. For example, children who fall from significant heights often suffer skeletal fractures, but abdominal and chest injuries rarely result from falling from significant heights.

Physical Examination

Physical examination of the child with a traumatic injury should be approached with an evaluation of the ABCs (primary survey) first. Assess patency of airway and establish effectiveness of breathing (as discussed earlier in the chapter). Examine the child's respiratory effort, breath sounds, and color. Next, evaluate the circulation. Note the pulse rate and quality. Observe the color, skin temperature, and perfusion. If bleeding has occurred, the child's circulation may become compromised.

After assessing and intervening for airway, breathing, and circulation, proceed to the secondary survey. Assess for disability. Rapidly assess critical neurologic function. Determine the level of consciousness, pupillary reaction, and verbal and motor responses to auditory and painful stimuli. If the patient is a young infant, palpate the anterior fontanel: a full and bulging fontanel signals increased intracranial pressure. The traumatized child's neurologic status may range from completely normal to comatose.

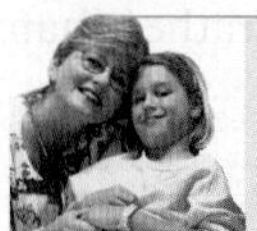

Unequal pupils or a fixed and dilated pupil is considered a neurosurgical emergency. Immediately report this finding.

Following ABCs and D (disability) is E (exposure). Expose the child to observe the entire body for signs of injury, whether blunt or penetrating. Perform a systematic, thorough inspection of the child's body. Note active bleeding and extremity deformity, as well as evidence of any lacerations and abrasions. Observe for movement and any complaints of immobility or pain with movement. Inspect the abdomen for redness, skin discoloration, or distention. Auscultate for bowel sounds in all four quadrants. If the child is verbal, ask if he or she has any pain in the stomach. If the child is younger, ask, "Do you have a tummy ache?" If the child reports abdominal pain, ask the child to point to where it hurts. Note any guarding of the abdomen, which is an indication of abdominal pain. In the case of potential bowel injury, only light palpation is acceptable. Always assess the least tender areas first and palpate the more sensitive areas last.

Laboratory and Diagnostic Testing

As in other pediatric emergencies, never delay life-saving measures to wait for laboratory or diagnostic test results. In addition to routine laboratory tests, common laboratory and diagnostic tests for the pediatric trauma patient include:

- Type and cross-match: to assess the child's blood type before blood products are given
- Prothrombin time and partial thromboplastin time: to evaluate for clotting dysfunction
- Amylase and lipase: to identify pancreatic injury
- Liver function tests: to assess for liver injury
- Pregnancy test (in any female who has reached puberty)
- CT scan, ultrasound, or MRI of the head, abdomen, or extremities: to evaluate the extent of the injury

Nursing Management

Nursing management of the pediatric trauma victim focuses initially on the ABCs.

Providing Immediate Care

If head or spinal injury is suspected, open the airway using the jaw-thrust maneuver with cervical spine stabilization (see Fig. 32.4). The revised AHA guidelines for basic life support recommend that if the airway cannot be opened using the jaw-thrust maneuver, it may be opened using the head tilt–chin lift maneuver. The rationale for this change in guidelines is that the jaw thrust is often a difficult maneuver to perform. Since opening the airway is the priority, AHA has made this allowance even if the cervical spine is at risk (AHA, 2005d). In addition, new AHA recommendations advise that stabilization of the head and neck of a trauma victim should be provided manually rather than with an immobilization device.

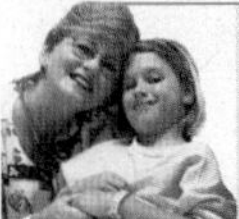

Infants and young children require unique cervical spine management because they have prominent occiputs that result in flexion of the neck in the supine position. To maintain the optimal neutral spinal position in the young child, use a special pediatric backboard with a head indentation, or use a folded towel to elevate the child's torso.

Clear the airway of obstruction using a large-bore suction device such as a Yankauer. If the child is breathing on his or her own, give the child oxygen at the highest flow possible (such as by a non-rebreathing mask). If the child is not breathing on his or her own, intervene using the AHA guidelines discussed earlier in this chapter.

If a BVM device is available, connect it to the oxygen source and use the bag to ventilate the child. Observe the chest rise and be careful not to overventilate, as this results in abdominal distention. Deliver breaths at the rate recommended by the AHA, one breath every 3 seconds. Do not hyperventilate. In the not-too-distant past, head injury in children was managed using hyperventilation. This resulted in **hypocapnia** (decreased amounts of carbon dioxide in the blood). The physiologic effect of hypocapnia is the induction of vasoconstriction, which in turn results in tissue ischemia. Therefore, current management of head injury in children excludes hyperventilation. The only exception to this rule is in an acute situation, if the child is showing signs of a possible brain stem herniation, hyperventilation may be used initially and briefly.

Assess the child for a strong central pulse. If the child has no pulse, initiate CPR immediately. When perfusion is compromised, administer IV fluid resuscitation. Trauma victims are more likely to require colloids or blood products due to blood loss from the injury.

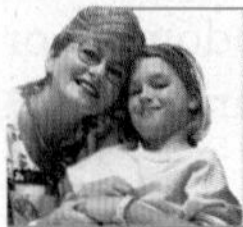

Patients with head injury who are demonstrating signs of shock such as poor perfusion and bradycardia should receive fluid volume resuscitation.

References

Books and Journals

Agarwal, S., Swanson, S., Murphy, A., et al. (2005). Comparing the utility of a standard pediatric resuscitation cart with a pediatric resuscitation cart based on the Broselow tape: A randomized, controlled, crossover trial involving simulated resuscitation scenarios. *Pediatrics, 116*(3), 741.

Alterman, D. M., Daley, B. J., Kennedy, A. P., et al. (2006). *Considerations in pediatric trauma.* Retrieved 10/16/06 from http://www.emedicine.com/med/topic3223.htm.

American Academy of Pediatrics. (2000). *Childhood emergencies in the office, hospital and community.* Elk Grove, IL: American Academy of Pediatrics.

American Academy of Pediatrics. (2001). Falls from heights: Windows, roofs, balconies. *Pediatrics, 107*(5), 1188–1191.

American Academy of Pediatrics. (2001). Injuries associated with infant walkers. *Pediatrics, 108*(3), 790–792.

American Academy of Pediatrics. (2002). Skateboard and scooter injuries. *Pediatrics, 109,* 542–543.

American Academy of Pediatrics. (2005). *The injury prevention program: A guide to safety counseling in office practice.* Retrieved 6/24/06 from http://www.aap.org/family/tippmain.htm.

American Academy of Pediatrics. (2006). *Summer safety tips: Part I.* Retrieved 6/24/06 from http://www.aap.org/advocacy/releases/summertips.htm.

American Academy of Pediatrics. (2006). *Summer safety tips: Part II.* Retrieved 6/24/06 from http://www.aap.org/advocacy/releases/summertips-p2.htm.

American Academy of Pediatrics, Committee on Injury, Violence, and Poison Prevention. (2003). Policy statement: Poison treatment in the home. *Pediatrics, 112*(5), 1182–1185.

American Association of Critical Care Nurses. (2006). *Core curriculum for pediatric critical care nursing* (2nd ed.). St. Louis: Mosby.

American College of Surgeons. (1999). *Committee on trauma: Optimal care of the injured patient,* Chapter 14.

American College of Surgeons. (2004). *National Trauma Data Bank Pediatric Report 2004.* Chicago: American College of Surgeons.

American Heart Association. (2001a). *Basic cardiac life support for healthcare providers.* Dallas: American Heart Association.

American Heart Association. (2001b). *Pediatric advanced life support provider manual.* Dallas: American Heart Association.

American Heart Association. (2003). Recommended guidelines for uniform reporting of data from drowning. *Circulation, 108,* 2565–2584.

American Heart Association. (2005a). Highlights of the 2005 American Heart Association guidelines for cardiopulmonary resuscitation and emergency cardiovascular care. *Currents in Emergency Cardiovascular Care, 16,* 4.

American Heart Association. (2005b). Part 6: Pediatric basic and advanced life support, *Circulation, 112,* III-73-III-90. Retrieved 1/24/06 from http://circ.ahajournal.org/cgi/content/full/112/22_suppl/III-73.

American Heart Association. (2005c). Part 10.3: Drowning. *Circulation, 112,* 133–135.

American Heart Association. (2005d). Part 11: Pediatric basic life support. *Circulation, 112,* 156–166.

American Heart Association. (2005e). Part 12: Pediatric advanced life support. *Circulation, 112,* 167–187.

American Heart Association. (2006). 2005 AHA guidelines for cardiopulmonary resuscitation (CPR) and emergency cardiovascular care (ECC) of pediatric and neonatal clients: Pediatric advanced life support. *Pediatrics, 117*(5), e1005–e1028.

American Medical Student Association. (2006). *Child abuse and neglect.* Retrieved 11/5/06 from http://www.amsa.org/programs/gpit/child.cfm.

Atkins, D. L., & Kenney, M. A. (2004). Automated external defibrillators: Safety and efficacy in children and young adolescents. *Pediatric Clinics of North America, 51*(5), 1443–1462.

Barry, J. D. (2005). Diagnosis and management of the poisoned child. *Pediatric Annals, 34*(12), 936–946.

Beckman, A., Sloan, B., Moore, G., et al. (2002). Should parents be present during emergency department procedures on children, and who should make that decision? A survey of emergency physician and nurse attitudes. *American Emergency Medicine, 9*(2), 154–158.

Behrman, R. E., Kliegman, R. M., & Jenson, H. B. (2004). *Nelson textbook of pediatrics* (17th ed.). Philadelphia: W. B. Saunders.

Belville, R. G., & Seupaul, R. A. (2005). MD pain measurement in pediatric emergency care: A review of the Faces Pain Scale-Revised. *Pediatric Emergency Care, 21*(2), 90–93.

Berger, S., Utech, L., & Hazinski, M. F. (2004). Lay rescuer automated external defibrillation programs for children and adolescents. *Pediatric Clinics of North America, 51*(5), 1463–1478.

Bernard, L. M. (2002). Emergency nurses' role in pediatric injury prevention. *Nursing Clinics of North America, 37*(1), 135–143.

Brenner, R., Trumble, A., Smith, G., et al. (2001). Where children drown, United States, 1995. *Pediatrics, 108*(1), 85–89.

Brophy, M., Sinclair, S. A., Hostetler, G., & Xiang, H. (2006). Pediatric eye injury-related hospitalizations in the United States. *Pediatrics, 117*(6), 2267.

Centers for Disease Control and Prevention, National Center for Health Statistics. (2005a). *Emergency department visit data from the National Hospital Ambulatory Medical Care Survey.* Retrieved 6/24/06 from http://www.cdc.gov/nchs/about/otheract/injury/injury_emergency.htm.

Centers for Disease Control and Prevention. (2005b). Child passenger safety: National child passenger safety week. Retrieved 9/27/05 from http://www.cdc.gov/ncipc/duip/spotlite/chldseat.htm#airbag.

Centers for Disease Control and Prevention, National Center for Injury Prevention and Control. (2005c). Injuries among children and adolescents. Retrieved 9/20/05 from www.cdc.gov/ncipc/factsheets/children.htm.

Centers for Disease Control and Prevention. (2005d). Pertussis. Retrieved 11/30/05 from www.cdc.gov/ncidod/dbmd/diseaseinfo/pertussis_t.htm.

Centers for Disease Prevention and Control, National Center for Injury Prevention and Control. (2006a). *Injuries among children and adolescents.* Retrieved 6/24/06 from http://www.cdc.gov/ncipc/factsheets/children.htm.

Centers for Disease Control and Prevention, National Center for Injury Prevention and Control. (2006b). *National Child Passenger Safety Week, February 12–18, 2006.* Retrieved 6/24/06 from www.cdc.gov/ncipc/duip/spotlite/chldseat.htm#airbag.

Centers for Disease Control and Prevention, National Center for Injury Prevention and Control (2006c). *Poisoning prevention: Prevention tips.* Retrieved 6/21/06 from http://www.cdc.gov/ncipc/factsheets/poisonprevention.htm.

Centers for Disease Control and Prevention, National Center for Injury Prevention and Control (2006d). *Water-related injuries: Fact sheet.* Retrieved 10/29/06 from http://www.cdc.gov/ncipc/factsheets/drown.htm.

Centers for Disease Control and Prevention, National Center for Injury Prevention and Control (2006e). *WISQARS injury mortality reports, 1999–2003.* Retrieved 10/29/06 from http://webappa.cdc.gov/sasweb/ncipc/mortrate10_sy.html.

Coffman, S. (2003). Bicycle injuries and safety helmets in children: Review of research. *Orthopaedic Nursing 22*(1), 9–15.

Common Sense about Kids and Guns. (2005). *Fact file.* Retrieved 9/28/05 from http://www.kidsandguns.org/study/fact_file.asp.

Crain, E. F., & Gershal, J. C. (2004). *Clinical manual of emergency pediatrics* (4th ed.). New York: McGraw-Hill.

Crawley-Coha, T. (2002). Childhood injury: A status report, part 2. *Journal of Pediatric Nursing, 17*(2), 133–136.

Davis, D. P. (2005). Quantitative capnometry as a critical resuscitation tool. *Journal of Trauma Nursing, 12*(2), 40–42.

DeBoer, S., Seaver, M., & Broselow, J. (2005). Color coding to reduce errors—the Broselow-Luten system streamlines pediatric emergency treatment. *American Journal of Nursing, 105*(8), 68–71.

Decina, L. E., Lococo, K. H., & Block, A. W. (2005). *Misuse of restraints: Results of a workshop to review field data results.* Retrieved 9/29/05 from http://www.nhtsa.dot.gov/people/injury/research/TSF_MisuseChildRetraints/809851.html.

Doniger, S. J., & Sharieff, G. Q. (2006). Pediatric dysrhythmias. *Pediatric Clinics of North America, 53*(1), 85–106.

Donoghue, A., Baren, J., & Winograd, S. M. (2004). Rapid sequence intubation in pediatrics. *Pediatric Emergency Medicine Reports, 105* (12). Retrieved 4/10/06 from Health Reference Center Academic via Thomson Gale.

Fallot, A. (2005). Respiratory distress: Evaluating and treating common pulmonary emergencies in the office. *Pediatric Annals, 34*(11), 885–891.

Farah, M. (2006). *Pediatrics, tachycardia.* Retrieved 1/24/06 from http://www.emedicine.com/emerg/topic408.htm.

Fish, F. A. (2004). Ventricular fibrillation: Basic concepts. *Pediatric Clinics of North America, 51*(5), 1211–1222.

Fortenberry, J. D., & Mariscalco, M. (2006). General principles of poisoning management. In J. A. McMillan (Ed.), *Oski's pediatrics: Principles and practice.* Philadelphia: Lippincott Williams & Wilkins.

Frost, P. (2005). Pediatric resuscitation: Recognizing and managing children at risk. *Nursing Spectrum/Nurseweek CE: Course—NW0560.*

Frost, P., & Wise, B. (2006). *Kids in crisis: Pediatric emergencies.* Retrieved 6/24/06 from http://www2.nursingspectrum.com/CE/Self-Study_modules/syllabus.html?CCID=1089.

Garzon, D. L. (2005). Contributing factors to preschool unintentional injury. *Journal of Pediatric Nursing, 20*(6), 441–447.

Glassbrenner, D. (2005). *Child restraint use in 2004, overall results.* Retrieved 10/29/06 from http://www-nrd.nhtsa.dot.gov/pdf/nrd-30/NCSA/RNotes/2005/809845.pdf.

Gresham, L. S., Zirkle, D. L., Tolchin, S., et al. (2001). Partnering for injury prevention: Evaluation of a curriculum-based intervention program among elementary school children. *Journal of Pediatric Nursing, 16*(2), 79–87.

Grossman, D. (2000). The history of injury control and the epidemiology of child and adolescent injuries. *The Future of Children: Unintentional Injuries in Childhood, 10,* (1).

Hazinski, M. F. (2005). Major changes in the 2005 AHA guidelines for CPR and ECC: reaching the tipping point for change. *Circulation, 112,* 206–211.

Himle, M. B., & Miltenberger, R. G. (2004). Preventing unintentional firearm injury in children: The need for behavioral skills training. *Education & Treatment of Children, 27* (2), 161–177.

Hingley, A. T. (2000). *Preventing childhood poisoning.* Retrieved 6/20/06 from http://www.kidsource.com/kidsource/content3/fda.poisoning.all.safety.html.

Hofer, C. K., Ganter, M., Tucci, M., et al. (2002). How reliable is length-based determination of body weight and tracheal tube size in the paediatric age group? The Broselow tape reconsidered. *British Journal of Anaesthesia, 88*(2), 283–285.

Holleran, R. S. (2002). The problem of pain in emergency care. *Nursing Clinics of North America, 37*(1), 67–78.

Hudgins, R. J., & Boydston, W. R. (2003). *Pediatric head injury for the primary care physician.* Retrieved 6/24/06 from http://www.choa.org/default.aspx?id=882.

Idris, A. H., Berg, R. A., Bierens, J., et al. (2003). Recommended guidelines for uniform reporting data from drowning. *Circulation, 108,* 2565–2600.

Johnston, C. C., Bournaki, M. C., Gagnon, A. J., et al. (2005). Self-reported pain intensity and associated distress in children aged 4–18 years on admission, discharge, and one-week follow up to emergency department. *Pediatric Emergency Care, 21*(5), 342–346.

Langlois, J. A., Rutland-Brown, W., & Thomas, K. E. (2005). The incidence of traumatic brain injury among children in the United States: Differences by race. *Journal of Head Trauma Rehabilitation, 20*(3), 229–238.

Lee, J., Ahmad, S., & Gale, C. (2005). Detection of coins ingested by children using a handheld metal detector: A systematic review. *Emergency Medicine Journal, 22*(12), 839–844.

Litovitz, T., Klein-Schwartz, W., White, S., et al. (2001). 2000 Annual Report of the American Association of Poison Control Centers Toxic Exposure Surveillance System. *American Journal of Emergency Medicine, 19*(5), 337–396.

Mace, S. E. (2005). The fifth vital sign: Pulse oximetry in noninvasive respiratory monitoring. *Pediatric Emergency Medicine Reports, 10*(3), 25–35.

MacLachlan, S. (2003). *Blunt pediatric trauma, emergency medical rounds.* Retrieved 10/1/06 from http://www.cgi.ualberta.ca/emergency/rounds/files/PedsTraumaMachlachlan2003.ppt#256,1, Blunt Pediatric Trauma.

Madden, M. A. (2005). Pediatric poisonings: Recognition, assessment, and management. *Critical Care Nursing Clinics of North America, 17*(4), 395–404.

Mannenbach, M., & Bechtel, K. (2005). Patterns of injury that should raise suspicion for child abuse. *Pediatric Emergency Medicine Reports.* Retrieved 4/10/06 from Health and Wellness Resource Center.

Marino, B. S., & Fine, K. S. (2007). *Blueprints pediatrics* (4th ed.). Philadelphia: Lippincott Williams & Wilkins.

Mariscalco, M. M. (2006). Shock. In J. A. McMillan (Ed.), *Oski's pediatrics: Principles and practice.* Philadelphia: Lippincott Williams & Wilkins.

Matteucci, M. J. (2005). One pill can kill: Assessing the potential for fatal poisonings in children. *Pediatric Annals, 34*(12), 965–968.

McKiernan, C. A., & Lieberman, S. A. (2005). Circulatory shock in children: An overview. *Pediatrics in Review, 26*(12), 451–460.
Meadows-Oliver, M. (2004). Syrup of ipecac: New guidelines from the AAP. *Journal of Pediatric Health Care, 18,* 109–110.
Minto, G., & Woodward, W. (2005). Drowning and immersion injury. *Anaesthesia and Intensive Care Medicine, 6*(9), 321–323.
Monachino, A. M. (2005). Pediatric code readiness: Practice is the key. *Journal for Nurses in Staff Development, 21*(3), 126–131.
Morantz, C., & Torrey, B. (2003). Update on automated defibrillator use in children. *American Family Physician, 68*(8), 1667.
Moses, S. (2005). *Fluid resuscitation in trauma.* Retrieved 1/9/06 from http://www.fpnotebook.com/ER46.htm.
Nadkarni, V., Larkin, G., Peberdy, M., et al. (2006). First documented rhythm and clinical outcome from in-hospital cardiac arrest among children and adults. *Journal of the American Medical Association, 29*(1), 50–57.
National Highway Traffic Safety Administration. (2006). *2004 motor vehicle occupant protection facts.* Retrieved 10/29/06 from http://www.nhtsa.dot.gov/people/injury/airbags/MVOP2004/images/2004MVOPFactsLo.pdf.
National Safety Council. (2006). *Water safety.* Retrieved 11/3/06 from http://www.nsc.org/library/facts/drown.htm.
Nibert, L., & Ondrejka, D. (2005). Family presence during pediatric resuscitation: An integrative review for evidence-based practice. *Journal of Pediatric Nursing, 20*(2), 145–146.
Osterhoudt, K. C. (2000). The toxic toddler: Drugs that can kill in small doses. *Contemporary Pediatrics, 3,* 73 [electronic version]. Retrieved 6/20/06 from http://www.contemporarypediatrics.com/contpeds/article/articleDetail.jsp?id=139730.
Osterhoudt, K. C., Durbin, D., Alpern, E. R., & Henretig, F. M. (2004). Risk factors for emesis after therapeutic use of activated charcoal in acutely poisoned children. *Pediatrics, 113*(4), 806–810.
Perondi, M. B. M., Reis, A. G., Paiva, E. F., et al. (2004). A comparison of high-dose and standard-dose epinephrine in children with cardiac arrest. *New England Journal of Medicine, 350,* 1722–1730.
Prentiss, K. A., Mick, N. W., Cummings, B. M., et al. (2007). *Emergency management of the pediatric client.* Philadelphia: Lippincott Williams & Wilkins.
Probst, B. D., Lyons, E., Leonard, D., et al. (2005). Factors affecting emergency department assessment and management of pain in children. *Pediatric Emergency Care, 21*(5), 298–305.
Rezendes, J. L. (2006). Bicycle helmets: Overcoming barriers to use and increasing effectiveness. *Journal of Pediatric Nursing, 21*(1), 35–44.
RNCeus. (2006). *Abnormal breath sounds.* Retrieved 10/25/06 from www.rnceus.com/resp/respabn.html.
Robertson, J., & Shilkofski, N. (2005). *The Harriet Lane handbook* (17th ed.). Philadelphia: Mosby.
Rosman, N. P. (2006). Acute head trauma. In J. A. McMillan (Ed.), *Oski's pediatrics: Principles and practice.* Philadelphia: Lippincott Williams & Wilkins.
Ross, J. (2006). *Summer injuries: Near drowning.* Retrieved 4/25/06 from http://rnweb.com/rnweb/article/articleDetail.jsp?id=168160.
Safe Kids. (2006b). *Facts about childhood falls.* Retrieved 10/29/06 from http://www.usa.safekids.org/content_documents/Falls_facts.pdf.
Safe Kids. (2006c). *Facts about drowning.* Retrieved 5/19/06 from http://www.usa.safekids.org/content_documents/Drowning_facts.pdf.
Safe Kids. (2006d). *Facts about injuries to child pedestrians.* Retrieved 10/29/06 from http://www.usa.safekids.org/content_documents/Ped_facts.pdf.
Safe Kids. (2006e). *Facts about injuries to children riding bicycles.* Retrieved 11/3/06 from www.usa.safekids.org/content_documents/Bike_facts.pdf.
Safe Kids. (2006f). *Falls safety.* Retrieved 11/5/06 from http://www.safekids.org/tips/tips_falls.html.
Safe Kids. (2006g). *Fire and burns safety.* Retrieved 11/5/06 from http://www.safekids.org/tips/tips_fire.htm.
Safe Kids. (2006h). *Motor vehicle safety.* Retrieved 11/5/06 from http://www.safekids.org/tips/tips_car.htm.
Safe Kids. (2006i). *Pedestrian safety.* Retrieved 11/5/06 from http://www.safekids.org/tips/tips_ped.htm.
Safe Kids (2006j). *Poisoning safety.* Retrieved 6/20/06 from http://www.safekids.org/tips/tips_poison.html.
Safe Kids (2006k). *Water and drowning safety.* Retrieved 11/5/06 from www.safekids.org/tips/tips_water.html.
Saluja, G., Brenner, R. A., Trumble, A. C., et al. (2006). Swimming pool drownings among U.S. residents aged 5–24 years: Understanding racial/ethnic disparities. *American Journal of Public Health, 96*(4), 728–733.
Samson, R. A., Berg, R. A., Bingham, R., et al. (2003). Use of automated external defibrillators in children: An update: An advisory statement from the pediatric advanced life support task force, international liaison committee on resuscitation. *Circulation, 107,* 3250–3255.
Schweich, P. J. (2006). Selected topics in emergency medicine. In J. A. McMillan (Ed.), *Oski's pediatrics: Principles and practice.* Philadelphia: Lippincott Williams & Wilkins.
Stephenson, M. (2005). Danger in the toy box. *Journal of Pediatric Health Care, 19,* 187–189.
Strange, G., Ahrens, W., McQuillen, K., et al. (2004). *Pediatric emergency medicine: Just the facts.* New York: McGraw-Hill.
Taketokmo, C. K., Hodding, J. H., & Kraus, D. M. (2005). *Lexi-comp's pediatric dosage handbook* (12th ed.). Hudson, OH: Lexi-comp.
Tinsworth, D., & McDonald, J. (2001). *Special study: Injuries and deaths associated with children's playground equipment.* Washington D.C.: U.S. Consumer Product Safety Commission.
Tomashek, K. M., Hsia, J., & Iyasu, S. (2003). Trends in postneonatal mortality attributable to injury, United States, 1988–1998. *Pediatrics, 111,* 1219–1225.
U.S. Department of Transportation, National Highway Traffic Safety Administration, National Center for Statistics and Analysis. (2005). *Technical report DOT HS 809 843: Motor vehicle traffic crashes as a leading cause of death in the U.S., 2002—a demographic perspective.* Springfield, VA: National Technical Information Service. Retrieved 6/24/06 from http://www-nrd.nhtsa.dot.gov/pdf/nrd-30/NCSA/Rpts/2005/809843.pdf.
Verive, M., Heidemann, S., & Fiore, M. (2004). *Near drowning.* Retrieved 10/29/06 from http://www.emedicine.com/ped/topic2570.htm.
Wang, M., Griffith, P. Sterling, J., et al. (2000). A prospective population-based study of pediatric trauma clients with mild alterations in consciousness (Glasgow Coma Scale score of 13–14). *Neurosurgery, 5*(46), 1093–1099.
White, M. G. (2003). *Capnometer & capnometry.* Retrieved 11/3/06 from http://breathing.com/articles/capnometry.htm.
Wilson, M. H., & Levin-Goodman, R. (2006). Injury control and prevention. In J. A. McMillan (Ed.), *Oski's pediatrics: Principles and practice.* Philadelphia: Lippincott Williams & Wilkins.
World Health Organization. (2006). *Facts about injuries: Drowning.* Retrieved 10/29/06 from http://www.who.int/violence_injury_prevention/publications/other_injury/en/drowning_factsheet.pdf.

Websites

www.aap.org/healthtopics/safety.cfm American Academy of Pediatrics safety information
www.aapcc.org American Association of Poison Control Centers
www.cdc.gov/ncipc/factsheets/childpas.htm Centers for Disease Control and Prevention: National Center for Injury Prevention and Control, Child Passenger Safety Fact Sheet
www.cdc.gov/ncipc/factsheets/teenmvh.htm Centers for Disease Control and Prevention: National Center for Injury Prevention and Control, Teen Drivers Fact Sheet
www.cpsc.gov/cpscpub/pubs/pois_prv.html U.S. Consumers Product Safety Commission, Poison Prevention Publications
www.ipl.org/div/kidspace/poisonsafe/kjump.html Kidspace @ the Internet Public Library
www.jnj.com/news/jnj_news/20020308_0811.htm Johnson & Johnson News
www.kidshealth.org Nemours Foundation
www.nrd.nhtsa.dot.gov/departments/nrd-30/ncsa National Highway Traffic Safety Administration, National Center for Statistics and Analysis
www.poisonprevention.org/materials.htm Poison Prevention Week Council
www.rnceus.com/index.html#_parent#_parent Nursing CEUs and information
www.safekids.org Safe Kids Worldwide

Chapter WORKSHEET

● MULTIPLE CHOICE QUESTIONS

1. An unresponsive toddler is brought to the emergency department. Assessment reveals mottled skin color, respiratory rate of 10 breaths per minute, and a brachial pulse of 52 beats per minute. What is the priority nursing action?

a. Prepare the defibrillator and draw up code medications.

b. Provide 100% oxygen with a bag-valve-mask and start chest compressions.

c. Start chest compressions and provide 100% oxygen via non-rebreather mask.

d. Begin an IV fluid infusion and administer epinephrine IV.

2. A 10-year-old child in respiratory distress requires intubation. Which sizes of tracheal tubes will the nurse prepare?

a. 9.5 mm and 10.0 mm

b. 8.5 mm and 9.0 mm

c. 6.0 mm and 6.5 mm

d. 6.5 mm and 7.0 mm

3. A preschooler presents to the emergency department with a history of vomiting, diarrhea, and fever over the past few days. She is receiving 100% oxygen via non-rebreather mask. Vital signs are temperature 104.5° F, pulse 144 bpm, respiratory rate 22 breaths per minute, and BP 70/50 mm Hg. She is listless and difficult to arouse and has weak peripheral pulses and prolonged capillary refill. What nursing intervention takes priority?

a. Administering acetaminophen rectally for the high fever

b. Administering IV antibiotics for the infection

c. Preparing the child for tracheal intubation

d. Giving an IV bolus of normal saline 20 mL/kg

4. Assessment of a 12-year-old who crashed his bicycle without a helmet reveals the following: temperature 99.2° F, pulse 100 bpm, respiratory rate 24 breaths per minute with easy work of breathing, and BP 102/70 mm Hg. What is the priority action by the nurse?

a. Assess neurologic status while observing for obvious injuries.

b. Administer IV fluid bolus of normal saline at 20 mL/kg.

c. Remove the cervical collar if he complains that it bothers him.

d. Listen for bowel sounds while assessing for pain.

5. An 18-month old child is brought to the emergency department via ambulance after an accidental ingestion. What is the priority nursing action?

a. Take the child's vital signs.

b. Give oral syrup of ipecac.

c. Insert a nasogastric tube.

d. Start an IV line.

● CRITICAL THINKING EXERCISES

1. A school-age child presents to the emergency department for evaluation. He had been feeling faint off and on and today fainted at school. On the cardiac monitor an abnormal cardiac rhythm is noted. At present the child is stable. What questions would be most appropriate for the nurse to ask when obtaining the child's health history? What objective assessments should the nurse make?

2. Charlie is a 2-year-old who is admitted to the hospital after accidentally ingesting a medication. His mother, who brought Charlie to the hospital, is upset and crying. How does Charlie's age and stage of development affect his risk for accidental ingestion? How should the nurse respond to the mother's distress? Develop a discharge teaching plan for Charlie and his family related to poison prevention.

3. A 7-month-old is brought to the acute care facility with a chief complaint of difficulty breathing. The infant's mother says that his cold has gotten worse and he won't eat. What additional questions should the nurse ask about the infant's health history? How would the nurse appropriately manage this infant's airway?

● STUDY ACTIVITIES

1. Spend a day in the pediatric emergency department or urgent care center and document the role of the triage nurse.
2. Observe the pediatric emergency medical team at work or observe a pediatric code in the hospital. Compare and contrast the measures performed for the child with those that would be performed for an adult in a similar emergency situation.
3. Develop a teaching project related to injury prevention and present it at a local elementary, middle, or high school. Ensure that the education is geared toward the children's developmental level.
4. Interview the parents of a child who has experienced an emergency situation about how they felt during and after the emergency. Present the information to your classmates.
5. When providing care to a child in an emergency, the nurse performs the following assessments. Place them in the proper sequence.

   a. Pupillary reaction
   b. Presence of cough or sputum
   c. Heart rate and capillary refill
   d. Presence of bruises and abrasions
   e. Work of breathing

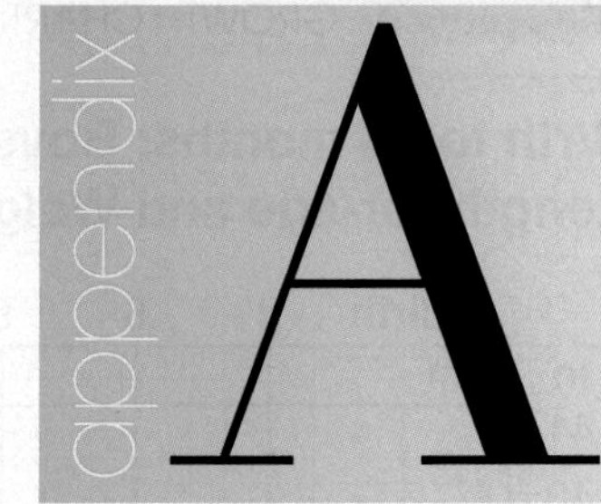

Growth Charts

Birth to 36 months: Boys
Length-for-age and Weight-for-age percentiles

NAME ______________________

RECORD # __________

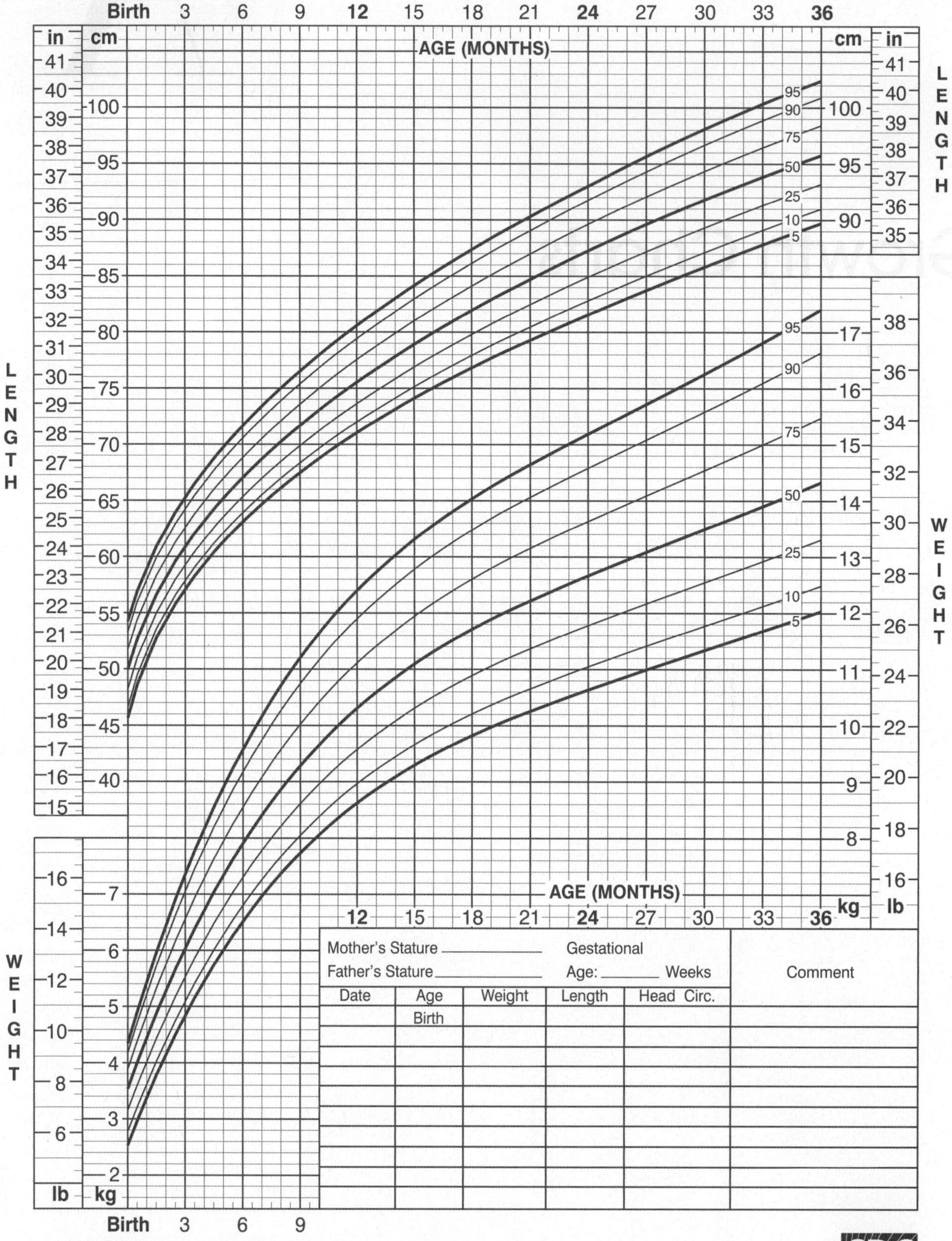

Mother's Stature ______			Gestational		Comment
Father's Stature ______			Age: ______ Weeks		
Date	Age	Weight	Length	Head Circ.	
	Birth				

Published May 30, 2000 (modified 4/20/01).
SOURCE: Developed by the National Center for Health Statistics in collaboration with the National Center for Chronic Disease Prevention and Health Promotion (2000).
http://www.cdc.gov/growthcharts

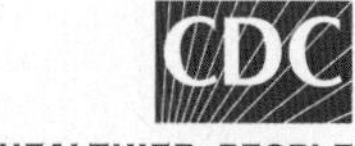

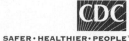

SAFER • HEALTHIER • PEOPLE™

Birth to 36 months: Girls
Length-for-age and Weight-for-age percentiles

NAME ______

RECORD # ______

Mother's Stature ______ Gestational

Father's Stature ______ Age: ______ Weeks

Date	Age	Weight	Length	Head Circ.	Comment
	Birth				

Published May 30, 2000 (modified 4/20/01).
SOURCE: Developed by the National Center for Health Statistics in collaboration with the National Center for Chronic Disease Prevention and Health Promotion (2000).
http://www.cdc.gov/growthcharts

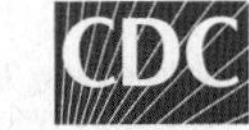

SAFER • HEALTHIER • PEOPLE™

Birth to 36 months: Boys
Head circumference-for-age and Weight-for-length percentiles

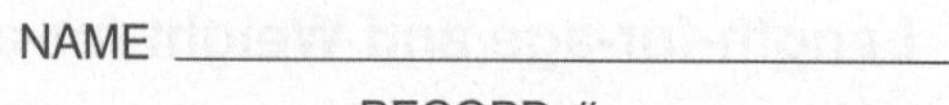

Birth 3 6 9 12 15 18 21 24 27 30 33 36

AGE (MONTHS)

in cm — HEAD CIRCUMFERENCE — cm in

cm: 30 32 34 36 38 40 42 44 46 48 50 52

in: 12 13 14 15 16 17 18 19 20

Head circumference percentiles: 95 90 75 50 25 10 5

Weight percentiles: 95 90 75 50 25 10 5

kg: 1 2 3 4 5 6 7 8 9 10 11 12 13 14 15 16 17 18 19 20 21 22

lb: 2 4 6 8 10 12 14 16 18 20 22 24 26 28 30 32 34 36 38 40 42 44 46 48 50

WEIGHT

LENGTH

cm: 46 48 50 52 54 56 58 60 62 64 66 68 70 72 74 76 78 80 82 84 86 88 90 92 94 96 98 100

in: 18 19 20 21 22 23 24 26 27 28 29 30 31 32 33 34 35 36 37 38 39 40 41

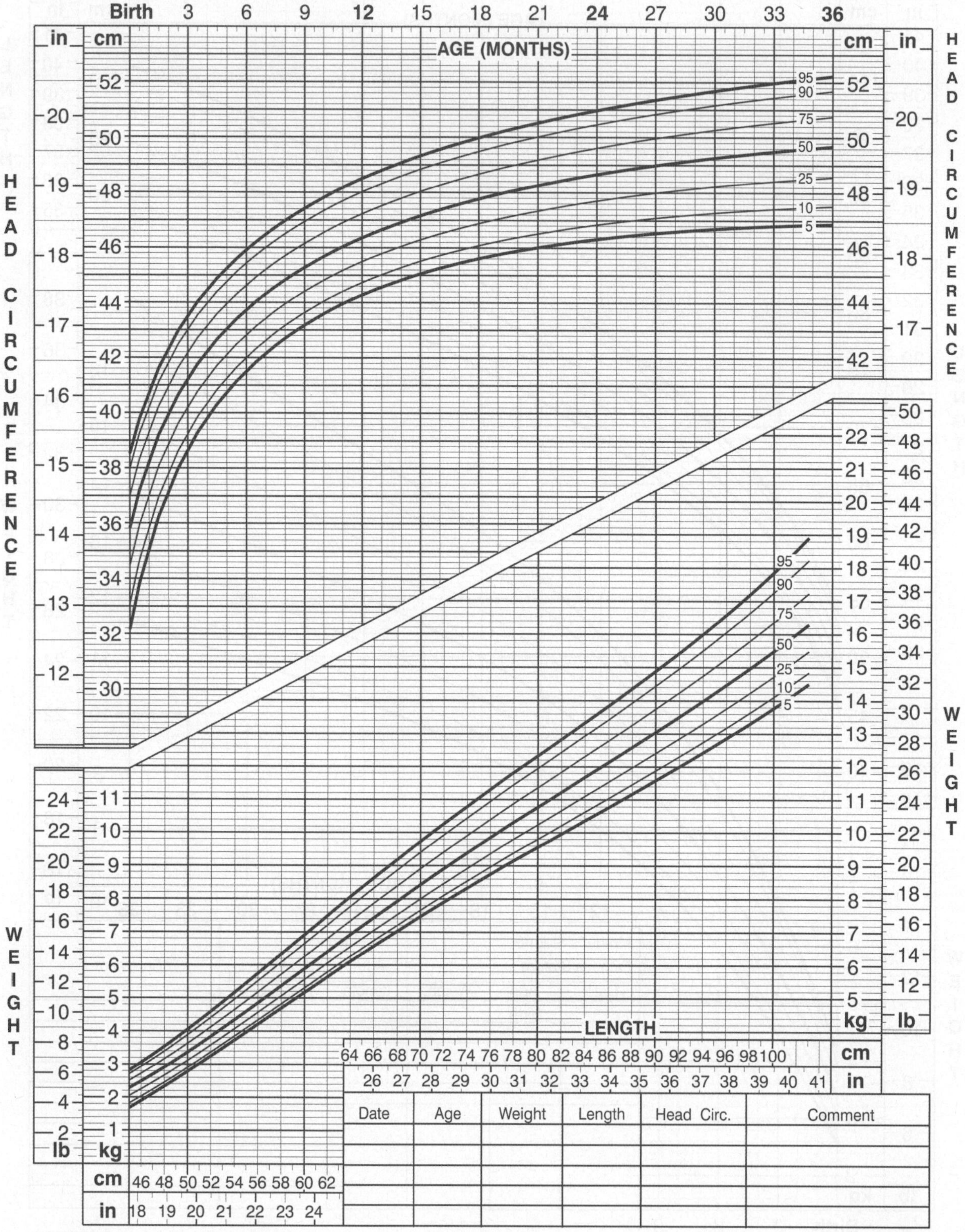

Date	Age	Weight	Length	Head Circ.	Comment

Published May 30, 2000 (modified 10/16/00).
SOURCE: Developed by the National Center for Health Statistics in collaboration with the National Center for Chronic Disease Prevention and Health Promotion (2000).
http://www.cdc.gov/growthcharts

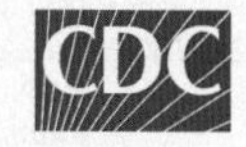

SAFER • HEALTHIER • PEOPLE™

Birth to 36 months: Girls
Head circumference-for-age and Weight-for-length percentiles

NAME ______________

RECORD # ______________

Date	Age	Weight	Length	Head Circ.	Comment

Published May 30, 2000 (modified 10/16/00).
SOURCE: Developed by the National Center for Health Statistics in collaboration with the National Center for Chronic Disease Prevention and Health Promotion (2000).
http://www.cdc.gov/growthcharts

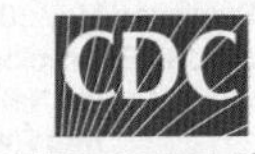

SAFER • HEALTHIER • PEOPLE™

2 to 20 years: Boys
Stature-for-age and Weight-for-age percentiles

NAME ________________

RECORD # ________

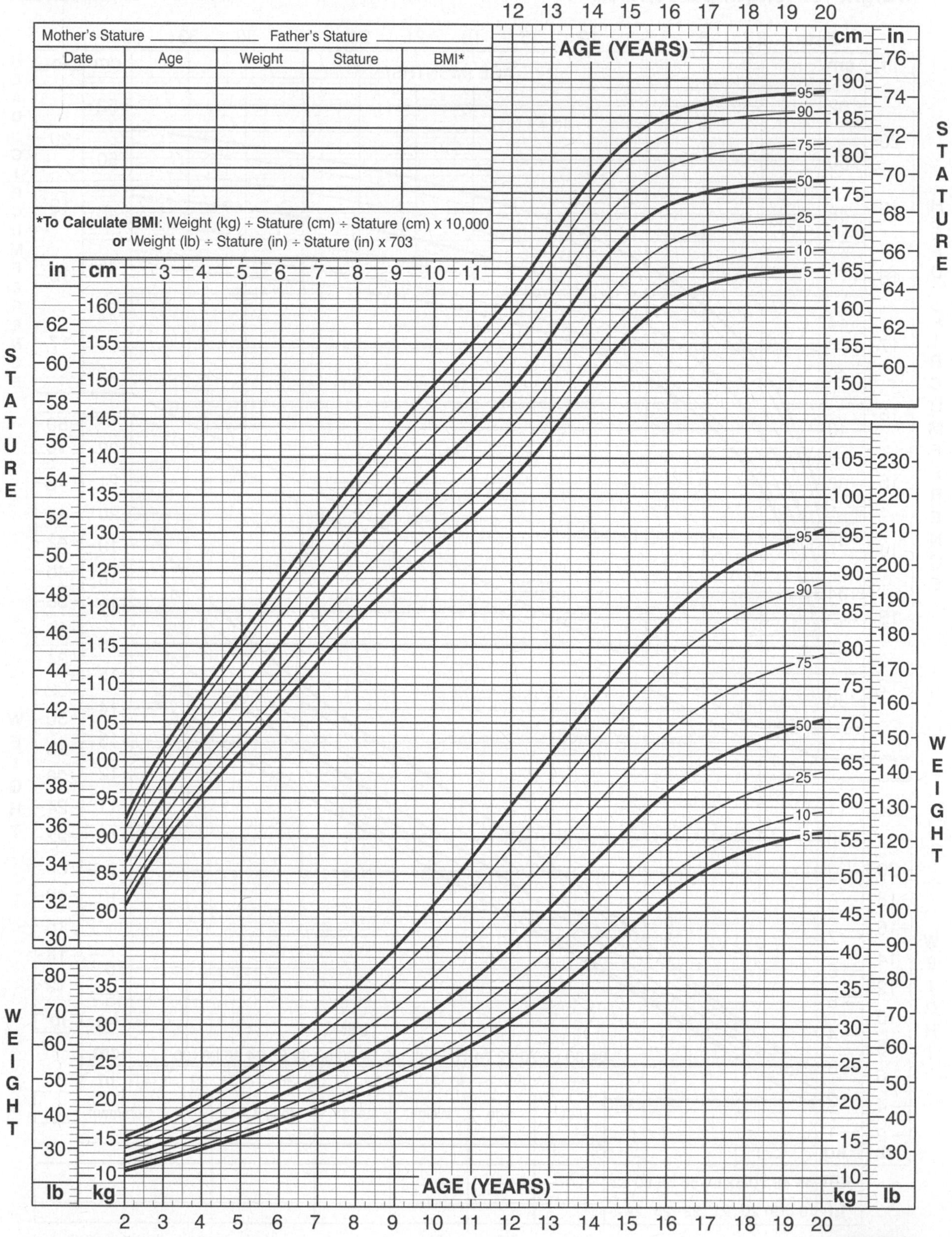

Mother's Stature ____________ Father's Stature ____________

Date	Age	Weight	Stature	BMI*

***To Calculate BMI**: Weight (kg) ÷ Stature (cm) ÷ Stature (cm) x 10,000
or Weight (lb) ÷ Stature (in) ÷ Stature (in) x 703

AGE (YEARS)

STATURE

WEIGHT

in cm

kg lb

AGE (YEARS)

2 3 4 5 6 7 8 9 10 11 12 13 14 15 16 17 18 19 20

Published May 30, 2000 (modified 11/21/00).
SOURCE: Developed by the National Center for Health Statistics in collaboration with the National Center for Chronic Disease Prevention and Health Promotion (2000).
http://www.cdc.gov/growthcharts

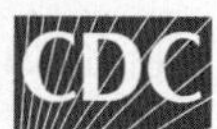

SAFER • HEALTHIER • PEOPLE™

2 to 20 years: Girls
Stature-for-age and Weight-for-age percentiles

NAME ____________________

RECORD # ____________________

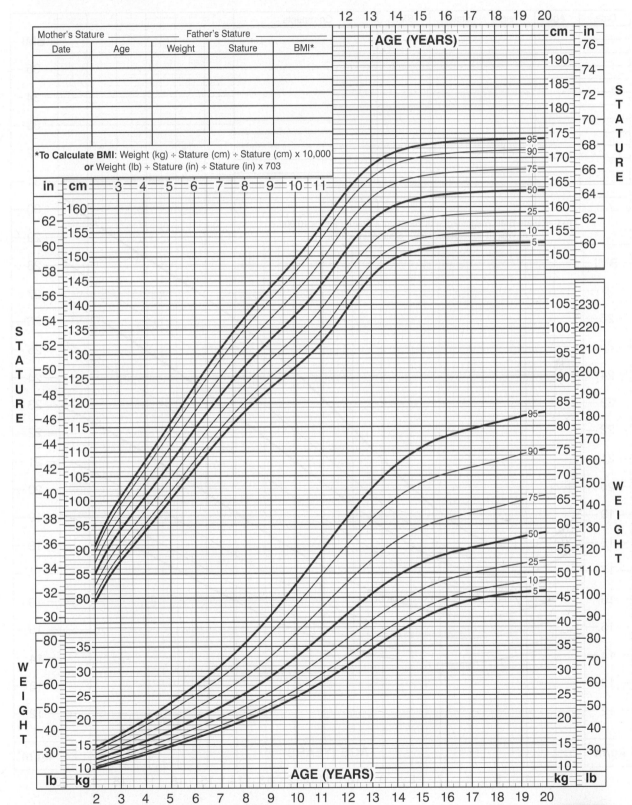

Mother's Stature ______________ Father's Stature ______________

Date	Age	Weight	Stature	BMI*

*To Calculate BMI: Weight (kg) ÷ Stature (cm) ÷ Stature (cm) x 10,000
or Weight (lb) ÷ Stature (in) ÷ Stature (in) x 703

AGE (YEARS)

STATURE

WEIGHT

in cm

kg lb

95 90 75 50 25 10 5

2 3 4 5 6 7 8 9 10 11 12 13 14 15 16 17 18 19 20

Published May 30, 2000 (modified 11/21/00).
SOURCE: Developed by the National Center for Health Statistics in collaboration with the National Center for Chronic Disease Prevention and Health Promotion (2000).
http://www.cdc.gov/growthcharts

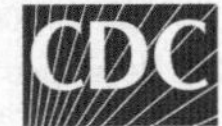

SAFER • HEALTHIER • PEOPLE™

2 to 20 years: Boys
Body mass index-for-age percentiles

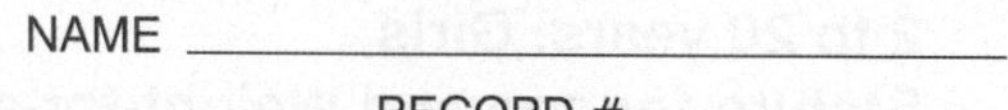

Date	Age	Weight	Stature	BMI*	Comments

***To Calculate BMI**: Weight (kg) ÷ Stature (cm) ÷ Stature (cm) x 10,000
or Weight (lb) ÷ Stature (in) ÷ Stature (in) x 703

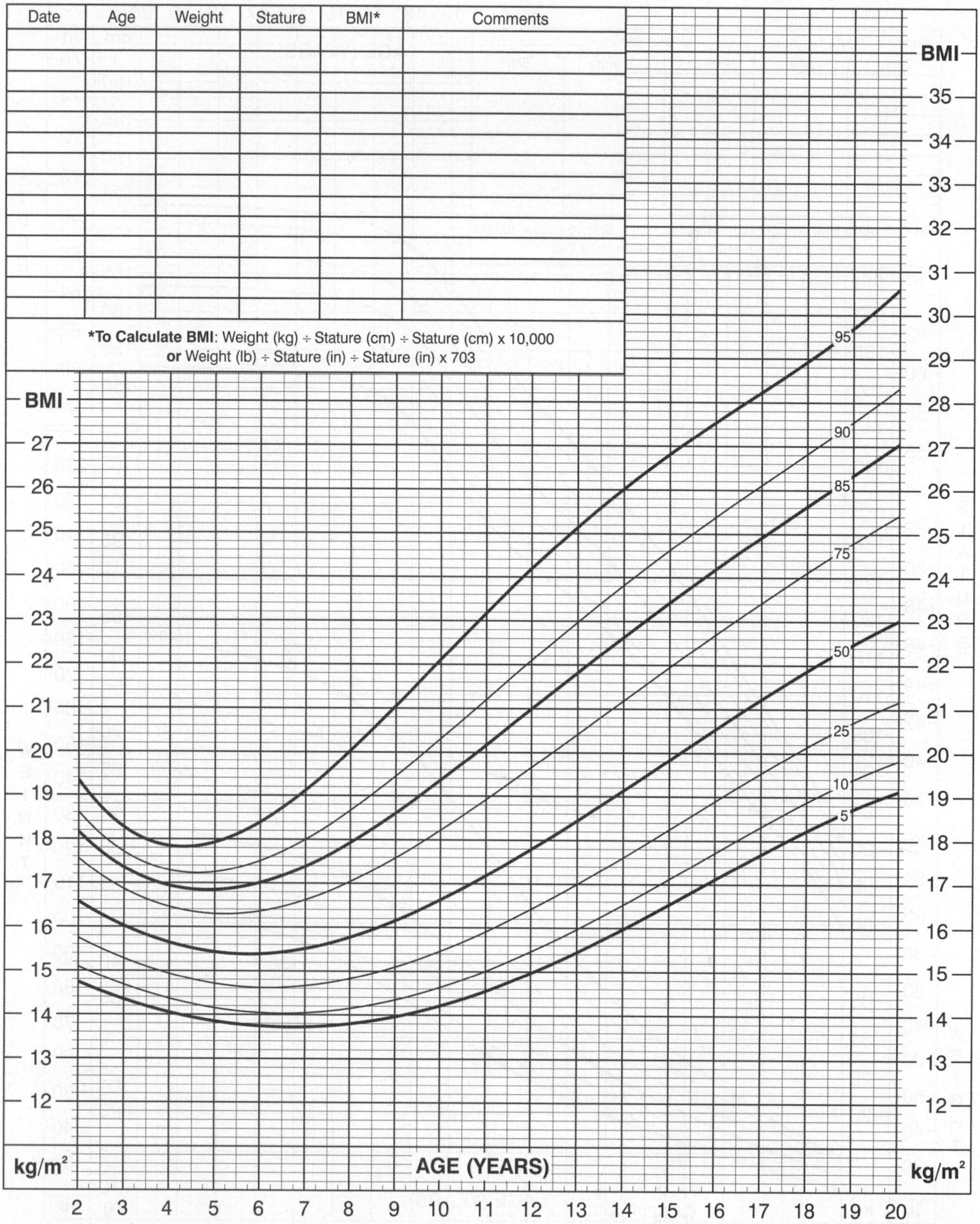

BMI — 12, 13, 14, 15, 16, 17, 18, 19, 20, 21, 22, 23, 24, 25, 26, 27, 28, 29, 30, 31, 32, 33, 34, 35

Percentile curves: 5, 10, 25, 50, 75, 85, 90, 95

kg/m² — AGE (YEARS) — kg/m²

2 3 4 5 6 7 8 9 10 11 12 13 14 15 16 17 18 19 20

Published May 30, 2000 (modified 10/16/00).
SOURCE: Developed by the National Center for Health Statistics in collaboration with the National Center for Chronic Disease Prevention and Health Promotion (2000).
http://www.cdc.gov/growthcharts

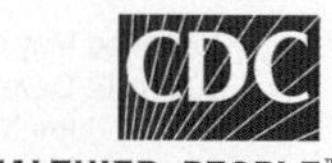

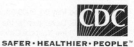

SAFER • HEALTHIER • PEOPLE™

2 to 20 years: Girls
Body mass index-for-age percentiles

NAME ______________________

RECORD # ______________

Date	Age	Weight	Stature	BMI*	Comments

***To Calculate BMI**: Weight (kg) ÷ Stature (cm) ÷ Stature (cm) x 10,000
or Weight (lb) ÷ Stature (in) ÷ Stature (in) x 703

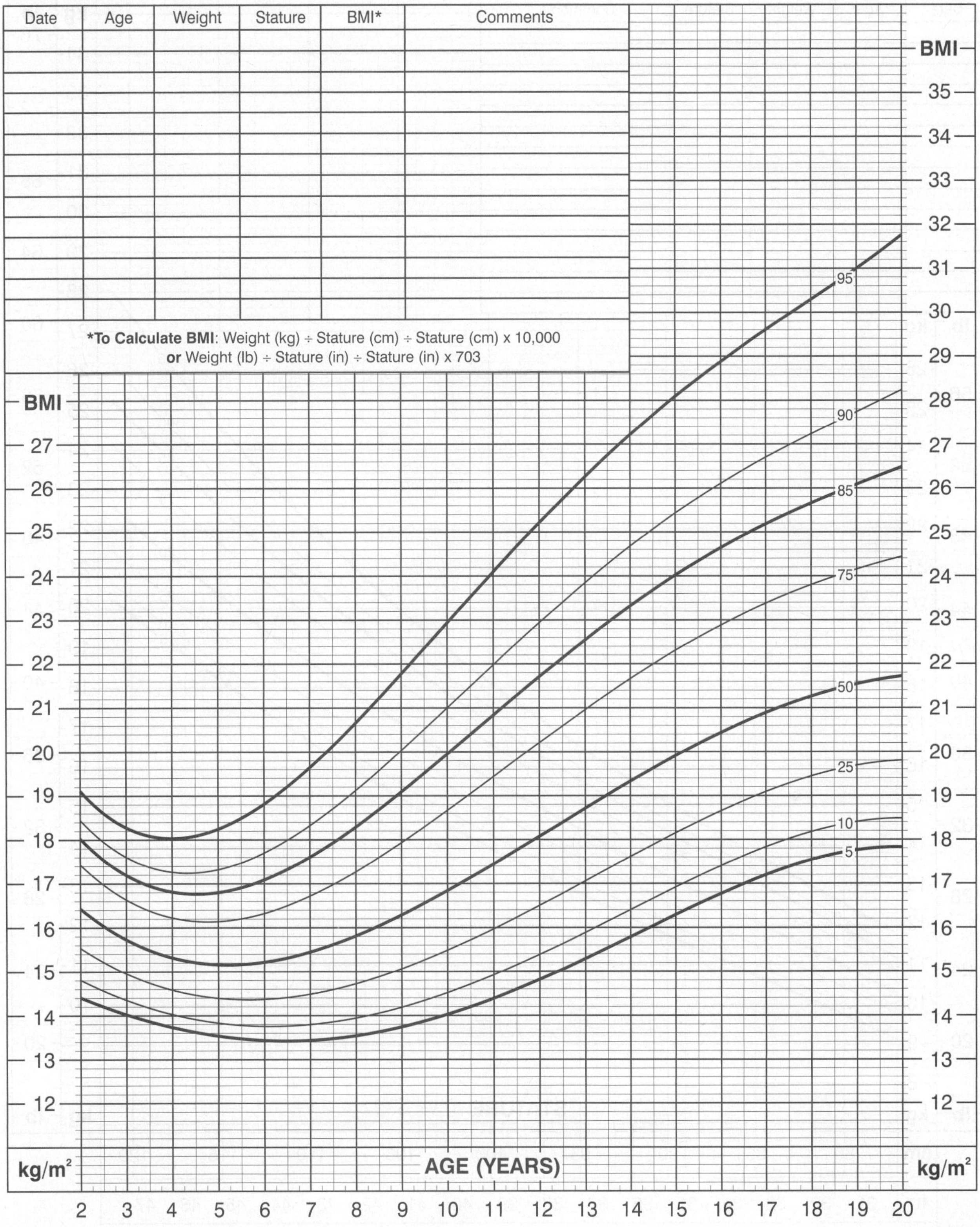

BMI
35
34
33
32
31
30
29
28
27
26
25
24
23
22
21
20
19
18
17
16
15
14
13
12

95
90
85
75
50
25
10
5

kg/m²

AGE (YEARS)

2 3 4 5 6 7 8 9 10 11 12 13 14 15 16 17 18 19 20

Published May 30, 2000 (modified 10/16/00).
SOURCE: Developed by the National Center for Health Statistics in collaboration with
the National Center for Chronic Disease Prevention and Health Promotion (2000).
http://www.cdc.gov/growthcharts

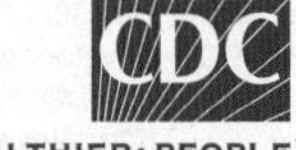

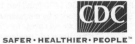

SAFER • HEALTHIER • PEOPLE™

NAME ______________________

RECORD # ______________

Weight-for-stature percentiles: Boys

Date	Age	Weight	Stature	Comments

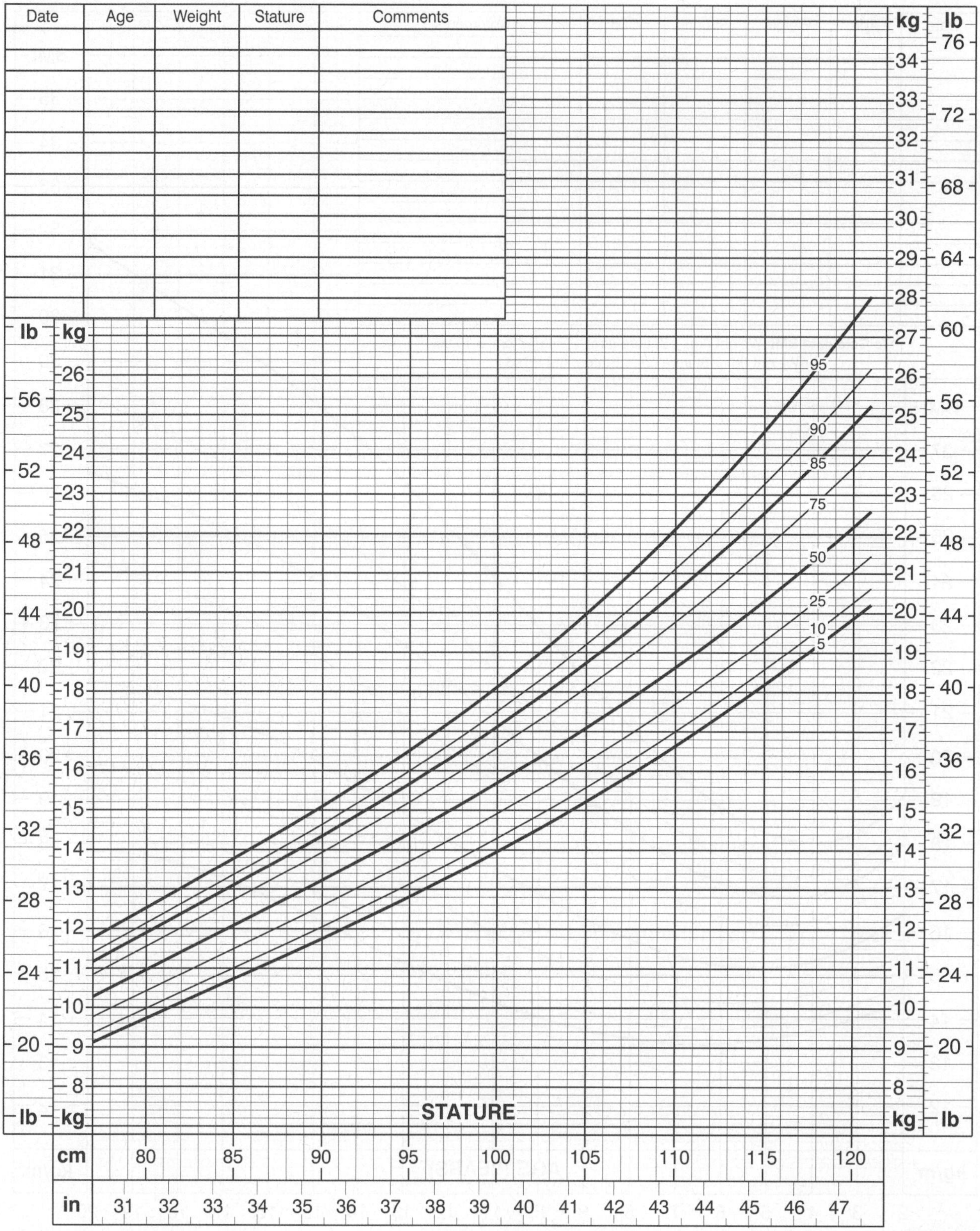

Published May 30, 2000 (modified 10/16/00).
SOURCE: Developed by the National Center for Health Statistics in collaboration with the National Center for Chronic Disease Prevention and Health Promotion (2000).
http://www.cdc.gov/growthcharts

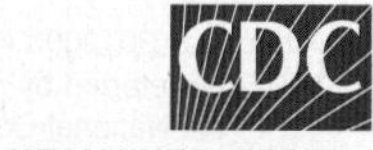

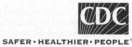

SAFER • HEALTHIER • PEOPLE™

NAME ______________________

Weight-for-stature percentiles: Girls

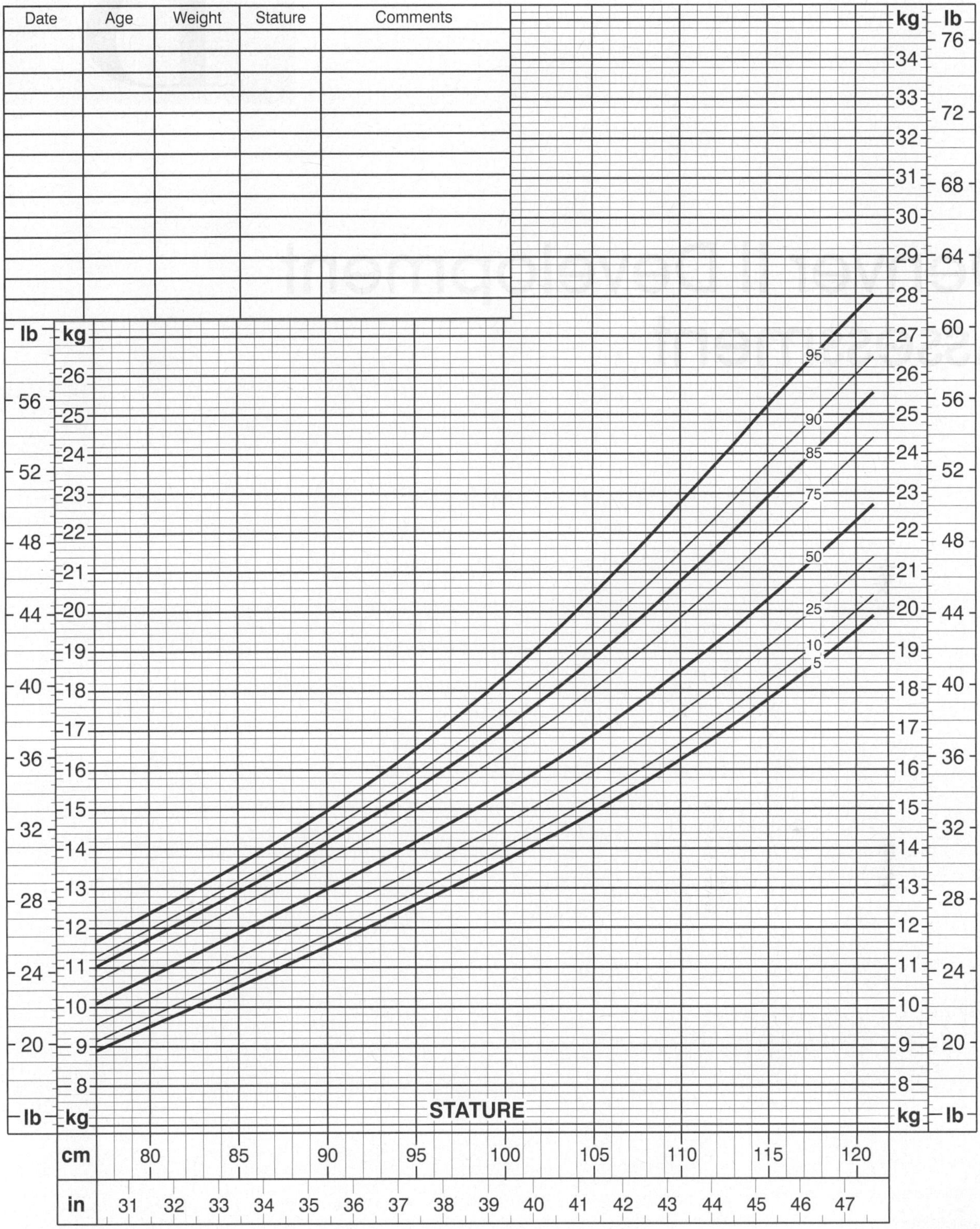

RECORD # ____________

Date	Age	Weight	Stature	Comments

Published May 30, 2000 (modified 10/16/00).
SOURCE: Developed by the National Center for Health Statistics in collaboration with the National Center for Chronic Disease Prevention and Health Promotion (2000).
http://www.cdc.gov/growthcharts

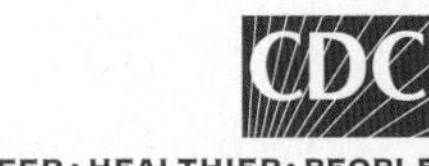

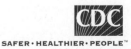

For additional information on growth charts for children with Down syndrome, please go to http://thepoint.lww.com.

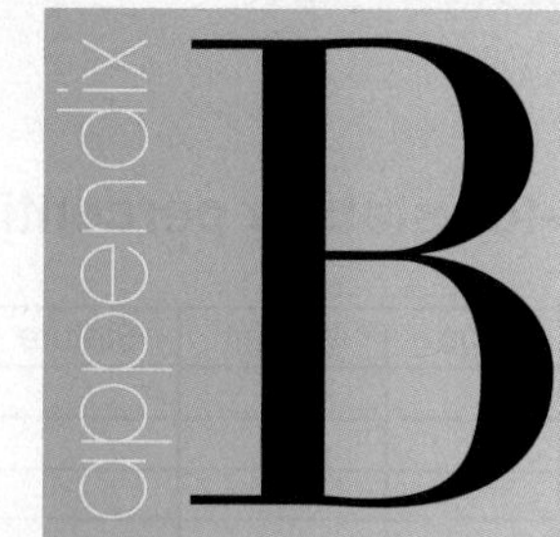

Denver II Development Assessment

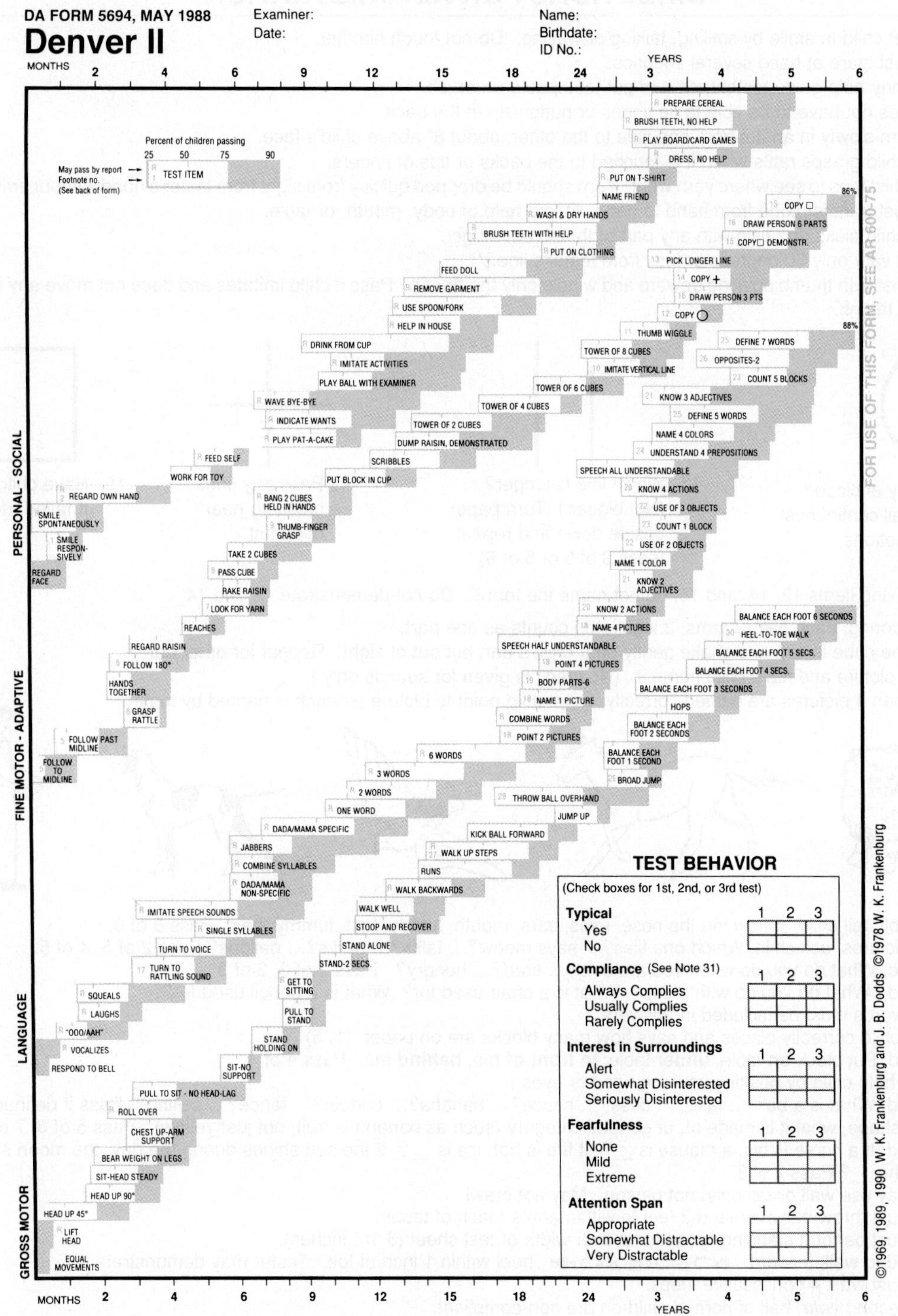

DA FORM 5694, MAY 1988

Denver II

Examiner:
Date:

Name:
Birthdate:
ID No.:

MONTHS 2 4 6 9 12 15 18 24 | YEARS 3 4 5 6

Percent of children passing: 25 50 75 90

May pass by report → R
Footnote no. → 1
(See back of form)
TEST ITEM

PERSONAL SOCIAL

PREPARE CEREAL
BRUSH TEETH, NO HELP
PLAY BOARD/CARD GAMES
DRESS, NO HELP
PUT ON T-SHIRT
NAME FRIEND
WASH & DRY HANDS
BRUSH TEETH WITH HELP
PUT ON CLOTHING
FEED DOLL
REMOVE GARMENT
USE SPOON/FORK
HELP IN HOUSE
DRINK FROM CUP
IMITATE ACTIVITIES
PLAY BALL WITH EXAMINER
WAVE BYE-BYE
INDICATE WANTS
PLAY PAT-A-CAKE
FEED SELF
WORK FOR TOY
REGARD OWN HAND
SMILE SPONTANEOUSLY
SMILE RESPONSIVELY
REGARD FACE

FINE MOTOR - ADAPTIVE

COPY □ (86%)
DRAW PERSON 6 PARTS
COPY □ DEMONSTR.
PICK LONGER LINE
COPY +
DRAW PERSON 3 PTS
COPY ○
THUMB WIGGLE
TOWER OF 8 CUBES
IMITATE VERTICAL LINE
TOWER OF 6 CUBES
TOWER OF 4 CUBES
TOWER OF 2 CUBES
DUMP RAISIN, DEMONSTRATED
SCRIBBLES
PUT BLOCK IN CUP
BANG 2 CUBES HELD IN HANDS
THUMB-FINGER GRASP
TAKE 2 CUBES
PASS CUBE
RAKE RAISIN
LOOK FOR YARN
REACHES
REGARD RAISIN
FOLLOW 180°
HANDS TOGETHER
GRASP RATTLE
FOLLOW PAST MIDLINE
FOLLOW TO MIDLINE

LANGUAGE

DEFINE 7 WORDS (88%)
OPPOSITES-2
COUNT 5 BLOCKS
KNOW 3 ADJECTIVES
DEFINE 5 WORDS
NAME 4 COLORS
UNDERSTAND 4 PREPOSITIONS
SPEECH ALL UNDERSTANDABLE
KNOW 4 ACTIONS
USE OF 3 OBJECTS
COUNT 1 BLOCK
USE OF 2 OBJECTS
NAME 1 COLOR
KNOW 2 ADJECTIVES
KNOW 2 ACTIONS
NAME 4 PICTURES
SPEECH HALF UNDERSTANDABLE
POINT 4 PICTURES
BODY PARTS-6
NAME 1 PICTURE
COMBINE WORDS
POINT 2 PICTURES
6 WORDS
3 WORDS
2 WORDS
ONE WORD
DADA/MAMA SPECIFIC
JABBERS
COMBINE SYLLABLES
DADA/MAMA NON-SPECIFIC
IMITATE SPEECH SOUNDS
SINGLE SYLLABLES
TURN TO VOICE
TURN TO RATTLING SOUND
SQUEALS
LAUGHS
"OOO/AAH"
VOCALIZES
RESPOND TO BELL

GROSS MOTOR

BALANCE EACH FOOT 6 SECONDS
HEEL-TO-TOE WALK
BALANCE EACH FOOT 5 SECS.
BALANCE EACH FOOT 4 SECS.
BALANCE EACH FOOT 3 SECONDS
HOPS
BALANCE EACH FOOT 2 SECONDS
BALANCE EACH FOOT 1 SECOND
BROAD JUMP
THROW BALL OVERHAND
JUMP UP
KICK BALL FORWARD
WALK UP STEPS
RUNS
WALK BACKWARDS
WALK WELL
STOOP AND RECOVER
STAND ALONE
STAND-2 SECS.
GET TO SITTING
PULL TO STAND
STAND HOLDING ON
SIT-NO SUPPORT
PULL TO SIT - NO HEAD-LAG
ROLL OVER
CHEST UP-ARM SUPPORT
BEAR WEIGHT ON LEGS
SIT-HEAD STEADY
HEAD UP 90°
HEAD UP 45°
LIFT HEAD
EQUAL MOVEMENTS

TEST BEHAVIOR

(Check boxes for 1st, 2nd, or 3rd test)

Typical	1	2	3
Yes			
No			

Compliance (See Note 31)	1	2	3
Always Complies			
Usually Complies			
Rarely Complies			

Interest in Surroundings	1	2	3
Alert			
Somewhat Disinterested			
Seriously Disinterested			

Fearfulness	1	2	3
None			
Mild			
Extreme			

Attention Span	1	2	3
Appropriate			
Somewhat Distractable			
Very Distractable			

FOR USE OF THIS FORM, SEE AR 600-75

MONTHS 2 4 6 9 12 15 18 24 | 3 4 5 6 YEARS

DIRECTIONS FOR ADMINISTRATION

1. Try to get child to smile by smiling, talking or waving. Do not touch him/her.
2. Child must stare at hand several seconds.
3. Parent may help guide toothbrush and put toothpaste on brush.
4. Child does not have to be able to tie shoes or button/zip in the back.
5. Move yarn slowly in an arc from one side to the other, about 8" above child's face.
6. Pass if child grasps rattle when it is touched to the backs or tips of fingers.
7. Pass if child tries to see where yarn went. Yarn should be dropped quickly from sight from tester's hand without arm movement.
8. Child must transfer cube from hand to hand without help of body, mouth, or table.
9. Pass if child picks up raisin with any part of thumb and finger.
10. Line can vary only 30 degrees or less from tester's line.
11. Make a fist with thumb pointing upward and wiggle only the thumb. Pass if child imitates and does not move any fingers other than the thumb.

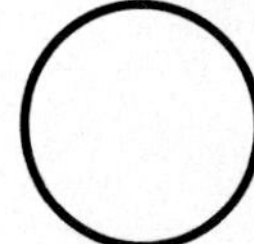

12. Pass any enclosed form. Fail continuous round motions.

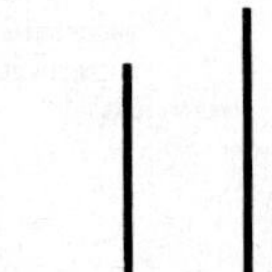

13. Which line is longer? (Not bigger.) Turn paper upside down and repeat. (pass 3 of 3 or 5 of 6)

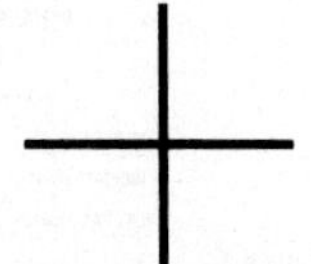

14. Pass any lines crossing near midpoint.

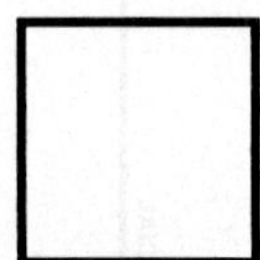

15. Have child copy first. If failed, demonstrate.

When giving items 12, 14, and 15, do not name the forms. Do not demonstrate 12 and 14.

16. When scoring, each pair (2 arms, 2 legs, etc.) counts as one part.
17. Place one cube in cup and shake gently near child's ear, but out of sight. Repeat for other ear.
18. Point to picture and have child name it. (No credit is given for sounds only.) If less than 4 pictures are named correctly, have child point to picture as each is named by tester.

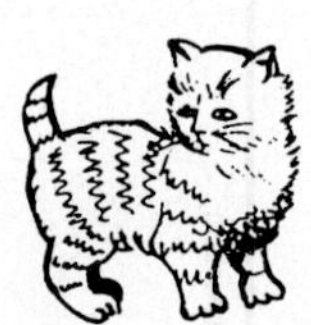
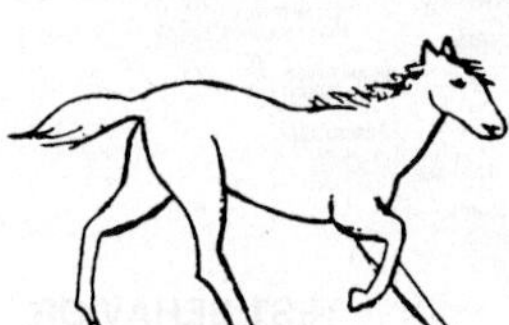
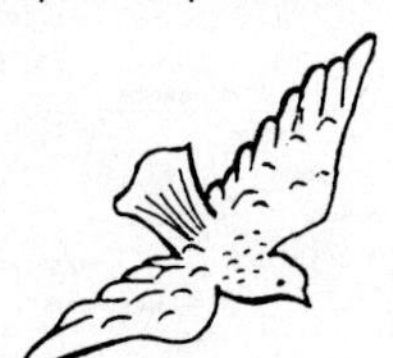
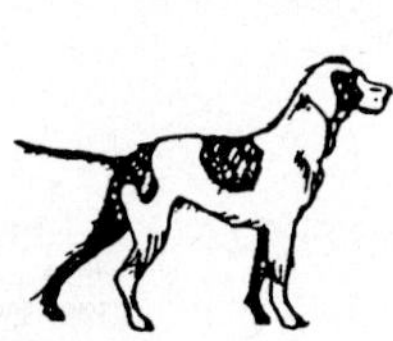
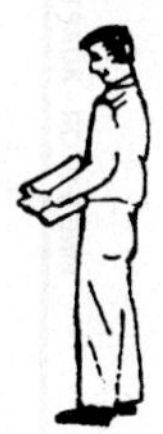

19. Using doll, tell child: Show me the nose, eyes, ears, mouth, hands, feet, tummy, hair. Pass 6 of 8.
20. Using pictures, ask child: Which one flies?... says meow?... talks?... barks?... gallops? Pass 2 of 5, 4 of 5.
21. Ask child: What do you do when you are cold?... tired?... hungry? Pass 2 of 3, 3 of 3.
22. Ask child: What do you do with a cup? What is a chair used for? What is a pencil used for? Action words must be included in answers.
23. Pass if child correctly places and says how many blocks are on paper. (1, 5).
24. Tell child: Put block **on** table; **under** table; **in front of** me, **behind** me. Pass 4 of 4. (Do not help child by pointing, moving head or eyes.)
25. Ask child: What is a ball?... lake?... desk?... house?... banana?... curtain?... fence?... ceiling? Pass if defined in terms of use, shape, what it is made of, or general category (such as banana is fruit, not just yellow). Pass 5 of 8, 7 of 8.
26. Ask child: If a horse is big, a mouse is __? If fire is hot, ice is __? If the sun shines during the day, the moon shines during the __? Pass 2 of 3.
27. Child may use wall or rail only, not person. May not crawl.
28. Child must throw ball overhand 3 feet to within arm's reach of tester.
29. Child must perform standing broad jump over width of test sheet (8 1/2 inches).
30. Tell child to walk forward, ⊂⊃⊂⊃⊂⊃⊂⊃→ heel within 1 inch of toe. Tester may demonstrate. Child must walk 4 consecutive steps.
31. In the second year, half of normal children are non-compliant.

OBSERVATIONS:

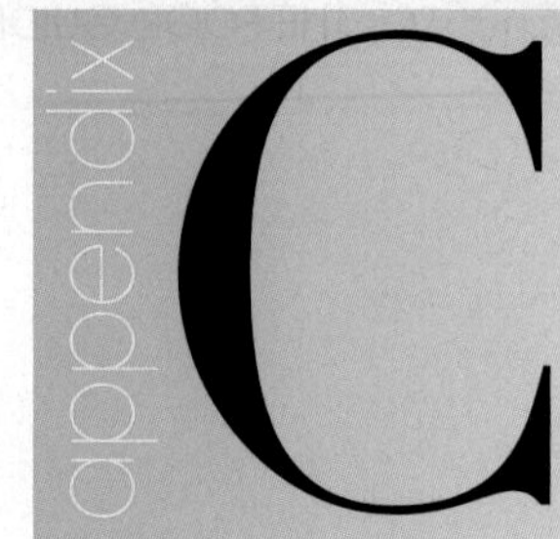

The Food Guide Pyramid

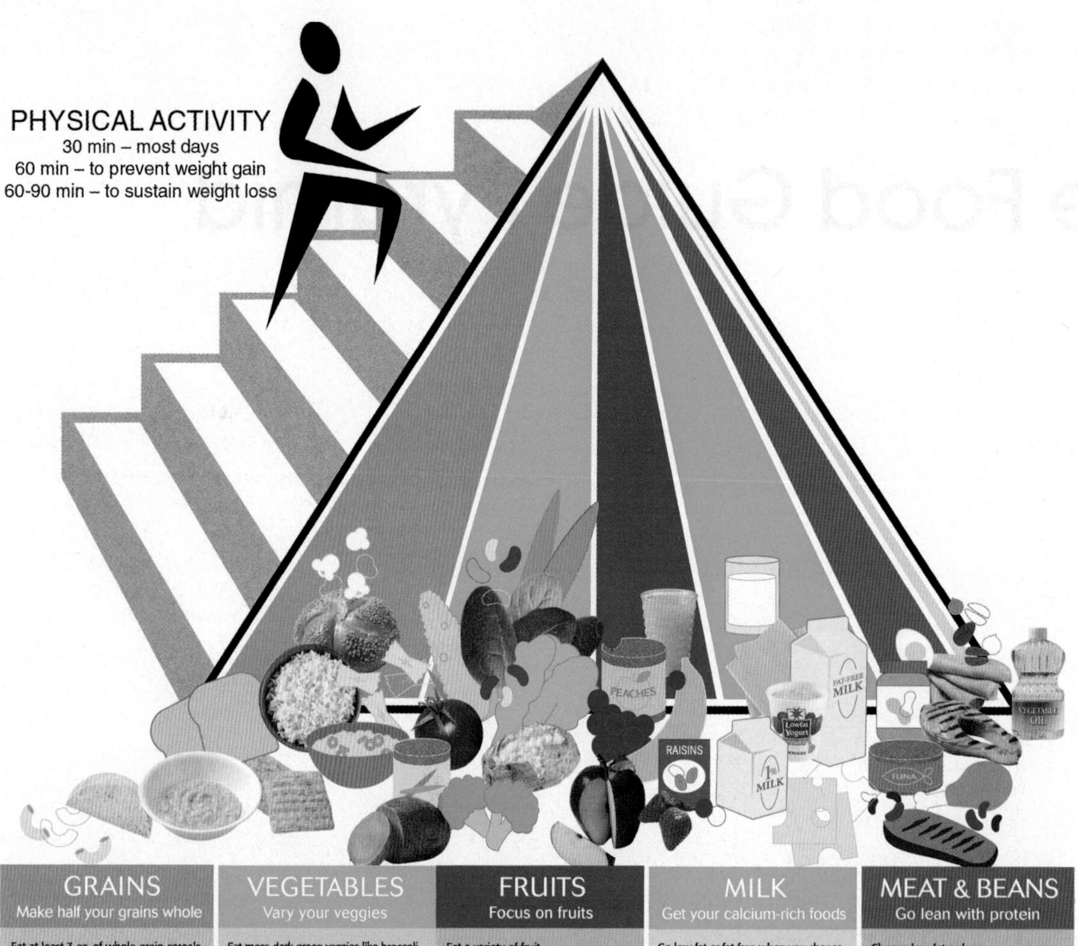
PHYSICAL ACTIVITY
30 min – most days
60 min – to prevent weight gain
60-90 min – to sustain weight loss
PEACHES
RAISINS
FAT-FREE MILK
Lowfat Yogurt
1% MILK
TUNA
VEGETABLE OIL

GRAINS Make half your grains whole	VEGETABLES Vary your veggies	FRUITS Focus on fruits	MILK Get your calcium-rich foods	MEAT & BEANS Go lean with protein
Eat at least 3 oz. of whole-grain cereals, breads, crackers, rice, or pasta every day 1 oz. is about 1 slice of bread, about 1 cup of breakfast cereal, or 1/2 cup of cooked rice, cereal, or pasta	Eat more dark-green veggies like broccoli, spinach, and other dark leafy greens Eat more orange vegetables like carrots and sweetpotatoes Eat more dry beans and peas like pinto beans, kidney beans, and lentils	Eat a variety of fruit Choose fresh, frozen, canned, or dried fruit Go easy on fruit juices	Go low-fat or fat-free when you choose milk, yogurt, and other milk products If you don't or can't consume milk, choose lactose-free products or other calcium sources such as fortified foods and beverages	Choose low-fat or lean meats and poultry Bake it, broil it, or grill it Vary your protein routine – choose more fish, beans, peas, nuts, and seeds
For a 2,000-calorie diet, you need the amounts below from each food group. To find the amounts that are right for you, go to MyPyramid.gov.				
Eat 6 oz. every day	Eat 2 1/2 cups every day	Eat 2 cups every day	Get 3 cups every day; for kids aged 2 to 8, it's 2	Eat 5 1/2 oz. every day

Find your balance between food and physical activity

- Be sure to stay within your daily calorie needs.
- Be physically active for at least 30 minutes most days of the week.
- About 60 minutes a day of physical activity may be needed to prevent weight gain.
- For sustaining weight loss, at least 60 to 90 minutes a day of physical activity may be required.
- Children and teenagers should be physically active for 60 minutes every day, or most days.

Know the limits on fats, sugars, and salt (sodium)

- Make most of your fat sources from fish, nuts, and vegetable oils.
- Limit solid fats like butter, margarine, shortening, and lard, as well as foods that contain these.
- Check the Nutrition Facts label to keep saturated fats, *trans* fats, and sodium low.
- Choose food and beverages low in added sugars. Added sugars contribute calories with few, if any, nutrients.

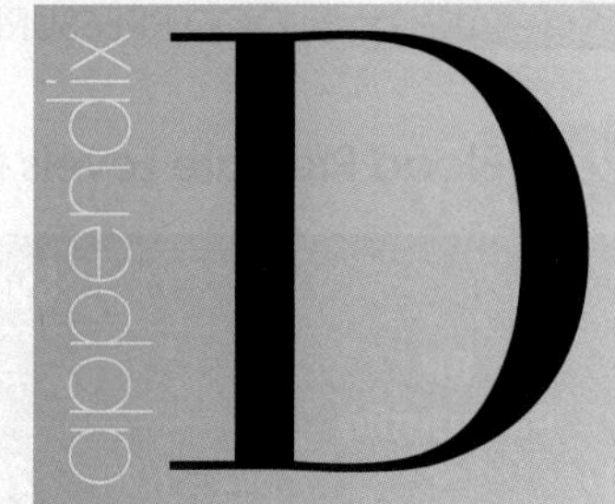

Blood Pressure Charts for Children and Adolescents

Table D.1 Blood Pressure Levels for Boys by Age and Height Percentile

Age (Year)	BP Percentile ↓	Systolic BP (mmHg) ← Percentile of Height →							Diastolic BP (mmHg) ← Percentile of Height →						
		5th	*10th*	*25th*	*50th*	*75th*	*90th*	*95th*	*5th*	*10th*	*25th*	*50th*	*75th*	*90th*	*95th*
1	50th	80	81	83	85	87	88	89	34	35	36	37	38	39	39
	90th	94	95	97	99	100	102	103	49	50	51	52	53	53	54
	95th	98	99	101	103	104	106	106	54	54	55	56	57	58	58
	99th	105	106	108	110	112	113	114	61	62	63	64	65	66	66
2	50th	84	85	87	88	90	92	92	39	40	41	42	43	44	44
	90th	97	99	100	102	104	105	106	54	55	56	57	58	58	59
	95th	101	102	104	106	108	109	110	59	59	60	61	62	63	63
	99th	109	110	111	113	115	117	117	66	67	68	69	70	71	71
3	50th	86	87	89	91	93	94	95	44	44	45	46	47	48	48
	90th	100	101	103	105	107	108	109	59	59	60	61	62	63	63
	95th	104	105	107	109	110	112	113	63	63	64	65	66	67	67
	99th	111	112	114	116	118	119	120	71	71	72	73	74	75	75
4	50th	88	89	91	93	95	96	97	47	48	49	50	51	51	52
	90th	102	103	105	107	109	110	111	62	63	64	65	66	66	67
	95th	106	107	109	111	112	114	115	66	67	68	69	70	71	71
	99th	113	114	116	118	120	121	122	74	75	76	77	78	78	79
5	50th	90	91	93	95	96	98	98	50	51	52	53	54	55	55
	90th	104	105	106	108	110	111	112	65	66	67	68	69	69	70
	95th	108	109	110	112	114	115	116	69	70	71	72	73	74	74
	99th	115	116	118	120	121	123	123	77	78	79	80	81	81	82
6	50th	91	92	94	96	98	99	100	53	53	54	55	56	57	57
	90th	105	106	108	110	111	113	113	68	68	69	70	71	72	72
	95th	109	110	112	114	115	117	117	72	72	73	74	75	76	76
	99th	116	117	119	121	123	124	125	80	80	81	82	83	84	84
7	50th	92	94	95	97	99	100	101	55	55	56	57	58	59	59
	90th	106	107	109	111	113	114	115	70	70	71	72	73	74	74
	95th	110	111	113	115	117	118	119	74	74	75	76	77	78	78
	99th	117	118	120	122	124	125	126	82	82	83	84	85	86	86
8	50th	94	95	97	99	100	102	102	56	57	58	59	60	60	61
	90th	107	109	110	112	114	115	116	71	72	72	73	74	75	76
	95th	111	112	114	116	118	119	120	75	76	77	78	79	79	80
	99th	119	120	122	123	125	127	127	83	84	85	86	87	87	88
9	50th	95	96	98	100	102	103	104	57	58	59	60	61	61	62
	90th	109	110	112	114	115	117	118	72	73	74	75	76	76	77
	95th	113	114	116	118	119	121	121	76	77	78	79	80	81	81
	99th	120	121	123	125	127	128	129	84	85	86	87	88	88	89
10	50th	97	98	100	102	103	105	106	58	59	60	61	61	62	63
	90th	111	112	114	115	117	119	119	73	73	74	75	76	77	78

Table D.1 Blood Pressure Levels for Boys by Age and Height Percentile (continued)

Age (Year)	BP Percentile ↓	Systolic BP (mmHg)							Diastolic BP (mmHg)						
		← Percentile of Height →							← Percentile of Height →						
		5th	10th	25th	50th	75th	90th	95th	5th	10th	25th	50th	75th	90th	95th
	95th	115	116	117	119	121	122	123	77	78	79	80	81	81	82
	99th	122	123	125	127	128	130	130	85	86	86	88	88	89	90
11	50th	99	100	102	104	105	107	107	59	59	60	61	62	63	63
	90th	113	114	115	117	119	120	121	74	74	75	76	77	78	78
	95th	117	118	119	121	123	124	125	78	78	79	80	81	82	82
	99th	124	125	127	129	130	132	132	86	86	87	88	89	90	90
12	50th	101	102	104	106	108	109	110	59	60	61	62	63	63	64
	90th	115	116	118	120	121	123	123	74	75	75	76	77	78	79
	95th	119	120	122	123	125	127	127	78	79	80	81	82	82	83
	99th	126	127	129	131	133	134	135	86	87	88	89	90	90	91
13	50th	104	105	106	108	110	111	112	60	60	61	62	63	64	64
	90th	117	118	120	122	124	125	126	75	75	76	77	78	79	79
	95th	121	122	124	126	128	129	130	79	79	80	81	82	83	83
	99th	128	130	131	133	135	136	137	87	87	88	89	90	91	91
14	50th	106	107	109	111	113	114	115	60	61	62	63	64	65	65
	90th	120	121	123	125	126	128	128	75	76	77	78	79	79	80
	95th	124	125	127	128	130	132	132	80	80	81	82	83	84	84
	99th	131	132	134	136	138	139	140	87	88	89	90	91	92	92
15	50th	109	110	112	113	115	117	117	61	62	63	64	65	66	66
	90th	122	124	125	127	129	130	131	76	77	78	79	80	80	81
	95th	126	127	129	131	133	134	135	81	81	82	83	84	85	85
	99th	134	135	136	138	140	142	142	88	89	90	91	92	93	93
16	50th	111	112	114	116	118	119	120	63	63	64	65	66	67	67
	90th	125	126	128	130	131	133	134	78	78	79	80	81	82	82
	95th	129	130	132	134	135	137	137	82	83	83	84	85	86	87
	99th	136	137	139	141	143	144	145	90	90	91	92	93	94	94
17	50th	114	115	116	118	120	121	122	65	66	66	67	68	69	70
	90th	127	128	130	132	134	135	136	80	80	81	82	83	84	84
	95th	131	132	134	136	138	139	140	84	85	86	87	87	88	89
	99th	139	140	141	143	145	146	147	92	93	93	94	95	96	97

BP, blood pressure

* The 90th percentile is 1.28 SD, 95th percentile is 1.645 SD, and the 99th percentile is 2.326 SD over the mean.

U.S. Department of Health and Human Services, National Institutes of Health, National Heart, Lung, and Blood Institute (NHLBI).

Table D.2 Blood Pressure Levels for Girls by Age and Height Percentile

Age (Year)	BP Percentile ↓	Systolic BP (mmHg) ← Percentile of Height →							Diastolic BP (mmHg) ← Percentile of Height →						
		5th	10th	25th	50th	75th	90th	95th	5th	10th	25th	50th	75th	90th	95th
1	50th	83	84	85	86	88	89	90	38	39	39	40	41	41	42
	90th	97	97	98	100	101	102	103	52	53	53	54	55	55	56
	95th	100	101	102	104	105	106	107	56	57	57	58	59	59	60
	99th	108	108	109	111	112	113	114	64	64	65	65	66	67	67
2	50th	85	85	87	88	89	91	91	43	44	44	45	46	46	47
	90th	98	99	100	101	103	104	105	57	58	58	59	60	61	61
	95th	102	103	104	105	107	108	109	61	62	62	63	64	65	65
	99th	109	110	111	112	114	115	116	69	69	70	70	71	72	72
3	50th	86	87	88	89	91	92	93	47	48	48	49	50	50	51
	90th	100	100	102	103	104	106	106	61	62	62	63	64	64	65
	95th	104	104	105	107	108	109	110	65	66	66	67	68	68	69
	99th	111	111	113	114	115	116	117	73	73	74	74	75	76	76
4	50th	88	88	90	91	92	94	94	50	50	51	52	52	53	54
	90th	101	102	103	104	106	107	108	64	64	65	66	67	67	68
	95th	105	106	107	108	110	111	112	68	68	69	70	71	71	72
	99th	112	113	114	115	117	118	119	76	76	76	77	78	79	79
5	50th	89	90	91	93	94	95	96	52	53	53	54	55	55	56
	90th	103	103	105	106	107	109	109	66	67	67	68	69	69	70
	95th	107	107	108	110	111	112	113	70	71	71	72	73	73	74
	99th	114	114	116	117	118	120	120	78	78	79	79	80	81	81
6	50th	91	92	93	94	96	97	98	54	54	55	56	56	57	58
	90th	104	105	106	108	109	110	111	68	68	69	70	70	71	72
	95th	108	109	110	111	113	114	115	72	72	73	74	74	75	76
	99th	115	116	117	119	120	121	122	80	80	80	81	82	83	83
7	50th	93	93	95	96	97	99	99	55	56	56	57	58	58	59
	90th	106	107	108	109	111	112	113	69	70	70	71	72	72	73
	95th	110	111	112	113	115	116	116	73	74	74	75	76	76	77
	99th	117	118	119	120	122	123	124	81	81	82	82	83	84	84
8	50th	95	95	96	98	99	100	101	57	57	57	58	59	60	60
	90th	108	109	110	111	113	114	114	71	71	71	72	73	74	74
	95th	112	112	114	115	116	118	118	75	75	75	76	77	78	78
	99th	119	120	121	122	123	125	125	82	82	83	83	84	85	86
9	50th	96	97	98	100	101	102	103	58	58	58	59	60	61	61
	90th	110	110	112	113	114	116	116	72	72	72	73	74	75	75
	95th	114	114	115	117	118	119	120	76	76	76	77	78	79	79
	99th	121	121	123	124	125	127	127	83	83	84	84	85	86	87
10	50th	98	99	100	102	103	104	105	59	59	59	60	61	62	62
	90th	112	112	114	115	116	118	118	73	73	73	74	75	76	76

Table D.2 Blood Pressure Levels for Girls by Age and Height Percentile (continued)

Age (Year)	BP Percentile ↓	Systolic BP (mmHg) ← Percentile of Height →							Diastolic BP (mmHg) ← Percentile of Height →						
		5th	10th	25th	50th	75th	90th	95th	5th	10th	25th	50th	75th	90th	95th
	95th	116	116	117	119	120	121	122	77	77	77	78	79	80	80
	99th	123	123	125	126	127	129	129	84	84	85	86	86	87	88
11	50th	100	101	102	103	105	106	107	60	60	60	61	62	63	63
	90th	114	114	116	118	118	119	120	74	74	74	75	76	77	77
	95th	118	118	119	121	122	123	124	78	78	78	79	80	81	81
	99th	125	125	126	128	129	130	131	85	85	86	87	87	88	89
12	50th	102	103	104	105	107	108	109	61	61	61	62	63	64	64
	90th	116	116	117	119	120	121	122	75	75	75	76	77	78	78
	95th	119	120	121	123	124	125	126	79	79	79	80	81	82	82
	99th	127	127	128	130	131	132	133	86	86	87	88	88	89	90
13	50th	104	105	106	107	109	110	110	62	62	62	63	64	65	65
	90th	117	118	119	121	122	123	124	76	76	76	77	78	79	79
	95th	121	122	123	124	126	127	128	80	80	80	81	82	83	83
	99th	128	129	130	132	133	134	135	87	87	88	89	89	90	91
14	50th	106	106	107	109	110	111	112	63	63	63	64	65	66	66
	90th	119	120	121	122	124	125	125	77	77	77	78	79	80	80
	95th	123	123	125	126	127	129	129	81	81	81	82	83	84	84
	99th	130	131	132	133	135	136	136	88	88	89	90	90	91	92
15	50th	107	108	109	110	111	113	113	64	64	64	65	66	67	67
	90th	120	121	122	123	125	126	127	78	78	78	79	80	81	81
	95th	124	125	126	127	129	130	131	82	82	82	83	84	85	85
	99th	131	132	133	134	136	137	138	89	89	90	91	91	92	93
16	50th	108	108	110	111	112	114	114	64	64	65	66	66	67	68
	90th	121	122	123	124	126	127	128	78	78	79	80	81	81	82
	95th	125	126	127	128	130	131	132	82	82	83	84	85	85	86
	99th	132	133	134	135	137	138	139	90	90	90	91	92	93	93
17	50th	108	109	110	111	113	114	115	64	65	65	66	67	67	68
	90th	122	122	123	125	126	127	128	78	79	79	80	81	81	82
	95th	125	126	127	129	130	131	132	82	83	83	84	85	85	86
	99th	133	133	134	136	137	138	139	90	90	91	91	92	93	93

BP, blood pressure

* The 90th percentile is 1.28 SD, 95th percentile is 1.645 SD, and the 99th percentile is 2.326 SD over the mean.

U.S. Department of Health and Human Services, National Institutes of Health, National Heart, Lung, and Blood Institute (NHLBI).

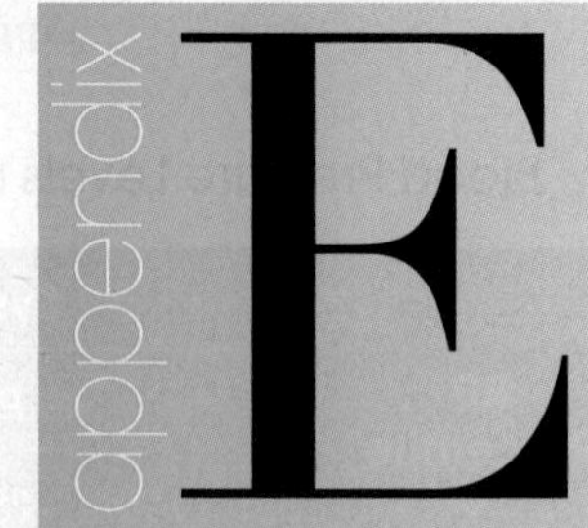

Down Syndrome Health Care Guidelines

Table E.1 Down Syndrome Health Care Guidelines (1999 Revision) Record Sheet

Sheet #1: Birth to Age 12 Years

Name:____________________ Birthday:____________________

	Age, in years															
Medical Issues	***At Birth or at Diagnosis***	*6-mo*	*1*	*1½*	*2*	*2½*	*3*	*4*	*5*	*6*	*7*	*8*	*9*	*10*	*11*	*12*
Karyotype & Genetic Counseling																
Usual Preventative Care																
Cardiology	Echo															
Audiologic Evaluation	ABR or OAE															
Ophthalmologic Evaluation	Red reflex															
Thyroid (TSH & T_4)	State screening															
Nutrition																
Dental Exam[1]																
Celiac Screening[2]																
Parent Support																
Developmental & Educational Services	Early Intervention															
Neck X-rays & Neurological Exam[3]							X-ray									
Pneumococcal Conjugate Vaccine Series																

Instructions: Perform indicated exam/screening and record date in blank spaces. The grey or shaded boxes mean no action is to be taken for those ages.

[1]Begin Dental Exams at 2 years of age, and continue every 6 months thereafter.

[2]IgA antiendomysium antibodies and total IgA.

[3]Cervical spine x-rays: flexion, neutral and extension, between 3–5 years of age. Repeat as needed for Special Olympic participation. Neurological examination at each visit.

Table E.2 Down Syndrome Health Care Guidelines (1999 Revision) Record Sheet

Sheet #2: 13 Years to Adulthood

Name:________________________ Birthday:________________________

Medical Issues	Age, in years							
	13	14	15	16	17	18	19	20–29
Usual Preventative Care								
Audiologic Evaluation								
Ophthalmologic Evaluation								
Thyroid (TSH & T_4)								
Nutrition								
Dental Exam[1]								
Parent Support								
Developmental & Educational Services								
Neck X-rays & Neurological Exam[2]								
Pelvic exam[3]								
Assess Contraceptive Need[3]								

Instructions: Perform indicated exam/screening and record date in blank spaces. The shaded boxes mean no action is to be taken for those ages.

[1]Begin Dental Exams at 2 years of age, and continue every 6 month thereafter.

[2]Cervical spine x-rays: flexion, neutral and extension, between 3–5 years of age. Repeat as needed for Special Olympics participation. Neurological examination at each visit.

[3]If sexually active.

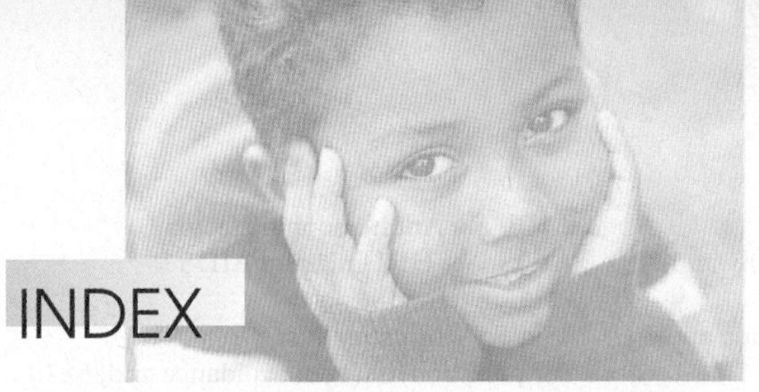

INDEX

Note: A *b* following a page number indicates a boxed features, a *d* indicates a display, an *f* indicates a figure, and a *t* indicates a table.

C

E

F

H

J

K

L

M

O

W